MELLONI'S
ILLUSTRATED
MEDICAL
DICTIONARY

Third Edition

Ida G. Dox, Ph.D.

Communicator in the Medical Sciences
Medical Lexicographer
Bethesda, Maryland

B. John Melloni, Ph.D.

Special Expert in Biomedical Communication (Retired)
National Library of Medicine
National Institutes of Health
Bethesda, Maryland

Co-Director of the Archives of Medical Visual Resources
The Francis A. Countway Library of Medicine
Harvard University Medical School
Boston, Massachusetts

Gilbert M. Eisner, M.D., F.A.C.P.

Adjunct Professor of Physiology and Biophysics
Clinical Professor of Medicine
Georgetown University School of Medicine
Washington, DC

Clinical Professor of Medicine
George Washington University School of Medicine
Washington, DC

Senior Attending Physician
Washington Hospital Center
Washington, DC

MELLONI'S
ILLUSTRATED
MEDICAL
DICTIONARY

Third Edition

The Parthenon Publishing Group Inc.

The Third Edition of Melloni's Illustrated Medical Dictionary is published by:

The Parthenon Publishing Group Inc.
One Blue Hill Plaza
Pearl River
New York 10965
Tel: (914) 735 9363
Fax: (914) 735 1385

This edition is published by arrangement with HarperCollins Publishers, Inc.
The first and second editions of this book were published by Williams and Wilkins

THIRD EDITION

ISBN 1-85070-479-1

Library of Congress Cataloging-in-Publication Data
Dox, Ida.
  Melloni's illustrated medical dictionary / Ida Dox, Biagio John Melloni, Gilbert
    M. Eisner. — 3rd. ed.
    p. cm.
   ISBN 1-85070-479-1
    1. Medicine—Dictionaries.   I. Melloni, Biagio John.   II. Eisner, Gilbert M.
  III. Title.   IV. Title: Illustrated medical dictionary.
   [DNLM: 1. Dictionaries, Medical   W 13 D752m]
  R121.D76   1993b
  610'.3–dc20
  DNLM/DLC
  for Library of Congress   92–48306
                                          CIP

Reprinted 1994

CONTENTS

PREFACE

The rapid expansion and accumulation of knowledge required in the health sciences has created the need for a dictionary of health-science terminology that helps the health conscious reader to quickly and easily assimilate this terminology. For the past decade, two editions of *Melloni's Illustrated Medical Dictionary* have successfully provided a choice between existing comprehensive volumes that require an in-depth scientific background and the glossary type that are limited in scope to a particular discipline.

This edition is an improved and updated version of the previous one. Many of the excellent suggestions received from readers have been incorporated with the confidence that they will make the book more useful. The structure and philosophy of the original book, however, remain the same. This new edition is a compilation of over 26,000 terms comprising the common core of information for all the health sciences, as well as a large number of terms most frequently used in the distinctive language of subspecialties. We anticipate that the third edition of *Melloni's Illustrated Medical Dictionary* will be used as a reference by members of the general public interested in brief, accurate, and "to the point" explanations of current medical terms.

To keep up with recent developments, and in consultation with experts in scientific and health science fields, a large number of terms have been added to this edition. For example, the 5th Report of the International Committee on Taxonomy of Viruses was consulted for the definitions of viruses. Definitions of those terms retained from the previous edition were carefully scrutinized. Some were modified, updated, or expanded; others, no longer appropriate, were deleted.

No effort was spared to preserve the format of the original book, which proved to be of considerable value to the reader and contributed to its receiving the Best Medical Book Award from the AMI, BFA, and HeSCA. As in previous editions of the dictionary, a number of departures from the formats of other dictionaries have been used to present a wide range of information in a concise manner. In one particular aspect, the book is unique: it is the first dictionary of its size and scope to incorporate approximately 2,500 illustrations as visual components of the textual definitions of its terms.

The illustrations are expressly designed to be simple and specific for enhanced understanding of the meaning of the definitions and improved retention of their content. Each illustration is integrated with a specific term and its definition for the dual purpose of further elucidating the term while, by visually "completing" the definition, precluding the need for a lengthier one. This integration of illustration and text is intensified by judicious use of color to identify, highlight, and correlate each illustration with the respective term and its definition. To further highlight the relationship, the illustrated terms are printed in color in the body of the text.

In keeping with the "quick access" philosophy of the dictionary, phonetic pronunciations of defined terms are printed on tinted paper and placed at the beginning of the book. The advantage of this approach is twofold: it allows quicker access to the terms being sought for pronunciation and allows unencumbered scanning of similar words. Prefixes, suffixes, and combining forms also are grouped at the beginning of the book, as are abbreviations and symbols.

To facilitate location of a desired term, the first and last terms of those alphabetized on a page are printed in color at the outside of the bottom margin of each page. Each term on the page is printed in a type that is larger and bolder than that used for its definition. When a term has more than one definition, each is clearly distinguished by a boldface number.

Main entry and subentry formatting of major anatomic terminology groupings, such as arteries, bones, muscles, nerves, and veins, has been replaced by illustrated tables alphabetized within the text. Terms comprising certain arbitrary groupings, such as diseases, syndromes, signs, symptoms, acids, etc., have been individually alphabetized as main entries. Tables of measurements, conversions, dosages, etc. are graphically presented on the pages where the subject terms of the respective calculations are located.

The most important and commonly used chemical compounds and drugs have been included as defined entries. Some of the more widely used brand names are cited at the end of the definitions, but are not included as defined entries.

Synonyms of defined terms are cited at the end of the definitions and are also included as cross-reference entries to the defined terms. Similarly, contemporary terms for syndromes are cross-referenced to respective long-familiar eponyms.

The terms included in this dictionary have been selected with the intended audience in mind. Arbitrary inclusions and exclusions were avoided through an extensive review of the current professional literature and by constant consultation with health science specialists. To reflect contemporary developments, terms that were only recently introduced but are gaining wide acceptance have been included. A limited number of obsolete terms were retained for historical perspective. A substantial number of colloquialisms were also included and, by liberal use of cross references, are closely interrelated with their professional equivalents.

Special attention has been given to the vocabulary used in the definitions. The definitions are simply, clearly, and concisely worded and usually do not begin with a broad conceptual statement. Whenever possible, the use of words that would require additional references has been avoided. When the understanding of one entry is complemented by that of another, appropriate cross references provide the necessary correlation.

If this dictionary enables the reader to grasp clearly the meaning of terms of the health-science vocabulary in the least possible time, through words and pictures, it will have realized its purpose.

Suggestions for the increased usefulness of the book are appreciated and, indeed, encouraged. These should be addressed to Ida G. Dox, Ph.D., 9308 Renshaw Drive, Bethesda, Maryland 20817.

ACKNOWLEDGMENTS

Although dozens of our colleagues at various institutions have generously contributed their time and expertise in helping to shape the definitions in this dictionary, we are particularly indebted to Drs. Rona Eisner, Joseph Bellanti, Melvin Blecher, Mortimer Lorber, Wesley Norman, and Jacques Quen.

For their excellent contributions to the illustrative section, we wish to thank H. Paul Melloni and Dr. June L. Melloni. We are also indebted to Peter J. Melloni and Roy G. Melloni, who meticulously produced all the color overlays for the book, a most laborious task.

Finally, to those readers who took the time to write and suggest changes and ideas, we express our gratitude.

ILLUSTRATION CREDITS

The authors acknowledge the following publications as sources from which the listed original illustrations for this dictionary were derived by permission.

American Family Physician, American Academy of Family Physicians, Kansas City, MO.
  Adrenal glands, ampulla, anesthesia, antibody, bone cement, tables of bones (lunate), constrictor muscles of pharynx, descensus testes, dialysis, diverticulum, dog tick, ductus arteriosus, fetal membrane, flexion, glaucoma, hookworm, hymenopterans, Jackson-Pratt ® drain, omphalomesenteric cyst, ovary, pancreas, pleura, proglottid, prostatic message, *Pyemotes ventricosus*, rheumatoid arthritis, spur, strain, tooth designation.

Bellanti JA: *Immunology* (II), ed 2. Philadelphia, WB Saunders Co, 1978.
  Afferent, hilum, lymph node.

Dorland's Illustrated Medical Dictionary, ed 25. Philadelphia, WB Saunders Co, 1974.
  Auricle.

Grollman S: *The Human Body: Its Structure and Physiology*, ed 3. New York, MacMillan Publishing Co, Inc, 1974.
  Nerve (vestibular and cochlear), osseous labyrinth, pathway, retina.

Kruger GO: *Textbook of Oral Surgery*, ed 4. St. Louis, The CV Mosby Co, 1974.
  Alveolectomy, impaction.

Langley L, Telford I, Christian J: *Dynamic Anatomy and Physiology*, ed 4. New York, McGraw-Hill Book Co, 1974.
  Acromion, aperture of sinus (sphenoid and maxillary), table of bones (femur and sphenoid), calvaria, chamber, ciliary body, ethmoidal infundibulum, navicular bone, optic axis, sacrum, vertebral arch, vertebral body.

Melloni BJ et al: *Anatomy and Physiology* (I and III). New York, McGraw-Hill Book Co, 1971.
  Air cells, basion, table of bones (ethmoid), canaliculus, cephalic index, cochlear duct, concha, conjunctiva, crista ampullaris, lacrimal gland, lacrimal sac, mastoid, nasal septum, opisthion, orbit, ossicles, scala, spinal ganglia of cochlea, visual pathways.

Melloni BJ: The internal ear. *What's New* 199:14–19, (Spring) 1957.
  Ear, semicircular canals.

—. Anatomy of hearing. *What's New* 219:26, (Fall) 1960.
  Cochlear duct.

—. Anatomy of sight. *What's New* 222:25–28 (Feb.–Mar.) 1961.
  Retina, optic chiasm.

—. How the aqueous humor circulates. *Am Fam Phys* 5:2, 1972.
  Chamber of the eye (anterior and posterior).

—. Plants of medical importance. *Am Fam Phys* 8:6, 1973.
  Hemlock; jimsonweed; poison ivy, oak, and sumac; marijuana; ragweed.

—. Focus on cells: osteocytes. *Am Fam Phys* 10:3, 1974
  Osteocyte.

Smith DR: *General Urology*, ed 10. Los Altos, Lange Medical Publishers, 1981.
  Benign.

Vidic B, Melloni BJ: Applied anatomy of the oral cavity and related structures. In Kornblut AD, deFries HO (eds): The *Otolaryngological Clinics of North America* 12:1, Philadelphia, WB Saunders Co, 1979.
  Buccal vestibule, facial vein, retromandibular vein.

ABBREVIATIONS AND SYMBOLS

A

A symbol for (a) the element argon; (b) type of human blood; (c) mass number
Å symbol for Angstrom unit
a (a) accommodation; (b) anode; (c) area; (d) artery; (e) type of human blood
AI, AII, AIII angiotensin I, II, and III
Ab antibody
ABG arterial blood gas
Ac symbol for the element actinium
a.c. Latin *ante cibum* (before meals)
ACh acetylcholine
ACLS advanced cardiac life support
ACTH adrenocorticotrophic hormone
A.D. Latin *auris dextra* (right ear)
A.D.A. (a) American Dental Association; (b) American Diabetes Association
ADAMHA Alcohol, Drug Abuse, and Mental Health Administration
ADH (a) antidiuretic hormone; (b) alcohol dehydrogenase
ad lib. Latin *ad libitum* (as much as desired)
ADP adenosine diphosphate
AFIP Armed Forces Institute of Pathology
Ag 1. antigen **2.** symbol for the element silver (Latin *argentium*)
A.H.A. American Hospital Association
AHF antihemophilic factor
AHG antihemophilic globulin
AI (a) aortic incompetence; (b) aortic insufficiency; (c) apical impulse; (d) artificial insemination; (e) artificial intelligence
AID (a) autoimmune disease; (b) artificial insemination donor
A.K. above the knee (site of amputation)
Al symbol for the element aluminum
ALA aminolevulinic acid
Ala alanine
ALG antilymphocyte globulin
ALS (a) antilymphocyte serum; (b) amyotrophic lateral sclerosis; (c) advanced life support
A.M.A. American Medical Association
AMI acute myocardial infarction
AML acute myelogenous leukemia
AMP adenosine monophosphate (see adenylic acid)
ANA antinuclear antibody
A.N.A. American Nurses' Association
ANF (a) antinuclear factor (see antinuclear antibody; (b) atrial natriuretic factor
AP (a) angina pectoris; (b) arterial pressure
APC (a) a mixture containing aspirin, phenacetin, and caffeine; (b) atrial premature contraction
APL anterior pituitary-like hormone
AR assisted respiration
ARDS (a) acute respiratory distress syndrome; (b) adult respiratory distress syndrome
Arg arginine
AS aortic stenosis
A.S. Latin *auris sinistra* (left ear)
As symbol for the element arsenic
A.S.B. American Society of Bacteriologists
ASC altered state of consciousness
ASD atrial septal defect
ASH asymmetric septal hypertrophy
Asn asparagine
ASO anti-streptolysin O
A.S.P. American Society of Parasitologists
Asp aspartic acid
A.S.R.T. American Society of Radiologic Technologists
AT 10 Dihydrotachysterol
ATG antithymic globulin
ATN acute tubular necrosis
at. no. atomic number
ATP adenosine triphosphate
ATPase adenosine triphosphatase
at. wt. atomic weight
A.U. Latin *aures unitas* (both ears)
Au symbol for the element gold (Latin *aurum*)
A-V (a) atrio-ventricular, as in A-V valve of the heart; (b) arteriovenous, as in A-V fistula

B

B 1. (a) base (of prism); (b) bursa-equivalent (see lymphocyte) **2.** symbol for (a) bacillus; (b) the element boron
Ba symbol for the element barium
BAL British antilewisite (see dimercaprol)
BBB bundle-branch block
B.B.B. blood-brain barrier
BCG bacillus Calmette-Guèrin (see under vaccine)
BCLS basic cardiac life support
Be symbol for the element beryllium
b.e. barium enema
BHN Brinell hardness number
Bi symbol for the element bismuth
b.i.d. Latin *bis in die* (twice daily)
Bk symbol for the element berkelium
BLS basic life support
b.m. bowel movement
BMG benign monoclonal gammopathy
BMR basal metabolic rate (see basal metabolism)
BNA *Basle Nomina Anatomica*
BNDD Bureau of Narcotics and Dangerous Drugs
BP blood pressure
b.p. boiling point
BPH benign prostatic hypertrophy
Bq symbol for becquerel (unit of radioactivity)
Br symbol for the element bromine
B.S. (a) blood sugar; (b) breath sounds
BSA body surface area
BSP Bromsulphalein® (see sulphobromophthalein sodium)
BTU British thermal unit
BUN blood urea nitrogen

C

C 1. Celsius or centigrade (temperature scale) **2.** symbol for (a) large calorie; (b) the element carbon
c (a) small calorie; (b) cylinder
c̄ Latin *cum* (with)
CA (a) cancer; (b) cardiac arrest
Ca 1. cathode **2.** symbol for the element calcium
ca (a) cancer; (b) Latin *circa* (about)
CABG coronary artery bypass graft
CABS coronary artery bypass surgery
CAD coronary artery disease
Cal large calorie
cal small calorie
cAMP cyclic AMP (adenosine-3′,5′-cyclic monophosphate)
cap (a) Latin *capiat* (let him take); (b) capsule
CAPD chronic ambulatory peritoneal dialysis
CAT computerized axial tomography
Cb symbol for the element columbium
CBC complete blood count
CBF cerebral blood flow
C.C. chief complaint
cc cubic centimeter
CCK cholecystokinin
CCU (a) coronary care unit; (b) critical care unit (same as ICU)
Cd symbol for the element cadmium
cd candella
CDC Centers for Disease Control
Ce symbol for the element cerium
CEA carcinoembryonic antigen
CF (a) citrovorum factor; (b) cystic fibrosis
Cf symbol for the element californium
cGMP cyclic GMP (3′-5′-guanosine cyclic monophosphate)
CG chorionic gonadotropin
CGS, cgs centimeter-gram-second unit
CHD coronary heart disease
Ch.D. Latin *Chirurgiae Doctor* (Doctor of Surgery)
CHF congestive heart failure
C-H length crown-heel length
CHO carbohydrate
C-R length crown-rump length
CI color index
Ci curie
CIPD chronic intermittent peritoneal dialysis
Cl symbol for the element chlorine
Cm symbol for the element curium
cm centimeter
C.M.A. certified medical assistant
CMI cell-mediated immunity
CMV cytomegalovirus
CN the cyanide radical
C.N.M. certified nurse midwife
CNS central nervous system
C.N.S. clinical nurse specialist
CO cardiac output
Co symbol for the element cobalt
CoI coenzyme I (now called NAD)
CoII coenzyme II (now called NADP)
CoIII coenzyme III
CoA coenzyme A
COLD chronic obstructive lung disease
COPD chronic obstructive pulmonary disease
Coq. Latin *coque* (boil)
c.p. chemically pure
CPC clinicopathologic conference
CPK creatine phosphokinase
c.p.m. counts per minute
CPR cardiopulmonary resuscitation
c.p.s. cycles per second
Cr symbol for the element chromium
CRF corticotropin-releasing factor
C.R.N.A. certified registered nurse anesthetist
C.R.T.T. certified respiratory therapy technician
Cs symbol for the element cesium
CSF cerebrospinal fluid
C.S.T. certified surgical technologist
CT (a) computed tomography; (b) Coomb's test
Cu symbol for the element copper (*cuprum*)
CVA cerebrovascular accident
CVP central venous pressure
CVS cardiovascular system
cx cervix
cyl (a) cylinder; (b) cylindrical lens
cys cysteine

D

D 1. (a) deciduous; (b) density of gases; (c) Latin *dexter* (right); (d) diopter **2.** symbol for (a) deuterium; (b) dose
d deuteron
DA developmental age
dag decagram
dB, db decibel
D.C. (a) direct current; (b) Doctor of Chiropractic

DCA deoxycorticosterone acetate
DD developmental disability
D.D.S. Doctor of Dental Surgery
DES diethylstilbestrol
D. et S. Latin *detur et signetur* (let it be given and labeled)
DFP diisopropyl fluorophosphate
D.H.E. 45 dihydroergotamine
DIC disseminated intravascular coagulation
dil Latin *dilue* (dilute, dissolve)
DIT diiodotyrosine
DJD degenerative joint disease
dl deciliter
DM diastolic murmur
dm decimeter
D.M.D. Doctor of Dental Medicine
DMSO dimethylsulfoxide
DNA deoxyribonucleic acid
DNase, DNAse deoxyribonuclease
DNP dinitrophenol
DNR do not resuscitate (no code)
D.N.Sc. Doctor of Nursing Science
D.O. (a) Doctor of Optometry; (b) Doctor of Osteopathy; (c) disto-occlusal
D.O.A., DOA dead on arrival (admission)
DOC (a) deoxycorticosterone; (b) deoxycholic acid
DOCA deoxycorticosterone acetate
DPG diphosphoglycerate
DPT diphteria-pertussis-tetanus
D.P. (a) Doctor of Pharmacy; (b) Doctor of Podiatry; (c) displaced person
D.P.H. Doctor of Public Health
D.P.M. Doctor of Podiatric Medicine
DPN diphosphopyridine nucleotide (now called NAD)
DPNH reduced diphosphopyridine nucleotide (now called NADH)
D.R. delivery room
D.S.N. Doctor of Science in Nursing
DT's delirium tremens
DUB dysfunctional uterine bleeding
D.V.M. Doctor of Veterinary Medicine

E

e symbol for the natural logarithm that has a value of 2.7
EBV Epstein-Barr virus
Eo+, Eo symbol for oxidation-reduction potential
ECF extracellular fluid
ECG electrocardiogram
E. coli *Escherichia coli*
ECT electroconvulsant therapy
EDB ethylene dibromide
ED₅₀ dose producing desired effect in 50% of subjects tested
EDTA ethylenediaminetetraacetic acid
EEG electroencephalogram
E.E.N.T. eye-ear-nose-throat
EFA essential fatty acid
EKG electrocardiogram (German *elektrokardiogram*)
EKY electrokymogram
EM (a) electron microscope; (b) electron micrograph
EMF electromotive force
EMG electromyogram
E.M.T. emergency medical technician (paramedic)
emu electromagnetic unit
ENG electronystagmography
E.N.T. ear-nose-throat
EOG electro-oculography
EPSP excitatory postsynaptic potential
ER endoplasmic reticulum
E.R. emergency room
Er symbol for the element erbium
ERG electroretinogram
ERPF effective renal plasma flow
ERV expiratory reserve volume
Es symbol for the element einsteinium
ESF erythropoiesis-stimulator factor (erythropoietin)
ESP extrasensory perception
ESR (a) erythrocyte sedimentation rate; (b)

electron spin resonance
ESRD end-stage renal disease
EST electroshock therapy
esu electrostatic unit
Eu symbol for the element europium
ev electron-volt

F

F **1.** Fahrenheit (temperature scale) **2.** Symbol for (a) factor; (b) farad; (c) visual field; (d) the element fluorine; (e) force
f Symbol for focal length
F₁, F₂, F₃, F₄, etc. first, second, third, fourth, etc. filial generation (see generation, filial)
FA fatty acid
Fab fragment antigen binding
F.A.C.C. Fellow of the American College of Cardiologists
F.A.C.D. Fellow of the American College of Dentists
F.A.C.F.P. Fellow of the American College of Family Physicians
F.A.C.O.G. Fellow of the American College of Obstetricians and Gynecologists
F.A.C.P. Fellow of the American College of Physicians
F.A.C.S. Fellow of the American College of Surgeons
F.A.C.S.M. Fellow of the American College of Sports Medicine
FAD flavin adenine dinucleotide
F.C.A.P. Fellow of the College of American Pathologists
FDA Food and Drug Administration
Fe symbol for the element iron (Latin *ferrum*)
FEV forced expiratory volume
FF filtration factor
FFA free fatty acid
FFP fresh-frozen plasma
F.H. family history
FHR fetal heart rate
FHT fetal heart tones
FIGlu formiminoglutamic acid
Fm symbol for the element fermium
FMF familial Mediterranean fever
FMN flavin mononucleotide
F.N.P. family nurse practitioner
Fr symbol for the element francium
FRC functional residual capacity
FRF follicle-stimulating hormone-releasing factor
FSH follicle-stimulating hormone
FUO fever of unknown origin
fx fracture

G

G gingiva
g **1.** (a) gender; (b) gram **2.** symbol for acceleration of gravity
Ga symbol for the element gallium
GABA gamma-aminobutyric acid
Gc gonococcus; gonorrhea
Gd symbol for the element gadolinium
Ge symbol for the element germanium
GFR glomerular filtration rate
GH growth hormone
GH-RF growth-hormone-releasing factor
GI gastrointestinal
Gl gland
Gln glutamic acid
Glu glutamine
Gly glycine
gm gram
GM counter Geiger-Müller counter (see counter, Geiger)
GMP cuanosine monophosphate (guanosine 5′-phosphoric acid)
GN glomerulonephritis
GnRH gonadotropin-releasing factor
GOT glutamic oxaloacetic transaminase (see under transaminase)
GPT glutamic pyruvic transaminase (see under transaminase)

gr grain (unit of weight)
GRF growth hormone-releasing factor
GSH reduced form of glutathione
GSSG oxidized glutathione
gt Latin *gutta* (drop)
GTH gonadotropic hormone
GTP guanosine triphosphate
GTT glucose tolerance test
gtt Latin *guttae* (drops)
GU genitourinary
GVH graft-versus-host
GYN gynecology

H

H **1.** hyperopia **2.** symbol for (a) hydrogen; (b) henry; (c) oersted
H⁺ symbol for hydrogen ion
¹H symbol for hydrogen-1
²H symbol for hydrogen-2
³H symbol for hydrogen-3
h (a) height; (b) horizontal; (c) hundred; (d) Plank's constant
H and P history and physical examination
H and E stain Hematoxylin and eosin stain (see under stain)
HAV hepatitis A virus
Hb hemoglobin
HBAg hepatitis B antigen (hepatitis-associated antigen)
HBcAg hepatitis B core antigen
HbCO symbol for carboxyhemoglobin
HbO₂ symbol for oxyhemoglobin
HbS symbol for sickle cell hemoglobin (now called hemoglobin S)
HBsAG hepatitis B surface antigen
HBV hepatitis B virus
hCG human chorionic gonadotropin
HCl (a) hydrochloric acid; (b) hydrogen chloride
Hct hematocrit
HCVD hypertensive cardiovascular disease
h.d. Latin *hora decubitus* (at bedtime)
HDL high density lipoprotein
He symbol for the element helium
Hf symbol for the element hafnium
Hfr high frequency
Hg symbol for mercury (Latin *hydrargyrum*)
Hgb hemoglobin
hGH human growth hormone
His histidine
HH hiatal hernia
HL half-life
HI latent hyperopia
HLA human lymphocyte antigen
Hm manifest hyperopia
HMD hyaline membrane disease
HMO health maintenance organization
hPL human placental lactogen
h.s. Latin *hora somni* (at bedtime)
HSV herpes simplex virus
Ht total hyperopia
5-HT 5-hydroxytryptamine (serotonin)
HTLV (a) human T-lymphotropic retrovirus; (b) human T-cell leukemia/lymphoma virus
Hz hertz

I

I **1.** intensity of magnetism **2.** symbol for (a) electric current; (b) the element iodine
¹²⁵I symbol for the radioactive isotope of iodine, with a half-life of 57.4 days
¹³¹I symbol for the radioactive isotope of iodine, with a half-life of 8.05 days
IABP intra-aortic balloon pump
IANC International Anatomical Nomenclature Committee
IC inspiratory capacity
ICD International Classification of Diseases of the World Health Organization
ICDA International Classification of Diseases, adapted for use in the United States
ICP intracranial pressure
ICS intercostal space

ICSH interstitial cell stimulating hormone
ICU intensive care unit
id. Latin *idem* (the same)
I.D., i.d. intradermal
IDDM insulin-dependent diabetes mellitus
IDP inosine 5′-diphosphate
IE immunoelectrophoresis
Ig immunoglobulin
IgA immunoglobulin A (gamma A globulin)
IgE immunoglobulin E (gamma E globulin)
IgG immunoglobulin G (gamma G globulin)
IgM immunoglobulin M (gamma M globulin)
IH infectious hepatitis
IHSS idiopathic hypertrophic subaortic stenosis
Ile isoleucine
I.M., i.m. intramuscular (usually pertaining to an injection)
In symbol for the element indium
INH isonicotinic acid hydrazide (see isoniazid)
IOP intraocular pressure
I.P., i.p. intraperitoneal
IPPB intermittent positive-pressure breathing
IQ intelligence quotient (see under quotient)
Ir symbol for the element iridium
IRV inspiratory reserve volume
I.S. intercostal space
ITP idiopathic thrombocytopenic purpura
IU international unit
I.V., i.v. intravenous
IVC inferior vena cava
IVP intravenous pyelogram

J

JG juxtaglomerular
JGA juxtaglomerular apparatus
JKᵃ antigen of the Kidd blood group
JKᵇ antigen of the Kidd blood group
JRA juvenile rheumatoid arthritis

K

K 1. (a) antigen of the Kell blood group; (b) Kelvin (temperature scale) 2. symbol for (a) dissociation constant; (b) the element potassium (Latin *kalium*)
k 1. cathode (kathode) 2. symbol for constant
ka cathode (kathode)
kcal large calorie
kev kilo-electron volt (1000 electron volts)
kg kilogram
KHN Knoop hardness number
kl kiloliter
Kr symbol for the element krypton
17-KS 17-ketosteroids
KUB x-rays of kidneys, ureters, bladder
KVO keep vein open

L

λ symbol for wavelength (lambda)
L 1. *Lactobacillus* 2. symbol for (a) inductance; (b) lambert (unit of brightness); (c) lethal
l 1. (a) left; (b) length; (c) lumber 2. symbol for liter
La symbol for the element lanthanum
LAO left anterior-oblique projection
LATS long-acting thyroid stimulator (see under stimulator)
LBBB left bundle-branch block
LBW low birth weight
LD (a) lethal dose; (b) learning disability
LD₅₀ median dose that will kill within a stated period of time 50% of the animals inoculated
LDH (a) lactic acid dehydrogenase; (b) lactate dehydrogenase
LDL low-density lipoprotein
LE lupus erythematosus
L.E. left eye
Le Lewis blood group

LES lower esophageal sphincter
Leu leucine
L.G.A. large for gestational age
LGV lymphogranuloma venereum
LH lutenizing hormone
LH-RF lutenizing hormone-releasing factor
Li symbol for the element lithium
L.M. licentiate in midwifery
LP (a) light perception; (b) lumbar puncture
L.P.N. licensed practical nurse
LRF lutenizing hormone-releasing factor
LSD lysergic acid diethylamide
LSH lutein-stimulating hormone
Lu symbol for the element lutetium
LV left ventricle
LVH left ventricular hypertrophy
L.V.N. licensed vocational nurse
Lw symbol for the element lawrencium
Lys lysine

M

μ symbol for micron
μμ micromicron
μCi microcurie (formerly μC)
μg microgram
μμg micromicrogram
μ mole micromole
M 1. (a) metal; (b) *Micrococcus*; (c) Latin *misce* (mix); (d) molar; (e) muscle; (f) myopia; (g) morgan 2. symbol for (a) blood factor; (b) molecular weight
ᴍ molar concentration
m meter
mμ millimicron
M.A. mental age
ma milliampere
MAO monoamine oxidase
MAOI monoamine oxidase inhibitor
MAP mean arterial pressure
MASH mobile army surgical hospital
Mb, MbCO, MbO myoglobin and its combinations with carbon monoxide and oxygen
MBC maximum breathing capacity
MBD minimal brain dysfunction
M.C. Medical Corps
mc millicurie (now mCi)
mcg microgram
mCi millicurie
MCT mean circulation time
MCV mean cell volume
Md mendelivium
MD muscular dystrophy (preferably called progressive muscular dystrophy)
M.D. Latin *Medicinae Doctor* (Doctor of Medicine)
MDA 3,4-methylene dioxyamphetamine
Me methyl radical CH₃⁻
MED minimal effective dose
MEFR maximal expiratory flow rate
mEq, meq milliequivalent
Met methionine
MetHb methemoglobin
M. et sig. Latin *misce et signa* (mix and label)
mev mega electron volt
MG myasthenia gravis
Mg symbol for the element magnesium
mg milligram
MI myocardial infarction
MICU medical intensive care unit
MID minimal infective dose
MIP maximum inspiratory pressure
MIT monoiodotyrosine
ml milliliter
MLD, mld minimal lethal dose
MLD₅₀ minimal dose lethal for 50% of experimental animals tested for assay of a toxic substance
mᴍ millimole
mm millimeter
Mn symbol for the element manganese
M.O. Medical Officer
Mo symbol for the element molybdenum
mol. wt. molecular weight
MOM milk of magnesia
mOsm, mosm milliosmole
m.p. melting point

MPC maximum permissible concentration
MPD maximal permissible dose
mppcf millions of particles per cubic foot
mr milliroentgen
M.R.A. medical record administrator (formerly medical record librarian)
mrad millirad
MRD, mrd minimal reacting dose
mrem millirem
mRNA messenger RNA
MS multiple sclerosis
msec millisecond
MSH melanocyte-stimulating hormone
M.T. (a) major tranquilizer; (b) medical technologist
MV megavolt
mv millivolt
MW molecular weight
My myopia

N

N symbol for (a) newton (unit of force); (b) the element nitrogen; (c) an antigenic determinant of erythrocytes
ɴ normal (concentration)
n 1. nasal 2. symbol for (a) refractive index; (b) neutron
NA *Nomina Anatomica*
Na symbol for the element sodium (Latin *natrium*)
NAD nicotinamide adenine dinucleotide
NADH reduced nicotinamide adenine dinucleotide
NADP, NAD phosphate nicotinamide adenine dinucleotide phosphate
nCi nanocurie
N.A.P.N.E.S. National Association for Practical Nurse Education and Services
NAS-NRC National Academy of Science-National Research Council
Nb symbol for the element niobium
NCI National Cancer Institute
Nd symbol for the element neodymium
NE norepinephrine
Ne symbol for the element neon
NEI National Eye Institute
NEFA nonesterified fatty acids
NF National Formulary
ng nanogram
NGU nongonococcal urethritis
NHLBI National Heart, Lung, and Blood Institute
Ni symbol for the element nickel
NIA National Institute on Aging
NIAAA National Institute on Alcohol Abuse and Alcoholism
NIADDK National Institute of Arthritis, Diabetes, and Digestive and Kidney Diseases
NIAID National Institute of Allergy and Infectious Diseases
NICHHD National Institute of Child Health and Human Development
NICU neonatal intensive care unit
NIDA National Institute on Drug Abuse
NIDDM noninsulin-dependent diabetes mellitus
NIDR National Institute of Dental Research
NIEHS National Institute of Environmental Health Sciences
NIGMS National Institute of General Medical Services
NIH National Institutes of Health
NIMH National Institute of Mental Health
NINCDS National Institute of Neurological and Communicative Disorders and Stroke
NLM National Library of Medicine
N.L.N. National League of Nursing
N.L.N.E. National League of Nursing Education
nm nanometer
n.m. nuclear membrane
NMR nuclear magnetic resonance
No symbol for the element nobelium
no number (numero)
Np symbol for the element neptunium
NPN nonprotein nitrogen

NPO   Latin *non-per-os* (nothing by mouth)
NREM   non-rapid eye movement
nsec   nanosecond
NSU   nonspecific urethritis
NZB   New Zealand black mouse

O

O   1. (a) Latin *octarius* (pint); (b) Latin *oculus* (eye)   2. symbol for (a) a blood type of the ABO group in which the serum does not contain agglutinogen; (b) oxygen
O-   ortho-
O₃   ozone
OAA   oxaloacetic acid
OB   obstetrics
OB/GYN   obstetrics and gynecology
OBS   organic brain syndrome
O.D.   (a) Latin *oculus dexter* (right eye); (b) optical density; (c) Doctor of Optometry; (d) overdose
OGTT   oral glucose tolerance test
omn. hor.   Latin *omni hora* (every hour)
OMPA   octamethyl pyrophosphoramide
OOB   out of bed
OPD   Outpatient Department
OPV   oral poliovirus vaccine
OR   operating room
O.S.   Latin *oculus sinister* (left eye)
Om   osmol
Os   symbol for the element osmium
O.T.   occupational therapy
OTC   over the counter
O.U.   Latin *oculus uterque* (both eyes)
oz   ounce

P

P   1. pharmacopeia   2. symbol for the element phosphorus
p   1. (a) pulse; (b) pupil   2. symbol for proton
p-   *para-* (chemical prefix)
P₁   symbol for the first parental generation; P₁ individuals are the parents of the F₁ generation (see filial generation)
Pa   symbol for (a) pascal (unit of pressure); (b) the element protactinium
PA   (a) pernicious anemia; (b) posterior-anterior; (c) pulmonary artery
P.A.   physician assistant
PABA   *p*-aminobenzoic acid
PA_CO₂   symbol denoting partial pressure of carbon dioxide (CO_2) in arterial blood; normal value is approximately 40 mmHg
p. ae.   Latin *partes aequales* (equal parts)
PAH   *p*-aminohippuric acid
PAMP   pulmonary arterial mean pressure
PA_O₂   partial pressure of oxygen in arterial blood
PAS   (a) *p*-aminosalicyclic acid; (b) periodic acid-Schiff (stain)
PASA   *p*-aminosalicyclic acid
PAT   paroxysmal atrial tachycardia
Pb   symbol for the element lead (Latin *plumbum*)
PBI   protein-bound iodine
p.c.   Latin *post cibum* (after meals)
PCG   phonocardiogram
P_CO₂, pCO₂   symbol for partial pressure of carbon dioxide
PCP   (a) phencyclidine (hallucinogen); (b) pulmonary capillary pressure
PCV   packed cell volume
Pd   symbol for the element palladium
PDGF   platelet-derived growth factor
PDM   periodontal membrane
PDR   *Physician's Desk Reference*
PE   pulmonary embolism
PEEP   positive end-expiratory pressure
Ped   pediatrics
PET   positron emission tomography
Pf   platelet factor
PFT   pulmonary function test
PG   prostaglandins
PGA, PGB, etc.   prostaglandin A, B, etc.

pg   picogram
PGH   (a) pituitary growth hormone; (b) prostaglandin H
pH   symbol for the degree of alkalinity or acidity of a solution; denotes the negative logarithm to the base 10 of the hydrogen-ion concentration pH = −log (H+); a solution with pH 7 is neutral; values below 7 indicate a degree of acidity; values above 7 indicate a degree of alkalinity; normal pH of blood serum is approximately 7.4
PHA   phytohemagglutinin
Pharm.D.   Doctor of Pharmacy
Ph.D.   Doctor of Philosophy
Phe   phenylalanine
Ph.G.   Graduate of Pharmacy
PHS   Public Health Service
PI   present illness
PID   pelvic inflammatory disease
PIF   prolactin-inhibiting factor
PK   (a) psychokinesis; (b) pyruvate kinase
PKU   phenylketonuria
Pm   symbol for the element promethium
PMI   point of maximum impulse (see impulse, cardiac)
PMN   polymorphonuclear leukocyte
PMS   premenstrual syndrome
PND   (a) paroxysmal nocturnal dyspnea; (b) postnasal drip
PNS   peripheral nervous system
p.o.   Latin *per os* (by mouth)
Po   symbol for the element polonium
Po₂, pO₂   symbol for partial pressure of oxygen
POMR, POR   problem-oriented medical record
PP   pyrophosphate
PPD   purified protein derivation
P-Pf   pellagra-preventing factor
PPLO   pleuropneumonia-like organisms
ppm   parts per million
ppt   precipitate
Pr   1. presbyopia   2. symbol for the element praseodymium
p.r.   Latin *per rectum* (by rectum)
p.r.n.   Latin *pro re nata* (when necessary)
Pro   proline
psi   pounds per square inch
PSP   phenolsulfonphthalein
P.T.   (a) physical therapy; (b) prothrombin time
Pt   symbol for the element platinum
pt   (a) patient; (b) pint
PTH   parathyroid hormone
Pu   symbol for the element plutonium
PVC   (a) polyvinyl chloride; (b) premature ventricular contraction
PVP   polyvinylpyrrolidone
PWC   pulmonary wedge pressure
PZI   protamine zinc insulin

Q

Q   1. (a) coulomb (unit of electrical quantity); (b) quadrant   2. symbol for (a) the first downward deflection of the QRS complex of the electrocardiogram; (b) the seventh in a series
Q₁₀   symbol for the increase in rate of a process as a result of raising the temperature 10°C
Q_CO₂   symbol for the carbon dioxide given off (in microliters) per milligram of tissue per hour at standard pressure and temperature
Q_O₂   symbol for oxygen consumption (in microliters) per milligram of tissue per hour at standard pressure and temperature
q.d.   Latin *quaque die* (everyday)
q.h.   Latin *quaque hora* (every hour)
q.i.d.   Latin *quater in die* (four times a day)
q.l.   Latin *quantum libet* (as much as desired)
q.q.h.   Latin *quaque quarta hora* (every four hours)
q.s.   Latin *quantum sufficit* (sufficient amount)
qns   quantity not sufficient
qt   quart

R

R   1. respiration.   2. symbol for (a) electrical resistance; (b) gas constant; (c) registered trademark (usually enclosed in a circle, ®); (d) organic radical; (e) roentgen
r   1. (a) radius; (b) ratio; (c) refraction   2. symbol for (a) oxidation-reduction potential; (b) radius
RA   (a) rheumatoid arthritis; (b) right atrium
Ra   symbol for the element radium
RAI   radioactive iodine
RAO   right anterior-oblique projection
RAS   reticular activating system
RAST   radioallergosorbent test
Rb   symbol for the element rubidium
RBBB   right bundle-branch block
RBC   red blood cell
RBF   renal blood flow
R.D.   registered dietician
RDA   recommended dietary allowance
R.D.H.   registered dental hygienist
RDS   respiratory distress syndrome
R.E.   right eye
Re   symbol for the element rhenium
REM   rapid eye movement
rep   roentgen-equivalent-physical (see under roentgen)
RER   rough endoplasmic reticulum
RES   reticuloendothelial system
RF   (a) rheumatoid factor; (b) risk factor
RH   (a) relative humidity; (b) releasing factor
RHD   rheumatic heart disease
RISA   radioiodinated serum albumin
R.N.   registered nurse
Rn   radon
RNA   ribonucleic acid
RNase, RNAase   ribonuclease
RNP   ribonucleoprotein
ROM   range of motion
ROS   review of systems (in health history)
R.Ph.   registered pharmacist
r.p.m.   revolutions per minute
RPR test   rapid plasma reagin test
r.p.s.   revolutions per second
R.Q.   respiratory quotient
RR   recovery room
rRNA   ribosomal ribonucleic acid
R.R.T.   registered respiratory therapist
RS   Reiter's syndrome
RSV   Rous sarcoma virus
RTA   renal tubular acidosis
RV   residual volume
R_x   symbol for (a) prescription; (b) treatment

S

S   1. (a) heart sound; (b) Latin *signa* (signature); (c) Latin *sinister* (left); (d) svedberg (unit of sedimentation)   2. symbol for the element sulfur
s   (a) Latin *semis* (half); (b) sine
S-A   sinoatrial or sinoauricular
SAH   subarachnoid hemorrhage
sat.   saturated
Sb   symbol for the element antimony (Latin *stibium*)
SBE   subacute bacterial endocarditis
Sc   symbol for the element scandium
Sc.D.   Doctor of Science
S.C.M.   state certified midwife
S.D.   (a) skin dose; (b) standard deviation
Se   symbol for the element selenium
SEM   scanning electron microscope
SER   smooth endoplasmic reticulum
Ser   serine
s.g.   specific gravity
SGOT   serum glutamic oxaloacetic transaminase (see under transaminase)
SGPT   serum glutamic pyruvic transaminase (see under transaminase)
SH   serum hepatitis (see viral hepatitis, type B)
SHR   spontaneously hypertensive rat
SI   International System of Units, from the French *Système International d'Unités* (see

under system)

Si symbol for the element silicon

sib. sibling

SIDS sudden infant death syndrome

Sig. Latin *signa* (write or set mark upon)

sin sine

SLE systemic lupus erythematosus

Sm symbol for the element samarium

Sn symbol for the element tin (Latin *stannum*)

sol solution

solv Latin *solve* (dissolve)

S.O.S. Latin *si opus sit* (if there is need)

sp. gr. specific gravity

SQ subcutaneous

Sr symbol for the element strontium

SRF somatotropin-releasing factor (growth hormone-releasing factor)

sRNA soluble ribonucleic acid (transfer ribonucleic acid)

SRS, SRS-A slow-reacting substance (slow-reacting substance of anaphylaxis)

ss Latin *semis* (half)

SSS (a) specific soluble substance; (b) sick-sinus syndrome

ST surgical technologist

stat. Latin *statim* (immediately)

STD sexually transmitted disease

STH somatotropin (growth hormone)

STS serologic test for syphilis

sum Latin *sumat* (let him take) or *sumendum* (to be taken)

SVC superior vena cava

SVG saphenous vein graft

T

T 1. (a) tension; (b) thymus derived (see lymphocyte T) 2. symbol for absolute temperature

t (a) temperature; (b) Latin *ter* (three times)

t½ (a) biologic half-life, the time it takes for the body to eliminate 50% of a drug; (b) half-life, the time required for one-half of a given number of radioactive atoms to disintegrate

T₂ diiodotyrosine

T₃ thyroid hormone triiodothyronine

T₄ thyroid hormone tetraiodothyronine (thyroxin)

Ta symbol for the element tantalum

T.A. toxin-antitoxin

T and A tonsillectomy and adenoidectomy

TAT (a) tetanus antitoxin; (b) thematic apperception test

Tb symbol for the element terbium

t.b. tubercle bacillus

TB, TBC tuberculosis

TBG thyroxin-binding globulin

tbsp tablespoon

TBW total body water

Tc symbol for the element technetium

t.d.s. Latin *ter die sumendum* (to be taken three times a day)

Te symbol for the element tellurium

TEM triethylenemelamine

TG triglyceride

Th symbol for the element thorium

THC tetrahydrocannabinol

Thr threonine

TIA transient ischemic attack

Ti symbol for the element titanium

t.i.d. Latin *ter in die* (three times a day)

tinct. Latin *tinctura* (tincture)

Tl symbol for the element thallium

TLC (a) total lung capacity; (b) thin layer chromatography

TLV threshold limit value

TM (a) transcendental meditation; (b) tympanic membrane

Tm symbol for (a) the element thulium; (b) tubular maximum

TMJ temporomandibular joint

Tn intraocular tension

TNT trinitrotoluene

TPN (a) triphosphopyridine nucleotide (former name for nicotinamide-adenine dinucleotide phosphate); (b) total parenteral nutrition

TPI *Treponema pallidum* immobilization test

tpr temperature, pulse, and respiration

tr Latin *tinctura* (tincture)

TRF thyrotropin-releasing factor

Tris tris(hydroxymethyl)aminomethate

trit Latin *trituratio* (triturate)

tRNA transfer RNA

Trp tryptophan (formerly abbreviated Try)

TSH thyroid-stimulating hormone

TSH-RF thyroid-stimulating hormone-releasing factor

tsp teaspoon

TURP transurethral resection of prostate

Tyr tyrosine

U

U symbol for (a) kilurane (1000 uranium units); (b) the element uranium

u (a) unit; (b) upper

UCS unconditional stimulus

UDP uridine diphosphate

UDP-galactose uridine diphosphate galactose

UDP-glucose uridine diphosphate glucose

UDPG uridine diphosphoglucose (uridine diphosphate glucose)

UHF ultrahigh frequency

ung., ungt. Latin *unguentum* (ointment)

Urd uridine

URI upper respiratory infection

USAN United States Adopted Names

USP United States Pharmacopeia

USPHS United States Public Health Service

UTI urinary tract infection

UTP uridine triphosphate

UV ultraviolet

V

V 1. (a) vision; (b) vitamin 2. symbol for the element vanadium

V$_{max}$ symbol for maximum velocity (in an enzymatic reaction)

v 1. vein 2. symbol for (a) velocity; (b) volt; (c) volume

V$_1$, V$_2$, V$_3$, V$_4$, V$_5$, V$_6$ precordial leads (see under lead)

VA Veterans' Administration

VAL valine

VC vital capacity

VCG vectocardiogram

VD venereal disease

VDH valvular disease of the heart

VISC vitreous infusion surgical cutter

VMA vanillylmandelic acid

V.N.A. Visiting Nurses Association

vol Volume

VR vocal resonance

VS (a) vital signs; (b) volumetric solution

VSD ventricular septal defect

V$_T$ tidal volume

v/v concentration expressed as volume (of solute) per volume (of solvent)

VWF von Willebrand's factor

W

W 1. wedge pressure 2. symbol for (a) energy; (b) the element tungsten (wolfram)

w watt

WBC white blood cell

WHO World Health Organization

WNL within normal limits

WPW Wolff-Parkinson-White syndrome

wt. weight

w/v weight (of solute) per volume (of solvent)

X

X 1. (a) exposure; (b) reactance; (c) sound particle displacement 2. symbol for Kienbock's unit of x-ray dosage

Xe symbol for the element xenon

Y

Y symbol for the element yttrium

Yb symbol for the element ytterbium

Z

Z symbol for (a) atomic number; (b) impedance

z (a) zero; (b) zone

Zn symbol for the element zinc

ZOE zinc oxide and eugenol (see under zinc)

ZPG zero population growth

Zr symbol for the element zirconium

ZPO zinc peroxide

PREFIXES, SUFFIXES, AND COMBINING FORMS

A

a-, an- without, lacking
ab- away from
abdomin-, abdomino- abdomen
acanth-, acantho- thorns, spines
acr-, acro- extremity, tip, end, summit
actin-, actino- ray
ad- to, motion toward, proximity
-ad direction toward
aden- gland
adip-, adipo- fat
aer-, aero- air or gas
all- other, different
ambi- both
amido- presence of the amide radical
amino- presence of the radical NH_2
amph-, amphi-, ampho- both, around
andro- male sex
antero- before
anthropo- human
anti- against, counteraction
-ase enzyme
ate neutralized or esterfied acid
azo- presence of the nitrogen group –N:N–

B

bi-, bin- two, twice
bio- life
bis- twice, doubled
-blast immature
blasto- early stage
bronch-, bronchi-, broncho- bronchus, trachea

C

cac-, caci-, caco- bad, ill
cardi-, cardio- heart
cario- caries
cent-, centi- one hundredth (10^{-2})
cephal-, cephalo- head
cerebr-, cerebri-, cerebro- brain
cheil-, cheilo- lips
chlor- green
chol-, chole-, cholo- bile
choledoch-, choledocho- common bile duct
chondro- cartilage
chorio- membrane
chrom-, chromat-, chromato-, chromo- color
chrys-, chryso- gold
chyl-, chylo- chyle
cine- movement
circum- on all sides
cis- location on the same or the near side
-clysis injection
colp-, colpo- vagina
con- together
contra- against
crani-, cranio- skull
cryo- cold
crypt-, crypto- hidden
cyan-, cyano- blue
cycl-, cyclo- circle, cycle
cyst-, cysto- bladder

D

dacry-, dacryo- tears
dactyl-, dactylo- finger, toe
deca-, deka- ten
deci- one tenth
dehydr-, dehydro- compound from which hydrogen has been removed

demi- half
dendr-, dendri-, dendro- tree-shaped
deoxy-, desoxy- compound derived by removal of one oxygen atom from another compound
derm-, derma-, dermat-, dermato- skin
desm-, desmo- ligament, fibrous band
deutero-, deuti-, deuto- second, secondary
dextro- on or toward the right
di- two
dia- through, throughout
diazo- a compound containing the —N═ N— or —N≡N⁺ group
didym-, didymo- testis
-didymus, -dymus conjoined twin
dihydro- addition of two hydrogen atoms
dipl-, diplo- double
dis- separation, removal
disc- disk
disco- placenta
dolicho- long
dors-, dorsi-, dorso- back
-dymus conjoined twins
dynamo- power, energy
dys- faulty, bad, improper

E

echin-, echino- spring
-ectasia, lectasis expansion
ect-, ecto- outer, external
-ectomy removal
eleo- oil
elytro- vagina
-emia blood
en- in, into, within
encephal-, encephalo- brain
end-, endo- inside, within
-ene presence of a carbon-carbon double bond
enter-, entero- intestines
entomo- insect
epi- upon
epiplo- omentum
erythr-, erythro- red
etio- cause
eu- good, well, normal
ex- out of, away from
exo- external, outward
extra- outside

F

-facient produces, brings about
femto- one quadrillionth (10^{-15})
ferri- containing iron in its highest valence (3)
ferro- divalent ion Fe^{++} in a compound
fibr-, fibro- fiber
fiss- split
for- opening
-fuge avoid, flee

G

galac-, galacta-, galacto- milk
galvano- direct electric current
gameto- gamete
gastr-, gastro- stomach
gem- twin substitutions of a single atom
-gen produce, originate
gen-, geno- producing
-genic causing
ger-, gerat-, gero-, geronto- old age
giga- one billion
gigant-, giganto- exceedingly large, excessive growth

gingivo- gums
gloss-, glosso- tongue
glyc-, glyco- sugar
gnath-, gnatho- jaw
-gnosis recognition
gonad-, gonado- testis, ovary
-gram something recorded
-graph record, something printed
gyn-, gyne-, gyneco-, gyno- female sex

H

hect- one hundred
hemangio- blood vessel
hem-, hemi- half
hem-, hema-, hemat-, hemato-, hemo- blood
hepat-, hepato- liver
heredo- heredity
heter-, hetero- other, different
hexa- six
hist-, histio-, histo- tissue
hol-, holo- whole
homeo-, homo- same, similar
hyal-, hyalo- glass, resembling glass
hydr-, hydro- water, hydrogen
hydroxy- presence of a hydrogen group (OH)
hygro- wet, moist
hyper- above, beyond, excessive
hypn-, hypno- sleep, hypnosis
hyp-, hypo- below, under, deficient
hypsi-, hypso- height
hyster-, hystero- uterus

I

i- immunoreactive
-ia, -iasis pathologic condition
-iatrics, -iatry medical treatment
-ic 1. chemical element that has the higher valence of two possible states 2. acid
-ics science, practice, treatment
-id 1. skin rash 2. family relationship 3. small specimen
-ide binary compound
ideo- idea
idio- peculiar to, individual
ileo- ileum
ilio- ilium
immuno- immunity
in- 1. without 2. inside 3. intensive action
infra- below, beneath
inter- between, among
intra- within
intro- in, into
irido- iris
ischio- ischium
-ism 1. abnormal condition 2. characteristic quality 3. process
is-, iso- identical, equal
-ite resembling, of the nature of
-itis inflammation

J

jejuno- jejunum
juxta- near

K

kal-, kali- potassium
kary-, karyo- nucleus of a living cell
kerato- cornea, thorny tissue

ket-, keto- presence of a ketone group (=CO)
kilo- one thousand
kin-, kine-, kineto- motion
koilo- concave
krymo-, kryo- cold

L

labio- lips
lact-, lacto- milk
laparo- abdomen
laryng-, laryngo- larynx
leio- smooth
-lepsis, -lepsy seizure
lept-, lepto- slender, thin
leuc-, leuco- white, colorless
leuk-, leuko- white, colorless
levo- on or toward the left
-lexis, -lexy speech
lien-, lieno- spleen
linguo- tongue
lip-, lipo- lipid, fat
lith-, litho- stone
-logy study
lymph-, lympho- lymph
-lysis dissolution, rupture, separation

M

macr-, macro- large
-mania mental aberration
mast-, masto- breast
mega- 1. one million 2. large
megal-, megalo-, -megaly large
mel- 1. limb 2. cheek 3. honey
melan-, melano- black
mening-, meningo- membrane
meno- menstruation
mento- chin
-mer smallest unit of a repeating chemical structure
mercapto- presence of a thiol group
mero- part, segment
mes-, meso- middle, intermediate
met-, meta- 1. behind 2. occurring later in a series 3. transformation 4. the 1,3 position in the benzene ring 5. a less hydrous acid
metr- uterus
micro- 1. small 2. one millionth
micromicro- one trillionth (10^{-12})
milli- one thousandth (10^{-3})
millimicro- one billionth (10^{-9})
mono- single
morpho- form, figure, structure
multi- many
myco-, myo- fungus
myelo- 1. bone marrow 2. spinal cord
my-, myo- muscle
myring-, myringo- tympanic membrane
myx-, myxo- mucus

N

nano- 1. small 2. one billionth (10^{-9})
narco- stupor
naso- nose
necr-, necro- dead
nemato- threadlike
neo- new
nephr-, nephro- kidney
neur-, neuro- nerve, nervous system
nitro- presence of the univalent group NO_2 in a compound
nitroso- presence of the radical —NO in a compound
noci- 1. injury 2. a harmful agent or influence
nor- 1. nitrogen without a radical 2. a change from a branched-chain compound to a straight-chain compound
noso- disease
nucle-, nucleo- 1. nucleus 2. nucleic acid

O

octa- eight
odont-, odonto- tooth
odyn-, odynia- pain
-oid resemblance, same shape
-ol alcohol, phenol
oleo- oil
olig-, oligo- few, little
-ology see -logy
-oma tumor or neoplasm
omo- shoulder
omphal-, omphalo- umbilicus
onco-, oncho- tumor
-onium positively charged ion
onych-, onycho-, onyx- fingernail, toenail
oo- egg, ovary
oophor-, oophoro- ovary
oothec-, ootheco- ovary
ophthalm-, ophthalmo- eye
-opia vision
orchi-, orchid-, orchio- testis
ortho- 1. straight, normal 2. correction 3. an acid in the highest form of hydration 4. adjacent carbon positions in a benzene ring
-ose 1. carbohydrate 2. a substance resulting from digestion of a protein
-osis 1. abnormal, diseased 2. increase 3. process
osmo- 1. osmosis 2. odor
ost-, oste-, osteo- bone
-ostomy see -stomy
ot-, oto- ear
-otomy see -tomy
-ous occurring in its lowest valency
ovari-, ovario- ovary
ovi-, ovo- egg
oxa- an oxygen bridge
oxo- oxygen
oxy- 1. pointed 2. acute 3. shield 4. presence of oxygen in a molecule

P

pachy- thick
-pagus conjoined twins
palato- palate
pale-, paleo- ancient, prehistoric
pan- all
pancreat-, pancreatico-, pancreato-, pancreo- pancreas
para- 1. alongside, accessory, deviation from normal 2. compound derived from two symetrically arranged substitutions in the benzene ring
parieto- wall of a body cavity
patho-, -pathy disease
ped-, pedi-, pedo- 1. child 2. foot
-penia deficiency
per- 1. throughout 2. highest possible amount of a specified chemical element or radical
peroxy- presence of an additional oxygen atom
-pexy fixation by stitching
phaco- lens
-phage, phago- something that eats or destroys
pharyng-, pharyngo- pharynx
phleb-, phlebo- vein
-phobia irrational or abnormal fear
phon-, phono- sound, voice
-phoresis transmission
-phoria constant tendency of an eye to turn from the normal position during binocular vision
-phos light
phot-, photo- light
-phrenia, phreno- 1. diaphragm 2. mind
physi-, physio- natural, physical
physo- 1. tendency to swell 2. air, gas
phyt-, phyto- plants
pico- one trillionth (10^{-12})
pili-, pilo- hair
plani-, plano- flatness
-plasia formation

-plasty shaping, repair of
platy- flatness
pleio- many
pleo- more
pleur-, pleuro- 1. side 2. pleura 3. rib
-ploid multiple in form
pluri- several
pneo- breath, respiration
pneum-, pneuma-, pneumat-, pneumato- 1. pressure of air or gas 2. breath, breathing
pneumo-, pneumon-, pneumono- lungs
pod-, podo- foot
-poesis, -poiesis production, make
poikilo- varied, irregular
polio- gray matter of nervous system
poly- 1. many 2. excessive
post- 1. behind 2. subsequent to
pre- before in time or space
pro- before
proct-, procto- anus, rectum
prostat-, prostato- prostate
prot-, proto- first in a series
pseud-, pseudo- false, deceptive resemblance
psych-, psycho- mind, mental process
psychro- cold
-ptosis downward displacement
ptyal-, ptyalo- saliva
pyel-, pyelo- renal pelvis
pyo- pus
pyro- fire

Q

quadr-, quadri- four
quinque- five

R

rachi-, rachio- spine
radio- radiation emission
re- again, against, behind
recto- rectum
reno- kidney
retro- behind
rhabd-, rhabdo- 1. rod-shaped 2. striated
-rhage-, -rhagia profuse flow
rheo- flow, current
rhin-, rhino- nose
rhod-, rhodo- reddish-rose color
-rrhaphy a joining by sutures
-rrhea, -rrhoea discharge
-rrhexis rupture

S

sacr-, sacro- sacrum
salping-, salpingo- tube
sarco- flesh
scat-, scato- feces
schist-, schisto- split, cleft
schiz-, schizo- division, cleavage
scirrh-, scirrho- hard
scler-, sclero- sclera
-scope observe, inspect
-scopy observation, inspection
scoto- darkness
semi- partly
ser-, sero- serum
sial-, sialo- saliva, salivary gland
sidero- iron
somat-, somatico-, somato- body
spermat-, spermato- semen
spermio-, spermo- semen, spermatozoa
spheno- wedge-shaped
sphygm-, sphygmo- pulse
spiro- 1. coil-shaped 2. breathing
splanch-, splanchno- viscera
splen-, spleno- spleen
spodo- waste material
spondyl-, spondylo- vertebra, vertebral column
spor-, sporo- spore
staphyl-, staphylo- bunch of grapes

Prefixes, Suffixes, and Combining Forms

stearo- fat
steat-, steato- fat
steno- narrowness, constriction
stereo- three-dimensionality
sterno- sternum
steth-, stetho- chest
stomat-, stomato-, stomo- mouth, opening
-stomy surgical opening
strepto- twisted, curved, flexible
stylo- point
sub- under, less than
sulf-, sulfo- presence of a sulfur atom (the spelling sulph- is no longer used)
super- 1. above, superior 2. excess
supra- above
sympath-, sympatheto-, sympathico-, sympatho- sympathetic nervous system
syn- together, joined
syring-, syringo- tube

T

tachy- rapid, accelerated
tel-, tele- distance
tel-, telo- 1. final form 2. an end
teno-, tenon- tendon
tera- one trillion
terato- deformed fetus
tetr-, tetra- four
therm-, thermo- heat
thi-, thio- replacement of oxygen by sulfur
-thiol presence of a thiol group (—SH)
thorac-, thoraco- chest
throm-, thrombo- blood clot, thrombus
-thymia the mind, emotions
thymo- 1. thymus 2. the mind, soul, emo-

tions
thyr-, thyro- thyroid gland
-tome cutting instrument
tomo- a section
-tomy cutting, incising
tox-, toxic-, toxico- poison
trachel-, trachelo- the neck
tracheo- the trachea
trans- 1. across, through, beyond 2. located on opposite sides of a molecule 3. transfer of a chemical group from one compound to another
tri- three
trich-, trichi-, tricho- hair
tris- in chemistry, three of the constituents that follow
troph-, tropho- nutrition
-trophy nutrition
-tropia abnormal deviation in the line of vision
-tropic 1. turning toward 2. having an affinity for
tuber- swelling
typhlo- cecum

U

ultra- surpassing of a specific range
uni- single
ure-, urea-, ureo- urea, urine
uretero- ureter
ureth-, urethro- urethra
uri-, uric-, urico- uric acid
urin-, urino- urine
uro- urine

V

vago- vagus nerve
varic-, varico- varix, varicosity
vas- vessel, fluid-conveying duct
vasculo-, vaso- blood vessels
vene- poison
veni-, veno- veins
ventr-, ventro- abdomen
ventriculo- ventricle
vesic-, vesica- 1. bladder 2. blister
vivi- alive, living

X

xanth-, xantho- yellow
xeno- different
xer-, xero- dryness

Y

-yl in chemistry, a radical, especially a univalent hydrocarbon radical
-ylene a bivalent hydrocarbon radical

Z

zo-, zoo- animals
zyg-, zygo- a yoke, especially a joining together in the manner of a yoke
-zygous a zygotic constitution
-zym-, zymo- enzyme
-zyme enzyme

PRONUNCIATION

The majority of main entry terms have been included for pronunciation. Although many of these terms have more than one acceptable pronunciation, only one has been assigned to each term. The choice was based on common usage.

Pronunciation of terms is reproduced by a simple phonetic respelling in accordance with the following key:

The stressed syllable in a word is followed by a boldface prime (′), lesser emphasis by a lightface prime (′).

In the absence of a diacritical mark, a vowel ending a syllable is long (as in ta′bl), a vowel within a syllable is short (as in cat).

The macron (‾) is used to indicate a long vowel within a syllable (as in ko·vāl′ent).

The breve (˘) is used to indicate a short vowel ending a syllable (as in ku′bĭ·tal).

A

abaissement (ah·bās·maw′)
abarognosis (a′bar′og·no′sis)
abarticulation (ab′ar·tik′u·la′shun)
abdomen (ab′do·men)
abdominal (ab·dom′i·nal)
abdominocentesis (ab·dom′i·no·sen·te′sis)
abdominoscopy (ab·dom′i·nos′ko·pe)
abducens (ab·du′senz)
abducent (ab·du′sent)
abduction (ab·duk′shun)
abembryonic (ab′em·bre·on′ik)
aberrant (ab·er′ant)
abetalipoproteinemia (a·ba′tah·lip′o·pro·te·in·e′me·ah)
abient (ab′e·ent)
abiogenesis (ab′e·o·jen′ĕ·sis)
abiotrophy (ab′e·ot′ro·fe)
abirritant (ab·ir′ri·tant)
ablation (ab·la′shun)
ablepharia (ah′blef·a′re·ah)
ablepsia (ah·blep′se·ah)
abluent (ab′lu·ent)
ablution (ab·lu′shun)
ablutomania (ab·lu′to·ma′ne·ah)
abneural (ab·nu′ral)
abortient (ah·bor′shent)
abortifacient (ah·bor′tĭ·fa′shent)
abortive (ah·bor′tiv)
abruptio placentae (ab·rup′she·o pla·sen′te)
absorptiometer (ab·sorp′she·om′ĕ·ter)
abstergent (ab·ster′jent)
abulia (ah·bu′le·ah)
abutment (ah·but′ment)
acalculia (ah′kal·ku′le·ah)
acantha (ah·kan′thah)
acanthesthesia (ah·kan′thes·the′ze·ah)
acanthion (ah·kan′the·on)
Acanthocephala (ah·kan′tho·sef′ah·lah)
acanthocephaliasis (ah·kan′tho·sef′ah·li′ah·sis)
acanthocheilonemiasis (ah·kan′tho·ki′lo·ne·mi′ah·sis)
acanthocyte (ah·kan′tho·sīt)
acanthocytosis (ah·kan′tho·si·to′sis)
acantholysis (ak′an·thol′i·sis)
acanthoma (ak′an·tho′mah)
acanthosis (ak′an·tho′sis)
acari (ak′ah·ri)
acariasis (ak′ah·ri′ah·sis)
acaricide (ah·kar′i·sīd)
acarid (ak′ah·rid)
Acaridae (ah·kar′ĭ·de)
Acarina (ak′ah·ri′nah)
acarodermatitis (ak′ah·ro·der′mah·ti′tis)
acarology (ak′ah·rol′o·je)
acarus (ak′ah·rus)
acatalasia (a′kat·ah·la′ze·ah)
acataphasia (a·kat′ah·fa′ze·ah)

acathamathesia (a·kath′ah·mah·the′ze·ah)
acaudal (a·kaw′dal)
acaudate (a·kaw′dāt)
acauline (a·kaw′līn)
accole′ (ak′o·la′)
accouchement (ah·koosh·maw′)
accrementition (ak′re·men·tish′un)
accretio cordis (ah·kre′she·o kor′dis)
accretion (ah·kre′shun)
acephalocyst (ah·sef′ah·lo′sist)
acervuline (ah·ser′vu·līn)
acervuloma (ah·ser′vu·lo′mah)
acervulus (ah·ser′vu·lus)
acescence (ah·ses′ens)
aceta (ah·se′tah)
Acetabularia (as′ĕ·tab′u·la′re·ah)
acetabuloplasty (as′ĕ·tab′u·lo·plas′te)
acetabulum (as′ĕ·tab′u·lum)
acetaldehyde (as′et·al′dĕ·hīd)
acetamide (as′et·am′ĭd)
acetaminophen (as′et·am′ĭ·no·fen)
acetanilide (as′ĕ·tan′ĭ·lid)
acetazolamide (as′et·ah·zol′ah·mīd)
acetic (ah·se′tik)
acetify (ah·set′ĭ·fi)
Acetobacter (ah·se′to·bak′ter)
acetolysis (as′ĕ·tol′ĭ·sis)
acetonemia (as′ĕ·to·ne′me·ah)
acetonuria (as′ĕ·to·nu′re·ah)
acetum (ah·se′tum)
acetyl (as′ĕ·til)
acetylcholine (as′ĕ·til·ko′lēn)
acetylcysteine (as′ĕ·til·sis′te·in)
acetylene (ah·set′ĭ·len)
acetylstrophanthidin (as′ĕ·til·stro·fan′thĭ·din)
achalasia (ak′ah·la′ze·ah)
acheiria (ah·ki′re·ah)
achillodynia (ak′i·lo·din′e·ah)
achillorrhaphy (ak′i·lor′ah·fe)
achillotomy (ak′ĭ·lot′o·me)
achlorhydria (ak′klor·hi′dre·ah)
achloropsia (ah′klo·rop′se·ah)
achluphobia (ah·kloo·fo′be·ah)
acholia (ah·ko′le·ah)
acholuria (ah·ko·lu′re·ah)
achondroplasia (ah·kon′dro·pla′ze·ah)
achordate (a·kor′dāt)
achoresis (ak′o·re′sis)
achromasia (ak′ro·ma′se·ah)
achromate (ah·kro′māt)
achromatin (ah·kro′mah·tin)
achromatophilia (ah·kro′mah·to·fil′e·ah)
achromatopsia (ah′kro·mah·top′se·ah)
achromatosis (ah·kro·mah·to′sis)
achromocyte (ah·kro′mo·sīt)
achromotrichia (ah·kro′mo·trik′e·ah)
achylia (ah·ki′le·ah)
acidemia (as′i·de′me·ah)
acidophil (as′id·o·fil′)
acidosis (as′ĭ·do′sis)
acidulous (ah·sid′u·lus)

aciduria (as′ĭ·du′re·ah)
acidyl (as′ĭ·dil)
acinar (as′ĭ·nar)
acini (as′ĭ·ni)
acinus (as′ĭ·nus)
aclasis (ah′klah·sis)
acleistocardia (ah·klīs′to·kar′de·ah)
acmesthesia (ak′mes·the′ze·ah)
acneform (ak′ne·form)
acocanthera (ak′o·kan·the′rah)
acognosia (ak′og·no′se·ah)
aconative (ah·kon′a·tiv)
acorea (ah′ko·re′ah)
acoria (ah·ko′re·ah)
acousma (ah·koos′mah)
acousmatagnosia (ah·koos′ma·tag·no′se·ah)
acousmatamnesia (ah·koos′mat·am·ne′ze·ah)
acoustic (ah·koos′tik)
acousticophobia (ah·koos′tĕ·ko·fo′be·ah)
acoustics (ah·koos′tiks)
acrid (ak′rid)
acridine (ak′rĭ·din)
acroagnosis (ak′ro·ag·no′sis)
acroanesthesia (ak′ro·an′es·the′ze·ah)
acroataxia (ak′ro·ah·tak′se·ah)
acrocephalosyndactyly (ak′ro·sef′ah·lo·sin·dak′tĭ·le)
acrocephaly (ak′ro·sef′ah·le)
acrochordon (ak′ro·kor′don)
acrocyanosis (ak′ro·si·ah·no′sis)
acrodynia (ak′ro·din′e·ah)
acroesthesia (ak′ro·es·the′ze·ah)
acrogeria (ak′ro·je′ri·ah)
acrognosis (ak·rog·no′sis)
acrokeratosis verruciformis (ak′ro·ker′ah·to′sis ver·roo′se·form′is)
acromegaly (ak′ro·meg′ah·le)
acromial (ah·kro′me·al)
acromion (ah·kro′me·on)
acromphalus (ah·krom′fah·lus)
acropachy (ak′ro·pak′e)
acroparesthesia (ak′ro·par′es·the′ze·ah)
acroposthitis (ak′ro·pos·thi′tis)
acrosome (ak′ro·sōm)
acrotrophodynia (ak′ro·trof′o·din′e·ah)
actin (ak′tin)
actinium (ak·tin′e·um)
Actinobacillus (ak′tĭ·no·bah·sil′lus)
actinodermatitis (ak′tĭ·no·der′mah·ti′tis)
actinolite (ak·tin′o·līt)
actinometer (ak′tĭ·nom′ĕ·ter)
Actinomyces (ak′tĭ·no·mi′sēz)
actinomycin (ak′tĭ·no·mi′sin)
actinomycosis (ak′tĭ·no·mi·ko′sis)
actinophage (ak·tin′o·fāj)
actomyosin (ak′to·mi′o·sin)
acuity (ah·ku′ĭ·te)
acusis (ah·ku′sis)
acyanoblepsia (ah·si′ah·no·blep′se·ah)
acyanotic (ah·si′ah·not′ik)
acyesis (ah′si·e′sis)

acyl (as′il)
acylation (as′ĕ·la′shun)
acystia (ah·sis′te·ah)
Acystosporidia (ah·sis′to·spo·rid′e·ah)
adactyly (a·dak′tĭ·le)
adducent (ah·du′sent)
adenase (ad′ĕ·nās)
adenasthenia (ad′en·as·the′ne·ah)
adenectomy (ad′ĕ·nek′to·me)
adenectopia (ad′ĕ·nek·to′pe·ah)
adenine (ad′ĕ·nīn)
adenitis (ad′ĕ·ni′tis)
adenoacanthoma
  (ad′ĕ·no·ak′an·tho′mah)
adenoblast (ad′ĕ·no·blast)
adenocarcinoma (ad′ĕ·no·kar′sĭ·no′mah)
adenocele (ad′ĕ·no·sēl′)
adenocystoma (ad′ĕ·no·sis·to′mah)
adenodiastasis (ad′ĕ·no·di·as′tah·sis)
adenoepithelioma
  (ad′ĕ·no·ep′ĭ·the′le·o′mah)
adenofibroma (ad′ĕ·no·fi·bro′mah)
adenohypophyseal
  (ad′ĕ·no·hi′po·fiz′e·al)
adenohypophysis (ad′ĕ·no·hi·pof′ĭ·sis)
adenoid (ad′ĕ·noid)
adenoidectomy (ad′ĕ·noid·ek′to·me)
adenolipoma (ad′ĕ·no·lĭ·po′mah)
adenolipomatosis
  (ad′ĕ·no·lip′o·mat·to′sis)
adenolymphocele (ad′ĕ·no·lim′fo·sēl)
adenolymphoma (ad′ĕ·no·lim·fo′mah)
adenoma (ad′ĕ·no′mah)
adenomatosis (ad′ĕ·no·mah·to′sis)
adenomatous (ad′ĕ·nom′ah·tus)
adenomyoma (ad′ĕ·no·mi·o′mah)
adenomyosis (ad′ĕ·no·mi·o′sis)
adenomyxoma (ad′ĕ·no·mik·so′mah)
adenopathy (ad′ĕ·nop′ah·the)
adenosarcoma (ad′ĕ·no·sar·ko′mah)
adenosclerosis (ad′ĕ·no·skle·ro′sis)
adenose (ad′ĕ·nos)
adenosine (ah·den′o·sēn)
adenosis (ad′ĕ·no′sis)
adenotome (ad′ĕ·no·tōm)
adenovirus (ad′ĕ·no·vi′rus)
adenyl (ad′ĕ·nil)
adenylate (ah·den′ĭ·lāt)
adenylic (ad′ĕ·nil′ik)
adhesiotomy (ad·he′ze·ot′o·me)
adiadochokinesia
  (ah·di′ah·do′ko·ki·ne′se·ah)
adiaphoresis (ah·di′ah·fo·re′sis)
adipometer (ad′ĭ·pom′ĕ·ter)
adiponecrosis (ad′ĭ·po·nĕ·kro′sis)
adipose (ad′ĭ·pōs)
adiposis (ad′ĭ·po′sis)
adiposity (ad′ĭ·pos′ĭ·te)
aditus (ad′ĭ·tus)
adjuvant (ad′ju·vant)
adnexa (ad·nek′sah)
adrenal (ah·dre′nal)
adrenalectomy (ah·dre′nal·ek′to·me)
adrenaline (ah·dren′ah·lēn)
adrenarche (ad′ren·ar′ke)
adrenergic (ad′ren·er′jik)
adrenocortical (ad′re′no·kor′te·kal)
adrenocorticomimetic
  (ad·re′no·kor′te·ko·mi·met′ic)
adrenocorticotrophic
  (ad·re′no·kor′te·ko·trof′ik)
adrenocorticotrophin
  (ad·re′no·kor′te·ko·trof′in)
adrenolytic (ad′ren·o·lit′ik)
adrenomegaly (ad·ren′o·meg′ah·le)
adrenoprival (ad·ren′o·pri′val)
adrenosterone (ad′re·no′ster·ōn)
adrenotrophin (ad·ren′o·trof′in)
adrenotropism (ad′re·not′ro·pizm)
adventitial (ad′ven·tish′al)
Aedes aegypti (a·ē′dez e·jip′te)
aeration (a′er·a′shun)
aerobe (a′er·ōb)
aerobiosis (a′er·o·bi·o′sis)
aeropathy (a′er·op′ah·the)
aerophagia (a′er·o·fa′je·ah)
aerophil (a′er·o·fil′)
aerosinusitis (a′er·o·si′nus·i′tis)

aerotitis (a′er·o·ti′tis)
affect (af′fekt)
afferent (af′er·ent)
afibrinogenemia
  (ah·fi′brin·o·jĕ·ne′me·ah)
agalactia (ah′gah·lak′she·ah)
agalorrhea (ah·gal′o·re′ah)
agammaglobulinemia
  (a·gam′ah·glob′u·lĭ·ne′me·ah)
aganglionosis (ah·gang′gle·on·o′sis)
agar (ahg′ar)
agenesis (ah·jen′ĕ·sis)
agenitalism (ah·jen′ĕ·tal·izm)
agenosomia (ah·jen′o·so′me·ah)
ageusia (ah·gu′ze·ah)
agglutination (ah·gloo′tĭ·na′shun)
agglutinin (ah·gloo′tĭ·nin)
agglutinogen (ag′loo·tin′o·jen)
agglutinoid (ah·gloo′tĭ·noid)
aglaucopsia (ah′glaw·kop′se·ah)
aglomerular (ah′glo·mer′u·lar)
aglucone (ah·gloo′kōn)
agnogenic (ag′no·jen′ik)
agnosia (ag·no′ze·ah)
agonist (ag′o·nist)
agoraphobia (ag′o·rah·fo′be·ah)
agranulocytes (ah·gran′u·lo·sīts)
agranulocytopenia
  (ah·gran′u·lo·si·to·pe′ne·ah)
agranulocytosis (ah·gran′u·lo·si·to′sis)
agraphia (ah·graf′e·ah)
akaryocyte (ah·kar′e·o·sīt)
akinesia (ah·kĭ·ne′ze·ah)
akinesthesia (ah·kin′es·the′ze·ah)
ala (a′lah)
alae (a′le)
alanine (al′ah·nēn)
alastrim (ah·las′trim)
alba (al′bah)
albinism (al′bĭ·nizm)
albuginea (al′bu·jin′e·ah)
albuminiferous (al·bu′mĭ·nif′er·us)
albuminocytologic
  (al·bu′mĭ·no·si′to·loj′ik)
albuminoid (al·bu′mĭ·noid)
albuminuria (al′bu·mĭ·nu′re·ah)
aldehyde (al′dĕ·hīd)
aldolase (al′do·lās)
aldopentose (al′do·pen′tōs)
aldosterone (al·dos′ter·ōn)
aldosteronism (al′do·ster′ōn·izm)
aleukemia (ah′lu·ke′me·ah)
alexia (ah·lek′se·ah)
algesia (al·je′ze·ah)
algesthesia (al′jes·the′ze·ah)
alginate (al′jĭ·nāt)
aliphatic (al′ĕ·fat′ik)
aliquot (al′ĕ·kwot)
alkalemia (al′kah·le′me·ah)
alkalescent (al′kah·les′ent)
alkali (al′kah·li)
alkaline (al′kah·līn)
alkaloid (al′kah·loid)
alkalosis (al′kah·lo′sis)
alkaptonuria (al′kap·to·nu′re·ah)
allantoin (ah·lan′to·in)
allantois (ah·lan′to·is)
allele (ah·lēl′)
allergen (al′er·jen)
allergenic (al′er·jen′ik)
alloarthroplasty (al′o·arth′ro·plas′te)
allochromasia (al′o·kro·ma′ze·ah)
allocortex (al′o·kor′teks)
allogamy (al·log′ah·me)
allogeneic (al′o·jĕ·ne′ik)
allograft (al′o·graft)
allolalia (al′o·la′le·ah)
allomerism (ah·lom′er·izm)
allomorphism (al′o·mor′fizm)
alloploid (al′o·ploid)
allosome (al·o·sōm)
allosterism (al·los′ter·izm)
alloxan (al′ok·san)
alochia (ah·lo′ke·ah)
aloes (al′ōz)
aloform (al′o·form)
alogia (ah·lo′je·ah)
alopecia (al′o·pe′she·ah)

alpha (al′fah)
Alphavirus (al′fah vi′rus)
Alternaria (awl′ter·na′re·ah)
alum (al′um)
alveolar (al·ve′o·lar)
alveolectomy (al′ve·o·lek′to·me)
alveoli (al·ve′o·li)
alveolus (al·ve′o·lus)
alveus (al′ve·us)
Alzheimer (altz′hi·mer)
amalgam (ah·mal′gam)
Amanita (am′ah·ni′tah)
amantadine (ah·man′tah·dēn)
ambenonium (am′be·no′ne·um)
amblyacousia (am′ble·a·koo′zhuh)
amblyopia (am′ble·o′pe·ah)
amblyoscope (am′ble·o·skōp)
ambulatory (am′bu·lah·to′re)
amebiasis (am′e·bi′ah·sis)
ameboma (am′e·bo′mah)
ameiosis (a′mi·o′sis)
amelanotic (ah′mel·ah·not′ik)
amelia (ah·me′le·ah)
amelioration (ah·mēl′yo·ra′shun)
ameloblast (ah·mel′o·blast′)
ameloblastofibroma
  (am′e·lo·blas′to·fi·bro′ma)
ameloblastoma (ah·mel′o·blas·to′ma)
ameloblastosarcoma
  (am′ĕ·lo·blas′to·sar·ko′mah)
amelogenesis (am′ĕ·lo·jen′ĕ·sis)
amenorrhea (ah·men′o·re′ah)
ametropia (am′ĕ·tro′pe·ah)
amide (am′īd)
amination (am′ĭ·na′shun)
amine (ah·mēn′)
aminoaciduria (ah·me′no·as′ĭ·du′re·ah)
aminophylline (ah·me′no·fil′in)
aminopyrine (ah·me′no·pi′rin)
amnesia (am·ne′ze·ah)
amnesiac (am·ne′ze·ak)
amniocentesis (am′ne·o·sen·te′sis)
amnion (am′ne·on)
amniorrhea (am′ne·o·re′ah)
amniorrhexis (am′ne·o·rek′sis)
amnioscopy (am′ne·os′ko·pe)
amniotomy (am′ne·ot′o·me)
amorphous (ah·mor′fus)
amphetamine (am·fet′ah·min)
amphiarthrosis (am′fe·ar·thro′sis)
amphipathic (am′fe·path′ik)
amphitrichous (am·fit′rĕ·kus)
amphixenosis (am·fiks·en·o′sis)
amphophil (am′fo·fil)
amphoric (am·for′ik)
ampule (am′pūl)
ampulla (am·pul′lah)
amygdala (ah·mig′dah·lah)
amygdalae (ah·mig′dah·le)
amyl (am′il)
amylase (am′ĭ·lās)
amylogenesis (am′ĭ·lo·jen′ĕ·sis)
amyloid (am′ĭ·loid)
amyloidosis (am′ĭ·loi·do′sis)
amylophagia (am′ĭ·lo·fa′je·ah)
amyotonia (a′mi·o·to′ne·ah)
amyotrophic (ah·mi′o·trof′ik)
amyotrophy (ah′mi·ot′ro·fe)
anabolism (ah·nab′o·lizm)
anacidity (an′ah·sid′ĭ·te)
anacrotic (an′ah·krot′ik)
anacusis (an′ah·ku′sis)
anaerobe (an·a′er·ōb)
anaerobic (an′a·er·o′bik)
anaerogenic (an·a′er·o·jen′ik)
anagenesis (an′ah·jen′ĕ·sis)
analeptic (an′ah·lep′tik)
analgesia (an′al·je′ze·ah)
analgesic (an′al·je′zik)
analogous (ah·nal′o·gus)
analogue (ah·nah·log)
analysand (ah·nal′ĭ·sand)
anaphoresis (an′ah·fo·re′sis)
anaphylactic (an′ah·fi·lak′tik)
anaphylaxis (an′ah·fi·lak′sis)
anaplasia (an′ah·pla′ze·ah)
anastole (ah·nas′to·le)
anastomose (ah·nas′to·mōs)

anastomosis (ah·nas'to·mo'sis)
anatomic (an'ah·tom'ik)
ancylostomiasis (an'sĭ·los'to·mi'ah·sis)
androgen (an'dro·jen)
androgynous (an·droj'ĕ·nus)
androsterone (an·dros'ter·ōn)
anechoic (an·ĕ·ko'ik)
anemia (ah·ne'me·ah)
anergic (an·er'jik)
anergy (an'er·je)
anesthesia (an'es·the'ze·ah)
anesthesiologist (an'es·the'ze·ol'o·jist)
anesthesiology (an'es·the'ze·ol'o·je)
anesthetic (an'es·thet'ik)
anesthetist (an·nes'thĕ·tist)
anesthetize (ah·nes'thĕ·tīz)
anestrus (an·es'trus)
aneuploid (an'u·ploid)
aneuploidy (an'u·ploi'de)
aneurysm (an'u·rizm)
aneurysmectomy (an'u·riz·mek'to·me)
angiectasia (an'je·ek·ta'se·ah)
angiitis (an'je·i'tis)
angioblast (an'je·o·blast)
angiocardiography
   (an'je·o·kar'de·og'rah·fe)
angiocardiopathy
   (an'je·o·kar'de·op'ah·the)
angioedema (an'je·o·e·de'mah)
angiogram (an'je·o·gram')
angiography (an'je·og'rah·fe)
angiokeratoma (an'je·o·ker'ah·to'mah)
angioma (an'je·o'mah)
angiomatosis (an'je·o·mah·to'sis)
angioneurosis (an'je·o·nu·ro'sis)
angiopathy (an'je·op'ah·the)
angioplasty (an'je·o·plas'te)
angiopoietic (an'je·o·poi·et'ik)
angiospasm (an'je·o·spazm)
angiostenosis (an'je·o·ste·no'sis)
angiotensin (an'je·o·ten'sin)
angiotensinogen (an'je·o·ten·sin'o·jen)
angiotome (an'je·o·tōm)
angiotrophic (an'je·o·trof'ik)
angstrom (ang'strem)
anhydrase (an·hi'drās)
anhydride (an·hi'drīd)
anhydrous (an·hi'drus)
aniline (an'ĭ·lĭn)
anion (an'i·on)
aniridia (an'ĭ·rid'e·ah)
aniseikonia (an'ĭ·si·ko'ne·ah)
anisochromasia (an·i'so·kro·ma'ze·ah)
anisocoria (an'ĭ·so·ko're·ah)
anisocytosis (an·ĭ·so·si·to'sis)
anisometropia (an·i'so·mĕ·tro'pe·ah)
ankyloblepharon (ang'kĭ·lo·blef'ah·ron)
ankylosis (ang'kĭ·lo'sis)
anlage (ahn'lah·geh)
anneal (ah·nēl')
anodontia (an'o·don'she·ah)
anodyne (an'o·dīn)
anomalopia (ah·nom'ah·lo'pe·ah)
anomaly (ah·nom'ah·le)
Anopheles (ah·nof'ĕ·lēz)
anophthalmos (an'of·thal'mos)
anopsia (an·op'se·ah)
anorchidism (an·or'ki·dizm')
anoretic (an'o·ret'ik)
anorexia (an'o·rek'se·ah)
anorexiant (an'o·rek'se·ant)
anoscope (a'no·skōp)
anosmia (ah·oz'me·ah)
anosognosia (an·o'sog·no'zhe·ah)
anovular (an·ov'u·lar)
anoxemia (an'ok·se'me·ah)
ansa (an'sah)
ansae (an'se)
antecubital (an'te·ku'bĭ·tal)
antemetic (ant'e·met'ik)
antenatal (an'te·na'tal)
antepartum (an'te·par'tum)
anteversion (an'te·ver'zhun)
anthelminthic (ant'hel·min'thik)
anthracemia (an'thrah·se'me·ah)
anthraconecrosis
   (an'thrah·ko·nĕ·kro'sis)
anthracosilicosis (an'thrah·ko·sil'ĭ·ko'sis)

anthracosis (an·thrah·ko'sis)
antrax (an'thraks)
anthrone (an'thrŏn)
anthropogeny (an'thro·poj'ĕ·ne)
anthropology (an'thro·pol'o·je)
anthropozoonosis
   (an'thro·po·zo'o·no'sis)
antiangiogenesis (an'tĭ·an'je·o·jen'ĕ·sis)
anticholinergic (an'tĭ·ko'lin·er'jik)
anticholinesterase (an'tĭ·ko·lin·es'ter·ās)
anticoagulant (an'tĭ·ko·ag'u·lant)
anticodon (an'tĭ·ko'don)
anticonvulsant (an'tĭ·kon·vul'sant)
antidepressant (an'tĭ·de·pres'sant)
antidiarrheal (an'tĭ·di'ah·re'al)
antidiuresis (an'tĭ·di'u·re'sis)
antidiuretic (an'tĭ·di'u·ret'ik)
antidote (an'tĭ·dōt)
antiemetic (an'tĭ·e·met'ik)
antifibrinolysin (an'tĭ·fi'bri·nol'ĭ·sin)
antihelix (an'tĭ·he'liks)
antihemagglutinin
   (an'tĭ·hem·ah·gloo'tĭ·nin)
antihemolysin (an'tĭ·he'mol'ĭ·sin)
antimetabolite (an'tĭ·mĕ·tab'o·līt)
antinauseant (an'tĭ·naw'ze·ant)
antiperistalsis (an'tĭ·per'ĭ·stal'sis)
antiprothrombin (an'tĭ·pro·throm'bin)
antipruritic (an'tĭ·proo·rit'ik)
antipyretic (an'tĭ·pi·ret'ik)
antirachitic (an'tĭ·rah·kit'ik)
antiscorbutic (an'tĭ·skor·bu'tik)
anti-streptolysin (an'tĭ·strep·tol'ĭ·sin)
antithrombin (an'tĭ·throm'bin)
antitragus (an'tĭ·trag'us)
antitreponemal (an'tĭ·trep'·o·ne'mal)
antitrypsin (an'tĭ·trip'sin)
antitussive (an'tĭ·tus'iv)
antral (an'tral)
antrectomy (an·trek'to·me)
antroscope (an'tro·skōp)
antrostomy (an·tros'to·me)
antrotomy (an·trot'o·me)
antrum (an'trum)
anulus (an'u·lus)
anuresis (an'u·re'sis)
anuria (ah·nu're·ah)
aorta (a·or'tah)
aortic (a·or'tik)
aortitis (a·or·ti'tis)
aortogram (a·or'to·gram')
aortography (a'or·tog'rah·fe)
aortopathy (a'or·top'ah·the)
aortotomy (a'or·tot'o·me)
apatite (ap'ah·tīt)
aperistalsis (ah'per·ĭ·stal'sis)
apex (a'peks)
apexcardiogram (a'peks·kar'de·o·gram)
aphakia (ah·fa'ke·ah)
aphalangia (ah'fah·lan'je·ah)
aphasia (ah·fa'ze·ah)
aphonia (ah·fo'ne·ah)
aphrodisia (af'ro·diz'e·ah)
aphrodisiac (af'ro·diz'e·ak)
aphtha (af'thah)
aphthae (af'the)
aphthous (af'thus)
apices (a'pĭ·sēz)
apicoectomy (a'pĕ·ko·ek'to·me)
apicostomy (a'pĕ·kos'to·me)
apituitarism (ah'pĭ·tu'ĭ·tar·izm)
aplanasia (ap'lah·na'ze·ah)
aplasia (ah·pla'zhe·ah)
apnea (ap·ne'ah)
apneumatic (ap'nu·mat'ik)
apneumatosis (ap'nu·mah·to'sis)
apocrine (ap'o·krin)
apoferritin (ap'o·fer'ĭ·tin)
aponeurorrhaphy (ap'o·nu·ror'ah·fe)
aponeurosis (ap'o·nu·ro'sis)
appendectomy (ap'en·dek'to·me)
appendiceal (ap·en·dis'e·al)
appendices (ah·pen'dĭ·sēz)
appendicitis (ah·pen'dĭ·si'tis)
appendicolithiasis
   (ah·pen'dĭ·ko·lĭ·thi'ah·sis)
appendix (ah·pen'diks)
apperception (ap'er·sep'shun)

appersonation (ap'er·sah·na'shun)
applique (ap'lĭ·ka')
apraxia (ah·prak'se·ah)
aptyalism (ap'ti·a'lizm)
apyknomorphous (ah·pik'no·mor'fus)
apyretic (ah'pi·ret'ik)
apyrexia (ah'pi·rek'se·ah)
apyrexial (ah'pi·rek'se·al)
aqueous (a'kwe·us)
arabinose (ah·rab'ĭ·nōs)
arachnid (ah·rak'nid)
Arachnida (ah·rak'ni·dah)
arachnodactyly (ah·rak'no·dak'tĭ·le)
arborize (ar'bo·rīz)
arbovirus (ar'bo·vi'rus)
archenteron (ar·ken'ter·on)
arctation (ark·ta'shun)
arcuate (ar'ku·āt)
arcus (ar'kus)
areata (ar'e·a'tah)
areatus (ar'e·a'tus)
areflexia (ah're·flek'se·ah)
Arenavirus (ah're·nah·vi'rus)
areola (ah·re'o·lah)
argentaffin (ar·jen'tah·fin)
argentaffinoma (ar'jen·taf'ĭ·no'mah)
argentation (ar'jen·ta'shun)
argentous (ar·jen'tus)
arginase (ar'ji·nas)
arginine (ar'ji·nin)
argon (ar'gon)
arrhenoblastoma (ah·re'no·blas·to'mah)
arrhythmia (ah·rith'me·ah)
arsenous (ar'sĕ·nus)
arsphenamine (ars·fen'ah·min)
arteriolar (ar·te·re'o·lar)
arteriole (ar·te're·ōl)
arteriolitis (ar·tēr'ĭ·o·li'tis)
arteriolonecrosis (ar·te·re·o'lo·ne·kro'sis)
arterionecrosis (ar·te're·o·ne·kro'sis)
arterioplasty (ar·te're·o·plas'te)
arteriorrhaphy (ar·te're·o·or'ah·fe)
arteriosclerosis (ar·te're·o·sklĕ·ro'sis)
arteriosclerotic (ar·te're·o·sklĕ·rot'ik)
arteriostenosis (ar·te're·o·stĕ·no'sis)
arteriotomy (ar'te·re·ot'o·me)
arteriovenous (ar·te're·o·ve'nus)
arteritis (ar'tĕ·ri'tis)
arthralgia (ar·thral'je·ah)
arthrectomy (ar·threk'to·me)
arthritic (ar·thrit'ik)
arthritis (ar·thri'tis)
arthrogram (ar'thro·gram)
arthrography (ar·throg'rah·fe)
arthrogryposis (ar'thro·grĭ·po'sis)
arthronosos (ar'thro·no'sos)
arthropathy (ar·throp'ah·the)
arthroplasty (ar'thro·plas'te)
arthropod (ar'thro·pod)
arthropyosis (ar'thro·pi·o'sis)
arthroscope (ar'thro·skōp)
arthroscopy (ar·thros'ko·pe)
arthrosis (ar·thro'sis)
arthrospore (ar'thro·spōr)
arthrosynovitis (ar'thro·sin'o·vi'tis)
arthrotomy (ar·throt'o·me)
arytenoid (ar·e'te·noid)
arytenoidectomy (ar'ĕ·te'noid·ek'to·me)
ascariasis (as'kah·ri'ah·sis)
Ascaris (as'kah·ris)
ascites (ah·si'tēz)
ascitic (ah·sit'ik)
ascomycete (as·ko'mi·sēt)
asepsis (a·sep'sis)
asialia (ah'si·a'le·ah)
asparaginase (as·par'ah·jin·ās)
asparagine (as·par'ah·jēn)
aspartame (ah·spar'tām)
aspergilloma (as'per·jil·o'mah)
Aspergillus (as'per·jil'us)
aspermatogenic (ah·sper'mah·to·jen'ik)
asphygmia (as·fig'me·ah)
asphyxia (as·fik'se·ah)
asphyxiant (as·fik'se·ant)
asphyxiation (as·fik'se·a'shun)
aspidium (as·pid'e·um)
asporogenous (as'po·roj'ĕ·nus)
astasia (as·ta'zhe·ah)

Pronunciation

asteatosis (as'te·ah·to'sis)
astereognosis (ah·ster'e·og·no'sis)
asterion (as·te're·on)
asterixis (as'ter·ik'sis)
asthenia (as·the'ne·ah)
asthenocoria (as·the'no·ko're·ah)
asthenopia (as'the·no'pe·ah)
asthenospermia (as'the·no·sper'me·ah)
asthma (az'mah)
astigmatism (ah·stig'mah·tizm)
astigmatometer (as'tig·mah·tom'e·ter)
astigmometer (as'tig·mom'e·ter)
astroblast (as'tro·blast)
astroblastoma (as'tro·blas·to'mah)
astrocele (as'tro·sel)
astrocyte (as'tro·sit)
astrocytoma (as'tro·si·to'mah)
astrocytosis (as'tro·si·to'sis)
astroglia (as·trog'le·ah)
asynclitism (ah·sin'klǐ·tizm)
asynergia (a'sin·er'je·ah)
asystole (ah·sis'to·le)
atactilia (a'tak·til'e·ah)
ataraxia (at'ah·rak'se·ah)
atavism (at'ah·vism)
ataxia (ah·tak'se·ah)
atelectasis (at'e·lek'tah·sis)
ateliosis (ah·te'le·o'sis)
atelocardia (at'ĕ·lo·kar'de·ah)
atelocheilia (at'ĕ·lo·ki'le·ah)
atelognathia (at'ĕ·log·na'the·ah)
atherogenesis (ath'er·o·jen'ĕ·sis)
atherogenic (ath'er·o·jen'ik)
atheroma (ath'er·o'mah)
atheromatous (ath'er·o'mah·tus)
atherosclerosis (ath'er·o·sklĕ·ro'sis)
athetoid (ath'ĕ·toid)
athetosis (ath'ĕ·to'sis)
athrepsia (ah·threp'se·ah)
athymia (ah·thi'me·ah)
atocia (ah·to'se·ah)
atomicity (ah'tŏ·mis'ĭ·te)
atomization (at'om·ĭ·za'shun)
atony (at'o·ne)
atopognosis (ah·top'og·no'sis)
atopy (at'o·pe)
atresia (ah·tre'ze·ah)
atretoblepharia (ah·tre'to·blĕ·fa're·ah)
atrial (a'tre·al)
atrichia (ah·trik'e·ah)
atriomegaly (a'tre·o·meg'ah·le)
atrioseptopexy (a'tre·o·sep'to·pek'se)
atriotomy (a'tre·ot'o·me)
atrioventricular (a'tre·o·ven·trik'u·lar)
atrium (a'tre·um)
atrophic (ah·trof'ik)
atrophied (at'ro·fēd)
atrophoderma (at'ro·fo·der'mah)
atrophy (at'ro·fe)
atropine (at'ro·pēn)
atropinism (at'ro·pin'izm)
attenuant (ah·ten'u·ant)
attrition (ah·trish'un)
audiometry (aw'de·om'ĕ·tre)
auditory (aw'dĭ·to're)
aura (aw'rah)
auricle (aw'rĕ·kl)
auricular (aw·rik'u·lar)
auscultate (aws'kul·tāt)
auscultation (aws'kul·ta'shun)
auscultatory (aws·kul'tah·to're)
autism (aw'tizm)
autistic (aw·tis'tik)
autoagglutination (aw'to·ah·gloo'tĭ·na'shun)
autoagglutinin (aw'to·ah·gloo'tĭ·nin)
autocatalysis (aw'to·kah·tal'ĭ·sis)
autochthonous (aw·tok'tho·nus)
autoclave (aw'to·klāv)
autodigestion (aw'to·di·jes'chun)
autoerotism (aw'to·er'o·tizm)
autogamy (aw·tog'ah·me)
autogenous (aw·toj'ĕ·nus)
autohemolysin (aw'to·he'mol'ĭ·sin)
autohemolysis (aw'to·he·mol'ĭ·sis)
autohypnosis (aw'to·hip·no'sis)
autoimmunize (aw'to·im'u·nīz)
autoinoculation (aw'to·in·ok'u·la'shun)

autologous (aw·tol'o·gus)
autonomic (aw'to·nom'ik)
autopepsia (aw'to·pep'se·ah)
autopsy (aw'top·se)
autosome (aw'to·sōm)
autotopagnosia (aw'to·top'ag·no'se·ah)
autotoxin (aw'to·tok'sin)
auxotroph (aw'to·trōf)
avascular (ah·vas'ku·lar)
avirulent (a·vir'u·lent)
avitaminosis (a·vi'tah·mĭ·no·sis)
avoirdupois (av'er·dŭ·poiz)
avulsion (ah·vul'shun)
axenic (a·zen'ik)
axilla (ak·sil'ah)
axillary (ak'sĭ·lar'e)
axofugal (ak·sof'u·gal)
axolemma (ak·so·lem'ah)
axon (ak'son)
axoplasm (ak'so·plazm)
azobilirubin (az'o·bil·ĭ·roo'bin)
azoospermia (a·zo'o·sper'me·ah)
azotemia (az'o·te'me·ah)
azotification (az·o'tĭ·fi·ka'shun)
azygos (as'ĭ·gos)
azygous (az'ĭ·gus)

B

Babesia (bah·be'ze·ah)
babesiosis (bah·be'ze·o'sis)
bacillary (bas'ĭ·la're)
bacillemia (bas'ĭ·le'me·ah)
bacilli (bah·sil'i)
bacilliform (bah·sil'ĭ·form)
bacilluria (bas'ĭ·lu're·ah)
bacillus (bah·sil'lus)
bacitracin (bas'ĭ·tray'sin)
bacteremia (bak'ter·e'me·ah)
bactericide (bak·tēr'ĭ·sīd)
bacteriform (bak·tēr'ĕ·form)
bacteriology (bak·te're·ol'o·je)
bacteriolysin (bak·te're·ol'ĭ·sin)
bacteriolytic (bak·te're·o·lit'ik)
bacteriophage (bak·te're·o·fāj')
bacteriopsonin (bak·te're·op'so·nin)
bacteriostasis (bak·te're·os'tah·sis)
bacteriostat (bak·te're·o·stat')
bacterium (bak·te're·um)
bacteriuria (bak·te're·u're·ah)
Bacteroides (bak'tĕ·roi'dez)
bagassosis (bag'ah·so'sis)
balanitis (bal'ah·ni'tis)
balanoblennorrhea (bal'ah·no·blen'o·re'ah)
balanoplasty (bal'ah·no·plas'te)
balanoposthitis (bal'ah·no·pos·thi'tis)
balanopreputial (bal'ah·no·pre·pu'she·al)
ballism (bal'izm)
ballistocardiogram (bal·lis'to·kar'de·o·gram')
ballottement (bah·lot'ment)
balneotherapeutics (bal'ne·o·ther·ah·pu'tiks)
baragnosis (bar'ag·no'sis)
barbital (bar'bĭ·tal)
barbiturate (bar·bit'u·rāt)
barbituric (bar'bit·u'rik)
barbiturism (bar·bit'u·rizm)
bariatrician (bar'e·ah·trish'un)
bariatrics (bar'e·at'riks)
barium (ba're·um)
baroreceptor (bar'o·re·sep'tor)
bartholinitis (bar'to·lin·i'tis)
bartonellosis (bar'to·nel·lo'sis)
basicranial (ba'se·kra'ne·al)
basilar (bas'ĭ·lar)
basilateral (ba'se·lat'er·al)
basion (ba'se·on)
basophilia (ba'so·fil'e·ah)
basophilic (ba·so·fil'ik)
becquerel (bek·rel')
bedewing (be·doo'ing)
bejel (bej'el)
belladonna (bel'ah·don'ah)
belle indifference (bel'ahn·dif'er·awns')
benign (be·nīn')

benzalkonium (ben'zal·ko'ne·um)
benzene (ben'zēn)
benzimidazole (ben'zim·ĭ·da'zōl)
benzoate (ben'zo·āt)
benzoin (ben'zoin)
benzyl (ben'zil)
beriberi (ber'e·ber'e)
berkelium (berk'le·um)
beryllium (ber·il'le·um)
bestiality (bes·te·al'ĭ·te)
beta (ba'tah)
betel (be'tl)
bezoar (be'zōr)
biauricular (bi'aw·rik'u·lar)
bicameral (bi·kam'er·al)
bicipital (bi·sip'ĭ·tal)
bicornous (bi·kor'nus)
bicornuate (bi·kor'nu·āt)
bicuspid (bi·kus'pid)
bifid (bi'fid)
bifurcate (bi·fur'kāt)
bigeminy (bi·jem'ĭ·ne)
biliary (bil'e·a·re)
bilifuscin (bil'ĭ·fus'in)
bilious (bil'yus)
biliousness (bil'yus·nes)
bilirubin (bil'ĭ·roo'bin)
bilirubinemia (bil'ĭ·roo·bĭ·ne'me·ah)
bilirubinuria (bil'ĭ·roo·bĭ·nu're·ah)
biliuria (bil'ĭ·u're·ah)
biliverdin (bil'ĭ·ver'din)
Billroth (bil'roth)
bilobate (bi·lo'bāt)
bilobular (bi·lob'u·lar)
binary (bi'na·re)
binaural (bi·naw'ral)
bioassay (bi'o·as·sa')
biogenesis (bi'o·jen'ĕ·sis)
biokinetics (bi'o·kĭ·net'iks)
biometrician (bi'o·mĕ·trish'un)
biometry (bi·om'ĕ·tre)
bion (bi'on)
biopsy (bi'op·se)
biospectrometry (bi'o·speck·trom'e·tre)
biosynthesis (bi'o·sin'thĕ·sis)
biotelemetry (bi'o·tel·em'ĕ·tre)
biotin (bi'o·tin)
bipara (bip'ar·ah)
biparietal (bi'pah·ri'ĕ·tal)
biparous (bip'ah·rus)
bipennate (bi·pen'āt)
birefringence (bi're·frin'jens)
bismuth (biz'muth)
biuret (bi'u·ret)
bivalence (bi·va'lens)
biventer (bi'ven·ter)
Blalock (bla'lok)
blastocele (blas'to·sēl)
blastocyst (blas'to·sist)
blastogenesis (blas'to·jen'ĕ·sis)
blastomere (blas'to·mēr)
Blastomyces (blas'to·mi'sēz)
blastomycosis (blas'to·mi·ko'sis)
blastula (blas'tu·lah)
blennadenitis (blen'ad·ĕ·ni'tis)
blennorrhea (blen'no·re'ah)
blennorrheal (blen'no·re'al)
blepharectomy (blef'ah·rek'to·me)
blepharitis (blef'ah·ri'tis)
blepharochalasis (blef'ah·ro·kal'ah·sis)
blepharoconjunctivitis (blef'ah·ro·kon·junk'tĭ·vi'tis)
blepharon (blef'ah·ron)
blepharophimosis (blef'ah·ro·fi·mo'sis)
blepharoplasty (blef'ah·ro·plas'te)
blepharoptosis (blef'ah·ro·to'sis)
blepharospasm (blef'ah·ro·spazm)
blepharotomy (blef'ah·rot'o·me)
bolus (bo'lus)
bombesin (bom'bĕ·sin)
borborygmus (bor'bo·rig'mus)
Borrelia (bŏ·rel'e·ah)
bosselation (bos'ĕ·la'shun)
botryoid (bot're·oid)
botryomycosis (bot're·o·mi·ko'sis)
bougienage (boo·zhe·nahzh')
bouton (boo·taw')
bovine (bo'vīn)

brachia (bra′ke·ah)
brachial (bra′ke·al)
brachiotomy (bra·ke·ot′o·me)
brachium (bra′ke·ŭm)
brachycephalism (brak′e·sef′ah·lizm)
brachydactyly (brak′e·dak′tĭ·le)
brachytherapy (brak′e·ther′a·pe)
bradycardia (brad′e·kar′de·ah)
bradycrotic (brad′e·krot′ik)
bradykinesia (brad′e·kĭ·ne′se·ah)
bradykinin (brad′e·ki′nin)
bradypnea (brad′ip′ne·ah)
brei (bri)
bromcresol (brom·kre′sol)
bromide (bro′mīd)
bromine (bro′mēn)
bromphenol (brom·fe′nol)
bronchi (brong′ki)
bronchiectasis (brong′ke·ek′tah·sis)
bronchiogenic (brong′ke·o·jen′ik)
bronchiole (brong′ke·ōl)
bronchiolectasis (brong′ke·o·lek′tah·sis)
bronchiolitis (brong′ke·o·li′tis)
bronchiostenosis (brong′ke·o·stĕ·no′sis)
bronchocele (brong′ko·sēl)
bronchoegophony (brong′ko·e·gof′o·ne)
bronchography (brong·kog′rah·fe)
broncholith (brong′ko·lith)
bronchomalacia (brong′ko·mah·la′she·ah)
bronchophony (brong·kof′o·ne)
bronchoplasty (brong′ko·plas′te)
bronchoplegia (brong′ko·ple′je·ah)
bronchoscope (brong′ko·skōp)
bronchoscopy (brong·kos′ko·pe)
bronchospirography
   (brong′ko·spi·rog′rah·fe)
bronchospirometer
   (brong′ko·spi·rom′ĕ·ter)
bronchostenosis (brong′ko·ste·no′sis)
bronchus (brong′kus)
Brucella (broo·sel′ah)
brucellosis (broo′sel·lo′sis)
bruit (brwe)
bruxism (bruk′sizm)
bruxomania (bruk′so·ma′ne·ah)
bubo (bu′bo)
buccal (buk′al)
buccolingual (buk′ko·ling′gwal)
bulbopontine (bul′bo·pon′tīn)
bulbourethral (bul′bo·u·re′thral)
bulimia (bu·lim′e·ah)
bulla (bul′ah)
bullae (bul′e)
bunion (bun′yun)
buphthalmos (buf·thal′mos)
burette (bu·ret′)
bursa (ber′sah)
bursae (ber′se)
bursectomy (ber·sek′to·me)
bursitis (ber·si′tis)
bursotomy (ber·sot′o·me)
busulfan (bu·sul′fan)

C

cachexia (kah·kek′se·ah)
cacosmia (kak·oz′me·ah)
cadaver (kah·dav′er)
cadaverine (kah·dav′er·in)
cafe au lait (ka·fe′ o la′)
caisson (ka′sun)
calcaneus (kal·ka′ne·us)
calcareous (kal·ka′re·us)
calcicosis (kal′sĭ·ko′sis)
calcine (kal′sin)
calcinosis (kal′sĭ·no′sis)
calciphilia (kal′sĭ·fil′e·ah)
calcitonin (kal′sĭ·to′nin)
calciuria (kal′sĭ·u′re·ah)
calcodynia (kal′ko din′e·ah)
calculus (kal′ku·lus)
calculi (kal′ku·li)
calefacient (kal′e·fa′shent)
caliceal (kal·i·se′al)
calices (kal′ĭ·sēz)
caliculus (kah·lik′u·lus)
caliectasis (ka′li·ek′tah·sis)

calipers (kal′ĭ·perz)
calix (ka′liks)
callous (kal′us)
callus (kal′us)
calvaria (kal·va′re·ah)
Campylobacter (kam′pĭ·lo·bak′ter)
canaliculi (kan′ah·lik′u·li)
canaliculus (kan′ah·lik′u·lus)
cancellous (kan′sĕ·lus)
cancroid (kang′kroid)
cancrum (kang′krum)
candela (kan·del′ah)
Candida (kan′dĭ·dah)
candidiasis (kan′dĭ·di′ah·sis)
canker (kang′ker)
cannabis (kan′ah·bis)
cannula (kan′u·lah)
canthoplasty (kan′tho·plas′te)
canthorrhaphy (kan·thor′ah·fe)
canthotomy (kan·thot′o·me)
canthus (kan′thus)
capacitance (kah·pas′ĭ·tans)
capillariomotor (kap′ĭ·lār′e·o·mo′tor)
capillary (kap′ĭ·lār′e)
capilli (kah·pil′li)
capillus (kah·pil′lus)
capita (kap′ĭ·tah)
capitellum (kah′pĭ·tel′um)
capitulum (kah·pit′u·lum)
capsid (kap′sid)
caput (kap′ut)
carbamide (kar·bam′īd)
carbaminohemoglobin
   (kar·bam′ĭ·no·he′mo·glo′bin)
carbamoyl (kar′bah·moil)
carbamoylglutamic
   (kar·bam′o·il·gloo′tah·mik)
carbarsone (kar′bar·sōn)
carbohydrases (kar′bo·hi′drās)
carbonyl (kar′bo·nil)
carboxyhemoglobin
   (kar·bok′se·he′mo·glo′bin)
carboxyhemoglobinemia
   (kar·bok′se·he′mo·glo′bin·e′me·ah)
carboxyl (kar·bok′sil)
carboxylase (kar·bok′sĭ·lās)
carboxypeptidase (kar·bok′se·pep′tĭ·dās)
carbuncle (kar′bung·kl)
carcinogen (kar·sin′o·jen)
carcinogenesis (kar′sĭ·no·jen′ĕ·sis)
carcinogenic (kar′sĭ·no·jen′ik)
carcinoid (kar′sĭ·noid)
carcinoma (kar′sĭ·no′mah)
carcinomatous (kar′sĭ·nom′ah·tus)
cardia (kar′de·ah)
cardiatelia (kar′de·ah·te′le·ah)
cardiectasis (kar′de·ek′tah·sis)
cardiectomy (kar′de·ek′tŏ·me)
cardiectopia (kar′de·ek·to′pe·ah)
cardiocentesis (kar′de·o·sen·te′sis)
cardiogram (kar′de·o·gram)
cardiography (kar′de·og′rah·fe)
cardioinhibitory (kar′de·o·in·hib′ĭ·to·re)
cardiokinetic (kar′de·o·kĭ·net′ik)
cardiolipin (kar′de·o·lip′in)
cardiology (kar·de·ol′o·je)
cardiomegaly (kar′de·o·meg′ah·le)
cardiomyoliposis (kar′de·o·mi′o·li·po′sis)
cardiomyopathy (kar′de·o·mi·op′ah·the)
cardiopathy (kar′de·op′ah·the)
cardiopericardiopexy
   (kar′de·o·per′ĭ·kar′de·o·pek·se)
cardioplasty (kar′de·o·plas′te)
cardiorrhexis (kar′de·o·rek′sis)
cardioverter (kar′de·o·ver′ter)
carina (kah·ri′nah)
carnosine (kar′no·sin)
carotene (kar′o·tēn)
carotenemia (kar′o·te·ne′me·ah)
cartilaginous (kar′tĭ·laj′ĭ·nus)
caruncle (kar′ung·kl)
caseation (ka′se·a′shun)
caseous (ka′se·us)
catabolite (kah·tab′ŏ·līt)
catacrotism (kah·tak′ro·tizm)
catalepsy (kat′ah·lep′se)
catamnesis (kat′am·ne′sis)
cataphasia (kat′ah·fa′ze·ah)

cataplasia (kat′ah·pla′se·ah)
cataplexy (kat′ah·plek·se)
cataract (kat′ah·rakt)
catarrh (kah·tahr′)
catatonia (kat·ah·to′ne·ah)
catechol (kat′ĕ·kol)
catecholamines (kat′ĕ·kol′ah·mēnz)
catharsis (kah·thar′sis)
cathepsin (kah·thep′sin)
cathepsis (kah·thep′sis)
catheterization (kath′ĕ·ter·i·za′shun)
catheterize (kath′ĕ·ter·īz)
cathexis (kah·thek′sis)
cation (kat′i·on)
cauda (kaw′dah)
caudad (kaw′dad)
caudae (kaw′de)
caudal (kaw′dal)
caudate (kaw′dāt)
caul (kawl)
cauterization (kaw′ter·i·za′shun)
cautery (kaw′ter·e)
caveolae (ka·ve·o′le)
cavitary (kav′ĭ·ta′re)
cavus (kav′us)
cecum (se′kum)
celiac (se′le·ak)
cellulose (sel′u·lōs)
celom (se′lom)
celomic (se·lom′ik)
Celsius (sel′se·us)
cementoblast (se·men′to·blast)
cementocyte (se·men′to·sit)
cementoma (se′men·to′mah)
cementum (se·men′tum)
centesis (sen·te′sis)
centibar (sen′ti·bar)
centrad (sen′trad)
centrage (sen′traj)
centrifugal (sen·trif′u·gal)
centrifuge (sen′tri·fūj)
centrilobular (sen′tri·lob′u·lar)
centromere (sen′tro·mēr)
cephalad (sef′ah·lad)
cephalalgia (sef′ah·lal′je·ah)
cephalic (sĕ·fal′ik)
cephalin (sef′ah·lin)
cephalization (sef′al·i·za′shun)
cephalocentesis (sef′ah·lo·sen·te′sis)
cephalodynia (sef′ah·lo·din′e·ah)
cephalogyric (sef′ah·lo·ji′rik)
cephalosporin (sef′ah·lo·spōr′in)
ceramide (ser′ah·mid)
cerebellopontine (ser′ĕ·bel′o·pon′tēn)
cerebellorubral (ser′ĕ·bel′o·ru′bral)
cerebellum (ser′ĕ·bel′um)
cerebromeningitis (ser′ĕ·bro·men′in·ji′tis)
cerebrosclerosis (ser′e·bro′skle·ro′sis)
cerebrose (ser′e·brōs)
cerebroside (ser′e·bro·sīd)
cerium (se′re·um)
ceruloplasmin (se·roo′lo·plaz′min)
cerumen (sĕ·roo′men)
cervix (ser′viks)
cesium (se′ze·um)
Cestoda (ses·to′dah)
cestode (ses′tōd)
chalasia (kah·la′ze·ah)
chalazion (kah·la′ze·on)
chalone (kal′ōn)
chancre (shang′ker)
chancroid (shang′kroid)
cheilectomy (ki·lek′to·me)
cheilion (ki′li·on)
cheilitis (ki·li′tis)
cheilognathouranoschisis (ki′lo·na′tho·
   u·rah·nos′ki·sis)
cheiloplasty (ki′lo·plas′te)
cheiloschisis (ki·los′ki·sis)
cheilosis (ki·lo′sis)
cheiroscope (ki′ro·skōp)
chelate (ke′lāt)
chelation (ke·la′shun)
chemocautery (ke′mo·kaw′ter·e)
chemodectoma (ke′mo·dek·to′mah)
chemokinesis (ke′mo·ki·ne′sis)
chemolysis (ke·mol′i·sis)
chemonucleolysis (ke′mo·nu′kle·ol′i·sis)

chemoprophylaxis (ke'mo·pro'fi·lak'sis)
chemoreceptor (ke'mo·re·sep'tor)
chemosis (ke·mo'sis)
chemotaxis (ke'mo·tak'sis)
chemotherapeutics (ke'mo·ther·ah·pu'tiks)
chemotherapy (ke'mo·ther'ah·pe)
chiasma (ki·as'mah)
chigoe (chig'o)
chilblain (chil'blān)
chimera (ki·me'rah)
chirognostic (ki'rog·nos'tik)
chirokinesthesia (ki'ro·kin'es·the'ze·ah)
chiroplasty (ki'ro·plas'te)
chiropractic (ki'ro·prak'tik)
chiropractor (ki'ro·prak'tor)
chitin (ki'tin)
chitobiose (ki'to·bi'ōs)
chitosamine (ki'to·sah·mēn)
Chlamydia (klah·mid'e·ah)
chloasma (klo·az'mah)
chloracne (klor·ak'ne)
chloralism (klo'ral·izm)
chloralose (klo'rah·lōs)
chlorambucil (klo·ram'bu·sil)
chloramphenicol (klo'ram·fen'i·kol)
chlordiazepoxide (klōr'di·az'ē·pok'sīd)
chlorhydria (klōr·hi'dre·ah)
chloridometer (klo'ri·dom'ē·ter)
chloriduria (klo'ri·du're·ah)
chloroform (klo'ro·form)
chloroma (klo·ro'mah)
chlorometry (klo·rom'ē·tre)
chlorophyllin (klo'ro·fil·in)
chloroplast (klo'ro·plast)
chloropsia (klo·rop'se·ah)
chloroquine (klo'ro·kwin)
chlorosis (klo·ro'sis)
chlorothiazide (klo'ro·thi'ah·zīd)
chlorpromazine (klōr·pro'mah·zēn)
chlorpropamide (klōr·pro'pah·mīd)
chlortetracycline (klōr'tet·rah·si'klēn)
chloruresis (klōr'u·re'sis)
choana (ko'a·nah)
cholagogue (ko'lah·gog)
cholangiectasis (ko·lan'je·ek'tah·sis)
cholangiocarcinoma (ko·lan'je·kar'si·no'mah)
cholangiography (ko·lan'je·og'rah·fe)
cholangiole (ko·lan'je·ōl)
cholangioscopy (ko·lahn·je·os'ko·pi)
cholangiostomy (ko'lan·je·os'to·me)
cholangiotomy (ko'lan·je·ot'o·me)
cholangitis (ko'lan·ji'tis)
cholanopoiesis (ko'lah·no·poi·e'sis)
cholecyst (ko'le·sist)
cholecystagogic (ko'le·sis'tah·goj'ik)
cholecystagogue (ko'le·sis'tah·gog)
cholecystectasia (ko'le·sis'tek·ta'ze·ah)
cholecystectomy (ko'le·sis·tek'to·me)
cholecystic (ko'le·sis'tik)
cholecystitis (ko'le·sis·ti'tis)
cholecystogram (ko'le·sis'to·gram)
cholecystography (ko'le·sis·tog'rah·fe)
cholecystokinase (ko'le·sis'to·ki'nās)
cholecystokinetic (ko'le·sis'to·ki·net'ik)
cholecystokinin (ko'le·sis'to·kin'in)
cholecystolithiasis (ko'le·sis'to·li·thi'ah·sis)
cholecystorrhaphy (ko'le·sis·tor'ah·fe)
cholecystotomy (ko'le·sis·tot'o·me)
choledochal (kol'ē·dok·al)
choledochectomy (kol'ē·do·kek'to·me)
choledochitis (kol'ē·do·ki'tis)
choledochoduodenostomy (ko·led'o·ko·du'o·dē·nos'to·me)
choledochography (ko·led'o·kog'rah·fe)
choledocholith (ko·led'ŏ·ko·lith')
choledocholithiasis (ko·led'ŏ·ko·li·thi'ah·sis)
choledocholithotomy (ko·led'ŏ·ko·li·thot'o·me)
choledochoplasty (ko·led'o·ko·plas'te)
choledochorrhaphy (ko·led'o·kor'ah·fe)
choledochoscope (ko·led'o·ko·skōp')
choledochoscopy (ko·le·do·kos'ko·pe)
choledochotomy (ko·led'o·kot'o·me)
choledochous (ko·led'o·kus)

cholelith (ko'le·lith)
cholelithiasis (ko'le·li·thi'ah·sis)
cholelithotomy (ko'le·li·thot'o·me)
cholemesis (ko·lem'ē·sis)
cholemia (ko·le'me·ah)
cholemic (ko·le'mik)
cholepoiesis (ko'le·poi·e'sis)
cholera (kol'er·ah)
choleresis (kol·er·e'sis, ko·ler'ē·sis)
cholerrhagia (kol'e·ra'ji·ah)
cholestasia (ko'le·sta'ze·ah)
cholestasis (ko'le·sta'sis)
cholestatic (ko'le·stat'ik)
cholesteatoma (ko'le·ste'ah·to'mah)
cholesteremia (ko·les'ter·e'me·ah)
cholesterol (ko·les'ter·ol)
cholesterolosis (ko·les'ter·ol·o'sis)
cholic (ko'lik)
cholinergic (ko'lin·er'jik)
cholinester (ko'lin·es'ter)
cholinesterase (ko'lin·es'ter·ās)
cholinomimetic (ko'li·no·mi·met'ik)
cholorrhea (kol·or·re'ah)
cholylcoenzyme (ko'lil·ko·en'zīm)
chondral (kon'dral)
chondralgia (kon·dral'je·ah)
chondrectomy (kon·drek'to·me)
chondrin (kon'drin)
chondritis (kon·dri'tis)
chondroblastoma (kon'dro·blas·to'mah)
chondroclast (kon'dro·klast)
chondrocostal (kon'dro·kos'tal)
chondrocyte (kon'dro·sīt)
chondrodystrophia (kon'dro·dis·tro'fe·ah)
chondroitin (kon·dro'i·tin)
chondroma (kon·dro'mah)
chondromalacia (kon'dro·mah·la'she·ah)
chondropathy (kon·drop'ah·the)
chondrophyte (kon'dro·fit)
chondroplasty (kon'dro·plas'te)
chondrosarcoma (kon'dro·sar·ko'mah)
chondrosternal (kon'dro·ster'nal)
chorda (kor'dah)
chordae (kor'di)
chordee (kor'de)
chordoma (kor·do'mah)
chorea (ko·re'ah)
choreic (kŏ·re'ik)
choreiform (kŏ·re'i·form)
choreoathetosis (ko're·o·ath'ē·to'sis)
chorioamnionitis (ko're·o·am'ne·o·ni'tis)
chorioangioma (ko're·o·an'je·o'mah)
choriomeningitis (ko're·o·men'in·ji'tis)
chorion (ko're·on)
chorionic (ko're·on'ik)
choristoma (ko'ris·to'mah)
choroid (ko'roid)
choroideremia (ko'roi·der·e'me·ah)
choroiditis (ko'roid·i'tis)
choroidocyclitis (ko·roi'do·sik·li'tis)
chromaffin (kro·maf'in)
chromaffinoma (kro'maf·i·no'mah)
chromaffinopathy (kro'maf·i·nop'ah·the)
chromatogenous (kro'mah·toj'ē·nus)
chromatography (kro'mah·tog'rah·fe)
chromatolysis (kro'mah·tol'i·sis)
chomatophilic (kro'mah·to·fil'ik)
chromatopsia (kro'mah·top'se·ah)
chromesthesia (kro'mes·the'ze·ah)
chromidium (kro·mid'e·um)
chromogen (kro'mo·jen)
chromometer (kro·mom'ē·ter)
chromomycosis (kro'mo·mi·ko'sis)
chromonema (kro'mo·ne'mah)
chromonemata (kro'mo·ne'mah·tah)
chromophil (kro'mo·fil)
chromophore (kro'mo·for)
chromosome (kro'mo·sōm)
chronaxia (kro·nak'se·ah)
chronaxie (kro'nak·se)
chronic (kron'ik)
chronognosis (kron'og·no'sis)
chronotaraxis (kro·no·tar·ak'sis)
chronotropism (kro·not'ro·pizm)
chrysiasis (krī·si'ah·sis)
chrysotherapy (kris'o·ther'ah·pe)
chyle (kil)
chylomicron (ki'lo·mi'kron)

chylomicronemia (ki'lo·mi'kron·e'me·ah)
chylopoiesis (ki'lo·poi·e'sis)
chylothorax (ki'lo·tho'raks)
chyluria (ki·lu're·ah)
chyme (kīm)
chymopoiesis (ki'mo·poi·e'sis)
chymotrypsin (ki'mo·trip'sin)
chymotrypsinogen (ki'mo·trip·sin'o·jen)
cicatrectomy (sik'ah·trek'to·me)
cicatrix (sik'ah·triks)
cicatrization (sik'ah·tri·za'shun)
ciliarotomy (sil'e·ar·ot'o·me)
cimbia (sim'be·ah)
cimetidine (si·met'i·dēn)
cinchona (sin·ko'nah)
cinchonism (sin'ko·nizm)
circadian (ser'kah·de·an, ser·ka'di·an)
circinate (ser'si·nāt)
circumocular (ser'kum·ok'u·lar)
circumvallate (ser'kum·val'āt)
circumvolute (ser'kum·vo'lūt)
cirrhosis (sir·ro'sis)
cisterna (sis·ter'nah)
cistron (sis'tron)
citrate (sit'rāt)
claudication (klaw'di·ka'shun)
claustrum (klaws'trum)
cleoid (kle'oid)
clidarthritis (kli·dar·thri'tis)
clidotomy (kli·dot'o·me)
climacter (kli·mak'ter)
climacteric (kli·mak'ter·ik)
clinocephaly (kli'no·sef'ah·le)
clinodactyly (kli'no·dak'ti·le)
clinoid (kli'noid)
clinoscope (kli'no·skōp)
clitoridectomy (kli'to·ri·dek'to·me)
clitoris (klit'o·ris)
clivus (kli'vus)
cloaca (klo·a'kah)
clofibrate (klo·fi'brāt)
clonorchiosis (klo'nor·ki'ah·sis)
Clonorchis (klo·nor'kis)
Clostridium (klo·strid'e·um)
coagglutinin (ko'ah·gloo'ti·nin)
coagulant (ko·ag'u·lant)
coagulase (ko·ag'u·lās)
coagulate (ko·ag'u·lāt)
coagulin (ko·ag'u·lin)
coaptation (ko'ap·ta'shun)
coarctation (ko'ark·ta'shun)
cocci (kok'si)
Coccidia (kok·sid'e·ah)
Coccidioides (kok·sid'e·oi'dēz)
coccidioidomycosis (kok·sid'e·oi'do·mi·ko'sis)
coccidiosis (kok'sid·e·o'sis)
coccoid (kok'oid)
coccus (kok'us)
coccygeal (kok·sij'e·al)
coccyges (kok'si·jes)
coccyx (kok'siks)
cochlea (kok'le·ah)
codecarboxylase (ko'de·kar·bok'sil·ās)
codon (ko'don)
coitus (ko'i·tus)
colchicine (kol'chi·sin)
colibacilluria (ko'li·bas'i·lu're·ah)
colic (kol'ic)
collagenosis (kol·laj'ē·no'sis)
colliculi (kŏ·lik'u·li)
colliculus (kŏ·lik'u·lus)
colligative (kol'i·ga'tiv)
collimation (kol'li·ma'shun)
colliquation (kol'i·kwa'shun)
colliquative (kŏ·lik'wah·tiv)
collum (kol'lum)
coloboma (kol'o·bo'mah)
colocolic (kol'o·kol'ik)
cololysis (ko·lol'i·sis)
colonoscopy (ko'lon·os'ko·pe)
colopexy (ko'lo·pek'se)
coloproctitis (ko'lo·prok·ti'tis)
colorimetry (kul'or·im'e·tre)
colorrhagia (kol'or·ra'je·a)
colorrhea (ko'lo·re'ah)
colostomy (ko·los'to·me)
colostrorrhea (ko·los'tro·re'ah)

colostrum (kŏ·los'trum)
colpocleisis (kol'po·kli'sis)
colpoperineorrhaphy
 (kol'po·per'ĭ·ne·or'ah·fe)
colpopoiesis (kol'po·poi·e'sis)
colpoptosis (kol'po·to'sis)
colporrhaphy (kol'por'ah·fe)
colporrhexis (kol·po·rek'sis)
colposcope (kol'po·skōp)
colposcopy (kol·pos'ko·pe)
colpoxerosis (kol'po·ze·ro'sis)
columbium (ko·lum'be·um)
columella (kol'u·mel'ah)
comedo (kom'ĕ·do)
comedones (kom·ĕ·do'nēz)
comes (ko'mēz)
comites (kom'ĭ·tēz)
commensal (kŏ·men'sal)
comminuted (kom'ĭ·nūt'ed)
commissure (kom'ĭ·shūr)
commissurotomy (kom'ĭ·shūr·ot'o·me)
communicans (kŏ·mu'nĭ·kanz)
communis (kŏ·mu'nis)
compos mentis (kom'pos men'tis)
concameration (kon·kam'er·a'shun)
concatenate (kon·kat'ĕ·nāt)
concha (kon'chah)
conchae (kon'che)
concussion (kon·kush'un)
condom (kon'dum)
condylar (con'dĭ·lar)
condylarthrosis (kon'dil·ar·thro'sis)
condyle (kon'dīl)
condyloma (kon'dĭ·lo'mah)
condylomatous (kon'dĭ·lo'mah·tus)
condylotomy (kon'dĭ·lot'o·me)
confluent (kon'floo·ent)
congener (kon'jĕ·ner)
conglutination (kon·gloo'tĭ·na'shun)
conglutinin (kon·gloo'tĭ·nin)
conidia (ko·nid'e·ah)
conidiophore (ko·nid'e·o·fōr)
conidiospore (ko·nid'e·o·spōr)
conidium (ko·nid'e·um)
coniofibrosis (ko'ne·o·fi·bro'sis)
conjugase (kon'ju·gās)
consanguineous (kon'sang·gwin'e·us)
consensual (kon·sen'shu·al)
constipation (kon'stĭ·pa'shun)
consultant (kon·sul'tant)
contagion (kon·ta'jun)
contiguity (kon'tĭ·gu'ĭ·te)
continence (kon'tĭ·nens)
contracture (kon·trak'tūr)
contrecoup (kon·tr·koo')
contusion (kon·tu'zhun)
convalescence (kon'vah·les'ens)
convolution (kon·vo·lu'shun)
convulsion (kon·vul'shun)
coproantibodies (kop'ro·an'tĭ·bod'ēz)
coprolalia (kop'ro·la'le·ah)
coprolith (kop'ro·lith)
coproporphyrin (kop'ro·por'fir·in)
coracoid (kor'ah·koid)
cordate (kor'dāt)
cordopexy (kor'do·pek'se)
corecleisis (kor'e·kli'sis)
corectasis (kor·ek'ta·sis)
corectopia (kor·ek·to'pe·ah)
coreometer (ko're·om'ĕ·ter)
corestenoma (ko're·ste·no'mah)
cornea (kor'ne·ah)
corneosclera (kor'ne·o·skle'rah)
corneum (kor'ne·um)
cornu (kor·nu)
cornua (kor'nu·ah)
corona (ko·ro'nah)
coronion (ko·ro'ne·on)
coronoid (kor'o·noid)
corpora (kor'po·rah)
corpus (kor'pus)
cortex (kor'teks)
cortical (kor'tĭ·kal)
corticifugal (kor'tĭ·sif'u·gal)
corticipetal (kor'tĭ·sip'e·tal)
corticopontine (kor'tĭ·ko·pon'tīn)
corticosteroid (kor'tĭ·ko·ste'roid)
corticothalamic (kor'tĭ·ko·thah·lam'ik)

corticotropin (kor'tĭ·ko·tro'pin)
cortisol (kor'tĭ·sol)
cortisone (kor'tĭ·sōn)
Corynebacterium (ko·ri'ne·bak·te're·um)
coryza (kŏ·ri'zah)
cosmesis (koz·me'sis)
costochondral (kos'to·kon'dral)
costotome (kos'to·tōm)
cotyledon (kot'ĭ·le'don)
coup (koo)
coxsackievirus (kok·sak'e·vi'rus)
craniomalacia (kra'ne·o·mah·la'she·ah)
craniopharyngioma
 (kra'ne·o·fah·rin'je·o'mah)
craniorrhachischisis
 (kra'ne·o·rah·kis'kĭ·sis)
cranioschisis (kra'ne·os'kĭ·sis)
craniostosis (kra'ne·os·to'sis)
craniotabes (kra'ne·o·ta'bēz)
creatine (kre'ah·tēn)
creatinine (kre·at'ĭ·nēn)
creatinuria (kre·at'ĭ·nu're·ah)
cremaster (kre·mas'ter)
crenocyte (kre'no·sīt)
crepitation (krep'ĭ·ta'shun)
crepitus (krep'ĭ·tus)
cresol (kre'sol)
cricoid (kri'koid)
cricoidectomy (kri'koi·dek'to·me)
cricothyroid (kri·ko·thi'roid)
cricotracheotomy (kri'ko·tra·ke·ot'o·me)
crinogenic (kri'no·jen'ik)
crista (kris'tah)
cristae (kris'te)
croup (kroop)
cruciate (kroo'she·āt)
crura (kroo'rah)
crus (kroos)
cryanesthesia (kri'an·es·the'ze·ah)
cryesthesia (kri'es·the'ze·ah)
cryoaerotherapy (kri'o·a'er·o·ther'ah·pe)
cryocautery (kri'o·kaw'ter·e)
cryogenics (kri'o·jen'iks)
cryoglobulin (kri'o·glob'u·lin)
cryoglobulinemia
 (kri'o·glob'u·lin·e'me·ah)
cryoscopy (kri·os'ko·pe)
cryosurgery (kri'o·sur'jer·e)
cryothalamectomy
 (kri'o·thal'ah·mek'to·me)
crypt (kript)
cryptococcin (krip'to·kok'sin)
cryptococcosis (krip'to·kok·o'sis)
cryptomerorachischisis
 (krip'to·me'ro·rah·kis'kĭ·sis)
cryptophthalmos (krip'tof·thal'mos)
cryptorchid (krip·tor'kid)
cryptosporidiosis (krip'to·spor·id'e·o'sis)
cryptozoite (krip'to·zo'īt)
cubitus (ku'bĭ·tus)
cuirass (kwe·ras')
cul-de-sac (kul'dĕ·sahk)
culdocentesis (kul'do·sen·te'sis)
culdoscope (kul'do·skōp)
culdoscopy (kul·dos'ko·pe)
Culex (ku'leks)
culicide (ku'lĭ·sīd)
culicifuge (ku·lis'ĭ·fūj)
cunei (ku'ne·i)
cuneiform (ku·ne'ĭ·form)
cuneus (ku'ne·us)
cuniculus (ku·nik'u·lus)
cunnilingus (kun'ĭ·ling'gus)
cupric (ku'prik)
cupula (ku'pu·lah)
curare (koo·rah're)
curettage (ku'rĕ·tahzh')
curette (ku·ret')
curie (ku're)
curium (ku're·um)
cutaneous (ku·ta'ne·us)
cuvet (ku·vet')
cyanmethemoglobin
 (si'an·met'he·mo·glob'bin)
cyanocobalamin (si'ah·no·ko·bal'ah·min)
cyanophil (si·an'o·fil)
cybernetics (si'ber·net'iks)
cyclarthrodial (sik'lar·thro'de·al)

cyclarthrosis (sik'lar·thro'sis)
cyclitis (sik·li'tis)
cyclizine (si'klĭ·zēn)
cyclochoroiditis (si'klo·ko'roid·i'tis)
cyclodialysis (si'klo·di·al'ĭ·sis)
cyclodiathermy (si'klo·di'ah·ther'me)
cyclokeratitis (si'klo·ker·ah·ti'tis)
cyclophorometer (si'klo·fo·rom'ĕ·ter)
cyclophosphamide (si'klo·fos'fah·mīd)
cycloplegia (si'klo·ple'je·ah)
cycloplegic (si'klo·ple'jik)
cyclothymia (si'klo·thīm'e·ah)
cyclotomy (si·klot'o·me)
cyclotron (si'klo·tron)
cylindruria (sil'in·droo're·ah)
cystadenocarcinoma
 (sis·tad'e·no·kar'sĭ·no'mah)
cystadenoma (sis'tad·e·no'mah)
cystathionine (sis'tah·thi'o·nīn)
cystathioninuria
 (sis'tah·thi'o·nīn·u're·ah)
cystectasia (sis·tek·ta'ze·ah)
cysteine (sis·te'in)
cysticercosis (sis'tĭ·ser·ko'sis)
cysticercus (sis'tĭ·ser'kus)
cysticotomy (sis'tĭ·kot'o·me)
cystine (sis'tēn)
cystinosis (sis'tĭ·no'sis)
cystinuria (sis'tĭ·nu're·ah)
cystitomy (sis·tit'o·me)
cystolith (sis'to·lith)
cystolithectomy (sis'to·lĭ·thek'to·me)
cystolithiasis (sis'to·lĭ·thi'ah·sis)
cystoma (sis·to'mah)
cystometer (sis·tom'e·ter)
cystometrogram (sis'to·met'ro·gram)
cystoplegia (sis'to·ple'je·ah)
cystoptosia (sis'top·to'se·ah)
cystopyelitis (sis'to·pi·e·li'tis)
cystorrhagia (sis'to·ra'je·ah)
cystoscope (sis'to·skōp)
cystoscopy (sis·tos'ko·pe)
cystospasm (sis'to·spazm)
cystoureteritis (sis'to·u·re'ter·i'tis)
cystourethritis (sis'to·u're·thri'tis)
cystourethrocele (sis'to·u·re'thro·sēl)
cytidine (si'tĭ·dēn)
cytoclasis (si·tok'lah·sis)
cytocyst (si'to·sist)
cytokines (si'to·kīnz)
cytolysin (si·tol'ĭ·sin)
cytomegalovirus (si'to·meg'ah·lo·vi'rus)
cytomorphology (si'to·mor·fol'o·je)
cytopemphis (si'to·pem'fis)
cytopoiesis (si'to·poi·e'sis)
cytosine (si'to·sēn)
cytosol (si'to·sol)
cytotrophoblast (si'to·trof'o·blast)
cytotropic (si'to·trop'ik)
cytozoon (si'to·zo'on)

D

dacryagogue (dak're·ah·gog)
dacryoadenitis (dak're·o·ad'ĕ·ni'tis)
dacryocystalgia (dak're·o·sis·tal'je·ah)
dacryocystitis (dak're·o·sis·ti'tis)
dacryocystogram (dak're·o·sis'to·gram)
dacryocystorhinostenosis
 (dak're·o·sis'to·ri'no·stĕ·no'sis)
dacryocystorhinostomy
 (dak're·o·sis'to·ri·nos'to·me)
dacryocystotomy (dak're·o·sis·tot'o·me)
dacryolith (dak're·o·lith')
dacryolithiasis (dak're·o·lĭ·thi'ah·sis)
dacryoma (dak're·o'mah)
dacryon (dak're·on)
dacryops (dak're·ops)
dacryorrhea (dak're·o·re'ah)
dacryosolenitis (dak're·o·so·lĕ·ni'tis)
dactinomycin (dak'tĭ·no·mi'sin)
dactyl (dak'til)
dactyledema (dak'til·ĕ·de'mah)
dactylogryposis (dak'tĭ·lo·grĭ·po'sis)
dactyloid (dak'tĭ·loid)
dactylolysis (dak'tĭ·lol'ĭ·sis)
dactylomegaly (dak'tĭ·lo·meg'ah·le)

dapsone (dap′sōn)
deacidification (de·ah·sid′ĭ·fĭ·ka′shun)
deafferentation (de·af′er·en·ta′shun)
deamidate (de·am′ĭ·dāt)
deaminase (de·am′ĭ·nās)
deaminate (de·am′ĭ·nāt)
debilitate (de·bil′ĭ·tāt)
débridement (da·brēd·maw′)
decarboxylase (de′kar·bok′sĭ·lās)
decarboxylation (de′kar·bok·sĭ·la′shun)
decerebrate (de·ser′ĕ·brāt)
decerebration (de′ser·ĕ·bra′shun)
decidua (de·sid′u·ah)
deciduous (de·sid′u·us)
deciliter (des′ĭ·le′ter)
decimeter (des′ĭ·me′ter)
decoction (de·kok′shun)
decortication (de′kor·tĭ·ka′shun)
decrudescence (de′kroo·des′ens)
decubitus (de·ku′bĭ·tus)
decussate (de·kus′āt)
defecation (def′e·ka′shun)
defemination (de·fem′ĭ·na′shun)
defervescence (def′er·ves′ens)
defibrillation (de·fib′rĭ·la′shun)
defibrillator (de·fib′rĭ·la′tor)
defluvium (de·floo′ve·um)
defurfuration (de·fur′fu·ra′shun)
deglutition (deg′loo·tish′un)
degu (da′gu)
dehalogenase (de·hal′o·jĕ·nās)
dehiscence (de·his′ens)
deja vu (da·zhah′ voo′)
deliquesce (del′ĭ·kwes′)
deliquescent (del·ĭ·kwes′ent)
demasculinization
  (de·mas′ku·lin·ĭ·za′shun)
dementia (de·men′she·ah)
demifacet (dem′e·fas′et)
demilune (dem′e·lūn)
demipenniform (dem′e·pen′ĭ·form)
demulcent (de·mul′sent)
demyelination (de·mi′ĕ·li·na′shun)
demyelinization (de·mi′ĕ·lin·ĭ·za′shun)
denaturation (de·na′chur·a′shun)
denatured (de·na′churd)
dendriform (den′drĭ·form)
dendrite (den′drīt)
dengue (deng′e)
denidation (den′ĭ·da′shun)
dentifrice (den′tĭ·fris)
dentigerous (den·tij′er·us)
dentin (den′tin)
dentinoma (den′tĭ·no′mah)
dentulous (den′tu·lus)
deoxidation (de·ok′sĭ·da′shun)
deoxidize (de·ok′sĭ·dīz)
deoxycholic (de·ok′sĭ·kol′ik)
deoxycorticosterone
  (de·ok′sĭ·kor′te·kos′ter·ōn)
deoxygenate (de·ok′sĭ·jĕ·nāt′)
deoxyribonuclease
  (de·ok′se·ri′bo·nu′kle·ās)
deoxyribonucleic
  (de·ok′se·ri′bo·nu·kle′ik)
deoxyribonucleoprotein
  (de·ok′se·ri′bo·nu′kle·o·pro′te·in)
deoxyribonucleoside
  (de·ok′se·ri′bo·nu′kle·o·sīd)
deoxyribinucleotide
  (de·ok′se·ri′bo·nu′kle·o·tīd)
deoxyribose (de·ok′se·ri′bōs)
deoxysugar (de·ok′se·shoog′ăr)
depancreatize (de·pan′kre·ah·tīz)
dephosphorylation (de·fos′for·i·la′shun)
depilation (dep′ĭ·la′shun)
depulization (de·pu′li·za′shun)
depurant (dep′u·rant)
Dermacentor (der′mah·sen′tor)
dermametropathism
  (der′mah·mĕ·trop′ah·thizm)
Dermatobia (der′mah·to′be·ah)
dermatome (der′mah·tōm)
dermatomycosis (der′mah·to·mi·ko′sis)
dermatomyositis (der′mah·to·mi′o·si′tis)
dermatophyte (der′mah·to·fīt)
dermatophytid (der′mah·tof′ĭ·tid)
dermatophytosis (der′mah·to·fi·to′sis)

descemetitis (des′ĕ·mĕ·ti′tis)
descensus (de·sen′sus)
desiccant (des′ĭ·kant)
desmolase (des′mo·lās)
desmopexia (des′mo·pek′se·ah)
desmosome (des′mo·sōm)
despumation (des′pu·ma′shun)
desquamation (des′kwah·ma′shun)
detumescence (de′tu·mes′ens)
deuteranopia (doo′ter·ah·no′pe·ah)
deuterium (doo·te′re·um)
deuteron (doo′ter·on)
deutoplasm (doo′to·plazm)
dextrans (dek′stranz)
dextraural (deks·traw′ral)
dextrocular (deks·trok′u·lar)
dextrorotatory (deks·tro·ro′tah·tōr·e)
diabetes (di′ah·be′tēz)
diabetic (di′ah·bet′ik)
diabetogenic (di′ah·bet′o·jen′ik)
diabetologist (di′ah·bĕ·tol′o·jist)
diadochokinesia (di·ad′ŏ·ko·ki·ne′se·ah)
diakinesis (di′ah·kĭ·ne′sis)
dialysance (di′ah·li′sans)
dialysate (di·al′ĭ·sāt)
diamine (di′ah·mēn)
diapedesis (di′ah·pĕ·de′sis)
diaphoretic (di′ah·fo·ret′ik)
diaphysis (di·af′ĭ·sis)
diarthrosis (di′ar·thro′sis)
diaschisis (di·as′kĭ·sis)
diastalsis (di′ah·stal′sis)
diastasis (di·as′tah·sis)
diastema (di′ah·ste′mah)
diastole (di·as′to·le)
diastolic (di′ah·stol′ik)
diataxia (di′ah·tak′se·ah)
diathermy (di′ah·ther′me)
diathesis (di·ath′ĕ·sis)
diatomaceous (di′ah·to·ma′shus)
diazepam (di·az′ĕ·pam)
diazoxide (di·az·ok′sīd)
dibasic (di·bā′sik)
dichotomy (di·kot′o·me)
dichromatism (di·kro′mah·tism)
dichromophil (di·kro′mo·fil)
dicrotic (di·krot′ik)
dicumarol (di·koo′mah·rol)
didactylism (di·dak′til·izm)
didymus (did′ĭ·mus)
diencephalon (di′en·sef′ah·lon)
digastric (di·gas′trik)
Digenea (di·je′ne·ah)
digit (dij′it)
digitalis (dij′ĭ·tal′is)
digitoxin (dij′ĭ·tok′sin)
digoxin (di·goks′in)
dihydrate (di·hi′drāt)
dihydroergotamine
  (di·hi′dro·er·got′ah·mēn)
diohydrostreptomycin
  (di·hi′dro·strep′to·mi′sin)
dihydrotachysterol
  (di·hi′dro·tak·is′tĕ·rol)
diiodotyrosine (di′i·o′do·ti′ro·sēn)
diisopropyl fluorophosphate
  (di′i·so·pro′pil floo·ah·ro·fos′fāt)
dilatation (dil·ah·ta′shun)
dilation (di·la′shun)
dilator (di·la′tor)
diltiazem (dil·ti′ah·zem)
diluent (dil′u·ent)
dilution (di·lu′shun)
dimenhydrinate (di′men·hi′drĭ·nāt)
dimercaprol (di′mer·kap′rol)
dinitrophenol (di·ni′tro·fe′nol)
dinucleotide (di·nu′kle·o·tīd)
diopter (di·op′ter)
dioptrics (di·op′triks)
dioptrometer (di·op·trom′ĕ·ter)
diotic (di·o′tik)
dipeptidase (di·pep′tĭ·dās)
dipeptide (di·pep′tīd)
diphenylhydantoin (di·fen′l·hi·dan′to·in)
diphosphopyridine (di·fos′fo·pir′ĭ·dēn)
diphtheria (dif·the′re·ah)
diphyllobothriasis (di·fil′o·both·ri′ah·sis)
Diphyllobothrium (di·fil′o·both′re·um)

diplacusis (dip′lah·ku′sis)
diplococci (dip′lo·kok′si)
diplococcus (dip′lo·kok′us)
diploe (dip′lo·e)
diplopia (dĭ·plo′pe·ah)
diplotene (dip′lo·tēn)
dipsosis (dip·so′sis)
dipyridamole (di′pi·rid′ah·mōl)
Dirofilaria (di′ro·fĭ·la′re·ah)
disaccharide (di·sak′ah·rīd)
discectomy (dis·sek′to·me)
discission (dis·sizh′un)
discutient (dis·ku′she·ent)
diskectomy (dis·kek′to·me)
diskitis (dis·ki′tis)
dismutase (dis·mu′tās)
dissect (dĭ·sekt′)
dissection (dĭ·sek′shun)
dissolution (dis′so·lu′shun)
dissolve (diz·zolv′)
disulfiram (di·sul′fi·ram)
diuresis (di′u·re′sis)
diuretic (di′u·ret′ik)
diverticula (di′ver·tik′u·lah)
diverticulectomy (di′ver·tik′u·lek′to·me)
diverticulitis (di′ver·tik·u·li′tis)
diverticulosis (di′ver·tik′u·lo′sis)
diverticulum (di′ver·tik′u·lum)
divulse (dĭ·vuls′)
dizygotic (di′zi·got′ik)
dolichocephalic (dol′i·ko·se·fal′ik)
dolichocephalism (dol′i·ko·sef′ah·lizm)
dopa (do′pah)
dopamine (do′pah·mēn)
dracontiasis (drak′on·ti′ah·sis)
Dracunculus (drah·kung′ku·lus)
drusen (droo′sen)
duodenal (du′o·de′nal)
duodenectomy (du′o·dĕ·nek′to·me)
duodenitis (du′od·ĕ·ni′tis)
duodenocholecystostomy
  (du′o·de′no·ko′le·sis·tos′to·me)
duodenocholedochotomy
  (du′o·de′no·ko′led·o·kot′o·me)
duodenoenterostomy
  (du′o·de′no·en′ter·os′to·me)
duodenojejunostomy
  (du′o·de′no·jĕ·joo·nos′to·me)
duodenolysis (du′o·dĕ·nol′i·sis)
duodenorrhaphy (du′o·dĕ·nor′ah·fe)
duodenoscopy (du′od·ĕ·nos′ko·pe)
duodenostomy (du′od·ĕ·nos′to·me)
duodenotomy (du′od·ĕ·not′o·me)
duodenum (du′o·de′num)
dura mater (dur′rah ma′ter)
dyad (di′ad)
dyne (dīn)
dysacusis (dis′ah·koo′sis)
dysarthria (dis·ar′thre·ah)
dysarthrosis (dis′ar·thro′sis)
dysautonomia (dis′aw·to·no′me·ah)
dyschezia (dis·ke′ze·ah)
dyschiria (dis·ki′re·ah)
dyschondrogenesis
  (dis′kon·dro·jen′ĕ·sis)
dyscrasia (dis·kra′ze·ah)
dysdiadochokinesia
  (dis′di·ad′ŏ·ko·ki·ne′se·ah)
dyseneia (dis′ĕ·ne′ah)
dysentery (dis′en·ter′e)
dyserethism (dis·er′e·thizm)
dysgammaglobulinemia
  (dis·gam′mah·glob′u·lĕ·ne′me·ah)
dysgeusia (dis·gu′ze·ah)
dysgnathia (dis·gna′the·ah)
dysgnosia (dis·no′se·ah)
dyshematopoiesis
  (dis·hem′ah·to′poi·e′sis)
dyshidrosis (dis·hid·ro′sis)
dyslalia (dis·la′le·ah)
dyslexia (dis·lek′se·ah)
dyslogia (dis·lo′je·ah)
dysmenorrhea (dis′men·o·re′ah)
dysostosis (dis·os·to′sis)
dyspareunia (dis′pah·roo′ne·ah)
dysphagia (dis·fa′je·ah)
dysphasia (dis·fa′ze·ah)
dysphoria (dis·fo′re·ah)

dysplasia   (dis·pla′se·ah)
dyspnea   (disp′ne·ah)
dyspraxia   (dis·prak′se·ah)
dyssynergia   (dis′sin·er′je·ah)
dyssynergy   (dis·sin′er·je)
dysthymia   (dis·thī′me·ah)
dystocia   (dis·to′se·ah)
dystontogenesis   (dis·ton·to·jen′ĕ·sis)
dystrophy   (dis′tro·fe)

E

ebonation   (e′bo·na′shun)
ebullism   (eb′u·lizm)
eburnation   (e′bur·na′shun)
eccentrochondroplasia
   (ek·sen′tro·kon′dro·pla′se·ah)
ecchondroma   (ek′kon·dro′mah)
ecchymoma   (ek′ĭ·mo′mah)
ecchymosis   (ek′ĭ·mo′sis)
eccrinology   (ek′rĭ·nol′o·je)
eccrisis   (ek′rĭ·sis)
eccyesis   (ek′si·e′sis)
ecdysis   (ek′dĭ·sis)
echidnase   (e·kid′nās)
echinococcosis   (e·ki′no·kok·o′sis)
echinosis   (ek′ĭ·no′sis)
Echinostoma   (ek′ĭ·nos′to·mah)
echinulate   (e·kin′u·lāt)
echocardiogram   (ek′o·kar′de·o·gram)
echocardiography   (ek′o·kar′de·og′ra·fe)
echoencephalography
   (ek′o·en·sef′ah·log′rah·fe)
echolalia   (ek′o·la′le·ah)
echopathy   (ek·op′ah·the)
echophonia   (ek′o·fon′e·ah)
echophony   (ek·of′o·ne)
echopraxia   (ek′o·prak′se·ah)
echovirus   (ek′o·vi′rus)
eclampsia   (ĕ·klamp′se·ah)
eclamptogenous   (ĕ·klam′toj′en·us)
ecmnesia   (ek·ne′ze·ah)
ectasia   (ek·ta′ze·ah)
ecthyma   (ek·thi′mah)
ectocardia   (ek·to·kar′de·ah)
ectochoroidea   (ek′to·ko·roi′de·ah)
ectocrine   (ek′to·krin)
ectoderm   (ek′to·derm)
ectogenous   (ek·toj′ĕ·nus)
ectomere   (ek′to·mēr)
ectopagia   (ek′to·pa′je·ah)
ectopia   (ek·to′pe·ah)
ectopic   (ek·top′ik)
ectoplasm   (ek′to·plazm)
ectostosis   (ek′to·sto′sis)
ektothrix   (ek′to·thriks)
ectozoon   (ek′to·zo′on)
ectrodactylism   (ek′tro·dak′tĭ·lizm)
ectrodactyly   (ek′tro·dak′tĭ·le)
ectrogeny   (ek·troj′ĕ·ne)
ectromelia   (ek′tro·me′la·ah)
ectropion   (ek·tro′pe·on)
ectrosyndactyly   (ek′tro·sin·dak′tĭ·le)
eczema   (ek′zĕ·mah)
eczematous   (ek·zem′ah·tus)
edema   (ĕ·de′ma)
edematous   (ĕ·dem′ah·tus)
edentate   (e·den′tāt)
edentulous   (e·den′tu·lus)
effect   (ĕ·fect′)
efferent   (ef′er·ent)
effervesce   (ef·er·ves′)
effleurage   (ef·loo·rahzh′)
effloresce   (ef′lo·res′)
effluvium   (ĕ·floo′ve·um)
effuse   (ĕ·fūs′)
effusion   (ĕ·fu′zhun)
ego   (e′go)
egomania   (e′go·ma′ne·ah)
egophony   (e·gof′o·ne)
eicosanoid   (i′ko·san′oid)
eidetic   (i·det′ik)
eikonometer   (i′ko·nom′ĕ·ter)
einsteinium   (īn·sti′ne·um)
ejaculate   (e·jak′u·lāt)
ejaculation   (e·jak′u·la′shun)

ejaculatory   (e·jak′u·lah·to′re)
elastance   (e·las′tans)
elastin   (e·las′tin)
elastomer   (e·las′to·mer)
elastosis   (e′las·to′sis)
electroanesthesia
   (e·lek′tro·an′es·the′ze·ah)
electrocardiogram
   (e·lek′tro·kar′de·o·gram)
electrocardiography
   (e·lek′tro·kar′de·og′rah·fe)
electrocauterization
   (e·lek′tro·kaw′ter·i·za′shun)
electrocautery   (e·lek′tro·kaw′ter·e)
electrocoagulation
   (e·lek′tro·ko·ag′u·la′shun)
electrocorticogram
   (e·lek′tro·kor′ti·ko·gram)
electrode   (e·lek′trōd)
electrodialysis   (e·lek′tro·di·al′ĭ·sis)
electroencephalogram
   (e·lek′tro·en·sef′ah·lo·gram)
electroencephalograph
   (e·lek′tro·en·sef′ah·lo·graf)
electroencephalography
   (e·lek′tro·en·sef′ah·log′rah·fe)
electrography   (e′lek·trog′rah·fe)
electrokymogram   (e·lek′tro·ki′mo·gram)
electrokymography
   (e·lek′tro·ki·mog′rah·fe)
electrolysis   (e′lek·trol′ĭ·sis)
electrolyte   (e·lek′tro·līt)
electromyogram   (e·lek′tro·mi′o·gram)
electromyography   (e·lek′tro·mi·og′rah·fe)
electron   (e·lek′tron)
electronystagmography
   (e·lek′tro·nis′tag·mog′rah·fe)
electrooculogram
   (e·lek′tro·ok′u·lo·gram)
electro-oculography
   (e·lek′tro-ok′u·log′rah·fe)
electrophoresis   (e·lek′tro·fo·re′sis)
electroretinogram
   (e·lek′tro·ret′ĭ·no·gram)
electrostethograph   (e·lek′tro·steth′o·graf)
elephantiasis   (el′ĕ·fan·ti′ah·sis)
elliptocytosis   (e·lip′to·si·to′sis)
eluate   (el′u·āt)
eluent   (e·lu′ent)
elution   (e·lu′shun)
elutriation   (e·lu′tre·a′shun)
elytrocleisis   (el′ĭ·tro·kli′sis)
emaciation   (e·ma′se·a′shun)
emaculation   (e·mak′u·la′shun)
embed   (em·bed′)
embolectomy   (em′bo·lek′to·me)
emboli   (em′bo·li)
embolism   (em′bo·lizm)
embolalia   (em′bŏ·lo·la′le·ah)
embolus   (em′bo·lus)
embrasure   (em·bra′zhur)
embrocation   (em·bro·ka′shun)
embryo   (em′bre·o)
embryoblast   (em′bre·o·blast)
embryogenesis   (em′bre·o·jen′ĕ·sis)
embryogenic   (em′bre·o·jen′ik)
embryogeny   (em′bre·oj′ĕ·ne)
embryology   (em′bre·ol′o·je)
embryoma   (em′bre·o′mah)
embryomorphous   (em′bre·o·mor′fus)
embryopathy   (em′bre·op′ah·the)
embryophore   (em′bre·o·fōr)
embryotoxon   (em′bre·o·tok′son)
emesis   (em′ĕ·sis)
emetic   (ĕ·met′ik)
emetocathartic   (em′ĕ·to·kah·thar′tik)
emmetropia   (em·ĕ·tro′pe·ah)
emollient   (e·mol′e·ent)
emphysema   (em′fi·se′mah)
empiricism   (em·pir′ĭ·sizm)
empyema   (em′pi·e′mah)
empyocele   (em′pi·o·sēl)
emulsion   (e·mul′shun)
emulsive   (e·mul′siv)
enameloma   (en·am′el·o′mah)
enanthem   (en·an′them)
enanthema   (en′·an·the′·mah)

enantiomer   (en·an′te·o·mer)
enantiomerism   (en·an′te·om′er·izm)
enantiomorph   (en·an′te·o·morf)
enantiopathy   (en·an′te·op′ah·the)
enarthrodial   (en′ar·thro′de·al)
enarthrosis   (en′ar·thro′sis)
encanthis   (en·kan′this)
encephalitis   (en·sef′ah·li′tis)
encephalocele   (en·sef′ah·lo·sēl)
encephalogram   (en·sef′ah·lo·gram)
encephalography   (en·sef′ah·log′rah·fe)
encephalomalacia
   (en·sef′ah·lo·mah·la′she·ah)
encephalomeningitis
   (en·sef′ah·lo·men′in·ji′tis)
encephalomyelitis
   (en·sef′ah·lo·mi′ĕ·li′tis)
encephalomyelocele
   (en·sef′ah·lo·mi·el′o·sēl)
encephalomyelopathy
   (en·sef′ah·lo·mi′ĕ·lop′ah·the)
encephalomyeloradiculopathy
   (en·sef′ah·lo·mi′ĕ·lo·rah·dik·u′lop′ah·
   the)
encephalopathy   (en·sef′ah·lop′ah·the)
encephalopsychosis
   (en·sef′ah·lo·si·ko′sis)
enchondroma   (en′kon·dro′mah)
enchondrosarcoma
   (en′kon′dro·sar·ko′mah)
enclitic   (en·klit′ik)
encopresis   (en·ko·pre′sis)
encyesis   (en′si·e′sis)
Endamoeba   (en′dah·me′bah)
endarterectomy   (end′ar·ter·ek′to·me)
endarterium   (end′ar·te′re·um)
endaural   (end·aw′ral)
end-diastolic   (end-di·ah·stol′ik)
endergonic   (end′er·gon′ik)
endoauscultation   (en′do·aws′kul·ta′shun)
endobronchial   (en′do·brong′ke·al)
endocardiography
   (en′do·kar·de·og′rah·fe)
endocardium   (en′do·kar′de·um)
endochondral   (en′do·kon′dral)
endocrine   (en′do·krīn)
endocrinology   (en′do·krĭ·nol′o·je)
endocrinopathy   (en′do·kri·nop′ah·the)
endocrinous   (en·dok′rĭ·nus)
endocytosis   (en′do·si·to′sis)
endoderm   (en′do·derm)
endodontics   (en′do·don′tiks)
endoenzyme   (en′do·en′zīm)
endogenous   (en·doj′ĕ·nus)
Endolimax   (en′do·li′maks)
endolymph   (en′do·limf)
endometrioma   (en′do·me′tre·o′mah)
endometriosis   (en′do·me′tre·o′sis)
endometrium   (en·do·me′tre·um)
endomysium   (en′do·mis′e·um)
endoneurium   (en′do·nu′re·um)
endonuclease   (en′do·nu′kle·ās)
endopeptidase   (en′do·pep′tĭ·dās)
endophthalmitis   (en′dof·thal·mi′tis)
endopolyploidy   (en′do·pol′e·ploi′de)
endorphin   (en·dor′fin)
endosalpinx   (en′do·sal′pinks)
endoscope   (en′do·skōp)
endoscopy   (en·dos′ko·pe)
endosteoma   (en·dos′te·o′mah)
endothelioma   (en′do·the′le·o′mah)
endothelium   (en′do·the′le·um)
endothrix   (en′do·thriks)
endotoxin   (en′do·tok′sin)
endotracheal   (en′do·tra′ke·al)
enediol   (ēn·di′ōl)
enema   (en′e·mah)
enkephalin   (en·kef′ah·lin)
enol   (e′nol)
enophthalmos   (en′of·thal′mus)
enostosis   (en′os·to′sis)
Entamoeba histolytica
   (en′tah·me′bah his·to·lit′ĭ·ka)
enteral   (en′ter·al)
enterobiasis   (en′ter·o·bi′ah·sis)
Enterobius vermicularis
   (en′ter·o′be·us ver·mik′u·la′ris)

enterocele (en'ter·o·sēl')
enterocleisis (en'ter·o·kli'sis)
enteroclysis (en'ter·ok'li·sis)
enterococcus (en'ter·o·kok'us)
enterocolostomy (en'ter·o·ko·los'to·me)
enterogastrone (en'ter·o·gas'trōn)
enterolith (en'ter·o·lith')
enteron (en'ter·on)
enteroparesis (en'ter·o·par'e·sis)
enteropathy (en'ter·op'ah·the)
enteropeptidase (en'ter·o·pep'ti·dās)
enteroptosia (en'ter·op·to'se·ah)
enterospasm (en'ter·o·spazm)
Enterovirus (en'ter·o·vi'rus)
enthesitis (en·thĕ·si'tis)
entopic (en·top'ik)
entozoa (en'to·zo'ah)
entozoon (en'to·zo'on)
entropion (en·tro'pe·on)
entropy (en'tro·pe)
enucleation (e·nu'kle·a'shun)
enuresis (en'u·re'sis)
enzymatic (en'zi·mat'ik)
enzyme (en'zīm)
eosin (e'o·sin)
eosinophil (e'o·sin'o·fil)
ependyma (ĕ·pen'di·mah)
ependymoma (ĕ·pen'di·mo'mah)
ephedrine (ĕ·fed'rin)
epicanthus (ep'i·kan'thus)
epicardia (ep'i·kar'de·ah)
epicardium (ep'i·kar'de·um)
epicondyle (ep'i·kon'dīl)
epicondylitis (ep'i·kon'di·li'tis)
epicranium (ep'i·kra'ne·um)
epidemiography (ep'i·de'me·og'rah·fe)
epidemiology (ep'i·de'me·ol'o·je)
epidermis (ep'i·der'mis)
epididymectomy (ep'i·did'i·mek'to·me)
epididymis (ep'i·did'i·mis)
epididymitis (ep'i·did'i·mi'tis)
epididymotomy (ep'i·did'i·mot'o·me)
epigastrium (ep'i·gas'tre·um)
epiglottis (ep'i·glot'is)
epiglottitis (ep'i·glot·ti'tis)
epileptoid (ep'i·lep'toid)
epimenorrhea (ep'i·men'o·re'ah)
epimerase (ĕ·pim'er·ās)
epimers (ep'i·merz)
epimysium (ep'i·mis'e·um)
epinephrine (ep'i·nef'rin)
epineurium (ep'i·nu're·um)
epiphora (ĕ·pif'o·rah)
epiphysiodesis (ep'i·fiz'e·od'ĕ·sis)
epiphyses (ĕ·pif'i·sēz)
epiphysis (ĕ·pif'i·sis)
epiplocele (ĕ·pip'lo·sēl)
epiploectomy (ep'ĕ·plo·ek'to·me)
episclera (ep'i·skle'rah)
episioperineoplasty
   (ĕ·piz'e·o·per'i·ne'o·plas'te)
episioperineorrhaphy
   (ĕ·piz'e·o·per'i·ne·or'ah·fe)
episiotomy (ĕ·piz'e·ot'o·me)
episome (ep'i·sōm)
epispadias (ep'i·spa'de·as)
epistasis (ĕ·pis'tah·sis)
epistaxis (ep'i·stak'sis)
epithalamus (ep'i·thal'ah·mus)
epithelioid (ep'i·the'le·oid)
epithelioma (ep'i·the'le·o'·mah)
epithelium (ep'i·the'le·um)
epitope (ep'i·tōp)
eponychia (ep'o·nik'e·ah)
eponychium (ep'o·nik'e·um)
eponym (ep'o·nim)
epoophoron (ep'o·of'o·ron)
epulis (ep·u'lis)
equilibration (e'kwĭ·lĭ·bra'shun)
equimolar (e'kwĭ·mo'lar)
equimolecular (e'kwi·mo·lek'u·lar)
equinus (e·kwi'nus)
erbium (er'be·um)
erectile (ĕ·rek'tīl)
erethism (er'ĕ·thizm)
ergocalciferol (er·go·kal·sif'er·ol)
ergodynamograph (er'go·di·nam'o·graf)

ergosterol (er·gos'tĕ·rol)
ergot (er'got)
ergotamine (er·got'ah·mēn)
ergotism (er'got·izm)
erubescence (er·u·bes'ens)
eructation (ĕ·ruk·ta'shun)
erysipelas (er'ĭ·sip'ĕ·las)
erysipeloid (er'ĭ·sip'ĕ·loid)
Erysipelothrix (er'ĭ·sip'ĕ·lo·thriks')
erysiphake (er·is'ĭ·fāk)
erythema (er'ĭ·the'mah)
erythrasma (er'ĭ·thras'mah)
erythrityl (ĕ·rith'rĭ·til)
erythroblast (ĕ·rith'ro·blast)
erythroblastemia (ĕ·rith'ro·blas·te'me·ah)
erythroblastopenia
   (ĕ·rith'ro·blas'to·pe'ne·ah)
erythroblastosis fetalis
   (ĕ·rith'ro·blas·to'sis fe'tal'is)
erythroclasis (er'ĕ·throk'lah·sis)
erythrocuprein (ĕ·rith'ro·koo'prin)
erythrocyte (ĕ·rith'ro·sīt)
erythrocythemia (ĕ·rith'ro·si·the'me·ah)
erythrocytolysin (ĕ·rith'ro·si·tol'ĭ·sin)
erythrocytorrhexis (ĕ·rith'ro·si·to·rek'sis)
erythrocytosis (ĕ·rith'ro·si·to'sis)
erythrogenin (ĕ·rith'ro·jen'in)
erythrogonium (ĕ·rith'ro·go'ne·um)
erythrokinetics (ĕ·rith'ro·ki·net'iks)
erythromelalgia (ĕ·rith'ro·mel·al'je·ah)
erythromelia (ĕ·rith'ro·mel'e·ah)
erythromycin (ĕ·rith'ro·mi'sin)
erythron (er'ĭ·thron)
erythroneocytosis
   (ĕ·rith'ro·ne'o·si·to'sis)
erythropenia (ĕ·rith'ro·pe'ne·ah)
erythrophagocytosis
   (ĕ·rith'ro·fag'o·si·to'sis)
erythropoiesis (ĕ·rith'ro·poi·e'sis)
erythropoietin (ĕ·rith'ro·poi'ĕ·tin)
erythroprosopalgia
   (ĕ·rith'ro·pros'o·pal'je·ah)
erythropyknosis (ĕ'rith'ro·pik·no'sis)
eschar (es'kar)
escharotic (es·kah·rot'ik)
Escherichia (esh'er·i'ke·ah)
esocataphoria (es'o·kat·ah·fo're·ah)
esodeviation (es'o·de've·a'shun)
esophagalgia (ĕ·sof'ah·gal'je·ah)
esophageal (ĕ·sof'ah·je'al)
esophagectasia (ĕ·sof'ah·jek·ta'se·ah)
esophagectomy (ĕ·sof'ah·jek'to·me)
esophagitis (ĕ·sof'ah·ji'tis)
esophagocardioplasty
   (ĕ·sof'ah·go·kar'de·o·plas'te)
esophagocele (ĕ·sof'ah·go·sēl)
esophagogastrectomy
   (ĕ·sof'ah·go·gas·trek'to·me)
esophagogastrostomy
   (ĕ·sof'ah·go·gas·tros'to·me)
esophagojejunostomy
   (ĕ·sof'ah·go·jĕ·ju·nos'to·me)
esophagomyotomy
   (ĕ·sof'ah·go·mi·ot'o·me)
esophagoplasty (ĕ·sof'ah·go·plas'te)
esophagoscope (ĕ·sof'ah·go·skōp)
esophagostenosis (ĕ·sof'ah·go·stĕ·no'sis)
esophagus (ĕ·sof'ah·gus)
esophoria (es'o·fo're·ah)
ester (es'ter)
esterase (es'ter·ās)
estradiol (es'trah·di'ol)
estriol (es'tre·ol)
estrogen (es'tro·jen)
estrone (es'trōn)
estrous (es'trus)
estrus (es'trus)
ethacrynic (eth·ah·krin'ik)
ethambutol (ĕ·tham'bu·tol)
ethchlorvynol (eth·klōr'vĭ·nol)
ether (e'ther)
etherification (e'ther·ĭ·fi·ka'shun)
ethmoid (eth'moid)
ethmoidectomy (eth'moi·dek'to·me)
ethmosphenoid (eth'mo·sfe'noid)
ethyl (eth'il)
ethylene (eth'ĭ·lēn)

ethylenediaminetetraacetic
   (eth'ĭ·lēn·di'ah·mēn·tet'ra·as·e'tik)
etiocholanolone (e'te·o·ko·lan'o·lōn)
etiologic (e'te·o·loj'ik)
etiology (e'te·ol'o·je)
Eubacterium (u'bak·te're·um)
eucholia (u·ko'le·ah)
euchromatin (u·kro'ma·tin)
eugenics (u·jen'iks)
eugenol (u'jen·ol)
euglobulin (u·glob'u·lin)
euglycemia (u'gli·se'me·ah)
eukaryote (u·kar'e·ōt)
eunuchoid (u'nŭ·koid)
eunuchoidism (u'nŭ·koi'dizm)
euploidy (u·ploi'de)
eupnea (ūp'ne·ah)
euthanasia (u'thah·na'zhe·ah)
evacuant (e·vak'u·ant)
evagination (e·vaj'ĭ·na'shun)
evanescent (ev'ah·nes'ent)
eventration (e·ven·tra'shun)
eversion (e·ver'zhun)
evert (e·vert')
evisceration (e·vis'er·a'shun)
evulsion (e·vul'shun)
exacerbation (eg·zas'er·ba'shun)
exanthema subitum
   (eg'zan·the'mah su'bĭ·tum)
exanthematous (eg'zan·them'ah·tus)
excipient (ek·sip'e·ent)
excise (ek·sīz')
excision (ek·sizh'un)
exclave (eks'klāv)
excoriation (eks·ko're·a'shun)
excrement (eks'krĕ·ment)
excreta (eks·kre'tah)
excrete (eks·krēt')
excretion (eks·kre'shun)
excretory (eks'kre·to·re)
exergonic (eks'er·gon'ik)
exflagellation (eks'flaj·ĕ·la'shun)
exhumation (eks'hu·ma'shun)
exitus (ek'sĭ·tus)
exocataphoria (ek'so·kat'ah·fo're·ah)
exocrine (ek'so·krin)
exocytosis (eks'o·si·to'sis)
exodontics (ek'so·don'tiks)
exogenous (eks·oj'ĕ·nus)
exonuclease (ek'so·nu'kle·ās)
exophoria (ek·so·fo're·ah)
exophthalmometer
   (ek'sof·thal·mom'ĕ·ter)
exophthalmos (ek'sof·thal'mus)
exosporium (ek'so·spo're·um)
exostoses (ek'sos·to'sēz)
exostosis (ek'sos·to'sis)
exotoxin (ek'so·tok'sin)
expectorant (ek·spek'to·rant)
expectoration (ek·spek'to·ra'shun)
expiratory (eks·pi'rah·to're)
explant (eks·plant')
exsanguinate (ek·sang'gwi·nāt)
exsiccant (ek·sik'ant)
exsiccate (ek'sĭ·kāt)
exsiccation (ek'sĭ·ka'shun)
exstrophy (ek'stro·fe)
exsufflation (ek'suf·fla'shun)
exteroceptor (eks'ter·o·sep'tor)
extirpation (ek'ster·pa'shun)
extorsion (eks·tor'shun)
extracranial (eks'trah·kra'ne·al)
extradural (eks'trah·du'ral)
extraperitoneal (eks'trah·per'ĭ·to·ne'al)
extrapolate (eks·trap'o·lāt)
extrapyramidal (eks·trah·pi·ram'ĭ·dal)
extrasystole (eks'trah·sis'to·le)
extrauterine (eks'trah·u'ter·īn)
extravasate (eks·trav'ah·sāt)
extravasation (eks'trav·ah·sa'shun)
extroversion (eks'tro·ver'zhun)
extrude (eks·trood')
extrusion (eks·troo'zhun)
extubate (eks·tu·bāt)
extubation (eks'tu·ba'shun)
exudate (eks'u·dāt)
exudation (eks'u·da'shun)

exudative (eks·u'dah·tiv)
exude (eks·ūd')

F

facet (fas'et)
facetectomy (fas'ĕ·tek'to·me)
facies (fa'she·ēz)
faciobrachial (fa'she·o·bra'ke·al)
faciocervical (fa'she·o·ser'vĕ·kal)
facioplegia (fa'she·o·ple'je·ah)
factitious (fak·tish'us)
factorial (fak·tor'e·al)
facultative (fak'ul·ta'tiv)
Fahrenheit (far'en·hīt)
falciform (fal'sĭ·form)
falx (falks)
farad (far'ad)
faraday (far'ah·da)
farcy (far'se)
farinaceous (far'ĭ·na'shus)
fascia (fash'e·ah)
fasciae (fash'e·e)
fascial (fash'e·al)
fascicle (fas'ĭ·kl)
fascicular (fah·sik'u·lar)
fasciculation (fah·sik'u·la'shun)
fasciculi (fah·sik'u·li)
fasciculus (fah·sik'u·lus)
fasciitis (fas'e·i'tis)
Fasciola hepatica
  (fah·si'o·lah hĕ·pat'ĭ·kah)
fascioliasis (fas'e·o·li'ah·sis)
Fasciolopsis (fas'e·o·lop'sis)
fascioplasty (fash'e·o·plas'te)
fasciorrhaphy (fash'e·or'ah·fe)
fastigium (fas·tij'e·um)
fatality (fa·tal'ĭ·te)
fatigability (fat'ĭ·gah·bil'ĭ·te)
fauces (faw'sez)
faveolus (fa·ve'o·lus)
favism (fa'vism)
favus (fa'vus)
febrifacient (feb'rĭ·fa'shent)
febrile (feb'ril)
fecal (fe'kal)
fecalith (fe'kah·lith)
fecaluria (fe'kah·lu're·ah)
feces (fe'sēz)
feculent (fek'u·lent)
fecundate (fe'kun·dāt)
fecundation (fe'kun·da'shun)
fecundity (fe·kun'dĭ·te)
fellatio (fĕ·la'she·o)
feminization (fem'ĭ·ni·za'shun)
femoral (fem'or·al)
femur (fe'mur)
fenestra cochleae (fe·nes'trah kok'le·e)
fenestra vestibuli (fe·nes'trah ves·tib'u·li)
fenestration (fen'es·tra'shun)
ferment (fer'ment)
ferment (fer·ment')
fermentable (fer·ment'ah·bl)
fermentative (fer·ment'ah·tiv)
fermium (fer'me·um)
ferning (fern'ing)
ferritin (fer'ĭ·tin)
ferrocyanide (fer'o·si'ah·nīd)
ferroporphyrin (fer'o·por'fĭ·rin)
ferruginous (fer·u'jĭ·nus)
fertility (fer·til'ĭ·te)
fervescence (fer·ves'ens)
festinant (fes'tĭ·nant)
festination (fes'tĭ·na'shun)
festoon (fes·toon')
festooning (fes·toon'ing)
fetal (fe'tal)
feticide (fe'tĭ·sid)
fetid (fĕ'tid)
fetishism (fĕt'ish·izm)
fetography (fe·tog'rah·fe)
fetology (fe·tol'o·je)
fetometry (fe·tom'ĕ·tre)
fetor hepaticus (fe'tor he·pat'ĭ·kus)
fetoscope (fe'to·skōp)
fetus (fe'tus)

fiberoptics (fi'ber·op'tiks)
fiberscope (fi'ber·skop)
fibril (fi'bril)
fibrillar (fi'brĭ·lar)
fibrillation (fi·brĭ·la'shun)
fibrilliform (fi·bril'ĭ·form)
fibrillogenesis (fi·bril'o·jen'ĕ·sis)
fibrin (fi'brin)
fibrination (fi'brĭ·na'shun)
fibrinogen (fi·brin'o·jen)
fibrinogenopenia
  (fi·brin'o·jen'o·pe'ne·ah)
fibrinoid (fi'brĭ·noid)
fibrinolysin (fi'brĭ·nol'ĭ·sin)
fibrinolysis (fi'brĭ·nol'ĭ·sis)
fibroadenoma (fi'bro·ad'ĕ·no'mah)
fibroadipose (fi'bro·ad'ĭ·pōs)
fibroblast (fi'bro·blast)
fibrocartilage (fi'bro·kar'tĭ·lij)
fibrochondroma (fi'bro·kon·dro'mah)
fibrocystoma (fi'bro·sis·to'mah)
fibroelastosis (fi'bro·e'las·to'sis)
fibroenchondroma
  (fi'bro·en'kon·dro'mah)
fibroepithelioma (fi'bro·ep'ĭ·the'le·o'mah)
fibroid (fi'broid)
fibrolipoma (fi'bro·lĭ·po'mah)
fibroma (fi·bro'mah)
fibromatosis (fi'bro·mah·to'sis)
fibromyoma (fi'bro·mi·o'mah)
fibromyositis (fi'bro·mi·o·si'tis)
fibronectin (fi'bro·nek'tin)
fibroplasia (fi'bro·pla'ze·ah)
fibrosarcoma (fi'bro·sar·ko'mah)
fibrosis (fi·bro'sis)
fibula (fib'u·lah)
fibulocalcaneal (fib'u·lo·kal·ka'ne·al)
filamentous (fil·ah·men'tus)
Filaria (fi·la're·ah)
filariasis (fil'ah·ri'ah·sis)
filariform (fi·lār'ĭ·form)
filaroides (fil'ah·roi'dēz)
filial (fil'e·al)
filiform (fil'ĭ·form)
fillet (fil'et)
filterable (fil'ter·ah·bl)
filtrable (fil'trah·bl)
filtrate (fil'trāt)
filum terminale (fi'lum ter·mĭ·na'le)
fimbria (fim'bre·ah)
fimbriae (fim'bre·e)
fimbriate (fim'bre·āt)
fimbriated (fim'bre·āt·ed)
fission (fish'un)
fissiparous (fĭ·sip'ah·rus)
fissuration (fish'er·a'shun)
fissure (fish'ūr)
fistula (fis'tu·lah)
fistulation (fis'tu·la'shun)
fistulatome (fis'tu·lah·tōm)
fistulectomy (fis'tu·lek'to·me)
fistulotomy (fis'tu·lot'o·me)
fistulous (fis'tu·lus)
flaccid (flak'sid)
flagella (flah·jel'ah)
flagellantism (flaj'ĕ·lan'tizm)
Flagellata (flaj'ĕ·la'tah)
flagellate (flaj'ĕ·lāt)
flagellum (flah·jel'um)
flange (flanj)
flatulence (fla'u·lens)
flatulent (flat'u·lent)
flatus (fla'tus)
flavin (fla'vin)
flavivirus (fla'vĭ·vi'rus)
flavobacterium (fla'vo·bak·te're·um)
flavoenzyme (fla'vo·en'zīm)
flexion (flek'shun)
flexure (flek'sher)
floccillation (flok'sĭ·la'shun)
flocculation (flok'u·la'shun)
flocculent (flok'u·lent)
flocculus (flok'u·lus)
flora (flo'rah)
florid (flor'id)
flowmeter (flo'me·ter)
floxuridine (floks·ur'ĭ·dēn)

fluctuant (fluk'tu·ant)
fluidglycerate (floo'id·glis'er·āt)
fluidram (floo'ĭ·dram')
flumina pilorum (floo'mĭ·nah pi·lo'rum)
fluocinolone acetonide
  (floo'o·sin'o·lōn ah'sĕ·to'nīd)
fluorescein (floo'o·res'e·in)
fluorescence (floo'o·res'ens)
fluoridate (floo'or·ĭ·dāt)
fluoridation (floo'or·ĭ·da'shun)
fluoride (floo'o·rīd)
fluorine (floo'or·ēn)
fluorometer (floo'or·om'ĕ·ter)
fluoroscope (floo'or·o·skōp)
fluoroscopy (floo'or·os'ko·pe)
fluorouracil (floo'or·ūr'ah·sil)
flux (fluks)
foci (fo'si)
focimeter (fo·sim'ĕ·ter)
folate (fo'lāt)
foliaceous (fo'le·a'shus)
foliate (fo'le·āt)
folic (fo'lik)
folinic (fo·lin'ik)
follicle (fol'ĭ·kl)
follicular (fo·lik'u·lar)
folliculitis (fo·lik'u·li'tis)
folliculoma (fo·lik'u·lo'mah)
fomentation (fo'men·ta'shun)
fomes (fo'mēz)
fontanel (fon'tah·nel')
foramen (fo·ra'men)
foramina (fo·ram'ĭ·nah)
forceps (for'seps)
forensic (fo·ren'zik)
formaldehyde (for·mal'dĕ·hīd)
formalin (for'mah·lin)
formication (for'mĭ·ka'shun)
formiminoglutamic
  (for·mim'ĭ·no·gloo·tam'ik)
formulary (for'mu·lār'e)
formyl (for'mil)
fornix (for'niks)
fossa (fos'ah)
fossae (fos'e)
fossette (fos·set')
fossula (fos'u·lah)
fossulae (fos'u·le)
fourchette (foor·shet')
fovea (fo've·ah)
foveate (fo've·āt)
foveation (fo've·a'shun)
foveola (fo·ve'o·lah)
foveolate (fo·ve'o·lāt)
fracture (frak'chur)
fragilitas ossium (frah·jil'ĭ·tas os'se·um)
fragility (frah·jil'ĭ·te)
francium (fran'se·um)
fremitus (frem'ĭ·tus)
frenectomy (fre·nek'to·me)
frenotomy (fre·not'o·me)
frenulum (fren'u·lum)
fricative (frik'ah·tiv)
fructokinase (fruk'to·ki'nās)
fructosan (fruk'to·san)
fructose (fruk'tōs)
fructosuria (fruk'to·su're·ah)
fuchsin (fook'sin)
fugue (fūg)
fulgurant (ful'gu·rant)
fulguration (ful'gu·ra'shun)
fulminate (ful'mĭ·nāt)
fumagillin (fu'mah·jil'in)
fundal (fun'dal)
fundi (fun'di)
fundiform (fun'dĭ·form)
fundus (fun'dus)
fungi (fun'ji)
fungus (fung'gus)
funic (fu'nik)
funicle (fu'nĭ·kl)
funicular (fu·nik'u·lar)
funiculitis (fu·nik'u·li·tis)
funiculus (fu·nik'u·lus)
funiform (fu'nĭ·form)
furfur (fur'fur)
furfures (fur'fu·rēz)

furfuraceous (fur'fu·ra'shus)
furosemide (fur'sĕ·mīd)
furuncle (fu'rung·kl)
furunculosis (fu·rung'ku·lo'sis)
fuscin (fu'sin)
fusospirochetal (fu'so·spi'rō·kē'tal)

G

gadolinium (gad'o·lin'e·um)
galactacrasia (gah·lak·tă·kra'se·ah)
galactagogue (gah·lak'tă·gog)
galactan (gah·lak'tan)
galactoblast (gah·lak'to·sēl)
galactocele (gah·lak'to·sēl)
galactokinase (gah·lak'to·ki'nās)
galactophore (gah·lak'to·fōr)
galactophorous (gal'ak·tof'o·rus)
galactophygous (gal'ak·tof'ĭ·gus)
galactopoiesis (gah·lak'to·poi·e'sis)
galactopoietic (gah·lak'to·poi·et'ik)
galactorrhea (gah·lak'to·re'ah)
galactosamine (gah·lak'to·sam'in)
galactosan (gah·lak'to·san)
galactoschesia (gah·lak'to·ske'se·ah)
galactoschesis (gal'ak·tos'kĕ·sis)
galactose (gah·lak'tōs)
galactosemia (gah·lak'to·se'me·ah)
galactosuria (gah·lak'to·su're·ah)
galactozymase (gah·lak'to·zi'mās)
galea aponeurotica
  (ga'le·ah ah'po·nu·rot'ĭ·kah)
gallamine (gal'ah·mīn)
gallium (gal'e·um)
gallstone (gawl'stōn)
galvanopalpation
  (gal'vah·no·pal·pa'shun)
galvanotonus (gal'vah·no·to'nus)
gamete (gam'ēt)
gametocyte (gah·met'o·sīt)
gametogenesis (gam'ĕ·to·jen'ĕ·sis)
gametogonia (gam'ĕ·to·go'ne·ah)
gametogony (gam'ĕ·tog'o·ne)
gamma (gam'ah)
gammopathy (gam·op'ah·the)
ganglia (gang'gle·ah)
gangliate (gang'glē·āt)
gangliectomy (gang'gle·ek'to·me)
ganglion (gang'gle·on)
ganglionectomy (gang'gle·o·nek'to·me)
ganglioneuroma (gang'gle·o·nu·ro'mah)
ganglionic (gang'gle·on'ik)
ganglioside (gang'gle·o·sīd)
gangliosidosis (gang'gle·o·si·do'sis)
gangosa (gang·go'sah)
gangrene (gang'grēn)
gangrenous (gang'grĕ·nus)
gaseous (gas'e·us)
gastrectomy (gas·trek'to·me)
gastrin (gas'trin)
gastrinoma (gas'trin·o'mah)
gastritis (gas·tri'tis)
gastroblenorrhea (gas'tro·blen'no·re'ah)
gastrocele (gas'tro·sēl)
gastrocnemius (gas'trok·ne'me·us)
gastrocolic (gas'tro·kol'ik)
gastrocoloptosis (gas'tro·ko'lop·to'sis)
gastrocolostomy (gas'tro·ko·los'to·me)
gastroduodenal (gas'tro·du'o·de'nal)
gastroduodenostomy
  (gas'tro·du'o·dĕ·nos'to·me)
gastroenteric (gas'tro·en·ter'ik)
gastroenteritis (gas'tro·en·ter·i'tis)
gastroenteroanastomosis
  (gas'tro·en'ter·o·ah·nas'to·mo'sis)
gastroenterology (gas'tro·en'ter·ol'o·je)
gastroenteropathy
  (gas'tro·en'ter·op'ah·the)
gastroenteroptosis
  (gas'tro·en'ter·op·to'sis)
gastroepiploic (gas'tro·ep'ĭ·plo'ik)
gastroesophageal (gas'tro·e·sof'ah·je'al)
gastroesophagitis (gas'tro·e·sof'ah·ji'tis)
gastrogavage (gas'tro·gah·vazh')
gastrograph (gas'tro·graf)
gastrohepatic (gas'tro·hĕ·pat'ik)

gastrohydrorrhea (gas'tro·hi'dro·re'ah)
gastrointestinal (gas'tro·in·tes'tĭ·nal)
gastromalacia (gas'tro·mah·la'she·ah)
gastromegaly (gas'tro·meg'ah·le)
gastropathy (gas·trop'ah·the)
gastrophrenic (gas'tro·fren'ik)
gastroplication (gas'tro·plĭ·ka'shun)
gastroptosis (gas'tro·to'sis)
gastropyloric (gas'tro·pi·lor'ik)
gastrorrhaphy (gas·tror'ah·fe)
gastroscope (gas'tro·skōp)
gastroscopy (gas·tros'ko·pe)
gastrospasm (gas'tro·spazm)
gastrula (gas'troo·lah)
gastrulation (gas'troo·la'shun)
Gaultheria (gawl·the're·ah)
gauntlet (gawnt'let)
gavage (gah·vahzh')
gelation (jĕ·la'shun)
gemellology (jem'el·ol'o·je)
geminate (jem'ĭ·nāt)
gemma (jem'ma)
gemmation (jĕ·ma'shun)
gemmule (jem'ūl)
genera (jen'er·ah)
generic (jĕ·ner'ik)
genesial (jĕ·ne'ze·al)
genesic (jĕ·nes'ik)
genesiology (jĕ·ne'ze·ol'o·je)
genetics (jĕ·net'iks)
geniculum (jĕ·nik'u·lum)
genioglossus (je'ne·o·glos'us)
geniohyoid (je'ne·o·hi'oid)
genioplasty (jĕ·ni'o·plas'te)
genitourinary (jen'ĭ·to·u'rĭ·nār·e)
genome (je'nōm)
genotype (jen'o·tīp)
gentamicin (jen'tah·mi'sin)
gentian (jen'shun)
genu valgum (je'nu val'gum)
genu varum (je'nu va'rum)
genus (je'nus)
geophagia (je·o·fa'je·ah)
geophagy (je·of'ah·je)
geotrichosis (je'o·tri·ko'sis)
Geotrichum (je·ot'rĭ·kum)
geriatrics (jer'e·at'riks)
germanium (jer'ma'ne·um)
geroderma (jer·o·der'mah)
gerodontics (jer'o·don'tiks)
gerodontology (jer'o·don·tol'o·je)
geromarasmus (jer'o·mah·raz'mus)
gerontal (jer·on'tal)
gerontology (jer'on·tol'o·je)
gestalt (ges·tawlt')
Giardia lamblia (je·ar'de·ah lam'ble·ah)
giardiasis (je'ar·di'ah·sis)
gibbosity (gĭ·bos'ĭ·te)
gibbous (gib'us)
gibbus (gib'us)
gigantism (ji·gan'tizm)
gingiva (jin'jĭ·vah)
gingivectomy (jin·jĭ·vek'to·me)
gingivitis (jin'jĭ·vi'tis)
gingivoplasty (jin'jĭ·vo·plas·te)
gingivostomatitis (jin'jĭ·vo·sto'mah·ti'tis)
ginglymus (jin'gli·mus)
gitalin (jit'ah·lin)
glabella (glah·bel'ah)
glabrous (gla'brus)
gladiolus (glah·di'o·lus)
glandes (glan'dēz)
glanders (glan'derz)
glandilemma (glan'dĭ·lem'ah)
glandule (glan'dūl)
glans (glanz)
glaucoma (glaw·ko'mah)
glenohumeral (gle·no·hu'mer·al)
glenoid (gle'noid)
glia (gli'ah)
gliacyte (gli'ah·sīt)
gliadin (gli'ah·din)
glial (gli'al)
glioblastoma (gli·o·blas·to'mah)
glioma (gli·o'mah)
gliomatosis (gli'o·mah·to'sis)
gliomatous (gli'o'mah·tus)

gliosis (gli·o'sis)
gliosome (gli'o·sōm)
globi (glo'bi)
globin (glo'bin)
globulin (glob'u·lin)
globulinuria (glob'u·lin·u're·ah)
globus hystericus (glo'bus his·ter'ĭ·kus)
globus pallidus (glo'bus pal'ĭ·dus)
glomangioma (glo·man'je·o'mah)
glomerular (glo·mer'u·lar)
glomerulonephritis
  (glo·mer'u·lo·nĕ·fri'tis)
glomerulosclerosis
  (glo·mer'u·lo·sklĕ·ro'sis)
glomerulus (glo·mer'u·lus)
glomus (glo'mus)
glossal (glos'al)
glossalgia (glos·sal'je·ah)
glossectomy (glos·sek'to·me)
Glossina (glos·si'nah)
glossolalia (glos'o·la'le·ah)
glossopharyngeal (glos'o·fah·rin'je·al)
glossoplegia (glos'o·ple'je·ah)
glossorrhaphy (glos·sor'ah·fe)
glottic (glot'ik)
glottis (glot'is)
glucagon (gloo'kah·gon)
glucan (gloo'kan)
glucocorticoid (gloo'ko·kor'tĭ·koid)
glucokinase (gloo'ko·ki'nās)
glucosamine (gloo'ko·sam'ēn)
glucosan (gloo'ko·san)
glucose (gloo'kōs)
glucoside (gloo'ko·sīd)
glucosuria (gloo'ko·su're·ah)
glucuronidase (gloo'ku·ron'ĭ·dās)
glucuronide (gloo·ku'ron·īd)
glutamic (gloo·tam'ik)
glutamine (gloo'tah·min)
glutaraldehyde (gloo'tah·ral'dĕ·hīd)
glutathione (gloo'tah·thi'ōn)
glutelin (gloo'tĕ·lin)
gluten (gloo'ten)
glutethimide (gloo·teth'ĭ·mīd)
glycemia (gli·se'me·ah)
glyceraldehyde (glis'er·al'dĕ·hīd)
glyceridase (glis'er·ĭ·dās)
glyceride (glis'er·īd)
glycerin (glis'er·in)
glycerol (glis'er·ol)
glycerose (glis'er·ōs)
glyceryl (glis'er·il)
glycine (gli'sēn)
glycinuria (gli'si·nu're·ah)
glycocalyx (gli'ko·ka'liks)
glycocholic (gli'ko·kol'ik)
glycogen (gli'ko·jen)
glycogenase (gli'ko·jĕ·nās)
glycogenesis (gli'ko·jen'ĕ·sis)
glycogenolysis (gli'ko·jĕ·nol'ĭ·sis)
glycogeusia (gli'ko·ju'se·ah)
glycol (gli'kol)
glycolysis (gli·kol'ĭ·sis)
glyconeogenesis (gli'ko·ne·o·jen'ĕ·sis)
glycoside (gli'ko·sīd)
glycosphingolipid (gli'ko·sfing'o·lip'id)
glycosuria (gli'ko·su're·ah)
glycyrrhiza (glis'ir·ri'zah)
glycyrrhizic (glis'ir·riz'ik)
gnathic (nath'ik)
gnathion (nath'e·on)
gnathoplasty (nath'o·plas'te)
gnathostatics (nath'o·stat'iks)
Gnathostoma spinigerum
  (nath·os'to·mah spi·nij'ĕ·rum)
gnathostomiasis (nath'o·sto·mi'ah·sis)
gnosis (no'sis)
goiter (goi'ter)
gomphosis (gom·fo'sis)
gonad (go'nad)
gonadectomy (go'nah·dek'to·me)
gonadoblastoma (gon'ah·do·blas·to'mah)
gonadogenesis (gon'ah·do·jen'ĕ·sis)
gonadotropic (gon'ah·do·trōp'ik)
gonadotropin (gon'ah·do·tro'pin)
goniometer (gon'ne·om'ĕ·ter)
gonion (go'ne·on)

gonioscope (go′ne·o·skōp)
gonioscopy (go′ne·os′ko·pe)
goniosynechia (go′ne·o·si·nek′e·ah)
goniotomy (go′ne·ot′o·me)
gonococcemia (gon′o·kok·se′me·ah)
gonococci (gon′o·kok′si)
gonorrhea (gon′o·re′ah)
gouge (gowj)
gout (gowt)
gramicidin (gram′i·si′din)
grammeter (gram′me·ter)
granulocyte (gran′u·lo·sīt)
granulocytopenia
 (gran′u·lo·si′to·pe′ne·ah)
granulocytosis (gran′u·lo·si·to′sis)
granuloma (gran′u·lo′mah)
granulomatosis (gran′u·lo′mah·to′sis)
granulomatous (gran′u·lom′ah·tus)
granulopoiesis (gran′u·lo·poi·e′sis)
gravid (grav′id)
gravida (grav′i·dah)
gravimeter (grah·vim′ĕ·ter)
gripe (grip)
grippe (grip)
griseofulvin (gris′e·o·ful′vin)
gryposis (grĭ·po′sis)
guaiacol (gwi′ah·kol)
guanethidine (gwan·eth′i·dēn)
guanidine (gwan′i·dēn)
guanidinemia (gwan′i·din·e′me·ah)
guanidinosuccinic
 (gwan′i·din·o·suk·sin′ik)
guanine (gwan′in)
gubernaculum (gu′ber·nak′u·lum)
gullet (gul′et)
gumma (gum′ah)
gummatous (gum′ah·tus)
gustatory (gus′tah·to′re)
gutta-percha (gut′ah-per′chah)
guttate (gut′āt)
gynandrism (ji·nan′drizm)
gynatresia (jin′ah·tre′ze·ah)
gynecoid (jin′ĕ·koid)
gynecologist (gi′nĕ·kol′o·jist)
gynecology (gi′nĕ·kol′o·je)
gynecomastia (jin′ĕ·ko·mas′te·ah)
gypsum (jip′sum)
gyri (ji′ri)
gyrus (ji′rus)

H

habena (hah·be′nah)
habenula (hah·ben′u·lah)
habitus (hab′ĭ·tus)
Haemaphysalis (hem′ah·fis′ah·lis)
Haemophilus (he·mof′ĭ·lus)
Haemosporidia (hem′o·spo·rid′e·ah)
hafnium (haf′ne·um)
halazone (hal·ah·zōn)
halide (hal′ĭd)
hallucal (hal′u·kal)
hallucination (hah·lu′sĭ·na′shun)
hallucinogen (hah·lu′sĭ·no·jen)
hallux valgus (hal′uks val′gus)
halogen (hal′o·jen)
halophil (hal′o·fīl)
halophile (hal′o·fīl)
halothane (hal′o·thān)
hamartoblastoma
 (ham·ar′to·blas·to′mah)
hamartoma (ham·ar·to′mah)
hamular (ham′u·lar)
hamulus (ham′u·lus)
hapalonychia (hap′ah·lo·nik′e·ah)
haplodont (hap′lo·dont)
haploid (hap′loid)
haplopia (hap·lo′pe·ah)
haplosis (hap·lo′sis)
hapten (hap′ten)
haptene (hap′tēn)
haptoglobin (hap′to·glo′bin)
haptometer (hap·tom′ĕ·ter)
haptophore (hap′to·fōr)
hashish (hash·ēsh)
haustral (hos′tral)

haustration (hos·tra′shun)
haustrum (hos′trum)
haversian (ha·ver′shan)
hebephrenia (heb′ĕ·fre′ne·ah)
hedonic (he·don′ik)
helicine (hel′ĭ·sēn)
helicotrema (hel′ĭ·ko·tre′mah)
heliopathy (he′le·o·path′e)
heliotaxis (he′le·o·tak′sis)
heliotropism (he′le·ot′ro·pizm)
helix (he′liks)
helminth (hel′minth)
helminthiasis (hel′min·thi′ah·sis)
helminthic (hel·min′thik)
helminthoid (hel·min′thoid)
helminthology (hel′min·thol′o·je)
heloma (he·lo′mah)
helosis (he·lo′sis)
helotomy (he·lot′o·me)
hemagglutination
 (hem′ah·gloo′tĭ·na′shun)
hemagglutinin (hem′ah·gloo′tin)
hemagogue (hem′ah·gog)
hemal (he′mal)
hemangiectasia (hem·an′je·ek·ta′se·ah)
hemangiectasis (hem·an′je·ek′tah·sis)
hemangioblast (hĕ·man′je·o·blast)
hemangioblastoma
 (hĕ·man′je·o·blas·to′mah)
hemangioendothelioma
 (hĕ·man′je·o·en′do·the′le·o′mah)
hemangioma (hĕ·man′je·o′mah)
hemangiomatosis
 (hĕ·man′je·o·mah·to′sis)
hemangiopericytoma
 (hĕ·man′je·o·per′ĕ·si·to′mah)
hemangiosarcoma
 (hĕ·man′je·o·sar·ko′mah)
hemarthrosis (hem·ar·thro′sis)
hematemesis (hem′ah·tem′ĕ·sis)
hematic (he·mat′ik)
hematin (hem′ah·tin)
hematinuria (hem′ah·tin·u′re·ah)
hematocele (hem′ah·to·sēl)
hematochezia (hem′ah·to·ke′ze·ah)
hematocolpometra
 (hem′ah·to·kol′po·me′trah)
hematocolpos (hem′ah·to·kol′pos)
hematocrit (he·mat′o·krit)
hematocystis (hem′ah·to·sis′tis)
hematocyturia (hem′ah·to·si·tu′re·ah)
hematogenous (hem′ah·toj′ĕ·nus)
hematoidin (hem·ah·toid′in)
hematology (hem′ah·tol′o·je)
hematoma (hem′ah·to′mah)
hematometra (hem′ah·to·me′trah)
hematometry (hem′ah·tom′ĕ·tre)
hematomyelia (hem′ah·to·mi·e′le·ah)
hematopenia (hem′ah·to·pe′ne·ah)
hematoporphyrin (hem′ah·to·por′fī·rin)
hematosalpinx (hem′ah·to·sal′pinks)
hematostaxis (hem′ah·to·stak′sis)
hematoxylin (hem′ah·tok′sĭ·lin)
hematozoa (hem′ah·to·zo′ah)
hematozoon (hem′ah·to·zo′on)
hematuria (hem′ah·tu′re·ah)
heme (hēm)
hemeralopia (hem′er·ah·lo′pe·ah)
hemiamblyopia (hem′e·am′ble·o′pe·ah)
hemianacusia (hem′e·an·ah·ku′ze·ah)
hemianalgesia (hem′e·an′al·je′ze·ah)
hemianesthesia (hem′e·an′es·the′ze·ah)
hemianopsia (hem′e·an·op′se·ah)
hemiatrophy (hem′e·at′ro·fe)
hemiballism (hem′e·bal′izm)
hemicentrum (hem′e·sen′trum)
hemichorea (hem′e·ko·re′ah)
hemidiaphoresis (hem′e·di′ah·fo·re′sis)
hemigastrectomy (hem′e·gas·trek′to·me)
hemikaryon (hem′e·kar′e·on)
hemilaminectomy
 (hem′e·lam′ĭ·nek′to·me)
hemimelia (hem′e·me′le·ah)
hemin (he′min)
heminephrectomy (hem′e·nĕ·frek′to·me)
hemiparesis (hem′e·par′e·sis)
hemiplegia (hem′e·ple′je·ah)
Hemiptera (he·mip′ter·ah)

hemisoantibody (hēm′ĭ·so·an′tĭ·bod·e)
hemizygosity (hem′e·zi·gos′ĭ·te)
hemizygous (hem′e·zi′gus)
hemoagglutinin (he′mo·ah·gloo′tĭ·nin)
hemochromatosis (he′mo·kro′mah·to′sis)
hemochromometer
 (he′mo·kro·mom′ĕ·ter)
hemoclasia (he′mo·kla′se·ah)
hemoclasis (he·mok′lah·sis)
hemocyanin (he′mo·si′ah·nin)
hemocytometer (he′mo·si·tom′ĕ·ter)
hemocytotripsis (he′mo·si′to·trip′sis)
hemodialysis (he′mo·di·al′ĭ·sis)
hemodialyzer (he′mo·di′ah·liz′er)
hemofuscin (he′mo·fūs′in)
hemoglobin (he′mo·glo′bin)
hemoglobinemia (he′mo·glo′bĭ·ne′me·ah)
hemoglobinometer
 (he′mo·glo′bĭ·nom′ĕ·ter)
hemoglobinopathy
 (he′mo·glo′bi·nop′ah·the)
hemoglobinuria (he′mo·glo′bĭ·nu′re·ah)
hemogram (he′mo·gram)
hemohistioblast (he′mo·his′te·o·blast′)
hemolysin (he·mol′ĭ·sin)
hemolysinogen (he′mo·li·sin′o·gen)
hemolysis (he·mol′ĭ·sis)
hemolytic (he′mo·lit′ik)
hemomanometer (he′mo·mah·nom′ĕ·ter)
hemopathy (he·mop′ah·the)
hemoperfusion (he′mo·per·fu′zhun)
hemopexin (he′mo·pek′sin)
hemophagocytosis (he′mo·fag′o·si·to′sis)
hemophilia (he′mo·fil′e·ah)
hemophiliac (he′mo·fil′e·ak)
hemophthalmia (he′mof·thal′me·ah)
hemopneumothorax
 (he′mo·nu′mo·tho′raks)
hemopoiesis (he′mo·poi·e′sis)
hemoporphyrin (he′mo·por′fī·rin)
hemoprecipitin (he′mo·pre·sip′ĭ·tin)
hemopsonin (he′mop·so′nin)
hemoptysis (he·mop′tĭ·sis)
hemopyelectasia
 (he′mo·pi·ĕ·lek·ta′se·ah)
hemorheology (he′mo·re·ol′o·je)
hemorrhage (hem′or·ij)
hemorrhagic (hem′o·raj′ik)
hemorrhagin (hem′o·ra′jin)
hemorrhoid (hem′o·roid)
hemorrhoidectomy (hem′o·roid·ek′to·me)
hemosiderin (he′mo·sid′er·in)
hemosiderosis (he′mo·sid′er·o′sis)
hemospermia (he′mo·sper′me·ah)
hemostasis (he′mo·sta′sis)
hemostat (he′mo·stat)
hemostyptic (he′mo·stip′tik)
hemothorax (he′mo·tho′raks)
hemotoxin (he′mo·tok′sin)
hemotympanum (he′mo·tim′pah·num)
heparin (hep′ah·rin)
heparinize (hep′er·ĭ·nīz)
hepatalgia (hep′ah·tal′je·ah)
hepatectomy (hep′ah·tek′to·me)
hepatitis (hep′ah·ti′tis)
hepatization (hep′ah·ti·za′shun)
hepatocyte (hep′ah·to·sīt)
hepatolienography
 (hep′ah·to·li′ĕ·nog′rah·fe)
hepatolysin (hep′ah·tol′ĭ·sin)
hepatoma (hep′ah·to′mah)
hepatomegaly (hep′ah·to·meg′ah·le)
hepatopathy (hep′ah·top′ah·the)
hepatorenal (hep′ah·to·re′nal)
hepatorrhaphy (hep′ah·tor′ah·fe)
hepatosplenography
 (hep′ah·to·splĕ·nog′rah·fe)
hepatosplenomegaly
 (hep′ah·to·sple′no·meg′ah·le)
hereditary (hĕ·red′ĭ·ter·e)
heredity (hĕ·red′ĭ·te)
heritable (her′ĭ·tah·bl)
hermaphrodism (her·maf′ro·dizm)
hermaphrodite (her·maf′ro·dīt)
hermaphroditism (her·maf′ro·di·tizm)
hernia (her′ne·ah)
herniorrhaphy (her′ne·or′ah·fe)
heroin (her′o·in)

herpangina (herp′an·ji′nah)
herpes (her′pēz)
Herpesviridae (her′pēz·vi′rī·de)
herpesvirus (her′pēz·vi′rus)
herpetiform (her·pet′ī·form)
heterochromatin (het′er·o·kro′mah·tin)
heteroecious (het′er·o·e′shus)
heterogametic (het′er·o·gah·met′ik)
heterogamy (het′er·og′ah·me)
heterogeneity (het′er·o·jĕ·ne′ī·te)
heterolalia (het′er·o·la′le·ah)
heterologous (het′er·ol′o·gus)
heterolysis (het′er·ol′ī·sis)
heteromeric (het′er·o·mer′ik)
heteromorphism (het′er·o·mor′fizm)
heteronymous (het′er·on′ī·mus)
heterophonia (het′er·o·fo′ne·ah)
heterophoria (het′er·o·fo′re·ah)
heterophthalmia (het′er·of·thal′me·ah)
Heterophyes (het′er·of′ī·ēz)
heterophyiasis (het′er·o·fi·i′ah·sis)
heterophyid (het′er·o·fi′id)
heteroplasia (het′er·o·pla′ze·ah)
heteroploidy (het′er·o·ploi′de)
heterosexuality (het′er·o·seks′u·al′ī·te)
heterotaxia (het′er·o·tak′se·ah)
heterozygote (het′er·o·zi′gōt)
hexacanth (hek′sah·kanth)
hexachlorophene (hek′sah·klo′ro·fēn)
hexokinase (hek′so·ki′nās)
hexosamine (hek′sōs·am′in)
hexosan (hek′so·san)
hexose (hek′sōs)
hexulose (hek′su·lōs)
hexylresorcinol (hek′sil·re·sor′sin·ol)
hiatus (hi·a′tus)
hidradenitis (hi′drad·ĕ·ni′tis)
hidradenoma (hi′drad·ĕ·no′mah)
hidrocystoma (hid′ro·sis·to′mah)
hidropoiesis (hid′ro·poi·e′sis)
hidrosis (hi·dro′sis)
hilum (hi′lum)
hippocampus (hip′o·kam′pus)
hippus (hip′us)
hirsute (her′soot)
hirsutism (her′soot·izm)
hirudin (hĭ·roo′din)
histamine (his′tah·mēn)
histidine (his′tī·din)
histiocyte (his′te·o·sīt)
histiocytosis (his′te·o·si·to′sis)
histocompatibility
   (his′to·kom·pat′ī·bil′ī·te)
histofluorescence (his′to·floo′o·res′ens)
histogenesis (his′to·jen′ĕ·sis)
histology (his·tol′o·je)
histone (his′tōn)
Histoplasma capsulatum
   (his′to·plaz′mah kap·su·la′tum)
histoplasmin (his′to·plaz′min)
histoplasmosis (his′to·plaz·mo′sis)
holandric (hol·an′drik)
holarthritis (hol′ar·thri′tis)
holoblastic (hol′o·blas′tik)
holocrine (hol′o·krīn)
holodiastolic (hol′o·di′ah·stol′ik)
holoenzyme (hol′o·en′zīm)
holography (hol·og′raf·e)
holosystolic (hol′o·sis·tol′ik)
homeopathy (ho′me·op′ah·the)
homeoplasia (ho′me·o·pla′ze·ah)
homeostasis (ho′me·o·sta′sis)
hominid (hom′ī·nid)
homoblastic (ho′mo·blas′tik)
homocysteine (ho′mo·sis·te′in)
homocystine (ho′mo·sis′tin)
homocystinuria (ho′mo·sis′tin·u′re·ah)
homogenate (ho·moj′ĕ·nāt)
homogeneous (ho′mo·je′ne·us)
homogenous (ho·moj′ĕ·nus)
homologue (hom′o·log)
homonomous (ho·mon′o·mus)
homonymous (ho·mon′ī·mus)
homopolymer (ho′mo·pol′ĕ·mer)
homopolypeptide (ho′mo·pol′e·pep′tīd)
homozoic (ho′mo·zo′ik)
homozygosis (ho′mo·zi·go′sis)
homozygosity (ho′mo·zi·gos′ī·te)

homozygote (ho′mo·zi′gōt)
homunculus (ho·munk′u·lus)
hordeolum (hor·de′o·lum)
horismascope (ho·riz′ma·skōp)
hormone (hor′mōn)
hormonogenic (hor′mo·no·jen′ik)
horripilation (hor′ī·pi·la′shun)
hospice (hos′pis)
humectant (hu·mek′tant)
humeral (hu′mer·al)
humerus (hu′mer·us)
humulin (hum′u·lin)
hyalin (hi′ah·lin)
hyaline (hi′ah·līn)
hyalitis (hi′ah·li′tis)
hyaloid (hi′ah·loid)
hyalomere (hi′ah·lo·mēr)
hyaluronic (hi′ah·lu·ron′ik)
hyaluronidase (hi′ah·lu·ron′ī·dās)
hybaroxia (hi′bă·rok′se·ah)
hybridization (hi′brid·i·za′shun)
hybridoma (hi′brĭ·do′mah)
hydatid (hi′dah·tid)
hydatidiform (hi′dah·tid′ī·form)
hydralazine (hi·dral′ah·zēn)
hydramnios (hi·dram′ne·os)
hydrargyria (hi′drar·jir′e·ah)
hydrargyrism (hi·drar′jī·rizm)
hydrarthrosis (hi′drar·thro′sis)
hydrencephalocele (hi′dren·sef′ah·lo·sēl)
hydrencephalomeningocele
   (hi′dren·sef′ah·lo·mĕ·ning′go·sēl)
hydriatic (hi′dre·at′ik)
hydroa (hid·ro′ah)
hydroblepharon (hi′dro·blef′ah·ron)
hydrocarbon (hi′dro·kar′bon)
hydrocele (hi′dro·sēl)
hydrocelectomy (hi′dro·se·lek′to·me)
hydrocephalic (hi′dro·sĕ·fal′ik)
hydrocephalus (hi′dro·sef′ah·lus)
hydrochloric (hi′dro·klor′ik)
hydrochloride (hi′dro·klo′rīd)
hydrochlorothiazide
   (hi′dro·klo′ro·thi′ah·zīd)
hydrocolloid (hi′dro·kol′loid)
hydrocolpocele (hi′dro·kol′po·sēl)
hydrocolpos (hi′dro·kol′pos)
hydrocortisone (hi′dro·kor′tī·sōn)
hydrocyanic (hi′dro·si′an·ik)
hydrogen (hi′dro·jen)
hydrogenation (hi′dro·jen·a′shun)
hydrolabyrinth (hi′dro·lab′ī·rinth)
hydrolase (hi′dro·lās)
hydrolysate (hi·drol′ī·zāt)
hydrolysis (hi·drol′ī·sis)
hydrolytic (hi′dro·lit′ik)
hydrolyze (hi′dro·līz)
hydrometer (hi·drom′ĕ·ter)
hydrometra (hi′dro·me′trah)
hydrometry (hi·drom′ĕ·tre)
hydromphalus (hi·drom′fah·lus)
hydromyelia (hi′dro·mi·e′le·ah)
hydronephrosis (hi′dro·nĕ·fro′sis)
hydronium (hi·dro′ne·um)
hydropericardium
   (hi′dro·per′ī·kar′de·um)
hydrophile (hi′dro·fīl)
hydrophilic (hi′dro·fil′ik)
hydrophobic (hi′dro·fo′bik)
hydropneumogony (hi′dro·nu·mo′go·ne)
hydropneumothorax
   (hi′dro·nu′mo·tho′raks)
hydrops (hi′drops)
hydropyonephrosis
   (hi′dro·pi′o·nĕ·fro′sis)
hydrorchis (hi·dror′kis)
hydrosalpinx (hi′dro·sal′pinks)
hydrosol (hi′dro·sol)
hydrospirometer (hi′dro·spi·rom′ĕ·ter)
hydrothorax (hi′dro·tho′raks)
hydrotropism (hi·drot′ro·pizm)
hydroureter (hi′dro·u′re·ter)
hydroxide (hi·drok′sīd)
hydroxyapatite (hi·drok′se·ap′ah·tīt)
hydroxyl (hi·drok′sil)
hyudroxylysine (hi·drok′se·li′sēn)
hydroxyphenyluria
   (hi·drok′se·fe·nil·u′re·ah)

hydroxyproline (hi·drok′se·pro′lin)
hydroxyprolinemia
   (hi·drok′se·pro′len·e′me·ah)
hygroma (hi·gro′mah)
hygrometer (hi·grom′ĕ·ter)
hymen (hi′men)
hymenal (hi′men·al)
hymenectomy (hi′men·ek′to·me)
Hymenolepis (hi′mĕ·nol′ĕ·pis)
Hymenoptera (hi′men·op′ter·ah)
hymenopteran (hi′men·op′ter·an)
hymenorrhapy (hi′men·or′ah·fe)
hymenotomy (hi′men·ot′o·me)
hyoglossal (hi′o·glos′al)
hyoid (hi′oid)
hyoscyamine (hi′o·si′ah·min)
hypacusis (hi′pah·ku′sis)
hypalgesia (hi′pal·je′ze·ah)
hypamnios (hi·pam′ne·os)
hypencephalon (hi′pen·sef′ah·lon)
hyperacidity (hi′per·ah·sid′ī·te)
hyperacusia (hi′per·ah·ku′ze·ah)
hyperacusis (hi′per·ah·ku′sis)
hyperaldosteronism
   (hi′per·al′do·ster′ōn·izm)
hyperalgesia (hi′per·al·je′ze·ah)
hyperalimentation
   (hi′per·al′ī·men·ta′shun)
hyperbaric (hi′per·bār′ik)
hyperbarism (hi′per·bar′izm)
hyperbilirubinemia
   (hi′per·bil′ī·roo′bĭ·ne′me·ah)
hypercalcemia (hi′per·kal·se′me·ah)
hypercalciuria (hi′per·kal′sĭ·u′re·ah)
hypercapnia (hi′per·kap′ne·ah)
hypercementosis (hi′per·se′men·to′sis)
hyperchloremia (hi′per·klo·re′me·ah)
hyperchlorhydria (hi′per·klōr·hi′dre·ah)
hypercholesterolemia
   (hi′per·ko·les′ter·ol·e′me·ah)
hypercholia (hi′per·ko′le·ah)
hyperchromatism (hi′per·kro′mah·tizm)
hyperchromia (hi′per·kro′me·ah)
hypercryalgesia (hi′per·kri′al·je′ze·ah)
hypercryesthesia (hi′per·kri′es·the′ze·ah)
hypercythemia (hi′per·si·the′me·ah)
hyperdipsia (hi′per·dip′se·ah)
hyperemesis (hi′per·em′ĕ·sis)
hyperemia (hi′per·e′me·ah)
hyperextension (hi′per·ek·sten′shun)
hyperflexion (hi′per·flek′shun)
hypergammaglobulinemia
   (hi′per·gam′ah·glob′u·lĭ·ne′me·ah)
hypergenitalism (hi′per·jen′ī·tal·izm)
hyperglobulinemia
   (hi′per·glob′u·lĭ·ne′me·ah)
hyperglycemia (hi′per·gli·se′me·ah)
hypergonadism (hi′per·go′nad·izm)
hyperhidrosis (hi′per·hi·dro′sis)
hyperinsulinism (hi′per·in′su·lin·izm)
hyperkalemia (hi′per·kah·le′me·ah)
hyperkeratosis (hi′per·ker′ah·to′sis)
hyperlipemia (hi′per·li·pe′me·ah)
hyperlipoproteinemia
   (hi′per·lip′o·pro′te·in·e′me·ah)
hyperlysinemia (hi′per·li′sin·e′me·ah)
hyperlysinuria (hi′per·li′sin·u′re·ah)
hypermastia (hi′per·mas′te·ah)
hypermenorrhea (hi′per·men′o·re′ah)
hypermyotonia (hi′per·mi′o·to′ne·ah)
hypernatremia (hi′per·nah·tre′me·ah)
hyperonychia (hi′per·o·nik′e·ah)
hyperopia (hi′per·o′pe·ah)
hyperorchidism (hi′per·or′kĭ·dizm)
hyperosmia (hi′per·oz′me·ah)
hyperostosis (hi′per·os·to′sis)
hyperoxaluria (hi′per·ok′sah·lu′re·ah)
hyperoxia (hi′per·ok′se·ah)
hyperpancreatism (hi′per·pan′kre·ă·tizm)
hyperparathyroidism
   (hi′per·par′ah·thi′roid·izm)
hyperphoria (hi′per·fo′re·ah)
hyperphosphaturia
   (hi′per·fos′fah·tu′re·ah)
hyperpigmentation
   (hi′per·pig′men·ta′shun)
hyperpituitarism (hi′per·pĭ·tu′ī·tah·rizm)
hyperplasia (hi′per·pla′ze·ah)

hyperpnea (hi'perp·ne'ah)
hyperprolactinemia
  (hi'per·pro·lak'tin·e'me·ah)
hyperprolinemia (hi'per·pro'li·ne'me·ah)
hyperpyretic (hi'per·pi·ret'ik)
hyperpyrexia (hi'per·pi·rek'se·ah)
hypersecretion (hi'per·se·kre'shun)
hypersensitive (hi'per·sen'si·tiv)
hypersensitization
  (hi'per·sen'si·ti·za'shun)
hypersialosis (hi'per·si'ah·lo'sis)
hypersomatotropism
  (hi'per·so·mat'ah·trop'izm)
hypersteatosis (hi'per·ste·ah·to'sis)
hypersthenuria (hi'per·sthě·nu're·ah)
hypertelorism (hi'per·te'lor·izm)
hypertension (hi'per·ten'shun)
hyperthecosis (hi'per·the·ko'sis)
hyperthelia (hi'per·the'le·ah)
hyperthermia (hi'per·ther'me·ah)
hyperthrombinemia
  (hi'per·throm'bi·ne'me·ah)
hyperthymia (hi'per·thi'me·ah)
hyperthyroidism (hi'per·thi'roi·dizm)
hypertrichosis (hi'per·trik·o'sis)
hypertriglyceridemia
  (hi'per·tri·glis'er·i·de'me·ah)
hypertrophy (hi·per'tro·fe)
hypertropia (hi'per·tro'pe·ah)
hyperuricemia (hi'per·u'ri·se'me·ah)
hyperuricosuria (hi'per·u·ri·ko·su're·ah)
hyperuricuria (hi'per·u·ri·ku're·ah)
hyperventilation (hi'per·ven'ti·la'shun)
hypervitaminosis (hi'per·vi'tah·mi·no'sis)
hypervolemia (hi'per·vo·le'me·ah)
hypervolia (hi'per·vo'le·ah)
hypha (hi'fah)
hyphae (hi'fe)
hyphema (hi·fe'mah)
hyphidrosis (hip'hid·ro'sis)
hypnagogic (hip'nah·goj'ik)
hypnagogue (hip'nah·gog)
hypnopompic (hip'no·pom'pik)
hypnosis (hip·no'sis)
hypnotic (hip·not'ik)
hypnotism (hip'no·tizm)
hypnotize (hip'no·tīz)
hypobaropathy (hi'po·bah·rop'ah·the)
hypocalcemia (hi'po·kal·se'me·ah)
hypocapnia (hi'po·kap'ne·ah)
hypochloremia (hi'po·klo·re'me·ah)
hypochlorhydria (hi'po·klor·hi'dre·ah)
hypochlorite (hi'po·klo'rīt)
hypochlorous (hi'po·klor'us)
hypocholesterolemia
  (hi'po·ko·les'ter·o·le'me·ah)
hypochondriac (hi'po·kon'dre·ak)
hypochondriasis (hi'po·kon·dri'ah·sis)
hypochondrium (hi'po·kon'dre·um)
hypochromatic (hi'po·kro·mat'ik)
hypochromia (hi'po·kro'me·ah)
hypochylia (hi'po·ki'le·ah)
hypocupremia (hi'po·ku·pre'me·ah)
hypodactylia (hi'po·dak·til'e·ah)
hypodermic (hi'po·der'mik)
hypodermoclysis (hi'po·der·mok'li·sis)
hypoesophoria (hi'po·es'o·fo're·ah)
hypoesthesia (hi'po·es·the'ze·ah)
hypofibrinogenemia
  (hi'po·fi·brin'o·jě·ne'me·ah)
hypogalactia (hi'po·gah·lak'she·ah)
hypogammaglobulinemia
  (hi'po·gam'ah·glob'u·li·ne'me·ah)
hypogastrium (hi'po·gas'tre·um)
hypogenitalism (hi'po·jen'i·tal·izm)
hypogeusia (hi'po·gu'ze·ah)
hypoglycemia (hi'po·gli·se'me·ah)
hypognathous (hi·pog'nah·thus)
hypogonadism (hi'po·go'nad·izm)
hypohidrosis (hi'po·hi·dro'sis)
hypokalemia (hi'po·ka·le'me·ah)
hypomenorrhea (hi'po·men'o·re'ah)
hyponatremia (hi'po·nah·tre'me·ah)
hyponychium (hi'po·nik'e·um)
hypoparathyroidism
  (hi'po·par'ah·thi'roid·izm)
hypophoria (hi'po·fo're·ah)
hypophosphatasia (hi'po·fos'fah·ta'ze·ah)

hypophyseal (hi'po·fiz'e·al)
hypophysectomize (hi'po·fi·sek'to·mīz)
hypophysial (hi'po·fiz'e·al)
hypophysis (hi·pof'i·sis)
hypopituitarism (hi'po·pi·tu'i·tah·rizm')
hypoplasia (hi'po·pla'ze·ah)
hypopnea (hi'po·ne'ah)
hypoproteinemia (hi'po·pro'ti·ne'me·ah)
hypoprothrombinemia
  (hi'po·pro·throm'bi·ne'me·ah)
hypopyon (hi·po'pe·on)
hyporiboflavinosis
  (hi'po·ri'bo·flah·vi·no'sis)
hyposalivation (hi'po·sal'i·va'shun)
hyposmia (hi·poz'me·ah)
hypospadias (hi'po·spa'de·as)
hypostasis (hi·pos'tah·sis)
hyposthenia (hi'pos·the'ne·ah)
hyposthenuria (hi'pos·thě·nu're·ah)
hypotaxia (hi'po·tak'se·ah)
hypotelorism (hi'po·tel'o·rizm)
hypotension (hi'po·ten'shun)
hypothalamus (hi'po·thal'ah·mus)
hypothenar (hi'poth'ě·nar)
hypothermia (hi'po·ther'me·ah)
hypothesis (hi·poth'ě·sis)
hypothrombinemia
  (hi'po·throm'bi·ne'me·ah)
hypothyroidism (hi'po·thi'roid·izm)
hypotonia (hi'po·to'ne·ah)
hypotropia (hi'po·tro'pe·ah)
hypovolemia (hi'po·vo·le'me·ah)
hypoxanthine (hi'po·zan'thēn)
hypoxemia (hi'pok·se'me·ah)
hypoxia (hi·pok'se·ah)
hypsarrhythmia (hip'sah·rith'me·ah)
hysteralgia (his'ter·al'je·ah)
hysteratresia (his'ter·ah·tre'ze·ah)
hysterectomy (his'tě·rek'to·me)
hysteresis (his'tě·re'sis)
hysteria (his·tēr'e·ah)
hysterocolposcope (his'ter·o·kol'po·skōp)
hysterogram (his'ter·o·gram)
hysterography (his'tě·rog'rah·fe)
hysteromyomectomy
  (his'ter·o·mi'o·mek'to·me)
hysteromyotomy (his'ter·o·mi·ot'o·me)
hystero-oophorectomy
  (his'ter·o-o'of·o·rek'to·me)
hysterosalpingectomy
  (his'ter·o·sal'pin·jek'to·me)
hysterosalpingogram
  (his'ter·o·sal·ping'o·gram)
hysterosalpingography
  (his'ter·o·sal'ping·gog'rah·fe)
hysteroscope (his'ter·o·skōp')

I

iatrogenic (i·at'ro·jen'ik)
iatrogeny (i·ah·troj'ě·ne)
ibuprofen (i·bu'pro·fen)
ichthyoid (ik'the·oid)
ichthyosis (ik·the·o'sis)
icteric (ik·ter'ik)
icterogenic (ik'ter·o·jen'ik)
icterus (ik'ter·us)
ictus (ik'tus)
id (id)
ideation (i'de·a'shun)
idioagglutinin (id'e·o·ah·gloo'ti·nin)
idioisoagglutinin
  (id'e·o·i'so'ah'glu'tin·in)
idiolysin (id'e·ol'i·sin)
idioneurosis (id'e·o·nu·ro'sis)
idionodal (id'e·o·no'dal)
idiopathic (id'e·o·path'ik)
idiophrenic (id'e·o·fren'ik)
idiosyncrasy (id'e·o·sin'krah·se)
idiosyncratic (id'e·o·sin·krat'ik)
idiot-savant (e·de·o'sah·vahn')
idoxuridine (i·doks·ur'i·dēn)
ileal (il'e·al)
ileitis (il'e·i'tis)
ileocecal (il'e·o·se'kal)
ileocecum (il'e·o·se'kum)

ileocolic (il'e·o·kol'ik)
ileocolitis (il'e·o·ko·li'tis)
ileocolostomy (il'e·o·ko·los'to·me)
ileostomy (il'e·os'to·me)
ileum (il'e·um)
ileus (il'e·us)
iliac (il'e·ak)
iliolumbar (il'e·o·lum'bar)
iliopectineal (il'e·o·pek·tin'e·al)
ilium (il'e·um)
imbibition (im'bi·bish'un)
imbrication (im'bri·ka'shun)
imidazole (im'id·az'ōl)
imide (im'id)
imino (i·me'no)
imipramine (i·mip'rah·mēn)
immersion (i·mer'shun)
immiscible (i·mis'i·bl)
immobilization (im·mo'bil·i·za'shun)
immobilize (im·mo'bil·īz)
immune (i·mūn')
immunity (i·mu'ni·te)
immunization (im'u·ni·za'shun)
immunize (im'u·nīz)
immunoagglutination
  (im'u·no·ah·gloo'ti·na'shun)
immunochemistry (im'u·no·kem'is·tre)
immunocompetence
  (im'u·no·kom'pě·tens)
immunocompromised
  (im'u·no·kom'pro·mīzd)
immunocyte (im'u·no·sīt)
immunoelectrophoresis
  (i·mu'no·e·lek'tro·fo·re'sis)
immunofluorescence
  (im'u·no·floo'o·res'ens)
immunogen (im'u·no·jen)
immunogenetics (im'u·no·jě·net'iks)
immunogenic (im'u·no·jen'ik)
immunoglobulin (im'u·no·glob'u·lin)
immunohematology
  (i·mu'no·hēm'ah·tol'o·je)
immunologic (im'u·no·loj'ik)
immunologist (im'u·nol'o·jist)
immunology (im'u·nol'o·je)
immunoprophylaxis
  (im'u·no·pro'fi·lak'sis)
immunosuppression
  (im'u·no·su·presh'un)
immunosuppressive (im'u·no·su·pres'iv)
immunotherapy (i·mu'no·ther'ah·pe)
impaction (im·pak'shun)
impairment (im·pār'ment)
impedance (im·pēd'ans)
imperforate (im·per'fo·rāt)
impermeable (im·per'me·ah·bl)
impetigo (im'pě·ti'go)
impetus (im'pě·tus)
implant (im·plant')
implant (im'plant)
impotence (im'pǒ·tens)
impregnate (im·preg'nāt)
impulse (im'puls)
inadequacy (in·ad'ě·kwah·se)
inanimate (in·an'i·māt)
inanition (in'ah·nish'un)
inarticulate (in'ar·tik'u·lāt)
inbreeding (in'brēd·ing)
incarcerated (in·kar'ser·āt'ed)
incest (in'sest)
incestuous (in·ses'tu·us)
incidence (in'si·dens)
incipient (in·sip'e·ent)
incise (in·sīz')
incision (in·sizh'un)
incisor (in·si'zer)
incisura (in·si·su'rah)
incoherent (in'ko·hēr'ent)
incompatible (in'kom·pat'i·bl)
incompetence (in·kom'pě·tens)
incontinence (in·kon'ti·nens)
incoordination (in'ko·or'di·na'shun)
incrustation (in'krus·ta'shun)
incubator (in'ku·ba·ter)
incurable (in·ku'rah·bl)
incus (ing'kus)
indican (in'di·kan)
indicanuria (in'di·kan·u're·ah)

indicator (in′dĭ·ka′ter)
indices (in′dĭ·sēz)
indigenous (in·dij′ĕ·nus)
indigestible (in′di·jes′tĭ·bl)
indigestion (in′di·jes′chun)
indigo (in′dĭ·go)
individuation (in′dĭ·vid′u·a′shun)
indole (in′dōl)
induce (in·dūs′)
induction (in·duk′shun)
inductorium (in·duk·to′re·um)
induration (in·du·ra′shun)
indwelling (in′dwel·ing)
inebriation (in·e′bre·a′shun)
inert (in·ert′)
inertia (in·er′she·ah)
infancy (in′fan·se)
infantile (in′fan·tīl)
infarct (in′farkt)
infarction (in·fark′shun)
infect (in·fekt′)
infection (in·fek′shun)
infectious (in·fek′shus)
infecundity (in′fe·kun′dĭ·te)
infertility (in′fer·til′ĭ·te)
infest (in·fest′)
infestation (in·fes·ta′shun)
infiltration (in′fil·tra′shun)
infirmity (in·fir′mĭ·te)
inflammation (in′flah·ma′shun)
inflammatory (in·flam′ah·to′re)
influenza (in′flu·en′zah)
influenzavirus (in′flu·en′zah·vi′rus)
infraclavicular (in′frah·klah·vik′u·lar)
infrahyoid (in′frah·hi′oid)
infranatant (in·frah·na′tant)
infraorbital (in·frah·or′bĭ·tal)
infratrochlear (in′frah·trok′le·ar)
infundibulum (in′fun·dib′u·lum)
inhalant (in·ha′lant)
inhalation (in′hah·la′shun)
inhale (in·hāl′)
inheritance (in·her′ĭ·tans)
inhibition (in′hĭ·bish′un)
ineon (in′e·on)
initiator (in·ĭ·she′a·tor)
inject (in·jekt′)
injectable (in·jeck′tah·bl)
injection (in·jek′shun)
injector (in·jek′tor)
innate (in′nāt)
innervation (in′er·va′shun)
innidiation (ĭ·nid′e·a′shun)
innocuous (ĭ·nok′u·us)
innominate (ĭ·nom′ĭ·nāt)
innoxious (ĭ·nok′shus)
inoculable (ĭ·nok′u·lah·bl)
inoculate (ĭ·nok′u·lāte)
inoculation (ĭ·nok′u·la′shun)
inorganic (in′or·gan′ik)
inosculate (in·os′ku·lāt)
inosine (in′o·sin)
inositol (in·o′sĭ·tol)
inotropism (in·ot′ro·pizm)
inpatient (in′pa·shent)
insanity (in·san′ĭ·te)
insectarium (in′sek·ta′re·um)
insecticide (in·sek′tĭ·sīd)
insectifuge (in·sek′tĭ·fūj)
insemination (in·sem′ĭ·na′shun)
insertion (in·ser′shun)
insidious (in·sid′e·us)
in situ (in si′tu)
insoluble (in·sol′u·bl)
insomnia (in·som′ne·ah)
insomniac (in·som′ne·ak)
inspiration (in′spĭ·ra′shun)
inspiratory (in·spi′rah·to′re)
inspissation (in′spis·sa′shun)
inspissator (in·spis′a·tor)
instinct (in′stinkt)
instrumentation (in′stroo·men·ta′shun)
insufficiency (in′sŭ·fish′en·se)
insufflate (in·suf′lāt)
insufflation (in′sŭ·fla′shun)
insufflator (in′sŭ·fla′tor)
insula (in′su·lah)
insulin (in′su·lin)

insulinase (in′su·lin·ās)
insulinoma (in′su·lin·o′mah)
insulinopenia (in′su·lin·o·pe′ne·ah)
integument (in·teg′u·ment)
interacinous (in′ter·as′ĭ·nus)
intercadence (in·ter·ka′dens)
intercalary (in·ter′kah·ler′e)
intercondylar (in′ter·kon′dĭ·lar)
intercondylic (in′ter·kon′dĭ·lik)
intercostal (in′ter·kos′tal)
intercourse (in′ter·kōrs)
intercuspation (in′ter·kus·pa′shun)
interdental (in′ter·den′tal)
interdigitation (in′ter·dij′ĭ·ta′shun)
interface (in′ter·fās)
interferon (in′ter·fēr′on)
interictal (in′ter·ik′tal)
interleukin (in′ter·loo′kin)
interlobar (in′ter·lo′bar)
interlobular (in·ter·lob′u·lar)
intermenstrual (in′ter·men′stru·al)
intermittence (in′ter·mit′ens)
intermittency (in′ter·mit′en·se)
intermuscular (in′ter·mus′ku·lar)
intern (in′tern)
interneuron (in′ter·nu′ron)
internist (in·ter′nist)
internodal (in′ter·no′dal)
internuclear (in′ter·nu′kle·ar)
interosseous (in′ter·os′e·us)
interphase (in′ter·fāz)
interproximal (in′ter·prok′sĭ·mal)
interradicular (in′ter·rah·dik′u·lar)
interscapular (in′ter·skap′u·lar)
interspinal (in·ter·spi′nal)
interstice (in·ter′stis)
interstitial (in′ter·stish′al)
intertriginous (in′ter·trij′ĭ·nus)
intertrigo (in′ter·tri′go)
intertrochanteric (in′ter·tro′kan·ter′ik)
intervertebral (in·ter·ver′tĕ·bral)
intervillous (in′ter·vil′us)
intestine (in·tes′tin)
intima (in′tĭ·mah)
intolerance (in·tol′er·ans)
intortor (in·tor′tor)
intoxication (in·tok′sĭ·ka′shun)
intra-abdominal (in′trah-ab·dom′ĭ·nal)
intra-articular (in′trah-ar·tik′u·lar)
intracapsular (in′trah·kap′su·lar)
intracardiac (in′trah·kar′de·ak)
intracatheter (in′trah·kath′ĕ·ter)
intracellular (in′trah·sel′u·lar)
intracranial (in′trah·kra′ne·al)
intracutaneous (in′trah·ku·ta′ne·us)
intradural (in′trah·du′ral)
intrahepatic (in′trah·he·pat′ik)
intraluminal (in′trah·lu′mĭ·nal)
intramedullary (in′trah·med′u·lār·e)
intramuscular (in′trah·mus′ku·lar)
intranasal (in′trah·na′sal)
intraneural (in′trah·nu′ral)
intraocular (in′trah·ok′u·lar)
intraoral (in′trah·o′ral)
intraorbital (in′trah·or′bĭ·tal)
intraosseous (in′trah·os′e·us)
intraperitoneal (in′trah·per′ĭ·to·ne′al)
intrathecal (in′trah·the′kal)
intrauterine (in′trah·u′ter·in)
intravascular (in′trah·vas′ku·lar)
intravenous (in′trah·ve′nus)
intraventricular (in′trah·ven·trik′u·lar)
intrinsic (in·trin′sik)
introitus (in·tro′ĭ·tus)
introjection (in′tro·jek′shun)
intromission (in′tro·mish′un)
introversion (in′tro·ver′shun)
introvert (in′tro·vert)
intubate (in′tu·bāt)
intubation (in′tu·ba′shun)
intumesce (in·tu·mes′)
intumescence (in·tu·mes′ens)
intumescent (in·tu·mes′ent)
intussuscept (in′tus·sus·sept′)
intussusception (in′tus·sus·sep′shun)
intussusceptum (in′tus·sus·sep′tum)
intussuscipiens (in′tus·sus·sip′e·ens)
inulin (in′u·lin)

in utero (in u′ter·o)
invaginate (in·vaj′ĭ·nāt)
invagination (in·vaj′ĭ·na′shun)
invasive (in·va′siv)
inversion (in·ver′zhun)
invertase (in·ver′tās)
invertebrate (in·ver′tĕ·brāt)
in vitro (in ve′tro)
in vivo (in ve′vo)
involucrum (in′vo·lu′krum)
involution (in′vo·lu′shun)
iodate (i′o·dāt)
iodide (i′o·dīd)
iodine (i′o·dīn)
iodoform (i·o′do·form)
iodopsin (i′o·dop′sin)
ion (i′on)
ionization (i′on·ĭ·za′shun)
iontophoresis (i·on·to·fo·re′sis)
ipecac (ip′ĕ·kak)
ipsilateral (ip′sĭ·lat′er·al)
iridectomy (ir′ĭ·dek′to·me)
iridencleisis (ir′ĭ·den·kli′sis)
irides (ir′ĭ·dēz)
iridesis (ĭ·rid′ĕ·sis)
iridium (ĭ·rid′e·um)
iridization (ir′ĭ·dĭ·za′shun)
iridocele (ĭ·rid′o·sēl)
iridocoloboma (ir′ĭ·do·kol′o·bo′mah)
iridoconstrictor (ir′ĭ·do·kon·strik′tor)
iridocyclectomy (ir′ĭ·do·si·klek′to·me)
iridocyclitis (ir′ĭ·do·si·kli′tis)
iridodilator (ir′ĭ·do·di·la′tor)
iridodonesis (ir′ĭ·do·do·ne′sis)
iridomalacia (ir′ĭ·do·mah·la′she·ah)
iridosclerotomy (ir′ĭ·do·skle·rot′o·me)
iris bombé (i′ris bom·ba′)
iritis (i·ri′tis)
irradiate (ĭ·ra′de·āt)
irradiation (ĭ·ra′de·a′shun)
irreducible (ir′re·dūs′ĭ·bl)
irrigate (ir′ĭ·gāt)
irrigation (ir′ĭ·ga′shun)
irritability (ir′ĭ·tah·bil′ĭ·te)
irritable (ir′ĭ·tah·bl)
irritant (ir′ĭ·tant)
irritation (ir′ĭ·ta′shun)
ischemia (is·ke′me·ah)
ischemic (is·kem′ik)
ischia (is′ke·ah)
ischium (is′ke·um)
islet (i′let)
isoagglutinin (i′so·ah·gloo′tĭ·nin)
isoallele (is′o·ah·lēl)
isoantibody (i·so·an′tĭ·bod′e)
isoantigen (i′so·an′tĭ·jen)
isocortex (i′so·kor′teks)
isogamete (i′so·gam′ēt)
isogamy (i·sog′ah·me)
isogeneic (i′so·jĕ·ne′ik)
isogenic (i′so·jen′ik)
isograft (i′so·graft)
isohemagglutinin
　(i′so·hēm′ah·gloo′tĭ·nin)
isohemolysin (i′so·he·mol′ĭ·sin)
isohemolysis (i′so·he·mol′ĭ·sis)
isoimmunization (i′so·im′u·ni·za′shun)
isolate (i′so·lāt)
isoleucine (i′so·lu′sin)
isomer (i′so·mer)
isomerase (i·som′er·ās)
isomerism (i·som′ĕ·rizm)
isometropia (i′so·mĕ·tro′pe·ah)
isoniazid (i′so·ni′ah·zid)
isophane (i′so·fān)
isopropyl (i′so·pro′pil)
isoproterenol (i′so·pro′tĕ·re′nol)
isopter (i·sop′ter)
isotonic (i′so·ton′ik)
isotope (i′so·tōp)
isotoxin (i′so·tok′sin)
isovalericacidemia
　(i′so·vah·ler′ik·as′ĭ·de′me·ah)
isovolumic (i′so·vol·u′mik)
isozyme (i′so·zīm)
isthmus (is′mus)
iter (i′ter)
ixodes (iks·o′dēz)

ixodiasis (iks′o·di′ah·sis)
ixodic (ik·sod′ik)
ixodidae (iks·od′ĭ·de)

J

jactitation (jak′tĭ·ta′shun)
jaundice (jawn′dis)
jaundiced (jawn′dist)
jejunal (je·joo′nal)
jejunectomy (je′joo·nek′to·me)
jejunitis (je′joo·ni′tis)
jejunocolostomy (je·joo′no·ko·los′to·me)
jejunoileitis (je·joo′no·il′e·i′tis)
jejunoileostomy (jě·joo′no·il′e·os′to·me)
jejunojejunostomy
  (je·joo′no·je′joo·nos′to·me)
jejunoplasty (je·joo′no·plas′te)
jejunostomy (je·joo·nos′to·me)
jejunum (je·joo′num)
joule (jool)
jugal (joo′gal)
jugulum (joo′gu·lum)
jugum (joo′gum)
junctura (junk·tu′rah)
juxtaglomerular (juks′tah·glo·mer′u·lar)
juxtamedullary (juks′tah·med′u·lar′e)
juxtapose (juks′tah·pōz)
juxtaposition (juks′tah·po·zish′un)
juxtapyloric (juks′tah·pi·lor′ik)

K

kala azar (kah′lah ah·zar′)
kaliopenia (ka′le·o·pe′ne·ah)
kaliuresis (ka′le·u·re′sis)
kaliuretic (ka′le·u·ret′ik)
kallikrein (kal′li·kre′in)
kaolin (ka′o·lin)
kappa (kap′ah)
karyochrome (kar′e·o·krōm)
karyocyte (kar′e·o·sīt)
karyogamy (kar′e·og′ah·me)
karyolysis (kar′e·ol′i·sis)
karyon (kar′e·on)
karyopyknosis (kar′e·o·pik·no′sis)
karyorrhexis (kar′e·o·rek′sis)
karyosome (kar′e·o·sōm)
karyotype (kar′e·o·tīp)
karyotyping (kar′e·o·tīp′ing)
keloid (ke′loid)
keloidosis (ke′loi·do′sis)
keloplasty (ke′lo·plas′te)
keratalgia (ker′ah·tal′je·ah)
keratectasia (ker′ah·tek·ta′ze·ah)
keratectomy (ker′ah·tek′to·me)
keratin (ker′ah·tin)
keratinization (ker′ah·tin′ĭ·za′shun)
keratinosome (ke·rat′ĭ·no·sōm)
keratinous (ke·rat′ĭ·nus)
keratitis (ker′ah·ti′tis)
keratoacanthoma
  (ker′ah·to·ak′an·tho′mah)
keratocele (ker′ah·to·sēl)
keratochromatosis
  (ker′ah·to·kro·mah·to′sis)
keratoconjunctivitis
  (ker′ah·to·kon·junk′tĭ·vi′tis)
keratoconometer
  (ker′ah·to·ko·nom′ĕ·ter)
keratoconus (ker′ah·to·ko′nus)
keratocyte (ker′ah·to·sīt)
keratodermia (ker′ah·to·der′me·ah)
keratogenous (ker′ah·toj′ĕ·nus)
keratohelcosis (ker′ah·to·hel·ko′sis)
keratoiridoscope (ker′ah·to·ir′ĭ·do·skōp)
keratoiritis (ker′ah·to·i·ri′tis)
keratoleptynsis (ker′ah·to·lep·tin′sis)
keratolysis (ker′ah·tol′i·sis)
keratomalacia (ker′ah·to·mah·la′she·ah)
keratome (ker′ah·tŏm)
keratometer (ker′ah·tom′ĕ·ter)
keratomycosis (ker′ah·to·mi·ko′sis)
keratonosus (ker′ah·ton′o·sus)
keratonyxis (ker′ah·to·nik′sis)

keratopathy (ker′ah·top′ah·the)
keratoplasty (ker′ah·to·plas′te)
keratoprosthesis (ker′ah·to·pros·the′sis)
keratorhexis (ker′ah·to·rek′sis)
keratoscope (ker′ah·to·skōp)
keratosis (ker′ah·to′sis)
keratotomy (ker′ah·tot′o·me)
kerion (ker′re·on)
ketoacidosis (ke′to·as′ĭ·do′sis)
ketoaciduria (ke′to·as′ĭ·du′re·ah)
ketone (ke′tōn)
ketonuria (ke′to·nu′re·ah)
ketose (ke′tōs)
ketosis (ke·to′sis)
kilogrammeter (kil′o·gram·me′ter)
kinanesthesia (kin′an·es·the′ze·ah)
kinase (ki′nās)
kinescope (kin′e·skōp)
kinesiology (kĭ·ne′se·ol′o·je)
kinesitherapy (kĭ·ne′sĭ·ther′ah·pe)
kinesthesia (kin′es·the′ze·ah)
kinetics (ki·net′iks)
kinetocardiogram
  (kĭ·ne′to·kar′de·o·gram)
kinetocardiograph
  (kĭ·ne′to·kar′de·o·graf)
kinetoplasm (kĭ·ne′to·plazm)
kinin (ki′nin)
Klebsiella pneumoniae
  (kleb′se·el′ah nu·mo′ne·e)
kleptomania (klep′to·ma′ne·ah)
koilonychia (koy·lo·nik′e·ah)
kraurosis vulvae (kraw·ro′sis vul′ve)
krypton (krip′ton)
kuru (koo′roo)
kwashiorkor (kwash·e·or′kor)
kymograph (ki′mo·graf)
kymoscope (ki′mo·skōp)
kynurenic (kin′u·re′nik)
kyphos (ki′fōs)
kyphoscoliosis (ki′fo·sko′le·o′sis)
kyphosis (ki·fo′sis)
kytorrhachic (ker′to·rak′ik)

L

labia (la′be·ah)
labile (la′bīl)
lability (lah·bil′ĭ·te)
labiochorea (la′be·o·ko·re′ah)
labiogingival (la′be·o·jin′jĭ·val)
labioplasty (la′be·o·plas′te)
labium (la′be·um)
labra (la′brah)
labrum (la′brum)
labyrinth (lab′ĭ·rinth)
labyrinthine (lab′ĭ·rin′thīn)
labyrinthitis (lab′ĭ·rin·thi′tis)
labyrinthotomy (lab′ĭ·rin·thot′o·me)
laceration (las′er·a′shun)
lacrimal (lak′rĭ·mal)
lacrimation (lak′rĭ·ma′shun)
lactagogue (lak′tah·gog)
lactase (lak′tās)
lactate (lak′tāt)
lactation (lak·ta′shun)
lacteal (lak′te·al)
lactescent (lak′tes′ent)
lactic (lak′tik)
lacticacidemia (lak′tik·as′ĭ·de′me·ah)
lactiferous (lak·tif′er·us)
lactifuge (lak′tĭ·fūj)
lactigenous (lak·tij′ĕ·nus)
lactogen (lak′to·gen)
lactogenic (lak′to·jen′ik)
lactoglobulin (lak′to·glob′u·lin)
lactone (lak′tōn)
lactose (lak′tōs)
lactosuria (lak′to·su′re·ah)
lactovegetarian (lak′to·vej′ĕ·ta′re·an)
lacuna (lah·ku′nah)
lacunae (lah·ku′ne)
Laennec (la′en·nek′)
lagophalmos (lag′of·thal′mos)
lallation (lah·la′shun)
lambda (lam′dah)
lambdoid (lam′doid)

lamella (lah·mel′ah)
lamellae (lah·mel′e)
lamina (lam′i·nah)
laminar (lam′i·nar)
laminectomy (lam′ĭ·nek′to·me)
laminotomy (lam′ĭ·not′o·me)
lancet (lan′set)
lanolin (lan′o·lin)
lanuginous (lah·nu′jĭ·nus)
lanugo (lah·nu′go)
laparohysterectomy
  (lap′ah·ro·his′ter·ek′to·me)
laparohysterotomy
  (lap′ah·ro·his′ter·ot′o·me)
laparoscope (lap′ah·ro·skōp)
laparoscopy (lap′ah·ros′ko·pe)
laparotomy (lap′ah·rot′o·me)
larva migrans (lar′vah mi′granz)
larvicide (lar′vĭ·sīd)
laryngeal (lah·rin′je·al)
laryngectomy (lar′in·jek′to·me)
laryngismus (lar′in·jiz′mus)
laryngitis (lar′in·ji′tis)
laryngocele (lah·ring′go·sel)
laryngocentesis (lah·ring′go·sen·te′sis)
laryngology (lar′ing·gol′o·je)
laryngoparalysis
  (lah·ring′go·pah·ral′ĭ·sis)
laryngopharyngeal
  (lah·ring′go·fah·rin′je·al)
laryngopharynx (lah·ring′go·far′inks)
laryngoscope (lah·ring′go·skōp)
laryngoscopy (lar′ing·gos′ko·pe)
laryngospasm (lah·ring′go·spazm)
laryngostenosis (lah·ring′go·stĕ·no′sis)
laryngostomy (lar′ing·gos′to·me)
laryngotome (lar′ring′go·tōm)
laryngotomy (lar′ing·got′o·me)
larynx (lar′inks)
lascivia (lah·siv′e·ah)
Lasegue (lah′sāg)
laser (la′zer)
lassitude (las′ĭ·tūd)
latah (lah′tah)
latent (la′tent)
lateral (lat′er·al)
laterotorsion (lat′er·o·tor′shun)
lateroversion (lat′er·o·ver′shun)
latissimus (lah·tis′ĭ·mus)
lattice (lat′is)
lavage (lah·vahzh′)
laxative (lak′sah·tiv)
lead (lēd)
lead (led)
leaflet (lēf′let)
lecithin (les′ĭ·thin)
lectin (lek′tin)
legionnaire (le′jun·ār′)
leiomyoma (li′o·mi·o′mah)
leiomyomatosis (li′o·mi′o·mah·to′sis)
leiomyosarcoma (li′o·mi′o·sar·ko′mah)
Leishmania (lēsh·mā′ne·ah)
leishmaniasis (lēsh′mah·ni′ah·sis)
leishmanid (lēsh′man·id)
lemniscus (lem·nis′kus)
lenitive (len′ĭ·tiv)
lente (len′te)
lenticonus (len′tĭ·ko′nus)
lenticular (len·tik′u·lar)
lenticulostriate (len·tik′u·lo·stri´āt)
lentiform (len′tĭ·form)
lentigines (len·tij′ĕ·nēz)
lentigo (len·ti′go)
leontiasis (le′on·ti′ah·sis)
leprid (lep′rid)
leproma (lep·ro′mah)
leprosarium (lep′ro·sa′re·um)
leprosy (lep′ro·se)
leptocyte (lep′to·sīt)
leptocytosis (lep′to·si·to′sis)
leptomeningeal (lep′to·mĕ·nin′je·al)
leptospira (lep′to·spi′rah)
leptospirosis (lep′to·spi·ro′sis)
leptotene (lep′to·tēn)
Leptotrichia (lep′to·trik′e·ah)
lesbian (lez′be·an)
lesion (le′zhun)
lethal (le′thal)

lethargy (leth′ar·je)
leucine (loo′sēn)
leukapheresis (loo′kah·fē·re′sis)
leukemia (loo·ke′me·ah)
leukemic (loo·ke′mik)
leukemogenesis (loo·ke′mo·jen′ĕ·sis)
leukemoid (loo·ke′moid)
leukoagglutinin (loo′ko·ah·gloo′tĭ·nin)
leukoblast (loo′ko·blast)
leukocyte (loo′ko·sīt)
leukocytoblast (loo′ko·si′to·blast)
leukocytogenesis (loo′ko·si′to·jen′ĕ·sis)
leukocytolysin (loo′ko·si·tol′ĭ·sin)
leukocytolysis (loo′ko·si·tol′ĭ·sis)
leukocytometer (loo′ko·si·tom′ĕ·ter)
leukocytopoiesis (loo′ko·si′to·poi·e′sis)
leukocytosis (loo′ko·si·to′sis)
leukocytotactic (loo′ko·si′to·tak′tik)
leukocytotaxia (loo′ko·si′to·tak′se·ah)
leukocytoxin (loo′ko·si′to·tok′sin)
leukoderma (loo′ko·der′mah)
leukodystrophy (loo′ko·dis′tro·fe)
leukoerythroblastosis
   (loo′ko·ĕ·rith′ro·blas·to′sis)
leukoencephalopathy
   (loo′ko·en·sef′ah·lop′ah·the)
leukokoria (loo′ko·ko′re·ah)
leukomyelopathy
   (loo′ko·mi·e·lop′ah·the)
leukonychia (loo′ko·nik′e·ah)
leukopedesis (loo′ko·pĕ·de′sis)
leukopenia (loo′ko·pe′ne·ah)
leukoplakia (loo′ko·pla′ke·ah)
leukopoiesis (loo′ko·poi·e′sis)
leukoprotease (loo′ko·pro′te·ās)
leukorrhea (loo′ko·re′ah)
leukosis (loo·ko′sis)
leukotaxine (loo′ko·tak′sēn)
leukotriene (loo′ko·tri′ēn)
levodopa (le′vo·do′pah)
levorotatory (le′vo·ro′tah·to′re)
levulosuria (lev′u·lo·su′re·ah)
lewisite (loo′ĭ·sīt)
libidinous (lĭ·bid′ĭ·nus)
libido (lĭ·be′do)
lichen planus (li′ken pla′nus)
lidocaine (li′do·kān)
ligament (lig′ah·ment)
ligand (li′gand)
ligase (li′gās)
ligate (li′gāt)
ligation (li·ga′shun)
ligature (lig′ah·chŭr)
lightening (līt′en·ing)
limbi (lim′bi)
limbic (lim′bik)
limbus (lim′bus)
liminal (lim′ĭ·nal)
liminometer (lim′ĭ·nom′ĕ·ter)
lyncomycin (lin′ko·mi′sin)
lindane (lin′dān)
linea (lin′e·ah)
lineae (lin′e·e·)
lingual (ling′gwal)
lingulla (ling′gu·lah)
linguopapilitis (ling′gwo·pap′ĭ·li·tis)
linin (li′nin)
linkage (lingk′ij)
linoleic (lin′o le′ik)
linolenic (lin′o·le′nik)
lipase (lip′ās)
lipedema (lip′ĕ·de′mah)
lipid (lip′id)
lipidoses (lip′ĭ·do′sēz)
lipidosis (lip·i·do′sis)
lipoatrophy (li′po·at′ro·fe)
lipocele (lip′o·sēl)
lipochondrodystrophy
   (lip′o·kon′dro·dis′tro·fe)
lipochrome (lip′o·krōm)
lipocyte (lip′o·sīt)
lipodystrophy (lip′o·dis′tro·fe)
lipofibroma (lip′o·fi′bro′mah)
lipofuscin (lip′o·fus′sin)
lipogenic (lip′o·jen′ik)
lipoid (lip′oid)
lipoidosis (lip′oi·do′sis)
lipolipoidosis (lip′o·lip′oi·do′sis)

lipoma (li·po′mah)
lipoprotein (lip′o·pro′te·in)
liposarcoma (lip′o·sar·ko′mah)
liquefacient (lik′wĕ·fa′shent)
liquefaction (lik′wĕ·fak′shun)
liquescent (lik·wes′ent)
Listeria (lis·ter′e·ah)
listeriosis (lis·ter′e·o′sis)
liter (le′ter)
lithagogue (lith′ah·gog)
lithocystotomy (lith′o·sis·tot′o·me)
lithodialysis (lith′o·di·al′ĭ·sis)
litholapaxy (li·thol′ah·pak′se)
lithonephrotomy (lith′o·nĕ·frot′o·me)
lithotomy (li·thot′o·me)
lithotresis (lith′o·tre′sis)
lithotrite (lith′o·trit)
lithuresis (lith′u·re′sis)
litmus (lit′mus)
livedo reticularis (li·ve′do rĕ·tik′u·la′ris)
lixiviation (liks′iv·e·a′shun)
lixivium (liks·iv′e·um)
lobectomy (lo·bek′to·me)
lobeline (lob′ĕ·lēn)
lobotomy (lo·bot′o·me)
lobule (lob′ūl)
lochia (lo′ke·ah)
lochiorrhea (lo′ke·o·re′ah)
lochioschesis (lo′ke·os′kĕ·sis)
loci (lo′si)
locular (lok′u·lar)
loculation (lok′u·la′shun)
locum tenens (lo′kum ten′ens)
locus (lo′kus)
logopathy (log·op′ah·the)
logoplegia (log′o·ple′je·ah)
logorrhea (log′o·re′ah)
lophotrichous (lo·fot′rĭ·kus)
lordoscoliosis (lor′do·sko′le·o′sis)
lordosis (lor·do′sis)
lordotic (lor·dot′ik)
loupe (loop)
loxoscelism (lok·sos′sĕ·lizm)
loxotomy (lok·sot′o·me)
lozenge (loz′enj)
lumbar (lum′ber)
lumbosacral (lum′bo·sa′kral)
lumbrical (lum′brĭ·kal)
lumbricoid (lum′brĭ·koid)
lumen (loo′men)
lumina (loo′min·ah)
luminescence (loo′mĭ·nes′ens)
lumirhodopsin (loo′mĭ·ro·dop′sin)
lumpectomy (lum·pek′to·me)
lunula (loo′nu·lah)
lupus (loo′pus)
lutein (loo′te·in)
luteinization (loo′te·in′ĭ·za′shun)
luteogenic (loo′te·o·jen′ik)
luteoma (loo′te·o·mah)
luteotrophic (loo′te·o·trof′ik)
luteotropic (loo′te·o·trop′ik)
luxation (luk·sa′shun)
lymph (limf)
lymphadenectasia
   (lim·fad′ĕ·nek·ta′ze·ah)
lymphadenectomy (lim·fad′ĕ·nek′to·me)
lymphadenitis (lim·fad′ĕ·ni′tis)
lymphadenography (lim·fad′ĕ·nog′rah·fe)
lymphadenoma (lim·fad′ĕ·no′mah)
lymphadenomatosis
   (lim·fad′ĕ·no·mah·to′sis)
lymphadenopathy (lim·fad′ĕ·nop′ah·the)
lymphagogue (lim′fah·gog)
lymphangiectasia (lim·fan′je·ek·ta′ze·ah)
lymphangiectomy (lim·fan′je·ek′to·me)
lymphangioendothelioma
   (lim·fan′je·en′do·the·le·o′mah)
lymphangiography (lim·fan′je·og′rah·fe)
lymphangioma (lim·fan′je·o′mah)
lymphangitis (lim′fan·ji′tis)
lymphatic (lim·fat′ik)
lymphectasia (lim′fek·ta′ze·ah)
lymphedema (lim′fĕ·de′mah)
lymphoblast (lim′fo·blast)
lymphoblastoma (lim′fo·blas·to′mah)
lymphocele (lim′fo·sēl)
limphocyte (lim′fo·sīt)

lymphocytoma (lim′fo·si·to′mah)
lymphocytopenia (lim′fo·si·to·pe′ne·ah)
lymphocytopoiesis (lim′fo·si′to·poi·e′sis)
lymphocytosis (lim′fo·si·to′sis)
lymphoepithelioma
   (lim′fo·ep′ĭ·the′le·o′mah)
lymphogranuloma venereum
   (lim′fo·gran′u·lo′mah ve·ne′re·um)
lymphoidectomy (lim′foi·dek′to·me)
lymphokine (lim′fo·kīn)
lymphoma (lim·fo′mah)
lymphomatosis (lim′fo·mah·to′sis)
lymphopathy (lim·fop′ah·the)
lymphopenia (lim·fo·pe′ne·ah)
lymphopoiesis (lim′fo·poi·e′sis)
lymphoreticular (lim′fo·rĕ·tik′u·lar)
lymphosarcoma (lim′fo·sar·ko′mah)
lymphostasis (lim·fos′tah·sis)
lyophil (lī′o·fil)
lyophilization (li·of′ĭ·lĭ·za′shun)
lysin (li′sin)
lysine (li′sēn)
lysis (li′sis)
lysogen (li′so·jen)
lysogenesis (li′so·jen′ĕ·sis)
lysogeny (li·soj′ĕ·ne)
lysokinase (li′so·ki′nās)
lisolecithin (li′so·les′ĭ·thin)
lysosome (li′so·sōm)
lysozyme (li′so·zīm)

M

macerate (mas′er·āt)
maceration (mas′er·a′shun)
macroamylase (mak′ro·am′ĭ·lās)
macrobrachia (mak′ro·bra′ke·ah)
macrocephalous (mak′ro·sef′ah·lus)
macrochilia (mak′ro·ki′le·ah)
macrodonidium (mak′ro·ko·nid′e·um)
macrocryoglobulinemia
   (mak′ro·kri·o·glob′u·lin·e′me·ah)
macrocyte (mak′ro·sīt)
macrocytosis (mak′ro·si·to′sis)
macrodactyly (mak′ro·dak′tĭ·le)
macroencephaly (mak′ro·en·sef′ah·le)
macrogenitosomia
   (mak′ro·jen′ĭ·to·so′me·ah)
macroglia (mak·rog′le·ah)
macroglobulinemia
   (mak′ro·glob′u·lĭ·ne′me·ah)
macroglossia (mak′ro·glos′e·ah)
macrognathia (mak′ro·na′the·ah)
macromastia (mak′ro·mas′te·ah)
macromelia (mak′ro·me′le·ah)
macromolecule (mak′ro·mol′ĕ·kūl)
macrophage (mak′ro·fāj)
macrophthalmia (mak′rof·thal′me·ah)
macropolycyte (mak′ro·pol′e·sīt)
macropsia (mah·krop′se·ah)
macrorhinia (mak′ro·rin′e·ah)
macrotia (mak·ro′she·ah)
macula (mak′u·lah)
maculae (mak′u·le)
macule (mak′ūl)
maculoerythematous
   (mak′u·lo·er·ĭ·the′mah·tus)
maculopapule (mak′u·lo·pap′ūl)
maculopathy (mak′u·lop′ah·the)
maduromycosis (mah·du′ro·mi·ko′sis)
magma (mag′mah)
magneton (mag′ne·ton)
malabsorption (mal′ab·sorp′shun)
malacia (mah·la′she·ah)
malady (mal′ah·de)
malaise (mal·āz)
malar (ma′lar)
malaria (mah·la′re·ah)
malarial (mah·la′re·al)
malathion (mal′ah·thi′on)
malignancy (mah·lig′nan·se)
malignant (mah·lig′nant)
malinger (mah·ling′ger)
malingerer (mah·ling′ger·er)
malleation (mal′e·a′shun)
malleoli (mal·le′o·li)
malleolus (mal·le′o·lus)

malleus (mal'e·us)
malnutrition (mal'nu·trish'un)
malocclusion (mal'o·kloo'zhun)
malpighian (mal·pig'i·an)
maltase (mawl'tās)
maltose (mawl'tōs)
mamelon (mam'ě·lon)
mammaplasty (mam'ah·plas'te)
mammary (mam'er·e)
mammilla (mah·mil'ah)
mammillaplasty (mam·mil'ah·plas'te)
mammillary (mam'i·ler'e)
mammogram (mam'o·gram)
mammography (mam·og'rah·fe)
mandible (man'dĭ·bl)
mandibular (man·dib'u·lar)
mandibulectomy (man'dib·u·lek'to·me)
maneuver (mah·noo'ver)
manganese (man'gah·nēs)
manganous (man'gah·nus)
mange (mānj)
mania (ma'ne·ah)
manic (man'ik)
mannitol (man'i·tol)
manometer (mah·nom'ě·ter)
manubrium (mah·nu'bre·um)
marasmus (mah·raz'mus)
Marfan (mar·fahn')
marrow (mar'o)
marsupialization (mar·su'pe·al·i·za'shun)
masculine (mas'ku·lin)
maser (ma'zer)
masochism (mas'o·kizm)
masochist (mas'o·kist)
massage (mah·sahzh')
masseter (mas·se'ter)
Mastadenovirus (mast'ad·ě·no·vi'rus)
mastectomy (mas·tek'to·me)
masticate (mas'tĭ·kāt)
mastication (mas'ti·ka'shun)
mastitis (mas·ti'tis)
mastodynia (mas'to·din'e·ah)
mastoidectomy (mas'toi·dek'to·me)
mastoideocentesis
    (mas·toi'de·o·sen'te'sis)
mastoidotomy (mas'toi·dot'ø·me)
masturbation (mas'tur·ba'shun)
matrices (ma'trĭ·sēz)
matrilineal (ma'trĭ·lin'e·al)
matrix (ma'triks)
matroclinous (mat'ro·kli'nus)
maturation (mah'chu·ra'shun)
maxilla (mak·sil'ah)
maxillary (mak'sĭ·ler·e)
maxillofacial (mak·sil'o·fa'shal)
measle (me'zel)
measles (me'zelz)
meatal (me·a'tal)
meatotome (me·at'o·tōm)
meatus (me·a'tus)
mechlorethamine (mek'lōr·eth'ah·mēn)
meclizine (mek'lĭ·zēn)
mecometer (me·kom'ě·ter)
meconium (mě·ko'ne·um)
medial (me'de·al)
median (me'de·an)
mediastinal (me'de·as·ti'nal)
mediastinopericarditis
    (me'de·as'tĭ·no·per'ĭ·kar·di'tis)
mediastinoscope (me'de·ah·sti'no·skōp)
mediastinoscopy (me'de·as'tĭ·nos'ko·pe)
mediastinum (me'de·as·ti'num)
medicament (med'ĭ·kah·ment)
medicamentosus (med'ĭ·kah·men·to'sus)
medicate (med'ĭ·kāt)
medication (med'ĭ·ka'shun)
medicinal (mě·dis'ĭ·nal)
medicochirurgical (med'ĭ·ko·ki·rur'jĭ·kal)
meditation (med'ĭ·ta'shun)
MEDLARS (med'larz)
MEDLINE (med'līn)
medroxyprogesterone
    (mě·drok'se·pro·jes'ter·ōn)
medulla (mě·dul'ah)
medulloblastoma (mě·dul'o·blas·to'mah)
megacolon (meg'ah·ko'lon)
megadyne (meg'ah·dīn)
megakaryoblast (meg'ah·kar'e·o·blast)

megakaryocyte (meg'ah·kar'e·o·sīt)
megakaryophthisis (meg'ah·kar·e·o·ti'sis)
megalocornea (meg'ah·lo·kor'ne·ah)
megalocystis (meg'ah·lo·sis'tis)
megalogastria (meg'ah·lo·gas'tre·ah)
megalomania (meg'ah·lo·ma'ne·ah)
megaloureter (meg'ah·lo·u·re'ter)
megavitamin (meg'ah·vi'tah·min)
megavolt (meg'ah·vōlt)
meglumine (meg'lu·mēn)
megohm (meg'ōm)
meibomianitis (mi·bo'me·ah·ni'tis)
meibomitis (mi'bo·mi'tis)
meiosis (mi·o'sis)
melalgia (mel·al'je·ah)
melancholia (mel'an·ko'le·ah)
melangeur (mě·law·zhur')
melanic (mel'an·ik)
melaniferous (mel'ah·nif'er·us)
melanin (mel'ah·nin)
melanoameloblastoma
    (mel'ah·no·ah·mel'o·blas·to'mah)
melanocyte (mel'ah·no·sīt)
melanodermatitis
    (mel'ah·no·der'mah·ti'tis)
melanogen (mě·lan'o·jen)
melanogenesis (mel'ah·no·jen'ě·sis)
melanoma (mel'ah·no'mah)
melanonychia (mel'ah·no·nik'e·ah)
melanopathy (mel'ah·nop'ah·the)
melanophore (mel'ah·no·fōr)
melanoplakia (mel'ah·no·pla'ke·ah)
melanosis (mel'ah·no'sis)
melanosome (mel'ah·no·sōm)
melanotic (mel'ah·not'ik)
melanuria (mel'an·u're·ah)
melatonin (mel'ah·to'nin)
melena (mě·le'nah)
meliodosis (me'le·oi·do'sis)
mellitus (mě·li'tus)
melphalen (mel'fah·len)
membrane (mem'brān)
membranelle (mem'brah·nel')
membranous (mem'brah·nus)
menacme (me·nak'me)
menadione (men'ah·di'ōn)
menarche (mě·nar'ke)
Meniere (men'e·ār')
meningeal (mě·nin'je·al)
meninges (mě·nin'jez)
meningioma (mě·nin'je·o'mah)
meningism (mě·nin'jizm)
meningismus (men'in·jis'mus)
meningitis (men'in·ji'tis)
meningocele (mě·ning'go·sel)
meningococcemia
    (mě·ning'go·kok·se'me·ah)
meningococcus (mě·ning'go·kok'us)
meningoencephalitis
    (mě·ning'go·en·sef'ah·li'tis)
meningoencephalocele
    (mě·ning'go·en·sef'ah·lo·sēl)
meningoencephalopathy
    (mě·ning'go·en·sef'ah·lop'ah·the)
meningohydroencephalocele
    (mě·ning'go·hi'dro·en·sef'ah·lo·sēl)
meningomyelitis (mě·ning'go·mi'ě·li'tis)
meningomyelocele
    (me·ning'go·mi'ě·lo·sēl)
meninx (me'ninks)
meniscectomy (men'ĭ·sek'to·me)
menisci (men·is'si)
meniscitis (men'ĭ·si'tis)
meniscus (mě·nis'kus)
menolipsis (men'o·lip'sis)
menopausal (men'o·paw'zal)
menopause (men'o·pawz)
menorrhagia (men'o·ra'je·ah)
menorrhea (men'o·re'ah)
menoschesis (mě·nos'kě·sis)
menstruation (men'stroo·a'shun)
mensual (men'su·al)
mensuration (men'su·ra'·shun)
menthol (men'thol)
meperidine (mě·per'ĭ·dēn)
meprobamate (mě·pro'bah·māt)
mercaptan (mer·kap'tan)
mercaptomerin (mer·kap'to·mer'in)

mercurial (mer·ku're·al)
mercurialism (mer·ku're·al·izm)
mercuric (mer·ku'rik)
mercurous (mer'ku·rus)
mercury (mer'ku·re)
merocrine (mer'o·krīn)
mesangial (mes·an'je·al)
mesangium (mes·an'je·um)
mesaortitis (mes'a·or·ti'tis)
mesaxon (mes·ak'son)
mescaline (mes'kah·lēn)
mesencephalon (mes'en·sef'ah·lon)
mesenchyme (mes'en·kīm)
mesentery (mes'en·ter'e)
mesial (me'ze·al)
mesiodistal (me'ze·o·dis'tal)
mesiolabioincisal
    (me'ze·o·la'be·o·in·si'zal)
mesiolinguoincisal
    (me'ze·o·ling'gwo·in·si'zal)
mesoappendix (mes·o·ah·pen'diks)
mesocecum (mes·o·se'kum)
mesocolon (mes'o·ko'lon)
mesoderm (mes'o·derm)
mesogastrium (mes'o·gas'tre·um)
mesognathion (mes'o·na'the·on)
mesometrium (mes'o·me'tre·um)
meson (mes'on)
mesonephros (mes'o·nef'ros)
mesorchium (mes·or'ke·um)
mesoropter (mes'o·rop'ter)
mesosalpinx (mes'o·sal'pinks)
mesosome (mes'o·sōm)
mesotendineum (mes'o·ten·din'e·um)
mesothelium (mes'o·the'le·um)
mesovarium (mes'o·va're·um)
metabolism (mě·tab'o·lizm)
metabolite (mě·tab'o·līt)
metachromasia (met'ah·kro·ma'ze·ah)
metacryptozoite (met'ah·krip'to·zo'īt)
metafemale (met'ah·fe'māl)
metakinesis (met'ah·kĭ·ne'sis)
metaldehyde (met·al'dě·hīd)
metalloporphyrin (me·tal'o·por'fĭ·rin)
metamale (met'ah·māl)
metamorphosis (met'ah·mor'fŏ·sis)
metamyelocyte (met'ah·mi'ě·lŏ·sīt')
metanephrine (met'ah·nef'rēn)
metanephros (met'ah·nef'rōs)
metaphase (met'ah·fāz)
metastasis (mě·tas'tah·sis)
metastasize (me·tas'tah·sīz)
metatarsus (met'ah·tar'sus)
metathalamus (met'ah·thal'ah·mus)
metencephalon (met'en·sef'ah·lon)
metestrum (mě·tes'trum)
methadone (meth'ah·dōn)
methamphetamine (meth'am·fet'ah·mēn)
methane (meth'ān)
methanol (meth'ah·nol)
methantheline (meth·an'the·lēn)
methaqualone (me·thah'kwah·lōn)
methemalbumin (met'hem·al·bu'min)
methemoglobin (met·he'mo·glo'bin)
methenamine (meth·en'ah·mēn)
methionine (mě·thi'o·nēn)
methotrexate (meth'o·trek'sāt)
methoxyflurane (mě·thok'se·floo'rān)
methscopolamine (meth'sko·pol'ah·mēn)
methyl (meth'il)
methylate (meth'ĭ·lāt)
methylcholanthrene (meth'il·ko·lan'thrēn)
methyldopa (meth'il·do'pah)
methylene (meth'ĭ·lēn)
methylmalonic (meth'il·mah·lon'ik)
methylphenidate (meth'il·fen'ĭ·dāt)
methylprednisolone
    (meth'il·pred'ni·so·lōn)
methyprylon (meth'i·pri'lon)
metritis (mě·tri'tis)
metrodynamometer
    (me'tro·di'nah·mom'ě·ter)
metronoscope (mě·tron'o·skōp)
metropathia hemorrhagica
    (me'tro·path'e·ah hem'ōr·ra'jĭ·kah)
metropathy (mě·trop'ah·the)
metrostaxis (me'tro·stak'sis)
metyrapone (mě·tēr'ah·pōn)

micelle (mi·sel')
microaneurysm (mi'kro·an'u·rizm)
microangiopathy (mi'kro·an'je·op'ah·the)
microbe (mi'krōb)
microbial (mi·kro'be·al)
microbiology (mi'kro·bi·ol'o·je)
microcirculation (mi'kro·sir'ku·la'shun)
micrococcus (mi'kro·kok'us)
microcoulomb (mi'kro·koo'lom)
microcurie (mi'kro·ku're)
microcyte (mi'kro·sīt)
microdactyly (mi'kro·dak'tĭ·le)
microfarad (mi'kro·far'ad)
microglia (mi·krog'le·ah)
microglossia (mi'kro·glos'e·ah)
micrognathia (mi'kro·na'the·ah)
microhm (mi'krōm)
microliter (mi'kro·le'ter)
microlithiasis (mi'kro·lĭ·thi'ah·sis)
micromelia (mi'kro·me'le·ah)
micron (mi'kron)
microphage (mi'kro·fāj)
micropipette (mi'kro·pi·pet')
micropsia (mi·krop'se·ah)
micropuncture (mi'kro·punk'chur)
microscope (mi'kro·skōp)
Microsporum (mi·kros'po·rum)
microsyringe (mi'kro·ser·inj')
microtome (mi'kro·tōm)
microtubules (mi'kro·tu'būlz)
microvilli (mi'kro·vil'i)
micturate (mik'tu·rāt)
micturition (mik'tu·rish'un)
midwifery (mid'wif·er·e)
migraine (mi'grān)
miliaria (mil'e·a're·ah)
miliary (mil'e·a·re)
milieu (me·lyuh')
milium (mil'e·um)
millicurie (mil'ĭ·ku're)
milliequivalent (mil'ĭ·kwiv'ah·lent)
milligram (mil'ĭ·gram)
milliliter (mil'ĭ·le'ter)
millimeter (mil'ĭ·me·ter)
millimicrogram (mil'ĭ·mi'kro·gram)
millimicron (mil'ĭ·mi'kron)
millimole (mil'ĭ·mōl)
milliosmole (mil'ĭ·oz'mōl)
millirad (mil'ĭ·rad)
millirem (mil·ĭ·rem)
milliroentgen (mil'ĭ·rent'gen)
millisecond (mil'ĭ·sek'ond)
millivolt (mil'ĭ·vōlt)
mimesis (mi·me'sis)
miosis (mi·o'sis)
miracidia (mi·rah·sid'e·ah)
miracidium (mi·rah·sid'e·um)
miscarriage (mis·kar'ij)
misce et signa (mis'e et sig'nah)
miscible (mis'ĭ·bl)
mithridatism (mith'rĭ·dă'tizm)
miticide (mi'tĭ·sīd)
mitochondria (mi'to·kon'dre·ah)
mitosis (mi·to'sis)
mitotic (mi·tot'ik)
mitral (mi'tral)
mitrale (mi·tra'le)
mittelschmerz (mit'el·shmärts)
mnemonics (ne·mon'iks)
Möbius (me'be·us)
modality (mo·dal'ĭ·te)
modiolus (mo·di'o·lus)
modulation (mod'u·la·shun)
moiety (moi'ĕ·te)
mol (mol)
molal (mo'lal)
molality (mo·lal'ĭ·te)
molar (mo'lar)
molarity (mol·ar'ĭ·te)
mole (mōl)
molecular (mo·lek'u·lar)
molecule (mol'ĕ·kūl)
molluscum contagiosum
    (mŏ·lus'kum kon·ta·je·o'sum)
monad (mon'ad)
monarthritis (mon'ar·thri'tis)
monarticular (mon'ar·tik'u·lar)
monaural (mon·aw'rl)

mongolism (mon'go·lizm)
mongoloid (mon'go·loid)
Monilia (mo·nil'e·ah)
moniliasis (mon·ĭ·li'ah·sis)
monoamine (mon'o·am'ēn)
monoblast (mon'o·blast)
monochromatic (mon'o·kro·mat'ik)
monocrotic (mon'o·krot'ik)
monocular (mon·ok'u·lar)
monocyte (mon'o·sīt)
monocytopenia (mon'o·si'to·pe'ne·ah)
monodactylism (mon·o·dak'til·izm)
monoiodotyrosine
    (mon'o·i'o·do·ti'ro·sēn)
monokine (mon'o·kīn)
monomer (mon'o·mer)
mononeuritis (mon'o·nu·ri'tis)
mononucleosis (mon'o·nu'kle·o'sis)
monorchid (mon·or'kid)
monorchism (mon·or'kid·izm)
monosaccharide (mon'o·sak'ah·rīd)
monosodium (mon'o·so'de·um)
monosomy (mon'o·so'me)
monotrichous (mon·ot'rĭ·kus)
monovalent (mon'o·va'lent)
monozygotic (mon'o·zi·got'ik)
mons (monz)
morbidity (mor·bid'ĭ·te)
Morbillivirus (mor'bil'ĭ·vi'rus)
mordant (mor'dant)
moribund (mor'ĭ·bund)
morphea (mor·fe'ah)
morphine (mor'fēn)
morphogenesis (mor'fo·jen'ĕ·sis)
morphology (mor·fol'o·je)
Morquio (mor·ke'o)
mortality (mor·tal'ĭ·te)
mortuary (mor'tu·a're)
morula (mor'u·lah)
morulation (mor'u·la'shun)
mosaic (mo·za'ik)
mosaicism (mo·za'ĭ·sizm)
moulage (moo·lahzh')
moxa (mok'sah)
moxibustion (mok'sĭ·bus'chun)
mucid (mu'sid)
mucilage (mu'sĭ·lij)
mucin (mu'sin)
mucocele (mu'ko·sēl)
mucocutaneous (mu'ko·ku·ta'ne·us)
mucoid (mu'koid)
mucolipidosis (mu'ko·lip'ĭ·do'sis)
mucopolysaccharide
    (mu'ko·pol'e·sak'ah·rīd)
mucopolysaccharidosis
    (mu'ko·pol'e·sak'ah·rĭ·do'sis)
mucopurulent (mu'ko·pu'roo·lent)
mucormycosis (mu'kor·mi·ko'sis)
mucosa (mu·ko'sah)
mucosanguineous
    (mu'ko·sang·gwin'e·us)
mucoserous (mu'ko·se'rus)
mucosin (mu·ko'sin)
mucous (mu'kus)
mucus (mu'kus)
multifactorial (mul'tĭ·fak·to're·al)
multifid (mul'tĭ·fid)
multifocal (mul'tĭ·fo'kal)
multigravida (mul'tĭ·grav'ĭ·dah)
multilobular (mul'tĭ·lob'u·lar)
multilocular (mul'tĭ·lok'u·lar)
multinuclear (mul'tĭ·nu'kle·ar)
multipara (mul·tip'ah·rah)
multiparity (mul'tĭ·par'ĭ·te)
multiparous (mul'tip'ah·rus)
multipolar (mul'tĭ·po'lar)
multivalence (mul'tĭ·va'lens)
multivalent (mul'tĭ·va'lent)
muramidase (mu·ram'ĭ·dās)
murein (mu're·in)
muscae volitantes (mus'ke vol·ĭ·tan'tēz)
muscarine (mus'kah·rin)
muscle (mus'el)
musculoaponeurotic
    (mus'ku·lo·ap'o·nu·rot'ik)
musculocutaneous
    (mus'ku·lo·ku·ta'ne·us)

musculoskeletal (mus'ku·lo·skel'ĕ·tal)
musculotropic (mus'ku·lo·trop'ik)
mutagen (mu'tah·jen)
mutant (mu'tant)
mutase (mu'tās)
mutation (mu·ta'shun)
myasthenia gravis
    (mi'as·the'ne·ah grah'vis)
mycelium (mi·se'le·um)
mycete (mi'sēt)
Mycetozoa (mi·se'to·zo'ah)
mycid (mi'sid)
Mycobacterium (mi'ko·bak·te're·um)
mycodermatitis (mi'ko·der'mah·ti'tis)
mycodermomycosis
    (mi'ko·der'mo·mi·ko'sis)
mycology (mi·kol'o·je)
Mycoplasma (mi'ko·plaz'mah)
mycosis (mi·ko'sis)
mydriasis (mĭ·dri'ah·sis)
mydriatic (mid're·at'ik)
myelencephalon (mi'ĕ·len·sef'ah·lon)
myelin (mi'ĕ·lin)
myelinated (mi'ĕ·lĭ·nāt'ed)
myelitis (mi'ĕ·li'tis)
myeloblast (mi'ĕ·lo·blast)
myeloblastoma (mi'ĕ·lo·blas·to'mah)
myeloblastosis (mi'ĕ·lo·blas·to'sis)
myelocele (mi·el'o·sēl)
myelocyst (mi'ĕ·lo·sist)
myelocystocele (mi'ĕ·lo·sis'to·sēl)
myelocyte (mi'ĕ·lo·sīt)
myelocytosis (mi'ĕ·lo·si·tō'sis)
myelofibrosis (mi'ĕ·lo·fi·bro'sis)
myeloid (mi'ĕ·loid)
myeloma (mi'ĕ·lo'mah)
myelomeningitis (mi'ĕ·lo·men'in·ji'tis)
myeloneuritis (mi'ĕ·lo·nu·ri'tis)
myelophthisis (mi'ĕ·lo·ti'sis)
myelopoiesis (mi'ĕ·lo·poi·e'sis)
myeloproliferative
    (mi'ĕ·lo·pro·lif'er·ah·tiv)
myelosis (mi'ĕ·lo'sis)
myesthesia (mi'es·the'ze·ah)
myiasis (mi·i'ah·sis)
mylohyoid (mi'lo·hi'oid)
myocardial (mi'o·kar'de·al)
myocarditis (mi'o·kar·di'tis)
myocardium (mi'o·kar'de·um)
myoclonus (mi·ok'lo·nus)
myofibril (mi'o·fi'bril)
myofibroma (mi'o·fi·bro'mah)
myofibrosis (mi'o·fi·bro'sis)
myogen (mi'o·jen)
myoglobin (mi'o·glo'bin)
myoglobinuria (mi'o·glo'bin·u're·ah)
myoglobulin (mi'o·glob'u·lin)
myokymia (mi'o·kim'e·ah)
myoma (mi·o'mah)
myomectomy (mi'o·mek'to·me)
myometrium (mi'o·me'tre·um)
myon (mi'on)
myoneural (mi'o·nu'ral)
myopathy (mi·op'ah·the)
myopericarditis (mi'o·per'ĭ·kar·di'tis)
myopia (mi·o'pe·ah)
myopic (mi·op'ik)
myorrhexis (mi'o·rek'sis)
myosarcoma (mi'o·sar·ko'mah)
myosclerosis (mi'o·skler·ro'sis)
myosin (mi'o·sin)
myositis (mi'o·si'tis)
myotonia (mi'o·to'ne·ah)
myringectomy (mir'in·jek'to·me)
myringoplasty (mĭ·ring'go·plas'te)
myringotome (mĭ·ring'go·tōm)
myringotomy (mir'in·got'o·me)
myxadenoma (miks'ad·ĕ·no'mah)
myxedema (mik'sĕ·de'mah)
myxedematous (mik'sĕ·dēm'ah·tus)
myxocyte (mik'so·sīt)
myxofibroma (mik'so·fi·bro'mah)
myxolipoma (mik'so·lĭ·po'mah)
myxoma (mik·so'mah)
myxomatosis (mik'so·mah·to'sis)
myxoneuroma (mik'so·nu·ro'mah)
myxosarcoma (mik'so·sar·ko'mah)
myxovirus (mik'so·vi'rus)

N

nadolol (na·do′lol)
nafcillin (naf·sil′in)
naloxone (nal·oks′ōn)
nanocurie (na′no·ku′re)
nanogram (na′no·gram)
nanomelia (na′no·me′le·ah)
nanometer (na′no·me′ter)
nanosecond (na′no·sek′ond)
naphthalene (naf′thah·lēn)
naphthol (naf′thol)
narcissism (nar′si·sizm)
narcolepsy (nar′ko·lep′se)
narcosis (nar·ko′sis)
narcotic (nar·kot′ik)
nares (na′rēz)
naris (na′ris)
nasal (na′zal)
nascent (nas′ent)
nasion (na′ze·on)
nasofrontal (na′zo·frun′tal)
nasolabial (na′zo·la′be·al)
nasolacrimal (na′zo·lak′ri·mal)
nasopharyngeal (na′zo·fah·rin′je·al)
nasopharyngitis (na′zo·far′in·ji′tis)
nasopharyngoscope
 (na′zo·fah·rin′go·skōp)
nasopharynx (na′zo·far′inks)
nasoscope (na′zo·skōp)
nasosinusitis (na′zo·si′nu·si′tis)
nates (na′tēz)
natriuresis (na′tre·u·re′sis)
natriuretic (na′tre·u·ret′ik)
nausea (naw′se·ah)
nauseant (naw′se·ant)
nauseate (naw′se·āt)
nauseous (naw′shus)
nebulization (neb′u·li·za′shun)
nebulizer (neb′u·līz′er)
Necator (ne·ka′tor)
necatoriasis (ne·ka′to·ri′ah·sis)
necrobiosis (nek′ro·bi·o′sis)
necrocytosis (nek′ro·si·to′sis)
necrology (ně·krol′o·je)
necrolysis (ně·krol′i·sis)
necrophilia (nek′ro·fil′e·ah)
necrose (nek′rōs)
necrosis (ně·kro′sis)
necrotic (ně·krot′ik)
Neisseria (nīs·se′re·ah)
Nemathelminthes (nem′ah·thel·min′thēz)
Nematoda (nem′ah·to′dah)
nematode (nem′ah·tōd)
nematodiasis (nem′ah·to·di′ah·sis)
nematoid (nem′ah·toid)
nematology (nem′ah·tol′o·je)
neocystostomy (ne′o·sis·tos′to·me)
neologism (ne·ol′o·jism)
neomorph (ne′o·morf)
neomycin (ne′o·mi′sin)
neonatal (ne′o·na′tal)
neonate (ne′o·nāt)
neonatologist (ne′o·na·tol′o·jist)
neonatology (ne′o·na·tol′o·je)
neoplasia (ne′o·pla′ze·ah)
neoplasm (ne′o·plazm)
nephelometer (nef′ě·lom′ě·ter)
nephrectomy (ně·frek′to·me)
nephritis (ně·fri′tis)
nephroblastoma (nef′ro·blas·to′mah)
nephrocalcinosis (nef′ro·kal′si·no′sis)
nephrogram (nef′ro·gram)
nephrography (ně·frog′rah·fe)
nephrolith (nef′ro·lith)
nephrolithiasis (nef′ro·li·thi′ah·sis)
nephrolithotomy (nef′ro·li·thot′o·me)
nephrology (ně·frol′o·je)
nephromalacia (nef′ro·mah·la′she·ah)
nephromere (nef′ro·mēr)
nephron (nef′ron)
nephropathy (ně·frop′ah·the)
nephropexy (nef′ro·pek′se)
nephrophthisis (ně·frof′thi·sis)
nephroptosia (nef′rop·to′se·ah)
nephropyelitis (nef′ro·pi′ě·li′tis)
nephropyeloplasty (nef′ro·pi′ě·lo·plas′te)

nephropyosis (nef′ro·pi·o′sis)
nephrorrhagia (nef′ro·ra′je·ah)
nephrosclerosis (nef′ro·sklě·ro′sis)
nephrosis (ně·fro′sis)
nephrostome (nef′ro·stōm)
nephrostomy (ně·fros′to·me)
nephrotic (ně·frot′ik)
nephrotome (nef′ro·tōm)
nephrotomogram (nef′ro·to′mo·gram)
nephroureterectomy
 (nef′ro·u·re′ter·ek′to·me)
nesslerize (nes′ler·īz)
neural (nu′ral)
neuralgia (nu·ral′je·ah)
neurasthenia (nu′ras·the′ne·ah)
neurilemma (nu′ri·lem′ah)
neurilemoma (nu′ri·lem·mo·mah)
neuritis (nu·ri′tis)
neuroanatomy (nu′ro·ah·nat′o·me)
neurobiology (nu′ro·bi·ol′o·je)
neuroblastoma (nu′ro·blas·to′mah)
neurocladism (nu·rok′lah·dizm)
neuroectoderm (nu′ro·ek′to·derm)
neuroendocrinology
 (nu′ro·en′do·kri·nol′o·je)
neuroepithelioma
 (nu′ro·ep′i·the′le·o′mah)
neuroepithelium (nu′ro·ep′i·the′le·um)
neurofibril (nu′ro·fi′bril)
neurofibroma (nu′ro·fi·bro′mah)
neurofibromatosis
 (nu′ro·fi′bro·mah·to′sis)
neurogenic (nu′ro·jen′ik)
neuroglia (nu·rog′le·ah)
neurogliocyte (nu·rog′le·o·sīt)
neurogliomatosis (nu′ro·gli′o·mah·to′sis)
neurohormone (nu′ro·hor′mōn)
neurohypophyseal (nu′ro·hi′po·fiz′e·al)
neurohypophysis (nu′ro·hi·pof′i·sis)
neurology (nu·rol′o·je)
neurolysis (nu·rol′i·sis)
neuromyasthenia (nu′ro·mi′as·the′ne·ah)
neuromyelitis optica
 (nu′ro·mi′ě·li′tis op′ti·kah)
neuromyopathy (nu′ro·mi′op′ah·the)
neuromyositis (nu′ro·mi′o·si′tis)
neuron (nu′ron)
neuropathogenesis
 (nu′ro·path′o·jen′ě·sis)
neuropathy (nu·rop′ah·the)
neurophysin (nu′ro·fi′sin)
neuroplasty (nu′ro·plas′te)
neuropodia (nu′ro·po′de·ah)
neuropodium (nu′ro·po′de·um)
neuropore (nu′ro·pōr)
neurorrhaphy (nu·ror′ah·fe)
neurosarcocleisis (nu′ro·sar′ko·kli′sis)
neurosecretion (nu′ro·se·kre′shun)
neuroses (nu·ro′sēz)
neurosis (nu·ro′sis)
neurosplanchnic (nu′ro·splangk′nik)
neurosurgery (nu′ro·ser′jer·e)
neurotransmitter (nu′ro·tranz′mit·er)
neurotrophasthenia
 (nu′ro·tro′fas·the′ne·ah)
neurulation (nu′roo·la′shun)
neutrino (nu·tre′no)
neutron (nu′tron)
neutropenia (nu′tro·pe′ne·ah)
neutrophil (nu′tro·fil)
neutrophilia (nu′tro·fil′e·ah)
nevi (ne′vi)
nevus (ne′vus)
niacin (ni′ah·sin)
niche (nich)
nicking (nik′ing)
nicotinamide (nik′o·tin′ah·mīd)
nicotine (nik′o·tēn)
nicotinomimetic (nik′o·tin′o·mi·met′ik)
nidation (ni·da′shun)
nidus (ni′dus)
nifedipine (ni·fed′i·pēn)
nihilism (ni′i·lizm)
ninhydrin (nin·hi′drin)
nitrite (ni′trīt)
nitrofurantoin (ni′tro·fu·ran′to·in)
nitrofurazone (ni′tro·fu′rah·zōn)
nitrogen (ni′tro·jen)

nitrogenous (ni·troj′ě·nus)
nitroglycerin (ni·tro·glis′er·in)
nitrosamine (ni′trōs·ah′mēn)
nitrosyl (ni′tro·sil)
nitrous (ni′trus)
Nocardia (no·kar′de·ah)
nocardiosis (no·kar·de·o′sis)
nociperception (no′se·per·sep′shun)
nodose (no′dōs)
nodule (nod′ūl)
noma (no′mah)
Nomina Anatomica
 (no′mi·nah an·ah·tom′i·kah)
nonapeptide (non′ah·pep′tīd)
non compos mentis
 (non kom′pos men′tis)
noninvasive (non′in·va′siv)
nonparous (non·par′us)
norepinephrine (nor′ep·i·nef′rin)
norethandrolone (nor′eth·an′dro·lōn)
norethindrone (nor·eth′in·drōn)
norethynodrel (nor′ě·thi′no·drel)
normetanephrine (nor·met′ah·nef′rin)
normoblast (nor′mo·blast)
normocyte (nor′mo·sīt)
normokalemia (nor′mo·kah·le′me·ah)
normotensive (nor′mo·ten′siv)
normothermia (nor′mo·ther′me·ah)
normotonic (nor′mo·ton′ik)
nosocomial (nos′o·ko′me·al)
nosology (no·sol′o·je)
notochord (no′to·kord)
noxa (nok′sah)
nubile (nu′bil)
nucha (nu′kah)
nuchal (nu′kal)
nuclear (nu′kle·ar)
nuclease (nu′kle·ās)
nucleated (nu′kle·āt′ed)
nuclei (nu′kle·i)
nucleic (nu′kle′ik)
nucleocapsid (nu′kle·o·kap′sid)
nucleohistone (nu′kle·o·his′tōn)
nucleoli (nu·kle′o·li)
nucleolonema (nu′kle·o′lo·ne′mah)
nucleolus (nu·kle′o·lus)
nucleon (nu′kle·on)
nucleophil (nu′kle·o·fil′)
nucleoprotein (nu′kle·o·pro′te·in)
nucleosidase (nu′kle·o·si′dās)
nucleoside (nu′kle·o·sīd)
nucleotidase (nu′kle·o·ti·dās)
nucleotide (nu′kle·o·tīd)
nucleus (nu′kle·us)
nuclide (nu′klīd)
nulligravida (nul·i·grav′i·dah)
nullipara (nuh·lip′ah·rah)
nulliparity (nul′i·par′i·te)
nulliparous (nuh·lip′ah·rus)
nummular (num′u·lar)
nutrition (nu·trish′un)
nyctalopia (nik′tah·lo′pe·ah)
nymphomania (nim′fo·ma′ne·ah)
nystagmic (nis·tag′mik)
nystagmography (nis′tag·mog′rah·fe)
nystagmus (nis·tag′mus)
nystatin (nis′tah·tin)

O

obese (o·bēs′)
obesity (o·bēs′i·te)
oblique (ŏ·blēk)
oblongata (ob′long·ga′tah)
obsession (ob·sesh′un)
obstetric (ob·stet′rik)
obstetrical (ob·stet′ri·kal)
obstetrician (ob′stě·trish′un)
obstetrics (ob·stet′riks)
obstipation (ob′sti·pa′shun)
obstruction (ob·struk′shun)
obstruent (ob′stroo·ent)
obtundent (ob·tun′dent)
obturator (ob′tu·ra′tor)
occipital (ok·sip′i·tal)
occipitotemporal (ok·sip′i·to·tem′po·ral)
occiput (ok′si·put)

occlude (ŏ·klood)
occlusion (ŏ·kloo′zhun)
occult (ŏ·kult)
ochronosis (o′kro·no′sis)
ocrylate (ok′rĭ·lāt)
octapeptide (ok′tah·pep′tīd)
octavalent (ok′tah·va′lent)
ocular (ok′u·lar)
oculist (ok′u·list)
oculomotor (ok′u·lo·mo′tor)
oculus (ok′u·lus)
ocutome (ok′u·tŏm)
odditis (od·di′tis)
odontectomy (o′don·tek′to·me)
odontexesis (o′don·teks′e·sis)
odontoblast (o·don′to·blast)
odontoblastoma (o·don′to·blas·to′mah)
odontoclast (o·don′to·klast)
odontogenesis (o·don′to·jen′ĕ·sis)
odontogenic (o·don′to·jen′ik)
odontoid (o·don′toid)
odontoma (o·don·to′mah)
odontoscope (o·don′to·skōp)
odoriferous o′dŏr·if′er·us)
odynacusis (o′din·ah·ku′sis)
odynometer (o′din·om′ĕ·ter)
odynophagia (o′din·o·fa′je·ah)
oersted (er′sted)
oestrid (es′trid)
ohm (ōm)
olecranon (o·lek′rah·non)
olefin (o′le·fin)
olein (o′le·in)
olfaction (ol·fak′shun)
olfactory (ol·fak′to·re)
oligocholia (ol′ĭ·go·ko′le·ah)
oligochylia (ol′ĭ·go·ki′le·ah)
oligochymia (ol′ĭ·go·ki′me·ah)
oligodactyly (ol′ĭ·go·dak′tĭ·le)
oligodendroglia (ol′ĭ·go·den·drog′le·ah)
oligodendroglioma
   (ol′ĭ·go·den′dro·gli·o′mah)
oligohydramnios (ol′ĭ·go·hi·dram′ne·os)
oligomenorrhea (ol′ĭ·go·men′o·re′ah)
oliguria (ol′ĭ·gu′re·ah)
omega (o·ma′gah)
omental (o·men′tal)
omentectomy (o′men·tek′to·me)
omentopexy (o·men′to·pek′se)
omentorrhaphy (o′men·tor′ah·fe)
omentum (o·men′tum)
omni hora (om′ni ho′rah)
omnivorous (om·niv′ŏ·rus)
omohyoid (o′mo·hi′oid)
omothyroid (o′mo·thi′roid)
omphalocele (om′fah·lo·sēl)
omphalomesenteric
   (om′fah·lo·mes′en·ter′ik)
omphalorrhea (om′fah·lo·re′ah)
omphalotomy (om′fah·lot′o·me)
onanism (o′nah·nizm)
Onchocerca (ong′ko·ser′kah)
onchocerciasis (ong′ko·ser·ki′ah·sis)
oncogenesis (ong′ko·jen′ĕ·sis)
oncogenic (ong′ko·jen′ik)
oncology (ong·kol′o·je)
oncosis (ong·ko′sis)
Oncovirinae (ong′ko·vir′ĭ·ne)
oncovirus (ong′ko·vi′rus)
oneosis (o′ne·o′sis)
onychectomy (on′ĭ·kek′to·me)
onychia (o·nik′e·ah)
onychogryposis (on′ĭ·ko·grĭ·fo′sis)
onychoid (on′ĭ·koid)
onychomalacia (on′ĭ·ko·mah·la′she·ah)
onychomycosis (on′ĭ·ko·mi·ko′sis)
onychopathy (on′ĭ·kop′ah·the)
onychophagia (on′ĭ·ko·fa′je·ah)
onychotomy (on′ĭ·kot′o·me)
oocyesis (o′o·si·e′sis)
oocyst (o′o·sist)
oocyte (o′o·sīt)
oogenesis (o′o·jen′ĕ·sis)
oogonium (o′o·go′ne·um)
oophorectomy (o′of·o·rek′to·me)
oophoritis (o′of·o·ri′tis)
oophorocystectomy
   (o·of′o·ro·sis·tek′to·me)

oophoropathy (o·of′o·rop′ah·the)
oophorosalpingectomy
   (o·of′o·ro·sal′pin·jek′to·me)
opacity (o·pas′ĭ·te)
opaque (o·pāk′)
operable (op′er·ah·bl)
operate (op′er·āt)
operation (op·er·a′shun)
opercula (o·per′ku·lah)
operculated (o·per′ku·la·ted)
operculum (o·per′ku·lum)
operon (op′er·on)
ophthalmia (of·thal′me·ah)
ophthalmic (of·thal′mik)
ophthalmoblenorrhea
   (of·thal′mo·blen′o·re′ah)
ophthalmodiaphanoscope
   (of·thal′mo·di·ah·fan′o·skōp)
ophthalmodonesis (of·thal′mo·do·ne′sis)
ophthalmodynamometer
   (of·thal′mo·di′nah·mom′ĕ·ter)
ophthalmologist (of′thal·mol′o·jist)
ophthalmology (of′thal·mol′o·je)
ophthalmometer (of′thal·mom′ĕ·ter)
ophthalmomycosis (of·thal′mo·mi·ko′sis)
ophthalmomyotomy
   (of·thal′mo·mi·ot′o·me)
ophthalmophacometer
   (of·thal′mo·fa·kom′ĕ·ter)
ophthalmoplegia (of·thal′mo·ple′je·ah)
ophthalmorrhea (of·thal′mo·re′ah)
ophthalmoscope (of·thal′mo·skōp)
ophthalmotonometer
   (of·thal′mo·to·nom′ĕ·ter)
opiate (o′pe·āt)
opioid (o′pe·oid)
opisthion (o·pis′the·on)
opisthotonos (o′pis·thot′o·nos)
opium (o′pe·um)
opponens (o·po′nenz)
opsin (op′sin)
opsonin (op′so·nin)
optic (op′tik)
optical (op′tĭ·kal)
optician (op·tish′an)
opticocinerea (op′tĭ·ko·sĭ·ne′re·ah)
optics (op′tiks)
optometer (op·tom′ĕ·ter)
optometry (op·tom′ĕ·tre)
oral (o′ral)
orbit (or′bit)
orbital (or′bĭ·tal)
orcein (or·se′in)
orchialgia (or′ke·al′je·ah)
orchidectomy (or′kĭ·dek′to·me)
orchiectomy (or′ke·ek′to·me)
orchiepididymitis (or′ke·ep′ĭ·did′ĭ·mi′tis)
orchiopexy (or′ke·o·pek′se)
orchtitis (or·ki′tis)
organelle (or′gan·el′)
organism (or′gah·nizm)
organotropism (or·gah·not′ro·pizm)
orgasm (or′gazm)
orifice (or′ĭ·fis)
origin (or′ĭ·jin)
ornithine (or′nĭ·thin)
ornithosis (or′ni·tho′sis)
oropharynx (o′ro·far′inks)
orrhorrhea (or·o·re′ah)
orthocrasia (or′tho·kra′se·ah)
orthodontics (or′tho·don′tiks)
orthodontist (or′tho·don′tist)
orthognathic (or′tho·na′thik)
orthometer (or·thom′ĕ·ter)
orthopedics (or′tho·pe′diks)
orthopedist (or′tho·pe′dist)
orthopercussion (or′tho·per·kush′un)
orthophosphate (or′tho·fos′fāt)
Orthopoxvirus (or′tho·poks′vi·rus)
orthoptics (or·thop′tiks)
orthoptist (or·thop′tist)
orthoscopy (or·thos′ko·pe)
orthothanasia (or′tho·thah·na′ze·ah)
orthotics (or·thot′iks)
orthotist (or′tho·tist)
orthotonos (or·thot′o·nos)
oscillograph (o·sil′o·graf)
oscillometer (os′ĭ·lom′ĕ·ter)

oscilloscope (ŏ·sil′o·skōp)
oscula (os′ku·lah)
osculum (os′ku·lum)
Osler (ōs′ler)
osmium (oz′me·um)
osmol (oz′mōl)
osmolality (oz′mo·lal′ĭ·te)
osmolarity (oz′mo·lār′ĭ·te)
osmophore (oz′mo·fōr)
osmoreceptor (oz′mo·re·sep′tor)
osmosis (oz·mo′sis)
osmotic (oz·mot′ik)
osphresiology (os′fre·ze·ol′o·je)
osseous (os′e·us)
ossicle (os′sĭ·kl)
ossicular (ŏ·sik′u·lar)
ossiculectomy (os′ĭ·ku·lek′to·me)
ossiculotomy (os′ĭ·ku·lot′o·me)
ossification (os′ĭ·fĭ·ka′shun)
ossify (os′ĭ·fi)
ostealgia (os′te·al′je·ah)
osteitis (os′te·i′tis)
osteoarthritis (os′te·o·ar·thri′tis)
osteoarthropathy
   (os′te·o·ar·throp′ah·the)
osteoblast (os′te·o·blast′)
osteoblastoma (os′te·o·blas·to′mah)
osteochondritis (os′te·o·kon·dri′tis)
osteochondrodystrophy
   (os′te·o·kon′dro·dis′tro·fe)
osteochondroma (os′te·o·kon·dro′mah)
osteochondromatosis
   (os′te·o·kon′dro·mah·to′sis)
osteochondrosarcoma
   (os′te·o·kon′dro·sar·ko′mah)
osteochondrosis (os′te·o·kon·dro′sis)
osteoclasis (os·te·ok′lah·sis)
osteoclast (os′te·o·klast)
osteoclastoma (os′te·o·klas·to′mah)
osteocyte (os′te·o·sīt)
osteodystrophy (os′te·o·dis′tro·fe)
osteofibroma (os′te·o·fi·bro′mah)
osteogenesis (os′te·o·jen′ĕ·sis)
osteoid (os′te·oid)
osteology (os′te·ol′o·je)
osteolysis (os′te·ol′ĭ·sis)
osteoma (os′te·o′mah)
osteomalacia (os′te·o·mah·la′she·ah)
osteomyelitis (os′te·o·mi′ĕ·li′tis)
osteomyelodysplasia
   (os′te·o·mi′ĕ·lo·dis·pla′ze·ah)
osteomyelography
   (os′te·o·mi′ĕ·log′rah·fe)
osteon (os′te·on)
osteonecrosis (os′te·o·nĕ·kro′sis)
osteopath (os′te·o·path)
osteopathy (os′te·op′ah·the)
osteopetrosis (os′te·o·pĕ·tro′sis)
osteophlebitis (os′te·o·fle·bi′tis)
osteoporosis (os′te·o·po·ro′sis)
osteorrhaphy (os′te·or′ah·fe)
osteosarcoma (os′te·o·sar·ko′mah)
osteosclerosis (os′te·o·skle·ro′sis)
osteotabes (os′te·o·ta′bēz)
osteotome (os′te·o·tŏm)
osteotomoclasis (os′te·o·to·mok′lah·sis)
osteotomy (os′te·ot′o·me)
ostium (os′te·um)
otalgia (o·tal′je·ah)
othemorrhea (o′them·o·re′·ah)
otic (o′tik)
otitis (o·ti′tis)
otoblennorrhea (o′to·blen′o·re′ah)
otocleisis (o′to·kli′sis)
otoconia (o′to·ko′ne·ah)
otodynia (o′to·din′e·ah)
otolaryngologist (o′to·lar′in·gol′o·jist)
otolaryngology (o′to·lar′in·gol′o·je)
otologist (o·tol′o·jist)
otology (o·tol′o·je)
otomycosis (o′to·mi·ko′sis)
otopathy (o·top′ah·the)
otopyorrhea (o′to·pi′o·re′ah)
otorhinolaryngology
   (o′to·ri′no·lar′in·gol′o·je)
otorhinology (o′to·ri·nol′o·je)
otorrhagia (o′to·ra′je·ah)
otorrhea (o′to·re′ah)

otosclerosis (o'to·skle·ro'sis)
otoscope (o'to·skōp)
ouabain (wah·bah'in)
ova (o'vah)
ovarian (o·va're·an)
ovary (o'vah·re)
overdose (o'ver·dōs)
oviduct (o'vĭ·dukt)
oviparous (o·vip'ah·rus)
ovoviviparous (o'vo·vi·vip'ah·rus)
ovulation (o'vu·la'shun)
ovule (o'vūl)
ovum (o'vum)
oxaloacetic (oks'ah·lo·ah·se'tik)
oxalosis (ok'sah·lo'sis)
oxalosuccinic (ok'sah·lo·suk·sin'ik)
oxaluria (ok'sah·lu're·ah)
oxidation (ok'sĭ·da'shun)
oxide (ok'sīd)
oxidize (ok'sĭ·dīz)
oxycellulose (ok'sĭ·sel'u·lōs)
oxygen (ok'sĭ·jen)
oxyhemoglobin (ok'se·he'mo·glo'bin)
oxytetracycline (ok'se·tet'rah·si'klēn)
oxytocia (ok·se·to'se·ah)
oxytocic (ok·se·to'sik)
oxytocin (ok·se·to'sin)
oxyuriasis (ok'se·u·ri'ah·sis)
oxyuricide (ok'se·u'rĭ·sīd)
ozone (o'zōn)

P

pacchionian (pak'e·o'ne·an)
pacemaker (pās'ma·ker)
pachyblepharon (pak'e·blef'ah·ron)
pachycholia (pak'e·ko'le·ah)
pachydactyly (pak'e·dak'tĭ·le)
pachyderma laryngis
  (pak'e·der'mah lah·rin'jis)
pachydermoperiostosis
  (pak'e·der'mo·per'e·os·to'sis)
pachygyria (pak'e·ji're·ah)
pachylosis (pak'e·lo'sis)
pachymeningitis (pak'e·men'in·ji'tis)
pachymeningopathy
  (pak'e·men'in·gop'ah·the)
pachyonychia (pak'e·o·nik'e·ah)
pachyperitonitis (pak'e·per'ĭ·to·ni'tis)
pachysalpingitis (pak'e·sal'pin·ji'tis)
pachysomia (pak'e·so'me·ah)
pachytene (pak'e·tēn)
pagophagia (pa'go·fa'je·ah)
palatal (pal'ah·tal)
palate (pal'at)
palatine (pal'ah·tīn)
palatoglossal (pah'ah·to·glos'al)
palatopharyngeal (pal'ah·to·fah·rin'je·al)
palatopharyngoplasty
  (pal'ah·to·fah·rin'go·plas'te)
palatoplasty (pal'ah·to·plas'te)
palatoplegia (pal'ah·to·ple'je·ah)
palindrome (pal'in·drōm)
palindromia (pal'in·dro'me·ah)
paliphrasia (pal'ĭ·fra'ze·ah)
pallesthesia (pal·es·the'ze·ah)
palliate (pal'e·āt)
palliative (pal'e·ah·tiv)
pallidectomy (pal'ĭ·dek'to·me)
pallidotomy (pal'ĭ·dot'o·me)
pallium (pal'e·um)
pallor (pal'or)
palmar (pal'mar)
palpable (pal'pah·bl)
palpate (pal'pāt)
palpation (pal·pa'shun)
palpebra (pal'pĕ·brah)
palpebrae (pal'pĕ·bre)
palpebral (pal'pĕ·bral)
palsy (pawl'ze)
panacea (pan'ah·se'ah)
panagglutinin (pan'ah·gloo'tĭ·nin)
panangiitis (pan'an·je·i'tis)
panarthritis (pan'ar·thri'tis)
pancarditis (pan'kar·di'tis)
pancolectomy (pan'ko·lek'to·me)
pancreas (pan'kre·as)

pancreatectomy (pan'kre·ah·tek'to·me)
pancreathelcosis (pan'kre·ath'el·ko'sis)
pancreaticoduodenostomy
  (pan'kre·at'ĭ·ko·du'o·de·nos'to·me)
pancreaticogastrostomy
  (pan'kre·at'ĭ·ko·gas·tros'to·me)
pancreaticojejunostomy
  (pan'kre·at'ĭ·ko·je'ju·nos'to·me)
pancreatin (pan'kre·ah·tin)
pancreatitis (pan'kre·ah·ti'tis)
pancreatoduodenectomy
  (pan'kre·ah·to·du'o·dĕ·nek'to·me)
pancreatolith (pan'kre·at'o·lith)
pancreatolithectomy
  (pan'kre·ah·to·lĭ·thek'to·me)
pancreatolithiasis
  (pan'kre·ah·to·lĭ·thi'ah·sis)
pancreatolithotomy
  (pan'kre·ah·to·lĭ·thot'o·me)
pancreatropic (pan·kre'ah·trop'ik)
pancreozymin (pan'kre·o·zi'min)
pancytopenia (pan'si·to·pe'ne·ah)
pandemic (pan·dem'ik)
panendoscope (pan·en'do·skōp)
panendoscopy (pan'en·dos'ko·pe)
panhypopituitarism
  (pan·hi'po·pĭ·tu'ĭ·tar·izm)
panhysterectomy (pan'his·ter·ek'to·me)
panhysterosalpingectomy
  (pan·his'ter·o·sal'pin·jek'to·me)
panniculitis (pan·nik'u·li'tis)
panniculus (pah·nik'u·lus)
pannus (pan'us)
Panorex (pan'or·eks)
panosteitis (pan·os·te·i'tis)
pansystolic (pan·sis·tol'ik)
papain (pah·pa'in)
papaverine (pah·pav'er·in)
papilla (pah·pil'ah)
papillary (pap'ĭ·ler'e)
papilledema (pap'il·ĕ·de'mah)
papilliform (pap·pil'ĭ·form)
papillitis (pap'ĭ·li'tis)
papilloadenocystoma
  (pah·pil'o·ad'ĕ·no·sis·to'mah)
papillocarcinoma
  (pah·pil'o·kar'sĭ·no'mah)
papilloma (pap'ĭ·lo'mah)
papillomatosis (pap'ĭ·lo'mah·to'sis)
Papillomavirus (pap'ĭ·lo'mah·vi'rus)
papilloretinitis (pah·pil'o·ret'ĭ·ni'tis)
papular (pap'u·lar)
papulation (pap'u·la'shun)
papule (pap'ūl)
papulopustular (pap'u·lo·pus'tu·lar)
papulosis (pap·u·lo'sis)
papulovesicular (pap'u·lo·ve·sik'u·lar)
parabiosis (par'ah·bi·o'sis)
parablepsia (par'ah·blep'se·ah)
paracentesis (par'ah·sen·te'sis)
paracentral (par'ah·sen'tral)
parachordal (par'ah·kor'dal)
paracoccidioidomycosis
  (par'ah·kok·sid'e·oi'do·mi·ko'sis)
paracusis (par'ah·ku'sis)
paracyesis (par'ah·si·e'sis)
paradidymis (par'ah·did'ĭ·mis)
paradipsia (par'ah·dip'se·ah)
paraffin (par'ah·fin)
paraformaldehyde
  (par'ah·for·mal'de·hīd)
paraganglia (par'ah·gang'gle·ah)
paraganglioma (par'ah·gang'gle·o'mah)
paraganglion (par'ah·gang'le·on)
paragene (par'ah·jēn)
parageusia (par'ah·gu'se·ah)
paragonimiasis (par'ah·gon'ĭ·mi'ah·sis)
Paragonimus (par'ah·gon'ĭ·mus)
paralalia (par'ah·la'le·ah)
paraldehyde (par·al'dĕ·hīd)
parallax (par'ah·laks)
parallelepiped (par'ah·lel'ĕ·pi'ped)
paralysis (pah·ral'ĭ·sis)
paralytic (par'ah·lit'ik)
paramecium (par'ah·me'she·um)
paramenia (par'ah·me'ne·ah)
parameter (pah·ram'ĕ·ter)
parametritis (par'ah·mĕ·tri'tis)

parametrium (pah'ah·me'tre·um)
paramyloidosis (par·am'ĭ·loi·do'sis)
paramyotonia (par'ah·mi'o·to'ne·ah)
Paramyxovirus (par'ah·mik'so·vi'rus)
paranoia (par'ah·noi'ah)
paranoiac (par'ah·noi'ak)
paranoid (par'ah·noid)
paranucleus (par'ah·nu'kle·us)
paraparesis (par'ah·par'e·sis)
paraperitoneal (par'ah·per'ĭ·to·ne'al)
paraphasia (par'ah·fa'ze·ah)
paraphimosis (par'ah·fi·mo'sis)
paraplegia (par'ah·ple'je·ah)
paraproctitis (par'ah·prok·ti'tis)
paraproteinemia
  (par'ah·pro'te·in·e'me·ah)
parapsychology (par'ah·si·kol'o·je)
paraquat (par'a·kwat)
parasite (par'ah·sīt)
parasitic (par'ah·sit'ik)
parasiticide (par'ah·sit'ĭ·sīd)
parasitism (par'ah·si'tizm)
parasitology (par'ah·si·tol'o·je)
parasitosis (par'ah·si·to'sis)
paraspadia (par'ah·spa'de·ah)
parasympathetic (par'ah·sim·pah·thet'ik)
parasympathomimetic
  (par'ah·sim'pah·tho·mĭ·met'ik)
parasystole (par'ah·sis'to·le)
parathion (par'ah·thi'on)
parathormone (par'ah·thor'mōn)
parathyroid (par'ah·thi'roid)
parathyrotropic (par'ah·thi·ro·trop'ik)
paratope (par'ah·tōp)
paraungual (par'ah·ung'gwal)
parectasia (par'ek·ta'se·ah)
paregoric (par'ĕ·gor'ik)
parenchyma (pah·reng'kĭ·mah)
parenteral (pah·ren'ter·al)
paresis (pah·re'sis)
paresthesia (par'es·the'ze·ah)
parietal (pah·ri'ĕ·tal)
parkinsonian (par'kin·so'ne·an)
parkinsonism (par'kin·son·izm)
paroniria (par'o·ni're·ah)
paronychia (par'o·nik'e·ah)
paroophoron (par'o·of'o·ron)
parosmia (par·oz'me·ah)
parotid (pah·rot'id)
parotidectomy (pah·rot'ĭ·dek'to·me)
parotitis (par'o·ti'tis)
parous (pa'rus)
paroxysm (par'ok·sizm)
pars (parz)
partes (par'tēz)
parthenogenesis (par'thĕ·no·jen'ĕ·sis)
particulate (par·tik'u·lāt)
parturient (par·tu're·ent)
parturifacient (par'tu·re·fa'shent)
parturition (par'tu·rish'un)
pascal (pas·kal')
passive (pas'iv)
passivity (pas·siv'ĭ·te)
pasteurellosis (pas'ter·ĕ·lo'sis)
pasteurization (pas'ter·ĭ·za'shun)
pasteurize (pas'ter·īz)
patella (pah·tel'ah)
patellapexy (pah·tel'ah·pek'se)
patellectomy (pat'ĕ·lek'to·me)
patency (pa'ten·se)
patent (pa'tent)
pathogen (path'o·jen)
pathogenesis (path'o·jen'ĕ·sis)
pathogenic (path'o·jen'ik)
pathognomonic (path'o·no·mon'ik)
pathologic (path'o·loj'ik)
pathologist (pah·thol'o·jist)
pathology (pah·thol'o·je)
pathomimesis (path'o·mĭ·me'sis)
pathoneurosis (path'o·nu·ro'sis)
pathophysiology (path'o·fiz'e·ol'o·je)
patroclinous (pat'ro·kli'nus)
patten (pat'n)
patulous (pat'u·lus)
peau d'orange (po' do·rahnj')
pecten (pek'ten)
pectin (pek'tin)
pectora (pek'tor·ah)

Pronunciation

pectoral (pek'to·ral)
pectoralgia (pec'to·ral'je·ah)
pectoralis (pek'to·ra'lis)
pectoriloquy (pek'to·ril'o·kwe)
pectus (pek'tus)
pederasty (ped'er·as'te)
pediatrician (pe'de·ah·trish'un)
pediatrics (pe'de·at'riks)
pedicel (ped'i·sel)
pedicle (ped'i·kl)
pediculicide (pe·dik'u·li·sīd)
pediculosis (pe·dik'u·lo'sis)
pediculus (pe·dik'u·lus)
pedigree (ped'i·gre')
pedodontics (pe·do·don'tiks)
pedology (pe·dol'o·je)
pedophilia (pe·do·fil'e·ah)
peduncle (pě·dung'kl)
pedunculate (pě·dung'ku·lāt)
peduncolotomy (pě·dung'ku·lot'o·me)
pellagra (pě·la'grah)
pellagroid (pě·lag'roid)
pellicle (pel'i·kl)
pelves (pel'ves)
pelvimeter (pel·vim'ě·ter)
pelvimetry (pel·vim'·ě·tre)
pelviotomy (pel've·ot'o·me)
pelvis (pel'vis)
pelvospondylitis (pel·vo·spon'dĭ·li'tis)
pemphigoid (pem'fĭ·goid)
pemphigus (pem'fĭ·gus)
penectomy (pě·nek'to·me)
penetrance (pen'ě·trans)
penicillamine (pen'ĭ·sil'ah·mēn)
penicillin (pen'ĭ·sil'in)
penicillinase (pen'ĭ·sil'ĭ·nās)
penile (pe'nīl)
penis (pe'nis)
pennate (pen'āt)
pentabasic (pen'tah·ba'sik)
pentatomic (pen'tah·tom'ik)
pentavalent (pen'tah·va'lent)
pentobarbital (pen'to·bar'bī·tal)
pentose (pen'tōs)
pepsin (pep'sin)
pepsinogen (pep·sin'o·jen)
pepsinogenous (pep·sin·oj'ě·nus)
peptidase (pep'ti·dās)
peptide (pep'tīd)
peptolysis (pep·tol'ĭ·sis)
peptone (pep'tōn)
peptonemia (pep'to·ne'me·ah)
peptonuria (pep'to·nu're·ah)
per annum (per a'num)
perception (per·sep'shun)
perchloride (per·klo'rīd)
percolation (per'ko·la'shun)
percuss (per·kus')
percussion (per·kush'un)
percussor (per·kus'or)
percutaneous (per'ku·ta'ne·us)
perforans (per'fo·ranz)
perforation (per'fo·ra'shun)
perfusate (per·fu'zāt)
perfusion (per·fu'zhun)
perianal (per'e·a'nal)
periaortic (per'e·a'or'tik)
periaortitis (per'e·a'or·ti'tis)
periapical (per'e·ap'ĭ·kal)
periarteritis (per'e·ar'tě·ri'tis)
periarthritis (per'e·ar·thri'tis)
pericardial (per'ĭ·kar'de·al)
pericardicentesis (per'ĭ·kar'de·sen·te'sis)
pericardiectomy (per'ĭ·kar'de·ek'to·me)
pericardiocentesis
    (per'ĭ·kar'de·o·sen·te'sis)
pericardiophrenic (per'ĭ·kar'de·o·fren'ik)
pericardiorrhaphy (per'ĭ·kar'de·or'ah·fe)
pericardiostomy (per'ĭ·kar'de·os'to·me)
pericarditis (per'ĭ·kar·di'tis)
pericardium (per'ĭ·kar'de·um)
pericardotomy (per'ĭ·kar·dot'o·me)
pericholangitis (per'ĭ·ko'lan·ji'tis)
pericholecystitis (per'ĭ·ko'le·sis·ti'tis)
perichondrial (per'ĭ·kon'dre·al)
perichondrium (per'ĭ·kon'dre·um)
pericolpitis (per'ĭ·kol·pi'tis)
pericranium (per'ĭ·kra'ne·um)

pericyte (per'ĭ·sīt)
peridesmic (per'ĭ·dez'mik)
peridesmitis (per'ĭ·dez·mi'tis)
peridesmium (per'ĭ·dez'me·um)
periesophagitis (per'e·ě·sof'ah·ji'tis)
periganglionic (per'ĭ·gang'gle·on'ik)
perihepatitis (per'ĭ·hep'ah·ti'tis)
perikaryon (per'ĭ·kar'e·on)
perilymph (per'ĭ·limf)
perimeter (pě·rim'ě·ter)
perimetrium (per·ĭ·me'tre·um)
perimetry (pě·rim'ĭ·tre)
perimysium (per'ĭ·mis'e·um)
perinatal (per'ĭ·na'tal)
perineal (per'ĭ·ne'al)
perineorrhaphy (per'ĭ·ne·or'ah·fe)
perinephric (per'ĭ·nef'rik)
perinephritis (per'ĭ·ně·fri'tis)
perineum (per'ĭ·ne'um)
perineural (per'ĭ·nu'ral)
perineurium (per'ĭ·nu're·um)
periodical (per'e·od'ĭ·kal)
periodontal (per'e·o·don'tal)
periodontics (per'e·o·don'tiks)
periodontist (per'e·o·don'tist)
periodontitis (per'e·o·don·ti'tis)
periodontium (per'e·o·don'she·um)
periodontosis (per'e·o·don·to'sis)
periorchitis (per'e·or·ki'tis)
periosteal (per'e·os'te·al)
periosteoma (per'e·os·te·o'mah)
periosteomyelitis
    (per'e·os·te·o·mi'ě·li'tis)
periosteotomy (per'e·os'te·ot'o·me)
periosteum (per'e·os'te·um)
periostitis (per'e·os·ti'tis)
peripapillary (per'ĭ·pap'ĭ·ler·e)
peripheral (pě·rif'er·al)
periphery (pě·rif'er·e)
periproctitis (per'ĭ·prok·ti'tis)
perirectal (per'ĭ·rek'tal)
perisalpinx (per'ĭ·sal'pinks)
peristalsis (per'ĭ·stal'sis)
peristole (pě·ris'tŏ·le)
perisynovial (per'ĭ·si·no've·al)
perithelioma (per'ĭ·the'le·o'mah)
perithelium (per'ĭ·the'le·um)
peritoneocentesis
    (per'ĭ·to'ne·o·sen·te'sis)
peritoneoclysis (per'ĭ·to'ne·o·kli'sis)
peritoneoscope (per'ĭ·to'ne·o·skōp')
peritoneoscopy (per'ĭ·to'ne·os'ko·pe)
peritoneum (per'ĭ·to·ne'um)
peritonitis (per'ĭ·to·ni'tis)
peritonsillitis (per'ĭ·ton'si·li'tis)
peritrichous (pě·rit'rĭ·kus)
periumbilical (per'e·um·bil'ĭ·kal)
periungual (per'e·ung'gwal)
periureteritis (per'e·u're·tě·ri'tis)
perleche (per·lesh')
permanganate (per·man'gah·nāt)
permanganic (per·man'gan·ik)
permeable (per'me·ah·bl)
permease (per'me·ās)
pernicious (per·nish'us)
peroneal (per'o·ne'al)
peroral (per·o'ral)
peroxidase (pě·rok'sĭ·dās)
peroxide (pě·rok'sīd)
peroxisome (pě·roks'ĭ·sōm)
peroxyacetyl (pě·roks'ĭ·ah·se'til)
perspiration (per'spĭ·ra'shun)
persuasion (per·swa'zhun)
pertussis (per·tus'is)
pervaporation (per·vap'or·a'shun)
perversion (per·ver'shun)
pervert (per'vert)
pes equinus (pes e·kwi'nus)
pessary (pes'ah·re)
pesticide (pes'tĭ·sīde)
pestilence (pes'tĭ·lens)
pestle (pes'l)
petechia (pe·te'ke·ah)
petechiae (pe·te'ke·e)
petiole (pet'e·ōl)
petit mal epilepsy (pě·te' mahl ep'ĭ·lep'se)
petrifaction (pet'rĭ·fak'shun)
petrissage (pa'trĭ·sahzh')

petrolatum (pet'ro·la'tum)
petrosal (pě·tro'sal)
petrous (pet'rus)
peyote (pa·o'te)
Peyronie (pa·ron·ē')
phacoanaphylaxis (fak'o·an'ah·fi·lak'sis)
phacocele (fak'o·sēl)
phacocystitis (fak'o·sis·ti'tis)
phacoerysis (fak'o·er·e'sis)
phacolysis (fak·kol'ĭ·sis)
phacomalacia (fak'o·mah·la'she·ah)
phacometachoresis
    (fak'o·met'ah·ko·re'sis)
phacometecesis (fak'o·met'ě·se'sis)
phacoscope (fak'o·skōp)
phagedenic (faj'ě·de'nik)
phagocyte (fag'o·sīt)
phagocytic (fag'o·sit'ik)
phagocytin (fag'o·si'tin)
phagocytoblast (fag'o·si'to·blast)
phagocytose (fag'o·si'tōs)
phagocytosis (fag'o·si·to'sis)
phagosome (fag'o·sōm)
phagotype (fag'o·tīp)
phalangeal (fah·lan'je·al)
phalanges (fah·lan'gēz)
phalanx (fa'lanks)
phallectomy (fal·ek'to·me)
phallic (fal'ik)
phallus (fal'us)
phantasm (fan'tazm)
pharmaceutics (fahr'mah·su'tiks)
pharmacodiagnosis
    (fahr'mah·ko·di'ag·no'sis)
pharmacogenetics
    (fahr'mah·ko·jě·net'iks)
pharmacognosy (fahr'mah·kog'no·se)
pharmacokinetics
    (fahr'mah·ko·kĭ·net'iks)
pharmacologist (fahr'mah·kol'o·jist)
pharmacology (fahr'mah·kol'o·je)
pharmacopedia (fahr'mah·ko·pe'de·ah)
pharmacopeia (fahr'mah·ko·pe'ah)
pharmacopoeia (fahr'mah·ko·pe'·ah)
pharmacy (fahr'mah·se)
pharyngalgia (far'in·gal'je·ah)
pharyngectomy (far'in·jek'to·me)
pharyngismus (far'in·jiz'mus)
pharyngitis (far'in·ji'tis)
pharyngocele (fah·ring'go·sēl)
pharyngodynia (fah·ring'go·din'e·ah)
pharyngoesophageal
    (fah·ring'go·e·sof'ah·je'al)
pharyngoglossal (fah·ring'go·glos'al)
pharyngolaryngitis
    (fah·ring'go·lar'in·ji'tis)
pharyngopalatine (fah·ring'go·pal'ah·tīn)
pharyngoplegia (fah·ring'go·ple'je·ah)
pharyngoscope (fah·ring'go·skōp)
pharyngoscopy (far'ing·gos'ko·pe)
pharyngospasm (fah·ring'go·spazm)
pharyngostenosis (fah·ring'go·stě·no'sis)
pharyngotomy (far'ing·got'o·me)
pharyngotonsillitis
    (fah·ring'go·ton'si·li'tis)
pharyngoxerosis (fah·ring'go·ze·ro'sis)
pharynx (far'inks)
phenacetin (fě·nas'ě·tin)
phencyclidine (fen·si'kli·dēn)
phenformin (fen·for'min)
phenobarbital (fe'no·bar'bī·tal)
phenocopy (fe'no·kop'e)
phenolphthalein (fe'nol·thal'e·in)
phenolsulfonphthalein
    (fe'nol·sul'fōn·thal'e·in)
phenomena (fě·nom'ě·nah)
phenomenon (fě·nom'ě·non)
phenothiazine (fe'no·thi'ah·zēn)
phenotype (fe'no·tīp)
phenoxybenzamine
    (fě·nok'se·ben'zah·mēn)
phentolamine (fen·tol'ah·mēn)
phenylalanine (fen'il·al'ah·nīn)
phenylbutazone (fen'il·bu'tah·zōn)
phenylephrine (fen'il·ef'rin)
phenylhydrazine (fen'il·hi'drah·zēn)
phenylketonuria (fen'il·ke'to·nu're·ah)
phenylpropanolamine

(fen'il·pro'pah·nol'ah·mēn)
phenylthiourea (fen'il·thi'o·u·re'ah)
pheochrome (fe'o·krōm)
pheochromocyte (fe'o·kro'mo·sīt)
pheochromocytoma
(fe·o·kro'mo·si·to'mah)
pheromones (fer'o·mōnz)
philtrum (fil'trum)
phimosis (fi·mo'sis)
phlebectomy (flĕ·bek'to·me)
phlebitis (flĕ·bi'tis)
phlebography (flĕ·bog'rah·fe)
phlebolith (fleb'o·lith)
phleborrhagia (fleb'o·ra'je·ah)
phleborrhexis (fleb'o·rek'sis)
phlebosclerosis (fleb'o·sklĕ·ro'sis)
phlebostasis (flĕ·bos'tah·sis)
phlebothrombosis (fleb'o·throm·bo'sis)
phlebotomy (flĕ·bot'o·me)
phlegm (flem)
phlegmon (fleg'mon)
phlegmonous (fleg'mon·us)
phlyctena (flik·te'nah)
phlyctenae (flik·te'ne)
phobia (fo'be·ah)
phocomelia (fo'ko·me'le·ah)
phonasthenia (fo'nas·the'ne·ah)
phonation (fo·na'shun)
phoneme (fo'nēm)
phonemic (fo·ne'mik)
phonetic (fo·net'ik)
phonetics (fo·net'iks)
phoniatrics (fo'ne·at'riks)
phonoangiography (fo'no·an'je·og'rah·fe)
phonocardiogram (fo'no·kar'de·o·gram)
phonocardiography
(fo'no·kar'de·og'rah·fe)
phonometer (fo·nom'ĕ·ter)
phonopathy (fo·nop'ah·the)
phonopneumomassage
(fo'no·nu'mo·mah·sahj')
phoropter (fo·rop'ter)
phosgene (fos'jēn)
phosphatase (fos'fah·tās)
phosphate (fos'fāt)
phosphatidic (fos'fah·ti'dik)
phosphatidylcholine (fos·fat'ĭ·dil·ko'lēn)
phosphatidylethanolamine
(fos·fat'ĭ·dil·eth'ah·nol·am'ēn)
phosphaturia (fos'fah·tu're·ah)
phosphene (fos'fēn)
phosphine (fos'fēn)
phosphoarginine (fos'fo·ar'jĭ·nēn)
phosphocreatine (fos'fo·kre'ah·tin)
phosphodiesterase (fos'fo·di·es'ter·ās)
phosphoenolpyruvic
(fos'fo·e'nol·pi·ru'vik)
phosphofructokinase
(fos'fo·fruk'to·ki'nās)
phosphoglucomutase
(fos'fo·gloo'ko·mu'tās)
phospholipase (fos'fo·lip'ās)
phospholipid (fos'fo·lip'id)
phosphoprotein (fos'fo·pro'te·in)
phosphor (fos'for)
phosphorated (fos'fo·rāt'ed)
phosphorescence (fos'fo·res'ens)
phosphorescent (fos'fo·res'ent)
phosphoribosyltransferase
(fos'fo·ri'bo·sil·trans'fer·ās)
phosphoric (fos'for·ik)
phosphorolysis (fos'fo·rol'ĭ·sis)
phosphorous (fos'fŏ·rus)
phosphorus (fos'fŏ·rus)
phosphorylase (fos·fōr'ĭ·lās)
phosphorylation (fos'fōr·ĭ·la'shun)
phosphotransferase (fos'fo·trans'fer·ās)
phot (fōt)
photochromogens (fo'to·kro'mo·jenz)
photocoagulation (fo'to·ko·ag'u·la'shun)
photocoagulator (fo'to·ko·ag'u·la'tor)
photodermatitis (fo'to·der'mah·ti'tis)
photoelectrometer (fo'to·e·lek·trom'ĕ·ter)
photoelectron (fo'to·e·lek'tron)
photogen (fo'to·jen)
photokinesis (fo'to·ki·ne'sis)
photoluminescent (fo'to·lu'mĭ·nes'ent)
photolysis (fo·tol'ĭ·sis)

photomacrography (fo'to·mak·rog'rah·fe)
photometry (fo·tom'ĕ·tre)
photon (fo'ton)
photophthalmia (fo'to·of·thal'me·ah)
photopsin (fo·top'sin)
photoretinitis (fo'to·ret'ĭ·ni'tis)
photoscan (fo'to·skan)
photosynthesis (fo'to·sin'thĕ·sis)
phototaxis (fo'to·tak'sis)
photothermal (fo·to·ther'mal)
phototropism (fo·tot'ro·pizm)
phrenic (fren'ik)
phrenicectomy (fren'ĭ·sek'to·me)
phreniclasia (fren'ĭ·kla'ze·ah)
phrenicotomy (fren'ĭ·kot'o·me)
phrenocolic (fren'o·kol'ic)
phrenosin (fren'o·sin)
phrenotropic (fren'o·trop'ik)
phthalein (thal'e·in)
phthiriasis (thi·ri'ah·sis)
Phthirus pubis (thir'rus pu'bis)
phthisic (tiz'ik)
phthisiology (tiz'e·ol'o·je)
phthisis (ti'sis)
phycomycosis (fi'ko·mi·ko'sis)
phylum (fi'lum)
phymatosis (fi·mah·to'sis)
physiatrics (fiz'e·at'riks)
physiatrist (fiz'e·at'rist)
physiognomy (fiz'e·og'no·me)
physiologic (fiz'e·o·loj'ik)
physiology (fiz'e·ol'o·je)
physique (fĭ·zēk')
physohematometra
(fi'so·hem'ah·to·me'trah)
physostigmine (fi'so·stig'mēn)
phytin (fi'tin)
phytohemagglutinin
(fi'to·hem'ah·gloo'tĭ·nin)
pia mater (pi'ah ma'ter)
pica (pi'kah)
pickwickian (pik·wik'e·an)
picogram (pi'ko'gram)
picrotoxin (pik'ro·tok'sin)
piedra (pe·a'drah)
piesesthesia (pi·e'zes·the'ze·ah)
piezochemistry (pi·e'zo·kem'is·tre)
piezoelectricity (pi·e'zo·e'lek·tris'ĭ·te)
pigment (pig'ment)
pigmentation (pig'men·ta'shun)
pilaster (pi·las'ter)
pileus (pi'le·us)
pili (pi'li)
pillar (pil'ar)
pilocarpine (pi'lo·kar'pin)
pilocystic (pi'lo·sis'tik)
pilomatrixoma (pi'lo·ma·trik·so'mah)
pilomotor (pi'lo·mo'tor)
pilonidal (pi'lo·ni'dal)
pilosebaceous (pi'lo·sĕ·ba'shus)
pilus (pi'lus)
pineal (pin'e·al)
pinealectomy (pin'e·al·ek'to·me)
pinealocyte (pin'e·ah·lo·sīt')
pinguecula (ping·gwek'u·lah)
pinna (pin'nah)
pinocytosis (pi'no·si·to'sis)
pipette (pi·pet')
pisiform (pi'sĭ·form)
pituicyte (pĭ·tu'ĭ·sīt)
pituitary (pĭ·tu'ĭ·tār'e)
pityriasis (pit'ĭ·ri'ah·sis)
Pityrosporum (pit'ĭ·ros'po·rum)
placebo (plah·se'bo)
placenta (plah·sen'tah)
placental (plah·sen'tal)
placentascan (plah·sen'tah·skan)
placentation (plas'en·ta'shun)
placentitis (plas'en·ti'tis)
placentography (plas'en·tog'rah·fe)
placode (plak'ōd)
pladarosis (plad·ah·ro'sis)
plagiocephaly (pla'je·o·sef'ah·le)
plagioprosopia (pla'je·o·pro·so'pe·ah)
plague (plāg)
planchet (plan'shet)
plano (pla'no)
planoconcave (pla'no·kon'kav)

planoconvex (pla'no·kon'veks)
plantain (plan'tān)
plantalgia (plan·tal'je·ah)
plantar (plan'tar)
plaque (plak)
plasma (plaz'mah)
plasmacytoma (plaz'mah·si·to'mah)
plasmacytosis (plaz'mah·si·to'sis)
plasmalemma (plaz'mah·lem'ah)
plasmapheresis (plaz'mah·fĕ·re'sis)
plasmin (plaz'min)
plasminogen (plaz·min'o·jen)
plasmodia (plaz·mo'de·ah)
plasmodium (plaz·mo'de·um)
plasmolysis (plaz·mol'ĭ·sis)
plastid (plas'tid)
platelet (plāt'let)
plateletpheresis (plāt'let·fĕ're·sis)
platybasia (plat'e·ba'se·ah)
platycephalous (plat'e·sef'ah·lus)
platyhelminth (plat'e·hel'minth)
platypellic (plat'e·pel'ik)
platyrrhine (plat'e·rīn)
pledget (plej'et)
pleiotropic (pli'o·trop'ik)
pleiotropism (pli·ot'ro·pizm)
pleiotropy (pli·ot'ro·pe)
pleocytosis (ple'·o·si·to'sis)
pleomastia (ple'o·mas'te·ah)
pleomorphism (ple'o·mor'fism)
pleoptics (ple·op'tiks)
plerocercoid (ple'ro·ser'koid)
plethysmography (pleth'iz·mog'rah·fe)
plethysmometry (pleth'iz·mom'ĕ·tre)
pleura (ploor'ah)
pleuralgia (ploor·al'je·ah)
pleurisy (ploor'ĭ·se)
pleurocentesis (ploor'o·sen·te'sis)
pleurodynia (ploor'o·din'e·ah)
pleurogenic (ploor'o·jen'ik)
pleurography (ploo·rog'rah·fe)
pleurolith (ploor'o·lith)
plexus (plek'sus)
plica (pli'kah)
plicae (pli'se)
plication (pli·ka'shun)
plicotomy (pli·kot'o·me)
plombage (plom·bahzh')
plumbum (plum'bum)
pluricausal (ploo·rĭ·kaw'zal)
pluripotent (ploo·rip'o·tent)
pneumatization (nu'mah·tĭ·za'shun)
pneumatocele (nu·mat'o·sēl)
pneumaturia (nu'mah·tu're·ah)
pneumoarthrography
(nu'mo·ar·throg'rah·fe)
pneumocephalus (nu'mo·sef'ah·lus)
pneumocholecystitis
(nu'mo·ko'le·sis·ti'tis)
pneumococci (nu'mo·kok'si)
pneumoconiosis (nu'mo·ko'ne·o'sis)
Pneumocystis carinii
(nu'mo·sis'tis ka·ri'ne·i)
pneumocystosis (nu'mo·sis·to'sis)
pneumocyte (nu·mo·sīt')
pneumoencephalography
(nu'mo·en·sef'ah·log'rah·fe)
pneumography (nu·mog'rah·fe)
pneumohemothorax
(nu'mo·he·mo·tho'raks)
pneumohydrothorax
(nu'mo·hi'dro·tho'raks)
pneumolith (nu'mo·lith)
pneumolysis (nu·mol'ĭ·sis)
pneumomycosis (nu'mo·mi·ko'sis)
pneumonectomy (nu'mo·nek'to·me)
pneumonia (nu·mo'ne·ah)
pneumonic (nu·mon'ik)
pneumonitis (nu'mo·ni'tis)
pneumopericardium
(nu'mo·per·ĭ·kar'de·um)
pneumoperitoneum
(nu'mo·per'ĭ·to·ne'um)
pneumoperitonitis (nu'mo·per'ĭ·to·ni'tis)
pneumoroentgenography
(nu'mo·rent'gen·og'rah·fe)
pneumorrhachis (nu'mo·ra'kis)
pneumothorax (nu'mo·tho'raks)

Pneumovirus (nu′mo·vi·rus)
podagra (po·dag′rah)
podiatrist (po·di′ah·trist)
podiatry (po·di′ah·tre)
poditis (po·di′tis)
podocyte (pod′o·sīt)
pododynamometer
  (pod′o·di′nah·mom′ě·ter)
poikilocyte (poi′kĭ·lo·sīt)
poikiloderma (poi′kĭ·lo·der′mah)
polarity (po·lar′ĭ·te)
polarization (po′lar·ĭ·za·shun)
poliodystrophy (po′le·o·dis′tro·fě)
polioencephalitis (po′le·o·en·sef′ah·li′tis)
poliomyelitis (po′le·o·mi′ě·li′tis)
poliomyelopathy
  (po′le·o·mi′ě·lop′ah·the)
poliovirus (po′le·o·vi′rus)
pollen (pol′en)
pollenosis (pol′ě·no′sis)
pollutant (pol·lu′tant)
pollution (pol·lu′shun)
polyadenitis (pol′e·ad′ě·ni′tis)
polyamine (pol′e·am′ēn)
polyarteritis (pol′e·ar′tě·ri′tis)
polyarthritis (pol′e·ar·thri′tis)
polybasic (pol′e·ba′sik)
polycholia (pol′e·ko′le·ah)
polychondritis (pol′e·kon·dri′tis)
polychromatic (pol′e·kro·mat′ik)
polychromatophil (pol′e·kro·mat′o·fil)
polychromatophilia
  (pol′e·kro′mah·to·fil′e·ah)
polycystic (pol′e·sis′tik)
polycythemia (pol′e·si·the′me·ah)
polydactyly (pol′e·dak′tĭ·le)
polydipsia (pol′e·dip′se·ah)
polydysplasia (pol′e·dis·pla′ze·ah)
polyenoic (pol′e·e·no′ik)
polygene (pol′e·jēn)
polygraph (pol′e·graf)
polyhydramnios (pol′e·hi·dram′ne·os)
polyhydric (pol′e·hi′drik)
polyhypermenorrhea
  (pol′e·hi′per·men′o·re′ah)
polyhypomenorrhea
  (pol′e·hi′po·men′o·re′ah)
polyleptic (pol′e·lep′tik)
polylogia (pol′e·lo′je·ah)
polymastia (pol′e·mas′te·ah)
polymer (pol′ĭ·mer)
polymerase (pol·im′er·ās)
polymerization (pol′ĭ·mer′ĭ·za′shun)
polymethylmethacrylate
  (pol′e·meth′il·meth·ak′rĭ·lāt)
polymicrolipomatosis
  (pol′e·mi′kro·lip′o·mah·to′sis)
polymorph (pol′e·morf)
polymorphonuclear
  (pol′e·mor′fo·nu′kle·ar)
polymyalgia (pol′e·mi·al′je·ah)
polymyositis (pol′e·mi′o·si′tis)
polymyxin (pol′e·mik′sin)
polyneuritis (pol′e·nu·ri′tis)
polyneuropathy (pol′e·nu·rop′ah·the)
polynucleotidase (pol′e·nu′kle·o′tĭ·dās)
polynucleotide (pol′e·nu′kle·o·tīd)
polyopia (pol′e·o′pe·ah)
polyp (pol′ip)
polypectomy (pol′ĭ·pek′to·me)
polypeptide (pol′e·pep′tīd)
polyploidy (pol′e·ploi′de)
polypoid (pol′e·poid)
polyribosome (pol′e·ri′bo·sōm)
polysaccharide (pol′e·sak′ah·rĭd)
polysomy (pol′e·so′me)
polyspermia (pol′e·sper′me·ah)
polytetrafluoroethylene
  (pol′e·tet′rah·floo′o·ro·eth′ĭ·lēn)
polyunsaturated (pol′e·un·sach′ě·ra·ted)
polyuria (pol′e·u′re·ah)
pompholyx (pom′fo·liks)
pomphus (pom′fus)
pons (ponz)
pontic (pon′tik)
pontile (pon′tīl)
pontine (pon′tīn)
popliteal (pop·lit′e·al)

porcine (por′sīn)
porphobilinogen (por′fo·bi·lin′o·jen)
porphyria (por·fē′re·ah)
porphyrin (por′fĭ·rin)
porphyrinuria (por′fĭ·rĭ·nu′re·ah)
portacaval (por′tah·ka′val)
portal (por′tal)
positron (poz′ĭ·tron)
postcibal (pōst·si′bal)
postclimacteric (pōst′kli·mak′ter·ik)
posthioplasty (pos′the·o·plas′te)
posthitis (pos·thi′tis)
postmortem (pōst·mor′tem)
postpartum (pōst·par′tum)
postprandial (pōst·pran′de·al)
postsynaptic (pōst′sĭ·nap′tik)
postulate (pos′tu·lāt)
potassium (po·tas′e·um)
potency (po′ten·se)
potentiation (po·ten′she·a′shun)
potentiometer (po·ten′she·om′ě·ter)
potion (po′shun)
poultice (pōl′tis)
povidone (po′vĭ·dōn)
poxvirus (poks·vi′rus)
pragmatagnosia (prag′mat·ag·no′ze·ah)
preagonal (pre·ag′o·nal)
preagonic (pre·ah·gon′ik)
prealbumin (pre′al·bu′min)
preanesthetic (pre′an·es·thet′ik)
precancerous (pre·kan′ser·us)
precipitant (pre·sip′ĭ·tant)
precipitate (pre·sip′ĭ·tāt)
precipitation (pre·sip′ĭ·ta′shun)
precipitin (pre·sip′ĭ·tin)
preclinical (pre·klin′ĭ·kal)
precocious (pre·ko′shus)
precocity (pre·kos′ĭ·te)
precognition (pre′kog·nish′un)
preconscious (pre·kon′shus)
precordial (pre·kor′de·al)
precordium (pre·kor′de·um)
precuneus (pre·ku′ne·us)
precursor (pre′kur·sor)
prediabetes (pre·di′ah·be′tēz)
prediastole (pre′di·as′to·le)
predisposition (pre′dis·po·zish′un)
prednisolone (pred·nis′o·lōn)
prednisone (pred′nĭ·sōn)
predormitum (pre·dor′mĭ·tum)
preeclampsia (pre′e·klamp′se·ah)
preexcitation (pre·ek′si·ta′shun)
pregnancy (preg′nan·se)
pregnane (preg′nān)
pregnanediol (preg′nān·di′ol)
pregnanetriol (preg′nān·tri′ol)
pregnene (preg′nēn)
prehensile (pre·hen′sil)
prehormone (pre·hor′mōn)
preleukemia (pre·lu·ke′me·ah)
preluxation (pre·luk·sa′shun)
premalignant (pre′mah·lig′nant)
premature (pre·mah·tūr′)
prematurity (pre′mah·tu′rĭ·te)
premedication (pre′med·ĭ·ka′shun)
premelanosome (pre·mel′ah·no·sōm)
premenstrual (pre·men′stroo·al)
premolar (pre·mo′lar)
premunition (pre′mu·nish′un)
preoperative (pre·op′er·ah·tiv)
prepallium (pre·pal′e·um)
prepatellar (pre′pah·tel′ar)
prepuberty (pre·pu′ber·te)
prepuce (pre′pūs)
preputiotomy (pre·pu′she·ot′o·me)
presbycusis (pres′bě·ku′sis)
presbyopia (pres′bě·o′pe·ah)
presenility (pre′sě·nil′ĭ·te)
presomite (pre·so′mīt)
pressor (pres′or)
presynaptic (pre′sĭ·nap′tik)
presystole (pre·sis′to·le)
presystolic (pre′sis·tol′ik)
prevalence (prev′ah·lens)
prevertebral (pre·ver′tě·bral)
priapism (pri′ah·pizm)
primigravida (pri′mĭ·grav′ĭ·dah)
primipara (pri·mip′ah·rah)

primordial (pri·mor′de·al)
primordium (pri·mor′de·um)
proband (pro′band)
probang (pro′bang)
probenecid (pro·ben′ě·sid)
proboscis (pro·bos′kis)
proboscises (pro·bos′kĭ·sēz)
procainamide (pro·kān′ah·mīd)
procaine (pro′kān)
precaryote (pro·kar′e·ōt)
procercoid (pro·ser′koid)
process (pros′es)
prochlorperazine (pro′klōr·per′ah·zēn)
prochondral (pro·kon′dral)
procollagen (pro·kol′ah·jen)
proctalgia (prok·tal′je·ah)
proctatresia (prok′tah·tre′ze·ah)
proctectasia (prok′tek·ta′ze·ah)
proctectomy (prok·tek′to·me)
proctencleisis (prok′ten·kli·sis)
proctitis (prok·ti′tis)
proctoclysis (prok·tok′lĭ·sis)
proctocolonoscopy
  (prok′to·ko′lon·os′ko·pe)
proctocolpoplasty (prok′to·kol′po·plas′te)
protocystocele (prok′to·sis′to·sēl)
proctocystotomy (prok′to·sis′tot′o·me)
proctodeum (prok′to·de′um)
proctologist (prok′tol′o·jist)
proctology (prok·tol′o·je)
proctoparalysis (prok′to·pah·ral′ĭ·sis)
proctoperineoplasty
  (prok′to·per′ĭ·ne′o·plas′te)
proctopexy (prok′to·pek′se)
proctoplasty (prok′to·plas′te)
proctoplegia (pok′to·ple′je·ah)
proctoptosia (prok′top·to′se·ah)
proctoptosis (prok′top·to′sis)
proctorrhagia (prok′to·ra′je·ah)
proctorrhaphy (prok·tor′ah·fe)
proctoscope (prok′to·skōp)
proctoscopy (prok·tos′ko·pe)
proctosigmoidectomy
  (prok′to·sig′moi·dek′to·me)
proctosigmoidoscopy
  (prok′to·sig′moi·dos′ko·pe)
proctostat (prok′to·stat)
proctostenosis (prok′to·stě·no′sis)
proctostomy (prok·tos′to·me)
proctotomy (prok·tot·o·me)
prodrome (pro′drōm)
proenzyme (pro·en′zīm)
proerythroblast (pro′ě·rith′ro·blast)
proerythrocyte (pro′ě·rith′ro·sīt)
progeria (pro·je′re·ah)
progesterone (pro·jes′tě·rōn)
progestin (pro·jes′tin)
progestogen (pro·jes′to·jen)
proglottid (pro·glot′id)
prognathism (prog′nah·thizm)
prognosis (prog·no′sis)
prognosticate (prog·nos′tĭ·kāt)
prohormone (pro·hor′mōn)
proinsulin (pro·in′su·lin)
prokaryosis (pro′kar·e·o′sis)
prolactin (pro·lak′tin)
prolapse (pro·laps′)
prolymphocyte (pro·lim′fo·sīt)
promastigote (pro·mas′tĭ·gōt)
promegaloblast (pro·meg′ah·lo·blast)
prometaphase (pro·met′ah·fāz)
promethazine (pro·meth′ah·zēn)
promontory (prom′on·to′re)
promyelocyte (pro·mi′ě·lo·sīt)
pronate (pro′nāt)
pronation (pro·na′shun)
pronephroi (pro·nef′ro·i)
pronephros (pro·nef′ros)
pronormoblast (pro·nor′mo·blast)
propagation (prop′ah·ga′shun)
proparacaine (pro·par′ah·kān)
propenyl (pro·pe′nil)
properdin (pro′per·din)
prophage (pro′fāj)
prophase (pro′fāz)
prophylactic (pro′fi·lak′tik)
prophylaxis (pro′fi·lak′sis)
proposita (pro′poz′ĭ·tah)

Pronunciation

propositi (pro·poz'ĭ·ti)
propositus (pro·poz'ĭ·tus)
propranolol (pro·pran'o·lōl)
proprioceptor (pro'pre·o·sep'tor)
proptosis (prop·to'sis)
propylthiouracil (pro'pil·thi'o·u'rah·sil)
pro re nata (pro re na'tah)
posection (pro·sek'shun)
prosencephalon (pros'en·sef'ah·lon)
prosody (pros'o·de)
prosopagnosia (pros'a·pag·no'se·ah)
prostaglandin (pros'tah·glan'din)
prostatalgia (pros'tah·tal'je·ah)
prostate (pros'tāt)'
prostatectomy (pros'tah·tek'to·me)
prostatitis (pros'tah·ti'tis)
prostatocystitis (pros·ta'to·sis·ti'tis)
prostatocystotomy
   (pros·ta'to·sis·tot'o·me)
prostatomegaly (pros'ta·to·meg'ah·le)
prostatomyomectomy
   (pros·ta'to·mi'o·mek'to·me)
prostatorrhea (pros'tah·to·re'ah)
prostatovesiculectomy
   (pros'tah·to·vĕ·sik'u·lek'to·me)
prostatovesiculitis
   (pros'tah·to·vĕ·sik'u·li'tis)
prosthesis (pros·the'sis)
prosthetics (pros·thet'iks)
prosthodontics (pros'tho·don'tiks)
protaminase (pro·tam'ĭ·nās)
protamine (pro'tah·mēn)
protease (pro'te·ās)
protein (pro'te·in)
proteinase (pro'te·in·ās)
proteinosis (pro'te·in·o'sis)
proteinuria (pro'te·in·u're·ah)
proteolysis (pro'te·ol'ĭ·sis)
proteolytic (pro'te·o·lit'ik)
Proteus mirabillis (pro'te·us mir·ahb'ĭ·lis)
prothrombin (pro·throm'bin)
protodiastolic (pro'to·di'ah·stol'ik)
proton (pro'ton)
protoplasm (pro'to·plazm)
protoporphyria (pro'to·por·fir'e·ah)
protoporphyrin (por'to·por'fĭ·rin)
prototroph (pro'to·trof)
prototype (pro'to·tīp)
protozoan (pro'to·zo'an)
protuberance (pro·tu'ber·ans)
provirus (pro·vi'rus)
provitamin (pro·vi'tah·min)
proximal (prok'sĭ·mal)
proximoataxia (prok'sĭ·mo·ah·tak'se·ah)
prurient (proor'e·ent)
prurigo (proo·ri'go)
pruritis (proo·ri'tus)
psammoma (sah·mo'mah)
pseudarthrosis (soo'dar·thro'sis)
pseudesthesial (soo'des·the'ze·al)
pseudoallele (soo'do·ah·lēl')
pseudoaneurysm (soo'do·an'u·rizm)
pseudocoarctation
   (soo'do·ko'ark·ta'shun)
pseudocryptorchism
   (soo'do·krip·tor'kiz·um)
pseudocyesis (soo'do·si'e·sis)
pseudocyst (soo'do·sist)
pseudofracture (soo'do·frak'chur)
pseudoglaucoma (soo'do·glaw·ko'mah)
pseudogout (soo'do·gowt)
pseudohemophilia (soo'do·he'mo·fil'e·ah
pseudohermaphroditism
   (soo'do·her·maf'ro·dīt·izm)
pseudohypoparathyroidism
   (soo'do·hi'po·par'ah·thi'roi·dizm)
Pseudomonas (soo'do·mo'nas)
pseudomyopia (soo'do·mi·o'pe·ah)
pseudomyxoma (soo'do·mik·so'mah)
pseudoneoplasm (soo'do·ne'o·plazm)
pseudopodium (soo'do·po'de·um)
pseudopolyp (soo'do·pol'ip)
pseudopterygium (soo'do·ter·ij'e·um)
pseudoxanthoma elasticum
   (soo'do·zan·tho'mah e·las'tĭ·kum)
psilosis (si·lo'sis)
psittacosis (sit·ah·ko'sis)
psoas (so'as)
psoralen (sor'ah·len)

psoriasis (so·ri'ah·sis)
psoriatic (so·re·at'ik)
psyche (si'ke)
psychiatric (si·ke·at'rik)
psychiatrist (si·ki'ah·trist)
psychiatry (si·ki'ah·tre)
psychic (si'kik)
psycho (si'ko)
psychoanalysis (si'ko·ah·nal'ĭ·is)
psychoanalyst (si'ko·an'ah·list)
psychodysleptic (si'ko·dis·lep'tik)
psychogenesis (si'ko·jen'ĕ·sis)
psychogeriatrics (si'ko·jer'e·at'riks)
psychology (si·kol'o·je)
psychoneurosis (si'ko·nu·ro'sēz)
psychopath (si'ko·path)
psychopathy (si·kop'ah·the)
psychopharmaceuticals
   (si'ko·fahr'mah·su'tĭ·kalz)
psychopharmacology
   (si'ko·fahr'mah·kol'o·je)
psychosexual (si'ko·seks'u·al)
psychosis (si·ko'sis)
psychosomatic (si'ko·so·mat'ik)
psychosurgery (si'ko·ser'jer·e)
psychotherapy (si'ko·ther'ah·pe)
psychotic (si·kot'ik)
psychotomimetic (si·kot'o·mi·met'ik)
psychotropic (si·ko·trop'ik)
pterion (te're·on)
pterygium (tĕ·rij'e·um)
pterygoid (ter'ĭ·goid)
ptomaine (to'mān)
ptosis (to'sis)
ptotic (tot'ik)
ptyalin (ti'ah·lin)
pubarche (pu·bar'ke)
puberal (pu'ber·al)
pubertal (pu'ber·tal)
puberty (pu'ber·te)
pubes (pu'bēz)
pubescence (pu·bes'ens)
pubescent (pu·bes'ent)
pubis (pu'bis)
pubomadesis (pu'bo·mah'de·sis)
pudenda (pu·den'dah)
pudendum (pu·den'dum)
puerile (pu'er·il)
puerpera (pu·er'per·ah)
puerperium (pu'er·pe're·um)
Pulex irritans (pul'leks ir'ĭ·tanz)
pulmonary (pul'mo·ner'e)
pulmonic (pul·mon'ik)
pulpectomy (pul·pek'to·me)
pulpitis (pul·pi'tis)
pulpotomy (pul·pot'o·me)
pulsimeter (pul·sim'ĕ·ter)
puncta (punk'tah)
punctum (punk'tum)
puncture (punk'chur)
purgation (pur·ga'shun)
purine (pu·rēn)
Purkinje (pur·kin'je)
purpura (pur'pu·rah)
purulence (pu'roo·lens)
purulency (pu'roo·len'se)
purulent (pu'roo·lent)
pustular (pus'tu·lar)
pustulation (pus'tu·la'shun)
pustule (pus'tūl)
putamen (pu·ta'men)
putrefaction (pu'trĕ·fak'shun)
putrefactive (pu'trĕ·fak'tiv)
pyarthrosis (pi'ar·thro'sis)
pyelectasia (pi'ĕ·lek·ta'ze·ah)
pyelogram (pi'ĕ·lo·gram)
pyelography (pi'ĕ·log'rah·fe)
pyelolithotomy (pi'ĕ·lo·li·thot'o·me)
pyelonephritis (pi'ĕ·lo·nĕ·fri'tis)
pyelonephrolithotomy
   (pi'ĕ·lo·nef'ro·li·thot'o·me
pyeloplasty (pi'ĕ·lo·plas'te)
pyeloscopy (pi'ĕ·los·ko·pe)
pyelostomy (pi'ĕ·los'to·me)
pyelotomy (pi'ĕ·lot'o·me)
pyemia (pi·e'me·ah)
Pyemotes ventricosus
   (pi·ĕ·mo'tez ven·tri·ko'sus)
pyesis (pi·e'sis)

pyknic (pik'nik)
pyknomorphous (pik'no·mor'fus)
pyknosis (pik·no'sis)
pylephlebitis (pi'le·fle·bi'tis)
pylethrombophlebitis
   (pi'le·throm'bo·fle·bi'tis)
pylethrombosis (pi'le·throm·bo'sis)
pyloric (pi·lor'ik)
pyloristenosis (pi·lor'ĭ·stĕ·no'sis)
pylorogastrectomy
   (pi·lo'ro·gas·trek'to·me)
pyloromyotomy (pi·lo'ro·mi·ot'o·me)
pyloroplasty (pi·lo'ro·plas'te)
pylorospasm (pi·lo'ro·spazm)
pylorus (pi·lo'rus)
pyocele (pi'o·sēl)
pyoderma gangrenosum
   (pi'o·der'mah gang'gre·no'sum)
pyogenic (pi'o·jen'ik)
pyohemothorax (pi'o·he'mo·tho'raks)
pyolabyrinthitis (pi'o·lab'ĭ·rin·thi'tis)
pyomyositis (pi'o·mi'o·si'tis)
pyonephrolithiasis
   (pi'o·nef'ro·li·thi'ah·sis)
pyonephrosis (pi'o·nĕ·fro'sis)
pyopericarditis (pi'o·per'ĭ·kar·di'tis)
pyoperitonitis (pi'o·per'ĭ·to·ni'tis)
pyopneumopericardium
   (pi'o·nu'mo·per'ĭ·kar'de·um)
pyopneumoperitoneum
   (pi'o·nu'mo·per'ĭ·to·ne'um)
pyopneumothorax (pi'o·nu'mo·tho'raks)
pyopoiesis (pi'o·poi·e'sis)
pyorrhea (pi'o·re'ah)
pyosalpinx (pi'o·sal'pinks)
pyramid (pēr'ah·mid)
pyramidal (pĭ·ram'ĭ·dal)
pyretic (pi·ret'ik)
pyrexia (pi·rek'se·ah)
pyridine (pēr'ĭ·dēn)
pyridoxal (pēr'ĭ·dok'sal)
pyridoxine (pēr'ĭ·dok'sēn)
pyrimidine (pi·rim'ĭ·dēn)
pyrogallol (pi'ro·gal'ol)
pyrogen (pi'ro·jen)
pyrolysis (pi·rol'ĭ·sis)
pyrophosphate (pi'ro·fos'fāt)
pyrosis (pi·ro'sis)
pyrrole (pēr'ol)
pyruvate (pi'roo·vāt)
pyuria (pi·u're·ah)

Q

quadrant (kwahd'rant)
quadrantanopsia
   (kwahd'ran·tah·nop'se·ah)
quadrate (kwahd'rāt)
quadriceps (kwahd'rĭ·seps)
quadrigeminal (kwahd'rĭ·jem'ĭ·nal)
quadrilocular (kwahd'rĭ·lok'u·lar)
quadripara (kwahd·rip'ah·rah)
quadriplegia (kwahd'rĭ·ple'je·ah)
quadriplegic (kwahd'ĭ·ple'jik)
quadrivalent (kwahd'rĭ·va'lent)
quantitative (kwahn'tĭ·ta·tiv)
quaque hora (kwah'ke ho'rah)
quarantine (kwor'an·tēn)
quartan (kwor'tan)
quartile (kwor'tīl)
quasidominance (kwa'zi·dom'ĭ·nans)
quaternary (kwah'ter·ner'e)
Queckenstedt (kwek'en·stet)
quenching (kwench'ing)
quinacrine (kwin'ah·krin)
quinhydrone (kwin·hi'drōn)
quinidine (kwin'ĭ·din)
quinine (kwi'nīn)
quinone (kwi·nōn')
quinquina (kin·ke'nah)
quinsy (kwin'ze)
quintipara (kwin·tip'ah·rah)
quotidian (kwo·tid'e·an)
quotient (kwo'shent)

R

rabid (rab'id)
rabies (ra'bēz)
racemic (ra·se'mik)
racemose (ras'e·mōs)
rachicentesis (ra'ke·sen·te'sis)
rachiopathy (ra'ke·op'ah·the)
rachiotome (ra'ke·o·tōm)
rachiotomy (ra'ke·ot'o·me)
rachischisis (ra·kis'kǐ·sis)
rachitis (ra·ki'tis)
rachitogenic (rah·kit'o·jen'ik)
radarkymography (ra'dar·ki·mog'rah·fe)
radectomy (ra·dek'to·me)
radial (ra'de·al)
radiation (ra·de·a'shun)
radical (rad'ǐ·kal)
radiculalgia (rah·dik'u·lal'je·ah)
radicular (rah·dik'u·lar)
radiculectomy (rah·dik'u·lek'to·me)
radiculomyelopathy
    (rah·dik'u·lo·mi'ě·lop'ah·the)
radiculoneuropathy
    (rah·dik'u·lo·nu·rop'ah·the)
radioactivity (ra·de·o·ak·tiv'ǐ·te)
radiobiology (ra'de·o·bi·ol'o·je)
radiodermatitis (ra'de·o·der·mah·ti'tis)
radioepidermitis (ra'de·o·ep'ǐ·der·mi'tis)
radiofrequency (ra'de·o·fre'kwen·se)
radiograph (ra'de·o·graf')
radiography (ra'de·og'rah·fe)
radioimmunoassay
    (ra·de·o·im'u·no·as'a)
radioimmunodiffusion
    (ra'de·o·im'u·no·dif·fu'zhun)
radioimmunoelectrophoresis
    (ra·de·o·im'u·no·e·lek'tro·fo·re'sis)
radioiodine (ra'de·o·i'o·dīn)
radioisotope (ra'de·o·i'so·tōp)
radioligand (ra'de·o·li'gand)
radiology (ra'de·ol'o·je)
radiolucency (ra'de·o·lu'sen·se)
radiomimetic (ra'de·o·mi·met'ik)
radionuclide (ra'de·o·nu'klīd)
radiopacity (ra'de·o·pas'ǐ·te)
radiopaque (ra'de·o·pāk')
radiopelvimetry (ra'de·o·pel·vim'ě·tre)
radioreceptor (ra'de·o·re·sep'tor)
radioscopy (ra'de·os'ko·pe)
radiotherapy (ra'de·o·ther'ah·pe)
radiothermy (ra'de·o·ther'me)
radioulnar (ra'de·o·ul'nar)
radium (ra'de·um)
radius (ra'de·us)
radix (ra'diks)
radon (ra'don)
rale (rahl)
rami (ra'mi)
ramose (ra'mos)
ramous (ra'mus)
ramus (ra'mus)
ranine (ra'nīn)
ranula (ran'u·lah)
raphe (ra'fe)
raptus (rap'tus)
rarefaction (rār'ě·fak'shun)
raspatory (ras'pah·to·re)
rauwolfia serpentina
    (raw·wol'fe·ah ser·pen·ti'nah)
Raynaud (ra·nō')
reabsorption (re'ab·sorp'shun)
reagin (re'ah·jin)
rebase (re·bās')
recanalization (re·kan·al·ǐ·za'shun)
receptaculum (re'sep·tak'u·lum)
receptor (re·sep'tor)
recess (re'ses)
recessive (re·ses'iv)
recidivation (re·sid'ǐ·va'shun)
Recklinghausen (rek'ling·how'zen)
recombination (re'kom·bǐ·na'shun)
recon (re'kon)
recrement (rek'rě·ment)
recruitment (re·kroot'ment)
rectoabdominal (rek'to·ab·dom'ǐ·nal)

rectocele (rek'to·sēl)
rectosigmoid (rek'to·sig'moid)
rectourethral (rek'to·u·re'thral)
rectouterine (rek'to·u'ter·in)
rectovaginal (rek'to·vaj'ǐ·nal)
rectovesical (rek'to·ves'ǐ·kal)
rectum (rek'tum)
recumbent (re·kum'bent)
recuperate (re·ku'per·āt)
recurrence (re·kur'ens)
recurvation (re'kur·va'shun)
redox (red'oks)
reducible (re·du'sǐ·bl)
reductase (re·duk'tās)
reduction (re·duk'shun)
reflection (re·flek'shun)
reflex (re'fleks)
reflux (re'fluks)
refraction (re·frak'shun)
refractometer (re'frak·tom'ě·ter)
refractory (re·frak'to·re)
refracture (re·frak'chur)
refusion (re·fu'zhun)
regeneration (re·jen'er·a'shun)
regimen (rej'ǐ·men)
regression (re·gresh'un)
regurgitation (re·gur'jǐ·ta'shun)
rehabilitation (re'hah·bil'ǐ·ta'shun)
rehalation (re'hah·la'shun)
reimplantation (re'im·plan·ta'shun)
reinfection (re'in·fek'shun)
reinnervation (re'in·er·va'shun)
relapse (re·laps')
relaxant (re·lak'sant)
relaxin (re·lak'sin)
remediable (re·me'de·ah·bl)
remedy (rem'ě·de)
remission (re·mish'un)
remittent (re·mit'ent)
renal (re'nal)
renaturation (re·na'chur·a'shun)
renin (re'nin)
rennet (ren'et)
rennin (ren'in)
renography (re·nog'rah·fe)
renomegaly (re'·no meg'ah·le)
renovascular (re'no·vas'ku·lar)
reoviruses (re'o·vi'rus·ez)
repellent (re·pel'ent)
replantation (re·plan·ta'shun)
replication (rep'lǐ·ka'shun)
repolarization (re·po'lar·ǐ·za'shun)
repression (re·presh'un)
repressor (re·pres'or)
reproduction (re·pro·duk'shun)
repulsion (re·pul'shun)
reradiation (re'ra·de·a'shun)
resect (re·sekt')
resectable (re·sek'tah·bl)
resection (re·sek'shun)
reserpine (res·er·pēn)
resident (rez'ǐ·dent)
residual (re·zid'u·al)
residue (rez'ǐ·du)
residuum (re·zid'u·um)
resilience (re·zil'e·ens)
resinous (rez'ǐ·nus)
resistance (re·zis'tans)
resolvent (re·zol'vent)
resonance (rez'o·nans)
resorcinol (rě·zor'sǐ·nol)
resorption (re·sorp'shun)
respiration (res'pǐ·ra'shun)
respirator (res'pǐ·ra'tor)
respiratory (res'pǐ·rah·to·re)
respire (rě·spīr')
restenosis (re'stě·no'sis)
restiform (res'tǐ·form)
restoration (res'to·ra'shun)
restraint (re·strānt')
resuscitation (re'sus'ǐ·ta'shun)
resuscitator (re·sus'ǐ·ta'tor)
retardate (re·tar'dāt)
retardation (re'tar·da'shun)
rete (re'te)
retention (re·ten'shun)
reticulin (rě·tik'u·lin)

reticulocyte (rě·tik'u·lo·sīt')
reticulocytopenia
    (rě·tik'u·lo·si·to·pe'ne·ah)
reticuloendothelial
    (rě·tik'u·lo·en'do·the'le·al)
reticuloendothelioma
    (rě·tik'u·lo·en'do·the·le·o'mah)
reticuloendothelium
    (rě·tik'u·lo·en'do·the'le·um)
reticulum (rě·tik'u·lum)
retina (ret'ǐ·nah)
retinacula (ret'ǐ·nak'u·lah)
retinaculum (ret'ǐ·nak'u·lum)
retinitis (ret'ǐ·ni'tis)
retinoblastoma (ret'ǐ·no·blas·to'mah)
retinochoroiditis (ret'ǐ·no·ko·roi·di'tis)
retinoic (ret'ǐ·no'ik)
retinoid (ret'ǐ·noid)
retinomalacia (ret'ǐ·no·mah·la'she·ah)
retinopathy (ret'ǐ·nop'ah·the)
retinopiesis (ret'ǐ·no·pi·e'sis)
retinoscope (ret'ǐ·no·skōp')
retinoscopy (ret'ǐ·nos'ko·pe)
retractile (re·trak'til)
retroflexion (ret'ro·flek'shun)
retrognathia (ret'ro·nath'e·ah)
retrograde (ret'ro·grād)
retroillumination (ret'ro·ǐ·lu'mǐ·na'shun)
retrolental (ret'ro·len'tal)
retromandibular (ret'ro·man·dib'u·lar)
retroperitoneal (ret'ro·per'ǐ·to·ne'al)
retroperitoneum (ret'ro·per'ǐ·to·ne'um)
retrosternal (ret'ro·ster'nal)
retrouterine (ret'ro·u'ter·in)
retroversion (ret'ro·ver'zhun)
retrovirus (ret'ro·vi'rus)
reunient (re·u'ne·ent)
reversion (re·ver'zhun)
Reye (ri)
rhabdomyolysis (rab'do·mi·ol'ǐ·sis)
rhabdomyoma (rab'do·mi·o'mah)
rhabdomyosarcoma
    (rab'do·mi'o·sar·ko'mah)
rhagades (rag'ah·dēz)
rhagadiform (ra·gad'ǐ·form)
rhenium (re'ne·um)
rheobase (re'o·bās)
rheostat (re'o·stat)
rheotaxis (re'o·tak'sis)
rhesus (re'sus)
rheumatic (roo·mat'ik)
rheumatid (roo'mah·tid)
rheumatism (roo'mah·tizm)
rheumatoid (roo'mah·toid)
rhinalgia (ri·nal'je·ah)
rhinencephalon (ri'nen·sef'ah·lon)
rhineurynter (ri'nu·rin'ter)
rhinitis (ri·ni'tis)
rhinochiloplasty (ri'no·ki'lo·plas'te)
rhinodacryolith (ri'no·dak're·o·lith)
rhinokyphosis (ri'no·ki·fo'sis)
rhinolith (ri'no·lith)
rhinology (ri·nol'o·je)
rhinomycosis (ri'no·mi·ko'sis)
rhinopathy (ri·nop'ah·the)
rhinopharyngitis (ri'no·far'in·ji'tis)
rhinophyma (ri'no·fi'mah)
rhinoplasty (ri'no·plas'te)
rhinorrhea (ri'no·re'ah)
rhinosalpingitis (ri'no·sal·pin·ji'tis)
rhinoscleroma (ri'no·skle·ro'mah)
rhinoscope (ri'no·skōp)
rhinostenosis (ri'no·stě·no'sis)
Rhinovirus (ri'no·vi'rus)
rhizome (ri'zōm)
rhizomeningomyelitis
    (ri'zo·mě·nin'go·mi'ě·li'tis)
rhizotomy (ri·zot'o·me)
rhodopsin (ro·dop'sin)
rhombencephalon (rom'ben·sef'ah·lon)
rhombocele (rom'bo·sēl)
rhomboid (rom'boid)
rhonchus (rong'kus)
Rhus (rus)
rhytidoplasty (rit'ǐ·do·plas'te)
riboflavin (ri'bo·fla'vin)
ribonuclease (ri'bo·nu'kle·ās)

ribonucleic (ri'bo·nu·kle'ik)
ribonucleoprotein
 (ri'bo·nu'kle·o·pro'te·in)
ribonucleoside (ri'bo·nu'kle·o·sīd)
ribonucleotide (ri'bo·nu'kle·o·tīd)
ribose (ri'bōs)
ribosome (ri'bo·sōm)
riboviruses (ri'bo·vi'rus·ez)
ricin (ri'sin)
rickets (rik'ets)
Rickettsia (rĭ·ket'se·ah)
rickettsiosis (rĭ·ket'se·o'sis)
rigidity (rĭ·jid'ĭ·te)
rigor mortis (rig'or mor'tis)
rima (ri'mah)
ristocetin (ris'to·se'tin)
riziform (riz'ĭ·form)
roentgen (rent'gen)
roentgenism (rent'gen·izm)
roentgenkymography
 (rent'gen·ki·mog'rah·fe)
roentgenogram (rent·gen'o·gram')
roentgenography (rent'gen·og'rah·fe)
roentgenologist (rent'gĕ·nol'o·jist)
roentgenology (rent'gĕ·nol'o·je)
roentgenometry (rent'gĕ·nom'ĕ·tre)
roentgenoscopy (rent'gĕ·nos'ko·pe)
rongeur (rawn·zhur')
Rorschach (ror'shahk)
rosacea (ro·za'she·ah)
rosanilin (ro·zan'ĭ·lin)
roseola (ro·ze'o·lah)
rostellum (ros·tel'um)
rostrad (ros'trad)
rostral (ros'tral)
rotation (ro·ta'shun)
rotator (ro'ta·tor)
roughage (ruf'ij)
Roux-en-Y (roo en wi)
rubefacient (roo'bĕ·fa'shent)
rubella (roo·bel'ah)
rubeola (roo·be'o·lah)
Rubivirus (roo'bĭ·vi'rus)
Ruffini (roo·fe'ne)
ruga (roo'gah)
rugae (roo'je)
rugose (roo'gōs)
rugosity (roo·gos'ĭ·te)
ruminant (roo'mĭ·nant)
rumination (roo'mĭ·na'shun)
rupture (rup'chur)

S

saccharide (sak'ah·rīd)
saccharin (sak'ah·rin)
saccule (sak'ūl)
sacral (sa'ral)
sacralgia (sa·kral'je·ah)
sacrectomy (sa·krek'to·me)
sacrococcygeal (sa'kro·kok·sij'e·al)
sacroiliac (sa'kro·il'e·ak)
sacrum (sa'krum)
sadism (sa'dizm)
sadomasochism (sa'do·mas'o·kizm)
sagittal (saj'ĭ·tal)
salicylamide (sal'ĭ·sil·am'īd)
salicylate (sal'ĭ·sil'āt)
salicylazosulfapyridine
 (sal'ĭ·sil'ah·zo·sul'fah·pir'ĭ·dēn)
salicylic (sal'ĭ·sil'ik)
salient (sa'le·ent)
saline (sa'lēn)
saliva (sah·li'vah)
salivant (sal'ĭ·vant)
salivary (sal'ĭ·ver·e)
salivate (sal'ĭ·vāt)
salivation (sal'ĭ·va'shun)
Salmonella (sal'mo·nel'ah)
salmonellosis (sal'mo·nel·o'sis)
salpingectomy (sal'pin·jek'to·me)
salpingemphraxis (sal'pin·jem·frak'sis)
salpingian (sal·pin'je·an)
salpingitis (sal'pin·ji'tis)
salpingocele (sal·ping'go·sēl)
salpingocyesis (sal'ping·go·si·e'sis)

salpingography (sal'ping·gog'rah·fe)
salpingolysis (sal'ping·gol'ĭ·sis)
salpingo-oophorectomy
 (sal·ping'go·o'of·o·rek'to·me)
salpingo-oophoritis
 (sal·ping'go·o'of·o·ri'tis)
salpingo-oothecitis
 (sal·ping'go·o'o·the·si'tis)
salpingoperitonitis
 (sal·ping'go·per'ĭ·to·ni'tis)
salpingopharyngeal
 (sal·ping'go·fah·rin'je·al)
salpingostomy (sal'ping·gos'to·me)
salpinx (sal'pinks)
salubrious (sah·lu'bre·us)
saluretic (sal'u·ret'ik)
salve (sav)
sanatorium (san'ah·to're·um)
sanguineous (sang·gwin'e·us)
sanguinolent (sang·gwin'o·lent)
sanguinopurulent
 (sang'gwĭ·no·pu'roo·lent)
sanitarium (san'ĭ·ta're·um)
sanitary (san'ĭ·ta're)
sanitation (san·i·ta'shun)
saphenectomy (saf'ĕ·nek'to·me)
saphenous (sah·fe'nus)
saponification (sah·pon'ĭ·fĭ·ka'shun)
saprogenic (sap'ro·jen'ik)
saprophytic (sap'ro·fit'ik)
saprozoic (sap'ro·zo'ik)
sarcocele (sar'ko·sēl)
sarcoid (sar'koid)
sarcoidosis (sar'koi·do'sis)
sarcolemma (sar'ko·lem'ah)
sarcoma (sar·ko'mah)
sarcomatous (sar·ko'mah·tus)
sarcomere (sar'ko·mēr)
sarcoplasm (sar'ko·plazm)
sarcosome (sar'ko·sōm)
sarcostosis (sar'kos·to'sis)
saturate (sach'ĕ·rāt)
saturnism (sat'ur·nizm)
satyriasis (sat'ĭ·ri'ah·sis)
sauriasis (saw·ri'ah·sis)
scabicide (ska'bĭ·sīd)
scabies (ska'bēz)
scalene (ska'lēn)
scalpel (skal'pl)
scaphocephalism (skaf'o·sef'ah·lizm)
scapula (skap'u·lah)
scarification (skar'ĭ·fĭ·ka'shun)
scarlatina (skahr'lah·te'nah)
scatology (skah·tol'o·je)
scatoma (skah·to'mah)
schistocystis (shis'to·sis'tis)
schistocyte (shis'to·sīt)
schistocytosis (shis'to·si·to'sis)
Schistosoma (shis'to·so'mah)
schistosomiasis (shis'to·so·mi'ah·sis)
schizogony (skĭ·zog'o·ne)
schizoid (skiz'oid)
Schizomycetes (skiz'o·mi·se'tēz)
schizont (skiz'ont)
schizophasia (skiz'o·fa'ze·ah)
schizophrenia (skiz'o·fre'ne·ah)
schizotrichia (skiz'o·trik'e·ah)
sciage (se·azh')
sciatic (si·at'ik)
sciatica (si·at'ĭ·kah)
scinticisternography
 (sin'tĭ·sis·ter·nog'rah·fe)
scintillation (sin'tĭ·la'shun)
scintillator (sin'tĭ·la'tor)
scintiscan (sin'tĭ·skan)
scirrhoid (skir'oid)
scirrhous (skir'us)
scirrhus (skir'us)
sclera (skle'rah)
sclerectomy (skle·rek'to·me)
scleredema (skle'rĕ·de'mah)
scleritis (skle·ri'tis)
sclerodactyly (skle'ro·dak'tĭ·le)
scleroderma (skle'ro·der'mah)
sclerodermatitis (skle'ro·der'mah·ti'tis)
scleroiritis (skle'ro·i·ri'tis)
scleroma (skle·ro'mah)
scleromalacia (skle'ro·mah·la'she·ah)

scleronychia (skle'ro·nik'e·ah)
sclero-oophoritis (skle'ro·o·of'o·ri'tis)
sclerophthalmia (skle'rof·thal'me·ah)
scleroplasty (skle'ro·plas'te)
sclerosis (skle·ro'sis)
sclerostomy (skle·ros'to·me)
sclerotic (skle·rot'ik)
sclerotome (skle'ro·tōm)
sclerous (skle'rus)
scoleces (sko'lĕ·sēz)
scolex (sko'leks)
scoliosis (sko'le·o'sis)
scopolamine (sko·pol'ah·mēn)
scotochromogens (sko'to·kro'mo·jenz)
scotoma (sko·to'mah)
scotopic (sko·top'ik)
scrapie (skra'pe)
scrofula (skrof'u·lah)
scrotectomy (skro·tek'to·me)
scrotitis (skro·ti'tis)
scrotocele (skro'to·sēl)
scrotum (skro'tum)
scurvy (skur've)
scybalum (sib'ah·lum)
sebaceous (sĕ·ba'shus)
seborrhea (seb'o·re'ah)
sebum (se'bum)
secobarbital (se'ko·bar'bĭ·tal)
secretagogue (se·krēt'ah·gog)
secrete (se·krēt')
secretin (se·kre'tin)
secretion (se·kre'shun)
secretory (se·kre'to·re)
secundigravida (se·kun'dĭ·grav'ĭ·dah)
secundines (se·kun'dīnz)
secundipara (se'kun·dip'ah·rah)
sedate (se·dāt')
sedation (se·da'shun)
sedative (sed'ah·tiv)
sediment (sed'ĭ·ment)
sedimentation (sed'ĭ·men·ta'shun)
segmentation (seg'men·ta'shun)
seizure (se'zhur)
selenium (sĕ·le'ne·um)
semelincident (sem'el·in'sĭ·dent)
semen (se'men)
semenuria (se'mĕ·nu're·ah)
semicomatose (sem'e·ko'mah·tōs)
semiconscious (sem'e·kon'shus)
seminiferous (se'mĭ·nif'er·us)
seminoma (se'mĭ·no'mah)
semipermeable (sem'e·per'me·ah·bl)
semisulcus (sem'e·sul'kus)
semisupination (sem'e·soo'pĭ·na'shun)
senile (se'nīl)
senilism (se'nīl·izm)
senility (sĕ·nil'ĭ·te)
sentiment (sen'tĭ·ment)
sepsis (sep'sis)
septa (sep'tah)
septal (sep'tal)
septectomy (sep·tek'to·me)
septicemia (sep'tĭ·se'me·ah)
septotomy (sep·tot'o·me)
septum (sep'tum)
sequel (se'kwel)
sequester (se·kwes'ter)
sequestration (se'kwes·tra'shun)
sera (se'rah)
serine (ser'ēn)
seriscission (ser'ĭ·sizh'un)
seroconversion (se'ro·kon·ver'shun)
serology (se·rol'o·je)
seroma (sēr·o'mah)
seromucous (se'ro·mu'kus)
serosa (se·ro'sah)
serosanguinous (se'ro·sang·gwin'e·us)
serosynovitis (se'ro·sin'o·vi'tis)
serotonin (ser'o·to'nin)
serous (se'rus)
serpiginous (ser·pij'ĭ·nus)
serpigo (ser·pi'go)
serration (sĕ·ra'shun)
serrefine (sār·fēn')
serum (se'rum)
serums (se'rumz)
sesamoid (ses'ah·moid)
sessile (ses'il)

sexuality (seks′u·al′ĭ·te)
Sezary (sa·zah·re′)
sheath (shēth)
Shigella (shĭ·gel′ah)
shigellosis (shĭ·gel·o′sis)
shingles (shing′glz)
shiver (shiv′er)
shock (shok)
sialadenitis (si′al·ad′ĕ·ni′tis)
sialectasis (si′al·ek·ta′sis)
sialic (si·al′ik)
sialoadenectomy
  (si′ah·lo·ad′ĕ·nek′to·me)
sialoangiectasis (si′ah·lo·an′je·ek′tah·sis)
sialoangiitis (si′ah·lo·an′je·i′tis)
sialodochitis (si′ah·lo·do·ki′tis)
sialogogue (si·al′o·gog)
sialogram (si·al′o·gram)
sialography (si′ah·log′rah·fe)
sialolith (si·al′o·lith)
sialolithiasis (si′ah·lo·lĭ·thi′ah·sis)
sialolithotomy (si′ah·lo·lĭ·thot′o·me)
sialorrhea (si′ah·lo·re′ah)
sialoschesis (si′ah·los′kĕ·sis)
sialosyrinx (si′ah·lo·si′rinks)
sibilus (sib′ĭ·lus)
sibling (sib′ling)
siccant (sik′ant)
siderocyte (sid′er·o·sīt)
sideroderma (sid′er·o·der′mah)
siderofibrosis (sid′er·o·fi·bro′sis)
sideropenia (sid′er·o·pe′ne·ah)
siderosis (sid′er·o′sis)
sigmoid (sig′moid)
sigmoidectomy (sig′moi·dek′to·me)
sigmoidopexy (sig·moi′do·pek′se)
sigmoidoscope (sig·moi′do·skōp)
sigmoidoscopy (sig′moi·dos′ko·pe)
sigmoidotomy (sig′moi·dot′o·me)
silica (sil′ĭ·kah)
silicious (si·lish′us)
silicon (sil′ĭ·kon)
silicone (sil′ĭ·kōn)
silicosis (sil′ĭ·ko′sis)
simulation (sim′u·la′shun)
simulator (sim′u·la′tor)
Simulium (si·mu′le·um)
sinciptal (sin·sip′ĭ·tal)
sinciput (sin′si·put)
sinister (sin·is′ter)
sinoatrial (si′no·a′tre·al)
sinus (si′nus)
sinusitis (si′nŭ·si′tis)
sinusoid (si′nŭ·soid)
siphon (si′fun)
Sjogren (sho′gren)
skeletal (skel′ĕ·tal)
skeleton (skel′ĕ·ton)
slough (sluf)
smegma (smeg′mah)
sodium (so′de·um)
sodomy (sod′o·me)
Solanaceae (so′lah·na′se·e)
solanaceous (so′lah·na′shus)
solidus (sol′ĭ·dus)
somatogenic (so′mah·to·jen′ik)
somatology (so′mah·tol′o·je)
somatomedin (so′mah·to·me′din)
somatoplasm (so·mat′o·plazm)
somatostatin (so′mah·to·stat′in)
somatotherapy (so′mah·to·ther′ah·pe)
somatotonia (so′mah·to′ne·ah)
somatotropic (so′mah·to·trop′ik)
somatotropin (so′mah·to·tro′pin)
somatotype (so·mat′o·tīp)
somite (so′mīt)
somnambulism (som·nam′bu·lizm)
somniloquism (som·nil′o·kwizm)
somnolence (som′no·lens)
somnolent (som′no·lent)
sopor (so′por)
sorbitol (sor′bĭ·tol)
souffle (soof′fl)
sparganum (spar′gah·num)
spargosis (spar·go′sis)
spasm (spazm)
spasmodic (spaz·mod′ik)
spasmogenic (spaz′mo·jen′ik)

spasmolysis (spaz·mol′ĭ·sis)
spasmolytic (spaz′mo·lit′ik)
spastic (spas′tik)
spasticity (spas·tis′ĭ·te)
spatula (spach′ŭ·lah)
spay (spa)
species (spe′shēz)
specificity (spes′ĭ·fis′ĭ·te)
specimen (spes′ĭ·men)
spectrometer (spek·trom′ĕ·ter)
spectrophotometer (spek′tro·fo·tom′ĕ·ter)
spectroscope (spek′tro·skōp)
spectrum (spek′trum)
speculum (spek′u·lum)
spermatic (sper·mat′ik)
spermatid (sper′mah·tid)
spermatocele (sper′mah·to·sēl)
spermatocide (sper′mah·to·sīd)
spermatocyst (sper′mah·to·sist′)
spermatocystectomy
  (sper′mah·to·sis·tek′to·me)
spermatocyte (sper′mah·to·sīt)
spermatogenesis (sper′mah·to·jen′ĕ·sis)
spermatogonium (sper′mah·to·go′ne·um)
spermatolysin (sper′mah·tol′ĭ·sin)
spermatolysis (sper′mah·tol′ĭ·sis)
spermatorrhea (sper′mah·to·re′ah)
spermatoschesis (sper′mah·tos′kĕ·sis)
spermatozoa (sper′mah·to·zo′ah)
spermatozoon (sper′mah·to·zo′on)
spermiation (sper′me·a′shun)
spermiogenesis (sper′me·o·jen′ĕ·sis)
spermolith (sper′mo·lith)
sphenoid (sfe′noid)
spherocyte (sfēr′o·sīt)
spherocytosis (sfēr′o·si·to′sis)
spherule (sfēr′ūl)
sphincter (sfingk′ter)
sphincteralgia (sfingk′ter·al′je·ah)
sphincteritis (sfingk′ter·i′tis)
sphincterotomy (sfingk′ter·ot′o·me)
sphingolipid (sfing′go·lip′id)
sphingolipidosis (sfing′go·lip′ĭ·do′sis)
sphingomyelin (sfing′go·mi′ĕ·lin)
sphygmography (sfig·mog′rah·fe)
sphygmoscope (sfig′mo·skōp)
spica (spi′kah)
spicule (spik′ūl)
spina (spi′nah)
spinae (spi′ne)
spinal (spi′nal)
spindle (spin′dl)
spine (spīn)
spinnbarkeit (spin′bahr·kīt)
spiradenoma (spi′rad·ĕ·no′mah)
spirillosis (spi′rĭ·lo′sis)
Spirillum (spi·ril′um)
spirochete (spi′ro·kēt)
spirochetosis (spi′ro·ke·to′sis)
spirometer (spi·rom′ĕ·ter)
spironolactone (spi·ro′no·lak′tōn)
spissated (spis′āt·ed)
splanchnectopia (splank′nek·to′pe·ah)
splanchnic (splank′nik)
splanchnicectomy (splank′nĕ·sek′to·me)
splanchnicotomy (splank′nĕ·kot′o·me)
splanchnocele (splank′no·sēl)
spleen (splēn)
splenectomy (sple·nek′to·me)
splenic (splen′ik)
splenitis (sple·ni′tis)
splenium (sple′ne·um)
splenocele (sple′no·sēl)
splenohepatomegaly
  (sple′no·hep′ah·to·meg′ah·le)
splenolysis (sple·nol′ĭ·sis)
splenomalacia (sple′no·mah·la′she·ah)
splenomegaly (sple′no·meg′ah·le)
splenopathy (sple·nop′ah·the)
splenoptosis (sple·nop·to′sis)
splenorrhagia (sple′no·ra′je·ah)
splenosis (sple·no′sis)
splenotomy (sple·not′o·me)
splenotoxin (sple′no·tok′sin)
spodogenous (spo·doj′ĕ·nus)
spodophagous (spo·dof′ah·jus)
spondylarthritis (spon′dil·ar·thri′tis)
spondylitis (spon′dĭ·li′tis)

spondylolisthesis (spon′dĭ·lo·lis′the·sis)
spondylolysis (spon′dĭ·lol′ĭ·sis)
spondylopathy (spon′dĭ·lop′ah·the)
spondyloschisis (spon′dĭ·los′kĭ·sis)
spondylosis (spon′dĭ·lo′sis)
spongiocyte (spun′je·o·sīt)
spontaneous (spon·ta′ne·us)
sporangia (spo·ran′je·ah)
sporangiophore (spo·ran′je·o·fōr)
sporangium (spo·ran′je·um)
sporicide (spo′rĭ·sīd)
sporotrichosis (spo′ro·tri·ko′sis)
sporozoan (spo′ro·zo′an)
sporulation (spōr′u·la′shun)
sprue (sproo)
sputa (spu′tah)
sputum (spu′tum)
squalene (skwal′ēn)
squamous (skwa′mus)
stabile (sta′bil)
stability (stah·bil′ĭ·te)
stabilizer (sta′bil·i′zer)
stammering (stam′er·ing)
stannic (stan′ik)
stannous (stan′us)
stapedectomy (sta′pĕ·dek′to·me)
stapedial (stah·pe′de·al)
stapediotenotomy
  (stah·pe′de·o·tĕ·not′o·me)
stapediovestibular
  (stah·pe′de·o·ves·tib′u·lar)
stapedius (sta·pe′de·us)
stapes (sta′pēz)
staphylococcal (staf′ĭ·lo·kok′al)
staphylococcemia
  (staf′ĭ·lo·kok·se′me·ah)
staphylococci (staf′ĭ·lo·kok′si)
staphylococcus (staf′ĭ·lo·kok′us)
staphyloderma (staf′ĭ·lo·der′mah)
staphylolysin (staf′ĭ·lol′ĭ·sin)
staphyloma (staf′ĭ·lo′mah)
staphyloplasty (staf′ĭ·lo·plas′te)
staphyloptosia (staf′ĭ·lop·to′se·ah)
staphyloptosis (staf′ĭ·lop·to′sis)
stasis (sta′sis)
statistics (stah·tis′tiks)
statoconia (stat′o·ko′ne·ah)
steapsin (ste·ap′sin)
stearate (ste′ah·rāt)
stearic (ste′ah·rik)
stearin (ste′ah·rin)
steatitis (ste′ah·ti′tis)
steatocryptosis (ste′ah·to·krip·to′sis)
steatocystoma (ste′ah·to·sis·to′mah)
steatogenous (ste′ah·toj′ĕ·nus)
steatolysis (ste′ah·tol′ĭ·sis)
steatoma (ste′ah·to′mah)
steatomatosis (ste′ah·to·mah·to′sis)
steatonecrosis (ste′ah·to·nĕ·kro′sis)
steatopathy (ste′ah·top′ah·the)
steatopygia (ste′ah·to·pij′e·ah)
steatorrhea (ste′ah·to·re′ah)
steatosis (ste′ah·to′sis)
stegnosis (steg·no′sis)
stellate (stel′āt)
stellectomy (stel·ek′to·me)
stenion (sten′e·on)
stenochoria (sten′o·ko′re·ah)
stenosis (stĕ·no′sis)
stenostomia (sten′o·sto′me·ah)
stenotic (stĕ·not′ik)
stercobilin (ster′ko·bi′lin)
stercolith (ster′ko·lith)
stercoraceous (ster′ko·ra′shus)
stereoarthrolysis (stēr′e·o·ar·throl′ĭ·sis)
stereocampimeter
  (stēr′e·o·kam·pim′ĕ·ter)
stereocilia (stēr′e·o·sil′e·ah)
stereoisomer (stēr′e·o·i′so·mer)
stereoisomerism (stēr′e·o·i·som′er·izm)
stereology (stēr′e·ol′o·je)
stereopsis (stēr′e·op′sis)
stereoroentgenography
  (stēr′e·o·rent′gen·og′rah·fe)
stereoscope (stēr′e·o·skōp)
stereotaxis (stēr′e·o·tak′sis)
stereotaxy (stēr′e·o·tak′se)
stereotypy (stēr′e·o·ti′pe)

sterile (ster'il)
sterility (ste·ril'ĭ·te)
sterilization (ster'ĭ·lĭ·za'shun)
sterilizer (ster'ĭ·līz'er)
sternal (ster'nal)
sternoclavicular (ster'no·klah·vik'u·lar)
sternocleidomastoid
   (ster'no·kli'do·mas'toid)
sternotomy (ster·not'o·me)
sternum (ster'num)
steroid (ste'roid)
steroidogenesis (ste·roi'do·jen'ĕ·sis)
sterol (ste'rol)
stethoscope (steth'o·skōp)
sthenometry (sthen·om'ĕ·tre)
stigma (stig'mah)
stigmata (stig'mah·tah)
stilbestrol (stil·bes'trol)
stimuli (stim'u·li)
stimulus (stim'u·lus)
stoichiometry (stoi'ke·om'ĕ·tre)
stomatalgia (sto'mah·tal'je·ah)
stomatitis (sto·mah·ti'tis)
stomatocyte (sto'mah·to·sīt)
stomatology (sto'mah·tol'o·je)
stomatomalacia
   (sto'mah·to·mah·la'she·ah)
stomatomycosis (sto'mah·to·mi·ko'sis)
stomatopathy (sto'mah·top'ah·the)
stomatorrhagia (sto'mah·to·ra'je·ah)
stomodeum (sto'mo·de'um)
strabismal (strah·biz'mal)
strabismus (strah·biz'mus)
strabotomy (strah·bot'o·me)
stramonium (strah·mo'ne·um)
strata (stra'tah)
stratum (stra'tum)
strephosymbolia (stref'o·sim·bo'le·ah)
strepitus (strep'ĭ·tus)
Streptobacillus (strep'to·bah·sil'us)
streptococcal (strep'to·kok'al)
streptococcemia (strep'to·kok·se'me·ah)
streptococci (strep'to·kok'si)
Streptococcus (strep'to·kok'us)
streptococcus (strep'to·kok'us)
streptodermatitis (strep'to·der·mah·ti'tis)
streptodornase (strep'to·dor'nās)
streptokinase (strep'to·ki'nās)
streptolysin (strep·tol'ĭ·sin)
Streptomyces (strep'to·mi'sēz)
streptomycete (strep'to·mi'sēt)
streptomycin (strep'to·mi'sin)
streptotrichosis (strep'to·tri·ko'sis)
stria (stri'ah)
striate (stri'āt)
stricture (strik'chur)
strident (stri'dent)
stridor (stri'dor)
strobila (stro·bi'lah)
strobilae (stro·bi'le)
strobolaryngoscope
   (stro'bo·lah·ring'go·skōp)
stroboscope (stro'bo·skōp)
stromuhr (strōm'oor)
Strongyloides (stron'jĭ·loi'dēz)
strongyloidiasis (stron'jĭ·loi·di'ah·sis)
strontium (stron'she·um)
strophanthin (stro·fan'thin)
struma (stroo'mah)
strumitis (stroo·mi'tis)
strychnine (strik'nīn)
strychninism (strik'nin·izm)
Strychnos (strik'nos)
stupefacient (stu'pĕ·fa'shent)
stupefaction (stu'pĕ·fak'shun)
stuporous (stu'por·us)
stuttering (stut'er·ing)
stye (sti)
stylet (sti'let)
styloglossus (sti'lo·glos'us)
stylus (sti'lus)
styptic (stip'tik)
subarachnoid (sub'ah·rak'noid)
subarcuate (sub·ar'ku·āt)
subareolar (sub'ah·re'o·lar)
subatomic (sub'ah·tom'ik)
subcapsular (sub·kap'su·lar)
subcarbonate (sub·kar'bo·nāt)

subcartilaginous (sub'kar·tĭ·laj'ĭ·nus)
subclavian (sub·kla've·an)
subclavicular (sub'klah·vik'u·lar)
subconjunctival (sub'kon·junk·ti'val)
subconscious (sub·kon'shus)
subcorneal (sub·kor'ne·al)
subcortex (sub·kor'teks)
subcostal (sub·kos'tal)
subcutaneous (sub'ku·ta'ne·us)
subcutis (sub·ku'tis)
subdural (sub·du'ral)
subfamily (sub·fam'ĭ·le)
subfertility (sub'fer·til'ĭ·te)
sublation (sub·la'shun)
sublethal (sub·le'thal)
sublimate (sub'lĭ·mat)
sublimation (sub'lĭ·ma'shun)
subliminal (sub·lim'ĭ·nal)
sublingual (sub·ling'gwal)
subluxation (sub'luk·sa'shun)
submandibular (sub'man·dib'u·lar)
submaxillary (sub·mak'sĭ·ler'e)
suboccipital (sub'ok·sip'ĭ·tal)
subphylum (sub·fi'lum)
subscapular (sub·skap'u·lar)
subscription (sub·skrip'shun)
substernal (sub·ster'nal)
substitution (sub'stĭ·tu'shun)
substrate (sub'strāt)
substratum (sub·stra'tum)
subthalamus (sub·thal'ah·mus)
subungual (sub·ung'gwal)
subvirile (sub·vir'il)
subvitrinal (sub·vit'rĭ·nal)
subvolution (sub·vo·lu'shun)
succagogue (suk'ah·gog)
succedaneum (suk'sĕ·da'ne·um)
succinic (suk·sin'ik)
succinylcholine (suk'sĭ·nil·ko'lēn)
succinyl (suk'sĭ·nil)
succorrhea (suk·o·re'ah)
succussion (sŭ·kush'un)
sucrose (su'krōs)
sudoresis (su'do·re'sis)
sudoriferous (su'do·rif'er·us)
sudorific (su'do·rif'ik)
suffocate (suf'o·kāt')
suffusion (sŭ·fu'zhun)
sulci (sul'ki)
sulcus (sul'kus)
sulfa (sul'fah)
sulfadiazine (sul'fah·di'ah·zēn)
sulfamerazine (sul'fah·mer'ah·zēn)
sulfamethazine (sul'fah·meth'ah·zēn)
sulfanilamide (sul'fah·nil'ah·mīd)
sulfate (sul'fāt)
sulfhemoglobin (sulf'he·mo·glo'bin)
sulfhemoglobinemia
   (sulf'he·mo·glo'bin·e'me·ah)
sulfide (sul'fīd)
sulfisoxazole (sul'fĭ·sok'sah·zōl)
sulfmethemoglobin
   (sulf'met·he'mo·glo'bin)
sulfobromophthalein
   (sul'fo·bro'mo·thal'e·in)
sulfonamides (sul·fon'ah·mīdz)
sulfonylurea (sul'fon·il·u·re'ah)
sulfosalicylic (sul'fo·sal'ĭ·sil'ik)
sulfur (sul'fur)
sulfuric (sul·fur'ik)
sulfurous (sul'fur·us)
sumac (soo'mak)
superacidity (soo'per·ah·sid'ĭ·te)
superalimentation
   (soo'per·al'ĭ·men·ta'shun)
superalkalinity (soo'per·al'kah·lin'ĭ·te)
superciliary (soo'per·sil'e·a·re)
superego (soo'per·e'go)
superfecundation
   (soo'per·fe'kun·da'shun)
superinfection (soo'per·in·fek'shun)
supernatant (soo'per·na'tant)
supernumerary (soo'per·nu'mer·ar'e)
supersaturate (soo'per·sat'u·rāt)
superscription (soo'per·skrip'shun)
supination (soo'pĭ·na'shun)
supinator (soo'pĭ·na'tor)
suppository (sup·poz'ĭ·to·re)

suppression (sŭ·presh'un)
suppuration (sup'u·ra'shun)
supraclavicular (soo'prah·klah·vik'u·lar)
supracondylar (soo'prah·kon'dĭ·lar)
supradiaphragmatic
   (soo'prah·di'ah·frag·mat'ik)
suprahyoid (soo'prah·hi'oid)
suprainguinal (soo'prah·in'gwĭ·nal)
supraorbital (soo'prah·or'bi·tal)
supraspinal (soo'prah·spi'nal)
supraspinous (soo'prah·spi'nus)
suprasternal (soo'prah·ster'nal)
supraventricular (soo'prah·ven·trik'u·lar)
supravergence (soo'prah·ver'jens)
supraversion (soo'prah·ver'zhun)
surfactant (sur·fak'tant)
surgeon (sur'jun)
surgery (sur'jer·e)
surrogate (sur'o·gāt)
susceptibility (sus·sep'tĭ·bil'ĭ·te)
susceptible (sus·sep'tĭ·bl)
suspension (sus·pen'shun)
suspensory (sus·pen·so're)
sustentacular (sus'ten·tak'u·lar)
sustentaculum (sus'ten·tak'u·lum)
suture (su'chur)
Svedberg (sved'berg)
swab (swahb)
swallow (swahl'o)
sycoma (si·ko'mah)
sycosiform (si·ko'sĭ·form)
sycosis (si·ko'sis)
symbiont (sim'be·ont)
symbiosis (sim'be·o'sis)
symblepharon (sim·blef'ah·ron)
symblepharopterygium
   (sim·blef'ah·ro·ter·ij'e·um)
symmetry (sim'ĕ·tre)
sympathetic (sim'pah·thet'ik)
sympathicotripsy (sim·path'ĭ·ko·trip'se)
sympathicotropic (sim·path'ĭ·ko·trop'ik)
sympathoadrenal (sim'path·o·ah·dre'nal)
sympathoblast (sim·path'o·blast)
sympathogonia (sim'pah·tho·go'ne·ah)
sympatholytic (sim'pah·tho·lit'ik)
sympathomimetic
   (sim'pah·tho·mĭ·met'ik)
symphysiorrhaphy (sim·fiz'e·or'ah·fe)
symphysiotomy (sim·fiz'e·ot'o·me)
symphysis (sim'fĭ·sis)
symptom (simp'tum)
symptomatic (simp'to·mat'ik)
symptomatology (simp'tom·ah·tol'o·je)
synalgia (sin·al'je·ah)
synapse (sin'aps)
synapsis (sĭ·nap'sis)
synarthrosis (sin'ar·thro'sis)
syncanthus (sin·kan'thus)
synchondrosis (sin'kon·dro'sis)
synchysis (sin'ki·sis)
synclitism (sin'klit·izm)
syncope (sin'ko·pe)
syncytiotrophoblast
   (sin·sit'e·o·trof'o·blast)
syncytium (sin·sish'e·um)
syndactyly (sin'dak·tĭ·le)
syndesmectomy (sin'des·mek'to·me)
syndesmitis (sin'des·mi'tis)
syndesmology (sin'des·mol'o·je)
syndesmopexy (sin·des'mo·pek'se)
syndesmoplasty (sin·des'mo·plas'te)
syndesmorrhaphy (sin'des·mor'ah·fe)
syndesmosis (sin'des·mo'sis)
syndesmotomy (sin'des·mot'o·me)
syndrome (sin'drōm)
synechiotomy (sin·ek'e·ot'o·me)
synectenterotomy
   (sin'ek·ten'ter·ot'o·me)
syneresis (sin·er'ĕ·sis)
synergism (sin'er·jizm)
synergist (sin'er·jist)
synesthesialgia (sin'es·the'ze·al'je·ah)
syngamy (sing'gah·me)
syngeneic (sin'jĕ·ne'ik)
syngensioplastic (sin'jen·ze·o·plas'tik)
synostosis (sin'os·to'sis)
synovia (si·no've·ah)
synovianalysis (sĭ·no've·ah·nal'ĭ·sis)

Pronunciation

synovitis (sin′o·vi′tis)
synthesis (sin′thĕ·sis)
synthesize (sin′thĕ·sīz)
synthetase (sin′thĕ·tās)
syntrophism (sin′tro·fizm)
syntrophoblast (sin·trof′o·blast)
syphilid (sif′ĭ·lid)
syphilis (sif′ĭ·lis)
syphilitic (sif′ĭ·lit′ik)
syphiloid (sif′ĭ·loid)
syphilology (sif′ĭ·lol′o·je)
syphiloma (sif′ĭ·lo′mah)
syringadenoma (sĭ·ring·ad′ĕ·no′mah)
syringadenosus (sĭ·ring·ad′ĕ·no′sus)
syringe (si·rinj′)
syringitis (sir′in·ji′tis)
syringobulbia (sĭ·ring′go·bul′be·ah)
syringocystoma (sĭ·ring′go·sis·to′mah)
syringoma (sĭ·ring·go′mah)
syringomyelia (si·ring′go·mi·e′le·ah)
syringomyelitis (sĭ·ring′go·mi′ĕ·li′tis)
springomyelocele (sĭ·ring′go·mi′ĕ·lo·sēl)
syrinx (sir′inks)
syssarcosis (sis′sar·ko′sis)
systematic (sis′tĕ·mat′ik)
systematization (sis·tem′ah·tĭ·za′shun)
systematized (sis′tĕ·mah·tīzd)
systemic (sis·tem′ik)
systole (sis′to·le)
systolic (sis·tol′ik)
systremma (sis·trem′ah)

T

Tabanus (tah·ba′nus)
tabefaction (ta′bĕ·fak′shun)
tabes (ta′bēz)
tabescent (tah·bes′ent)
taboparesis (ta′bo·pah·re′sis)
tache (tahsh)
tachistesthesia (tah·kis′tes·the′ze·ah)
tachistoscope (tah·kis′to·skōp)
tachography (tah·kog′rah·fe)
tachyarrhythmia (tak′e·ah·rith′me·ah)
tachycardia (tak′e·kar′de·ah)
tachycrotic (tak′e·krot′ik)
tachylogia (tak′e·lo′je·ah)
tachyphagia (tak′e·fa′je·ah)
tachyphylaxis (tak′e·fi·lak′sis)
tachypnea (tak′ip·ne′ah)
tachysterol (tak·is′tĕ·rol)
tachysystole (tak′e·sis′to·le)
tactile (tak′til)
tactometer (tak·tom′ĕ·ter)
Taenia (te′ne·ah)
talalgia (tal·al′je·ah)
talcosis (tal·ko′sis)
taliped (tal′ĕ·ped)
talipes (tal′ĕ·pēz)
talocalcaneal (ta′lo·kal·ka′ne·al)
talocrural (ta′lo·kroo′ral)
talonavicular (ta′lo·nah·vik′u·lar)
talus (ta′lus)
tambour (tam·boor′)
tampon (tam′pon)
tamponade (tam′pon·ād)
tantalum (tan′tah·lum)
tantrum (tan′trum)
tapetum (tah·pe′tum)
tapeworm (tāp′wurm)
taphophobia (taf′o·fo′be·ah)
tapinocephalic (tap′ĭ·no·sĕ·fal′ik)
tapinocephaly (tap′ĭ·no·sef′ah·le)
tapotement (tah·pōt·maw′)
tarantula (tah·ran′tu·lah)
tardive (tahr′div)
tarsadenitis (tahr′sad·ĕ·ni′tis)
tarsal (tahr′sal)
tarsectomy (tahr·sek′to·me)
tarsi (tahr′si)
tarsitis (tahr·si′tis)
tarsoclasis (tahr·sok′lah·sis)
tarsomalacia (tahr′so·mah·la′she·ah)
tarsometatarsal (tahr′so·met′ah·tahr′sal)
tarsoplasty (tahr′so·plas′te)
tarsorrhaphy (tahr·sor′ah·fe)

tarsotomy (tahr·sot′o·me)
tarsus (tahr′sus)
tartar (tahr′tahr)
tartrate (tahr′trāt)
Taussig (taw′sig)
tautomerism (taw·tom′er·izm)
taxis (tak′sis)
technetium (tek·ne′she·um)
technician (tek·nish′an)
technique (tek·nēk′)
technologist (tek·nol′o·jist)
tectorial (tek·to′re·al)
tectorium (tek·to′re·um)
tectum (tek′tum)
tegmen (teg′men)
tegmentum (teg·men′tum)
tela (te′lah)
telae (te′le)
telangiectasia (tel·an′je·ek·ta′ze·ah)
telangioma (tel′an·je·o′mah)
telelectrocardiogram (tel′e·lek′tro·kar′de·o·gram)
telelectrocardiograph (tel′e·lek′tro·kar′de·o·graf)
telemetry (tĕ·lem′ah·tre)
telencephalon (tel′en·sef′ah·lon)
telepathy (tĕ·lep′ah·the)
telereceptor (tel′ĕ·re·sep′tor)
tellurium (tĕ·lu′re·um)
telocentric (tel′o·sen′trik)
telodendron (tel′o·den′dron)
telogen (tel′o·jen)
telomere (tel′o·mēr)
telophase (tel′o·fāz)
temperament (tem′per·ah·ment)
temperature (tem′per·ah·chur)
template (tem′plāt)
tempolabile (tem′po·la′bīl)
temporal (tem′po·ral)
temporomandibular (tem′po·ro·man·dib′u·lar)
tempostabile (tem′po·sta′bīl)
tenacious (te·na′shus)
tenacity (te·nas′ĭ·te)
tenaculum (te·nak′u·lum)
tenalgia (ten·al′je·ah)
tendinitis (ten′dĭ·ni′tis)
tendinoplasty (ten′dĭ·no·plas′te)
tendolysis (ten·dol′ĭ·sis)
tendon (ten′dun)
tendonitis (ten′do·ni′tis)
tendoplasty (ten′do·plas′te)
tendotomy (ten·dot′o·me)
tenectomy (tĕ·nek′to·me)
tenesmic (te·nez′mik)
tenesmus (te·nez′mus)
tenia (te′ne·ah)
teniacide (te′ne·ah·sīd)
teniae (te′ne·e)
teniafuge (te′ne·ah·fūj)
tenial (te′ne·al)
teniasis (te·ni′ah·sis)
tenodesis (ten·od′ĕ·sis)
tenonectomy (ten·o·nek′to·me)
tenophyte (ten′o·fīt)
tenoplasty (ten′o·plas′te)
tenorrhaphy (ten·or′ah·fe)
tenosynovectomy (ten′o·sin′o·vek′to·me)
tenosynovitis (ten′o·sin′o·vi′tis)
tenotomy (ten·ot′o·me)
tension (ten′shun)
tentorium (ten·to′re·um)
tephromalacia (tef′ro·mah·la′she·ah)
teratocarcinoma (ter′ah·to·kar′si·no′mah)
teratogen (ter′ah·to·jen)
teratogenesis (ter′ah·to·jen′ĕ·sis)
teratology (ter′ah·tol′o·je)
teratoma (ter′ah·to′mah)
teres (te′rēz)
ternary (ter′nah·re)
terra (ter′ah)
tertian (ter′shun)
testes (tes′tēz)
testicle (tes′tĭ·kl)
testicular (tes·tik′u·lar)
testis (tes′tis)
testitis (tes·ti′tis)
testosterone (tes·tos′tĕ·rōn)

tetanize (tet′ah·nīz)
tetanode (tet′ah·nōd)
tetanoid (tet′ah·noid)
tetanolysin (tet′ah·nol′ĭ·sin)
tetanospasmin (tet′ah·no·spaz′min)
tetanotoxin (tet′ah·no·tok′sin)
tetanus (tet′ah·nus)
tetany (tet′ah·ne)
tetartanopsia (tet′ar·tah·nop′se·ah)
tetracycline (tet′rah·si′klēn)
tetradactyl (tet′rah·dak′til)
tetrahydrocannabinol (tet′rah·hi′dro·kah·nab′ĭ·nol)
tetraplegia (tet′rah·ple′je·ah)
tetraploid (tet′rah·ploid)
tetrose (tet′rōs)
thalami (thal′ah·mi)
thalamic (thah·lam′ik)
thalamocortical (thal′ah·mo·kor′tĭ·kal)
thalamotegmental (thal′ah·mo·teg·men′tal)
thalamotomy (thal′ah·mot′o·me)
thalamus (thal′ah·mus)
thalassemia (thal′ah·se′me·ah)
thalidomide (thah·lid′o·mīd)
thallium (thal′e·um)
thallotoxicosis (thal′o·tok′sĭ·ko′sis)
thallus (thal′us)
thanatoid (than′ah·toid)
thanatology (than′ah·tol′o·je)
thanatopsia (than′ah·top′se·ah)
theca (the′kah)
thecae (the′ke)
thecitis (the·si′tis)
thecoma (the·ko′mah)
thelarche (the·lar′ke)
thelerethism (thel·er′ĕ·thizm)
thelitis (the·li′tis)
thelorrhagia (the·lo·ra′je·ah)
thenar (the′nar)
theophylline (the·of′ĭ·lēn)
theorem (the′o·rem)
therapeutic (ther′ah·pu′tik)
therapeutics (ther′ah·pu′tiks)
therapist (ther′ah·pist)
therapy (ther′ah·pe)
thermal (ther′mal)
thermalgesia (ther′mal·je′ze·ah)
thermanalgesia (therm′an·al·je′se·ah)
thermatology (ther′mah·tol′o·je)
thermoanesthesia (ther′mo·an′es·the′ze·ah)
thermocautery (ther′mo·kaw′ter·e)
thermochemistry (ther′mo·kem′is·tre)
thermocoagulation (ther′mo·ko·ag′u·la′shun)
thermocouple (ther′mo·kup·l)
thermodiffusion (ther′mo·dĭ·fu′zhun)
thermodilution (ther′mo·di·lu′shun)
thermodynamics (ther′mo·di·nam′iks)
thermoesthesia (ther′mo·es·the′ze·ah)
thermogenesis (ther′mo·jen′ĕ·sis)
thermography (ther·mog′rah·fe)
thermohyperesthesia (ther′mo·hi′per·es·the′ze·ah)
thermohypesthesia (ther′mo·hip′es·the′ze·ah)
thermoinhibitory (ther′mo·in·hib′ĭ·tor′e)
thermolabile (ther′mo·la′bil)
thermolysis (ther·mol′ĭ·sis)
thermomassage (ther′mo·mah·sahzh′)
thermometer (ther·mom′ĕ·ter)
thermophile (ther′mo·fīl)
thermophore (ther′mo·for)
thermoplacentography (ther′mo·plas′en·tog′rah·fe)
thermoplastic (ther′mo·plas′tik)
thermoplegia (ther′mo·ple′je·ah)
thermoreceptor (ther′mo·re·sep′tor)
thermoregulation (ther′mo·reg′u·la′shun)
thermoset (ther′mo·set)
thermostable (ther′mo·sta′bil)
thermotaxis (ther′mo·tak′sis)
thermotherapy (ther′mo·ther′ah·pe)
thesaurosis (the′saw·ro′sis)
thesis (the′sis)
thiaminase (thi·am′ĭ·nās)
thiamine (thi′ah·mēn)

thiazides (thi'ah·zīdz)
thigmesthesia (thig'mes·the'ze·ah)
thigmotaxis (thig'mo·tak'sis)
thiobarbiturates (thi'o·bar·bit'u·rātz)
thioguanine (thi'o·gwah'nēn)
thiol (thi'ol)
thionine (thi'o·nēn)
thiopental (thi'o·pen'tal)
thiosemicarbazone
(thi'o·sem'e·kar'bah·zōn)
thiosulfate (thi'o·sul'fāt)
thiosulfuric (thi'o·sul·fur'ik)
thiotepa (thi'o·te'pah)
thiouracil (thi'o·u'rah·sil)
thiourea (thi'o·u're·ah)
thoracectomy (tho'rah·sek·to'me)
thoracentesis (tho'rah·sen·te'sis)
thoracic (tho·ras'ik)
thoracoabdominal
(tho'rah·ko·ab·dom'ĭ·nal)
thoracomyodynia
(tho'rah·ko·mi'o·din'e·ah)
thoracoplasty (tho'rah·ko·plas'te)
thoracopneumoplasty
(tho'rah·ko·nu'mo·plas'te)
thoracoscopy (thor'rah·kos'ko·pe)
thoracostomy (tho'rah·kos'to·me)
thoracotomy (tho'rah·kot'o·me)
thorax (tho'raks)
threonine (thre'o·nēn)
threose (thre'ōs)
threshold (thresh'old)
throat (thrōt)
throe (thro)
thrombasthenia (throm'bas·the'ne·ah)
thrombectomy (throm·bek'to·me)
thrombelastograph (thromb'e·las'to·graf)
thrombi (throm'bi)
thrombin (throm'bin)
thrombinogen (throm·bin'o·jen)
thromboangiitis (throm'bo·an'je·i'tis)
thromboblast (throm'bo·blast)
thrombocytasthenia
(throm'bo·si'tas·the'ne·ah)
thrombocyte (throm'bo·sīt)
thrombocythemia
(throm'bo·sĭ·the'me·ah)
thrombocytopathy
(throm'bo·si·top'ah·the)
thrombocytopenia
(throm'bo·si·to'pe'ne·ah)
thrombocytosis (throm'bo·si·to'sis)
thromboembolectomy
(throm'bo·em'bo·lek'to·me)
thromboembolism (throm'bo·em'bo·lizm)
thromboendarterectomy
(throm'bo·end'ar·ter·ek'to·me)
thrombogenic (throm'bo·jen'ik)
thrombolysis (throm·bol'i·sis)
thrombophlebitis (throm'bo·fle·bi'tis)
thromboplastin (throm'bo·plas'tin)
thrombopoiesis (throm'bo·poi·e'sis)
thrombosis (throm·bo'sis)
thromboxane (throm·boks'ān)
thrombus (throm'bus)
thulium (thu'le·um)
thymectomy (thi·mek'to·me)
thymidine (thi'mĭ·dēn)
thymine (thi'mēn)
thymocyte (thi'mo·sīt)
thymoma (thi·mo'mah)
thymopathy (thi·mop'ah·the)
thymosin (thi'mo·sin)
thymus (thi'mus)
thyroaplasia (thi'ro·ah·pla'ze·ah)
thyrocricotomy (thi'ro·kri·kot'o·me)
thyroglobulin (thi'ro·glob'u·lin)
thyroglossal (thi'ro·glos'al)
thyrohyoid (thi'ro·hi'oid)
thyroid (thi'roid)
thyroidectomy (thi'roi·dek'to·me)
thyroiditis (thi'roi·di'tis)
thyromegaly (thi'ro·meg'ah·le)
thyronine (thi'ro·nēn)
thyroparathyroidectomy
(thi'ro·par'ah·thi'roi·dek'to·me)
thyropathy (thi·rop'ah·the)
thyroprival (thi'ro·pri'val)
thyroprotein (thi'ro·pro'te·in)
thyroptosis (thi'rop·to'sis)

thyrotomy (thi·rot'o·me)
thyrotoxicosis (thi'ro·tok·sĭ·ko'sis)
thyrotropic (thi'ro·trop'ik)
thyrotropin (thi·rot'ro·pin)
thyroxin (thi·rok'sin)
tibia (tib'e·ah)
tibiofibular (tib'e·o·fib'u·lar)
timbre (tim'ber)
timolol (ti'mo·lōl)
tinctura (tink·tu'rah)
tincture (tink'tūr)
tine (tīn)
tinea (tin'e·ah)
tinnitus (tĭ·ni'tus)
tintometer (tin·tom'ĕ·ter)
tissue (tish'u)
titanium (ti·ta'ne·um)
titer (ti'ter)
titrate (ti'trāt)
titration (ti·tra'shun)
toadstool (tōd'stool)
tobramycin (to'brah·mi'sin)
tocodynamometer
(to'ko·di'nah·mom'ĕ·ter)
tocopherol (to·kof'er·ol)
Togaviridae (to'gah·vir'ĭ·de)
tolazamide (tol·az'ah·mīd)
tolbutamide (tol·bu'tah·mīd)
tolerance (tol'er·ans)
tolerogen (tol'er·o·jen)
tolnaftate (tol·naf'tāt)
toluene (tol'u·ēn)
tomogram (to'mo·gram)
tomograph (to'mo·graf)
tomography (to·mog'rah·fe)
tomomania (to'mo·ma'ne·ah)
tongue (tung)
tonic (ton'ik)
tonicity (to·nis'ĭ·te)
tonoclonic (ton'o·klon'ik)
tonofibril (ton'o·fi'bril)
tonofilament (ton'o·fil'ah·ment)
tonography (to·nog'rah·fe)
tonometer (to·nom'ĕ·ter)
tonometry (to·nom'ĕ·tre)
tonsil (ton'sil)
tonsillar (ton'sĭ·lar)
tonsillectomy (ton'sĭ·lek'to·me)
tonsillitis (ton'sĭ·li'tis)
tonsilloadenoidectomy
(ton'sil·o·ad'ĕ·noi·dek'to·me)
tonsillotome (ton·sil'o·tōm)
topagnosis (top'ag·no'sis)
topalgia (to·pal'je·ah)
topectomy (to·pek'to·me)
topesthesia (top'es·the'ze·ah)
tophaceous (to·fa'shus)
tophi (to'fi)
tophus (to'fus)
topoanesthesia (top'o·an'es·the'ze·ah)
topognosis (top'og·no'sis)
topogometer (top'o·gom'ĕ·ter)
topography (to·pog'rah·fe)
torpor (tor'por)
torque (tork)
torsion (tor'shun)
torticollis (tor'tĭ·kol'is)
torus (to'rus)
totipotency (to'te·po'ten·se)
Tourette (too·ret')
tourniquet (toor·nĭ·ket)
toxemia (tok·se'me·ah)
toxic (tok·sik)
toxicant (toks'ĭ·kant)
toxicity (tok·sis'ĭ·te)
toxicoderma (tok'sĭ·ko·der'mah)
toxicodermatitis (tok'sĭ·ko·der·mah·ti'tis)
toxicogenic (tok'sĭ·ko·jen'ik)
toxicoid (tok'sĭ·koid)
toxicologist (tok'sĭ·kol'o·jist)
toxicology (tok'sĭ·kol'o·je)
toxicopathy (tok'sĭ·kop'ah·the)
toxiferous (tok·sif'er·us)
toxin (tok'sin)
toxocariasis (tok'so·kār·i'ah·sis)
toxoid (tok'soid)
toxophore (tok'so·for)
toxoplasmosis (tok'so·plaz·mo'sis)
trabecula (trah·bek'u·lah)
trabeculae (trah·bek'u·le)

trabecular (trah·bek'u·lar)
trabeculation (trah·bek'u·la'shun)
tracer (trās'er)
trachea (tra'ke·ah)
tracheal (tra'ke·al)
trachealgia (tra'ke·al'je·ah)
tracheitis (tra'ke·i'tis)
trachelorrhaphy (tra'kĕ·lor'ah·fe)
tracheobronchial (tra'ke·o·brong'ke·al)
tracheobronchitis (tra'ke·o·brong·ki'tis)
tracheobronchoscopy
(tra'ke·o·brong·kos'ko·pe)
tracheocele (tra'ke·o·sēl)
tracheoesophageal
(tra'ke·o·e·sof'ah·je'al)
tracheolaryngeal (tra'ke·o·lah·rin'je·al)
tracheomalacia (tra'ke·o·mah·la'she·ah)
tracheophony (tra'ke·of'o·ne)
tracheoplasty (tra'ke·o·plas'te)
tracheorrhagia (tra'ke·o·ra'je·ah)
tracheoschisis (tra'ke·os'ki·sis)
tracheoscopy (tra'ke·os'ko·pe)
tracheostenosis (tra'ke·o·stĕ·no'sis)
tracheostoma (tra'ke·os'to·mah)
tracheostomy (tra'ke·os'to·me)
tracheotome (tra'ke·o·tōm)
trachoma (trah·ko'mah)
tracing (trās'ing)
tract (trakt)
traction (trak'shun)
tractotomy (trak·tot'o·me)
tragacanth (trag'ah·kanth)
tragus (tra'gus)
trait (trāt)
trajector (trah·jek'tor)
trance (trans)
tranquilizer (tran'kwĭ·līz'er)
transacetylation (trans·as'ĕ·til·a'shun)
transaminse (trans·am'ĭ·nās)
transamination (trans'am·ĭ·na'shun)
transcription (tran·skrip'shun)
transdiaphragmatic
(trans'di·ah·frag·mat'ik)
transducer (trans·du'ser)
transduction (trans·duk'shun)
transferase (trans'fer·ās)
transference (trans·fer'ens)
transferrin (trans·fer'in)
transformation (trans'for·ma'shun)
transfusion (trans·fu'zhun)
transient (tran'shent)
transiliac (trans·il'e·ak)
transillumination (trans'ĭ·lu'mĭ·na'shun)
transition (tran'sĭ·shun)
translation (trans·la'shun)
translocation (trans'lo·ka'shun)
translucent (trans·lu'sent)
transmethylase (trans·meth'ĭ·lās)
transmethylation (trans'meth·i·la'shun)
transmission (trans·mish'un)
transmural (trans·mu'ral)
transmutation (trans'mu·ta'shun)
transpeptidase (trans·pep'tĭ·dās)
transphosphorylation
(trans·fos'for·ĭ·la'shun)
transpiration (tran'spi·ra'shun)
transpire (tran'spīr)
transplacental (trans'plah·sen'tal)
transplant (trans'plant)
transplantation (trans'plan·ta'shun)
transposition (trans'po·zish'un)
transposon (trans·po'zon)
transseptal (trans·sep'tal)
transsexual (trans·seks'u·al)
transsynaptic (trans·sĭ·nap'tik)
transthoracic (trans'tho·ras'ik)
transtracheal (trans·tra'ke·al)
transudate (trans'u·dāt)
transudation (trans'u·da'shun)
transurethral (trans'u·re'thral)
transvaginal (trans·vaj'ĭ·nal)
transversion (trans·ver'zhun)
transvestism (trans·ves'tizm)
transvestite (trans·ves'tīt)
trapezium (trah·pe'ze·um)
trauma (traw'mah)
traumatic (traw·mat'ik)
traumatize (traw'mah·tīz)
traumatogenic (traw'mah·to·jen'ik)
traumatology (traw'mah·tol'o·je)

Trematoda (trem′ah·to′dah)
trematode (trem′ah·tōd)
tremens (tre′menz)
tremor (trem′or)
Trendelenburg (tren·del′en·berg)
trephination (tref′ĭ·na′shun)
trephine (trĕ·fīn′)
trephining (trĕ·fīn′ing)
Treponema (trep′o·ne′mah)
treponemiasis (trep′o·ne·mi′ah·sis)
triad (tri′ad)
triage (tre·ahzh′)
triamcinolone (tri′am·sin′o·lōn)
triamterene (tri·am′ter·ēn)
triatomic (tri′ah·tom′ik)
tribasic (tri·ba′sik)
triceps (tri′seps)
trichatrophy (trik′ah·tro′fe)
trichiasis (trĭ·ki′ah·sis)
Trichinella (trik′i·nel′ah)
trichinosis (trik′i·no′sis)
trichloroethylene (tri′klo·ro·eth′i·lēn)
trichloromethane (tri·klo′ro·meth′ān)
trichobezoar (trik′o·be′zōr)
trichoclasia (trik′o·kla′ze·ah)
trichocryptosis (trik′o·krip·to′sis)
trichocyst (trik′o·sist)
trichoepithelioma
  (trik′o·ep′ĭ·the·le·o′mah)
trichoesthesia (trik′o·es·the′ze·ah)
trichogen (trik′o·jen)
trichology (tri·kol′o·je)
Trichomonas (trik′o·mo′nas)
trichomoniasis (trik′o·mo·ni′ah·sis)
trichomycosis (trik′o·mi·ko′sis)
trichonodosis (trik′o·no·do′sis)
trichopathy (trĭ·kop′ah·the)
trichophytobezoar (trik′o·fi′to·be′zor)
Trichophyton (tri·kof′i·ton)
trichophytosis (trik′o·fi·to′sis)
trichorrhea (trik′o·re′ah)
trichorrhexis (trik′o·rek′sis)
trichosis (tri·ko′sis)
Trichosporon (tri·kos′po·ron)
trichosporosis (trik′o·spo·ro′sis)
trichostasis (trĭ·kos′tah·sis)
Trichostrongylus (trik′o·stron′jĭ·lus)
trichotillomania (trik′o·til′o·ma′ne·ah)
trichuriasis (trik′u·ri′ah·sis)
Trichuris (trik·u′ris)
triethylenemelamine
  (tri·eth′ĭ·lēn·mel′ah·mēn)
trifocal (tri′fo·kal)
trifurcation (tri′fur·ka′shun)
trigeminal (tri·jem′ĭ·nal)
triglyceride (tri·glis′er·īd)
trigone (tri′gōn)
trigonitis (trig′o·ni′tis)
trihydrate (tri·hi′drāt)
trilaminar (tri·lam′ĭ·nar)
trilogy (tril′o·je)
trimester (tri·mes′ter)
trimethoprim (tri·meth′o·prim)
trimorphous (tri·mor′fus)
trinitrotoluene (tri′ni·tro·tol′u·ēn)
triolein (tri·o′le·in)
triose (tri′ōs)
triphosphopyridine (tri·fos′fo·pir′ĭ·dēn)
triploid (trip′loid)
triplopia (trip·lo′pe·ah)
tripoli (trip′o·le)
triradius (tri·ra′de·us)
trisaccharide (tri·sak′ah·rīd)
trismus (triz′mus)
trisomy (tri′so·me)
tritanopia (tri′tah·no′pe·ah)
triturable (trit′ŭr·ah·bl)
trituration (trit′ŭ·ra′shun)
triturium (trĭ·tu′re·um)
trivalent (tri′va·lent)
trocar (tro′kar)
trochanter (tro·kan′ter)
troche (tro′ke)
trochlea (trok′le·ah)
trochlear (trok′le·ar)
Trombicula (trom·bik′u·lah)
trombiculiasis (trom·bik′u·li′ah·sis)
Trombiculidae (trom·bik′u·li′de)
trophic (trof′ik)
trophoblast (trof′o·blast)

trophoneurosis (trof′o·nu·ro′sis)
trophopathia (trof′o·path′e·ah)
trophotropism (tro·fot′ropizm)
trophozoite (trof′o·zo′īt)
tropia (tro′pe·ah)
tropine (tro′pin)
tropism (tro′pizm)
tropocollagen (tro′po·kol′ah·jen)
troponin (tro′po·nin)
trough (trof)
truncate (trun′kāt)
truncus (trun′kus)
truss (trus)
Trypanosoma (tri′pan·o·so′mah)
trypanosomiasis (tri·pan′o·so·mi′ah·sis)
trypsin (trip′sin)
trypsinogen (trip·sin′o·jen)
tryptic (trip′tik)
tryptophan (trip′to·fan)
tsetse (tset′se)
tsutsugamushi (soot′soo·gah·moosh′e)
tubal (too′bal)
tubectomy (too·bek′to·me)
tubercle (too′ber·kl)
tubercula (too·ber′ku·lah)
tubercular (too·ber′ku·lar)
tuberculation (too·ber′ku·la′shun)
tuberculin (too·ber′ku·lin)
tuberculoma (too·ber′ku·lo′mah)
tuberculosis (too·ber′ku·lo′sis)
tuberculum (too·ber′ku·lum)
tuberosity (too′bĕ·ros′ĭ·te)
tuberous (too′ber·us)
tubocurarine (too′bo·ku·rah′rēn)
tuboovarian (too′bo·o·va′re·an)
tubular (too′bu·lar)
tubule (too′bŭl)
tubulization (too′bu·lĭ·za′shun)
tubulorrhexis (too′bu·lo·rek′sis)
tularemia (too′lah·re′me·ah)
tumefacient (too′mah·fa′shent)
tumefaction (too′me·fak′shun)
tumid (too′mid)
tumor (too′mor)
tumorigenesis (too′mor·ĭ·jen′ĕ·sis)
tumorous (too′mor·us)
tungsten (tung′sten)
tunica (too′nĭ·kah)
turbid (tur′bid)
turbidity (tur·bid′ĭ·te)
turbinate (tur′bĭ·nāt)
turbinectomy (tur′bĭ·nek′to·me)
turgescence (tur·jes′ens)
turgid (tur′jid)
turgor (tur′gor)
tussis (tus′is)
twinge (twinj)
tyloma (ti·lo′mah)
tympanectomy (tim′pah·nek′to·me)
tympanic (tim·pan′ik)
tympanocentesis (tim′pah·no·sen·te′sis)
tympanomastoiditis
  (tim′pah·no·mas′toi·di′tis)
tympanometry (tim′pah·nom′ĕ·tre)
tympanoplasty (tim′pah·no·plas′te)
tympanosclerosis (tim′pah·no·skle·ro′sis)
tympanosquamosal
  (tim′pah·no·skwah·mo′sal)
tympanum (tim′pah·num)
tympany (tim′pah·ne)
typhemia (ti·fe′me·ah)
typhlitis (tif·li′tis)
typhoid (ti′foid)
typhous (ti′fus)
typhus (ti′fus)
tyramine (ti′rah·mēn)
tyrosinase (ti·ro′sin·ās)
tyrosine (ti′ro·sēn)
tyrosinosis (ti′ro·si·no′sis)

U

ubiquinone (u·bik′wĭ·nōn)
ulalgia (u·lal′je·ah)
ulcer (ul′ser)
ulcerate (ul′sĕ·rāt)
ulceration (ul′sĕ·ra′shun)

ulcerative (ul′ser·ah·tiv)
ulcerogenic (ul′ser·o·jen′ik)
ulcerous (ul′ser·us)
ulerythema (u′ler·ĭ·the′mah)
ulna (ul′nah)
ulnar (ul′nar)
ulnoradial (ul′no·ra′de·al)
ultrafiltration (ul′trah·fil·tra′shun)
ultraligation (ul′trah·li·ga′shun)
ultramicrometer (ul′trah·mi·krom′ĕ·ter)
ultramicroscopic (ul′trah·mi′kro·skop′ik)
ultramicrotome (ul′trah·mi′kro·tōm)
ultrasonography (ul′trah·son·og′rah·fe)
ultrasonosurgery (ul′trah·son·o·sur′jer·e)
ultrasonotomy (ul′trah·so·not′o·me)
ultrasound (ul′trah·sownd)
ultrastructure (ul′trah·struk′chur)
ultraviolet (ul′trah·vi′o·let)
ululation (ul′u·la′shun)
umbilical (um·bil′ĭ·kal)
umbilicus (um·bil′ĭ·kus)
umbo (um′bo)
umbones (um·bo′nēz)
unciform (un′sĭ·form)
Uncinaria (un′sĭ·na′re·ah)
uncinariasis (un′sin·ah·ri′ah·sis)
unconscious (un·kon′shus)
uncus (ung′kus)
undecylenic (un·des′i·len′ik)
undescended (un′dĕ·sen′ded)
undifferentiated (un′dif·er·en′she·a·ted)
undulate (un′du·lāt)
unerupted (un′e·rup′ted)
ungual (ung′gwal)
unguent (ung′gwent)
ungues (ung′gwēz)
unguis (ung′gwis)
uniaxial (u′ne·ak′se·al)
unicellular (u′nĭ·sel′u·lar)
unigravida (u′nĭ·grav′ĭ·dah)
uninephrectomized
  (u·ne·nĕ·frek′to·mīzd)
uninuclear (u′nĭ·nu′kle·ar)
uniocular (u′ne·ok′u·lar)
unioval (u′ne·o′val)
unipennate (u′ne·pen′āt)
unipolar (u′nĭ·po′lar)
univalent (u′nĭ·va′lent)
unmyelinated (un·mi′ĕ·lĭ·nāt′ed)
unsaturated (un·sat′u·rāt′ed)
unstable (un·sta′bl)
unstriated (un·stri′a·ted)
urachal (u′rah·kal)
urachus (u′rah·kus)
uracil (u′rah·sil)
uranostaphyloplasty
  (u′rah·no·staf′i·lo·plas′te)
uranostaphyloschisis
  (u′rah·no·staf′i·los′ki·sis)
uranyl (u′rah·nil)
urate (u′rāt)
urea (u·re′ah)
urease (u′re·ās)
urecchysis (u·rek′i·sis)
uredema (u′rĕ·de′mah)
uredo (u·re′do)
urelcosis (u′rel·ko′sis)
uremia (u·re′me·ah)
uremic (u·re′mik)
ureolysis (u′re·ol′i·sis)
uresis (u·re′sis)
ureter (u·re′ter)
ureteral (u·re′ter·al)
ureterectasia (u·re′ter·ek·ta′se·ah)
ureterectomy (u·re′ter·ek′to·me)
ureteric (u′rĕ·ter′ik)
ureterocele (u·re′ter·o·sēl)
ureteroenterostomy
  (u·re′ter·o·en′ter·os′to·me)
ureterogram (u·re′ter·o·gram)
ureterography (u·re′ter·og′rah·fe)
ureterolith (u·re′ter·o·lith)
ureterolithiasis (u·re′ter·o·lĭ·thi′ah·sis)
ureterolithotomy (u·re′ter·o·lĭ·thot′o·me)
ureterolysis (u·re′ter·ol′i·sis)
ureteroneocystostomy
  (u·re′ter·o·ne′o·sis·tos′to·me)
ureteronephrectomy
  (u·re′ter·o·nĕ·frek′to·me)
ureteropyelitis (u·re′ter·o·pi′ĕ·li′tis)

ureteropyeloneostomy
(u·re'ter·o·pi'ě·lo·ne·os'to·me)
ureteropyeloplasty
(u·re'ter·o·pi'ě·lo·plas'te)
ureteropyosis (u·re'ter·o·pi·o'sis)
ureterostenosis (u·re'ter·o·stě·no'sis)
ureterostomy (u're·ter·os'to·me)
ureterotomy (u're·ter·ot'o·me)
ureterovesicostomy
(u·re'ter·o·ves'ĭ·kos'to·me)
urethane (u'rě·thān)
urethra (u·re'thrah)
urethral (u·re'thral)
urethralgia (u'rě·thral'je·ah)
urethrectomy (u'rě·threk'to·me)
urethremorrhagia (u·re'threm·o·ra'je·ah)
urethrism (u'rě·thrizm)
urethrismus (u·rě·thriz'mus)
urethritis (u'rě·thri'tis)
urethrocele (u·re'thro·sēl)
urethrocystitis (u·re'thro·sis·ti'tis)
urethrocystopexy (u·re'thro·sis'to·pek'se)
urethrography (u'rě·throg'rah·fe)
urethroplasty (u·re'thro·plas'te)
urethrorrhea (u·re'thro·re'ah)
urethroscope (u·re'thro·skōp)
urethroscopy (u'rě·thros'ko·pe)
urethrospasm (u·re'thro·spazm)
urethrostenosis (u·re'thro·stě·no'sis)
urethrostomy (u·rě·thros'to·me)
urethrotome (u·re'thro·tōm)
urethrotomy (u'rě·throt'o·me)
uric (u'rik)
uricosuria (u'rĭ·ko·su're·ah)
uridine (u'rĭ·děn)
uridrosis (u'rĭ·dro'sis)
uridyltransferase (u'rid·il·trans'fer·ās)
urinalysis (u'rĭ·nal'ĭ·sis)
urinary (u'rĭ·nār'e)
urinate (u'rĭ·nāt)
urination (u'rĭ·na'shun)
urine (u'rin)
uriniferous (u'rĭ·nif'er·us)
urinometer (u'rĭ·nom'ě·ter)
uroacidimeter (u'ro·as'ĭ·dim'ě·ter)
urobilin (u'ro·bi'lin)
urobilinemia (u'ro·bi'lĭ·ne'me·ah)
urobilinogen (u'ro·bi·lin'o·jen)
urocele (u'ro·sēl)
urodynia (u'ro·din'e·ah)
uroerythrin (u'ro·er'ĭ·thrin)
uroflometer (u'ro·flo'me·ter)
urogastrone (u'ro·gas'trōn)
urography (u·rog'rah·fe)
urokinase (u'ro·ki'nās)
urolith (u'ro·lith)
urolithiasis (u'ro·lĭ·thi'ah·sis)
urologic (u'ro·loj'ik)
urology (u·rol'o·je)
uropathy (u·rop'ah·the)
uroplania (u'ro·pla'ne·ah)
uropod (u'ro·pod)
uropoiesis (u'ro·poi·e'sis)
uroporphyrin (u'ro·por'fĭ·rin)
uroschesis (u·ros'kě·sis)
urosepsis (u'ro·sep'sis)
urticaria (ur'tĭ·ka're·ah)
uterine (u'ter·in)
uterocystostomy (u'ter·o·sis·tos'to·me)
uteroplasty (u'ter·o·plas'te)
uterus (u'ter·us)
utricle (u'trĭ·kl)
utricular (u·trik'u·lar)
utriculosaccular (u·trik'u·lo·sak'u·lar)
uvea (u've·ah)
uveitis (u've·i'tis)
uvula (u'vu·lah)
uvulectomy (u'vu·lek'to·me)
uvulitis (u'vu·li'tis)
uvulotomy (u'vu·lot'o·me)

V

vaccinate (vak'sĭ·nāt)
vaccination (vak'sĭ·na'shun)
vaccine (vak'sēn)
vaccinia (vak·sin'e·ah)

vacuant (vak'u·ant)
vacuolate (vak'u·o·lāt')
vacuolation (vak'u·o·la'shun)
vacuole (vak'u·ōl)
vacuum (vak'u·um)
vagal (va'gal)
vagectomy (vah·jek'to·me)
vagina (vah·ji'nah)
vaginal (vaj'ĭ·nal)
vaginalectomy (vaj'ĭ·nah·lek'to·me)
vaginalitis (vaj'ĭ·nah·li'tis)
vaginate (vaj'ĭ·nāt)
vaginectomy (vaj'ĭ·nek'to·me)
vaginismus (vaj'ĭ·niz'mus)
vaginitis (vaj'ĭ·ni'tis)
vaginocele (vaj'ĭ·no·sēl)
vaginodynia (vaj'ĭ·no·din'e·ah)
vaginofixation (vaj'ĭ·no·fiks·a'shun)
vaginolabial (vaj'ĭ·no·la'be·al)
vaginomycosis (vaj'ĭ·no·mi·ko'sis)
vaginopathy (vaj'ĭ·nop'ah·the)
vaginoperineal (vaj'ĭ·no·per'ĭ·ne'al)
vaginoperineorrhaphy
(vaj'ĭ·no·per'ĭ·ne·or'ah·fe)
vaginoperineotomy
(vaj'ĭ·no·per'ĭ·ne·ot'o·me)
vaginoplasty (vah·ji'no·plas'te)
vagitis (vah·ji'·tus)
vagolysis (va·gol'ĭ·sis)
vagolytic (va'go·lit'ik)
vagomimetic (va'go·mĭ·met'ik)
vagotomy (va·got'o·me)
vagotonia (va'go·to'ne·ah)
vagus (va'gus)
valence (va'lens)
valine (val'in)
valla (val'ah)
vallecula (vah·lek'u·lah)
vallum (val'um)
valve (valv)
valvoplasty (val'vo·plas'te)
valvotomy (val·vot'o·me)
valvular (val'vu·lar)
valvulitis (val'vu·li'tis)
valvulotome (val'vu·lo·tōm)
vanadium (vah·na'de·um)
vanilla (vah·nil'ah)
vanillin (va·nil'lin)
vanillylmandelic (van'ĭ·lil·man·del'ik)
vapor (va'por)
vaporizer (va'por·i'zer)
variant (var'e·ant)
varices (var'ĭ·sēz)
varicocele (var'ĭ·ko·sēl)
varicocelectomy (var'ĭ·ko·sě·lek'to·me)
varicography (var'ĭ·kog'rah·fe)
varicophlebitis (var'ĭ·ko·fle·bi'tis)
varicose (var'ĭ·kōs)
varicosity (var'ĭ·kos'ĭ·te)
varicotomy (var'ĭ·kot'o·me)
varicula (vah·rik'u·lah)
variola (vah·ri'o·lah)
varioloid (va're·o·loid)
varix (var'iks)
vas (vas)
vasa (va'sah)
vascular (vas'ku·lar)
vascularity (vas'ku·lar'ĭ·te)
vascularization (vas'ku·lar·ĭ·za'shun)
vasculature (vas'ku·lah·tūr)
vasculitis (vas'ku·li'tis)
vasculogenesis (vas'ku·lo·jen'ě·sis)
vasectomy (vah·sek'to·me)
vasocongestion (vas'o·kon·jest'yun)
vasoconstriction (vas'o·kon·strik'shun)
vasoconstrictor (vas'o·kon·strik'tor)
vasodilation (vas'o·di·la'shun)
vasodilator (vas'o·di·lāt'or)
vasodistention (vas'o·dis·ten'shun)
vasoganglion (vas'o·gang'gle·on)
vasohypertonic (vas'o·hi'per·tŏn'ik)
vasohypotonic (vas'o·hi'po·ton'ik)
vasoinhibitor (vas'o·in·hib'ĭ·tor)
vasoinhibitory (vas'o·in·hib'ĭ·tor·e)
vasoligation (vas'o·li·ga'shun)
vasomotor (vas'o·mo'tor)
vasoparalysis (vas'o·pah·ral'ĭ·sis)
vasopressin (vas'o·pres'in)

vasopressor (vas'o·pres'or)
vasosensory (vas'o·sen'so·re)
vasospasm (vas'o·spazm)
vasostimulant (vas'o·stim'u·lant)
vasotomy (vah·sot'o·me)
vasotonic (vas'o·ton'ik)
vasovesiculectomy
(vas'o·vě·sik'u·lek'to·me)
vectorcardiogram
(vek'tor·kar'de·o·gram')
vectorcardiography
(vek'tor·kar'de·og'rah·fe)
vegetarian (vej'ě·tār'e·an)
vegetation (vej'ě·ta'shun)
Veillonella (va'yon·el'ah)
velopharyngeal (vel'o·fah·rin'je·al)
velum (ve'lum)
vena (ve'nah)
venae (ve'ne)
venectomy (ve·nek'to·me)
veneer (vě·nēr')
venenous (ven'ě·nus)
venereal (ve·ne're·al)
venereology (ve·nēr'e·ol'o·je)
venesection (ven'ě·sek'shun)
venipuncture (ven'ĭ·punk'tūr)
venoclysis (ven·ock'lĭ·sis)
venography (ve·nog'rah·fe)
venom (ven'um)
venous (ve'nus)
ventilation (ven'tĭ·la'shun)
ventral (ven'tral)
ventricle (ven'trĭ·kl)
ventricular (ven·trik'u·lar)
ventriculi (ven·trik'u·li)
ventriculitis (ven·trik'u·li'tis)
ventriculocisternostomy
(ven·trik'u·lo·sis'ter·nos'to·me)
ventriculocordotomy
(ven·trik'u·lo·kor·dot'o·me)
ventriculography (ven·trik'u·log'rah·fe)
ventriculus (ven·trik'u·lus)
venule (ven'ūl)
verapamil (ver·ap'ah·mil)
verbigeration (ver·bij'er·a'shun)
vergence (ver'jens)
vermicide (ver'mĭ·sīd)
vermiculation (ver·mik'u·la'shun)
vermiculose (ver·mik'u·lōs)
vermiform (ver'mĭ·form)
vermilionectomy (ver·mil'yon·ek'to·me)
vermin (ver'min)
verminous (ver'mĭ·nus)
vermis (ver'mis)
vermix (ver'miks)
vernix (ver'niks)
verruca (vě·roo'kah)
verruciform (vě·roo'sĭ·form)
verrucose (ver'oo·kōs)
verrucosis (ver'oo·ko'sis)
verruga (vě·roo'gah)
versicolor (ver'sĭ·kol'or)
version (ver'zhun)
vertebra (ver'tě·brah)
vertebrae (ver'tě·bre)
vertebral (ver'tě·bral)
vertebrate (ver'tě·brāt)
vertebrectomy (ver'tě·brek'to·me)
vertex (ver'teks)
vertigo (ver'tĭ·go)
verumontanitis (ver'u·mon'tah·ni'tis)
verumontanum (ver'u·mon·ta'num)
vesical (ves'ĭ·kl)
vesicant (ves'ĭ·kant)
vesicate (ves'ĭ·kāt)
vesication (ves'ĭ·ka'shun)
vesicle (ves'ĭ·kl)
vesicobullous (ves'ĭ·ko·bul'us)
vesicula (vě·sik'u·lah)
vesiculae (vě·sik'u·le)
vesicular (vě·sik'u·lar)
vesiculation (vě·sik'u·la'shun)
vesiculectomy (vě·sik'u·lek'to·me)
vesiculitis (vě·sik'u·li'tis)
vesiculopapular (vě·sik'u·lo·pap'u·lar)
vesiculoprostatitis
(vě·sik'u·lo·pros'tah·ti'tis)
vesiculopustular (vě·sik'u·lo·pus'tu·lar)

vesiculotomy (vĕ·sik′u·lot′o·me)
vestibular (ves·tib′u·lar)
vestibule (ves′tĭ·būl)
vestibuloplasty (ves·tib′u·lo·plas′te)
vestibulotomy (ves·tib′u·lot′o·me)
vestibulourethral (ves·tib′u·lo·u·re′thral)
vestige (ves′tij)
vestigia (ves·tij′e·ah)
vestigial (ves·tij′e·al)
vestigium (ves·tij′e·um)
veterinarian (vet′er·ĭ·nār′e·an)
veterinary (vet′er·ĭ·nār′e)
viability (vi′ah·bil′ĭ·te)
viable (vi′ah·bl)
vial (vi′al)
vibration (vi·bra′shun)
vibrissa (vi·bris′ah)
vibrotherapeutics (vi′bro·ther′ah·pu′tiks)
vicarious (vi·kar′e·us)
vicinal (vis′ĭ·nal)
vigilambulism (vij′il·am′bu·lizm)
vigilance (vij′ĭ·lans)
villi (vil′i)
villikinin (vil′ĭ·ki′nin)
villositis (vil′o·si′tis)
villous (vil′us)
villus (vil′lus)
vinblastine (vin·blas′tēn)
vincristine (vin·kris′tēn)
vincula (ving′ku·lah)
vinculum (ving′ku·lum)
violaceous (vi′o·la′shus)
Viperidae (vi·per′ĭ·de)
viral (vi′ral)
viremia (vi·re′me·ah)
virgin (vir′jin)
virginity (vir·jin′ĭ·te)
virile (vir′il)
virilism (vir′ĭ·lizm)
virility (vi·ril′ĭ·te)
virilization (vir′ĭ·lĭ·za′shun)
virion (vi′re·on)
viroid (vi′roid)
virologist (vi·rol′o·jist)
virology (vi·rol′o·je)
viromicrosome (vi′ro·mi′kro·sōm)
viropexis (vi′ro·pek′sis)
virucide (vi′ru·sīd)
virulence (vir′u·lens)
viruliferous (vir′u·lif′er·us)
viruria (vi·ru′re·ah)
virus (vi′rus)
viscance (vis′kans)
viscera (vis′er·ah)
visceral (vis′er·al)
visceralgia (vis′er·al′je·ah)
visceromegaly (vis′er·o·meg′ah·le)
visceroptosis (vis′er·op·to′sis)
viscid (vis′id)
viscidity (vĭ·sid′ĭ·te)
viscosimeter (vis′ko·sim′ĕ·ter)
viscosity (vis·kos′ĭ·te)
viscosurgery (vis′ko·sur′jer·e)
viscous (vis′kus)
viscus (vis′kus)
vision (vizh′un)
visualize (vizh′u·al·īz)
visuoauditory (vizh′u·o·aw′dĭ·tor′e)
vital (vi′tal)
vitality (vi·tal′ĭ·te)
vitallium (vi·tal′e·um)
vitals (vi′talz)
vitamin (vi′tah·min)
vitelline (vĭ·tel′in)
vitiliginous (vit′ĭ·lij′ĭ·nus)
vitiligo (vit′ĭ·li′go)
vitreoretinopathy
(vit′re·o·ret′ĭ·nop′ah·the)
vitreous (vit′re·us)
vitrification (vit′rĭ·fĭ·ka′shun)
vitriol (vit′re·ol)
vivarium (vi·var′e·um)
vividialysis (viv′ĭ·di·al′ĭ·sis)
vividiffusion (viv′ĭ·dĭ·fu′zhun)

vivification (viv′ĭ·fi·ka′shun)
viviparous (vi·vip′ah·rus)
viviperception (viv′ĭ·per·sep′shun)
vivisection (viv′ĭ·sek′shun)
vocal (vo′kal)
volar (vo′lar)
volatile (vol′ah·til)
volatilization (vol′ah·til·ĭ·za′shun)
volatilize (vol′ah·til·īz)
volume (vol′ūm)
volumetric (vol′u·met′rik)
voluntary (vol′un·tār′e·)
volvulus (vol′vu·lus)
vomer (vo′mer)
vomitus (vom′ĭ·tus)
vortex (vor′teks)
vortices (vor′tĭ·sēz)
vorticose (vor′tĭ·kōs)
voyeur (voi·yer′)
voyeurism (voi′yer·izm)
vulcanize (vul′kah·nīz)
vulgaris (vul·ga′ris)
vulva (vul′vah)
vulvectomy (vul·vek′to·me)
vulvitis (vul·vi′tis)
vulvocrural (vul·vo·kroo′ral)
vulvouterine (vul′vo·u′ter·in)
vulvovaginal (vul′vo·vaj′ĭ·nal)
vulvovaginitis (vul′vo·vaj′ĭ·ni′tis)

W

Waardenburg (wahrd′en·berg)
waddle (wah′dl)
warfarin (war′fah·rin)
wart (wort)
wavelength (wāv′length)
wean (wēn)
wheal (hwēl)
wheeze (hwēz)
whey (hwa)
whipworm (hwip′werm)
whitehead (hwĭt′hed)
whitlow (hwit′lo)
whoop (hoop)
whorl (hwerl)
wintergreen (win′ter·grēn)
womb (woom)
workaholic (werk′ah·hol′ik)
wound (woond)
wrist (rist)
wryneck (ri′nek)
Wuchereria (voo′ker·e′re·ah)
wuchereriasis (voo·ker′e·ri′·ah·sis)

X

xanthelasma (zan′thel·az′mah)
xanthemia (zan·the′me·ah)
xanthene (zan′thēn)
xanthic (zan′thik)
xanthine (zan′thēn)
xanthinuria (zan′thin·u′re·ah)
xanthochromia (zan′tho·kro′me·ah)
xanthochromic (zan′tho·kro′mik)
xanthocyanopsia
(zan′tho·si′ah·nop′se·ah)
xanthodont (zan′tho·dont′)
xanthogranuloma (zan′tho·gran′u·lo′mah)
xanthoma (zan·tho′mah)
xanthomatosis (zan′tho·mah·to′sis)
xanthomatous (zan·tho′mah·tus)
xanthophyll (zan′tho·fil)
xanthopsia (zan·thop′se·ah)
xanthopterin (zan·thop′ter·in)
xanthosine (zan′tho·sēn)
xanthosis (zan·tho′sis)
xanthurenic (zan′thu·re′nik)
xanthyl (zan′thil)
xenogeneic (zen′o·jen·a′ik)
xenogenic (zen′o·jen′ik)

xenograft (zen′o·graft)
xenoimmune (zen′o·i·mūn′)
xenon (ze′non)
xenophthalmia (zen′of·thal′me·ah)
Xenopsylla (zen′op·sil′ah)
xerocheilia (ze′ro·ki′le·ah)
xeroderma (ze′ro·der′mah)
xerography (ze·rog′rah·fe)
xeromammography
(ze′ro·mam·mog′rah·fe)
xeromenia (ze′ro·me′ne·ah)
xerophthalmia (ze′rof·thal′me·ah)
xeroradiography (ze′ro·ra′de·og′rah·fe)
xerosis (ze·ro′sis)
xerostomia (ze′ro·sto′me·ah)
xerotic (ze·rot′ik)
xiphodynia (zif′o·din′e·ah)
xiphoid (zif′oid)
xylene (zi′lēn)
xylometazoline (zi′lo·met′ah·zo′lēn)
xylose (zi′lōs)
xylulose (zi′lu·lōs)
xylyl (zi′lil)

Y

yaws (yawz)
yeast (yēst)
Yersinia (yer·sin′e·ah)
yersiniosis (yer·sin′e·o·sis)
yogurt (yo′goort)
yolk (yōk)
ytterbium (ĭt·ter′be·um)
yttrium (ĭt′tre·um)

Z

zeaxanthin (ze′ah·zan′thin)
Zeitgeber (zīt′ga·ber)
zinc (zingk)
zirconium (zir·ko′ne·um)
zona (zo′nah)
zonesthesia (zo′nes·the′ze·ah)
zonula (zōn′u·lah)
zonular (zōn′u·lar)
zonulolysis (zōn′u·lol′ĭ·sis)
zooanthroponosis
(zo′o·an′thro·po·no′sis)
zoogenic (zo′o·jen′ik)
zoogonous (zo·og′ŏ·nus)
zooid (zo′oid)
zoologist (zo·ol′o·jist)
zoology (zo·ol′o·je)
zoonosis (zo′o·no′sis)
zoophilic (zo′o·fil′ik)
zoospore (zo′o·spōr)
zootoxin (zo′o·tok′sin)
zoster (zos′ter)
zosteroid (zos′ter·oid)
zwitterion (tsvit′er·i′on)
zygodactyly (zi′go·dak′tĭ·le)
zygoma (zi′go·mah)
zygomatic (zi′go·mat·ik)
Zygomycetes (zi′go·mi·se′tēz)
zygosis (zi·go′sis)
zygosity (zi·gos′ĭ·te)
zygote (zi′gōt)
zygotene (zi′go·tēn)
zymase (zi·mās)
zymogen (zi′mo·jen)
zymogenesis (zy′mo·jen′ē·sis)
zymogenic (zy′mo·jen′ik)
zymoid (zi′moid)
zymology (zi·mol′o·je)
zymolysis (zi·mol′ĭ·sis)
zymolytic (zi′mo·lit′ik)
zymoplastic (zi′mo·plas′tik)
zymosan (zi′mo·san)
zymose (zi′mōs)
zymosis (zi·mo′sis)
zymotic (zi·mot′ik)

MELLONI'S
ILLUSTRATED
MEDICAL
DICTIONARY

Third Edition

HOW TO USE THIS DICTIONARY

Each illustration is integrated with a specific term and its definition on that page. Brown correlates the respective illustration (or any of its parts) with the appropriate entry in the text below.

clubbed digits

Digitalis purpurea

Brown-McHardy pneumatic dilator

dinitrophenol

digitoxin

pneumatic bag

dimenhydrinate

sia. See under aplasia.

digest 1. To break up food into simpler, assimilable compounds by the muscular and chemical action of the digestive tract. **2.** To absorb mentally.

digestant An agent that aids the process of digestion.

digestion The process taking place in the alimentary canal whereby the nutritive components of food are converted into substances that can be absorbed by the intestine; the decomposition of materials into simpler compounds.

digestive Relating to digestion.

digit A finger or toe.

clubbed d.'s A bulbous enlargement of the fingertips, seen in some cases of heart disease and certain pulmonary disorders. Also called drumstick or clubbed fingers.

digital 1. Pertaining to, performed by, or resembling a digit or digits, especially a finger. **2.** Possessing digits.

digitalis 1. Foxglove, a plant of the genus *Digitalis*. **2.** Digitalis (USP), a drug obtained from the dried leaves of *Digitalis purpurea*, used in the treatment of heart disease, especially for congestive heart failure and some supraventricular tachyarrhythmias.

digitalization The treatment of an individual with digitalis or a related cardiac glycoside, to achieve a desired therapeutic effect.

digitate Having fingerlike processes.

digitation A finger-like process.

digitoxin A glycoside obtained from *Digitalis purpurea*; used in the treatment of congestive heart failure.

digitus, *pl.* **digiti** Latin for finger.

digoxin A glycoside obtained from the leaves of *Digitalis lanata*; used in the treatment of congestive heart failure.

DiGuglielmo's syndrome Erythremic myelosis; see under myelosis.

dihydrate A compound having two molecules of water.

dihydroergotamine (D.H.E. 45) A crystalline compound produced by the hydrogenation of ergotamine; used in the treatment of migraine headache.

dihydrostreptomycin Compound made by the hydrogenation of streptomycin and having antibiotic properties.

dihydrotachysterol (AT 10) A synthetic sterol that produces effects similar to those of vitamin D.

diiodotyrosine (T_2, DIT) A precursor of the thyroid hormone thyroxin. Also called iodogorgoic acid.

diisopropylfluorophosphate (DFP) A potent cholinergic agent; used in the treatment of glaucoma

and strabismus.

dilatation 1. The condition of being enlarged, occurring normally, artifically, or as a result of disease; said of a tubular structure, a cavity, or an opening; **2.** Dilation (1).

gastric d. Acute distention of the stomach with fluid and air; commonly seen following surgery or trauma.

dilation 1. The act of stretching or dilating. **2.** Dilatation (1).

dilator Instrument for enlarging a passage or cavity.

dildo, dildoe An object having the approximate size and shape of an erect penis; used to produce sexual pleasure by vaginal insertion.

diltiazem A calcium channel blocking agent used in the treatment of angina pectoris; especially useful in Prinzmetal's angina.

diluent A substance which reduces the concentration of a solution.

dilution 1. The process of reducing the concentration of a solution or substance. **2.** A weakened solution or substance; an attenuated mixture.

dimenhydrinate Drug used in preventing and treating motion sickness; Dramamine®.

dimension Any measurable distance.

vertical d. In prosthodontics, the distance between two points on the face, one above and one below the mouth, usually in the midline; it may be measured when the opposing occlusal surfaces are in maximum contact (occlusal vertical dimension) or in rest position, when the jaws are not in contact (rest vertical dimension).

dimer A chemical compound composed of molecules that consist of two identical simpler molecules.

dimercaprol A compound used as an antidote for lewisite and other arsenic poisoning. Also called British antilewisite (BAL).

dimethyl sulfoxide (DMSO) An industrial solvent occasionally used in medicine as a skin penetrant to facilitate absorption of medications from the skin. Also called methyl sulfoxide.

dimorphism The property of occurring in two forms.

dinitrophenol (DNP) A drug that causes an increase in rate of metabolism by interruption of the coupling of oxidation and phosphorylation; not used clinically because of its toxicity.

dinucleotide One of the compounds into which nucleic acid splits on hydrolysis; it may split into two mononucleotides.

diopter (D) The unit used to designate the refractive power of a lens or an optical system.

dioptometer An instrument for measuring refrac-

tion and accommodation of the eye. Also called dioptrometer.

dioptric 1. Relating to the unit of refractive power of lenses. **2.** Refractive.

dioptrics The science of the refraction of light.

dioptrometer See dioptometer.

diotic In audiology, denoting an arrangement in which each ear receives the same signal.

dioxide An oxide containing two atoms of oxygen per molecule.

dioxin A hydrocarbon; a pesticide contaminant thought to produce cancer and birth defects.

dipeptidase One of the protein-splitting enzymes that causes the breakdown of a dipeptide into its two constituent amino acids.

dipeptide Two amino acids linked by a peptide bond.

diphenhydramine hydrochloride An antihistamine used in the prevention and treatment of motion sickness, postoperative nausea, nausea and vomiting of pregnancy, and some allergies; Benadryl®.

diphenylhydantoin An anticonvulsant agent, used primarily to treat epilepsy; Dilantin®.

2,3-diphosphoglycerate (DPG) A chemical present in the red blood cells that binds to hemoglobin and has a great effect on its oxygen affinity; in its absence, hemoglobin unloads less oxygen in passing through tissue capillaries.

diphosphonates Synthetic substances similar to the pyrophosphates in structure but not biologically hydrolyzed; in vitro, they prevent hydroxyapatite crystal formation; it has been suggested that they coat the bone surface and prevent bone resorption.

diphosphopyridine nucleotide (DPN) Old term for nicotinamide adenine dinucleotide (NAD).

diphtheria An acute contagious disease caused by a bacillus, *Corynebacterium diphtheriae*; marked by inflammation of the upper respiratory tract, fibrin formation (false membrane) of the mucous membranes, and elaboration of soluble exotoxin which acts on the heart and cranial or peripheral nerve cells.

diphtheroid 1. Resembling diphtheria. **2.** A bacterium resembling the organism that causes diphtheria.

diphyllobothriasis Infestation with *Diphyllobothrium latum* (broadfish tapeworm), caused by ingestion of inadequately cooked, infected fish.

Diphyllobothrium A genus of tapeworms (family Diphyllobothriidae). Formerly called *Dibothriocephalus*.

D. latum Intestinal parasite transmitted to man by ingestion of undercooked infected fresh water

synonym of defined term

synonym cross reference to defined term

boldface numbers distinguish multiple definitions

abbreviation or symbol for defined term

first and last entry on page to facilitate location of desired term

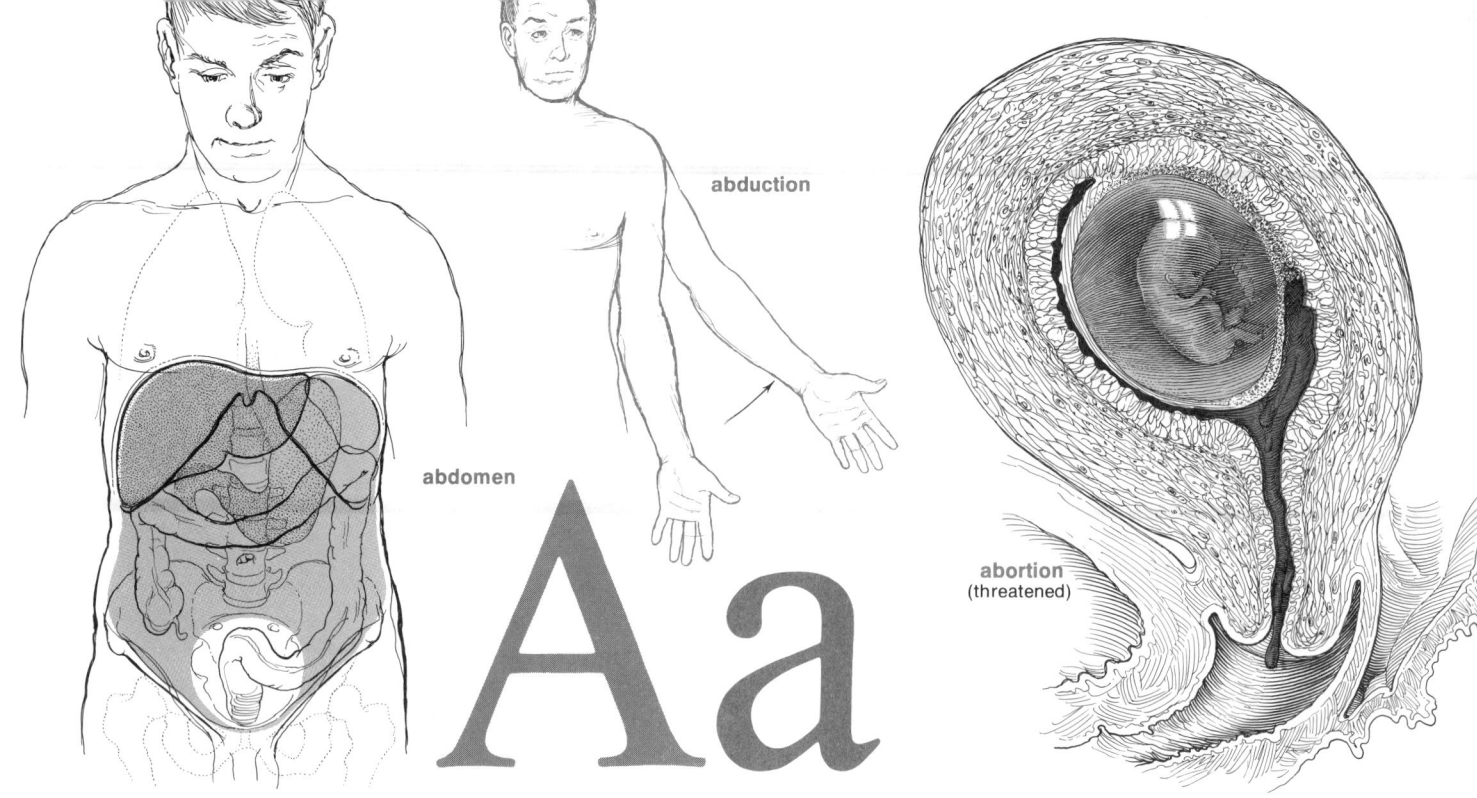

abdomen

abduction

abortion
(threatened)

Aa

α Alpha. For terms beginning with α, see under specific term.

abaissement French for a lowering or depression.

abarognosis Loss of sense of weight estimation.

abarthrosis See diarthrosis.

abarticular Not affecting, or far from, a joint.

abarticulation 1. Dislocation. 2. Diarthrosis.

abasia Inability to walk due to impaired motor coordination.

abasic Related to or afflicted with abasia.

abaxial, abaxile Not located on the axis of the body or any structure.

abdomen Area of the body between the thorax and pelvis containing the viscera. Also called belly.

  acute a. An incapacitating condition characterized by intense abdominal pain, which may or may not be associated with fever, nausea, vomiting, and shock.

abdominal Pertaining to the abdomen.

abdominalgia Pain in the abdomen

  periodic a. Disorder of unknown cause, marked by abdominal pain, recurring fever, inflamed peritoneum, and sometimes purpura. Also called Mediterranean fever; benign paroxysmal peritonitis.

abdominocentesis Puncturing of the abdominal wall for drainage purposes.

abdominoplasty Removal of loose skin and subcutaneous tissue from the abdominal wall.

abdominoposterior Denoting position of the fetus in the uterus in which its abdomen is turned toward the mother's back.

abdominoscopy Examination of the abdomen, especially visual examination of the abdominal organs.

abdominovaginal Relating to the abdomen and the vagina.

abdominovesical Relating to the abdomen and urinary bladder

abducens Denoting the sixth cranial nerve.

abducent Denoting structures that serve to abduct a part.

abduct To draw away from the median line of the body or from an adjacent part or limb.

abduction Movement of a part away from the middle line; act of turning outward.

abductor A structure, such as a muscle, that draws a part away from an axis of the body; opposite of adductor.

abembryonic Located away from the embryo.

aberrant Deviating from the normal or expected course, as a duct taking an unusual direction.

aberration 1. A deviation from the normal. 2. Unequal refraction of light rays passing through a lens, resulting in the formation of an imperfect image.

  chromatic a. Aberration resulting from unequal refraction of wavelengths; typical example is a display of colors around an object viewed through a simple lens. Also called newtonian and color aberration.

  chromosome a. A departure from the normal number of chromosomes or chromosome structure; e.g., in Down syndrome there are 47 chromosomes, in Turner's syndrome there are 45.

abetalipoproteinemia A familial condition marked by the presence in the blood of large numbers of acanthocytes and a marked decrease in serum beta-lipoproteins; may be associated with steatorrhea and progressive neurologic disease.

abient Having the tendency to avoid, or move away from, a stimulus.

abiogenesis The origin of living matter from nonliving matter; a theory of spontaneous generation.

abiogenetic Of or relating to spontaneous generation.

abiology The study of nonliving or inorganic things.

abiosis Lifelessness.

abiotrophy General term denoting degenerative changes of tissues due to genetic causes.

abirritant 1. Relieving irritation. 2. A substance having this property.

ablate To remove.

ablatio placentae Abruptio placentae.

ablation 1. Detachment. 2. Surgical removal or amputation.

ablepharia, ablepharon Congenital absence of the eyelids, partial or total.

ablepharous Without eyelids.

ablepsia, ablepsy Blindness.

abluent A substance that has cleansing properties.

ablution The act of cleansing.

ablutomania Abnormal concern with cleanliness.

abneural Away from the central nervous system or from the dorsal aspect.

abnormal Not normal; departing from the usual position, structure, or condition.

abnormality The condition or state of being abnormal.

ABO blood group International (Landsteiner) classification of human blood types according to their compatibility in transfusion; typed as A, B, AB, or O. Also called ABO factors.

aboral Distant from or opposite to the mouth.

abort 1. To terminate pregnancy before the fetus is viable. 2. To arrest the usual course of a disease. 3. To cease growth or development; to cause to remain rudimentary.

abortient 1. Aborting. 2. An abortifacient; a drug

that produces abortion.

abortifacient Anything that produces abortion.

abortigenic Abortifacient.

abortion 1. Interruption of pregnancy before the fetus has attained a stage of viability, usually before 24 weeks of gestation; characteristic symptoms are vaginal bleeding and expulsive uterine contractions. 2. The arrest of a disease or natural process before completion.

  accidental a. Abortion due to an injury.

  complete a. Elimination of the entire contents of the uterus (fetus, placenta, and membranes).

  elective a. Induced abortion without specific medical indication.

  habitual a. See recurrent abortion.

  incomplete a. Expulsion of the fetus while all or part of the placenta remains in the uterus.

  induced a. Intentionally caused abortion.

  inevitable a. Condition characterized by severe vaginal bleeding and uterine contractions, accompanied by cervical dilatation that has advanced beyond any hope of preventing the expulsion of the uterine contents.

  missed a. Abortion in which the fetus dies and is retained in utero for two months or longer.

  recurrent a. Loss of three or more successive pregnancies. Also called habitual abortion.

  septic a. Abortion in which the embryo and maternal genital tract are infected.

  spontaneous a. Termination of a previable conception without apparent cause.

  therapeutic a. Termination of a pregnancy for medical or psychiatric reasons.

  threatened a. Slight vaginal bleeding with or without feeble uterine contractions, in the absence of cervical dilatation.

abortive 1. Causing abortion. 2. Cutting short, arresting; said of a disease. 3. Failing to reach completion; partially developed.

aboulia See abulia.

abrachia Absence of arms.

abrade To rub or wear away the external layer by friction, as to scrape away the epidermis from a part; to excoriate.

abrasion 1. A superficial injury, in which the skin or mucous membrane is scraped away. 2. The process of wearing down of a tooth by friction; usually applied to excessive wear such as that caused by the use of an abrasive dentifrice.

abrasive 1. Producing abrasion. 2. A material used in dentistry for grinding or polishing.

abreaction A form of psychotherapy, called catharsis by Freud, in which emotional release is attained by recalling a forgotten (repressed), painful experience.

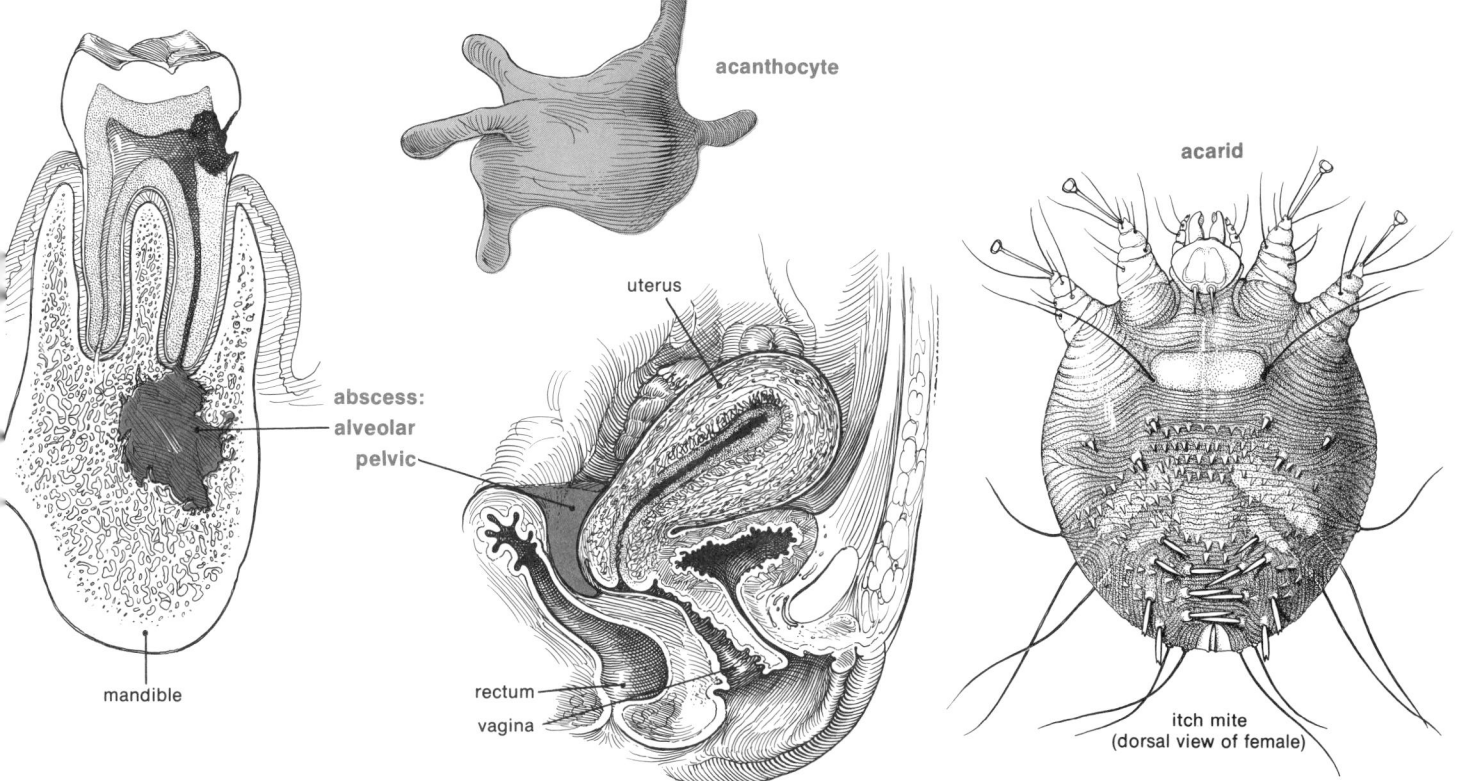

acanthocyte

abscess:
alveolar
pelvic

uterus

mandible

rectum
vagina

acarid

itch mite
(dorsal view of female)

abruptio placentae Premature separation of the normally implanted placenta from its uterine attachment after the twentieth week of gestation. Also called placental abruption; ablatio placentae.

abruption, placental Abruptio placentae.

absence A brief loss of consciousness; see epilepsy, petit mal.

abscess Localized accumulation of pus.

acute a. One of short duration, producing a throbbing pain and fever. Also called hot abscess.

alveolar a. A collection of pus in the tooth socket, resulting from dental caries; it causes a constant, severe, throbbing pain and swelling.

amebic a. One occurring as a complication of amebic dysentery, usually in the liver, and containing a brown pasty fluid.

appendicular a. An abscess in the area of the vermiform appendix.

chronic a. A long-standing collection of pus without inflammation. Also called cold abscess.

cold a. See chronic abscess.

extradural a. Abscess situated between the skull and the outer covering of the brain (dura mater); it is usually an extension of infection of the middle ear or frontal sinus.

gingival a. A localized, painful, inflammatory lesion of the gingiva, usually arising from a periodontal pocket.

hot a. See acute abscess.

mammary a. An abscess in the breast, generally seen during the lactation period or on weaning.

metastatic a. Secondary abscess caused by organisms carried in the bloodstream from a primary abscess.

orbital a. An abscess within the ocular orbit, frequently an extension of purulent sinusitis.

palmar a. A collection of pus in the palm of the hand, resulting from a puncture injury.

pelvic a. An abscess located in the pelvic cavity, usually in the rectouterine pouch.

periapical a. An abscess occuring in the alveolus near the apex of a tooth root, usually due to death of the tooth pulp.

periodontal a. A localized, purulent inflammation in the gingiva corium, infrabony pockets, or periodontal membrane; it may be acute or chronic.

periurethral a. One involving the tissues around the urethra, causing strained, painful urination.

psoas a. One occurring in the sheath of the psoas muscle secondary to tuberculosis of the lower spine or to regional enteritis. Also called iliac abscess.

pulp a. One within the pulp cavity of a tooth.

stitch a. An abscess around a suture.

subdiaphragmatic a. An abscess between the diaphragm and the liver or between the diaphragm and the spleen and stomach. Also called subphrenic abscess.

subphrenic a. See subdiaphragmatic abscess.

abscissa The horizontal coordinate which, together with a vertical one (ordinate), forms a frame of reference for the plotting of data.

absolute Complete; unrestricted; unadulterated.

absorb 1. To take in as through pores or interstices. **2.** To incorporate or take up gases, liquid, light rays, or heat. **3.** To neutralize an acid.

absorbable Capable of being absorbed.

absorbent Anything that can incorporate a substance into itself.

absorptiometer 1. An instrument used to measure the solubility of gas in a liquid. **2.** An instrument for measuring the layer of liquid between two glass plates; used as a hematoscope in the analysis of blood.

absorption 1. The taking up of substances by the skin or other tissues. **2.** The taking up of part or all of the energy of incident radiation by the medium through which radiation passes, resulting in reduction of radiation intensity.

abstergent 1. Cleansing or purgative. **2.** An agent having such properties.

abstinence A refraining from the indulgence in something, as sexual intercourse or stimulants, by one's own choice. Also called self-denial.

abstract 1. A preparation containing the soluble elements of a drug mixed with lactose. **2.** A summary of a book or literary article.

abulia Pronounced diminution of will power; inability to make decisions. Also written aboulia.

abuse 1. Improper use, particularly excessive use of anything. **2.** Maltreatment.

child a. Physical maltreatment of a child, usually by parents.

drug a. Excessive use, generally self-administered, of any drug, most commonly an agent that acts on the central nervous system, without regard for accepted medical practice.

abutment 1. A supporting structure. **2.** In dentistry, a natural tooth or root used to anchor and support a partial denture appliance.

intermediate a. A natural tooth, without other natural teeth in proximal contact, which is used as an abutment, in addition to the primary or terminal abutments.

acacia The dried gummy exudate from a tropical tree of the genus *Acacia*; used in the preparation of medicinal drugs. Also called gum arabic.

acalculia A form of aphasia characterized by inability to do simple arithmetic.

acantha A spinous process.

acanthamebiasis Infection with *Acanthamoeba*

castellani, a free-living ameba found in moist soil and water; may cause fatal inflammation of the brain and its membranes (meningoencephalitis).

acanthesthesia Condition in which there is a sensation of pressure with a sharp point.

acanthion A projection on the anterior nasal spine.

Acanthocephala A phylum of parasitic worms having a proboscis with hooked spines for attachment to the host.

acanthocephaliasis Infestation with acanthocephalids.

acanthocephalid Any worm of the phylum Acanthocephala.

Acanthocheilonema A genus of parasitic worms, commonly called filaria; the adults live mainly in the body cavities or the subcutaneous tissues, while the larvae exist in the peripheral blood.

acanthocheilonemiasis Infestation with *Acanthocheilonema perstans*.

acanthocyte An abnormal red blood cell having several protoplasmic projections that give it a thorny appearance.

acanthocytosis Familial condition marked by the presence in the blood of large numbers of acanthocytes.

acanthoid Having the shape of a spine; spinous.

acanthokeratodermia See hyperkeratosis.

acantholysis Disintegration of the epidermis.

acanthoma Carcinoma of the epidermis.

acanthosis Thickening of the prickle-cell layer of the skin.

acapnia See hypocapnia.

acari Plural of acarus.

acariasis 1. Any disease caused by mites. **2.** Infestation with mites.

sarcoptic a. See scabies.

acaricide Any agent that destroys mites.

acarid A mite or tick; any member of the order Acarina.

Acaridae A family of small mites (order Acarina), some of which cause skin eruptions in humans.

Acarina An order of the class Arachnida, which includes mites and ticks.

acarinosis Acariasis.

acarodermatitis A skin rash caused by mites.

acaroid Resembling a mite.

acarology The study of mites and ticks.

acarophobia Abnormal fear of mites (acari), or of small particles.

acarus, *pl.* acari A mite or tick.

acaryote See akaryocyte.

acatalasia Genetic disorder marked by deficiency of the enzyme catalase; manifestations range from mild (ulcers of tooth sockets) to severe (recession of

Glycine (Gly) · Alanine (Ala) · Valine (Val) · Isoleucine (Ileu) · Leucine (Leu) · Lysine (Lys) · Arginine (Arg) · Asparagine (Asn) · Glutamine (Gln) · Cysteine (Cys)

tooth sockets and gangrene of the gums). Two principal types have been identified: (a) Japanese type, in which the small amount of residual catalase is physiochemically normal, suggesting a mutation of a regulator (controller) gene; (b) Swiss type, in which the catalase is abnormal, suggesting a structural gene mutation. Formerly called acalalesemia.

acataphasia Loss of the power to formulate one's thoughts correctly.

acathamathesia Loss of the power of understanding.

acaudal, acaudate Without a tail.

acauline A term applied to a group of stemless fungi.

accelerant Accelerator.

acceleration Increased speed of action, as of pulse or respiration.

accelerator Anything (drug, device, nerve, or muscle) that increases speed of action or function.

accentuator A substance that increases the action of a tissue stain

acceptor A substance that unites with a chemical group or ion of another substance (the donor), thus allowing a chemical reaction to proceed.

accessory Supplementary; having a subordinate function to a similar but more important structure.

accessory sign Any sign that usually, but not always, accompanies a disease.

accident An unexpected, unintentional, undesirable event, or an unforeseen complication in the course of a disease.

   cerebrovascular a., cerebral vascular a. (CVA) Occlusion or rupture of a blood vessel in the brain. Also called stroke.

acclimatization, acclimation Adjustment of an individual or plant to a new environment.

accolé form See under form.

accommodation Alteration in the convexity of the lens of the eye to attain maximal sharpness of a retinal image of an object, distant or near.

accommodative Relating to accommodation.

accouchement French for childbirth or labor.

accrementition 1. Reproduction by budding. 2. Growth by gradual external addition.

accretio cordis Adhesion of the pericardium to adjacent structures, such as the chest wall, pleura, or diaphragm.

accretion Slow accumulation of deposits, as on the surface of a tooth.

acellular Having no cells.

acenesthesia Loss of the normal sense of physical existence.

acentric 1. Not centrally located. 2. Denoting a chromosome fragment lacking a centromere.

acephalocyst A cyst filled with liquid that is one of the stages in the development of a sterile tapeworm; it does not give origin to daughter cysts which contain tapeworm heads (scoleces).

acervuline Occurring in cluster forms.

acervuloma Intracranial tumor or meningioma containing acervulus.

acervulus Sandlike matter occurring in the pineal body and near the choroid plexus; composed of calcium carbonate. Also called brain sand.

acescence 1. Slight acidity. 2. The process of becoming sour.

acetabular Of or relating to the acetabulum.

Acetabularia A genus (phylum Chlorophyta) of single-celled algae which may grow as tall as 10 cm and which possess a distinctive cap; used in the study of molecular biology.

acetabulectomy Surgical removal of the acetabulum.

acetabuloplasty Surgical restoration of the acetabulum.

acetabulum The cup-shaped cavity in the lateral surface of the hipbone in which the head of the femur fits. Also called hip socket.

acetaldehyde A colorless liquid, CH_3CHO, with a pungent odor; an intermediate in yeast fermentation of carbohydrate and in alcohol metabolism in man. Also called acetic aldehyde.

acetamide A colorless crystalline substance, CH_3CONH_2; an amine of acetic acid, used as a solvent.

acetaminophen N-Acetyl-p-aminophenol; a white crystalline powder, used to reduce pain and fever by inhibition of prostaglandin synthesis.

acetanilide A white crystalline substance, obtained from the action of acetic acid upon aniline; formerly used to relieve pain and fever.

acetate Any acetic acid salt.

acetazolamide A diuretic that inhibits the action of carbonic anhydrase in the kidney, promoting the loss of bicarbonate and sodium; the effect is to produce a mild acidosis and to alkalinize the urine; used in glaucoma to reduce intraocular pressure. Diamox®.

acetic Relating to, or containing, vinegar.

acetic acid A colorless, organic acid with a pungent odor.

   glacial a. a. A caustic liquid containing 99.5% acetic acid; used to remove corns and warts.

acetify To convert to vinegar or acetic acid.

acetoacetic acid A colorless syrupy acid, $CH_3COCH_2 \cdot COOH$; one of the ketone bodies, oc-

curring in excessive quantities in the urine of diabetics.

Acetobacter A genus of bacteria (family Pseudomonadaceae) having elongated or rod-shaped forms, sometimes flagellated; important in the production of vinegar.

acetolysis The splitting of an organic compound by the introduction of the elements of acetic acid.

acetomorphine Heroin.

acetone A colorless, volatile, extremely flammable liquid with an ethereal odor, CH_3COCH_3; generally used as an organic solvent.

acetonemia The presence of relatively large amounts of acetone or acetone bodies in the blood, as occurs when there is incomplete oxidation of large amounts of fat, as in ketoacidosis or starvation.

acetonemic Characterized by acetonemia.

acetonuria The presence of acetone in the urine; it occurs in poorly controlled diabetes mellitus and in starvation from incomplete oxidation of fats.

acetophenetidin See phenacetin.

acetum, pl. **aceta** 1. Vinegar. 2. A solution of a drug made with acetic acid.

acetyl A radical or combining form of acetic acid, CH_3CO.

acetylation The introduction of a radical group of acetic acid (acetyl) into an organic compound.

acetylcholine (ACh) The acetic acid ester of choline, $CH_3CO—OCH_2CH_2—N(CH_3)_3OH$; the chemical transmitter of the nerve impulse across a synapse; also released by the endings of parasympathetic nerves (cholinergic nerves) upon stimulation; produces cardiac slowing, vasodilation, increased gastrointestinal activity, and other parasympathetic effects; it is hydrolyzed and inactivated by the enzyme cholinesterase; available as acetylcholine bromide and acetylcholine chloride.

acetylcholinesterase See cholinesterase.

acetyl coenzyme A, acetyl-CoA An important metabolic intermediate of the tricarboxylic acid cycle; formed when an acetyl group is attached to coenzyme A by a thioester bond during oxidation of fatty acid, amino acids, or pyruvate.

acetylcysteine An agent used in the treatment of some bronchopulmonary disorders to reduce the viscosity of mucus; Mucomyst®.

acetylene A colorless, flammable, explosive gas, C_2H_2, with a disagreeable garlic odor; made by the action of water on calcium carbide; formerly used as an anesthetic.

acetylsalicylic acid An antipyretic, analgesic agent of value in the treatment of arthritis and other inflammatory conditions. Also called aspirin.

Serine (Ser) | Threonine (Thr) | Proline (Pro) | Aspartic acid (Asp) | Glutamic acid (Glu)

Methionine (Met) | Tryptophan (Try) | Phenylalanine (Phe) | Tyrosine (Tyr) | Histidine (His)

acetylstrophanthidin A synthetic cardiac glycoside with the most rapid onset of action of all the digitalis preparations.

achalasia Failure to relax; referring especially to sphincter muscles of the esophagus.

ache A dull pain.

acheiria Congenital lack of one or both hands.

Achilles A mythical Greek hero who was invulnerable except in the heel.

  A. bursa See bursa of calcaneal tendon.

  A. tendon See tendon, calcaneal.

achillodynia Pain in or about the calcaneal tendon (Achilles tendon). Also called achillobursitis.

achillorrhaphy Repair of a torn calcaneal tendon (Achilles tendon).

achillotenotomy Achillotomy.

achillotomy Surgical division of the calcaneal tendon (Achilles tendon).

  plastic a. elongation of the calcaneal tendon by plastic surgery.

achlorhydria Absence of hydrochloric acid in the stomach. Also called gastric anacidity.

achloropsia A form of color blindness restricted to green.

achluphobia A morbid fear of darkness.

acholia Deficiency of bile.

acholic Lacking bile.

acholuria Absence of bile pigments from the urine.

achondroplasia, achondroplasty Congenital abnormality in the process of ossification in cartilage, resulting in dwarfism and deformity. Also called chondrodystrophia; chondrodystrophy.

achordate, achordal Without a notochord; denoting animal forms classified below the chordates.

achoresis Reduction of the capacity of a hollow organ, as of the bladder, caused by permanent contraction.

achromasia 1. Absence of normal pigmentation of skin. 2. Lack of staining reaction in a cell.

achromate A totally color blind individual who sees colors as different shades of gray.

achromatic 1. Colorless. 2. Refracting light without separating it into its component colors. 3. Staining poorly. 4. Characterized by color blindness.

achromatin The part of the cell nucleus that is only faintly stained by dyes.

achromatophilia The condition of being resistant to the action of stains.

achromatopsia Total color blindness. Also called achromatopia.

achromatosis Lack of natural pigmentation, as in the iris or the skin.

achromatous Colorless.

achromia See leukoderma.

achromocyte Phantom corpuscle; see under corpuscle.

achromotrichia Lack or loss of color in the hair.

achylia A rare condition marked by the absence of gastric juices.

achylous 1. Without gastric juice or other digestive secretion. 2. Without chyle.

acicular Needle-shaped; said of some crystals or leaves.

acid A compound capable of donating a hydrogen ion (proton) to a base; any substance that turns litmus indicators red and combines with a base to form a salt. For individual acids, see specific names.

  amino a. Any organic acid containing one or more amino groups (NH_2) and a carboxyl group (CO_2H); forms the essential components of proteins.

  chenic a., chenodeoxycholic a. A natural bile acid in humans; it reduces the stone-forming tendency of bile and dissolves cholesterol gallstones by decreasing the hepatic secretion of cholesterol.

  dibasic a. An acid containing molecules with two displaceable hydrogen ions.

  essential fatty a. (EFA) A polyunsaturated fatty acid indispensable for nutrition; its absence causes a specific deficiency disorder and it cannot be fabricated by the body (must be obtained from the diet); e.g., linoleic acid and linolenic acid. Originally called vitamin F.

  fatty a. Any of a large group of organic acids made up of molecules containing a carboxyl group at the end of a long hydrocarbon chain; the carbon content may vary from C_2 to C_{34}.

  inorganic a. An acid composed of molecules that do not contain carbon atoms; e.g., hydrochloric acid, boric acid.

  monobasic a. An acid containing molecules with one displaceable hydrogen ion.

  nonessential fatty a. The main form of circulating lipid.

  nonesterified fatty a. (NEFA) The main form of circulating fatty acid used for energy.

  organic a. An acid composed of molecules containing carbon atoms; e.g., ascorbic acid, amino acid.

  polybasic a. An acid containing molecules with three or more displaceable hydrogen ions.

  polyunsaturated fatty a. Any unsaturated fatty acid with two or more double bonds; e.g., linoleic acid (two double bonds) and arachidonic acid (four double bonds).

  resin a.'s A class of organic compounds derived

from certain plant resins; e.g., abietic acid and pimaric acid. Also called rosin acids.

  saturated fatty a. A fatty acid in which the carbon chain is connected by single bonds, and is incapable of accepting any more hydrogen, i.e., all the available valence bonds of the carbon chain are filled with hydrogen atoms; e.g., stearic acid and palmitic acid.

  unsaturated fatty a. A fatty acid in which the carbon chain has at least one double bond, and is capable of accepting additional hydrogen atoms; e.g., oleic acid.

acidemia An increase in the hydrogen ion concentration of the blood; a fall below normal in pH (in humans, a fall below pH 7.4). Cf. acidosis.

acid-fast Denoting bacteria that, once stained with acids such as basic fuchsin, are not decolorized by acid-alcohol.

acidifiable Capable of being made acid.

acidify 1. To make acid. 2. To become acid.

acidity 1. The quality or state of being acid. 2. The acid content of a fluid.

acidophil Eosinophilic leukocyte; see under leukocyte.

acidosis A process tending to produce an increase in hydrogen ion concentration in body fluids; if uncompensated, it produces a lowering of pH. Commonly used synonymously with acidemia.

  compensated a. Condition in which the pH of blood is kept normal through respiratory or renal mechanisms, although the blood bicarbonate may be out of the usual range.

  lactic a. Accumulation of lactic acid in the body causing decreased bicarbonate concentration.

  metabolic a. Acidosis caused by excessive production or ingestion of acid other than carbonic acid (H_2CO_3) or by loss of base.

  renal tubular a. (RTA) Acidosis caused by defective elimination of acid or by excessive loss of bicarbonate by the kidneys; characterized by an elevated plasma chloride and a lowered plasma bicarbonate concentration.

  respiratory a. Acidosis caused by failure to eliminate carbon dioxide (CO_2) adequately; the retained CO_2 in the blood yields carbonic acid (H_2CO_3) and its dissociation increases the hydrogen ion concentration; retention of CO_2 may occur because of a ventilatory problem, as in advanced emphysema, a muscular problem, or a central nervous system disorder.

acidosteophyte A sharp-pointed outgrowth of bone.

acidotic Relating to, or suffering from, acidosis.

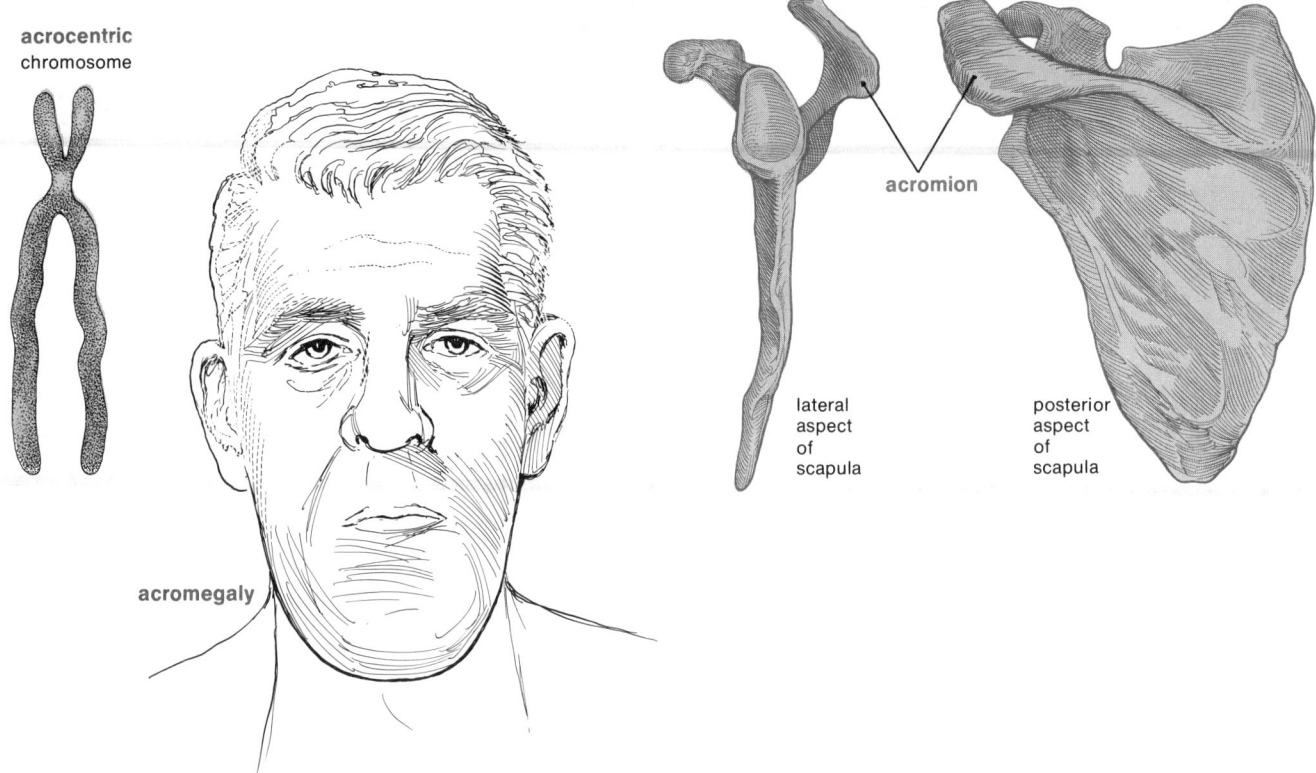

acrocentric
chromosome

acromion

lateral
aspect
of
scapula

posterior
aspect
of
scapula

acromegaly

acidulous Slightly sour or acid.

aciduria Abnormal amounts of acids in the urine.

  orotic a. Genetic disorder associated with defective metabolism of pyrimidine, resulting in megaloblastic anemia, retarded physical and mental growth, and excretion of orotic acid in the urine.

aciduric Capable of living under acid conditions; said of some bacteria.

acidyl A term used to denote any acid radical.

acinar Of or relating to an acinus.

acini Plural of acinus.

acinitis Inflammation of an acinus.

acinous Resembling a bunch of grapes or made up of minute sacs (acini).

acinus, *pl* **acini** 1. A minute saclike dilatation. 2. The smallest division of a gland.

aclasis Continuity of structure provided by pathologic tissue which arises from, and is continuous with, normal tissue.

acleistocardia Condition in which the foramen ovale of the heart fails to close.

acmesthesia Sensation of a pinprick in the skin.

acne An eruption caused by inflammation of the sebaceous glands.

  a. ciliaris Acne on the free edges of the eyelids.

  a. medicamentosa Acne that is aggravated by certain drugs.

  a. rosacea See rosacea.

  a. vulgaris Chronic acne, occurring commonly on the face, chest, and back of adolescents and young adults.

  cystic a. Acne vulgaris in which the lesions are minute abscesses containing sebum and keratin.

acneform, acneiform Resembling acne.

acocanthera A poisonous substance extracted from the leaves and stems of *Acocanthera venenata;* used by some natives of Africa as an arrow poison.

acognosia, acognosy The study or knowledge of remedies.

acolous Without limbs.

acomia Baldness.

aconative Without volition.

cis-**aconitic acid** A production of dehydration of citric acid; an intermediate in the tricarboxylic acid cycle.

acorea Congenital absence of the pupil of the eye.

acoria Lack of a feeling of satisfaction after eating.

acousma Sensation of hearing imaginary sounds. Also called acouasm.

acousmatagnosia Failure to recognize sounds. Also called mind deafness.

acousmatamnesia Inability to recall sounds.

acoustic Of or relating to sound or to the sense of hearing.

acousticophobia Abnormal fear of sounds.

acoustics The branch of science concerned with the study of sound, its generation, propagation, and perception.

acquired Developed after birth, in contrast to congenital or hereditary.

acquired immune deficiency syndrome See AIDS.

acral Relating to the extremities or peripheral parts.

acrania Congenital absence of the skull, or a portion of it.

acrid Pungent or sharp to the taste or smell.

acridine A coal tar derivative, $C_{13}H_9N$, occurring in colorless crystals and having a strong, irritating odor. Also called dibenzopyridine.

acritical Without a crisis.

acroagnosis Absence of sensory recognition of a limb.

acroanesthesia Lack of sensation in the extremities.

acroataxia Lack of muscular coordination of the fingers and toes.

acrocentric Denoting a chromosome whose centromere is situated close to one end.

acrocephalic Relating to or affected with acrocephaly.

acrocephalosyndactyly, acrocephalosyndactylism Congenital malformation consisting of a high-domed skull and complete or partial webbing of the digits. Also called Apert's syndrome.

acrocephaly Congenital malformation marked by a high-domed skull.

acrochordon A small, soft, pedunculated growth, occurring usually on the neck or eyelids.

acrocyanosis A chronic circulatory disorder intensified by cold and emotion, and characterized by cold, cyanotic, sweaty hands and feet; the skin is a mottled blue and red.

acrodermatitis Inflammation of the skin of the hands or feet.

  a. chronica atrophicans Dermatitis of the extremities accompanied by atrophy of the skin.

  a. vesiculosa tropica Dermatitis of the fingers, occurring in hot climates, in which the skin becomes glossy with numerous small vesicles.

acrodolichomelia Abnormal largeness of hands and feet.

acrodynia A disorder affecting infants and young children, marked by irritability, stomatitis, loss of teeth, insomnia, and redness of the fingers, toes, cheeks, nose, and buttocks. Also called pink disease; erythredema.

acroesthesia 1. Abnormally increased sensitivity. 2. Pain in the extremities.

acrogeria Premature aging of the skin of the hands and feet.

acrognosis Sensory perception of the limbs and their parts in relation to one another.

acrohyperhidrosis Abnormally increased sweating of the hands and feet.

acrokeratosis verruciformis A condition marked by warty growths on the hands and feet.

acromegalic Relating to or afflicted wtih acromegaly.

acromegaly A disease marked by progressive enlargement of the head, face, hands, feet, and internal organs due to a disorder of the pituitary gland, with overproduction of growth hormone after the normal growth period has ended.

acromelalgia A disease affecting the extremities, especially the feet, and marked by dilation of the blood vessels, headache, vomiting, and redness, pain, and swelling of the toes and fingers.

acrometagenesis Congenital deformity of the extremities.

acromial Of or relating to the acromion.

acromicria Abnormal smallness of bones of the head, hands, and feet; the converse of acromegaly.

acromioclavicular Of or relating to the acromion and clavicle.

acromiocoracoid Of or relating to the acromion and the coracoid process.

acromiohumeral Of or relating to the acromion and humerus.

acromion The flattened process extending laterally from the spine of the scapula and forming the most prominent point of the shoulder.

acromioscapular Pertaining to the acromion and the body of the scapula.

acromiothoracic Relating to the acromion of the scapula (shoulder blade) and the thorax. Also called thoracicoacromial.

acromphalus Abnormal protuberance of the navel.

acromycosis Any disease of the limbs caused by a fungus.

acromyotonia Rigidity of the hands or feet, resulting in spasmodic deformity.

acropachy Thickening (clubbing) of the tips of fingers and toes with proliferation of bone tissue and swelling. Also called pachyacria.

acroparesthesia A vasomotor-trophic disorder marked by attacks of numbness and prickly or tingling sensations in the extremities, chiefly the tips of the fingers and toes.

acrophobia Morbid fear of high places.

acroposthitis Inflammation of the prepuce.

acrosclerosis Thickening of the skin and subcutaneous tissue of the hands and feet due to swelling and thickening of fibrous tissue; scleroderma of the hands and feet.

sperm

acrosome

actomyosin

Actinomyces israelii

actin

acupuncture
(sites)

myosin

thyroid
cartilage

Adam's
apple

acrosome The dense structure covering the anterior half of the head of a spermatozoon; it contains the enzyme hyaluronidase which aids the penetration of the egg by the sperm during fertilization.

acrotic 1. Of, affecting, or located on the surface of the body. 2. Pulseless.

acrotrophodynia Neuritis of the extremities as a result of exposure to prolonged cold and moisture.

acrylic Denoting any derivative of acrylic acid, used in the construction of dental and medical prostheses. See also resin.

actin A muscle protein which, together with myosin, is responsible for muscular contraction.

actinic Referring to those rays of the electromagnetic spectrum that produce chemical effects.

actinism The property of radiation that produces chemical changes or activity.

actinium A radioactive element, symbol Ac, atomic number 89, atomic weight 227; found in uranium ores and possessing no stable isotopes.

Actinobacillus A genus of small, gram-negative, aerobic bacteria (family Brucellaceae) that cause disease in cattle and hogs; some species attack humans.

   A. mallei See *Pseudomonas mallei.*

   A. pseudomallei See *Pseudomonas pseudomallei.*

actinodermatitis Inflammation of the skin caused by radiation.

actinogenesis See radiogenesis.

actinolite Any substance that undergoes marked changes in the presence of light.

actinometer Any of several instruments for measuring the intensity and chemical effects of actinic rays.

Actinomyces A genus of nonmotile, nonacidfast bacteria (family Actinomycetaceae), occurring in groups of radiating club-shaped rods superficially resembling fungi; some varieties are used in the production of antibodies. Also called ray fungus.

   A. bovis A species that causes actinomycosis (lumpy jaw) in cattle and hogs.

   A. israelii A species that is the causal agent of human actinomycosis.

Actinomycetaceae A family of bacteria (order Actinomycetales) having filamentous shapes with a tendency to branch and resembling both bacteria and fungi; some varieties are pathogenic.

actinomycin An antibacterial substance found in some soil bacteria.

actinomycosis Disease of cattle and hogs, occasionally of humans, marked by slow-growing granulomas from which pus-discharging abscesses develop; located chiefly in the jaws and neck, less frequently in the lungs and alimentary tract; *Actin-*

omyces israelii is the cause in humans, *Actinomyces bovis* in animals. Also called lumpy jaw.

actinophage Any virus that destroys actinomycetes.

actinotherapy The treatment of disease, especially of the skin, with ultraviolet light.

action 1. The performance of an act, movement, or function. 2. The transmission of energy.

   ball valve a. The periodic or intermittent blockage of a tubular structure by a foreign body.

   cumulative a. Suddenly increased intensity, as the effect of a drug that had been previously administered with moderate or negligible effect.

   sparing a. The lowering of the requirement for an essential food factor in the diet caused by the presence of another food factor which, by itself, is not essential.

   specific dynamic a. The increase in heat production during digestion; from 4 to 6% for carbohydrates to 30% for proteins.

activation 1. Stimulation. 2. The act of making radioactive.

activator 1. A substance that stimulates the action of another. 2. An agent that accelerates a reaction.

   allosteric a. An activator that enhances enzyme activity when bound to a site other than the active site of the enzyme molecule.

active Capable of functioning or changing; requiring energy, as contrasted with passive.

activity 1. The condition of being active. 2. The intensity of a radioactive element. 3. The release of electrical energy by nerve tissue.

actomyosin A unique contractile protein with a linear molecular shape, formed by the union of actin and myosin; responsible for the contraction of muscle fibers.

acuity Acuteness, distinctness.

   visual a. clearness of vision; dependent on the size and sharpness of the image on the retina, the sensitivity of the nerves, and the interpretative ability of the brain.

aculeate Thorny; covered with sharp points.

acupressure Brief compression of a nerve with the fingers at a special point (pressure point) to relieve pain elsewhere in the body.

acupuncture A modality developed in China for certain types of anesthesia and treatment of various disorders by insertion of fine stainless steel needles into specific areas of the body; it is thought to work through the body's autonomic nervous system. Also called neuronyxis.

acusis Normal hearing.

acute Denoting a disease or symptoms of abrupt onset or lasting a relatively short period of time; opposite of chronic.

acute brain syndrome Sudden, often reversible, impairment of brain function secondary to other conditions such as drug ingestion or systemic metabolic disorders; manifested by faulty perception and interpretation, usually associated with delirium.

acyanoblepsia Inability to see the color blue. Also called blue blindness.

acyanotic Not marked by cyanosis.

acyclic 1. In chemistry, denotes an organic compound with an open chain structure. 2. Not occurring during the series of events that recur regularly.

acyclovir Antiviral agent for the treatment of herpes simplex and related viral infections.

acyl Any radical derived from an organic acid by removal of the hydroxyl group.

acylation Introduction of an acyl radical into a compound.

acystia Congenital absence of the urinary bladder.

Acystosporidia An order of parasitic sporozoa that includes the genus *Plasmodium,* the malarial parasite.

adactyly Congenital absence of fingers or toes.

adamantinoma See Ameloblastoma.

Adam's apple The thyroid cartilage of the larynx which forms a subcutaneous projection in the midline of the neck. Also called laryngeal prominence.

Adams-Stokes syndrome A syndrome characterized by fainting and sometimes convulsions due to prolonged asystole; seen usually when there is a failure of effective contraction in the course of complete heart block or when heart block supervenes on a sinus rhythm; sometimes Cheynes-Stokes respiration may occur. Also called Stokes-Adams or Morgagni-Adams-Stokes syndrome.

adaptation 1. Adjustment of the pupil of the eye to variations in the intensity of light. 2. Alteration by which an organism becomes fit for a new environment. 3. Decreased response of a sense organ to repeated stimuli.

   dark a. Eye adjustment to reduced illumination (sensitivity to light is greatly increased).

   light a. Eye adjustment to increased illumination (sensitivity to light is reduced).

adder European viper; see under viper.

addict One who has strong psychologic and physiologic dependence upon some practice which has progressed beyond voluntary control.

addiction Strong habituation to some practice, beyond voluntary control.

   drug a. Compulsive use of a habit-forming drug, the deprivation of which gives rise to symptoms of distress, or withdrawal symptoms, and compulsion to take the drug again. Also called pharmacopsychosis.

addisonian 1. Characterized by features of Addiadenine

islet cell adenoma

adenomyosis

adduction

adenohypophysis

son's disease. **2.** Relating to Addison's disease.

Addison's anemia See anemia, pernicious.

Addison's disease Primary adrenocortical insufficiency; adrenocortical insufficiency caused by destruction of the adrenal cortex, a disease characterized by chronic deficiency of hormones concerned with mineral metabolism and glycostasis; findings include striking skin pigmentation, anemia, hypotension with small heart, severe dental caries, and stiffness of the cartilages of the ear; hyponatremia is present and, later, there may be azotemia and hyperkalemia. Also called addisonism.

additive **1.** Any substance that is added to another material to fulfill a specific purpose, i.e., to improve it, strengthen it, etc. **2.** The quality of two drugs (e.g., epinephrine and norepinephrine) that act on the same receptors whereby doses of one drug can substitute for those of the other, in proportion to their relative potency.

adducent Bringing toward or together; performing adduction; denoting some adductor muscles.

adduct To pull or draw toward the median line of the body.

adduction Movement of a part toward or beyond the median line; act of turning inward.

adductor A structure, such as a muscle, that draws a part toward an axis of the body; opposite of abductor.

adenase An enzyme that converts adenine into hypoxanthine; present in the liver, pancreas, and spleen.

adenasthenia Abnormal reduction in the activity of a gland.

adendritic Denoting a nerve call without dendrites, such as certain cells in the spinal ganglia.

adenectomy Surgical removal of a gland.

adenectopia The presence of a gland somewhere other than its normal position.

adenine A white, crystalline purine derivative, $C_5H_5N_5$; one of the constituents of ribonucleic acid (RNA) and deoxyribonucleic acid (DNA).

a. arabinoside (Ara-A) A substance that acts intracellularly to inhibit viral replication; used in the treatment of some viral infections such as those caused by cytomegalovirus.

a. nucleotide See adenylic acid.

adenitis Inflammation of a lymph node or gland.

adenoacanthoma A malignant tumor made up of a glandular tissue.

adenoblast Embryonic cell from which glandular tissue develops.

adenocarcinoma A malignant tumor with cells arranged in a glandlike pattern.

papillary a. See carcinoma, papillary.

renal a. See carcinoma, renal cell.

adenocystoma A benign, epithelial, glandlike tumor associated with cysts.

adenodiastasis The presence of glands or glandular tissue in other than their normal sites.

adenoepithelioma A tumor made up of glandular and epithelial tissues.

adenofibroma A benign tumor made up of connective tissue with some glandular elements.

adenofibrosis Formation of a fibrous tissue in a gland.

adenohypophyseal, adenohypophysial Of or relating to the anterior portion of the pituitary gland.

adenohypophysis The anterior, glandular portion of the hypophysis (pituitary gland); it produces the following hormones: prolactin, follicle stimulating (FSH), luteinizing (LH), adrenocorticotropic (ACTH), thyroid-stimulating (TSH), melanocyte stimulating (MSH), and somatotropin or growth (STH or GH) hormones.

adenoid **1.** Resembling a gland. **2.** Pharyngeal tonsil.

adenoidectomy Surgical removal of the adenoids.

adenoiditis Inflammation of the pharyngeal tonsil.

adenoids Enlargement of the pharyngeal tonsil.

adenolipoma Benign tumor of fat tissue containing some glandular elements.

adenolipomatosis Condition marked by the presence of several subcutaneous adenolipomas, especially in the neck, axilla, and groin.

adenolymphocele Cystic enlargement of a lymph node.

adenolymphoma Papillary cystadenoma lymphomatosum; see under cystadenoma.

adenoma Benign tumor of epithelial tissue with a glandlike structure.

acidophilic a. Adenoma of the anterior portion of the pituitary gland; made up of acidophil cells and causing acromegaly and gigantism.

a. sebaceum A tumor of the face made up of sebaceous glands; appears as a collection of reddish and yellowish papules and is associated with mental deficiency.

basophilic a. A tumor of the anterior lobe of the pituitary gland; composed of basophil cells and associated with Cushing's syndrome.

bronchial a. Former term for a group of low-grade malignant tumors arising in the bronchi. They include carcinoid and mucoepidermoid tumors.

chromophil a. An acidophilic or a basophilic adenoma.

chromophobe a. A tumor composed of chromophobe cells in the anterior pituitary gland, associated with hypopituitarism.

colloid a., macrofollicular a. Former names for a colloid-containing follicular adenoma.

follicular a. A benign tumor of the thyroid gland that produces pouch-like dilatations (acini); these may vary in size from small and rudimentary to large and cystic containing abundant colloid.

eosinophilic a. A tumor of the eosinophilic cells of the anterior pituitary gland, causing gigantism and acromegaly.

islet cell a. A tumor of the pancreas, made up of tissue similar in structure to that of the islets of Langerhans.

tubular a. Benign, usually pedunculated, polyp of the colon mucosa; risk of its becoming cancerous correlates with size.

villous a. A benign, potentially malignant, tumor of the mucosa of the large intestine.

adenomatoid Resembling an adenoma.

adenomatosis Condition marked by the formation of multiple glandular tumors.

familial polyendocrine a. The presence of tumors in several endocrine glands.

pulmonary a. The presence in the alveoli and distal bronchi of abundant mucus and mucus-secreting columnar epithelial cells of neoplastic origin; characterized by the production of very large amounts of sputum.

adenomatous Relating to an adenoma or a glandular overgrowth.

adenomyoma A benign tumor composed of muscle tissue, found in the uterus and uterine ligaments.

adenomyosis The presence of adenomatous growths in smooth muscle, as the invasion of the uterine musculature by endometrium.

adenomyxoma A benign tumor made up of glandular and mucous tissue.

adenopathy Disease of glands, especially of the lymphatic glands.

adenosarcoma A malignant tumor containing glandular tissue.

adenosclerosis Hardening of a gland or lymph node.

adenose Relating to a gland.

adenosine An organic compound, $C_{10}H_{13}N_5O_4$, derived from nucleic acids; composed of adenine and a pentose sugar.

a. diphosphate (ADP) A product of the hydrolysis, and the substrate for the biosynthesis, of adenosine triphosphate (ATP).

a. monophosphate (AMP) See adenylic acid.

a. triphosphatase (ATPase) An enzyme, present

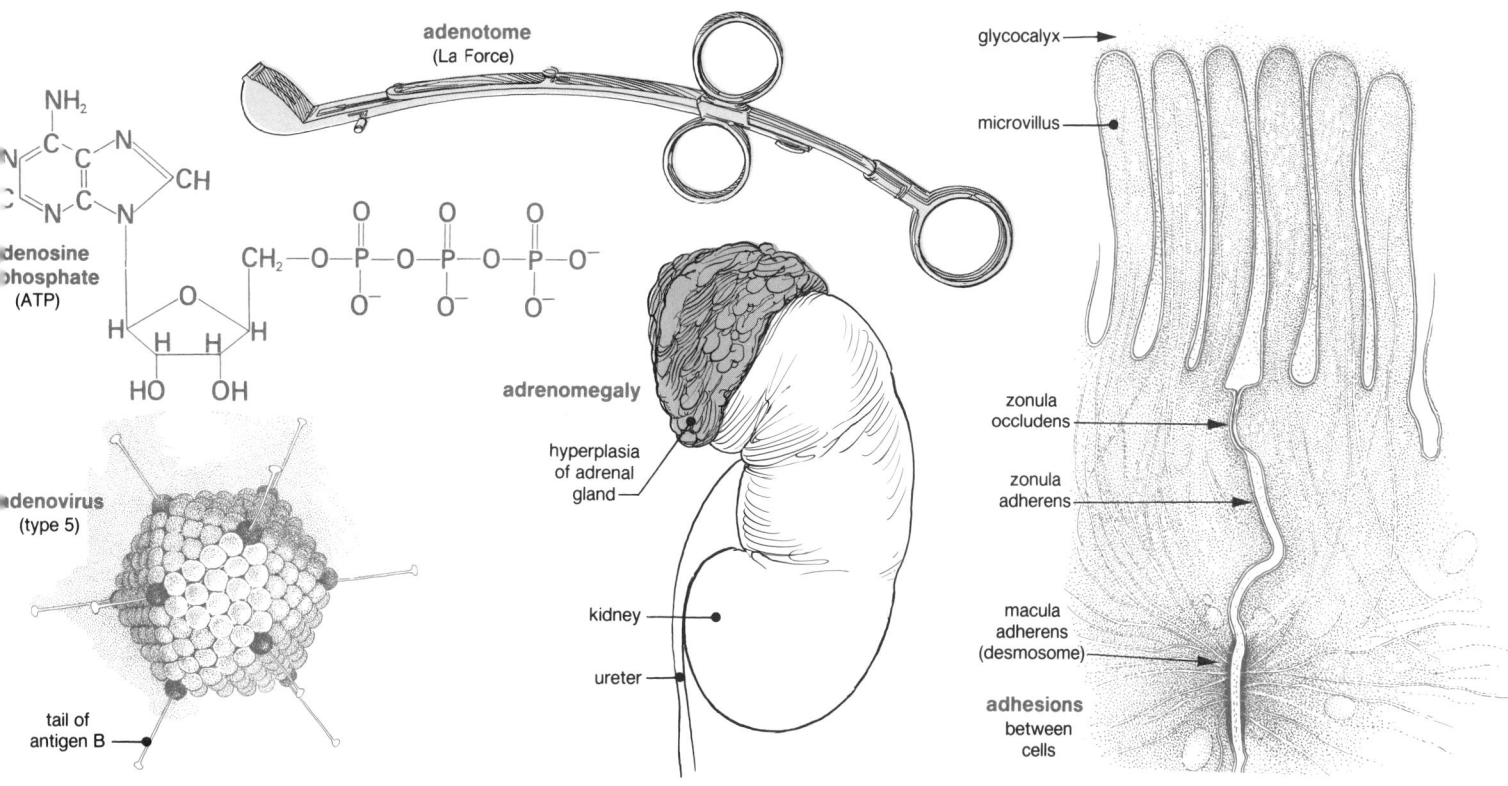

adenotome
(La Force)

adenosine
phosphate
(ATP)

adenovirus
(type 5)

tail of
antigen B

adrenomegaly

hyperplasia
of adrenal
gland

kidney

ureter

glycocalyx

microvillus

zonula
occludens

zonula
adherens

macula
adherens
(desmosome)

adhesions
between
cells

in muscle tissue, that promotes the splitting off of a phosphate group from adenosine triphosphate.

a. triphosphate (ATP)   Organic compound present in all cells; upon hydrolysis, it yields the energy required by a multitude of biologic processes.

adenosis   Any disease of the glands, especially one affecting the lymph nodes.

adenotome   A surgical instrument for the removal of adenoids.

adenotonsillectomy   Surgical removal of adenoids and tonsils.

Adenoviridae   A family of viruses (70 to 90 nm in diameter) which contain double-stranded DNA and develop in cell nuclei of mammals and birds; some members have been extensively used in experimental studies of cancer; includes viruses causing epidemic keratoconjunctivitis, pharyngitis, tonsillitis, and pneumonia. Also called adenovirus family.

adenovirus   A virus of the family Adenoviridae.

adenyl   A radical, $C_5H_4N_4$, that is a constituent of adenine.

adenylate cyclase   An enzyme located in cell membranes which, in the presence of magnesium, converts adenosine triphosphate (ATP) to 3′5′-cyclic AMP (cAMP); the enzyme is activated by a hormone interacting with a specific receptor (first messenger) on the cell membrane; the cyclic AMP acts as a second messenger within the cell.

adenylic acid   One of the hydrolysis products of all nucleic acids, occurring in all tissues and participating in high-energy phosphate transfer. Also called adenosine monophosphate (AMP); adenine nucleotide.

adhesion   1. The union of two surfaces. 2. A fibrous band that abnormally unites two parts.

fibrinous a.   Adhesion composed of fine strands of fibrin.

fibrous a.   Adhesion composed of a group of fibrinous adhesions.

primary a.   Adhesion or healing of a wound without suppuration or the formation of granulations. Also called healing by first intention.

adhesiotomy   Surgical division of adhesions.

adiadochokinesia, adiadochokinesis   Inability to perform rapid alternating movements (e.g., pronation and supination).

adiaphoresis   Deficiency of perspiration.

adiaphoretic   Characterized by or causing adiaphoresis.

adipectomy   See lipectomy.

adipic acid   Acid formed by the oxidation of fats.

adipocele   See lipocele.

adipocere   A waxy substance formed on decomposing dead bodies under humid conditions.

adipometer   Instrument for measuring the thickness of a skin fold to estimate amount of subcutaneous fat.

adiponecrosis   Death of fat tissue.

adipose   Of or related to fat; fatty.

adiposis   Excessive accumulation of fat in the body, either local or general.

adiposity   A bodily state in which the proportion of the body weight composed of fat is excessive; the body weight may not exceed normal (feature that distinguishes it from obesity).

aditus   A general anatomic term denoting approach or entrance to an organ.

adjustment   Modification made on a completed denture after its insertion in the mouth.

adjuvant   That which aids or assists, as a substance which enhances the response to an antigen.

Freund's complete a.   A mixture of mineral oil, plant waxes, and killed tubercle bacilli; used with antigen to increase antibody production.

Freund's incomplete a.   Freund's complete adjuvant minus the tubercle bacilli.

adnerval   Near or in the direction of a nerve.

adnexa   Parts accessory to the main organ. Also called appendages.

a. uteri   The ovaries and uterine tubes.

adolescence   The stage in human growth from the onset of puberty to the attainment of full physical development.

adolescent   1. Of or relating to adolescence. 2. A person during the period of adolescence.

adoral   Toward or near the mouth.

adrenal   1. Located near the kidney. 2. The adrenal gland. See under gland.

adrenalectomy   Surgical removal of the adrenal glands.

adrenaline   See epinephrine.

adrenarche   1. Puberty induced by hyperactivity of the adrenal cortex. 2. A physiologic change in which the function of the adrenal cortex is increased, occurring at approximately the age of nine years.

adrenergic   Term applied to nerve fibers of the sympathetic nervous system that, upon stimulation, release the chemical transmitter norepinephrine (and possibly small amounts of epinephrine) at their post-ganglionic endings.

alpha a.   Those actions of the adrenergic system mediated through receptors responsible for vasoconstriction, dilation of the iris of the eye and pilomotor contraction.

beta a.   Those actions of the adrenergic system mediated through receptors responsible for acceleration of the heart beat (beta 1) and bronchodilation (beta 2).

adrenocortical   Relating to the adrenal cortex.

adrenocorticomimetic   Having a function similar to that of the adrenal cortex.

adrenocorticotrophic, adrenocorticotropic   Stimulating the function or growth of the cortex of the adrenal gland.

adrenocorticotrophin, adrenocorticotropin   Adrenocorticotropic hormone; see under hormone.

adrenogenic   Produced or originating in the adrenal glands.

adrenogenital syndrome   Metabolic disorder caused by hyperfunction of the adrenal cortex, usually associated with premature virilization and, in the female, with pseudohermaphroditism and sexual infantilism; caused by a congenital deficiency in the ability to form cortisol with a compensatory increase in ACTH serving to cause hypersecretion of other adrenal steroids.

adrenogram   X-ray image of an adrenal gland.

adrenolytic   1. Inhibiting the action of sympathetic (adrenergic) nerves. 2. Having an inhibitory influence on the action of, or response to, epinephrine (adrenaline).

adrenomegaly   Enlargement of the adrenal glands.

adrenoprival   Absence of adrenal function.

adrenosterone   A male sex hormone (androgen), $C_{19}H_{24}O_3$, present in the adrenal cortex.

adrenotrophin, adrenotropin   Adrenocorticotropic hormone; see under hormone.

adrenotropism   The predominance of adrenal influence in endocrine function.

adsorb   To attach one substance to the surface of another.

adsorbate   A substance adhered to the surface of another by adsorption.

adsorbent   A substance that attracts and holds on its surface another substance.

adsorption   The process by which gas molecules or small particles in solution are attracted by, and attached to, the surface of another substance.

adulterant   1. Anything added to a substance which makes it impure or inferior. 2. Any of various materials added to a hallucinogenic drug in the hope of enhancing its potency.

adulteration   1. Addition of foreign substances to a product. 2. Alteration of a substance by the addition of material of cheaper and inferior qualities.

adult respiratory distress syndrome (ARDS)   Condition occurring shortly after trauma; characterized by edema of the alveolae and surrounding tissues, acute respiratory failure, and shock; precipitated by microembolism and loss of surfactant. Also called posttraumatic pulmonary insufficiency;

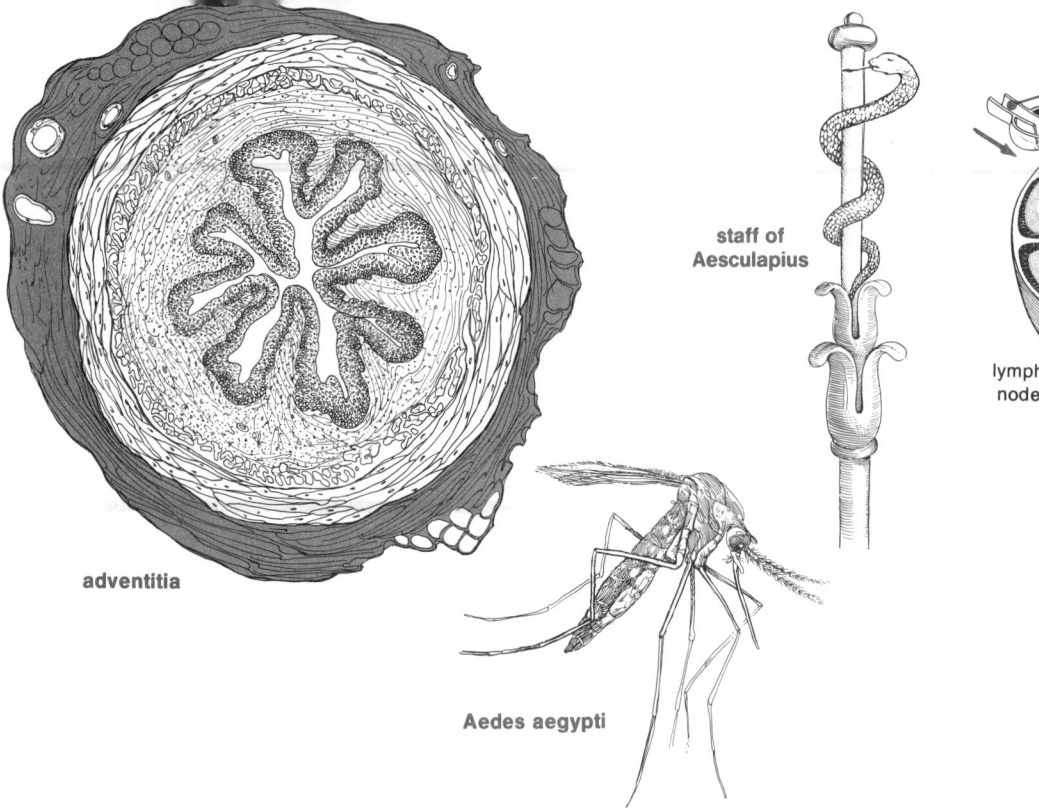

adventitia

staff of Aesculapius

afferent lymphatic vessels

lymph node

Aedes aegypti

red blood cells

agglutination

---

shock lung.

advancement Surgical procedure in which the tendon of a muscle is detached and reattached at an advanced point; used to correct strabismus.

adventitia The outer, loose connective tissue covering of a structure such as a blood vessel, thoracic duct, or ureter. Also called extima.

adventitial Relating to the outer layer of a blood vessel.

adynamia Weakness; asthenia.

Aedes aegypti An important species of mosquito, the carrier of yellow fever and dengue; may also transmit filariasis and encephalitis; generally breeds near houses. Also called tiger mosquito.

aerated Containing air, carbon dioxide, or oxygen.

aeration 1. The act of airing. 2. The saturation of a fluid with a gas. 3. The oxygenation of blood in the lungs.

aerobe Any organism capable of growing in the presence of air.

aerobic Growing only in the presence of air. Also called aerobiotic.

aerobiosis Life in an oxygen-containing environment.

aerodontalgia Toothache brought on by reduction of atmospheric pressure.

aerogenic Gas producing, such as certain bacteria.

aeropathy Disease caused by drastic changes in atmospheric pressure; e.g., aerotitis media, caisson disease.

aerophagia, aerophagy The swallowing of air; usually accompanies emotional disorders.

aerophil, aerophilic Air loving; an organism that requires air for proper growth.

aerophobia Abnormal fear of drafts or of fresh air.

aerosinusitis Inflammatory condition of paranasal sinuses caused by difference between pressures within the sinuses and that of the atmosphere. Also called barosinusitis.

aerosol Relatively stable suspension of liquids or solids in air, oxygen, or inert gases which is dispersed in the form of a fine mist, usually for therapeutic purposes.

aerotitis media Inflammation of the middle ear caused by a sudden increase in atmospheric pressure, as on descent in an aircraft from a high altitude, when obstruction of the auditory tube does not permit equalization of pressures within and without the middle ear. Also called aviator's ear.

Aesculapius The Roman god of healing.
  staff of A. A rod encircled by a single snake; symbol of the medical profession and emblem of

the American Medical Association, the Royal Army Medical Corps, and the Royal Canadian Army Medical Corps.

afebrile Without fever.

affect 1. Feeling or emotion. 2. The outward manifestation of one's feelings; one's feeling-tone as perceptible to others.

affective Referring to affect.

afferent Conveying a fluid or a nerve impulse toward an organ or area.

afferent loop syndrome Chronic partial obstruction of the duodenum and jejunum following gastrojejunostomy, resulting in distention and pain after eating.

affinity In chemistry, the attractive force of two substances for each other.

afibrinogenemia Marked deficiency of fibrinogen in the blood.

aflatoxin Toxin produced by the fungus *Aspergillus flavus;* found in stored grains and peanuts; causes liver cancer.

afterbirth The placenta and fetal membranes expelled from the uterus after childbirth.

afterdischarge The discharge of impulses from a reflex center after stimulation has ceased.

afterload In cardiac muscle, the force against which the ventricle ejects once contraction of the muscle fibers begins; for the left ventricle this is equivalent to aortic diastolic pressure.

afterpains Cramps due to uterine contractions after delivery.

aftersensation Sensation persisting after the stimulus that caused it has been removed.

agalactia Condition in which milk in the breasts is absent after childbirth.

agalorrhea Absence or arrest of milk flow.

agammaglobulinemia Condition marked by virtual absence of gamma globulin in the blood, inability to form antibody, and frequent attacks of infectious diseases.

agar A gelatinous material prepared from seaweed; used as a culture medium for bacteria.
  blood a. Bouillon solidified with 1% agar and mixed with blood.
  chocolate a. Agar mixed with fresh blood and then heated, which gives it a chocolate brown color; used as a culture medium for *Neisseria.*
  Endo a. A medium containing agar, lactose, peptone, dipotassium phosphate, sodium sulfite, basic fuchsin, and distilled water; used for bacteriologic testing of water.
  Sabouraud's a. Bouillon solidified with 1% agar, mixed with 1% Chassaing's peptone and 4% maltose or mannite; used for growth of fungi. Also called French proof agar.

age The period of time during which a person has lived.
  biologic a. Age as a measurement of the degree of physical maturity of an individual; for children, usually determined by a roentgenogram of the bones (bone age).
  bone a. See biologic age.
  chronologic a. The time from the date of birth; calendar age.
  menstrual a., gestational a. Age of an embryo or fetus beginning on the first day of the mother's last normal menstruation.
  mental a. The age level of intellectual ability as measured by standarized tests.

agenesis, agenesia Absence or abnormal development of a part.

agenosomia Congenital absence or defective development of the genitals and protrusion of the abdominal organs through an incomplete abdominal wall.

agent Anything capable of producing an effect upon an organism.
  adrenergic blocking a. Drug that slows the stimulating effects of sympathetic nerves, epinephrine, norepinephrine, and other adrenergic amines by blocking receptor sites of cells.
  alkylating a. Any compound, such as nitrogen mustard, that contains alkyl groups and is toxic to cells (both normal and malignant); used to treat cancer.
  blocking a. A drug that interferes with the function of the autonomic nervous system by blocking transmission at a receptor site, a synapse, or a neuromuscular junction. Also called blocker.
  calcium channel-blocking a. Drug that slows muscle contraction by blocking passage of calcium across the membrane of muscle cells; also slows nerve impulses through heart muscle.
  chelating a. A compound that combines with metals to form a complex (chelate); used in medicine to render poisonous metal compounds nonpoisonous.
  Eaton a. One of the main causes of primary atypical pneumonia. Also called *Mycoplasma pneumoniae.*
  sclerosing a. Any compound used in the treatment of varicose veins.

Agent Orange Herbicide containing the carcinogenic chemical dioxin.

ageusia Absence of taste perception.

agglutination 1. The clumping of cells or microorganisms when exposed to a specific immune serum. 2. The process of joining together in the healing of a wound.
  group a. The clumping together of several related

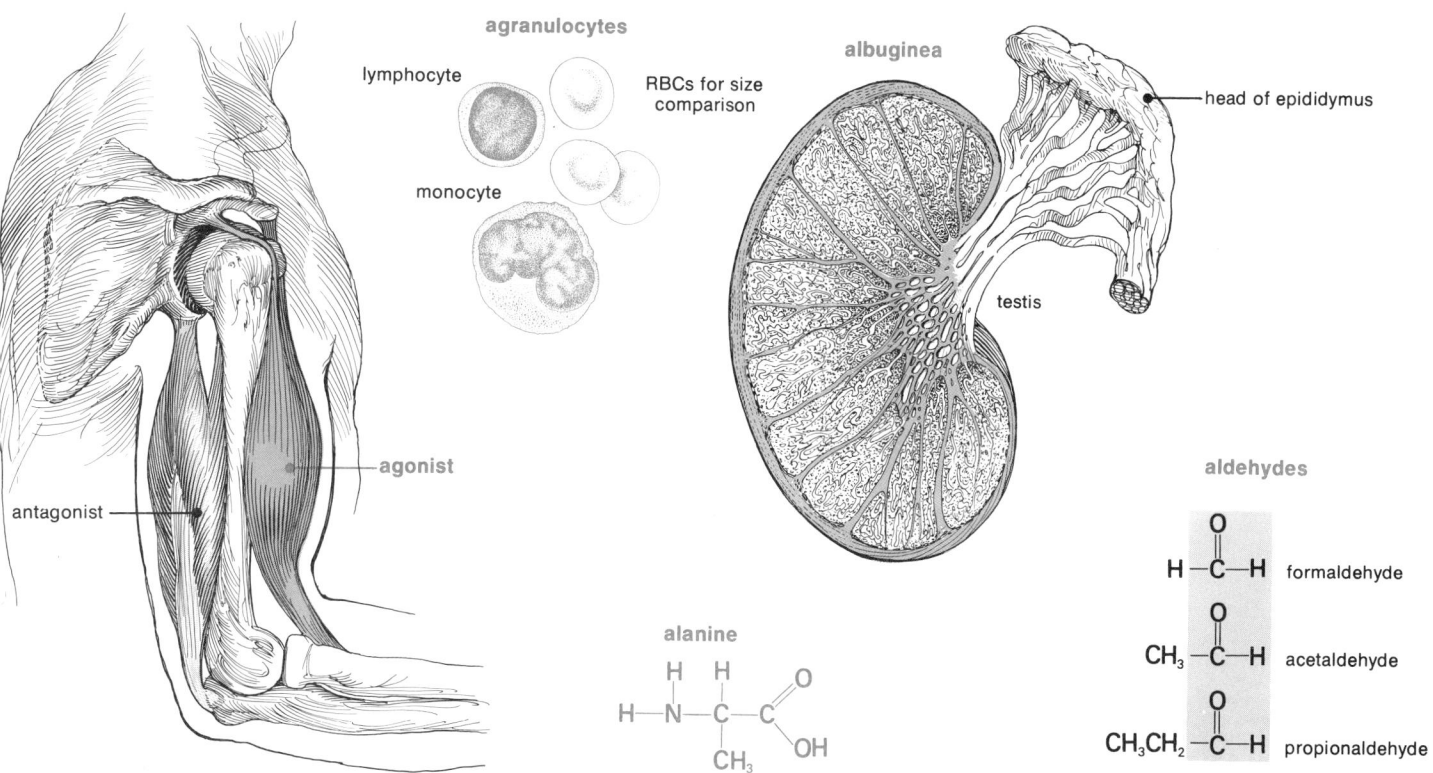

agranulocytes

lymphocyte

monocyte

RBCs for size comparison

albuginea

head of epididymus

testis

aldehydes

$$H-\overset{\overset{\displaystyle O}{\|}}{C}-H \quad \text{formaldehyde}$$

$$CH_3-\overset{\overset{\displaystyle O}{\|}}{C}-H \quad \text{acetaldehyde}$$

$$CH_3CH_2-\overset{\overset{\displaystyle O}{\|}}{C}-H \quad \text{propionaldehyde}$$

alanine

$$H-\overset{\overset{\displaystyle H}{|}}{N}-\overset{\overset{\displaystyle H}{|}}{\underset{\underset{\displaystyle CH_3}{|}}{C}}-\overset{\overset{\displaystyle O}{\|}}{C}-OH$$

agonist

antagonist

varieties of bacteria in the presence of serum specific for one of that group.

agglutinin An antibody that causes particulate antigens, such as bacteria or other cells, to adhere to one another, forming clumps.

cold a. Agglutinin that causes clumping of human group O red blood cells at temperatures from 0 to 5°C.

agglutinogen An antigenic substance that stimulates the formation of a particular antibody (agglutinin) that causes clumping of cells containing the antigen.

agglutinogenic Causing the production of an agglutinin.

agglutinoid An agglutinin that has lost its ability to produce clumping but can still combine with its corresponding agglutinogen.

aglomerular Having no glomeruli.

aglycone, aglucone The noncarbohydrate group of a glycoside.

agnogenic Of unknown cause.

agnosia Loss of ability to comprehend the meaning of sensory stimulation, such as auditory, visual, olfactory, tactile, and gustatory sensations.

agonist **1.** A muscle in a state of contraction opposing the action of another muscle (antagonist) which at the same time relaxes. **2.** A drug that can interact with receptors (specific sites in certain cells) and initiate a drug response; e.g., acetylcholine.

agoraphobia Abnormal fear of open spaces, especially of leaving the closed environment of home.

agranulocytes A group of so-called nongranular white blood cells that contain nonspecific (azurophilic) granules; it includes the lymphocyte and the monocyte; normally, it constitutes from 37 to 42% of the total white blood cell population. Also called agranular leukocytes.

agranulocytosis A state marked by a great reduction of granular white blood cells (polymorphonuclear leukocytes); often used to describe a syndrome including the hematologic change plus constitutional symptoms and the development of infected ulcers in the mouth (agranulocytic angina), throat, intestinal tract, and sometimes the skin; the acute form is most frequently drug induced but may be seen in acute leukemia; the chronic form is of unknown etiology and is seen more frequently in women. Also called agranulocytopenia.

agraphia Loss of the power to communicate ideas in writing, due to a cerebral lesion.

AIDS (acquired immune deficiency syndrome) The clinical state caused by human immunodeficiency virus (HIV). The HIV infection, acquired by sexual contact or from contaminated blood products,

progresses as follows: *Acute stage,* viruses enter helper T-cells (infected person can then infect others). About 3–5 weeks later, symptoms may appear (fever, muscle and joint pain, rash, hives, diarrhea) and last 2–3 weeks. *Asymptomatic stage,* T cells produce antibodies to kill the virus; in 5–6 months, antibodies can be detected in blood tests. The infected person may have no symptoms for several years but the virus population increases and destroys T cells, slowly at first, rapidly later. A helper T cell (T-4) population of less than 500 cells/mm³ is a bad prognostic sign. Defenses begin to fail and symptoms, formerly called AIDS related complex or ARC, appear (weight loss, fatigue, fever, diarrhea, swollen lymph nodes). *Full-blown AIDS,* final stage of the disease, immune defenses break down and other diseases attack the body (*Pneumocystis carinii* pneumonia; Kaposi's sarcoma; nervous system diseases; and fungal, bacterial, and parasitic infections).

air The mixture of gases that make up the earth's atmosphere.

alveolar a. Air remaining in the lungs after a normal expiration in which the O_2 and CO_2 tensions are in equilibrium with those of the arterial blood.

residual a. Residual volume; see under volume.

tidal a. Air that enters and leaves the lungs during normal respiration. Also called tidal volume.

akinesia Loss or impairment of voluntary muscular action.

akinesthesia Lack of perception of movement.

ala, *pl.* **alae** **1.** Any winglike structure. **2.** Axilla.

alanine (Ala) An amino acid of the pyruvic acid family; found widely in proteins.

alanine aminotransferase An enzyme that transfers amino groups from an *a*-amino acid to (usually) a 2-keto acid. Also called glutamic pyruvic transaminase (GPT).

alar Of or relating to any winged structure or to the armpit.

alastrim A contagious eruptive disease resembling a mild form of smallpox.

Albers-Schönberg disease See osteopetrosis.

albinism Absence of pigment in the skin, hair, and irises; may be partial or complete. Also called congenital leukoderma.

albino A person marked by albinism.

Albright's syndrome A polyostotic fibrous dysplasia of bone marked by dense overgrowth of bone and cystic transformation, most commonly involving several areas of the skeleton; accompanied by pigment spots on the skin and sexual precocity (principally in females).

albuginea A thick connective tissue capsule surrounding the testis and ovary.

albumin, albumen A protein in many animal and vegetable tissues, including human plasma, soluble in water and coagulable by heat; a principal constituent of egg white.

Bence-Jones a. See protein, Bence-Jones.

radioiodinated serum a. (RISA), **iodinated** ¹³¹I

serum a. Human serum albumin iodinated with ¹³¹I which emits beta and gamma radiation; used for determining blood and plasma volumes and cardiac output, and for detection of brain tumors.

albuminocytologic dissociation See under dissociation.

albuminoid **1.** Resembling albumin. **2.** Scleroprotein.

albuminuria Urinary excretion of albumin in excess of the normal daily amount. See also proteinuria.

alcohol **1.** A colorless, flammable fluid, ROH, obtained from fermented sugars and starches; used as a solvent, antiseptic, preservative of specimens, and in the preparation of drugs and intoxicating beverages. **2.** CH_3CH_2OH; the alcohol of wine, whiskey, etc.; produced by several microorganisms fermenting different substrates. Aslo called ethanol; ethyl or grain alcohol.

absolute a. Alcohol containing not more than 1% of water (by weight).

acid a. 70% ethyl alcohol containing 1% hydrochloric acid.

a. dehydrogenase (ADH) An enzyme present in the liver which promotes the dehydrogenation of ethyl alcohol to acetaldehyde.

denatured a. Alcohol that has been rendered unfit to drink by the addition of other chemicals.

methyl a. CH_3OH; a colorless, flammable liquid, soluble in water or ether; used as an industrial solvent and in the manufacture of formaldehyde; can cause severe acidosis and blindness when ingested. Also called methanol; wood alcohol; pyroxylic spirit.

rubbing a. A mixture of about 70% of absolute alcohol and varying quantities of water, denaturants, and perfumed oils; used as a rubefacient.

wood a. See methyl alcohol.

alcoholic **1.** Relating to or containing alcohol. **2.** Denoting a person addicted to alcohol.

alcoholism A pathologic condition, mainly of the nervous and gastroenteric systems, caused by excessive consumption of alcohol.

acute a. Condition caused by excessive drinking of alcoholic beverages. Also called drunkenness; intoxication.

chronic a. Addiction to alcohol, often accompanied by damage to the health of the individual.

aldehyde **1.** Any of a group of organic compounds

aldosterone (aldehyde form)

alginic acid

embryo

hindgut

allantois

yolk sac

allantoin

allergen

ragwee

obtained from oxidation of the primary alcohols and containing the group CHO. **2.** Acetaldehyde.

a. dehydrogenase An enzyme, important in the metabolism of ethyl alcohol, which promotes the oxidation of acetaldehyde to acetic acid.

aldolase An enzyme in muscle extract that catalyzes the reversible cleavage of fructose 1,6-diphosphate to yield dihydroxyacetone phosphate and glyceraldehyde.

aldopentose A sugar containing five carbon atoms and the aldehyde group —CHO.

aldosterone A potent electrolyte-regulating hormone secreted by the zona glomerulosa of the adrenal gland which causes retention of sodium in the body by enhancing sodium reabsorption by the cells of the distal tubule of the kidney, in addition to the cells of the gastrointestinal tract, and the sweat and salivary glands; reabsorption of sodium is usually accompanied by increased secretion of potassium ions.

aldosteronism Excessive secretion of aldosterone by the adrenal cortex. Also called hyperaldosteronism.

primary a. A syndrome in which (a) a tumor in the cortex of the adrenal gland (Conn's syndrome), or (b) hyperplasia of the adrenal gland without obvious cause, is responsible for excessive aldosterone secretion; the syndrome is characterized by hypertension, hypokalemic alkalosis, and weakness.

secondary a. Aldosteronism caused by excessive stimulation of the adrenal gland, frequently associated with fluid-retaining states.

Aldrich syndrome See Wiskott-Aldrich syndrome.

aldrin A highly toxic chlorinated hydrocarbon used as an insecticide.

aleukemia Deficiency of white corpuscles in the blood; denoting leukemic diseases in which the white blood cell count in peripheral blood is normal or deficient.

aleukemic Relating to or characterized by aleukemia.

alexia Inability to grasp the meaning of written or printed words.

algesia Increased sensitivity to pain.

algesiometer See odynometer.

algesthesia Perception of pain.

alginate An irreversible hydrocolloid salt of alginic acid which is extracted from marine kelp; used primarily for making dental impressions, particularly for partial dentures.

alginic acid A colloidal polysaccharide obtained from marine kelp; used in the making of alginate, a widely used dental impression material.

algophobia A morbid fear of pain.

algorithm Any procedure (either mechanical or through step-by-step instructions) designed to solve a particular type of problem.

alignment In dentistry, the line along which the teeth, natural or artificial, are arranged.

aliment Food.

alimentary Of or relating to food or nutrition.

alimentation The process of providing nourishment. Also called feeding.

aliphatic Relating to, or denoting, the fatty series of hydrocarbon compounds in which the carbon atoms are arranged in open chains rather than closed rings. Also called fatty; oily.

aliquot A portion; e.g., one of the equal parts into which a solution or a solid may be divided.

alkalemia A decrease in the hydrogen ion concentration of the blood; an increase beyond normal of pH (in man, a pH greater than 7.43). Cf. alkalosis.

alkalescent Becoming alkaline.

alkali Any of a group of basic compounds capable of combining with fatty acids to form soaps.

alkalimetry The measurement of the degree of alkalinity in a substance.

alkaline Relating to, containing, or having the reaction of an alkali (base).

alkalinity The state of being alkaline.

alkalize, alkalinize To make alkaline.

alkaloid A class of compounds present in certain plants that strongly affect human physiology; e.g., morphine (opium poppy), quinine (cinchona bark), reserpine (snake root), caffeine (tea leaves and coffee beans), cocaine (coca leaves), LSD (ergot fungus), nicotine (tobacco leaves).

alkalosis A process tending to produce a decrease in hydrogen ion concentration in the body fluids; if uncompensated, it leads to a rise in pH. Commonly used synonymously with alkalemia.

hypokalemic a. Alkalosis characterized by a low serum potassium concentration; characteristic of the most commonly seen form of metabolic alkalosis.

metabolic a. The state resulting from excessive retention of alkali or excessive loss of acid; common causes include prolonged vomiting or gastric drainage, diuretic therapy, and excessive adrenal corticosteroid secretion or administration; characterized by an elevation of the plasma bicarbonate concentration and a tendency to an alkaline arterial pH; when the arterial pH is actually more alkaline than normal, the condition should, strictly speaking, be called alkalemia.

respiratory a. The state resulting from hyperventilation and reduction of pCO_2 in body fluids.

alkalotic Relating to, or marked by, alkalosis.

alkapton See homogentisic acid.

alkaptonuria A hereditary condition in which homogentisic acid (alkapton) is not broken down to simpler compounds in the body but is excreted in the urine, which gives it a dark brown color when exposed to air. Also called homogentisuria.

allantoin A nitrogenous crystalline substance, $C_4H_6N_4O_3$; present in allantoic fluid, fetal urine, and some plants.

allantois A diverticulum that extends from the hindgut of the embryo, appearing at about the 16th day of development.

allele One of a series of two or more contrasting genes that occupy the same position in homologous chromosomes and determine the heredity of a particular trait; the term is shortened from allelomorph.

allelic Relating to two or more different genes that occupy the same position in homologous chromosomes.

allelism The existence of two or more contrasting genes that occupy the same position in homologous chromosomes.

allelomorph See allele.

allergen A substance that stimulates an allergic reaction in the body.

allergenic Capable of stimulating an allergic reaction.

allergic disease A disease resulting from allergy or any response stimulated by an allergen; can range from superficial lesions, as urticaria, to deep-seated lesions, as polyarteritis nodosa.

allergy Altered reactivity to a substance, which can result in pathologic reactions upon subsequent exposure to that particular substance. Also called hypersensitivity.

bronchial a. Asthma.

contact a. Cutaneous reaction caused by direct contact with a substance to which the person is hypersensitive.

delayed a. Reaction occurring several hours after contact with an allergen.

drug a. Unusual sensitivity to a drug or chemical.

immediate a. Reaction occurring within minutes after contact with an allergen.

alloantibody An antibody from one individual which reacts with an antigen present in another individual of the same species.

alloantigen An antigen produced by one individual which incites the formation of antibodies in another individual of the same species. Also called homologous antigen; isoantigen.

alloarthroplasty Surgical construction of an artificial joint.

allochromasia Change in the color of skin or hair.

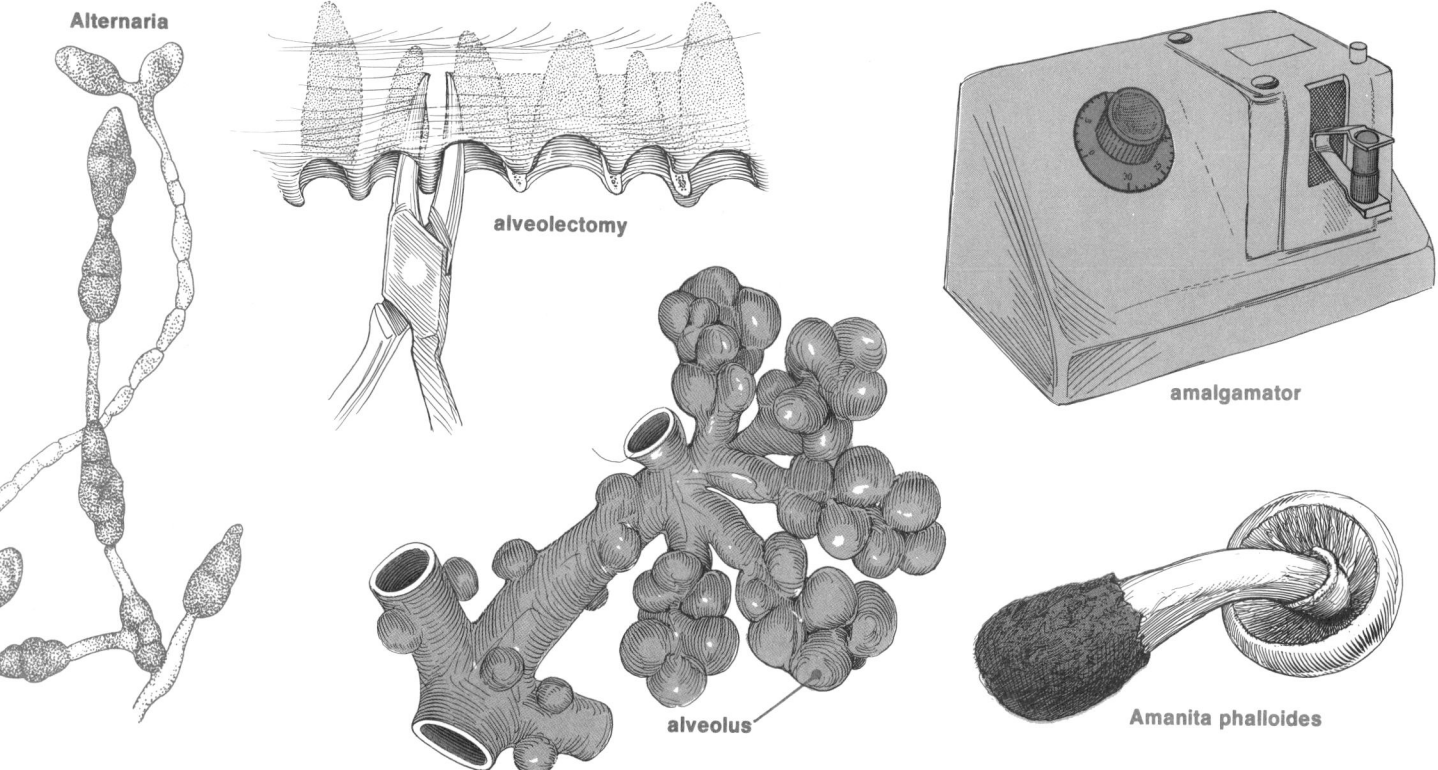

Alternaria

alveolectomy

amalgamator

alveolus

Amanita phalloides

allocortex The primitive part of the cerebral cortex, such as the olfactory cortex, which is not laminated.

allogamy Fertilization by the union of the ovum from one organism with the spermatozoon from another. Also called cross-fertilization.

allogeneic, allogenic Relating to genetically dissimilar individuals of a single species.

allograft A graft derived from a genetically dissimilar individual of the same species. Also called allogeneic graft.

allolalia Any speech defect that originates in the brain.

allomerism The state of having different chemical composition but the same crystalline form.

allomorphism A change in the shape of cells caused by mechanical factors.

alloplasia See heteroplasia.

alloplast An inert foreign body implant.

alloploid An organism arising from the combination of two or more sets of chromosomes from different ancestral species. Also called allopolyploid.

allosome A chromosome that differs from the ordinary chromosome (autosome); a sex chromosome.

allosterism Alteration of an enzyme's activity by regulatory molecules that are noncompetitively bound to sites other than the active or catalytic site of the enzyme molecule.

allotransplantation The transplantation of tissue from one individual to another of the same species but without the identical genetic makeup.

allotype Any of several genetically determined antigenic variants of a given class of immunoglobulins.

alloxan A reddish, crystalline substance, $C_4H_2N_2O$; a product of oxidation of uric acid; capable of destroying the islets of Langerhans and, hence, inducing experimental diabetes.

alloy A mixture of two or more metals.

alochia Absence of vaginal discharges (lochia) after childbirth.

aloes A purgative, brownish-yellow powder derived from plants of the genus *Aloe*.

aloform A wing-shaped structure, as the pterygoid bone of the skull.

alogia Speechlessness caused by mental confusion or retardation.

alopecia Baldness.

 a. areata, a. circumscripta Complete loss of hair in patches, chiefly on the scalp.

 a. capitis totalis Complete hair loss from the scalp.

 a. hereditaria Premature loss of hair, an inherited trait. Also called alopecia simplex.

 a. senillis Loss of hair normally occurring in old age. Also called senile alopecia.

 a. totalis, a. universalis Total loss of hair from all parts of the body.

alpha **1.** The first letter of the Greek alphabet, α; used to denote the first in order of importance. **2.** In chemistry, denotes a location immediately adjacent to the functional group of atoms in a molecule. For terms beginning with alpha, see under specific term.

Alphaherpesvirinae Subfamily of viruses (family Herpesviridae) that includes the herpesvirus; latent infections occur frequently (not exclusively) in ganglia. Also called herpes simplex virus group.

Alphavirus A genus of arthropod-borne viruses (family Togaviridae) that cause diseases such as encephalomyelitis of horses and humans; formerly classified as arbovirus, group A.

Alport's syndrome Hereditary nephritis associated with deafness.

alter To castrate a male animal.

alternans Alternating.

 electrical a. Regular alternating variation in the wave amplitude of the electrocardiogram.

Alternaria A genus of soil molds having dark-colored conidia; prevalent in air and usually considered to be a common laboratory contaminant; a common allergen in bronchial asthma.

alum Any double sulfate of a trivalent metal (aluminum, iron, etc.) and a univalent metal (sodium, potassium, etc.); used as an astringent and a styptic.

aluminum A silvery-white, metallic element of extremely light weight; symbol Al, atomic number 13, atomic weight 26.97; its compounds are used therapeutically as antacids and astringents.

 a. chloride A white or yellowish-white powder, $AlCl_3 \cdot 6H_2O$; used in 10 to 25% solution as an antiperspirant, a deodorant, or astringent.

 a. hydroxide, a. hydrate A white tasteless powder, $Al(OH)_3$; used externally as a drying powder because it takes up water, and internally as an antacid. Also called hydrated alumina.

 a. hydroxide gel A preparation containing from 3.6 to 4.4% of aluminum oxide (AlO_3) in the form of aluminum hydroxide; used to reduce stomach acidity; also prepared in tablet form, which is the dried aluminum hydroxide gel.

alveolalgia Dry socket; see under socket.

alveolar Of or relating to an alveolus.

alveolectomy Surgical removal of diseased tissue from the alveolar process, following the removal of teeth, in preparation for the fitting of a dental prosthesis.

alveoli Plural of alveolus.

alveolingual Relating to the surface of the alveolar process adjacent to the tongue.

alveolitis Inflammation of alveoli.

alveolotomy The surgical opening of a tooth socket for drainage and treatment purposes.

alveolus, pl. aveoli **1.** See tooth socket. **2.** An air sac of the lungs. **3.** One of the honeycomb pits in the mucous membrane of the stomach.

alveus **1.** A canal. **2.** The layer of white fibers in the brain which covers the area of the hippocampus adjacent to the lateral ventricle.

Alzheimer's disease Progressive brain disease usually occurring in persons over 50 years of age, marked by generalized atrophy of the brain; chief symptoms include memory loss, disorientation, impaired judgment, difficulty in walking, and speech disorders; death occurs in 5–10 years.

amalgam An alloy of mercury and other metals, used in dentistry for filling cavities in the teeth.

amalgamate To make an amalgam by dissolving a metal in mercury.

amalgamation The process of dissolving a metal in mercury to form an alloy.

amalgamator In dentistry, a device for mixing amalgam mechanically.

Amanita A genus of fungi.

 A. phalloides Poisonous mushroom which, upon ingestion, causes severe gastrointestinal symptoms, followed by damage to the kidneys, liver, and central nervous system. Also called death cup; death angel.

amantadine hydrochloride An antiviral agent used in preventing illness in individuals exposed to respiratory infection from influenza virus; also used in treating Parkinson's disease; Symmetrel®.

amaurosis Complete loss of vision.

 a. centralis Blindness caused by disease of the central nervous system.

 a. fugax Temporary blindness lasting a few minutes.

 toxic a. Blindness due to inflammation of the optic nerve caused by the presence in the system of a poisonous agent such as alcohol, tobacco, lead, etc.

amaurotic Relating to, or suffering from, blindness.

ambenonium chloride A chemical compound that inhibits the production of the enzyme cholinesterase; used in the treatment of chronic progressive muscular weakness (myasthenia gravis); Mytelase Chloride®.

ambidextrous Being equally skillful with both hands.

ambisexual Of, relating to, or affecting both sexes.

ambisexuality The state of having characteristics

Ambrosia elatior

embryo 2.5 mm in length

yolk s

amnion

amniocentesis

ameba

of both sexes.

ambivalence The existence of contrasting emotional feelings, such as love and hate, about a person or object.

amblyacousia A slight degree of hearing impairment.

amblyopia Diminished vision without a detectable lesion or disease of the eye.

amblyoscope A device consisting primarily of two angled tubes which can be made to swivel to different degrees of convergence or divergence: used for training an amblyopic eye to share equally with the other eye in binocular vision.

Ambrosia elatior Common ragweed that produces highly allergenic pollen capable of causing hay fever and asthma in some individuals; pollination period is from August through October.

ambulatory, ambulant Capable of walking about; said of a patient who is not confined to bed.

ameba Any protozoan of the genus *Amoeba*.

amebiasis The condition of being infected with *Amoeba histolytica*.

amebic Pertaining to, resembling, or caused by amebas.

amebicide Anything that destroys amebas.

ameboid Resembling an ameba.

ameboma A tumor-like mass sometimes formed in the wall of the colon due to chronic infestation with amebas.

ameiosis A type of cell division in which gametes are formed without reduction in chromosome number.

amelanotic Denoting certain types of unpigmented skin growths.

amelia Congenital absence of a limb or limbs.

amelification The development of tooth enamel.

amelioration Improvement; lessening of the severity of symptoms.

ameloblast The epithelial cell in the developing tooth that produces layers of matrix which become calcified to form rods of tooth enamel; when it completes its function of enamel formation, the ameloblast becomes part of the enamel cuticle (Nasmyth's membrane). Also called adamantoblast.

ameloblastofibroma A benign tumor composed of epithelial cells of a developing tooth (ameloblasts) and dense connective tissue.

ameloblastoma A tumor derived from epithelial tissue characteristic of the enamel organ, occurring mainly in the molar region of the mandible. Also called adamantinoma.

ameloblastosarcoma A malignant neoplasm derived from odontogenic tissue and containing a large number of ameloblasts.

amelogenesis Enamel formation.

amenorrhea Absence of menstruation.

amenorrheal, amenorrheic Relating to, or accompanied by, absence of menstruation.

ametropia A refractive disorder of the eye in which parallel rays of light do not focus on the retina, but either in front of it (myopia) or behind it (hyperopia).

axial a. Ametropia caused by the lengthening of the eyeball on the optic axis.

amide An organic compound derived from ammonia by the substitution of an acyl radical for hydrogen.

amination The formation of an amine.

amine Any of a group of organic compounds derived from ammonia by replacement of one or more hydrogen atoms by hydrocarbon radicals.

aminoacetic acid See glycine.

amino acid See under acid.

aminoacidemia The presence of amino acids in the blood as a result of congenital metabolic disease.

aminoaciduria The presence of excessive amounts of amino acids in the urine, or the presence of amino acids not usually found in the urine.

ρ-aminobenzoic acid (PABA) Para-aminobenzoic acid; a factor of the vitamin B complex; it is an essential growth factor for bacteria.

γ-aminobutyric acid (GABA) Gamma-aminobutyric acid; a substance in the brain, especially in the basal ganglia and neocortex, that plays a role in cortical transmission.

ε-aminocaproic acid (EACP) Epsilon-aminocaproic acid; compound that inhibits dissolution of fibrin in the blood; used to prevent bleeding.

aminoglycoside An antibiotic containing amino sugars linked by glycoside; it blocks protein synthesis in bacterial ribosomes.

ρ-aminohippuric acid (PAH) Para-aminohippuric acid; a substance used in clearance studies to determine the total amount of plasma flowing through the kidney.

δ-aminolevulinic acid (ALA) Delta-aminolevulinic acid; an intermediate in the biosynthesis of porphyrin; excessive levels are found in urine in acute intermittent porphyria.

aminopeptidase Enzyme promoting the breakdown of peptides; it aids in protein digestion.

aminophylline A xanthine derivative containing 85% anhydrous theophylline and 15% ethylenediamine; used to treat asthma.

aminopyrine Compound used to reduce fever and pain in rheumatism, neuritis, and tuberculosis. Also called amidopyrine; pyramidon.

ρ-aminosalicylic acid (PAS, PASA) Para-aminosalicylic acid; a crystalline compound which retards the growth of bacteria; used as an adjunct in the treatment of tuberculosis.

amitosis Direct division of a cell simply by elongation and division of the nucleus and cytoplasm into two new cells, unlike the ordinary process of cell reproduction (mitosis).

ammonia A colorless, volatile, pungent, alkaline gas, NH_3, soluble in water, forming ammonia water; formed in the body as a product of protein metabolism; usually converted to urea by the liver or excreted by the kidney to facilitate H^+ excretion.

ammoniacal Of or relating to ammonia.

ammoniated Combined with or containing ammonia.

ammonium A chemical ion (NH_4).

a. chloride A white crystalline compound, NH_4Cl; used as an expectorant and as an acidifying agent. Also called sal ammoniac.

amnesia Impairment of memory.

anterograde a. Inability to recall events after injury or disease.

retrograde a. Amnesia for events preceding injury or disease.

amnesiac An individual suffering from loss of memory.

amnestic, amnesic Causing amnesia.

amniocentesis Withdrawal of amniotic fluid, usually performed through the abdominal wall using a needle.

amniography Roentgenography of the pregnant uterus after injection of an opaque solution into the amniotic fluid.

amnion The thin, tough, innermost layer of the membranous sac that surrounds the fetus and contains amniotic fluid. Also called the "bag of waters."

amnionitis Inflammation of the amnion.

amniorrhea The premature escape of amniotic fluid (liquor amnii).

amniorrhexis Rupture of the amniotic membrane.

amnioscopy Direct observation of the amniotic fluid, through the intact amniotic sac, with an endoscope introduced through the cervical canal.

amniotomy Surgical rupture of the fetal membranes for the purpose of inducing labor.

Amoeba A genus of one-celled protozoans existing in water, soil, or as parasites, having a changeable shape, and moving by means of pseudopodia; some species cause disease in man.

amorphia, amorphism The state or condition of being without a definite form.

amorphous Lacking a definite shape or structure.

ampere The unit of electric current strength, equal to the current yielded by one volt of electromotive force against one ohm of resistance.

amphetamine Any of a group of synthetic chem-

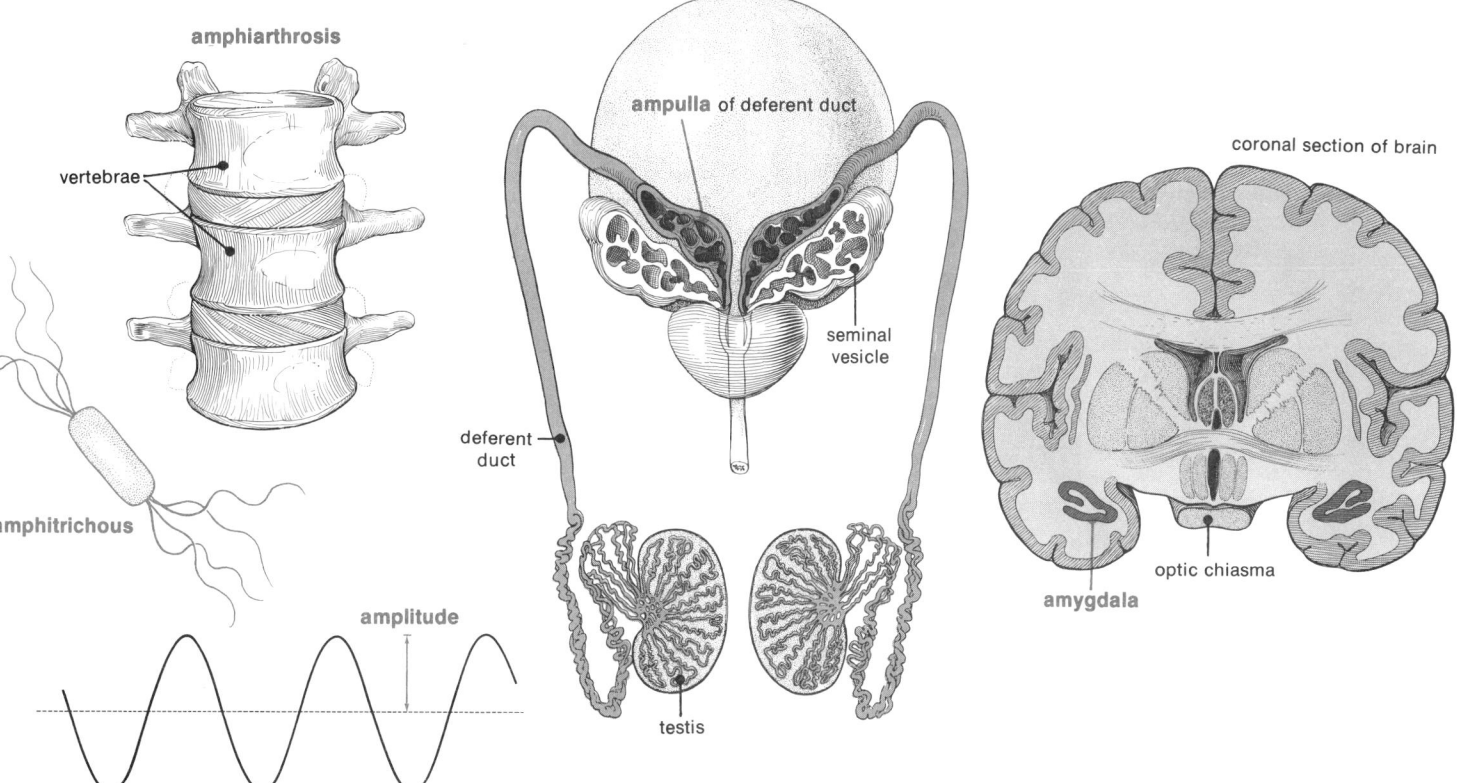

amphiarthrosis

vertebrae

amphitrichous

amplitude

ampulla of deferent duct

seminal vesicle

deferent duct

testis

coronal section of brain

optic chiasma

amygdala

icals that stimulate the central nervous system; pharmacologically classified as sympathomimetic amines. Slang names: speed, uppers, bennies.

amphiarthrosis A joint or articulation that allows only slight motion, e.g., between the bodies of the vertebrae. Also called amphiarthrodial joint.

amphipathic Relating to molecules possessing groups with characteristically different properties, e.g., molecules that are hydrophobic at one end and hydrophilic at the other end.

amphitrichous, amphitrichate Having flagella or a flagellum at both ends, as in certain microorganisms.

amphixenosis A transmissible disease of vertebrates caused by a microorganism, such as *Trypanosoma cruzi*, which can inhabit either man or animal as its maintenance host. Cf. anthropozoonosis; zooanthroponosis.

amphophil Denoting certain cells that stain readily with either acid or basic dyes.

amphoric The quality of a sound sometimes heard in auscultation, described as that produced by blowing over the mouth of a bottle.

amplitude One of three measurements of the vibration of a sound wave (others are frequency and wavelength); the vertical vibrations that reflect the intensity of sound.

ampule, ampoule, ampul A small glass container sealed to preserve the sterile condition of its contents, which are used primarily for subcutaneous, intramuscular, or intravenous injections.

ampulla A saclike dilation of a canal, as seen in the semicircular canals of the inner ear.

  a. of deferent duct, a. of vas deferens The dilation of the duct just before it is joined by the duct of the seminal vesicle.

  a. of Vater The short dilated tube formed by the union of the pancreatic and common bile ducts just before they empty into the duodenum. Also called greater papilla.

  phrenic a. The normal expansion of the lower end of the esophagus.

ampullitis Inflammation of an ampulla, especially of the dilated end of the deferent duct of the testis.

amputation Removal of a limb or any appendage of the body.

  Lisfranc's a. Amputation of the foot between the tarsus and metatarsus. Also called Lisfranc's operation.

  root a. Surgical removal of the apical portion of the root of a tooth.

  Syme's a. Removal of the foot at the ankle joint; both malleoli are removed. Also called Syme's operation.

amputee A person with one or more amputated limbs.

  double a. A person with two amputated limbs.

amygdala, *pl.* **amygdalae** 1. Any almond-shaped anatomic structure, such as a tonsil. 2. One of two ovoid masses of gray matter, located in the front part of the temporal lobe of the brain, in the roof of the terminal portion of the inferior horn of the lateral ventricle. Also called amygdaloid nuclear complex.

amygdalase A glucoside-splitting enzyme.

amygdaloid Almond-shaped.

amyl A univalent organic radical (C_5H_{11}).

  a. nitrate A flammable and volatile yellow liquid, $C_5H_{11}NO_2$; used as a motor depressant, and inhaled to relieve pain in angina pectoris.

amylase An enzyme that promotes the splitting of starches.

  pancreatic a. Amylase present in pancreatic juice. Also called amylopsin.

  salivary a. Amylase present in saliva. Also called ptyalin.

α-amylase See α-1,4-glucan-4-glucanohydrolase.

β-amylase See α-1,4-glucan maltohydrolase.

amylin The insoluble constituent or cellulose of starch.

amylogenesis Starch formation.

amyloid 1. Resembling starch. 2. An abnormal protein-polysaccharide complex deposited extracellularly in various organs or tissues as a product of certain disease processes.

amyloidosis Accumulation of an abnormal protein, amyloid, in various tissues of the body.

  primary a. Amyloidosis that is not caused by another disease, usually involving the tongue, intestinal tract, lungs, skin, and skeletal and heart muscles.

  secondary a. Amyloidosis resulting from a chronic disease, such as tuberculosis, rheumatoid arthritis, osteomyelitis, etc.; usually affecting the liver, kidneys, and spleen.

amylopectin A polysaccharide found in the insoluble component of starch.

amylophagia Abnormal craving for starch. Also called starch eating.

amylopsin Pancreatic amylase; see under amylase.

amylose The relatively soluble component of starch.

amyotonia Lack of muscular tone.

  a. congenita Amyotonia occurring in infants, affecting only the musculature innervated by spinal nerves. Also called Oppenheim's syndrome.

amyotrophic Relating to muscular degeneration or atrophy.

amyotrophy Wasting or degeneration of muscles.

anabolic Promoting or exhibiting anabolism.

anabolism The process by which living tissues build complex compounds from substances of a simple constitution; an energy-consuming constructive metabolic process; the reverse of catabolism.

anabolistic Having constructive metabolic properties, such as the ability to build complex molecules out of simple ones.

anacephaly Without a skull and with little brain tissue.

anacidity Lack of acidity; especially, lack of hydrochloric acid in the gastric juice.

anaclitic Having a psychologic dependence on others, as the normal dependence of an infant on its mother or mother substitute.

anacrotic Having an abnormal pulse, evidenced in a pulse tracing in which the ascending line of the curve has a small additional wave or shoulder, as in aortic stenosis. Also called anadicrotic.

anacusis, anakusis Total deafness.

anadicrotic See anacrotic.

anaerobe An organism that does not grow when freely exposed to air.

  facultative a. A microorganism that can grow in either the presence or absence of free oxygen.

anaerobic Growing in the absence of oxygen.

anaerogenic Producing no gas.

anagenesis Regeneration of tissue or structure.

anal Relating to or near the anus.

analeptic A central nervous system stimulant; a restorative medication.

analgesia Absence of sensibility to pain; during labor, analgesia may be induced by intermittent administration of certain inhalation anesthetics in concentrations lower than those required for surgical anesthesia.

analgesic 1. Relieving pain. 2. A medication that relieves pain without affecting consciousness; the most commonly used analgesic is aspirin (acetylsalicylic acid).

analgia Absence of pain.

analogous Similar in function or appearance, but not in origin or development.

analogue 1. An organ or part similar in function to one in another organism of a different species but different in structure or development. 2. A chemical compound similar in structure to another but dissimilar in composition.

analysand A patient who is being treated with psychoanalysis.

analysis, *pl.* **analyses** 1. The separation of a substance into its simple constituents. 2. Psychoanalysis.

  adsorption a. See chromatography.

  chromatographic a. See chromatography.

  dermatoglyphic a. Analysis of the variety of pat-

15

anaphase human somatic cell

46 chromosomes move toward centrioles

androsterone

anastomosis of intestine to stomach and of intestine to intestine

stomach

colon

small intestine

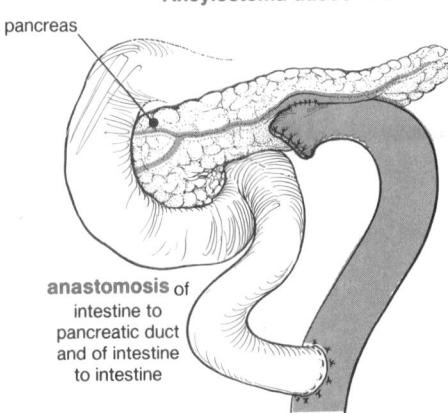

mouth parts

Ancylostoma duodenale

pancreas

anastomosis of intestine to pancreatic duct and of intestine to intestine

tern configurations of epidermal ridges for abnormal characteristics.

gastric a. Aspiration and study of the stomach contents; may be performed in the basal state, after a test meal, or after administration of a secretion-promoting agent.

gravimetric a. Determination by weight of the exact proportions of the components of a substance.

qualitative a. Determination of the nature of the constituents of a substance.

quantitative a. Determination of the quantity, as well as the nature, of the components of a substance.

spectrum a. Determination of the components of a gas by means of a spectroscope.

volumetric a. Quantitative analysis by weight.

analyst 1. One who performs an analysis. **2.** See psychoanalyst.

analyzer, analyzor 1. A polarizing filter used to determine the direction of polarization of a beam of light. **2.** One of two filters in an instrument used for the study of a polarized beam of light (polariscope).

breath a. A simple device for detecting whether or not a person is intoxicated; the subject blows into a balloon and if the proportion of alcohol in the breath is sufficiently high, a chemical reactant in the device changes color.

wave a. An apparatus by means of which complex wave forms are separated into their component frequencies.

anamnesis 1. The act of recalling to memory. **2.** The history of a patient's illness.

anaphase The third stage of cell division by mitosis, during which the two chromatids of each chromosome separate and migrate along the spindle fibers toward opposite poles.

anaphoresis 1. The motion of electrically charged particles in solution toward a positive pole or anode. **2.** Reduction of sweat secretion.

anaphylactic Characterized by a markedly abnormal or extreme sensitivity to a biologically foreign protein.

anaphylactogenic 1. A substance that produces an exaggerated or severe reaction to the presence of a foreign protein. **2.** Anything that reduces immunity.

anaphylactoid Resembling anaphylaxis.

anaphylaxis An immediate, severe hypersensitivity reaction, sometimes fatal, induced by a second injection of an antigen.

exercise-induced a. A shock-like syndrome associated with vigorous exercise; the first symptoms are usually itching and swelling, especially of the neck.

anaplasia 1. The loss of normal differentiation of cells, as in tumor cells. **2.** A reversion of cells to an embryonic state in which reproductive activity is very pronounced.

anaplastic 1. Of or relating to anaplasia. **2.** Of or relating to plastic surgery.

anaplasty Plastic surgery.

anarthria Loss of ability to articulate properly.

anasarca Generalized massive edema in subcutaneous tissue; may be due to cardiac, renal, or hepatic disease, and to starvation.

anastole Retraction of the margins of a wound.

anastomose 1. To open one into the other; said of blood vessels. **2.** To create by surgery a channel between tubular structures, as intestines or blood vessels.

anastomosis 1. A connection between tubular structures. **2.** The surgical or pathologic formation of a channel between tubular structures, as blood vessels or intestines.

anastomotic Relating to an anastomosis.

anatomic, anatomical 1. Relating to anatomy. **2.** Relating to structure as opposed to function.

anatomist A specialist in anatomy.

anatomy The science of the body structure of an organism and its parts.

comparative a. The study of the bodies of different animals in relation to one another.

dental a. The branch of anatomy concerned with the external and internal structure of teeth and the surrounding tissues.

developmental a. See embryology.

gross a. Study of structures as seen without the aid of a microscope.

microscopic a. See histology.

pathologic a. The study of diseased or injured tissues.

topographic a. The study of the location of the various organs and parts of the body and their relations to one another and to the surface of the body.

anchorage 1. The surgical fixation of a prolapsed organ. **2.** In dentistry, a tooth or part of a tooth to which a bridge, crown, filling, etc. is attached; in orthodontics, the teeth used as support for an appliance.

ancillary Subordinate; auxiliary.

anconitis Inflammation of the elbow joint.

Ancylostoma A genus of nematode parasites that attach themselves to the mucosa of the duodenum where they suck the blood of the host, causing anemia; they enter the body of man in the larval stage, usually through the skin of the feet and ankles.

A. duodenale A variety of hookworm characterized by the presence of two pairs of teeth; species predominate in southern Europe, coastal North Africa, northern India, and Japan. Also called "Old World" hookworm; *Uncinaria duodenalis.*

ancylostomiasis Hookworm disease; infestation with the parasite *Ancylostoma duodenale* or *Necator americanus,* causing anemia by the destruction of red blood cells; in children the infection may result in mental and physical retardation. Also called miner's, brickmaker's, or mountain anemia; uncinariasis.

cutaneous a. The appearance of small itchy vesicles at the site of entrance of the *Ancylostoma* larvae, usually on the feet, prior to the manifestation of intestinal symptoms. Also called ancylostomiasis dermatitis; ground itch.

androgen A hormone that stimulates the development of male sex characteristics.

androgenic Relating to an androgen or producing male characteristics.

androgynous Relating to female pseudohermaphroditism (a true female with masculine characteristics).

android Manlike.

andropathy Any disease peculiar to the male sex.

androsterone An androgen (male sex hormone) derived from testosterone metabolism.

anechoic Denoting absence of echoes in an area studied with ultrasonography.

anemia Any condition in which the concentration of hemoglobin in the blood is below the normal for the age and sex of the patient; usually there is also a reduction in the number of red blood cells per mm^3 and in the volume of packed red blood cells per 100 ml of blood.

Addison's a. See pernicious anemia.

aplastic a. Anemia characterized by bone marrow insufficiency or failure to produce a normal number of cells for discharge into the blood stream; usually but not always, associated with a hypocellular bone marrow and frequently with reduction of all the formed elements of the blood (pancytopenia).

congenital hypoplastic a. Chronic pure red blood cell aplasia; a form of anemia occurring in young infants and marked primarily by depletion of erythroid tissue in the bone marrow, resulting in pallor, listlessness, and poor appetite; minor associated congenital abnormalities are often observed. Also called erythroid hypoplasia.

congenital spherocytic a. See spherocytosis.

Cooley's a., Mediterranean a. Beta thalassemia; see under thalassemia.

hemolytic a. Anemia resulting from abnormal destruction of red blood cells in the body.

hypochromic a. Anemia characterized by a decrease in the hemoglobin content of the red blood cells, i.e., reduced mean corpuscular hemoglobin

caudal anesthesia

spinal anesthesia

angina pectoris

typical distribution of pain

abdominal aneurysm

concentration (MCHC).

hypochromic microcytic a. Anemia characterized by a decrease in the hemoglobin concentration of red blood cells and by smaller than normal cells, i.e., decreased mean corpuscular volume (MCV); usually caused by iron deficiency.

iron deficiency a. Hypochromic microcytic anemia due to inadequate iron supply.

macrocytic a. Any anemia in which the average size of circulating red blood cells is greater than normal, i.e., the mean corpuscular volume (MCV) is increased. See also megaloblastic anemia.

Marchiafava-Micheli a. Paroxysmal nocturnal hemoglobinuria; see under hemoglobinuria.

megaloblastic a. Any anemia usually caused by deficiency of vitamin B$_{12}$ or folic acid; characterized by macrocytic erythrocytes and an increased number of megaloblasts in the bone marrow; includes pernicious anemia and the anemias caused by folic acid deficiency, such as sprue, "blind loop" syndrome, and megaloblastic anemia of pregnancy.

myelophthisic a., myelopathic a. Anemia resulting from the destruction of blood cell-forming (hemopoietic) tissues by space-occupying lesions.

normochromic a. Anemia in which the hemoglobin concentration in the red blood cells is within the normal range, i.e., the mean corpuscular hemoglobin concentration (MCHC) is from 32 to 36%.

nutritional a. Anemia resulting from lack of some essential materials in the diet, as iron or vitamins.

pernicious a. (PA) A chronic progressive, megaloblastic anemia, occurring mostly in individuals in the fifth decade or older; caused by a lack of secretion of the intrinsic factor present in normal gastric juice, which is necessary for adequate absorption of vitamin B$_{12}$; it is frequently associated with neurologic damage. Also called Addison's anemia.

primary refractory a. Any of several persistent, frequently advanced anemias, that is not the result of any other primary disease (e.g., chronic disease of the liver or kidneys) and that does not respond to any treatment except blood transfusions. Also called aregenerative or hypoplastic anemia; progressive hypocythemia.

refractory a. Aplastic anemia.

sickle cell a. A hereditary chronic anemia, found primarily in blacks, in which a large portion of the red blood cells have a crescent or sickle shape, due to the presence of an abnormal hemoglobin (hemoglobin S). Also called sickle cell disease; drepanocytosis.

sideroblastic a., sideroachrestic a. Anemia in which the young erythrocytes in bone marrow contain iron (sideroblasts) and the iron content of reticuloendothelial tissues is increased.

anemic Of or pertaining to anemia.

anencephaly A congenital developmental defect consisting of absence of the vault of the skull, with an exposed, poorly developed, degenerated brain, resulting from the neural tube's failure to close in the cephalic area; the affected infant usually dies within a few days after birth.

anephric Without kidneys.

anergic 1. Relating to a diminished or absent response to specific antigens. **2.** Marked by abnormal lack of energy.

anergy 1. Lack of response to the injection of an antigen. **2.** Inability to react; sluggishness.

aneroid Not using or containing fluid.

anesthesia Partial or total loss of sensation, with or without loss of consciousness, due to injury or disease, or induced by the administration of a drug.

caudal a. Anesthesia produced by the injection of an anesthetic solution into the caudal part of the spinal canal.

crossed a. Anesthesia on one side of the body caused by a lesion on the opposite side of the brain.

epidural a. Anesthesia produced by the injection of an anesthetic agent into the extradural space.

field block a. Anesthesia produced by injecting the anesthetic solution in such a way as to create a wall around the operative field.

general a. A state of unconsciousness and complete loss of sensation produced by the administration of an anesthetic, either by inhalation, intravenously, or intramuscularly. Also called surgical anesthesia.

intraneural a. Local anesthesia produced by injecting the anesthetic solution into a nerve trunk.

local a. Anesthesia of a limited area of the body.

nerve block a. Anesthesia produced by injecting the anesthetic solution around and near a nerve.

rectal a. General anesthesia produced by introducing the anesthetic solution into the rectum.

regional a. Any of four types of anesthesia: spinal, epidural, caudal, or nerve block.

saddle block a. Anesthesia of the area of the buttocks, perineum, and inner thighs produced by injection of the anesthetic agent low in the dural sac.

spinal a. 1. Anesthesia of the lower part of the body produced by injecting an anesthetic agent in the subarachnoid space around the spinal cord. **2.** Anesthesia due to injury or disease of the spinal cord.

anesthesiologist A physician who specializes in anesthesiology.

anesthesiology The branch of science concerned with the study and administration of anesthesia.

anesthetic A drug that produces anesthesia.

anesthetist A person trained to administer anesthetics.

anesthetize To render insensible with an anesthetic.

anestrus The interval of sexual quiescence between two estrous cycles in mammals or prolonged failure of estrus in a mature animal.

aneuploid An organism having an abnormal number of chromosomes.

aneuploidy The state of having an abnormal number of chromosomes.

aneurysm A circumscribed sac-like bulging of a blood vessel, usually an artery.

abdominal a. Aneurysm of the abdominal aorta.

berry a. A small berry-like sacculation of a cerebral artery, usually at the circle of Willis.

dissecting a. Aneurysm in which blood forces its way between the layers of an arterial wall, causing them to separate; the blood may enter through an intimal tear or by interstitial hemorrhage.

exogenous a. Aneurysm due to trauma to the affected vessel. Also called traumatic aneurysm.

false a. A blood clot within the wall of an artery.

fusiform a. A spindle-shaped dilatation of an artery.

mycotic a. Aneurysm caused by growth of microorganisms within the vessel wall.

ventricular a. Dilatation of the ventricular wall of the heart.

aneurysmal Of or relating to an aneurysm.

aneurysmectomy Excision of an aneurysm.

angiectasia, angiectasis Dilatation of a blood vessel or a lymph vessel.

angiitis, angitis Inflammation of a blood or lymph vessel.

hypersensitivity a. Inflammation of a blood vessel as a manifestation of an allergic reaction to a specific substance.

angina A severe strangling pain.

abdominal a. Pain occurring in the abdominal area as a result of ischemia of the intestine.

a. decubitus Attack of angina pectoris precipitated by the recumbent position, usually occurring at night.

a. pectoris Constricting pain in the chest due to insufficient blood supply to the heart muscle, usually precipitated by effort and relieved rapidly by rest or nitrites; the pain is usually retrosternal and frequently radiates to the precordium, the left shoulder and arm, or the neck.

crescendo a. See unstable angina.

Ludwig's a. Painful inflammation and pus formation in the area of the submaxillary gland, usually resulting from a tooth infection.

Prinzmetal's a. A variant of angina pectoris occurring at rest, and associated with elevation of the ST segment of the electrocardiogram, as opposed to

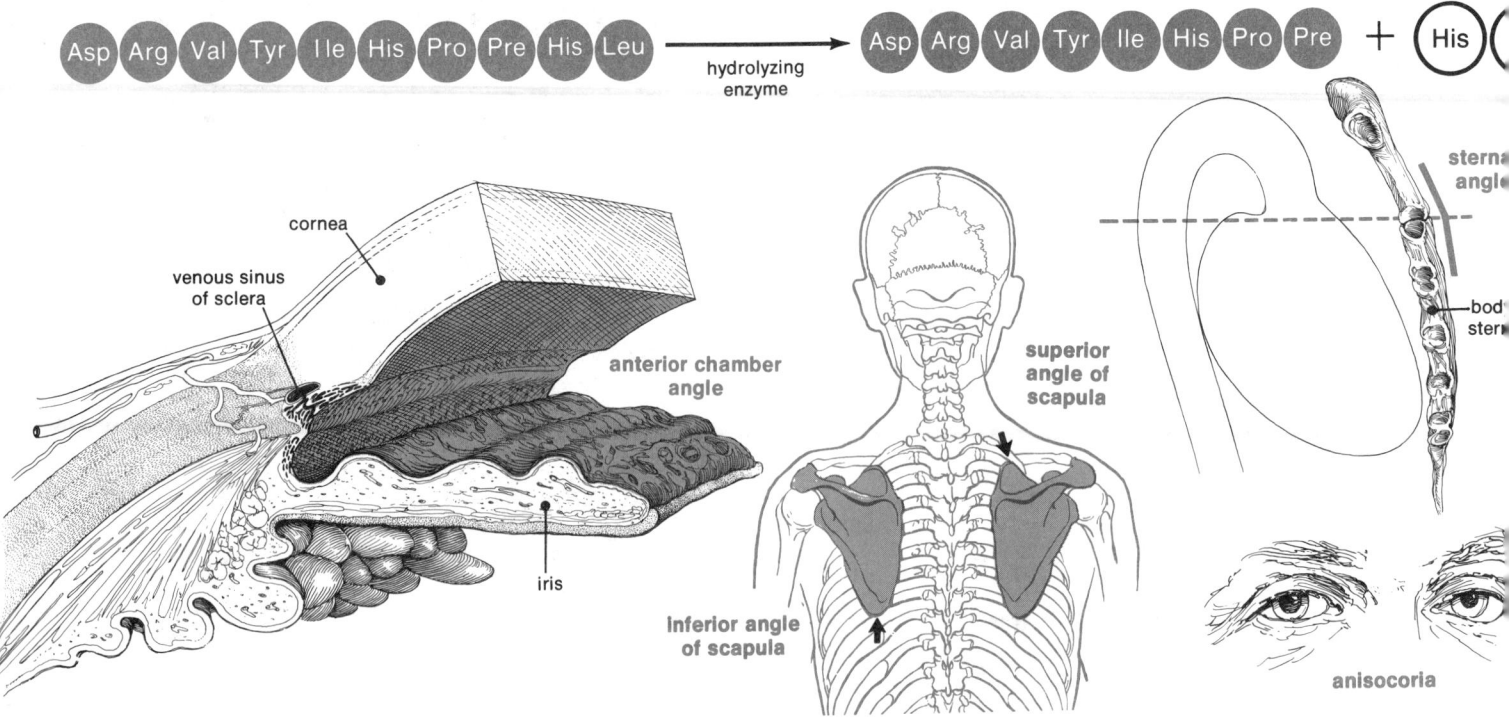

angiotensin I (decapeptide)

Asp Arg Val Tyr Ile His Pro Pre His Leu → (hydrolyzing enzyme) → **angiotensin II (octapeptide)** Asp Arg Val Tyr Ile His Pro Pre + His

cornea

venous sinus of sclera

anterior chamber angle

iris

superior angle of scapula

inferior angle of scapula

sternal angle

body sternum

anisocoria

---

the depression usually occurring in angina pectoris. Also called variant angina.

unstable a. Severe chest pain that increases in frequency or duration, starts at rest or during sleep, or recurs after myocardial infarction or bypass surgery. Also called crescendo angina.

variant a. See Prinzmetal's angina.

Vincent's a. See pharyngitis, fusospirochetal.

anginal Relating to, or of the nature, of angina.

angioblast 1. Embryonic tissue from which blood cells and blood vessels are formed. **2.** A vessel-forming cell.

angioblastoma See hemangioblastoma.

angiocardiography X-ray examination of the heart and great vessels following the intravenous injection of radiopaque material.

angiocardiopathy Any disease of the heart and blood vessels.

angioedema Allergic reaction manifested by well-demarcated localized swellings of the skin and subcutaneous tissues.

angiogenesis The formation of blood vessels.

angiogram A roentgenogram of a vessel obtained by outlining the structure with a radiopaque material.

angiography 1. Description of vessels. **2.** X-ray examination of blood vessels after injection of a radiopaque material.

selective a. The injection of radiopaque solution through a catheter into the vessels of the specific area of the body to be studied.

angiokeratoma A skin disorder consisting of a varying number of multiple violaceous (violet or purple discoloration) lesions. Also called telangiectatic wart.

angiokeratosis The occurrence of angiokeratoma.

angiology The study of blood and lymph vessels.

angioma A tumor composed of dilated blood vessels (hemangioma) or lymph vessels (lymphangioma).

cavernous a. See hemangioma, cavernous.

cherry a. See hemangioma, senile.

angiomatosis A condition marked by the presence of multiple angiomas.

retinocerebral a. See von Hippel-Lindau disease.

angiomatous Resembling a tumor made up of dilated vessels (angioma).

angiopathy Disease of blood vessels or lymphatics.

angioplasty Surgical reconstruction of a blood vessel.

percutaneous transluminal a. Enlargement of the lumen of a narrowed artery (coronary or renal) with a balloon-tip catheter; the catheter is introduced through the skin into the vessel to the narrowed seg-

ment where the balloon is inflated, thus dilating the lumen.

angiopoietic Causing the formation of blood vessels.

angiospasm Spasmodic contraction of a blood vessel. Also called vasospasm.

angiostenosis Constriction or narrowing of one or more blood vessels.

angiotensin A peptide formed by the action of the enzyme renin on a globulin in the blood plasma; renin splits off from its substrate a decapeptide known as angiotensin I (AI), which is then changed by a converting enzyme to the octapeptide angiotensin II (AII), a potent vasoconstrictor and stimulator of aldosterone synthesis and release; a heptapeptide, angiotensin III (AIII), has also been found which is a stimulator of aldosterone synthesis and release but has little or no vasoconstrictor activity.

angiotensinogen An a_2-globulin, also known as renin substrate; it has no pressor activity in the intact form but is acted upon by the enzyme renin which splits off a decapeptide unit, angiotensin I.

angiotome A segment of the vascular system of the embryo.

angiotrophic Relating to nutrition of blood and lymphatic vessels. Also called vasotrophic.

angle The figure formed by two lines or planes diverging from a common point; the space between two lines or planes diverging from a common point.

acromial a. The palpable point where the lateral border of the acromion joins, and becomes continuous with, the spine of the scapula.

a. of convergence The angle between the line of vision and the median line.

a. of the jaw The angle formed by the lower edge of the body of the mandible and the posterior edge of the ramus.

a. of Louis See sternal angle.

anterior chamber a. The angle formed at the junction of the iris and cornea. Also called iridocorneal or filtration angle; angle of the iris.

carrying a. The angle made by the axes of the arm and forearm when the forearm is extended.

cavosurface a. The angle formed by the junction of the wall of a prepared cavity and the surface of a tooth.

cerebellopontine a. The space at the junction of the cerebellum and pons.

critical a. The angle of incidence (angle made with the perpendicular by a light ray passing from one medium to another) which results in a refracted ray; if the angle of incidence is greater than 90°, the ray is reflected.

filtration a. Anterior chamber angle.

inferior a. of scapula The angle formed by the junction of the lateral and medial borders of the scapula.

line a. The angle formed by the junction of any two surfaces of a tooth.

point a. The meeting of three tooth surfaces at a point, forming a corner.

pontine a. Cerebellopontine angle.

sternal a. The angle or ridge on the anterior surface of the sternum (breastbone) at the junction of its body and manubrium. Also called angle of Louis.

superior a. of scapula The angle formed by the junction of the superior and medial borders of the scapula. Formerly called medial angle.

angstrom, Angström (Å, A) A unit of length equal to a ten-thousandth of a micron; 10^{-7} mm; used especially to measure the length of light waves or other electromagnetic radiation and cytologic ultrastructures.

anhedonia Inability to experience pleasure.

anhidrosis Marked deficiency of sweat.

anhidrotic, anidrotic Anything that diminishes the secretion of sweat.

anhydrase An enzyme that promotes the removal of water from a compound.

anhydrous Without water.

aniline An oily, colorless or brown compound derived from benzene; used in the preparation of dyes.

anion A negatively charged ion that is characteristically attracted to the positively charged anode; indicated as a superior minus sign, e.g., C1−.

anionic Relating to or containing a negatively charged ion; attracted to the anode or positively charged pole when a current is passed through a solution.

aniridia Complete or partial absence of the iris. Also called irideremia.

anisakiasis Infection of the lining of the stomach and small intestine, acquired by eating raw fish infected with Anisakidae parasites.

aniseikonia A defect of vision in which the image of an object seen by one eye is of a different size than the one seen by the other eye.

anisochromasia Condition in which only the periphery of the red blood cells is colored while the central portion is almost colorless, as in certain types of anemias caused by iron deficiency.

anisocoria A condition in which the pupils of the two eyes differ in size.

anisocytosis Abnormal variation in size of the red blood cells.

anisometropia Difference in the refractive power of the two eyes.

ankle The joint between the foot and the leg

trachea
esophagus
hypoglossal n
C1
C2
C3
antagonist
agonist

Anopheles
(head structures)

anoscope

**ansa
cervicalis**

phrenic n.

anteflexion

uterus

formed by the articulation of the tibia and fibula above with the talus below; the area of this joint.

ankyloblepharon Adhesion of the upper and lower eyelids.

ankyloglossia Tongue-tie.

ankylosed Denoting an abnormally immobilized joint.

ankylosis Abnormal immobility and fixation of a joint.

artificial a. See arthrodesis.

bony a. Abnormal fusion of the bones forming a joint. Also called true ankylosis.

dental a. Fixation of a tooth to its socket as a result of ossification of the surrounding membranes.

fibrous a. Ankylosis caused by the presence of fibrous bands between the bones forming the joint.

true a. See bony ankylosis.

ankylotic Marked by or relating to ankylosis.

anlage Primordium (2); the embryonic structure from which the adult organ is developed.

anneal To soften a metal by controlled heating and cooling; the process makes a metal more easily adapted and bent.

annealing In dentistry, the heating of gold leaf for the purpose of removing contaminants prior to its insertion into a cavity.

annular Circular or ring-shaped.

annulus See anulus.

anode The positive pole of a galvanic battery. Also called positive electrode.

anodontia Congenital absence of one or more teeth.

anodyne An agent that has pain-relieving qualities.

anogenital Relating to the anus and genitalia.

anomaly Anything marked by considerable deviation from the normal.

Ebstein's a. Distortion and downward displacement of the tricuspid valve, resulting in impaired function of the right ventricle.

Pelger-Huët nuclear a. Inherited anomaly of neutrophilic leukocytes characterized by nonlobulation of their nuclei.

anomia Inability to name, or to recall the names of objects. Also called optic aphasia.

Anopheles A genus of mosquitoes of the family Culicidae, some members of which transmit the malaria parasite to man.

anophthalmos Congenital absence of a true eyeball.

anopsia 1. Failure to use one eye, as in strabismus. 2. Hypertropia.

anorchidism, anorchism Congenital absence of the testis, unilaterally or bilaterally.

anoretic 1. Having no appetite. 2. An agent that

tends to depress appetite.

anorexia Loss of appetite.

a. nervosa Condition marked by great loss of appetite leading to emaciation and metabolic derangement, attended by serious neurotic symptoms centered around an inordinate fear of becoming fat; occurs predominantly in white, adolescent females.

anorexiant Anything that results in appetite loss (anorexia).

anoscope An instrument for inspecting the anus and lower rectum.

anosigmoidoscopy Visual examination of the anus, rectum, and sigmoid colon with the aid of an instrument.

anosmia Absence of the sense of smell.

anosognosia Unawareness, real or assumed, of a physical illness or defect.

anovular, anovulatory Denoting a menstrual period not accompanied by ovulation.

anoxemia Deficiency of oxygen in the arterial blood. Also called hypoxemia.

anoxia Hypoxia.

ansa, *pl.* **ansae** Any looplike structure.

a. cervicalis A nerve loop in the cervical plexus consisting of fibers from the first three cervical nerves, some of which accompany the hypoglossal nerve for a short distance.

a. hypoglossi Ansa cervicalis.

Henle's a. Nephronic loop; see under loop.

ant An insect of the family Formicidae.

fire a. An aggressive South American ant (genus *Solenopsis*), now commonly seen in the southern United States, whose sting can cause severe allergic reactions, including difficulty in breathing, sweating, nausea, itching, and periods of unconsciousness; it is the only insect in the United States whose sting produces a pustule (a pus-containing eruption).

antacid An agent that reduces the acidity of the gastric juice or other secretions; the most commonly used agents include aluminum hydroxide, magnesium hydroxide, and calcium carbonate.

antagonism Mutual resistance or opposition as between muscles, drugs, bacteria, etc.

antagonist 1. A muscle that opposes the action of another, its agonist. 2. A drug that, by producing no biological effects, inhibits the action of another drug when both interact with the same cell receptors (special sites of the cell membrane).

competitive a. See antimetabolite.

antebrachial Of or relating to the forearm.

antecardium See precordium.

antecibum (a.c.) Latin for before meals.

antecubital Located in front of the elbow.

anteflexion A type of displacement characterized by an abnormal bending forward of the upper part

of an organ.

antelocation Denoting the forward displacement of an organ, e.g., the uterus, as a whole.

antemortem Before death.

antenatal Occurring before birth. Also called prenatal.

antepartum Before childbirth.

anterior 1. In front. 2. Toward the belly. 3. In lower animals, the caudal end.

anterior tibial compartment syndrome Ischemic myositis and necrosis of the muscles of the anterior compartment of the leg resulting from vascular insufficiency secondary to specific vessel disease or injury, or to segmental spasm of the anterior tibial artery; seen in some young people following unaccustomed strenous activity.

anteroinferior Located in front and below.

anterolateral In front and to one side.

anteromedial In front and toward the middle.

anteroposterior 1. Relating to both front and back. 2. Directed from the front to the back.

anterosuperior In front and above.

anteversion The leaning forward of an organ, such as the uterus, as a whole, without bending.

anteverted Tilted forward.

anthelix See antihelix.

anthelminthic, anthelmintic, antihelminthic Able to destroy or expel intestinal worms.

anthracemia The presence of *Bacillus anthracis* in the blood.

anthraconecrosis Degeneration and transformation of tissue into a dry black mass. Also called black gangrene.

anthracosilicosis Fibrous hardening of the lungs due to continuous inhalation of coal and stove dust.

anthracosis Disease caused by accumulation of carbon in the lungs.

anthracotic Marked by anthracosis.

anthrax An acute infectious disease of wild and domesticated animals which may be transmitted to man either directly or by contact with hides or hair infected with the anthrax bacillus; the characteristic lesion in man resembles a carbuncle.

cutaneous a. 1. A skin disease appearing on the exposed areas of the face, neck, hands, or arms; it begins as a papule that becomes vesicular, then necrotic with a purple to black crust surrounded by extensive edema. Also called malignant pustule; anthrax boil. 2. A localized disease of cattle and horses marked by swellings due to infection of skin abrasions and wounds with the anthrax bacillus. Also called carbuncular fever.

gastroenteric a. See intestinal anthrax.

intestinal a. A form of internal anthrax marked by headache, fever, vomiting, bloody diarrhea, pros-areas where antigens are trapped

variable region

fragment antigen binding (Fab)

S-S

hinge

interchain disulfide (S-S) bridge

fragment crystalline (Fc)

H   H

constant region

structure of an**antibody**

Y-shaped
antibody

T-shaped
antibody

tration, and frequently hemorrhage from mucous membranes; death usually occurs. Also called gastroenteric anthrax.

pulmonary a. pneumonia caused by inhalation of dust containing the anthrax bacillus; marked by chills, fever, rapid respiration, cough, pain in the back and legs, and extreme prostration. Also called wool-sorter's pneumonia.

anthrone A substance used as a reagent to detect the presence of carbohydrates.

anthropogeny, anthropogenesis The scientific study of man's origin and development, both individual and racial.

anthropology The branch of science concerned with the origin, development, and behavior of man.

anthropometry The study of comparative measurements of the human body for use in anthropologic classification.

anthropozoonosis Disease of man acquired from lower vertebrates that harbor the pathogenic organisms, e.g., trichinosis, rabies, etc. Cf. zooanthroponosis; amphixenosis.

antiallergic Denoting anything that prevents, or alleviates, an allergic reaction.

antiandrogen A substance that can diminish the effects of masculinizing (androgenic) hormones.

antiangiogenesis The prevention of new vessel sprouts from penetrating into an early tumor implant; a technique, currently experimental, for prevention of cancer growth.

antiarrhythmic Countering an irregular heartbeat.

antibacterial Destructive to or preventing the growth of bacteria, e.g., spermine, the principle self-sterilizing factor in semen.

antibiosis The association of two organisms whereby one is affected detrimentally.

antibiotic Any substance, as penicillin or streptomycin, derived from fungi or bacteria, that destroys or inhibits the growth of microorganisms.

broad-spectrum a. An antibiotic which is effective against a variety of microorganisms, particularly against both gram-negative and gram-positive bacteria.

antibody (Ab) A three-lobed globulin containing two short and two long chains of protein, found in the blood and other body fluids, that can be incited by the presence of antigen (microorganisms, foreign proteins, etc.); it has a destructive influence on the antigen that stimulated its formation, thus producing immunity; the structure has considerable flexibility and is "hinged," so that it can pivot from a taut T-shape to a forked Y-shape.

antinuclear a. An antibody that acts against components of cell nuclei; found in systemic lupus erythematosus and certain collagen diseases.

blocking a. Antibody that, by combining with antigen, stops further activity of that antigen.

complement-fixing a. Antibody that, when combined with antigen, activates complement.

humoral a. See immunoglobulin.

natural a.'s Antibodies which occur naturally in the body without known antigen stimulation.

neutralizing a. Antibody that, by binding to an infective agent, limits its infectivity.

anticholinergic Inhibiting the action of a parasympathetic nerve.

anticholinesterase An agent that inhibits the action of cholinesterase.

anticoagulant Any substance that prevents coagulation of blood.

anticodon The three-base sequence of transfer RNA which pairs with a codon in messenger RNA.

anticomplement A substance that neutralizes the action of complement (material in normal serum that helps to destroy pathogens).

anticonvulsant Any substance that serves to prevent or arrest convulsion.

antidepressant 1. Counteracting depression. 2. Any agent used in treating pathologic depressive states. Also called psychic energizer; thymoleptic.

antidiuretic An agent that causes reduction of urine formation.

antidotal Relating to an antidote.

antidote An agent that counteracts the effects of an ingested poison, either by inactivating it or by opposing its action following absorption.

antidromic Conducting an impulse in a reverse direction of the normal.

antiemetic 1. Preventing or arresting nausea. 2. A drug that prevents or relieves nausea and vomiting by exerting its effects on the vestibular apparatus of the ear, the chemoreceptor trigger zone, the cerebral cortex, or the vomiting center of the brain.

antienzyme A substance that neutralizes the action of an enzyme.

antifibrinolysin A substance that retards the disintegration of fibrin in blood clots.

antigen (Ag) A foreign substance which stimulates an immune response; the immune response may be in the form of antibody formation and/or cell-mediated immunity.

carcinoembryonic a. (CEA) A glycoprotein component of normal embryonic gastrointestinal tissues; usually found in the adult only in certain carcinomas, especially colonic carcinoma. Also called oncofetal antigen.

endogenous a. Any antigen found within an individual.

exogenous a. Any antigen originating from the individual's environment, e.g., pollen.

hepatitis-associated a. (HAA) Hepatitis B surface antigen.

hepatitis B core a. (HBc Ag) Antigen of the DNA core of the hepatitis B virus (Dane particle), present in hepatocyte nuclei of patients with viral hepatitis, type B.

hepatitis B surface a. (HBs Ag) Antigen of the outer lipoprotein coat of the hepatitis B virus (Dane particle), found in the serum and the hepatocyte protoplasm of patients with viral hepatitis, type B; its presence in the blood indicates an infectious state. Also called hepatitis-associated antigen.

heterologous a. An antigen common to more than one species. Also called heterogenetic antigen.

HL-A a.'s Original name for human lymphocyte histocompatibility antigens; "A" stands for locus A (a specific area on a chromosome); now, HLA is the system designation and locus A is HLA-A. See human lymphocyte antigens.

homologous a. An antigen produced by one individual which incites the formation of antibodies in another individual of the same species; specifically, a genetically controlled antigenic determinant that distinguishes one individual of a given species from another. Also called isoantigen; alloantigen.

human lymphocyte a.'s (HLA) System designation for the gene products of four linked loci (sites) on the sixth chromosome. These loci are known as A, B, C and D; more than 50 alleles (variations of the gene) are located at loci HLA-A and HLA-B. Human lymphocyte antigens are responsible for rejection of tissue transplants and for certain diseases.

oncofetal a. Carcinoembryonic antigen.

T a. Antigen present in nuclei of cells infected by certain tumor viruses; thought to be an early virus-specific protein.

antigenic Pertaining to or having the properties of an antigen, especially that of inciting the formation of antibody.

antigenicity The property of being antigenic.

antihelix The curved prominence on the external ear parallel to and in front of the helix. Also called anthelix.

antihemagglutinin A substance that checks the action of hemagglutinin.

antihemolysin An agent that inhibits the action of a hemolysin.

antihidrotic Antisudorific.

antihistamine Any of several drugs used to counteract the action of histamine in the treatment of allergic symptoms.

antihistaminic Tending to neutralize the action of histamine; said of an agent having such an effect and used to relieve the symptoms of allergy.

antihypertensive Anything that reduces the

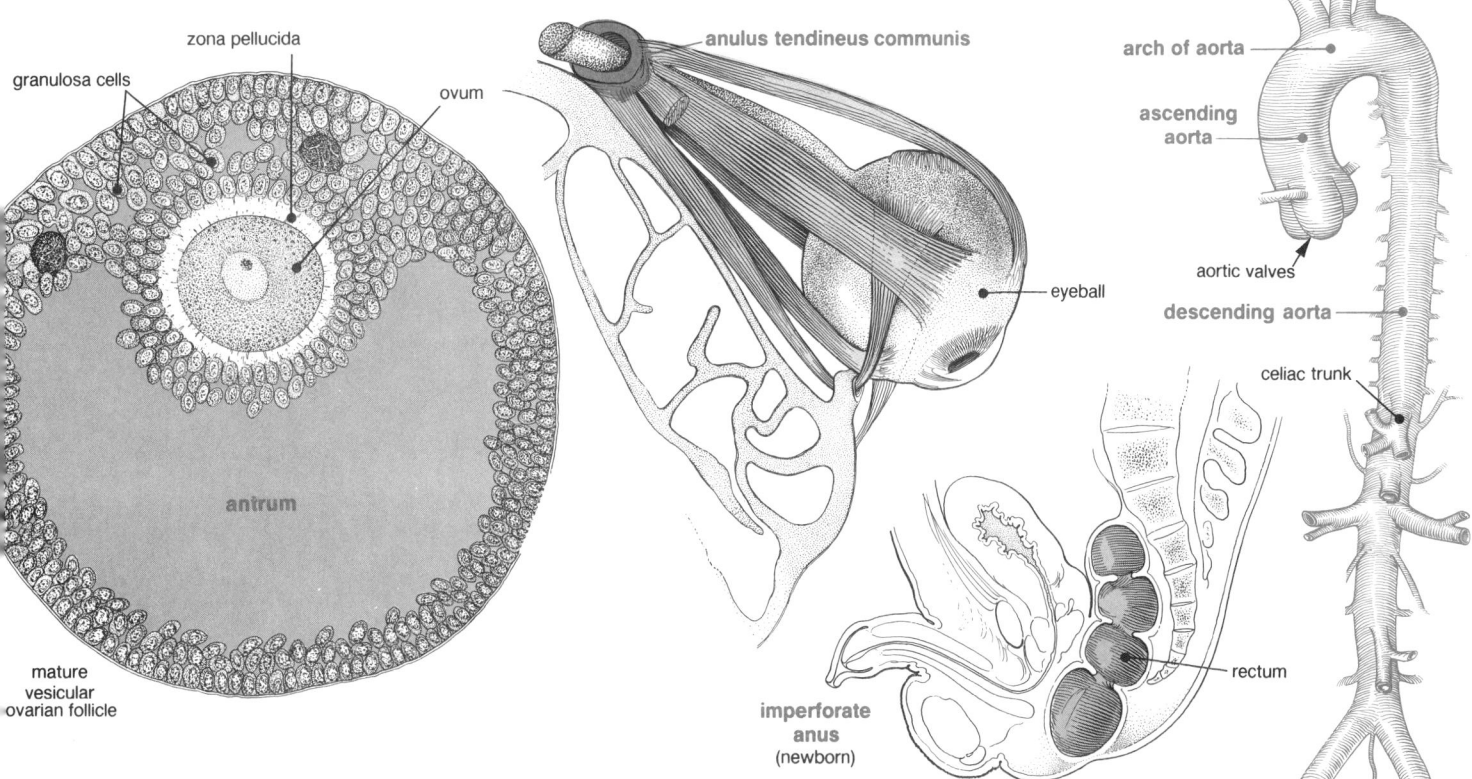

granulosa cells
zona pellucida
ovum
antrum
mature vesicular ovarian follicle

anulus tendineus communis
eyeball
imperforate anus (newborn)

arch of aorta
ascending aorta
aortic valves
descending aorta
celiac trunk
rectum

blood pressure.

anti-inflammatory Relieving inflammation.

antimalarial Denoting an agent that prevents or cures malaria.

antimetabolite In general, a substance that is chemically similar to an essential metabolite but interferes with, or prevents, its effective utilization. Also called competitive antagonist.

antimitotic Anything that arrests mitosis.

antimonic Relating to or containing antimony.

antimony A toxic, irritating, grayish, metallic element; symbol Sb, atomic number 51, atomic weight 121.77.

antimuscarinic Blocking muscarinic or post-ganglionic activity of parasympathetic nerves.

antimycotic Fungicide.

antinauseant 1. Preventing nausea. 2. An agent having such properties.

antinuclear Destructive to a cell nucleus.

antioxidant A substance that prevents oxidation.

antiperistalsis Reverse peristaltic action of the intestines by which their contents are forced upwards.

antiphagocytic Inhibiting ingestion and digestion by cells (phagocytosis).

antiprothrombin A substance that inhibits the conversion of prothrombin into thrombin, thus preventing coagulation of blood.

antipruritic Relieving itching.

antipyretic 1. Reducing or tending to relieve fever. 2. A medicine that reduces or relieves fever.

antirachitic Tending to cure rickets.

antirheumatic Tending to prevent or cure rheumatism.

antiscorbutic Curing or preventing scurvy.

antisecretory Inhibiting secretions.

antiseptic A germicide or, under special conditions, a bacteriostat; generally used on living tissue.

antiserum A human or animal serum containing specific antibodies.

antispasmodic An agent that prevents or relieves involuntary muscular contractions.

anti-streptolysin O (ASO) An antibody against a hemolysin produced by beta-hemolytic streptococci; a high or rising titer indicates recent beta hemolytic streptococcus infection.

antisudorific Arresting the secretion of sweat. Also called antihidrotic.

antithrombin A substance that counteracts the action of thrombin, thus preventing coagulation of blood.

antitoxin Antibody produced in the blood and other body fluids in response to the poison of a microorganism, usually bacterial exotoxins.

antitragus A projection on the external ear opposite the tragus and behind the opening of the external auditory canal.

antitreponemal Destructive to treponemes (bacteria of the genus *Treponema*).

antitrypsin A substance that inhibits the action of the proteolytic enzyme trypsin.

antitussive 1. Tending to relieve cough. 2. A cough remedy.

antivitamin Any substance that prevents the biologic functioning of a vitamin.

antivivisection Opposition to experimentation on living animals.

antivivisectionist One who is opposed to experimentation on living animals.

antral Relating to an antrum (body cavity).

antrectomy Surgical removal of the walls of an antrum, especially the mastoid antrum.

antroscope An instrument for examining an antrum or hollow space, especially the maxillary antrum.

antrostomy The formation of an opening or stoma, sometimes permanent, into any antrum for draining purposes.

antrotomy Incision into an antrum.

antrum A bodily chamber or cavity.

follicular a. The fluid-filled cavity within the developing ovarian follicle.

pyloric a. The dilated pyloric end of the stomach; it marks the beginning of the pyloric canal.

tympanic a. A cavity in the mastoid part of the temporal bone extending from the middle ear chamber and communicating with the mastoid air cells.

anulus A ring-shaped structure.

a. inguinalis profundus The orifice in the transversalis fascia forming the internal opening of the inguinal canal. Also called deep or abdominal inguinal ring.

a. inguinalis superficialis The orifice in the aponeurosis of the external oblique muscle forming the external opening of the inguinal canal. Also called superficial, subcutaneous, or external inguinal ring.

a. tendineus communis A fibrous ring in the ocular orbit that surrounds the optic foramen and part of the superior orbital fissure; it serves as the origin of four eye muscles. Also called ligament of Zinn.

anuresis Total retention of urine in the bladder; failure to urinate.

anuretic Relating to anuresis.

anuria Complete suppression of urine; in clinical use, denoting less than 100 ml urine daily for an adult of average size.

anuric Relating to anuria.

anus The lower opening of the digestive tract.

imperforate a. Congenital absence of anal orifice.

anvil See incus.

anxiety A state of apprehension, uneasiness, and fear out of proportion to the real threat; the chief characteristic of the neuroses, commonly accompanied by somatic symptoms.

a. syndrome Rapid heart beat, difficulty in breathing, and profuse sweating accompanied by panic.

castration a. Fear of loss of genital organs or genital function, as punishment for forbidden sexual or aggressive feelings. Also called castration complex.

separation a. A feeling of danger, apprehension, and distress upon separation from a needed person.

aorta The largest blood vessel in the body; the main trunk of the systemic arterial circulation, arising from the upper part of the left ventricle from which it receives blood for delivery to all tissues except the lungs.

abdominal a. The terminal part of the aorta, extending from the diaphragm to the pelvis where it divides into the common iliac arteries.

arch of the a. The curvature by which the aorta changes its course from cephalad to caudad and from which arise the brachiocephalic trunk, left common carotid, and left subclavian arteries.

ascending a. The first part of the aorta between its origin from the heart and the arch; it is about 3 cm in diameter.

descending a. The part of the aorta between the arch and the bifurcation.

aortic Relating to the aorta.

aortic arch syndrome Condition seen in any of a group of disorders marked by narrowing and occlusion of one or more of the large arterial vessels originating from the aortic arch (brachiocephalic trunk, left subclavian, and left common carotid arteries); such narrowing and occlusion lead to diminished or absent pulse in the neck and arms; caused by inflammatory and/or atheromatous changes with secondary thrombosis. See also pulseless disease.

aortitis Inflammation of one or more of the layers of the wall of the aorta.

rheumatoid a. Aortitis associated with rheumatoid arthritis.

aortogram X-ray image of the aorta, utilizing contrast material.

aortography Roentgenography of the aorta after the injection of a radiopaque medium.

retrograde a. Aortography after forcing the radiopaque material through one of the aortic branches, in a direction opposite the bloodstream.

translumbar a. Roentgenography after injection of the radiopaque material into the abdominal aorta.

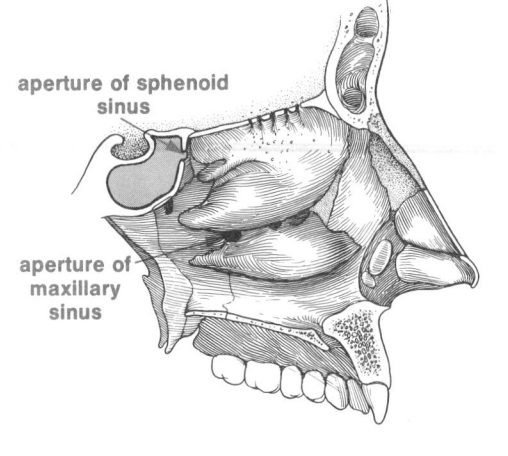

aperture of sphenoid sinus

aperture of maxillary sinus

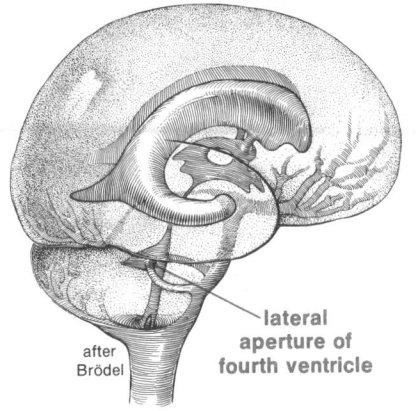

after Brödel

lateral aperture of fourth ventricle

apex (cochlea)

aponeurosis (plantar)

aponeurosis (pharyngeal)

aortoiliac occlusive disease Gradual obstruction of the terminal portion of the aorta by atherosclerosis; associated clinical features include intermittent claudication of the lower back, buttocks, thighs, or calves, and atrophy of the limbs; there may also be trophic changes and impotence. Also called Leriche's syndrome.

aortopathy Disease of the aorta.

aortotomy Incision into the aorta.

apathy Indifference; lack of emotion.

apatite A calcium phosphate present in bone and teeth.

aperiodic Occurring irregularly.

aperistalsis Absence of the normal contractions of the intestines.

apertognathia Open bite; see under bite.

aperture 1. An opening, hole, or gap. 2. An opening, usually adjustable, in an optical instrument which limits the amount of light passing through the lens.

  a. of maxillary sinus A large, irregular aperture through which the maxillary sinus communicates with the nasal cavity.

  a. of sphenoid sinus An orifice in the anterior wall of the sphenoid sinus through which the sinus opens into the nasal cavity.

  lateral a. of fourth ventricle One of two lateral openings on the roof of the fourth ventricle of the brain, communicating with the subarachnoid cavity. Also called foramen of Luschka.

  median a. of fourth ventricle An opening in the midline of the roof of the fourth ventricle of the brain, communicating with the subarachnoid cavity. Also called foramen of Magendi.

apex *pl.* **apices** The tip or pointed end of a conical structure, as the heart or lung.

  orbital a. The posterior part of the orbit.

  root a. The tip of the root of a tooth.

apexcardiogram A graphic record of the chest wall movements produced by the apex beat of the heart.

Apgar score See under score.

aphagia See dysphagia.

aphakia Absence of the lens of the eye.

aphalangia Absence of toes and fingers.

aphasia A general term for language disorders (reading, writing, speaking, or comprehension of written or spoken words) due to brain dysfunction, not a result of disease of the vocal organs or of intellectual deficiency.

  amnesic a. Inability to remember words.

  ataxic a. Motor aphasia.

  auditory a. A form of aphasia in which the individual distinguishes words from other sounds but does not understand them. Also called word deafness.

  expression a. Motor aphasia

  fluent a. Aphasia marked by effortless speech, with correct grammar but lacking in meaning.

  global a. Complete loss of the power to communicate verbally.

  mixed a. A mixture of sensory and motor aphasia.

  motor a. Loss of the ability to communicate by writing, speaking, or signs.

  nonfluent a. Aphasia marked by poorly articulated speech produced with great difficulty.

  optic a. Inability to name an object recognized by sight. Also called anomia.

  receptive a. Sensory aphasia.

  sensory a. Inability to understand spoken or written words, gestures, or signs.

  syntactical a. Inability to arrange words into coordinated sentences, so that what is spoken becomes nonsense.

  visual a. Alexia.

aphasic, aphasiac Relating to or afflicted with aphasia.

apheresis Removal of blood from a donor and reinfusion after selected blood components are removed and retained. Also called pheresis.

aphonia Loss of the voice.

  hysteric a. Inability to speak due to hysteria.

aphonic Relating to aphonia.

aphrodisiac Any agent that intensifies sexual desire.

aphtha *pl.* **aphthae** A small white patch on a mucous membrane, commonly seen in the mouth.

aphthous Relating to or having aphthae.

apical Relating to the apex of a structure, as the tip of the root of a tooth, the top of a lung, or the cardiac apex.

apicoectomy Surgical removal of the apical portion of a tooth root. Also called apicectomy.

apicostomy The surgical formation of an opening through the alveolar bone to the tip of a tooth root.

apituitarism State in which the pituitary body has ceased to function.

aplanasia Absence of spherical or monochromatic aberration. Also called aplanatism.

aplanatic Denoting an optical system or lens free from spherical or monochromatic aberration.

aplasia 1. Complete or partial failure of a tissue or an organ to develop. 2. In hematology, defective development, or failure to regenerate.

  congenital thymic a. A syndrome characterized by numerous clinical features, all related to some failure in development of the third and fourth pharyngeal pouches; the parathyroid glands are either underdeveloped or absent, often leading to tetany due to parathyroid insufficiency; the thymus is similarly underdeveloped or absent, leading to an increased vulnerability to those infections usually resisted by the cell-mediated portion of the immune response. Also called DiGeorge's syndrome; thymic alymphoplasia.

aplastic 1. Pertaining to defective development. 2. Relating to defective regenerative processes.

apnea Cessation of respiration.

  sleep a. Episodes of apnea during sleep and lasting more than 15 seconds; may be central, associated with cessation of respiratory drive, or obstructive, caused by obstruction of airflow at the nose or mouth.

apneumatic Denoting a collapsed lung.

apneumatosis Congenital airless state of the lungs (atelectasis).

apocrine Relating to a gland in which some of the apical portion of the gland is discharged along with the secretory product; seen in axillary sweat glands.

apodia Congenital absence of feet.

apoenzyme A protein that requires a coenzyme to function as an enzyme; the protein portion of an enzyme.

apoferritin A protein of the small intestine; it combines with iron to form ferritin, which is thought to regulate the absorption of iron in the intestinal tract.

apolar Without poles or processes, as certain nerve cells.

apomorphine hydrochloride A white crystalline derivative of morphine; used as an emetic, expectorant, and hypnotic.

aponeurorrhaphy See fasciorrhaphy.

aponeurosis A pearly white, iridescent, fibrous sheet, composed of closely packed, mostly parallel collagenous bundles; serves as a connection between a muscle and its attachment.

  epicranial a. Aponeurosis of the scalp, covering the upper part of the skull. Also called galea aponeurotica.

apoplexy Rupture of a vessel into an organ.

apoptosis Cell death occurring naturally (unlike necrosis) from internal perturbations.

apparatus 1. A group of instruments or devices used together or in succession to perform a specific task. 2. A group of organs or structures that collectively perform a common function.

  central a. The centrosome and centrosphere.

  Golgi a. A ubiquitous heterogeneous organelle in a cell consisting of a bowl-shaped, reticular network of saccules, vesicles, and vacuoles; in most cells it is located near the nucleus; it temporarily stores and packages secretory products. Also called Golgi body; Golgi complex.

  juxtaglomerular a. (JGA) The juxtaglomerular

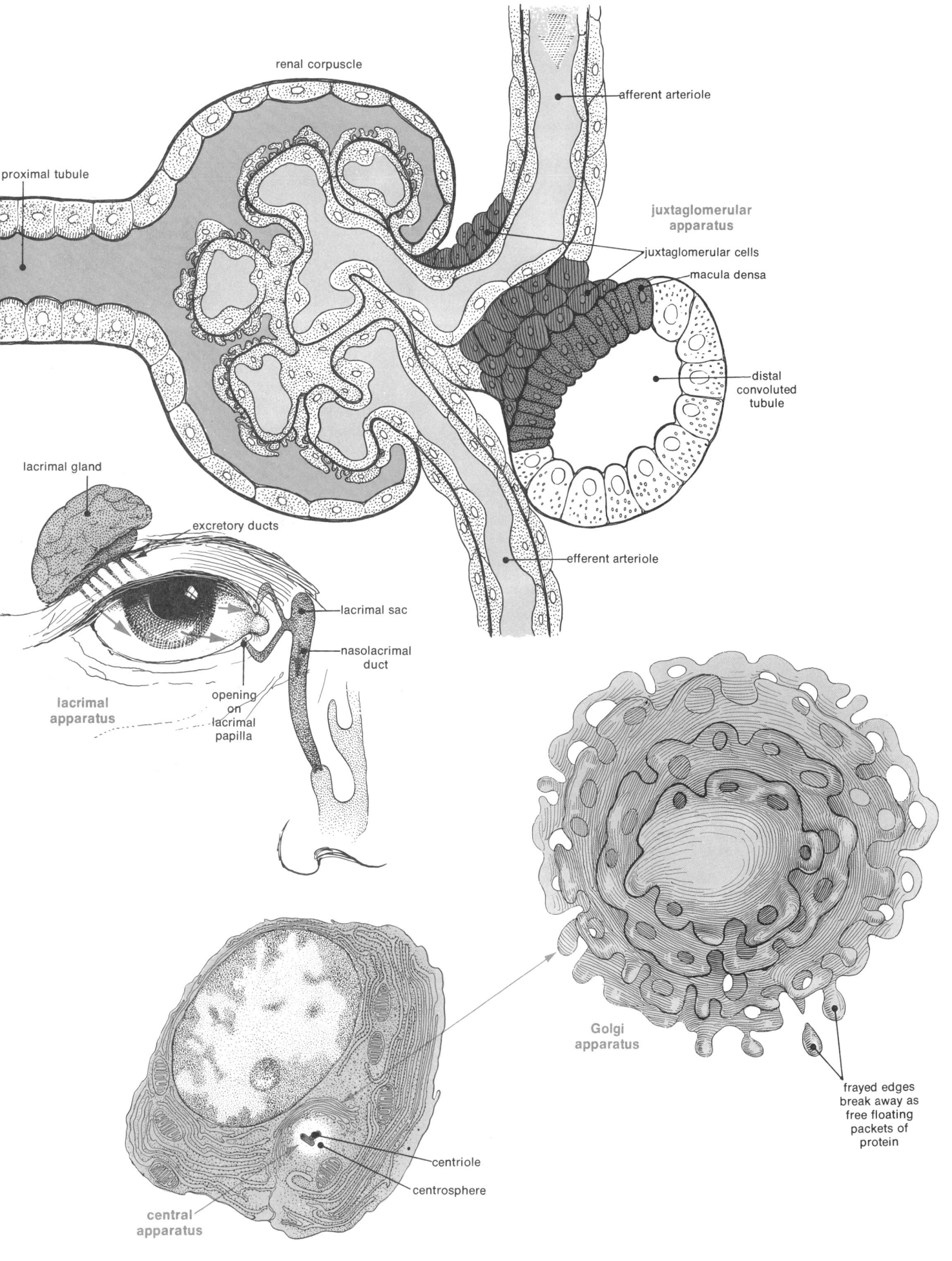

renal corpuscle

afferent arteriole

proximal tubule

juxtaglomerular apparatus

juxtaglomerular cells

macula densa

distal convoluted tubule

lacrimal gland

excretory ducts

lacrimal sac

nasolacrimal duct

efferent arteriole

lacrimal apparatus

opening on lacrimal papilla

Golgi apparatus

centriole

centrosphere

central apparatus

frayed edges break away as free floating packets of protein

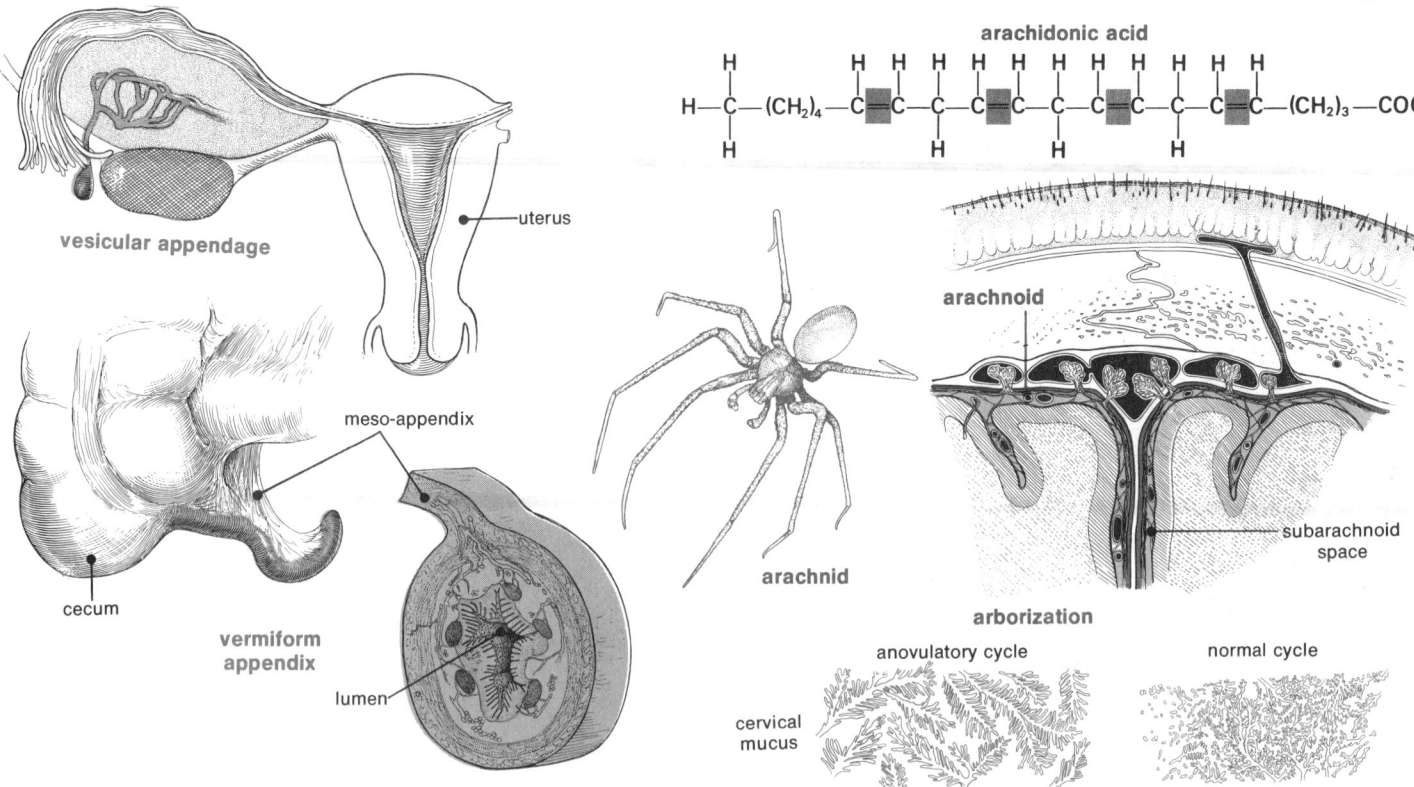

vesicular appendage

uterus

meso-appendix

cecum

vermiform appendix

lumen

arachidonic acid

$$H-C-(CH_2)_4-C=C-C-C=C-C-C=C-C-C=C-C-(CH_2)_3-COOH$$

arachnid

arachnoid

subarachnoid space

arborization

anovulatory cycle

normal cycle

cervical mucus

---

body (granular epithelioid cells in the terminal part of the afferent arteriole of the kidney) together with the macula densa (the thickened epithelial cells in the wall of the distal convoluted tubule where it contacts the afferent arteriole).

lacrimal a. The tear-forming and tear-conducting system, consisting of the lacrimal gland and ducts and associated structures.

Tiselius a. A device used to separate proteins from solution and to determine the molecular weight and the isoelectric point.

Van Slyke a. Apparatus used to measure the amount of respiratory gases in blood.

Warburg's a. Apparatus used to measure the oxygen consumption of incubated tissue slices.

appendage Any part in close but subordinate relation to a main structure. Also called appendix.

testicular a. A minute, oval, cystlike body on the upper end of the testis, a remnant of the embryonic mullerian duct. Also called hydatid of Morgagni; Morgagni's appendix.

vesicular a. A fluid-filled cystlike structure attached to the fimbriated end of the uterine tube, a remnant of the embryonic mullerian duct. Also called hydatid of Morgagni; Morgagni's appendix.

appendectomy Surgical removal of an appendix, especially the vermiform appendix.

appendiceal Of or relating to an appendix.

appendicitis Inflammation of the vermiform appendix.

appendicolithiasis The presence of stones in the vermiform appendix.

appendicular Relating to the appendix.

appendix *pl.* **appendices** An appendage, especially the vermiform appendix.

a. ceci Vermiform appendix.

epiploic a. One of several small peritoneal sacs extending from the serous coat of the large intestine, except the rectum. Also called appendix epiploica; epiploic appendage.

Morgagni's a. 1. Testicular appendage. 2. Vesicular appendage see under appendage.

vermiform a. The slender, worm-shaped tubular structure extending from the blind end of the cecum. Also called appendix vermiformis.

apperception Comprehension based on previous knowledge or memories of past experiences.

appersonation, appersonification A delusion of assuming the character of another individual.

appetite The natural desire for food.

applanation Flattening of a small area of the cornea with a special tonometer to measure the force applied and, thereby, the pressure within the eyeball.

appliance 1. A device designed for a particular

function, e.g., to stabilize a fractured bone. 2. A device for moving or for splinting teeth.

applicator A slender rod of wood or other material with a small piece of cotton attached to one end; used for making local applications of medicine.

appliqué form See under form.

apposition The placing in contact of two adjacent and opposing surfaces.

apraxia Inability to execute purposeful movements in absence of paralysis, due to a defect in cortical integration.

apraxic, apractic Relating to apraxia.

aptyalism, aptyalia Absence or deficiency of saliva. Also called asialism.

APUD Acronym for amine precursor uptake and decarboxylation; refers to epithelial cells of the gastrointestinal tract, pancreas, bile ducts, and bronchi which synthesize such polypeptide hormones as gastrin, secretin, and glucagon.

apyretic Without fever.

apyrexia Absence of fever.

apyrexial Of or relating to apyrexia.

aqua *pl.* **aquae** Latin for water.

aquatic Relating to or living in water.

aqueduct A canal.

a. of Sylvius See cerebral aqueduct.

cerebral a. A small canal connecting the third and fourth ventricles of the brain. Also called aqueduct of Sylvius.

vestibular a. A thin bony canal leading from the medial wall of the vestibule of the internal ear to the posterior surface of the petrous portion of the temporal bone, where it communicates with the cerebrospinal space; it houses the endolymphatic duct.

aqueous Watery.

aqueous humor See under humor.

arabinose A sugar, $C_5H_{10}O_5$, used in culture media.

arachidonic acid A polyunsaturated fatty acid, $C_{20}H_{32}O_2$; a precursor of prostaglandins essential in nutrition.

arachnid Any member of the class of arthropods, Arachnida.

Arachnida A class of arthropods (subphylum Chelicerata) that includes such forms as spiders, scorpions, mites, and ticks, characteristically having four pairs of legs.

arachnidism Systemic poisoning following the bite of a spider, especially of the black widow and brown recluse spiders.

arachnodactyly A hereditary condition marked by excessive length and slenderness of the bones of the fingers and toes; may be accompanied by relaxed joint ligaments and is usually associated with a connective tissue disorder.

arachnoid 1. Having the appearance of a cobweb. 2. The middle of the three membranes covering the brain and spinal cord, between the dura mater and the pia mater; attached to the dura mater but separated from the pia mater by the subarachnoid space.

arachnoidal Relating to the middle of the three membranes covering the brain and spinal cord (arachnoid).

arachnoiditis Inflammation of the arachnoid.

adhesive a. Inflammation of the arachnoid and adjacent pia mater, sometimes causing obliteration of the subarachnoid space.

arachnophobia An inordinate fear of spiders.

arborescent Treelike; branching.

arborization Denoting: 1. The branching of nerve fibers and capillaries. 2. The tree-shaped pattern sometimes formed by the dried smear of cervical mucus.

arborize To ramify or branch.

arbovirus Any arthropod-borne virus of the genera *Alphavirus* and *Flavivirus* (family Togaviridae).

arc 1. Anything shaped like an arch or a bow. 2. The luminous line formed by the electric current crossing a gap between two electrodes.

mercury a. An electric discharge through mercury vapor in a vacuum tube, producing ultraviolet rays.

reflex a. The path followed by a nerve impulse in the production of a reflex act.

arch Any of several curved structures of the body.

aortic a.'s of the embryo A series of six arterial channels encircling the embryonic pharynx (gut) in the mesenchyme of the pharyngeal arches; they never exist all at the same time.

a. of the aorta The curved portion of the aorta between the ascending and descending parts of the thoracic aorta. Also called aortic arch.

a.'s of the foot The two sets of arches (longitudinal and transverse) formed by the bones of the foot.

branchial a. Pharyngeal arch.

cortical a.'s of kidney The portion of kidney substance (cortex) located between the bases of the pyramids and the renal capsule.

costal a. An arch formed by the borders of the inferior aperture of the thorax, comprised of the costal cartilages of ribs seven to ten.

dental a. 1. The composite structure of the natural teeth and the alveolar bone. 2. The curved contour of the remains of the alveolar ridge after the loss of some or all of the natural teeth.

glossopalatine a. Anterior pillars of the fauces; see under pillar.

longitudinal a. The anteroposterior arch of the foot, formed by the seven tarsal and five metatarsal

aortic arches

4 week old embryo

aortic arch

heart

metatarsal bone

longitudinal arch

calcaneus

1 2 3 4

pharyngeal arches

vertebral arch

costal arch

cervical vertebra

pubic arch

zygomatic arch

bones and the ligaments binding them together.

neural a. See vertebral arch.

palatoglossal a. One of two folds of mucous membrane extending from the posterior edge of the soft palate to the lateral wall of the pharynx, behind the palatine tonsil.

pharyngeal a. One of a series of five mesodermal arches (bars) in the neck region of the embryo from which several structures of the head and neck develop. Formerly called branchial arch.

pharyngopalatine a. Posterior pillars of the fauces; see under pillar.

pubic a. Arch on the pelvis formed by the convergence of the inferior rami of the ischium and pubic bones on either side.

supercilliary a. An arched prominence above the upper margin of the orbit.

tendinous a. of pelvis A condensation of parietal pelvic fascia which arches from the posterior surface of the pubis to the spine of the ischium.

transverse a. The arch of the foot formed by the proximal parts of the metatarsal bones anteriorly and the distal row of the tarsal bones posteriorly.

vertebral a., neural a. The arch on the dorsal side of a vertebra which, with the vertebral body, forms the foramen in which the spinal cord is lodged.

zygomatic a. The arch formed by the zygomatic process of the temporal bone and the temporal process of the zygomatic bone.

archenteron The primitive digestive cavity of the embryo at the gastrula stage. Also called primary gut.

arctation Stricture; narrowing.

arcuate Arched.

arcus *pl.* **arcus** Any arch-shaped structure; an arch.

a. juvenilis A grayish-white ring around the cornea, occurring in the young.

a. senilis An opaque grayish ring around the cornea, occurring in the aged. Also called gerontoxon.

area A distinct part of a surface or space.

aortic a. Area on the chest over the cartilage of the second right rib.

apical a. Area about: **1.** The tip of the root of a tooth. **2.** The apex of a lung. **3.** The chest wall corresponding to the apex of the heart (normally the apex beat is in approximately the fifth left intercostal space in the midclavicular line).

a. of cardiac dullness Normally a small triangular area on the lower left side of the sternum which, on percussion of the chest, produces a dull sound; it corresponds to the portion of the heart not covered by lung tissue.

a. cribrosa An area of the renal papilla containing

20 or more pores through which the urine oozes into the minor calyces.

auditory a. Region of the cerebral cortex concerned with hearing, occupying the transverse temporal gyri and the superior temporal gyrus.

basal seat a. The portion of oral structures that is available to support a denture.

Broca's speech a. Area comprised of the triangular and opercular portions of the inferior frontal gyrus; it governs the motor aspects of speech and is better developed in the left hemisphere of right-handed persons.

Brodmann's a.'s The 47 areas of the cerebral cortex mapped out according to the arrangement of their cellular components.

controlled a. In radiography, the space in a room containing the radiation source.

frontal a. Portion of the cerebral cortex in front of the central sulcus (fissure of Rolando).

Little's a. A highly vascular area of the anterior portion of the nasal septum; frequent site of nosebleed.

macular a. The part of the retina that contains a yellow pigment, is used for central vision, and appears to be free of vessels when viewed with an ophthalmoscope.

mirror a. The reflecting surface of the lens of the eye and the cornea when illuminated with the slit lamp.

motor a. Portion of the cerebral cortex comprised of the anterior wall of the central sulcus (fissure of Rolando) and adjacent portions of the precentral gyrus; its stimulation with electrodes causes contraction of voluntary muscles. Also called precentral cortex area; primary motor area.

postcentral a. postrolandic a. The sensory area of the cerebral cortex, just posterior to the central sulcus (fissure of Rolando); it receives sensory stimuli from the whole body.

posterior palatal seal a. The soft tissue along the junction of the soft and hard palate on which pressure can be applied by a denture to help its retention.

precentral cortex a. See motor area.

premotor a. Area immediately in front of the motor area, concerned with integrated movements.

pulmonic a. Area of the chest at the second left intercostal space where flow sounds across the pulmonic valves are usually heard best.

subcallosal a. An area of the cortex in the medial aspect of each cerebral hemisphere, located immediately in front of the lamina terminalis and caudoventral to the subcallosal gyrus. Also called parolfactory area of Broca.

tricuspid a. Area of auscultation for murmurs

originating from the right atrioventricular valve (tricuspid); the lower left sternal area.

visual a. Area of the occipital lobe of the cerebral cortex concerned with vision; it consists of: (a) sensory or striate part, occupying the walls of the calcarine sulcus (occasionally extending around the occipital pole onto the lateral surface of the hemisphere); concerned with recognition of size, form, motion, color, illumination, and transparency; (b) psychic or parastriate part, surrounding the sensory portion; associates visual impressions and past experiences for recognition and identification.

areatus, areata Denoting circumscribed areas or patches.

areflexia A condition in which the reflexes are absent.

Arenaviridae Family of viruses (50 to 300 nm in diameter) which contain single-standed RNA, multiply in cytoplasm, and appear sandy on electron-microscopy; includes viruses causing lymphocytic choriomeningitis and Lassa fever. Also called arenavirus group.

Arenavirus Genus of viruses (family Arenaviridae) that includes the Lassa and the lymphocytic choriomeningitis viruses. Also called lymphocytic choriomeningitis group.

areola **1.** One of the minute spaces in a tissue. **2.** A ringlike pigmented area around a central point, as the pigmented area around the nipple on the breast.

areolar Relating to an areola.

argentaffin, argentaffine Denoting cells that have an affinity for silver salts.

argentaffinoma A tumor of the gastrointestinal mucosa, believed to arise from the Kulchitsky glands; found most often in the appendix but also in the small intestine, stomach, and rectum. Also called carcinoid.

argentation Staining with a silver salt such as silver nitrate.

argentous Relating to or containing silver, denoting a compound containing silver in its lower valency.

argentum Latin for silver.

arginase A liver enzyme that promotes the splitting of the amino acid arginine into urea and ornithine.

arginine (Arg) $C_6H_{14}N_4O_2$, an essential amino acid, derived from the digestion or hydrolysis of protein.

argon A colorless, odorless, gaseous element, constituting about 1% of the earth's atmosphere; symbol Ar, atomic number 18, atomic weight 39.6.

Argyll-Robertson pupil, Argyll-Robertson symptom See under pupil.

sinus arrhythmia

EXPIRATION INSPIRATION EXPIRATION

interlobular vein

interlobular artery

glomerulus

arcuate vein

arcuate artery

arteriola recta spuria

arteriola recta vera

collecting duct

interlobar artery

interlobar vein

nephronic loop

general structure of a muscular artery

TUNICA INTIMA:

endothelium

basement membrane

subendothelial connective tissue

TUNICA MEDIA:

internal elastic membrane

smooth muscle

external elastic membrane

ADVENTITIA

argyria Chronic silver poisoning causing a permanent grayish discoloration of the skin, conjunctiva, cornea, and internal organs due to the prolonged use of preparations containing silver compounds.

argyrosis Argyria.

arhythmia See arrhythmia.

ariboflavinosis See hyporiboflavinosis.

arm The upper limb of the human body, especially between the shoulder and the elbow.

armpit See axilla.

arrest To prevent or stop function, progress, growth, or motion.

cardiac a. Acute failure of the heart to provide adequate circulation to the brain and other vital organs.

cardiopulmonary a. Failure of circulation and pulmonary ventilation.

sinus a. Condition in which the sinoatrial (S-A) node of the heart fails to send impulses to the atria, resulting in a temporary cessation of cardiac contraction.

arrhenoblastoma An extremely rare tumor of the ovary that causes masculinization.

arrhythmia Irregularity, especially of the heart beat.

sinus a. A variation in the rhythm of the heart beat usually related to breathing (slower during expiration, more rapid during inspiration). Also called juvenile arrhythmia because it is commonly found in children.

arrhythmic Without rhythm.

arrhythmogenic Causing irregular heartbeats.

arsenic A highly poisonous metallic element; symbol As, atomic number 33, atomic weight 74.9; some of its compounds are used in medicine.

arsenous Relating to or containing arsenic; denoting a compound of arsenic in a low valency.

arsphenamine An organic compound of the arseno-type; its discovery by Ehrlich in 1907 represented a major advance in the treatment of syphilis. Also called Salvarsan ®; diarsenol.

arteria *pl.* **arteriae** Latin for artery.

arterial Relating to the arteries.

arteriectomy Surgical removal of a segment of an artery.

arteriogram X-ray image of an artery into which a radiopaque material has been introduced.

arteriography **1.** X-ray visualization of an artery or arteries after injection of a radiopaque substance. **2.** A treatise on, or description of, the arteries. **3.** Sphygmography.

arteriola *pl.* **arteriolae** Arteriole.

arteriolae rectae spuriae The straight vessels which arise from the juxtaglomerular efferent arterioles of the kidney and parallel the nephronic (Henle's) loop. Also called vasa recta spuria.

arteriolae rectae verae The true vasa recta; the straight vessels which arise directly from the arcuate arteries of the kidney and parallel the nephronic (Henle's) loop.

arteriolar Relating to an arteriole or arterioles.

arteriole The smallest subdivision of the arterial tree preceding the capillary; it possesses muscular walls which, by contracting and relaxing, can alter the flow of blood into the body tissues.

arteriolitis Inflammation of the arterioles.

arteriolonecrosis Degeneration or destruction of arterioles, as in malignant hypertension.

arteriomotor Causing contraction or dilation of arteries.

arterionecrosis Death of arterial tissues.

arterioplasty Replacement of a segment of an artery.

arteriorrhaphy Suture of an artery.

arteriorrhexis Rupture of an artery.

arteriosclerosis Disease of the arteries resulting in the thickening and loss of elasticity of the arterial walls. Also known as arterial sclerosis; hardening of the arteries.

a. obliterans The arteriosclerotic narrowing of the lumen of the arteries supplying the extremities.

Mönckeberg's a. A form of arteriosclerosis marked by the formation of ringlike calcifications in the middle layer of arterial walls, especially of small arteries. Also called medial calcific sclerosis; medial calcinosis.

arteriosclerotic Relating to or marked by arteriosclerosis.

arteriospasm Spasm of an artery.

arteriostenosis Constriction of an artery or arteries.

arteriotomy Incision into the lumen of an artery.

arteriovenous Relating to both arteries and veins.

arteritis Inflammation of an artery.

a. deformans Chronic inflammation of the inner layer of an artery (intima).

a. obliterans Inflammation of the inner layer of an artery causing the closure of the artery's lumen.

temporal a., cranial a. Disease of older persons involving the temporal arteries, and frequently leading to blindness by involvement of the ophthalmic and retinal arteries.

artery A vessel that transports blood away from the heart to different parts of the body; in the normal state after birth, all arteries conduct oxygenated blood except the pulmonary arteries which transport unoxygenated blood from the heart to the lungs.

ARTERY	ORIGIN	BRANCHES	DISTRIBUTION
alveolar a., anterior superior anterior dental a. *a. alveolaris superior anterior*	infraorbital a.	dental	incisor and cuspid teeth of maxilla, mucous membrane of maxillary sinus
alveolar a., inferior inferior dental a. mandibular a. *a. alveolaris inferior*	maxillary a.	mental, incisor, lingual, mylohyoid	mandible and mandibular teeth, gingiva, mucosa of mouth, lower lip, chin, mylohyoid muscle
alveolar a., posterior superior posterior dental a. *a. alveolaris superior posterior*	maxillary a.	dental, antral, alveolar, muscular	molar and bicuspid teeth of upper jaw, mucosa of maxillary sinus, gingiva
angular a. *a. angularis*	facial a.	muscular, lacrimal	muscles and skin of side of nose, lacrimal sac
aorta *aorta*	left ventricle at aortic valves		see specific branches
ascending aorta *aorta ascendens*	left ventricle at aortic valves	right coronary, left coronary	
arch of aorta *arcus aortae*	continuation of ascending aorta at level of the upper border of the right second sternocostal articulation	brachiocephalic, left common carotid, left subclavian; continues as thoracic aorta at fourth thoracic vertebra	
thoracic aorta *aorta thoracica*	continuation of arch of aorta at fourth thoracic vertebra	*visceral portion:* pericardial, bronchial, esophageal, mediastinal; *parietal portion:* posterior intercostal, subcostal, superior phrenic; continues as abdominal aorta at the aortic hiatus of diaphragm	
abdominal aorta *aorta abdominalis*	continuation of thoracic aorta at the aortic hiatus of diaphragm, usually at level of last thoracic vertebra	*visceral portion:* celiac, superior mesenteric, inferior mesenteric, middle suprarenal, renal, testicular, ovarian; *parietal portion:* inferior phrenic, lumbar, middle sacral; continues as common iliac arteries at fourth lumbar vertebra	
appendicular a. *a. appendicularis*	ileocolic a.		vermiform appendix
arch, deep palmar		see palmar arch, deep	
arch, plantar		see plantar arch	

ARTERY	ORIGIN	BRANCHES	DISTRIBUTION
arch, superficial palmar	see palmar arch, superficial		
arcuate a. of foot metatarsal a. *a. arcuata pedis*	dorsal a. of foot	second, third, and fourth metatarsal arteries	instep of foot
arcuate a.'s of kidney *aa. arcuatae renis*	interlobar a.	interlobular, afferent, arteriole	parenchyma of kidney
auditory a., internal	see labyrinthine artery		
auricular a., deep *a. auricularis profunda*	maxillary a.	temporomandibular	cuticular lining of external acoustic meatus, outer surface of tympanic membrane, temporomandibular joint
auricular a., posterior *a. auricularis posterior*	external carotid a.	stylomastoid, auricular, occipital, parotid	middle ear, mastoid cells, auricle, parotid gland, digastric, stapedius, and neck muscles
axillary a. *a. axillaris*	continuation of subclavian a. beginning at outer border of first rib	*first part:* highest thoracic; *second part:* thoracoacromial, lateral thoracic; *third part:* subscapular, posterior humeral circumflex, anterior humeral circumflex	pectoral muscles, muscles of shoulder and upper arm, acromion, shoulder joint, sternoclavicular joint, breast
basilar a. *a. basilaris*	from junction of two vertebral arteries	pontine, labyrinthine, anterior inferior cerebellar, superior cerebellar, posterior cerebral	pons, internal ear, cerebellum, pineal body, ventricles, posterior part of cerebrum
brachial a. *a. brachialis*	continuation of axillary a. at distal margin of tendon of teres major muscle	deep brachial, nutrient of humerus, superior ulnar collateral, inferior ulnar collateral, muscular	muscles of shoulder, arm, forearm, and hand; elbow joint
brachial a. deep superior profunda a. *a. profunda brachii*	brachial a.	nutrient, deltoid, middle collateral, radial collateral, muscular	humerus, elbow joint, muscles of upper arm including triceps and deltoid
brachiocephalic trunk innominate a. *truncus brachiocephalicus*	beginning of arch of aorta	right common carotid, right subclavian, lowest thyroid, thymic	right side of head, neck and upper arm, thyroid and thymus glands
bronchial a.'s *aa. bronchiales*	*right side:* first aortic intercostal; *left side:* thoracic aorta		bronchial tubes, alveolar tissue of lungs, bronchial lymph nodes, esophagus

artery | artery

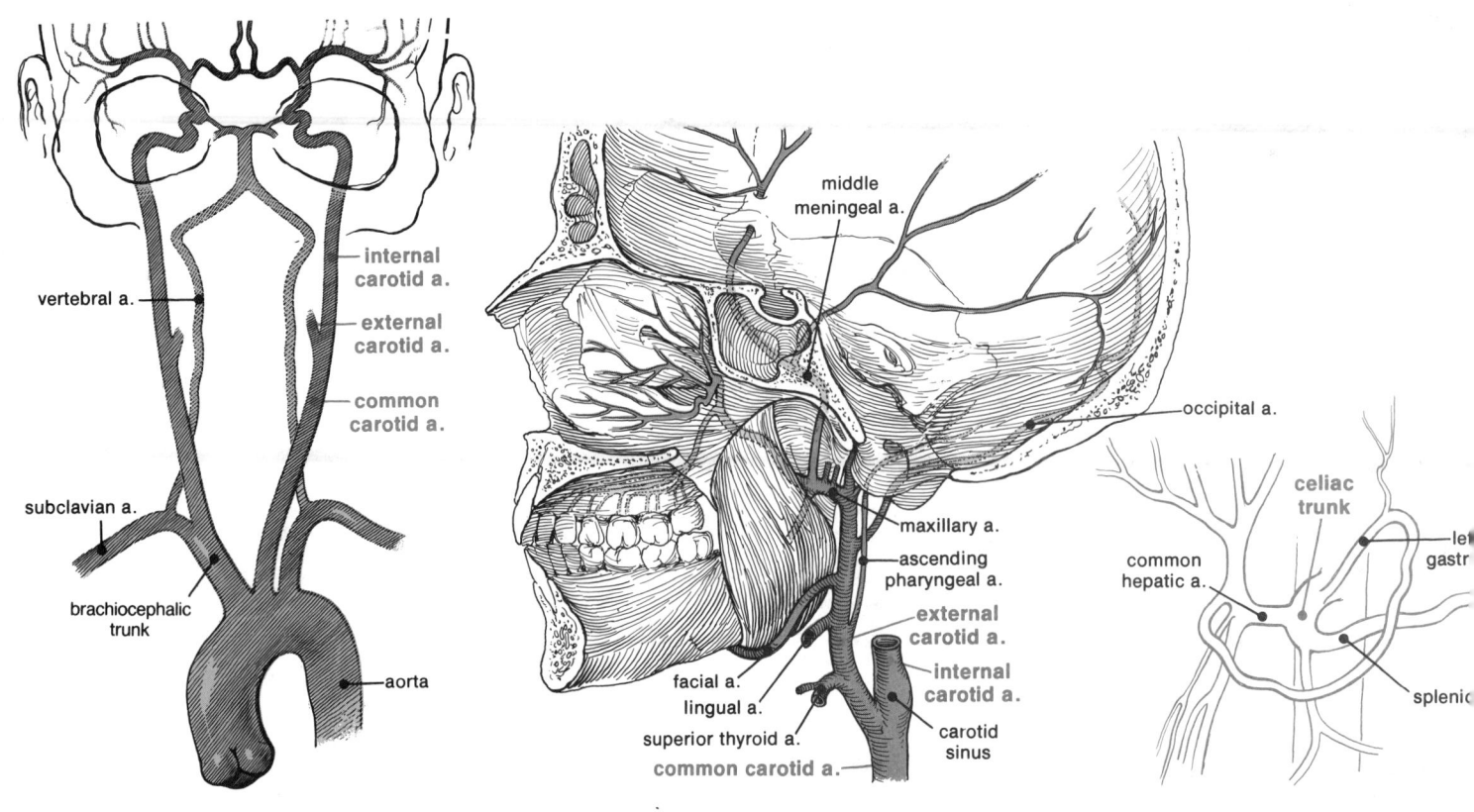

ARTERY	ORIGIN	BRANCHES	DISTRIBUTION
buccal a. buccinator a. *a. buccalis*	maxillary a.	muscular	buccinator muscle, mucosa of maxillary gums, mucosa and skin of cheeks
a. of bulb of penis *a. bulbi penis*	internal pudendal a.	bulbourethral	bulb of penis, posterior part of corpus spongiosum, bulbourethral gland
a. of bulb of vaginal vestibule *a. bulbi vestibuli vaginae*	internal pudendal a.		bulb of vestibule, erectile tissue of vagina
calcaneal a's., medial internal calcaneal a's. *rami calcanei mediales*	posterior tibial a.		skin and fat in back of calcaneal tendon and heel; muscles on tibial side of sole
capsular a.'s, middle	see suprarenal arteries, middle		
carotid a., common *a. carotis communis*	*right side:* bifurcation of the brachiocephalic trunk; *left side:* highest part of arch of aorta	external carotid, internal carotid	head
carotid a., external *a. carotis externa*	common carotid a.	*anterior part:* superior thyroid, lingual; *posterior part:* occipital, posterior auricular; *medial part:* ascending pharyngeal; *terminal part:* superficial temporal, maxillary	anterior aspect of face and neck, side of head, skull, dura mater, posterior part of scalp
carotid a., internal *a. carotis interna*	common carotid a.	*cervical part:* carotid sinus; *petrous part:* caroticotympanic, pterygoid canal; *cavernous part:* cavernous sinus, tentorial, inferior hypophyseal, meningeal, trigeminal, and trochlear; *cerebral part:* superior hypophyseal, ophthalmic, anterior choroidal, anterior and middle cerebral, posterior communicating	middle ear, brain, hypophysis, trigeminal ganglion, meninges, orbit
celiac trunk celiac artery *truncus celiacus*	abdominal aorta, just caudal to aortic hiatus of diaphragm	left gastric, common hepatic, splenic	esophagus, stomach, duodenum, spleen, pancreas, liver, gallbladder, greater omentum

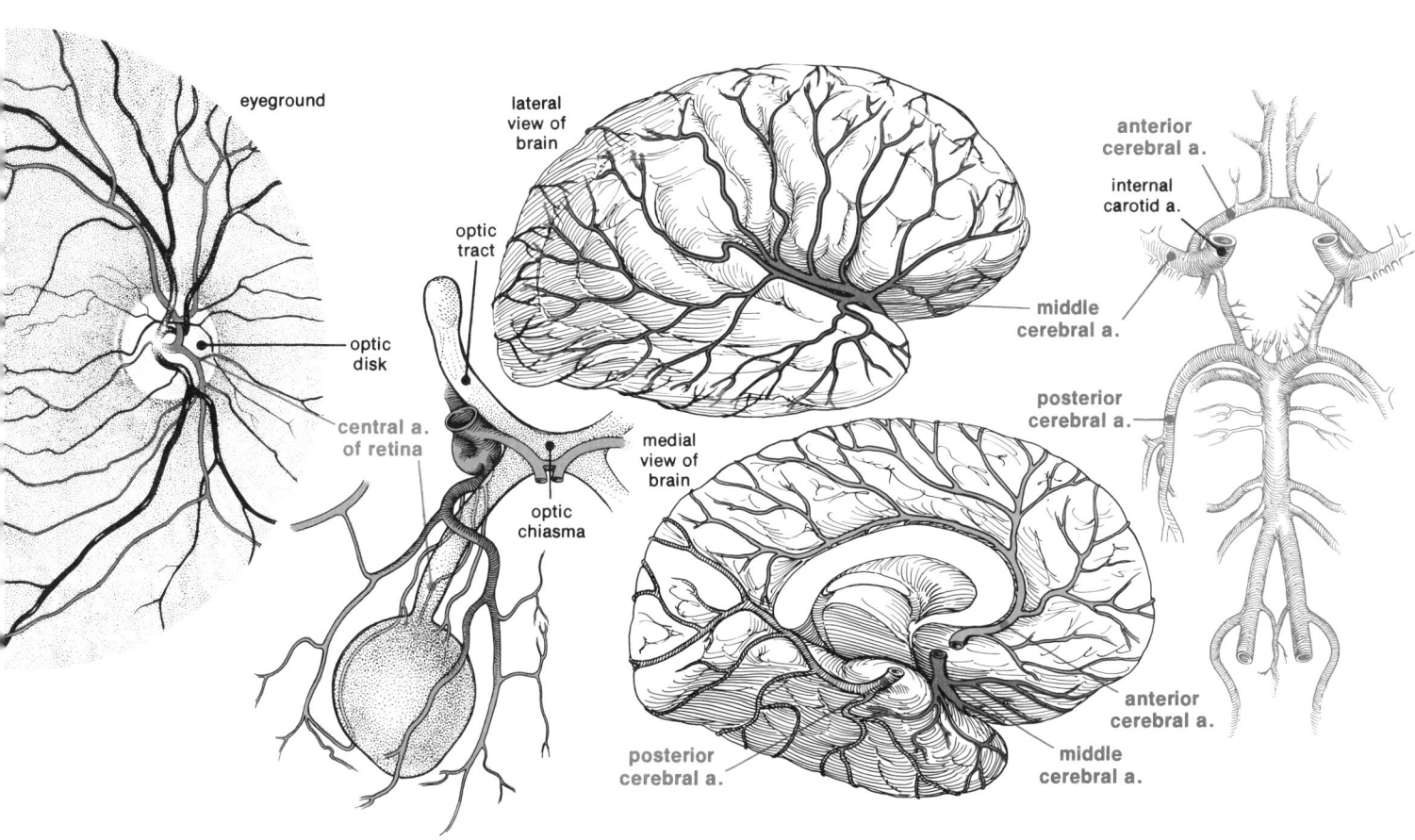

eyeground

lateral view of brain

optic tract

optic disk

optic chiasma

optic

central a. of retina

medial view of brain

anterior cerebral a.

internal carotid a.

middle cerebral a.

posterior cerebral a.

anterior cerebral a.

middle cerebral a.

posterior cerebral a.

ARTERY	ORIGIN	BRANCHES	DISTRIBUTION
central a. of retina *a. centralis retinae*	ophthalmic a. or lacrimal a.	nasal, temporal	retina
cerebellar a., anterior inferior *a. cerebelli inferior anterior*	basilar a.	labyrinthine a.	anterior part of inferior surface of cerebellum
cerebellar a., posterior inferior *a. cerebelli inferior posterior*	vertebral	medial, lateral	inferior surface of cerebellum, medulla oblongata, choroid plexus of fourth ventricle
cerebellar a., superior *a. cerebelli superior*	basilar a. near its termination	medial, lateral	superior surface of cerebellum, vermis of cerebellum, pineal body, pia mater, pons, superior medullary velum, choroid plexus of third ventricle
cerebral a., anterior *a. cerebri anterior*	internal carotid at the medial extremity of the lateral cerebral sulcus	*precommunicating part:* anterior communicating short, long (recurrent), and anterocentral; *postcommunicating part:* medial, frontobasal, callosomarginal, paracentral, precuneal, parietooccipital	hypothalamus, caudate nucleus, internal capsule, choroid plexus, lateral ventricle, corpus striatum, corpus callosum, frontal lobe, parietal lobe, olfactory lobe
cerebral a., middle *a. cerebri media*	internal carotid	*sphenoidal part:* anterolateral central; *insular part:* insula, lateral frontobasal, anterior, medial, and posterior temporal; *terminal part:* central, precentral, and postcentral sulcus, anterior and posterior parietal, angular gyrus	lentiform nucleus, internal capsule, caudate nucleus, corpus striatum, insula, motor, premotor, sensory, and auditory areas, lateral surface of cerebral hemisphere
cerebral a., posterior *a. cerebri posterior*	terminal bifurcation of basilar a.	*precommunicating part:* posteromedial central; *postcommunicating part:* posterolateral central, thalamus, peduncular, posteromedial, and posterolateral choroidal; *terminal part:* lateral occipital, medial occipital	thalamus, third ventricle, globus pallidus, cerebral peduncle, colliculi, pineal body, medial and lateral geniculate bodies, uncus, parahippocampal, medial and lateral occipitotemporal gyri, occipital lobe

artery | artery

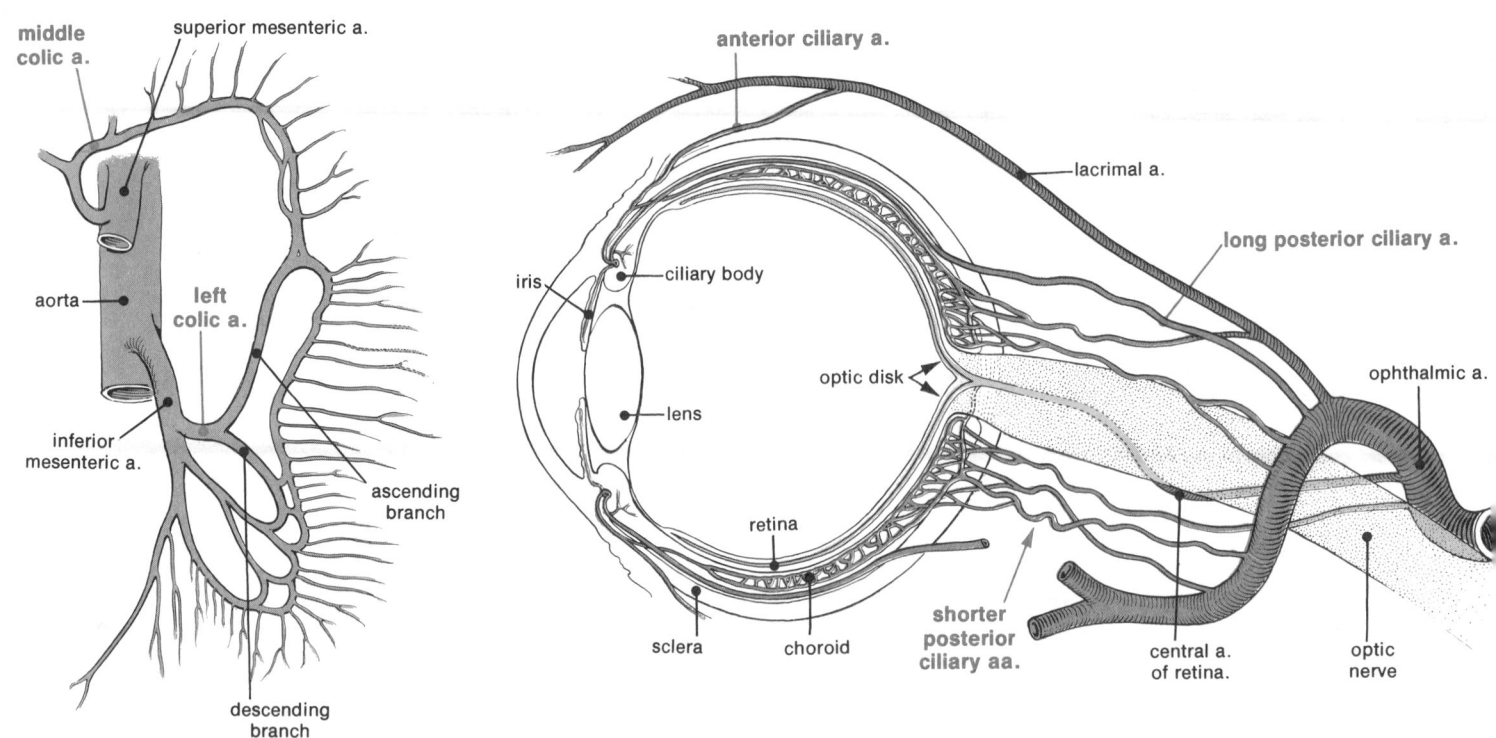

Labels for the colic artery diagram (left):
middle colic a.
superior mesenteric a.
aorta
left colic a.
inferior mesenteric a.
ascending branch
descending branch

Labels for the eye diagram (right):
anterior ciliary a.
lacrimal a.
long posterior ciliary a.
ophthalmic a.
iris
ciliary body
optic disk
lens
retina
shorter posterior ciliary aa.
central a. of retina.
optic nerve
sclera
choroid

ARTERY	ORIGIN	BRANCHES	DISTRIBUTION
cervical a., ascending *a. cervicalis ascendens*	inferior thyroid a.	spinal	muscles of neck, vertebral canal, vertebrae
cervical a., deep *a. cervicalis profunda*	costocervical trunk	spinal, muscular	spinal cord, deep neck muscles
cervical a., superficial *a. cervicalis superficialis*	transverse cervical	ascending, descending	trapezius and neighboring muscles
cervical a., transverse *a. transversa colli* *a. transversa cervicis*	thyrocervical trunk	superficial cervical, dorsal scapular	trapezius, levator m. of scapula, supraspinous m.
choroid a., anterior *a. choroidea anterior*	internal carotid a.		internal capsule, choroid plexus of the inferior horn of lateral ventricle, optic tract, cerebral peduncle, base of brain, lateral geniculate body, caudate nucleus
choroid a., posterior *a. choroidea posterior*	posterior cerebral a.		choroid plexuses of lateral and third ventricles
ciliary a.'s, anterior *aa. ciliares anterior*	ophthalmic a. or lacrimal a.	episcleral, conjunctival	conjunctiva, iris
ciliary a.'s, long posterior (two in number) *aa. ciliares posterior longae*	ophthalmic a.	iris, muscular	iris, ciliary body
ciliary a.'s, short posterior (6–12 in number) *aa. ciliares posterior breves*	ophthalmic a. or one of its branches		choroid and ciliary processes of eyeball
circumflex a., anterior humeral	see humeral circumflex artery, anterior		
circumflex a., lateral femoral	see femoral circumflex artery, lateral		
circumflex a., medial femoral	see femoral circumflex artery, medial		
circumflex a., posterior humeral	see humeral circumflex artery, posterior		
circumflex a., scapular	see scapular circumflex artery		
circumflex iliac a., deep	see iliac circumflex artery, deep		
circumflex iliac a., superficial	see iliac circumflex artery, superficial		
clitoris, deep a. of *a. profunda clitoridis*	internal pudendal a.		corpus cavernosum of clitoris
clitoris, dorsal a. of *a. dorsalis clitoridis*	internal pudendal a.		glans and prepuce of clitoris
coccygeal a.	see sacral artery, middle		
colic a., left *a. colica sinistra*	inferior mesenteric a.	ascending, descending	descending colon, left part of transverse colon

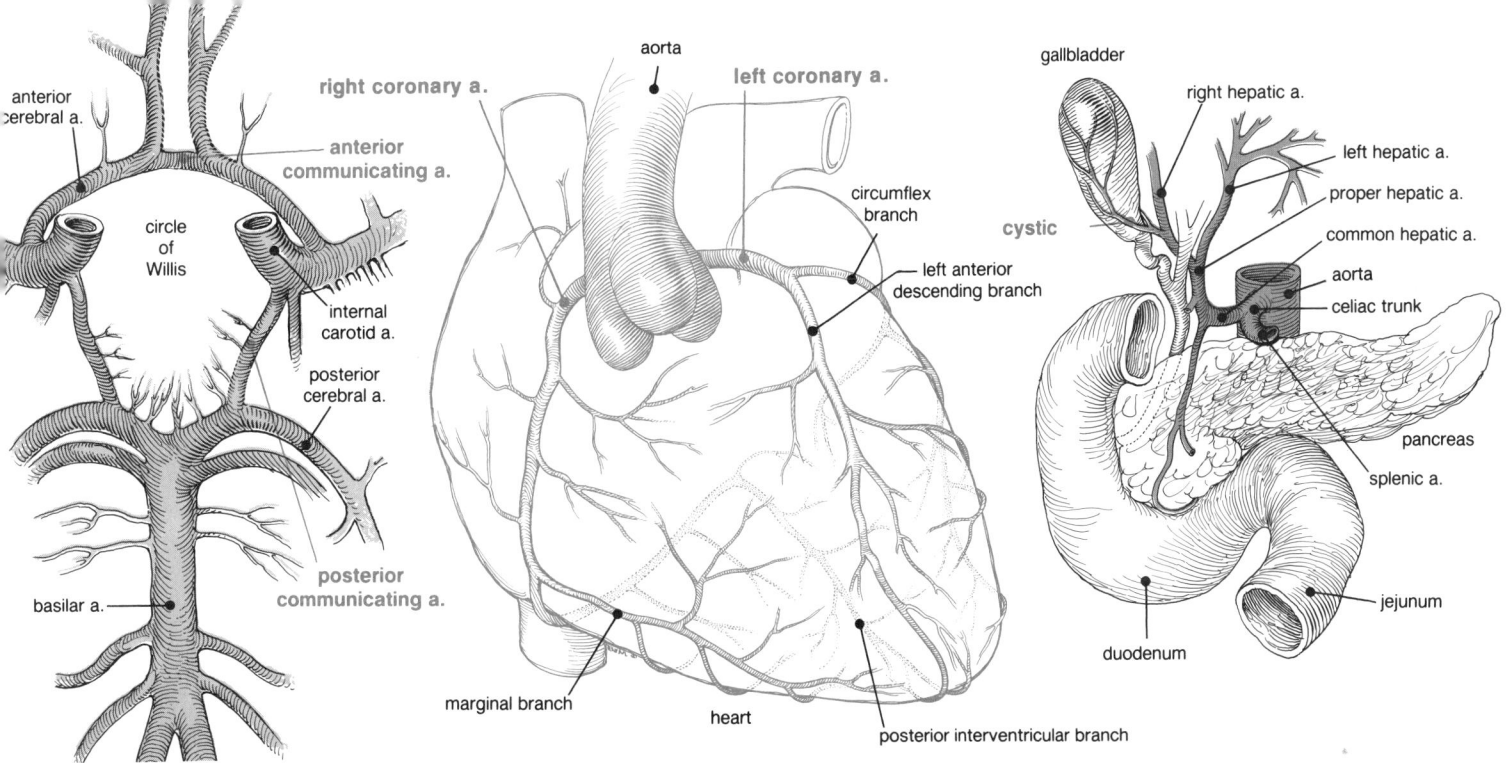

anterior cerebral a.

right coronary a.

aorta

left coronary a.

gallbladder

right hepatic a.

anterior communicating a.

circle of Willis

internal carotid a.

posterior cerebral a.

basilar a.

posterior communicating a.

circumflex branch

cystic

left anterior descending branch

marginal branch

heart

posterior interventricular branch

left hepatic a.

proper hepatic a.

common hepatic a.

aorta

celiac trunk

pancreas

splenic a.

jejunum

duodenum

ARTERY	ORIGIN	BRANCHES	DISTRIBUTION
colic a., middle *a. colica media*	superior mesenteric a., just caudal to the pancreas	right, left	transverse colon
colic a., right *a. colica dextra*	superior mesenteric a. or ileocolic a.	descending, ascending	ascending colon
collateral a., inferior ulnar anastomotica magna a. *a. collateralis ulnaris inferior*	brachial a., about 5 cm proximal to elbow	posterior, anterior, anastomotic	triceps, elbow joint, round pronator muscle
collateral a., middle *a. collateralis media*	deep brachial a.	muscular, anastomotic	elbow joint, triceps and anconeus muscles
collateral a., radial *a. collateralis radialis*	deep brachial a.	muscular, anastomotic	triceps, elbow joint, brachioradial and brachial muscles
collateral a., superior ulnar inferior profunda a. *a. collateralis ulnaris superior*	brachial a., distal to middle of arm	muscular, articular, anastomotic	elbow joint, triceps muscle of arm
communicating a., anterior *a. communicans anterior cerebri*	anterior cerebral a. (connects the two anterior cerebral arteries)	anteromedial	anterior perforated substance of the brain
communicating a., posterior *a. communicans posterior cerebri*	connects the internal carotid a. with posterior cerebral a.	hypophyseal	base of brain between infundibulum and optic tract; internal capsule, anterior third of thalamus; third ventricle
conjunctival a.'s, anterior *aa. conjunctivales anterior*	anterior ciliary a.'s		conjunctiva
conjunctival a.'s, posterior *aa. conjunctivales posterior*	medial palpebral a.		conjunctiva
coronary a., left *a. coronaria sinistra*	aorta at left (posterior) aortic sinus (of Valsalva)	sinoatrial nodal, anterior interventricular (anterior descending), left atrial, circumflex	sinoatrial node, interventricular septum, left atrium, left and right ventricles
coronary a., right *a. coronaria dextra*	aorta at right (anterior) aortic sinus (of Valsalva)	marginal, sinoatrial nodal, right atrial, posterior interventricular (posterior descending), atrioventricular nodal	sinoatrial node, atrioventricular node, right atrium, interventricular septum, right and left ventricles
costocervical trunk superior intercostal a. *truncus costocervicalis*	subclavian a.	deep cervical; continues as the highest intercostal a.	deep neck muscles, first and second intercostal spaces, spinal cord
cremasteric a. external spermatic a. *a. cremasterica*	inferior epigastric a.		cremaster muscle, coverings of spermatic cord
cystic a. *a. cystica*	right hepatic a.	superficial, deep	gallbladder

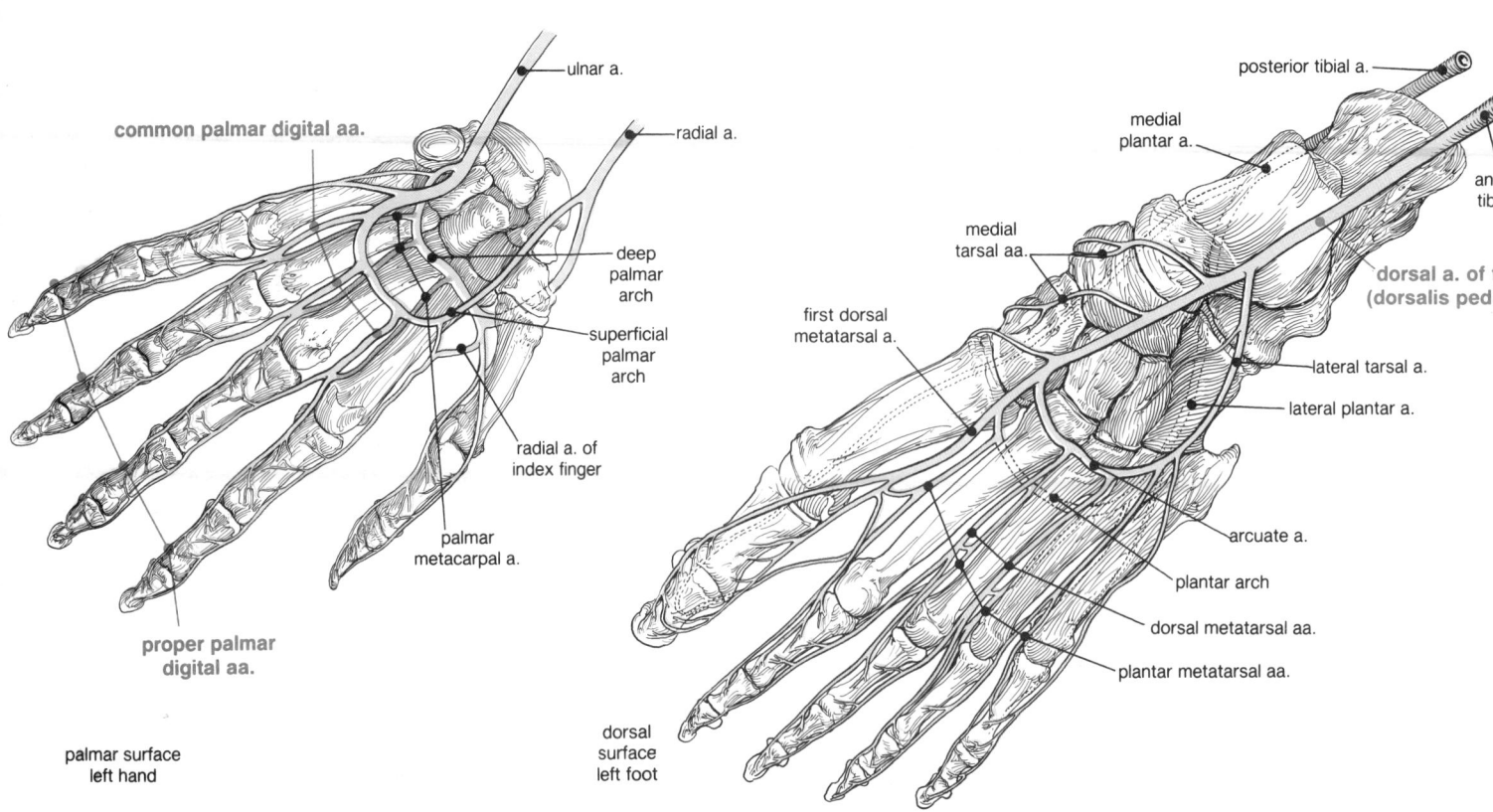

common palmar digital aa.

ulnar a.

radial a.

deep palmar arch

superficial palmar arch

radial a. of index finger

palmar metacarpal a.

proper palmar digital aa.

palmar surface left hand

posterior tibial a.

medial plantar a.

medial tarsal aa.

first dorsal metatarsal a.

ant tibi

dorsal a. of f (dorsalis pedi

lateral tarsal a.

lateral plantar a.

arcuate a.

plantar arch

dorsal metatarsal aa.

plantar metatarsal aa.

dorsal surface left foot

ARTERY	ORIGIN	BRANCHES	DISTRIBUTION
deep a. of clitoris	see clitoris, deep artery of		
deep a. of penis	see penis, deep artery of		
deferential a. a. of ductus deferens *a. ductus deferentis*	umbilical a. (embryonic), superior vesical a.	ureteric	ductus deferens, bladder, seminal vesicles, ureter, testicle
dental a., anterior	see alveolar artery, anterior superior		
dental a., inferior	see alveolar artery, inferior		
dental a., posterior	see alveolar artery, posterior superior		
diphragmatic a., inferior	see phrenic artery		
digital a.'s, collateral	see digital arteries, proper palmar		
digital a.'s, common palmar (three in number) volar digital a.'s *aa. digitales palmares communes*	superficial palmar arch	proper palmar, digital	fingers
digital a.'s, common plantar *aa. digitales plantares communes*	plantar metatarsal a.'s	proper plantar, digital	toes
digital a.'s of foot, common	see metatarsal arteries, plantar		
digital a.'s, proper palmar collateral digital a.'s *aa. digitales palmares propriae*	common palmar digital a.'s	dorsal	the sides of each finger, matrix of fingernails
digital a.'s, proper plantar *aa. digitales plantares propriae*	common plantar digital a.'s		toes
dorsal a. of clitoris	see clitoris, dorsal artery of		
dorsal a. of foot dorsalis pedis a. dorsal pedal a. *a. dorsalis pedis* (anatomoses with lateral plantar a. to form plantar arterial arch)	continuation of anterior tibial a. at ankle joint	lateral tarsal, medial tarsal, arcuate, dorsal metatarsal, deep plantar, dorsal digital (continues to first intermetatarsal space where it divides into first dorsal metatarsal and deep plantar arteries)	foot
dorsal a. of penis	see penis, dorsal artery of		
dorsalis pedis a.	see dorsal artery of foot		
a. of ductus deferens	see deferential artery		
duodenal a.	see pancreaticoduodenal artery, inferior		
epigastric a., deep	see epigastric artery, inferior		

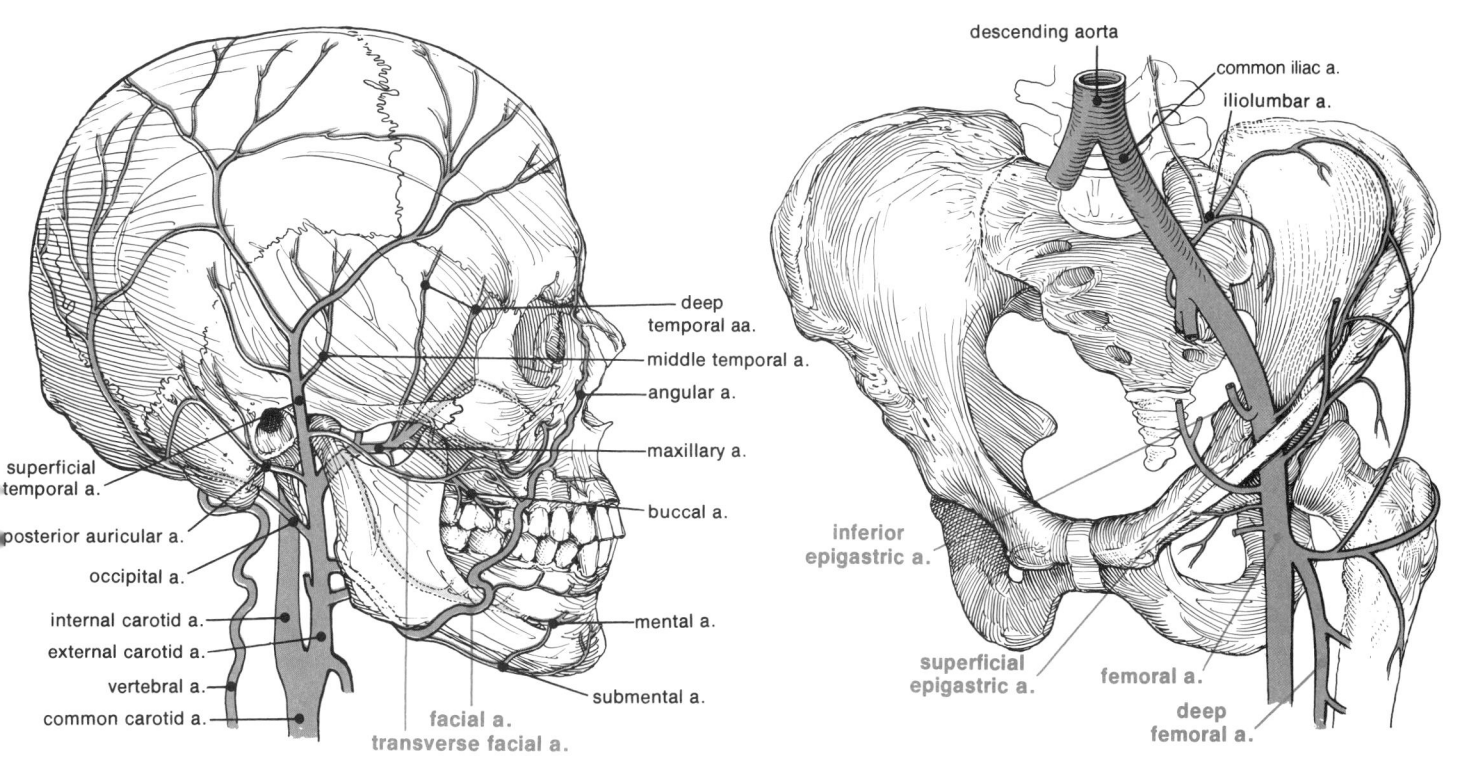

Labels on left skull diagram:
- deep temporal aa.
- middle temporal a.
- angular a.
- maxillary a.
- buccal a.
- superficial temporal a.
- posterior auricular a.
- occipital a.
- internal carotid a.
- external carotid a.
- vertebral a.
- common carotid a.
- mental a.
- submental a.
- facial a.
- transverse facial a.

Labels on right pelvis diagram:
- descending aorta
- common iliac a.
- iliolumbar a.
- inferior epigastric a.
- superficial epigastric a.
- femoral a.
- deep femoral a.

ARTERY	ORIGIN	BRANCHES	DISTRIBUTION
epigastric a., inferior deep epigastric a. *a. epigastrica inferior*	external iliac, immediately above inguinal ligament	cremasteric, pubic, muscular, round ligament of uterus	cremaster and abdominal muscles, peritoneum
epigastric a., superficial *a. epigastrica superficialis*	femoral a. about 1 cm below inguinal ligament		lower part of abdominal wall, superficial lingual lymph nodes
episcleral a., superior *a. epigastrica superior*	internal thoracic a.	cutaneous, muscular, peritoneal, phrenic, hepatic	skin, muscles, and fascia of upper part of abdominal wall; diaphragm, peritoneum, faliciform ligament of liver
episcleral a. *a. episcleralis*	anterior ciliary a.		iris, ciliary body
esophageal a.'s (four to five in number) *aa. esophagei*	thoracic aorta; inferior thyroid and left gastric a.'s		esophagus
ethmoidal a., anterior *a. ethmoidalis anterior*	ophthalmic a.	meningeal, nasal	anterior and middle ethmoid air cells, frontal sinus, dura mater, nasal cavity
ethmoidal a., posterior *a. ethmoidalis posterior*	ophthalmic a.	meningeal, nasal	posterior ethmoid air cells, dura mater, nasal cavity
facial a. external maxillary a. *a. facialis*	external carotid a.	*cervical portion:* ascending palatine, tonsillar, glandular, submental; *facial portion:* inferior labial, superior labial, lateral nasal, angular, muscular	face, tonsil, palate, labial glands and muscles of lips, submandibular gland, ala and dorsum of nose, muscles of expression
facial a., deep	see maxillary artery		
facial a., transverse *a. transverse faciei*	superficial temporal a. while still in parotid gland	glandular, muscular, cutaneous	parotid gland and duct, masseter muscle, skin of face
femoral a. *a. femoralis*	continuation of external iliac a. immediately distal to inguinal ligament	superficial epigastric, superficial circumflex iliac, external pudendal, descending genicular, deep femoral, muscular	integument of abdominal wall, groin, and perineum; muscles of thigh, external genitals, inguinal lymph nodes
femoral a., deep profunda femoris a. *a. profunda femoris*	femoral a.	medial femoral circumflex, lateral femoral circumflex, perforating muscular	muscles of thigh, hip joint, head and shaft of femur, gluteal muscles

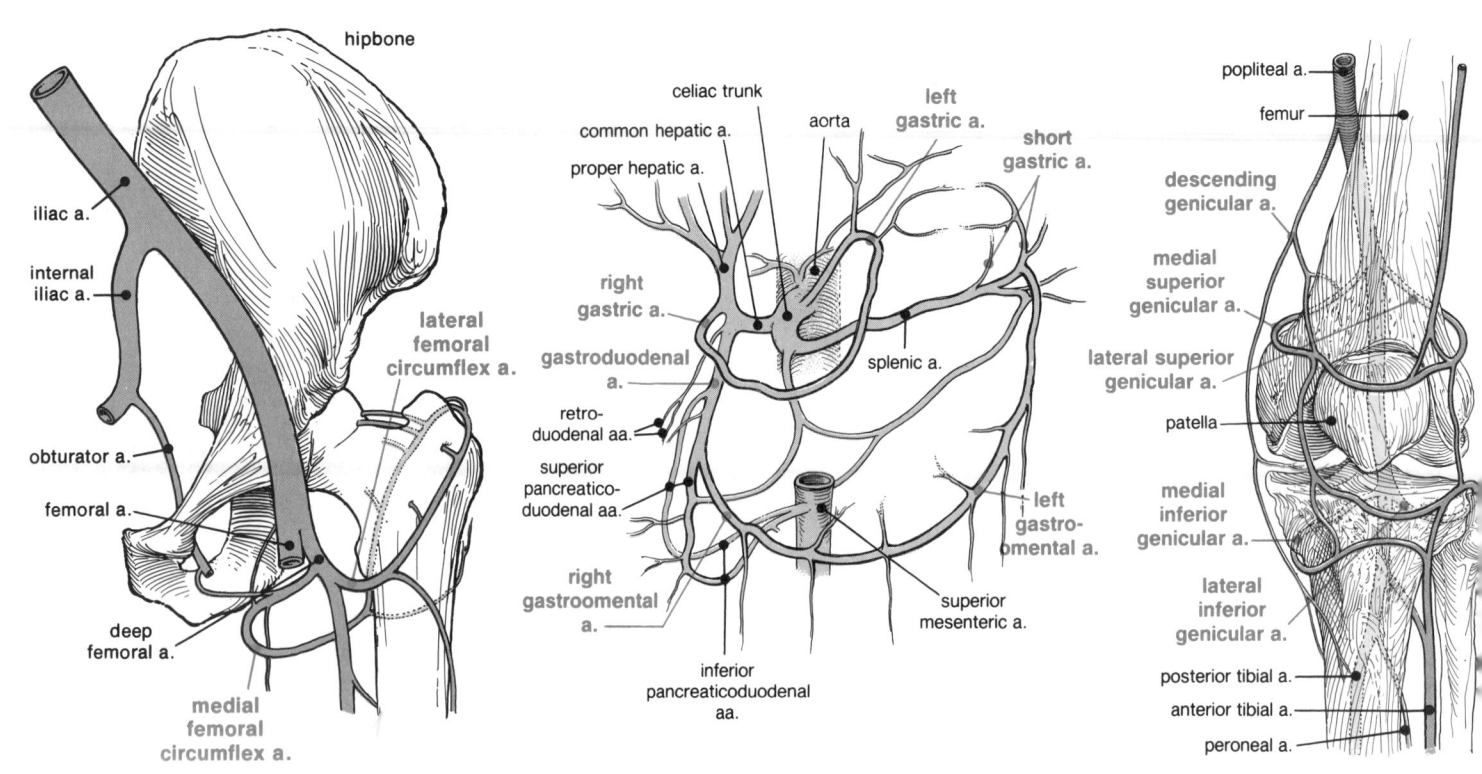

ARTERY	ORIGIN	BRANCHES	DISTRIBUTION
femoral circumflex a., lateral lateral circumflex a. of thigh *a. circumflexa femoris lateral*	deep femoral a.	ascending, descending, transverse	hip joint, thigh muscles
femoral circumflex a., medial medial circumflex a. of thigh *a. circumflexa femoris medial*	deep femoral a.	deep, ascending, transverse, acetabular	hip joint, thigh muscles
fibular a.	see peroneal artery		
frontal a.	see supratrochlear artery		
gastric a., left *a. gastrica sinistra*	celiac trunk	esophageal	lesser curvature of stomach, abdominal part of esophagus; left lobe of liver (at times)
gastric a., right *a. gastrica dextra*	common hepatic a. or proper hepatic a.		pyloric end of stomach
gastric a.'s, short *aa. gastricae breves*	splenic a.		fundus of stomach
gastroduodenal a. *a. gastroduodenalis*	common hepatic a.	right gastroepiploic, superior pancreaticoduodenal, retroduodenal	stomach, duodenum, pancreas, greater omentum
gastroomental a., left gastroepiploic a., left *a. gastroomentalis sinistra*	splenic a.	gastric, omental (epiploic)	stomach, greater omentum
gastroomental a., right gastroepiploic a., right *a. gastroomentalis dextra*	gastroduodenal a.	gastric, omental (epiploic)	stomach, greater omentum
genicular a., descending descending a. of the knee highest genicular a. *a. genus descendens*	femoral a.	saphenous, articular	knee joint and adjacent parts
genicular a., highest	see genicular artery, descending		
genicular a., lateral inferior *a. genus lateralis inferior*	popliteal a.		knee joint, gastrocnemius muscle
genicular a., lateral superior *a. genus lateralis superior*	popliteal a.		lower part of femur, knee joint, patella, contiguous muscles
genicular a., medial inferior *a. genus medialis inferior*	popliteal a.		proximal end of tibia, knee joint
genicular a., medial superior *a. genus medialis superior*	popliteal a.		femur, knee joint, patella, contiguous muscles

artery | artery

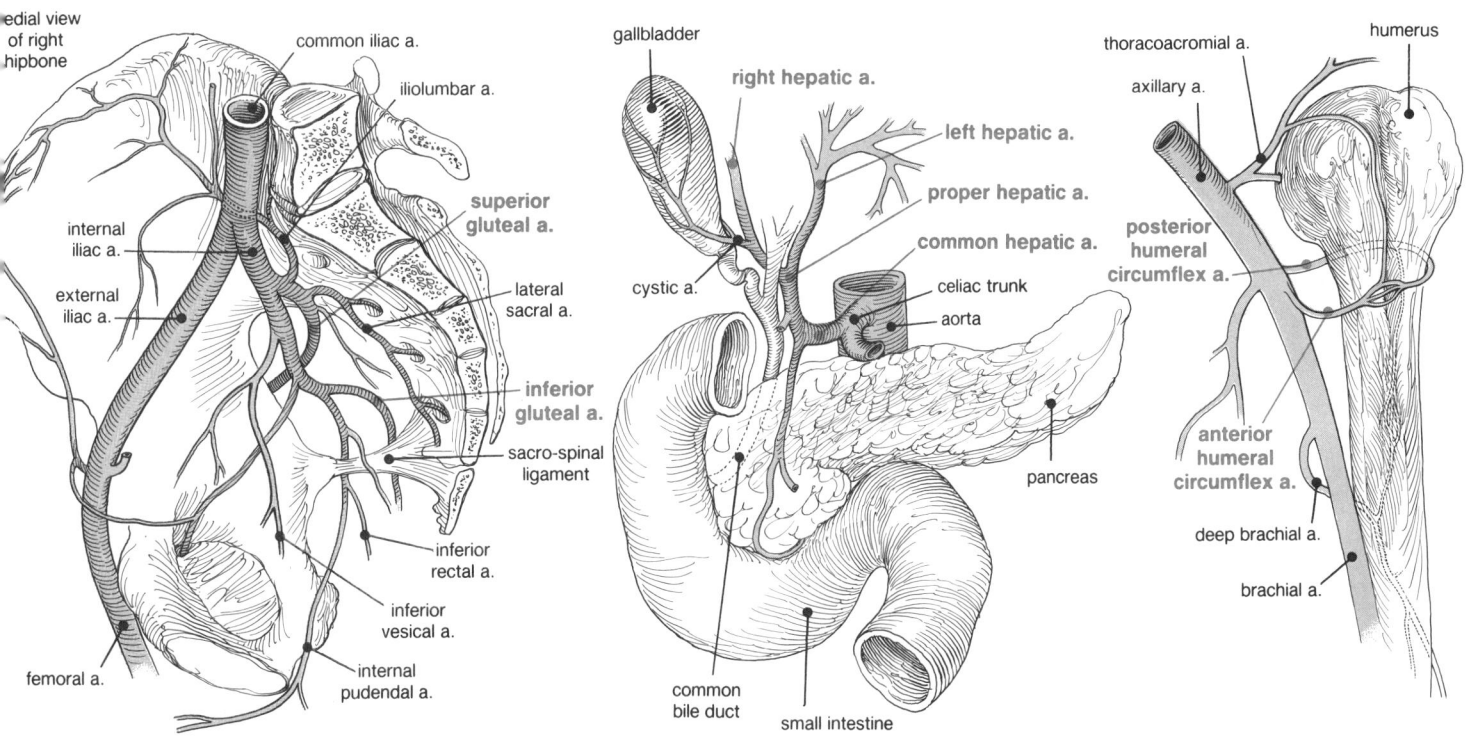

ARTERY	ORIGIN	BRANCHES	DISTRIBUTION
genicular a., middle azygos articular a. *a. genus media*	popliteal a.		ligaments and synovial membrane of knee joint
gluteal a., inferior *a. glutea inferior*	internal iliac a.	sciatic, coccygeal, muscular, articular, cutaneous	buttock and back of thigh
gluteal a., superior *a. glutea superior*	internal iliac a.	superficial, deep, nutrient	muscles of hip and buttock; ilium, skin on dorsal surface of sacrum, hip joint
hemorrhoidal a., inferior	see rectal artery, inferior		
hemorrhoidal a., middle	see rectal artery, middle		
hemorrhoidal a., superior	see rectal artery, superior		
hepatic a., common *a. hepatica communis*	celiac trunk	gastroduodenal, proper hepatic, right gastric	stomach, greater omentum, pancreas, duodenum, liver, gallbladder
hepatic a., left *a. hepatica sinista*	proper hepatic a.	caudate lobe, medial segmental, lateral segmental	liver
hepatic a., proper *a. hepatica propria*	common hepatic a.	left hepatic, right hepatic, right gastric	liver, gallbladder, pyloric part of stomach
hepatic a., right *a. hepatica dextra*	proper hepatic a.	cystic, caudate lobe, anterior (left) segmental, posterior (right) segmental, caudate process	liver and gallbladder
humeral circumflex a., anterior *a. circumflexa humeri anterior*	axillary a.	pectoral, muscular, ascending	head of humerus, shoulder joint, long head of biceps, muscle of arm, deltoid, coracobrachial, tendon of greater pectoral muscle
humeral circumflex a., posterior *a. circumflexa humeri posterior*	axillary a. at distal border of subscapular muscle	muscular, articular, nutrient	shoulder joints, neck of humerus, deltoid, teres minor, and triceps muscles
hyaloid a. *a. hyaloidea* (usually disappears in the last month of intrauterine life)	central a. of retina		vitreous body, lens of eye
hypogastric a.	see iliac artery, internal		
ileal a.'s *aa. ilei*	superior mesenteric a.		ileum

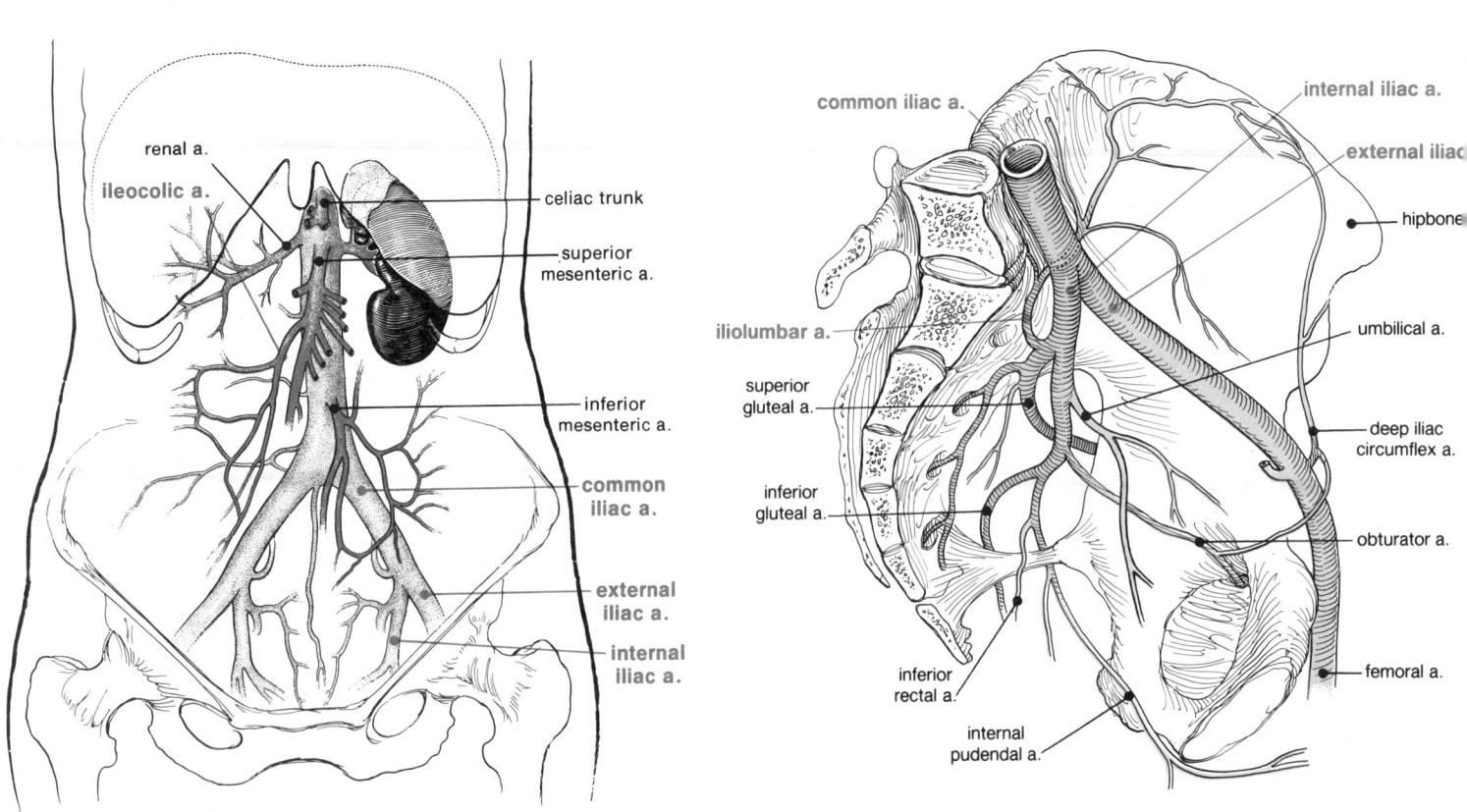

ARTERY	ORIGIN	BRANCHES	DISTRIBUTION
ileocolic a. *a. ileocolica*	superior mesenteric a.	superior (anastomoses with right colic a.), inferior (anastomoses with end of superior mesenteric a.), colic, anterior cecal, posterior cecal, appendicular, ileal	cecum, vermiform appendix ascending colon, distal part of ileum
iliac a., common *a. iliaca communis*	abdominal aorta	internal and external iliac	pelvis, genital and gluteal regions, perineum, lower abdominal wall
iliac a., external *a. iliaca externa*	continuation of common iliac a.	inferior epigastric, deep iliac circumflex, muscular	lower part of abdominal wall, external genitals, psoas major, cremaster, ductus deferens in male, round ligament of uterus in female
iliac a., internal hypogastric a. *a. iliaca interna*	common iliac a.	*anterior trunk:* obturator, superior gluteal, inferior gluteal, umbilical, inferior vesical, uterine, vaginal, middle rectal, internal pudendal; *posterior trunk:* iliolumbar, lateral sacral	wall and viscera of pelvis, external genitals, region of anus, medial aspect of thigh
iliac circumflex a., deep *a. circumflexa ilium profounda*	external iliac a.	ascending	psoas, iliac, sartorius, and neighboring muscles; overlying skin, oblique and transverse abdominal muscles
iliac circumflex a., superficial *a. circumflexa ilium superficialis*	femoral		skin of groin, superficial lingual lymph nodes
iliolumbar a. *a. ilioumbalis*	internal iliac a.	lumbar, iliac	greater psoas muscle, quadratus muscle of loins, gluteal, and abdominal muscles; ilium, cauda equina
infraorbital a. *a. infraorbitalis*	maxillary	orbital, anterior superior alveolar	orbit, maxilia, maxillary sinus and teeth, lower eyelid, extrinsic eye muscles, cheek, side of nose
innominate a.		see brachiocephalic trunk	
intercostal a.'s, anterior intercostal a.'s *aa. intercostales anterior*	internal thoracic a.	pectoral, glandular	first five or six intercostal spaces, pectoral muscles, mammary gland

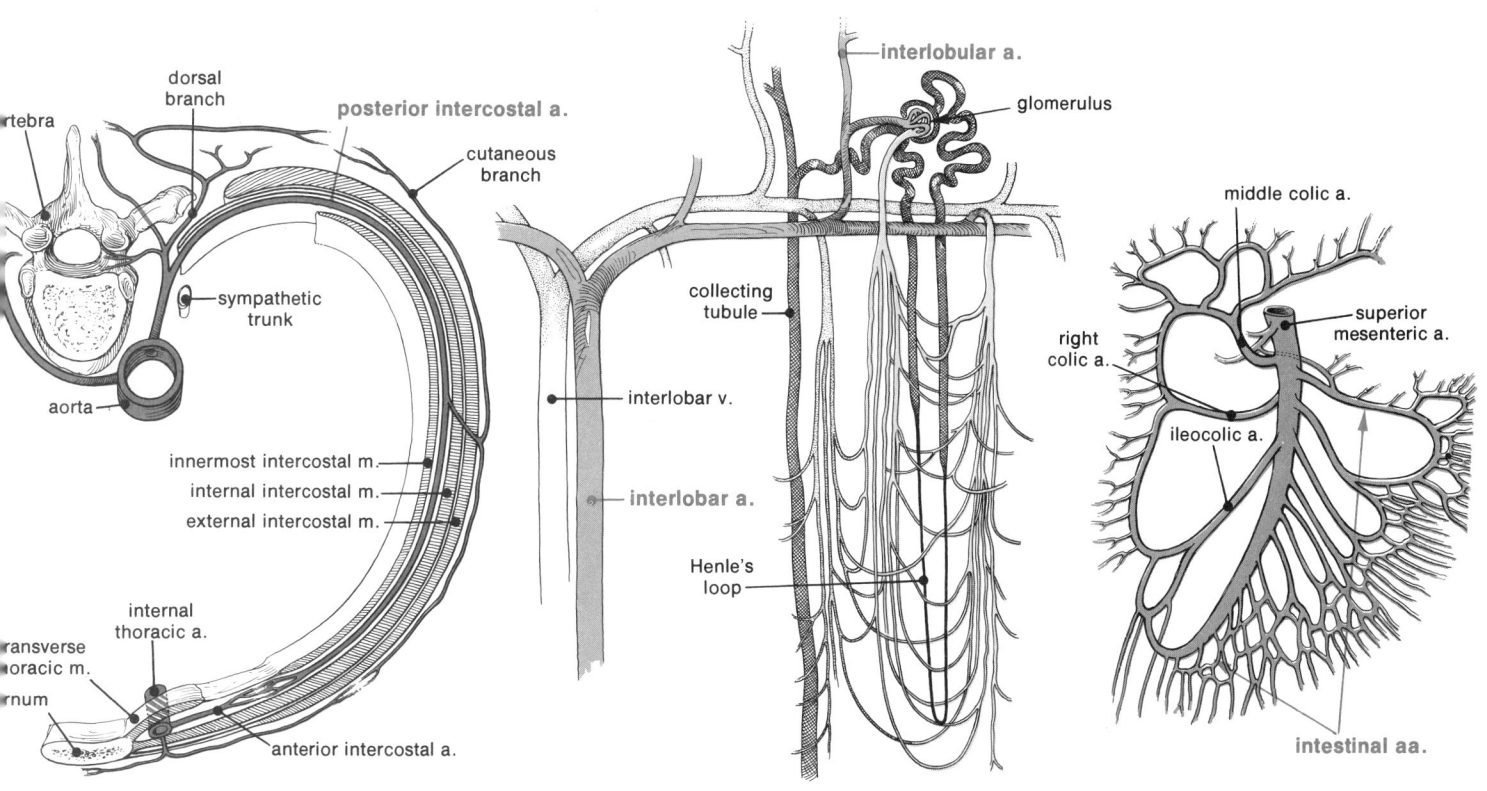

ARTERY	ORIGIN	BRANCHES	DISTRIBUTION
intercostal a.'s, highest *a. intercostalis suprema*	costocervical trunk	first and second posterior intercostal	first and second intercostal spaces, spinal cord, back muscles
intercostal a.'s I-II, posterior *aa. intercostales posteriores I-II*	highest intercostal a.	dorsal, spinal	upper part of thoracic wall
intercostal a.'s III-XI, posterior *aa. intercostales posteriores III-XI*	thoracic aorta	dorsal, collateral intercostal, lateral cutaneous, muscular	thoracic wall
interlobar a.'s of kidney *aa. interlobares renis*	six segmental branches of renal a.	arcuate	corticomedullary zone of kidney
interlobular a.'s of kidney *aa. interlobulares renis*	arcuate a.'s of kidney	afferent glomeruli	renal glomeruli
interlobular a.'s of liver *aa. interlobulares hepatis*	right or left hepatic a.'s		between hepatic lobules
interosseous a., anterior volar interosseous a. *a. interossea anterior*	common interosseous a.	median, muscular, nutrient	deep parts of front of forearm; radius, ulna
interosseous a., common *a. interossea communis*	ulnar a., immediately distal to tuberosity of radius	posterior and anterior interosseous	forearm, radius, ulna
interosseous a., posterior dorsal interosseous a. *a. interossea posterior*	common interosseous a.	recurrent interosseous	deep parts of back of forearm
interosseous a.'s palmar	see metacarpal arteries, palmar		
interosseous a., recurrent *a. interossea recurrens*	posterior interosseous a.		back of elbow joint
intestinal a.'s (12–15 in number) *aa. jejunales et ilei* *aa. intestinales*	superior mesenteric a.		jejunum, ileum
labial a., inferior *a. labialis inferior*	facial a. near angle of mouth		labial glands, mucous membrane, muscles of lower lip
labial a., superior *a. labialis superior*	facial a.	septal, alar	upper lip, nasal septum, ala of nose
labyrinthine a. internal auditory a. *a. labyrinthi*	basilar a. or anterior inferior cerebellar a.	vestibular, cochlear	internal ear
lacrimal a. *a. lacrimalis*	ophthalmic a. close to optic canal	lateral palpebral, zygomatic, recurrent meningeal, long posterior ciliary	lacrimal gland, conjunctiva, superior and lateral recti muscles, cheek, ciliary processes, eyelids

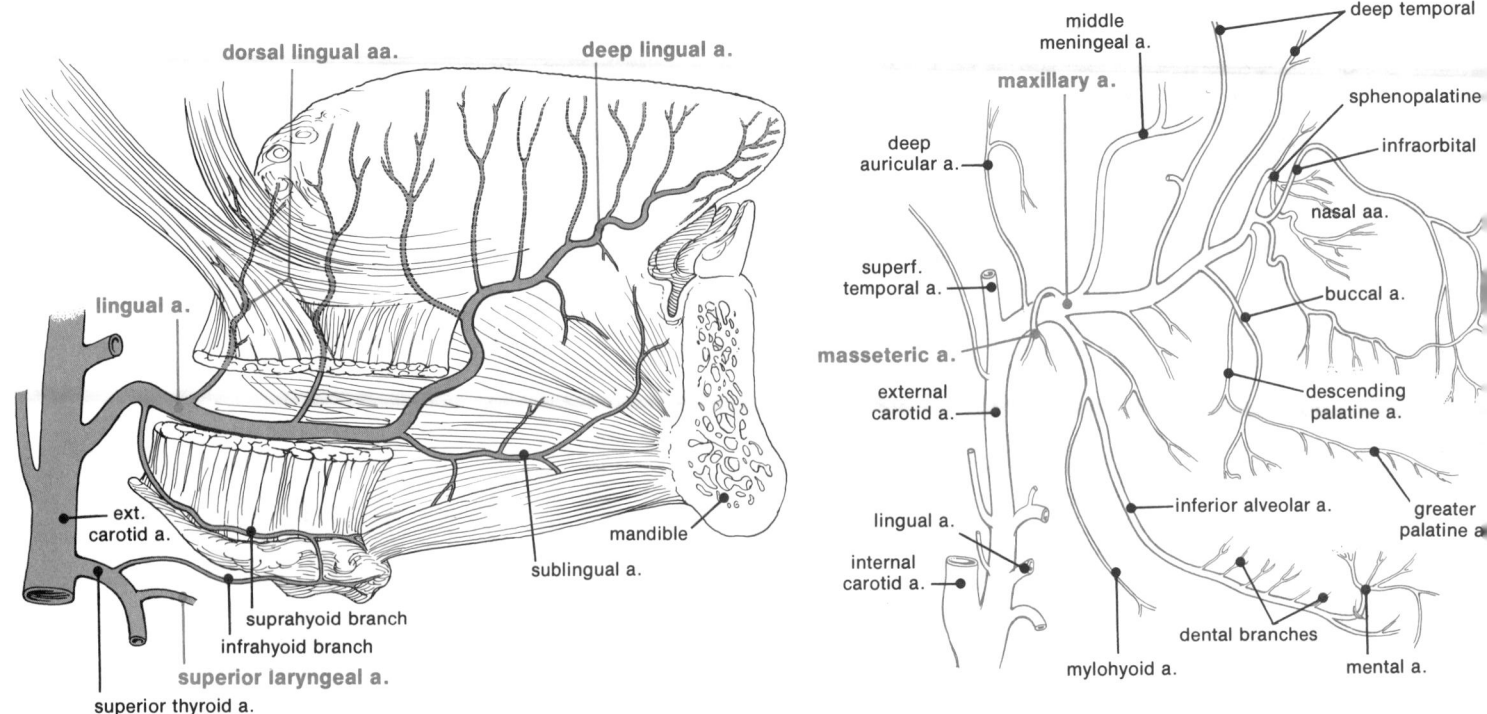

ARTERY	ORIGIN	BRANCHES	DISTRIBUTION
laryngeal a., inferior *a. laryngea inferior*	inferior thyroid a.		muscles of larynx, mucous membrane of larynx
laryngeal a., superior *a. laryngea superior*	superior thyroid a. (occasionally from external carotid a.)		muscles, mucous membrane, and glands of larynx
lienal a.	see splenic artery		
lingual a. *a. lingualis*	external carotid a.	suprahyoid, dorsal lingual, sublingual, deep lingual	muscles and mucosa of tongue, sublingual gland, gingiva, tonsil, epiglottis
lingual a., deep ranine a. *a. profunda linguae*	lingual a. (terminal portion)		intrinsic lingual muscles, lingual mucosa
lingual a.'s, dorsal *a. lingualis, rami dorsales*	lingual a.		mucous membrane of posterior part of tongue; palatoglossal arch, tonsil, epiglottis
lumbar a.'s (4–5 in number) *aa. lumbales*	abdominal aorta	dorsal, spinal	lumbar vertebrae, back muscles, abdominal wall
lumbar a., lowest *a. lumbalis ima*	median sacral a.		sacrum, iliac muscle
malleolar a., anterior lateral external malleolar a. *a. malleolaris anterior lateral*	anterior tibial a.		lateral side of ankle
malleolar a., anterior medial internal malleolar a. *a. malleolaris anterior medial*	anterior tibial a.		medial side of ankle
malleolar a., posterior medial internal malleolar a. *a. malleolaris posterior medial*	posterior tibial		medial side of ankle
mammary a., external	see thoracic artery, lateral		
mammary a., internal	see thoracic artery, internal		
mandibular a.	see alveolar artery, inferior		
masseteric a. *a. masseterica*	maxillary		masseter muscle
maxillary a. internal maxillary a. deep facial a. *a. maxillaris*	external carotid a.	*mandibular portion:* deep auricular, anterior tympanic, inferior alveolar, middle meningeal, accessory	ear, teeth, dura mater, trigeminal ganglion, temporal, masseter, buccinator, and eye muscles, lacrimal gland,

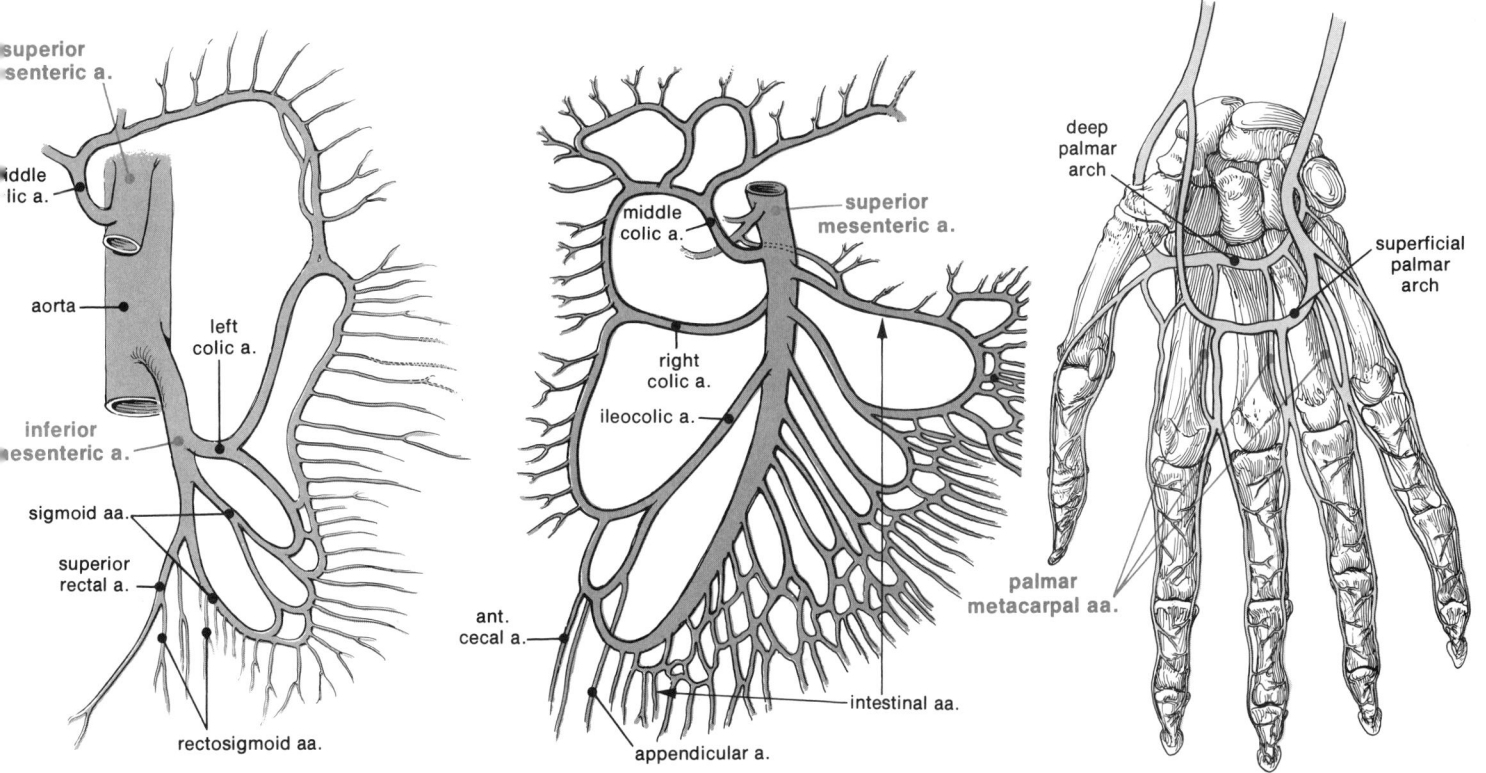

ARTERY	ORIGIN	BRANCHES	DISTRIBUTION
maxillary a. (cont'd)		meningeal; *pterygoid portion:* deep temporal, pterygoid, masseteric, buccal; *pterygopalatine portion:* posterior superior alveolar, infraorbital, greater palatine, artery of the pterygoid canal, pharyngeal, sphenopalatine	palatine tonsil, soft palate, upper pharynx, auditory tube, nasal cavity, sinuses
maxillary a., external	see facial artery		
maxillary a., internal	see maxillary artery		
median a. *a. mediana*	anterior interosseous a.		accompanies and supplies median nerve to palm
medullary a.'s *aa. medullares*	vertebral a. and its branches		medulla oblongata
meningeal a., anterior *a. meningea anterior*	anterior ethmoidal a. or internal carotid a.		dura mater of anterior cranial fossa
meningeal a., middle *a. meningea media*	maxillary a.	frontal, parietal, petrosal, superior tympanic, ganglionic	cranial bones, dura mater, tensor tympani muscle, semilunar ganglion, orbit
meningeal a., posterior *a. meningea posterior*	ascending pharyngeal a.		bone and dura mater of posterior cranial fossa
mesenteric a., inferior *a. mesenterica inferior*	abdominal aorta	left colic, sigmoid, superior rectal	transverse, descending, and sigmoid colon, upper part of rectum
mesenteric a., superior *a. mesenterica superior*	abdominal aorta	inferior pancreaticoduodenal, intestinal, ileocolic, right colic, middle colic	small intestine, proximal half of colon
metacarpal a.'s dorsal (three in number) *aa. metacarpeae dorsales*	dorsal carpal branch, dorsal carpal network (rete), or radial a.	dorsal digital	back of second, third, and fourth fingers
metacarpal a.'s, palmar palmar interosseous a.'s. *aa. metacarpeae palmares*	deep palmar arch		interosseous muscles, metacarpal bones, second, third, and fourth lumbrical muscles
metatarsal a., first dorsal *a. metatarsalis dorsalis I*	dorsal a. of foot	branch to medial side of great toe, branch to adjoining sides of the second and great toes	medial border of great toe and adjoining sides of great and second toes

artery | artery

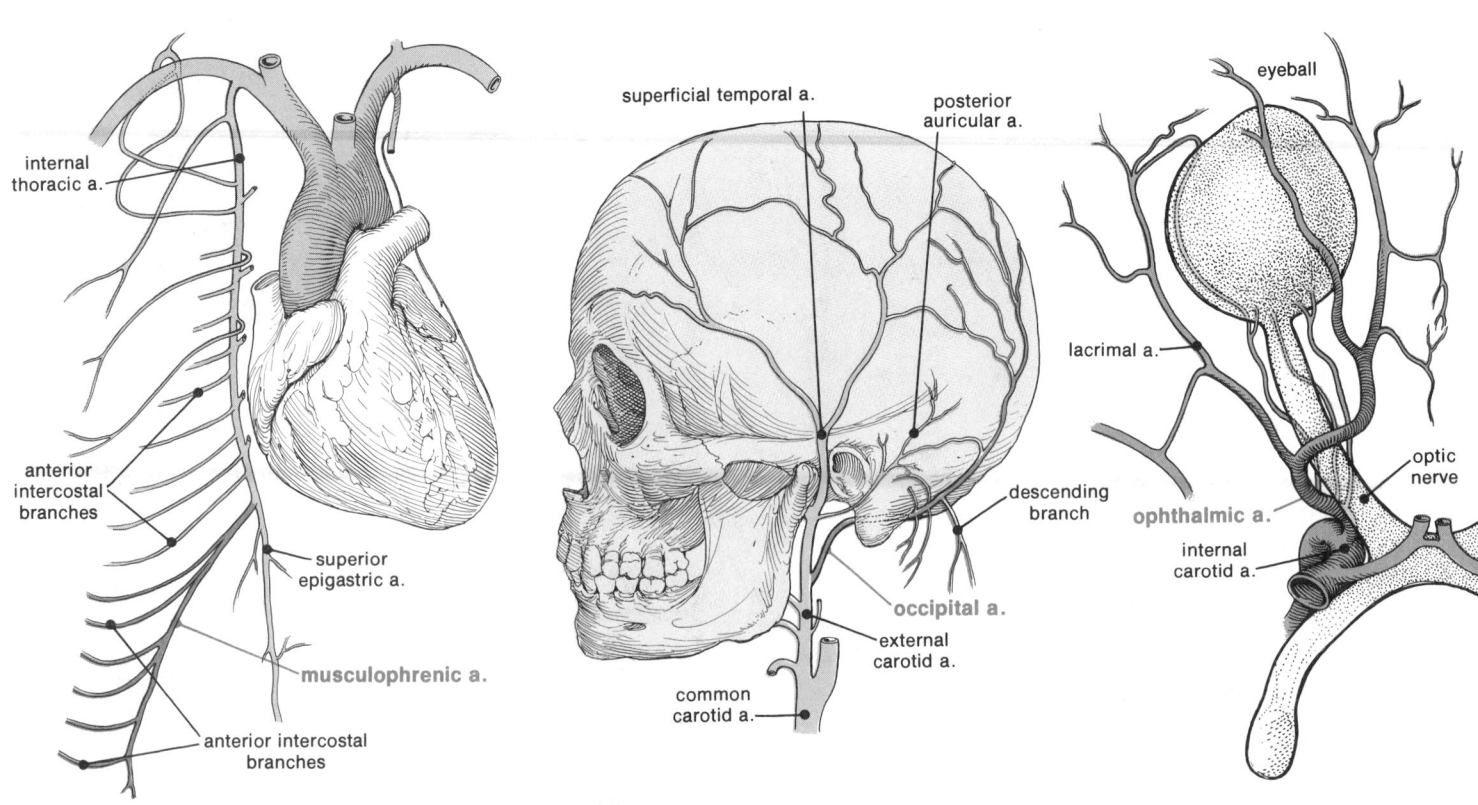

internal thoracic a.

anterior intercostal branches

superior epigastric a.

musculophrenic a.

anterior intercostal branches

superficial temporal a.

posterior auricular a.

descending branch

occipital a.

external carotid a.

common carotid a.

eyeball

lacrimal a.

optic nerve

ophthalmic a.

internal carotid a.

ARTERY	ORIGIN	BRANCHES	DISTRIBUTION
metatarsal a.'s, plantar (four in number) digital a.'s of foot, common *aa. metatarseae plantares*	plantar arch	plantar digital, anterior perforating	plantar surface and adjacent sides of toes
musculophrenic a. *a. musculophrenica*	internal thoracic a.	anterior intercostal	diaphragm, seventh, eighth, and ninth intercostal spaces, pericardium
mylohyoid a. *a. mylohyoideus*	inferior alveolar a.		mylohyoid muscle
nasal a., dorsal *a. dorsalis nasi*	ophthalmic a.		skin of nose, lacrimal sac
nasal a., lateral *a. nasalis lateralis*	facial a.		lateral nasal wall
nasal a., posterior lateral *a. nasalis posterioris lateralis*	sphenopalatine a.		posterior parts of conchae and lateral nasal wall
nasal a., posterior septal *a. nasalis posterioris septi*	sphenopalatine a.		nasal septum
nutrient a. of fibula *a. nutricia fibulae*	peroneal a.		substance of fibula
nutrient a.'s of humerus *aa. nutriciae humeri*	deep brachial a. about middle of arm		substance of humerus
nutrient a. of tibia (largest nutrient a. of bone in body) *a. nutricia tibiae*	posterior tibial a.		substance of tibia
obturator a. *a. obturatoria*	internal iliac a.	pubic, acetabular, obturator, anterior, posterior	bladder, ilium, pelvic muscles, hip joint
occipital a. *a. occipitalis*	external carotid a.	muscular, sternocleidomastoid, auricular, meningeal, descending, terminal	dura mater, diploë, mastoid air cells, muscles of neck and scalp
ophthalmic a. *a. ophthalmica*	internal carotid a.	*orbital portion:* lacrimal, supraorbital, posterior ethmoidal, anterior ethmoidal, medial palpebral supratrochlear, dorsal nasal; *ocular portion:* central artery of the retina, short posterior ciliary, long posterior ciliary, anterior ciliary, muscular	orbit and surrounding parts

muscles and bulb of the eye |

artery | artery

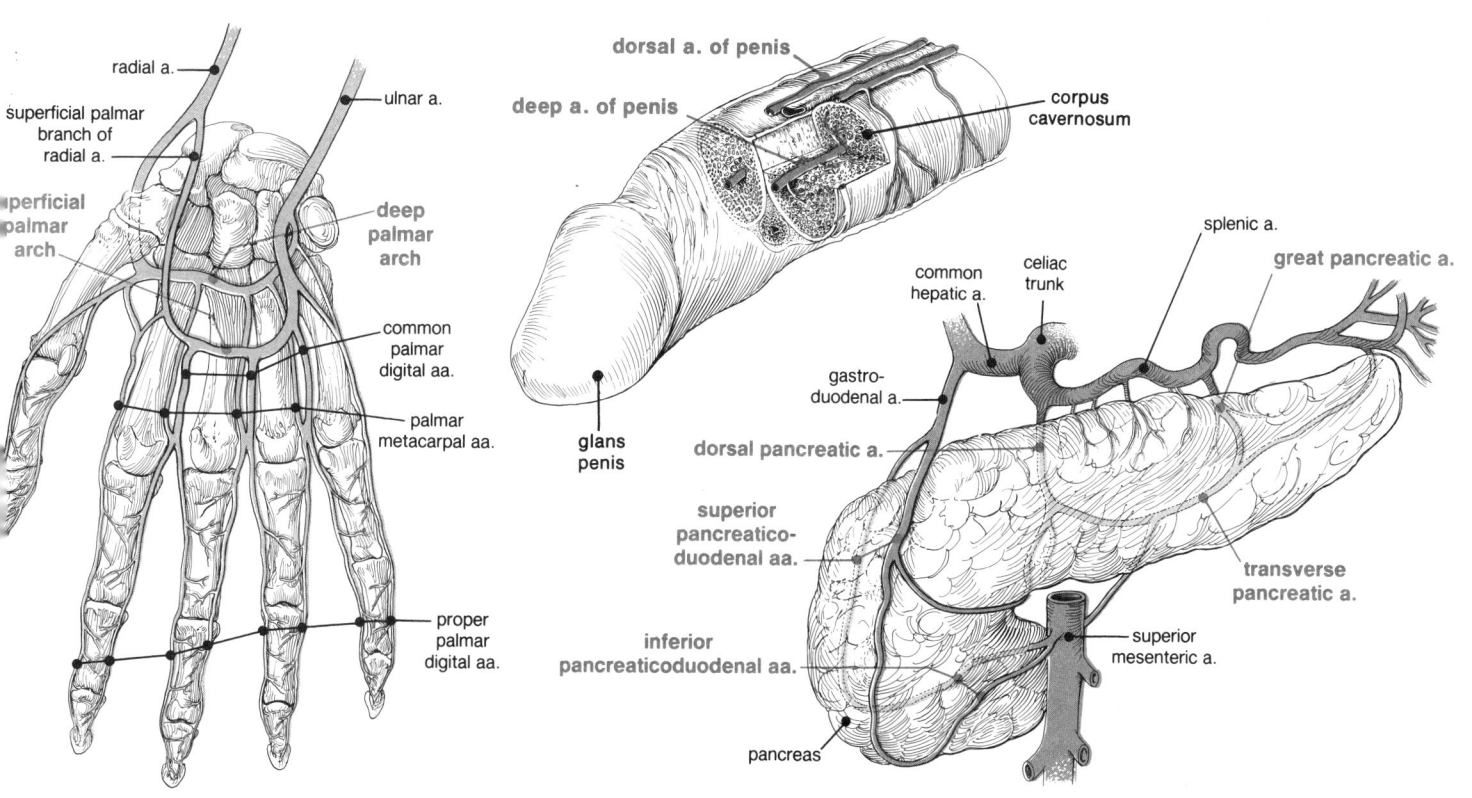

ARTERY	ORIGIN	BRANCHES	DISTRIBUTION
ovarian a.'s *aa. ovaricae*	ventral surface of abdominal aorta slightly below the renal a.'s	ureteric; anastomoses with uterine a.	ovary, ureter, uterus, round ligament
palatine a., ascending *a. palatina ascendens*	facial		soft palate, palatine glands, auditory tube
palatine a., descending *a. palatina descendens*	maxillary a.	greater palatine, lesser palatine	soft palate, hard palate, tonsil, gums
palatine a., greater *a. palatina major*	descending palatine a.		hard palate, gums, palatine glands
palatine a.'s, lesser *aa. palatinae minores*	descending palatine a.		soft palate, palatine tonsil
palmar arch, deep *arcus palmaris profundus*	radial a.	palmar metacarpal; anastomoses with deep palmar branch of ulnar	carpal extremities of metacarpal bones, interosseous muscles
palmar arch, superficial *arcus palmaris superficialis*	ulnar a.	common palmar digital	palm
palpebral a.'s, lateral *aa. palpebrales laterales*	lacrimal a.	superior, inferior	eyelids, conjunctiva
palpebral a.'s, medial *aa. palpebrales mediales*	ophthalmic a. near the pulley of the superior oblique muscle	superior, inferior	eyelids, conjunctiva, nasolacrimal duct
pancreatic a., dorsal *a. pancreatica dorsalis*	splenic a.	right, left (inferior pancreatic a.)	pancreas
pancreatic a., great *a. pancreatica magna*	splenic a.		pancreas
pancreatic a., inferior *a. pancreatica inferior*	dorsal pancreatic a.		pancreas, greater omentum
pancreaticoduodenal a., inferior duodenal a. *a. pancreaticoduodenalis inferior*	superior mesenteric a. or from its first intestinal branch		head of pancreas, descending and inferior parts of duodenum
pancreaticoduodenal a., superior *a. pancreaticoduodenalis superior*	gastroduodenal a.	ventral and dorsal pancreaticoduodenal arcade	pancreas, three parts of duodenum
penis, deep a. of a. of corpus cavernosum *a. profunda penis*	internal pudendal a.		corpus cavernosum of penis
penis, dorsal a. of *a. dorsalis penis*	internal pudendal a.		glans and prepuce of penis, integument and fibrous sheath of corpus cavernosum

43

ARTERY	ORIGIN	BRANCHES	DISTRIBUTION
perforating a.'s *aa. perforantes*	deep femoral a.	first, second, and third perforating	back of thigh, femur
pericardiacophrenic a. *a. pericardiacophrenica*	internal thoracic a.		diaphragm, pericardium, pleura
perineal a. superficial perineal a. *a. perinealis*	internal pudendal a.	transverse perineal, posterior scrotal/labial	perineum, external genitalia, bulbocavernous and ischiocavernous muscles
peroneal a. fibular a. *a. peronea*	posterior tibial a.	muscular, nutrient (fibula), perforating, communicating, posterior lateral malleolar, lateral calcaneal	soleus and other deep calf muscles, lateral side and back of ankle and heel
pharyngeal a., ascending *a. pharyngea ascendens*	external carotid a.	pharyngeal, palatine, prevertebral, inferior tympanic, posterior meningeal	wall of pharynx, soft palate, tonsil, ear, meninges, muscles of back of head and neck
phrenic a.'s phrenic a.'s, inferior diaphragmatic a., inferior *aa. phrenicae*	abdominal aorta or celiac trunk	superior suprarenal	diaphragm, adrenal gland
phrenic a.'s, superior *aa. phrenicae superior*	thoracic aorta		diaphgram
plantar a., deep communicating a. *ramus plantaris profundus*	dorsal a. foot	first plantar metatarsal; with lateral plantar a., forms plantar arch	undersurface and adjacent sides of first and second toes
plantar a., lateral *a. plantaris lateral*	posterior tibial a.	calcaneal, muscular, cutaneous; continues to form plantar arch by uniting with deep plantar branch of the dorsal artery of foot	muscles of foot, skin of toes and lateral side of foot
plantar a., medial internal plantar a. *a. plantaris medialis*	posterior tibial a.	deep, superficial	flexor muscle of toes, abductor muscle of great toe, skin of inner side of sole
plantar arch *arcus plantaris*	lateral plantar a.	perforating, plantar metatarsal	interosseous muscles, toes
popliteal a. *a. poplitea*	continuation of femoral a. at the adductor hiatus	muscular, sural, cutaneous, medial superior genicular, lateral superior genicular, middle genicular, medial inferior genicular; lateral inferior genicular; it divides at the distal border of the popliteus and continues as anterior and posterior tibial arteries	muscles of thigh in region of knee, femur, patella, and tibia
princeps pollicis a.	see principal artery of thumb		
principal a. of thumb princeps pollicis a. *a. princeps pollicis*	radial a.	radial a. to index finger	sides of thumb, dorsal interosseous muscles of hand
profunda a., inferior	see collateral artery, superior ulnar		
profunda a., superior	see brachial artery, deep		
a. profunda brachii	see brachial artery, deep		
profunda femoris a.	see femoral artery, deep		
profunda linguae a.	see lingual artery, deep		
a. of pterygoid canal vidian a. *a. canalis pterygoidei*	maxillary a. or internal carotid a.	pharyngeal, tubal	sphenoid sinus
pudendal a.'s, external external pudic a.'s *aa. pudendae externae*	femoral a.	anterior scrotal or anterior labial; inguinal	skin of scrotum and perineum in male; labium major in female
pudendal a., internal *a. pudenda interna*	internal iliac a.	muscular, inferior rectal, perineal, artery of the bulb, urethral, deep artery of the penis or clitoris, dorsal artery of the penis or clitoris	penis, scrotum, clitoris, muscles of perineum, anal canal

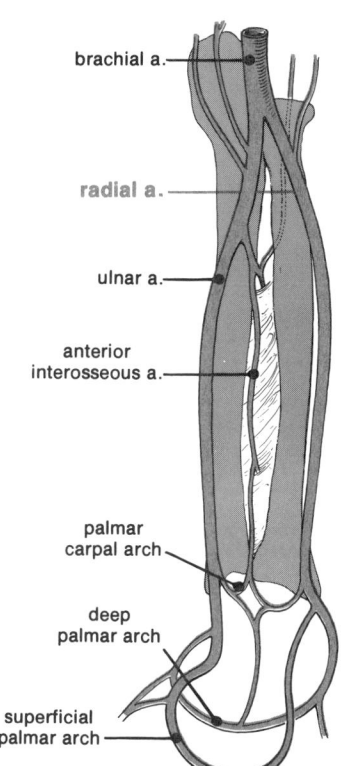

ARTERY	ORIGIN	BRANCHES	DISTRIBUTION
pulmonary a., left *a. pulmonis sinistra*	pulmonary trunk	branches named according to the segment which they supply; e.g., apical segmental, anterior segmental	left lung
pulmonary a., right *a. pulmonis dextra*	pulmonary trunk	branches named according to the segment which they supply; e.g., posterior segmental, apical segmental	right lung
pulmonary trunk *truncus pulmonis*	conus of right ventricle	right and left pulmonary	lungs
radial a. *a. radialis*	brachial a.	*forearm group:* recurrent radial, muscular; *wrist group:* palmar carpal, superficial palmar, dorsal carpal; *hand group:* first dorsal metacarpal, principal a. of thumb, radial a. of index finger, deep palmar arch, palmar metacarpal, perforating, recurrent	muscles of forearm and hand, radius, skin of back of hand and palmar surface of thumb, outer aspect of index finger, intercarpal articulations
radial a. of index finger radialis indicis a. *a. radialis indicis*	radial a.		radial (lateral) side of index finger
radialis indicis a.	see radial artery of index finger		
ranine a.	see lingual artery, deep		
rectal a., inferior inferior hemorrhoidal a. *a. rectalis inferior*	internal pudendal a.		muscles and skin of anal region, rectum, external sphincter muscle
rectal a., middle middle hemorrhoidal a. *a. rectalis media*	internal iliac a.		rectum, prostate, seminal vesicles, vagina
rectal a., superior superior hemorrhoidal a. *a. rectalis superior*	continuation of inferior mesenteric a.	superior rectal artery branches; anastomoses with middle and inferior rectal arteries	rectum
recurrent a., anterior tibial *a. recurrens tibialis anterior*	anterior tibial a.		front and sides of knee joint, anterior tibial muscle
recurrent a., anterior ulnar *a. recurrens ulnaris, ramus anterior*	ulnar a., immediately distal to elbow joint		brachial and round pronator muscles
recurrent a., posterior tibial *a. recurrens tibialis posterior*	anterior tibial a.		tibiofibular joint, knee joint, popliteus muscle

ARTERY	ORIGIN	BRANCHES	DISTRIBUTION
recurrent a., posterior ulnar *a. recurrens ulnaris, ramus posterior*	ulnar a.		elbow joint and neighboring muscles and skin
recurrent a., radial *a. recurrens radialis*	radial a., immediately distal to elbow		elbow joint, supinator, brachioradial, and brachial muscles
recurrent a., ulnar *a. recurrens ulnaris*	ulnar a.	anterior, posterior	brachial and round pronator muscles
renal a. *a. renalis*	abdominal aorta	inferior suprarenal, ureteral, anterior, posterior	kidney, adrenal gland, ureter
retroduodenal a.'s *aa. retroduodenales*	gastroduodenal a., just above level of duodenum	pancreatic, duodenal	first two parts of duodenum, head of pancreas, bile duct
sacral a.'s, lateral *aa. sacrales laterales*	internal iliac	superior and inferior spinal branches	muscles and skin on dorsal surface of sacrum; sacral canal
sacral a., middle *a. sacralis mediana*	dorsal side of aorta, slightly above its bifurcation	middle sacral artery branches; anastomose with lumbar branch of iliolumbar and lateral sacral arteries	rectum, sacrum, coccyx
scapular circumflex a. *a. circumflexa scapulae*	subscapular a.		subscapular, teres major, teres minor, and deltoid muscles; shoulder joint, long head of triceps
scapular a., dorsal *a. scapularis dorsalis*	thyrocervical trunk, transverse cervical a. or subclavian a.	muscular	levator muscle of scapula, trapezius and rhomboid muscles
scapular a., transverse	see suprascapular artery		
sciatic a.	see gluteal artery, inferior		
sigmoid a.'s *aa. sigmoideae*	inferior mesenteric	branches of sigmoid arteries; anatomose cranially with left colic artery and caudally with superior rectal artery	caudal part of descending colon, iliac colon, sigmoid (pelvic colon)
spermatic a., external	see cremasteric artery		
spermatic a.'s, internal	see testicular arteries		
sphenopalatine a. nasopalatine a. *a. sphenopalatina*	maxillary a.	posterior lateral nasal, posterior septal	frontal, maxillary, ethmoidal, and sphenoidal sinuses, nasal septum
spinal a., anterior ventral spinal a. *a. spinalis anterior*	vertebral a. near termination		anterior side of medulla oblongata and spinal cord, filum terminale, meninges
spinal a., posterior dorsal spinal a. *a. spinalis posterior*	posterior inferior cerebellar a. or vertebral a. at side of medulla oblongata	ascending	medulla oblongata, posterior part of spinal cord, and cauda equina, meninges, fourth ventricle
splenic a. lienal a. *a. lienalis*	celiac trunk	pancreatic, short gastric, left gastroomental, splenic, dorsal pancreatic, caudal pancreatic, great pancreatic	spleen, pancreas, stomach, greater omentum
sternocleidomastoid a. sternomastoid a. *a. sternocleidomastoidea*	occipital a. close to its commencement		sternocleidomastoid muscle
stylomastoid a. *a. stylomastoidea*	posterior auricular a.	mastoid, stapedial, posterior tympanic	middle ear chamber, stapes, stapedius muscle, mastoid cells, semicircular canals
subclavian a. *a. subclavia*	*right side:* brachiocephalic trunk; *left side:* arch of aorta	vertebral, thyrocervical, internal thoracic, costocervical, dorsal scapular; it becomes the axillary artery at the outer border of the first rib	neck, thoracic wall, muscles of upper arm and shoulder, spinal cord and brain
subcostal a. twelfth thoracic a. *a. subcostalis*	thoracic aorta	dorsal, spinal	upper abdominal wall below twelfth rib

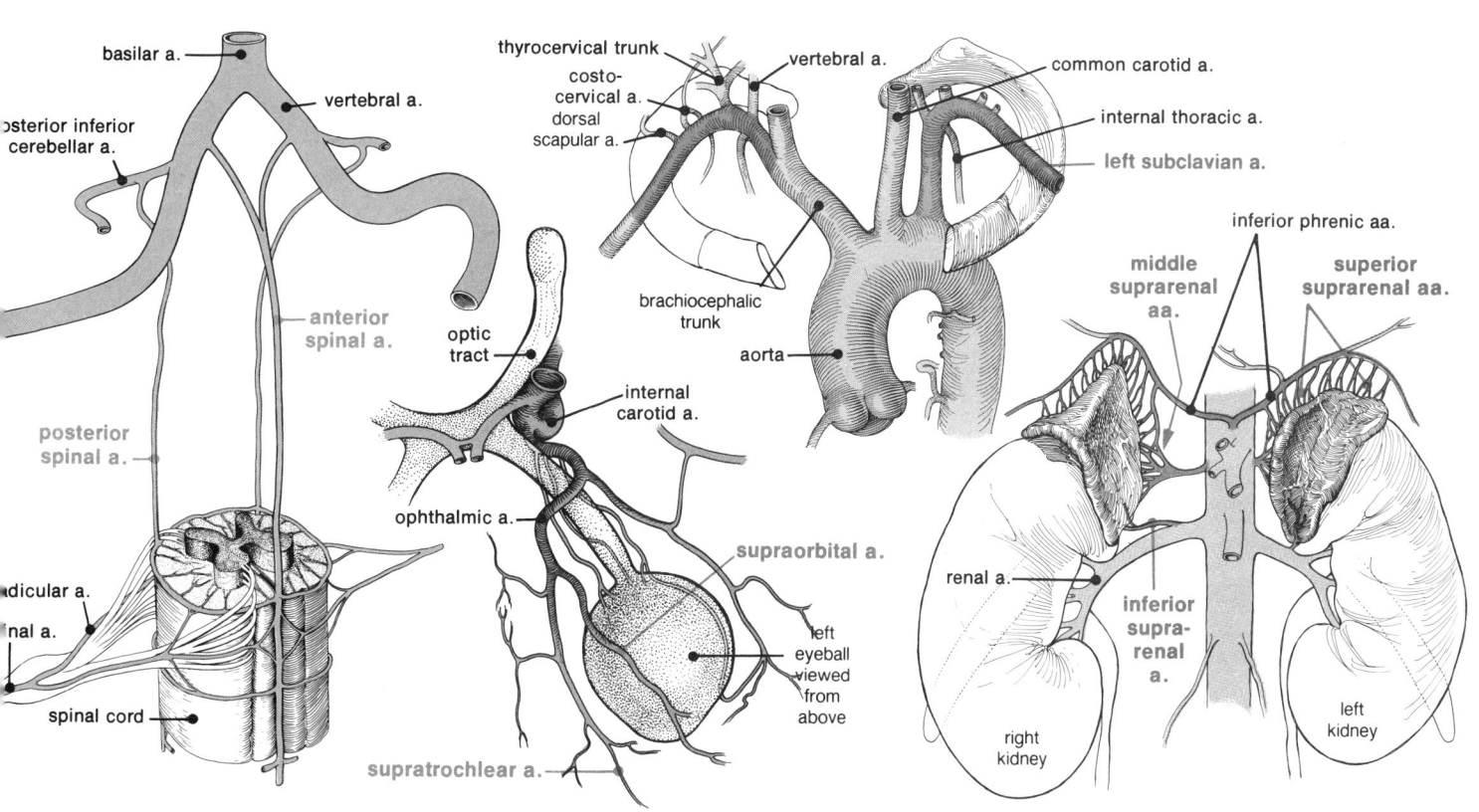

ARTERY	ORIGIN	BRANCHES	DISTRIBUTION
sublingual a. *a. sublingualis*	lingual a.		sublingual gland, mylohyoid, geniohyoid and genioglossus muscles; mucous membrane of mouth and gums
submental a. *a. submentalis*	facial a. (occasionally external maxillary a.)	superficial, deep	mylohyoid, digastric, and platysma muscles: sublingual salivary gland, skin under chin, lip
subscapular a. *a. subscapularis*	axillary a.	circumflex scapular, thoracodorsal	scapular region, shoulder joint
superficial perineal a.		see perineal artery	
supraorbital a. frontal a. *a. supraorbitalis*	ophthalmic a. as it crosses the optic nerve	superficial, deep	skin, muscles, and pericranium of forehead; superior rectus muscle of eyeball, levator muscle of upper eyelid, diplöe
suprarenal a., inferior *a. suprarenalis inferior*	renal a.		adrenal gland
suprarenal a.'s, middle middle capsular a.'s *aa. suprarenales mediae*	abdominal aorta, at level of superior mesenteric a.	anastomoses with suprarenal branches of inferior phrenic and renal arteries	adrenal gland
suprarenal a., superior *a. suprarenalis superior*	inferior phrenic a.		adrenal gland
suprascapular a. transverse scapular a. *a. suprascapularis*	thyrocervical trunk	acromial, suprasternal articular, nutrient	clavicle, scapula, skin of chest, skin over acromion, acromioclavicular and shoulder joints, supraspinous and intraspinous muscles
supratrochlear a. frontal a. *a. supratrochlearis* *a. frontalis*	ophthalmic a.		skin, muscles, and pericranium of forehead
sural a.'s inferior musclar a.'s *aa. surales*	popliteal a. opposite the knee joint		gastrocnemius, soleus, and plantar muscles; neighboring skin
tarsal a., lateral tarsal a. *a. tarsea lateralis*	dorsal a. of foot		muscles and articulations of tarsus

ARTERY	ORIGIN	BRANCHES	DISTRIBUTION
tarsal a.'s, medial *aa. tarseae mediales*	dorsal a. of foot		skin and joints of medial border of foot
temporal a.'s, deep (two in number) *aa. temporales profundae*	maxillary a.		temporal muscle
temporal a., middle *a. temporalis media*	superficial temporal a. immediately above zygomatic arch		temporal muscle
temporal a., superficial *a. temporalis superficialis*	external carotid a.	transverse facial, middle temporal, zygomaticoorbital, anterior auricular, frontal, parietal, parotid	temporal, masseter, frontal, and orbicular muscles; external auditory meatus, auricle, skin of face and scalp, parotid gland, temporomandibular joint
testicular a.'s spermatic a.'s, internal *aa. testiculares*	ventral surface of abdominal aorta, slightly caudal to the renal a.'s	ureteral, epididymal (anastomose with ductus deferens a.)	epididymis, testis, ureter, cremaster muscle
thoracic a., highest *a. thoracica suprema*	axillary a. or thoracoacromial a.		pectoral muscles, parietes of the thorax, anterior serratus and intercostal muscles
thoracic a., internal internal mammary a. *a. thoracica interna*	subclavian a.	pericardiacophrenic, mediastinal, thymic, sternal, anterior intercostal, perforating, musculophrenic, superior epigastric	anterior thoracic wall, diaphragm, structures in mediastinum such as pericardium and thymus gland
thoracic a., lateral long thoracic a. external mammary a. *a. thoracica lateralis*	thoracoacromial, subscapular, or axillary a.	lateral mammary (in female)	pectoral, anterior serratus, and subscapular muscles; axillary lymph nodes, mammary gland (in female)
thoracic a., twelfth		see subcostal artery	
thoracoacromial a. acromiothoracic a. *a. thoracoacromialis*	axillary a.	pectroal, acromial, clavicular, deltoid	pectoral, deltoid, and subclavius muscles; mammary gland, coracoid process, sternoclavicular joint, arcromion
thoracodorsal a. *a. thoracodorsalis*	subscapular a.		subscapular, latissimus dorsi, anterior serratus, and intercostal muscles
thyrocervical trunk *truncus thyrocervicalis*	first portion of subclavian a.	inferior thyroid, suprascapular, transverse cervical	thyroid gland, scapular region, deep neck
thyroid a., inferior *a. thyroidea inferior*	thyrocervical trunk	inferior laryngeal, tracheal, esophageal, ascending cervical, muscular	larynx, trachea, esophagus, thyroid gland, neck muscles
thyroid a., lowest *a. thyroidea ima*	arch of aorta or brachiocephalic trunk		thyroid gland; thymus
thyroid a., superior *a. thyroidea superior*	external carotid a.	infrahyoid, sternocleidomastoid, superior laryngeal, cricothyroid	muscles and mucosa of larynx, pharynx, esophagus; thyroid gland, muscles attached to thyroid cartilage and hyoid bone; sternocleidomastoid and neighboring muscles and integument
tibial a., anterior *a. tibialis anterior*	popliteal a. at bifurcation	posterior tibial recurrent, fibular, anterior tibial recurrent, muscular, anterior medial malleolar, anterior lateral malleolar; continues as dorsal a. of foot at ankle joint	muscles of leg; knee joint, ankle, foot, skin of front of leg
tibial a., posterior *a. tibialis posterior*	popliteal a.	peroneal, nutrient (tibial), muscular, posterior medial malleolar, communicating, medial calcaneal, medial plantar, lateral plantar	muscles and bones of leg; ankle joint, foot
tibial recurrent a., anterior *a. recurrens tibialis anterior*	anterior tibial a.		anterior tibial muscle, knee joint, patella, long extensor muscle of toes
tibial recurrent a., posterior *a. recurrens tibialis posterior*	anterior tibial a.		popliteal muscle, knee joint, tibiofibular joint

ARTERY	ORIGIN	BRANCHES	DISTRIBUTION
tympanic a., anterior tympanic a. *a. tympanica anterior*	maxillary a.	posterior, superior, ossicular	tympanic membrane, middle ear chamber, ossicles
tympanic a., inferior *a. tympanica inferior*	ascending pharyngeal a.		medial wall of the middle ear chamber
tympanic a., posterior *a. tympanica posterior*	stylomastoid a.	mastoid, stapedial	middle ear chamber, posterior part of tympanic membrane
tympanic a., superior *a. tympanica superior*	middle meningeal a.	frontal, parietal	middle ear chamber, tensor tympani muscle
ulnar a. *a. ulnaris*	brachial a., slightly distal to elbow	*forearm portion:* anterior ulnar recurrent, posterior ulnar recurrent, common interosseous, muscular; *wrist portion:* palmar carpal, dorsal carpal; *hand portion:* deep palmar, superficial palmar arch, common palmar digital	hand, wrist, forearm
umbilical a. *a. umbilicalis*	internal iliac a.	ductus deferens, superior vesical; continues as lateral umbilical ligament	urinary bladder, ureter, testes, seminal vesicles, ductus deferens
urethral a. *a. urethralis*	internal pudendal		urethra, corpus cavernosum of penis
uterine a. fallopian a. *a. uterina*	medial surface of internal iliac	cervical, ovarian, tubal, vaginal, ligamentous, ureteric	uterus, uterine tube, round ligament, part of vagina, ovary
vaginal a. *a. vaginalis*	internal iliac a. or uterine a.	rectal, vesical, vestibular	vagina, fundus of urinary bladder and part of rectum, vestibular bulb
vertebral a. *a. vertebralis*	subclavian a.	*cervical portion:* spinal, muscular; *cranial portion:* meningeal, posterior spinal, anterior spinal, posterior inferior cerebellar, medullary	bodies of vertebrae, deep muscles of neck, falx cerebelli, spinal cord, cerebellum, brain stem
vesical a., inferior *a. vesicalis inferior*	internal iliac a.		fundus of bladder, prostate, seminal vesicles
vesical a.'s, superior *aa. vesicales superior*	umbilical a.		ureter, bladder, urachus
vidian a.	see pterygoid canal, artery of		
zygomaticoorbital a. *a. zygomatico-orbitalis*	superficial temporal a. (occasionally from the middle temporal a.)		orbicular muscle of eye

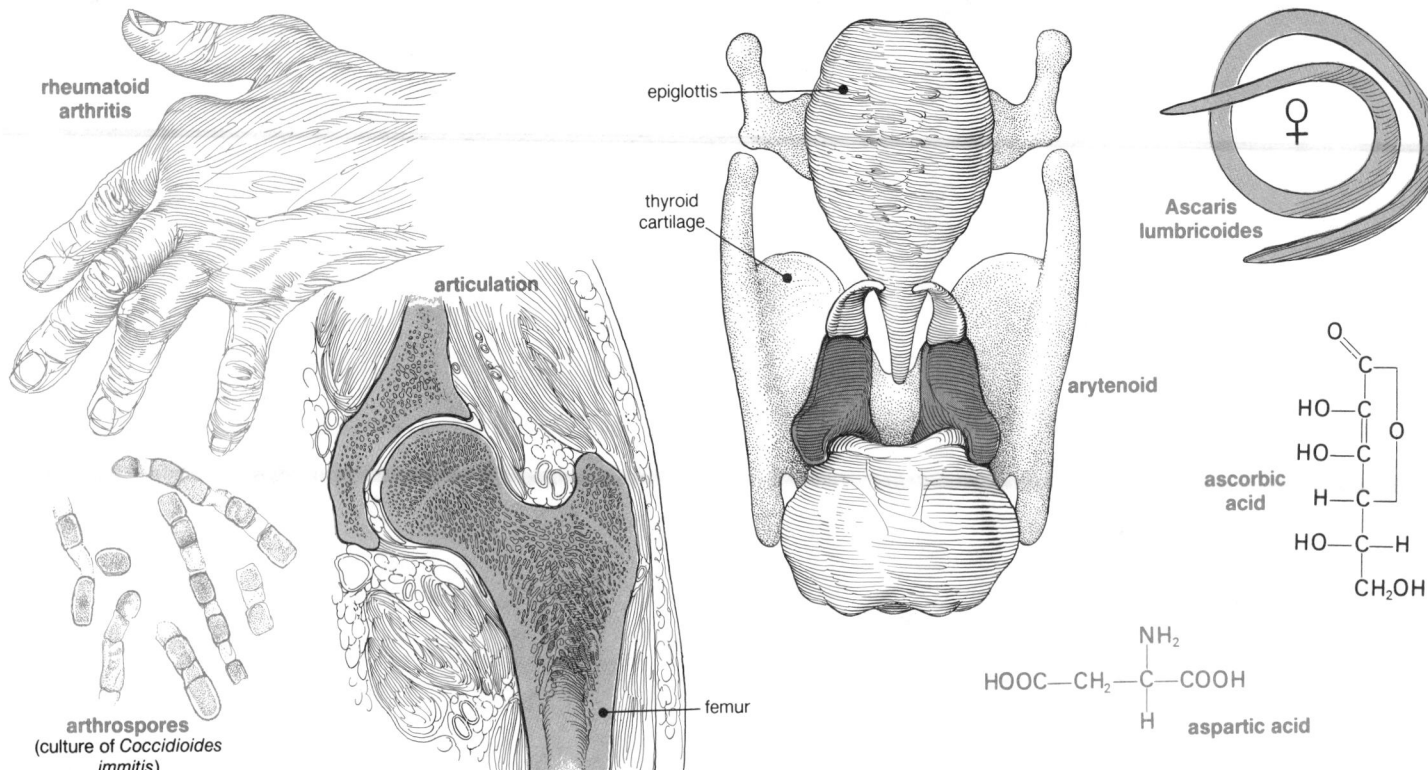

rheumatoid arthritis

articulation

epiglottis

thyroid cartilage

arytenoid

femur

arthrospores
(culture of *Coccidioides immitis*)

Ascaris lumbricoides

$$HO-\underset{H}{\overset{O}{\underset{|}{C}}}$$

ascorbic acid

aspartic acid

$$HOOC-CH_2-\underset{\underset{H}{|}}{\overset{\overset{NH_2}{|}}{C}}-COOH$$

arthralgia   Pain in a joint. Also called arthrodynia.
arthrectomy   Removal of a joint.
arthritic   Relating to or suffering from arthritis.
arthritis   Inflammation of the joints.
   atrophic a.   Rheumatoid arthritis.
   degenerative a.   See degenerative joint disease.
   gonococcal a.   A form associated with gonorrhea, involving one or several joints, especially of the knees, ankles, and wrists; *Neisseria gonorrhoeae* can be isolated from the joint fluid.
   hypertrophic a.   See degenerative joint disease.
   juvenile rheumatoid a.   (JRA) An uncommon, crippling disease of children involving the large joints and cervical spine with enlargement of lymph nodes, liver, and spleen. Also called Still's disease.
   rheumatoid a.   (RA) Chronic disease of unknown cause involving most connective tissues of the body with predilection for small joints, especially those of the fingers; marked by proliferative inflammation of the synovial membranes leading to deformity, ankylosis, and invalidism. Also called atrophic arthritis; chronic proliferative arthritis.
   suppurative a.   Purulent infection involving, as a rule, a single large joint; caused by any of several microorganisms, especially *Streptococcus hemolyticus*, *Staphylococcus aureus*, pneumococcus, and meningococcus; it usually follows injury to the affected joint. Also called pyogenic arthritis.
   syphilitic a.   Condition characterized by: (a) mild chronic effusion into the knee joints (Clutton's joints) occurring during puberty in congenital syphilis; (b) painful, stiff, tender joints with transient swelling occurring with secondary syphilis; inflammation of adjacent periosteum usually occurs.
   tuberculous a.   Arthritis caused by the tubercle bacillus; usually mono-articular, involving any joint in the body, especially the knee, hip, and spine, with destruction of contiguous bone.
arthrocentesis   Puncture of a joint followed by the withdrawal of fluid, usually by suction through the puncture needle.
arthrodesis   Surgical fixation of a joint. Also called artificial ankylosis.
arthrodia   A joint that permits a gliding motion, as between the articular processes of the vertebrae. Also called gliding joint.
arthrodial   Relating to arthrodia.
arthrodynia   Arthralgia.
arthrodysplasia   Malformation of a joint or joints.
arthrogram   X-ray image of a joint.
arthrography   1. Roentgenography of a joint. 2. A treatise on joints.
arthrogryposis   Permanent or persistent flexure of a joint.

   a. multiplex congenita   Congenital contraction of several joints of the extremities.
arthronosos   Disease of the joints.
arthropathy   Any disease of the joints.
   diabetic a.   Arthrosis occurring in diabetes as a result of disease of the trophic nerves innervating the joint.
   neuropathic a.   Any joint disease having a nervous origin.
   tabetic a.   A form of neuropathic joint disease marked by chronic, progressive degeneration and enlargement of a joint, with effusion of fluids into the synovial space. Also called Charcot's disease.
arthroplasty   Surgical restoration of joint function, either by repairing damaged joint surfaces or by inserting an artificial joint.
arthropod   Any of several invertebrate animals (phylum Arthropoda) having a segmented external covering and jointed limbs; e.g., scorpions, crabs, centipedes.
arthropyosis   The production of pus within a joint. Also called arthro-empyesis.
arthroscope   Instrument used to view the interior of a joint and correct certain abnormalities.
arthroscopy   Direct visualization of a joint, such as the knee joint, by means of an arthroscope.
arthrosis   1. A joint. 2. A degenerative condition of a joint.
arthrospore   A sporelike cell produced by the fragmentation of any part of the segmented filamentous mycelium, as seen in *Coccidioides immitis*.
arthrosynovitis   Inflammation of the synovial membrane of a joint.
arthrotomy   Incision into a joint.
articular   Relating to an articulation or a joint.
articulate   1. To unite or connect by means of a joint. 2. To utter distinct speech sounds. 3. Having joints; jointed. 4. Capable of speaking in clear, expressive language.
articulation   1. A joint, as between bones. 2. The process of producing a speech sound.
artifact   Anything that has been artificially changed from its normal state, as a histologic tissue that has been mechanically altered.
arytenoid   1. One of a pair of small pyramidal cartilages situated in the back of the larynx. 2. Relating to the arytenoid cartilages.
arytenoidectomy   Surgical removal of an arytenoid cartilage in the larynx.
asbestos   An incombustible fibrous mineral form of magnesium and calcium silicate.
asbestosis   Fibrosis of the lungs caused by prolonged inhalation of asbestos particles and resulting in chronic shortness of breath; a pneumoconiosis.
ascariasis   Infestation with the large roundworm

Ascaris lumbricalis, characterized by a larval pulmonary stage and an adult intestinal stage.
ascaridiasis   Ascariasis.
Ascaris   A genus of roundworms (order Nematoda) that are intestinal parasites.
   A. lumbricoides   A species, reddish and tapered at both ends, found in the small intestines, especially of children.
ascites   Accumulation of free serous fluid in the abdominal cavity in clinically detectable amounts, seen sometimes as a result of cirrhosis of the liver, kidney disease, intraabdominal cancer, and severe congestive heart failure. Also called hydroperitoneum; abdominal dropsy.
ascitic   Relating to ascites.
ascomycete   Any of numerous fungi that contain spore-producing saclike structures (asci).
ascorbic acid   A white crystalline substance, $C_6H_8O_6$; found in citrus fruits, green leafy vegetables, and tomatoes; used in the treatment and/or prevention of scurvy. Also called vitamin C.
asepsis   Absence of disease-causing microorganisms.
aseptic   Not septic; free of contamination.
aseptic necrosis   See under necrosis.
asexual   Without sex.
asialia   Lack of saliva.
asparaginase   An enzyme that promotes the breakdown of asparagine to aspartic acid and ammonia; has been used to treat acute leukemia.
asparagine   (Asn) A nonessential amino acid found in asparagus shoots and other plants.
aspartame   A nutritive sweetener composed of two amino acids; approximately 180 times sweeter than sucrose (table sugar).
aspartase   An enzyme that promotes the conversion of aspartic acid to fumaric acid.
aspartic acid   (Asp) A nonessential amino acid found mostly in sugar cane and sugar-beet molasses.
aspergilloma   A mass of fungus mycelium in a pulmonary cavity (intracavitary fungus ball) caused by fungi of the genus *Aspergillus*.
aspergillosis   Infection of the lungs and bronchi with *Aspergillus* fungi; usually affects debilitated patients; may also occur as an allergic reaction.
Aspergillus   A genus of fungi (family Ascomycetes); it contains several disease-causing species.
aspermatogenic   Failing to produce spermatozoa.
asphygmia   Temporary absence of pulse.
asphyxia   Suffocation due to interference with the oxygen supply of the blood.
   a. neonatorum   Asphyxia occurring in the newborn.
asphyxiant   Anything that causes asphyxia or suf-

aspiration

astrocytes

fibrous type

protoplasmic type

bladder

aspirator

uterus

vagina

sagittal section of adult female pelvis

anterior asynclitism

posterior asynclitism

focation.

asphyxiate 1. To cause asphyxia. 2. To undergo asphyxia; to suffocate.

asphyxiation Asphyxia.

aspidium The rhizome and leaf of the male fern (*Dryopteris filix-mas*); formerly used in the treatment of tapeworm infestation.

aspirate To remove fluid from a bodily cavity by means of a suction device.

aspiration 1. Intake of foreign material into the lungs during the act of breathing. 2. Withdrawal, by suction, with an aspirator of fluid or gases from a body cavity.

aspirator An instrument for removing fluids from a body cavity by suction.

aspirin Common name for acetylsalicylic acid.

asporogenous Not propagating by spores.

assay 1. Analysis of a substance to determine its purity, potency, weight, etc. 2. To examine.

assimilate To consume and incorporate into the tissues.

assimilation The process of converting food substances into tissues.

association Relationship between persons or ideas.

astasia Inability to stand, in the absence of organic disorders.

asteatosis Condition marked by deficient activity of the sebaceous glands.

  a. cutis Dry-scaly skin with scanty sebaceous gland secretion.

aster See astrosphere.

astereognosis Failure to recognize objects or to appreciate their form by feeling them. Also called stereoanesthesia.

asterion A craniometric point on either side of the skull at the junction of the lambdoid, occipitomastoid, and parietomastoid sutures.

asterixis A flapping movement or tremor, best seen in the outstretched hands, characteristic of certain metabolic disorders, particularly hepatic coma. Also called liver flap.

asthenia Loss of strength; weakness.

  neurocirculatory a. Condition marked by breathlessness, palpitation, chest pain, giddiness, and fatigue, in absence of organic heart disease.

asthenocoria Sluggish reaction of the pupil to light stimulus.

asthenopia General term denoting distress arising from the use of the eyes. See also eyestrain.

asthenospermia Reduction of motility of spermatozoa.

asthma Disease characterized by an increased responsiveness of the trachea and bronchi to various stimuli, manifested by recurrent attacks of widespread narrowing of the airways, difficult breathing, wheezing, and cough; most commonly an allergic reaction to some extrinsic allergen or may be triggered by infection (infectious asthma), or associated with emotional stress.

  allergic a. The common form of asthmas characterized by spasm of the muscular walls of the small bronchial tubes, with swelling and edema of the mucous membrane; believed to be an allergic reaction.

  atopic a. Allergic asthma.

episode, caused by pulmonary congestion secondary to left heart failure.

  intrinsic a. Asthma caused by an endogenous disturbance rather than by environmental factors.

  spasmodic a. A form of asthma caused by spasm of the bronchioles.

astigmatic Relating to or marked by astigmatism.

astigmatism 1. Faulty vision caused by imperfections in the curvature of the cornea which prevent light rays from focusing at a single point on the retina; instead they are focused separately; occasionally due to defects in the curvature of the lens of the eye; may accompany myopia or hyperopia. 2. In an electron-beam tube, a focus defect in which electrons from a single source point of a specimen come to focus at different points; the main cause of image deterioration in electron microscopy. 3. A refractive defect of an optical system, such as a lens or mirror, that prevents sharp focusing.

astigmometer, astigmatometer An instrument for measuring the degree of astigmatism.

astragalus See talus.

astrapophobia A morbid fear of lightning.

astringent 1. Causing contraction of the tissues and arresting discharges. 2. An agent that produces such an effect.

astroblast An immature astrocyte.

astroblastoma A relatively rare, rapidly growing brain tumor made up of astroblasts; two-thirds of cases occur in the cerebrum of middle-aged adults; the cerebellum is the second most frequent site.

astrocele Centrosphere.

astrocyte The largest neuroglial cell having a star-shaped cell body with numerous processes radiating outward; many of the processes end on blood vessels as perivascular feet.

astrocytoma A non-capsulated brain tumor arising from astrocytes.

astrocytosis An increase in the number of astrocytes; usually occurring close to degenerative lesions, abscesses, or brain tumors.

astroglia A cell of non-neuronal tissue (neuroglia cell) consisting of a small body and several long straight processes.

astrokinetic Relating to the movements of the centrosome in a dividing cell.

astrosphere A group of fibrillar cytoplasmic rays extending outward from the centrosome and centrosphere of a dividing cell. Also called aster; attraction sphere.

asymmetry Dissimilarity in corresponding parts.

asymptomatic Free of symptoms.

asynclitism In obstetrics, state in which the fetal head does not lie exactly between the sacral promontory and symphysis but is deflected either anteriorly, near the symphysis, or posteriorly, near the promontory, with its occipitofrontal plane oblique to any given maternal pelvic plane. Formerly called obliquity.

  anterior a., anterior parietal presentation Deflection of the fetal head posteriorly; the sagittal suture approaches the sacral promontory and the anterior parietal bone presents itself to the examining fingers. Formerly called Nägele's obliquity.

  posterior a., posterior parietal presentation Deflection of the fetal head anteriorly; the sagittal suture lies close to the symphysis and the posterior parietal bone presents itself to the examining fingers. Formerly called Litzmann's obliquity.

asynergia, asynergy Lack of coordination among the parts that normally work together.

asystole Absence of muscular contractions of the heart.

atactilia Lack of the sense of touch.

ataractic Tranquilizing; said of some drugs.

ataraxia Emotional tranquility.

atavism The reappearance of a trait in an individual after being absent for several generations.

ataxia Lack of muscular coordination.

  a. telangiectasia Hereditary progressive cerebellar ataxia associated with recurrent pulmonary infections and ocular and cutaneous telangiectases (permanent dilatation of capillaries and small arteries).

  cerebellar a. Ataxia resulting from disease of the cerebellum.

  Friedreich's a., hereditary spinal a. Hereditary disease occurring in children, marked by degeneration of the dorsal and lateral columns of the spinal cord, attended by progressive ataxia, nystagmus, and absence or diminution of deep tendon reflexes.

  vasomotor a. Disorder of the vasomotor centers, causing spasm of the smaller blood vessels.

atelectasis A shrunken and airless state of the lung, or a portion of it, due to failure of expansion or resorption of air from the alveoli; it may be acute or chronic, complete or incomplete.

  primary a. Failure of the lungs to expand ade-

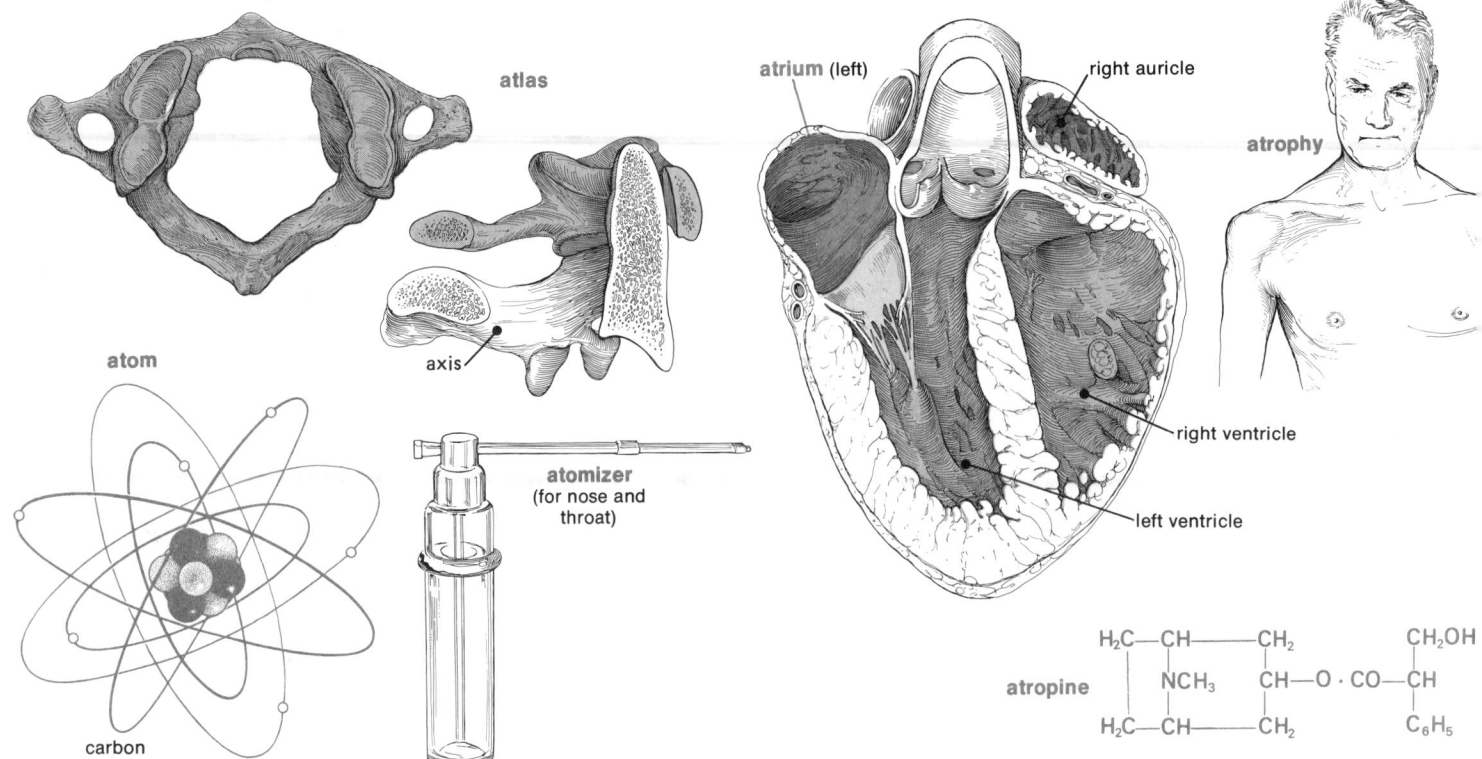

atlas

atom

carbon

axis

atomizer
(for nose and
throat)

atrium (left)

right auricle

atrophy

right ventricle

left ventricle

atropine

$$H_2C-CH-\!\!\!-\!\!\!-CH_2 \qquad\qquad CH_2OH$$
$$\qquad\quad NCH_3 \qquad CH-O\cdot CO-CH$$
$$H_2C-CH-\!\!\!-\!\!\!-CH_2 \qquad\qquad C_6H_5$$

quately after birth; may be due to fetal hypoxia, prematurity, excessive intrapulmonary secretions, or intercurrent pneumonia; lack of surfactant, especially in premature infants, is a prime cause.

secondary a. Pulmonary collapse, especially of infants, due primarily to hyaline membrane disease.

ateliosis Incomplete development. Also called infantilism.

atelognathia Defective development of the lower jaw.

Atgam Anti-thymocyte gammaglobulin; used to suppress the immune response in organ transplantation.

atheroembolism Cholesterol and debris released from ulcerated plaques of a large artery, carried in the bloodstream and lodged in small arteries.

atherogenesis The formation of atheroma in the arterial walls.

atherogenic Having the capacity to contribute to the formulation of atheroma.

atheroma A degenerative cholesterol-containing plaque in the inner layer of an artery.

atheromatous Relating to atheroma.

atherosclerosis A form of arteriosclerosis marked by the deposition of lipids in the inner layer of arterial walls, resulting in the formation of elevated fatty-fibrous plaques (atheromas); the process usually begins during the first two decades of life and increases in severity with the rising age level.

athetoid Resembling athetosis.

athetosis Condition marked by constant, slow, involuntary writhing movements of the hands, fingers, and sometimes the feet.

athlete's foot See tinea pedis.

athrepsia Marasmus.

athymia 1. Lack of emotion. 2. Absence of the thymus.

athyroidism Condition caused by absence, or deficient functioning, of the thyroid gland.

athyrosis Athyroidism.

atlantoaxial Relating to the atlas and the axis; as the articulation of these two vertebrae.

atlanto-occipital Relating to the atlas and the occipital bone.

atlanto-odontoid Relating to the atlas (first cervical vertebra) and the odontoid process of the axis (second cervical vertebra).

atlas The first cervical vertebra articulating with the occipital bone above and the second vertebra (axis) below.

atmos A unit of air pressure equal to one dyne per cm². Also called aer.

atmosphere 1. The layer of gases surrounding the earth; composed of 20.94% oxygen, 0.04% carbon dioxide, 78.03% nitrogen, and 0.99% inert gases. 2.

A unit of air pressure.

atocia Sterility in the female.

atom The smallest chemical unit, consisting of a cloud of electrons moving rapidly around a positively charged, dense, central nucleus composed of protons and neutrons; an atom is classified by the number of protons (proton or atomic number, Z) and the number of neutrons (neutron number, N) contained in its nucleus.

atomicity 1. The state of being composed of atoms. 2. The number of replaceable atoms or groups in the molecule of a substance.

atomization The process of reducing a fluid to a spray.

atomizer A device for delivering a liquid as a fine spray.

atonia See atony.

atonic Lacking normal tone or strength; said of a muscle.

atony Lack of normal tone. Also called atonia.

uterine a. Loss of muscular tone of the uterus, which may result in failure of progress of labor or postpartum hemorrhage.

atopic Displaced; not in the usual or normal place.

atopognosis, atopognosia Inability to localize tactile stimuli; loss of ability to correctly locate a sensation.

atopy Denoting an allergy characteristic of humans and tending to be inherited; e.g., hay fever, asthma.

atresia Absence or closure of a normal body opening or canal.

a. ani Imperforate anus.

biliary a. A condition of infants who are born without functioning bile ducts; unless they receive a liver transplant, these children usually die after several years because of resultant cirrhosis.

esophageal a. Congenital failure of the full esophageal lumen to develop.

tricuspid a. Absence of the opening between the right atrium and right ventricle.

atresic Imperforate; lacking an opening.

atretoblepharia Symblepharon.

atrial Relating to an atrium.

atrichia Congenital or acquired absence of hair.

atrichosis Atrichia.

atriomegaly Enlargement of an atrium.

atrioseptopexy A heart operation to correct a defect in the interatrial septum.

atriotomy Surgical incision of an atrium.

atrioventricular Relating to both an atrium and ventricle of the heart.

atrium 1. One of the two (right and left) upper chambers of the heart; after birth, in the normal human the right atrium receives blood from the vena cavae and the left atrium receives blood from

the pulmonary veins; the blood passes from each atrium to the respective ventricle. 2. A shallow depression in the nasal cavity; the anterior extension of the middle meatus, located above the vestibule.

Atropa A genus of herbs (family Solanacea).

A. belladonna A poisonous plant, commonly called nightshade, from which belladonna and atropine are derived.

atrophia Atrophy.

a. cutis See atrophoderma.

atrophic Characterized by atrophy.

atrophied Wasted; shrunken.

atrophoderma Atrophy of the skin. Also called atrophia cutis.

a. pigmentosum See xeroderma pigmentosum.

a. senile The characteristic dry condition of the skin in old age.

atrophy A wasting, progressive degeneration and loss of function of any part of the body.

Leber's hereditary optic a. A hereditary condition of rapid onset, affecting primarily young adult males; marked by bilateral degeneration of the optic disk occasionally involving only the papillomacular bundle. Also called Leber's disease.

peroneal muscular a. A hereditary disorder appearing during adolescence or adulthood; marked by degeneration of peripheral nerves and roots, resulting in weakness and wasting of the distal muscles of the extremities, especially the legs; the wasting does not extend above the elbows or above the middle third of the thighs. Also called Charcot-Marie-Tooth disease.

Pick's a. Localized atrophy of the cerebral cortex.

progressive muscular a. An inheritable disease, transmitted as an autosomal recessive trait, with an early onset and a progressive course; marked by degeneration of the anterior horn cells of the spinal cord, resulting in wasting and paralysis of the muscles of the extremities and trunk. Also called Duchenne-Aran disease.

atropine An alkaloid with antimuscarinic actions obtained from *Atropa belladonna*; used to dilate the pupil, as an antispasmodic, and to inhibit gastric secretion; other effects include inhibition of salivary, bronchial, and sweat secretion, increase in heart rate, and inhibition of the urinary bladder.

atropinism Poisoning caused by an overdose of belladonna derivatives (atropine and scopolamine) or by accidental ingestion of plants such as jimson weed.

attachment 1. A device by which something is stabilized. 2. In dentistry, a mechanical device for the fixation of a dental prosthesis, such as a clasp, retainer, or cap.

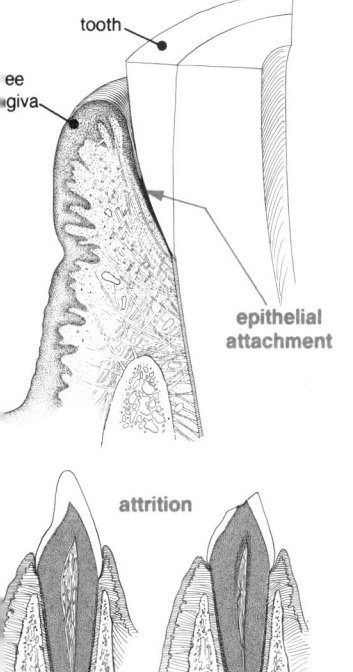

tooth

ee giva

epithelial attachment

attrition

Hertz (Hz)
decibels (dB)

x left ear
o right ear

audiogram illustrating average hearing (top two lines), a mild conductive hearing loss (middle two lines) and a severe hearing loss (bottom two lines)

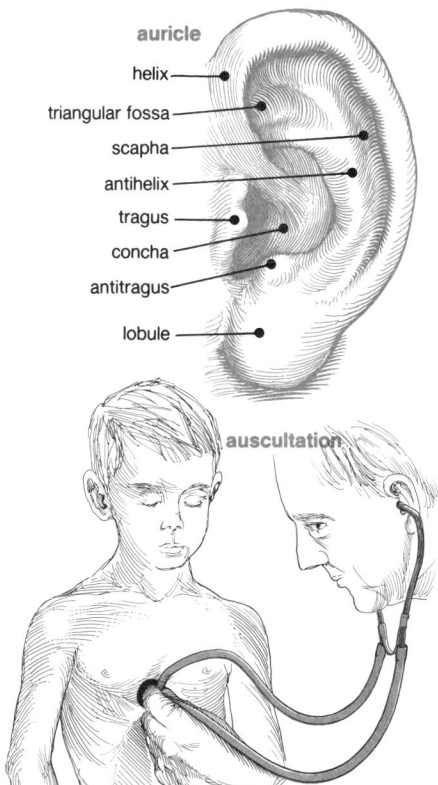

auricle
helix
triangular fossa
scapha
antihelix
tragus
concha
antitragus
lobule

auscultation

epithelial a. A collar of epithelial cells which adheres to the tooth, at the base of the gingival sulcus, and is continuous with the free marginal gingiva.

precision a. A device used in fixed and removable partial dentures, consisting of closely fitting male and female parts; the precise retention of the denture depends upon resistance between parallel walls of the two parts forming the attachment. Also called internal, key-and-keyway, parallel, or slotted attachment.

attack The occurrence or establishment of a destructive process.

drop a. Sudden falling without warning.

heart a. Occlusion of an artery supplying the heart, usually accompanied by pain and frequently by irritability of the myocardium and/or congestive heart failure. See also myocardial infarction; coronary thrombosis.

panic a. Intense fear, sweating, dizziness, chest pains, and trembling occurring in nonthreatening settings.

transient ischemic a. (TIA) Episode of neurologic dysfunction without permanent damage, commonly lasting from a few seconds to 10 minutes, caused by insufficient blood supply to a specific part of the brain; an episode persisting 24 hours or more is considered more likely to be a stroke.

vagal a. Condition characterized by slow pulse, labored breathing, and sometimes convulsions.

attenuant Any agent that: (a) dilutes a fluid, (b) rarifies a gas, (c) reduces the virulence of a pathogenic microorganism, or (d) reduces the strength of a drug.

attenuation 1. Dilution or weakening. 2. Reduction of virulence of a microorganism.

attraction The force acting between two bodies that draws them together.

capillary a. The force that causes a fluid to move up and along a fine, hairlike tube.

chemical a. The force causing atoms of different elements to unite.

magnetic a. The force that tends to draw iron and steel toward a magnet and resist their separation.

neurotropic a. The tendency of a regenerating axon to direct itself toward the motor end-plate.

attrition 1. Wearing away by friction. 2. In dentistry, the normal wearing away of the biting surfaces of teeth due to mastication.

atypical Differing from the normal or usual type; not typical.

audiogenic 1. Sound producing. 2. Caused by sound.

audiogram A chart plotted from the results of hearing tests with the audiometer.

audiology The study and measaurement of hearing and the treatment of deafness.

audiometer An instrument for determining the acuity of hearing.

audiometry The measuring of hearing acuity with the audiometer.

Bekesy a. Testing of hearing with the audiometer while the patient controls the intensity of the tone.

audition 1. The sense of hearing. 2. The act of hearing.

auditory Relating to the special sense of hearing.

aura The peculiar sensation that precedes an epileptic seizure, recognized by the individual.

auditory a. Noises or buzzing in the ears sometimes heard by a patient prior to an epileptic attack.

olfactory a. Olfactory sensation which sometimes precedes an epileptic seizure.

visual a. Flashes of light sometimes seen by an individual immediately prior to an attack of epilepsy.

aural 1. Relating to the ear. 2. Relating to an aura.

auriasis See chrysiasis.

auric Relating to gold.

auricle 1. External portion of the ear. Also called pinna. 2. Pouchlike appendage projecting from the upper anterior portion of each atrium of the heart.

auricular 1. Relating to the ear. 2. Relating to an auricle of the heart.

auriculoventricular Atrioventricular.

auris *pl.* **aures** Latin for ear.

a. dextra (A.D.) right ear.

a. sinistra (A.S.) left ear.

aures unitas (A.U.) both ears.

auscult To auscultate.

auscultate To examine the chest or abdomen by listening.

auscultation The act of listening to the sounds made by the internal organs for diagnostic purposes.

auscultatory Of or relating to auscultation.

autism Emotional disturbance characterized by morbid self-absorption and inability to relate to other people, usually diagnosed in early childhood (early infantile autism).

autistic Morbidly self-centered.

autoagglutination The spontaneous clumping together or agglutination of red blood cells.

autoagglutinin A serum factor that causes the individual's own cellular elements (red blood cells, platelets, etc.) to agglutinate.

autoanalysis Attempted analysis, or psychoanalysis, of oneself. Also called self-analysis.

autoantibody Antibody that is produced in, and reacts with, an antigen in the same person or animal.

cold a. An antibody that reacts at zero to 5°C.

warm a. An antibody that reacts best at 37°C.

autoantigen An antigen that incites the production of autoantibodies.

autocatalysis A reaction that gradually accelerates due to the catalytic property of one of the products of the reaction.

autoclave 1. A container used for sterilization by pressured steam. 2. To sterilize in an autoclave.

autocrine Denoting a mode of hormone action whereby the hormone binds to receptors on the cell that produced it, affecting the function of that cell.

autodigestion Degeneration of tissues due to separation from blood supply; applied especially to spontaneous digestion of the walls of the stomach after death. Also called autolysis; self-digestion.

autoerotism, autoeroticism Self-arousal and self-gratification of sexual desire.

autogamy A process of fertilization within the cell, as in certain protozoans; the nucleus divides, giving rise to two pronuclei which immediately unite.

autogenous 1. Self-producing. 2. Having its origin within the body.

autograft Autogenous graft; see under graft.

autohemolysin An antibody that acts upon the red blood cells of the individual in whose blood it was formed.

autohemolysis Destruction of the red blood cells of an individual by the action of hemolytic agents in his blood.

autohemotherapy Treatment by withdrawal and injection of the person's own blood.

autohypnosis Self-induced hypnosis. Also called self-hypnosis.

autoimmune disease Any disease characterized by tissue injury caused by an apparent immunologic reaction of the host with his own tissues; distinguished from autoimmune response, with which it may or may not be associated.

autoimmunize To immunize an individual against his own antigens.

autoinfection Infection with organisms already present in the body. Also called self-infection.

autoinoculation The spread of an infection from one site of the body to another.

autointoxication A condition caused by absorption of waste products or any toxin produced by the body.

autologous Related to self; derived from the subject itself.

autology Study of one's own self.

autolysis See autodigestion.

autolyze To cause the disintegration of tissues or cells within the organism in which the autolyzing agent is produced.

1	2	3	4	5	6	7	8
9	10	11	12	13	14	15	16
17	18	19	20	21	22	XX	

autosomes

augmented limb leads

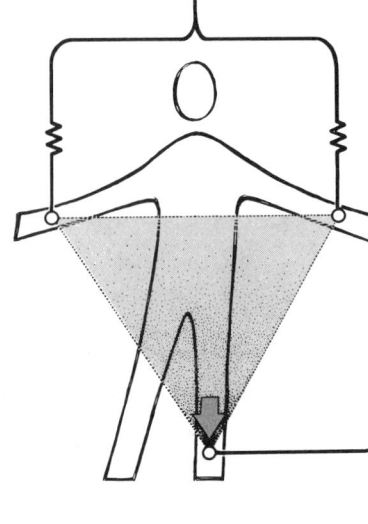

aVR

aVL

aVF

automatism 1. Involuntary or automatic action. 2. A condition in which activity is carried out by the patient without his conscious knowledge, often inappropriate to circumstances.

autonomic Independent; self-controlling.

autopepsia Self-digestion, as of the gastric mucosa by its own secretion.

autopsy Examination of a dead body, usually to determine the cause of death. Also called necropsy; postmortem diagnosis or examination.

autoradiograph Image on photographic film produced by the emission of radioactive substances in tissues, showing the location and relative concentration of these substances; made by placing the structure in close contact with photographic emulsion. Also called radioautograph.

autoradiography A cytochemical procedure for localizing sites of radioactivity within tissue sections.

autoregulation The intricate adaptive mechanisms that maintain a relatively constant blood flow to an organ despite changes in arterial pressure.

autosensitize To develop sensitivity to one's own serum or tissue.

autosome Any member of the 22 pairs of nonsex chromosomes.

autotopagnosia The impaired recognition of any part of the body; may occur with lesions of the posteroinferior portion of the parietal lobe.

autotoxic Marked by autointoxication.

autotoxin Any poison acting upon the body from which it originates.

autotransfusion Transfusion of the patient's own blood.

autotransplantation The transferring of tissue from one part of the patient's body to another.

autovaccination Vaccination with vaccine prepared from the patient's own body.

autoxidation, auto-oxidation The spontaneous combination of a substance with oxygen at ordinary temperatures and without a catalyst, as in the rusting of iron.

auxotroph A mutant microorganism that can be cultivated only by supplementing a minimal medium with growth factors or amino acids, not required by wild-type strains.

avascular Without blood vessels, normally or otherwise.

aVF One of three unipolar augmented limb leads. See lead.

avirulent Not virulent; not causing disease.

avitaminosis Any condition caused by deficiency of one or more vitamins in the diet.

aVL One of three unipolar augmented limb leads. See lead.

avoirdupois A system of weight measurements in which 16 ounces make a pound, one ounce contains 16 drachms, and one drachm equals approximately 27.3 grains; one pound in this system contains 7000 troy grains or 453.6 grams; used for the British Pharmacopia prior to the introduction of metric weights.

aVR One of three unipolar augmented limb leads. See lead.

external border
of greater pectoral
muscle

clavicle

humerus

axilla

scapula

smaller pectoral
muscle

odontoid
process

atlas

left
hipbone

coccyx

pelvic
axis

ischium

lens of eye

cornea

optic
axis

visual
line

spinous
process

axis

neurilemma

myelin

node of Ranvier

axoplasm

axon

neurofibril

axolemma

avulsion   Pulling or tearing away; forcible separation.

axenic   Germ free, said of animals reared in a bacteria-free environment; denoting a pure culture.

axial   **1.** Relating to or forming an axis. **2.** In dentistry, relating to the long axis of a tooth. **3.** Relating to or situated in the central part of the head, neck, and trunk. **4.** Denoting a region of the body that includes the head, neck, and trunk.

axilla   The pyramidal region at the junction of the arm and the chest; it contains the axillary vessels, lymphatics, brachial plexus, and muscles. Also called armpit.

axillary   Of or relating to the axilla (armpit).

axis *pl.* **axes**   **1.** The second cervical vertebra. Also called epistropheus. **2.** Any of the imaginary lines used as points of reference, about which a body or a part may rotate. **3.** Any of various centrally located structures, as the notochord of the embryo.

   electrical a.   The direction of the electromotive forces originating in the heart.

   long a.   A line passing lengthwise through the center of a structure.

   mandibular a.   A line passing through both mandibular condyles around which the mandible rotates.

   optic a.   **1.** A line passing through the centers of the cornea and lens, or the closest approximation of this line. **2.** In doubly refracting crystals, the direction in which light is not doubly refracted.

   pelvic a.   A hypothetical curved line passing through the center point of each of the four planes of the pelvis.

   rotational a.   Fulcrum line; see under line.

   visual a.   Visual line; see under line.

axofugal   Directed away from an axon.

axolemma, axilemma   The thin sheath enclosing the axon of a nerve fiber.

axon   The long cytoplasmic process of a neuron (nerve cell). Also called neuroaxon.

axonal   Of or relating to an axon.

axoplasm   The cytoplasm of an axon containing mitochondria, microtubules, neurofilaments, agran-

ular endoplasmic reticulum, and some multivesicular bodies.

azidothymidine (AZT)   See zidovudine.

azobilirubin   A red-violet pigment resulting from the condensation of diazotized sulfanilic acid and bilirubin in the van den Bergh reaction for determination of bilirubin.

azoospermia   Absence of spermatozoa in the semen, causing sterility.

azotemia   An excess of urea or other nitrogenous substances in the blood.

   prerenal a.   Elevation of blood urea nitrogen resulting from primary alterations outside of the kidney, such as a reduction of renal blood flow due to congestive heart failure or hypotension, rather than renal disease per se.

azotification   The action of bacteria upon nitrogenous matter in the soil. Also called nitrification.

azygos   A single or unpaired anatomical structure, such as the azygos vein.

azygous   Unpaired.

Bacillus subtilis

bacteriophage T4

950 Å — head

nucleic acid (in most cases double-stranded DNA)

protein coat

core — tail sheath

tail fibers

tail sheath contracts, forcing core through cell wall

viral DNA entering bacterium — cytoplasm of bacterium

Douglas bag

bacterium (Escherichia coli)

Bb

β Beta. For terms beginning with *β*, see under specific term.

Babesia A genus (family Babesidae, order Haemosporidia) of irregularly shaped parasites of the red blood cells, causing babesiosis in most domestic animals.

babesiosis Any disease caused by a species of *Babesia* spread by ticks and afflicting many domestic animals.

Babinski's sign Extension of the large toe with fanning of the small toes upon stimulation of the sole of the foot, a normal response up to six months of age but abnormal thereafter; a positive response is pathognomonic of corticospinal disease; although upper extremity and head signs were also described by Babinski, the term is usually applied to the Babinski toe sign. Also called Babinski's reflex or phenomenon; extensor plantar response.

baby An infant.

blue b. An infant with a congenital heart defect in which the ductus arteriosus or foramen ovale of the heart fails to close, causing a mixing of venous and arterial blood in the left ventricle and a blood supply inadequate in oxygen; the skin usually has a bluish tint.

bacillary, bacillar Relating to or caused by a bacillus.

bacillemia The presence of rod-shaped bacteria (bacilli) in the blood.

bacilli Plural of bacillus.

bacilliform Shaped like a bacillus; rod-shaped.

bacilluria The passage of urine containing rod-shaped bacteria (bacilli).

Bacillus A genus of rod-shaped bacteria (family Bacillaceae).

B. antracis The causative agent of anthrax.

B. botulinus See *Clostridium botulinum.*

B. cereus A saprophytic, spore-forming bacillus with peritrichous flagella; thought to be responsible for some outbreaks of food poisoning.

B. coli See *Escherichia coli.*

B. hemolyticus *Clostridium haemolyticum.*

B. histolyticus *Clostridium histolyticum.*

B. leprae See *Mycobacterium leprae.*

B. polymyxa A saprophytic, gram-negative bacillus that produces the antibiotic polymyxin.

B. subtilis A widely distributed saprophytic, spore-forming, gram-positive bacillus found in soil and decomposing organic matter; a source of antibiotics. Also called grass or hay bacillus.

B. tetani See *Clostridium tetani.*

B. tuberculosis See *Mycobacterium tuberculosis.*

bacillus *pl.* **bacilli** Any of various rod-shaped bacteria.

Bang's b. See *Brucella abortus.*

Doderlein's b. A gram-positive bacterium commonly found in the vagina; believed to be identical to *Lactobacillus acidophilus.*

Ducrey's b. See *Haemophilus ducreyi.*

Friedlander's b. See *Klebsiella pneumoniae.*

gas b. See *Clostridium perfringens.*

grass b. See *Bacillus subtilis.*

Hansen's b. See *Mycobacterium leprae.*

Koch's b. 1. *Mycobacterium tuberculosis.* 2. *Vibrio cholerae.*

Koch-Weeks b. See *Haemophilus influenzae.*

Pfeiffer's b. See *Haemophilus influenzae.*

tubercle b. (t.b.) *Mycobacterium tuberculosis.*

Weeks' b. See *Haemophilus influenzae.*

Welch's b. See *Clostridium perfringens.*

bacitracin An antibiotic substance obtained from a microorganism belonging to the *Bacillus subtilis* group; used as a topical application.

back The posterior portion of the trunk.

backache Pain in the back, especially in the lumbosacral or lower part of the back.

backbone 1. Vertebral column; see under column. 2. Atoms in a polymer that are common to all its molecules. 3. The main chain of a polypeptide.

background 1. The natural radiation of the earth and its atmosphere, and that coming from outer space. 2. The presence of sound or radiation at a fairly constant low level.

backing A metal support used in dentistry to attach a facing to a prosthesis.

bacteremia The presence of viable bacteria in the blood stream.

bacteria Plural of bacterium.

bacterial Relating to bacteria.

bactericidal Capable of destroying bacteria.

bactericide Any substance that destroys bacteria.

bacteriform Resembling bacteria.

bacteriologic Relating to bacteriology.

bacteriologist A specialist in bacteriology.

bacteriology The branch of microbiology concerned with the study of bacteria, especially in relation to medicine and agriculture.

bacteriolysin An antibody that combines with the bacterial cells (antigen) that caused its formation and later destroys the cells.

bacteriolytic Capable of dissolving bacteria.

bacteriophage A very delicate bacterial virus with considerable variation in structure which may attack and destroy bacterial cells under certain conditions; it contains a nucleic acid core (usually DNA, but may also be RNA) and a protein coat; it is the simplest replicating structure currently known to exist. Also called phage.

bacteriophagia, bacteriophagy The destruction of bacteria by any agent that causes disintegration.

bacteriopsonin An opsonin or antibody that acts upon bacteria.

bacteriostasis The retardation of the growth and reproduction of bacteria.

bacteriostat Any chemical agent that inhibits bacterial growth.

bacteriostatic Inhibiting the growth and reproduction of bacteria. Cf. bactericidal.

Bacterium A group of bacteria formerly classified as a genus of the family Bacteriaceae, later reclassified as *Acetobacter.*

bacterium *pl.* **bacteria** Any of various one-celled microorganisms of the plant kingdom, existing as free-living organisms or as parasites, multiplying by subdivision, and having a large range of biochemical (including pathogenic) properties. They are classified according to their shape into: (a) bacilli (rod-shaped), (b) cocci (spherical), (c) spirilla (spiral-shaped), and (d) vibrios (comma-shaped); they are further classified on the basis of staining characteristics, colony morphology, and metabolic behavior.

enteric b. A bacterium indigenous to the intestines, usually a nonpathogenic gram-negative rod.

L-forms of bacteria Small, filterable bacterial forms with defective or absent cell walls (caused by antibiotics, specific antibodies, or lysosomal enzymes) which retain the ability to multiply.

bacteriuria The presence of bacteria in the urine.

Bacteroides A genus of bacteria (family Bacteroidaceae) composed of gram-negative, nonmotile, anaerobic bacilli normally inhabiting the mouth, intestinal tract, and genital organs of man; some species are pathogenic.

B. fragilis The most commonly seen species of all anaerobes and a potential pathogen in humans.

B. melaninogenicus A species characterized by production of dark pigment; occasionally pathogenic in humans.

bad trip Colloquialism for an unpredictable effect of psychedelic drugs which produces unpleasant or disastrous perceptual distortions; recurrent reactions may appear up to many months after the last use of the drug (flashback).

bag 1. Pouch. 2. The udder of a cow. 3. Slang term for scrotum.

Ambu b. A self-reinflating bag used to produce positive pressure respiration during resuscitation.

b. of waters Colloquialism for the amniotic sac and fluid in which the fetus is suspended.

Douglas b. A device for measuring oxygen consumption of an individual, consisting of a 100-liter canvas or plastic bag with an attached mouthpiece

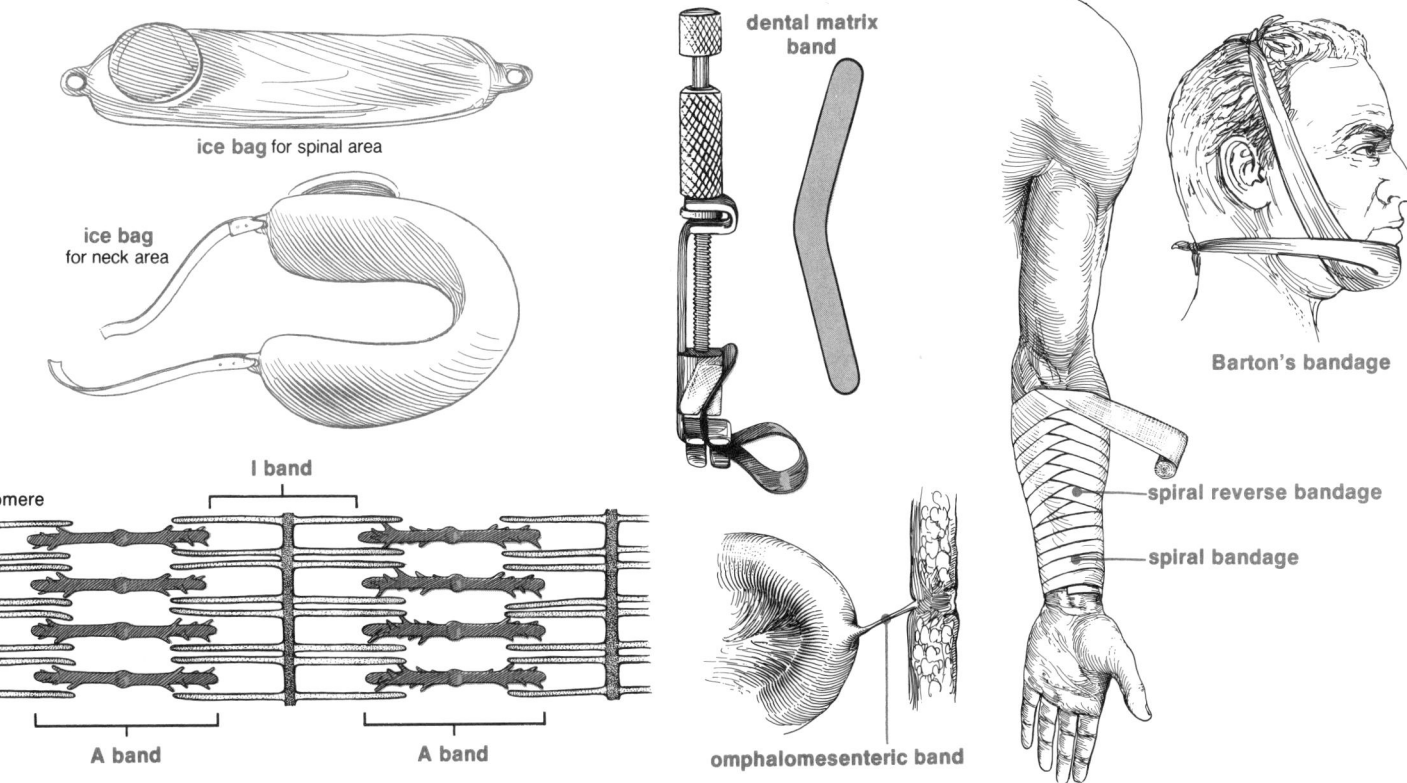

ice bag for spinal area

ice bag for neck area

dental matrix band

Barton's bandage

spiral reverse bandage

spiral bandage

I band

sarcomere

A band   A band

omphalomesenteric band

which houses inspiratory and expiratory valves; room air is breathed in and all expired air is collected in the bag for analysis of the oxygen and carbon dioxide content.

ice b. Rubber bag into which crushed ice is put to produce local cooling; available in a variety of shapes to fit specific parts of the body.

bagassosis A chronic respiratory disorder caused by continued inhalation of the dust of bagasse (the crushed, juiceless residue of sugar cane).

balance 1. A weighing device. 2. A state of bodily stability produced by the harmonious functional performance of its parts. 3. In chemistry, equality of the reacting components on each side of a chemical equation.

acid-base b. The normal ratio of acid and base elements in the blood plasma. Also called acid-base equilibrium.

fluid b. State of the body in relation to the intake and loss of water.

nitrogen b. State of the body in relation to the intake and loss of nitrogen; positive nitrogen balance occurs when the amount of nitrogen excreted is smaller than the amount ingested, as during the growing age of children; negative nitrogen balance occurs when the amount of nitrogen excreted is greater than the amount ingested, as during malnutrition or febrile illnesses.

balanitis Inflammation of the glans penis.

balanoblennorrhea Inflammation of the glans penis due to gonorrhea.

balanoplasty Any reconstructive operation upon the glans penis.

balanoposthitis Inflammation of the glans penis and the adjacent surface of the prepuce.

balanopreputial Relating to the glans penis and the prepuce.

baldness Absence or decrease in the amount of hair. Also called alopecia.

ballism, ballismus 1. Violent or jerking movements as observed in chorea. 2. Paralysis agitans.

ballistocardiogram A graphic record of the movements of the body with each cardiac contraction and ejection of blood from the ventricles; used as a noninvasive means to calculate cardiac output and examine cardiac dynamics.

ballistocardiograph A device for taking a ballistocardiogram, consisting of a recording system and a table suspended from the ceiling or an apparatus resting on the patient's body.

balloon 1. To expand a cavity with air to facilitate its examination. 2. To distend an organ or vessel with gas or fluid. 3. A spherical, inflatable, nonporous sac, as the one near the tip of a Foley catheter.

ballottement 1. A method of physical examina-

tion to determine the size and mobility of an organ in the body, particularly in the presence of fluid. 2. A method of diagnosis of pregnancy: the examining finger is inserted into the vagina and a sudden tap is given on the uterus; the fetus, if present, rises in the amniotic fluid and rebounds to its original position, striking the wall of the uterus which is felt by the examining finger.

balm An ointment or a soothing application.

balneology The branch of medical science concerned with mineral waters and their therapeutic use, especially as a bath.

balneotherapeutics, balneotherapy The treatment of disease by means of baths of mineral waters.

balsam The gummy exudate of some trees and shrubs, used in pharmacologic preparations.

band 1. Any appliance or structure that encircles or binds another. 2. Any ribbon-shaped anatomic structure.

A b. The broad, dark band produced by the thick (100 Å) myosin filaments which traverse the central part of the sarcomere.

absorption b.'s Areas of darkness in the spectrum indicating the regions where light was absorbed by the medium (gas, liquid or solid) through which it passed.

chromosome b. Part of a chromosome which is distinguishable from its adjacent segments by a difference in staining intensity.

I b. A light band extending toward the center of the sarcomere from each Z line of the striated muscle fibers, composed of thin (50 Å) longitudinally oriented actin filaments.

Maissiati's b. Iliotibial tract; see under tract.

omphalomesenteric b. An abnormal persistent band from the intestine to the navel, a remnant of the embryonic omphalomesenteric (vitelline) duct that failed to obliterate; it occasionally results in small bowel obstruction when intestines loop around it.

orthodontic b. A thin strip of metal closely encircling the crown of a tooth in a horizontal plane.

Z b. Z line. See under line.

bandage 1. A piece of gauze or other material used for protecting an injured part, for immobilizing an injured limb, for keeping dressings in place, etc. 2. To cover by wrapping with a strip of material.

Barton's b. A figure-of-eight bandage for the support of the lower jaw.

capeline b. A double-headed roller bandage used to cover the head or an amputation.

elastic b. A bandage made of an elastic material, used to exert mild continuous pressure.

figure-of-eight b. A roller bandage applied in

such a way that the turns cross like the figure eight.

Galen's b. A broad head bandage with the ends split into three sections; after the bandage is placed on the head, the anterior ends are tied behind the neck, the posterior ends, on the forehead, and the middle ends, under the chin.

plaster b. A bandage that is impregnated with plaster of Paris; used for immobilization.

reverse b. One applied to a limb in such a way that the roller is half-twisted with each revolution.

roller b. Bandage material rolled into a compact cylinder.

spiral b. One applied spirally around a limb.

spiral reverse b. A bandage that is folded on itself as it is applied around a limb, i.e., with alternate obverse and reverse turns.

T-b. A bandage shaped like the letter T, generally used to keep dressings on the perineum.

Velpeau's b. A bandage used to support the arm and hold it across the chest.

bandaging The application of a bandage.

banding The staining of chromosomes to make characteristic cross bands visible, thus facilitating identification of chromosome pairs, allocation of phenotypic features to the specific chromosome segment, and classification of clinical syndromes.

G b. Banding with Giemsa dye stain.

Q b. Banding with quinacrine fluorescent stain.

bank A place for collecting and storing biological products.

blood b. A bank for blood and blood products.

sperm b. A bank where sperm is preserved frozen for future use in artificial insemination.

Banti's syndrome Chronic congestive splenomegaly; see under splenomegaly.

bar 1. The international unit of pressure; one megadyne (10^6 dyne) per cm² or 0.987 atmosphere. 2. A piece of metal connecting two or more parts of a removable partial denture.

Passavant's b. See ridge, Passavant's.

barbital A colorless or white crystalline powder, $C_8H_{12}N_2O_3$; a barbituric acid derivative used as a sedative.

barbiturate 1. A salt of barbituric acid. 2. Any derivative of barbituric acid used as a sedative.

barbituric acid A crystalline substance, $CH_2(CONH)_2CO$, not itself a sedative, but from which barbiturates (sedative drugs) are derived.

bariatrician A physician who specializes in reducing the weight of obese patients.

bariatrics The branch of medicine concerned with the care and treatment of overweight people.

barium A soft silvery-white metallic element; symbol Ba, atomic number 56, atomic weight 137.36.

b. sulfate A fine, white, almost insoluble powder,

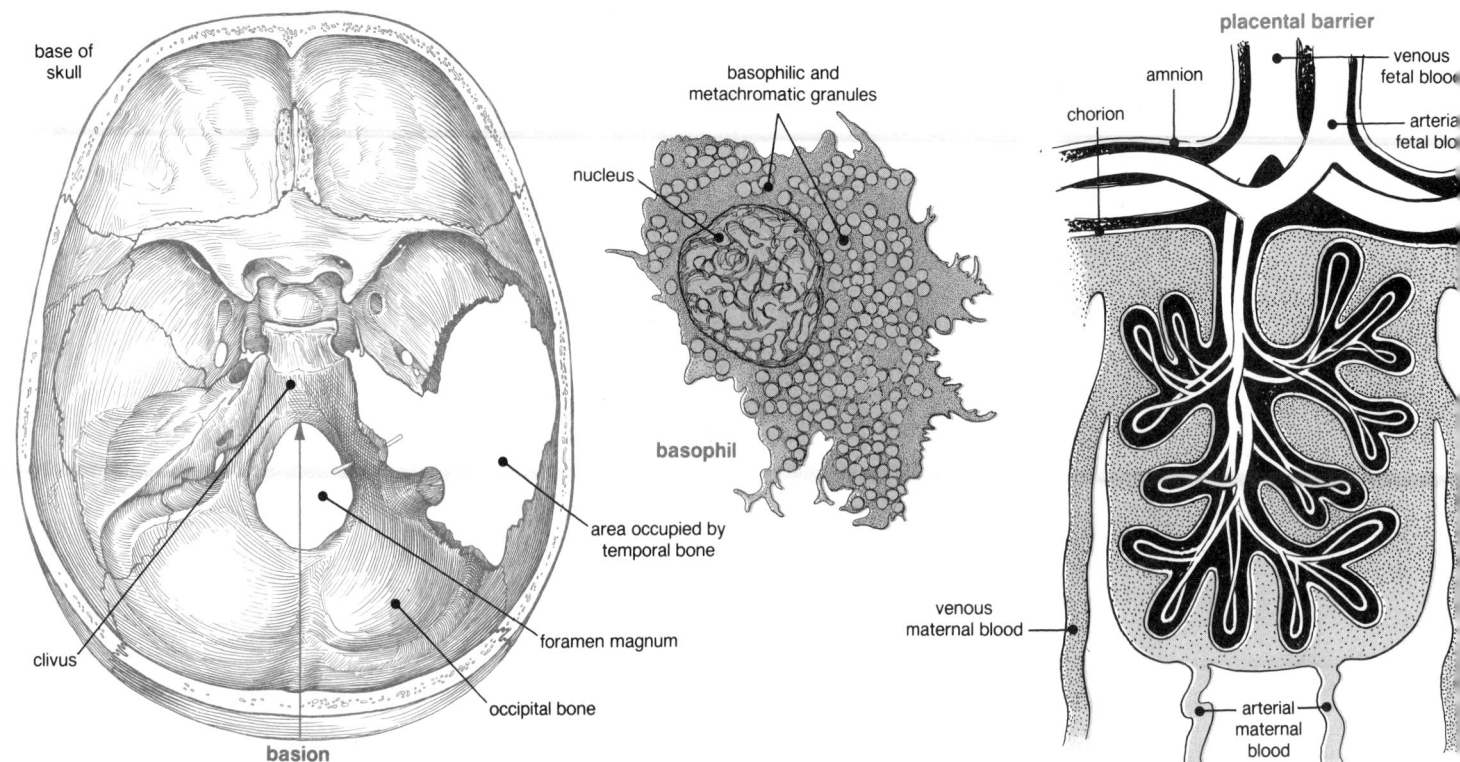

base of skull

basion

clivus

occipital bone

foramen magnum

area occupied by temporal bone

nucleus

basophilic and metachromatic granules

basophil

placental barrier

chorion

amnion

venous fetal blood

arterial fetal blood

venous maternal blood

arterial maternal blood

BaSO₄; used as a radiopaque contrast medium when given orally or as an enema for x-ray visualization of the gastrointestinal tract.

baroceptor See baroreceptor.

baroreceptor A sensory nerve terminal (sense organ) that responds to changes in pressure. Also called pressoreceptor; baroceptor.

barosinusitis See aerosinusitis.

barotrauma Injury caused by pressure, generally to the middle ear or paranasal sinuses, due to the difference between atmospheric pressure and that within the affected cavity.

bar reader A device that provides for the placement of a bar (opaque septum) between a printed page and the viewer's eyes so as to occlude different areas of the page for each of the eyes; used principally for the diagnosis and training of simultaneous binocular vision.

barrel A cylinder or hollow shaft.

  vaginal b. The vaginal cavity extending from the uterus to the vulva.

barren Denoting a woman who is incapable of producing offspring (sterile).

barrier An impediment or obstacle.

  blood-air b. The tissues in the lung, measuring about 0.2 µ in thickness, separating the blood from the air and through which the exchange of gases occurs; comprised of squamous endothelium (lining the capillary), a basal lamina layer, and an attenuated pneumocyte type I cell (squamous alveolar cell in contact with the air).

  blood-brain b. (B.B.B.) The barrier of tissues interposed between the blood and the neurons in the brain; consists of the walls of the capillaries, the layers of the perivascular sheath, the neuroglia, and the ground substance of the brain. Also called hematoencephalic barrier.

  blood-testis b. The tight junction barrier of the Sertoli cells in the seminiferous tubules of the testis that restricts substances from getting to the lumen where the spermatozoa (sperm) are developing, thereby protecting them, especially from the vascular supply.

  hemato-encephalic b. See blood-brain barrier.

  placental b. The semipermeable epithelial layer of the placenta separating the maternal blood from the fetal blood.

  protective b. In radiology, material such as lead or concrete, used for absorbing ionizing radiation for protective purposes.

bartholinitis Inflammation of the greater vestibular glands (Bartholin's glands).

Bartonella bacilliformis A species of gram-negative encapsulated bacillus that causes bartonellosis; transmitted to man by the bite of sandflies.

bartonellosis Disease occurring mainly in Peru, caused by an arthropod-borne bacillus (*Bartonella bacilliformis*), usually marked by a febrile stage with anemia (Oroya fever) followed several weeks later by a nodular cutaneous eruption (verruga peruana); occasionally one stage of the disease occurs without the other. Also called Carrion's disease. See also Oroya fever (under fever); verruga peruana.

Bartter's syndrome Disorder marked by juxtaglomerular cell hyperplasia, secondary hyperaldosteronism, hypokalemic alkalosis, and a marked increase in prostaglandin production and in plasma renin levels in the absence of hypertension.

basal Of or relating to a base.

base 1. The foundation or supporting part of anything. 2. The chief ingredient of a mixture. 3. A substance that turns litmus indicators blue and combines with an acid to form a salt. 4. A hydrogen ion acceptor. 5. The part opposite the apex, as the base of the heart.

  acrylic resin b. A denture base made of acrylic resin.

  cement b. A dressing placed at the bottom of deep cavities to protect the dental pulp from thermal shock and to serve as a floor for a permanent filling.

  denture b. The framework of a partial denture that rests on the ridge. Also called saddle.

Basedow's disease Exophthalmic goiter; see under goiter.

baseplate A temporary form corresponding to the base of a denture, used for making jaw relation plates, or for arranging artificial teeth. Also called record, temporary, or trial base.

basic Of or relating to a base. See also basilar.

basicranial Of or relating to the base of the skull.

basilar Of or relating to a base, as the basilar membrane of the cochlear duct.

basilateral Relating to the base and side or sides of a structure.

basion The middle point on the anterior margin of the foramen magnum (occipital foramen).

basis Latin base.

  b. cordi The base of the heart.

  b. cranii The base of the skull; the inner surface is called basis cranii interna; the outer surface is termed basis cranii externa.

Basle Nomina Anatomica (BNA) A system of anatomic nomenclature adopted by an anatomic association; it is superseded by *Nomina Anatomica*.

basocytosis Abnormal increase in the number of basophils in the blood. Also called basophilic leukocytosis.

basophil A cell, especially a white blood cell (basophilic leukocyte), containing large granules that stain readily with basic dyes.

basophilia 1. Abnormal increase of basophilic leukocytes in the blood. 2. The presence of basophilic red blood cells in the blood.

basophilic Staining easily with basic dyes.

bath 1. The immersion of the body, or part of it, in water or any other medium. 2. The apparatus in which the body is immersed.

  contrast b. The alternate immersion of a bodily part in hot and cold water (usually at half-hour intervals), to increase blood circulation to the part.

  douche b. The local application of a stream of water.

  Finnish b. A bath sauna.

  sitz b. A bath in which only the hips and buttocks of the patient are immersed in a tub of water.

  tepid b. A bath in water at a temperature of approximately 86°F.

  water b. 1. The immersion of the body, or part of it, in water. 2. The immersion in water of a liquid-containing vessel to heat or cool the liquid.

Batten-Mayou disease Cerebral sphingolipidosis; see under sphingolipidosis.

battered child syndrome Multiple injuries inflicted upon a child by an older individual, usually an adult and often a parent.

Battle's sign Discoloration behind the ear, seen in fracture of the base of the skull.

beaded Having the appearance of a string of beads, as in rachitic rosary.

beaker A wide mouth glass cylinder with a pouring lip, used in laboratories for mixing and heating substances.

bearing down The expulsion effort of a woman during the second stage of labor.

beat 1. To pulsate. 2. To strike. 3. A pulsation, as of the heart.

  apex b. The beat of the apex of the heart during ventricular systole; normally felt at the left fifth intercostal space, at the midclavicular line.

  capture b. A conducted heart beat occurring after a period of atrioventricular (A-V) dissociation.

  double b. Coupled pulse; see under pulse.

  dropped b. A nonconducted heart beat; one that fails to appear due to an atrioventricular (A-V) block.

  ectopic b. A heart beat originating at some point in the heart other than the sinoatrial node.

  escape b. An automatic heart beat following an interval longer than the dominant cycle, i.e., after the normal beat has defaulted.

  fusion b. A heart beat arising from the simultaneous activation of either the atria or ventricles of the heart by two impulses from different sites.

  premature b. An ectopic heart beat that depends on, and is coupled to, the preceding beat, occurring

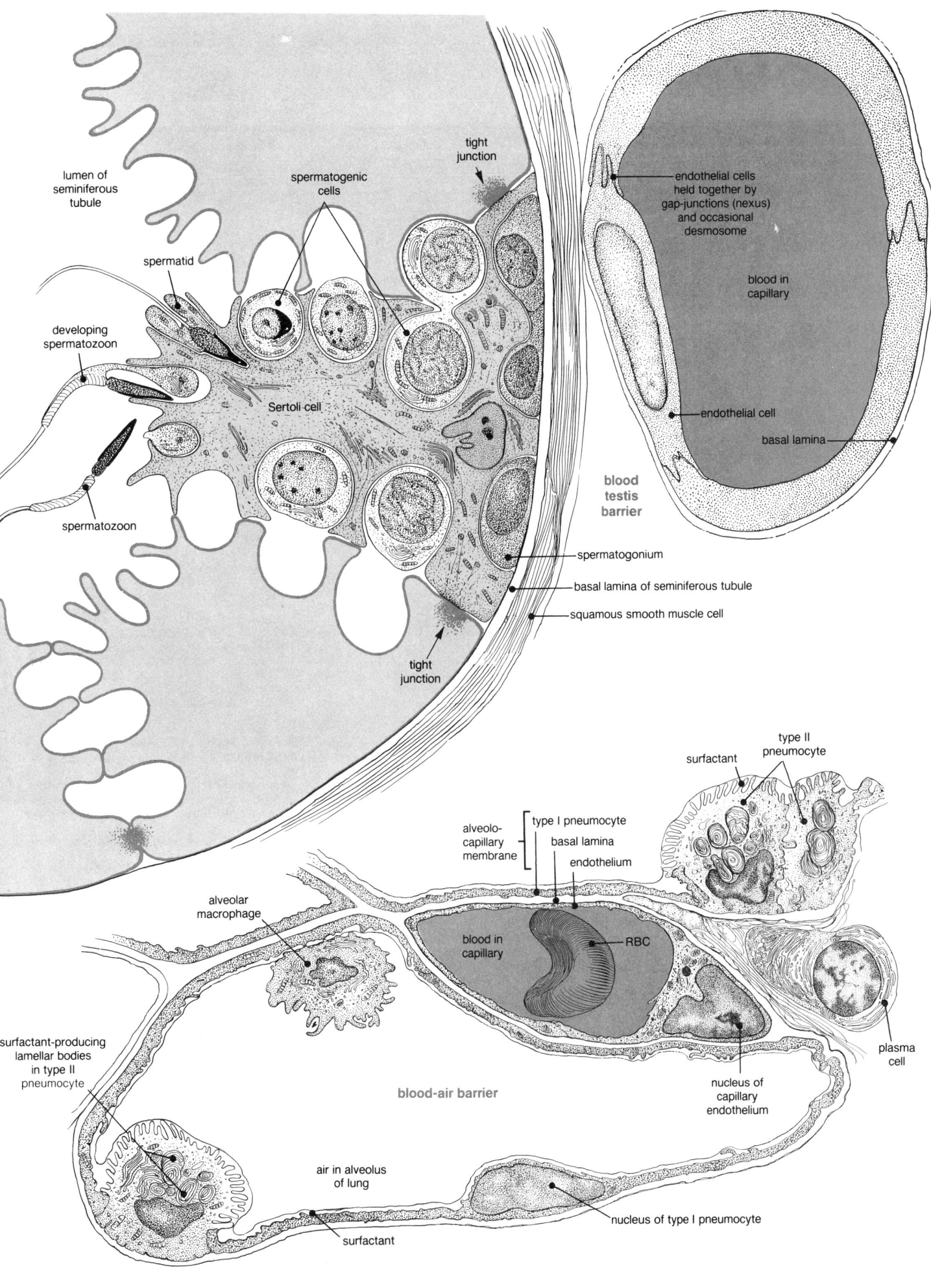

lumen of
seminiferous
tubule

spermatogenic
cells

tight
junction

spermatid

developing
spermatozoon

Sertoli cell

endothelial cells
held together by
gap-junctions (nexus)
and occasional
desmosome

blood in
capillary

spermatozoon

endothelial cell

basal lamina

blood
testis
barrier

spermatogonium

basal lamina of seminiferous tubule

squamous smooth muscle cell

tight
junction

type II
pneumocyte

surfactant

alveolo-
capillary
membrane

type I pneumocyte

basal lamina

endothelium

alveolar
macrophage

blood in
capillary

RBC

surfactant-producing
lamellar bodies
in type II
pneumocyte

plasma
cell

nucleus of
capillary
endothelium

blood-air barrier

air in alveolus
of lung

nucleus of type I pneumocyte

surfactant

59

bedbug
(cimex lectularis)

section of
normal prostate

bladder

benign
tumor of
prostate

benzene

model

structural
formula

benzocaine

benzoic acid

benzyl alcohol

before the next dominant beat.

becquerel (Bq) New unit of radioactivity proposed as a replacement for the curie (Ci); the radioactivity of a material decaying at the rate of one disintegration per second, 3.7×10^{10} Bq = 1 Ci; 1 Bq = 27.03×10^{-12} Ci.

bed **1.** A piece of furniture for resting and sleeping. **2.** In anatomy, a base or layer of tissue upon which a structure rests.

  capillary b. The total mass of capillaries and their volume capacity.

  Gatch b. A hinged bed in which the patient's head and knees may be elevated.

bedbug A blood-sucking insect. *Cimex lectularius* (family Cimicidae), about 5 mm long when fully grown, with a flat, reddish-brown body and a disagreeable odor; its bite produces urticarial wheals with central hemorrhagic points; it often infests human dwellings and usually hides during the day in bed frames, torn mattresses, between floorboards, and under the edges of wallpaper.

bedewing, corneal A swelling of the corneal epithelium characterized by irregular reflections from a multitude of droplets when seen with the slit lamp.

bedpan A pan with a wide flat rim which serves as a receptacle for the excreta of bedridden individuals.

bedsore Ulcer of the skin, and sometimes of the muscles, occurring in pressure areas of bedridden patients who are allowed to lie in the same position for long periods of time. Also called decubitus ulcer.

bed-wetting An involuntary release of urine during sleep, usually of concern if continued beyond the age of toilet training; may be of nervous or emotional origin, or due to infection or inflammation of the urinary tract. Also called nocturnal enuresis.

bee An insect of the genus *Apis,* of which the honeybee is the most common stinging insect; it leaves its stinger and venom sac attached to the victim.

beeswax Wax secreted by the honeybee; one of the ingredients of many dental waxes.

behavior The manner in which a person acts or functions.

  compensatory b. A behavior in which individuals suffering from anxiety disorders who are intolerant of themselves often exhibit a compensatory attitude of intolerance of others.

behavioral Relating to behavior.

behaviorism A school of psychologic theory concerned with the observable, tangible, and objective facts of behavior, rather than with subjective phenomena such as thoughts, emotions, or impulses.

behavior modification Treatment that attempts to modify selective symptoms by techniques such as systematic desensitization and biofeedback.

Behçet's disease, Behçet's syndrome Recurrent ulceration of the genitals and oral cavity with inflammation of the iris, ciliary body, and choroid and the formation of a puslike fluid in the anterior chamber of the eye; pyodermas are common and involvement of the central nervous system occurs in a variety of forms.

bejel Nonvenereal infection with a treponeme very similar to *Treponema pallidum*; occurs mainly in arid climates.

bel A unit of sound intensity, being the logarithm to the base 10 of the ratio of two levels of sound; the difference in intensity between a sound that is barely audible and one 10 times louder is 1 bel; named after Alexander Graham Bell.

belching Popular term for eructation.

belladonna **1.** A poisonous plant, *Atropa belladonna*, with purple flowers and black berries. Also called deadly nightshade. **2.** An atropine preparation derived from the leaves and roots of the belladonna plant; formerly widely used as an anticholinergic agent. The drug, whose name means beautiful woman in Italian, was once used to dilate the pupils of the eyes to render a female more attractive.

belle indifference French term meaning a constant unjustified state of complacency and indifference, often seen in patients with conversion hysteria.

belly **1.** Abdomen. **2.** The prominent fleshy part of a muscle.

bellyache Colic.

bellybutton Umbilicus; navel.

Bence Jones albumin, Bence Jones protein See protein, Bence Jones.

bends A manifestation of caisson disease, consisting of severe pain in the joints and muscles, especially of the limbs and hip, which are maintained in a semiflexed position (hence the name); produced by liberation of gas bubbles in the tissues. See also caisson disease.

benign Denoting a condition capable of disturbing the function of an organ, without endangering the life of the individual; not malignant.

benzalkonium chloride A compound used as an antiseptic and germicide.

benzene A thin, colorless, highly flammable liquid, C_6H_6; a coal-tar derivative, used in the manufacture of numerous chemical products. Commonly called benzol.

benzene ring See under, ring.

γ-benzene hexochloride See lindane.

benzimidazole A compound occurring as part of the vitamin B_{12} molecule.

benzoate An ester or salt of benzoic acid.

benzocaine A surface anesthetic of the skin and mucous membranes, widely used for relief of sunburn, pruritus, and burns; an ethyl ester of aminobenzoic acid.

benzoic acid A white crystalline acid occurring naturally in the resin benzoin; used in fungicides and dentifrices.

benzoin A resin obtained as a gum from a tree, *Styrax benzoin,* sometimes used as an inhalant expectorant in the treatment of laryngitis and bronchitis; tincture of benzoin is also used as a base to provide a sticky surface for adhesive tape.

benzyl A hydrocarbon radical.

  b. alcohol $C_6H_5CH_2OH$; a substance used as a local anesthetic.

Berger's disease See nephropathy, IgA.

beriberi Disease resulting from a dietary deficiency of thiamine (vitamin B_1).

  cardiovascular b. Disease manifested principally by high output cardiac failure and edema; the acute fulminating form is called shoshin. Also called wet beriberi.

  dry b. A chronic form in which polyneuropathy is prominent.

  infantile b. A form occurring during the first year of life, usually with prominent cardiovascular manifestations; most commonly occurs in the first months of life in small, breast-fed infants; reflects severe thiamine deficiency in the mother.

  wet b. See cardiovascular beriberi.

berkelium A synthetic, transuranium radioactive element; symbol Bk, atomic number 97, atomic weight 247; it has nine isotopes with half-lives from three hours to 1,380 years.

Bernheim's syndrome Right heart failure without pulmonary congestion in the presence of left ventricular enlargement.

berylliosis Condition caused by either inhalation of, or contact with, fumes or particles of beryllium salts; marked by granulomatous growths in the lungs or skin.

beryllium A high melting point, corrosion-resistant metallic element; symbol Be, atomic number 4; atomic weight 9.013; used as a reflector in nuclear reactors and, in a copper alloy, for electrical contracts and nonsparking tools. Formerly called glucinum.

bestiality Sexual relations between a human and an animal.

beta **1.** The second letter of the Greek alphabet, β. **2.** The second item in a system of classification, as of chemical compounds. For terms beginning with beta, see under specific term.

Betaherpesvirinae Subfamily of viruses (family

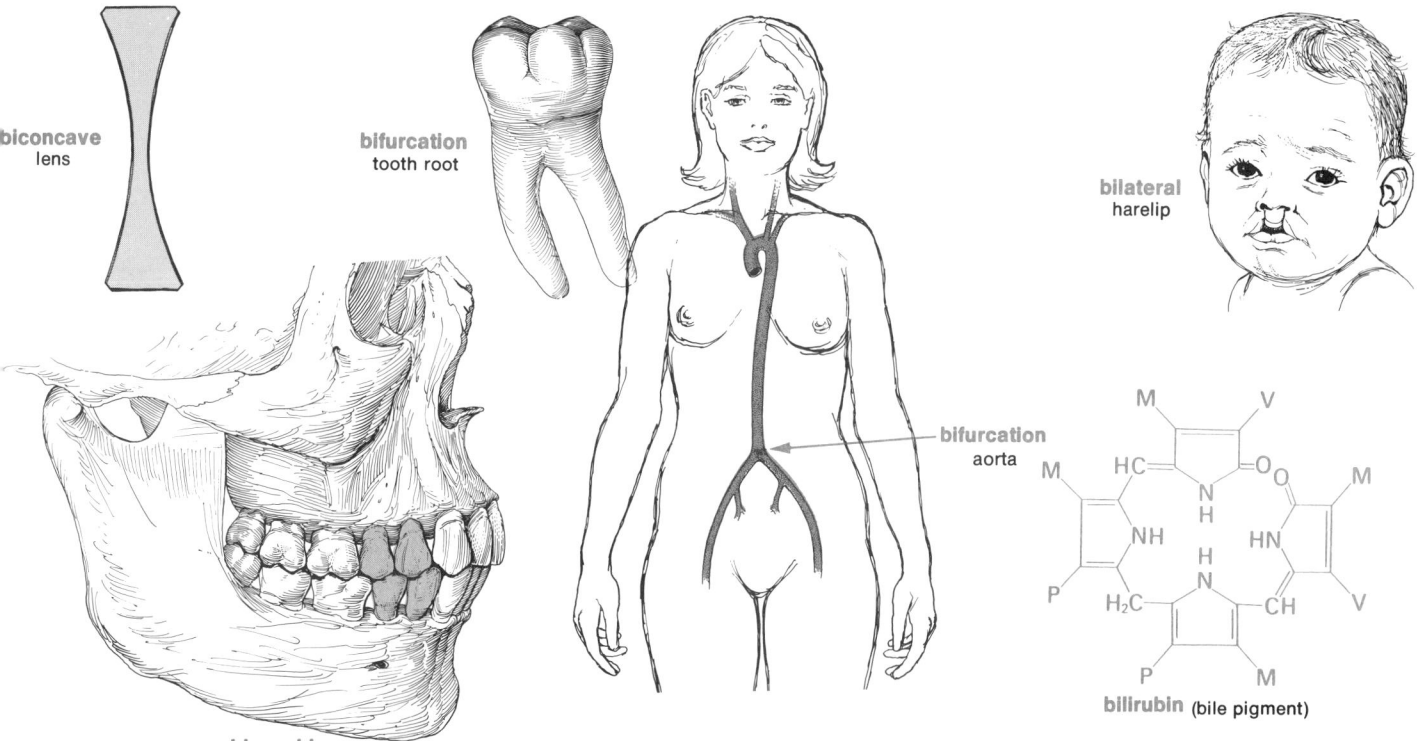

biconcave
lens

bifurcation
tooth root

bilateral
harelip

bifurcation
aorta

bilirubin (bile pigment)

bicuspids

Herpesviridae) which cause enlargement of infected cell and inclusion bodies containing DNA in nucleus and cytoplasm; may remain latent in salivary glands, kidneys, lymphoreticular cells and other tissues. Also called cytomegalovirus group.

betel A climbing plant of East India, *Piper betle*; a species of pepper, the leaves and nuts of which are chewed to produce both stimulant and narcotic effects.

bezoar A hard mass found chiefly in the alimentary canal of ruminants and occasionally in man, composed of hair and/or vegetable fibers; it was formerly thought to have magical properties and was used as an antidote for poison.

bias 1. In statistics, the distortion in the results of a study arising from systematic errors in sampling or analysis. 2. An unvarying voltage applied to an electrode.

biauricular 1. Having two auricles. 2. Relating to both auricles.

bibasic See dibasic.

bibulous Absorbent.

bicameral Composed of two chambers or cavities; said of an abscess.

bicarbonate A compound containing the radical group HCO_3.

biceps Denoting a muscle with two heads or points of origin.

bicipital 1. Having two heads. 2. Of or relating to a biceps muscle.

biconcave Having a depression on both sides or surfaces.

biconvex Protruding on both sides or surfaces.

bicornous, bicornuate, bicornate Having two horns or horn-shaped structures.

bicuspid Having two cusps or points, such as the premolars or the left atrioventricular (mitral) valve of the heart.

bifid Divided into two parts, as a bifid ureter.

bifocal Having two focal lengths.

bifocals Eyeglasses in which each lens has two focal lengths, used for both distant and near vision.

bifurcate To divide or separate into two parts.

bifurcation Division or separation into two parts or branches.

bigeminal Occurring in pairs.

bigeminy Doubling, especially the occurrence of two pulse beats in rapid succession followed by a pause before the next two beats. Also written bigemini.

bilateral Relating to or having two sides.

bile A bitter, yellowish brown or brownish green liquid, secreted by the liver, stored in the gallbladder, and discharged into the duodenum; it aids in digestion mainly by emulsifying fats. Also called gall.

Bilharzia Former name for a genus of trematode worms or flukes now called *Schistosoma*.

bilharziasis, bilharziosis See schistosomiasis.

biliary Relating to bile and the bile ducts.

bilifuscin A dark green-brown pigment present in bile and bile salts.

bilious 1. Of, relating to, or containing bile. Also called biliary. 2. A vague popular term denoting a disturbed condition of the digestive system.

biliousness A vaguely defined condition marked by indigestion, excessive gas, and often constipation and headache, popularly attributed to gallbladder dysfunction.

bilirubin An orange-red pigment formed from hemoglobin during destruction of erythrocytes by the reticuloendothelial system; in the presence of liver disease or excessive destruction of red blood cells, accumulation of bilirubin in the blood and tissues causes jaundice.

bilirubinemia The presence of bilirubin in the blood, usually referring to an increased level.

bilirubinuria The occurrence of the pigment bilirubin in the urine.

biliuria The presence of bile or bile salts in the urine.

biliverdin, biliverdine A green bile pigment formed from the oxidation of bilirubin.

bilobate Composed of two lobes.

bilobular Having two lobules.

bimanual Performed with both hands, e.g., bimanual palpation.

bimodal Having two distinct modes or peaks; said of a graphic curve.

bimolecular Relating to or affecting two molecules.

binary Composed of two parts.

binaural Relating to both ears.

bind 1. To secure, as with ligature or band. 2. To bandage. 3. To unite molecules. 4. To constipate.

binder A broad abdominal bandage.

binge and purge syndrome Bulimia.

binocular 1. Relating to both eyes. 2. Used by both eyes at the same time, as a microscope.

binomial 1. Having two names. 2. In mathematics, an expression pertaining to two terms connected by a plus or minus sign (as $m + n$ or $10 - 5$).

binuclear, binucleate Possessing two nuclei.

bioassay Estimation of a substance's potency by comparing its effects on living organisms or on tissue preparations with those of a standard.

bioastronautics The study of the effects of space travel on living organisms.

bioavailability The degree to which the active ingredient of a drug is absorbed by the body in the form which is physiologically active; it is an indication of both the relative amount of an administered drug that reaches the general circulation and the rate at which this occurs.

biocatalyst Enzyme.

biochemistry The chemistry of living matter or organisms. Also called biologic chemistry.

biodynamics The science concerned with energy as it relates to living organisms and their environment.

bioenergetics The study of energy changes produced within living tissues.

bioengineering Application of engineering principles to solve biomedical problems, e.g., design and construction of devices, using suitable materials, for implantation within the body (plastic heart valves, metal pins and plates, electrodes, etc.), or of life-supporting apparatus for external use (heart-lung machine, artificial kidney, etc.). Also called biomedical engineering.

bioequivalence The application of the bioavailability concept whereby it can be assumed that a drug has the same therapeutic efficacy as another drug if it achieves the same maximum concentration, the same rate of absorption, and the same total amount of absorption as a recognized standard.

bioethics The branch of ethics concerned with the moral and social implications of practices and developments in medicine and the life sciences.

biofeedback A technique which uses electronic monitoring to give an individual immediate and continuing signals on changes in bodily functions of which he is not usually conscious, such as fluctuations in blood pressure; the subject endeavors to learn to control the function.

biogenesis Huxley's term given to the view that living things originate only from things already living, as opposed to spontaneous generation.

biokinetics The study of the growth changes and movements within developing organisms.

biologic, biological Relating to biology.

biologist A specialist in biology.

biology The science concerned with the study of living organisms, their structure, function, growth, etc.

  cell b. The science concerned with the study of the cell; it seeks an explanation of the physiochemical and metabolic processes of protoplasm. Also called cytology.

biomedical Relating to biomedicine.

biomedical engineering See bioengineering.

biomedicine The aspects of biologic sciences that relate to clinical medicine.

biometrician A specialist in biometry.

biometry The statistical study of biologic information.

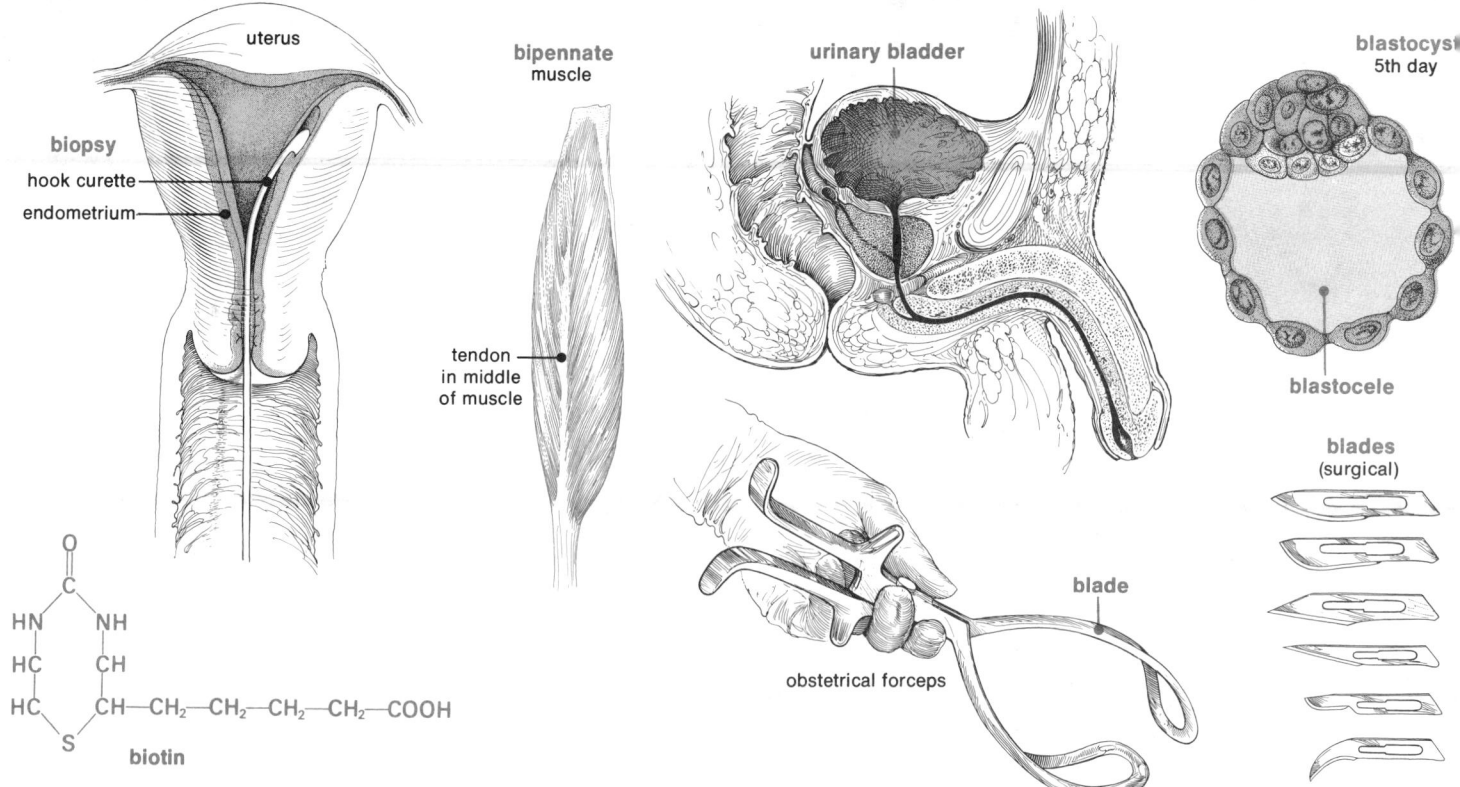

uterus

biopsy
hook curette
endometrium

bipennate muscle

tendon in middle of muscle

urinary bladder

blastocyst 5th day

blastocele

blades (surgical)

blade

obstetrical forceps

biotin

biotin chemical structure:
$$O = C$$
$$HN \quad NH$$
$$HC \quad CH$$
$$HC \quad CH—CH_2—CH_2—CH_2—CH_2—COOH$$
$$S$$

biomicroscope A binocular microscope, used with a narrow beam of light (slit lamp) for examining the living eye.

biomicroscopy 1. A microscopic inspection of the living tissues in the body. 2. Inspection of the cornea or the lens by means of a slit lamp and corneal microscope combination.

biomolecules Molecules present in living matter.

bion Any living organism.

bionics The application of biologic principles to the design of electronic systems.

bionosis Any disease caused by living organisms.

biophysics The science of the physical forces acting on the cells of the living body.

  dental b. The relationship between the biologic behavior of the structures of the mouth and the physical action of a dental prosthesis.

biopsy The removal and examination (gross and microscopic) of tissue from the living body for the purpose of diagnosis.

  needle b. Obtaining of biopsy material by aspiration through a needle.

  surface b. Examination of cells scraped from a surface, as from the cervix of the uterus.

  surgical b. Obtaining of biopsy tissue by surgery.

biorhythm 1. The cyclic occurrence of a biologic process. 2. A self-sustaining pattern of behavior that occurs in cycles, is relatively independent of the environment's ambient temperature, and which deviates (at least slightly) from the external geophysical cycle which it parallels.

biospectrometry The determination of the quantity of various substances in living tissues by means of a spectroscope. Also called clinical spectrometry.

biospectroscopy Examination of specimens of living tissue with the spectroscope. Also called clinical spectroscopy.

biostatistics The study concerned with the acquisition, analysis, and interpretation of data relating to human mortality, morbidity, natality, and demography.

biosynthesis The formation of chemical substances by or in living organisms.

biotechnology The application of human and engineering data to problems relating to the adjustment of man and the machine. Also called ergonomics.

biotelemetry The recording and measuring, without wires, of the vital processes of an organism located at a point remote from the measuring device.

biotic Relating to the life processes. Also called biologic.

biotin A vitamin acting as a coenzyme, found chiefly in liver, yeast, and egg yolk. Formerly called vitamin H.

biotoxin Any toxic substance formed in the body tissues.

biotransformation The interaction between a drug and the living organism which results in a chemical change in the drug molecule. Also called drug metabolism.

biotransport The translocation of a solute through a biologic barrier without being altered.

biotype See physique.

bipara A woman who has given birth twice. Also called secundipara.

biparietal Relating to both parietal bones of the skull.

biparous Having borne twins.

biped An animal with two feet.

bipennate, bipenniform Having a double feather arrangement; said of certain muscles from the arrangement of their fibers on each side of a tendon.

bipolar 1. Having two poles. 2. Relating to both ends of a cell.

bipositive Having two positive charges or valences, as the calcium ion, Ca^{++}.

birefringence The splitting of light in two slightly different directions to form two rays. Also called double refraction.

birth The act of being born.

birthmark A circumscribed growth present at birth, as a hemangioma.

biscuit In dentistry (in association with porcelain), the fired article before it is glazed; referred to as low, medium, or high biscuit, depending on the stage of vitrification.

bisexual 1. Having the reproductive organs of both sexes. 2. A hermaphrodite. 3. Denoting a person who engages in sexual relations with both sexes.

bis in die (b.i.d.) Latin for twice a day.

bismuth A crystalline, brittle metallic element; symbol Bi, atomic number 83, atomic weight 209.

  b. subcarbonate $(BiO)_2CO_3$; a white or pale yellow powder, used as an astringent and antacid. Also called bismuth oxycarbonate.

bisulfite Any compound containing the inorganic acid group HSO_3.

bite 1. To grip or tear with the teeth. 2. To pierce the skin with the teeth or a stinger. 3. The amount of pressure produced in closing the jaws. See also record, interocclusal. 4. The contact of the mandibular teeth with the maxillary teeth in any functional relation.

  close b. Small interarch distance; see under distance.

  open b. Condition in which some of the apposing teeth (usually the anterior teeth) fail to make contact when the jaws are fully closed. Also called aperto-

gnathia.

bitemporal Relating to both temples.

bite plane See under plane.

biuret paper, reagent, test See under nouns.

bivalence, bivalency Combining power double that of a hydrogen atom; a valence of 2.

bivalent 1. Having valence 2 or the combining power of two hydrogen atoms. Also called divalent. 2. In genetics, composed of two homologous chromosomes.

biventer Having two bellies, said of some muscles, e.g., the digastric muscle.

blackhead A plug of sebaceous material in the orifice of a hair follicle. Also called comedo.

blackout Temporary loss of consciousness.

black widow One of the world's most dangerous spiders, *Latrodectus mactans*; the extremely poisonous female is about one and a half inches long with a shiny black body and a red hourglass patch on its abdomen; the male is about one-fourth the size of the female and has yellow-brown markings; name acquired from the fact that the female eats its mate.

bladder A distendable musculomembranous sac that serves as a receptacle for fluid, especially the urinary bladder.

  atonic b. One that is unable to contract due to paralysis of the motor nerves that innervate it.

  autonomic b. Condition marked by periodic involuntary urination.

  cord b. Dysfunction of the bladder due to a lesion of its nerve supply.

  gall b. See gallbladder.

  ileal b. A surgically created bladder consisting of an isolated segment of ileum which is opened to the exterior through the abdominal wall and into which the ureters are attached.

  nervous b. A constant desire to urinate, with incomplete emptying of the bladder.

  neurogenic b. Any disturbance of bladder function caused by impairment of the nerve supply.

  reflex neurogenic b. Condition in which the person has no awareness of filling or ability to contract the bladder voluntarily; caused by a lesion in sacral nerves 2, 3 and 4.

  urinary b. The reservoir for urine, which it receives from the kidneys through the ureters and discharges through the urethra.

blade 1. The cutting end of an instrument. 2. The long arm of instruments such as certain forceps.

  shoulder b. See scapula.

blastocele The fluid-filled cavity of a blastocyst.

blastocyst The embryo at the time of its implantation into the uterine wall, consisting of a single layer of outer cells (trophoblast), a fluid-filled cavity (blastocele), and a mass of inner cells (embryoblast).

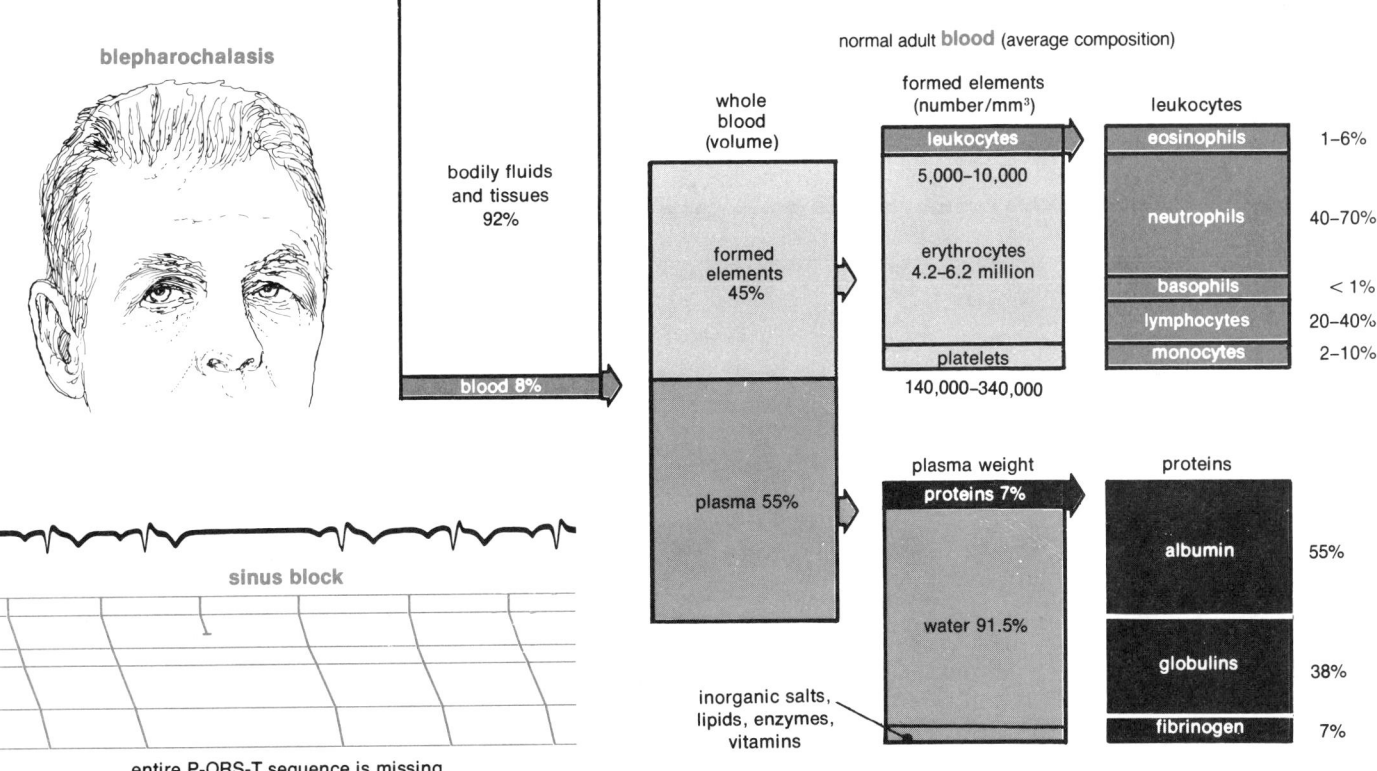

blepharochalasis

sinus block

entire P-QRS-T sequence is missing

normal adult **blood** (average composition)

bodily fluids and tissues 92%

blood 8%

whole blood (volume)

formed elements 45%

plasma 55%

formed elements (number/mm³)

leukocytes 5,000–10,000

erythrocytes 4.2–6.2 million

platelets 140,000–340,000

leukocytes

eosinophils	1–6%
neutrophils	40–70%
basophils	< 1%
lymphocytes	20–40%
monocytes	2–10%

plasma weight
proteins 7%
water 91.5%
inorganic salts, lipids, enzymes, vitamins

proteins

albumin	55%
globulins	38%
fibrinogen	7%

Also called blastodermic vesicle.

blastogenesis 1. Reproduction by budding. 2. The development of an embryo during cleavage and germ layer formation. 3. The transformation of small lymphocytes of human blood in tissue culture into large blastlike cells capable of undergoing mitosis.

blastomere One of the cells into which the fertilized egg divides.

Blastomyces A genus of pathogenic fungi (family Moniliaceae).

B. coccidioides See *Coccidioides immitis*.

B. dermatitidis A species that is the cause of North American blastomycosis.

blastomycosis A fungal infection of the skin and internal organs.

North American b. A chronic disease caused by a yeastlike fungus (*Blastomyces dermatitidis*), originating in the respiratory system, especially the lungs, and disseminating to the skin and sometimes to bone and other organs.

South American b. See paracoccidioidomycosis.

blastopore A small opening into the archenteron (primitive digestive cavity) of the embryo at the gastrula stage.

blastospore A spore developed by budding from a fungal filament or hypha.

blastula Early stage in the development of an embryo; a spherical structure consisting of a single layer of cells that enclose a fluid-filled cavity.

blastulation Formation of the blastocyst or blastula.

bleaching 1. Removal of color by means of chemical agents. 2. In dentistry, a method for returning a discolored tooth to its normal color.

bleaching agent Any chemical used for brightening discolored teeth.

bleb A blister.

bleeder A person afflicted with hemophilia or any other bleeding disease.

bleeding The escape of blood.

dysfunctional uterine b. Bleeding from the uterus due to endocrine imbalance rather than a localized disorder.

blennadenitis Inflammation of the mucous glands.

blennorrhea A profuse mucous discharge from the vagina or urethra.

blennorrheal, blennorrhagic Relating to blennorrhea.

blepharectomy Surgical removal of all or a portion of an eyelid.

blepharitis Inflammation of the eyelids.

blepharochalasis Condition of the upper eyelids marked by excessive tissue which hangs over the lid margin when the eye is open. Also called false ptosis.

blepharoconjunctivitis Inflammation of the eyelid and of the conjunctiva, especially of the palpebral conjunctiva.

blepharon Eyelid.

blepharophimosis A condition in which the aperture of the eyelids is narrow. Also called blepharostenosis.

blepharoplasty Any restorative surgical procedure of the eyelids. Also called tarsoplasty.

blepharoptosis Drooping of the upper eyelid.

blepharospasm Spasmodic winking, or contraction of the muscles of the eyelid.

blepharotomy An incision on an eyelid.

blind loop syndrome Syndrome which may occur after operations of the small intestine which form a blind loop; stagnation of intestinal contents results in increased bacterial growth with malabsorption of vitamin B$_{12}$, fat, and other nutrients.

blindness Lack or loss of sight.

color b. Inability to distinguish differences between some colors.

day b. See hemeralopia.

legal b. Loss of vision to a degree as defined by legal statute to constitute blindness; maximal correction of acuity of 20/200 or less, and diameter of visual field of 20 degrees or less.

letter b. A form of aphasia in which letters, though seen, relate no meaning to the mind.

night b. Impaired vision in subdued light, generally due to a deficiency of vitamin A. Also called nyctalopia.

snow b. Temporary blindness caused by excessive exposure to sunlight reflected from snow.

word b. Inability to recognize written or printed words as conveyors of ideas.

blink To close and open the eyelids rapidly; an involuntary act by which the tears are spread over the conjunctivas, keeping them moist.

blister Common name for vesicle (2) and bulla (1).

bloat, bloating Distention of the abdomen with gas.

block 1. To obstruct or to prevent passage through. 2. To experience difficulty in recollection due to an unconscious emotional factor. 3. An obstruction. 4. In psychoanalysis, the difficulty in recollection due to an unconscious emotional factor.

alveolar-capillary b. Impaired diffusion of gases, especially oxygen, between the capillaries and alveoli of the lungs.

arborization b. A form of intraventricular block, thought to be due to widespread blockage in the Purkinje fibers of the heart.

atrioventricular (A-V) **b.** Disorder of the atrioventricular bundle, causing disruption in the transmission of impulses from atria to ventricles; usually classified in three degrees; (a) in first degree A-V block, conduction time of the impulses is prolonged but all impulses reach the ventricles; (b) in second degree A-V block, some impulses are blocked and do not reach the ventricles so that ventricular beats are dropped; (c) in third degree A-V block, (complete block), no impulses can reach the ventricles.

bundle-branch b. (BBB) A form of intraventricular block due to impaired conduction in one of the main branches of the atrioventricular bundle (bundle of His).

caudal b. See under anesthesia.

epidural b. See under anesthesia.

heart b. Atrioventricular block.

intra-atrial b. Impaired conduction through the atria.

intraventricular (I-V) **b.** Impaired conduction through the ventricles.

peri-infarction b. Delayed conduction through the myocardium at the site of an old myocardial infarct.

saddle b. See under anesthesia.

sinus b., sinoatrial (S-A) b., sinoauricular b. Failure of the nervous impulse to leave the sinus node.

blockade 1. Intravenous injection of harmless material, such as colloidal dyes, for the purpose of rendering the reticuloendothelial cells temporarily functionless. 2. Obstruction of nerve impulse transmission by a drug.

adrenergic b. Inhibition by a drug of the responses of effector cells to adrenergic sympathetic nerve impulses (sympatholytic), and to adrenaline (adrenolytic).

cholinergic b. Interruption by a drug of nerve impulse transmission at autonomic ganglionic synapses (ganglionic blockade), at myoneural junctions (myoneural blockade), and at postganglionic parasympathetic effector cells.

ganglionic b. Interruption by a drug of nerve impulse transmission at autonomic ganglionic synapses.

blocker Blocking agent; see under agent.

blood The fluid circulated by the heart through the vascular system of vertebrates; consisting of plasma (a pale yellow fluid) in which are suspended red and white blood cells and platelets; it carries oxygen and nutrients to all the body tissues and waste products to the excretory systems.

occult b. Blood in the feces in amounts too small to be seen but detectable by laboratory tests.

blood count 1. The number of red or white blood cells in 1 mm³ of blood. 2. The determination of these numbers.

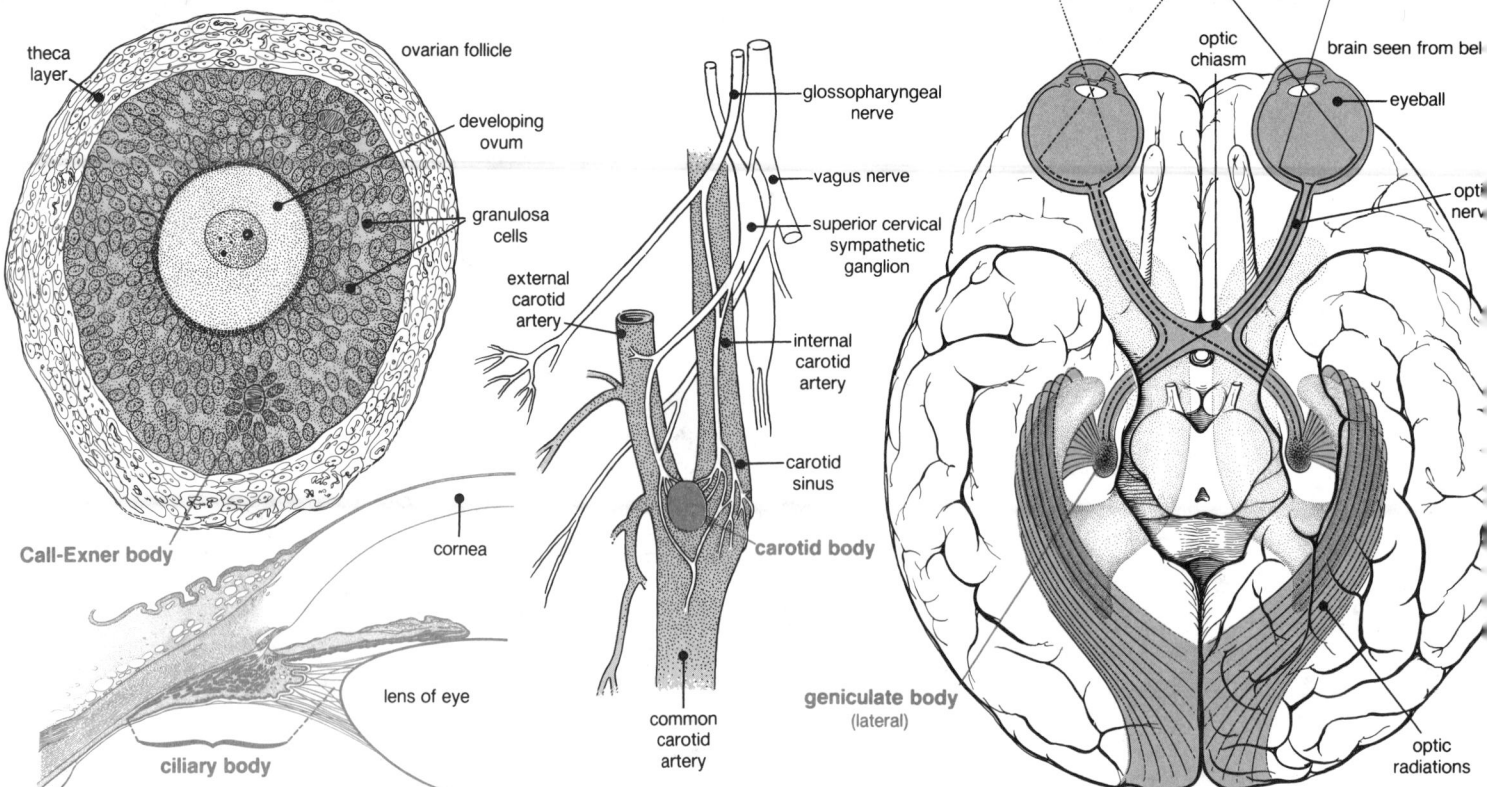

theca layer

ovarian follicle

developing ovum

granulosa cells

Call-Exner body

cornea

lens of eye

ciliary body

glossopharyngeal nerve

vagus nerve

superior cervical sympathetic ganglion

external carotid artery

internal carotid artery

carotid sinus

carotid body

common carotid artery

geniculate body (lateral)

optic chiasm

brain seen from bel

eyeball

opti nerv

optic radiations

complete b. c. (CBC) One usually comprised of a hemoglobin determination, a hematocrit, a red blood cell count, a white blood cell count, and a differential white blood cell count.

differential b. c. The percentage of various types of white blood cells in a specific volume of blood. Also called differential white blood cell count.

blood group (N) Any of various immunologically distinct and genetically determined classes of human blood, identified clinically by characteristic agglutination reactions. Also called blood type. For individual blood groups, see specific names.

blood grouping The classification of blood samples according to their agglutinating characteristics.

bloodletting The removal of blood from a vein for therapeutic purposes.

bloodshot The reddish appearance of a part, as the conjunctiva, due to the congested state of the blood vessels.

blood substitute Any of various fluid substances (human plasma, serum albumin, dextran solution, etc.) used for transfusion.

blood type See blood group.

blot The appearance of a material transferred from an electrophoresis gel to a treated paper or membrane.

Northern b. A blot of RNA fragments.

Southern b. A blot of DNA fragments.

Western b. A blot of proteins.

blush Localized density observed in x-ray examination of blood vessels, due to increased vascularity in a tumor or to leakage of blood.

body 1. The whole material structure of man or animal. 2. The main part of anything.

adrenal b. Adrenal gland.

aortic b.'s Small bilateral structures on a branch of the aorta near its arch; they contain chemoreceptors which are stimulated by decreases in blood oxygen tension.

Aschoff b.'s The specific lesions of acute rheumatic carditis occurring as nodules within the connective tissue of the myocardium; a fully developed body consists of nonspecific phagocytes, myocardial histiocytes, multinucleated cells, and fibroblastic proliferation. Also called Aschoff nodules.

Auer b.'s Elongated structures found in the cytoplasm of immature myeloid cells in acute myelocytic leukemia.

Barr b. Sex chromatin body.

basal b. Cylindrical thickening at the base of each cilium or flagellum; consists of nine triplets of microtubules arranged within the periphery of the cell membrane; triplets are continuous with the doublets of each cilium or flagellum.

Call-Exner b.'s Extracellular multilaminated

bodies containing an accumulation of densely staining material; they are located among the granulosa cells in maturing ovarian follicles.

carotid b. A neurovascular ellipsoidal structure, 3 to 6 mm in diameter, situated on each side of the neck at the bifurcation of the common carotid artery; it is part of the visceral afferent system that helps to regulate respiration; it contains chemoreceptor endings that monitor the oxygen and carbon dioxide content of the blood circulating through the carotid body. Also called carotid glomus.

cell b. The portion of a nerve cell that surrounds and includes the nucleus, exclusive of any projections. Also called soma.

chromaffin b.'s See paraganglia.

ciliary b. The circular structure at the front of the eye between the outer edge of the iris and the ora serrata of the retina; it consists of six layers including the ciliary muscle (which, through the suspensory ligament, permits the lens to accommodate for near and far vision) and a layer of vessels and processes (the most vascular portion of the eye).

Councilman b. 1. A globule formed from necrosis of a hepatocyte (liver cell), seen in yellow fever. Also called Councilman's lesion. 2. The degenerated hyaline hepatocyte in viral hepatitis.

elementary b. 1. See particle, elementary. 2. A platelet. 3. Old term for a virion or virus particle.

geniculate b.'s Four paired oval masses located in the posteroinferior aspect of the thalamus (two lateral and two medial); the lateral are relay nuclei in the visual pathway; the medial serve as relay nuclei in the auditory pathway to the cerebral cortex.

Golgi b. See apparatus, Golgi.

Heinz b.'s Irregularly shaped, refractile granules in red blood cells (usually located at or close to the periphery of the cell), occurring as a result of polymerization and precipitation of denatured hemoglobin molecules.

hematoxylin b.'s Relatively large, deeply staining bodies occasionally found lying free in the tissues in certain diseases, believed to be the remnants of an injured cell nucleus; the structures are so named because of their affinity for hematoxylin stain; found most commonly in systemic lupus erythematosus, especially in renal glomeruli and blood vessel walls. Also called hematoxyphil bodies.

hematoxyphil b.'s See hematoxylin bodies.

Howell-Jolly b.'s Small, round, well defined nuclear remnants commonly found near the periphery of red blood cells following splenectomy; occasionally present in megaloblastic anemia and leukemia.

hyaline b. See Councilman body.

hyaline b.'s of the pituitary Cells filled with hyaline material occasionally occurring in the posterior

lobe of the hypophysis. Also called herring bodies.

inclusion b.'s Structures frequently observed in either the nucleus or the cytoplasm (occasionally in both) of cells infected with certain viruses.

juxtaglomerular b. A group of cells around the renal glomerular arterioles containing cytoplasmic granules believed to be composed of renin.

ketone b.'s Acetoacetic acid, acetone, and β-hydroxybutyrate present in excess in the blood and urine of diabetics. Also called acetone bodies; ketones.

Leishman-Donovan b.'s (L-D bodies) The ovoid, nonflagellated form of the parasite *Leishmania donovani*, usually packed in clusters within the cells of their mammalian host, causing visceral leishmaniasis (kala azar).

lipid b. See droplet, lipid.

Mallory b.'s Large accumulation of eosinophilic material in damaged liver cells; seen in certain diseases, especially those caused by alcoholism. Also called alcoholic hyaline bodies.

malpighian b. Renal corpuscle; see under corpuscle.

mamillary b. One of two small pea-shaped bodies of the hypothalamus located behind the infundibulum in the interpeduncular space; it receives fibers from the fornix and projects to the anterior thalamic nuclei.

Negri b.'s Bodies containing the rabies virus in the cytoplasm of nerve cells. Also called Negri corpuscles.

Nissl b.'s Clusters of ribosomes and endoplasmic reticulum in the cell body and dendrites of a nerve cell; they stain deeply with basic dyes.

pacchionian b.'s Arachnoid granulations; see under granulation.

para-aortic b.'s Small masses of chromaffin tissue (derived from neural ectoderm) found near the sympathetic ganglia along the abdominal aorta; they secrete epinephrine. Also called Zuckerkandl's bodies.

pineal b. A small gland-like structure, located on the roof of the third ventricle of the brain, overhanging the two superior quadrigeminal bodies. Also called epiphysis cerebri; pineal gland.

pituitary b. See hypophysis.

polar b. One of the three cells formed by the ovum during its maturation.

psammoma b.'s Minute spheres, resembling grains of sand, composed of concentrically laminated mineral deposits; found in papillary cancer.

quadrigeminal b.'s Four paired (a superior and an inferior pair) eminences forming the dorsal part of the midbrain. Also called corpora quadrigemina.

residual b.'s Pockets of undigestible ingested

red blood cells

Howell-Jolly bodies

Heinz body

glomerulus

afferent arteriole

juxtaglomerular body

distal convoluted tubule

urinary space

efferent arteriole

ketone bodies

OH   O
| ‖
CH₃—CH—CH₂—C—O⁻

β-hydroxybutyrate

O   O
‖   ‖
CH₃—C—CH₂—C—O⁻

acetoacetate

O
‖
CH₃—C—CH₃

acetone

regions of the body

parietal
frontal
temporal
orbital
nasal
oral
clavicular
sternocleidomastoid
lateral neck
infraclavicular
sternal
deltoid
anterior antebrachial
anterior brachial
anterior brachial
posterior brachial
palm of hand
anterior cubital
posterior cubital
axillary
mammary
anterior cubital
hypochondriac
anterior antebrachial
epigastric
posterior antebrachial
lumbar
umbilical
dorsal region of hand
inguinal
pubic
urogenital
femoral triangle
anterior femoral
anterior knee
anterior crural
posterior crural
dorsal region of foot
calcaneal

axon

dendrite

Nissl bodies

cell body of neuron

hypothalamus

pineal body

mamillary body

pituitary body

polar body

ovum

granulosa cells

lacrimal gland

sclera

lens of eye

vitreous body

nuclei from female skin

sex chromatin bodies

vertebral body

lumbar vertebra

transverse process

spinous process

vertebral foramen

spinous process

osteon

spongy bone

compact bone

periosteum

tongue

pharyngeal wall

soft palate

bolus being swallowed

epiglottis

trachea

esophagus

| H | O | | CH₃ | O | | | H | O | CH₃ | O | | |
glycine   alanine   **peptide bond**

---

material in a cell; e.g., aging pigments (lipofuscin).

restiform b. Cerebellar peduncle, inferior; see under peduncle.

sex chromatin b. A small, darkly stained mass of chromatin located almost always just inside the nuclear membrane; it appears in 40 to 80% of the cells of a normal female and represents one of the two X chromosomes. Also called Barr body.

trachoma b.'s Distinctive bodies found in cells of the conjunctiva of a trachomatous eye.

vertebral b. The cylindrical ventral portion of the vertebra; adjacent vertebral bodies are joined by fibrocartilaginous disks.

vitreous b. The transparent, gelatinous mass, of a consistency slightly firmer than egg white, filling the eyeball behind the lens. Also called corpus vitreum; vitreous.

wolffian b. See mesonephros.

Zuckerkandl's b.'s See para-aortic bodies.

boil An abscess or pyogenic infection of a sweat gland or hair follicle, usually caused by *Staphylococcus aureus*. Also called furuncle.

bolus 1. A soft mass of food moved as a unit in the process of swallowing. **2.** A volume of material injected rapidly as a single unit into a fluid channel.

bomb An apparatus containing a radioactive material for application of rays to a desired area of the body.

bombard To subject a specific area of the body to the action of rays.

bombesin A peptide neurotransmitter.

bond In chemistry, any of several forces holding atoms or ions together in a molecule.

covalent b. A bond resulting from the sharing of one, two, or three pairs of electrons by neighboring atoms.

ionic b. A bond formed by the transfer of one or more electrons from one kind of atom to another; characteristic of salts. Also called electrovalent bond.

peptide b. A covalent bond linking two amino acids, formed when the carboxyl group of one is linked to the amino group of the other. Also called

peptide linkage.

bone The hard, semirigid, calcified connective tissue forming the skeleton of vertebrates. For specific bones, see table of bones.

alveolar b. The thin plate forming the walls of the tooth sockets.

cancellous b. See spongy bone.

cheek b. Zygomatic bone; see table of bones.

compact b. A type in which the bony substance is densely packed and the spaces and channels are narrow. Also called dense bone.

dense b. See compact bone.

heel b. See calcaneus.

hip b. See hipbone.

innominate b. Former name for hipbone.

jaw b. See jawbone.

shin b. See tibia.

spongy b. Bone having a latticework appearance and relatively large marrow spaces. Also called cancellous bone.

thigh b. See femur.

atlas

vertebral foramen

odontoid process

axis

sagittal section of atlas and axis

ethmoid bone

inferior nasal concha

scaphoid

lunate

carpal bones

triangular

PROXIMAL ROW

pisiform

trapezium

trapezoid

capitate

hamate

DISTAL ROW

vertebra

thoracic cage viewed from above

sternum

scapula

clavicle

first rib

BONE	LOCATION	DESCRIPTION	ARTICULATIONS
ankle b.	see talus		
anvil b.	see incus		
astragalus	see talus		
atlas *atlas*	neck	first cervical vertebra	occipital (above), axis (below)
axis epistropheus *axis*	neck	second cervical vertebra	atlas (above), third cervical vertebra (below)
backbones	see vertebrae		
calcaneus heel b. *calcaneus*	foot	largest of the tarsal b.'s situated at back of foot, forming heel; somewhat cuboidal	talus, cuboid
capitate b. magnum b. *os capitatum*	wrist	largest of carpal b.'s, occupies center of wrist	second, third, and fourth metacarpal b.'s; lunate, trapezoid, scaphoid, hamate
carpal b.'s *ossa carpi*	wrist	eight in number, arranged in two rows: scaphoid, lunate, triangular, and pisiform; trapezium, trapezoid, capitate, and hamate	
cheekbone	see zygomatic bone		
clavicle collar b. *clavicula*	shoulder	long curved b. placed nearly horizontally above first rib	sternum, scapula, cartilage of first rib
coccyx *os coccygis*	lower back	from three to five triangular rudimentary vertebrae with only the first not fused	sacrum
concha, inferior nasal inferior turbinate b. *concha nasalis inferior*	skull	thin, irregular, scroll-shaped b. extending horizontally along lateral wall of nasal cavity	ethmoid, maxilla, palatine

bone | bone

plantar aspect of left foot

navicular bone · **medial cuneiform bone** · metatarsus · phalanges

calcaneus · cuboid · lateral cuneiform bone · intermediate cuneiform bone

orbit · ethmoid bone · crista galli

maxillary sinus · nasal cavity · inferior nasal concha · maxillary molar

hipbone · anterior crest · tibia · interosseous membrane · fibula

head of femur in acetabulum · neck · greater trochanter · lesser trochanter · femur (posterior view) · intracondylar fossa · lateral condyle · medial condyle

tibial tuberosity · styloid process · tibia · fibula (anterior view) · medial malleolus · lateral malleolus

BONE	LOCATION	DESCRIPTION	ARTICULATIONS
cuboid *os cuboideum*	foot	pyramidal b. on lateral side of foot, proximal to fourth and fifth metatarsal b.'s	calcaneus, lateral cuneiform, fourth and fifth metatarsal b.'s, navicular
cuneiform b., intermediate second cuneiform b. *os cuneiforme intermedium*	foot	wedge-shaped; smallest of the three cuneiforms, positioned beween medial and lateral ones	navicular, medial cuneiform, lateral cuneiform, second metatarsal
cuneiform b., lateral external cuneiform b. *os cuneiforme lateral*	foot	intermediate-sized cuneiform located in center of front row of tarsal b.'s	navicular, intermediate cuneiform, cuboid; second, third, and fourth metatarsals
cuneiform b., medial internal cuneiform b. *os cuneiforme mediale*	foot	largest of the three cuneiforms, at medial side of foot between the navicular and base of first metatarsal	navicular, intemediate cuneiform, first and second metatarsal
elbow b.	see ulna		
epistropheus	see axis		
ethmoid b. *os ethmoidale*	skull	unpaired, T-shaped b. forming part of nasal septum and roof of cavity; curled processes form superior and middle conchae	sphenoid, frontal, both nasal, lacrimal, and palatine b.'s; maxillae, inferior nasal conchae, vomer
fabella *fabella*	knee	sesamoid b. in lateral head of gastrocnemius muscle behind lateral condyle of femur	femur
femur thigh b. *femur*	thigh	longest and heaviest b. in the body, situated between hip and knee	hipbone, patella, tibia
fibula splint b. *fibula*	leg	lateral b. of leg	tibia, talus
flank b.	see ilium		

frontal bone

parietal bone

temporal bone

zygomatic bone

maxilla

greater horn

lesser horn

body

hyoid bone
(anterior view)

head of humerus in glenoid fossa

scapula

humerus
(posterior view)

lateral epicondyle

medial epicondyle

olecranon of ulna

ilium

hipbone
(lateral view)

acetabulum

pubis

obturator foramen

ischium

malleus

short process

incus

long process

stapes

ossicles of middle ear

BONE	LOCATION	DESCRIPTION	ARTICULATIONS
frontal b. forehead b. *os frontale*	skull	flat b. forming anterior part of skull	ethmoid, sphenoid, maxillae, and both nasal, parietal, lacrimal, and zygomatic b.'s
greater multangular b.		see trapezium bone	
hamate b. unciform b. *os hamatum*	wrist	most medial b. of distal row of carpals; distinguished by hooklike process (hamulus) that projects from its palmar surface	lunate, triquetrum, capitate, fourth and fifth metacarpals
hammer b.		see malleus	
hipbone innominate b. *os coxae*	pelvis and hip	large, broad, irregularly shaped b. that forms greater part of pelvis; consists of three parts: ilium, ischium, and pubis	femur, sacrum, with its fellow of opposite side at pubic symphysis.
humerus arm b. *humerus*	arm	longest and largest b. of upper limb, situated between shoulder and elbow	scapula, radius and ulna
hyoid b. lingual b. *os hyoideum*	neck	U-shaped b. in front of neck between mandible and larynx	suspended from tips of skull's styloid processes by ligaments
ilium flank b. *os ilium*	pelvis	broad expanded upper part of the hipbone, divisible into a body and an ala	sacrum, femur, ischium, pubis
incus anvil b. *incus*	ear	middle b. of auditory ossicles	malleus, stapes
inferior tubinate b.		see concha, inferior nasal	
innominate b.		see hipbone	
ischium *os ischii*	pelvis	inferior and dorsal part of the hipbone, divisible into a body and a ramus	femur, ilium, pubis

bone | bone

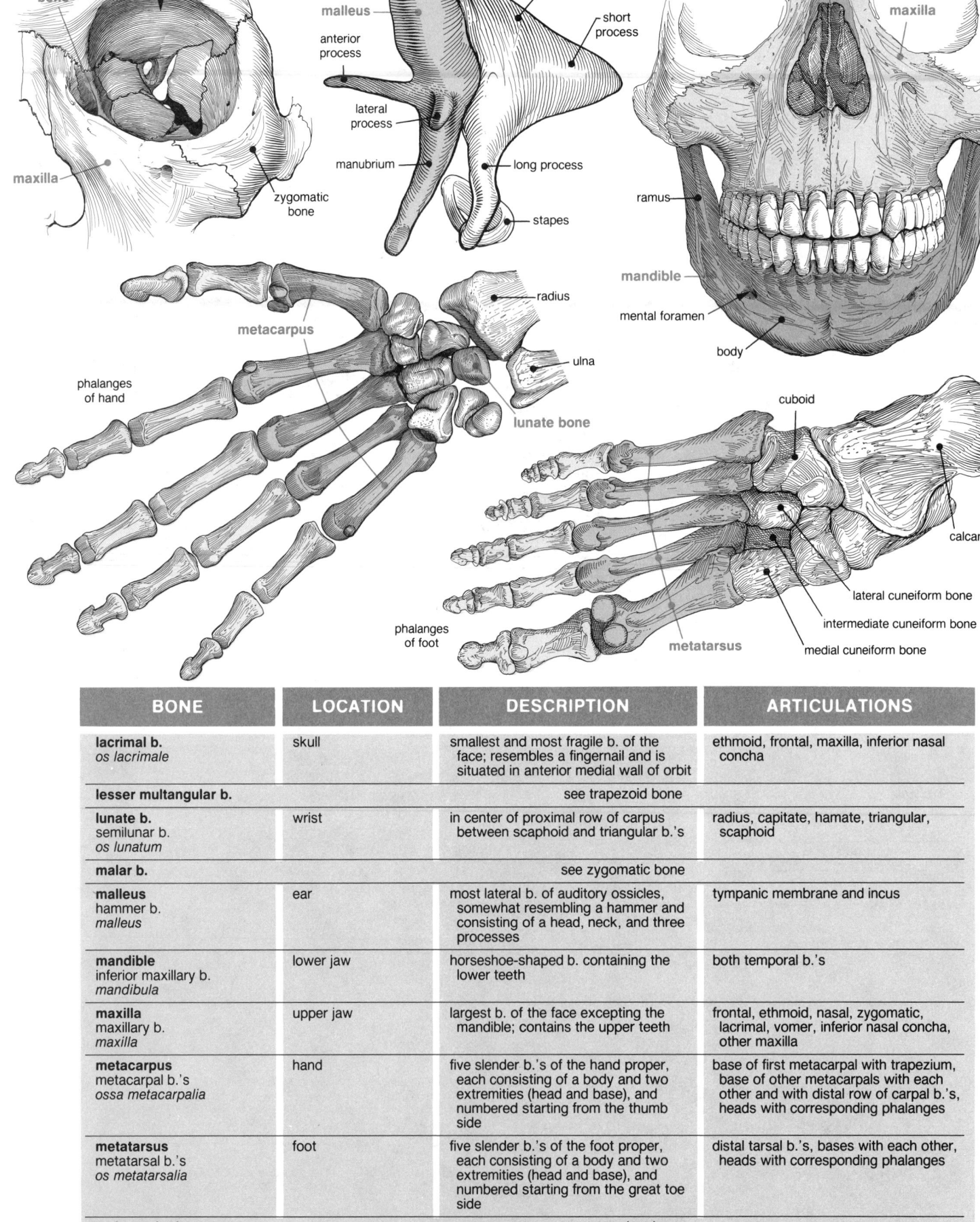

BONE	LOCATION	DESCRIPTION	ARTICULATIONS
lacrimal b. *os lacrimale*	skull	smallest and most fragile b. of the face; resembles a fingernail and is situated in anterior medial wall of orbit	ethmoid, frontal, maxilla, inferior nasal concha
lesser multangular b.			see trapezoid bone
lunate b. semilunar b. *os lunatum*	wrist	in center of proximal row of carpus between scaphoid and triangular b.'s	radius, capitate, hamate, triangular, scaphoid
malar b.			see zygomatic bone
malleus hammer b. *malleus*	ear	most lateral b. of auditory ossicles, somewhat resembling a hammer and consisting of a head, neck, and three processes	tympanic membrane and incus
mandible inferior maxillary b. *mandibula*	lower jaw	horseshoe-shaped b. containing the lower teeth	both temporal b.'s
maxilla maxillary b. *maxilla*	upper jaw	largest b. of the face excepting the mandible; contains the upper teeth	frontal, ethmoid, nasal, zygomatic, lacrimal, vomer, inferior nasal concha, other maxilla
metacarpus metacarpal b.'s *ossa metacarpalia*	hand	five slender b.'s of the hand proper, each consisting of a body and two extremities (head and base), and numbered starting from the thumb side	base of first metacarpal with trapezium, base of other metacarpals with each other and with distal row of carpal b.'s, heads with corresponding phalanges
metatarsus metatarsal b.'s *os metatarsalia*	foot	five slender b.'s of the foot proper, each consisting of a body and two extremities (head and base), and numbered starting from the great toe side	distal tarsal b.'s, bases with each other, heads with corresponding phalanges
multangular b., greater			see trapezium bone
maltangular b., lesser			see trapezoid bone
nasal b. *os nasale*	skull	one of two small oblong paired b.'s positioned side by side to form bridge of nose	frontal, ethmoid, opposite nasal, maxilla

bone | bone

BONE	LOCATION	DESCRIPTION	ARTICULATIONS
navicular b. navicular b. of foot scaphoid b. of foot *os naviculare* *os naviculare pedis*	foot	situated at medial side of tarsus between talus and cuneiform b.'s	talus, three cuneiforms, occasionally with cuboid
navicular b. of hand		see scaphoid bone	
occipital b. *os occiptale*	skull	unpaired saucer-shaped b. forming posterior part of base of cranium pierced by the foramen magnum	both parietals and temporals; sphenoid, atlas
palatine b. palate b. *os palatinum*	skull	one of two, somewhat L-shaped paired b.'s, the two forming the posterior part of hard palate, part of floor and lateral wall of nasal cavity, and part of floor of the orbit	sphenoid, ethmoid, maxilla, vomer, opposite palatine, inferior nasal concha
parietal b. *os parietale*	skull	paired b.'s between frontal and occipital b.'s forming sides and roof of cranium	opposite parietal, frontal, occipital, temporal, sphenoid
patella knee cap *patella*	knee	flat, rounded, triangular b. (sesamoid), situated in front of knee joint	femur
pelvis		a body ring resembling a basin, composed of two hipbones, sacrum, and coccyx	
phalanges of foot *ossa digitorum pedis*	foot	miniature long b.'s, two in great toe and three in each of other toes	proximal row of phalanges with corresponding metatarsal b.'s and middle phalanges; middle phalanges with proximal and distal phalanges; ungual phalanges with middle phalanges
phalanges of hand *ossa digitorum manus*	hand	miniature long b.'s, two in thumb and three in each of other fingers	proximal row of phalanges with corresponding metacarpal b.'s and middle phalanges; middle phalanges with proximal and distal phalanges; ungual phalanges with middle phalanages
pisiform b. *os pisiforme*	wrist	most medial of proximal row of carpus; smallest carpal b.	triangular
pubis *os pubis*	pelvis	anterior lower portion of hipbone	ilium, ischium, femur

costotransverse capsule

transverse process

lamina

superior articular facet

floating ribs

thoracic rib

pedicle

costocentral capsule

spinal canal

body of vertebra

ribs

sternum

scapula

humerus

clavicle

ribs

costal cartilages

vertebral column

BONE	LOCATION	DESCRIPTION	ARTICULATIONS
pyramidal b.	see triangular bone		
radius *radius*	forearm	lateral b. of forearm; proximal end is small and forms small part of elbow; distal end is large and forms large part of wrist joint	humerus, ulnar, lunate, scaphoid
ribs *costae*	chest	12 pairs of thin, narrow, arch-shaped b.'s forming posterior and lateral walls of chest	all posteriorly with vertebral column; upper seven pairs anteriorly with sternum, through intervention of costal cartilages; lower five pairs anteriorly with costal cartilages; lowest two pairs free at ventral extremities (floating)

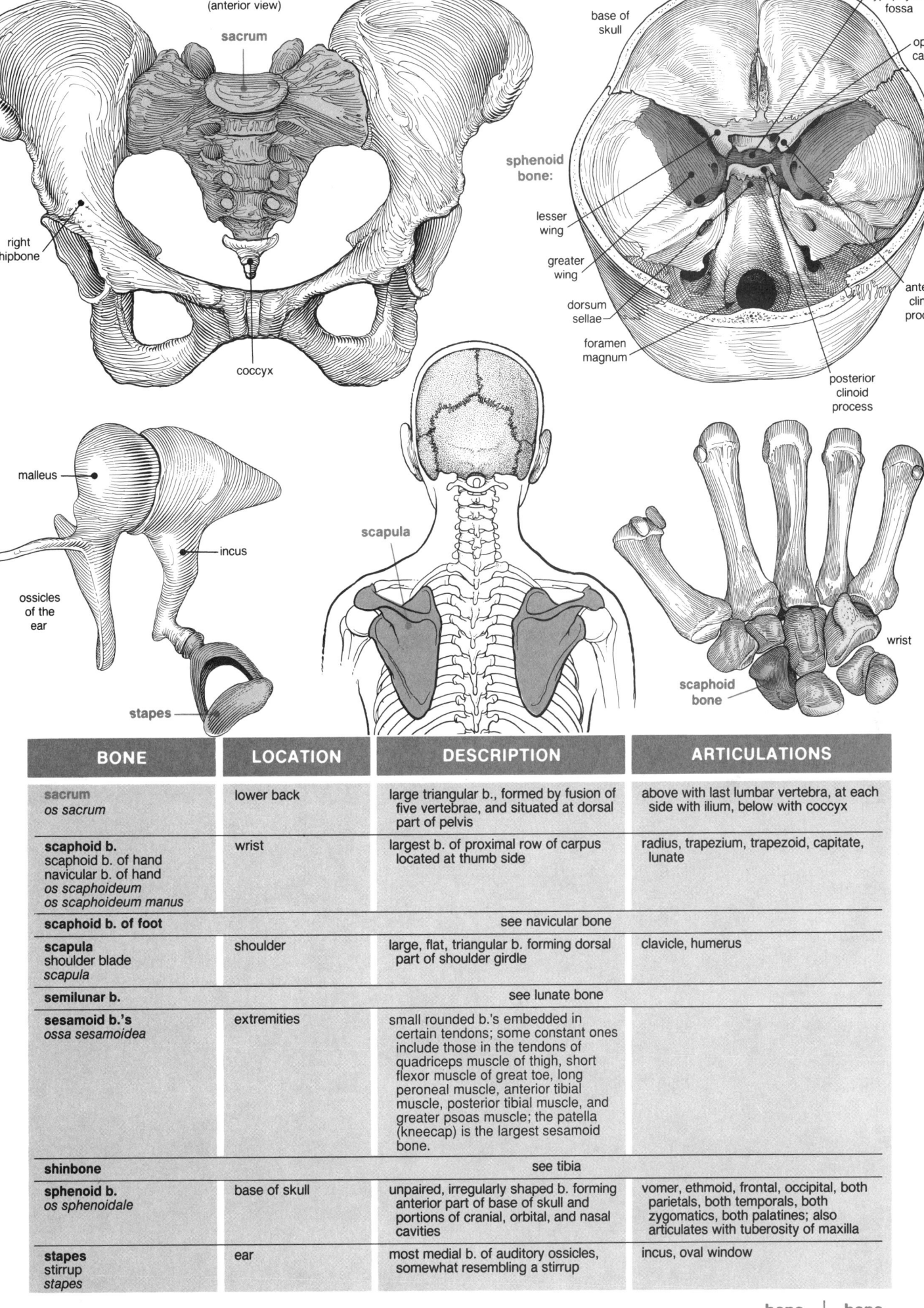

pelvis
(anterior view)

sacrum

right
hipbone

coccyx

base of
skull

hypophyseal
fossa

optic
canal

sphenoid
bone:

lesser
wing

greater
wing

dorsum
sellae

foramen
magnum

anterior
clinoid
process

posterior
clinoid
process

malleus

incus

ossicles
of the
ear

stapes

scapula

scaphoid
bone

wrist

BONE	LOCATION	DESCRIPTION	ARTICULATIONS
sacrum *os sacrum*	lower back	large triangular b., formed by fusion of five vertebrae, and situated at dorsal part of pelvis	above with last lumbar vertebra, at each side with ilium, below with coccyx
scaphoid b. scaphoid b. of hand navicular b. of hand *os scaphoideum* *os scaphoideum manus*	wrist	largest b. of proximal row of carpus located at thumb side	radius, trapezium, trapezoid, capitate, lunate
scaphoid b. of foot	see navicular bone		
scapula shoulder blade *scapula*	shoulder	large, flat, triangular b. forming dorsal part of shoulder girdle	clavicle, humerus
semilunar b.	see lunate bone		
sesamoid b.'s *ossa sesamoidea*	extremities	small rounded b.'s embedded in certain tendons; some constant ones include those in the tendons of quadriceps muscle of thigh, short flexor muscle of great toe, long peroneal muscle, anterior tibial muscle, posterior tibial muscle, and greater psoas muscle; the patella (kneecap) is the largest sesamoid bone.	
shinbone	see tibia		
sphenoid b. *os sphenoidale*	base of skull	unpaired, irregularly shaped b. forming anterior part of base of skull and portions of cranial, orbital, and nasal cavities	vomer, ethmoid, frontal, occipital, both parietals, both temporals, both zygomatics, both palatines; also articulates with tuberosity of maxilla
stapes stirrup *stapes*	ear	most medial b. of auditory ossicles, somewhat resembling a stirrup	incus, oval window

bone | bone

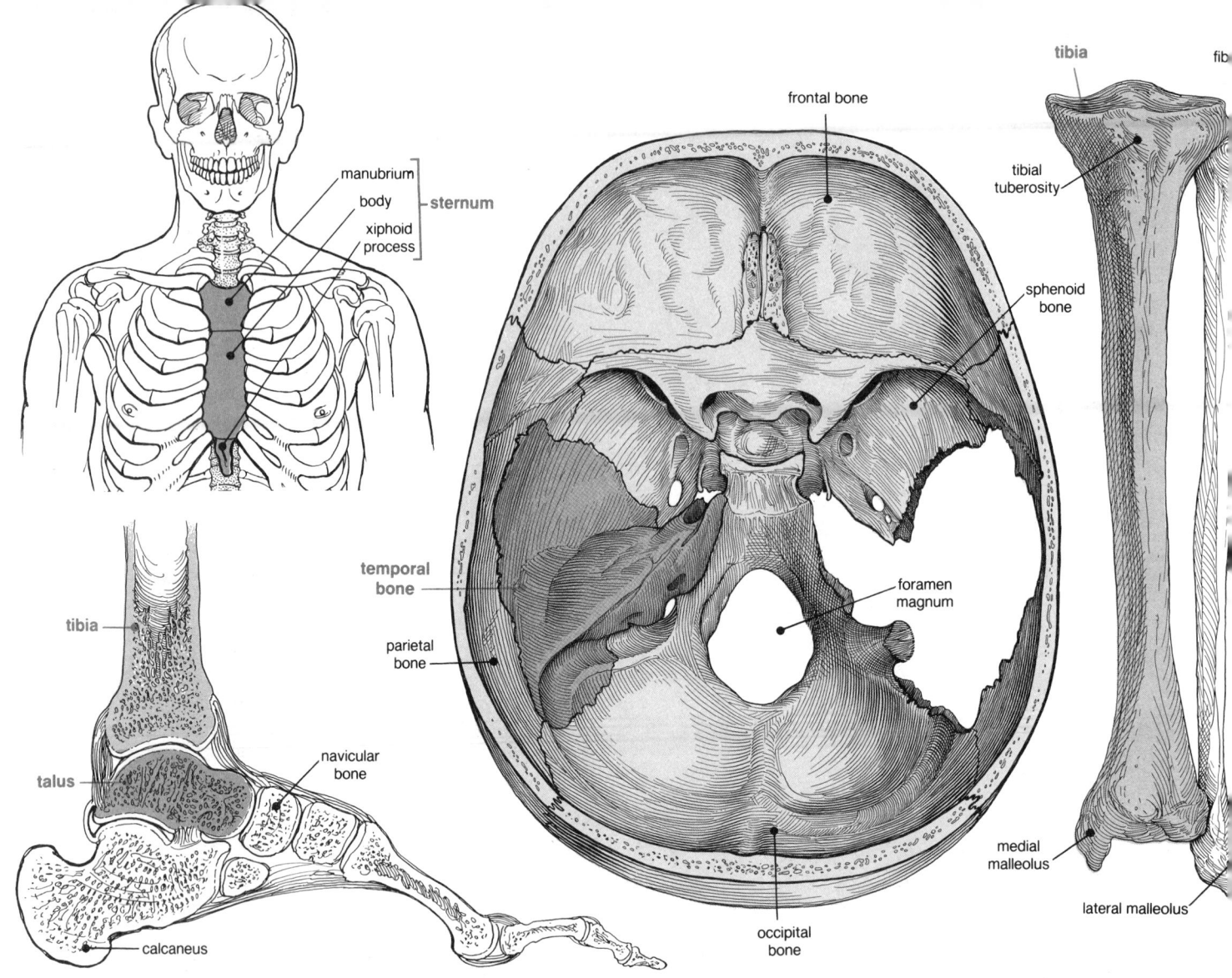

manubrium
body
xiphoid process
— sternum

frontal bone

tibia

fib

tibial tuberosity

sphenoid bone

temporal bone

parietal bone

foramen magnum

tibia

talus

navicular bone

calcaneus

occipital bone

medial malleolus

lateral malleolus

BONE	LOCATION	DESCRIPTION	ARTICULATIONS
sternum breastbone *sternum*	chest	elongated, flattened, dagger-shaped b. forming ventral wall of thorax; consists of three parts: manubrium, body, xiphoid process	both clavicles and first seven pairs of costal cartilages
stirrup b.	see stapes		
sutural b.'s wormian b.'s *ossa suturalis*	skull	irregular, isolated b.'s occasionally found along cranial sutures, especially lambdoid suture	usually occipital and parietal b.'s
talus ankle b. astragalus *talus*	ankle	second largest of the tarsal b.'s; supports tibia and rests on calcaneus	tibia, fibula, calcaneus, navicular
temporal b. *os temporale*	skull	irregularly shaped b. consisting of three parts: squamous, petrous, and tympanic; forms part of side and base of cranium	occipital, parietal, zygomatic, sphenoid, mandible
tibia shinbone *tibia*	leg	situated at medial side of leg between ankle and knee joint; second longest b. in the body	above with femur and fibula; below with fibula and talus
tapezium b. greater multangular b. *os trapezium*	wrist	most lateral of four b.'s of distal row of carpus	scaphoid, first metacarpal, trapezoid, second metacarpal
trapezoid b. lesser multangular b. *os trapezoideum*	wrist	smallest b. in distal row of carpus	scaphoid, second metacarpal, trapezium, capitate
triangular b. pyramidal b. triquetral b. *os triquetrum*	wrist	pyramidal shape; second from little finger side of proximal row of carpus	lunate, pisiform, hamate, triangular articular disk

bone | bone

posterior view of the vertebral column

cervical vertebrae

thoracic vertebrae

lumbar vertebrae

cervical vertebra

superior view

lateral view

thoracic vertebra

superior view

lateral view

lumbar vertebra

lateral view

superior view

cervical vertebrae

thoracic vertebrae

lumbar vertebrae

sagittal view of the vertebral column

BONE	LOCATION	DESCRIPTION	ARTICULATIONS
triquetral b.	see triangular bone		
turbinate b., inferior	see choncha, inferior nasal		
turbinate b., middle	not a separate bone; see ethmoid bone		
turbinate b., superior	not a separate bone; see ethmoid bone		
ulna elbow b. *ulna*	forearm	medial b. of forearm; lies parallel with radius	humerus, radius
unciform b.	see hamate bone		
vertebrae, cervical backbones *vertebrae*	back of neck	seven segments of vertebral column; smallest of the true vertebrae; possess a foramen in each transverse process	first vertebra with skull, all others with adjoining vertebrae
vertebrae, lumbar backbones *vertebrae*	lower back	five segments of vertebral column; largest b.'s of movable part of vertebral column	with adjoining vertebrae; fifth vertebra with sacrum
vertebrae, thoracic backbones *vertebrae*	back	12 segments of vertebral column; possess facets on the sides of all the bodies and the first 10 also have facets on the transverse processes	with adjoining vertebrae, heads of ribs, tubercles of ribs (except 11th and 12th)
vomer *vomer*	skull	thin, flat b. forming posterior and inferior part of nasal septum	ethmoid, sphenoid, both maxillae, both palatine bones; also articulates with septal cartilage of nose
wormian b.'s	see sutural bones		
zygomatic b. malar b. cheekbone *os zygomaticum*	skull	forms prominence of cheek and lower, lateral aspects of orbit	frontal, sphenoid, temporal, maxilla

brush border

sinus bradycardi[a]

normal

orthopedic cervical **brace**

Borrelia

bulbous bougie

boutons termineaux

borate A salt of boric acid.

borax Sodium borate, $Na_2B_4O_7$; used in dentistry in the casting of fluxes and to retard the setting reaction of gypsum products.

borborygmus Rumbling noise produced by movement of gas in the intestines.

border Edge or margin.

brush b. A border of many fine, closely packed microvilli, as seen on the free surface of the cuboidal cells of the proximal convoluted tubules of the kidney.

denture b. 1. The boundary of a denture base. 2. The area of a denture base at the junction of the polished surface with the impression (tissue) surface. Also called denture edge.

striated b. A border of many fine, closely packed microvilli on the free surface of the columnar absorptive cells of the intestine; it greatly increases the surface area of intestinal epithelium. Also called striated free border.

vermillion b. The exposed reddish portion of the upper and lower lips.

Bordetella A genus of gram-negative pathogenic coccobacilli.

B. pertussis The causative agent of whooping cough in man. Formerly called *Hemophilus pertussis*.

boric acid A white or crystalline compound, H_3BO_3; used as an antiseptic.

Bornholm disease Epidemic pleurodynia; see under pleurodynia.

boron A soft, brown nonmetallic element; symbol B, atomic number 5, atomic weight 10.82.

Borrelia A genus of bacteria (family Treponemataceae), several species of which are the cause of relapsing fever throughout the world. Formerly called *Spironema*, the organisms are now included by many authorities in the genus *Treponema*.

B. burgdorferi The cause of Lyme disease, transmitted by the tick *Ixodes dammini*.

borreliosis Infection with *Borrelia* bacteria.

boss 1. A round swelling. 2. A hump on the back.

bosselation Condition marked by the presence of one or more round protuberances or swellings.

Bothriocephalus *Diphyllobothrium*.

botryoid Resembling a bunch of grapes.

bottle A receptacle with a narrow neck.

wash b. 1. A fluid-containing bottle with two tubes passing through its cork, arranged in such a way that blowing through one tube forces a stream of fluid through the other; used for washing chemical materials. 2. A fluid-containing bottle with a tube passing to the bottom through which gases are forced for the purpose of purifying the gases.

botulism Poisoning caused by the toxin of *Clos-*

tridium botulinum in improperly preserved food.

bougie A flexible cylindrical instrument used in the diagnosis and treatment of strictures of tubular structures, such as the esophagus or urethra; it also serves to measure the degree of narrowing.

b. à boule Bulbous bougie.

bulbous b. A bougie with a bulb-shaped tip.

filliform b. A very slender bougie.

bougienage Examination or treatment (dilation) of a tubular structure by means of a bougie or cannula.

bouillon 1. A clear thin broth. 2. A culture medium prepared from beef.

bouton A swelling or thickening.

b. de Bagdad Cutaneous leishmaniasis; see under leishmaniasis.

b. en chemise Abscesses of the intestinal mucosa, seen in amebic dysentery.

b.'s termineaux The numerous enlarged synaptic axon terminals of a neuron which make contact with the receptive end of another neuron (either with the cell body, a dendrite, or its axon). Also called terminal buttons; synaptic knobs; end-feet.

bovine Relating to cattle.

bowel The intestine.

Bowen's disease Squamous cell carcinoma occurring as pink-to-brown papules at multiple sites on the skin within the epidermis.

bowleg See genu varum.

brace A device for supporting a bodily part.

orthodontic b.'s General term for orthodontic appliances designed to move teeth into a more esthetic and/or functional position; composed of bands fitted to the teeth with attachments or brackets to hold spring wires; often the wires are supplemented by rubber bands.

brachial Relating to the arm.

brachium *pl.* **brachia** 1. The arm, especially above the elbow. 2. Any armlike structure.

brachybasia The slow, shuffling gait indicative of motor nerve disease.

brachycephalic Characterized by brachycephalism.

brachycephalism A deformity in which the skull has an abnormally flattened anteroposterior plane, due to premature closure of the coronal suture.

brachydactyly Abnormal shortness of fingers and toes.

brachytherapy Radiotherapeutic treatment applied with the x-ray source near the tissues being irradiated. Also called plesiotherapy.

bracket In orthodontics, a small piece of metal fixed on the band surrounding a tooth; used to fasten the arch wire to the band.

bradycardia Abnormal slowness of the heartbeat,

a rate usually less than 60 beats per minute.

sinus b. Bradycardia resulting from the sinus node originating impulses at a slow rate; usually due, in part at least, to vagal inhibition of the sinus node; seen often in patients with high vagal tone, in trained athletes, in hypothyroidism, and secondary to increased intracranial tension.

bradycrotic Marked by a slow pulse.

bradykinesia Abnormal slowness of movement.

bradykinin A potent vasodilator polypeptide hormone produced by the action of kallikrein on an alpha 2-globulin.

bradypnea Abnormally slow rate of breathing, as in shock.

braille A system of writing and printing for the blind, consisting of raised dots representing letters and numerals; invented by Louis Braille, a French teacher of the blind.

brain The portion of the central nervous system contained within the skull; composed of the cerebrum, cerebellum, pons, and medulla oblongata. Also called encephalon.

brain stem The part of the brain connecting the forebrain (prosencephalon) and the spinal cord; it consists of the midbrain (mesencephalon), pons, and medulla oblongata.

bran A by-product of the milling of wheat to produce flour; consists mainly of the coat of the grain; used as a bulk cathartic.

branchial Relating to gills.

branchiogenic, branchiogenous Originating from the embryonic branchial arches or the ridges between the branchial clefts.

brawny Dark and swollen.

breakdown, nervous A vague popular euphemism for a mental disorder, usually implying an acute and marked change in behavior and inability to function.

breast 1. Mammary gland. 2. Chest.

chicken b. See pectus carinatum.

keel b. See pectus carinatum.

pigeon b. See pectus carinatum.

breastbone See sternum.

breath 1. The inhaled and exhaled air in respiration. 2. The air exhaled, as evidenced by vapor.

breathing The act of taking in and expelling air from the lungs.

intermittent positive pressure b. (IPPB) The intermittent inflation of the lungs with air or an oxygen mixture at an adjustable pressure and rate of flow.

mouth b. The process of inhaling and exhaling air chiefly through the mouth rather than the nose.

shallow b. A weak type of breathing, as seen in acute pulmonary disease.

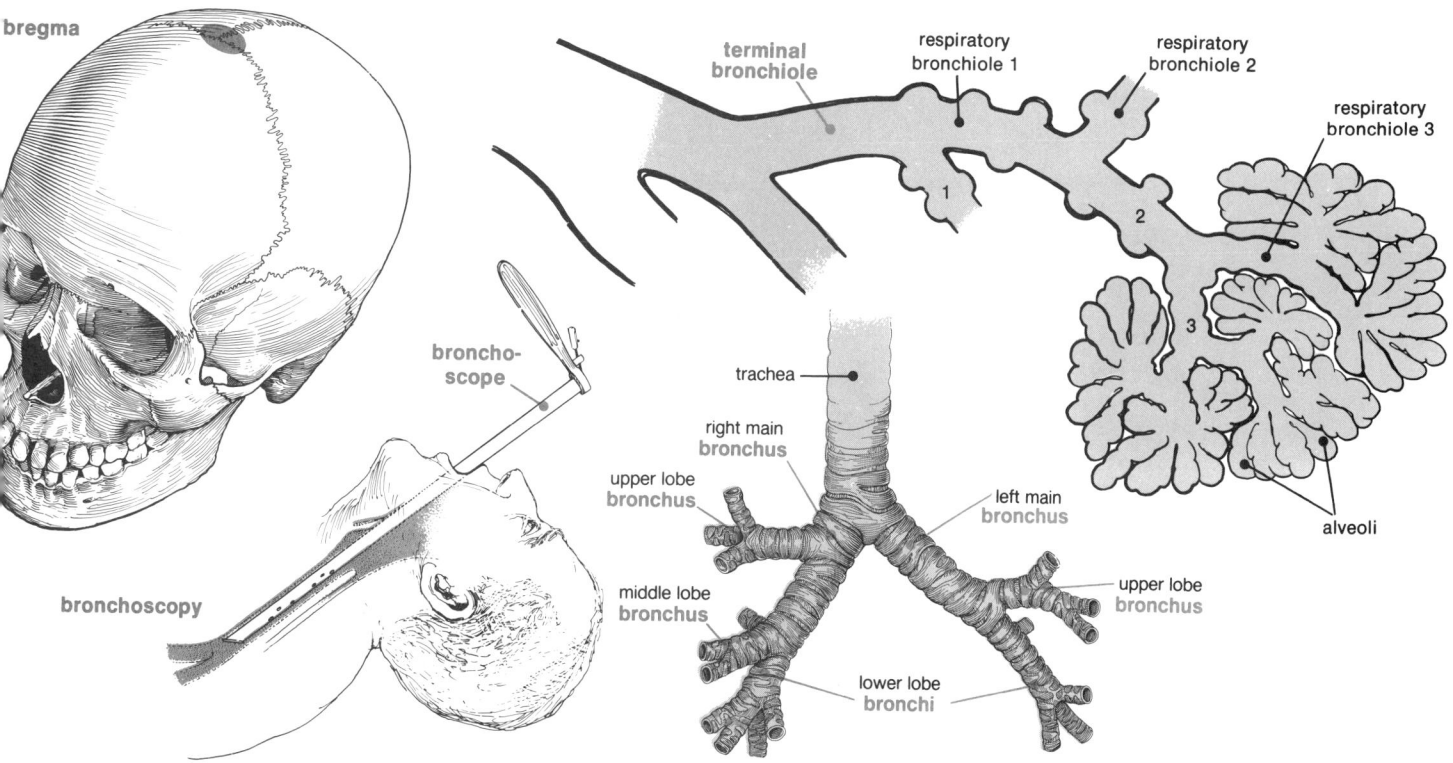

bregma

bronchoscope

bronchoscopy

terminal bronchiole

respiratory bronchiole 1

respiratory bronchiole 2

respiratory bronchiole 3

alveoli

trachea

right main bronchus

upper lobe bronchus

left main bronchus

middle lobe bronchus

upper lobe bronchus

lower lobe bronchi

---

breed 1. To develop new or improved strains in animals or plants. 2. A strain of animal or plant.

bregma The point on the skull where the sagittal and coronal sutures meet. Also called sinciput.

brei A suspension of minced tissue, used especially in metabolic experimentation.

bridge 1. In dentistry, a nonremovable prosthesis consisting of one or more artificial teeth suspended between and attached to abutments (terminal natural crowns or roots). 2. The upper part of the human nose, between the eyes.

Bright's disease A term applied in the past to a variety of acute and chronic renal diseases, especially those thought to represent forms of glomerulonephritis.

Brill's disease See Brill-Zinsser disease.

Brill-Zinsser disease The occurrence of typhus in persons who suffered an infection of primary epidemic typhus in the past; caused by *Rickettsia prowazekii* which, according to Zinsser, remain viable in the body of the patient; recrudescence or relapse occurs years after the original infection. Also called Brill's disease; recrudescent typhus.

British antilewisite (BAL) See dimercaprol.

broach A small instrument used in the examination or treatment of the root canal of a tooth.

Broadbent's sign Pulsation observed in the left posterior axillary line, occurring synchronously with cardiac systole; a sign of adherent pericardium.

broad-spectrum Widely effective. See also antibiotic, broad-spectrum.

bromcresol green A slightly yellow crystalline compound, $C_{21}H_{14}Br_4O_5S$, slightly soluble in water; soluble in alcohol, ether, and ethyl alcohol; used as an indicator of pH: yellow at pH 3.8, blue-green at pH 5.4.

bromcresol purple A pale yellow crystalline compound, $C_{21}H_{16}Br_2O_5S$; soluble in alcohol and dilute alkalis; used as an indicator of pH: yellow at pH 5.2, purple at pH 6.8.

bromide A binary compound of bromine and another element or organic radical; a salt of hydrobromic acid.

bromine A heavy, corrosive, reddish, volatile, nonmetallic liquid element, with a highly irritating vapor; symbol Br, atomic number 35, atomic weight 79.916.

bromism Bromide poisoning marked by headache, skin eruptions, apathy, and muscular weakness.

bromphenol blue An indicator of pH.

Brompton cocktail See mixture, Brompton.

bronchi Plural of bronchus.

bronchial Relating to the bronchi.

bronchiectasis, bronchiectasia An irreversi-ble, abnormal dilatation of the bronchi or bronchioles; the extent of the disorder may range from a mild involvement of a single pulmonary segment to gross distortion of the entire bronchial tree.

bronchiogenic Of bronchial origin.

bronchiole Any of the thin-walled extensions of a bronchus.

  terminal b. The last bronchiole without alveoli in its wall.

bronchiolectasis, bronchiolectasia Chronic dilatation of the terminal bronchioles.

bronchiolitis Inflammation of the bronchioles.

  acute obliterating b. A form of fibrosis of the lung due to fibrous induration of the walls of the terminal bronchioles.

bronchiostenosis Narrowing of the bronchi.

bronchitis Inflammation of the mucous membrane of the bronchi.

bronchoalveolar See bronchovesicular.

bronchocavernous Relating to a bronchus and a pulmonary cavity.

bronchocele A circumscribed dilatation of a bronchus.

bronchoconstrictor An agent that causes narrowing of the lumen of a bronchus.

bronchodilator An agent that causes dilatation of the lumen of a bronchus.

bronchoegophony An exaggerated egophony (bleating quality of voice heard in auscultation).

bronchogenic Of bronchial origin.

bronchogram The radiogram obtained by bronchography.

bronchography Radiographic examination of the bronchi after injection of a radiopaque material.

broncholith A bronchial calculus (stone).

broncholithiasis Presence of bronchial calculi.

bronchomalacia Degeneration of the supporting tissues of the bronchi and trachea.

bronchomotor An agent that changes the caliber of bronchi.

bronchopathy Disease of the bronchial tubes.

bronchophony Exaggerated resonance of the voice heard in auscultation over a bronchus surrounded by consolidated lung tissue.

bronchoplasty Surgical repair of a defect in the trachea or the bronchi.

bronchoplegia Paralysis of the muscular fibers in the walls of the bronchi.

bronchopneumonia Inflammation of the lungs, usually following infection of the bronchi. Also called lobular or bronchial pneumonia.

bronchopulmonary Relating to the bronchi and the lungs.

bronchorrhea Abnormally profuse secretion from the bronchi.

bronchoscope A thin tubular instrument used for inspecting the interior of the trachea and bronchi.

bronchoscopy The endoscopic examination and treatment of the tracheobronchial tree and lungs, by means of the bronchoscope used as a speculum.

bronchospasm Spasmodic constriction of the bronchial tubes. Also called bronchoconstriction.

bronchospirography The measuring of the airflow in one lung only, or one lobe of a lung.

bronchospirometer A device for measuring separately the air capacity of each lung.

bronchospirometry The determination of the respiratory capacity of a lung by the use of a bronchospirometer.

bronchostenosis Narrowing of the lumen of a bronchial tube.

bronchovesicular Relating to the bronchial tubes and air sacs in the lungs.

bronchus *pl.* **bronchi** Either of two main branches of the trachea leading to the bronchioles and serving to convey air to and from the lungs.

Brown-Sequard syndrome Damage of a lateral half of the spinal cord, causing motor and sensory disturbances below the level of the lesion, i.e., motor paralysis and loss of joint position sense and vibration sense on the same side of the body and loss of pain and temperature sensation on the opposite side.

Brucella A genus of bacteria (family Brucellaceae) composed of gram-negative, rod-shaped to coccoid parasitic cells; they cause primary infections of the genital organs, mammary glands, and respiratory and intestinal tracts.

  B. abortus A species causing abortion in cattle and undulant fever (brucellosis) in man. Also called Bang's bacillus.

  B. melitensis A species causing undulant fever in man and abortion in goats.

  B. suis A species resembling *Brucella melitensis*; the cause of abortion in swine and brucellosis in man.

brucellosis An infectious disease caused by bacteria of the genus *Brucella* and transmitted by animals; characterized by remittent fever, general weakness, aches, and pains, sometimes becoming chronic. Also called undulant, Malta, Mediterranean, or abortus fever; melitensis.

Brudzinski's signs 1. Brudzinski's neck sign: flexion of both legs and thighs upon forcible flexion of the neck. 2. Brudzinski's contralateral leg sign: (a) flexion of one thigh at the hip causes a similar movement of the other thigh; (b) when one thigh and leg are flexed and the other extended, lowering of the flexed leg causes flexion of the extended one. Brudzinski's signs are seen in meningitis.

Brugia A genus of parasitic filarial worms trans-

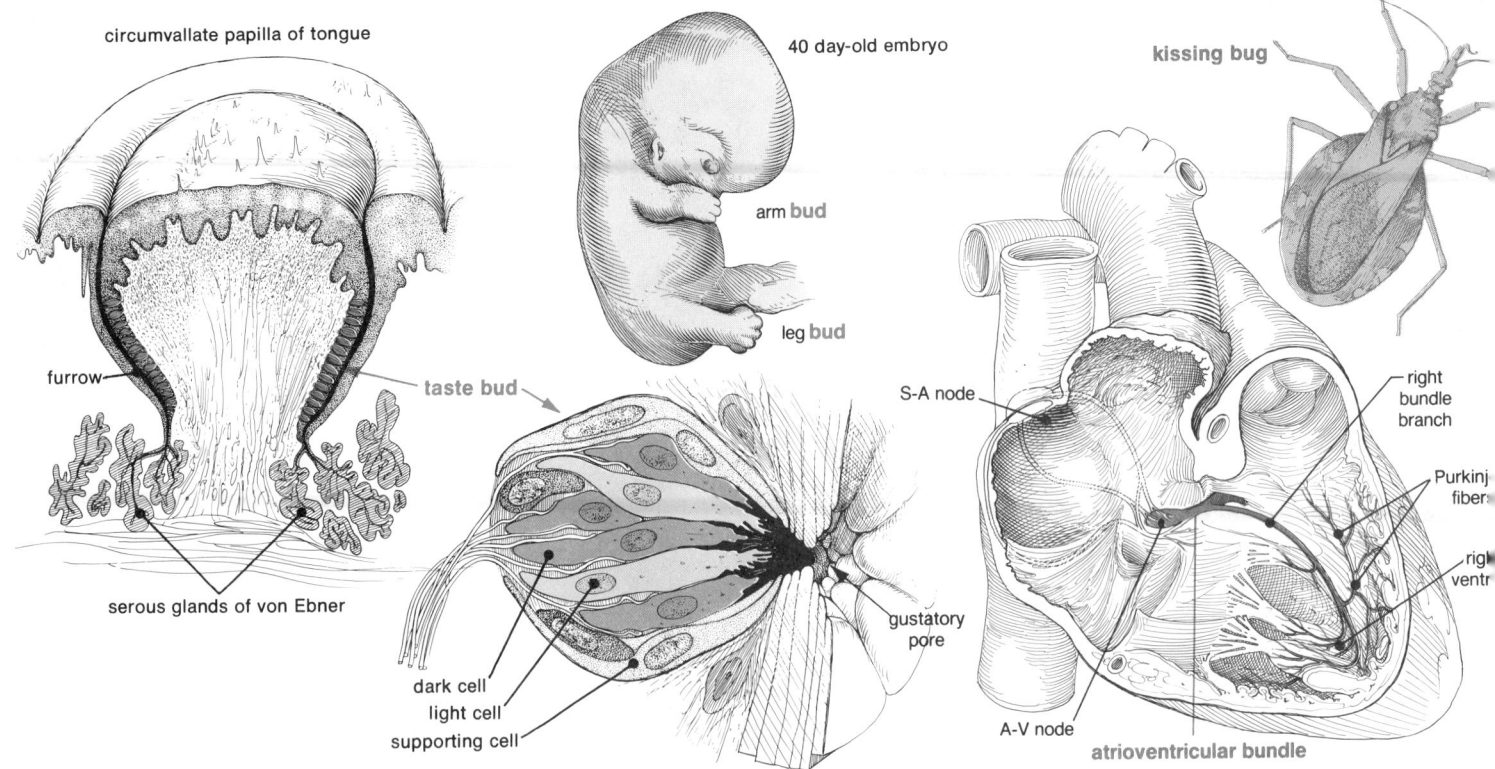

circumvallate papilla of tongue

furrow

serous glands of von Ebner

taste bud

40 day-old embryo

arm bud

leg bud

dark cell

light cell

supporting cell

gustatory pore

kissing bug

S-A node

A-V node

atrioventricular bundle

right bundle branch

Purkinj fiber

rig ventr

mitted to man and other mammals by mosquitoes.

B. malayi The species causing filariasis and elephantiasis in Southeast Asia. Formerly called Malayan filaria; *Wuchereria malayi.*

bruise Hematoma without laceration; usually a superficial lesion but can occur in deeper structures; a contusion.

bruit Sound or murmur, especially an abnormal one heard during auscultation; from the French word for noise.

abdominal b. A murmur heard on auscultation of the abdomen, generally traceable to the aorta or one of its major branches.

aneurysmal b. A blowing murmur heard over an aneurysm.

b. de canon The abnormally loud first heart sound heard intermittently in complete heart block; cannon sound.

b. de Roger Roger's murmur; see under murmur.

carotid b. A murmur heard over a carotid artery.

diastolic b. Bruit occurring during the diastolic phase of the heart cycle after the second heart sound; this usually connotes an abnormal valve function.

epigastric b. A murmur heard in the epigastrium during auscultation of the abdomen.

systolic b. Bruit heard during the systolic phase of the heart cycle between the first and second heart sounds.

thyroid b. A vascular murmur heard over a hyperactive thyroid gland.

bruxism Forceful clenching and grinding of the teeth, especially during sleep.

bruxomania Unconscious grinding of the teeth while awake.

bubo Enlargement and inflammation of a lymph node, especially in the groin or axilla.

malignant b. One associated with bubonic plague.

tropical b. See lymphogranuloma venereum.

venereal b. Bubo in the groin associated with venereal disease.

bubonic Relating to an enlarged suppurating lymph node in the groin or axilla.

buccal Pertaining to the cheek.

buccolingual 1. Denoting the plane of a posterior tooth from its buccal surface across to its lingual surface. 2. Relating to the cheek and the tongue.

bucco-occlusal Relating to the buccal and occlusal surfaces of a posterior tooth; usually denoting the line angle formed by the junction of the two surfaces.

buccopharyngeal Relating to both the mouth and pharynx.

buckling, scleral Technique for repair of detachment of the retina in which the deep sclera and the

choroid are infolded over the retinal tear to promote adherence of the retina to the choroid layer of the eye.

bud Any small organic part resembling a plant bud.

bronchial b. One of the outgrowths from the primordial bronchus, giving rise to the bronchial tree.

lung b.'s Two lateral outpocketings of the respiratory primordium of the foregut that gives rise to the tracheobronchial tree.

metanephric b. An outgrowth from the mesonephric duct, giving rise to the lining of the ureter, pelvis, and calyces of the kidney, and the straight collecting tubules.

taste b. One of numerous flask-shaped minute organs, located on the tongue, the under surface of the soft palate, and the posterior surface of the epiglottis; composed of modified epithelial supporting cells which surround a mass of spindle-shaped gustatory cells and the fibrils of the nerves of taste (chorda tympani and glossopharyngeal). Also called gustatory caliculus; taste bulb.

tooth b. The primordial structures from which a tooth develops.

Budd-Chiari syndrome Hepatic vein occlusion; see under occlusion.

budding See gemmation.

Buerger's disease See thromboangiitis obliterans.

buffer 1. Any substance that maintains the relative concentrations of hydrogen and hydroxyl ions in a solution by neutralizing any added acid or alkali. 2. To add a buffer to a solution; to maintain body fluids at a relatively constant pH when acid or alkali is added to or lost from the body.

buffering A process by which hydrogen ion concentration is maintained constant.

biologic b. Ionic shifts between intra- and extracellular spaces which protect extracellular pH.

renal b. Removal of excess acid or base by the kidney.

respiratory b. Increases or decreases in respiratory rate which act to increase or decrease CO_2 and, subsequently, H_2CO_3 and HCO_3.

bug Any of various insects of the order Hemiptera.

assassin b. See kissing bug.

bed b. See bedbug.

cone-nose b. See kissing bug.

kissing b. An insect (family Reduviidae) similar to the ordinary bedbug but with a cone-shaped anterior end; usually found in bedrooms where it feeds at night on the blood of its sleeping and unsuspecting hosts; acquired its name because of its inclination to bite the lips of sleeping people. Also called cone-nose or assassin bug.

red b. See chigger.

bulb 1. Any globular structure. 2. The medulla oblongata.

aortic b. A dilatation at the beginning of the aorta.

b. of the corpus spongiosum See bulb of penis.

b. of penis The expanded posterior portion of the corpus spongiosum penis.

carotid b. See sinus, carotid.

duodenal b. See cap, duodenal.

jugular b. A dilatation of the internal jugular vein just before it joins the subclavian vein.

Krause's end-b. A spherical sense organ located at the termination of some sensory nerve fibers; it responds to the sensation of cold. Also called Krause's corpuscle.

olfactory b. The expanded anterior end of the olfactory tract.

bulbar 1. Relating to or resembling a bulb. 2. Relating to the medulla oblongata.

bulbopontine Relating to the part of the brain composed of the pons and the portion of the medulla oblongata over it.

bulbourethral Relating to the bulb of the urethra, the enlarged posterior portion of the corpus spongiosum of the penis.

bulimia Repeated episodes of solitary binge eating, often followed by self-induced vomiting or massive laxative use to avoid weight gain; these episodes usually alternate with periods of fasting; seen primarily in young white females.

bulkage Any substance, such as bran, that stimulates peristalsis by increasing the bulk of the intestinal contents.

bulla *pl.* **bullae** 1. A blister or circumscribed elevation on the skin containing serous fluid, larger than one centimeter in size, e.g., as in a second degree burn. 2. A bubble-like structure. Cf. vesicle.

pulmonary b. A large air-filled bulla on the surface or within the lung; seen in certain diseases.

bullous 1. Characterized by the presence of blisters (bullae). 2. Of the nature of bullae.

bundle A group of nerve or muscle fibers.

atrioventricular (A-V) b. A bundle of specialized muscular fibers located in the membranous interventricular septum of the heart; the only direct muscular connection between the atria and the ventricles; it originates at the atrioventricular (A-V) node in the floor of the right atrium, extends downward in the septum, divides into right and left branches, and ends in numerous strands (Purkinje system) in the papillary and ventricular muscles. Also called bundle of His; fasciculus atrioventricularis.

b. of His See atrioventricular bundle.

posterior longitudinal b. Medial longitudinal fasciculus; see under fasciculus.

bunion

burnishers

prepatellar bursitis

after Netter

burette

button

sprue

inlay

burs

bunion Painful condition of the big toe, marked by lateral angulation of the toe (hallux valgus), enlargement of the head of the metatarsal bone, and a swollen, inflamed overlying bursa; caused by poorly fitted shoes. Cf. hallux valgus.

bunionectomy Treatment of a bunion by surgical means; e.g., by fusing the first metatarsal and proximal phalanx after removing adjacent portions of both bones.

buphthalmos A condition marked by an increase of intraocular fluid with enlargement of the eyeball and protrusion of the cornea. Also called congenital glaucoma; hydrophthalmos.

bur A rotary dental instrument with one cutting end designed in any of several shapes and a shaft at the other end which is inserted into a hand piece; used for excavating decay from a tooth, shaping cavity forms, or any surface reduction of tooth substance.

burette, buret A calibrated, uniform-bore glass tube with a stopcock at its lower end, used in the laboratory for accurate fluid dispensing.

burn 1. To injure by fire, heat, or a chemical. 2. The lesion thus produced.
  brush b. Injury to the skin by friction of a rapidly moving object. Also called rope or mat burn.
  chemical b. A burn caused by a caustic agent.
  first degree b. Reddening of skin without blistering; only epidermis is affected.
  flash b. A burn caused by brief exposure to radiant heat of high intensity.
  radiation b. A burn due to overexposure to x-rays, radium, ultraviolet rays, etc.
  second degree b. Blistering of skin; epidermis and dermis are involved.
  thermal b. A burn produced by contact with heat.
  third degree b. Destruction of full thickness of skin; may involve subcutaneous fat, muscle, and bone.

burner The part of a lamp or stove that is lighted to produce a flame.
  Bunsen b. A gas burner used in the laboratory, consisting of a metal tube with adjustable air holes at the base.

Burnett's syndrome See milk-alkali syndrome.

burnisher A dental instrument with rounded edges for smoothing, polishing, or stretching the metallic surface of a tooth restoration.

bursa *pl.* **bursae** A closed sac lined with specialized connective tissue and containing a viscid fluid; usually present over bony prominences, between and beneath tendons, and between certain movable structures; it serves to facilitate movement by diminishing friction.
  Achilles b. See bursa of calcaneal tendon (tendo calcaneus).

  adventitious b. An abnormal bursa developed as a result of irritation.
  anserine b. A bursa located at the medial aspect of the knee, under, and near the insertion of, the gracilis and semitendinous tendons.
  b. of calcaneal tendon, b. of tendo calcaneus A bursa located at the heel, between the calcaneus bone and calcaneal tendon (Achilles tendon). Also called Achilles or retrocalcaneal bursa.
  b. of Fabricius A saclike outgrowth of the cloaca in chicks, similar to the human thymus; contains lymphoid follicles and produces lymphocytes which are active in humoral immunity; it atrophies after six months. See also B lymphocytes, under lymphocyte.
  deep infrapatellar b. A bursa located below the patella (kneecap) between the lower portion of the patellar ligament and the tibia.
  deep trochanteric b. A bursa located in the hip between the greater trochanter of the femur and the gluteus maximus muscle. Also called trochanteric bursa of gluteus maximus muscle.
  gastrocnemius b. A bursa composed of two portions (lateral and medial) and located in the back of the knee, under the two heads of the gastrocnemius muscle; the medial portion is usually connected with the semimembranous bursa (of clinical importance because when distended with fluid, it is the usual cause of a popliteal cyst).
  iliopectineal b. A bursa located on the anterior surface of the hip joint capsule, between the iliofemoral and pubofemoral ligaments; it frequently communicates with the capsule of the joint.
  ischiogluteal b. A large bursa separating the gluteus maximus muscle from the ischial tuberosity; chronic ischiogluteal bursitis is caused by prolonged sitting on hard surfaces and is commonly known as weaver's bottom.
  olecranon b. A bursa located at the elbow between the skin and the tip of the olecranon process of the ulna.
  omental b. Lesser sac of peritoneum; see under sac.
  popliteal b. A bursa located on the posterolateral portion of the knee, under the popliteus muscle; it is often a continuation of the synovial sac of the knee.
  prepatellar b. A bursa situated anterior to the lower part of the patella (kneecap); chronic irritation causes prepatellar bursitis (housemaid's knee).
  quadriceps b. An extension of the synovial sac on the anterior aspect of the knee, between the femur and the quadriceps tendon. Also called suprapatellar bursa.
  radiohumeral b. A bursa located at the elbow, over the radiohumeral joint, between the extensor

digitorum and supinator muscles.
  semimembranous b. A bursa located in the medial aspect of the knee, between the semimembranous tendon and the medial head of the gastrocnemius muscle. See also gastrocnemius bursa.
  subacromial b. A bursa located between the acromium and the capsule of the shoulder joint; usually connected with the subdeltoid bursa.
  subdeltoid b. A bursa located between the deltoid muscle and the capsule of the shoulder joint; usually combined with the subacromial bursa.
  subscapular b. A bursa between the tendon of the subscapular muscle and the glenoid border of the scapula; it communicates with the shoulder joint.
  superficial acromial b. A bursa located at the shoulder between the acromium and the skin.
  superficial prepatellar b. A bursa on the anterior aspect of the knee, over the insertion of the patellar ligament into the tuberosity of the tibia. Also called pretibial bursa.

bursectomy Surgical removal of a bursa.

bursitis Inflammation of a bursa.
  prepatellar b. Inflammation of the bursa in front of the patella (kneecap), usually due to repeated trauma. Also called housemaid's knee.

bursotomy Incision into a bursa.

buttock One of two protuberances formed by the gluteal muscles.

button 1. Any knob-shaped or disk-shaped structure, lesion, or device. 2. A collection of cells obtained after centrifuging a fluid specimen containing a small number of cells. 3. In dentistry, the excess metal remaining from casting; located at the end of the sprue.
  peritoneal b. A device for draining ascitic fluid.
  terminal b.'s Boutons terminaux.

bypass A shunt; a diverted flow.
  cardiopulmonary b. Procedure whereby the flow of blood is diverted from the heart and lungs to permit surgery within the heart, ascending aorta or coronary arteries; venous blood normally emptying into the right atrium is diverted from the venae cavae to an extracorporeal circuit, passed through an oxygenator where gases are exchanged, and returned to the arterial circulation.
  coronary b. Technique used in the treatment of coronary arterial disease; a graft (usually a reversed saphenous-vein graft) is sutured to the aorta and the distal segment of a coronary artery, beyond the diseased portion to provide circulation through the remainder of the vessel. Also called coronary artery bypass graft.

byssinosis A form of chronic inflammatory and fibrotic disease caused by inhalation of dust in cotton, flax, and hemp mills; chief symptom is acute airway obstruction. Also called cotton-mill fever.

caffeine

calcitonin

metatarsal

phalanges

caduceus

calcaneus

dental calculi

renal calculi

cacao An evergreen tropical tree. *Theobroma cacao.* Also called chocolate tree.

cachectic Relating to cachexia.

cachet A wafer capsule formerly used by pharmacists to enclose unpalatable drugs.

cachexia Severe malnutrition, weakness, and muscle wasting resulting from a chronic disease.

cacosmia An olfactory hallucination; a perception of unpleasant odors that do not exist.

cadaver Corpse; a dead body.

cadaverine An amine, $C_5H_{14}N_2$, found in decomposing animal tissue.

cadmium A soft, bluish-white metallic element; symbol Cd, atomic number 48, atomic weight 112.40; found in nature associated chiefly with zinc; used in the manufacture of storage batteries, in plating, and in alloys; inhalation may produce pulmonary edema; excessive absorption may also produce interstitial nephritis.

caduceus The winged staff of Mercury, with two oppositely entwined serpents; emblem of the U.S. Army Medical Corp.

cafe au lait In dermatology, a term used to express a shade of brown; from French, coffee with milk. See also under spot.

caffeine A bitter alkaloid compound found in coffee, tea, and cola beverages; used medicinally as a stimulant and diuretic.

caffeinism The chronic results of excessive consumption of beverages containing caffeine, characterized by rapid beating of the heart, irritability, and insomnia.

cage 1. Any enclosure used to confine. 2. Any structure resembling a cage.

  Faraday c. A cage screened from external electrical waves, used in electroencephalography.

  thoracic c. The bones and musculature of the chest which enclose the thoracic organs.

caisson disease A disorder occurring in divers, tunnel workers, or individuals exposed to increased atmospheric pressures; the high pressure causes the gases to dissolve in the blood and body tissues; when the individual returns too suddenly to normal pressure, the dissolved gases return to their original gaseous form and are trapped as bubbles within blood vessels and tissues; symptoms include pain in the joints, respiratory distress, and sometimes coma and death. Also called decompression sickness.

calamine 1. A mineral, hydrous zinc silicate. 2. A powder composed of zinc oxide (not less than 98%) with about 0.5% of ferric oxide, used in lotions and ointments to relieve itching in inflammatory skin disorders. See also lotion, calamine.

calcaneal, calcanean Pertaining to the calcaneus (heel bone).

calcaneus The quadrangular bone articulating with the talus above and the cuboid anteriorly. Also called heel bone.

calcareous Chalky; resembling or containing calcium or limestone.

calcicosis A lung disease (pneumoconiosis) caused by prolonged inhalation of limestone dust. Also called marble cutters' phthisis.

calciferol See vitamin D₂.

calciferous 1. Containing lime. 2. Forming any of the salts of calcium.

calcific Caused by or producing calcification.

calcification 1. Normal deposition of mineral salts in the bone and tooth tissues, thus contributing to their hardening and maturation. 2. Pathologic hardening of organic tissue by deposits of calcium salts within its substance.

calcination The process of calcining.

calcine 1. To heat material to a high temperature causing loss of water, reduction, or oxidation. 2. In dentistry, the removal of water of crystallization from gypsum by heating in order to produce plaster of Paris.

calcinosis A disorder marked by the deposition of calcium salts in the skin and subcutaneous tissues, and sometimes in the tendons and muscles.

  c. cutis A calcium deposit on the skin, usually occurring secondary to a preexisting skin eruption.

  c. universalis Calcinosis involving widespread areas or the entire body.

calcipenia Condition characterized by deficiency of calcium in the tissues.

calciphilia Condition in which the tissues tend to absorb calcium salts from the blood, thus becoming calcified.

calcitonin A thyroid gland hormone which regulates calcium metabolism; it is secreted in response to a high level of blood calcium and acts to lower the level by inhibiting bone resorption. Also called thyrocalcitonin.

calcitriol Dihydroxycholecalciferol; the active form of vitamin B₃.

calcium A silvery, moderately hard metallic element; symbol Ca, atomic number 20, atomic weight 40.08; together with phosphate and carbonate, it gives bone most of its structural properties; it is an essential nutrient in regulating blood coagulation, muscular contraction, conduction of nerve impulses, cell membrane function, enzyme action, and in assuring cardiac rhythmicity; several of the salts of calcium are used in medicine.

  c. carbonate Chalk; an antacid and astringent; $CaCO_3$; 40% calcium by weight.

  c. fluoride A compound occurring naturally in bones and teeth; CaF_2.

  c. gluconate An odorless, tasteless, granular salt of calcium; 8% calcium by weight.

  c. hydroxide Slaked lime, $Ca(OH)_2$, used in dentistry as a topical stimulant for production of secondary dentin to reseal the pulp cavity.

  c. oxalate A white, crystalline, insoluble calcium compound, CaC_2O_4; found as sediment in acid urine and in urinary stones.

calcium-45 A radioactive calcium isotope (^{45}Ca) having a half-life of 164 days; may be used as a tracer in the study of bone metabolism.

calciuria Urinary excretion of calcium; occasionally used as a synonym for hypercalciuria.

calcodynia Pain in the heel.

calculus *pl.* **calculi** An abnormal stony concretion usually composed of mineral salts and formed most frequently in the cavities of the body which serve as reservoirs for fluids. Also called stone.

  arthritic c., articular c. A deposit of urates in or near a joint. Also called chalkstone.

  biliary c. Gallstone.

  dental c. A yellow to brown concretion adhering to the surface of a tooth, made up of calcium salts, microorganisms, and other debris. Also called tartar.

  mulberry c. A calculus composed mainly of calcium oxalate, shaped like a mulberry, and deposited in the bladder.

  renal c. A concretion in the kidney usually made up of calcium oxalate, calcium phosphate, or uric acid. Also called kidney stone.

  salivary c. A calculus in a salivary duct or gland.

  stag-horn c. A calculus with several branches occurring in the kidney pelvis.

  subgingival c. A dental calculus occurring below the margin of the gum.

  supragingival c. A dental calculus adherent to the exposed surface of a tooth.

  urinary c. A calculus in the kidney, ureter, bladder, or urethra.

  vesical c. A urinary stone lodged in the bladder. Also called bladder stone.

calefacient Anything that produces a localized sensation of warmth.

calf *pl.* **calves** The muscular back portion of the human leg; formed by the bellies of the gastrocnemius and soleus muscles.

caliber The diameter of a tube.

calibrate 1. To standardize systematically the graduations of a quantitative measuring apparatus. 2. To determine the diameter of a tube.

caliceal, calyceal Relating to the calix.

calicectasis See caliectasis.

calices Plural of calix.

caliculus A cup-shaped structure.

  gustatory c. Taste bud; see under bud.

Atwater-Ross human calorimeter
water intake
thermometer
oxygen
water exit
thermometer
stirrer
H₂SO₄   soda lime   H₂SO₄
bomb calorimeter
crucible containing food
calvaria
Schlemm's canal
iris
lens
superior
posterior
lateral
semicircular canals
stapes

caliectasis Distention of the pelvis and calices of a kidney. Also called calicectasis.

californium Radioactive element; symbol Cf, atomic number 98, atomic weight 249; half life 45 minutes.

calipers, caliper An instrument composed of two hinged legs, used for measuring diameters, such as the pelvic diameters, or intervals as on an electrocardiogram.

calisthenics 1. A system of light gymnastic exercises to improve muscular tone and to improve physical well-being. 2. The practice of such simple, systematic exercises.

calix *pl.* **calices** A cup-shaped cavity in an organ. Also written calyx.

major renal c. One of two or three cup-shaped subdivisions of the pelvis of the kidney.

minor renal c. One of several (seven to 13) cup-shaped subdivisions of the major renal calices.

Calkins' sign In obstetrics, the morphologic change of the uterus at delivery from a discoid to ovoid shape; due to a separation of the placenta from the uterine wall.

callosal Of or relating to the corpus callosum.

callosity See callus (1).

callous Hard and toughened; relating to callus.

callus 1. A circumscribed thickening of the skin. Also called callosity. 2. A hard bonelike substance which is formed between and around the fragments of broken bone and eventually accomplishes repair of the fracture.

central c. Provisional callus formed within the medullary cavity of fractured bone.

definitive c. The exudate formed between the fractured surfaces of a bone, which changes into true bone.

provisional c. Callus formed between and around the fractured surfaces of a bone, keeping the ends of the bone in apposition and becoming absorbed after repair is completed.

calor Latin for heat.

caloric 1. Relating to calories. 2. Relating to heat.

calorie Any of several units of heat.

large c. (Cal, kcal, C) The calorie used in metabolic studies as a measurement of energy-producing value of various foods according to the amount of heat they produce when oxidized in the body; specifically the amount of heat required to raise the temperature of one kilogram of water one degree centigrade (from 15°C to 16°C) at a pressure of one atmosphere. Also called kilocalorie.

small c. (cal, c) The unit of heat equal to the amount of heat required to raise the temperature of one gram of water one centigrade at a pressure of one atmosphere. Also called gram calorie.

calorific Heat generating.

calorigenic Producing or increasing heat.

calorimeter An apparatus for measuring the amount of heat given off by an individual or by a chemical reaction.

Atwater-Rosa human c. A large chamber in which an individual can reside for an extended period of time in order to measure the total output of bodily heat.

Benedict-Roth c. See apparatus, Benedict-Roth.

bomb c. A cylindrical apparatus for determining the potential energy of food; the food is ignited and the heat of combustion is calculated from the rise in temperature in the calorimeter.

calorimetry The measurement of the amount of heat given off by the body.

calvaria The upper part of the skull.

calvarium Term used incorrectly instead of calvaria.

calx 1. Lime or calcium oxide. 2. The heel.

calyceal See caliceal.

calycectasis See caliectasis.

calycle Caliculus.

calyculus Caliculus.

calyx See calix.

camera 1. An apparatus used for recording images, either photographically or electronically. 2. Any cavity of the body.

camphor A solid, crystalline, volatile substance obtained from an evergreen tree, *Cinnamomum camphora*, or prepared synthetically; used medicinally as an expectorant, stimulant, and diaphoretic.

Campylobacter Genus of motile spiral, gram-negative bacteria (family Spirillaceae); found in the intestinal tract and reproductive organs of animals and the intestinal tract of humans.

C. fetus intestinalis Subspecies causing abortion in cattle and sheep, as well as a human infection.

C. fetus jejuni Subspecies causing infectious diarrhea and acute inflammation of the stomach and intestines in humans; transmitted orally.

canal A tubular structure; a channel.

adductor c. An aponeurotic canal in the middle third of the thigh; it contains the femoral artery and vein, and the saphenous nerve. Also called Hunter's canal.

Alcock's c. See pudendal canal.

alimentary c. The mouth, esophagus, stomach, and intestines.

atrioventricular c. The canal in the embryonic heart leading from the common sinoatrial chamber to the ventricle.

auditory c. External auditory meatus; see under meatus.

birth c. The cavity of the uterus and vagina through which a child passes at birth. Also called parturient canal.

carotid c. A passage through the petrous part of the temporal bone, transmitting the internal carotid artery.

central c. 1. One extending throughout the entire length of the spinal cord. 2. One extending through the middle of each osteon of compact bone.

femoral c. The medial and smallest of the three compartments of the femoral sheath; it contains some lymphatic vessels and a lymph gland.

haversian c.'s See central canal (2).

Hunter's c. See adductor canal.

incisive c. incisor c. One of two canals opening on either side of the midline in the hard palate, just behind the incisor teeth; through each pass the terminal branches of the descending palatine artery and of the nasopalatine nerve.

inferior dental c. See mandibular canal.

inguinal c. An obliquely directed passage through the layers of the lower abdominal wall on either side, through which passes the spermatic cord in the male and the round ligament of the uterus in the female.

mandibular c. The canal within the mandible containing the inferior alveolar vessels and nerves, from which terminal branches reach the mandibular teeth. Also called inferior dental canal.

Müller's c. Paramesonephric duct; see under duct.

optic c. A short canal through the sphenoid bone at the apex of the orbit which transmits the optic nerve and ophthalmic artery into the orbital cavity. Also called optic foramen.

parturient c. Birth canal.

pterygoid c. The canal which passes through the root of the pterygoid process of the sphenoid bone.

pudendal c. The fibrous tunnel within the obturator fascia that lines the lateral wall of the ischiorectal fossa; it transmits the pudendal vessels and nerves. Also called Alcock's canal.

root c., pulp c. The portion of the pulp cavity within the root of a tooth which leads from the apex to the pulp chamber and contains the pulp tissue.

Schlemm's c. A ringlike canal in the anterior edge of the sclera, encircling the cornea; it serves as a drain of the excess aqueous humor of the anterior chamber of the eye. Also called scleral venous sinus.

semicircular c.'s The three bony canals (anterior, lateral, and posterior) in the internal ear in which the membranous semicircular ducts are located.

spinal c. The canal formed by the vertebrae, containing the spinal cord. Also called vertebral canal.

tympanic c. See scala tympani.

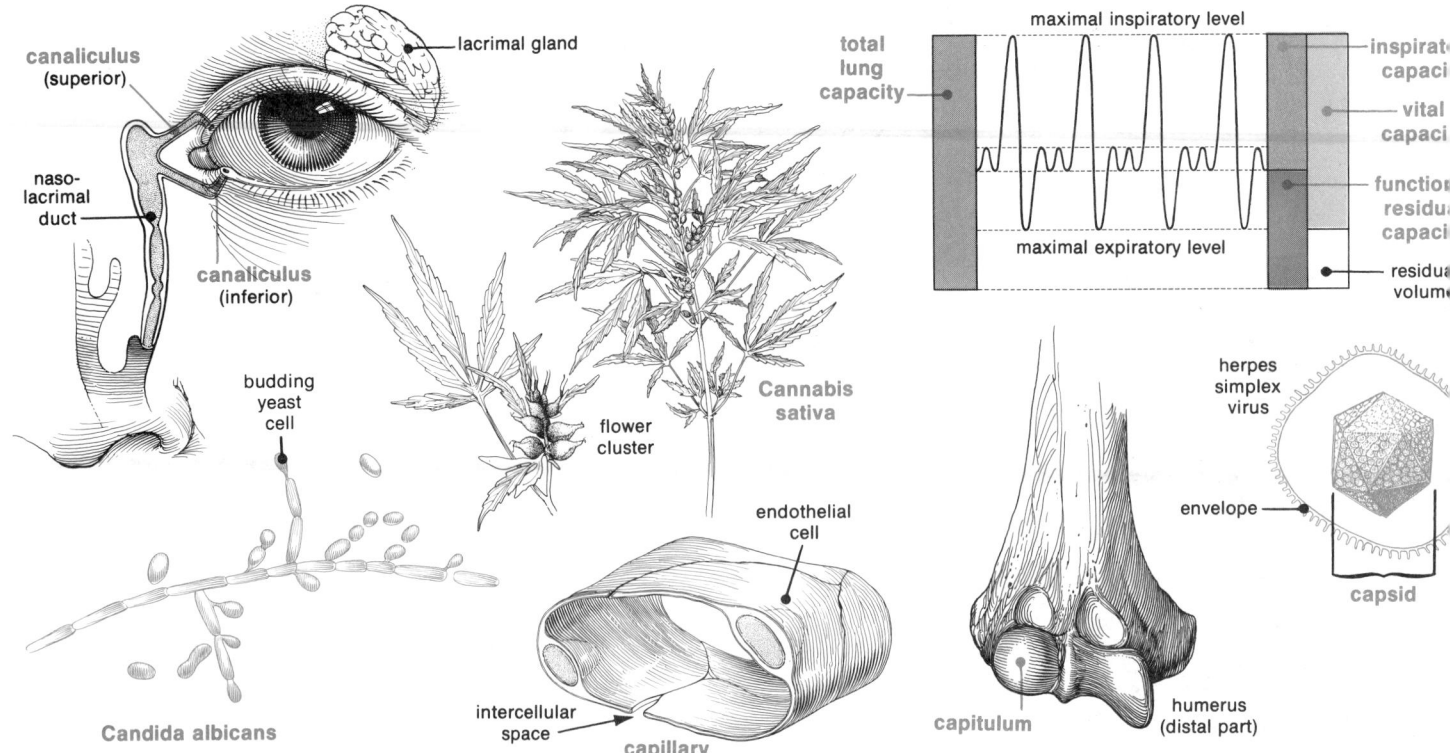

canaliculus (superior)

lacrimal gland

naso-lacrimal duct

canaliculus (inferior)

budding yeast cell

flower cluster

Cannabis sativa

total lung capacity

maximal inspiratory level

maximal expiratory level

inspirat capaci

vital capaci

functio residua capaci

residua volume

herpes simplex virus

envelope

capsid

endothelial cell

intercellular space

capillary

capitulum

humerus (distal part)

Candida albicans

vertebral c. See spinal canal.

vestibular c. See scala vestibuli.

canalicular Relating to a small canal or canaliculus.

canaliculization The formation of small canals in a tissue.

canaliculus pl. **canaliculi** A minute channel or canal.

bile canaliculi Canaliculi between liver cells, forming a mesh.

canaliculi dentales Dental tubules; see under tubule.

lacrimal c. One of two fine channels leading from the medial ends of the eyelids to the lacrimal sac.

canalis pl. **canales** Latin for canal or channel.

cancellated Having a netlike or spongelike structure, such as the spongy bone between the cortical plates and the alveolar bone proper of the mandible.

cancellous Denoting the spongy or honeycomb structure of some bone tissue; such as the ends of long bones.

cancer General term for any malignant tumor.

scirrhous c. See carcinoma, scirrhous.

cancericidal Capable of destroying carcinomas.

cancerophobia Abnormal fear of acquiring a malignant growth.

cancerous Relating to or of the nature of a malignant neoplasm.

cancroid 1. Like cancer. 2. A tumor of moderate malignancy.

cancrum An ulcer that spreads rapidly, occurring usually in the mucosa of the mouth or nose.

candela (cd) The unit of luminous intensity equal to the luminous intensity of five mm² of platinum at its solidification point (1773.5°C). Also called new or international candle.

Candida A genus of yeastlike fungi.

C. albicans A saprophytic species most commonly responsible for monilial infections, such as thrush, vaginitis, and sometimes systemic infection.

candidiasis Infection with microorganisms of the genus *Candida*.

candle Old term for the unit of luminous intensity; preferred term is candela.

canine 1. Relating to a dog. 2. Relating to a cuspid (canine tooth).

canker Aphthous stomatitis; see under stomatitis.

cannabis The dried flowering tops of the *Cannabis sativa* plants, commonly known as marijuana and hashish.

cannabism Condition caused by overuse of hashish or Indian hemp; marked by hallucinations and other subjective symptoms.

cannula A tube inserted into the body to withdraw or deliver fluid; it is used in conjunction with a

metal rod (trocar) which is fitted into its lumen to puncture the wall of the cavity or vessel and then withdrawn, leaving the cannula in place.

cannulation The insertion of a cannula into a bodily cavity or vessel.

Cantelli's sign See doll's eye sign.

cantharis pl. **cantharides** Toxic preparation from the dried beetle, *Cantharis vesicatoria*, mistakenly believed to have aphrodisiac qualities; formerly used as a counterirritant and to promote blister formation. Also called Spanish fly.

canthectomy Surgical excision of a canthus.

canthitis Inflammation of a canthus.

canthoplasty Plastic surgery of the canthus of the eye.

canthorrhaphy Suturing of the eyelids, usually at the outer canthus, to shorten the palpebral fissure.

canthotomy The surgical slitting of the canthus, usually for widening the space between eyelids. Also called cantholysis.

canthus The angle (nasal or temporal) formed by the junction of the upper and lower eyelids.

cap Any structure that serves as a cover.

acrosomal c. A thin covering over the anterior two-thirds of the nucleus of sperm.

cradle c. The grayish-yellow crust formed on the scalp of an infant, caused by seborrhea. Also called milk crust.

duodenal c. The first portion of the duodenum, extending 4 to 5 cm from the pylorus. Also called bishop's cap; pileus ventriculi; duodenal bulb.

enamel c. The enamel organ covering the top of a growing tooth papilla.

knee c. See patella.

metanephric c. One of the masses of mesodermal cells adhering to the ureteral bud of an embryo and developing into the uriniferous tubules of the kidney.

capacitance The quantity of electric charge that may be stored in a body. Formerly called capacity.

capacitation The series of physiologic and biochemical events through which spermatozoa become capable of penetrating ova when coming in contact with various fluids of the uterus and uterine tube.

capacitor An electric circuit element capable of temporarily holding a charge of electricity. Formerly called condenser.

capacity 1. The maximum potential amount a cavity or receptacle can contain. 2. A measure of ability.

cranial c. The cubic content of the skull.

functional residual c. (FRC) The amount of air remaining in the lungs during normal quiet respiration.

heat c. The quantity of heat needed to raise the temperature of a substance 1°C.

inspiratory c. (IC) The maximal volume of air that can be inspired after a normal expiration. Formerly called complemental air.

maximum breathing c. (MBC) The volume of air breathed per minute when a person breathes as deeply and as quickly as possible for 15 seconds.

residual c. Residual volume; see under volume.

total lung c. (TLC) The amount of air contained in the lungs at the end of a maximal inspiration; the vital capacity plus residual volume. Formerly called total lung volume.

vital c. (VC) The greatest volume of air that can be exhaled forcefully following maximal inspiration. Also called breathing or respiratory capacity.

capillariomotor Causing dilatation or constriction of the capillaries.

capillarity The interaction between surfaces of a liquid and solid that causes the liquid to rise or fall as in capillary tubes.

capillary A blood vessel intermediate between the arteriole and venule, whose walls consist of a single layer of cells; oxygen and chemicals filter through the capillary into the tissues, while carbon dioxide and other metabolic wastes pass from the tissue into the capillary.

capillus pl. **capilli** A hair of the head.

capitellum A small rounded end or head, as the elbow end of the humerus.

capitulum A small head-shaped eminence or rounded articular extremity of a bone.

Caplan's syndrome Pulmonary nodules due to lesions which appear to be a combination of rheumatoid arthritis and pneumoconiosis.

capping Covering.

pulp c. The procedure of placing a covering over the exposed vital pulp of a tooth.

capsid Protein coat of a virus.

capsule 1. A small, soluble, gelatinous container used to enclose a dose of an oral medicine. 2. A fibrous or membranous sac surrounding a part, an organ, or a tumor. 3. A mucopolysaccharide layer surrounding certain bacteria.

Bowman's c. Glomerular capsule.

c. of the lens A transparent, brittle but highly elastic membrane closely surrounding the lens of the eye.

Crosby c. An attachment at the end of a flexible tube, used to obtain a peroral biopsy of intestinal mucosa.

Glisson's c. Former name for the fibrous capsule of liver; a thin layer of loose connective tissue enveloping the bile duct, hepatic artery, and portal vein.

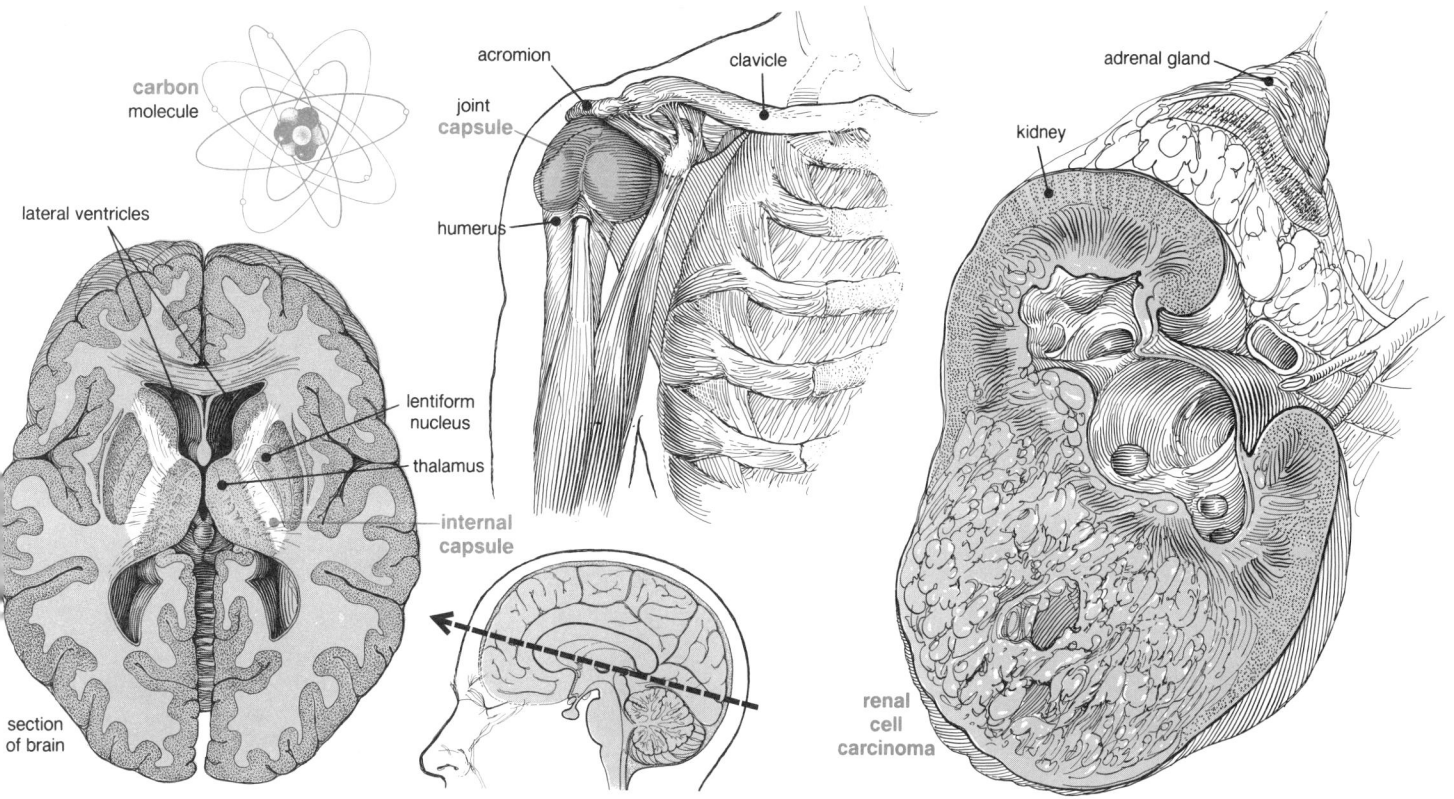

carbon molecule

acromion   clavicle   joint capsule   humerus

adrenal gland   kidney

lateral ventricles   lentiform nucleus   thalamus   internal capsule

section of brain

renal cell carcinoma

glomerular c. A double walled membranous envelope surrounding a minute tuft of non-anatsomosing capillaries (glomerulus); it is the invaginated pouch-like beginning of a renal tubule.

internal c. A broad band of white fibers located in each cerebral hemisphere, between the caudate nucleus and thalamus on the medial side and the lentiform nucleus on the lateral side; generally divided into an anterior limb, a genu, a posterior limb, a retrolentiform part, and a sublentiform part; along with the caudate and lentiform nuclei, it forms the corpus striatum, an important unit of the extrapyramidal system.

joint c. A saclike structure enclosing the cavity of a synovial joint, composed of an outer fibrous layer and an inner synovial membrane.

capsulitis Inflammation of the capsule of an organ or part.

capsuloplasty Surgical repair of a joint capsule, or replacement of a portion or all of the capsule.

capsulotomy The surgical cutting of a capsule, as of the capsule of the crystalline lens in a cataract operation.

caput *pl.* **capita** 1. The head. 2. Any headlike prominence of an organ or structure.

carbamide An isomer of urea in anhydrous form. See urea.

carbaminohemoglobin Carbon dioxide in combination with hemoglobin in the blood.

carbamoyl The organic group NH_2CO-.

carbamoylglutamic acid An intermediate in the carbamoylation of ornithine to citrulline in the urea cycle.

carbarsone A crystalline odorless acid, containing 28.85% arsenic in its anhydrous state; used in the treatment of protozoan infections such as amebiasis.

carbohydrases A general term for enzymes that promote the digestion of carbohydrates.

carbohydrates Any of the group of organic compounds composed of carbon, hydrogen, and oxygen, with a 2 to 1 ratio of hydrogen to oxygen; e.g., sugars, starches, cellulose.

carbolic Relating to phenol.

carbon A tetravalent organic element; symbol C, atomic number 6, atomic weight 12.011.

c. dioxide CO_2; the product of the combustion of carbon with a large supply of air. Also called carbonic acid gas.

c. monoxide CO; a colorless, odorless, poisonous gas with a strong affinity for hemoglobin; formed by the imperfect combustion of carbon with a limited supply of air.

c. tetrachloride CCl_4; a colorless oily liquid; formerly used as a local anesthetic, anthelminthic, and cleaning agent but no longer recommended because of its toxicity to the liver and kidney. Commonly called carbon tet. Also called tetrachloromethane.

carbon-12 An isotope of carbon, ^{12}C; its atomic weight, 12.000, was adopted in 1961 as the atomic weight unit (awu).

carbon-14 A radioactive carbon isotope with atomic weight 14 and a half-life of 5600 years.

carbonic acid Carbon dioxide plus water, H_2OCO_2.

carbonize To convert into charcoal; to char.

carbonyl The organic bivalent radical = CO, characteristic of the ketones and aldehydes.

carboxyhemoglobin (HbCO) Carbon monoxide in combination with oxygen, present in the blood in carbon monoxide poisoning.

carboxyl The characteristic monovalent group—COOH of nearly all organic acids.

carboxylase An enzyme that catalyzes the removal of carbon dioxide from the carboxyl group (COOH) of organic acids.

carboxypeptidase An enzyme of intestinal juice that acts on the peptide bond of amino acids having a free carboxyl.

dipeptidyl c. Enzyme that splits C-terminal dipeptides from a variety of substances. Also called angiotensin converting enzyme (ACE).

carbuncle Painful infection of the skin and subcutaneous tissues with production and discharge of pus and dead tissue, similar to a boil (furuncle) but more severe, and with multiple sinus formation; usually caused by *Staphylococcus aureus*.

renal c. An abscess in the cortex of the kidney, usually resulting from the union of several smaller abscesses; it may occasionally rupture into the collecting system or it may rupture through the renal capsule, causing perirenal abscess.

carbuncular Relating to carbuncles.

carcinogen A cancer-producing agent.

carcinogenesis The origin, development, or production of cancer.

carcinogenic Anything that causes cancer.

carcinoid A small yellow tumor occurring in the intestinal tract, chiefly in the appendix, and in the lungs. Also called argentaffinoma.

carcinoid syndrome A group of symptoms associated with carcinoid tumors, chiefly skin flushes, diarrhea, lesions of the heart valves, and bronchial constriction; caused by release from the tumor of one or more biologically active substances.

carcinoma A malignant cellular tumor which tends to invade surrounding tissues and/or spread to other parts of the body by metastasis, causing eventual death.

alveolar cell c. A rare type of carcinoma derived either from the lining cells of the pulmonary alveoli or from the terminal bronchioles; occurring in the peripheral parts of the lung in the form of single nodules or multiple nodules that coalesce to form a diffuse mass. Also called terminal bronchiolar carcinoma.

basal cell c. A malignant tumor derived from the basal layer of the skin or from structures derived from basal cells; it invades locally but rarely metastasizes and occurs most frequently on the face and scalp. Also called basal cell epithelioma.

bronchogenic c. Carcinoma arising from a bronchus; the most common form of carcinoma of the lung.

c. in situ. Carcinoma that is still confined to its site of origin, before it spreads to other tissues.

clear cell c. of kidney The predominant form of renal cell carcinoma; composed of cells having unstainable cytoplasm.

colloid c. A form of adenocarcinoma in which the degenerative process results in the formation of several areas of mucinous or hyaline material. Also called mucinous carcinoma.

embryonal c. A highly malignant neoplasm of the testis appearing as a small grayish-white nodule or mass, sometimes associated with hemorrhage and necrosis.

epidermoid c. Squamous cell carcinoma.

hepatocellular c. Liver cancer strongly associated with hepatitis B. Also called hepatoma.

intraductal c. Malignant neoplasm consisting of proliferating epithelial cells of a duct, especially in the breast, which eventually fill the lumen.

medullary c. A soft, fleshy, usually large tumor consisting chiefly of epithelial cells with little fibrous stroma. Also called medullary or encephaloid cancer.

melanotic c. Malignant melanoma; see under melanoma.

mucinous c. See colloid carcinoma.

oat cell c. A small-celled carcinoma usually originating in a bronchus. Also called small cell carcinoma.

papillary c. A finger-like malignant tumor.

primary c. Carcinoma at the site of origin.

renal cell c. The most common malignant tumor of the kidney. Also called hypernephroma.

scirrhous c. A stony-hard tumor having a great amount of fibrous tissue, usually occurring in the breast. Also called scirrhous cancer; fibrocarcinoma.

squamous cell c. A malignant epithelial tumor which may originate from normal epithelium, probably made susceptible by chronic radiodermatitis, senile keratosis, burn scars, or leukoplakia; squamous cell carcinomas of the skin occur more fre-

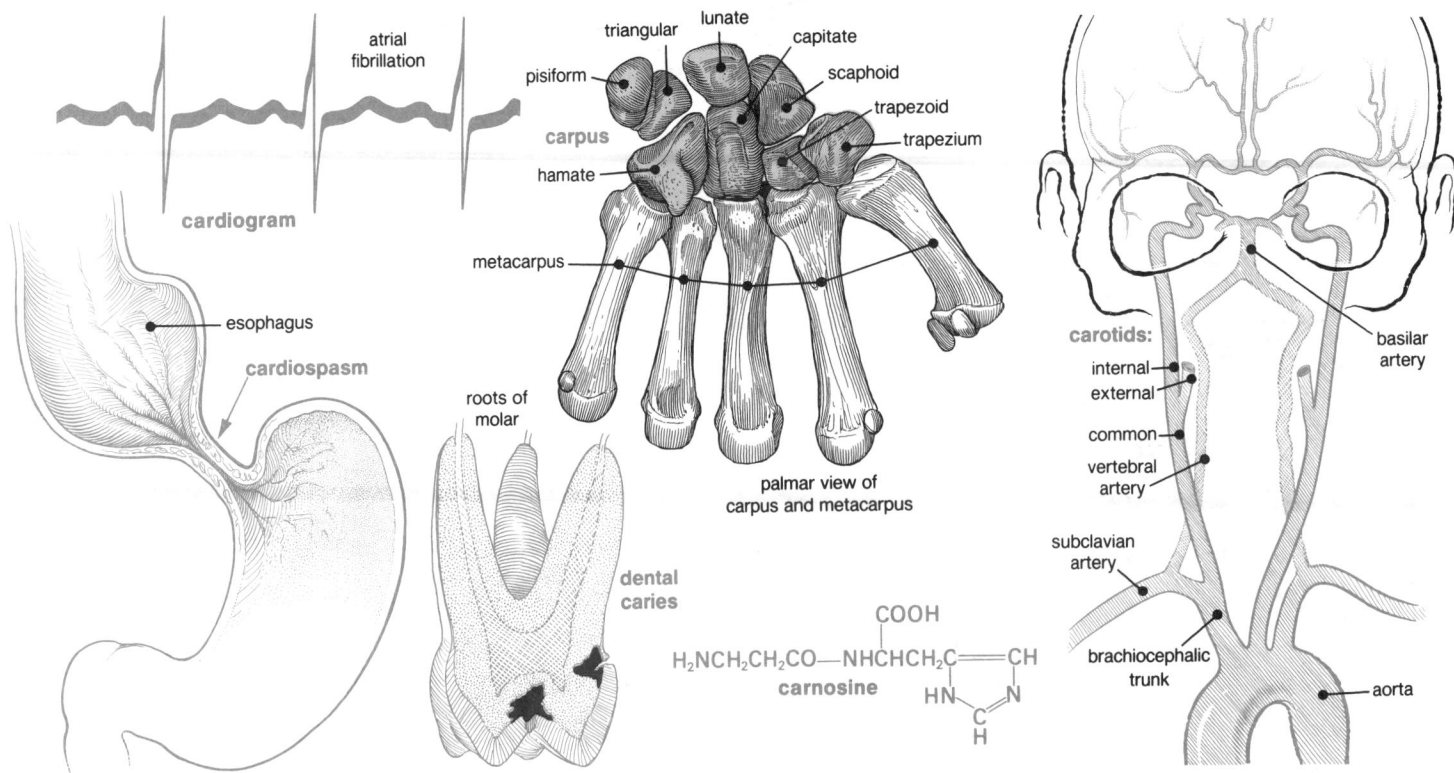

cardiogram

cardiospasm

esophagus

roots of molar

dental caries

carpus

triangular — lunate — capitate
pisiform — scaphoid
hamate — trapezoid
metacarpus — trapezium

palmar view of
carpus and metacarpus

$H_2NCH_2CH_2CO-NHCHCH_2C$

COOH

carnosine

carotids:
internal
external
common
vertebral artery
subclavian artery
brachiocephalic trunk

basilar artery
aorta

---

quently in persons over 40 years old. Also called epidermoid or prickle cell carcinoma.

terminal bronchiolar c. See alveolar cell carcinoma.

transitional c. A malignant neoplasm derived from transitional epithelium; usually occurring in the bladder, ureters, renal pelves, and nasopharynx.

carcinomatoid Resembling a carcinoma.

carcinomatosis Condition resulting from the spread of carcinoma to multiple sites in the body.

carcinomatous Having characteristics of carcinoma.

cardia The esophageal opening of the stomach.

cardiac 1. Pertaining to the heart. 2. Relating to esophageal opening of the stomach. 3. Denoting a person with heart disease.

cardiatelia Incomplete development of the heart.

cardiectomy Surgical removal of the cardiac portion of the stomach.

cardiectopia Development of the heart in a position other than the normal.

cardioaccelerator An agent that hastens the heart's action.

cardiocentesis Surgical puncture of the heart.

cardiodynamics The study of the movements and forces involved in the action of the heart.

cardioesophageal Relating to the esophagus and adjacent part of the stomach.

cardiogenic Originating in the heart.

cardiogram A graphic record of the activity of the heart, made with the cardiograph; the term is commonly used instead of electrocardiogram.

cardiograph Instrument used to record graphically the movements of the heart.

cardiography The recording of the heart movements with a cardiograph.

cardioinhibitory Retarding the action of the heart.

cardiokinetic Having an influence on the action of the heart.

cardiolipin A substance obtained from beef heart muscle; used as an antigen in tests for syphilis.

cardiolith A calculus within the heart.

cardiologist A specialist in the diagnosis and treatment of diseases of the heart.

cardiology The branch of medicine concerned with the heart and its diseases.

cardiomegaly Enlargement of the heart. Also called megalocardia.

cardiomyoliposis Fatty degeneration of the muscle of the heart.

cardiomyopathy Disease of the muscular wall of the heart. Also called myocardiopathy.

cardiomyotomy Cardiotomy.

cardionatrin I Atrial natriuretic factor; see under

factor.

cardionecrosis Necrosis of the heart.

cardioneurosis Cardiac neurosis; see under neurosis.

cardiopathy Any disease of the heart.

cardiopericardiopexy The operative procedure of spreading sterile magnesium silicate within the pericardial sac for the purpose of creating adhesive pericarditis, thus increasing the blood supply of the heart muscle.

cardioplasty Plastic surgery of the junction of the esophagus and stomach for the relief of spasm of the esophagus or upper end of the stomach (cardiospasm).

cardioplegia Temporary interruption of the heart's activity for the purpose of performing surgery upon the heart.

cardiopulmonary Relating to the heart and lungs.

cardiorenal Relating to the heart and kidneys; also called cardionephric and nephrocardiac.

cardiorrhexis Rupture of the heart wall.

cardioselectivity The quality of having a relatively greater effect on heart tissue than on other tissues.

cardiospasm Spasmodic constriction of the distal portion of the esophagus, at its junction with the stomach, with accompanying dilatation of the rest of the esophagus. Also called achalasia cardia.

cardiotomy 1. Surgical incision into the heart wall. 2. Incision into the esophageal opening (cardia) of the stomach.

cardiotonic Having a favorable or tonic effect on the heart; strengthening the heart action.

cardiotoxic Having a toxic effect on the heart.

cardiovascular Relating to the heart and blood vessels.

cardioversion Restoration of the heart's normal rhythm by means of electrical shock, the technique is used for treatment in selected cases of supraventricular tachycardia, ventricular tachycardia, and atrial fibrillation.

cardioverter Device used to administer electrical countershock to restore the normal heart rhythm.

carditis Inflammation of the heart.

care, medical General term for the application of specific training to the identification, treatment, or prevention of illness.

primary m. c. Care provided by the health professional who is approached first for treatment.

secondary m. c. Medical care by a physician at the request of the primary caregiver.

tertiary m. c. Consultative care by a specialist in a medical center.

caries Molecular death and breakdown of a bone.

contact c. Caries occurring in the proximal surface of the tooth adjacent to a restoration.

dental c. Localized, progressive decay of the teeth that starts on the surface and, if untreated, extends to the pulp with subsequent infection.

carina Any ridgelike structure, as the central ridge formed by the bifurcation of the trachea.

cariogenesis The process of caries formation.

cariogenic Producing caries; said of certain foods.

cariostatic Anything that inhibits the progress of dental caries.

carious Relating to or having caries.

carmine red A specific stain for glycogen and mucus in which the active ingredient is carminic acid; also used for staining embryos, small animals, and large blocks of tissue.

carneous Fleshy.

Carnivora The order of flesh-eating mammals.

carnosine A nitrogenous base made up of alanine and histadine, found in skeletal muscle.

Caroli's disease A disorder characterized by segmental saccular dilatation of the intrahepatic bile ducts, a marked predisposition to biliary calculous disease, cholangitis, and lung abscesses; the disease is familial and is probably inherited as a mendelian recessive.

carotene A provitamin capable of conversion into vitamin A; the yellow pigment of carrots and other yellow foods.

carotenemia Increased carotene in the blood causing a yellowish pigmentation of the skin. Also called carotinemia; xanthemia.

carotid 1. Either of the two principal arteries of the neck (carotid artery). 2. Relating to either of the carotid arteries.

carotid sinus syndrome Slow heartbeat, low blood pressure, fainting, and occasional convulsions due to overstimulation of the carotid sinus.

carotinemia See carotenemia.

carpal Relating to the bones of the wrist (carpus).

carpal tunnel syndrome A complex of symptoms caused by any condition (usually thickening of the synovia of the flexor tendons) that compresses the median nerve in the carpal tunnel of the wrist; marked by pain and numbness in the area of the hand innervated by the median nerve; the duration and degree of nerve compression determine the patient's complaints; in late stages there is atrophy of thenar muscles.

carpometacarpal Relating to the wrist bones and the metacarpus (the five bones between the wrist and fingers).

carpopedal Relating to the wrists and feet, as the spasm of tetany.

carpus The wrist; the eight bones of the wrist.

carrier
for amalgam

epiglottic cartilage

hyoid bone

thyroid
cartilage

corniculate
cartilage

arytenoid
cartilage

cricoid cartilage

caruncle

costal
cartilages

walking cast

hanging cast

carrier **1.** An individual who, although showing no symptoms of disease, harbors infectious organisms in his body and spreads the infection to others. **2.** An individual who carries a normal gene and an abnormal recessive gene which is not expressed obviously, although it may be detectable by appropriate laboratory tests. **3.** A substance in a cell which is capable of accepting an atom or a subatomic particle, thus facilitating transport of organic solutes. **4.** In dentistry, an instrument for carrying plastic amalgam to the cavity into which it is inserted.
  chronic c. A person who harbors disease-producing organisms for some time after recovery.
  passive c. One who harbors infectious organisms without having had the disease.
Carrion's disease See bartonellosis.
cartilage A tough, nonvascular connective tissue making up most of the fetal skeleton and present in the adult in the articular parts of bones and certain tubular structures; there are three main varieties: hyaline cartilage (most widely distributed type), elastic cartilage, and fibrous cartilage.
  accessory c.'s of nose See lesser alar cartilages.
  articular c. A type of hyaline cartilage forming a thin sheet upon the joint surface of bones.
  arytenoid c. One of two triangular cartilages located in the back of the larynx.
  c. of nasal septum A somewhat quadrilateral plate of cartilage completing the separation of the nasal cavities in front.
  corniculate c. One of two minute cones of yellow elastic cartilage in the larynx, located at the apex of each arytenoid cartilage.
  costal c. One of 24 bars of hyaline cartilage serving to prolong the ribs anteriorly and contributing to the elasticity of the chest wall.
  cricoid c. The ring-shaped and lowermost of the cartilages of the larynx.
  cuneiform c. One of two small rod-shaped laryngeal cartilages on either side in the aryepiglottic fold.
  elastic c. Yellow fibrocartilage, a variety of cartilage containing bundles of yellow elastic fibers with little or no white fibrous tissue; found chiefly in the external ear, the auditory tube, and some laryngeal cartilages.
  epiglottic c. A thin, leaflike lamina of yellow fibrocartilage located behind the root of the tongue and the body of the hyoid bone, forming the central portion of the epiglottis.
  epiphyseal c. The layer of cartilage between the shaft and the epiphysis of a long bone; present during the growing years, after which the cartilage ossifies and growth in length ceases.
  fibrous c. Fibrocartilage.
  greater alar c.'s Two cartilaginous plates sup-

porting the nostrils. Also called lower lateral cartilages of nose.
  hyaline c. An elastic bluish-white translucent type of cartilage covered with a membrane (perichondrium) except when coating the articular ends of bones.
  lateral c. One of two triangular plates of cartilage located below the inferior margin of the nasal bone. Also called upper lateral cartilage.
  lesser alar c.'s Two to four cartilages located posterior to the greater alar cartilage on either side. Also called accessory cartilages of nose.
  lower lateral c.'s of nose See greater alar cartilages.
  thyroid c. The largest of the cartilages of the larynx; its anterior prominence is called Adam's apple.
  tracheal c. One of from 16 to 20 incomplete cartilaginous rings forming the trachea.
  upper lateral c. See lateral cartilage.
cartilaginous Consisting of cartilage.
caruncle A small fleshy protuberance.
  lacrimal c. A small reddish protuberance at the medial junction of the eyelids.
  urethral c. A small, fleshy, painful growth occurring at the orifice of the female urethra.
carver A dental instrument used to shape wax or amalgam.
cascara sagrada The dried bark of a tree, *Rhamnus purshiana* or buckthorn; used as a laxative.
case An instance or occurrence of disease.
  index c. See proband.
caseation Necrosis of tissues into a cheeselike mass.
casein The chief protein of milk.
caseinogen The precursor of casein; a substance present in milk which, when activated by rennin, is converted into casein.
caseous Resembling cheese, as certain necrotic tissue.
cassette **1.** A lighttight camera cartridge or metal plate holder for daylight loading of x-ray or photographic film. **2.** A cartridge containing magnetic tape. **3.** A cartridge containing both a film loop and a synchronized magnetic tape.
cast **1.** A solid mold of a hollow, usually tubular, structure of the body. **2.** A rigid dressing, usually made of gauze and plaster of Paris, used for immobilization of a bodily part.
  blood c. A cast composed of a thick material containing various elements of blood, formed in kidney tubules or bronchioles and caused by bleeding into the structures.
  cellular c. A renal cast containing red and white

blood cells or epithelial cells.
  epithelial c. A cast containing cells from the inner lining of renal tubules, found in the urine.
  fatty c. A renal cast composed chiefly of fat globules.
  granular c. A colorless renal cast composed of particles of cellular debris.
  hanging c. A plaster cast applied to immobilize a fracture as well as deliver a traction force via the weight of the cast; commonly used for the treatment of fractures of the lower part of the humerus.
  hyaline c. A relatively transparent renal cast consisting mainly of precipitated protein.
  leukocyte c. A renal cylindrical plug of tightly packed leukocytes.
  mucous c. See cylindroid.
  red blood cell c. A renal cast containing red blood cells due to entry of the red cells via the glomeruli or the upper parts of the nephron.
  renal c. Urinary cast.
  urinary c. A cast discharged in the urine.
  walking c. A plaster cast extending from below the knee to the toes with an added attachment, such as a boot, to allow a natural gait.
  waxy c. A light yellow cylinder with a tendency to split transversely, found in the urine in cases of oliguria or anuria.
castrate **1.** To remove the testes or the ovaries. **2.** One from whom the gonads have been removed.
castration Removal of the testes or ovaries.
  functional c. Atrophy of the gonads by prolonged treatment with sex hormones.
catabolic Promoting or exhibiting catabolism.
catabolism The breakdown of chemical compounds into more elementary principles by the body; an energy-producing metabolic process, the reverse of anabolism.
catabolite A product of catabolism.
catacrotism Anomaly of the pulse marked by one or more minor expansions of the artery following the main beat.
catalepsy A trance-like condition with rigidity of muscles allowing the body (including extremities) to assume a position for an indefinite period of time.
catalyst A substance, usually present in small amounts, that influences the rate of a chemical reaction without being changed in the process.
  negative c. One that retards a chemical reaction.
  organic c. An enzyme that catalyzes specific reactions.
  positive c. A catalyst that accelerates a chemical reaction.
catalyze To modify the rate of a chemical reaction; to act as a catalyst.
catamnesis A patient's medical history following

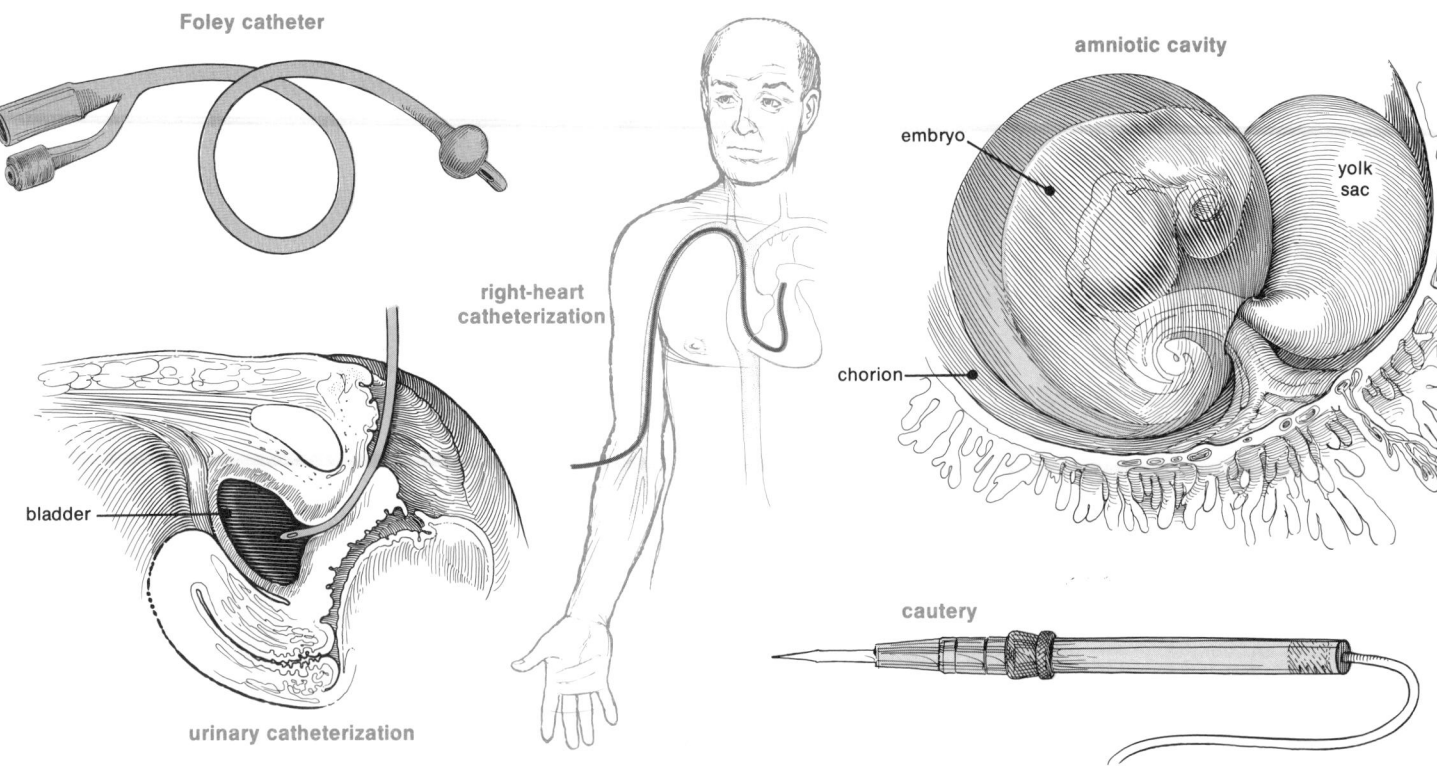

Foley catheter

right-heart
catheterization

amniotic cavity

embryo

yolk
sac

chorion

bladder

urinary catheterization

cautery

---

an illness; the "follow-up" history.

cataphasia A speech disorder consisting of involuntary repetition of the same word.

cataplasia, cataplasis Degenerative reversion of cells or tissues to an embryonic state.

cataplexy A sudden and temporary loss of muscle tone and of postural reflexes, causing limpness of the body or a part, usually triggered by an emotional surge, such as gales of laughter, sudden elation, anger, etc.

 narcolepsy c. Transient loss of muscle tone in conjunction with intermittent attacks of uncontrollable sleep.

cataract Loss of transparency of the lens of the eye and/or its capsule, resulting in partial or total blindness.

 immature c. An early stage of a cataract.

 mature c. A cataract in which the entire lens substance has become opaque and can be easily separated from its capsule.

 radiation c. A cataract caused by continued exposure to radioactive materials.

 senile c. A cataract occurring in old age.

 stationary c. One that has ceased to progress.

 traumatic c. A cataract caused by an injury or foreign body.

catarrh Inflammation of a mucous membrane, especially of the nose and throat, with a discharge.

catatonia A type of schizophrenia characterized by generalized inhibition, mutism, stupor, negativism, or waxy flexibility (withdrawn type), or occasionally by excessive and sometimes violent motor activity and excitement (excited type).

cat-cry syndrome See cri-du-chat syndrome.

catechol A chemical compound, 1,2-dihydroxybenzene, $C_6H_6O_2$; of interest mainly because of the importance of its aminated derivatives.

catecholamines Amine compounds derived from catechol, such as epinephrine and norepinephrine, which have sympathomimetic activity and are concerned with nervous transmission, vascular tone, and many metabolic activities.

catgut A tough, thin thread made from the dried intestines of sheep, used as absorbable surgical ligatures and sutures.

catharsis 1. Purging or cleansing, especially of the bowels. 2. Therapeutic discharge of emotional tension by recalling of past events.

cathartic 1. A drug that promotes evacuation of intestinal contents in a more or less fluid state by increasing motor activity of the intestine, either directly or reflexly; distinguished from a laxative which produces a milder effect. Also called purgative. 2. Relating to a catharsis.

cathepsin Any intracellular protein-splitting en-

zyme that acts on the interior peptide bonds of a protein, causing its decomposition; cathepsins are widely distributed in animal tissues, especially the liver, kidney, and spleen.

cathepsis Protein hydrolysis by the action of cathepsins.

catheter A slender, flexible tube made of rubber, metal, or plastic; used to introduce or remove fluids from a bodily channel or hollow organ.

 balloon tip c. A twin-lumen catheter with a distendible balloon at the end.

 Fogarty c. A catheter having an inflatable balloon near the tip; used to remove thrombi from large veins and stones from the biliary ducts.

 Foley c. A catheter equipped with a small balloon near the tip which can be inflated to retain the catheter in place.

 pacing c. A catheter equipped with electrodes at the tip, passed into the right atrium or ventricle to function as a heart pacer.

 Swan-Ganz c. A thin, soft catheter with a balloon at the end to measure pulmonary arterial pressure; introduced into the basilic vein and carried by the bloodstream through the heart into a small artery in the lung.

 two-way c. A twin-channeled catheter for irrigation.

catheterization Introduction of a catheter into a bodily passage.

 cardiac c. Passage of a catheter into the heart by way of a blood vessel; first attempted by Forsmann on himself in 1928.

 left-heart c. Introduction of a radiopaque catheter into the brachial or femoral artery and passage in a retrograde direction through the artery to the aorta and, frequently, across the aortic valve into the left ventricle.

 right-heart c. Passage of a radiopaque flexible catheter into a vein, usually the basilic; the catheter is manipulated under fluoroscopic control through the venous system to the right atrium, and eventually into the right ventricle and pulmonary artery.

catheterize To introduce a catheter into a bodily canal or passage.

cathexis Attachment of emotional energy and significance to a person, object, or idea.

cathode (Ca, k, ka) The negatively charged electrode of an electron tube, galvanic cell (primary cell) or storage battery (secondary cells). Also called negative electrode.

cation A positively charged ion that is characteristically attracted to the negatively charged cathode; indicated as a plus sign, e.g., H^+.

CATLINE (catalog-online) A segment of MEDLARS that contains references to books and serials

catalogued at the National Library of Medicine; available at medical libraries in the MEDLARS network for immediate access to authoritative cataloging information; also used as a source of information for ordering books and journals and to provide reference and interlibrary loan services.

cat-scratch disease Regional inflammation of lymph nodes of unknown origin, frequently following the scratch or bite of a cat. Also called cat-scratch fever.

cauda pl. **caudae** A tail or tapered end of a structure.

 c. equina The bundle of nerves (sacral and coccygeal) in which the spinal cord ends.

caudad Directed posteriorly or toward the tail.

cauda equina syndrome Dull pain and anesthesia of the buttocks, genitalia, and/or thigh with impaired bladder and bowel function; caused by compression of the spinal nerve roots.

caudal Relating to the lower part.

caudate Possessing a tail or a tail-like appendage.

caul The portion of fetal membranes surrounding the head of the fetus at birth when the membranes remain intact until completion of delivery.

causalgia A painful, burning sensation, accompanied by trophic changes in the skin and nails, due to a peripheral nerve injury, usually of the median or sciatic nerves.

caustic Corrosive; capable of burning.

cauterization The act of cauterizing; the application of a caustic substance or electric current for the purpose of scarring or destroying aberrant tissue.

cauterize To apply a cautery.

cautery An agent used for scarring or destroying tissue.

caval Of or relating to the vena cava.

caveolae Minute vesicles that develop by invagination of the plasmalemma of the cell surface; they usually pinch off to form free vesicles within the cytoplasm and serve as a mechanism for cell ingestion.

cavern A cavity, especially one caused by disease, as seen in tuberculous lungs.

cavernitis Inflammation of a corpus cavernosum of the penis.

 fibrous c. See Peyronie's disease.

cavernous Relating to or having cavities.

cavernous sinus syndrome A syndrome caused by thrombosis of the cavernous sinus, characterized by edema of eyelids and conjunctivae, protrusion of the eyeball (proptosis), and paralysis of the third, fourth, and sixth cranial nerves. Also called Foix's syndrome.

cavitary 1. Relating to or having cavities. 2. Any parasite having a body cavity and living inside the

cranial cavity

nasal cavity

oral cavity

spinal canal

pleural cavity

lung

heart

sternum

pericardial cavity

dentin

pulp cavity

cecum

ileum

ileocecal junction

cavus

host's body.

cavitation Formation of cavities, as in the lungs in pulmonary tuberculosis.

cavity 1. A hollow space within the body; a chamber. 2. Loss of tooth structure due to decay.

   abdominal c. The bodily cavity between the diaphragm above and the pelvis below.

   amniotic c. The space within the amnion.

   body c. The cavity of the body containing the organs.

   buccal c. 1. The space between the lips and the gums and teeth. 2. Decay on the buccal surface of a tooth.

   compound c. A cavity involving two or more surfaces of a tooth.

   cranial c. The space within the skull.

   distal c. A cavity located on the surface of a tooth away from the midline.

   glenoid c. Glenoid fossa; see under fossa.

   medullary c. of bone The elongated cavity within the shaft of a long bone.

   nasal c. An irregular space extending from the

base of the cranium to the roof of the mouth and divided in two by a thin vertical septum (nasal septum).

   oral c. The cavity of the mouth.

   pelvic c. The short, wide, curved canal within the bony framework of the minor pelvis; it contains the pelvic colon, rectum, bladder, and some of the organs of reproduction.

   pericardial c. The potential cavity between the two layers of the membrane enveloping the heart (pericardium).

   pleural c. The potential space between the two layers of the pleura (parietal and visceral).

   proximal c. A cavity occurring on the mesial or distal surface of a tooth.

   pulp c. The central chamber of a tooth containing blood vessels, lymphatic vessels, and nerve fibers; the entire space occupied by the pulp.

   splanchnic c. One of the three major cavities of the body; cranial, thoracic, or abdominal.

   tympanic c. The cavity of the middle ear, located in the temporal bone and containing the ear ossicles.

   visceral c. Splanchnic cavity.

cavogram A roentgenogram of the vena cava.

cavosurface Relating to a prepared cavity and the surface of a tooth.

cavum Latin for cavity or hollow.

cavus The condition in which the longitudinal arch of the foot is exaggerated, due to contraction of the plantar fascia or to a deformed bony arch.

cecostomy Surgical creation of an opening into the cecum through the abdominal wall.

cecum The cul-de-sac that forms the beginning of the large intestine; the blind gut.

celiac Relating to the abdominal cavity.

celiac disease Disorder characterized by intolerance to gluten (a protein present in the grains of wheat, rye, oats, and barley), abnormal structure of the small intestine, and poor absorption of food. Also called nontropical sprue; gluten-induced enteropathy; sprue. Cf. tropical sprue.

celiohysterectomy Surgical removal of the uterus through an incision in the abdomen. Also called abdominal hysterectomy.

typical mammalian cell

centrosome
lysosome
centriole
Golgi apparatus
mitochondrion
cytoplasm

nucleus
nucleolus
microtubule
rough endoplasmic reticulum with attached ribosomes
cell membrane

smooth endoplasmic reticulum
forming vacuole

air cells

band cells

RBCs for size comparison

alpha cell of pancreas

beta cell of pancreas

celioscopy   See laparoscopy.

cell   1. The smallest unit of living matter capable of independent functioning, composed of protoplasm and surrounded by a semipermeable plasma membrane. 2. A receptacle.

acidophilic c.   A cell whose cytoplasm or its granules have an affinity for acid dyes such as eosin.

acinar c.   One of the secreting cells lining an acinus or alveolus of a compound acinous gland, such as the pancreas. Also called acinous cell.

adipose c.   See fat cell.

air c.   An air-containing space of one of the air sinuses of the skull.

alpha c. of pancreas   A cell of the islet of Langerhans (islet of pancreas) marked by fine cytoplasmic granules; known to produce glucagon (hyperglycemic-glycogenolytic factor); it stains red with phloxine.

alveolar c.   Type I pneumocyte; see under pneumocyte.

amacrine c.   A special inhibitory retinal cell, regarded as a modified nerve cell.

anaplastic c.   an undifferentiated cell characteristic of carcinoma.

aneuploid c.   A cell with an unbalanced number of chromosomes.

antigen-sensitive c.   See immunocompetent cell.

argentaffin c.'s   Cells having an affinity for silver salts and therefore capable of being stained by them; located throughout the gastrointestinal tract.

B c.'s   B lymphocytes; see under lymphocyte.

balloon c.   A large, degenerated cell.

band c.   Any granulocytic leukocyte in which the nucleus has a simple, nonlobulated, elongated shape, resembling a band; it represents a normal stage prior to the development of a mature segmented granulocytic leukocyte (polymorphonuclear white blood cell). Also called stab cell.

basal c.   A cell appearing in the deepest layer of a stratified epithelium; an early keratinocyte.

basophil c. of anterior lobe of hypophysis   The beta cell of the anterior lobe of the hypophysis (pituitary gland).

beta c. of anterior lobe of hypophysis   A cell that contains basophil granules and is thought to furnish the gonadotrophic hormones.

beta c. of pancreas   The predominant cell of the islet of Langerhans (islet of pancreas), marked by coarse cytoplasmic granules that represent a precursor of insulin; it stains blue with the Gomori stain.

Betz c.'s   The large pyramidal cells of the fifth layer of the motor cortex.

bipolar c.   A neuron having two processes (afferent and efferent), as those in the retina.

blast c.   1. An immature precursor cell (e.g., ery-

throblast, lymphoblast, neuroblast); a primitive cell, the least differentiated of a line of blood-forming elements. 2. A leukemic cell of indeterminable type.

blood c.   One of the formed elements of the blood; an erythrocyte or leukocyte.

burr c.   An elongated erythrocyte with multiple long, sharp, spinelike projections from the cell surface; seen in hemolytic anemias, especially those associated with uremia and carcinoma.

cartilage c.'s   Cells situated in the smooth walled spaces or lacunae of cartilage. Also called chondrocytes.

chief c. of parathyroid gland   The principal cell of the parathyroid gland.

chief c. of stomach   An enzyme-producing cell of a gastric gland in the stomach. Also called zymogenic cell.

chromaffin c.   A cell whose cytoplasm exhibits fine brown granules when stained with a dichromate; occurring in the adrenal medulla and paraganglia of the sympathetic nervous system and some other tissues.

chromophobe c.   A cell of the adenohypophysis (anterior pituitary) which has little affinity for histologic dyes.

clear c.   Any cell containing non-stainable, or faintly stainable material.

cleavage c.   Blastomere.

columnar c.   A cell in which the height is significantly greater than the width, usually epithelial; it may be a tall columnar or low columnar.

committed c.   Any cell committed to the production of antibodies specific for a given antigen-determinant, such as primed cell, memory cell, and antibody-producing cell.

cone c. of retina   One of the visual receptors sensitive to color.

cuboid c.   A cell which resembles a cube, i.e., all its diameters are approximately the same size.

daughter c.   Any cell resulting from the division of a parent cell.

dentin c.   Odontoblast.

dust c.   Alveolar macrophage; see under macrophage.

endothelial c.   One of the thin, flat cells (squamous) forming the lining (endothelium) of the blood and lymph vessels and the inner layer of the endocardium.

epithelial c.   One of a variety of cells that form epithelium.

epithelioid c.   The chief cell of granular growths formed in certain inflammatory diseases.

eukaryotic c.   A cell with a true nucleus, a cell with a nuclear membrane.

fat c.   A very large connective tissue cell (60 to 80 μ) in which neutral fat is stored; the cytoplasm is

usually compressed into a thin envelope, with the nucleus at one point in the periphery. Also called adipose cell.

fibroblast c.   A spindle-shaped connective tissue cell responsible for elaborating collagen and reticular fibers; the most common cell type found in connective tissue.

foam c.   A macrophage exhibiting a peculiar vacuolated appearance due to the presence of lipids in a multitude of small vacuoles; notably seen in xanthoma. Also called xanthoma cell.

fusiform c.'s of cerebral cortex   Spindle-shaped cells in the sixth layer of the cerebral cortex.

ganglion c.   A large nerve cell in a ganglion peripheral to the central nervous system. Also called gangliocyte.

Gaucher c.   An abnormal cell found in spleen, liver, lymph nodes and bone marrow in Gaucher's disease; it is a round or polyhedral pale reticuloendothelial cell 20 to 80 μ in diameter containing a glucocerebroside.

germ c.   The ovum or spermatozoon.

germinal c.'s   Cells from which other cells are derived or proliferated, especially the dividing cells in the embryonic neural tube.

ghost c.   A cell in its last stages of degeneration, appearing as a shadow.

gitter c.   A honeycombed, compound granule cell; a microglial cell.

glitter c.   A large leukocyte seen in the urine exhibiting brownian movement in the cytoplasm; associated with urinary tract infection.

goblet c.'s   Unicellular mucous glands found in the epithelium of certain mucous membranes, especially of the respiratory and intestinal tracts.

Golgi's c.'s   Type I: nerve cells with very long axons that leave the gray matter of the central nervous system to terminate in the periphery. Also called Golgi type I neuron. Type II: nerve cells with short axons that ramify in the gray matter and terminate near the cell body. Also called Golgi type II neuron.

granule c.   One of many small cells in the granular layer of the cerebellar cortex.

granulosa c.'s   Special epithelial cells displaying high mitotic activity which surround the ovum in a primary follicle and, in a vesicular follicle, form the stratum granulosum, corona radiata, and cumulus oophorus; they secrete a refractile substance that forms the protective zona pellucida around the ovum; during the early stages of follicular maturation, they secrete an inhibitory substance (polypeptide) that maintains the primary oocyte in an arrested stage of meiotic prophase. Also called follicular cells.

granulosa lutein c.'s   Giant glandular cells that

alveolar cells

cuboid cell

cone foot

cone cell
of retina

columnar cells

intestinal villus

mitochondria

lamellae

endothelial cell
(squamous)

fat cell

capillary

lymphocytes in
medullary cord
of lymph node

build-up
of mucin

goblet cell

secondary
vesicular
follicle
of ovary

ovum

fully
formed

greatly
distended

discharged

theca lutein cells

blood clot

granulosa cells

corpus luteum

granulosa lutein cells

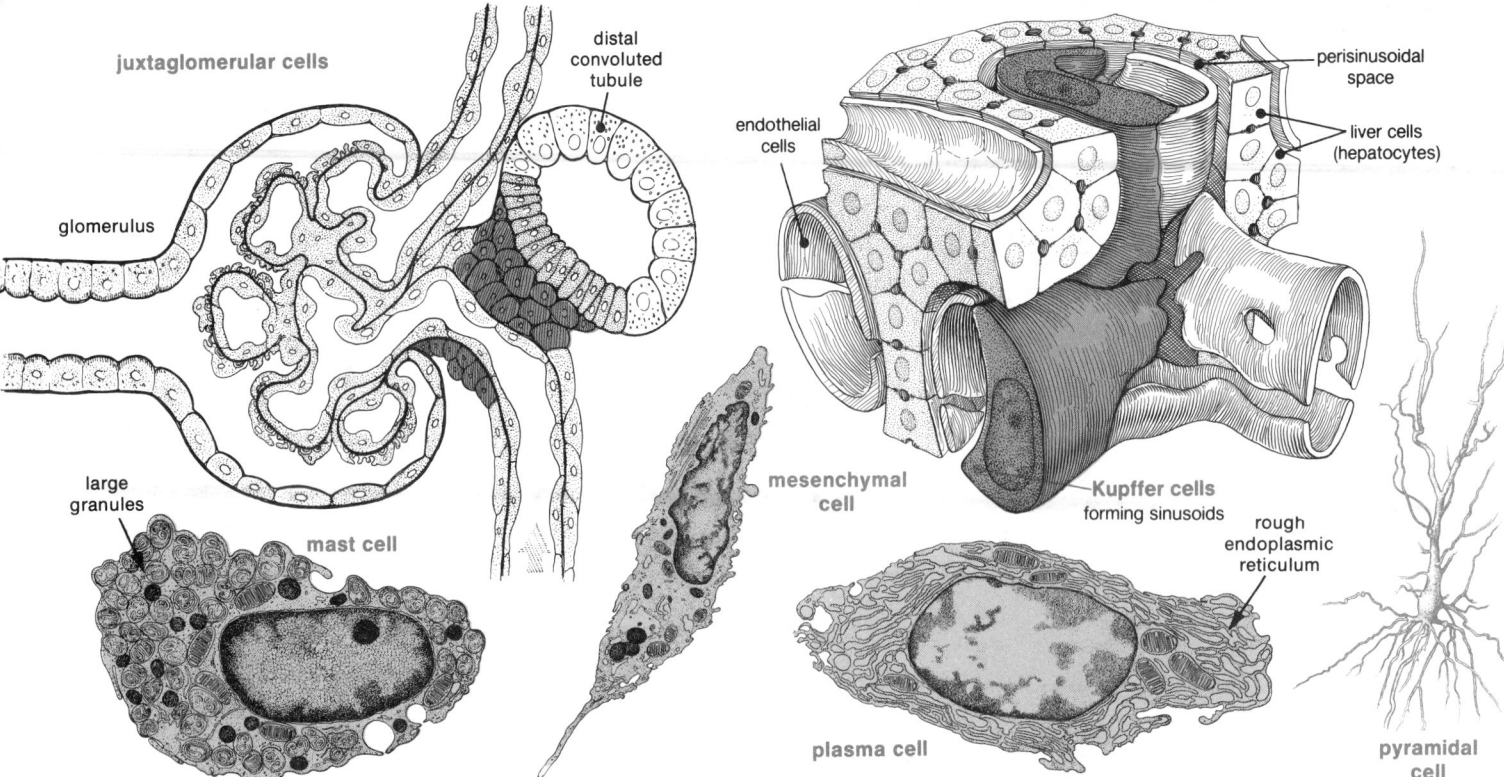

juxtaglomerular cells

distal convoluted tubule

glomerulus

endothelial cells

perisinusoidal space

liver cells (hepatocytes)

large granules

mast cell

mesenchymal cell

Kupffer cells forming sinusoids

rough endoplasmic reticulum

plasma cell

pyramidal cell

comprise the major part of the wall of a ruptured vesicular follicle (corpus luteum) in the ovary; formed by hypertrophy of the follicular granulosa cells of the old vesicular follicle; they produce the sex steroid progesterone. Also called follicular lutein cells.

great alveolar c. Type II pneumocyte; see under pneumocyte.

hair c.'s Pear-shaped epithelial cells with delicate hairlike microvilli (stereocilia) one to 100μ in length on the free surface; they are present in neuroepithelial sensory areas of the utricle, saccule, ampullae, and the spiral organ of Corti.

HeLa c.'s The first documented, continuously cultured human malignant cells, derived from a cervical carcinoma; used in the cultivation of viruses.

helmet c. An irregular, contracted, somewhat triangular erythrocyte; seen in microangiopathic anemia.

helper c. Helper T-lymphocyte; see under lymphocyte.

Hürthle c. An enlarged, granular thyroid follicular epithelial cell with acidophilic cytoplasm, as seen in Hashimoto's disease.

immunocompetent c. Any cell which can form antibodies or elaborate cells which form antibodies when stimulated by antigen, e.g., inducible cell. Also called antigen-sensitive cell.

inducer c. An unprimed cell which can become a primed cell or an antibody-producing cell when stimulated by antigen. Also called virgin lymphocyte; antigen-inducible cell.

interstitial c.'s 1. Cells of the connective tissue of the ovary or testis which are believed to produce internal secretion of those structures; in the seminiferous tubules of the testis they are known as Leydig's cells. 2. Cells in the medullary portions of the kidney which are thought to be sites of production of prostaglandins and possibly of another lipid substance with antihypertensive properties.

islet c. One of the cells in the islet (island) of Langerhans of the pancreas.

juxtaglomerular c.'s A group of secretory cells forming the middle layer of the wall of the afferent arteriole just before it enters the glomerulus in the kidney; thought to play a role in production of the hormone renin.

killer c.'s, Kc.'s Small cells, believed to be derived from T lymphocytes (thymus-dependent lymphocytes), which are able to attack target cells (e.g., tumor cells) after IgG antibodies have reacted with an antigen on the target cell; complement is not needed to kill the cell.

Kulchitsky c.'s The argentaffin cells of the intes-

tinal glands.

Kupffer c.'s Reticuloendothelial cells of the liver; fixed macrophages or reticuloendothelial cells lining the capillary system which conveys blood from the interlobular branches of the portal vein to the central vein; they are phagocytic in character and are active in freeing the bloodstream of foreign particles.

Langhans' giant c.'s 1. Multinucleated giant cells in tuberculosis and other granulomas; the nuclei are located in an arciform manner at the periphery of the cells. 2. Rounded cells with clear cytoplasm and light-staining nuclei forming the cytotrophoblast.

L.E. c. Abbreviation for lupus erythematosus cell, a leukocyte containing an amorphous round body which is a phagocytosed nucleus from another cell which has been traumatized and exposed to serum antinuclear globulin; a large purple-red homogenous inclusion body is seen occupying most of the cytoplasm of the phagocytosing cell; L.E. cells are formed in vitro in the blood of individuals with systemic lupus erythematosus, or by the action of the individual's serum on normal leukocytes.

lepra c.'s Large mononuclear phagocytes (macrophages) with foamlike cytoplasm; associated with lepromatous lesions which contain the acid-fast organisms of leprosy.

Leydig's c. An endocrine interstitial cell located between the seminiferous tubules of the testis.

lupus erythematosus c. See L.E. cell.

lymph c., lymphoid c. Lymphocyte.

Marchand's c.'s The phagocytes in the adventitia of blood vessels. Also called adventitial cells.

mast c.'s Large cells with coarse cytoplasmic granules containing heparin (anticoagulant) and histamine (vasodilator) occurring in most loose connective tissue, especially along the path of blood vessels; the cells act as mediators of inflammation on contact with antigen; sometimes called tissue mast cells or histogenous mast cells to distinguish them from the hematogenous mast cells (basophilic leukocytes) circulating in the blood.

memory c.'s Short-memory and long-memory cells which can mount an accelerated antibody response to antigen.

mesangial c. An intercapillary cell of the renal glomerulus located mostly near that part of the capillary facing the center of the glomerulus; it borders directly on the endothelial cell.

mesenchymal c. A cell present in mesenchyme and capable of differentiating into any of the special types of connective tissue or supporting tissues, smooth muscle, vascular endothelium, or blood cells.

mesothelial c. One of the flat cells of the simple

squamous epithelium (mesothelium) lining the pleural, pericardial, peritoneal, and scrotal cavities.

mother c. See parent cell.

myeloid c. Any young cell that develops into a mature granulocyte.

myoepithelial c. One of the smooth muscle cells of ectodermal origin, with processes that spiral around some of the epithelial cells of sweat, mammary, lacrimal and salivary glands; their contraction forces the secretion of the glands toward the ducts.

nerve c. See neuron.

neuroglial c. Any of the nonneuronal cells of nervous tissue including the oligodendroglia, astrocytes, microglia, and ependymal cells. Also called glial cell.

neurosecretory c. A nerve cell that elaborates a chemical substance, as those of the hypothalamus.

oat c. A cell resembling an oat grain; seen in lung cancer.

olfactory c. One of the slender sensory nerve cells surmounted by sensitive hairs, present in the olfactory mucous membrane at the roof of the nose; the receptor for the sense of smell.

osteochondrogenic c. A young cell of the inner layer of periostium, capable of developing into a bone or a cartilage cell.

oxyphilic c.'s 1. Parietal cells. 2. Acidophilic cells present in the parathyroid glands; they increase in number with age.

Paneth's c.'s Pyramidal-shaped cells occurring in small groups near the base of the crypts of Lieberkühn; believed to secrete digestive enzymes throughout the small intestine.

parent c. A cell that gives rise to a new generation of daughter cells by cell division. Also called mother cell.

parietal c. One of the cells present in the periphery of the gastric glands; it lies upon the basement membrane covered by the chief cells and secretes hydrochloric acid which reaches the lumen of the gland through fine channels.

plasma c. A cell that stores and releases antibody and is believed to be of primary importance in antibody synthesis; characterized by RNA-rich cytoplasm and an eccentrically placed nucleus; the cytoplasm contains an extensive system of endoplasmic reticulum studded with ribosomes; the cell is derived embryologically from a bursal equivalent tissue and is therefore also referred to as a B cell; in certain diseases, such as chronic lymphocytic leukemia, there is a proliferation of this cell type.

primed c. A cell that has been primed by antigen for antibody production.

prokaryotic c. A cell in which the nuclear substance, lacking an envelope (plasmalemma), is in

rod
cell
of
retina

membrane
lamellae
containing
rhodopsin

ganglion cell
amacrine cell
bipolar cell
horizontal cell

cone cell
of retina

Schwann's
cell

jelly-roll
configuration
of myelin
sheaths

axon

nucleus

developing
sperm

sickle
cells

stellate
cell

Sertoli
cell

sustentacular
cells

taste bud

direct contact with the rest of the protoplasm; includes most viruses and bacteria.

Purkinje's c.'s The large nerve cells of the cerebellar cortex with flask-shaped bodies forming a single cell layer between the molecular and granular layers; their dendrites are arranged in the molecular layer in a plane transverse to the folia, and their axons penetrate the granular layer to form the only pathways out of the cerebellar cortex; they terminate in the central cerebellar nuclei. Also called Purkyně cells.

pus c. A neutrophilic leukocyte; a necrotic granulocyte characteristic of suppurative inflammation.

pyramidal c. A nerve cell of the cerebral cortex; usually somewhat triangular with an apical dendrite directed toward the surface of the cortex and several smaller dendrites at the base; the axon is given off at the base of the cell and descends to deeper layers.

red blood c. (RBC) See erythrocyte.

Renshaw c. An inhibitory interneuron in the ventral horn of the spinal cord that acts as a negative feedback monitor of motorneurons.

respiratory c. Type I pneumocyte; see under pneumocyte.

reticular c. A primitive mesenchymal cell providing the framework of such structures as bone marrow, lymph nodes, and spleen.

reticuloendothelial c. Phagocytic cell similar to the leukocyte but attached to vascular and lymphatic channels rather than being circulatory.

rod c. of retina One of the visual photoreceptor cells of the retina sensitive to gray shades.

Schwann's c. A special cell which surrounds a peripheral axon forming a myelin sheath.

septal c. Type II pneumocyte; see under pneumocyte.

Sertoli c.'s The elaborate nonspermatogenic sustentacular cells in the seminiferous tubules of male gonads (testes) extending from the basal lamina to the lumen; they house the developing spermatogenic cells in deep recesses and produce sex hormone-binding globulin and androgens.

sickle c. An abnormal crescent-shaped red blood cell; the shape is due to the presence of hemoglobin S. Also called drepanocyte; meniscocyte.

smudge c. Any leukocyte that becomes so degenerated that the cytoplasm disappears, leaving a naked nucleus that stains poorly and exhibits no characteristic chromatin pattern; rarely found in normal blood but seen in large numbers in acute myeloblastic and lymphoblastic anemia, and in chronic lymphatic leukemia.

sperm c. Spermatozoon.

squamous c. A flat, scalelike epithelial cell.

squamous alveolar c. Type I pneumocyte, see under pneumocyte.

stab c. See band cell.

stellate c.'s of the cerebral cortex A star-shaped interneuron cell located in the second, third, and fourth layers of the cortex of the brain.

stem c.'s Cells that can produce cells which are able to differentiate.

suppressor c.'s See suppressor T cells.

suppressor T c.'s Cells of the lymphoid system which turn off immune responses (humoral and cell-mediated) once they are started, by inhibiting the production of sensitized antibodies and antibody-forming cells; also play an active role in development of tolerance to self and heterologous antigens.

sustentacular c. One of the supporting cells of an epithelium, as seen in the spiral organ of Corti, taste bud, and olfactory epithelium.

T c.'s T lymphocytes; see under lymphocyte.

target c. 1. An abnormal erythrocyte which when stained shows a dark center surrounded by a light band encircled by a darker ring, resembling a bull's eye target; found in a variety of anemias including thalassemia and other hemoglobinopathies. Also

prosthesis

cross section of tooth and surrounding structures

dentin

centromeres

bone cement

cementum

chromoson

femur

pulp cavity

dentin

enamel

longitudinal section of tooth

nucleus

centriole

centrosphere

microtubular triplets

called Mexican hat cell. **2.** A cell displaying a foreign (nonself) antigen recognized by an effector T lymphocyte. **3.** A cell containing specific receptors for circulating messengers such as hormones.

tart c. A granulocyte that has an engulfed nucleus of another cell which is still well preserved.

taste c. A neuroepithelial cell that perceives gustatory stimuli, situated at the center of a taste bud.

theca lutein c.'s Lutein cells located within the folds of the glandular corpus luteum of the ovary and derived from the theca interna; they produce estrogens. Also called paraluteal cells.

Tiselius electrophoresis c. The cell or container in a Teselius apparatus containing the solution to be electrophoretically analyzed.

transitional c. **1.** A monocyte. **2.** Any cell thought to represent a phase of development from one form to another.

type I c. Type I pneumocyte; see under pneumocyte.

type II c. Type II pneumocyte; see under pneumocyte.

wasserhelle c.'s The water-clear cells of the parathyroid gland.

white blood c.'s (WBC) Formed elements in the blood that include granular leukocytes, lymphocytes, and monocytes.

cellular Relating to, resembling, composed of, or derived from cells.

cellularity The number and quality of the cells constituting a tissue.

cellule **1.** A small cavity or compartment. **2.** A minute cell.

cellulite Popular term for fat deposits beneath the skin.

cellulitis A diffuse spreading infection, especially of the subcutaneous tissue.

cellulose A carbohydrate polymer, $C_6H_{10}O_5$; the main constituent of the cell walls of plants; an important source of bulk in the diet because it is not affected by the digestive enzymes.

celom The body cavity of the embryo, between the two layers of the mesoderm after one unites with the ectoderm and the other with the endoderm.

celomic Relating to the body cavity or celom.

Celsius (C) Denoting a temperature scale that indicates the freezing point of water as 0°C and the boiling point at 100°C under normal atmospheric pressure. Also called centigrade.

cement **1.** Cementum. **2.** Any of several materials used in dentistry, neurosurgery, and orthopedic surgery as luting and sealing agents, temporary restorations, and bases.

bone c. A luting agent for filling interstices of bone; it is widely used in the fixation of hip and knee implants.

intercellular c. A substance holding together cells especially epithelial cells.

muscle c. See myoglia.

cementoblast One of the cells active in the formation of cementum.

cementocyte A cell occupying a lacunar space in the cementum of a tooth; it generally possesses protoplasmic processes that radiate from the cell body into the canaliculi of the cementum; it is derived from cementoblasts trapped within newly formed cementum.

cementoma Periapical ossifying fibroma, an asymptomatic periapical lesion marked by the proliferation of fibrous connective tissue at the apex of a tooth; it is generally replaced by a calcified mass resembling cementum.

cementum A specialized, bonelike, fibrous tissue covering the anatomic roots of human teeth which serves primarily as an attachment area of the tooth to its surrounding structures; it is more resistant to resorption than bone, thus making orthodontic movement of teeth possible.

cellular c. Cementum possessing cementocytes, primarily located in the apical portion of the tooth.

center **1.** The middle; the central part of an organ or structure. Also called core. **2.** A specialized region in which a process, such as ossification, begins. **3.** A collection of neurons governing a particular function. **4.** An agency designed to serve the community.

germinal c. A light staining oval mass in the center of a secondary lymphatic nodule consisting primarily of large lymphoid cells; a site of antibody synthesis.

ossification c. Any region in which the process of ossification first begins in a tissue.

reflex c. Any part of the nervous system where the reception of a sensory impression is automatically followed by a motor impulse.

respiratory c.'s Regions in the medulla and pons which coordinate the activity of respiration.

speech c. A unilateral area in the inferior frontal gyrus, associated with articulate speech.

vasomotor c.'s Areas of the central nervous system (in the tuber cenereum, medulla oblongata, and spinal cord) that control the constriction and dilatation of peripheral blood vessels.

vomiting c. A center in the lower part of the medulla oblongata, stimulation of which may cause vomiting.

centesis The puncturing of a cavity.

centibar A unit of atmospheric pressure; one-hundredth of a bar.

centigrade (C) **1.** Divided into or consisting of 100 gradations. **2.** Denoting a temperature scale in which the interval between the freezing and boiling points of water is divided into 100 degrees; normal human body temperature is approximately 37°C. Also called Celsius.

centigram (cg) One hundredth of a gram.

centiliter (cl) One hundredth of a liter.

centimeter (cm) One hundredth of a meter.

centimorgan (cM) One hundredth of a morgan.

centrad **1.** Toward the center. **2.** A unit of ophthalmic prism strength, equal to one hundredth of the radius of the circle; symbolized by an inverted delta (∇).

centrage Condition in which the center of the various refracting and reflecting surfaces of an optical system lie on a straight line.

central core disease A congenital myopathy usually manifested before the first month of life; characterized by proximal muscle weakness, most severe in the lower limbs, resulting in delayed walking; on biopsy the central core of muscle fibers stains abnormally.

centric Of or relating to a center.

centrifugal Directed away from a center or axis; efferent.

centrifuge **1.** An apparatus which, by means of centrifugal force, separates substances of different densities or simulates gravitational effects. **2.** To separate substances by a centrifuge.

centrilobular Occurring at or near the center of a lobule.

centriole Any of two short, cylindrical organelles (usually at right angles to each other) containing nine pairs of parallel microtubules about a central cavity, located in the centrosome and considered to play an important role in cell division; usually associated with the Golgi apparatus in a nondividing cell. Sometimes called attraction particle.

centripetal Directed toward a center or axis; afferent.

centromere The constricted part of the chromosome to which the spindle fibers attach during mitosis; chromosome movement occurs about this point. Also called kinetochore.

centrosome Two associated centrioles, which play an important role in cell division (mitosis).

centrosphere A clear, gel-like zone of a cell which contains the centrosome.

centrum *pl.* **centra** The center of an anatomical structure.

cephalad Toward the head.

cephalalgia See headache.

cephalhematoma Accumulation of blood under the periosteum of the skull of a newborn infant; it usually occurs over one or both parietal bones, appears hours or days after delivery, increases in

cerebroside

pineal body
colliculi
cerebral aqueduct
cerebellum
pons
fourth ventricle
central canal

falx cerebri
dura
nous sinus
uitary gland
henoid sinus
thmoid sinus
cerebellum
tentorium cerebelli
mesencephalon
cerebrum
internal carotid a.

frontal lobe
temporal lobe
trigeminal n.
cerebellum
inferior aspect of brain
cerebrum

size, and disappears after a few weeks; caused by injury to the periosteum during labor.

cephalic Relating to the head.

cephalin A member of a large group of lipids known as phospholipids; found in most animal tissues, especially the brain and spinal cord; important in the blood clotting process.

cephalization 1. The gradual evolutionary concentration in the brain of important functions of the nervous system. 2. The concentration of growth tendency at the anterior end of the embryo.

cephalocentesis The draining of fluid from the brain by means of a hollow needle or trocar and cannula.

cephalodynia Headache.

cephalogyric Referring to circular movements of the head.

cephalomegaly Abnormal enlargement of the head.

cephalosporin Any broadspectrum antibiotic derived from the fungus *Cephalosporium;* the newer antibiotics are semisynthetic.

ceramide General term used to designate any *N*-acyl fatty acid derivative of a sphingosine.

cercaria, *pl.* **cercariae** A larval stage of trematode parasites. Cercariae leave their first host, usually a snail, to infest fish or vegetation, or to directly penetrate human skin.

cereal 1. An edible grain, the plant producing it, or the food prepared from it. 2. Of or relating to such grain.

cerebellar Of or relating to the cerebellum.

cerebellar syndrome A cerebellar deficiency manifested chiefly by slurred speech, slow and clumsy movement of the limbs and staggering gait.

cerebellopontile Relating to both the cerebellum and pons.

cerebellorubral Relating to the cerebellum and the red nucleus.

cerebellum The part of the central nervous system situated below and posterior to the cerebrum and above the pons and medulla; it has a somewhat oval shape and is morphologically divided into two lateral hemispheres and a middle portion; its function is to maintain equilibrium and coordination.

cerebral Of or relating to the brain.

cerebration Conscious or unconscious mental activity.

cerebritis Diffuse inflammation of the brain without suppuration.

cerebron See phrenosin.

cerebropathy See encephalopathy.

cerebropsychosis Mental disorder caused by, or associated with, a lesion of the brain.

cerebrosclerosis Sclerosis of the brain substance. Also called encephalosclerosis.

cerebrose A hexose (monosaccharide having six carbon atoms) present in brain tissue.

cerebroside A phosphorous-free glycolipid containing galactose (occasionally glucose), an unsaturated amino-alcohol, and a fatty acid.

cerebrospinal Relating to the brain and spinal cord.

cerebrotomy Surgical incision of the brain substance.

cerebrovascular Denoting the blood supply of the brain.

cerebrum The brain, excluding the medulla, pons, and cerebellum.

cerium A metallic element; symbol Ce, atomic number 58, atomic weight 140.25.

certifiable 1. Applied to any disease required by

scolex

cestode

lens

iris

posterior chamber of eye

anterior chamber of eye

uterus

cervix

polypeptide chain

radical   radical   radical   radical

chancre

law to be reported to the health authorities. **2.** Denoting a person exhibiting sufficiently severe psychotic behavior to require hospitalization. **3.** Having satisfied the requirements for certification.

certification **1.** The notification of reportable infectious disease cases to health authorities as required by law. **2.** The attainment of a document attesting that a person may officially practice in certain professions; verification of qualifications. **3.** The court procedure by which a patient is committed to an institution.

ceruloplasmin A plasma protein that carries more than 95% of the body's circulating copper; it is thought that the copper carried by ceruloplasmin goes into the cellular manufacture of cytochrome oxidase. Ceruloplasmin is deficient in Wilson's disease (hepatolenticular degeneration).

cerumen The soft brownish-yellow waxlike secretion of the ceruminous glands lining the canal of the external ear. Also called earwax.

ceruminolytic Any agent that softens or dissolves earwax in the external ear canal.

ceruminosis Excessive formation of earwax.

cervical **1.** Relating to the neck. **2.** Relating to the uterine cervix.

cervical disk syndrome Pain, numbness, and muscular spasm of the neck, radiating to the shoulders, caused by irritation and compression of the cervical nerve roots by a protruding intervertebral disk.

cervical fusion syndrome See Klippel-Feil syndrome.

cervical rib syndrome Pain and tingling along the forearm and hand due to pressure upon the brachial plexus and subclavian artery by a rudimentary cervical rib, fibrous band, first thoracic rib, or tight scalene muscle. Also called Naffziger's syndrome.

cervicectomy Amputation of the uterine cervix. Also called trachelectomy.

cervicitis Inflammation of the uterine cervix.

cystic c. A cervix containing multiple nabothian cysts.

cervicobrachial Relating to the neck and the arm.

cervix (cx) Any neck-shaped anatomic structure, as the narrow end of the bladder.

uterine c. The neck of the uterus; the lower part of the uterus extending from the isthmus into the vagina.

cesarean hysterectomy See under hysterectomy.

cesarean section See under section.

cesium Element of the alkali metal group, symbol Cs, atomic number 55, atomic weight 132.91.

Cestoda A class of Platyhelminthes or flatworms, which includes the tapeworm; term derived from the Latin *cestoda*, meaning ribbon shaped.

cestode A tapeworm.

Chaddock's signs Reflexes usually obtained in pyramidal tract lesions. **1.** Chaddock's toe sign: extension of the toe on stroking the lateral malleolus and the lateral dorsum of the foot. **2.** Chaddock's wrist sign: flexion of the wrist with fanning of the fingers upon stroking the wrist on the side of the little finger.

Chadwick's sign Dark bluish discoloration of the lining of the vagina and cervix; considered an early sign of pregnancy. Also called Jacquemier's sign.

chafe **1.** To irritate or wear away by rubbing. **2.** Irritation.

Chagas disease Disease characterized by great enlargement of the heart, which becomes very heavy but rather feeble in action, and by apical aneurysms; caused by the protozoan parasite *Trypanosoma cruzi* and transmitted by the bite of a blood-sucking arthropod; the parasite multiplies in the gut of the arthropod, is discharged in its feces, and infects man through contamination of the bite wound as a result of the arthropod defecating immediately after sucking the blood; the disease also may be transmitted by transfusion or inoculation with contaminated blood. Also called American trypanosomiasis.

chain **1.** In chemistry, a group of atoms bonded together in a linear fashion. **2.** In bacteriology, a group of microorganisms attached end-to-end.

closed c. A chain formed by atoms linked together in the shape of a ring.

heavy c., H c. A large polypeptide chain of the immunoglobulin molecule, linked to light chains by disulfide bonds.

J c. A polypeptide chain present in certain immunoglobulin molecules, particularly IgM and IgA, which allows them to form polymers.

lateral c. See side chain.

light c., L c. Either of two small polypeptide chains, designated lambda and kappa, of the immunoglobulin molecule.

polypeptide c. A repeating peptide chain formed by amino acids, each of which contributes an identical group to the backbone of the chain plus a distinguishing radical as a side group.

side c. A group of atoms linked to a closed chain. Also called lateral chain.

sympathetic c. See trunk, sympathetic.

chalasia, chalasis The relaxation of a group of muscles, especially muscles that work together.

chalazion A cyst in a tarsal (meibomian) gland that is seen merely as a lump in an otherwise normal eyelid. Also called meibomian cyst.

chalone A substance that inhibits cell division and is synthesized by mature cells of the tissue upon which it acts.

chamber A closed space.

anterior c. of the eye The space between the cornea and the iris; it is filled with aqueous humor.

hyperbaric c. A chamber in which the air pressure may be raised to higher than normal atmospheric pressure.

ionization c. A gas-filled enclosure fitted with electrodes between which an electric current passes when the gas is ionized by radiation.

posterior c. of the eye The space between the iris and the lens; it is filled with aqueous humor.

pulp c. The space in the crown or body of a tooth occupied by the pulp; principally the area of the pulp cavity within the coronal portion of the tooth and into which the root canals open.

Thoma's counting c. Thoma-Zeiss hemocytometer; see under hemocytometer.

vitreous c. The cavity of the eyeball behind the lens containing the vitreous body.

chancre The first lesion of syphilis present at the site of entrance of the syphilitic infection; it appears as a hard, reddish ulcer with an eroded center covered by a yellowish secretion. Also called hard, hunterian, indurated, or true chancre; hard sore.

soft c., simple c. See chancroid.

chancroid An infectious, nonsyphilitic, pus-discharging, venereal ulcer caused by *Haemophilus ducreyi*. Also called soft or simple chancre; soft sore.

change of life See menopause.

channel Canal.

chap **1.** To cause the skin to crack or split. **2.** A split or crack.

character **1.** The combination of features or traits that distinguishes an individual or object from another. **2.** One such feature, attribute, or trait.

charcoal A black porous material obtained by burning wood with a restricted amount of air.

activated c. Medicinal charcoal, charcoal that has been treated to increase its adsorptive power; used as an antidote and to reduce hyperacidity.

Charcot-Marie-Tooth disease Peroneal muscular atrophy; see under atrophy.

Charcot's disease Tabetic arthropathy; see under arthropathy.

charleyhorse A popular name for a cramp or stiffness of muscles, especially of the leg or arm following injury or excessive activity.

chart **1.** Information or data depicted in the form of graphs or tables. **2.** The health record of a patient. **3.** To enter information into the patient's record or to record data in graphic form.

optic chiasma

optic tract

optic nerve

eyeball

chigger

funnel chest

chestpiece (section)

Chediak-Higashi syndrome A rare hereditary condition found in infants; symptoms include decreased pigmentation of the skin, hair, and eyes, cytoplasmic inclusions of the leukocytes, and susceptibility to pyogenic infections; early death is common.

cheek A fleshy protuberance on either side of the face, forming the lateral walls of the mouth. Also called bucca; mala.

cheekbite Interocclusal record; see under record.

cheek biting The interposing of cheek tissue between the teeth of the upper and lower dentitions, occasionally resulting in hyperkeratotic lesions and irritations of the buccal mucosa.

cheekbone Zygomatic bone; see table of bones.

cheilectomy 1. Surgical removal of a portion of the lip. 2. Cutting away of bony irregularities on the rim of a joint cavity.

cheilion The corner or angle of the mouth.

cheilitis Inflammation of the lip.

   actinic c., solar c. Inflammation of the lip characterized by a scaly crust on the vermillion border, usually due to overexposure to sunlight.

cheilognathouragnoschisis Congenital malformation consisting of a cleft that extends from the palate, through the gum, to the upper lip.

cheiloplasty Plastic surgery of the lips. Also called labioplasty.

cheiloschisis Cleft lip; see under lip.

cheilosis A noninflammatory condition of the lip marked by fissuring and chapping; characteristic of riboflavin deficiency.

cheiroscope A binocular instrument used for antisuppression training of the eyes in strabismus.

chelate 1. A compound containing a metal ion connected by coordinate bonds to two or more nonmetal ions in the same molecule. 2. To effect chelation.

chelation The coordinate bond formation between a metal ion and two or more nonmetal ions in the same molecule.

chemical 1. Relating to chemistry. 2. A substance produced by the interaction of elements.

chemise A piece of linen used to secure a tampon around a catheter that has been inserted into a wound.

chemistry The science concerned with the atomic and molecular composition of the different types of matter and the laws that govern their mutual reactions.

   analytic c. The breaking up of compounds to determine and study their composition.

   biologic c. See biochemistry.

   inorganic c. The branch of chemistry concerned with substances not containing carbon.

   organic c. The study of substances containing carbon.

   physiologic c. See biochemistry.

chemobiotic Denoting a compound containing an antibiotic and another therapeutic chemical.

chemocautery The destruction of tissue by the application of a caustic substance.

chemoceptor See chemoreceptor.

chemodectoma A tumor of the chemoreceptor system, such as the carotid body, glomus jugulare, and aortic arch bodies.

chemodectomatosis Occurrence in the lungs of multiple minute tumors of the chemoreceptor type.

chemodifferentiation Differentiation at the molecular level which usually precedes and controls morphologic differentiation of cells in the developing embryo.

chemokinesis Increased activity of an organism stimulated by a chemical substance.

chemoluminescence 1. Light produced by the transformation of chemical energy. 2. Radiation producing chemical action.

chemolysis Chemical decomposition.

chemonucleolysis Dissolution of the center of an intervertebral disk by injecting it with an enzyme, e.g., chymopapain.

chemopallidectomy Injection of a chemical substance in the globus pallidum in the brain; an operation performed for the relief of rigidity in parkinsonism.

chemopallidothalamectomy Destruction of portions of brain tissue (globus pallidus and thalamus) by injection of a chemical.

chemoprophylaxis Prevention of a specific disease by the use of a chemical.

chemoreceptor An end organ, such as a taste bud, or sense organ, such as the carotid body, sensitive to chemical stimuli. Also called chemoceptor.

chemosensitive Sensitive to changes in the chemical composition of substances.

chemosis Eye disorder marked by swelling of the conjunctiva around the cornea.

chemosurgery The use of chemical substances to destroy tissues.

chemotaxis Movement of an organism toward or away from a chemical substance, especially the unidirectional migration of white blood cells toward an attractant.

chemotherapeutics The branch of therapeutics dealing with the treatment of disease with chemicals.

chemotherapy Treatment or prevention of disease by means of chemical substances.

chenodeoxycholic acid One of the acids present in bile which participate in digestive processes.

cherubism The characteristic facial features of individuals affected with familial fibrous dysplasia of the jaws; chubbiness and upturned eyes.

chest See thorax.

   barrel c. A short and round chest with ribs in a horizontal position; seen in cases of advanced emphysema.

   flail c. An unstable chest wall due to multiple rib fractures causing a paradoxical motion (moving inward on inspiration and outward on expiration). Also called flapping chest wall.

   funnel c. See pectus excavatum.

chestpiece The portion of the stethoscope placed against the patient's body for the determination and study of sounds, within the body.

Chiari-Frommel syndrome Condition characterized by prolonged milk secretion and atrophy of the uterus following pregnancy.

chiasma, chiasm An X-shaped crossing.

   optic c. The point of crossing of the fibers of the optic nerves.

chickenpox An acute contagious disease, usually of young children, caused by the varicella-zoster virus (family Herpesviridae); marked by a skin eruption, fever, and mild constitutional symptoms; incubation period is from 11 to 24 days. Also called varicella.

chigger Any of various six-legged larvae of mites, the most common being *Trombicula alfreddugesi;* the chigger usually attaches itself to parts of the body that are snugly clothed, such as the waist and ankles; itching generally begins three to six hours after it has attached. Also called red bug; harvest mite.

chigoe The small tropical sand flea, *Tunga penetrans;* the egg-carrying female burrows under the skin of man, causing intense itching.

chilblain Condition resulting from excessive exposure to cold temperature, marked by inflammatory swelling of hands and feet accompanied by severe itching and burning sensations, and sometimes ulceration; usually affects individuals with a history of cold limbs in summer as well as in winter. Also called pernio. Cf. frostbite.

child A young person between the periods of infancy and adolescence.

   battered c. A child who has been subjected to physical abuse, usually by parents, with resulting injuries.

   hyperactive c. A child who is characterized by excessive energy, emotional instability, and short attention span, usually related to minimal brain dysfunction.

childbearing Pregnancy and parturition.

childbirth Parturition.

   natural c. A concept in the management of parturition in which prenatal education, exercises, and

chloramphenicol

chlorpromazine hydrochloride

chlordiazepoxide

chlorpropamide

chlorothiazide

chlortetracycline

flagellum

Chlamydomonas

contractile vacuole

eye spot

nucleus

pyrenoid

cell wall

psychologic conditioning largely replace anesthesia and surgical intervention at the time of labor. Also called physiologic childbirth.

chill 1. A moderate sensation of coldness. 2. A feeling of coldness accompanied by shivering and fever.

Chilomastix A genus of protozoa parasitic in the intestines; one species, *Chilomastix mesnili,* is believed to cause diarrhea.

chimera 1. In experimental embryology, an organism developed from combined portions of different embryos. 2. An individual who has received a genetically different transplant.

chin The central anterior prominence of the lower jaw. Also called mentum.

double c. Loose fatty flesh under the chin.

Chinese restaurant syndrome Transient syndrome consisting of chest pains, throbbing of the head, and feelings of tightness of facial muscles after ingesting monosodium L-glutamate, which is used in Chinese food; occurs in individuals who are unusually sensitive to this additive.

chirognostic Capable of distinguishing between right and left.

chirokinesthesia The subjective sensation of motions of the hand.

chiroplasty Plastic surgery of the hand.

chiropodist See podiatrist.

chiropody See podiatry.

chiropractic A philosophy of therapy in which disease is attributed to mild dislocations of the vertebral column, causing pressure on the nerves; the preferred method of treatment is by manipulation of the vertebrae.

chiropractor One who practices chiropractic.

chisel A metal instrument with a beveled cutting edge designed after the carpenter's chisel; used in dentistry for cutting or cleaving enamel.

chitin A transparent, horny organic substance (polysaccharide), constituting the chief component of insect exoskeletons, crustacean shells; and the cell walls of certain fungi.

chitobiose The disaccharide present in chitin.

chitosamine See glucosamine.

Chlamydia A genus of non-motile, gram-negative intracellular bacteria (family Chlamydiaceae), once considered viruses because of their intracellular parasitism; unlike viruses, they possess both RNA and DNA and multiply by binary fission.

C. psittaci A species causing a pulmonary infection.

C. trachomatis The cause of trachoma, inclusion conjunctivitis, lymphogranuloma venereum, urethritis, and proctitis.

Chlamydomonas A genus (phylum Chlorophyta) of single-celled algae that can reproduce both sexually and asexually; used in genetic studies.

chloasma The occurrence of irregularly shaped brownish spots or patches on the skin; commonly known as the mask of pregnancy when appearing on the face and neck of a pregnant woman and as liver spots in elderly people, although there is no association with disease of the liver.

chloracne A skin eruption, resembling acne, caused by constant contact with certain chlorinated compounds.

chloral A colorless oily liquid of pungent odor, CCl_3CHO; produced by the action of chlorine gas on alcohol.

c. hydrate A colorless crystalline compound, soluble in water and alcohol; used as a hypnotic and sedative.

chloralism Condition caused by the constant use of chloral as an intoxicant.

chloralose A crystalline substance used as a general anesthetic in laboratory animals.

chlorambucil A derivative of nitrogen mustard which retards proliferation and maturation of lymphocytes; used in the treatment of chronic lymphocytic leukemia and some lymphomas; Leukeran®.

chloramphenicol A broad-spectrum antibiotic originally obtained from *Streptomyces venezuellae* but now produced synthetically; effective against many strains of gram-positive and gram-negative pathogenic microorganisms; used selectively because of the occurrence (infrequently) of aplastic anemia; Chloromycetin®.

chlordane A chlorinated hydrocarbon used as an insecticide; may cause human poisoning by absorption through the skin, inhalation or ingestion.

chlordiazepoxide The nonproprietary name for Librium®, a drug widely used for treating anxiety, tension, and psychoneuroses.

chloremia 1. See chlorosis. 2. The presence of large amounts of chloride in the blood.

chlorhydria The presence of abnormally large amounts of hydrochloric acid in the stomach.

chloric Of or containing chlorine.

chloride Any compound of chlorine.

chloridometer An apparatus used in the turbidimetric analysis of chlorides.

chloriduria The presence of chloride in the urine.

chlorinate To combine with chlorine or a chlorine compound.

chlorinated Containing chlorine.

chlorine A greenish yellow, irritating, gaseous element; symbol Cl, atomic number 17, atomic weight 34.45; used as a disinfectant and bleaching agent.

chlorite Any salt of chlorous acid.

chloroethane See ethyl chloride.

chloroform A colorless, volatile, heavy liquid of sweetish taste, $CHCl_3$; formerly used as a general anesthetic.

chloroma A tumor arising from myeloid tissue and containing a pale green pigment; most frequently found in the periosteum and ligamentous structures of the skull; seen usually in children and young adults. Commonly called green cancer.

chlorometry The quantitative study of chlorine.

***p*-chlorophenoxyisobutyrate** See clofibrate.

chlorophillins Substances derived from chlorophyll, capable of absorbing odorous molecules and thus acting as deodorants.

chlorophyll, chlorophyl Any of a group of green pigments in plant cells that absorb light during the food making process of photosynthesis.

chloroplast A cytoplasmic organelle of all green plant cells; it contains chlorophyll.

chloropsia A condition in which all objects appear to have a tint of green. Also called green vision.

chloroquine phosphate Quinoline diphosphate; an agent used in the treatment of malaria, hepatic amebiasis, and certain skin diseases.

chlorosis A form of anemia occurring in adolescent girls; marked by a moderate reduction in red blood cells and a great reduction in hemoglobin content; attributed to insufficient intake of iron. Also called green sickness; chloremia.

chlorothiazide A commonly prescribed diuretic and antihypertensive drug; it inhibits renal tubular reabsorption of sodium and is used in treating hypertension and edema due to congestive heart failure, liver disease, and pregnancy; Diuril®.

chlorotic Relating to chlorosis.

chlorpromazine hydrochloride A phenothiazine derivative used orally, muscularly, or intravenously to depress conditioned reflexes and the hypothalamic centers; used as a major tranquilizer in psychoses, and in the management of postoperative nausea and in radiation sickness; Thorazine Hydrochloride®.

chlorpropamide An oral hypoglycemic agent in the sulfonylurea class; Diabinese®.

chlortetracycline An antibiotic substance obtained from *Streptomyces aureofaciens;* active against hemolytic streptococci, staphylococci, typhoid bacilli, brucellae, and certain viruses; it has been supplanted in use by other tetracycline compounds with fewer side effects; Aureomycin®.

chloruresis The presence of chloride in the urine.

chloruretic Relating to an agent that promotes an increase of chloride excretion in the urine.

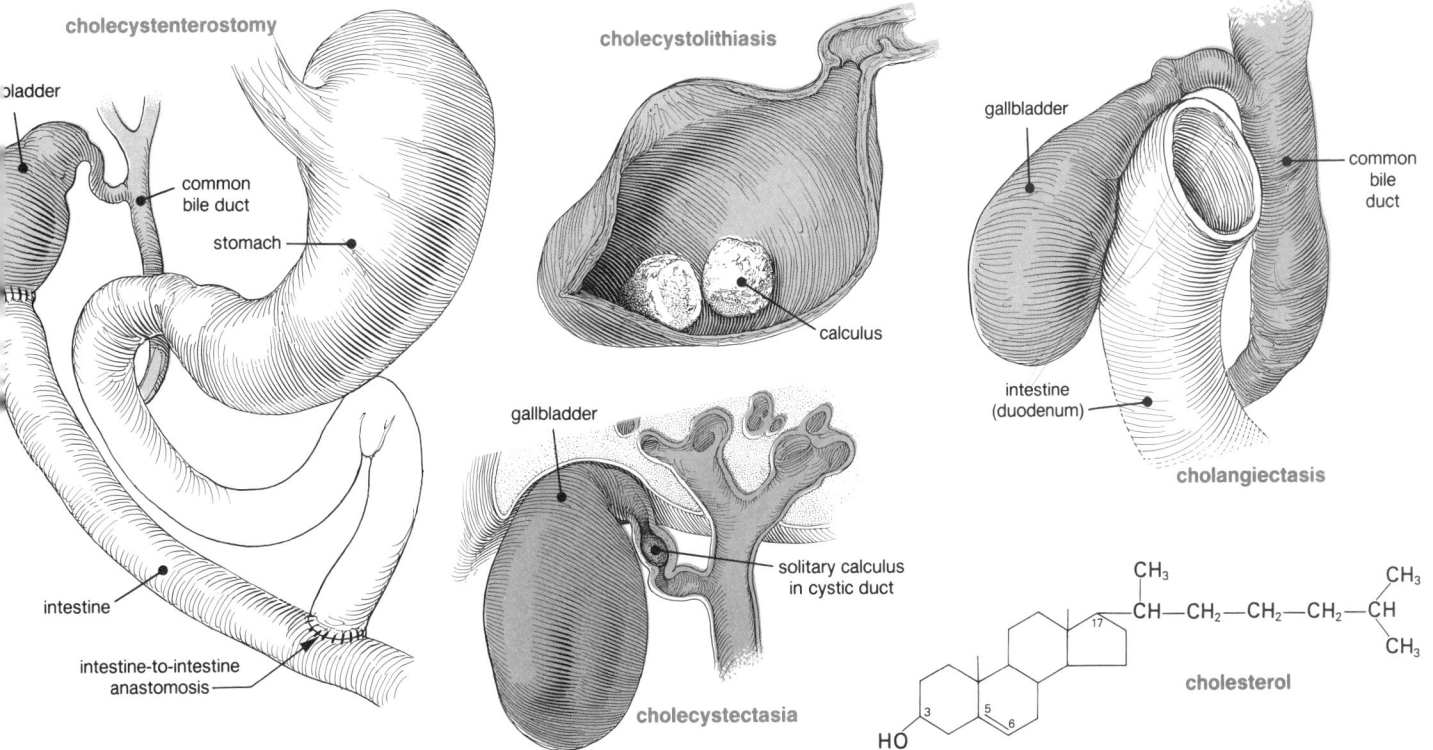

cholecystenterostomy

bladder

common
bile duct

stomach

intestine

intestine-to-intestine
anastomosis

cholecystolithiasis

calculus

gallbladder

solitary calculus
in cystic duct

cholecystectasia

gallbladder

common
bile
duct

intestine
(duodenum)

cholangiectasis

CH_3
CH—CH_2—CH_2—CH_2—CH
CH_3
CH_3

17

3

5

6

HO

cholesterol

choana The funnel-like opening of the nasal cavity into the nasopharynx on either side. Also called the posterior naris.

choanal Of or relating to a choana.

choke To interfere with or terminate breathing by obstructing or breaking the trachea.

cholagogue Any agent that promotes the flow of bile.

cholangiectasis Dilation of the bile duct.

cholangiocarcinoma Malignant tumor of the liver originating in the epithelium of the intrahepatic bile ducts.

cholangioenterostomy Surgical union of the bile duct to the intestine.

cholangiography Radiologic examination of the bile ducts after ingestion of a radiopaque substance.

cholangiole One of the minute terminal branches of the bile duct.

cholangiopancreatography X-ray examination of the bile ducts and pancreas.

endoscopic retrograde c. (ERCP) Use of an endoscope to pass a catheter for injection of radiopaque dye into pancreatic and bile ducts.

cholangioscopy Visual examination of the bile ducts with an endoscope.

cholangiotomy Surgical incision into a bile duct.

cholangitis Inflammation of the bile duct.

cholanopoiesis Synthesis by the liver of cholic acid or its conjugates, or of natural bile salts.

cholecalciferol See vitamin D_3.

cholechromopoiesis Synthesis of bile pigments by the liver.

cholecyst Gallbladder.

cholecystagogue An agent that stimulates gallbladder actiivty.

cholecystasia Dilatation of the gallbladder.

cholecystectomy Surgical removal of the gallbladder.

cholecystenterostomy Surgical joining of the gallbladder and the intestine.

cholecystic Relating to the gallbladder.

cholecystis Gallbladder.

cholecystitis Inflammation of the gallbladder.

cholecystoduodenostomy Surgical creation of a direct connection between the gallbladder and the duodenum.

cholecystogram An x-ray image of the gallbladder.

cholecystography X-ray visualization of the gallbladder after administration of a radiopaque substance, which is excreted by the liver and concentrated by the gallbladder.

cholecystojejunostomy Surgical establishment of a connection between the gallbladder and je-

junum.

cholecystokinase An enzyme that promotes the breakdown of cholecystokinin.

cholecystokinetic Causing release of the gallbladder contents.

cholecystokinin (CCK) A hormone secreted by the mucosa of the upper intestinal tract which stimulates contraction of the gallbladder.

cholecystolithiasis The presence of one or more stones in the gallbladder.

cholecystorraphy Suturing of the bladder.

cholecystostomy Surgical formation of an opening into the gallbladder with insertion of a drainage tube through the abdominal wall.

cholecystotomy Surgical incision into the gallbladder.

choledoch Common bile duct.

choledochal Of or relating to the common bile duct.

choledochectomy Surgical removal of a portion of the common bile duct.

choledochitis Inflammation of the common bile duct.

choledochoduodenostomy Surgical anastomosis between the common bile duct and the duodenum.

choledochoenterostomy Surgical formation of a connection between the common bile duct and any part of the intestine.

choledochography X-ray visualization of the common bile duct after administration of a radiopaque material.

choledocholith Stone in the common bile duct.

choledocholithiasis The presence of stones in the common bile duct.

choledocholithotomy Incision into the common bile duct for the removal of a stone.

choledochoplasty Reparative surgery of the common bile duct.

choledochorrhaphy Suturing of the common bile duct.

choledochoscope A device for inspecting the lumen of the common bile duct.

choledochoscopy Visual examination of the common bile duct by means of a choledochoscope.

choledochostomy Surgical formation of an opening into the common bile duct for drainage.

choledochotomy Surgical incision into the common bile duct.

choledochous Containing or conveying bile.

choledochus Common bile duct; see under duct.

cholelith Gallstone.

cholelithiasis The presence of gallstones.

cholelithotomy Surgical removal of a gallstone.

cholemesis, cholemesia The vomiting of bile.

cholemia The presence of bile in the blood.

cholemic Relating to the presence of bile in the blood.

choleperitonitis Inflammation caused by the presence of bile in the peritoneal cavity.

cholepoiesis The formation of bile.

cholera An acute infectious disease of man caused by the bacteria *Vibrio cholerae;* characterized by severe diarrhea, vomiting, cramps, and loss of huge amounts of fluid and electrolyte from the body; occurs endemically and epidemically in Asia. Also called Asiatic cholera.

choleresis Secretion of bile by the liver, distinguished from the expulsion of bile by the gallbladder.

cholerrhagia Excessive secretion of bile.

cholestasis, cholestasia Suppression or arrest of the flow of bile.

cholestatic Tending to arrest the flow of bile.

cholesteatoma A misnomer for a cystic mass in the middle ear composed of a lining of stratified squamous epithelium filled with material containing blood and cholesterol; associated with chronic middle ear infection.

cholesteremia Increased amounts of cholesterol in the blood.

cholesterol A white, waxy, crystalline organic alcohol; a universal tissue constituent, present in all animal fats and oils, in bile, brain tissue, blood, and egg yolk; it constitutes a large portion of the most common type of gallstone and is found in deposits in the vessel walls in atherosclerosis.

cholesterolosis Focal deposits of cholesterol in the tissues, especially the gallbladder mucosa.

cholic Relating to the bile.

cholic acid A digestive acid present in bile.

choline A compound synthesized by the body and found in most animal tissues; important in fat metabolism; a precursor of acetylcholine.

cholinergic 1. Stimulated by or capable of liberating acetylcholine; parasympathomimetic. 2. Simulating the effects of acetylcholine.

cholinester An ester of choline.

cholinesterase An enzyme present throughout the body tissues that promotes the hydrolysis of acetylcholine to form acetic acid and choline; it acts to remove acetylcholine discharged at the neuromuscular junction and prevent it from re-exciting the muscle. Also called acetylcholinesterase.

cholinomimetic Producing an effect similar to that of acetylcholine.

cholorrhea Excessive secretion of bile.

cholylcoenzyme A A condensation product of choline and coenzyme A.

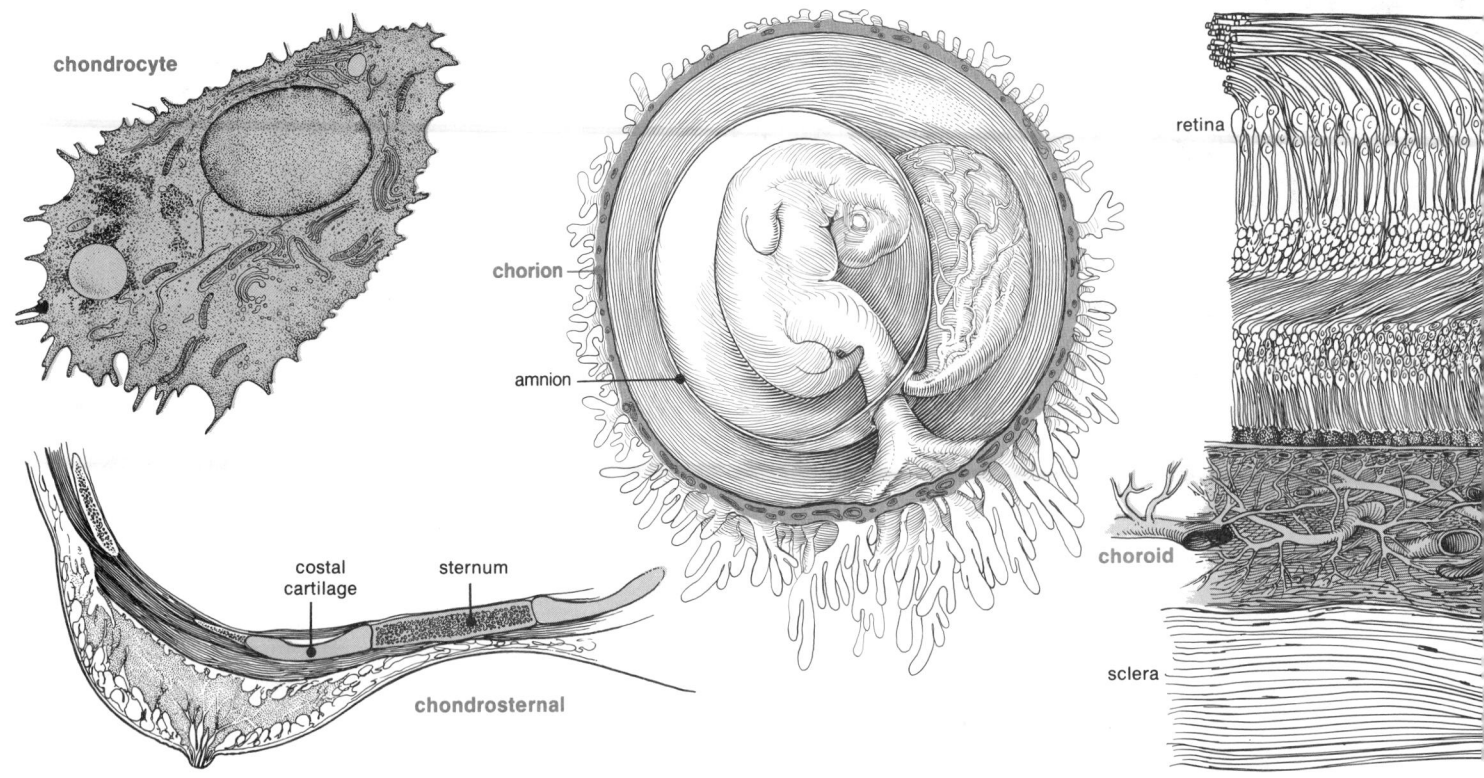

chondrocyte

chorion

amnion

retina

choroid

sclera

costal
cartilage

sternum

chondrosternal

chondral Relating to cartilage.

chondralgia Pain in a cartilage.

chondrectomy Removal of a cartilage.

chondrification Conversion into cartilage.

chondritis Inflammation of cartilage.

  costal c. Costochondritis, painful inflammation of the costal cartilages, occasionally mistaken for pain of cardiac origin.

chondroblast A cartilage-producing cell.

chondroblastoma A benign tumor of long bones occurring in children under the age of 20; it consists of tissue resembling fetal cartilage.

chondrocalcinosis Calcified deposits in articular cartilage and synovial fluid of large joints, producing arthritic pain and goutlike symptoms.

chondroclast A giant cell concerned with the absorption of cartilage.

chondrocostal Relating to the cartilage of the ribs.

chondrocyte A cartilage cell; since the cartilage has no blood vessels, the chondrocyte receives its nutrition by diffusion from the capillaries of the perichondrium.

chondrodermatitis nodularis chronica helicis The presence of painful nodules on the helix of the ear.

chondrodynia Chondralgia; pain in a cartilage.

chondrodystrophia, chondrodystrophy See achondroplasia.

chondrogenesis The formation of cartilage.

chondroitin A mucopolysaccharide present in chondrin; upon hydrolysis it yields acetic acid, glucuronic acid, and galactosamine.

chondroma A benign tumor composed of cartilage.

chondromalacia Softening of an articular cartilage, most commonly seen in the kneecap (patella).

chondromatosis The presence of multiple cartilaginous growths (chondromas).

chondro-osseous Relating to cartilage and bone.

chondropathy Any disease of cartilage.

chondrophyte A cartilaginous growth at the articular surface of a bone.

chondroplasty Reparative surgery of cartilage.

chondrosamine See galactosamine.

chondrosarcoma A malignant bone tumor derived from cartilage cells which erodes the bone and invades adjacent soft tissues.

chondrosternal Relating to (a) a sternal cartilage; (b) the rib cartilages and the sternum.

chondrotome A surgical knife used for cutting cartilage.

chorda *pl.* **chordae** 1. A tendon. 2. A stringlike

anatomic structure.

  chordae tendineae Tendinous strands extending from the papillary muscles to the leaflets of the atrioventricular valves of the heart.

  c. tympani A branch of the facial nerve that innervates the submandibular and sublingual glands and the anterior two-thirds on the tongue.

Chordata The phylum that includes all animals having a notochord at some developmental stage.

chordee Downward curvature of the penis due to fibrous bands on the undersurface of the corpora.

chorditis Inflammation of a chorda.

chordoma A rare tumor believed to arise from remnants of notochordal tissue; occurring along the vertebral column, especially the sacrococcygeal area and at the base of the skull.

chorea Any of a group of disorders characterized by brief, rapid, involuntary movements of the limbs, face, trunk, and head.

  acute c. A symptom complex occurring in children, marked by muscle weakness, incoordination, and involuntary movements intensified by voluntary effort; associated with acute rheumatic fever. Also called Syndenham's chorea; St. Vitus dance; infectious chorea.

  hereditary c. A hereditary, progressive, degenerative disease of the brain beginning in adult life and causing mental deterioration; characterized by involuntary jerky movements, usually of the trunk, shoulders, and lower limbs. Also called chronic progressive chorea; Huntington's chorea.

  senile c. Mild involuntary, usually unilateral, movements of the limbs occurring in the aged.

choreic Of or relating to chorea.

choreiform Resembling chorea (a spasmodic nervous disorder).

choreoathetoid Characterized by choreoathetosis.

choreoathetosis Abnormal involuntary movements of the body, a combination of choreic and athetoid patterns as twitching, writhing, contortions of face, heel walking, and bizarre postures.

chorioadenoma destruens A cellular, locally invasive tumor of the outermost fetal membrane (chorion); it penetrates and sometimes perforates the wall of the uterus, extending into adjacent tissues.

chorioamnionitis Inflammation of the fetal membranes.

chorioangioma A rare benign tumor arising from placental capillaries which appears as a solitary nodule in the placenta.

choriocarcinoma A malignant tumor arising from the outermost of the fetal membranes (chorion); rarely coexisting with the pregnancy but usu-

ally developing immediately afterward; it may result from either ectopic or normal pregnancies. Formerly called chorionepithelioma.

choriomeningitis Inflammation of the cerebral membranes (meninges) with involvement of the choroid plexuses, especially of the third and fourth ventricles.

  lymphocytic c. A disease affecting rodents, especially mice, sometimes transmitted to man; caused by an arenavirus (family Arenaviridae).

chorion The outermost membrane enclosing the fetus.

chorionepithelioma See choriocarcinoma.

chorionic Relating to the outermost of the fetal membranes (chorion).

chorioretinitis Inflammation of the middle layer of the eye (choroid) and the retina. Also called Jensen's disease; retinochoroiditis.

choristoma A growth composed of normal tissue occurring in abnormal locations.

choroid 1. The middle, vascular layer of the eyeball. 2. Resembling the chorion membrane enclosing the fetus.

choroideremia A hereditary disease marked by progressive degeneration of the vascular layer of the eye (choroid); the earliest symptom is night blindness followed by loss of peripheral vision and eventual total blindness.

choroiditis Inflammation of the vascular coat of the eye.

choroidocyclitis Inflammation of the vascular coat of the eye and the ciliary body.

Christmas disease Hemophilia B. See also factor IX.

chromaffin 1. Readily staining yellow or brown with chromium salts. 2. Denoting certain cells present mostly in the medulla of the adrenal glands and to a lesser extent along the ganglionated sympathetic chain (paraganglia) and the abdominal aorta (organs of Zuckerkandl).

chromaffinoma A tumor composed of chromaffin tissues.

chromaffinopathy Any disease of the chromaffin tissues.

chromate A salt of chronic acid.

chromatic Of or relating to color.

chromatids Two daughter strands joined by a single centromere, formed by the splitting of a chromosome in the prophase stage of mitosis; eventually each chromatid becomes a chromosome.

chromatin The portion of the cell nucleus that is easily stained by dyes, consisting of nucleic acids and proteins.

chromatism 1. Abnormal pigmentation. 2. Color

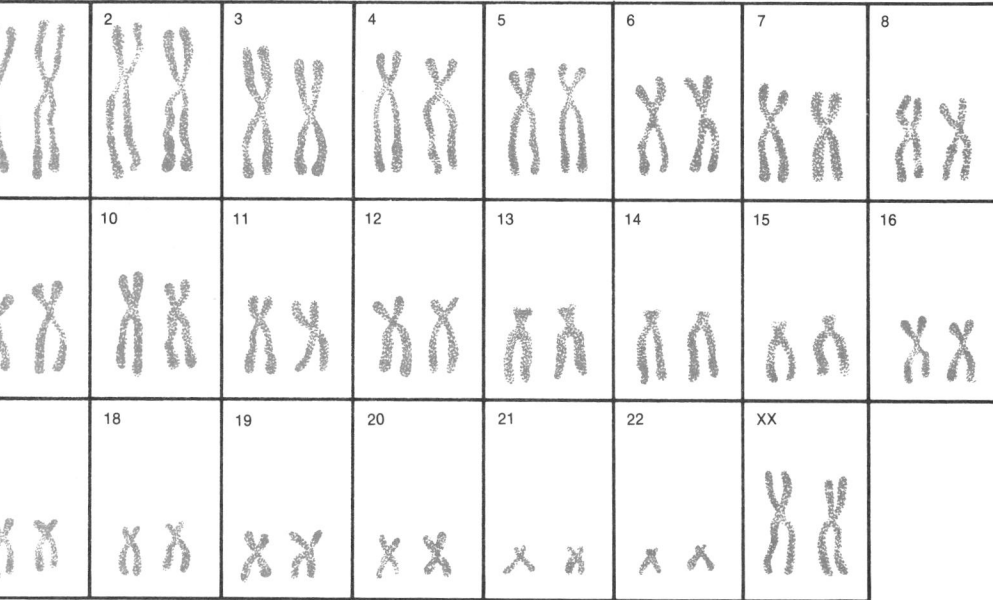

chromosomes arranged in pairs according to size

karyotype of a normal female

acrocentric chromosome

chromosome satellite

metacentric chromosome

submetacentric chromosome

distortion in an image produced by a lens. Also called chromatic aberration.

chromatogenous Producing pigmentation or color.

chromatogram The absorbent column containing the stratified constituents separated from a solution by chromatography.

chromatography A method of chemical analysis by means of which substances in solution are separated into constituent layers of different colors as they pass through an adsorbent (paper or powder) at different velocities. Also called adsorption analysis; chromatographic analysis.

  gas c. Differential separation of complex mixtures by vaporizing and diffusing the substance along with a carrier gas through an adsorbent.

  paper c. Partition chromatography in which one of the substances being separated adheres to, and forms a film on, filter paper; used in biochemistry to estimate traces of complex organic compounds. Also called paper partition chromatography.

  partition c. Separation of similar substances by repeated divisions between immiscible liquids.

  thin-layer c. (TLC) Chromatography through a thin layer of an inert material (e.g., cellulose) supported on a glass or plastic plate.

chromatolysis 1. The dissolution of the chromidial (chromophilic) substance (Nissl bodies) in the neuron following injury to the cell body or to the axon. 2. The destruction of the body of the cell by a specific lysin, leaving only the cell membrane.

chromatomere A group of membrane-limited round granules containing a substance thought to have lysosomal properties.

chromatometer See chromometer.

chromatophilic Staining easily.

chromatopsia Color vision, an abnormal condition in which all objects appear tinged with one particular color. Also called chromopsia.

chromatoptometry See chromometry.

chromesthesia 1. Condition in which colors are seen when other senses are stimulated. 2. The perception of other sensations, such as taste or smell, when colors are seen. 3. The color sense.

chromidium pl. **chromidia** A granule in the cell cytoplasm that stains deeply with basic dyes.

chromium A steel-gray metallic element; symbol Cr, atomic number 24, atomic weight 52.01.

Chromobacterium A genus of gram-negative flagellated bacteria (family Rhizobiaceae); it produces a violet pigment.

chromoblast An embryonic pigment cell.

chromoblastomycosis A chronic infection caused by *Phialophora* or *Cladosporium*, principally in the tropics; the lesion is usually a slow-growing nodule which ulcerates and becomes purplish red to gray and wartlike. Also called chromomycosis.

chromocyte A pigmented cell.

chromocytometer An instrument for determining the amount of hemoglobin in red blood cells.

chromogen 1. A substance capable of chemically changing into a pigment. 2. A pigment-producing organelle.

chromogenesis The production of pigment.

chromometer A scale used for testing color perception. Also called chromatometer.

chromometry The measuring of color perception. Also called chromatoptometry.

chromomycosis See chromoblastomycosis.

chromonema pl. **chromonemata** A coiled filament which extends the entire length of a chromosome and contains the genes.

chromophil, chromophile 1. A cell or tissue that stains readily. 2. Chromaffin.

chromophilia The property of being readily stained; said of certain cells.

chromophilic, chromophilous Staining readily.

chromophobe, chromophobic Denoting a cell or tissue that resists staining.

chromophobia 1. Resistance to stains. 2. Morbid dislike of colors.

chromophore Color radical, a molecular group that is capable of selective absorption of light, resulting in coloration of certain substances.

chromoprotein A compound, such as hemoglobin, composed of a pigment and a simple protein.

chromopsia See chromatopsia.

chromoscope An instrument or scale used in the study and testing of color phenomena as related to color perception.

chromosome One of a group of threadlike structures contained in the nucleus of a cell, composed primarily of genes, or the genetic material DNA; human cells normally have 46, or 23 pairs, of chromosomes; one of each pair is contributed by the mother, the other by the father at conception.

  acrocentric c. A chromosome with the centromere placed very close to one end so that the shorter arm is very small.

  c. satellite A small chromosomal segment separated from the main body of the chromosome by a secondary constriction; in man usually associated with the short arm of an acrocentric chromosome.

  metacentric c. A chromosome with a centrally placed centromere that divides the chromosome into two arms of approximately equal length.

  Philadelphia (Ph¹) c. An abnormal minute chromosome probably derived from a small acrocentric chromosome (no. 21 or 22) by loss of a large part of the long arm; found in cultured leukocytes of many patients afflicted with chronic myelocytic leukemia.

  sex c.'s Chromosomes responsible for the determination of sex; normally females have two X chromosomes, males have one X and one Y.

  submetacentric c. A chromosome with the centromere so placed that it divides the chromosome into two arms of unequal length.

  telocentric c. A chromosome with a terminal centromere; such chromosomes are unstable and arise by misdivision or breakage within the centromere region.

  X c. One of the sex chromosomes carried by the female in a double dose (two XX) and by the male in a single dose (one X and one Y).

  Y c. One of the sex chromosomes carried by the male in a single dose (one Y and one X).

chronaxie, chronaxy, chronaxia The unit which serves as the quantitative index of electric excitability; the time required by an electric current (of twice the minimum strength needed to elicit a threshold response) to pass through a motor nerve and cause a contraction in the associated muscle.

chronic Denoting a disease of slow progress and persisting over a long period of time; opposite of acute.

chronic brain syndrome Impairment of brain function, usually permanent, manifested by faulty memory, judgement, comprehension, and orientation; secondary to other conditions such as alcoholism, senility, cerebrovascular disease, etc.

chronic granulomatous disease A congenital hereditary susceptibility to severe infection caused by the inability of polymorphonuclear leukocytes to destroy bacteria. Also called congenital dysphagocytosis.

chronobiology The study of the duration of life and ways of prolonging it. See also geriatrics; gerontology.

chronognosis Perception of the passage of time.

chronograph An instrument used for graphically recording short periods of time, as the duration of an event or episode.

chronophotograph One of a series of photographs showing motion.

chronotaraxis Confusion relating to the passage of time.

chronotropism Modification of the rate of a regular periodic movement, as of the heart beat.

chrysiasis Deposition of gold in the tissues following administration of gold salts. Also called auriasis.

chrysotherapy The therapeutic administration of gold salts. Also called aurotherapy.

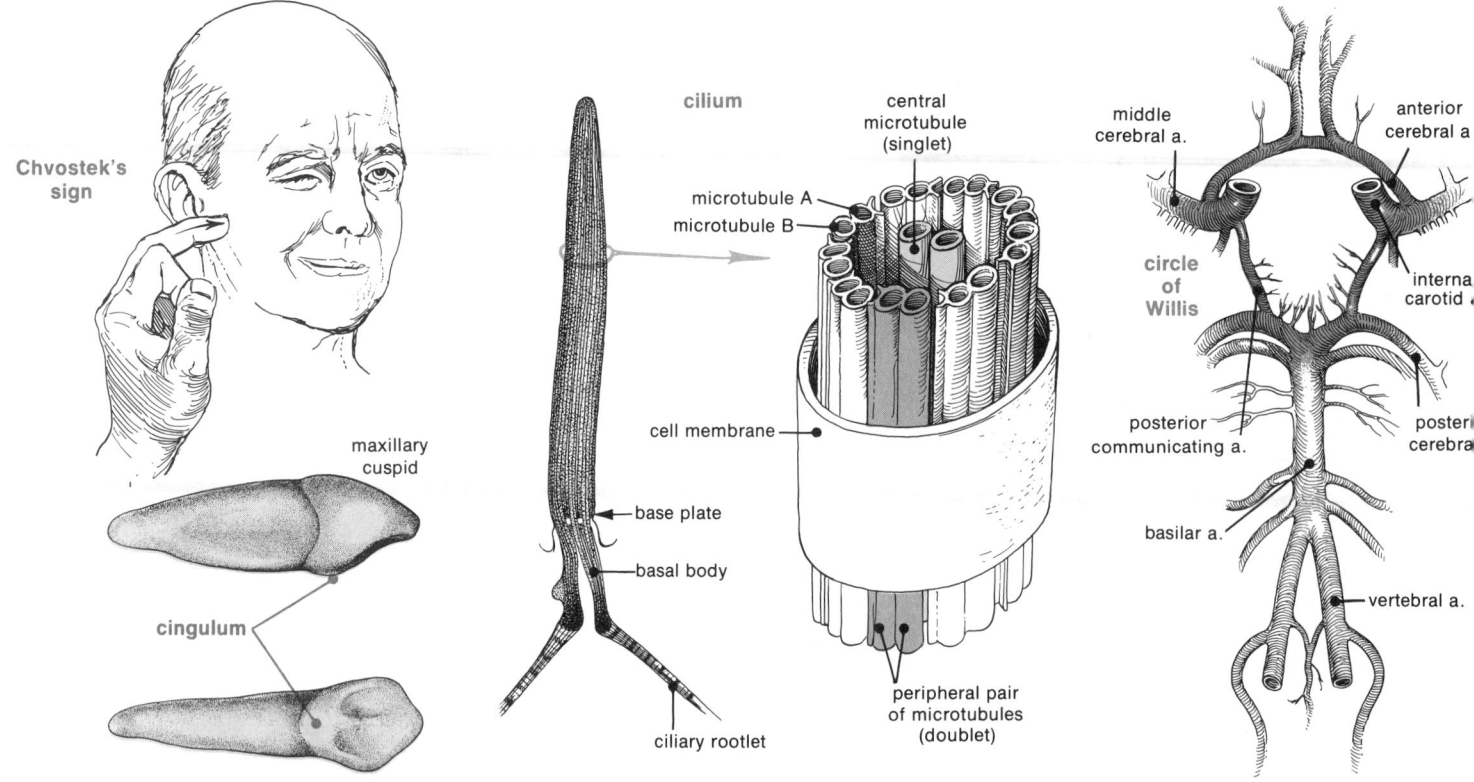

Chvostek's sign

maxillary cuspid

cingulum

cilium

central microtubule (singlet)

microtubule A
microtubule B

cell membrane

base plate

basal body

ciliary rootlet

peripheral pair of microtubules (doublet)

middle cerebral a.

anterior cerebral a

circle of Willis

interna carotid

posterior communicating a.

posteri cerebra

basilar a.

vertebral a.

Chvostek's sign A unilateral spasm of facial muscles elicited by a slight tap over the facial nerve; seen in tetany. Also called Weiss' sign.

chyle A milky fluid composed of lymph and digested fat, absorbed into the lymphatic capillaries (lacteals) from the intestine during digestion; it is transported by the thoracic duct to the left subclavian vein where it becomes mixed with the blood.

chylomicronemia Increased number of microscopic particles of fat (chylomicrons) in the blood.

chylomicrons Minute fat particles (about one μ in size) present in lymph which normally are quickly cleared from the blood.

chylopericardium A milky effusion into the pericardium due to injury or to obstruction of the thoracic duct.

chyloperitoneum Accumulation of a milky liquid in the peritoneal cavity. Also called chylous ascites.

chylopoiesis The formation of chyle.

chylothorax The collection of a milky fluid of lymphatic origin (chyle) in the pleural cavity.

chyluria The presence of chyle or lymph in the urine, giving it a white, turbid appearance.

chyme The semifluid mass of food passed from the stomach to the duodenum.

chymopoiesis The conversion of food into chyme. Also called chymification.

chymosin See rennin.

chymotrypsin A digestive enzyme (proteinase) present in pancreatic juice; proposed for use in the treatnent of inflammation and edema caused by trauma.

chymotrypsinogen Pancreatic enzyme that gives rise to chymotrypsin.

cicatrectomy Surgical removal of a scar.

cicatrix The fibrous tissue formed during the healing of a wound. Also called scar.

cicatrization The formation of scar tissue.

cilia Plural of cilium.

ciliarotomy An incision through the peripheral region of the anterior surface of the iris (ciliary zone).

ciliary Relating to (a) any hairlike process; (b) the eyelashes; (c) certain structures of the eye.

ciliated Having hairlike processes.

cilioretinal Relating to the ciliary body and the retina.

cilium *pl.* **cilia** **1.** A microscopic hairlike projection on a cell surface capable of vibratory or lashing movements. **2.** Eyelash.

cillosis Twitching of the eyelids. Also called ciliosis.

cimbia A band of white fibers across the ventral surface of the cerebral peduncle.

cimetidine A drug that blocks the actions of histamine on H₂ receptor sites, thus inhibiting secretion of stomach acid; effective in the treatment and prevention of peptic ulcer.

cinchona Any of various trees of the genus *Cinchona,* found in South America, whose bark contains quinine and a number of alkaloids.

cinchonism Toxic condition resulting from an overdose of cinchona or its alkaloids, marked by headache, deafness, giddiness, and ringing in the ears. Also called quininism.

cineangiocardiography The production of motion picture films showing, fluoroscopically, contrast medium passing through the heart chambers and great vessels.

cineangiography The production of motion picture films of the passage of a radiopaque substance through blood vessels.

cinefluorography The production of motion picture film of fluoroscopic observations.

cinegastroscopy Motion pictures of the interior of the stomach.

cinemicrography The producing of motion picture films through a microscope.

cineradiography The production of motion picture films of sequential images appearing on a fluoroscopic screen. Also called cineroentgenography.

cineroentgenography See cineradiography.

cingulum **1.** A band of association fibers in the brain that partly encircle the corpus callosum. **2.** A U-shaped enamel ridge on the lingual surface of incisor teeth.

cingulumotomy Creation of a precisely placed leukotome lesion in the cingulum of the frontal lobe to relieve intractable pain and emotional anguish.

circa (ca) Latin for approximately.

circadian Denoting the rhythm of biologic phenomena that cycle approximately every 24 hours; e.g., in persons who sleep at night ACTH (and cortisol) secretion begins to rise in the early morning hours, peaks at the time of awakening, and falls to low values in the evening.

circinate Ring-shaped.

circle A ring-shaped anatomic structure.

c. of Willis A circle of anastomosing arteries at the base of the brain. Also called circulus arteriosus.

circuit The path followed by an electric current.

circulation Movement through a circular course, as of the blood through bodily vessels.

collateral c. Circulation of blood taking place through small anastomosing vessels when the main course is obstructed.

coronary c. Circulation taking place through the system of blood vessels supplying the heart muscles.

enterohepatic c. Normal circulation of substances through the liver, into the bile, through the intestines, and back to the liver.

extracorporeal c. Temporary circulation of blood outside the body through a heart-lung machine, artificial kidney, etc.

fetal c. The blood supply to the fetus through the placenta and umbilical cord during intrauterine life.

lymph c. The flow of lymph through lymphatic vessels and glands.

placental c. The flow of blood through the placenta which transfers oxygen and nutritive materials from mother to fetus and carbon dioxide and waste products from fetus to mother.

portal c. Circulation of blood through capillaries in the liver from the portal to the hepatic veins.

pulmonary c. The flow of blood from the heart, through the pulmonary artery and lungs, and back to the heart through the pulmonary veins.

systemic c. General circulation, circulation throughout the whole body.

circulus *pl.* **circuli** Latin for circle.

circumcision The removal of a circular portion of the foreskin or prepuce.

circumduction The circular movement of a part, as of a limb or eye.

circumflex Denoting certain arched anatomic structures.

circumnuclear Surrounding a nucleus.

circumocular Surrounding the eye.

circumoral Around the mouth.

circumscribed Confined within bounds; encircled.

circumvallate Any structure surrounded by a raised ring.

circumvolute Coiled or twisted around a central axis.

cirrhosis A chronic disease of the liver marked by a loss of normal lobular architecture, with nodular regeneration of parenchymal cells separated by fibrous septa, and by vascular derangement and anastomoses; these structural abnormalities interfere with liver function and circulation, and ultimately cause death.

alcoholic c. Variable fatty change of liver cells in small, uniform, regenerative nodules which replace the lobular architecture of the entire liver; each nodule is surrounded by thin septa of connective tissue; the color varies between brown and yellow, determined by the amount of fatty deposition. Also called Laënnec's or portal cirrhosis.

biliary c. Any of several morphologically and etiologically different types of cirrhosis which have in common a long history of extra- or intra-hepatic suppression of bile flow, and an enlarged, firm, finely granular liver with a green hue; extensions of connective tissue septa into the lobular parenchyma are sparse, regenerative nodules are rare.

cardiac c. An extensive centrilobular fibrotic reaction, as in chronic passive hepatic congestion from

coronary circulation

aorta

left coronary a.

circumflex branch

right coronary a.

heart

rginal eries

posterior interventricular branch of right coronary a.

left anterior descending branch of left coronary a.

fetal circulation

ductus arteriosus

placenta

foramen ovale

umbilical v.

ductus venosus

umbilical a.

fetus

placenta

rine v.

maternal venule

placental circulation

umbilical artery

umbilical vein

umbilical cord

rine a.

myometrium of uterus

chorion

amnion

maternal arteriole

villus (contains fetal blood vessels)

ate a.

subchorial space (contains maternal blood)

ver

inferior vena cava

hepatic v.

portal circulation

splenic v.

portal v.

inferior mesenteric v.

superior mesenteric v.

pulmonary trunk

left atrium

pulmonary a.

pulmonary vv.

pulmonary circulation

lung

101

Labels in figure (top left): subclavian vein, thoracic duct, cisterna chyli, intestinal lymphatic trunk, lumbar lymphatic trunk

Labels (center top): lentiform nucleus, coronal section of cerebrum, insula, claustrum, optic chiasm

Labels (center bottom): cisterna, nucleus, plasma cell

Labels (right top): embryo, pharyngeal clefts, foregut, lung buds, trachea, esophagus, axon, presynaptic terminal bulb of axon, synaptic cleft, postsynaptic membrane

any cause.

cryptogenic c. Cirrhosis that often has an unknown cause, but may result from chronic or recurrent viral hepatitis or from autoimmune liver disease.

Laënnec's c. See alcoholic cirrhosis.

portal c. See alcoholic cirrhosis.

postnecrotic c. Cirrhosis caused by massive necrosis involving multiple lobules, with collapse of the reticular framework to form large scars alternating with large nodules of regenerated or residual liver.

primary biliary c. A type marked by fibrosis of bile ducts associated with jaundice, itching, and high levels of blood cholesterol; seen most commonly in females, usually in middle age, and thought to be an autoimmune disorder. Also called Hanot's cirrhosis.

cirrhotic Affected with cirrhosis.

cisplatin Anticancer drug, often used to treat cancer of the testes; major adverse effects include nausea and vomiting.

cisterna Any dilatation or enclosed space serving as a reservoir for lymph or other body fluid.

c. cerebellomedullaris See cisterna magna.

c. chyli The triangular dilatation at the beginning of the thoracic duct, situated in front of the second lumbar vertebra; it receives two lumbar lymphatic trunks and the intestinal lymphatic trunk. Also called receptaculum chyli.

c. magna The large subarachnoid space between the medulla oblongata and the under side of the cerebellum. Also called cisterna cerebellomedullaris.

subarachnoid c. One of several intercommunicating spaces at the base of the brain formed by the separation of the arachnoid from the pia mater.

cisternal Relating to any fluid-containing sac or cavity in the body.

cisternography X-ray examination of the subarachnoid spaces at the base of the brain after infusion of a radiopaque material.

cistron The smallest hereditary unit of function; the section of the DNA molecule that specifies a particular biochemical function.

citrate A salt of citric acid.

citric acid A colorless crystalline acid, $C_6H_8-O_7H_2O$, present in the juice of citrus fruits.

Citrobacter Bacteria (family Enterobacteriaceae) causing infections in debilitated patients.

clamp An instrument used to compress a part.

clap Slang expression for gonorrhea.

clarificant Any agent that clears a turbid liquid.

clasp In dentistry, one of the metal components of a partial denture; consists usually of two tapered retentive arms joined by a supportive body; serves to stabilize the denture.

class A biologic category ranking below a phylum and above an order.

classification A systematic grouping into categories.

Angle's c. A list of the several forms of malocclusion grouped into four main classes.

Duke's c. Classification of the degree of spread of carcinoma of the large bowel: A, confined within bowel; B, spread by direct continuity; no lymph node involvement; C_1, lymphatic invasion adjacent to the tumor and bowel wall; C_2, lymph node involvement at a nearby site; D, distant metastases.

Lancefield's c. The division of streptococci into several categories by means of specific precipitin reactions.

clastic Having a tendency to break or divide.

claudication Limping.

intermittent c. Condition marked by cramplike pains and weakness of legs induced by walking, and the disappearance of all discomfort when at rest; caused by narrowing of the arteries of the legs.

claustrophobia A morbid fear of confined spaces.

claustrum An anatomic structure resembling a barrier, as the thin layer of grey matter on the lateral surface of the external capsule of the brain, separating the insula from the lentiform nucleus.

c. virginale Hymen.

clava The swelling on the back side of the medulla oblongata, which contains the gracile nucleus. Also called gracile tubercle.

clavicle Either of two long, curved bones extending from the sternum to the acromion and forming the anterior half of the shoulder girdle; its medial end articulates with the sternum and the first rib, and is the only bony attachment between the upper extremity and the trunk. Also called collarbone.

clavicotomy Surgical division of a clavicle.

clavus Latin for corn.

clawfoot A disabling deformity of the foot in which the longitudinal arch is extremely high, the toes are clawed, and the forefoot is dropped; it may be congenital or acquired (from polio or diseases of the central nervous system). Also called pes cavus; cavus foot.

clearance 1. Removal of a substance from the blood by an excretory organ such as the kidney, usually expressed in terms of the milliliters of blood that would contain the amount of substance removed per minute; a virtual volume per unit of time; the standard clearance formula is $C = UV/P$: C = clearance in milliliters per minute; U = urine concentration of a substance; P = plasma concentration of the substance; V = urine flow in milliliters per minute. 2. The space existing between apposed structures.

immune c. Clearance of antigen from the blood resulting from complexing with antibodies.

inulin c. The most precise of the commonly used measures of glomerular filtration rate, since inulin is freely filtered but neither secreted nor reabsorbed by the tubules; requires infusion of inulin since this substance occurs naturally only in plants.

occlusal c. In dentistry, condition in which the upper and lower teeth pass one another horizontally without contact or interference.

osmolar c. The volume of blood which would contain the number of osmolar particles excreted by the kidney in one minute.

PAH c. Clearance of para-aminohippurate; an approximate measure of renal plasma flow; when combined with the extraction ratio, a more precise value is obtained.

cleavage 1. The first stages of cell division after the egg is fertilized. 2. The splitting up of a molecule into two or more simpler ones.

cleft A fissure

branchial c. See pharyngeal clefts.

pharyngeal c.'s A series of ectodermal grooves on the surface of an embryo, along the lateral walls of the pharyngeal gut, corresponding to the pharyngeal pouches; they usually appear during the fourth or fifth weeks of development. Also called branchial clefts.

synaptic c. The space, usually 200 to 300 A, between the presynaptic terminal knob and the apposing postsynaptic neuron.

Schmidt-Lantermann c. The funnel-shaped intrusion of cytoplasm in the myelin lamellae around the axon of a nerve cell; thought to play a role in the transport of nutrients through the supporting cell.

clenched fist sign The gesture of a patient with angina pectoris by pressing the chest with a clenched fist.

cleoid A dental carving instrument.

click A sharp sound.

ejection c. A sharp cardiac sound heard in early systole over the area of the aorta or the pulmonary artery when these vessels are dilated.

mitral c. The opening sound of the mitral valve.

systolic c. A sharp cardiac sound heard during systole; a midsystolic click (whether or not followed by a late systolic murmur) often indicates a floppy mitral valve leaflet.

clidal Of or relating to a clavicle.

clidarthritis 1. Gouty pain in the clavicle. 2. Inflammation of the articular portions of the clavicle.

clidocostal Pertaining to the clavicle and ribs.

clidotomy Surgical division of the clavicles of a dead fetus to facilitate its delivery.

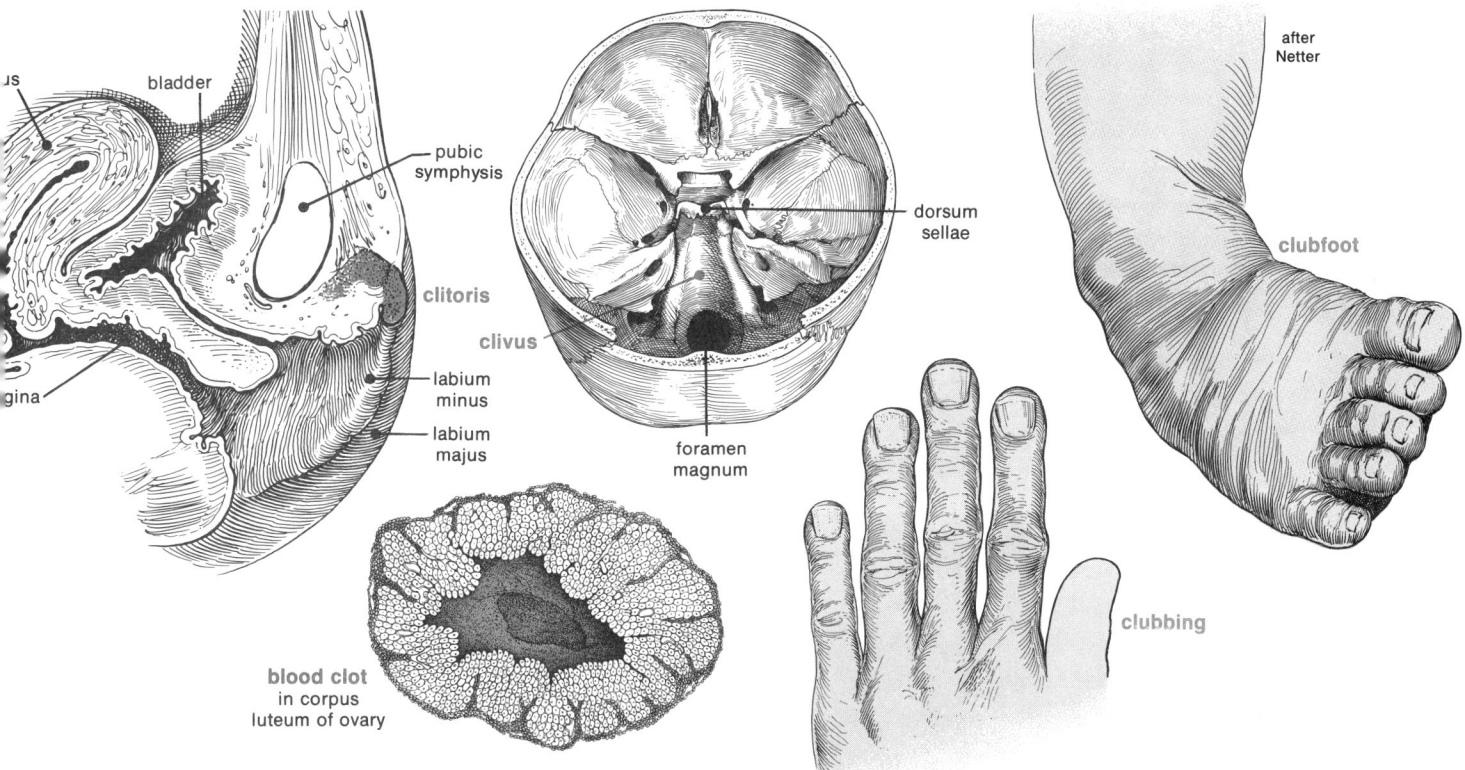

bladder
pubic symphysis
clitoris
clivus
labium minus
labium majus
dorsum sellae
foramen magnum
after Netter
clubfoot
vagina
blood clot in corpus luteum of ovary
clubbing

climacter See climacteric.

climacteric A critical period of life when physiologic changes take place; known as menopause for women and male climacteric for men. Also called climacterium; climacter.

climacterium See climacteric.

climatology The study of climate in relation to health and disease.

climatotherapy Treatment of disease by moving the patient to a suitable climate.

climax 1. The height or crisis of a disease. 2. Orgasm.

clinic 1. An institution where treatment is given to patients not requiring hospitalization. 2. Medical instruction given to students in which patients are examined and treated in their presence. 3. An establishment run by medical specialists working cooperatively.

clinical 1. Relating to the bedside observation of the course and symptoms of a disease. 2. Relating to a clinic.

clinician A practicing physician.

clinicopathologic Relating to the signs and symptoms of a disease and the laboratory study of specimens obtained through biopsy or autopsy.

clinicopathologic conference (CPC) A teaching conference in which the patient's case is discussed following which the pathologic data are presented.

clinocephaly Congenital deformity marked by flatness or concavity of the upper part of the skull. Also called saddle head.

clinodactyly Permanent curvature (lateral or medial) of one or more fingers; usually produced by a shift in alignment of the interphalangeal joint surface; seen most commonly in the little finger.

clinoid Resembling a bed; said of certain anatomic structures, as the clinoid process of the sphenoid bone.

clinoscope Instrument to measure cyclophoria (tendency of one eye to deviate).

clithrophobia Abnormal fear of being locked in.

clitoridectomy Surgical removal of the clitoris.

clitoris A small cylindric organ situated at the anterior part of the vulva, homologous with the penis.

clitorism 1. Prolonged, usually painful, erection of the clitoris. 2. Abnormally large clitoris.

clitoromegaly Enlargement of the clitoris.

clivus The internal slope at the base of the skull, from the front of the foramen magnum to the dorsum sellae, formed by the basilar portion of the occipital bone and the body of the sphenoid bone; it supports the pons and the medulla oblongata.

cloaca 1. The cavity into which the intestinal, urinary, and genital tracts open in certain animals.

2. The combined intestinal and genitourinary opening in the embryo.

clofibrate p-Chlorophenoxyisobutyrate; a lipid-lowering drug used in the treatment of hyperlipidemia; Atromid-S®.

clonal Of or relating to a clone.

clone, clon A colony of genetically identical cells derived from a single cell by asexual division.

clonic Characterized by alternate contraction and relaxation of muscles.

clonicotonic Characterized by rapid alternate contraction and relaxation (clonic) and continued tension (tonic); said of certain muscular spasms.

cloning 1. The developing of a colony of cells from one cell by repeated mitosis; all cells have the same genetic constitution. 2. The transplantation of a somatic cell nucleus into an ovum for the purpose of developing an embryo through asexual reproduction.

clonorchiosis Disease, prevalent in the Far East, caused by invasion of the bile ducts by *Clonorchis sinensis;* transmitted to man by ingestion of raw or undercooked freshwater fish infected with larvae.

Clonorchis A genus of flukes (family Opisthorchiidae) having both sets of sex organs in the same individual, in which self-fertilization often occurs; some species are parasitic in the liver of man.

C. sinensis A species that is the cause of clonorchiosis. Also called Chinese liver fluke.

clonus A spasm in which contraction and relaxation of a muscle alternate in rapid succession.

Clostridium A genus of bacteria (family Bacillaceae) characterized by gram-positive, motile (occasionally nonmotile), anaerobic, or aerotolerant rods; some species produce putrefaction of proteins.

C. bifermentans A species found in putrid meat, gaseous gangrene, and soil; some strains are pathogenic.

C. botulinum A species that produces botulinum toxin, the cause of food poisoning (botulism); there are five types (A to E), each of which elaborates an immunologically distinct form of exotoxin; the toxins of types A, B, and E cause human illness, with type A toxin being responsible for the severest and most common intoxications. Formerly called *Bacillus botulinus*.

C. difficile A cause of diarrhea in humans following treatment with certain antibiotics.

C. haemolyticum A species producing a hemolytic toxin; found in cattle afflicted with icterohemoglobinuria or red-water disease.

C. histolyticum A species found in soil and feces; causes necrosis of tissue; toxic to small laboratory animals. Formerly called *Bacillus histolyticus*.

C. novyi A species producing a powerful exo-

toxin; pathogenic for man and animals; classified into three immunologic types, A, B, and C.

C. perfringens A species consisting of short encapsulated rods; the chief cause of gas gangrene; also the cause of enterotoxemia in cattle, sheep, and man; found in soil and milk. Also called *Clostridium welchii;* gas bacillus. Formerly called Welch's bacillus.

C. septicum A species producing a lethal and hemolytic exotoxin; found in the intestines and in manured soil.

C. tetani A species consisting of motile rods with a drumstick shape, producing an exotoxin with affinity for motor nerve centers; the cause of tetanus or lockjaw; found in soil and wounds. Formerly called *Bacillus tetani*.

C. welchii See *Clostridium perfringens*.

closure 1. The act of closing or the state of being closed. 2. The conclusion of a reflex pathway.

clot 1. A thrombus. 2. To coagulate.

blood c. A solidified elastic mass of fibrin enmeshing platelets, red blood cells, and white blood cells; produced when whole blood coagulates.

clubbing Broadening and thickening of the soft tissues of the ends of fingers or toes, associated with a variety of chronic pulmonary conditions.

clubfoot One of the most common congenital deformities of the foot in which only the outer portion of the ball of the foot touches the ground; the ankle is plantar flexed, the foot is inverted, and the anterior half of the foot is directed toward the midline. Also called talipes equinovarus.

clump 1. To aggregate; to form a cluster. 2. A mass so formed.

clumping The clustering of bacteria or other cells suspended in a liquid.

clysis Infusion of fluid into the body.

coagglutinin A substance that causes agglutination of antigen only in the presence of univalent antibody; by itself it does not cause agglutination.

coagulable Capable of clotting.

coagulant 1. Causing coagulation or clotting. 2. A substance that causes clotting.

coagulase In microbiology, an extracellular enzyme or complex that promotes plasma coagulation and is clinically associated with disease production.

coagulate 1. To cause the conversion of a fluid into a semisolid mass. 2. To become such a mass.

coagulation 1. Clotting; the conversion of a fluid into a jellylike solid. 2. A clot.

coagulative Causing coagulation.

coagulin An antibody that causes coagulation of its antigen.

coagulopathy A disease affecting the blood-clotting process.

coarctation — aorta

Coccidioides

single

double

cuboid

cocci

cluster

sheet
(one cell
thick)

chain

cochlea

cocaine

consumption c. Condition marked by great reduction in the circulating levels of platelets and of certain coagulation factors; due to utilization of platelets in excessive blood clotting throughout the body.

coagulum *pl.* **coagula** A clot; a curd.

coaptation The fitting together of parts, as the ends of a broken bone.

coarct To press together; to constrict.

coarctation A narrowing or constriction, as of a blood vessel.

coat A membrane or a layer of tissue.

buffy c. 1. A light yellowish layer of platelets and white blood cells covering the packed red cells of centrifuged blood. **2.** A layer of similar composition, plus fibrin, that covers the blood clot when coagulation is delayed so that red cells have time to settle.

cobalamin A general term for a member of the vitamin B$_{12}$ group.

cobalt A hard, brittle, steel-gray metallic element; symbol Co, atomic number 27, atomic weight 58.94; cobalt ingestion has been associated with cardiomyopathy.

cobalt-60 A radioactive isotope of cobalt, used in radiotherapy.

cobralysin The substance in cobra venom that destroys red blood cells.

coca A tree, *Erythroxylon coca,* with leaves that contain cocaine and other alkaloids.

cocaine A crystalline narcotic alkaloid, colorless or white, extracted from coca leaves; used as a local anesthetic. Also called coke or snow (street expression).

cocainism The habitual use of cocaine.

cocainize To anesthetize by the administration of cocaine.

cocarboxylase See thiamine pyrophosphate.

cocarcinogen An agent that increases the activity of a carcinogen.

cocci Plural of coccus.

Coccidia An order of protozoans, some of which are pathogenic and parasitic in the epithelium of the small intestine.

Coccidioides A genus of zygomycetous fungi, some of which are parasitic in man.

C. immitis A species of fungi causing coccidioimycosis. Also called *Blastomyces coccidioides.*

coccidioidomycosis A disease caused by the fungus *Coccidioides immitis,* affecting primarily the lungs; it is frequently asymptomatic and rarely disseminated; the disease is endemic in desert areas of the United States; one form is known as desert or San Joaquin Valley fever.

coccidiosis Disease of certain vertebrates caused by any protozoans of the order Coccidia; in man,

the infection is self-limiting and accompanied by nausea and diarrhea.

coccobacillus An oval-shaped microorganism.

coccoid Resembling a spherical bacterium (coccus).

coccus *pl.* **cocci** A bacterium of round or oval shape.

coccyalgia See coccydynia.

coccydynia Pain in the coccygeal region, frequently caused by a fall upon the buttocks. Also called coccygodynia; coccyalgia.

coccygeal Relating to or located in the proximity of the coccyx.

coccygectomy Surgical removal of the coccyx.

coccygodynia See coccydynia.

coccyx *pl.* **coccyges** Three or four small, fused, rudimentary vertebrae that form the caudal extremity of the vertebral column.

cochlea The spiral cavity in the internal ear; the essential organ of hearing containing the membranous cochlear duct in which the spiral organ of Corti with its nerve endings is located.

cochlear Of or relating to the cochlea.

cochleare magnum (coch. mag.) Latin for tablespoon.

cochleovestibular Relating to the cochlea and the vestibule of the ear.

cochlitis Inflammation of the cochlea.

code 1. A systematic collection of rules. **2.** A system of symbols used for transmitting information.

genetic c. The pattern of three adjacent nucleotides in a DNA molecule that controls protein synthesis.

codecarboxylase A coenzyme of various amino acid decarboxylases. Also called pyridoxal phosphate.

codehydrogenase I See nicotinamide adenine dinucleotide.

codehydrogenase II See nicotinamide adenine dinucleotide phosphate.

codeine A white, crystalline narcotic alkaloid obtained from opium or morphine, used for the relief of cough and as an analgesic.

codon The group of three adjacent nucleotides that codes the insertion of one specific amino acid during protein synthesis; usually expressed in mRNA equivalents, e.g., GAG (guanine-adenine-guanine) for glutamic acid rather than CTC (cytosine-thymine-cytosine).

coefficient A numerical measure of the effect or change produced by variations of specified conditions, or of the ratio between two quantities.

c. of absorption 1. The milliliters of a gas that will saturate 100 ml of liquid, at standard temperature and pressure. **2.** In radiology, the constant for

radiation of a given wavelength, the value of which depends on the atomic number of the substance through which the radiation passes.

c. of relationship The probability that two persons with a common ancestor have a common gene that came from that ancestor.

correlation c. A measure of the closeness of the relationships between variables; a value of 1 represents perfect correlation and 0 represents no relationship; the sign of the correlation coefficient is positive when the variables move in the same direction (height vs. weight) and negative when they move in opposite directions (life expectancy vs. weight).

distribution c. The constant ratio in which a substance, soluble in two immiscible solvents, distributes itself in equilibrium between the two solvents; the basis of many chromatographic separation procedures. Also called partition coefficient.

filtration c. The volume of fluid passed in unit time through a unit area of membrane per unit pressure difference.

partition c. See distribution coefficient.

phenol c. See Rideal-Walker coefficient.

Poisseuille's viscosity c. The ratio of the shearing force per unit area between two parallel layers of a liquid in motion, to the velocity gradient between the layers; a numerical measure of the viscosity as determined by the capillary tube method; usually symbolized by η.

Rideal-Walker c. The ratio of bactericidal effectiveness of a germicide compared to that of phenol as a standard; the disinfecting power of the substance is obtained by dividing the figure indicating the degree of dilution of the germicide that destroys a microorganism in a given time by that indicating the degree of dilution of phenol which destroys the same organism in the same time under the same conditions. Also called phenol coefficient.

temperature c. The fractional change in any physical property per degree rise in temperature.

coelom Celom.

coenzyme A nonprotein organic compound, produced by living cells, which plays an intimate and frequently essential role in the activation of enzymes; e.g., thiamine, riboflavin.

c. III (ColII) A nucleotide containing nicotinamide which functions in oxidation of cysteine.

c. A (CoA) The "active" acetate.

coeur French for heart.

c. en sabot The characteristic x-ray appearance of the heart in tetralogy of Fallot; it vaguely resembles a wooden shoe.

cofactor A substance that is essential to bring about the action of an enzyme.

cognition 1. The intellectual process by which

colchicine

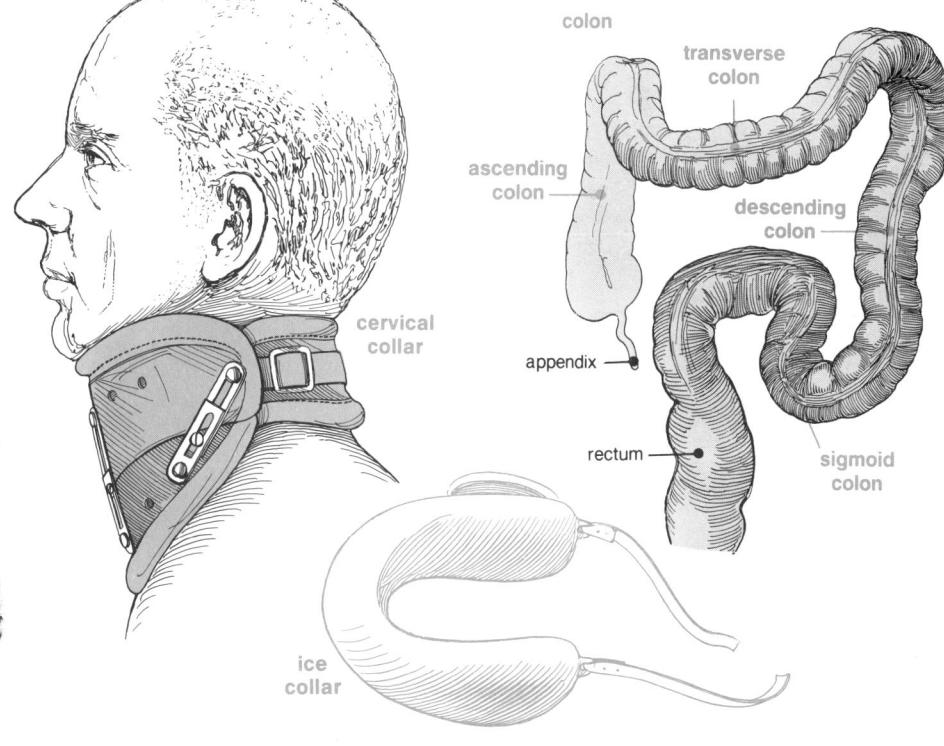

colon

transverse colon

ascending colon

descending colon

appendix

rectum

sigmoid colon

cervical collar

ice collar

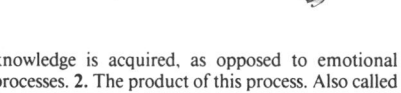

collagen

knowledge is acquired, as opposed to emotional processes. **2.** The product of this process. Also called comprehension; judgment; perception.

cohesion The mutual attraction by which the molecules of a substance are held together.

cohort In epidemiology, a group of persons who share a designated characteristic and who are traced over an extended period of time.

coin-counting A sliding movement of the tips of thumb and index finger against each other, occurring in paralysis agitans.

coition Coitus.

coitus Copulation; sexual intercourse.

  c. interruptus Sexual intercourse intentionally interrupted by withdrawal immediately prior to ejaculation. Also called interrupted or incomplete coitus.

cola See kola.

colchicine An alkaloid obtained from colchicum; used in the treatment of acute gout.

cold The common cold, a symptom complex due to a viral infection of the respiratory tract; marked by nasal discharge, sneezing, some malaise, and usually without fever.

  chest c. Bronchitis.

  head c. Acute rhinitis.

colectomy Surgical removal of the colon, or a segment of it.

colibacilluria The presence of *Escherichia coli* in a urine specimen that has been aseptically obtained. Also called coliuria.

colic **1.** Relating to the colon. **2.** Acute abdominal pain. **3.** A symptom complex seen in infants under three months of age, characterized by paroxysmal abdominal pain and frantic crying.

  biliary c. Severe pain caused by the passage of a gallstone through the bile duct.

  intestinal c. More or less severe pain caused by spasm of smooth muscle, as in gallstones, appendicitis, lead poisoning, or air-swallowing.

  lead c. Abdominal pain caused by lead poisoning.

  renal c. Pain caused by the impaction or passage of a stone along the ureter or renal pelvis.

  ureteral c. Severe pains caused by obstruction of the ureter.

coliform Resembling the colon bacillus (*Escherichia coli*).

colitis Inflammation of the colon.

  granulomatous c. A disease of the colon which produces lesions involving all layers, resembling the changes produced in the ileum by regional enteritis (inflammation of the intestine).

  mucous c. Irritable colon; see under colon.

  pseudomembranous c. See enterocolitis, pseu-

domembranous.

  spastic c. Irritable colon; see under colon.

  ulcerative c. A chronic disease of unknown cause marked by ulceration of the mucosa and submucosa of the colon with bleeding and malnutrition.

coliuria See colibacilluria.

collagen The supportive protein component of connective tissue, bone, cartilage, and skin; converted into gelatin by boiling.

collagenase An enzyme that promotes the breakdown of collagen.

collagen diseases A group of diseases having in common such histologic features as inflammatory damage to connective tissues and blood vessels with deposition of fibrinoid material; included in this group are such disorders as systemic lupus erythematosus, polyarteritis nodosa, dermatomyositis, scleroderma, and rheumatoid arthritis. Also called connective tissue diseases.

collagenosis Collagen diseases.

collapse **1.** A state of extreme prostration. **2.** The act of caving in.

collar **1.** A band or device, usually one encircling the neck. **2.** An encircling anatomic structure.

  cervical c. A device generally used to support, stabilize, immobilize, or hyperextend the neck in cases where a rigid cast or bracing is not indicated.

  ice c. A rubber bag designed to be filled with crushed ice and placed on the neck to produce cooling, as in postoperative care of tonsillectomies.

collarbone See clavicle.

collateral Secondary, auxiliary, or alternate.

colliculus *pl.* **colliculi** A small elevation, as in the roof of the midbrain.

colligative In physical chemistry, denotes dependence on the number of particles (molecules, atoms, or ions) present in a given space, rather than on their nature; applied to solutions.

collimation The controlling of the size of x-ray beam spread by use of lead plates placed in front of the primary roentgen ray beam.

collimator An apparatus, often consisting of a pair of lead plates, used to confine a beam of radiation within a specific area.

colliquation The degeneration of tissue with subsequent conversion into a liquid-like form (liquefaction).

  ballooning c. Liquefaction of the cell protoplasm leading to edematous swelling and softening. Also called ballooning degeneration.

colliquative **1.** Denoting an excessive watery discharge. **2.** Characterized by liquefaction of tissues.

collodion A colorless, flammable, syrupy solution of pyroxylin or gum cotton in ether and alcohol; used as a protective coat for cuts and surgical dress-

ings and as a support film on copper grids in election microscopy. Also called collodium.

collodium See collodion.

colloid **1.** A gluelike substance, such as gelatin, consisting of a suspension of submicroscopic particles in a continuous medium. **2.** A yellowish gelatinous material present in the tissues as a result of colloid degeneration.

collum **1.** Latin for neck. **2.** Any necklike structure.

  c. anatomicum humeri A narrow groove separating the head of the humerus from its tubercles; it affords attachment to the capsular ligament of the shoulder-joint. Also called anatomic neck of the humerus.

  c. chirurgicum humeri The constriction below the tubercles of the humerus; a frequent site of fractures. Also called surgical neck of the humerus.

  c. femoris A more or less conical portion of bone separating the head and shaft of the femur. Also called neck of femur.

  c. tali A constriction separating the head from the body of the ankle bone (talus). Also called neck of talus.

coloboma Any defect in which a portion of a structure, especially of the eye, is absent; it may be congenital, pathologic, or artificial.

colocolic Denoting a surgical joining of one part of the colon to another.

cololysis Freeing the colon from adhesions.

colon Portion of the large intestine extending from the cecum to the rectum.

  ascending c. The part of the colon extending upward on the right side of the abdomen from the cecum to the hepatic flexure.

  descending c. The part of the colon extending downward on the left side of the abdomen from the splenic flexure to the sigmoid colon.

  irritable c. (IC) A condition marked by abdominal pain, gas, constipation or diarrhea, and the passage of mucus; it usually starts in adolescence or early adult life, and the attacks frequently coincide with emotional stress. Also called irritable bowel syndrome; spastic or mucous colitis; spastic colon.

  lead pipe c. A term applied to the radiologic appearance of a scarred, contracted, and rigid colon, usually the consequence of advanced ulcerative colitis.

  sigmoid c. The S-shaped part of the colon in the pelvis between the descending colon and rectum.

  spastic c. See irritable colon.

  transverse c. The portion of the colon which crosses the abdomen from the hepatic flexure to the splenic flexure.

colonic Of or relating to the colon.

colonization **1.** Innidiation; metastasis. **2.** The act

colony
Trichophyton
mentagrophytes

colostomy

colon

vertebral
column
(adult)
cervical
vertebrae
(7)

thoracic
vertebrae
(12)

lumbar
vertebrae
(5)

sacral
vertebrae
(5)

coccygeal
vertebrae
(4)

cervix

colpomicroscope

of forming compact groups or colonies, e.g., the developing of colonies of the same type of microorganisms, or grouping and caring for individuals with a common disease such as leprosy.

colonorrhagia See colorrhagia.

colonorrhea See colorrhea

colonoscopy Examination of the upper portion of the rectum with an endoscope.

colony A visible group or growth of microorganisms on a solid medium, presumably arising from a single microorganism.

M-type c., mucoid c. A usually virulent colony marked by a well developed carbohydrate capsule which may act as a defense mechanism.

R-type c., rough c. A nonvirulent or slightly virulent colony having a granular growth, irregular margins, and flat surface.

S-type c., smooth c. A colony presenting a round, even, smooth surface; some capsule-forming species have a degree of virulence.

colopexy, colopexia Shortening of an elongated gastrocolic omentum by means of sutures to support a prolapsed transverse colon; procedure is also used in the correction of a prolapsed stomach.

coloproctitis Inflammation of the colon and rectum. Also called proctocolitis; rectocolitis.

color A visual perception characterized by the attributes of brightness, hue, and saturation, arising from stimulation of the retina by light.

complementary c.'s 1. Two colors in which the direct perception of one produces an afterimage of the other. **2.** Two primary colors which, when mixed, produce light gray or white.

monochromatic c. See pure color.

primary c.'s A set of three colors (red, blue, and yellow) from which all other colors can be produced by mixing.

pure c. Color produced by one wavelength. Also called monochromatic color.

color blindness See under blindness.

colorectal Relating to the colon and rectum.

colorimetry 1. The quantitative analysis of color, either in terms of hue, saturation, and brightness, or by comparison with known standards. **2.** The quantitative chemical analysis of a solution by color comparison with a standard solution.

colorrhagia Abnormal discharge from the colon. Also called colonorrhagia

colorrhea Diarrhea thought to originate in the colon. Also called colonorrhea.

colostomy Surgical establishment of a permanent opening into the colon through the abdominal wall.

colostrorrhea A copious secretion of colostrum (first milk secreted at the end of pregnancy).

colostrum A thin, sticky secretion of the breasts

occurring a few days before and after childbirth. Also called foremilk.

colotomy Incision of the colon.

colpalgia Pain in the vagina.

colpatresia Occlusion of the vagina.

colpectomy Surgical removal of the vagina.

colpitis Vaginitis.

c. emphysematosa Emphysematous vaginitis; see under vaginitis.

c. mycotica Mycotic vaginitis; see under vaginitis.

colpocele 1. A hernia into the vagina. Also called vaginocele; elytrocele. **2.** Colpoptosis.

colpocleisis Surgical closure of the vaginal lumen.

colpocystocele Prolapse of the bladder into the vagina.

colpodynia Neuralgic vaginal pain. Also called vaginodynia.

colpohysterectomy Removal of the uterus through the vagina.

colpohysterotomy Incision into the uterus through the vagina.

colpomicroscope A high-powered microscope with a built-in light source for direct visual examination of a stained cervix; it facilitates a histologic diagnosis in vivo.

colpomicroscopy Examination of cells of the cervix and vagina in situ with the aid of a colpomicroscope.

colpoperineorrhaphy Surgical repair of an injured vagina and torn perineum. Also called vaginoperineorraphy.

colpopexy Suture of a prolapsed vagina to the abdominal wall. Also called vaginofixation.

colpoplasty Reparative surgery of the vagina. Also called vaginoplasty.

colpopoiesis Surgical construction of an artificial vagina.

colpoptosis, colpoptosia Prolapse of the walls of the vagina.

colporrhaphy Surgical repair of a tear in the vagina.

colporrhexis The partial or total tearing loose of the uterine cervix from its vaginal attachment; an uncommon injury occurring during childbirth.

colposcope A low-powered microscope with a built-in light source for direct visual inspection of the uterine cervix and vagina. Also called vaginoscope.

colposcopy Examination of the uterine cervix and vagina by means of a colposcope.

colpospasm Spasm of the vaginal wall.

colpostenosis Narrowing of the vagina.

colpotomy Incision through the vaginal wall, usu-

ally for the purpose of draining a pelvic abscess.

colpoxerosis Abnormal dryness of the vaginal mucosa.

columbium An element, symbol Cb, now known as niobium.

columella 1. A small column. **2.** The lower portion of the nasal septum.

column A pillar-shaped anatomic structure.

anterior c. The anterior (ventral) portion of the gray matter on either side of the spinal cord.

enamel c. One of the groups of fibers which make up the tooth enamel.

lateral c. The portion of gray matter of the spinal cord, extending between the anterior and posterior columns; present only in the thoracic and upper lumbar regions.

posterior c. The posterior (dorsal) portion of the gray matter on either side of the spinal cord.

spinal c. See vertebral column.

vertebral c. The columnar arrangement of vertebrae, from the skull through the coccyx, which encloses and supports the spinal cord. Also called spinal column; backbone; spine.

coma A state in which psychologic and motor responses to stimulation are impaired.

deep c. Coma in which responses are completely lost.

diabetic c. Coma due to ketoacidosis caused by uncontrolled diabetes mellitus; symptoms leading to coma progress slowly (few days in adults, 12 to 14 hours in juveniles) and include dry mouth, thirst, and excessive urination, followed usually by nausea, vomiting, and abdominal pain; those immediately preceding the coma may be labored breathing, flushed complexion, and drowsiness.

hepatic c. Coma occurring in the terminal stages of cirrhosis of the liver, hepatitis, or other liver diseases; may be preceded by mental confusion, flapping tremor, or jaundice.

hyperosmolar nonketotic c. Diabetic coma without increased ketone bodies; caused by the dehydrating effect on brain cells of the hyperosmolarity of marked hyperglycemia.

moderately deep c. Coma in which only rudimentary responses of a reflex nature are present; e.g., corneal reflex.

comatose In a condition of coma.

combustion Burning; oxidation or other chemical change accompanied by the production of heat and light.

heat of c. See under heat.

comedo *pl.* **comedones** A plug of dried sebaceous material retained in the orifice of a hair follicle. Commonly called blackhead.

comedocarcinoma Carcinoma of the breast fill-anterior commissure of brain

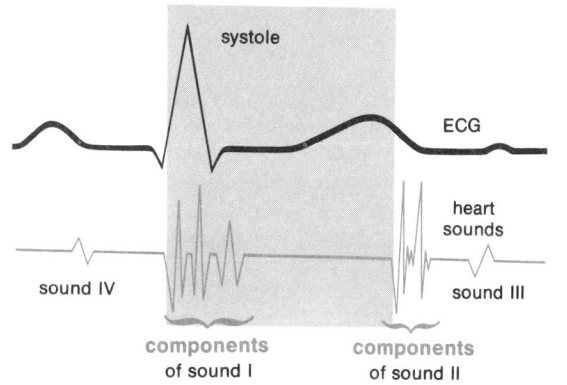

systole
ECG
sound IV
sound III
heart sounds
components of sound I
components of sound II

compound F
(hydrocortisone)

atrial complex   ventricular complex

G

composition of living cells (major elements)

element	O	C	H	N	Ca	P	K	Total
composition by weight (%)	65	18	10	3	1.5	1.0	0.35	98.85

ing the ducts with a necrotic cheesy material that can be extruded with slight pressure.

comes *pl.* **comites** A companion blood vessel of another vessel or nerve.

commensal Denoting two non-parasitic organisms that live together, one benefiting from the association while the other is neither benefited nor harmed.

comminuted Denoting a bone broken into several fragments.

comminution The process of breaking into small pieces.

commissure 1. Joining together; in the brain or spinal cord, bundles of nerve fibers crossing the midline from side to side. 2. A line formed by the junction of two bones in the skull. 3. The angle or corner of the eye, the lips, or the labia.

anterior c. of brain A bundle of white fibers crossing the midline in front of the third ventricle.

posterior c. of brain A bundle of white fibers crossing the midline posterior to the third ventricle, at its junction with the cerebral aqueduct.

commissurotomy Surgical division of the bands of a commissure.

mitral c. Surgical division of the fibrous band of the mitral valve in the heart to relieve mitral stenosis.

commitment The legal placing of a person in a mental hospital or any other protective custody.

communicable Capable of being transmitted or communicated; denoting the ease with which infection is transmitted from one person to another.

communicans Denoting a nerve that connects two others.

compatible 1. In pharmacology, denoting two or more substances that are capable of being mixed without undergoing undesirable chemical changes or loss of therapeutic properties. 2. Describing two samples of blood in which the serum of each does not agglutinate the red blood cells of the other; blood that causes no reaction when transfused.

compartment syndrome Injury occurring during exercise due to expansion and compression of a muscle group within its confined fascial space.

compensation 1. The act of offsetting a functional or structural defect. 2. A defense mechanism in which the individual, consciously or unconsciously, strives to make up for real or imagined deficiencies.

compensatory Serving to counterbalance or make up for.

competence 1. The closure of a heart valve so as to prevent leakage from one chamber to another. Also called integrity. 2. The quality or condition of being capable; especially, capable of normal adult

function and rational decision making. 3. The ability of a group of embryonic cells to react to a given morphogenic stimulus with resulting differentiation.

competition Process by which one substance inhibits the action of another, structurally similar, substance.

complaint An expression of pain or discomfort.

chief c. The symptom reported by the patient as responsible for his seeking medical attention.

complement (C) A multifactorial immune system consisting of 11 serologically nonspecific proteins present in fresh normal serum that are necessary for the destruction of cellular antigens in the presence of antibody.

complex 1. A group of interrelated parts or factors. 2. In psychiatry, a group of associated ideas (largely unconscious), having a strong emotional tone and influencing the personality. 3. In electrocardiography, a group of deflections corresponding to a base in the cardiac cycle.

atrial c. The P wave in the electrocardiogram.

brain wave c. A combination of fast and slow electrical activities of the brain.

castration c. See anxiety, castration.

Eisenmenger's c. Congenital heart condition consisting of a ventricular septal defect with pulmonary hypertension, resulting in right-to-left shunt through the defect; it may or may not be associated with overriding aorta.

immune c. A complex composed of antibody linked to antigen.

inferiority c. Feelings of inferiority due to real or imagined physical or social inadequacies; may be manifested by extreme shyness or timidity or by overcompensation through excessive ambition or aggressiveness.

major histocompatibility c. (MHC) The linked gene loci (on chromosome 6) coding for cell proteins that determine tissue type and transplant compatibility.

membrane attack c. The complex of complement components C5 through C9 that creates a hole in the membrane of cells or bacteria.

Oedipus c. The strong attachment and desire that a child (usually between the ages of three and six) develops for the parent of the opposite sex; the feelings are largely repressed because of fear of punishment by the parent of the same sex, who is regarded as a rival; resolution centers on identification with the same sex parent.

QRS c. An electrocardiographic display of ventricular contraction.

spike and wave c. In electroencephalography, a complex consisting of a dart and dome wave, usually seen in petit mal seizures.

superiority c. Exaggerated aggressiveness, an overcompensation for feelings of inferiority.

ventricular c. The QRS wave in the electrocardiogram.

vitamin B c. A group of water-soluble compounds found together in foodstuffs; some are believed to be chiefly concerned with release of energy from food (e.g., nicotinamide, riboflavin, thiamine, and biotin), others with the formation of red blood cells (e.g., vitamin B_{12} and folic acid).

complexion The appearance and general condition of the skin.

compliance The quality of yielding; the tendency of a hollow organ (e.g., the bladder) to distend.

lung c. Change of volume per change of pressure, an index of the mechanical properties of the lung.

component A constituent part.

composition 1. The act of combining parts or elements to form a whole. 2. In chemistry, the group of atoms that forms the molecule of a substance.

compos mentis Latin term meaning of sound mind.

compound 1. A substance consisting of two or more chemical elements or parts in union. 2. In pharmacy, a preparation containing a mixture of drugs. 3. In dentistry, a molding or impression material that softens when heated and solidifies without chemical change when cooled. 4. To prepare a pharmaceutical mixture.

acyclic c., aliphatic c. See open chain compound.

aromatic c. A cyclic compound with conjugated double bonds within the ring; e.g., benzene.

azo c. An organic compound containing the azo ($-N=N-$) group. Also called diazo compound.

binary c. A compound whose molecule is composed of two elements or atoms of different kinds; e.g., HCl.

closed chain c. See cyclic compound.

c. A The adrenal hormone, 11-dehydrocorticosterone.

c. B The adrenal hormone, corticosterone.

c. E The adrenal hormone, cortisone.

c. F The adrenal hormone, hydrocortisone. Also called cortisol.

c. S The adrenal hormone 11-deoxycortisol.

cyclic c. Any organic compound that has atoms linked together in the form of a ring. Also called closed chain compound.

endothermic c. A compound whose formation involves the absorption of heat.

exothermic c. A compound whose formation involves the emission of heat.

heterocyclic c. An organic compound that contains rings composed of dissimilar elements.

impression c., modeling c. One used to secure

ring compound

helix

concha of auricle

tragus

superior nasal concha

middle nasal concha

compression of bladder by anteflexed uterus

inferior nasal concha

light microscope

phase microscope

electron microscope

condensers

✳ specimen

an imprint of negative likeness of oral tissues.

inorganic c. Any compound that does not contain carbon.

modeling c. See impression compound.

nonpolar c. One composed of molecules possessing asymmetrical distribution of charge so that no positive or negative poles exist; e.g., hydrocarbons.

open chain c. An organic compound in which the carbon atoms are linked in a linear fashion. Also called acyclic, aliphatic, paraffin, or fatty compound.

organic c. Any compound containing carbon.

quaternary c. One that contains four elements.

ring c.'s A group of compounds in which the molecules are structured in such a way that the ends of the chain of carbon atoms are linked together in a closed ring.

saturated c. A compound in which all the atoms of the molecules are united by single bonds.

substitution c. A compound formed when elements of a molecule are replaced by other elements or radicals.

ternary c., tertiary c. A compound whose molecules contain three elements.

tray c. An impression-like compound which is more viscous when soft and more rigid when cooled.

unsaturated c. An organic compound containing C=C or C≡C combinations, capable of becoming saturated by the addition of other atoms.

compress A pad of gauze or other soft material used as a dressing or applied to a part of the body where localized pressure is necessary.

graduated c. A compress made of several layers of cloth gradually increasing in number so that it is thickest in the center.

wet c. A compress moistened with an antiseptic solution or with hot or cold water.

compression Pressing together.

cerebral c. Pressure on the brain by tumor, hemorrhage, depressed fracture of the skull, etc.

digital c. Pressure applied with the fingers over a blood vessel to check bleeding.

external cardiac c. Closed chest massage; see under massage.

compression molding In dentistry, the pressing of a plastic material to the negative form of a mold.

compression syndrome See crush syndrome.

Compton effect See effect, Compton.

compulsion An irresistible urge to do something contrary to the person's wishes or standards.

conation The volitional aspect of behavior which includes impulse, drive, and purposive striving; one of three elements of behavior, the other two being cognition (thinking) and affect (feeling).

concameration A series of connecting cavities.

concatenate Connected in a chainlike series.

concave Having a hollowed surface.

concavity A depression.

concavoconvex 1. Concave on one side and convex on the opposite. 2. Denoting a lens with greater concave than convex curvature.

concentration 1. The quantity of a specified substance in a unit amount of another substance. 2. A preparation that has had its strength increased by evaporation.

maximum permissible c. (MPC) The quantity of radiation considered to be relatively safe.

concentric Having a common center.

conception 1. The act of forming an idea. 2. The fertilization of an ovum or the act of becoming pregnant.

conceptus The product of conception. Also called embryo.

concha *pl.* **conchae** A shell-shaped structure such as the external ear or a turbinated bone in the nose.

bony inferior nasal c. A thin, spongy, curved bony plate forming the lower part of the lateral wall of the nasal cavity; it articulates with the ethmoid, maxilla, palatine, and lacrimal bones. Also called inferior turbinate bone.

bony superior nasal c. The upper and smaller of the two curved bony plates projecting from the inner wall of the ethmoid in the nasal cavity. Also called superior turbinate bone.

c. of auricle The large shell-shaped hollow of the external ear, between the tragus and antihelix.

c. bullosa Distention of the nasal conchae, especially of the middle one; seen in some cases of chronic rhinitis.

inferior nasal c. The bony inferior nasal concha and its overlying mucous membrane.

middle nasal c. The bony middle nasal concha and its overlying mucous membrane.

sphenoidal c. A thin curved bony plate forming part of the roof of the nasal cavity. Also called sphenoturbinal bone.

superior nasal c. The bony superior nasal concha and its overlying mucous membrane.

conchoidal Shell-like in shape.

concrement Concretion.

concrescence The growing together of normally separate parts, as the roots of a tooth.

concretion An aggregation of solid material; a calculus.

concussion 1. A violent jarring or shaking of a part of the body, as caused by a fall or a blow. 2. The morbid condition resulting from such a jarring.

brain c. The immediate and temporary disturbance of brain function as manifested by dizziness, cold perspiration, visual disturbances, and loss of consciousness.

condensation 1. The act of making more compact. 2. The changing of a gas to a liquid or a liquid to a solid. 3. In psychoanalysis, the representation of several ideas by a single dream-image or symbol. 4. In dentistry, compaction.

condense To compress, such as the restorative material into the prepared cavity of a tooth.

condenser 1. A device for cooling a gas to a liquid, or a liquid to a solid. 2. A dental instrument designed to compress restorative material into the prepared cavity of a tooth. 3. A simple or compound lens used to gather light rays and focus them on an object to be illuminated.

achromatic c. A condenser used in a microscope for bright field work and corrected for both spherical aberration and chromatic aberration.

dark-field c. An optical system used in microscopes, by means of which light is collected and directed upon the specimen while the remainder of the field is dark.

phase contrast c. A condenser that transmits light through rings so as to work in conjunction with a phase-altering pattern in the objective.

substage c. A lens or group of lenses that converges the illuminating beam for proper passage of light through the microscope.

condition In psychology, to train to respond to a specific stimulus in a specific way.

conditioning The process of training an individual or organism to respond to a specific stimulus in a specific way, usually by simultaneous presentation of unrelated stimuli one of which evokes the desired response.

instrumental c. See operant conditioning.

operant c., instrumental c. The procedure whereby a stimulus, once having evoked a response that produces a reward (or removes or prevents a punishment), is thereafter more likely to evoke that response.

physical c. An improvement in strength or efficiency of muscular performance by exercise.

condom A sheath, usually made of thin rubber, used to cover the penis during sexual intercourse to prevent conception or infection.

conductance A measure of the readiness with which a substance allows an electric charge to pass through it.

conduction The transmitting of energy (heat, electricity, etc.) or nerve stimuli from one point to another.

aberrant ventricular c. Abnormal spread of a supraventricular impulse in the ventricle, caused by delayed activation of one of the branches of the atrioventricular (His) bundle. Also called ventricular

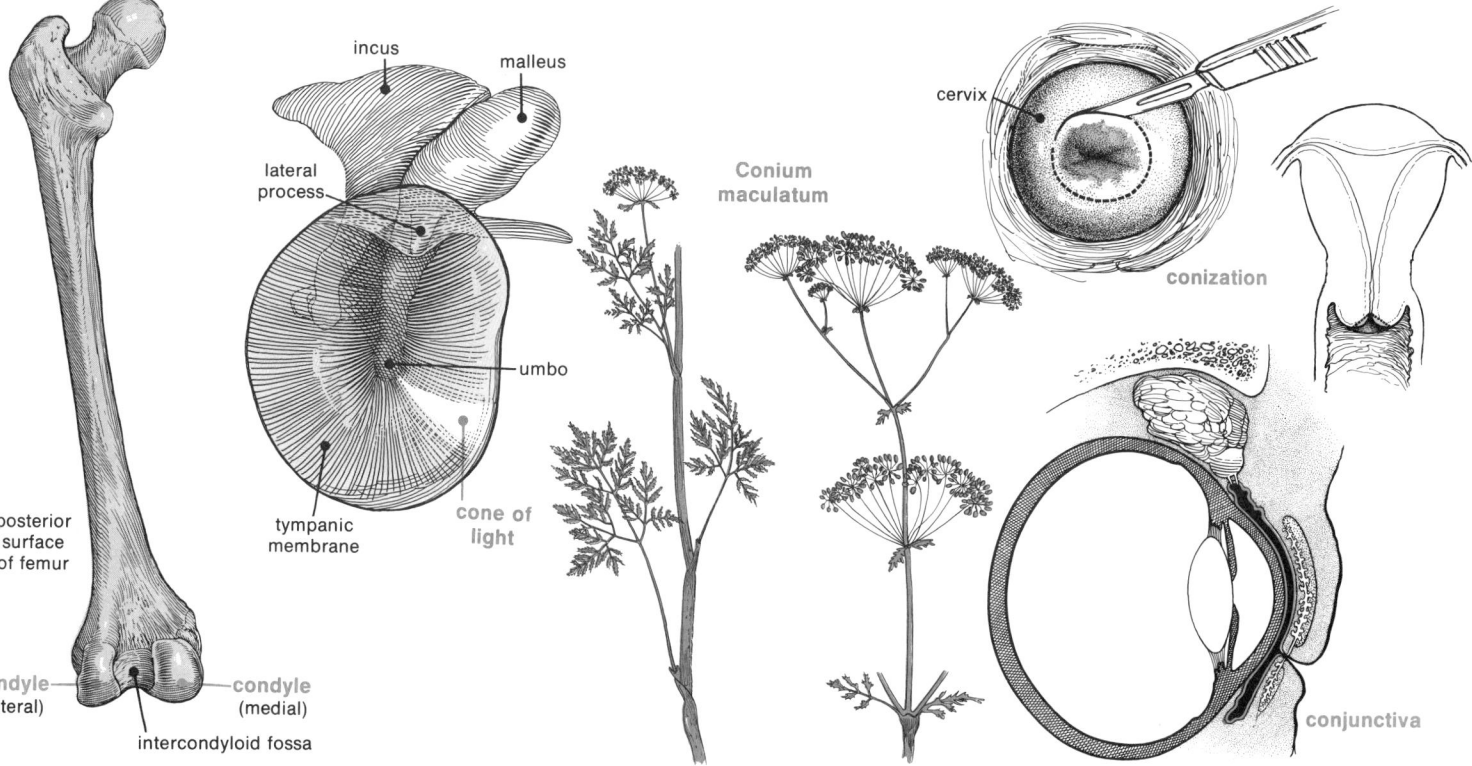

posterior surface of femur

incus

malleus

lateral process

umbo

cone of light

tympanic membrane

condyle (lateral)

condyle (medial)

intercondyloid fossa

Conium maculatum

cervix

conization

conjunctiva

aberration.

accelerated c. The partial or complete bypass of the normal conduction pathways by the sinus impulse, resulting in early activation of the ventricular muscle.

air c. Transmission of sound to the internal ear through the external auditory canal and the middle ear.

bone c. Transmission of sound to the internal ear through the bones of the skull.

concealed c. Partial transmission of an impulse through the A-V junction, which depolarizes only a portion of the junction, thus causing abnormal conduction of the next impulse.

delayed c. First degree atrioventricular (A-V) heart block. See under block.

intraventricular c. Conduction of the cardiac impulse through the ventricular muscle. Also called ventricular conduction.

nerve c. Transmission of an impulse through a nerve.

retrograde c. Transmission of an impulse through the cardiac muscle or the conduction system in a manner opposite to that of the normal impulse. Also called reconduction; ventriculoatrial conduction.

saltatory c. Conduction in which the nerve impulse jumps from one node of Ranvier to the next.

synaptic c. The propagation of a nerve impulse through a synapse.

ventricular c. See intraventricular conduction.

ventriculoatrial c. See retrograde conduction.

conductivity The ability to transmit or convey heat, electricity, sound, etc.

conductor 1. Any substance capable of transmitting heat, electricity, sound, etc. **2.** A grooved probe for guiding a surgeon's knife.

condylar Of or relating to a condyle.

condylarthrosis A joint in which an ovoid surface (condyle) fits into an elliptical cavity.

condyle A rounded knoblike prominence at the end of a bone by means of which it articulates with another bone.

condylectomy Surgical removal of a condyle.

condyloma A venereal wartlike growth at the junction of skin and mucous membrane of the anus, vulva, or the glans penis.

c. acuminatum Moist wart; see under wart.

c. latum A flat raised lesion of secondary syphilis appearing in moist areas such as the lips, the female genitalia, or the perianal region.

condylomatous Of or relating to a condyloma.

condylotomy Division of a condyle.

cone A figure or anatomic structure tapering to a point from a circular base.

c. of light The triangular reflection of light seen on inspection of the tympanic membrane.

medullary c. The tapered end of the spinal cord.

retinal c. One of about six or seven million photoreceptor cells which, with the rod cells, form the second of the 10 layers of the retina.

confabulation The replacement of memory lapses with detailed fabrications of imaginary experiences; sometimes occurring in organic brain diseases in which intellectual impairment takes place.

confection A sweetened pharmaceutical preparation. Also called confectio; electuary.

configuration 1. The shape or outline of something as determined by the arrangement of its parts. **2.** The spatial grouping of atoms in a molecule.

confinement The period of childbirth.

conflict The struggle between two opposing emotions, thoughts, needs, or courses of action.

confluence of the sinuses, confluens sinuum The junction of the sinuses of the dura mater (superior sagittal, straight, occipital, and two transverse), located in a slight depression at one side of the internal protuberance of the occipital bone.

confluent Running together, as the skin lesions of certain diseases which are not distinct but become merged.

conformation The spatial arrangement of atoms in a molecule achieved by rotation of groups about single, covalent bonds, without breaking any covalent bonds.

conformer A mold or shell fitted in a cavity to preserve its shape, as in the eye socket after removal of the eye prior to insertion of an artificial eye.

confusion Mental state in which a person is disoriented in regard to his environment; impaired capacity to think clearly and with customary speed.

congener 1. A drug which is part of a group of chemical compounds sharing the smae parent compound. **2.** One of two or more muscles with the same function.

congenital Present at birth.

congested Containing an abnormally large amount of blood.

congestion Abnormal accumulation of blood in a part.

hypostatic c. Accumulation of blood in the lowest part of an organ due to the action of gravity when the circulation is feeble.

passive venous c. Congestion of a part due to partial stagnation of blood in the capillaries and venules, resulting from faulty venous drainage or failure of the right ventricle of the heart.

conglutination 1. Abnormal adhesion. **2.** Agglutination or clumping of red blood cells in the presence of serum.

conglutinin A nonantibody protein with the capability of combining with the carbohydrate portion of complement and thus capable of clumping particles covered by the complement; found in normal bovine serum.

congo red A red azo dye, used in biologic stains and as an indicator (red in alkaline solutions and blue in acid solutions).

conidiophore A spore-bearing, specialized hyphal filament in fungi.

conidiospore A fungal spore produced on a specialized conidiophore.

conidium *pl.* **conidia** The reproductive spore of fungi produced asexually.

coniofibrosis Abnormal formation of fibrous tissue caused by the presence of dust.

coniosis Any disease caused by dust.

Conium maculatum A notoriously poisonous large herb of the carrot family. Also called poison hemlock; spotted parsley.

conization The removal of a conical piece of tissue, as from the cervix.

conjugase An enzyme, present in the liver and kidney of mammals, that splits folic acid conjugates into pteroylglutamic acid and glutamic acid.

conjugate Paired.

conjugation 1. Sexual reproduction of unicellular organisms whereby the two cells exchange genetic material. **2.** In chemistry, the combination of large molecules (e.g., proteins) with those of another substance.

conjunctiva The thin transparent mucous membrane lining the inner surface of the eyelids (palpebral conjunctiva) and the exposed surface of the anterior sclera up to the border of the cornea (bulbar conjunctiva); the epithelial layer of the conjunctiva is continuous with the corneal epithelium.

conjunctivitis Inflammation of the conjunctiva resulting from bacterial, viral, or allergic agents; e.g., acute catarrhal conjunctivitis is caused by a bacterium (usually pneumococcus), epidemic keratoconjunctivitis is caused by a virus (adenovirus 8), vernal catarrh is caused by hypersensitivity to exogenous allergens.

connective tissue diseases See collagen diseases.

connector In dentistry, the part of a fixed partial denture which unites its component parts; e.g., an artificial tooth.

Conn's syndrome Excessive secretion of the hormone aldosterone due to a tumor in the cortex of the adrenal gland; the typical findings include hypertension, hypokalemic alkalosis, weakness, and low plasma renin. Also called primary aldosteronism.

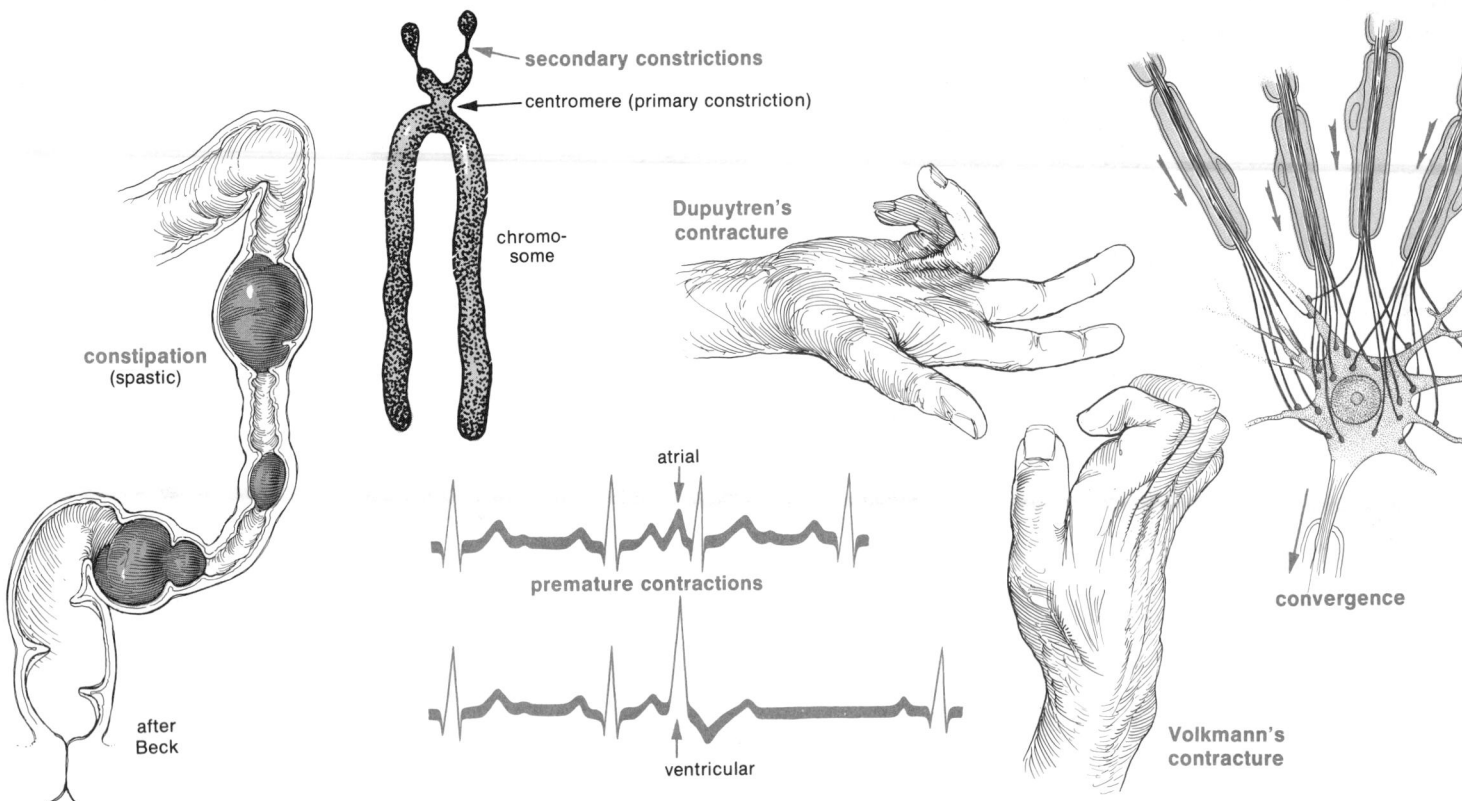

secondary constrictions

centromere (primary constriction)

chromo-some

constipation (spastic)

Dupuytren's contracture

atrial

premature contractions

after Beck

ventricular

convergence

Volkmann's contracture

consanguineous Related by blood.

consanguinity Kinship; blood relationship from common ancestry.

conscious Being aware of one's existence, actions, and environment.

consciousness State of awareness of and responsiveness to environment.

consciousness-raising A method of making individuals realize their potentials, in order to bring about change.

consensual Denoting an involuntary act. Also called reflex.

conservative Applied to a cautious method of treatment.

consolidation 1. Solidification into a dense mass; applied especially to the inflammatory solidification of the lung in pneumonia. 2. The mass so formed.

constant (k) A quantity which, under stated conditions, does not vary with changes in the environment.

    decay c. The mathematical expression for the number of atoms of radionuclide which will decay in a unit of time.

    dissociation c. (K) In chemistry, the constant that depends upon the equilibrium between the dissociated and undissociated forms of a compound.

    gas c. (R) The universal constant of proportionality, appearing in the equation of the general gas law, equal to the pressure of the gas times its volume divided by its temperature.

    Michaelis-Menten c. (K_m) One that expresses the concentration of the substrate at which half the maximum velocity of a reaction is achieved.

    Plank's c. (h) A constant expressing the ratio of the energy possessed by a quantum of energy to its frequency; its value is approximately 6.625×10^{-27} erg-sec.

constellation In psychiatry, a set of related ideas.

constipate To slow the action of the bowels.

constipation A decrease in the frequency of bowel movements, accompanied by a difficult prolonged effort in passing a very hard stool, followed by a sensation of incomplete evacuation.

constitution The physical make-up and state of health of the body.

constriction 1. A narrowing; a binding. 2. A subjective sensation of being tightly bound or squeezed.

    secondary c. The slender heterochromatic area of a chromosome which separates the satellite from the rest of the chromosome (the primary constriction is at the centromere).

constrictor Denoting a muscle that narrows a canal or opening.

consultand A prospective parent who seeks genetic counsel and whose genetic constitution is in question. Cf. proband; relative of interest.

consultant A physician who is called in an advisory capacity.

consultation A conference of two or more physicians to evaluate the diagnosis and treatment of the disease in a particular patient.

consumption Wasting away of tissues; previously a popular name for pulmonary tuberculosis.

contact 1. The point at which two adjacent bodies touch one another. 2. A person who has been exposed to the virus of an infectious disease.

contagion Transmission of a disease by direct or indirect contact.

contagious Transmissible by direct or indirect contact. Also called catching.

contagium The causative agent of an infectious disease.

contaminant That which contaminates; an impurity.

contamination 1. The process of soiling, as with infectious matter or unwanted radioactive matter. 2. In an experiment, allowing the variable that is to be validated to influence the variable used for validation. 3. An error of speech characterized by the fusion of part of one word with that of another.

content 1. That which is contained in an enclosed space. 2. The amount of a specified substance.

contiguity The state of being adjacent in time or space; immediately preceding or following.

continence Self-restraint, especially from sexual activity.

contour 1. Surface configuration. 2. To shape into a desired form, as a denture or a broken tooth.

contraception The prevention of conception.

contraceptive Any agent or device used for the prevention of conception.

contract To pull together; to reduce in size or increase tension by drawing together.

contractile Able to contract.

contractility The ability to shorten or increase tension, applied to a muscle.

contraction 1. The shortening or increase in tension of functioning muscle. 2. A heart beat. 3. A shrinkage or reduction in size.

    Braxton-Hicks c.'s, Braxton-Hicks sign Painless irregular contractions of the pregnant uterus, beginning during the first trimester and increasing in frequency as pregnancy advances; occasionally observed in hematometria and cases of soft myomas.

    hourglass c. The narrowing of the middle of a hollow organ.

    premature c. A premature heart beat.

contracture A permanent contraction due to

tonic spasm, muscle atrophy, or scars.

    Dupuytren's c. Shortening of the palmar fascia producing permanent flexion of one or more fingers.

    ischemic c. Contracture of a muscle resulting from circulatory interference, as by a tight bandage or from cold temperatures.

    organic c. Contracture that is permanent, usually due to fibrosis within the muscle.

    Volkmann's c. Contraction of the fingers and sometimes wrist following a severe injury or improper use of a tourniquet.

contraindication Any condition that renders undesirable the use of a medication or surgical procedure.

contralateral Located on the opposite side.

contrastimulant 1. Counteracting the effects of a stimulant. 2. Any agent producing such an effect.

contrecoup Occurring on the opposite side, as the fracture of a portion of the skull opposite to the point of impact.

control 1. To verify a scientific experiment by comparing with a standard or by conducting a parallel experiment, conditions being equal except for one factor. 2. A standard against which the results of an experiment are checked.

    birth c. Limitation of the number of children conceived by the voluntary use of contraceptive measures.

contusion A superficial injury or bruise.

    brain c. A localized injury to the surface of the brain, usually attended by extravasation of blood and sometimes swelling; symptoms vary according to the extent and location of the injury.

conus *pl.* **coni** A cone-shaped structure.

    c. arteriosus The upper, anterior portion of the right ventricle of the heart, ending in the pulmonary artery. Also called arterial cone.

    c. medullaris The tapered end of the spinal cord. Also called medullary cone.

convalescence A stage in recovery between the abatement of a disease or injury and complete health.

convection Heat transfer in liquids or gases by the movement of heated particles.

convergence 1. The turning toward or approaching a common point from different directions; e.g., the coordinated movement of the two eyes toward a near point, or the movement of the peripheral cells of the blastula toward the center during the gastrulation stage of the embryo. 2. The connecting of several presynaptic neurons with one postsynaptic neuron.

    negative c. Outward deviation of the visual axes. Also called divergence.

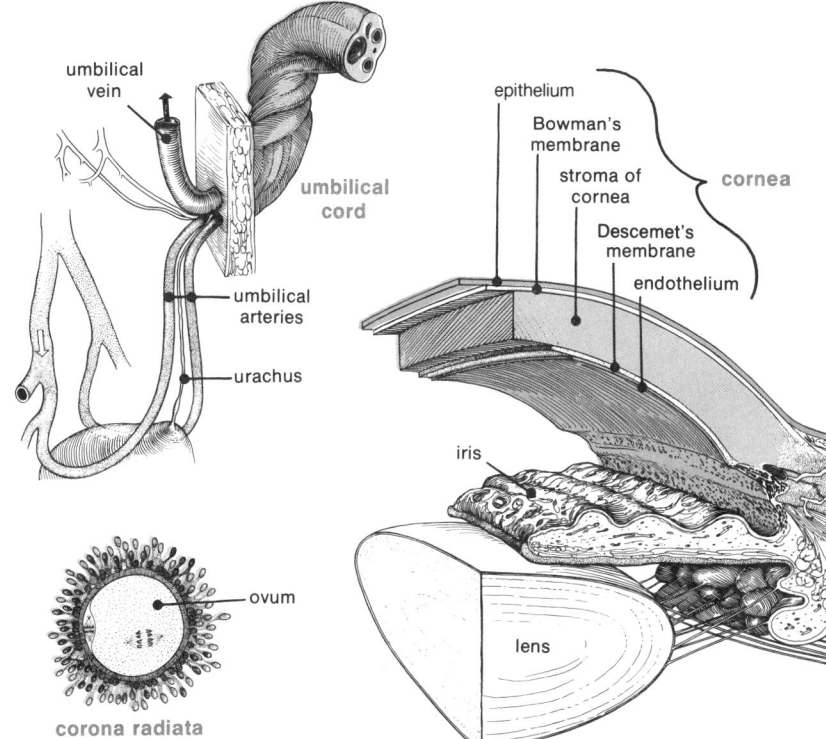

U.S. Customary Units to Metric Units	
...es to centimeters	................multiply by 10, then divide by 4
...ls to meters	....................multiply by 9, then divide by 10
...nds to kilograms	.................multiply by 5, then divide by 11
...ns to liters	......multiply by 4, then subtract 1/5 of the number of gallons

Temperature Units	
...rees Fahrenheit to degrees Centigrade	.... subtract 32, then multiply by 5/9
...ees Centigrade to degrees Fahrenheit	.......multiply by 9/5, then add 32
...ees Kelvin to degrees Centigrade	........................add 273

umbilical vein

umbilical cord

umbilical arteries

urachus

epithelium

Bowman's membrane

stroma of cornea

cornea

Descemet's membrane

endothelium

iris

ovum

lens

corona radiata

---

positive c. Inward deviation of the visual axes. Also called convergent squint.

convergent Moving or inclined toward a common point.

conversion 1. The act of changing. 2. In psychiatry, the symbolic physical manifestation of a psychic conflict.

convertin See factor VII.

convex An outwardly curved surface.

convexoconcave Denoting a lens that has a greater convex than concave curvature.

convoluted Rolled, coiled, or twisted.

convolution A twisting or infolding of an anatomic part upon itself. See also gyrus.

convulsant Causing convulsions.

convulsion A violent involuntary muscular contraction, or a series of such contractions producing jerking movements.

Cope's sign A sign of appendicitis: (a) tenderness over the area of the appendix on extending the thigh; (b) tenderness on compressing the femoral artery in the femoral (Scarpa's) triangle.

copolymer A plastic composed of two or more chemically different monomers or base units.

copolymerization The chemical joining of different monomers to form a compound of a high molecular weight.

copper A malleable, reddish-brown metallic element; symbol Cu, atomic number 29, atomic weight 63.54.

coproantibodies Antibodies present in the intestinal contents.

coprolalia The involuntary use of obscene words.

coprolith A mass of inspissated feces.

coproporphyrin A porphyrin compound normally present in feces; a decomposition product of bilirubin. Also called stereoporphyrin.

copulation Sexual intercourse; coitus.

cor Latin for heart.

c. biloculare A more or less two-chambered heart due to the absence or incomplete development of the interatrial and interventricular septa.

c. bovinum An abnormally large heart. Also called bucardia.

c. pulmonale Enlargement of the right ventricle of the heart, secondary to a disorder of the substance or blood vessels of the lung.

c. triloculare A three-chambered heart due to absence of either the interatrial or the interventricular septum.

coracoacromial Relating to the coracoid and acromial processes of the scapula (shoulder blade).

coracobrachial Relating to the coracoid process of the scapula and the arm.

coracoclavicular Relating to the coracoid process of the scapula and the clavicle.

coracohumeral Relating to the coracoid process of the scapula and the humerus.

coracoid Shaped like a raven's beak; denoting the thick, curved process at the superior border of the scapula (shoulder blade).

cord Any flexible, stringlike structure.

medullary c.'s Columns of dense lymphoid tissue (mostly packed lymphocytes) surrounded by sinuses in the medulla of lymph nodes.

spermatic c. The structure that extends from the internal inguinal ring to the testis.

spinal c. The elongated portion of the central nervous system that is enclosed by the vertebral column.

umbilical c. The structure connecting the placenta with the umbilicus of the fetus; it contains two arteries and one vein coiled around each other; in the newborn it measures about 61.4 cm in length and 12.7 mm in diameter.

vocal c. One of the four membranous bands in the larynx; the upper pair is called false vocal cords, the lower pair the true vocal cords (those that enter into voice production).

cordate Heart-shaped.

cordectomy Surgical removal of a cord, as of a vocal cord.

cordopexy Surgical fixation of a cord, especially a vocal cord.

cordotomy Severing of the sensory tracts of the spinal cord for the relief of intractable pain.

core 1. The central mass of a boil. 2. A metal casting designed to retain in position the artificial crown of a tooth. 3. A section of a mold used to record and maintain the relationships of parts, such as teeth or metallic restorations.

corecleisis, coreclisis Obliteration of the pupil.

corectasis Pathologic dilatation of the pupil.

corectopia Abnormal position of the pupil to one side of the center of the iris.

coreometer An instrument for measuring the size of the pupil. Also called pupillometer.

coreometry Measurement of the pupil of the eye. Also called pupillometry.

corepressor A small molecule, usually a product of a specific enzyme pathway, capable of combining with the inactive repressor to form an active complex which combines with the operator and prevents mRNA synthesis; a homeostatic mechanism for regulating enzyme production in repressible enzyme systems.

corestenoma A narrowing or partial closing of the pupil.

corium See dermis.

corn A circumscribed induration and thickening of the skin.

hard c. A corn over a toe joint covered by friction and/or pressure from ill-fitting shoes.

seed c. A wart on the foot.

soft c. A thickening of the skin between two toes caused by pressure and kept soft by moisture.

cornea The transparent anterior part of the outer coat of the eyeball that serves as the major refracting medium; it consists of five layers; corneas donated for transplantation are now routinely preserved at eye banks.

conical c. See keratoconus.

corneal Relating to the cornea.

corneitis See keratitis.

corneosclera The cornea and sclera considered as a unit that forms the outer layer of the eyeball.

corneous Hornlike.

corneum The superficial layer of the skin. Also called stratum corneum.

corniculate Having the shape of a small horn.

cornification Conversion into horny tissue or keratin.

cornu *pl.* **cornua** 1. A horn-shaped structure. 2. Any structure composed of bony tissue.

corona Any structure resembling a crown.

c. radiata An investment of follicular cells remaining attached to the ovum when released by the ovary; formerly the cumulus oophorus around the developing oocyte.

coronalis Coronal, relating to the coronal suture or plane.

coronary 1. Encircling in the manner of a crown, as the vessels supplying the heart muscle. 2. Coronary occlusion; a heart attack.

coroner An official whose duty is to investigate any death thought to be of other than natural causes.

coronion A craniometric point at the tip of the lower jaw.

coronoid 1. Shaped like a crow's beak; denoting certain processes of bones, as the coronoid process of the mandible (lower jaw). 2. Crown-shaped.

corpora Plural of corpus.

corporeal 1. Relating to or characteristic of the body. 2. Relating to a corpus.

corpulence, corpulency Obesity.

corpus *pl.* **corpora** Body; the main portion of a structure.

c. albicans A mass of white, collagenous scar tissue formed in the ovary after discharge of the ovum; it represents the remnants of a corpus luteum, either of the menstrual cycle or of pregnancy, and eventually disappears.

corpus callosum

corpus luteum

granulosa lutein cells

blood clot

theca lutein cells

Meissner's corpuscle

pacinian corpuscle

peripheral nerve

CH_2OH
$C=O$
OH

cortisone

c. callosum A mass of transverse fibers connecting the two hemispheres of the brain.

c. cavernosum One of the two parallel columns of erectile tissue of the penis or of the clitoris.

c. ciliare Ciliary body; see under body.

c. geniculatum laterale Lateral geniculate body; see body, geniculate.

c. geniculatum mediale Medial geniculate body; see body, geniculate.

c. luteum An endocrine body producing the hormone progesterone; it is composed of a mass of large cells containing a yellow pigment (lutein) and develops in the ovary, at the site of a ruptured ovarian follicle after discharge of the ovum; if pregnancy does not occur, the corpus luteum retrogresses to a mass of scar tissue (corpus albicans) which eventually disappears; if pregnancy occurs, it continues to grow until the 13th week before slowly retrogressing.

c. mamillare Mamillary body; see under body.

corpora quadrigemina Quadrigeminal bodies; see under body.

c. spongiosum The median column of erectile tissue of the penis, situated between and inferior to the corpora cavernosa and surrounding the urethra.

c. striatum The caudate and lentiform nuclei and the internal capsule considered as a whole situated in front and lateral to the thalamus in each hemisphere of the brain. Also called striate body.

c. vitreum Vitreous body; see under body.

corpuscle 1. A small body or mass. **2.** A cell capable of moving freely in the body. **3.** A primary particle such as a photon or electron.

blood c. Any blood cell.

colostrum c. One of numerous large, round bodies containing fat droplets, present in colostrum; thought to be modified leukocyte. Also called galactoblast.

Golgi-Mazzoni c. An encapsulated sensory nerve ending found in the subcutaneous tissue of the pulp of the fingers; similar to a pacinian corpuscle, but with a thinner capsule and with axons that ramify more extensively and end in flat expansions.

Krause's c. A spherical sense organ located at the termination of some sensory nerve fibers; it responds to the sensation of cold. Also called Krause's end-bulb.

malpighian c. See renal corpuscle.

Meissner's c. A small, oval, encapsulated receptor organ present in the dermal papillae of the skin, particularly prevalent on the palmar and plantar surfaces; signals fine, discriminative touch sensations. Also called tactile corpuscle of Meissner.

pacinian c. An encapsulated receptor organ that signals mechanical deformations as touch or vibratory sensations; characterized by an unmyelinated terminal axon covered by numerous concentric layers of connective tissue; found in subcutaneous tissue, fascial planes around joints and tendons, and in the mesentery about the pancreas; especially numerous in the palm of the hand, sole of the foot, and genital organs; it responds to deep pressure and vibrations.

phantom c. A red blood cell that is devoid of color due to losing its hemoglobin. Also called shadow corpuscle; achromocyte.

Purkinje's c.'s See cell, Purkinje's.

red blood c. See erythrocyte.

renal c. One of many invaginated pouchlike commencements of a renal tubule (glomerular or Bowman's capsule) with a central tuft of vessels (glomerulus). Also called malpighian body or corpuscle.

Ruffini's c.'s Ruffini's nerve endings; see under ending.

shadow c. See phantom corpuscle.

terminal c. Any specialized encapsulated nerve ending, such as the pacinian corpuscle.

white blood c. See cell, white blood.

correspondence The state of being in harmony.

retinal c. The faculty of vision by which an object seen with the two eyes (thus forming two retinal images) is perceived as one due to the coordinate functioning of retinal receptors.

corrosive Caustic; denoting an agent that causes a gradual wearing away or disintegration of a substance by chemical alteration.

cortex The external portion of an organ, such as the brain, kidney, or adrenal gland.

cortexone See deoxycorticosterone.

cortical Relating to a cortex.

corticifugal Conducting impulses away from the cerebral cortex.

corticipetal Conducting impulses toward the cerebral cortex.

corticoid Corticosteroid.

corticopontine Relating to the cerebral cortex and pons.

corticospinal Relating to the cerebral cortex and spinal cord.

corticosteroid Any of the hormones of the adrenal cortex or any synthetic substitute.

corticosterone See cortisone.

corticothalamic Relating to the cerebral cortex and thalamus.

corticotropin 1. A hormone produced by the anterior lobe of the pituitary gland that stimulates the secretion of cortisone and other hormones of the adrenal cortex. **2.** A pharmaceutical preparation made synthetically or extracted from the anterior pituitary of mammals, used to stimulate the activity of the adrenal cortex. Also called adrenocorticotrophin.

corticotropin-releasing factor (CRF) A factor released by the hypothalamus in response to a low plasma cortisol level, capable of causing secretion of ACTH by the anterior pituitary gland.

cortisol 17-Hydroxycorticosterone; a steroid hormone isolated from the adrenal cortex or produced synthetically; of the naturally occurring adrenal cortical hormones, cortisol is most capable of correcting by itself the effects of adrenalectomy; provides resistance to stresses and maintains a number of enzyme systems. Also called hydrocortisone.

cortisone A hormone from the adrenal cortex active in regulating carbohydrate metabolism and the nutrition of connective tissue; its release is regulated by the action of the adrenocorticotropic hormone (ACTH) of the pituitary gland; an excess of cortisone activity is responsible for Cushing's syndrome. Also called corticosterone.

Corynebacterium A genus of irregularly staining, gram-positive bacteria having a club shape and causing disease in plants and animals.

C. diphtheriae The species that causes diphtheria in man; produces a powerful exotoxin; found in the mucous membrane of the upper respiratory tract of infected persons.

coryza Acute inflammation of the nasal mucosa, attended by a discharge.

cosmesis Concern for the appearance of the patient, especially in surgical operations.

cosmetic Denoting any preparation or operative procedure intended to improve the appearance of a person.

costa *pl.* **costae** Latin for rib.

costal Relating to a rib.

costectomy Surgical removal of a rib.

costocentral See costovertebral.

costochondral Relating to a rib and its cartilage.

costochondritis Inflammation of the rib cartilages, causing pain over the anterior chest wall.

costoclavicular Relating to the ribs and a clavicle.

costoclavicular syndrome Vascular disorders of the upper limb due to intermittent compression of the neuromuscular bundle between the clavicle and the first rib.

costophrenic Relating to the ribs and the diaphragm.

costoscapular Relating to the ribs and a scapula.

costosternal Relating to the ribs and the sternum.

costotome

cotyledon

maternal side of placenta

Geiger counter
GM tube
shield

volume   voltage   counts/min
          on
          off   volts

solution of radioactive sample and detector (fluor)

photomultiplier tube

scintillation counter (liquid type)

amplifier

pulse outlet counter

electronic pulse

chlorine molecules

covalency

costotome An instrument used for cutting through a rib.

costotomy Division of a rib or costal cartilage.

costovertebral Relating to the ribs and the thoracic vertebrae. Also called costocentral.

cotransport The simultaneous transport of two substances across a membrane, in the same direction.

cotton 1. Any of various plants of the genus *Gossypium.* 2. The soft, white fiber covering the seeds of the cotton plant.

  absorbent c. Cotton from which fatty matter and impurities have been removed.

cotyledon One of 15 to 20 irregularly shaped compartments (lobes) into which the maternal surface of the placenta is divided; it houses numerous small villi.

cough A forceful and sudden expulsion of air from the lungs.

  whooping c. An acute respiratory illness of infants and young children usually caused by *Bordetella pertussis,* a gram-negative coccobacillus. Also called pertussis.

coulomb (Q) A unit of electrical quantity equal to the amount of charge transferred in one second by a steady current of one ampere.

counseling A professional service that provides an individual with a better understanding of his problems and potentialities.

  genetic c. A service by individuals knowledgeable in human genetics that provides information about inherited disorders so that people can make informed choices about family planning.

count 1. To list one by one in order to calculate a total. 2. The formulation of a total obtained by examining a sample.

  Arneth c. The percentage of distribution of polymorphonuclear neutrophils according to the number of lobes their nuclei contain.

  blood c. See blood count.

  complete blood c. See blood count, complete.

  differential blood c. See blood count, differential.

counter A computer or any apparatus for counting.

  Geiger c. An instrument used to detect, measure, and record the emission of radioactive particles; it consists of a negatively charged metallic cylinder in a vacuum tube containing a positively charged wire. Also called Geiger-Müller counter (GM counter).

  scintillation c. Device used to detect and count radioactive particles. Also called scintillator.

counterconditioning In behavior therapy, establishment of a second conditioned response to nullify a previously learned response.

countercurrent A current flowing in a direction opposite to another.

counterdrug A drug that counteracts or neutralizes an opposing agent.

counterextension Countertraction.

counterirritant A substance applied locally to produce superficial irritation in order to relieve a deep-seated inflammation.

counterpulsation A procedure used to aid the failing heart by automatically removing arterial blood just before and during ventricular ejection and returning it to the circulation during diastole.

countershock Electric shock applied to the heart to correct a disturbance of its rhythm.

counterstain A second stain, usually of a contrasting color, applied to a microscopy specimen to color parts not affected by the first stain.

countertraction A traction or pull which is antagonistic to the action of another traction; a back-pull.

countertransference The psychoanalyst's emotional reaction to his patient; it may be conscious or unconscious.

countertransport The passage of two substances across a cell membrane, simultaneously but in opposite directions, e.g., Na+ and H+ ions.

coup French for stroke or blow.

couple To copulate; said of lower animals.

coupling 1. Pairing or joining. 2. Bigeminal rhythm; heart beats occurring in pairs; a normal sinus beat followed by a premature beat.

  constant c. See fixed coupling.

  fixed c. The occurrence of several premature beats with a constant interval between each of them and the preceding normal beat. Also called constant coupling.

  variable c. The occurrence of several premature beats with different intervals between each of them and the preceding normal beat.

Courvoisier's sign See law, Courvoisier's.

covalency In chemistry, a bond marked by the sharing of electrons (usually in pairs) by two atoms in a chemical compound.

cover glass, coverslip A piece of thin glass used to cover a mounted specimen for examination under the microscope.

cowpox See vaccinia (1).

coxa *pl.* **coxae** Latin for hipbone and hip joint.

coxalgia Pain in the hip joint.

Coxiella burnetii The spoecies of *Coxiella* that causes Q fever in man.

coxodynia Coxalgia; pain in the hip joint.

coxsackievirus One of a group of viruses (genus *Enterovirus,* family Picornaviridae) having pathologic effects on the brain, heart, muscle, epithelium of respiratory tract, and skin; divided into two anti-

genically different groups (A and B); the name is derived from the town of Coxsackie, New York, where it was discovered while an outbreak of poliomyelitis was being investigated.

cramp 1. A painful spasm. 2. Intestinal colic. 3. An occupational neurosis.

  heat c. Pain in the abdomen and/or legs occurring in persons working in extreme hot weather.

  tailor's c. Spasm and neuralgic pain of the fingers, hand, and forearm. Also called tailor's spasm.

  writer's c. Spastic pain of the muscles of the thumb and two adjoining fingers induced by excessive writing. Also called mogigraphia; graphospasm.

cranial Of or relating to the skull.

craniectomy Surgical removal of a portion of the skull.

craniocele See encephalocele (3).

craniofacial Relating to both the skull and the face.

craniology The scientific study of the skull, especially human, in all its aspects.

craniomalacia Thinning and softening of the bones of the skull.

craniometer An instrument used to measure skulls.

craniometric Relating to skull measurement.

craniometry Measurement of the skull, especially human, after removal of the soft tissues.

craniopathy Any disease of the skull.

craniopharyngioma The second most frequent type of tumor of the hypophysis arising from remnants of the embryonic adenohypophysis (Rathke's pouch) and having a cystic or a solid form, frequently with calcium deposits. Also called Rathke's pouch tumor.

craniopuncture Puncture of the skull.

craniorrhachischisis Congenital fissure of the skull and vertebral column.

craniosacral Relating to the origins of the parasympathetic nervous system.

cranioschisis Congenital defect of the skull in which it fails to close completely, leaving a fissure.

craniosclerosis Abnormal thickening of the skull.

craniostenosis Congenital malformation of the skull due to premature fusion of the cranial sutures.

craniostosis Premature ossification of the skull.

craniotabes Localized softening of an infant's skull, usually due to severe rickets.

craniotome An instrument used for perforation and crushing of the skull of a fetus.

craniotomy 1. Surgical opening into the skull. 2. In obstetrics, puncturing of the head of a dead fetus and evacuation of the contents to facilitate its delivery.

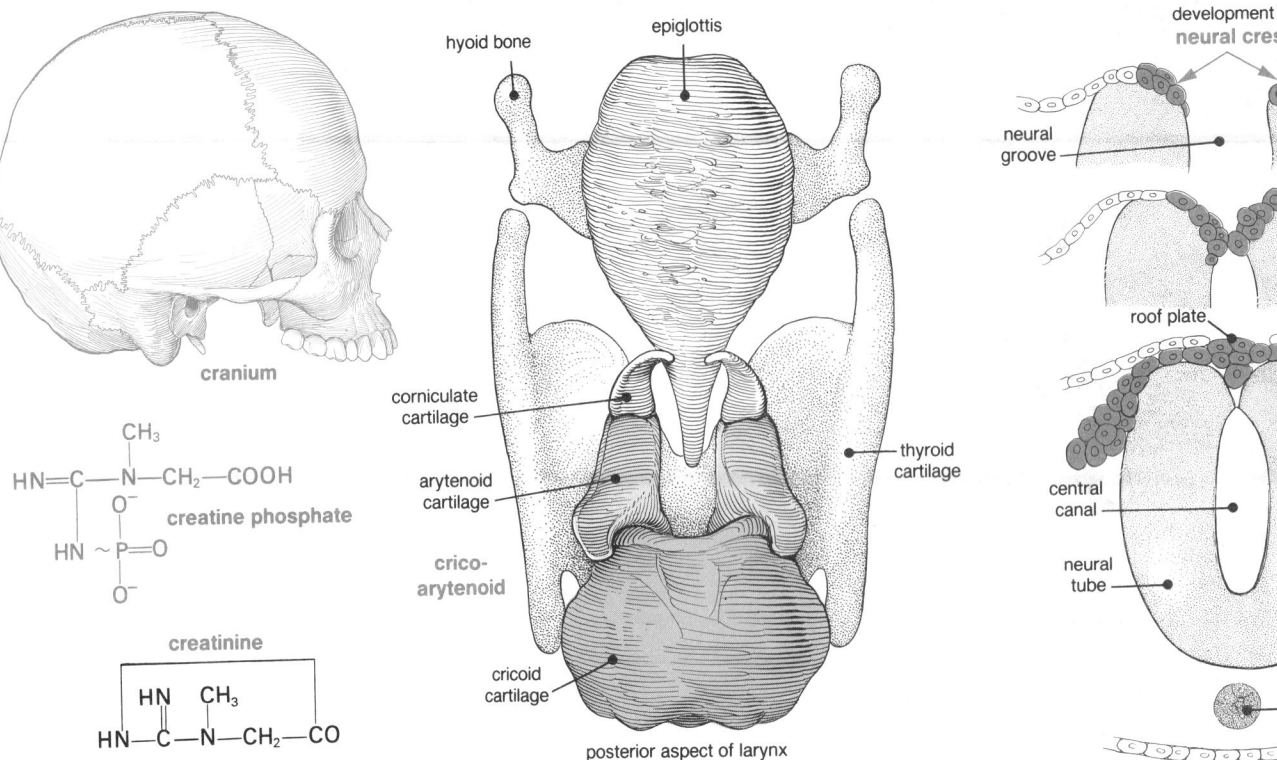

cranium

creatine phosphate

$HN=C-N-CH_2-COOH$
$\quad CH_3$
$\quad O^-$
$HN\sim P=O$
$\quad O^-$

creatinine

$HN \quad CH_3$
$HN-C-N-CH_2-CO$

hyoid bone
epiglottis
corniculate cartilage
arytenoid cartilage
crico-arytenoid
cricoid cartilage
thyroid cartilage

posterior aspect of larynx

development of neural crest
ectoderm
neural groove
roof plate
central canal
neural tube
notochord

---

cranium The bones of the head in general; specifically, the bones enclosing the brain. Also called the skull.

crater The most depressed area of an ulcer.

crateriform Hollowed like a bowl; in bacteriology, denoting a type of liquefaction of gelatin by bacteria in a stab culture.

crazing The formation of fine cracks on the surface of a structure, such as an artificial tooth, induced by release of internal stress.

cream 1. The fatty constituent of milk that tends to accumulate at the surface on standing. 2. Any of various substances resembling cream.

creatine, creatin A nitrogenous compound found mainly in muscle tissue.

c. phosphate Phosphocreatine; a creatine phosphoric acid compound; a source of energy in muscle contraction.

c. phosphokinase (CPK) An enzyme that promotes the formation of ATP (adenosine triphosphate) from phosphocreatine and ADP (adenosine diphosphate); essential to muscle contraction.

creatinine A normal metabolic waste, a product of creatine metabolism; excreted in the urine, primarily by filtration; since it is generally produced at a constant rate, the clearance rate and the serum level are widely used as an index of kidney function.

creatinine clearance Rate at which the kidney removes endogenous or exogenous creatinine from blood plasma; an approximate measure of glomerular filtration rate. Normal values are 100–125 ml/minute for males and 85–125 ml/minute for females of average size.

creatinuria The presence of increased amounts of creatine in the urine; usually a sign of a decrease in muscle mass, as in muscular dystrophy.

cremaster See table of muscles.

crenate, crenated Notched.

crenocyte An abnormal red blood cell with scalloped or notched edges.

crepitant Crackling.

crepitation 1. A grating sound like that produced when rubbing hair between the fingers, heard in certain diseases such as pneumonia. 2. Noise made by friction of the two ends of a fractured bone. 3. Sensation felt when palpating over an area in which there is subcutaneous gas.

crepitus 1. Crepitation. 2. A dry, crackling sound.

crescent, malarial A gametocyte of the malarial parasite *Plasmodium falciparum,* characterized by its crescentic shape. Also called sickle form.

cresol Any of three isomeric phenols (ortho-cresol, meta-cresol, and para-cresol); poisonous, colorless liquid or crystals, used as disinfectant.

CREST Acronym for a syndrome characterized by

---

calcinosis, Raynaud's phenomenon, esophageal involvement, sclerodactyly, and telengiactasia.

crest A bony ridge.

alveolar c. The margin of the bone surrounding each tooth.

c. of scapular spine The border of the spine of the scapula (shoulder blade).

ethmoidal c. One located in the medial side of the maxilla which articulates with the middle concha.

ganglionic c. See neural crest.

gingival c. The edge of the free gingiva separating the gingival sulcus from the external gingiva.

iliac c. The long curved upper border of the ilium.

infundibuloventricular c. See supraventricular crest.

intertrocanteric c. The ridge between the greater and lesser trochanters of the femur, marking the junction of the neck and shaft of the bone.

nasal c. The ridge along the middle of the floor of the nasal cavity.

neural c. A band of ectodermal cells dorsolateral to the embryonic neural tube that give origin to ganglia of the cranial and spinal nerves and ganglia of sympathetic trunk. Also called ganglionic crest.

bone.

spiral c. The serrated edge of the osseous spiral lamina of the cochlea.

supraventricular c. The muscular ridge separating the conus arteriosus from the remaining cavity of the right ventricle of the heart. Also called infundibuloventricular crest.

cretin A mentally retarded dwarf due to congenital thyroid deficiency; one afflicted with cretinism.

cretinism Condition characterized by stunted growth, apathy, distended abdomen, protruding swollen tongue, and arrested mental development, resulting from an inadequate production of thyroid hormones in early infancy.

cretinoid Exhibiting symptoms similar to those of cretinism.

Creutzfeldt-Jakob disease A spongiform encephalopathy characterized by dementia accompanied by myoclonus; the dementia progresses so rapidly that deterioration is usually seen daily; the individual afflicted with the disease moves inevitably from good health to total helplessness or death within a year; caused by prions (small, proteinaceous infectious particles). Also called Jakob-Creutzfeldt disease.

crevice A narrow crack.

gingival c. The space between the enamel of a tooth and the margin of the gums; in cases in which

---

the gums have receded, between the gums and the cementum.

crib death See sudden infant death syndrome.

cribriform Sievelike; perforated.

cricoarytenoid Relating to both the cricoid and arytenoid cartilages.

cricoid Ring-shaped, denoting the cartilage at the lower end of the larynx.

cricoidectomy Surgical removal of the cricoid cartilage.

cricothyroid Relating to the cricoid and thyroid cartilages.

cricotracheotomy Division of the cricoid cartilage and upper trachea.

cri-du-chat syndrome Hereditary condition marked by abnormal smallness of the head and jaw, severe mental deficiency, and a characteristic high-pitched catlike cry; caused by deletion of the short arm of chromosome 5. Also called cat-cry syndrome.

Crigler-Najjar disease See Crigler-Najjar syndrome.

Crigler-Najjar syndrome An inherited disease of infants, usually fatal, associated with deficiency of the bilirubin enzyme glucuronyl transferase in the liver. Also called Crigler-Najjar disease.

crinogenic Causing increased glandular secretion.

cripple 1. One who is partially or completely disabled. 2. To render disabled.

crisis 1. A sudden change in the course of an acute disease; e.g., a disease that terminates by crisis is one in which a change for the better occurs suddenly. 2. A paroxysmal attack of pain or distress in an organ as seen in tabes dorsalis.

addisonian c. Symptoms occurring in untreated or sudden onset of Addison's disease: included are nausea, vomiting, hypotension, and collapse. Also called adrenal crisis.

anaphylactoid c. Symptoms resembling those of life-threatening allergic reactions (e.g., to penicillin) arising from a breaking up of the body's colloid equilibrium; produced by injecting a variety of substances, such as peptones, into the body.

Dietl's c. Severe abdominal pain caused by a kinked ureter, occurring in individuals with a floating kidney.

oculogyric c. A crisis in which the eyeballs become fixed in one position (usually upward) for a length of time; occurring in encephalitis lethargica.

thyroid c. See thyrotoxic crisis.

thyrotoxic c. A sudden increase of the symptoms of thyrotoxicosis; rapid pulse, fever, nausea, diarrhea, a rise in the basal metabolic rate, and coma. Also called thyroid crisis or storm.

crista *pl.* **cristae** A sharp upstanding ridge or crest.

---

crista ampullaris

cross-bite

crus of incus (short)

crus of incus (long)

anterior posterior } crura of stapes

crucible former

crutches

cross section (trachea)

c. ampullaris An elevation on the inner surface of the ampulla of each semicircular duct that contains innervated hair cells responsive to movement of the endolymph.

c. galli The cock's comb; a perpendicular bony ridge on the upper surface of the ethmoid in the anterior cranial fossa projecting above the level of the cribriform plate; the anterior end of the falx cerebri is attached to it.

c. iliaca Iliac crest; see under crest.

crocodile tears syndrome Spontaneous secretion of tears occurring simultaneously with normal salivation during eating, caused by a lesion of the facial nerve; usually follows partial recovery from facial paralysis.

Crohn's disease Regional enteritis; see under enteritis.

cromolyn sodium The disodium salt of cromoglycic acid; used in the treatment of asthma and allergic rhinitis.

crossbite Condition in which the normal labiolingual or bucco-lingual relationship between the upper and lower teeth is reversed (the lower teeth are anterior and/or buccal to the upper teeth).

anterior c. Condition in which the upper incisors are locked lingual to the lower incisors.

crossbreed 1. Hybrid. **2.** To produce a hybrid by the mating of animals or plants of different breeds of varieties. Also called hybridize.

crossing over See under gene.

cross matching Cross-agglutination test; see under test.

cross section A section through an organ, usually at right angles to an axis.

croup A term commonly used to denote any kind of laryngitis with laryngeal spasm in children; marked by a hoarse, barking cough (croupy cough), and difficult breathing.

croup kettle A vessel with a long spout used to boil water and convey steam to a sick room.

croupy Of the nature of croup.

crown The topmost part of a structure, as of the head or tooth.

anatomical c. The portion of a tooth covered by enamel.

artificial c. A restoration of the major part or of the entire coronal part of a tooth which is affixed to the remains of a natural tooth structure; usually made of gold, porcelain, or plastic.

clinical c. The portion of a tooth visible in the oral cavity, beyond the margin of the gums. Also called physiologic crown.

dowel c. A crown replacing the entire coronal part of a tooth secured with the aid of a retention post extending into a filled root canal.

face c. A crown with a veneer for esthetics.

partial c. A crown that does not cover all the surfaces of a tooth; used as a retainer or single unit restoration.

crown and bridge The branch of prosthodontics concerned with crown restorations and the fixed type of tooth-borne partial denture prosthesis.

crowning The stage of childbirth in which the head of the baby is visible, its largest diameter being encircled by the stretched vulva.

cruciate Shaped like a cross; overlapping or crossing.

crucible A vessel or receptacle made of porcelain or graphite, used for melting materials at very high temperatures.

crucible former A stand which holds a sprued wax pattern of a dental restoration; it forms the base for the casting ring.

crura Plural of crus.

crural Relating to the leg or thigh.

crus *pl.* **crura 1.** Latin for leg. **2.** Any leglike structure.

common membranous c. The short duct formed by the united ends of the posterior and superior semicircular ducts.

common osseous c. The short canal formed by the union of the posterior and superior semicircular canals.

c. cerebri Cerebral peduncle; see under peduncle.

c. of the diaphragm Either of two fibromuscular bands (right and left) that connect the diaphragm with the lumbar vertebrae; the two crura encircle the aorta.

c. of the incus Either of two processes (short and long) of the incus.

c. of penis The tapering posterior portion of the corpus cavernosum penis.

c. of the stapes Either of two limbs (anterior and posterior) of the stapes.

crush To press between two bodies so as to cause injury.

crush syndrome Shock and renal failure following a severe crushing injury causing soft tissue trauma; acute tubular necrosis is thought to result from the myoglobin released from the damaged muscles. Also called compression syndrome.

crust 1. A hard outer layer or covering. **2.** A scab; the dried exudate of a lesion.

Crustacea A class of predominantly aquatic animals (phylum Arthropoda) having segmented bodies covered with an exoskeleton; it includes lobsters, crabs, shrimps, barnacles, wood lice, etc.

crustacean Belonging or relating to the class Crustacea.

crutch A supporting device, used singly or in pairs, designed to aid those who need help in walking.

Cruveilhier-Baumgarten syndrome Intrahepatic portal vein obstruction, usually due to cirrhosis of the liver, associated with patency of the umbilical vein, varicose paraumbilical veins, and a venous hum or thrill.

cry 1. An inarticulate expression of distress. **2.** To utter such a sound.

epileptic c. A vocal sound sometimes made by a person at the onset of an epileptic convulsion.

cryanesthesia Loss of the ability to feel cold.

cryesthesia Sensitiveness to cold temperatures.

cryobiology The study of the effect of low temperatures on living organisms.

cryocautery Destruction of tissue by freezing with substances such as liquid air or carbon dioxide snow.

cryoconization Removal of a cone of tissue from the wall of the lower cervical canal with a freezing instrument (cryoprobe).

cryoextraction The removal of a cataract by the use of an instrument that is supercooled to make frozen contact with the lens of the eye.

cryoextractor A copper pencil-shaped instrument with a small ball in its end that is placed in a freezing substance and used in the removal of a cataractous lens of the eye.

cryogenic Producing very low temperatures.

cryogenics The branch of physics concerned with the production and effects of very low temperatures.

cryoglobulin Abnormal gamma-globulin which precipitates when exposed to low temperatures (less than 37°C).

cryoglobulinemia The presence of cryoglobulin (abnormal protein) in the blood plasma.

cryometer An instrument for measuring very low temperatures.

cryopathy Any condition caused by cold.

cryoprecipitate Precipitate formed upon cooling of a solution.

cryopreservation Preservation of cells, tissues, or in vitro fertilized embryos by freezing.

cryoprotein A blood protein that precipitates from solution when cooled.

cryoscopy The determination of the freezing point of a solution compared with that of distilled water; based on the principle that the freezing point is depressed according to the concentration and nature of the solute.

cryostat Apparatus used to maintain low-temperature environments so that certain procedures (e.g., sectioning frozen tissues) may be carried out.

cryosurgery Surgery performed by the application of extreme cold temperatures.

cryothalamectomy Destruction of the thalamus

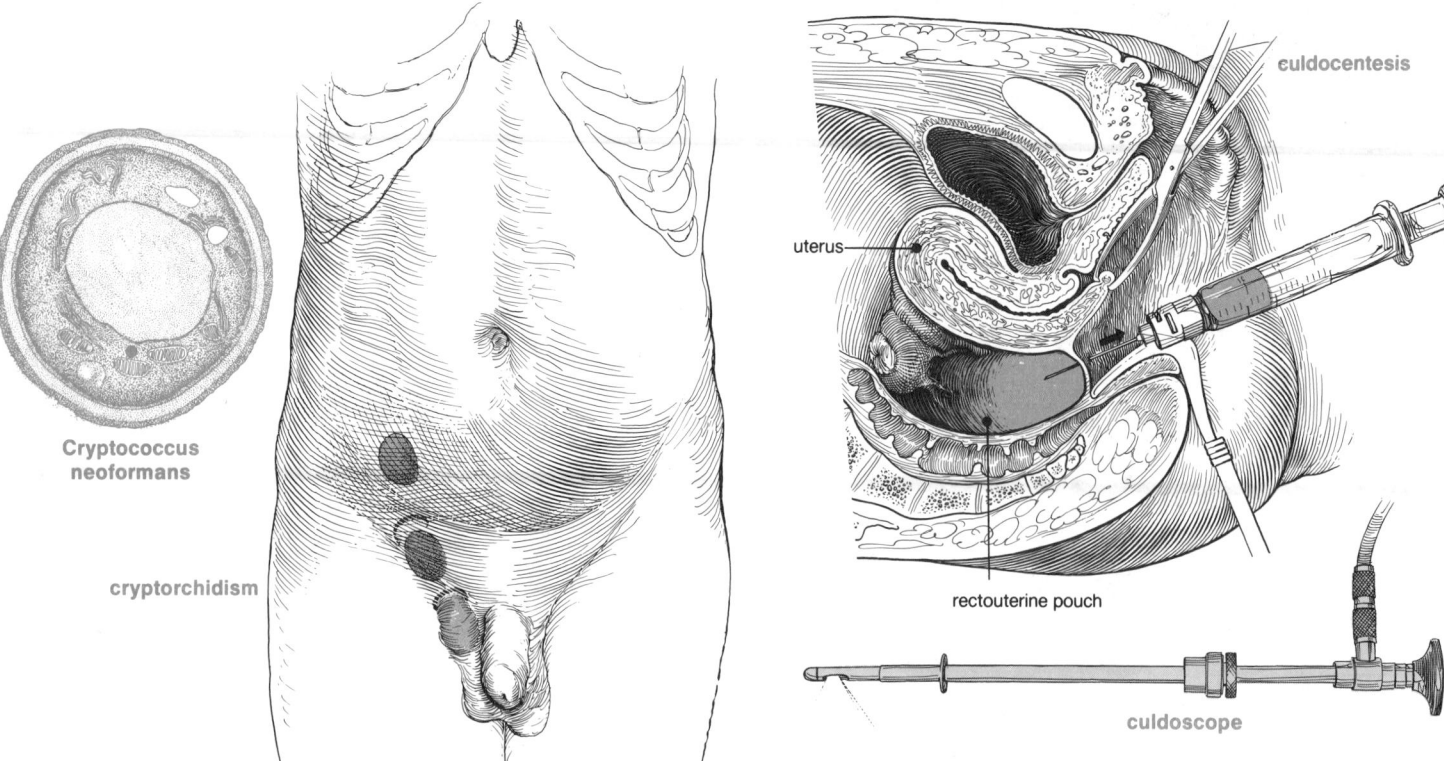

Cryptococcus
neoformans

cryptorchidism

culdocentesis

uterus

rectouterine pouch

culdoscope

by extreme cold temperatures for the treatment of
Parkinson's disease.

cryotherapy The therapeutic use of extremely low
temperatures, as of liquid nitrogen in the treatment
of chronic cervicitis.

crypt A glandular sac or pitlike depression.
   anal c. One of the furrows separating the folds of
mucous membrane in the upper anal canal.
   c.'s of Leiberkühn Simple tubular glands in the
mucous membrane of the intestines, believed to be
concerned with the secretion of digestive enzymes
and of some hormones. Also called intestinal glands.
   dental c. The space filled by a developing tooth.
   tonsillar c. One of several pits on the surface of
the palatine tonsil.

cryptitis Inflammation of a crypt or a follicle.
   anal c. Inflammation of the mucous membrane
of an anal crypt, especially painful during bowel
movements.
   urethral c. Inflammation of the mucous follicles
of the external orifice of the female urethra.

cryptococcin An antigen derived from the fungus
Cryptococcus neoformans.

cryptococcosis A chronic disseminated disease
caused by the fungus *Cryptococcus neoformans;* it
causes a respiratory infection often overlooked until
it spreads to other areas of the body, particularly the
central nervous system where it causes meningitis.
Also called torulosis.

Cryptococcus A genus of yeastlike fungi (family
Cryptococcaceae).
   C. neoformans Species commonly found in pi-
geon droppings and causing cryptococcosis in man.
Formerly called *Saccharomyces neoformans.*

cryptogenic, cryptogenetic Of obscure origin.

cryptolith A calculus in a crypt or pit of a structure.

cryptomenorrhea Monthly occurrence of the
signs of menstruation without a flow of blood, as in
imperforate hymen.

cryptomerorachischisis See spina bifida occulta.

cryptophthalmos Congenital anomaly marked
by the absence of eyelids; the skin is continuous
from the forehead to the cheek over a rudimentary
eye.

cryptorchid 1. Relating to an undescended testis.
2. An individual whose testis or testes have not
descended into the scrotum.

cryptorchidectomy Surgical removal of an undescended testis.

cryptorchidism, cryptorchism Condition in
which the descent of a testis is arrested at some point
in its normal path into the scrotum; the testis may
be situated anywhere between the renal and scrotal

areas.

cryptosporidiosis Infection with cryptosporidia,
usually characterized by diarrhea; most commonly
seen in immunocompromised individuals; milder
self-limited disease may be seen in immunocompetent individuals.

Cryptosporidium A genus of parasitic protozoans
(family Eimeriidae) found in the intestinal tract of
many animals and humans.

cryptozoite A stage in the cycle of the malarial
parasite, when it exists in bodily tissue, usually the
liver parenchyma, prior to entering the red blood
cell.

crystal 1. A solid substance composed of atomic
groupings (unit cells) having a geometric form which
is characteristic for different compounds. 2. One
unit cell of such a substance.
   Charcot-Leyden c.'s Elongated crystalline structures formed from eosinophils; found in the sputum
of patients with bronchial asthma. Also called Charcot-Neumann crystals.
   Charcot-Neumann c.'s See Charcot-Leyden
crystals.

crystalline 1. Transparent; clear. 2. Relating to or
made of crystal or composed of crystals.

crystallization Spontaneous grouping of the molecules of a substance into an orderly repetitive pattern; change in form to a solid phase, as when a
solute precipitates from solution.

crystallography The study of the structure and
phenomena of crystals.
   x-ray c. A technique for the three-dimensional
mapping of substances, too small to be viewed even
through an electron microscope, through the use of
x-ray diffraction techniques.

crystalloid 1. Resembling a crystal. 2. A noncolloidal substance which, when in solution, can diffuse
through a semipermeable membrane and is generally capable of being crystallized.
   c. of Charcot-Böttcher A slender crystal-shaped
inclusion peculiar to the Sertoli cell of the seminiferous epithelium.

crystalluria The presence of crystals in the urine.

cubital Of or relating to the forearm or to the ulna.

cubitus The elbow; the joint between the arm and
forearm.

cue A perceived stimulus to which a person responds.

cuff Bandlike structure surrounding a part.
   rotator c. A supportive structure covering the upper part of the shoulder joint capsule; formed by
tendons of four muscles (supraspinous, infraspinous,
teres minor, subscapular).

cul-de-sac *pl.* **culs-de-sac** A pouch or sac.
   conjunctival c. The recess, upper or lower,

formed by the junction of the ocular and palpebral
conjunctiva.
   c. of Douglas The peritoneal cavity between the
posterior wall of the uterus and the anterior wall of
the rectum. Currently called rectouterine pouch.

culdocentesis Aspiration of pus or any fluid
from the rectouterine pouch (cul-de-sac of Douglas)
through a transvaginal puncture.

culdoscope A lighted instrument used for the
visual examination of the pelvic cavity and its contents.

culdoscopy Viewing of the pelvic cavity and organs by introduction of an instrument (culdoscope)
through the posterior wall of the vagina.

Culex A genus of mosquitoes, including some species which carry and transmit several disease-causing
agents.
   C. pipiens The common house mosquito.
   C. tarsalis The mosquito that transmits St. Louis
and western equine encephalomyelitis.

culicide Any agent that kills mosquitoes.

culicifuge An agent that drives away mosquitoes
and gnats.

Cullen's sign Blue discoloration of the skin
around the navel as a result of intraperitoneal hemorrhage, as in ruptured ectopic pregnancy.

culture 1. The propagation of microorganisms in
a nutrient medium. 2. A colony of microorganisms
grown in a nutrient medium.
   pure c. A culture in which all the microorganisms are of one species.
   tissue c. The growth and maintenance of tissue
cells in vitro after removal from the body.

cum (c̄) Latin meaning with; used in prescription
writing.
   c. correction (CC) Latin for with correction; in
ophthalmology, wearing prescribed lenses.

cumulus oophorus A mass of granulosa (follicular) cells surrounding the developing ovum in the
ovarian follicle.

cuneate Wedge-shaped.

cuneiform Wedge-shaped.

cuneus *pl.* **cunei** The posterior portion of the
occipital lobe of each cerebral hemisphere.

cuniculus The burrow made in the skin by the
itch mite.

cunnilingus Oral stimulation of the vulva or clitoris.

cunnus Latin for vulva.

cup A cuplike structure.
   eye c. A small oblong cup that fits on the orbit;
used for the application of a medicated liquid or
wash to the eye. Also called eye bath.
   glaucomatous c. A deep depression of the optic
disk, occurring in glaucoma due to increased intra-

cupula of pleura

uterine curettage

mesiolingual cusp
mesiobuccal cusp
distolingual cusp
distal cusp
distobuccal cusp

endometrium

spinal curvature

curve of Spee

cuspid

heart of 30 day old embryo

atrioventricular endocardial cushions

atrioventricular canal

---

ocular pressure.

physiologic c. A normal depression on the surface of the optic disk.

cupola See cupula.

cupping 1. Formation of a cup-shaped depression. 2. Application of a cupping glass (glass vessel from which air has been exhausted) to the skin in order to draw blood to the surface.

c. of the optic disk Exaggerated depression at the center of the optic disk, as seen in glaucoma.

cupric Relating to or containing divalent copper.

c. sulfate Deep blue crystals used as irritant, astringent, and fungicide. Also called copper sulfate; blue vitriol.

cupula A dome-shaped structure. Also called cupola.

c. cristae ampullaris A gelatinous mass over the crista of the ampulla of the semicircular canal containing tufts of cilia from the underlying hair cells.

c. of pleura The domelike peak of the pleural sac covering the apex of the lung and located near the neck. Also called cervical pleura.

curare A resinous substance obtained from *Strychnos toxifera* and other plants, used as a poison on arrows; death results from paralysis of the muscles of respiration unless artificial respiration is provided; used medicinally, it is administered systemically as an effective muscle relaxant, acting by blocking nerve impulses at the myoneural junction.

curarization The administration of curare or related compounds to produce muscular relaxation or paralysis.

curarize To administer curare or related compounds to induce motor, but not sensory, paralysis.

curative 1. Serving to cure. 2. A remedy.

curd The coagulated part of milk.

cure 1. To restore to health. 2. A method of treatment or a remedy. 3. In dentistry, the procedure by which a plastic material (as that of a denture base) is hardened.

faith c. Cure based upon prayer.

radical c. A cure that completely eradicates a condition.

rest c. The treatment of a mental disorder by rest and change of environment.

curet See curette.

curettage Surgical scraping of the interior of a cavity with a curette to remove growths or diseased tissue, or to obtain tissue for examination (biopsy).

fractional c. Separate curettage of the uterine lining (endometrium) and the endocervix for diagnostic evaluation.

periapial c. Removal of diseased tissue surrounding the root of a tooth.

uterine c. Curettage of the uterus. See also D and C.

curette A spoon-shaped surgical instrument used to scrape the walls of a body cavity. Also written curet.

curie (Ci, c) A unit of radioactivity expressed in terms of particles emitted per second; one curie of a radioactive substance emits 37,000,000,000 particles per second; this value was established from what was originally thought to be the disintegration rate of 1 g of radium.

curium A synthetic radioactive element; symbol Cm, atomic number 96, atomic weight 247.

current A steady onward movement, as of water or electricity.

alternating c. (AC) An electric current that reverses direction of flow at regular intervals.

c. of injury The current that passes through a conductor connecting the injured and the uninjured portions of a nerve or other excitable tissue.

direct c. (DC) An electric current that flows in one direction only.

high frequency c. An alternating electric current having a frequency of at least 10,000 cycles per second.

stabile c. A current applied with both electrodes placed in a fixed position.

curvature A bending or curving.

greater c. of the stomach The left and inferior borders of the stomach.

lesser c. of the stomach The right border of the stomach.

spinal c. Deviation of the spine.

curve 1. A line that deviates from a straight course in a smooth, continuous, nonangular manner. 2. A line representing plotted data on a graph.

c. of Spee A curve formed by the upper dental arch meeting with the lower dental arch viewed buccally from the first bicuspid to the last molar.

distribution c. A curve in which the number of individuals is plotted along the ordinate and the property under investigation is plotted along the abscissa.

dye-dilution c. Indicator-dilution curve; a curve indicating the serial concentrations of a dye.

frequency c. A curve representing an approximation of the rate of occurrences of a periodic event. Also called gaussian or probability curve.

gaussian c. See frequency curve.

indicator-dilution c. See dye-dilution curve.

Price-Jones c. A curve representing variations in the diameters of red blood cells.

probability c. See frequency curve.

Starling c. A curve indicating cardiac output against atrial pressure.

strength-duration c. A curve indicating the re-

lationship between the intensity of an electrical stimulus and the time it must flow to be effective.

stress-strain c. A curve showing the ratio of deformation to load during testing of a material under tension.

cushingoid Having the characteristics of Cushing syndrome or disease; may also be caused by corticosteroid therapy.

Cushing's disease Adrenocortical overactivity caused by excessive secretion of pituitary adrenocorticotropic hormone (ACTH).

Cushing's syndrome A metabolic disorder caused by chronic excess of glucocorticoids; characterized by a round face, central obesity, prominent dorsal fat pad, florid complexion, abdominal striae, hypertension, and impaired carbohydrate tolerance among other findings.

cushion Any anatomic structure resembling a pad.

atrioventricular canal c.'s See atrioventricular endocardial cushions.

atrioventricular endocardial c.'s A pair of apposing masses of mesenchymal tissue in the embryonic heart; they appear at the superior and inferior borders of the atrioventricular canal in a 6 mm embryo; they grow together and fuse, dividing the canal into right and left atrioventricular orifices. Also called atrioventricular canal cushions.

Passavant's c. See ridge, Passavant's.

cusp 1. One of the triangular segments of a heart's valve. 2. A pronounced elevation on the occlusal surface (grinding surface) of a tooth.

cuspid A tooth having one cusp or point; one of the four anterior teeth situated between the upper and lower incisors and bicuspids; used primarily for biting and tearing; the longest and most stable tooth in the mouth. Also called canine or dog tooth; an upper cuspid is also called eye tooth.

cuspidor In dentistry, a bowl-shaped vessel adjacent to a dental chair, used for spitting into. Also called spittoon.

cut 1. To dilute; to reduce or adulterate the strength of, such as to adulterate heroin with milk sugar (lactose) or quinine. 2. Medical colloquialism meaning to operate.

cutaneous Relating to the skin.

cutdown A small opening over a vein to facilitate introduction of a needle or a cannula into the vessel.

cuticle 1. The epidermis. 2. The thin fold of skin overlying the base of a fingernail or toenail.

cuticularization The formation of skin over an abraded area.

cutis vera True skin or dermis. Also called corium.

cutter An instrument or tool for cutting.

vitreous infusion surgical c. (VISC) A miniatur-

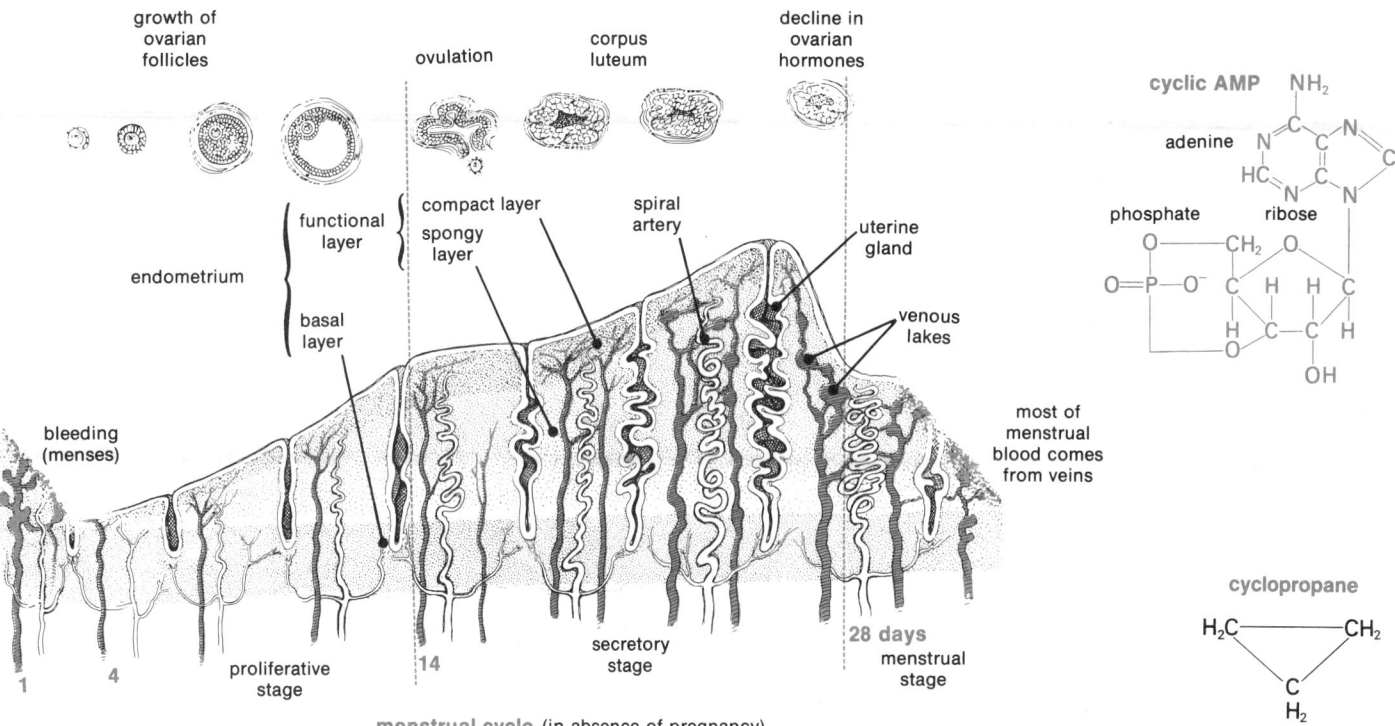

growth of ovarian follicles

ovulation

corpus luteum

decline in ovarian hormones

cyclic AMP

adenine

phosphate   ribose

endometrium

functional layer

compact layer

spongy layer

spiral artery

uterine gland

venous lakes

basal layer

bleeding (menses)

most of menstrual blood comes from veins

cyclopropane

proliferative stage

secretory stage

28 days

menstrual stage

menstrual cycle (in absence of pregnancy)

ized surgical instrument used in closed vitrectomy to enter the back of the eye through a minute incision and remove a portion of the vitreous body; it consists of a miniature assembly which simultaneously provides light to view the interior of the eye, cuts and sucks out tissue, and pours in a sterile solution.

cuvet, cuvette A glass container in which solutions are placed for photometric study.

cyanate A salt of cyanic acid.

cyanide Any of a group of compounds of hydrocyanic acid containing the radical –Cn or ion (CN)⁻.

  mercuric c. An extremely poisonous compound, $Hg(CN)_2$; used as an antiseptic.

  potassium c. An extremely poisonous compound, KCN; used as a reagent, fumigant, and insecticide.

cyanmethemoglobin Cyanide methemoglobin; a compound of cyanide with methemoglobin.

cyanocobalamin A substance having hematopoietic properties; used in the treatment of pernicious anemia. Also called vitamin B_{12}.

cyanophil, cyanophile Any cell or tissue element readily stainable with blue dyes.

cyanopsia A defect of vision in which all objects seem to be tinted blue.

cyanopsin A photosensitive substance, thought to have a spectral sensitivity similar to that of the cones of the retina of some animals.

cyanose tardive Term applied to the potentially cyanotic group of congenital heart diseases with an abnormal communication between systemic and pulmonary circulation; cyanosis is absent while the shunt is from left to right, but if the shunt reverses, as after exercise or late in the course of the disease, cyanosis appears. Also called delayed cyanosis.

cyanosis Bluish discoloration of the skin, lips, and nail beds caused by insufficient oxygen in the blood; it appears when the reduced hemoglobin in the small vessels is 5 g per 100 ml or more.

cyanotic Relating to or characterized by cyanosis.

cybernetics The comparative study of biologic and mechanoelectric systems of automatic control, such as the nervous system and electronic computers, for the purpose of explaining the nature of the brain.

cyclarthrodial Of or relating to a rotary joint.

cyclarthrosis A rotary joint.

cycle A time interval in which a regularly repeated sequence of events takes place.

  anovulatory c. A sexual cycle in which no ovum is produced.

  brain wave c. The complete series of changes in amplitude of a wave of the electroencephalogram before repetition occurs.

carbon dioxide c., carbon c. The natural processes through which carbon in the atmosphere, in the form of carbon dioxide, is converted into carbohydrates by photosynthesis, metabolized by living organisms, and ultimately returned to the atmosphere, again as carbon dioxide.

  cardiac c. The complete round of events that occur, in the heart with each beat.

  citric acid c. See tricarboxylic acid cycle.

  estrous c. The periodic series of physiologic changes that occur under the influence of sex hormones in higher animals.

  exogenous c. The phase in the development of a parasite spent in the body of the invertebrate host, as of the malarial parasite in the body of a mosquito.

  Krebs c. See tricarboxylic acid cycle.

  life c. The entire life of an organism.

  menstrual c. The periodic changes that take place in the female reproductive organs; the period in which an ovum matures, is ovulated, and enters the lumen of the uterus through the uterine tube; ovarian hormonal secretions effect endometrial changes such that, if fertilization occurs, nidation will be possible; in the absence of fertilization, ovarian secretions wane, the endometrium sloughs, and menstruation begins.

  nitrogen c. The continuous process in which nitrogen is deposited in the soil, assimilated by bacteria and plants, transferred to animals, and returned to the soil.

  ovarian c. The normal periodic changes that take place in the ovary during the production and discharge of an ovum.

  reproductive c. The series of physiologic changes that takes place in the female reproductive organs from the time of conception to delivery.

  tricarboxylic acid c. A series of enzymatic reactions involving the complete oxidation of acetyl units, providing the main source of energy in the mammalian body and taking place mostly during respiration. Also called Krebs or citric acid cycle.

  urea c. The series of chemical reactions that occur in the liver, resulting in the production of urea.

cyclectomy Surgical removal of a portion of the ciliary body.

cyclic Occurring periodically.

cyclic AMP Adenosine-3′,5′-cyclic monophosphate; ubiquitous in nature and the mediator of hormone actions in mammals. Also called genetic regulator.

cyclic GMP 3′,5′-Guanosine cyclic monophosphate; a nucleotide that serves as a second messenger, playing a role complementary to cyclic AMP's in regulating intracellular processes, one nucleotide promoting those the other inhibits; when the cyclic

GMP level goes up, the cyclic AMP level goes down and vice versa.

cyclitis Inflammation of the ciliary body.

  plastic c. Severe cyclitis with exudation of a material rich in fibrin that accumulates in the anterior and posterior chambers.

  purulent c. Acute cyclitis with a copious discharge of pus, usually involving the iris and choroid.

  serous c. Simple cyclitis with a relatively fluid discharge.

cyclizine hydrochloride An antihistamine used in preventing and relieving symptoms of motion sickness and postoperative nausea and vomiting; also relieves vertigo and other symptoms caused by vestibular disorders of the ear; Marezine®.

cyclochoroiditis Inflammation of the ciliary body and the choroid layer of the eye.

cyclodialysis The surgical creation of an opening between the anterior chamber of the eye and the suprachoroidal space to reduce intraocular pressure in glaucoma.

cyclodiathermy The partial destruction of the ciliary body by the application of heat for the reduction of intraocular pressure in the treatment of glaucoma.

cycloid 1. In psychiatry, a personality characterized by alternating states of elation and depression. 2. Resembling cyclothymia.

cyclokeratitis Inflammation of the ciliary body and the cornea.

cyclophoria Tendency of one eye to deviate on its anteroposterior axis.

cyclophorometer Instrument used to measure cyclophoria.

cyclophosphamide A white crystalline powder used as an antitumor agent; Cytoxan®.

cycloplegia Paralysis of the ciliary muscle and loss of the power of accommodation.

cycloplegic 1. Relating to paralysis of the ciliary muscle of the eye. 2. An agent that causes paralysis of the ciliary muscle.

cyclopropane A colorless, inflammable, explosive gas, C_3H_6; used as a general anesthetic. Also called trimethylene.

cyclosporine An immunosuppressive drug used in organ transplantation; it selectively inhibits T lymphocytes. Formerly called cyclosporin A.

cyclothymia Cyclic fluctuations of mood between elation and mild depression.

cyclotomy Surgical incision of the ciliary muscle of the eye.

cyesis Pregnancy.

cylinder (cyl) 1. A cylindrical lens. 2. A rodlike renal cast.

cylindroid A cylindrical mass in the urine resembling a hyaline cast. Also called mucous cast.

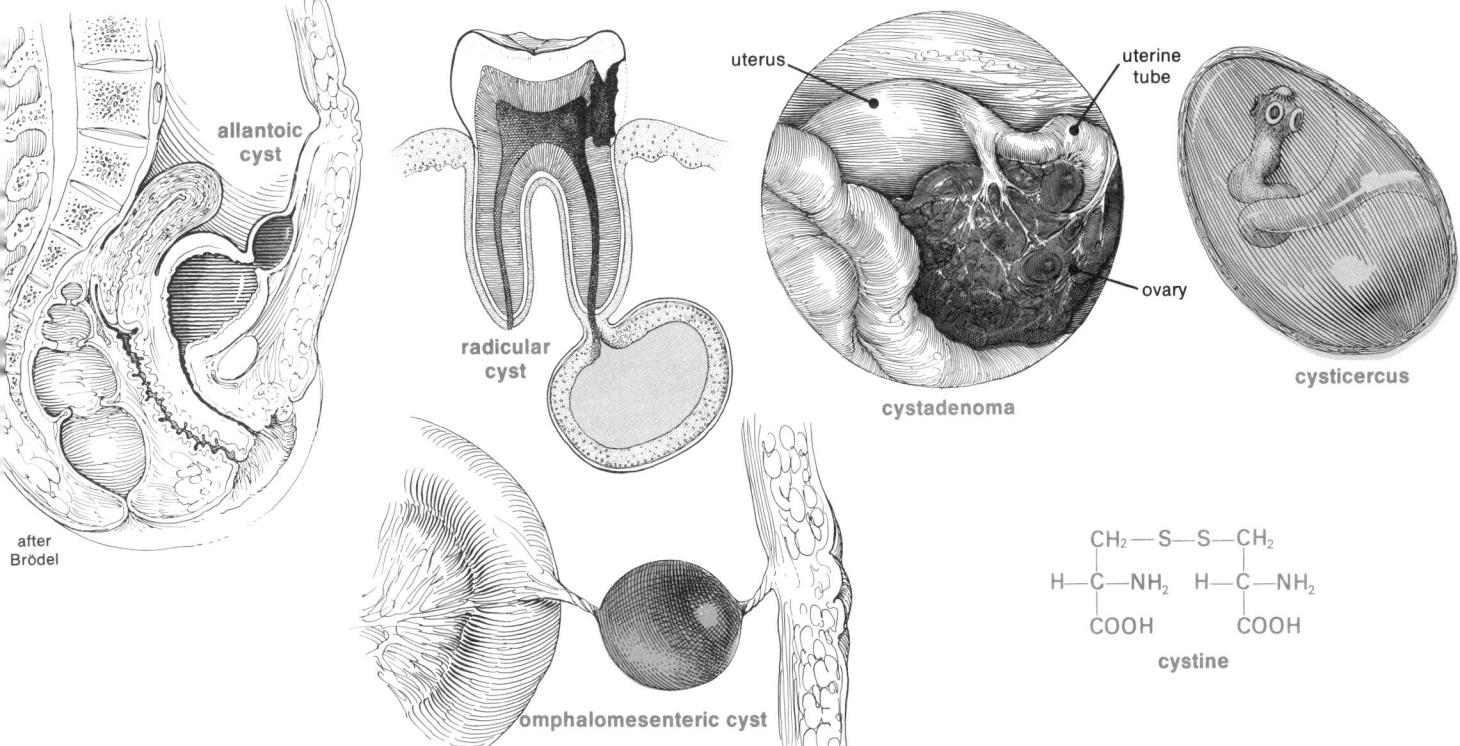

allantoic cyst

after Brödel

radicular cyst

uterus / uterine tube / ovary

cystadenoma

cysticercus

omphalomesenteric cyst

$$CH_2 - S - S - CH_2$$
$$H - C - NH_2 \quad H - C - NH_2$$
$$COOH \qquad COOH$$

cystine

cylindroma A relatively benign epithelial tumor appearing as multiple nodules, especially on the scalp and face.

cylindruria The presence of casts in the urine.

cynophobia Exaggerated fear of dogs.

cypridopathy Any venereal disease.

cypridophobia Abnormal fear of venereal disease or of sexual intercourse.

cyst 1. An abnormal sac within the body containing air or fluid. 2. A bladder.

allantoic c. A cystic dilation of the urachus. Also called urachal cyst.

alveolodental c. A cyst associated with an unerupted tooth, occurring either in the surrounding tissues (extracapsular) or within the developing tooth (intracapsular). Also called odontocele.

Baker's c. A collection of escaped synovial fluid in the tissues outside the knee joint.

Bartholin-gland c. The most common cyst of the vulva, resulting from retention of glandular secretions due to a blocked duct.

branchial c. A cyst resulting from the nonclosure of a bronchial cleft.

bursal c. A retention cyst in a bursa.

chocolate c. A cyst of the ovary containing a thick dark brown tenacious fluid; often seen in endometriosis. Also called Sampson cyst.

corpus luteum c. A cyst in the ovary formed from corpus luteum that remains cystic with excessive fluid content instead of regressing normally; commonly associated with disturbance of or delay in menstruation.

dermoid c. A common tumor of the ovary, usually bilateral, consisting of displaced ectodermal tissues; it has thick, bluish white, smooth walls with sebaceous and hairy contents.

dilatation c. See retention cyst.

distention c. See retention cyst.

echinococcus c. Hydatid cyst.

ependymal c. Cystic dilatation of the central canal of the spinal cord or of the cerebral ventricles. Also called neural cyst.

hydatid c. One formed, usually in the liver, by the larval stage of the tapeworm.

lacteal c. Milk cyst; a retention cyst in the breast resulting from obstruction of a lactiferous duct.

meibomian c. See chalazion.

milk c. See lacteal cyst.

mother c. The main echinococcus cyst containing smaller daughter cysts.

mucous c. Retention cyst resulting from closure of the duct of a mucous gland.

nabothian c. Retention cyst resulting from obstruction of a mucous gland of the uterine cervix. Also called nabothian follicle.

neural c. See ependymal cyst.

omphalomesenteric duct c. A cystic dilatation along the remnant of the embryonic omphalomesenteric (vitelline) duct.

ovarian c. Cystic tumor of the ovary.

periapical c. See radicular cyst.

piliferous c. Dermoid cyst containing hair.

pilonidal c. A hair-containing cyst in the dermis or subcutaneous tissues, usually connected to the surface of the skin by a sinus tract; generally situated in the sacrococcygeal region. Also called sacrococcygeal cyst.

pseudomucinous c. One containing a gelatinous material.

radicular c. One around the root of a nonvital tooth. Also called root or periapical cyst.

retention c. One resulting from obstruction of the duct of a gland. Also called dilatation, distention, or secretory cyst.

root c. See radicular cyst.

Sampson's c. See chocolate cyst.

sebaceous c. Tumor resulting from retention of the excretion of a sebaceous gland. Also called wen; steatoma; steatocystoma; sebocystoma; sebaceous tumor.

secretory c. See retention cyst.

serous c. One containing clear serous fluid.

solitary bone c. Cyst lined with a thin layer of connective tissue and containing serous fluid; usually seen in the shaft of a long bone of a child. Also called unicameral cyst; osteocytoma.

sublingual c. See ranula.

subsynovial c. Distention of a synovial follicle.

unicameral c. See solitary bone cyst.

urachal c. See allantoic cyst.

cystadenocarcinoma A malignant tumor derived from glandular epithelium, most frequently occurring as a partially solid mass with a cystic pattern; seen chiefly in the ovaries.

cystadenoma A cystic neoplasm lined with epithelial cells and filled with retained secretions.

papillary c. lymphomatosum A rare benign tumor of salivary gland origin; seen chiefly in the region of the parotid gland. Also called Warthin's tumor; adenolymphoma.

cystalgia Pain in the bladder.

cystathionine An intermediate in the conversion of methionine to cysteine.

cystathioninuria A rare, inherited disorder of amino acid metabolism resulting in an excessive secretion of cystathionine in the urine; associated with mental retardation.

cystectasia, cystectasy Dilatation of the bladder.

cystectomy Surgical removal of a portion of the urinary bladder.

cysteine (Cys) An amino acid, $C_3H_7NO_2S$, present in most proteins.

cystic 1. Relating to a cyst. 2. Relating to the gallbladder or urinary bladder.

cystic disease of breast See fibrocystic disease of breast.

cystic disease of renal medulla The presence of multiple cysts in the medulla of the kidney, seen primarily in two clinical syndromes: uremic medullary cystic disease (nephronophthisis) and sponge kidney (non-uremic medullary cystic disease); the former is an inherited disease in which medullary cysts are associated with glomerulosclerosis, interstitial fibrosis, and renal failure, often appearing in childhood; the latter is a relatively benign condition, usually diagnosed by intravenous pyelography, which may be associated with calculi or infections.

cysticercosis Infestation with the larvae of the cestode *Taenia solium* (pork tapeworm).

cysticercus The cystic or larval form of the tapeworm, consisting of a scolex or head enclosed in a fluid-filled sac or cyst.

cystic fibrosis of pancreas Congenital hereditary disease marked by dysfunction of any of the exocrine glands, resulting in a striking increase in the sodium and potassium concentration of sweat and overproduction of viscid mucus, which causes obstruction of the structures involved (pancreatic and bile ducts, intestines, and bronchi); it affects principally infants and children; common forms include meconium ileus in the newborn and chronic pulmonary disease and pancreatic insufficiency in older children. Also called mucoviscidosis; fibrocystic disease of pancreas.

cysticotomy Surgical incision into the cystic duct.

cystiform Resembling a cyst.

cystine A sulfur-containing amino acid present in many proteins.

cystinosis Failure of normal cystine (amino acid) metabolism due to a genetically determined enzyme deficiency; the cystine accumulates and precipitates widely in many tissues, including the renal tubular epithelium and bone marrow; one of many causes of Fanconi syndrome.

cystinuria 1. The presence of cystine in the urine. 2. A hereditary defect in renal tubular reabsorption of the amino acids (cystine, lysine, arginine, and ornithine), resulting in recurrent kidney stone formation.

cystitis Inflammation of the urinary bladder.

interstitial c. Nonbacterial chronic cystitis; it produces pain and an urge to void.

cystitomy 1. Capsulotomy. 2. Cystotomy. 3. Cholecystotomy.

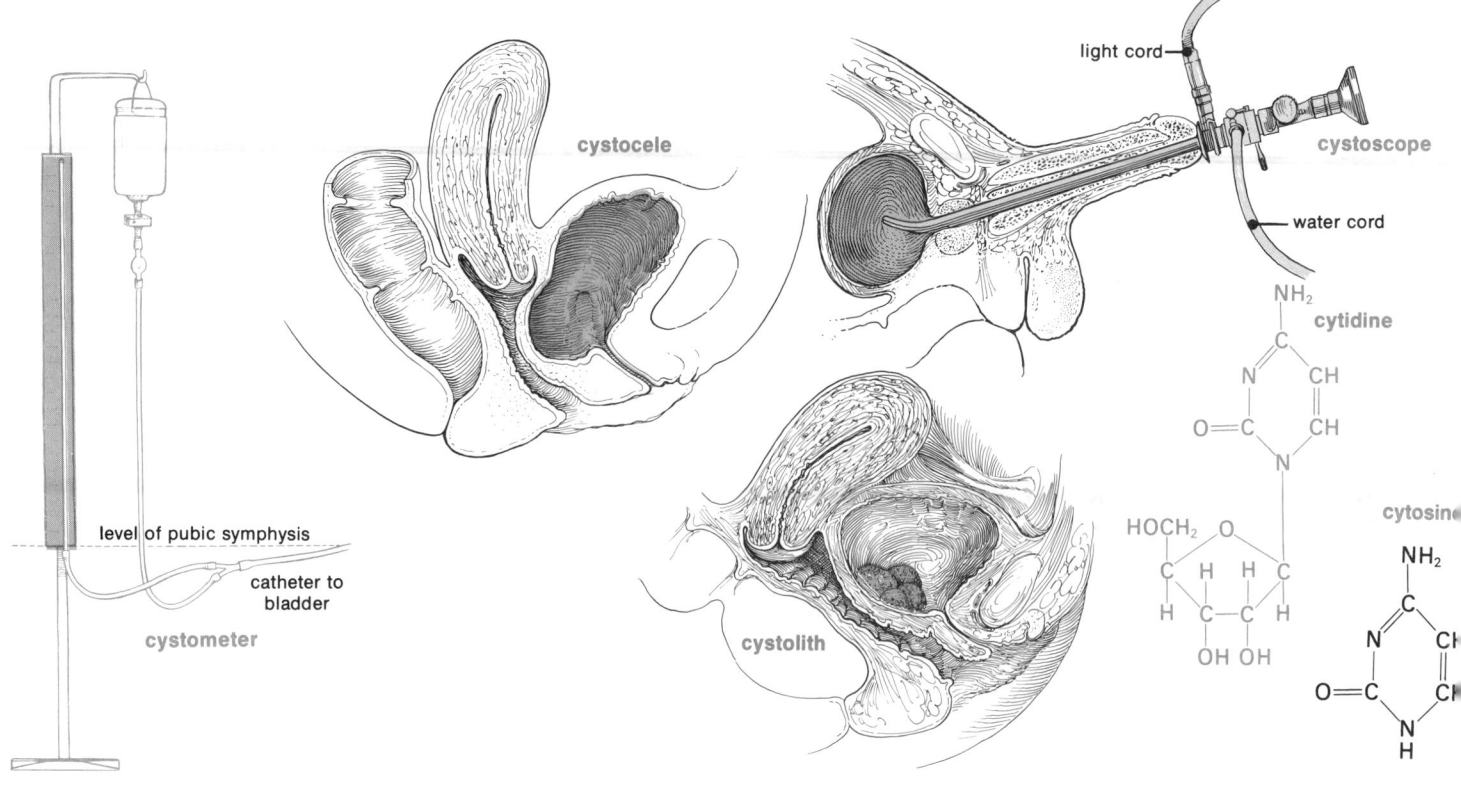

cystocele

cystoscope

cystoscope

water cord

light cord

cytidine

cytosine

level of pubic symphysis

catheter to bladder

cystometer

cystolith

cystocele Hernia formed by the downward and backward displacement of the urinary bladder toward the vaginal orifice, due most commonly to weakening of the musculature during childbirth. Also called vesicocele.

cystogram X-ray picture of the bladder, obtained after instilling radiopaque fluid into it through a catheter.

cystography Roentgenography of the bladder after introduction of a radiopaque fluid.

cystoid 1. Resembling a cyst. 2. A collection of soft material resembling a cyst, but without an enclosing capsule.

cystolith A bladder stone.

cystolithectomy Surgical removal of a bladder stone; erroneously used when referring to the removal of a gallbladder stone. Also called cystolithotomy.

cystolithiasis The presence of bladder stones.

cystolithic Of or relating to a bladder stone.

cystolithotomy See cystolithectomy.

cystoma A tumor containing cysts.

cystometer A diagnostic device that measures the tone of the detrusor muscle in the wall of the urinary bladder in relation to the volume of fluid in the bladder.

cystometrogram A graphic record of the pressure within the urinary bladder.

cystometry The continuous recording of the pressures within the urinary bladder by means of a cystometer; the procedure is used for determining the tone of the bladder when neurologic disturbance of the bladder wall is suspected.

cystoplasty Surgical repair of the bladder.

cystoplegia Paralysis of the bladder.

cystoptosia, cystoptosis Prolapse of a portion of the mucous membrane of the bladder into the urethra.

cystopyelitis Inflammation of the bladder and of the pelvis of the kidney.

cystorrhagia Bleeding from the bladder.

cystorrhea Discharge of mucus from the bladder. Also called vesical catarrh.

cystoscope A tubular instrument fitted with a light for examining the interior of the urinary bladder.

cystoscopy Visual examination of the interior of the urinary bladder by means of a cystoscope.

cystospasm Spasmodic contraction of the bladder.

cystostomy A temporary opening made into the bladder in order to divert urine from the urethra.

cystotomy Surgical incision of the urinary bladder. Also called vesicotomy.

cystoureteritis Inflammation of the bladder and a ureter or ureters.

cystourethritis Inflammation of the bladder and urethra.

cystourethrocele Prolapse of female urethra and neck of bladder.

cytidine A nucleoside consisting of cytosine attached through a β-glycosidic linkage to ribose.

cytoanalyzer A machine used to screen smears containing cells suspected of malignancy.

cytoarchitecture The arrangement of cells in a tissue, especially of the cerebral cortex.

cytobiology Cell biology.

cytocentrum Centrosome.

cytochemistry A branch of cell biology devoted to the chemical and physicochemical analysis of living matter.

cytochrome A respiratory enzyme capable of undergoing alternate reduction and oxidation; chemically related to hemoglobin.

  c. oxidase The terminal enzyme in the chain of events that constitutes cellular oxygen consumption.

  c. P-450 Pigment involved in extramitochondrial transport of electrons in the liver and in mixed function oxidation reactions; important in the metabolism of many drugs; found in adrenal mitochondria and in liver microsomes; so named because the CO compound of the reduced cytochrome has an absorption maximum of 450 nanometers.

cytocide Destructive to cells.

cytoclasis The fragmentation of cells.

cytocyst The remains of a cell enclosing a schizont (malarial parasite undergoing asexual division).

cytodendrite Dendrite.

cytodiagnosis Diagnosis of disease based on the study of cells.

cytogenesis The origin of cells.

cytogenetics The combined study of heredity and the structure and function of cells.

cytokines Any of several hormone-like factors which act as intercellular messengers to regulate many cell functions, especially those concerned with immunologic and inflammatory responses; produced by a variety of cell types, e.g., lymphocytes, macrophages, platelets, fibroblasts, and keratinocytes.

cytology Cell biology; the science concerned with the study of cells.

  exfoliative c. Examination, for the purpose of diagnosis, of cells recovered from secretions, exudate, or washings of a tissue, such as sputum, vaginal secretion, gastric washings, etc.

cytolysin An antibody that is capable of causing the dissolution of an animal cell.

cytolysis The destruction of a cell.

cytomegalic Characterized by greatly enlarged cells.

cytomegalic inclusion disease A viral infection presenting symptoms according to the organs affected; formerly believed to affect only children, but seen now in adults with debilitating diseases; caused by a cytomegalovirus.

cytomegalovirus (CMV) One of a group of highly specific human herpesviruses causing intranuclear inclusions and enlargement of cells of various organs; in humans, it causes cytomegalic inclusion disease. Also called herpesvirus 4.

cytometer A device used for counting and measuring blood cells.

cytomorphology The study of the configuration of cells.

cytopathic Characterized by a diseased condition of cells.

cytopathogenic Capable of producing a diseased condition in cells.

cytopathology The study and interpretation of cellular changes as an aid in diagnosing disease.

cytopenia Diminution of the cellular elements in the blood.

cytophagy The devouring or ingestion of cells by other cells (phagocytes).

cytophotometry The measuring of light absorbed by, or emitted from, stained cells or intracellular structures.

  flow c. Enumeration and separation of cells on the basis of their size and fluorescence intensity.

cytoplasm The protoplasm or substance of a cell surrounding the nucleus, carrying structures within which most of the life processes of the cell take place.

cytopoiesis The development of cells.

cytosine A pyrimidine base, $C_4H_5N_3O$; a disintegration product of nucleic acid.

cytosis 1. The presence of more than the usual number of cells. 2. Term used with a prefix to denote certain characteristics of cells.

cytosmear Cytologic smear; see under smear.

cytosol The soluble portion of the cytoplasm after all the particles, such as mitochondrial and endoplasmic reticular components, are removed.

cytosome The cell body without the nucleus.

cytostome The opening that serves as a mouth in certain complex protozoa.

cytotaxis, cytotaxia The movement of a cell toward or away from another cell in response to a specific stimulus.

cytotoxic Damaging to cells. Also called cytolytic.

cytotoxin An antibody that destroys or inhibits the functions of cells.

cytotrophoblast The inner, cellular, layer of the trophoblast developed from the single-layered trophoblast at the time of implantation of the blastocyst.

cytotropic Having an affinity for cells.

cytozoic Living in a cell.

cytozoon A protozoan parasitic in a cell.

frontal bone

dacryon

maxillary bone

lacrimal bone

ocular orbit

dacryocystitis

Datura stramonium

DDT

δ   Delta. For terms beginning with δ, see under specific term.

dacryadenitis   See dacryoadenitis.

dacryagogue   **1.** Promoting the flow of tears. **2.** Any agent that induces the lacrimal gland to secrete tears.

dacryoadenalgia   Pain or discomfort in a lacrimal gland.

dacryoadenitis   Inflammation of the lacrimal gland. Also called dacryadenitis.

dacryoblennorrhea   A chronic discharge of mucus from the lacrimal ducts, as in chronic dacryocystitis. Also called dacryocystoblennorrhea.

dacryocyst   The lacrimal sac.

dacryocystalgia   Pain or discomfort in a lacrimal sac.

dacryocystectomy   Surgical removal of the lacrimal sac.

dacryocystitis   Inflammation of the lacrimal sac, usually due to obstruction of the nasolacrimal duct; most often seen in infants and in menopausal women.

dacryocystocele   Protrusion of the lacrimal sac. Also called dacryocele.

dacryocystogram   An x-ray image of the lacrimal apparatus obtained after injection with a radiopaque substance.

dacryocystorhinostenosis   Narrowing of the nasolacrimal duct, obstructing the normal flow of tears to the nasal cavity.

dacryocystorhinostomy   The operative creation of a passage between the lacrimal sac and the nose to effect the drainage of tears when the nasolacrimal duct is occluded.

dacryocystotomy   Surgical incision of the lacrimal sac.

dacryohemorrhea   The shedding of tears mixed with blood.

dacryolith   A calculus or stone in the lacrimal apparatus (tear-forming and tear-conducting structures). Also called tear stone.

dacryolithiasis   The presence of calculi (dacryoliths) in the lacrimal passage.

dacryoma   **1.** A cyst caused by obstruction of the lacrimal duct. **2.** A tumor of the lacrimal apparatus.

dacryon   A cranial point where the lacrimal, frontal, and maxillary bones meet at the angle of the ocular orbit.

dacryops   **1.** A watery condition of the eye; the constant presence of excess tear fluid on the eye due to poor drainage caused by constriction of the lacrimal punctum. **2.** Dilatation of a lacrimal duct by contained fluid.

dacryopyorrhea   The shedding of tears containing pus.

dacryopyosis   Formation or discharge of pus in the lacrimal sac or duct.

dacryorrhea   An excessive flow of tears.

dacryosolenitis   Inflammation of the lacrimal or nasal duct.

dacryostenosis   Stricture of any lacrimal passage.

dactinomycin   An antineoplastic agent used in the treatment of Wilms' tumor in children and trophoblastic disease in women.

dactyl   A digit; a finger or toe.

dactylalgia   Pain in the fingers or toes.

dactyledema   Edema of a finger.

dactylitis   Inflammation of a digit.

dactylocampsis   Permanent flexion or bending of the fingers or toes.

dactylography   The study of fingerprints.

dactylogryposis   Contraction of the fingers or toes.

dactyloid   Finger-shaped.

dactylology   Use of the finger alphabet as a means of communication, as by deaf-mutes.

dactylolysis   **1.** Surgical correction of fused or webbed fingers or toes. **2.** Loss of a finger or toe.

   d. spontanea   Spontaneous loss of a digit; thought to be associated with the sickle-cell trait.

dactylomegaly   A condition in which fingers or toes are abnormally large. Also called macrodactylia.

dactyloscopy   The examination of fingerprints for purposes of personal identification.

dactylospasm   Spasmodic contraction of the fingers.

dactylus   A finger or a toe; usually a toe, as distinguished from digitus, a finger.

Dalrymple's sign   Abnormal wideness of the palpebral fissures, occurring in exophthalmic goiter.

dalton   A unit of molecular weight equivalent to the weight of a hydrogen atom; a water molecule weighs 18 daltons and a hemoglobin molecule weighs 64,500 daltons; the terms dalton and molecular weight are used interchangeably.

dam   A barrier preventing the flow of fluid; especially a thin rubber sheet used in dentistry and surgery to isolate the operative field from the access of bodily fluid. Also called rubber-dam.

   coffer d.   A thin sheet of rubber stretched around the neck of a tooth to keep it dry during dental restoration.

D and C   Abbreviation for dilatation and curettage; dilatation of the uterine cervix and scraping of the lining of the uterus (endometrium) with a curette.

dander   Dry skin shed by animals (dogs, cats, etc.); the cause of allergy in certain persons.

dandruff   Common name for the mild form of seborrheic dermatitis; see under dermatitis.

Dandy-Walker syndrome   Congenital hydrocephalus in infants due to obstruction or atresia of the median aperture of the fourth ventricle (foramen of Magendi) and the lateral aperture of the fourth ventricle (foramen of Luschka).

dapsone   A compound used in the treatment of leprosy and tuberculosis.

Datura stramonium   A species of an annual herb containing alkaloids that block the parasympathetic nerves. Also called jimsonweed; thorn apple.

daturine   See hyoscyamine.

DDT   Dichlorodiphenyltrichloroethane, a colorless, toxic insecticide.

deacidification   The act of removing or neutralizing an acid.

deactivation   The process of rendering inactive; making harmless or ineffective.

dead   Lifeless.

deaf   Afflicted with deafness; unable to hear.

deafferentation   The suppression or loss of afferent nerve impulses from a portion of the body.

deaf-mute   An individual who can neither hear nor speak.

deafmutism   Inability to speak due to congenital or early deafness.

deafness   Inability to hear, partial or complete.

   acoustic trauma d.   Loss of hearing caused by prolonged exposure to excessive noise.

   cerebral d.   Deafness caused by a lesion in the auditory area of the brain.

   conductive d.   Loss of hearing caused by disease of, or injury to, the tympanic membrane or ear ossicles.

   nerve d.   Deafness caused by damage to the cochlear division of the vestibulocochlear nerve.

   sudden d.   A sudden loss of hearing, thought to be related to systemic diseases including fat metabolism and hypercoagulation (diseases that block the circulation).

   toxic d.   Loss of hearing caused by certain chemical agents.

   word d.   Inability to understand the spoken word. Also called auditory aphasia.

dealcoholization   The removal of alcohol from a substance.

deamidate   To remove the amido group from an organic compound. Also called desamidate; deamidize.

deaminase   An enzyme that promotes the removal of the amino group from amino compounds such as amino acids.

deaminate   To remove, usually by hydrolysis, an amino group from an organic compound.

decarboxylase

$$\underset{\text{lysine}}{H_2C-CH_2-CH_2-CH_2-\underset{\overset{|}{NH_2}}{CH}-COOH} \rightarrow \underset{\text{cadaverine}}{H_2C-CH_2-CH_2-CH_2-\underset{\overset{|}{NH_2}}{CH_2}} + CO_2$$

range of human hearing
in
decibels

130	— jet engine
120	— punch press
110	
100	— rivet hammer
90	
80	— heavy traffic
70	
60	— normal conversation
50	
40	— quiet office
30	
20	— whisper
10	
0	— standard threshold of hearing

decidua vera
uterine cavity
decidua capsularis
chorionic villi
amnion
umbilical cord
embryo
decidua basalis
decidua marginalis
myometrium of uterus

deamination The removal of an amino group (NH₂) from an organic compound. Also called deaminization.

death The cessation of life.

  black d. The worldwide epidemic of the 14th century, believed to be pneumonic plague.

  brain d. Complete and irreversible cessation of cerebral cortex function.

  crib d. Popular name for sudden infant death syndrome.

  maternal d. The death of a woman from any cause while pregnant or within 42 days of termination of pregnancy, irrespective of the duration and the site of pregnancy.

  rapid d. See sudden death.

  sudden d. Death most commonly caused by myocardial infarction, subarachnoid hemorrhage secondary to ruptured aneurysm, intracerebral hemorrhage, rupture of the aorta or other great vessel secondary to trauma, or extradural hematoma. Also called rapid death.

death rattle The gurgling noise rarely heard in the throat of a dying person, caused by loss of the cough reflex and accumulation of mucus.

death struggle The rare signs of the final moments of death: a twitching or convulsion. Also called agony; death throe; psychorrhagia.

debilitate To make weak or feeble; to enervate.

debility The condition of abnormal bodily weakness; lack or loss of strength.

debouch 1. To open or empty into another part. 2. An outlet.

debridement Excision of devitalized tissue and the removal of all foreign matter from a wound surface.

decagram Ten grams.

decalcification 1. The loss of calcium salts from bones or teeth. 2. The removal of calcium ions from the blood to prevent or delay coagulation.

decalcify To remove calcium salts, especially from bones or teeth.

decalcifying 1. Denoting any agent or process that removes calcium salts from bones or teeth. 2. Denoting an agent that removes calcium ion from blood to render it incoagulable.

decaliter A measure of 10 liters; 2.64 gallons; roughly 10 quarts.

decant 1. To pour off the upper clear portion of a fluid without disturbing the sediment. 2. To pour fluid from one bottle into another.

decapitate To remove the head; to behead.

decapsulation The removal of a capsule or enveloping membrane.

decarboxylase Any enzyme that accelerates the removal of carbon dioxide (CO₂) from the carboxyl group of a compound, especially from α-amino acids; e.g., lysine decarboxylase.

decarboxylation Replacing of a carboxyl group from an organic compound, usually with hydrogen.

decay 1. The decomposition of organic compounds as a result of bacterial or fungal action. 2. In physics, spontaneous, progressive decrease of the number of atoms in a radioactive substance.

deceleration Decrease in velocity.

decerebrate 1. To remove the portion of the brain above the lower border of the quadrigeminal bodies. 2. An experimental animal so prepared. 3. A person who has sustained a brain injury which renders him physiologically comparable to a decerebrate animal.

decerebration Removal of a portion of brain in experimental animals.

decerebrize To remove the brain.

decibel (dB, db) A unit for measuring the ratio of two powers or intensities (electric or acoustic power); in measurement of acoustic intensities, it is equal to 10 times the common logarithm of the ratio of two levels of intensity, or to the smallest degree of loudness that is ordinarily heard by the human ear; at a distance of about four feet, an ordinary conversation produces a level of approximately 60 dB (on a scale from 1 to 130).

decidua The mucous membrane (endometrium) lining the uterus that undergoes modification in preparation for and during pregnancy and is cast off at parturition and during menstruation.

  d. basalis The endometrium between the implanted chorionic vesicle and the myometrium of the uterus; it becomes the maternal part of the placenta. Also called decidua serotina.

  d. capsularis The endometrium that seals the implanted chorionic vesicle from the uterine cavity; it undergoes rapid regression from about the fourth month of pregnancy. Also called decidua reflexa.

  d. marginalis The junction between the decidua basalis and the decidua capsularis.

  d. menstrualis The hyperemic endometrial mucosa of the nonpregnant uterus during the menstrual period.

  d. parietalis See decidua vera.

  d. reflexa See decidua capsularis.

  d. serotina See decidua basalis.

  d. vera The entire endometrium lining the uterus, except the parts surrounding the chorionic vesicle. Also called decidua parietalis.

deciduation The casting off of endometrial tissue during menstruation.

deciduoma A mass of decidual tissue in the uterus.

deciduous 1. Temporary; not permanent; denoting that which falls off at the end of a stage of development. 2. In dentistry, used to designate the primary dentition.

deciliter (dl) A measure of one-tenth (10⁻¹) of a liter.

decimeter (dm) A linear measure of one-tenth (10⁻¹) of a meter.

decinormal (0.1 N) One tenth of normal; denoting a solution having one-tenth of the normal strength. See also solution, normal.

decipara (para X) A woman who has borne 10 children.

declination 1. A sloping; a bending downward. 2. In ophthalmology, rotation of the eye about an anteroposterior axis.

decline 1. The stage of abatement of symptoms of an acute disease. 2. A period of involution. 3. A wasting disease.

declive Latin for hill or slope.

  d. cerebelli The sloping portion of the vermis of the middle lobe of the cerebellum, bounded anteriorly by the primary fissure and posteriorly by the postclival fissure. Also called clivus monticuli.

decoction 1. The process of boiling down or concentrating by boiling. 2. A medicine prepared by boiling.

decompensation 1. Failure of the heart to maintain adequate circulation in certain cardiac and circulation disorders. 2. Failure of usual coping mechanisms resulting in personality disintegration.

decompose 1. To decay. 2. To separate a compound into its basic elements.

decomposition 1. Organic decay; disintegration; lysis. 2. The separation of compounds into constituents by chemical reaction.

decompression The removal of pressure.

  bowel d. Relief of a distended portion of the intestine by passage of a long tube connected to suction or by establishing a direct opening, such as a cecostomy.

  cardiac d. Surgical incision into the pericardium for the release of accumulated fluid from the pericardial sac. Also called pericardial decompression.

  cerebral d. Removal of a section of the skull, with puncture of the dura mater, to relieve intracranial pressure.

  orbital d. Removal of bone from the orbit to relieve pressure behind the eyeball, as in exophthalmus.

  pericardial d. See cardiac decompression.

decongestant Any agent that reduces congestion or swelling.

right atrium

atrial septal defect

severe knock knee **deformity**

QRS deflections

R R

Q Q

S S

unilateral bowleg **deformity**

degenerative joint disease

Heberden's nodes

decongestive Reducing congestion or swelling.
decontamination **1.** Making safe by eliminating or neutralizing harmful agents (noxious chemicals, radioactive material). **2.** Removal of contamination.
decorticate To surgically remove the cortex of an organ or structure.
decortication Removal of the cortical substance (external layer) of an organ or structure, as the brain or kidney.
decrudescence Abatement of the intensity of symptoms of disease.
decubital Relating to a decubitus ulcer (bedsore).
decubitus The act of reclining; lying down.
decussate **1.** To cross or intersect so as to form an X. **2.** Crossed like the letter X.
decussation A point of crossing, especially of nerve tracts.
dedifferentiation **1.** The reversion of specialized cellular forms to a more primitive condition. **2.** The process in which specialized tissues are the site of origin of primitive elements of the same type.
defecation The discharge of feces from the bowels.
defect Malformation.
  atrial septal d. Defect in the septum between the atria of the heart.
  birth d. Congenital malformation; see under malformation.
  filling d. Any abnormality in the contour of the digestive tract, as seen in an X-ray image.
  ventricular septal d. (VSD) Defect in the septum between the ventricles of the heart.
defective Denoting a person deficient in some physical or mental attribute.
defemination The loss or decrease of feminine characteristics.
defense mechanism An unconscious process through which a person seeks relief from anxiety.
deferent Carrying down or away. Also called efferent.
deferentectomy See vasectomy.
deferentitis Inflammation of the ductus deferens. Also called vasitis; spermatitis.
defervescence The disappearance or subsidence of fever.
defibrillation The arrest of quivering movements of cardiac muscle fibers (fibrillation).
defibrillator **1.** Anything that arrests ventricular fibrillation and restores the normal heart beat. **2.** An apparatus capable of delivering an electric shock to arrest ventricular fibrillation.
defibrination The removal of fibrin from the blood to prevent it from clotting.
deficiency The state of being insufficient; a lack;

a shortage.
  antitrypsin d. Hereditary disorder that in its severe form is frequently associated with emphysema.
  mental d. See retardation, mental.
  pseudocholinesterase d. Hereditary disorder manifested by an excessive reaction to drugs that are usually hydrolyzed by serum pseudocholinesterase, especially some of the agents used to achieve muscular relaxation during anesthesia, such as succinylcholine.
  pyruvate kinase d. Hereditary disorder marked by lack of pyruvate kinase, causing hemolytic anemia.
deficit A deficiency in quantity or quality.
  pulse d. The difference between the number of heart beats (greater) and the number of beats counted at the wrist (less) due to failure of a very early ventricular contraction to propel sufficient blood to produce a palpable pulse.
definition **1.** The power of an optical system to produce a sharp image. **2.** The maximum ability of the eye to discriminate between two points.
deflection **1.** The act of turning aside, as of a light ray toward an opaque body. **2.** A wave of the electrocardiogram.
  intrinsicoid d. In electrocardiography, the sudden downstroke from maximum positivity.
defloration The act of rupturing the hymen. Also called deflowering.
deflorescence Disappearance of the skin eruption of any eruptive disease.
defluvium Hair loss.
deformation **1.** A change of form from the normal. **2.** A deformity; a bodily disfiguration or malformation.
deformity Any bodily disfigurement.
  gunstock d. Displacement of the forearm to one side resulting from condylar fracture at the elbow.
  lobster-claw d. A hand or foot with the middle digits fused or missing.
defundation Surgical removal of the fundus of the uterus.
defurfuration The falling off or shedding of fine scales from the skin. Also called branny desquamation.
degenerate **1.** Marked by deterioration. **2.** A person who is morally degraded.
degeneration **1.** Deterioration of physical, mental, or moral characteristics. **2.** The deterioration of tissues with corresponding functional impairment as a result of injury or disease; the process may advance to an irreversible stage and eventually cause death of the tissues (necrosis).
  atheromatous d. Localized accumulation of

lipid material (atheroma) in the inner layers of the arterial walls.
  ballooning d. Liquefaction of the cell protoplasm leading to edematous swelling and softening. Also called ballooning colliquation.
  basophilic d. Blue staining of connective tissue by the hematoxylin-eosin stain in conditions such as lupus erythematosus and senile skin.
  cerebromacular d. Cerebral sphingolipidosis; see under sphingolipidosis.
  fatty d. Any abnormal accumulation of fat within the parenchymal cells of organs or glands. Also called fatty change or metamorphosis.
  fibrinoid d. The formation of a dense, homogeneous, acidophilic substance in the tissues.
  hepatolenticular d. An inherited disorder characterized by abnormal metabolism of copper causing accumulation of the metal in the liver and in the lenticular nucleus of the brain, accompanied by deposition of a brown pigment at the corneal margins. Also called Wilson's disease.
  heredomacular d. See macular degeneration.
  hyaline d. A regressive process in which cellular cytoplasm becomes glossy and homogeneous due to injury that causes coagulation and denaturation of proteins.
  hydropic d. A reversible form of intracellular edema with accumulation of water within the cell.
  macular d. A hereditary condition marked by progressive degeneration of the macula and loss of vision. Also called Best's disease; heredomacular degeneration.
  mucoid medial d. Cystic medial necrosis; see under necrosis.
  reaction of d. The abnormal reaction of a degenerated nerve or muscle to an electric stimulus.
  secondary d. See wallerian degeneration.
  senile d. The normal degeneration of tissues in old age.
  wallerian d. Dissolution and resorption of the distal stump of a sectioned peripheral nerve. Also called secondary degeneration.
  Zenker's d. A form of hyaline degeneration in which the cytoplasm of striated muscle cells becomes clumped, homogeneous, and waxy; occurs in patients dying of febrile illnesses, as typhoid fever and diphtheria.
degenerative joint disease (DJD) A chronic disorder marked by degeneration of articular cartilage and hypertrophy of bone, accompanied by pain which appears with activity and subsides with rest; a common form of chronic joint disease in the middle-aged and the elderly. Also called osteoarthritis; degenerative or hypertrophic arthritis.

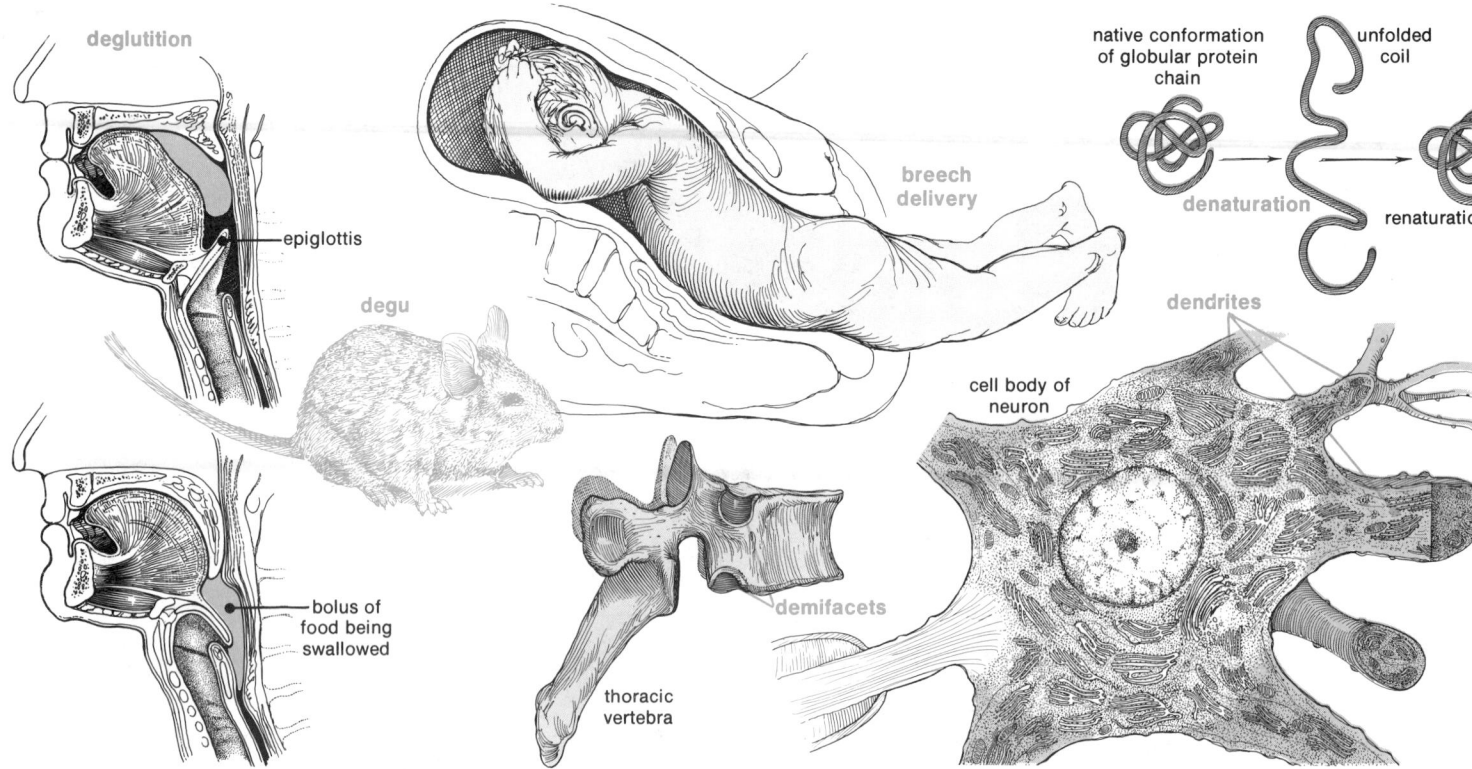

deglutition

epiglottis

bolus of food being swallowed

degu

breech delivery

native conformation of globular protein chain

denaturation

unfolded coil

renaturation

dendrites

cell body of neuron

demifacets

thoracic vertebra

deglutition The act of swallowing.

degranulation The loss of granules, as in the disappearance of the neutrophilic granules in a leukocyte immediately following particle ingestion.

degree 1. A division of a temperature scale. 2. A unit of angular measure equal to 1/360 of the circumference of a circle. 3. Severity; extent.

degu A ratlike animal from Chile possessing two anatomically separate thymus glands (cervical thymus and mediastinal thymus); used extensively by immunologists to study the thymus, which, in early life, sets up the immune defense mechanisms for the body. Also called trumpet-tailed rat.

degustation The act or sense of tasting.

dehalogenase Enzyme present in the thyroid gland that promotes the removal of iodine from mono- and diiodotyrosines.

dehiscence A rupturing or bursting, as the coming apart of the sides of a wound.

dehydrate To extract water from the body or from any substance; to make anhydrous.

dehydration Diminution of water content of the body or tissues.

dehydrogenase An enzyme that catalyzes the removal of hydrogen from a substrate and the transfer of the hydrogen to an acceptor.

dehydrogenation To remove hydrogen from a compound. Also called dehydrogenization.

dehypnotize To awaken from a hypnotic state.

déjà vu A feeling that a new experience or situation has happened before. Also called déjà vu phenomenon.

dejection 1. A state of mental depression. Also called melancholy. 2. Defecation.

delactation Weaning.

delamination A division into layers or laminae; specifically the splitting of blastoderm into ectoderm and entoderm.

de-lead To remove lead from bodily tissues.

deleterious Harmful.

deletion In genetics, loss of a segment of a chromosome through breakage; a chromosome aberration.

delimitation The process of putting bounds; preventing the spread of a disease.

deliquesce To become damp; to melt.

deliquescent Denoting a solid substance that becomes liquified by absorbing moisture from the atmosphere.

delirious In a state of mental confusion and excitement.

delirium A condition of temporary mental excitement and confusion, marked by hallucinations, delusions, anxiety, and incoherence.

d. tremens (DT's) acute mental disturbance due to withdrawal from alcohol, marked by sweating, tremor, anxiety, precordial pain, and both visual and auditory hallucinations.

deliver 1. To assist a woman in birth. 2. To remove; e.g., a tumor.

delivery Childbirth; labor.

abdominal d. Delivery of a child by cesarean section.

breech d. Extraction of an infant whose pelvis or lower extremity is the presenting part.

forceps d. Delivery in which an instrument is placed on the fetal head to exert traction on its body; classified according to the level of the head of the fetus at the time the instrument is applied, as follows: (a) high forceps, the application of forceps before engagement has taken place; (b) low forceps, the application of forceps when the head of the fetus has reached the perineal floor and is visible, and the sagittal suture of the fetal skull is in the anteroposterior diameter of the pelvis; (c) midforceps, the application of forceps after engagement has taken place but before the criteria of low forceps have been met.

postmortem d. Delivery of a child after death of its mother.

premature d. Expulsion of a fetus before full term, after the 28th week of gestation.

delouse To rid of infestation with lice.

delta 1. The fourth letter of the Greek alphabet, Δ, δ; used to denote the fourth in a series. 2. Any triangular anatomic space. 3. In chemistry, the capital (Δ) denotes a double bond between carbon atoms; the lower case (δ) denotes the location of a substituent on the fourth atom from the primary functional group in an organic molecule. 4. Symbol (Δ) for change. For terms beginning with delta, see under the specific term.

deltoid Triangular; shaped like the Greek letter delta, Δ. See table of muscles.

delusion A false belief maintained even against contradictory evidence or logical argument.

d. of grandeur Exaggerated belief in one's importance.

d. of persecution A false belief that one is being persecuted.

demarcation The marking of boundaries.

line of d. An inflamed area separating gangrenous and healthy tissue.

demasculinization The loss of male characteristics.

demented Afflicted with dementia or loss of reason.

dementia Deterioration of intellectual function due to organic factors; formerly used to denote madness or insanity.

d. praecox Obsolete term for schizophrenia.

senile d. Mental deterioration caused by atrophy of the brain due to aging.

demifacet The half of a facet on the side of some thoracic vertebrae for articulation with the head of a rib. Also called costal facet.

demilune 1. Crescent; semilunar. 2. The gametocyte of *Plasmodium falciparum*.

serous d. Five to 10 serous cells capping the terminal end of a mucous, tubuloalveolar secretory unit of mixed salivary glands. Also called crescent of Gianuzzi.

demineralization A reduction of the mineral constituent of the tissues through excessive elimination.

demipenniform Feather-shaped on one side only; said of certain muscles with a tendon on one side.

demography The study of human populations, especially their growth, geographical distribution, and vital statistics.

demonstrator A person who supplements the teachings of a professor by instructing small groups, preparing dissections, etc.

demophobia Morbid fear of crowds.

demulcent 1. Soothing; allaying irritation. 2. Any gummy or oily substance having such properties.

demyelination, demyelinization Destruction or loss of myelin from the sheath of a nerve.

denarcotize To remove or separate narcotic properties from an opiate.

denaturation Loss of characteristic biologic activity in protein molecules due to extremes of pH or temperature.

denatured Changed in nature; adulterated.

dendriform Branched like a tree; tree-shaped.

dendrite One of the cytoplasmic branches of nerve cells (neurons) which conducts the impulses received from the terminations of other neurons toward the cell body. Also called dendritic process.

dendritic Relating to or resembling dendrites or protoplasmic processes of the nerve cells.

dendroid Branched; treelike.

denervate To remove or sever the nerve supply to a bodily part.

dengue Epidemic disease of tropical and subtropical regions caused by a dengue virus (genus *Flavivirus*) and transmitted by *Aedes* mosquitoes; marked by severe headache, intense pain of the back and joints, high fever, and a spotty rash; after three or four days, all symptoms subside only to reappear 24 hours later with a characteristic skin eruption. Also called break-bone, 7-day, or dandy fever.

denial An unconscious defense mechanism, in which consciously intolerable thoughts, wishes, feelings, or needs are rejected or blocked out.

pulp cavity
dentin
enamel

deciduous dentition

partial denture

molars   bicuspids   cuspids   incisors   cuspids   bicuspids   molars

permanent dentition

denidation Disintegration and expulsion of the superficial uterine mucosa.

denitrify To remove nitrogen from a compound.

dens, *pl.* **dentes** 1. Latin for tooth. 2. A toothlike structure, as the odontoid process of the axis (second vertebra).

densimeter An instrument for determining the density of a fluid.

densitometer A type of densimeter for determining the degree of bacterial growth in a fluid by means of its turbidity.

photon d. A device used to measure the density of bone by passage of a beam of photons through the bone to be measured. Also called bone-mineral analyzer.

densitometry Technique for measuring the density of a substance, especially bone.

bone d. The use of a densitometer to pass a beam of photons through bone; the attenuation of the beam is the measure of the density of the bone.

density 1. The state of compactness. 2. The amount of matter per unit volume expressed in grams per cubic centimeter. 3. The measure of the degree of resistance to the speed of a transmission.

count d. See photon density.

optical d. The light-absorbing quality of a translucent substance.

photon d. In radioisotope scanning, the number of counted events per square centimeter or per square inch of imaged area. Also called count density.

vapor d. The ratio of the weight of a vapor or gas to an equal volume of hydrogen.

dental Of or relating to teeth.

dental floss Thread of nylon or silk used to remove debris from between teeth.

dentalgia Toothache.

dentate Notched; having toothlike projections.

denticle A calcified body in the pulp chamber of a tooth. Also called pulp stone.

denticulate Having toothlike projections.

dentiform Shaped like a tooth. Also called odontoid; dentoid.

dentifrice A compound, such as a paste or powder, used in conjunction with a toothbrush for cleaning the teeth.

dentigerous Containing teeth, as certain cysts.

dentin The hard tissue forming the main substance of teeth; it surrounds the tooth pulp and is covered by enamel on the crown and by cementum on the roots.

primary d. Dentin formed before the eruption of a tooth.

secondary d. Highly irregular dentin formed after tooth eruption due to irritation from caries or

injuries, or the normal wearing down of the teeth.

dentinal Relating to dentin.

dentine Dentin.

dentinoma An extremely rare encapsulated tumor composed of connective tissue and masses of dentin.

dentinum Latin for dentin.

dentist One who practices dentistry.

dentistry The science and art concerned with the diagnosis, prevention, and treatment of diseases of the tissues comprising the mouth, especially the restoration or replacement of defective teeth.

dentition The arrangement of the natural teeth in the dental arch.

deciduous d. Set of 20 teeth that begin to erupt when a child is about six months old. Also called primary dentition.

permanent d. Set of 32 teeth that begin to erupt when a child is about 6 years old.

primary d. See deciduous dentition.

retarded d. Delayed eruption or growth of one or more teeth, deciduous or permanent.

transitional d. Dentition containing deciduous and permanent teeth.

dentulous Possessing natural deciduous or permanent teeth.

denture An artifical substitute for missing natural teeth and surrounding tissues.

complete d. A dental prosthesis that replaces all the natural teeth and associated structures in a jaw.

fixed partial d. A partial denture that is supported by the teeth or roots and cannot be readily removed; often designated as a fixed bridge.

immediate d. A denture made before the anterior teeth are extracted and inserted immediately after extraction for cosmetic reasons.

partial d. A dental prosthesis replacing one or more teeth and held in place by remaining teeth and underlying tissues; may be removable or fixed.

denucleated Deprived of a nucleus.

denudation To make bare; to divest of covering.

deodorant An agent that counteracts undesirable odors.

deossification Removal of the mineral elements of bone.

deoxidation Removal of oxygen from a compound. Also called reduction.

deoxidize To remove oxygen from a chemical compound; to reduce.

deoxycholic acid (DOC) A digestive bile acid formed in the small intestine by the action of intestinal bacteria on cholic acid.

deoxycorticosterone (DOC) A steroid hormone occurring in the adrenal cortex; a precursor of corticosterone. Also called deoxycortone; cortexone.

d. acetate (DOCA, DCA) A salt-retaining steroid.

deoxycortone See deoxycorticosterone.

deoxygenate To deprive of oxygen.

deoxyribonuclease (DNase, DNAase) An enzyme that breaks down deoxyribonucleic acid (DNA) to nucleotides.

deoxyribonucleic acid (DNA) The molecular basis of heredity; see DNA.

deoxyribonucleoprotein A nucleoprotein that yields deoxyribonucleic acid (DNA) on hydrolysis.

deoxyribonucleoside A compound consisting of a purine or pyrimidine base combined with deoxyribose (a DNA sugar).

deoxyribonucleotide A substance composed of a purine or pyrimidine base bonded to deoxyribose (a DNA sugar), which in turn is bound to a phosphate group.

deoxyribose The pentose sugar constituent of deoxyribonucleic acid (DNA).

deoxysugar Any of several sugars containing less oxygen atoms than carbon atoms in the molecule, resulting in one or more carbons lacking an attached hydroxyl group.

depancreatize To remove the pancreas.

depersonalization A condition in which a person loses his sense of personal identity or feels his body to be unreal.

dephosphorylation The removal of a phosphate group from a compound through the action of an enzyme.

depigmentation Partial or complete loss of pigment.

depilate To remove hair, usually from the surface of the body.

depilation The removal of hair.

depilatory 1. An agent that removes or destroys hair from the body. 2. Capable of removing hair.

deplete To exhaust; to empty.

depletion 1. The process of emptying. 2. Exhausted condition caused by excessive loss of bodily fluids. 3. Excessive loss of bodily constituents necessary for normal functioning.

deplumation Abnormal loss of the eyelashes.

depolarization The elimination or neutralization of polarity.

deposit Sediment.

depravity 1. Moral deterioration or corruption. 2. A perverse act.

depressant Serving to reduce functional activity.

depressed 1. Sunk below level of surrounding parts. 2. Below normal functional level. 3. Dejected.

depression 1. Emotional dejection; morbid sadness accompanied by loss of interest in surroundings and lack of energy. 2. Area lower than the surrounding level.

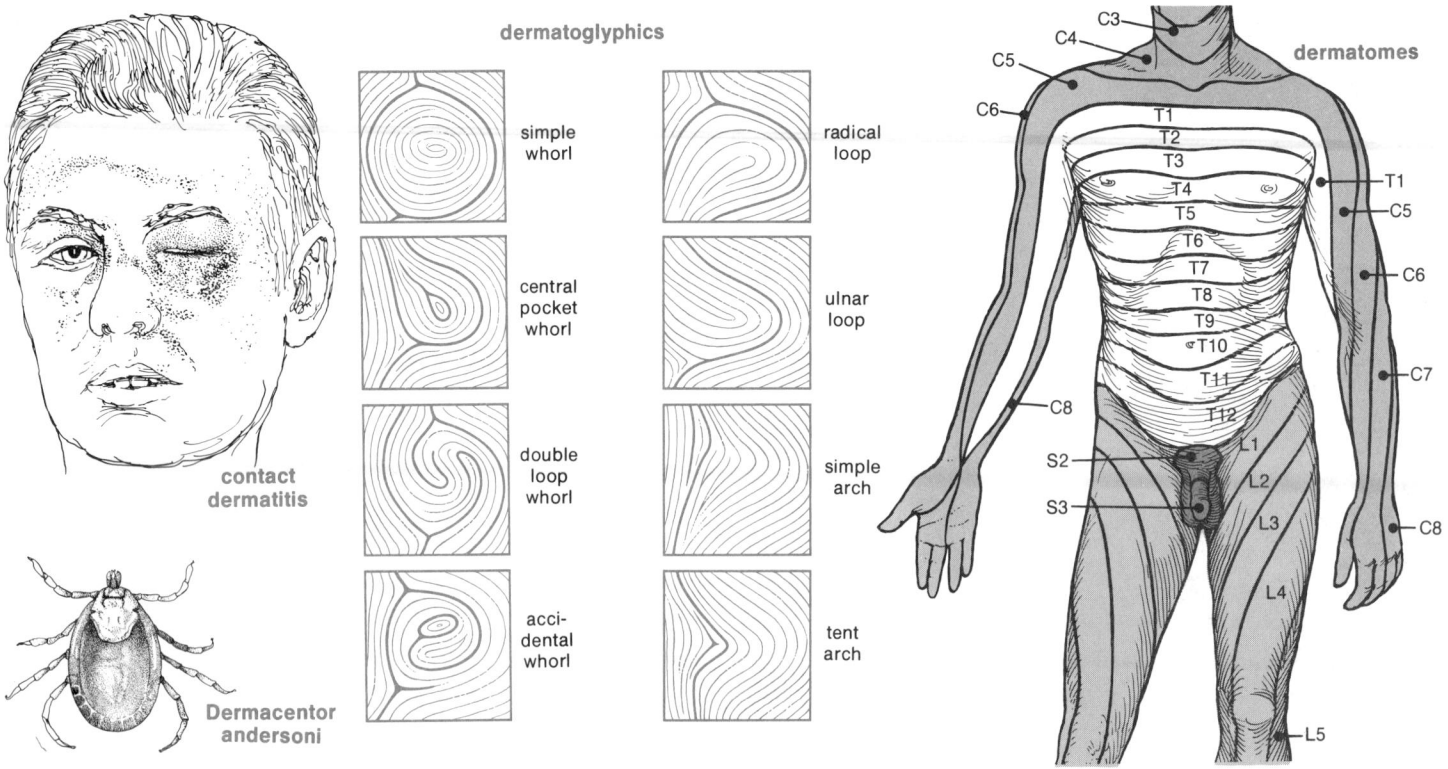

dermatoglyphics

simple whorl

central pocket whorl

double loop whorl

accidental whorl

radical loop

ulnar loop

simple arch

tent arch

contact dermatitis

Dermacentor andersoni

dermatomes

anaclitic d. Impairment of an infant's development (physical, intellectual, and social) which sometimes follows a sudden separation from its mother or mother substitute.

endogenous d. A major depressive disorder manifested by a cluster of symptoms occurring in the absence of predominant causative factors; e.g., dejected mood, psychomotor retardation, insomnia, weight loss, guilt feelings, and lack of reactivity to one's environment.

reactive d. Depression caused by an external predominant factor and relieved by the removal of that factor.

depressomotor 1. Serving to retard motor activity. 2. Anything that causes such an effect.

depressor 1. Anything that depresses or reduces functional activity, as certain nerves, muscles, or chemicals. 2. An instrument or device used to push structures out of the way during an examination or operation.

tongue d. A broad wooden blade used to push the tongue against the floor of the mouth during examination of the throat.

deprivation Loss or absence of stimuli, nurture, organs, powers, or attributes that are needed.

sensory d. A diminution of sensory stimuli.

depth A dimension downward or inward.

anesthetic d. The depth of depression of the central nervous system caused by an anesthetic drug; an indication of the potency of the anesthetic.

d. of focus The variation of the distance between an object and a lens or optical system without causing objectionable blurring.

depulization The destruction of fleas carrying the plague bacillus.

depurant 1. Anything that purifies. 2. An agent that promotes the excretion of waste matter.

derangement 1. Mental disorder. 2. Disarrangement of the regular order; disorder.

derivation 1. The source from which something originates. 2. The diversion of fluids from one part of the body to another.

derivative 1. In chemistry, a compound obtained from another and containing some of the elements of the original substance. 2. Resulting from derivation.

dermabrasion Operative procedure used to remove acne or chicken pox scars, tattoos, and superficial foreign bodies acquired during road or industrial accidents; the most popular method consists of freezing the skin, followed by mechanical removal of the epidermis and upper dermis with a high-speed rotary steel brush. Also called skin or surgical planing.

Dermacentor A genus of ticks (family Ixodidae).

D. andersoni The wood tick, a transmitter of Rocky Mountain spotted fever and tularemia and the cause of tick paralysis.

D. variabillis The American dog tick, the transmitter of spotted fever and tularemia.

dermadrome Any syndrome that includes cutaneous and internal symptoms.

dermal Of or relating to the skin.

dermalaxia Softening of the skin.

dermametropathism A method of diagnosing certain skin disorders by observing the markings when a blunt instrument is drawn across the skin.

dermatitis, pl. dermatitides Inflammation of the skin.

actinic d. A sensitivity reaction of the skin produced by exposure to sunlight, distinguished from sunburn.

atopic d. Any dermatitis caused by allergy. Also called atopic eczema.

chemical d. Dermatitis produced by contact with chemicals.

contact d. Dermatitis caused by contact with material to which a person is hypersensitive.

d. exfoliativa infantum, d. exfoliativa neonatorum A pustular dermatitis with abundant flaking and red coloration of the skin accompanied by fever, malaise, and occasionally gastrointestinal symptoms; it affects young infants and is frequently fatal. Also called Ritter's disease.

d. herpetiformis Chronic disorder marked by an eruption of itchy burning clusters of vesicles and papules occurring mostly on the forearms and abdomen. Also called Duhring's disease; hydroa herpetiforme.

d. medicamentosa An allergic reaction to medications taken internally or applied locally, manifested by the eruption of a rash.

d. venenata An edematous vesicular eruption caused by contact with a sensitizing substance such as poison ivy, cosmetics, etc.

exfoliative d. Generalized exfoliation, redness, and severe scaling of the skin with constitutional symptoms. Also called Wilson's disease.

industrial d. Any dermatitis caused by contact with materials used in industry.

ivy d. See poison ivy (2).

seborrheic d. A condition of unknown cause with a predilection for the scalp but also seen on the eyebrows, behind the ears, the chest, back, and pubic area; characterized by varying degrees of redness, scaling, and sometimes itching. Commonly known in its mild form as dandruff; seborrhea.

solar d. Dermatitis produced in persons allergic to sun's rays.

stasis d. Dermatitis occurring usually on the lower legs in association with varicose veins.

Dermatobia A genus of flies (family Oestridae) that includes the parasitic botflies.

dermatocele A localized loose condition of the skin.

dermatoconiosis Occupational dermatitis caused by irritation of the skin by dust.

dermatofibroma A benign skin tumor believed to be a capillary hemangioma that has become indurated, cellular, and fibrous. Also called sclerosing hemangioma; histiocytoma.

dermatofibrosarcoma protuberans A skin tumor composed of several small nodules covered with dark reddish blue skin; it tends to recur after removal.

dermatoglyphics 1. The variety of pattern configurations of epidermal ridges on the volar aspect of the hands and feet; the ridge configuration may be altered in some disorders. 2. The study of skin patterns, especially of the palms of the hands and soles of the feet.

dermatography, dermatographism See dermographia.

dermatoid Resembling skin.

dermatologist A specialist in disorders of the skin and related systemic diseases; also called skin specialist.

dermatology The medical specialty concerned with the diagnosis and treatment of skin diseases.

dermatome 1. Surgical instrument used in cutting thin slices of skin for grafting. 2. In embryology, the dorsolateral wall of a somite from which the skin is derived. 3. A skin area supplied by sensory fibers of a single spinal nerve.

dermatomegaly Congenital defect consisting of an excessive amount of skin which hangs in folds.

dermatomycosis Any cutaneous fungal infection.

dermatomyositis A form of polymyositis; a painful inflammation of the skin, subcutaneous tissue, and muscle; the muscles most affected are those of the pelvic and shoulder girdles and pharynx; in 15 to 20% of cases there is an associated neoplasm.

dermatonosology The classification of skin diseases. Also called dermonosology.

dermatopathology The study of skin diseases.

dermatopathy Any disease of the skin.

dermatophyte Any fungus capable of causing skin disease.

dermatophytid Secondary skin eruption, usually on the fingers and hands, following sensitization of fungi. Often called id. See also reaction, id.

dermatophytosis Any superficial fungal infection of the skin; e.g., athlete's foot.

dermatoplasty Skin grafting to correct defects or

descensus testis

tooth designation

apical region of contact between two intestinal cells

micro-villi

zonula occludens

zonula adherens

desmosome

replace loss of skin.

dermatosis, *pl.* **dermatoses** Any skin eruption.

dermatoskeleton See exoskeleton (2).

dermatotherapy The treatment of skin diseases.

dermatotropic Acting selectively on the skin. Also called dermotropic.

dermatrophia, dermatrophy Thinning or atrophy of the skin.

dermis The broad, dense connective tissue layer of the skin positioned snugly under the epidermis and composed mostly of collagenous fibers with some elastic and reticular fibers; it contains blood vessels, lymphatic channels, nerves, sebaceous glands, hair follicles, and sweat glands. Also called corium; true skin; cutis vera.

dermoblast One of the mesodermal cells that develops into the true skin or corium.

dermographia A sensitive condition of the skin in which wheals are formed by lightly drawing a pencil or blunt instrument over it. Also called dermography; dermatography; dermatographia; dermatographism.

    white d. Blanching of the skin on stroking.

dermoid 1. Resembling skin. 2. A congenital cyst or saclike growth containing fluid and hair, skin, teeth, or other dermal structures.

dermoskeleton See exoskeleton (2).

dermostosis Bony formations on the skin.

dermotoxin A substance that causes pathologic changes in the skin.

dermotropic See dermatotropic.

descemetitis Inflammation of the posterior limiting (Descemet's) membrane of the cornea.

descensus Falling; descent.

    d. testis Descent of the testis from the abdomen into the scrotum shortly before the end of intrauterine life.

desensitization 1. See immunotherapy (3). 2. In psychotherapy, the act of eliminating or reducing an emotional complex.

desensitize See hyposensitize.

desex To castrate.

desiccant 1. An agent possessing a high affinity for water, used to absorb moisture; a drying agent. 2. Promoting dryness.

desiccate To dry.

desiccator A closed vessel containing a dehydrating agent (calcium chloride, sulfuric acid, etc.) in which a substance or an apparatus is placed for drying and to be kept free from moisture.

designation Distinguishing name.

    cluster d. A numerical nomenclature for cell surface molecules (markers) that are typical of different cell lineages and that are recognized by specific monoclonal antibodies.

desmoid A nodule resulting from the proliferation of fibrous tissue of muscle sheaths, especially of the abdominal wall; usually occurring in women following pregnancy. Also called desmoid tumor.

desmopexia Shortening of the round ligaments of the uterus by suturing them to the abdominal wall for the correction of uterine displacement.

desmoplasia Disproportionate formation of fibrous tissue.

desmoplastic 1. Causing adhesions. 2. Causing fibrosis in the vascular stroma of a tumor.

desmopressin acetate (DDAVP) A synthetic analog of vasopressin used as an antidiuretic.

desmosome Two apposed, small, ellipsoidal plates, about 0.5 μ in diameter, along the interfaces between the plasma membrane of adjacent cells; it serves as a site of adhesion; visible only by electron microscopy. Also called macula adherens.

    half-d. A plate on one cell without a companion plate butting up against it, as found at the basal plasma membrane in some epithelia. Also called hemidesmosome.

despumation The removal of impurities or scum from the surface of a liquid.

desquamate To cast off or shed the outer layer of a surface, as the scaling off of the epidermis.

desquamation The shedding or peeling of the superficial layer of the skin (epidermis) in flakes or scales.

detachment 1. The state of being separated; e.g., the separation of the retina from its normally attached choroid. 2. In psychiatry, the condition of being free from emotional or social involvement.

deterioration 1. Worsening. 2. In psychiatry, the chronic, progressive impairment of emotional and intellectual functions.

determinant The determining factor that establishes the characteristics of an entity.

determination The estimation of the extent, quality, or character of anything.

determinism The doctrine that any event is the inevitable consequence of prior influences and hence can be completely explained by its antecedents.

De Toni-Fanconi syndrome See Lignac-De Toni-Fanconi syndrome.

detoxicate To remove the effects or counteract the toxic properties of a poison.

detoxication 1. The process of neutralizing the toxic properties of a substance. 2. The recovery from the toxic effects of a substance.

detumescence The return to the flaccid state or to the normal size of a swollen organ or part.

    d. of penis The return of the penis to the flaccid state from an erection.

deuteranopia A form of color blindness in which red, orange, yellow, and green cannot be differentiated when their brightnesses and saturations are equal; similarly, blue, violet, and blue-purple appear to differ only in brightness and saturation, but not in hue; a sex-linked hereditary defect, occurring in about one percent of males and only rarely in females.

deuterium (D) An isotope of hydrogen having an atomic weight of 2.0141, consisting of one proton and one neutron in the nucleus. Also called hydrogen-2 (^{2}H); heavy hydrogen.

    d. oxide (D$_2$O) See heavy water.

deuteron (d) A subatomic particle consisting of a proton and a neutron; the nucleus of deuterium (heavy hydrogen). Also called deuton; diplon.

deutoplasm The nonliving material in the cytoplasm, especially reserve food substance or yolk in the ovum.

Deutschländer's disease March foot; see under foot.

devascularization Removal of blood vessels from a part.

deviance A difference or departure from a norm or rule.

    psychiatric d. Divergence from accepted norms of mental health.

    role d. See social deviance.

    sexual d. Departure from accepted sexual norms. Formerly called perversion.

    social d. Departure from accepted social behavior. Also called role deviance.

deviation 1. A turning aside. 2. Departure from an accepted course of behavior.

    axis d. Deflection of the electrical axis of the heart to the right or left.

    parallel conjugate d. 1. Normally, the joint and equal movement of the two eyes in the same direction when shifted from one object to another. 2. Pathologically, failure of both eyes to turn to one side; the defect is compensated by rotating or tilting the head.

    primary d. In strabismus, the deviation of the defective eye when the normal eye is fixed on an object.

    secondary d. In strabismus, the deviation of the normal eye when the defective eye is made to fixate on an object.

    skew d. Special form of vertical imbalance of both eyes.

    standard d. (S.D.) In statistics, a measure of dispersion or variation in a distribution.

device Something made or constructed for a particular purpose.

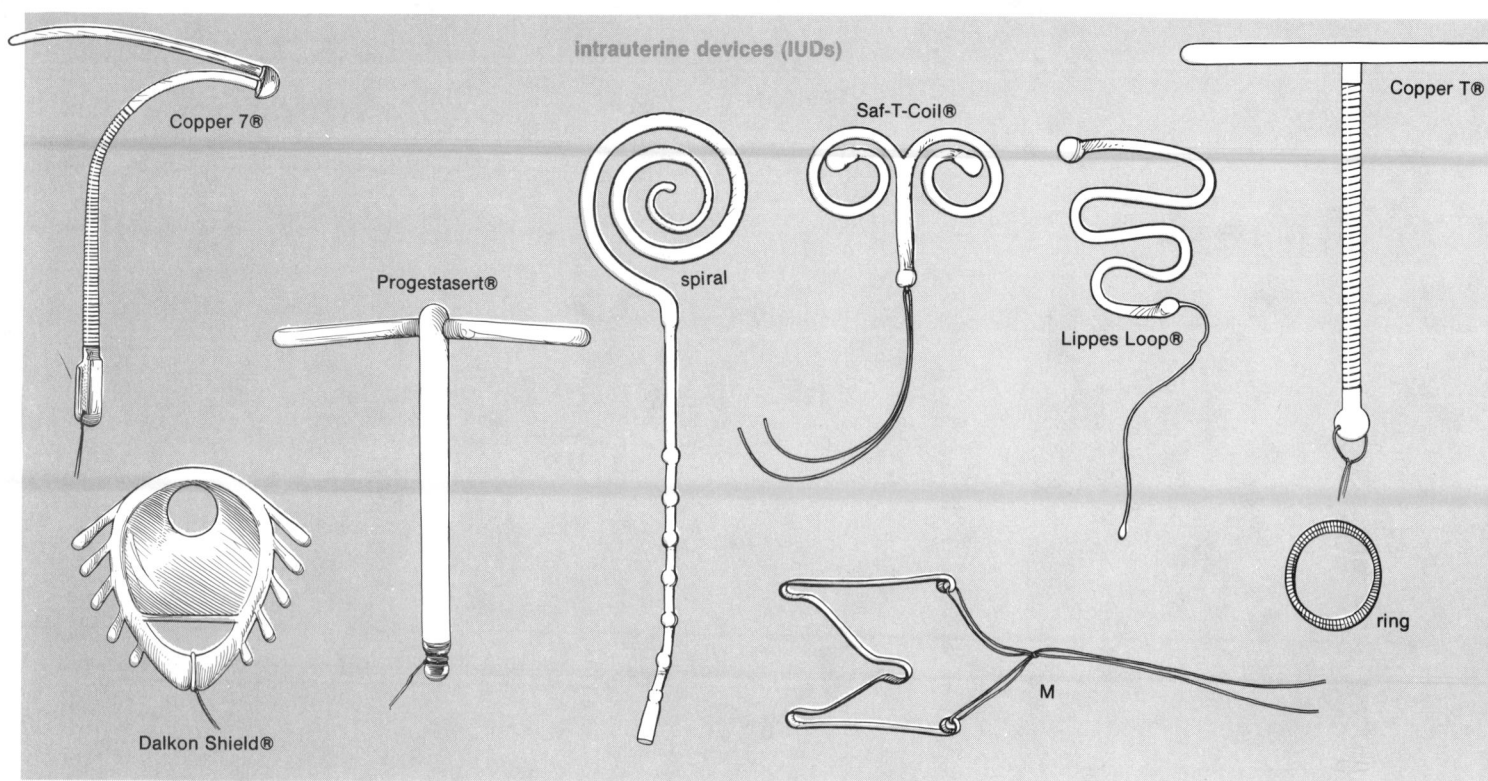

intrauterine devices (IUDs)

Copper 7®

Progestasert®

spiral

Saf-T-Coil®

Lippes Loop®

Copper T®

Dalkon Shield®

ring

M

intrauterine d. (IUD) A metal or plastic loop or spiral inserted into the uterus to prevent conception.

Devic's disease See neuromyelitis optica.

devitalization In dentistry, the destruction of the pulp of a tooth.

devitalized Without vitality; dead.

devolution 1. Degeneration; catabolism. 2. The opposite of evolution.

dexter (D) Latin for right.

dextrad Toward the right.

dextral 1. Of, related to, or located on the right side. 2. Right-handed.

dextran Any of various large polymers of glucose, used in solution as a plasma substitute.

dextrans Polysaccharides of glucose obtained from yeast and bacteria in which the glucose residues are bound in α-1,6 linkages; the linkage at the branch point (1, 2, 1, 3, 1, 4) and the spacing between the branch points is characteristic of the species of the organism from which the dextran was obtained; used as plasma substitutes.

dextrin A soluble carbohydrate formed by the hydrolysis of starch, the first stage in the formation of glucose; commercial dextrin is a white or yellow powder, used in solution as an adhesive.

dextrin 6-glucosyltransferase A bacterial enzyme that promotes the synthesis of dextrans from dextrins. Also called dextran dextrinase.

dextroamphetamine sulfate A sympathomimetic agent; a stimulant to the central nervous system and appetite depressant; Dexedrine®.

dextrocardia Abnormal location of the heart on the right side of the chest.

dextrocular 1. Relating to the right eye. 2. Denoting a condition in which better vision exists in the right eye.

dextromethorphan hydrobromide Medical preparation taken orally as a cough suppressant.

dextroposition Abnormal right-sided location of an organ normally located in the left side.

d. of heart Condition either congenital or acquired (as in collapse of the right lung), in which the major portion of the heart lies on the right side.

dextrorotatory Turning the plane of polarization to the right; bending rays of light clockwise; said of some crystals and solutions.

dextrose See glucose.

dextrothyroxin sodium *d*-Thyroxine, a thyroid hormone analog used to reduce the cholesterol content in the tissues.

dextroversion Displacement or turning toward the right.

diabetes General term for diseases characterized by excessive excretion of urine; when used alone the term refers to diabetes mellitus.

alloxan d. The production of diabetes mellitus in experimental animals by the administration of alloxan, an agent that damages the insulin-producing cells of the pancreas.

brittle d. Insulin-dependent diabetes mellitus which is very difficult to control, with frequent episodes of hyper- and hypoglycemia.

bronzed d. A disorder of iron metabolism marked by deposits of iron in the tissues, especially skin, pancreas, and liver; deposition in the skin causes a bronzed pigmentation; deposits in the pancreas lead to diabetes. Also called hemochromatosis.

d. insipidus A comparatively rare form of diabetes marked by excessive thirst and the passage of large amounts of dilute urine, due to inadequate production of antidiuretic hormone (vasopressin) by the posterior lobe of the hypophysis. Cf. nephrogenic diabetes insipidus.

d. mellitus (DM) The most common form of diabetes; a chronic systemic disease marked by: (a) disorders in the metabolism of insulin (a hormone produced by the pancreas) and of carbohydrate, protein, and fat, and (b) disorders in the structure and function of blood vessels, referred to as "complications of diabetes;" the primary manifestation of the disease is high concentration of sugar in the blood; spillover of sugar into the urine leads to excessive urination, thirst, and loss of weight; mellitus is Latin for honeyed, referring to the presence of sugar in the urine; has been classified into insulin-dependent, noninsulin-dependent, gestational, and diabetes associated with other diseases.

gestational d. Pregnancy-induced glucose intolerance limited to the pregnant condition.

insulin-dependent d. mellitus (IDDM) Diabetes mellitus characterized by insulin deficiency; may occur at any age, but is most common in childhood and adolescence, and is of sudden onset; affected persons need injections of insulin to survive. Also called type I diabetes mellitus; diabetes I.

juvenile d. Former term for insulin-dependent diabetes mellitus.

latent d. Impairment of glucose tolerance.

maturity-onset d. Former term for noninsulin-dependent diabetes mellitus.

nephrogenic d. insipidus Diabetes insipidus caused by inability of the kidney tubules to reabsorb water; does not respond to the administration of antidiuretic hormone. Also called vasopressin-resistant diabetes.

noninsulin-dependent d. mellitus (NIDDM) Diabetes mellitus characterized by the presence of insulin in the blood; insulin levels may be normal, elevated, or depressed; onset is usually slow and may occur at any age, but is most common in persons over 40 with a tendency to obesity. Also called type II diabetes mellitus; diabetes II.

type I diabetes mellitus See insulin-dependent diabetes mellitus.

type II diabetes mellitus See noninsulin-dependent diabetes mellitus.

vasopressin-resistant d. See nephrogenic diabetes insipidus.

diabetic 1. Relating to diabetes. 2. An individual afflicted with diabetes.

diabetogenic Causing diabetes.

diabetologist A specialist in the study and treatment of diabetes.

diacetylmorphine See heroin.

diadochokinesia, diadochokinesis The normal ability of alternating opposite muscular actions, such as extension and flexion of a limb.

diagnose To identify the nature of a disease; to make a diagnosis.

diagnosis The determination of the nature of a disease.

clinical d. A diagnosis based on the signs and symptoms of a disease.

d. by exclusion A diagnosis made by excluding all but one of the disease processes thought to be possible causes of the symptoms being considered.

differential d. The determination of which of two or more diseases with similar symptoms is the one with which the patient is afflicted; consideration or listing of diseases possibly responsible for a patient's illness, based on information available at the time, e.g., symptoms, signs, physical findings, and laboratory data.

laboratory d. A diagnosis made by a chemical, microscopic, bacteriologic, or biopsy study of secretions, discharges, blood, or tissue.

pathologic d. 1. A diagnosis (sometimes a postmortem diagnosis) made from a study of the lesions present. 2. A diagnosis of the pathologic conditions present, determined by a study and comparison of the symptoms.

physical d. A diagnosis based on information obtained through physical examination of the patient, using the techniques of inspection, palpation, percussion, and auscultation.

postmortem d. Examination of a dead body, usually to determine the cause of death. Also called autopsy.

diagnostician One who is experienced in determining the nature of diseases; formerly used to apply to physicians with extensive training and experience in medicine, comparable to internists of today.

diakinesis The terminal part of the prophase stage in meiosis during which the spireme threads break up into shorter and thicker chromosomes, and the

diatom

peritoneal dialysis

suboccipitobregmatic diameter

fetal skull at term

occipitofrontal diameter

occipitomental diameter

diapedesis

WBC

diazepam

diazoxide

nucleolus and nuclear membrane disappear.

dialysance The amount of blood (measured in milliliters) completely cleared of a substance by a dialyzing membrane in a period of time, usually one minute.

dialysate Fluid used in dialysis.

dialysis The separation of smaller molecules (crystalloids) from larger molecules (colloids) in a solution by selective diffusion through a semipermeable membrane.

chronic ambulatory peritoneal d. (CAPD) A technique in which peritoneal dialysis is performed on a nearly constant basis in ambulatory patients.

peritoneal d. Dialysis in which sterile dialyzing fluid is introduced into the abdominal cavity; the peritoneum acts as the semipermeable membrane.

dialysis disequilibrium syndrome Nausea, vomiting, hypertension, and central nervous system signs occasionally occurring within hours after starting hemodialysis for kidney failure; thought to be due to removal of metabolites (especially urea) from the extracellular fluid and blood at a much greater rate than from the brain cells, with subsequent cerebral edema.

dialyze To separate a substance from a solution by dialysis; to subject to dialysis.

dialyzer A semipermeable membrane used in dialysis.

diameter 1. A straight line passing through the center of a circle and terminating at opposite points of its periphery. 2. The distance along such a line. 3. The thickness or width of any structure or opening.

biparietal d. The greatest transverse diameter of a skull; it extends from one parietal bone to the other; in the fetus at term it usually measures 9.25 cm.

occipitofrontal d. The diameter of a skull which follows a line extending from the root of the nose to the prominent portion of the occipital bone.

occipitomental d. The distance of a skull from the chin to the most prominent portion of the occipital bone; in the fetal skull at term it usually measures 11.5 cm.

suboccipitobregmatic d. The diameter of a fetal skull at term which follows a line drawn from the middle of the large fontanel to the under surface of the occipital bone just where it joins the neck; it usually measures 9.5 cm.

diamine An organic compound containing two amino groups; e.g., $NH_2CH_2CH_2NH_2$, ethylene diamine.

diapause A period of biological dormancy, as the suspension of growth and decreased metabolism in insects during a specific stage in their life cycle.

diapedesis 1. The passage of blood or any of its corpuscles through the pores of blood vessels. 2. The process by which phagocytic cells leave the blood and accumulate at extravascular sites of tissue injury.

diaphoretic An agent that causes sweating, especially profuse sweating.

diaphragm 1. The musculomembranous structure which separates the thoracic and abdominal cavities. 2. Any dividing membrane.

contraceptive d. A flexible ring covered with rubber or other plastic material, fitted over the cervix of the uterus to prevent pregnancy.

pelvic d. The part of the pelvic floor formed by the paired levator ani and coccygeus muscles and their fasciae.

urogenital d. A deep musculomembranous fascia extending between the ischiopubic rami and surrounding the urogenital ducts.

diaphysis The shaft of a long bone.

diaphysitis Inflammation of the body or shaft of a long bone.

diaplacental Passing through the placenta.

diapophysis The upper articular surface of a transverse vertebral process.

diarrhea Abnormally frequent passage of loose stools; the evacuation of a single loose stool does not constitute diarrhea.

nocturnal d. Diarrhea occurring primarily at night; seen in diabetes mellitus.

traveler's d. Diarrhea affecting travelers usually during the first week of a trip and lasting one to three days.

diarthric Of or relating to two joints. Also called biarticular.

diarthrosis A joint that permits relatively free movement. Also called diarthrodial or synovial joint.

diaschisis A sudden functional disorder caused by a focal disturbance of the brain.

diastalsis The type of peristalsis of the small intestine in which a wave of inhibition precedes the wave of contraction.

diastase A mixture of amylolytic or starch-splitting enzymes that convert starch into dextrin and maltose; present in some germinating grains such as malt.

diastasis Separation of two bones normally joined together without existence of a true joint, as in separation of the epiphysis from the shaft of a long bone.

d. recti Separation of the abdominal rectus muscles from the midline, usually seen after pregnancy or abdominal surgery.

diastema Excessive space between two adjacent teeth.

diastole Rhythmic relaxation of the muscles of the heart chambers during which time they fill with blood.

diastolic Relating to a diastole.

diataxia Loss of muscular coordination on both sides of the body.

diathermy Local generation of heat in the body tissues by a high frequency electric current.

medical d. Production of sufficient heat to warm the tissues without destroying them.

short wave d. Heating of tissues by means of an oscillating current of high frequency; used in physiotherapy to relieve pain.

surgical d. High frequency diathermy used for the destruction of diseased tissues (electrocoagulation), cauterization, etc.

diathesis An inherited or congenital bodily predisposition to a disease, or metabolic or structural abnormality; susceptibility to certain disorders.

cystic d. A predisposition to the formation of cysts in an organ.

gouty d. A predisposition to gout; goutiness.

hemorrhagic d. A predisposition to spontaneous hemorrhage.

diatom A microscopic, unicellular alga with a hard silica-containing cell wall.

diatomaceous Consisting of the siliceous skeletons or shells of the unicellular diatoms.

diatomic 1. Consisting of two atoms. 2. Dibasic.

diazepam A benzodiazepine derivative, $C_{16}H_{13}ClN_2O$; used primarily as an antianxiety agent, e.g., for sedation prior to cardiac catheterization and endoscopy; also a useful adjunct in the treatment of muscular spasms; Valium®.

diazotize To treat an amine with nitrous acid.

diazoxide A nondiuretic thiazide derivative used intravenously to acutely lower blood pressure in the treatment of hypertensive crises; Hyperstat®.

dibasic Having two replaceable hydrogen atoms; denoting a compound with two hydrogen atoms replaceable by a monovalent metal. Also called bibasic.

dibenzopyridine See acridine.

Dibothriocephalus See *Diphyllobothrium*.

dicentric Having two centromeres, as certain abnormal chromosomes.

dichloride A chemical compound containing two chloride atoms per molecule.

dichorial, dichorionic Having two chorions (outermost fetal membrane).

dichotomy Division or cutting into two parts.

dichromate A chemical compound containing the radical Cr_2O_7=. Also called bichromate.

dichromatic 1. Having two colors. 2. Relating to

dicumarol

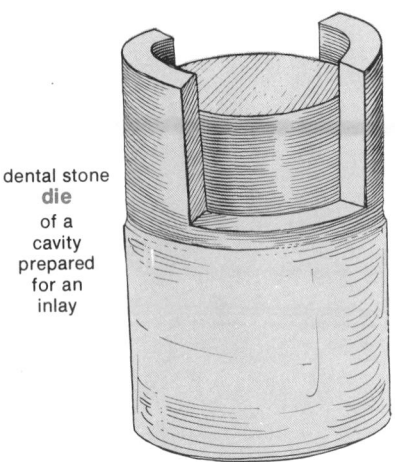

dental stone
die
of a
cavity
prepared
for an
inlay

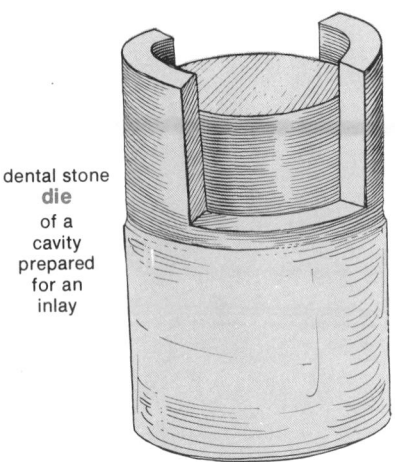

diffraction
of light waves

opaque
barrier

light waves

metencephalon

mesencephalon

myelencephalon

diencephalon

telencephalon

brain of human
embryo of
five weeks

the visual defect dichromatism.

dichromatism A defect in color perception; the spectrum is seen as comprised of only two colors separated by an achromatic or colorless band. Also called dichromatopsia; parachromatopsia; partial color blindness.

dichromism The property of exhibiting two colors, as certain crystals when seen from different directions, or certain solutions in varying degrees of concentration.

dichromophil, dichromophile Denoting tissues that take both acid and basic stains but in different areas.

dicrotic Double beat, denoting a pulse with two beats for each heart beat.

dictyokinesis The division of the Golgi apparatus of a cell during mitosis.

dictyoma Tumor of the retina.

dicumarol A coumarin derivative that inhibits the formation of prothrombin in the liver; a long-acting anticoagulant agent. Also called bishydroxycoumarin.

didactic Intended to instruct by means of lectures or textbooks rather than by clinical demonstrations with patients.

didactylism Having two fingers on a hand or two toes on a foot.

didymus A testis; from the Greek word *didymos*, meaning twin.

die A specialized model made from an impression, as the positive reproduction of a prepared tooth; usually made of metal or super hard dental stone.

diencephalon The portion of the embryonic brain between the mesencephalon and the telencephalon from which develop the thalamus, metathalamus, epithalamus, subthalamus, and hypothalamus; it encloses the third ventricle; together with the telencephalon it makes up the prosencephalon.

diener A laboratory assistant.

diet 1. Bodily nourishment. 2. Regulated nourishment, especially as prescribed for medical reasons. 3. To follow a specific dietary plan, especially for reduction of body weight by limitation of caloric intake.

balanced d. A diet containing the essential ingredients in proper proportion for adequate nutrition. Also called adequate diet.

bland d.'s Regular diets modified to be free from roughage or spicy, irritating foods; progressive regimen (bland 1, 2, 3, or 4), generally used in treatment of upper gastrointestinal disturbances.

clear liquid d. One used postoperatively for individuals unable to tolerate full liquids or solid food.

diabetic d.'s Any of nine balanced diets recommended by the American Diabetes Association for diabetic individuals; they are free of sugar and high carbohydrate foods and have caloric levels from 1200 to 3500; they are commonly divided in fifths, generally consisting of three meals and two snacks.

elimination d. A diet omitting foods suspected of causing allergic reactions; usually eliminated are eggs, milk, and wheat, less frequently, nuts, chocolate, and fish.

full liquid d. A diet composed of foods which are in liquid form at body temperature; it basically serves as a pre- or postoperative diet, and as a transition to a more liberal soft regimen.

Giordano-Giovannetti d. A renal diet providing 20–30 g of high biologic value protein. Also called Giovannetti diet.

high potassium d.'s Diets for individuals undergoing vigorous diuretic therapy; they provide approximately 100 mEq of potassium per day.

Kempner rice-fruit d. One consisting chiefly of rice and fruits with addition of minerals and vitamins and restriction of sodium; prescribed originally for arterial hypertension or chronic kidney disease.

low calcium d. A daily diet of from 100 to 200 mg of calcium; used in the treatment of hyperparathyroidism and urinary calcium stones, or as a test diet to determine urinary calcium excretion; diets of 250 mg of calcium are used in the treatment of certain individuals with hypercalcemia and/or hypercalciuria.

low cholesterol d. See low saturated fat diet.

low fat d. A diet containing minimal amounts of fats (40–50 g per day), as lean meat, fish, skimmed milk, cottage cheese, and cereal products; the caloric level may be varied through changes in protein and carbohydrate levels.

low residue d. A diet low in cellulose content, as fruits, vegetables, and unrefined cereals; vegetables are pureed to change the consistency of the cellulose.

low saturated fat d. A diet high in polyunsaturated fatty acids of vegetable origin, with restrictions on foods high in cholesterol and saturated fatty acids, such as eggs, butter, and meat. Also called cholesterol-lowering or low cholesterol diet.

low sodium d.'s Diets providing low levels of sodium for the treatment of congestive heart failure, and other conditions associated with edema; four levels of low sodium diets are commonly used: 250 mg, 500 mg, 1000 mg, and 2000 mg of sodium (a regular diet without added salt provides about 4 g of sodium).

reduction d.'s Diets for weight reduction, with caloric levels of 800, 1000, 1200, 1500, and 1800, that are adequate in protein and restricted in car-

bohydrate and fat; a level should be selected which allows for approximately one pound of weight loss per week.

regular d. One adequate to meet recommended daily allowances of the National Research Council; it contains approximately 80–100 g of protein, 4 g of sodium, 83 mEq of potassium, and 2000 cal.

renal d.'s Diets low in protein, sodium, and potassium; used in the treatment of renal failure. Cf. Giordano-Giovannetti diet.

salt-free d. Low sodium diet.

Sippy d. Bland diet.

soft d. A regular diet modified to include foods easily digested, excluding those high in indigestible cellulose and gas-forming fruits and vegetables; it contains approximately 75 g of protein, 4 g of sodium, 72 mEq of potassium, and 2000 cal.

dietetic 1. Of or relating to diet. 2. Specially prepared or processed food for regulated diets.

dietetics The study of diet in relation to health and disease.

diethylstilbestrol See stilbestrol.

dietitian A specialist in dietetics.

dietogenetics The study of the relationship between the genetic constitution of an individual, his diet, and various food requirements.

dietotherapy The treatment of disease by a regulated selection of food.

difference 1. A specific variation. 2. The amount by which one quantity varies from another.

arteriovenous oxygen d. The difference in the oxygen content of the arterial blood entering and the venous blood leaving a specified area or organ.

differential Relating to, showing, or dependent on a difference or distinction.

differentiation 1. In biology, the process of developing into specialized organs; said of embryonic tissues. 2. The act of distinguishing one disease from another. Also called differential diagnosis.

diffraction The interaction of matter with any wave motion (light and sound waves and all electromagnetic waves); e.g., the tendency of light rays to bend in the direction of an obstacle.

diffuse 1. Spread out; not circumscribed, localized, or limited. 2. To move by diffusion.

diffusion 1. The process of uniformly spreading out or scattering; the passage of the molecules of one substance between the molecules of another to form a mixture of the two substances. 2. Dialysis.

digastric Having two bellies, as the digastric muscle.

Digenea A subclass of flatworms or flukes (class Trematoda), parasitic in man and other mammals.

DiGeorge's syndrome Congenital thymic aplaclubbed digits

Digitalis purpurea

Browne-McHardy pneumatic **dilator**

dinitrophenol

pneumatic bag

digitoxin

$C_{18}H_{31}O_9$

dimenhydrinate

sia. See under aplasia.

digest 1. To break up food into simpler, assimilable compounds by the muscular and chemical action of the digestive tract. 2. To absorb mentally.

digestant An agent that aids the process of digestion.

digestion The process taking place in the alimentary canal whereby the nutritive components of food are converted into substances that can be absorbed by the intestine; the decomposition of materials into simpler compounds.

digestive Relating to digestion.

digit A finger or toe.

clubbed d.'s A bulbous enlargement of the fingertips, seen in some cases of heart disease and certain pulmonary disorders. Also called drumstick or clubbed fingers.

digital 1. Pertaining to, performed by, or resembling a digit or digits, especially a finger. 2. Possessing digits.

digitalis 1. Foxglove, a plant of the genus *Digitalis*. 2. Digitalis (USP), a drug obtained from the dried leaves of *Digitalis purpurea*, used in the treatment of heart disease, especially for congestive heart failure and some supraventricular tachyarrhythmias.

digitalization The treatment of an individual with digitalis or a related cardiac glycoside, to achieve a desired therapeutic effect.

digitate Having fingerlike processes.

digitation A finger-like process.

digitoxin A glycoside obtained from *Digitalis purpurea*; used in the treatment of congestive heart failure.

digitus, *pl.* **digiti** Latin for finger.

digoxin A glycoside obtained from the leaves of *Digitalis lanata*; used in the treatment of congestive heart failure.

DiGuglielmo's syndrome Erythremic myelosis; see under myelosis.

dihydrate A compound having two molecules of water.

dihydroergotamine (D.H.E. 45) A crystalline compound produced by the hydrogenation of ergotamine; used in the treatment of migraine headache.

dihydrostreptomycin Compound made by the hydrogenation of streptomycin and having antibiotic properties.

dihydrotachysterol (AT 10) A synthetic sterol that produces effects similar to those of vitamin D.

diiodotyrosine (T_2, DIT) A precursor of the thyroid hormone thyroxin. Also called iodogorgoic acid.

diisopropylfluorophosphate (DFP) A potent cholinergic agent; used in the treatment of glaucoma

and strabismus.

dilatation 1. The condition of being enlarged, occurring normally, artifically, or as a result of disease; said of a tubular structure, a cavity, or an opening; 2. Dilation (1).

gastric d. Acute distention of the stomach with fluid and air; commonly seen following surgery or trauma.

dilation 1. The act of stretching or dilating. 2. Dilatation (1).

dilator Instrument for enlarging a passage or cavity.

dildo, dildoe An object having the approximate size and shape of an erect penis; used to produce sexual pleasure by vaginal insertion.

diltiazem A calcium channel blocking agent used in the treatment of angina pectoris; especially useful in Prinzmetal's angina.

diluent A substance which reduces the concentration of a solution.

dilution 1. The process of reducing the concentration of a solution or substance. 2. A weakened solution or substance; an attenuated mixture.

dimenhydrinate Drug used in preventing and treating motion sickness; Dramamine®.

dimension Any measurable distance.

vertical d. In prosthodontics, the distance between two points on the face, one above and one below the mouth, usually in the midline; it may be measured when the opposing occlusal surfaces are in maximum contact (occlusal vertical dimension) or in rest position, when the jaws are not in contact (rest vertical dimension).

dimer A chemical compound composed of molecules that consist of two identical simpler molecules.

dimercaprol A compound used as an antidote for lewisite and other arsenic poisoning. Also called British antilewisite (BAL).

dimethyl sulfoxide (DMSO) An industrial solvent occasionally used in medicine as a skin penetrant to facilitate absorption of medications from the skin. Also called methyl sulfoxide.

dimorphism The property of occurring in two forms.

dinitrophenol (DNP) A drug that causes an increase in rate of metabolism by interruption of the coupling of oxidation and phosphorylation; not used clinically because of its toxicity.

dinucleotide One of the compounds into which nucleic acid splits on hydrolysis; it may split into two mononucleotides.

diopter (D) The unit used to designate the refractive power of a lens or an optical system.

dioptometer An instrument for measuring refrac-

tion and accommodation of the eye. Also called dioptrometer.

dioptric 1. Relating to the unit of refractive power of lenses. 2. Refractive.

dioptrics The science of the refraction of light.

dioptrometer See dioptometer.

diotic In audiology, denoting an arrangement in which each ear receives the same signal.

dioxide An oxide containing two atoms of oxygen per molecule.

dioxin A hydrocarbon; a pesticide contaminant thought to produce cancer and birth defects.

dipeptidase One of the protein-splitting enzymes that causes the breakdown of a dipeptide into its two constituent amino acids.

dipeptide Two amino acids linked by a peptide bond.

diphenhydramine hydrochloride An antihistamine used in the prevention and treatment of motion sickness, postoperative nausea, nausea and vomiting of pregnancy, and some allergies; Benadryl®.

diphenylhydantoin An anticonvulsant agent, used primarily to treat epilepsy; Dilantin®.

2,3-diphosphoglycerate (DPG) A chemical present in the red blood cells that binds to hemoglobin and has a great effect on its oxygen affinity; in its absence, hemoglobin unloads less oxygen in passing through tissue capillaries.

diphosphonates Synthetic substances similar to the pyrophosphates in structure but not biologically hydrolyzed; in vitro, they prevent hydroxyapatite crystal formation; it has been suggested that they coat the bone surface and prevent bone resorption.

diphosphopyridine nucleotide (DPN) Old term for nicotinamide adenine dinucleotide (NAD).

diphtheria An acute contagious disease caused by a bacillus, *Corynebacterium diphtheriae*; marked by inflammation of the upper respiratory tract, fibrin formation (false membrane) of the mucous membranes, and elaboration of soluble exotoxin which acts on the heart and cranial or peripheral nerve cells.

diphtheroid 1. Resembling diphtheria. 2. A bacterium resembling the organism that causes diphtheria.

diphyllobothriasis Infestation with *Diphyllobothrium latum* (broadfish tapeworm), caused by ingestion of inadequately cooked, infected fish.

Diphyllobothrium A genus of tapeworms (family Diphyllobothriidae). Formerly called *Dibothriocephalus*.

D. latum Intestinal parasite transmitted to man by ingestion of undercooked infected fresh water

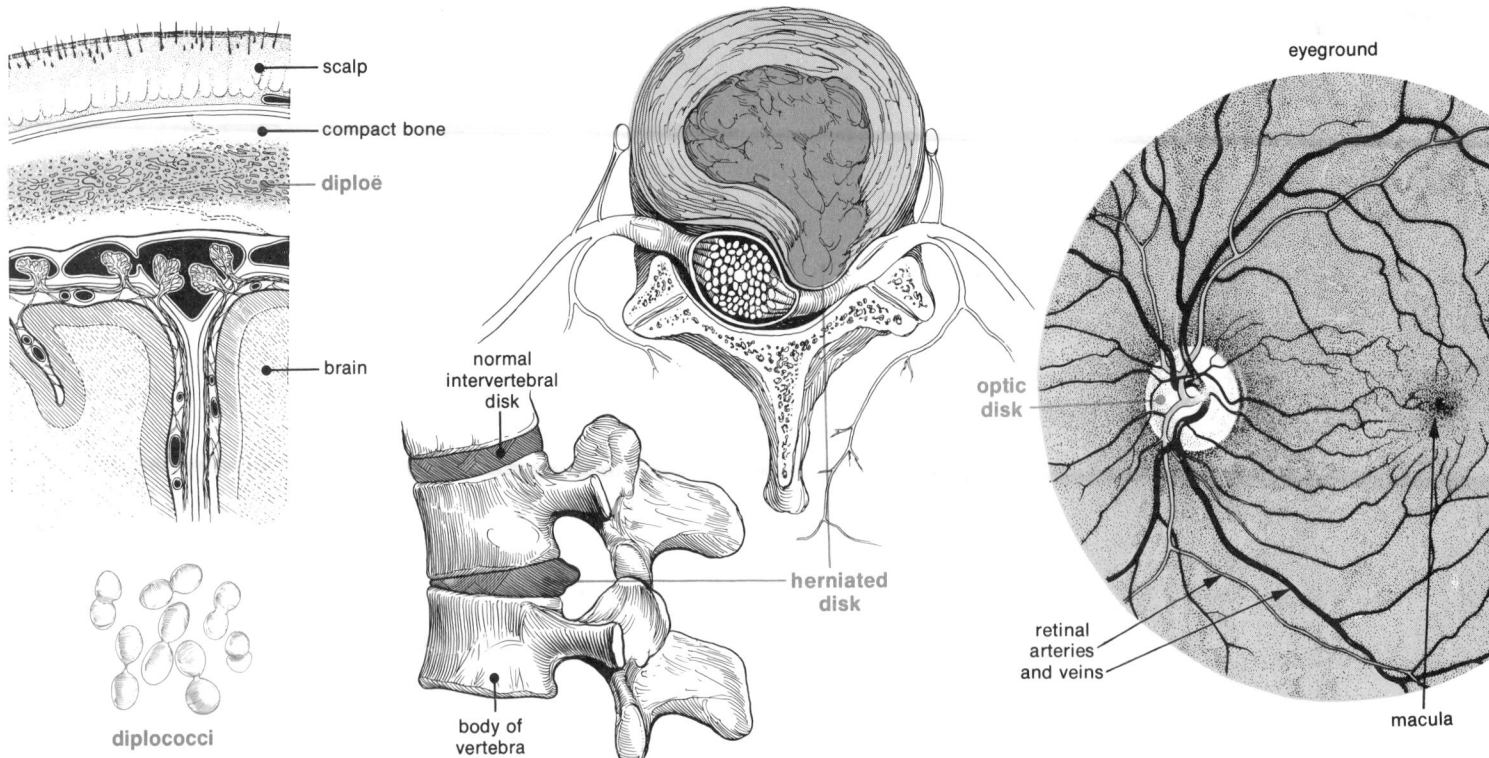

scalp
compact bone
diploë
brain

normal intervertebral disk

herniated disk

body of vertebra

diplococci

eyeground

optic disk

retinal arteries and veins

macula

fish. Also called fish tapeworm.

diplacusis Condition in which one sound is heard differently by the two ears, resulting in the perception of two sounds instead of one.

diplegia Paralysis of corresponding parts on both sides of the body. Also called bilateral paralysis.

   congenital facial d. See Möbius' syndrome.

diplobacteria Bacteria linked in pairs.

Diplococcus Former name for a genus of bacteria.

   D. gonorrhoeae See *Neisseria gonorrhoeae*.

   D. pneumoniae See *Streptococcus pneumoniae*.

diplococcus, *pl.* **diplococci** Any of various spherical or ovoid bacteria joined together in pairs.

diploë The spongy (cancellous) bone with a limited marrow cavity between the two tables (layers) of the cranial bones.

diploid Having two sets of chromosomes, the total number of chromosomes being twice that of a gamete.

diplopia Double vision.

diplotene In meiosis, the fourth of five stages of prophase in which the intimately paired homologous chromosomes begin to separate, forming a characteristic chiasma or X appearance; at this stage, blocks of genes are exchanged between homologous chromosomes.

dipsomania An insatiable, uncontrollable desire for alcoholic drinks.

dipsosis Abnormally excessive thirst.

dipyridamole A crystalline compound used to reduce platelet aggregation and as a dilator of coronary blood vessels.

Dirofilaria A genus of filaria (family Onchocercidae, superfamily Filarioidea) known to infest mammals; rarely found in humans.

   D. immitis The heartworm, a parasite in the pulmonary arteries of dogs.

disability 1. A legal loss of function and earning power. 2. Incapacity. 3. Any handicap.

   learning d. (LD) A complex of symptoms that involves impairment of some or all of the following functions: learning, language, perception, memory, and concentration; neurologic examination usually yields minor abnormalities, if any; diagnosis rests on psychological assessment of cognitive function.

disablement 1. A legal incapacity without loss of earning power. 2. Incapacitation.

disaccharide A class of sugars, including sucrose, lactose, and maltose, which yield two monosaccharides on hydrolysis.

disarticulation Amputation of a limb by separating the bones at the joint.

disc See disk.

discectomy Surgical removal of an intervertebral disk.

discharge 1. Material that is released as an excretion or a secretion. 2. To pour forth; to emit. 3. The activation of a nerve cell.

discission Surgical procedure in which the capsule of the lens of the eye is either punctured or cut.

discogenic Referring to a disorder originating in an intervertebral disk.

discography See diskography.

discoid 1. Having the shape of a disk. 2. A dental disk-shaped carving and excavating instrument.

discopathy Disease of a disk, especially of an intervertebral disk.

discrete Denoting certain lesions of the skin which are separate, not joined or confluent.

discutient Denoting an agent that causes the dispersal of a tumor or any pathologic accumulation.

disease Any abnormal condition, affecting either the whole body or any of its parts, which impairs normal functioning. For individual diseases, see specific names.

   allogeneic d. Either an acute or a chronic disease resulting primarily from a reaction to a graft.

   communicable d. Any disease transmissible by infection or contagion directly or through a carrier of the pathogen.

   congenital d. A disease present at birth.

   contagious d. A disease transmissible by direct or indirect contact.

   deficiency d. A disease due to a prolonged lack of vitamins, minerals, or any other essential dietary component.

   endemic d. A disease present in a specific locality more or less continuously.

   functional d. A disease occurring without an apparent physical cause.

   hereditary d. A disease transmitted genetically from a parent to offspring.

   infectious d. A disease caused by the presence of a pathologic microorganism.

   local d. Disorder confined to a specific part or organ, usually without generalized involvement.

   mental d. See disorder, mental.

   occupational d. A disease caused by the environment of a particular occupation.

   organic d. A disease in which structural changes in the body take place.

   periodic d. Any disease that recurs regularly.

   social d. Popular but incorrect term for veneral diseases, especially gonorrhea and syphilis.

   systemic d. A disease affecting several organs or the entire body.

   venereal d. (VD) Any disease acquired through sexual intercourse, as gonorrhea, syphilis, chancroid, etc.

disengagement In obstetrics, the emergence of the presenting part of the fetus from the vulva.

disequilibrium Lack of balance or stability.

disimpaction 1. Separation of an impacted bone fracture. 2. The breaking up of a fecal impaction.

disinfectant Any agent that kills disease-causing microorganisms; generally used on inanimate objects.

disinfection The destruction of infectious agents by chemical or physical means directly applied.

   terminal d. One in which the infectious agent is eliminated from personal clothing and possessions in the immediate environment of the patient.

disintegration 1. Breakdown or separation of component parts. 2. Disorganization of mental processes.

disk Any platelike structure. Also written disc.

   articular d. A circular fibrocartilaginous pad present in some synovial joints and attached to the joint capsule; e.g., the articular disk of the temporomandibular joint, which separates the cavity of the capsule into two separate compartments, thus reducing friction between the articulating surfaces of the bones.

   dental d. A small disk of paper or plastic, coated with cuttle-fish bone, emery, garnet, or sand; used in dentistry to cut, smooth, or polish teeth and dental restorations.

   herniated d. Posterior rupture of the inner portion of an intervertebral disk, causing pressure on the nerve roots with resulting pain; occurring most commonly in the lower back. Also called slipped, ruptured, or prolapsed disk.

   intercalated d. The double membrane separating cells of cardiac muscle fibers.

   intervertebral d. The fibrocartilaginous tissue between the bodies of adjacent vertebrae, consisting of a jellylike center surrounded by a fibrous ring.

   optic d. The pinkish white oval or circular area of the retina, which is the site of entrance of the optic nerve. Also called blind spot.

   ruptured d. See herniated disk.

   slipped d. See herniated disk.

   tactile d. The saucer-shaped termination of specialized sensory nerve fibers in contact with a modified cell in the deep layers of the epidermis. Also called meniscus tactus.

diskectomy The surgical removal, in part or whole, of an intervertebral disk.

diskitis Inflammation of a disk, especially of one between the vertebrae.

diskography Radiographic visualization of internormal position

displacement of uterus

displaced condylar head

dislocation of mandible

normal position

normal distention of ascending colon

extreme distention of ascending colon

colon

vertebral disk space after injection of a radiopaque substance. Also written discography.

disk syndrome Pain in the lower back, radiating to the thigh with occasional loss of ankle and knee reflexes, resulting from compression of spinal nerve roots by an intervertebral disk.

dislocate To shift from the usual or normal position, especially to displace a bone from its socket; to luxate.

dislocation **1.** Displacement of a limb or organ from the normal position. **2.** Specifically, a displacement of a bone from its socket or joint.

dismutase An enzyme that promotes the reaction of two identical molecules to produce two molecules in different oxidation states.

disorder A disturbance of function or health.

affective d. Manic-depressive psychosis; see under psychosis.

autosomal dominant d. A disorder occurring when only one abnormal gene is present and the corresponding gene (allele) on the homologous chromosome is normal. Also called autosomal dominant disease.

autosomal recessive d. A disorder that is apparent only when both corresponding genes (alleles) in homologous chromosomes are abnormal. Also called autosomal recessive disease.

bipolar d. Disorder marked by alternating moods of elation and depression.

borderline personality d. Behavioral pattern marked by impulsiveness, intense interpersonal relationships, and instability in mood and emotion.

character d. Deeply ingrained, maladaptive patterns of behavior unaccompanied by subjective feelings of anxiety or guilt.

functional d. Mental disorder not caused by organic disease.

genetic d. A disorder in which the genetic component expresses itself in a predictable manner without much influence from the environment.

immunoproliferative d. Proliferation of cells of the lymphoreticular system associated with auto-allergic disturbances or gamma-globulin abnormalities.

mendelian d. Pathologic condition determined at a single chromosomal gene locus, whether autosomal or on a sex chromosome, and transmitted in a dominant or recessive way.

mental d. Any psychiatric disorder listed in the *Standard Nomenclature of Diseases and Operations* of the American Medical Association, or in the *Diagnostic and Statistical Manual for Mental Disorders* of the American Psychiatric Association. Also called mental illness.

neuropsychologic d. Impairment of mental function due to a lesion in the brain; it may have a sudden onset and a short duration (acute) or it may be prolonged (chronic).

personality d. General term used to denote any long-standing maladaptive pattern of behavior; distinguished from neurotic and psychotic symptoms.

psychophysiologic d., psychosomatic d. Disturbances of visceral functioning secondary to long-continued emotional attitudes.

sleep d. Any disturbance of sleep, such as somnambulism.

disorganization Destruction or breakdown of tissues with resulting loss of function.

disorientation Loss of the sense of direction or location.

dispensary **1.** An office in any institution (hospital, school, etc.) from which medical supplies and medicines are distributed. **2.** A public institution that dispenses free medical aid. **3.** An outpatient department of a hospital.

dispensatory A book describing the sources, preparation, contents, and uses of medicines.

dispense To prepare and distribute medicines to the sick.

disperse To scatter.

dispersion **1.** The process of dispersing or the state of being dispersed. **2.** A suspension of solid, liquid, or gaseous particles of colloidal size in another medium.

coarse d. A suspension of relatively large particles in a liquid.

molecular d. One in which the dispersed particles are individual molecules; a true solution.

displacement **1.** The condition of being moved from a normal position. **2.** In chemistry, a reaction in which an atom, molecule, or radical group is removed from a compound and replaced with another. **3.** The weight of a fluid expelled by a floating body or by another fluid of greater density. **4.** A defense mechanism in which an emotion, such as anger, is unconsciously directed to an object or person other than the direct cause of frustration; e.g., an angry individual beating the wall with his fist.

dissect To cut apart, especially in the study of anatomy.

dissection **1.** The act of dissecting. **2.** A tissue that has been dissected.

disseminated Widely distributed throughout an organ, tissue, or the body; scattered; dispersed.

dissimulation The act of feigning health by a sick person.

dissociation **1.** Separation. **2.** Change of a com-

plex chemical compound into a simple one.

albuminocytologic d. Increase in the protein content of the cerebrospinal fluid without increase in cell count.

atrioventricular d. Independent action of the atria and ventricles of the heart.

complete A-V d. **1.** Atrioventricular dissociation not interrupted by ventricular captures. **2.** Complete atrioventricular block; independent beating of atria and ventricle caused by failure of impulses to reach the ventricles.

electromechanical d. Electrical activity in the heart without resulting mechanical contraction, as in cardiac rupture.

incomplete A-V d. Atrioventricular dissociation interrupted by ventricular captures.

interference d. Atrioventricular dissociation occasionally interrupted by ventricular captures.

dissolution **1.** Decomposition into component parts; disintegration. **2.** A dissolving. **3.** Autolysis.

dissolve **1.** To cause a substance to change from a solid to a dispersed state by placing it in contact with a solvent fluid. **2.** To melt; to reduce to a liquid state.

dissolvent Solvent; capable of dissolving another substance.

distad Toward the periphery.

distal **1.** Farthest from a point of reference. **2.** In dentistry, the location most distant from the median line of the jaw.

distal end The posterior part of a dental appliance.

distance The space between two points.

interocclusal d. The distance or space between the occlusal surfaces of the mandibular and maxillary teeth when the mandible is in the physiologic rest position. Also called free-way space.

map d. The distance between two gene loci in a chromosome; measured in centimorgans.

reduced interarch d. Condition in which the mandible rises too far before the teeth make contact. Also called overclosure.

small interarch d. A small space between the upper (maxillary) and lower (mandibular) dental arches. Also called close bite.

distemper Infectious viral disease of certain mammals, especially young dogs, often causing paralysis and death.

distensibility The ability to stretch.

distention, distension The state of being stretched or distended.

distill To subject a liquid mixture to vaporization and subsequent condensation with collection of components by differential cooling.

$$(CH_3CH_2)_2N-C(\overset{S}{\|})-S-S-C(\overset{S}{\|})-N(CH_2CH_3)_2$$

disulfiram

presynaptic neuron

divergence

postsynaptic neurons

urethral diverticulum

diverticulosis

Meckel's diverticulum

model of DNA

adenine

thymine

guanine

cytosine

molecular chain

distillation The vaporization of a liquid mixture by heat followed by separations of its components by condensation of the vapor.

distobuccal Relating to the distal and buccal surfaces of a posterior tooth; usually denoting the line angle formed by the junction of the two surfaces.

distobucco-occlusal Relating to the distal, buccal, and occlusal surfaces of a posterior tooth; usually denoting the point angle formed by the junction of the three surfaces.

distolabioincisal Relating to the distal, labial, and incisal surfaces of an anterior tooth; usually denoting the point angle formed by the junction of the three surfaces.

distolingual Relating to the distal and lingual surfaces of a tooth; usually denoting the line angle formed by the junction of the two surfaces.

distolinguoincisal Relating to the distal, lingual, and incisal surfaces of an anterior tooth; usually denoting the point angle formed by the junction of the three surfaces.

distomiasis Condition caused by the presence of flukes in the organs or tissues.

disto-occlusal Relating to the distal and occlusal surfaces of a posterior tooth; usually denoting the line angle formed by the junction of the two surfaces.

distortion 1. A deformed image caused by irregularities in a lens. 2. A mechanism aiding in the disguising or repression of unacceptable thoughts.

distraction 1. Mental or emotional disturbance. 2. Separation of joint surfaces without fracture or dislocation. 3. In orthodontics, unusually large distance of structures, such as teeth, from the median plane.

distress Physical or mental anguish or pain.

fetal d. Metabolic derangements in the fetus affecting the functions of vital organs to the point of temporary or permanent injury or death.

distribution 1. The arrangement of blood vessels and nerves in the different bodily parts. 2. The areas of the body supplied by the terminal branches of such structures.

disulfiram A counterdrug that produces an aversion to alcohol; Antabuse®.

diuresis Discharge of increased amounts of urine.

alcoholic d. Production of unusually large quantities of urine after consumption of alcoholic beverages.

osmotic d. Diuresis due to concentration in the kidney tubules of substances that limit the reabsorption of water.

solute d. Diuresis caused by increased concentration of solute in the blood or resulting from excretion of increased amounts of solute in the urine.

water d. Diuresis caused by diminution of antidiuretic hormone, resulting in excretion of increased amounts of urine without a marked change in the excretion of solute.

diuretic 1. Tending to promote the excretion of urine. 2. An agent that increases the amount of urine.

divalent See bivalent (1).

divergence 1. The act or state of spreading apart from a common point. 2. The spreading of branches of a presynaptic neuron to form synapses and cause activity with a number of postsynaptic neurons.

diverticular Of or relating to a diverticulum.

diverticulectomy Surgical removal of a diverticulum or of diverticula.

diverticulitis Inflammation and infection of a diverticulum; the most common symptom of intestinal diverticulitis is a crampy pain usually in the lower left side of the abdomen, associated with nausea and fever.

diverticulosis Presence of diverticula in the intestines, especially in the colon; it results from herniation of the mucosa through defects in the muscular wall, usually at the site of entry of blood vessels; usually asymptomatic; infection is termed diverticulitis.

diverticulum, *pl.* **diverticula** A saccular dilatation protruding from the wall of a tubular organ.

hypopharyngeal d. A diverticulum located in the hypopharynx between the inferior constrictor muscle and the cricopharyngeal muscle. Also called Zenker's or pharyngoesophageal diverticulum.

intestinal d. A herniation of the mucous membrane through a defect in the muscular layer of the intestinal wall.

Meckel's d. A congenital sacculation or appendage of the ileum.

pulsion d. A diverticulum formed by pressure from within, usually causing herniation of mucosa through a muscular layer.

traction d. One formed by the pulling force of adhesions, occurring mainly in the esophagus.

urethral d. An outpouching of the urethral lumen; in the female, it may vary in size from 3 mm to 8 cm in diameter; when large, the diverticulum may be buried along the entire length of the urethra.

vesicourachal d. A diverticulum of the bladder into the urachus resulting from persistent patency of part of the allantoic duct which prenatally extends from the bladder to the umbilical cord.

Zenker's d. See hypopharyngeal diverticulum.

division Separation.

heterotypic d. The first reduction division of meiosis.

homotypic d. The second reduction division of meiosis.

indirect nuclear d. Mitosis.

divulse To separate by tearing.

divulsion The removal of a part by tearing or pulling apart.

dizygotic Relating to fraternal (nonidentical) twins, i.e., twins derived from two separate zygotes.

dizygous Dizygotic.

dizziness An abnormal sensation of unsteadiness characterized by a feeling of movement within the head, without actual motion.

DNA Deoxyribonucleic acid, the molecular basis of heredity, present in chromosomes; it is the largest biologically active molecule presently known and is responsible for the replication of the key substances of life, proteins and nucleic acid; it consists of two long chains of alternate sugar (with attached base) and phosphate groups twisted into a double helix.

recombinant DNA Biologically active DNA that has been formed by the in vitro joining of segments of DNA from different species.

Z DNA A form of DNA that is twisted in the opposite direction from the usual DNA spiral; while its detailed function is not fully known, Z DNA may play a role in controlling gene expression.

doctor 1. A person holding a doctorate degree awarded by a college or university in any specialized field, as in music. 2. A person trained in and licensed to practice the healing arts, as a physician, dentist, or veterinarian. 3. To treat medically.

dolichocephalic, dolichocephalous Longheaded; having a disproportionately long head; denoting a skull with a cephalic index of below 80, or an individual with such a skull.

dolichopellic, dolichopelvic A disproportionately long pelvis, with a pelvic index above 95.

doll's eye sign Movement of the eyes in a direction opposite to a sudden movement of the head, caused by a lesion in the central mechanism for voluntary eye movement. Also called doll's head phenomenon; Cantelli's sign.

domain One of the regions of a peptide molecule having a coherent structure or functional significance that distinguishes it from other regions of the same molecule.

dominant In genetics, capable of expression to the exclusion of a contrasted (recessive) character.

donor 1. One who donates or contributes tissue, such as blood or an organ for transfusion or transplant. 2. In chemistry, a substance that donates part of itself to another substance (the receptor).

methyl d.'s Compounds that, in living tissue, can supply methyl groups for transfer to other com-

calculation of children's dosage

age	fraction of adult dosage
1 month	1/20
2 months	1/15
months	1/10
months	1/9
1 year	1/7
2 years	1/6
3 years	1/5
4 years	1/4
5–6 years	1/3
7–8 years	1/2
0–12 years	2/3
3–15 years	3/4

cigarette drain

Jackson-Pratt® drain

Down syndrome

1	2	3		4	5		6	7	8	9	10	11	12

13	14	15	16	17	18	19	20	21	22	XX	three chromo-somes in group 21

dopa 3,4-Dihydroxyphenylalanine, a crystalline amino acid; a precursor of norepinephrine, epinephrine, and melanin.

dopamine A compound produced by the decarboxylation of dopa; in parkinsonism, there is a depletion of dopamine in the basal ganglia of the brain, particularly in the caudate nucleus and putamen. Also called *o*-hydroxytyramine.

dopaminergic Involving the action of dopamine.

dope A narcotic or habit-forming drug taken for pleasure or to maintain an addiction.

dornase Streptodornase.

pancreatic d. A deoxyribonuclease preparation made from beef pancreas, used as an inhalation to reduce the tenacity of thick secretions.

dorsal Relating to the back or to the posterior part of an anatomic structure.

dorsiflexion Flexion or turning upward, as of the foot or toes.

dorsolumbar Relating to the back of the body in the region of the lower thoracic and upper lumbar vertebrae.

dorsum The back or the upper or posterior surface.

d. sellae The portion of the sphenoid bone that forms the posterior boundary of the sella turcica.

dosage 1. The giving of medication in prescribed amounts. 2. The determination of the proper amount of a dose.

dose (D) 1. A specified quantity of medication to be taken or administered at one time or stated intervals. 2. The amount of radiation administered to, or absorbed accidentally by, the tissues at one time.

booster d. A supplementary dose given sometime after the initial dose to maintain immunity.

curative d. The amount of a substance required to cure a disease or correct a deficiency.

daily d. The total amount of a medicine taken within 24 hours.

divided d. Fractional portions of a medicine administered at short intervals so that the full dose is given within a definite period.

erythema d. The minimal safe amount of radiation required to produce redness of the skin within 10 days to two weeks; represented by the Sabouraud meter as the B tint, the Holzknecht as 5(5H), the Hampson as 4, and the Kienbock as 10.

maintenance d. The amount of a medicine administered to keep the patient under the influence of the drug after larger previous amounts.

maximal permissible d. (MPD) The greatest amount of radiation to which a person may be exposed without causing harmful effects.

pounds.

minimal infective d. (MID) The smallest amount of infectious material that produce disease.

minimal lethal d. (MLD, mld) The smallest amount of a toxin required to kill an experimental animal.

sensitizing d. Anaphylaxis.

skin d. (S.D.) The quantity of radiation received on the skin surface.

dosimetry Determination of correct dosage.

dotage The mental weakness or senility of old age.

doublet 1. A combination of two similar structures, as a combination of two joined microtubules in a cilium or flagellum. 2. A pair of lenses mounted together to form a single lens system.

douche A stream of liquid, vapor, or gas directed into a cavity of the body, particularly the rinsing of the vagina with a liquid.

dovetail In dentistry, a fanned-out prepared cavity resembling the tail of a dove, made deliberately to prevent displacement of the restoration.

dowel A pin, usually made of metal, fitted into the root canal of a natural tooth to give support to an artificial crown.

down-regulation The rapid development of a resistant-to-treatment or tolerant state resulting from repeated administration of a pharmaceutically or physiologically active agent.

Down syndrome Congenital defect caused by a chromosomal abnormality; the affected person has three chromosomes (trisomy) instead of the normal two for the pair designated Number 21; marked by various degrees of mental retardation and characteristic physical features such as short flattened skull, slanting eyes, thickened tongue, broad hands and feet, and other anomalies. Also called mongolism; trisomy 21.

doxorubicin An anticancer drug.

dracontiasis Infection with *Dracunculus medinensis*.

Dracunculus A genus of nematodes resembling the true filaria worms but having a crustacean rather than an insect as an intermediate host.

drain 1. To draw off the fluid from a bodily cavity, especially to provide for its exit as soon as it is formed. 2. To discharge. 3. A device (tube or wick) used to remove fluid from a wound.

cigarette d. A cigarette-shaped gauze wick enclosed in a thin-walled rubber tube.

Jackson-Pratt® d. A flexible silicon rubber suction drain with small intraluminal ridges which prevent collapse of its lumen and with a radiopaque marker incorporated in the side; used to drain the subdural space after removal of a subdural hematoma. Also called subdural brain drain.

Penrose d. Cigarette drain.

stab d. A drain passed through a puncture wound some distance from the operative incision.

subdural brain d. See Jackson-Pratt® drain.

sump d. A drain composed of two tubes, the larger one containing a slender tube which is attached to a suction pump.

drainage 1. The continuous withdrawal of fluids from a cavity or wound. 2. The material withdrawn or discharged.

capillary d. Drainage effected by means of a wick of gauze, strands of hair, or other material.

closed d. Drainage of chest cavity carried out with protection against the entrance of outside air into the cavity.

open d. Drainage of chest through an opening in the chest wall without sealing off the outside air.

tidal d. Drainage of a paralyzed urinary bladder by an irrigation apparatus.

dram 1. An avoirdupois unit of weight equal to 27.34 grains or 0.062 ounce. 2. An apothecary unit of weight equal to 60 grains or 1/8 ounce.

drawer sign A sign elicited from a patient lying on his back with his knee flexed at 90 degrees while the examiner grasps the upper part of the patient's leg with both hands and pulls the head of the tibia; a forward movement indicates rupture of the anterior cruciate ligament; if the tibia can be pushed under the femoral condyle, the posterior cruciate ligament is ruptured. Also called Rocher's sign.

drawsheet A narrow sheet stretched crosswise under a patient in bed; used as an aid in moving or turning the patient.

dream A series of images experienced during sleep, usually with a definite sense of reality.

wet d. A dream, usually erotic, accompanied by emission of semen during sleep.

dress To apply a dressing.

dressing 1. Material or preparation applied to a wound or lesion for the purpose of preventing external infection, absorbing discharges, etc. 2. The application of such materials.

occlusive d. One that covers and seals a wound completely.

pressure d. A dressing consisting of gauze and abundant resilient material held in place with elastic bandage; thus pressure is applied on the wound to prevent accumulation of fluids.

dribble To flow in drops, as the urine from a distended bladder.

drift Unobtrusive and cumulative changes over time in the genetic composition of a population.

drill A cutting instrument for boring holes in bones or teeth by rotary motion.

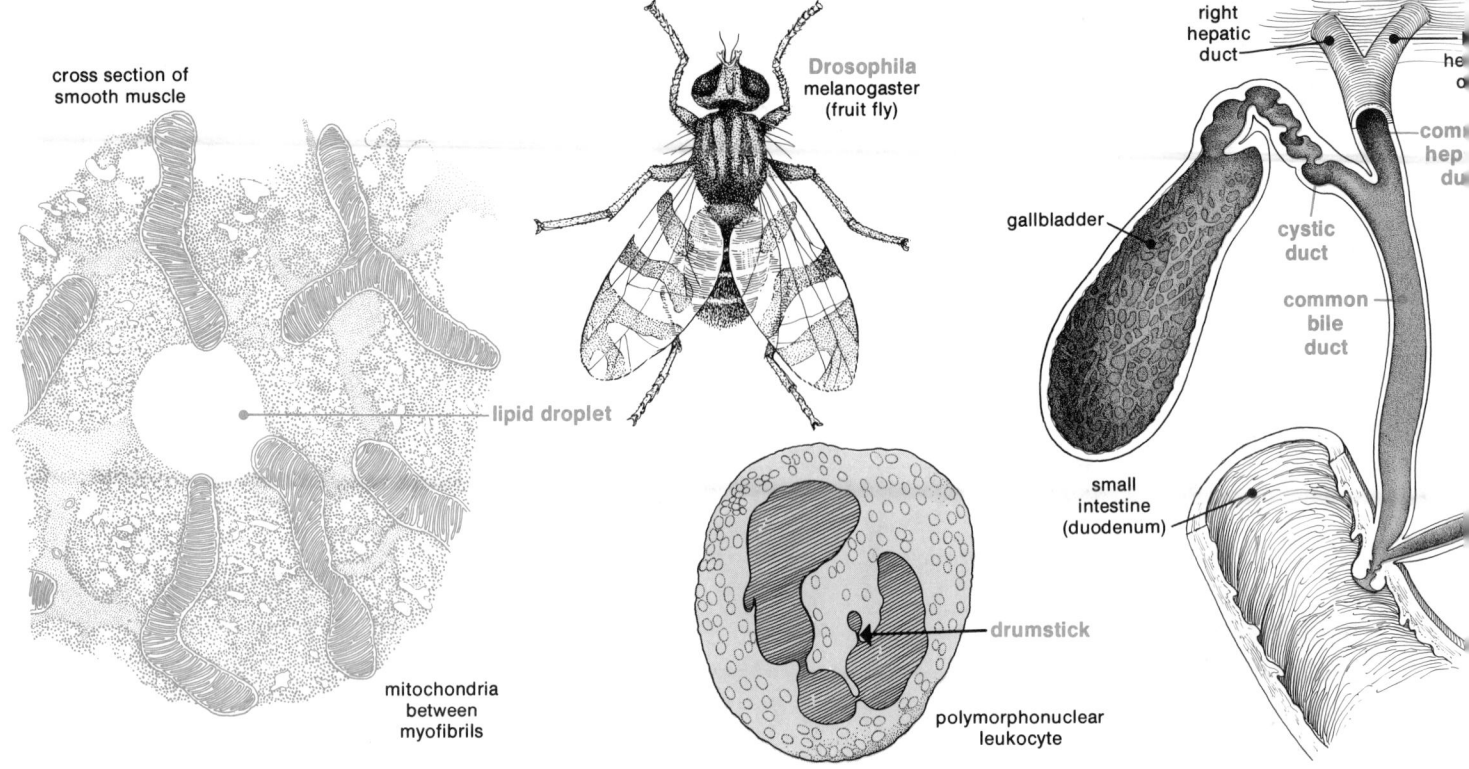

cross section of
smooth muscle

lipid droplet

mitochondria
between
myofibrils

Drosophila
melanogaster
(fruit fly)

drumstick

polymorphonuclear
leukocyte

right
hepatic
duct

gallbladder

cystic
duct

common
bile
duct

small
intestine
(duodenum)

drip 1. To fall in drops. 2. A liquid that falls in drops. 3. Colloquial expression referring to a discharge.

intravenous d. The continuous intravenous injection of a substance a drop at a time.

postnasal d. Excessive discharge of mucus from the posterior nares.

dromic Denoting nerve impulses conducted in a normal direction.

dromotropic Affecting conductivity of nerves.

drop 1. The smallest possible quantity of a liquid heavy enough to fall in a pear-shaped globule. 2. To fall in drops or to let fall in drops.

foot d. See footdrop.

hanging d. A drop of a fluid on the undersurface of the object glass examined under the microscope.

toe d. See footdrop.

wrist d. Wristdrop.

droplet A very small drop.

lipid d. A spherical body of lipid occurring freely in the cytoplasm of cells; it is not ordinarily membrane bound and is generally surrounded by mitochondria. Also called lipid body or inclusion.

drops Popular name for any liquid medicine administered with a dropper.

eye d. Ophthalmic solution; see under solution.

knock-out d. Popular name for chloral alcoholate; made by mixing chloral hydrate with any alcoholic drink and given with criminal intent to produce rapid unconsciousness.

dropsy 1. See hydrops. 2. Obsolete term used to describe heart failure, chronic renal disease, and other fluid-retaining states.

Drosophila A genus of flies containing about 900 species, including the fruit fly (D. melanogaster), which is used extensively in genetic studies.

drowse To be partially asleep.

drug 1. Any substance used as a medicine in the treatment or prevention of disease. 2. A narcotic or hallucinogen, whether or not used for medical purposes, employed usually illegally for altering mood, perception, or consciousness.

crude d. Any medicinal material before refining.

psychedelic d. A drug, usually self-administered, that causes marked changes in mood.

psychotropic d. Any drug that influences psychic functions, behavior, or experiences, such as chlorpromazine (Thorazine®).

sulfa d. Any of a group of synthetic organic compounds, related to sulfonamide, used as antibacterial agents.

drug dependence Condition in which the user of a drug considers the effects it produces, or the conditions associated with its use, essential to main-

tain an optimal state of well being.

drug-fast Relating to microorganisms that resist the action of a chemical.

drug misuse Inappropriate use of medicine either in inappropriate dosages or for purposes for which it was not intended.

drumstick A minute protrusion from the nucleus of a polymorphonuclear leukocyte, present in about two percent of these cells when two X chromosomes are present, as in normal females (XX) or in patients with Klinefelter's syndrome who have an extra sex chromosome (XXY).

drunkenness Acute alcoholism; see under alcoholism.

drusen Small, circular, yellow or white hyaline or colloid nodules occurring in the innermost layer of the vascular coat of the eye (choroid); usually they do not interfere with vision.

Dubin-Johnson syndrome Congenital familial defect in the excretory function of the liver resulting in mild jaundice, the presence of large amounts of bilirubin in the blood, and frequently a dark pigment in the liver cells. Also called chronic idiopathic jaundice.

Duchenne-Aran disease Progressive muscular atrophy; see under atrophy.

duct A tube or channel, usually for conveying the product of a gland to another part of the body.

accessory pancreatic d. The smaller of the two pancreatic ducts which enter the duodenum. Also called duct of Santorini.

Bartholin's d. See major sublingual duct.

cochlear d. A spirally arranged membranous tube within the cochlea of the internal ear.

common bile d. The duct formed by union of the hepatic duct and cystic duct; it conveys bile to the duodenum.

common hepatic d. The duct formed by the union of the right and left hepatic ducts.

cystic d. The duct leading from the gallbladder to the common bile duct.

deferent d. The duct that conveys sperm from the epididymis to the ejaculatory duct. Also called vas deferens; ductus deferens; spermatic duct.

ejaculatory d. The canal formed by the union of the deferent duct (vas deferens) and the excretory duct of the seminal vesicle; it opens into the prostatic urethra.

endolymphatic d. A duct in the labyrinth of the ear which connects the endolymphatic sac with the utricle and saccule.

excretory d. of the seminal vesicle The duct that drains the seminal vesicle and leads to the ejaculatory duct.

lactiferous d. One of about eighteen ducts which drain milk from the lobes of the mammary gland and open at the nipple. Also called milk duct.

major sublingual d. The duct that drains the sublingual salivary gland and opens at the sublingual papilla in the floor of the mouth. Also called Bartholin's duct.

mesonephric d. An embryonic duct that develops, in the male, into the deferent duct; in the female it is obliterated. Also called wolffian duct.

milk d. See lactiferous duct.

mullerian d. See paramesonephric duct.

nasolacrimal d. A duct conveying tears from the lacrimal sac to the nasal cavity.

omphalomesenteric d. A narrowed passage connecting the midgut of the embryo with the yolk sac. Also called vitelline duct; yolk stalk.

pancreatic d. The main excretory duct of the pancreas; it opens into the duodenum.

papillary d. of Bellini One of numerous ducts in the inner part of the renal medulla, formed by a succession of junctions of about seven straight collecting tubules.

paramesonephric d. Either of the two embryonic tubes that develop, in the female, into the uterine tubes, vagina, and uterus; it disappears in the male. Also called mullerian duct; Müller's canal.

paraurethral d. One of several ducts of the paraurethral (Skene's) glands. Also called Schüler's ducts.

parotid d. The duct that conveys saliva from the parotid gland to the mouth at the level of the upper second molar.

perilymphatic d. A minute canal connecting the perilymphatic space of the cochlea with the subarachnoid space.

semicircular d. One of three membranous tubes within the semicircular canal of the internal ear; it contributes to balance and orientation.

spermatic d. See deferent duct.

sublingual d., major The duct that drains the sublingual gland and opens into the floor of the mouth near the opening of the submandibular duct.

sublingual d.'s, minor The ducts (10 to 30) that drain the sublingual gland and open along the fold of mucous membrane (plica sublingualis) in the mouth. Also called Walther's ducts.

submandibular d. A duct about 5 cm long that drains the submandibular gland and opens at the tip of the sublingual papilla on the floor of the mouth adjacent to the frenulum of the tongue. Also called Wharton's duct.

sudoriferous d. The duct leading from the body of a sweat gland to the surface of the skin. Also called sweat duct.

drip | duct

136

section of cochlear duct

vestibular membrane

cochlear duct

semicircular duct

basilar membrane

spiral organ of Corti

deferent duct

bladder

seminal vesicle

prostate gland

prostate gland

ejaculatory duct

deferent duct

urethra

urethra

testes

thoracic duct

left subclavian vein

aorta

ductus arteriosus (patent)

pulmonary a.

common bile duct

accessory pancreatic duct

pancreas

pancreatic duct

small intestine (duodenum)

thoracic d. The largest lymphatic channel in the body; it conveys lymph into the left subclavian vein.

thyroglossal d. An embryonic duct extending along the midline of the neck; its lower part gives rise to the isthmus of the thyroid gland; normally the remainder disappears but occasionally it persists in the adult and forms a cyst or a fistula.

utriculosaccular d. A duct located in the internal ear extending from the utricle and joining the endolymphatic duct.

venous d. In the fetus, the continuation of the umbilical vein through the liver to the inferior vena cava; it obliterates after birth, becoming the ligamentum venosum.

vitelline d. See omphalomesenteric duct.

Wharton's d. See submandibular duct.

wolffian d. See mesonephric duct.

ductile Capable of being made into wire or hammered into thin plates, as certain metals; capable of being shaped or molded, as plastic.

duction The movement of an eye by the extrinsic muscles.

ductus, *pl.* **ductus** Latin for duct, a tubular structure.

d. arteriosus A communicating channel between the pulmonary artery and the aorta in the fetus; it normally obliterates shortly after birth.

d. deferens Deferent duct; see under duct.

patent d. arteriosus A ductus arteriosus that does not obliterate but remains patent after birth.

Duhring's disease See dermatitis herpetiformis.

dull 1. Not sharp; said of an instrument, pain, or sound. 2. Lacking mental alertness.

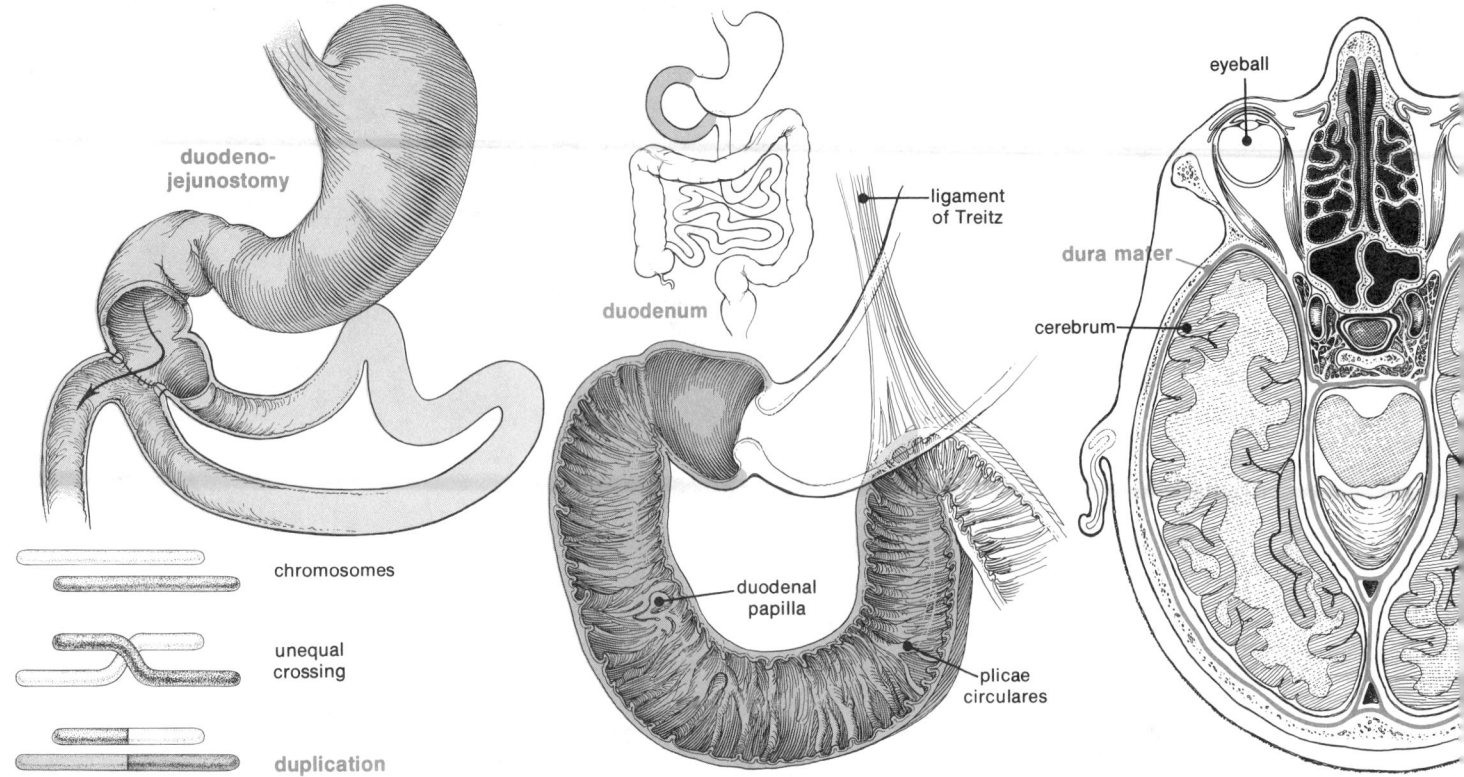

duodeno-
jejunostomy

chromosomes

unequal
crossing

duplication

ligament
of Treitz

duodenum

duodenal
papilla

plicae
circulares

eyeball

dura mater

cerebrum

dullness, dulness The quality of sound elicited by percussion over a solid part or organ, characterized by very little resonance.

shifting d. Dull sound produced by percussion, usually of the abdominal cavity, that shifts location as the patient is moved; indicative of the presence of free fluid.

dumb Colloquial term for mute.

dumping syndrome Symptoms occurring within 30 minutes after the end of a meal, including nausea, warmth, sweating, palpitation, pallor, headache, diarrhea, pain in the upper abdomen, and weakness; caused by excessively rapid emptying of the stomach, usually following loss of the pylorus in stomach resection. Also called postgastrectomy syndrome.

duodenal Of, relating to, or situated in the duodenum.

duodenectomy Surgical removal of the duodenal portion of the small intestine, total or partial.

duodenitis Inflammation of the duodenal portion of the small intestine.

duodenocholecystostomy Surgical formation of a passage between the gallbladder and the duodenum.

duodenocholedochotomy Surgical incision into the common bile duct and the adjoining portion of the duodenum.

duodenoenterostomy Surgical formation of a passage between the duodenum and another part of the small intestine.

duodenojejunostomy Surgical formation of a passage between the duodenum and the jejunum.

duodenolysis The operation of freeing the duodenum from adhesions.

duodenorrhaphy Suturing of the duodenum.

duodenoscopy Visual observation of the duodenum's interior by means of an endoscope.

duodenostomy Surgical formation of an orifice or passage into the duodenum.

duodenotomy Surgical incision into the duodenum.

duodenum The first portion of the small intestine; shaped like a horseshoe; it starts at the lower end of the stomach and extends to the jejunum; the term comes from the Latin *duodeni* (twelve), because this portion of the intestine is about 12 fingerbreadths (25–30 cm) in length.

duplication In genetics, a chromosome aberration consisting of the presence of an extra piece of chromosome, usually originated by unequal exchange of fragments between homologous chromosomes; the other chromosome has a segment missing (deletion).

dura See dura mater.

dural Relating to the dura mater.

dura mater A tough, fibrous, whitish membrane; the outermost of the three membranes covering the brain and spinal cord. Also called dura.

dwarf An abnormally small person. Also called nanus.

dwarfism In a broad sense, failure to achieve full growth potential; may be induced by ecological factors (e.g., dietary intake, systemic disease), by genetic factors, or by endocrine factors; lack of height is only one of the resulting features.

achondroplastic d. A form caused by congenital abnormality in the process of ossification of cartilage; affected individuals have a relatively elongated trunk, short extremities, and a large head.

pituitary d. Dwarfism accompanied by sexual infantilism and decreased function of the thyroid and adrenal glands; caused by lesions of the anterior portion of the pituitary gland early in childhood.

primordial d. Inadequate term designating a condition characterized by insufficient growth with normal functional development.

dyad 1. A pair. 2. A bivalent element or radical. 3. One pair of chromosomes after the disjunction of a tetrad at the first meiotic division.

dye Any coloring substance.

dynamics 1. The science of the relationship between motion and the forces causing it. 2. The emotional forces determining patterns of behavior.

dynamometer An apparatus for measuring the force of muscular contraction under controlled conditions.

dyne A unit of force equal to the force required to give a body of 1 g an acceleration of 1 cm per second squared.

dysacusis, dysacusia 1. Defect of hearing marked by inability to discriminate between sounds; distinguished from lack of sensitivity to sound. 2. Pain in the ear caused by sound.

dysarthria Impairment of ability to produce clear speech caused by muscular dysfunction secondary to central or peripheral nervous system disease.

dysarthrosis 1. Malformation of a joint. 2. Impairment of articulation. 3. A false joint.

dysautonomia Dysfunction of the autonomic nervous system.

familial d. Congenital nerve disorder affecting infants and children; characterized by indifference to pain, inability to shed tears, emotional instability, drooling, excessive sweating, and poor motor control. Also called Riley-Day syndrome.

dysbarism General term denoting physiologic changes resulting from changes in barometric pressure, such as the effects of rapid decompression.

dysbasia Difficult or distorted walking; it may be

organically or psychically determined.

dyscephalia, dyscephaly Malformation of the head and face.

dyschezia Difficult or painful defecation.

dyschiria Disorder in which the individual is unable to tell which side of his body has been touched.

dyschondrogenesis Defective development of cartilage.

dyschondroplasia See Ollier's syndrome.

dyschromia Any abnormality in the pigmentation (color) of the skin or hair.

dyscoria Irregularly shaped pupil.

dyscrasia A general morbid condition of the body.

bleeding d. A pathologic condition due to abnormal hemostasis, as hemophilia.

plasma cell d. General term to describe various pathologic conditions and biochemical abnormalities of cells that normally produce gamma globulin; e.g., the proliferative disorders of plasma cells.

dysdiadochokinesia Inability to make alternating movements in rapid succession, such as extending and flexing a limb.

dyseneia Defective articulation arising from defects in hearing.

dysentery Disease marked by frequent watery stools containing blood and mucus, attended by abdominal pain, dehydration, and sometimes fever.

amebic d. Dysentery due to infection with *Entamoeba histolytica*, which may cause ulceration of the colon; symptoms vary from slight abdominal discomfort and diarrhea alternating with constipation to profuse bleeding and discharge of mucus and pus.

bacillary d. Dysentery caused by bacteria of the genus *Shigella*.

dyserethism A slow response to stimuli.

dysergia Motor incoordination.

dysesthesia 1. Impairment or partial loss of sensation. 2. Painful or disagreeable sensation produced by ordinary stimuli.

dysfunction Abnormal or impaired functioning of an organ or bodily system.

minimal brain d. (MBD) Condition manifested by one or several of the following: short attention span, poor modulation of emotions, reading and/or writing disabilities, hyperactivity, poor coordination, and impulsiveness.

dysgammaglobulinemia Disorders or abnormalities of gamma globulins in the blood serum.

dysgenic Applying to factors that cause the deterioration of hereditary qualities.

dysgenics, dysgenesis The study of the factors causing defective or deficient embryonic develop-

chondroectodermal dysplasia
(Ellis-van Creveld syndrome)

postaxial polydactyly of hand

vell developed extra finger

underdeveloped fingernails

limited abduction in flexion

clinical signs of **congenital acetabular dysplasia**

asymmetrical skin fold

"climbing up the legs" characteristic way of rising from the floor in early **childhood muscular dystrophy**

---

ment. Also called cacogenics.

gonadal d. Defective gonadal development.

seminiferous tubule d. See Klinefelter's syndrome.

dysgerminoma A rare malignant ovarian tumor composed of undifferentiated germinal epithelium; the counterpart of seminoma of the testis. Also called ovarian seminoma.

dysgeusia A general term describing any distortion of normal taste perception.

dysgnathia Any abnormality of the maxilla or mandible.

dysgnosia Any disorder of the intellect.

dysgraphia 1. Difficulty in writing, usually due to ataxia, tremor, or motor neurosis. 2. Writer's cramp; see under cramp.

dyshematopoiesis, dyshemopoiesis Defective or imperfect blood formation.

dyshidrosis, dysidrosis 1. An abnormality of sweat production. 2. A deep eruption of blisters occurring primarily on the hands and feet, accompanied by intense itching. Also called pompholyx.

trichophytic d. Tinea pedis.

dyskeratoma Skin tumor containing cells that display abnormal keratinization.

warty d. A benign skin tumor with a central keratoic plug, occurring on the scalp, face, or neck.

dyskinesia Difficulty in performing voluntary movements.

dyslalia Impairment of speech due to defective speech organs.

dyslexia Alexia.

dyslogia Impairment of the thought processes and of speech.

dysmegalopsia Abnormal visual perception in which objects appear larger than they are.

dysmelia Congenital absence of a portion of one or more limbs.

dysmenorrhea Painful menstrual periods.

functional d. Primary dysmenorrhea.

primary d. Dysmenorrhea caused by a functional disturbance.

secondary d. Dysmenorrhea caused by inflammation, tumor, infection, or anatomic factors.

dysmetria Inability to stop a muscular movement at a desired point.

dysmorphism 1. Abnormality of shape. 2. Allomorphism.

dysontogenesis Abnormal development.

dysosmia A general term describing any distortion of normal smell perception.

dysostosis Defective bone formation.

craniofacial d. Ocular hypertelorism; see under hypertelorism.

mandibulofacial d. Hereditary abnormalities of the palpebral fissures, mandible and zygomatic bones, and lower lids, with malposition and malocclusion of teeth, low-set malformed ears, and high or cleft palate; called Franceschetti's syndrome when complete, and Treacher Collins' syndrome when partial.

d. multiplex See Hurler's syndrome.

dyspareunia Painful intercourse.

dyspepsia Indigestion.

dysphagia Difficulty in swallowing. Also called aphagia.

dysphasia Impairment of coordination in speech and inability to arrange words in their proper order, usually associated with brain injury.

dysphonia Difficulty or pain in speaking.

dysphoria An emotional state characterized by depression, restlessness, and malaise, usually accompanied by poor self-esteem.

dysplasia Abnormal development of bodily tissue.

chondroectodermal d. An inherited disorder marked by short extremities with normal trunk, polydactyly, and abnormal development of teeth and nails; frequently associated with congenital heart defects. Also called Ellis-van Creveld syndrome.

congenital acetabular d. Congenital dislocation of the hip; a complete or partial displacement of the femoral head out of the acetabulum; not related to trauma or to other musculoskeletal disease.

dentinal d. Hereditary abnormality of dentin formation marked by disarrangement of dentin tubules by masses of collagneous matrix, poorly developed tooth roots, and absence of pulp canals and chambers.

ectodermal d. General term denoting abnormal development of tissues derived from ectoderm.

fibromuscular d. Nonatherosclerotic disease of arteries, especially the renal arteries, causing constriction.

fibrous d. of bone Condition in which the marrow of one or more bones is replaced by fibrous tissue.

hereditary renal-retinal d. Inherited disorder marked by retinitis pigmentosa, diabetes insipidus, and progressive uremia.

polyostotic fibrous d. The occurrence of fibrous dysplasia in several bones, usually on one side of the body.

dysplastic Relating to or marked by abnormality of development.

dyspnea Difficult or labored breathing usually associated with serious disease of the heart or lungs.

paroxysmal nocturnal d. (PND) Acute dyspnea occurring suddenly at night, caused by pulmonary congestion and edema.

dyspraxia Impaired functioning of an organ or part.

dysproteinemia Abnormality in blood proteins.

dysstasia Difficulty in standing.

dyssyllabia Syllable stumbling.

dyssynergia, dyssynergy Disturbance of muscular coordination.

dysthymia Chronic mild depression.

dystocia Difficult childbirth.

fetal d. Difficult labor due to abnormalities of position or size of the fetus.

maternal d. Difficult labor due to uterine inertia or deformities of the birth canal.

dystonia Abnormal tonicity of musculature.

dystontogenesis Abnormal development and differentiation of tissues.

dystopia Malposition.

dystopic Out of place.

dystrophy Disorder caused by faulty nutrition or by lesions of the pituitary gland and/or brain.

adiposogenital d. Condition caused by lesions of the pituitary gland and the hypothalamus, marked by increase in fat, especially about the abdomen, hips, and thighs, with underdeveloped genital organs and loss of hair; usually manifested during puberty and often mistaken for obesity. Also called Fröhlich's syndrome.

cerebrooculorenal d. See oculocerebrorenal syndrome.

childhood muscular d. Inherited disorder affecting boys usually between two and five years of age; has an insidious beginning and is usually fatal by the third decade; first symptoms and signs appear in muscles of the pelvis and lower extremities, including a swaying gait, frequent falls, and difficulty arising from the floor. Also called Duchenne's dystrophy.

Duchenne's d. See childhood muscular dystrophy.

muscular dystrophy (MD) Inherited disease of muscles marked by progressive weakness and deterioration.

myotonic d. See myotonia atrophica.

progressive muscular d. Progressive, gradual muscular deterioration of unknown cause.

pseudohypertrophic d., pseudomuscular d. Degenerative disease of childhood, marked by enlargement and weakness, followed by wasting, of the muscles of the shoulder girdle and sometimes of the pelvic girdle.

dysuria Difficulty or pain in urination.

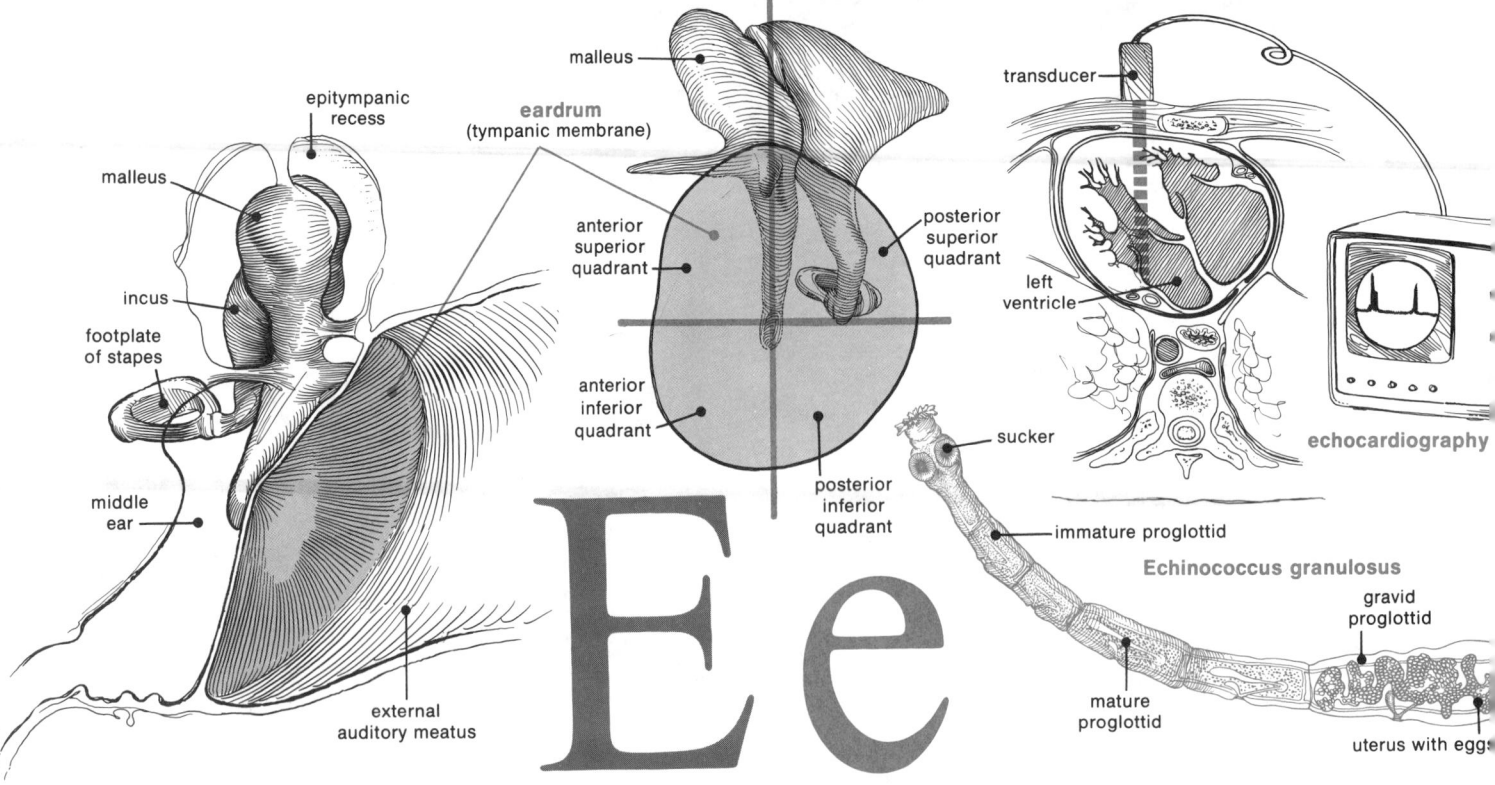

epitympanic recess

malleus

incus

footplate of stapes

middle ear

external auditory meatus

malleus

eardrum (tympanic membrane)

anterior superior quadrant

posterior superior quadrant

anterior inferior quadrant

posterior inferior quadrant

transducer

left ventricle

echocardiography

sucker

immature proglottid

Echinococcus granulosus

gravid proglottid

mature proglottid

uterus with eggs

Ee

ear The compound organ of hearing and equilibrium; it is sensitive to sound waves, to the effects of gravity, and to motion; the organ consists of the external ear, which includes the auricle (pinna) and the external auditory meatus, the middle ear or tympanic cavity, which contains the ossicles, and the internal ear, which includes the semicircular canals, vestibule, and cochlea.

aviators e. See aerotitis media.

cauliflower e. Boxer's ear, a thickened deformed ear caused by injury to the tissues due to repeated blows.

darwinian e. One with a protrusion on the helix.

glue e. Serous otitis media with very thick fluid in the middle ear chamber, characterized by a marked conductive hearing loss.

swimmer's e. Infection of the auditory canal associated with swimming; may be fungal or bacterial in nature.

earache Pain in the ear. Also called otalgia.

eardrum The tympanic membrane; a flattened cone-shaped fibrous sheet that separates the external auditory meatus from the middle ear chamber.

earth 1. Soil; the loose, friable substances forming the ground. **2.** An amorphous pulverizable mineral. **3.** A metallic oxide characterized by a high melting point; e.g., alumina, which was formerly classified as an element.

alkaline e. Any oxide of the elements in the family to which calcium and magnesium belong.

diatomaceous e. Purified siliceous earth composed mainly of shell wall remains of minute aquatic unicellular diatoms; used as an inert filler in many dental materials and as a mild abrasive and polishing agent. Also called infusorial earth.

infusorial e. Diatomaceous earth.

rare e. Any of those rare elements with atomic numbers from 57 to 71 that closely resemble one another chemically.

earth-eating The practice of eating dirt or clay.

earwax The soft brownish-yellow waxlike secretion of the ceruminous glands lining the canal of the external ear. Also called cerumen.

Eaton agent pneumonia Mycoplasmal pneumonia; see under pneumonia.

Eaton-Lambert syndrome Myasthenia syndrome usually associated with tumor, especially oat cell carcinoma of the lung; characterized by weakness and pain in the limbs with peculiarly slow movements and curare sensitivity; electromyography is diagnostic.

ebonation The removal of loose bone chips after an injury.

ebullism 1. The formation of water vapor in the tissues due to extreme reduction in barometric pressure occurring at altitudes above 60,000 feet. **2.** The bubbling of a fluid; a boiling. **3.** A sudden emotional outpouring, as of violence.

ebur Resembling ivory.

eburnation The transformation of bone into a dense ivory-like substance.

eccentric 1. Situated away from the center. **2.** Deviating from the established norm. **3.** One who deviates markedly from normal or conventional conduct or speech; abnormal in emotional reactions and in general behavior, with no intellectual defect; an erratic person.

eccentrochondroplasia Abnormal ossification, especially in long bones, in which osseous tissue is formed from areas other than the epiphysial cartilage.

ecchondroma A benign cartilaginous tumor; an outgrowth of normally situated cartilage projecting through the shaft of a bone. Also called ecchondrosis.

ecchondrosis See ecchondroma.

ecchymoma A slight hematoma due to a bruise.

ecchymosis A bruise; a "black and blue spot" on the skin caused by escape of blood from injured vessels.

ecchymotic Relating to an ecchymosis.

eccrine See exocrine.

eccrinology The study of secretions and excretions.

eccrisis 1. The excretion of a waste product. **2.** Any waste product.

eccritic Anything that promotes the excretion of waste products.

eccyesis Ectopic pregnancy or gestation.

ecdemic Indicating a disease brought into an area from without; not endemic.

ecdysis Desquamation or shedding of an outer covering. Also called molting.

echidnase Enzyme present in the venom of vipers that causes swelling and inflammation in the snake-bitten victim.

echinococcosis Infection caused by the larval form of *Echinococcus granulosus* or *Echinococcus multilocularis*, producing expanding cysts in the liver or lungs; anaphylactic reaction may occur from rupture of cyst fluid into the pleural or peritoneal cavity. Also called hydatid disease.

Echinococcus granulosus A species of tapeworm occurring in the adult form in dog's intestines; the larval forms occur in man, forming hydatid cysts in the liver and other tissues.

Echinodermata A phylum of radially symmetrical invertebrates often having a body covered with spines; it includes starfishes, sea urchins, sea lilies, etc.

echinosis Irregular appearance of red blood cells; having lost their smooth surface, they resemble the shell of a sea urchin.

Echinostoma Genus of flukes with a characteristic collar of spines, distributed widely in Southeast Asia; some species infect humans, causing diarrhea.

echinulate Having small spines; applied in bacteriology to cultures that spread out in pointed outgrowths.

echo Repetition of a sound; reflection of a sound wave to its point of origin.

echocardiogram Graphic display obtained from the application of ultrasonic procedures.

echocardiography The use of an ultrasonic apparatus that sends sound impulses toward the walls of the heart, which in turn bounce or echo the sounds back; the patterns produced are graphically displayed for interpretation; used for determining the movement patterns of the heart and its valves, chamber size, wall thickness, and the presence of pericardial fluid.

echoencephalography A method of examing the brain by recording the reflection of high frequency (ultrasonic) sound waves; it is used to obtain a safe, rapid, and painless estimate of the position of the midline of the third ventricle; useful in evaluating patients with suspected subdural or epidural hemorrhage or other conditions which might cause a brain shift.

echography Ultrasonography.

echolalia Compulsive or involuntary echo-like repetition of another's words or phrases.

echolocation The method by which certain animals, as bats and dolphins, orient themselves, i.e., by means of reflected sound waves produced by the high-frequency sounds that they emit.

echopathy A syndrome characterized by the senseless imitation of speech (echolalia) or gestures and postures (echopraxia) of others; may be seen during the catatonic phase of schizophrenia.

echophonia, echophony The echo of the voice sometimes heard in auscultation of the chest.

echopraxia The involuntary and meaningless imitation of movements made by another. Also called echomatism.

echovirus Virus of the genus *Enterovirus* (family Picornaviridae) associated with aseptic meningitis and gastroenteritis in man; the term is an acronym of enteric cytopathogenic human orphan virus.

eclampsia An acute disorder peculiar to pregnant and puerperal women, marked by convulsions during which there is a loss of consciousness usually

semicircular canals

cochlear nerve

internal ear

incus

cochlea

stapes

middle ear chamber

malleus

round window

tympanic membrane (eardrum)

external auditory meatus

auditory (eustachian) tube

ear

auricle

semicircular canals:

superior

posterior

lateral

endolymphatic duct

osseous labyrinth

endolymphatic sac

oval window

macula of utricle

crista ampullaris

vestibule

macula of saccule

footplate of stapes in oval window

facial nerve

vestibular ganglion: superior part

inferior part

cochlear nerve

scala tympani

cochlear duct

scala vestibuli

cochlea

cochlear duct

utricle

saccule

ampullae

ductus reuniens

membranous labyrinth

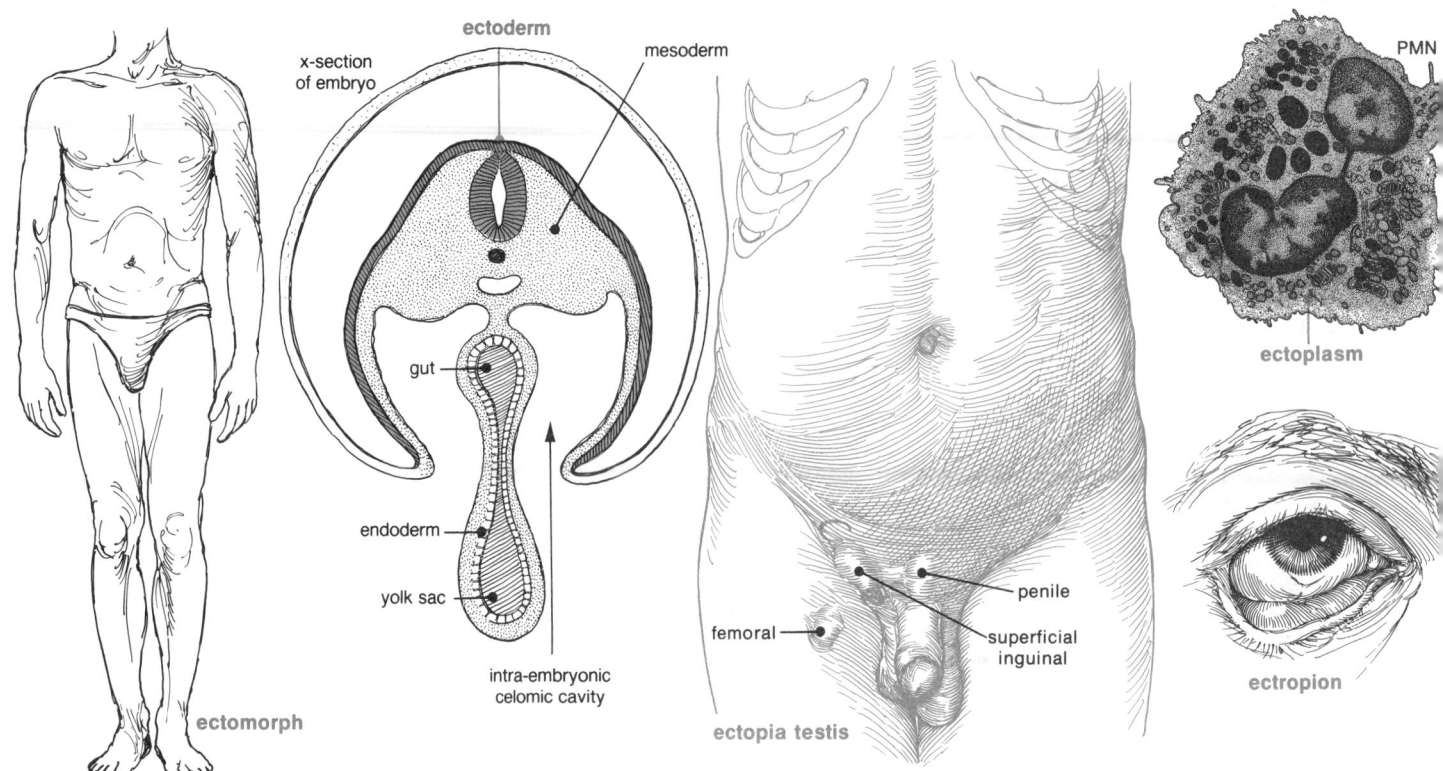

ectoderm
x-section of embryo
mesoderm
PMN
ectoplasm
gut
endoderm
yolk sac
intra-embryonic celomic cavity
ectomorph
femoral
penile
superficial inguinal
ectopia testis
ectropion

followed by more or less prolonged coma; associated with hypertension, edema, and/or proteinuria; in most cases clinical manifestations occur after the 24th week of gestation and disappear after delivery; a phase of toxemia of pregnancy. Also called eclamptogenic toxemia.

puerperal e. Eclampsia occurring after delivery.

eclamptic Relating to eclampsia.

eclamptogenous Denoting anything that causes convulsions. Also called convulsant.

ecmnesia Inability to remember recent events only.

E. coli Abbreviation for *Escherichia coli*.

ecology The science of the relationship between organisms and their evironment.

economy The functional arrangement of organs and structures within the body.

ecosite A parasite to which the host is immune under normal conditions. Also called ecoparasite.

ecosystem An ecological system; a community of organisms, together with its physical environment, considered as an entity.

ectasia, ectasis Dilatation of a hollow organ or a tubular structure.

ectatic Characterized by ectasia.

ecthyma A pustular eruption, usually seated upon a shallow ulcer, that evolves into a firm crust or scab; caused by staphylococci or streptococci; scarring is a characteristic sequela.

e. contagiosum A viral disease of sheep occasionally transmitted to man. Also called orf.

ectiris The anterior or outer endothelium of the iris.

ectoantigen, exoantigen 1. Any exciter of antibody formation, separate from its source. 2. An antigen formed from the ectoplasm of bacterial cells.

ectoblast Ectoderm.

ectocardia Abnormal position of the heart.

ectochoroidea The outer part of the choroid layer of the eye. Also called suprachoroid.

ectocornea The anterior or outer epithelium of the cornea.

ectocrine 1. A substance, synthesized or resulting from the decomposition of organisms, that affects plant life. 2. Ectohormone.

ectocyst The outer layer of a hydatid cyst.

ectoderm The outermost of the three germ layers of the embryo; it gives rise to the nervous system and to the epidermis and its derivatives, such as hair and the lens of the eye.

ectodermal, ectodermic Relating to the ectoderm.

ectodermatosis See ectodermosis.

ectodermosis A disorder arising from the mal-

development of any organ or tissue derived from the ectoderm. Also called ectodermatosis.

ectogenous Originating outside the body.

ectohormone A substance that is secreted by an organism into its immediate environment and modifies the functional activity of some distant organism; a parahormonal mediator of ecological importance. Also called ectocrine.

ectomere Any of the cells formed by division of the fertilized egg that participates in the formation of the ectoderm.

ectomorph A person with a lean and slightly muscular body; one in which tissues derived from the ectoderm predominate.

ectomorphic Slender and not muscular.

ectopagia The lateral fusion of conjoined twins.

ectoparasite A parasite that lives on the surface of the body of its host.

ectopia A congenital displacement or abnormal position of an organ.

e. testis A condition in which a testicle has strayed from the path of normal descent into the scrotum; it may be due to an abnormal connection of the distal end of the gubernaculum testis, a conection which leads the gonad to an abnormal position.

ectopic Located in, or arising from a place other than normal; e.g., heart beats arising from other than the S-A node.

ectopic ACTH syndrome Secretion of ACTH by nonendocrine tumors producing hypokalemic alkalosis and weakness.

ectoplacental Outside or surrounding the placenta.

ectoplasm Clear, thin cytoplasm at the periphery of a cell; it is more gelled than the rest of the cytoplasm in the cell; the clarity is due to the exclusion of all organelles except filaments.

ectopy Ectopia.

ectostosis Formation of bone beneath the perichondrium or the periostium.

ectothrix Denoting a type of fungal infection in which the hyphae grow both within and on the surface of the hair shaft. Cf. endothrix.

ectotoxin Exotoxin.

ectozoon Any parasitic animal living on the surface of the host.

ectrodactylism, ectodactyly Congenital absence of a digit or of digits.

ectrogeny Congenital absence of a part.

ectromelia 1. Congenital absence of one or more limbs. 2. A viral disease of mice causing, among other symptoms, gangrene and loss of feet; it causes high mortality in laboratory mouse colonies. Also

called mousepox.

ectropion Eversion or outward displacement of the margin of an eyelid.

ectrosyndactyly A congenital absence of one or more digits and the fusion of the others.

eczema General term for a group of acute or chronic inflammatory skin disorders characterized by redness, thickening, oozing, and the formation of papules, vesicles, and crusts; often accompanied by itching and burning.

allergic e. One caused by an allergic reaction.

atopic e. See dermatitis, atopic.

e. herpeticum A generalized widespread infection of the skin caused by the herpes simplex virus.

e. madidans A moist eruption. Also called weeping eczema.

e. marginatum See tinea cruris.

e. pustulosum Eczema in which the lesions become covered with pus crusts.

e. rubrum Eczema presenting excoriated oozing lesions accompanied by redness.

e. vesiculosum An eruption of vesicles.

nummular e. Eruption of coin-sized and coin-shaped patches of vesicular dermatitis, usually affecting the extensor surfaces of the hands, arms, and legs.

stasis e. Eczema of the legs, frequently with ulceration, caused by impaired circulation.

weeping e. See eczema madidans.

winter e. Dry scales on the skin due to evaporation of moisture from the skin surface.

eczematous Affected with or of the nature of eczema.

edema Swelling of any part of the body due to collection of fluid in the intercellular spaces of tissues.

angioneurotic e. Recurrent local edema due to increased vascular permeability of allergic or nervous origin; affecting most commonly the eyelids, lips, tongue, lungs, larynx, or extremities and occurring in persons having a variety of allergies. Also called giant urticaria.

Berlin's e. Edema of the macular area of the retina, giving it a white appearance, caused by a severe blow to the eyeball. Also called concussion edema.

cardiac e. Edema caused by heart disease with resulting increase in venous pressures.

cerebral e. Edema of the brain caused by tumors, infarction, generalized edema due to heart or kidney disease, or certain toxic conditions.

concussion e. See Berlin's edema.

dependent e. Swelling of dependent areas, especially the legs, due to accumulation of fluid.

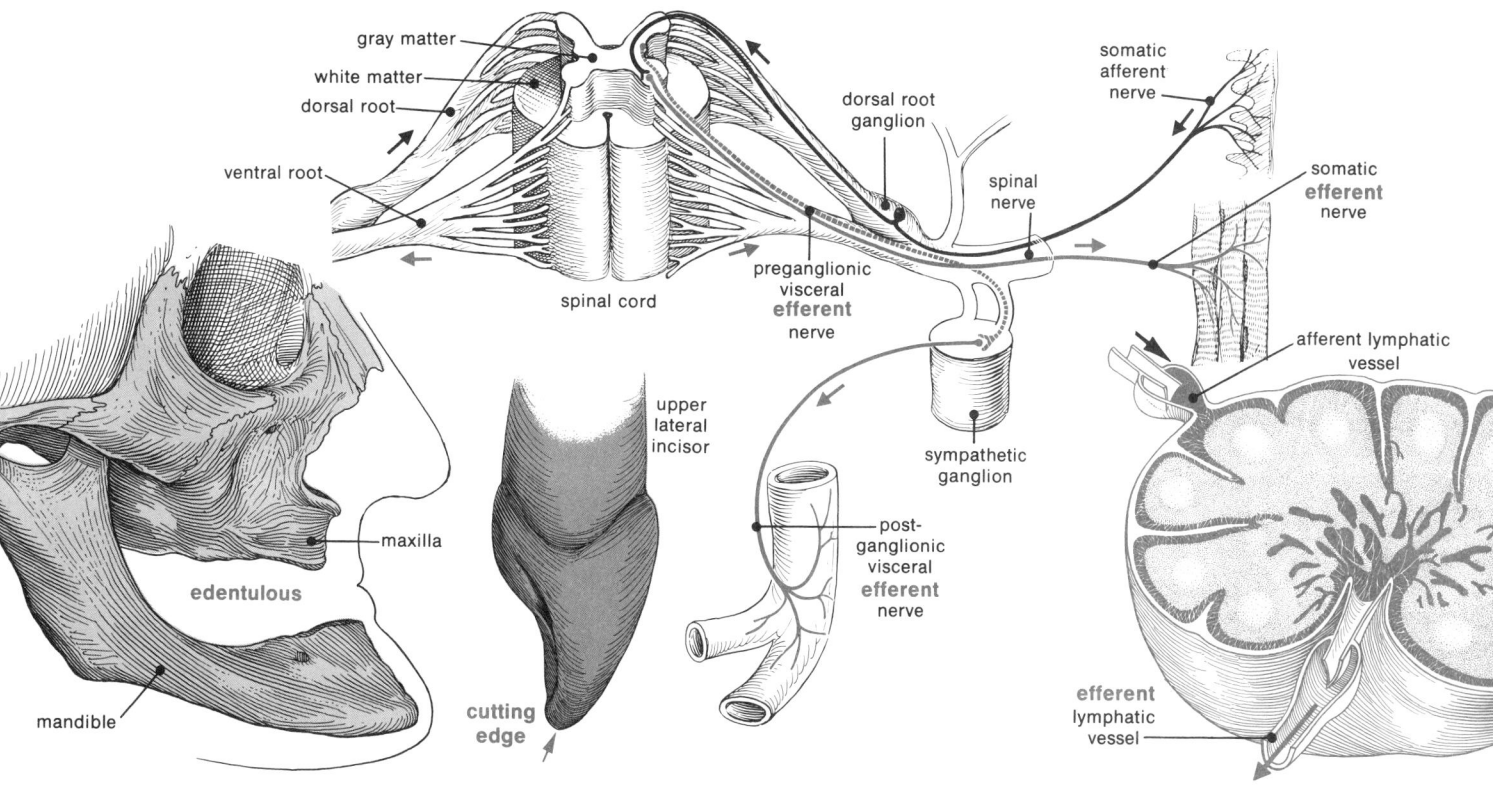

gray matter
white matter
dorsal root
ventral root
spinal cord
dorsal root ganglion
spinal nerve
preganglionic visceral **efferent** nerve
sympathetic ganglion
post-ganglionic visceral **efferent** nerve
somatic afferent nerve
somatic **efferent** nerve
afferent lymphatic vessel
efferent lymphatic vessel

maxilla
edentulous
mandible

upper lateral incisor
cutting edge

e. neonatorum A generalized, usually fatal, edema in the newborn.

famine e. See nutritional edema.

high altitude pulmonary e. (HAPE) An acute form of altitude sickness causing edema of the lungs.

idiopathic e. Recurrent sodium and fluid retention and swelling occurring in women in the absence of cardiac, hepatic, or renal disease; it occurs most commonly in obese, premenopausal adults; the etiology is not known, although altered capillary and/or lymphatic permeability have been suggested as causes.

menstrual e. The increase in weight and retention of water occurring during or just before menstruation.

nutritional e. Swelling caused by prolonged dietary deficiency; usually due at least in part to hypoproteinemia. Also called famine edema.

pitting e. Condition in which pressure on edematous area causes indentations that remain for a time after pressure is released.

pulmonary e. Escape of fluid into the air sacs and interstitial tissue of the lungs; causes include left ventricular failure, mitral stenosis, and chemicals which are pulmonary toxins.

edematous Characterized or affected by edema.
edentulous Toothless.
edge 1. A rim, margin, border, or ridge. 2. The sharpened side of a blade.

cutting e. 1. The beveled, knifelike working angle of a dental hand instrument. 2. The incisal edge of an anterior tooth.

e. strength In dentistry, the ability of a fine margin to resist fracture.

eduction The process of coming out, as the emerging from general anesthesia.

effect A result; something brought about by a force or an agent.

Bohr e. The effect of carbon dioxide (CO_2) on the oxygen affinity of blood, i.e., CO_2 in the tissues facilitates the removal of oxygen from hemoglobin, resulting in a greater availability of oxygen to the tissues.

Compton e. A change in wavelength of a bombarding photon with the displacement of an orbital electron.

cumulative e. The sudden pronounced effect resulting after several ineffective doses. Also called cumulative action.

Doppler e. The apparent change in frequency of sound or light waves when the observer and the source are in relative motion; the frequency increases when they approach one another and de-creases when they move away. Also called Doppler phenomenon.

Pasteur e. The slowing down of fermentation by oxygen, first observed by Pasteur.

side e. An effect other than that for which a drug or therapy is administered, especially an undesirable secondary effect.

toxic e. A drug-produced harmful effect on some biologic mechanism.

effector An end organ that, upon receiving a nerve impulse, distributes it, activating either secretion of a gland or contraction of a muscle.

allosteric e. Any small molecule that modifies enzyme activity by binding at sites other than the catalytically active sites.

efferent Conveying a fluid or a nerve impulse away from a central organ or area.

effervesce To emit gas bubbles to the surface, as a carbonated liquid.

effervescent 1. Bubbling; giving off gas. 2. Producing effervescence.

efficacy The ability to produce a desired effect; effectiveness.

efficiency The ability to accomplish a desired effect or product results with a minimum of unnecessary effort; competency.

visual e. A rating used in determining compensation for ocular injuries based on measurable functions of central acuity, field vision, and ocular motility.

effloresce 1. To lose water upon exposure to a dry atmosphere, thus becoming a powder. 2. To become covered with a powdery substance.

efflorescent Denoting a substance that gives up water on exposure to air at ordinary temperature.

effluvium 1. An exhalation, especially one that is foul-smelling or noxious. 2. An outflowing or shedding, especially subtle, as rising vapor or shedding of hair. 3. Gaseous waste.

effuse Spread out widely and thinly on a surface; denoting the surface character of a bacterial culture; spreading profusely.

effusion 1. The escape of fluid into a body cavity. 2. The fluid effused.

pleural e. Fluid filling the membranous sac covering the lung and lining of the chest.

egg 1. The female reproductive cell of birds and reptiles, expelled from the maternal body prior to the development of the embryo, or sometimes without fertilization. 2. Ovum. Also called oocyte.

ego The awareness of the existence of the self as different from others; in psychoanalytic theory, all those functions of the personality which enable it to experience itself and act in self-fulfilling yet socially acceptable fashion; it mediates between the other two parts of the personality structure (id and superego) and reality.

ego-dystonic Denoting those aspects of the personality which are alien or unacceptable to the self.

ego-syntonic Denoting those aspects of the personality which are acceptable to the self.

egocentric Marked by constant or extreme preoccupation with one's self.

egomania Pathologic preoccupation with one's self.

egophony A form of bronchophony; the bleating nasal quality of voice heard over an area of compressed lung above a pleural effusion or an area of consolidation; transmission of the spoken voice is altered so that long e ($\bar{e}$) sounds like long a ($\bar{a}$).

Ehlers-Danlos syndrome Inherited disorder marked by hyperelasticity of the skin, fragility of cutaneous blood vessels, overextension of joints, and the formation of pigmented nodules (raisin tumors) at the site of skin injury.

Ehrlichia A genus of nonmotile gram-negative bacteria (order Rickettsiales) causing disease in dogs and humans.

ehrlichiosis Infection with *Ehrlichia canis* causing symptoms similar to those of Rocky Mountain spotted fever, but without a rash; transmitted from dogs by ticks.

eicosanoid A 20-carbon unsaturated fatty acid derived from arachidonic acid; e.g., prostaglandins and leukotrienes.

eikonometer Any instrument used to measure the difference in sizes of the images seen by the two eyes (aniseikonia).

einsteinium A synthetic radioactive element; symbol Es, atomic number 99, atomic weight 254; first produced in 1955.

Eisenmenger's syndrome Strictly defined, a ventricular septal defect, overriding aorta, right ventricular hypertrophy, and a normal or dilated pulmonary artery; because these terms have been frequently used to describe cases with right to left shunt without all of the above components, they are not regarded as useful terms by cardiologists. Also called Eisenmenger's complex.

ejaculate To expel abruptly, especially to discharge semen in orgasm.

ejaculation Emission of the semen.

premature e. Emission of the semen prior to or immediately upon engaging in sexual intercourse.

ejaculatory Of or relating to ejaculation.

ejector Anything that removes any material forcefully.

saliva e. A device containing a perforated suc-

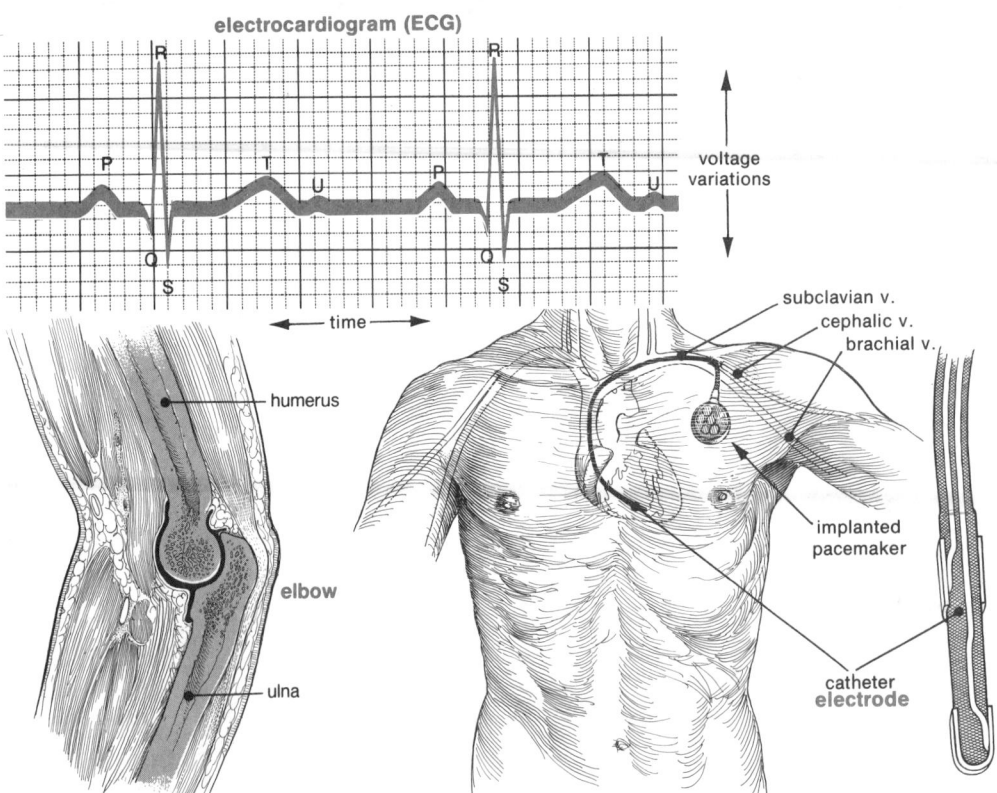

electrocardiogram (ECG)

voltage variations

time

humerus
elbow
ulna

subclavian v.
cephalic v.
brachial v.

implanted pacemaker

catheter **electrode**

electroencephalograms (EEG)

frontal-central
L
R

central-occipital
L
R

frontal-temporal
L
R

temporal-occipital
L
R

50 μV
1 second

---

tion tube used to remove fluids from the mouth.

elastance A measure of a structure's ability to return to its initial or original form following deformation; e.g., the measure of the ability of a hollow organ, such as the bladder, to revert toward its original dimensions upon removal of the distending force (urine).

elastic 1. Capable of being stretched, bent, or deformed in any way, and then return to original form. 2. A rubber band used in orthodontics to apply force to the teeth.

intermaxillary e. A rubber band placed between orthodontic appliances of upper and lower jaws to cause tooth movement as the jaw opens and closes.

intramaxillary e. A rubber band placed within an orthodontic appliance.

elastica A general term for elastic tissue, such as the elastic layer in the wall of an artery.

elasticin Elastin.

elasticity The quality of being elastic.

modulus of e. A measure of elasticity or stiffness of a material determined by dividing the stress by the corresponding strain value.

elastin A yellow scleroprotein present in elastic fibers that allows them to stretch about one and one-half times their original length.

elastomer Any of various polymers that can be stretched like rubber, and that will relax to their original dimensions when unstressed.

elastometer A device for measuring the elasticity of bodily tissues.

elastosis Degeneration of the elastic tissues.

e. dystrophica Angioid streaks of the retina due to degeneration of the basal lamina of the choroid; a manifestation of pseudoxanthoma elasticum.

e. perforans serpiginosa Circinate group of asymptomatic keratotic papules, marked by thickened epidermis around a central keratin plug overlying an accumulation of elastic tissue.

senile e. A dermatosis marked by degeneration of elastic tissue in the skin of the elderly or in those afflicted with chronic actinic effect.

elbow The joint between the arm and the forearm.

bend of the e. Cubital fossa; see under fossa.

miner's e. Inflammation of the bursa over the elbow (olecranon bursitis) caused by pressure.

point of the e. See olecranon.

tennis e. Soreness of the lateral aspect of the elbow and muscles of the forearm usually caused by excessive rotatory motions of the forearm as in playing tennis. Also called lateral epicondylitis.

tip of the e. See olecranon.

electroanalysis Quantitative separation of metals by means of an electric current.

---

electroanesthesia Anesthesia induced by an electric current.

electrobiology The study of electrical phenomena in the living organism.

electrocardiogram (ECG, EKG) A graphic record of the electric current produced by the contraction of the heart, obtained with an electrocardiograph; the voltage variations, resulting from the depolarization and repolarization of the heart muscle and producing electric fields, are plotted against time on paper tape.

electrocardiograph An instrument for recording the electric currents produced by heart muscle in the process of contraction; a galvanometer which records voltage variations; developed by Wilhem Einthoven in 1906.

electrocardiography A method of recording the electric current generated by the activity of the heart muscle by means of an electrocardiograph.

fetal e. Electrocardiography of a fetus while in the uterus.

electrocardioscope An oscilloscope for the continuous monitoring of the electrocardiogram (ECG).

electrocauterization Cauterization by means of an electrically heated platinum wire.

electrocautery An instrument for cauterizing tissue in which a platinum wire is heated by a current of electricity.

electrochemistry The science of chemical reactions produced by electricity; study of the electrical aspects of chemical reactions.

electrocoagulation The hardening of diseased tissues induced by high frequency currents; a form of surgical diathermy.

electrocontractility The capability of muscle tissue to contract in response to an electric stimulation.

electroconvulsant Denoting a type of therapy for emotional disorders in which an electric current is passed through the head of the patient to produce convulsions; See also therapy, electroshock.

electrocorticogram A record of electrical activity emanating from the cerebral cortex; obtained by placing electrodes in direct contact with the cortex.

electrocute To cause death by passing a high voltage electric current through the body.

electrode A conductor of electricity through which current enters or leaves a medium, such as gas, vacuum, nonmetallic solid, etc.

central terminal e. In electrocardiography, one in which the wire connections (to the right and left arms and to the left leg) are fastened together at one end and connected to the electrocardiograph to form the indifferent electrode.

exploring e. In unipolar electrocardiography,

---

one which is placed on the chest near the heart region and paired with an indifferent electrode.

glass e. An electrode made of a thin-walled glass bulb containing a platinum wire and filled with a standard buffer solution mixed with a little quinhydrone; used in determining hydrogen ion (pH) concentrations.

hydrogen e. An electrode considered the ultimate standard of reference in all hydrogen ion (pH) determinations; made by partly immersing platinum black in platinum and allowing it to absorb hydrogen to saturation.

indifferent e. In unipolar electrocardiography, an electrode having multiple terminals.

negative e. See cathode.

positive e. See anode.

electrodesiccation Destruction of tissue by dehydration using monopolar electric current through a needle electrode.

electrodialysis Dialysis by the application of an electric field across the semipermeable dialysis membrane, used especially to separate electrolytes.

electroencephalogram (EEG) A graphic record of the electric activity of the brain obtained by means of the electroencephalograph.

depth e. An electroencephalogram obtained by placing electrodes directly on subcortical structures.

low voltage e. An electroencephalogram in which no activity larger than 20 μv can be recorded between any two points on the scalp.

electroencephalograph An instrument used to record the electric currents produced in the brain.

electroencephalography The recording of the electric currents generated by the activity of the brain, especially the cerebral cortex, by means of an electroencephalograph.

electrogastrograph An instrument for recording the bioelectrical potentials associated with gastrointestinal activity.

electrogram Any electrically produced graph or tracing; e.g., the recording of the electrical activity of the heart made with the recording electrode placed directly on the surface of the cardiac muscle.

His bundle e. An electrogram usually made by placing a catheter electrode in the right ventricle; it records the A-V junctional electrical activity.

electrography The production of graphic records by means of electricity.

atrioventricular bundle e. Electrography of the atrioventricular bundle during cardiac catherization.

His bundle e. Atrioventricular bundle electrography.

electrokymogram (EKY) A graphic record of the heart's movements obtained by electrokymography.

electrolyte composition

electromyograms

normal muscle | muscle cramp | myotinic muscle | muscular dystrophy

intracellular fluid

serum

carbon atom
6 electrons
6 protons
6 neutrons

electron

albumin

globulins

paper electrophoresis

electroretinogram (ERG)

number of electrons in some atoms

element	symbol	atomic number	K	L	M	N	O	P	Q
hydrogen	H	1	1						
lithium	Li	3	2	1					
carbon	C	6	2	4					
nitrogen	N	7	2	5					
oxygen	O	8	2	6					
sodium	Na	11	2	8	1				
chlorine	Cl	17	2	8	7				
potassium	K	19	2	8	8	1			
calcium	Ca	20	2	8	8	2			
mercury	Hg	80	2	8	18	32	18	2	
radium	Ra	88	2	8	18	32	18	18	2

electrokymography 1. The registered recording of the movements of the heart and great vessels by means of the electrokymograph. 2. The science of interpreting electrokymograms.

electrolarynx A vibrating mechanism that makes it possible for a person to speak intelligibly after his larynx has been surgically removed.

electrolysis 1. Chemical decomposition of a compound produced by passing a current of electricity through it. 2. Decomposition or destruction of specific tissues of the body by means of electricity, e.g., removal of unwanted hair.

electrolyte Any substance which, when in solution, dissociates into ions, thus becoming capable of conducting an electric current.

electrolytic 1. Relating to or produced by electrolysis. 2. Relating to an electrolyte.

electrolyze To cause a chemical decomposition by means of an electric current.

electromyogram (EMG) A graphic record obtained by electromyography of the somatic electric currents associated with muscle activity.

electromyography The recording of the electric currents generated by muscular activity.

electron An elementary, subatomic particle of nature; it has a negative charge of 1 and a mass of 9.1×10^{-28} g.

valence e. An electron in an atom capable of participating in the formation of chemical bonds with other atoms.

electronarcosis The passing of an electric current through the brain to produce narcosis or unconsciousness.

electronegative 1. Possessing a negative electric charge. 2. Referring to those elements whose unchanged atoms have a tendency to attract electrons and become anions; e.g., oxygen and chlorine.

electron gun An electrode, as in a cathode-ray tube, that emits a controlled beam of accelerated electrons.

electronic 1. Of, relating to, or conducting electrons. 2. Relating to electronics.

electronics The study of electronic phenomena.

electron-volt (ev) The energy imparted to an electron by a potential of one volt; equal to 1.6×10^{-12} erg.

electronystagmography (ENG) The electronic recording of eye movements in nystagmus.

electrooculogram (EOG) A record of eye positions made by an electro-oculograph.

electro-oculography The production of records of eye position (electro-oculograms) by recording, during eye movement, the difference in electrical potential between two electrodes placed on the skin at either side of the eye.

electrophoresis The movement of charged particles in an electric field toward either the anode or the cathode; used as a means of separating substances in a medium.

paper e. The migration of charged particles along a strip of filter paper, saturated with a few drops of an electrolyte, when a potential gradient is placed across the paper.

thin-layer e. (TLE) The movement of charged particles through a thin layer of an inert material such as cellulose.

electrophysiology The study of electrical phenomena related to physiologic processes.

electroplate To plate or coat with a thin layer of metal by electrolysis or electrodeposition; in dentistry, impressions are plated to form metalized working dies.

electropositive 1. Relating to or possessing a positive electric charge. 2. Denoting an element whose atoms tend to release electrons to form a chemical bond; e.g., sodium, potassium, or calcium.

electroretinogram (ERG) The electrical potential of the retina recorded by a galvanometer from the surface of the eyeball and originated by a pulse of light; it depicts the integrity of the neuroepithelium of the retina.

electroscope An instrument for detecting the presence of electric charges.

electroshock See therapy, electroshock.

electrostethograph An electrical instrument for recording the respiratory and cardiac sounds of the chest.

electrotherapy, electrotherapeutics The treatment of disease by means of electricity.

electrothermal Relating to electricity and heat; especially, the production of heat electrically.

element 1. A substance made up of atoms having the same number of protons in each nucleus. 2. An irreducible substance or indivisible constituent of a composite entity.

electronegative e. An element having more than four valence electrons and tending to gain electrons in a chemical combination.

electropositive e. An element having less than four valence electrons and tending to release electrons in a chemical combination.

radioactive e. An element that spontaneously transforms into another element with emission of radioactivity.

trace e.'s Elements present in the body in minute amounts; important in metabolism or to form essential compounds.

eleothorax See oleothorax.

elephantiasis Hypertrophy and inflammation of the skin and subcutaneous tissues, especially of the legs and scrotum, due to obstructed lymphatic cir-

elevator

embolus

internal carotid a.

embryoblast

blastocyst

blastocele

5 week human embryo

6 week human embryo

7 week human embryo

culation, usually caused by a nematode worm (*Wuchereria bancrofti*).

elevator **1.** An instrument used as a lever to pry up a depressed bone fragment. **2.** An instrument for extracting teeth and roots that cannot be grasped with a forceps.

eliminant An agent that promotes the excretion or removal of waste.

elimination The expulsion of waste material from the body.

elixir A clear, sweetened solution of alcohol and water, used as a vehicle for medicine taken orally.

ellipsoid Any anatomic structure having an oval shape, especially (a) any one of the oval masses of cells surrounding the second part of the penicillate artery of the spleen, and (b) the outer portion of the inner rod segment of the retina.

elliptocytosis Inherited disorder in which a large number of red blood cells (25 to 90%) have an oval or elliptical shape. Also called ovalocytosis.

Ellis-van Creveld syndrome Chondroectodermal dysplasia; see under dysplasia.

elongation **1.** The act of increasing in length, or the condition of being lengthened. **2.** A measure of the ability of a metal to increase in length before breaking; indicates the ductility of a metal.

eluate The material separated by elution.

eluent The liquid used in elution.

elution Separation of substances by washing.

elutriation The process of purifying, separating, or removing by washing, decanting, and settling.

elytrocleisis Obliteration of the vaginal barrel, as with adhesions.

emaciation Excessive wasting of the body; extreme leanness.

emaculation The removal of blemishes from the skin.

emanation **1.** The act of giving off; exhalation. **2.** The gaseous product of disintegration of a radioactive substance.

emancipation In embryology, the gradual separation or segregation of different areas of the embryo into fields of specialized developmental potentialities.

emasculation Castration.

embalm To treat a dead body with preservatives to prevent its decay.

embed To surround a tissue specimen with a firm substance, such as wax, to facilitate the cutting of thin slices.

embolectomy Surgical removal of an embolus.

emboli Plural of embolus.

embolic Of or relating to an embolus or to embolism.

emboliform Resembling an embolus or a wedge.

embolism The sudden obstruction of a blood vessel by a clot or any foreign material (embolus) formed or introduced elsewhere in the circulatory system and carried to that point by the bloodstream.

　air e. The presence of air bubbles in the heart or blood vessel. Also called pneumathemia; gas embolism.

　crossed e. See paradoxical embolism.

　fat e. The presence of fat globules in the blood. Also called oil embolism.

　gas e. See air embolism.

　oil e. See fat embolism.

　paradoxical e. The presence in an artery of an embolus that originated in a vein, having passed to the arterial circulation through a septal defect in the heart. Also called crossed embolism.

　pulmonary e. (PE) The plugging of pulmonary arteries with fragments of a thrombus, most frequently from the leg after an operation.

　septic pulmonary e. The lodging in a pulmonary artery of an infected thrombus that has become detached from its site of origin.

embolization The introduction of certain substances into the circulation for the therapeutic occlusion of vessels.

embololalia The involuntary insertion of meaningless words in a sentence.

embolus A plug within a vessel (a blood clot or other substance such as air, fat, or a tumor) which is carried in the blood stream from another site until it lodges and becomes an obstruction to circulation.

　riding e., straddling e. One located at the bifurcation of an artery and blocking both branches.

　saddle e. One that straddles the bifurcation of the aorta and occludes both common iliac arteries. Also called pantaloon embolus.

embrasure The space produced by the diverging surfaces of adjacent teeth; it may be labial, buccal, lingual, incisal, occlusal, or gingival.

embrocation **1.** The rubbing of the body with liquid medication. **2.** The liquid used.

embryo An organism in the earliest stage of development; in man, from the time of conception to the end of the second month in the uterus.

embryoblast An aggregation of cells that stick together and collect at the embryonic pole of the blastocyst and that give rise to the tissues of the embryo. Also called inner cell mass.

embryogenesis The development of the embryo from the fertilized egg.

embryogenic, embryogenetic Producing an embryo; relating to the origin of an embryo.

embryogeny The origin of the embryo.

embryologist A scientist who specializes in embryology.

embryology The science concerned with the formation and development of living organisms from the fertilization of the ovum until birth; the study of the development of the embryo. Also called developmental anatomy.

embryoma General term for tumors believed to be derived from embryonic tissues.

　e. of kidney Wilm's tumor; see under tumor.

embryomorphous Relating to or similar to the structure of the embryo.

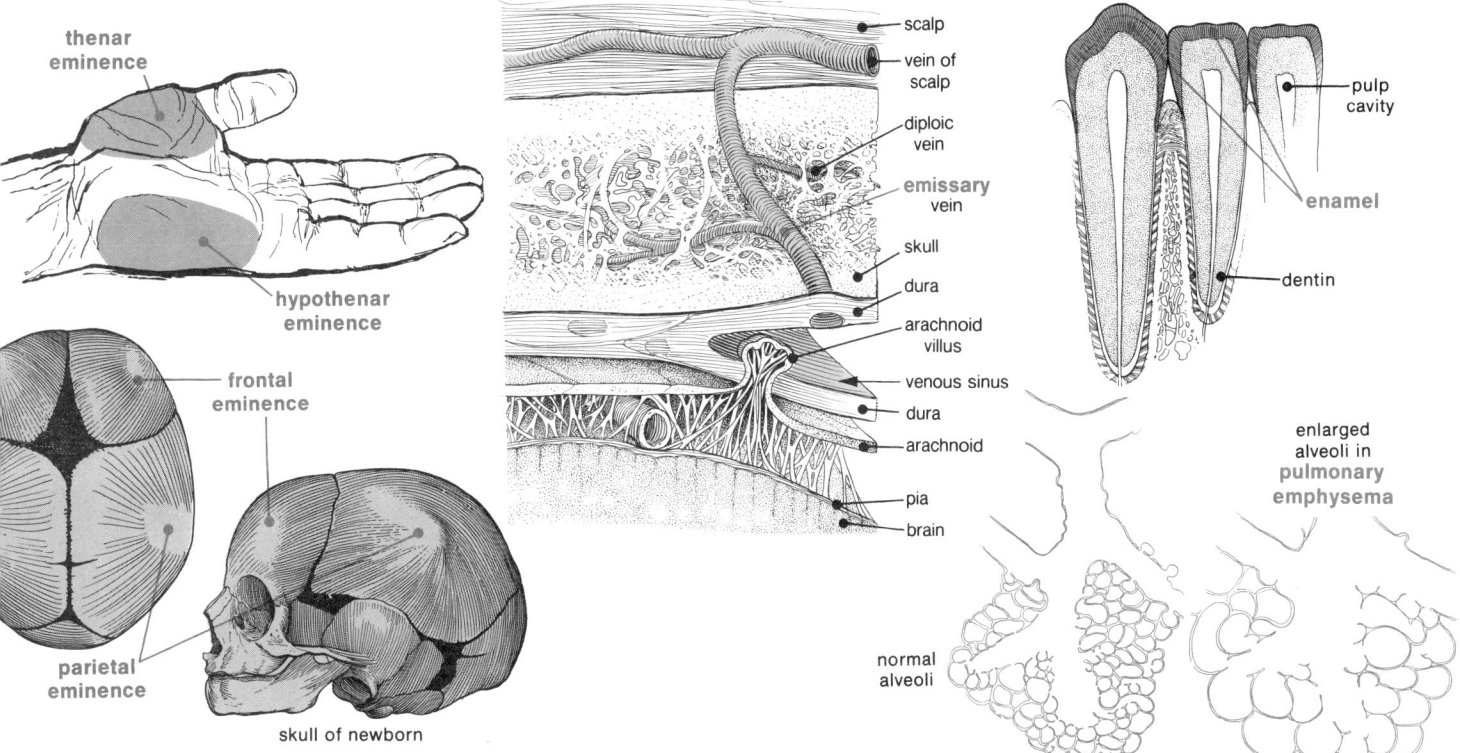

thenar eminence

hypothenar eminence

frontal eminence

parietal eminence

skull of newborn

scalp
vein of scalp
diploic vein
emissary vein
skull
dura
arachnoid villus
venous sinus
dura
arachnoid
pia
brain

pulp cavity
enamel
dentin

enlarged alveoli in **pulmonary emphysema**

normal alveoli

embryonic 1. Of, or relating to, an embryo. 2. Undeveloped; rudimentary.

embryonization Reversion of any tissue to a primitive or embryonic stage.

embryopathy A morbid condition in the embryo or fetus resulting from interference with normal development.

embryophore A membrane around the embryo of a tapeworm forming the inner layer of the egg shell.

embryotomy Any mutilating operation on the fetus to facilitate its removal when delivery is not possible.

embryotoxon A congenital opacity in the deep layers of the peripheral part of the cornea.

embryotroph 1. The nutriment supplied to the embryo. 2. The fluid adjacent to the blastodermic vesicle of deciduate placental mammals during implantation.

emedullate To extract bone marrow.

emergency A serious situation, developing suddenly and unexpectedly, and requiring immediate medical attention.

emergent 1. Developing suddenly and unexpectedly, and requiring prompt action. 2. Coming out; leaving a bodily cavity or other part.

emery A fine-grained abrasive composed of an extremely hard mineral; aluminum oxide combined with iron, magnesia, or silica.

emesis Vomiting.

emetic 1. Causing vomiting. 2. An agent that causes vomiting.

emetine A bitter-tasting alkaloid, $C_{29}H_{40}N_2O_4$; used parenterally as an amebicide.

emetocathartic 1. Both emetic and cathartic. 2. Any agent that induces vomiting and purging.

emigration A process of active motility, whereby motile white blood cells escape from small blood vessels to the surrounding tissues through the intercellular junctions of the vessel walls; monocytes, basophils, eosinophils, neutrophils, and lymphocytes are cells with the ability to emigrate.

eminence A circumscribed, elevated area or prominence, especially of a bone.

  frontal e. The rounded elevation on the skull on either side just above the eye.

  hypothenar e. The prominence on the ulnar side (medial part) of the palm produced by the short muscles of the little finger; one of three muscle divisions of the hand.

  parietal e. The prominence on either side of the skull just above the superior temporal line.

  thenar e. The elevation on the radial side (lateral part) of the palm of the hand produced by the short muscles of the thumb; one of three muscle divisions of the hand.

emiocytosis See exocytosis.

emissary Providing an outlet for a fluid, such as the veins that connect the venous sinuses within the skull with the veins of the scalp.

emission A discharge.

  nocturnal e. Discharge of semen during sleep.

emmenagogue 1. Increasing or producing menstrual flow. 2. Any agent producing such an effect.

emmenia Menses.

emmetropia The normal condition of the refractive system of the eye in which the light rays entering the eyeball focus exactly on the retina.

emollient 1. Soothing. 2. An agent that softens and soothes the skin or mucous membranes.

emotion Any strong feeling (joy, anger, fear).

emotional 1. Relating to an emotion. 2. Easily affected with emotions.

empathic Relating to or marked by empathy.

empathy The intimate understanding of, and identification with, the feelings of another person.

emphysema A swelling due to the abnormal presence of air in tissues or cavities of the body; the term usually refers to a condition of the lungs.

  centrilobular e. Emphysema in which the alveoli occupying the central area of each acinus become dilated and destroyed; generally more prominent in the upper lobes, but extending to all lung areas; commonly seen in chronic bronchitis.

  compensatory e., compensating e. Dilatation of a portion of a lung when another portion is unable to function properly.

  irregular e. A form in which the alveoli of the affected acinus are not uniformly involved; scar formation occurs almost invariably.

  mediastinal e. The presence of air in the mediastinal tissue.

  panlobular e. Emphysema marked by enlarged lungs with loss of vascular lung markings in areas of radiologic hyperlucency in the lower lobes; seen in individuals with homozygous α-1-antitrypsin deficiency.

  paraseptal e. Emphysema with blebs and bullae that are largely localized subpleurally.

  pulmonary e. Lung disease characterized by enlargement of the alveoli (air spaces distal to the terminal bronchioles) with loss of elastic fibers and rupture of their walls.

  subcutaneous a. The presence of air or gas in the subcutaneous tissues.

empirical, empiric Based upon practical experience.

empiricism The view that experience serves as a guide to medical practice or to the therapeutic use of any remedy; reliance on experience as the only source of knowledge.

empyema Pus in a body cavity, especially the pleural cavity.

empyocele Accumulation of pus in the scrotum. Also called suppurating hydrocele.

emulsify To convert into an emulsion.

emulsion A preparation composed of two liquids that do not mix, one being dispersed in the other in the form of small globules.

emulsive A substance that can be emulsified or by which a fat or resin can be emulsified.

emulsoid A dispersion in which the dispersed particles are relatively liquid and absorb some of the liquid in which they are dispersed. Also called emulsion colloid.

enamel The hard, vitreous substance that covers the anatomic crown of a tooth.

  mottled e. Defective structure of enamel due to excessive ingestion of fluoride during tooth formation; the affected teeth may have white, yellow, or brown spots which sometimes are pitted.

enameloma Spherical nodule of enamel attached to a tooth, usually on the root. Also called enamel pearl.

enanthem, enanthema Eruption on a mucous membrane, especially one accompanying an eruptive fever.

enantiomer One of a pair of molecules that are mirror images of each other; although they have the same chemical properties, certain of the physical and essentially all the physiologic properties are different.

enantiomerism In chemistry, isomerism in which the molecules in the configuration are related to one another like an object and its mirror image, thus not superimposable.

enantiomorph A crystal that is similar in form, but with the mirror image of another.

enantiopathy 1. Treating with antidotes or substances that produce effects opposite to those of the morbid state being treated. 2. The mutual antagonism of two morbid states.

enarthrodial Relating to a ball and socket joint (enarthrosis).

enarthrosis A joint that permits extensive movement in almost any direction, as seen in the hip and shoulder. Also called ball and socket joint.

encanthis 1. A small tumor at the inner canthus of the eye. 2. Inflammation of the lacrimal caruncle (the pink fleshy mound at the medial canthus).

encapsulated Encased in a capsule.

enceinte French for pregnant; from Late Latin

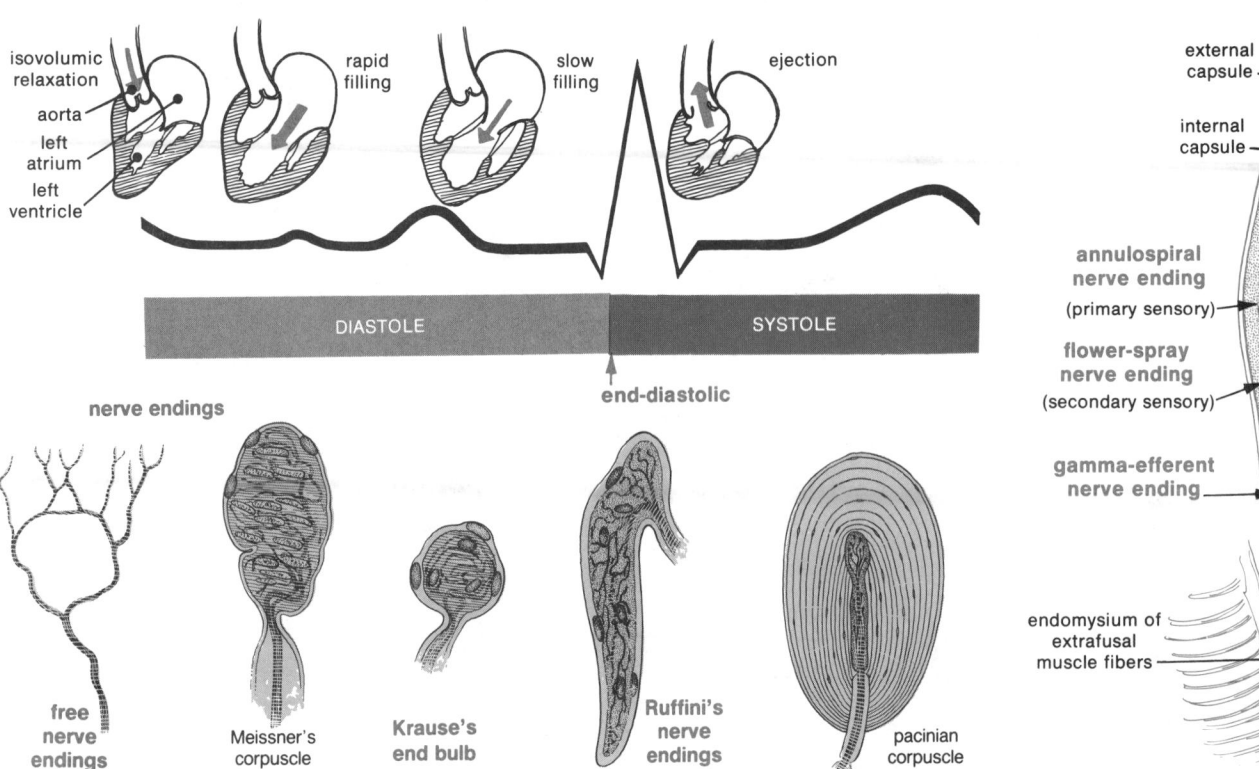

isovolumic relaxation
aorta
left atrium
left ventricle

rapid filling

slow filling

ejection

DIASTOLE

SYSTOLE

end-diastolic

nerve endings

free nerve endings (pain)

Meissner's corpuscle (touch)

Krause's end bulb (cold)

Ruffini's nerve endings (warmth)

pacinian corpuscle (pressure)

external capsule

internal capsule

neuro-muscular spindle

annulospiral nerve ending (primary sensory)

flower-spray nerve ending (secondary sensory)

gamma-efferent nerve ending

intra-fusal muscle fibers:

nuclear bag type

nuclear chain type

endomysium of extrafusal muscle fibers

incincta, without a girdle.

encephalemia Congestion of the brain.

encephalic 1. Of, or relating to, the brain. 2. In the skull.

encephalitic Relating to or afflicted with inflammation of the brain.

encephalitis Inflammation of the brain, classified when possible by reference to the etiologic agent or pathogenic mechanism; headache, nausea, vomiting, fever, and lethargy are common initial symptoms.

acute necrotizing e. Encephalitis with tissue destruction affecting chiefly the temporal lobes; usually caused by herpes simplex virus.

e. periaxialis diffusa A rapidly progressive disease occurring chiefly in children; marked by widespread demyelinization of the cerebral cortex, with convulsions, mental symptoms, motor and sensory disturbances, and gradual loss of sight; death usually occurs within three years after onset. Also called Schilder's disease.

encephalocele 1. The cranial cavity. 2. The ventricles of the brain. 3. Protrusion of brain tissue through a congenital defect of the skull. Also called craniocele.

encephalogram An x-ray picture of the head.

encephalography Roentgenography of the brain. Cf. echoencephalography.

encephalolith A cerebral calculus; a calculus in the brain.

encephalomalacia Softening of the brain.

encephalomeningitis See meningoencephalitis.

encephalomyelitis Acute inflammation of the brain and spinal cord. Also called myeloencephalitis.

benign myalgic e. Epidemic neuromyasthenia; see under neuromyasthenia.

encephalomyelocele Congenital bone defect of the occipital area with herniation of the meninges, medulla, and spinal cord.

encephalomyelopathy Any disease of the brain and spinal cord.

encephalomyeloradiculopathy Disease involving the brain, spinal cord, and roots of spinal nerves.

encephalon See brain.

encephalopathy Any disease of the brain. Also called cerebropathy.

hepatic e. Metabolic disorder of the nervous system marked by flapping tremor (asterixis), musty odor of the breath, and disturbances of consciousness which may progress to deep coma; associated with advanced disease of the liver or with passage of toxic substances from the portal to the systemic circulation via a portocaval shunt.

hypertensive e. A form associated with severe arterial hypertension; marked by headache, nausea, vomiting, papilledema, convulsions, and coma.

lead e. Inflammation of the brain, vomiting, stupor, convulsions, and coma caused by ingestion or absorption of lead compounds.

encephalopsychosis Any psychosis caused by physical damage to the brain.

enchondroma A benign tumor composed of cartilaginous tissue and occurring within a bone.

enchondrosarcoma A malignant bone tumor arising from a preexistent benign cartilaginous tumor within the bone (enchondroma).

enclave A mass of tissue totally enclosed within another.

enclitic Denoting the relation of the planes of the fetal head to those of the pelvis of the mother.

encoding Modification of stimuli received through the senses; first stage in the memory process.

encyesis A normal pregnancy in the uterus.

encysted Enclosed in a cyst or a membranous sac.

Endamoeba A genus of amebae not parasitic in man; the term is sometimes used incorrectly for *Entamoeba*.

endarterectomy Surgical removal of atheromas with the lining of an artery.

endarterial Within an artery; relating to the intima or inner layer of the arterial wall.

endarteritis Inflammation of the inner layer of an artery. Also called endoarteritis.

endarterium The intima or inner layer of the arterial wall.

endaural 1. Within the ear. 2. Through the ear canal.

end-bulb, end-bud One of the minute spherical bodies located at the termination of a sensory nerve fiber; present in certain parts of the skin, mucous membranes, muscles, joints, and connective tissue of internal organs.

Krause's e-b. Krause's corpuscle; see under corpuscle.

end-diastolic 1. Occurring at the termination of diastole, just before the next systole, as in end-diastolic pressure. 2. Interrupting the final stage of diastole, barely premature, as in end-diastolic extrasystole.

endemic Relating to any disease prevalent continually in a particular locality.

endergonic Indicating a chemical reaction that is accompanied by an absorption of free energy, regardless of the form of energy involved.

endermic, endermatic Through the skin, as the action of certain medicines when absorbed through the skin.

end-feet Bouton termineaux; see under bouton.

ending A termination, as of a nerve.

annulospiral nerve e. A coiled nerve ending around the nuclear region of a muscle fiber; sensitive to stretch.

flower-spray nerve e.'s Intricate series of nerve branches on the contractile part of the intrafusal muscle fibers; sensitive to increased tension.

free nerve e.'s Network of nerve endings found throughout the body, in skin, mucous membranes, and deep tissues; their fibers are both myelinated and non-myelinated.

gamma-efferent nerve e.'s The terminal part of motor fibers that innervate the intrafusal muscle fibers near their ends.

nerve e. Any one of the specialized terminations of sensory or motor nerve fibers.

Ruffini's nerve e.'s Sensory nerve endings that serve as joint receptors, mechanoreceptors, receptors for position sense, and skin receptors; characterized by whorls of fine fibers that end as numerous knobs. Also called Ruffini's corpuscles.

endoarteritis See endarteritis.

endoauscultation Auscultation of the heart or stomach by passing a stethoscopic tube or electronic amplifier into the esophagus or heart.

endobronchial Within the bronchial tubes. Also called intrabronchial.

endocardial 1. Relating to the endocardium. 2. In the heart.

endocardiography Recording of the electric currents traversing the heart muscle, prior to a heartbeat, with the exploring electrode within the heart chambers.

endocarditis A disease caused by infection of the lining membrane of the cardiac chambers, or of the intima of a great vessel.

abacterial thrombotic e. See nonbacterial thrombotic endocarditis.

atypical verrucous e. See Libman-Sacks syndrome.

bacterial e. Endocarditis due to bacteria or other microorganisms, causing deformity of the valve leaflets; it may be acute, usually caused by pyogenic organisms such as staphylococci, or subacute (chronic), usually due to *Streptococcus viridans* or *Streptococcus faecalis*.

marantic e. A nonbacterial type with deposition of clots.

nonbacterial thrombotic e. Endocarditis associated with verrucous lesions and clots, occurring in the last stages of many chronic infections and wasting diseases. Also called abacterial thrombotic endocarditis; terminal endocarditis.

rheumatic e. Endocarditis with special involvement of the valves associated with rheumatic fever.

terminal e. See nonbacterial thrombotic endo-

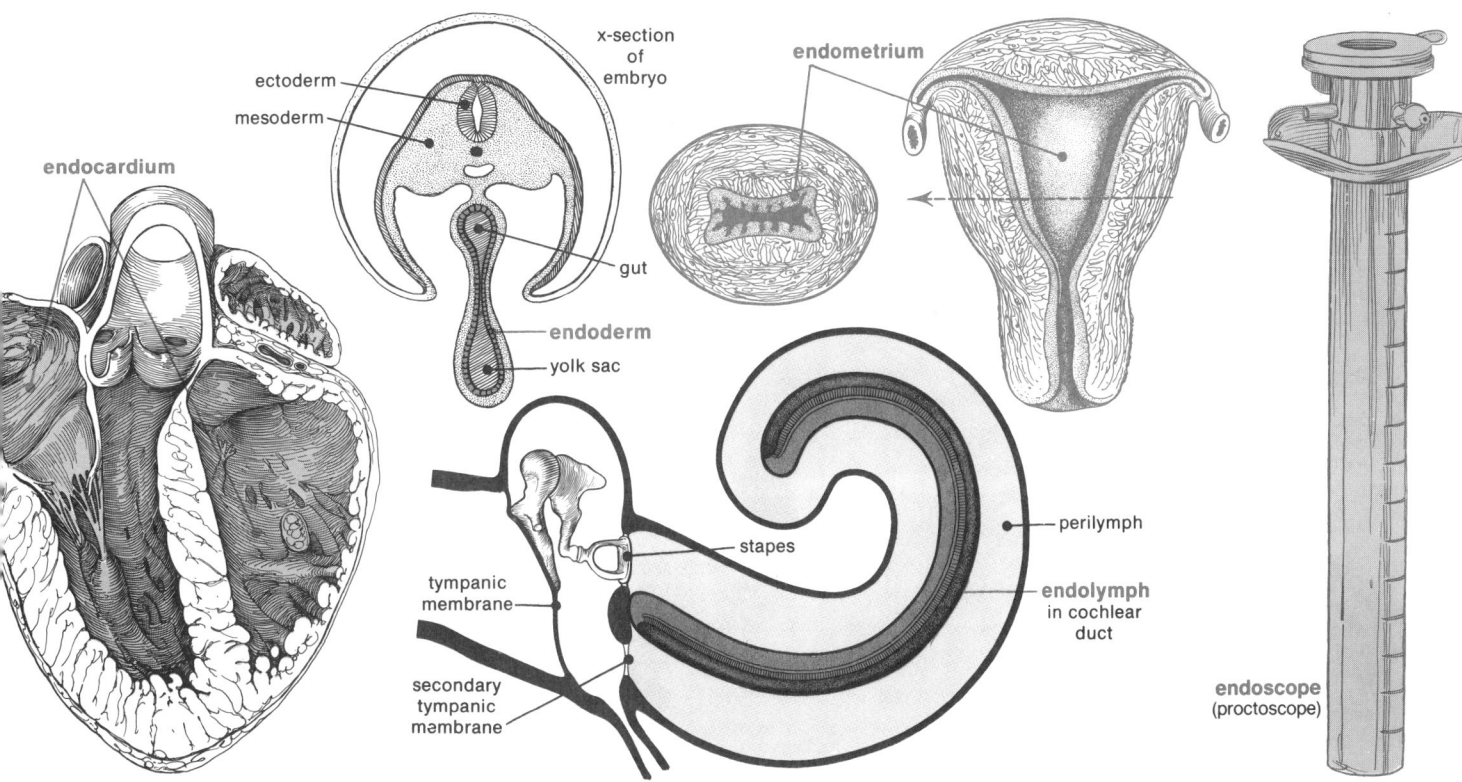

ectoderm
mesoderm
endocardium
x-section of embryo
endometrium
gut
endoderm
yolk sac
stapes
tympanic membrane
secondary tympanic membrane
perilymph
endolymph in cochlear duct
endoscope (proctoscope)

carditis.

vegetative e., verrucous e. A type associated with the formation of fibrinous clots on the ulcerated valves.

endocardium The serous membrane that lines the chambers of the heart.

endoceliac In any of the cavities of the body. Also called intracelial.

endocervical Within the uterine cervix. Also called intracervical.

endocervicitis Inflammation of the mucous membrane of the uterine cervix.

endochondral Within cartilage. Also called intracartilaginous.

endocranial 1. Within the skull. 2. Relating to the skull.

endocrine Secreting internally; denoting a gland whose secretions are discharged into the blood or lymph.

endocrinology The branch of science dealing with endocrine glands and their secretions.

endocrinopathy Any disease of the endocrine glands.

endocrinotherapy Treatment of disease with extracts of endocrine glands.

endocrinous Of, or relating to, any internal secretion.

endocytosis The uptake of particles by a cell through invagination of its plasma membrane.

endoderm The innermost of the three germ layers of the embryo; it gives rise to the lining of the gastrointestinal tract from pharynx to rectum and to neighboring glands such as the liver, pancreas, thyroid, etc. Also called entoderm.

endodontics The branch of dentistry concerned with the diagnosis and treatment of diseases of the tooth pulp and/or infection of the root canal and periapical areas.

endodontist A specialist in endodontics.

endoenzyme An enzyme that is retained by and acts within the cell that produced it.

endogenous Originating within the body.

endointoxication Poisoning by a toxin produced within the organism.

endolaryngeal Within the larynx.

Endolimax A genus of nonpathogenic amebae.

E. nana A species parasitic in the large intestine of man, other primates, and pigs.

endolymph The fluid contained in the membranous labyrinth of the internal ear; an isotonic solution that is of high potassium and low sodium concentration.

endometrial Relating to or containing endometrium.

endometrioma A mass of ectopic endometrium

in endometriosis.

endometriosis An abnormal condition in which the uterine mucous membrane invades other tissues in the pelvic cavity; the uterus and ovaries are the most common sites; other areas include the intestines, umbilicus, bladder, and ureters.

endometritis Inflammation of the membrane lining the interior of the uterus.

endometrium The mucosal layer lining the cavity of the uterus; its structure changes with age and with the menstrual cycle.

endomitosis See endopolyploidy.

endomorph A person having a body build characterized by prominence of the abdomen and other parts developed from the embryonic endodermal layer.

endomysium The microscopic sheath of delicate connective tissue that surrounds and separates individual muscle fibers.

endoneurium The delicate connective tissue sheath surrounding and separating individual nerve fibers. Also called Henle's sheath; connective tissue sheath of Retzius.

endonuclease A nuclease (phosphodiesterase) that cleaves polynucleotides into poly- or oligonucleotide fragments of varying size.

endoparasite A parasite that lives within the body of its host.

endopeptidase A proteolytic enzyme that is capable of hydrolyzing a peptide linkage at points within the chain, not near the ends; e.g., pepsin, trypsin, and ribonuclease.

endophlebitis Inflammation of the inner layer of a vein.

endophthalmitis Inflammation of the internal structures of the eye.

endoplasm The internal cytoplasm; it is less viscous than the ectoplasm.

endopolyploidy The reproduction of nuclear elements without accompanying spindle formation or cytoplasmic division, resulting in a polyploid nucleus. Also called endomitosis.

end-organ See organ, end.

endorphin One of a group of low-molecular weight peptides normally found in the brain and other parts of the body; capable of producing effects similar to those of opiates.

endosalpinx The mucous membrane that lines the interior of a uterine tube.

endoscope An instrument used to examine the interior of a hollow organ or a cavity; e.g., gastroscope, proctoscope, and cystoscope.

endoscopy Inspection of the interior of a canal or any air or food passage by means of an endoscope.

endoskeleton The internal supporting bony skel-

eton of vertebrates.

endosmosis The passage of a fluid through a membrane into a cavity or a cell containing fluid of a lesser density; osmosis in a direction toward the interior of a cell or a cavity.

endosonoscopy Ultrasonic scanning with transducers, used as miniature probes, in the gastrointestinal tract, bladder, etc.

endospore 1. A small, resistant, asexual spore, as that formed within the vegetative cells of some bacteria, particularly those belonging to the genera *Bacillus* and *Clostridium*. 2. The innermost layer of the wall of a spore.

endosteitis, endostitis Inflammation of the tissue lining the medullary cavity of a bone (endosteum).

endosteoma A benign tumor in the medullary cavity of a bone.

endosteum The membrane lining bone cavities.

endothelin A peptide, derived from the inner lining of blood vessels, that induces constriction of the vessels.

endothelioma Any tumor, benign or malignant, derived from the endothelial tissue of blood vessels, lymphatic vessels, or serous membranes.

endothelium A thin layer of cells lining serous cavities, blood vessels, and lymph vessels.

endothermic Denoting a chemical reaction that produces heat absorption.

endothermy Diathermy.

endothrix Within the hair shaft; denoting a type of fungal infection in which the hyphae grow only within the hair shaft, where they form long, parallel rows of arthrospores. Cf. ectothrix.

endotoxemia Presence of endotoxins in the blood, which may cause shock.

endotoxin A toxin produced and retained by bacterial cells and released only by destruction or death of the cells. Also called intracellular toxin.

endotracheal Within the trachea.

end-plate The terminal part of a motor nerve fiber that transmits nerve impulses to muscle.

end-product A chemical product that represents the final sequence of metabolic reactions.

end-stage renal failure (ESRF) Irreversible failure of kidney function.

enema 1. The infusion of a fluid into the rectum for cleansing or other therapeutic purposes. 2. The liquid so infused.

energetics The physics of energy and its changes.

energy (W) The exertion of power to effect physical change; dynamic force; the capacity to do work, taking the forms of kinetic energy, potential energy, rest energy, electrical energy, etc.

binding e. The energy released in binding a group

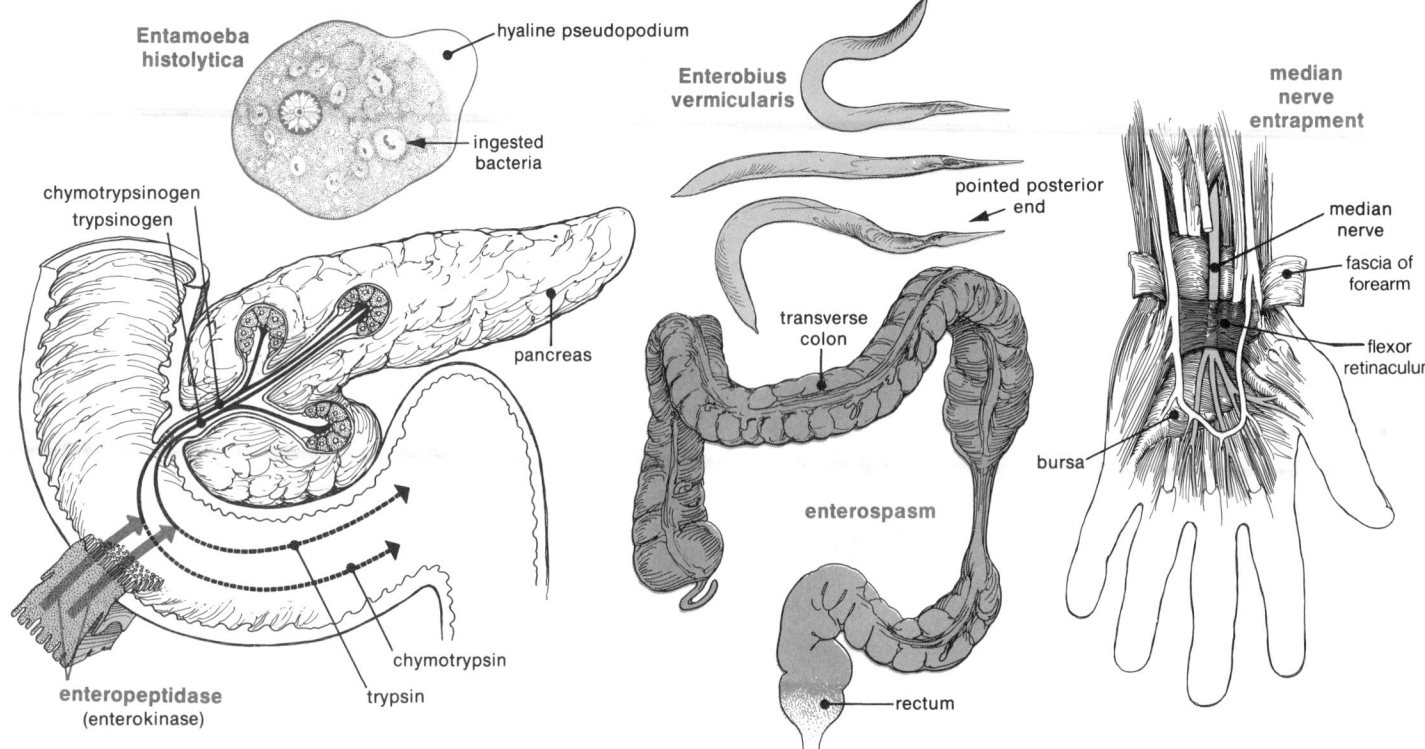

Entamoeba histolytica — hyaline pseudopodium, ingested bacteria

chymotrypsinogen, trypsinogen, pancreas

enteropeptidase (enterokinase), chymotrypsin, trypsin

Enterobius vermicularis — pointed posterior end

transverse colon, enterospasm, rectum

median nerve entrapment — median nerve, fascia of forearm, flexor retinaculum, bursa

---

of protons and neutrons into an atomic nucleus.

chemical e. Energy emanating from a chemical reaction or absorbed in the formation of a chemical compound.

conservation of e. The principle that the total amount of energy remains constant, none being lost or created in the conversion of one type of force into another.

e. of activation The amount of energy needed by molecules in order to initiate a reaction.

free e. A thermodynamic function, symbolized as ΔG, that expresses the maximum amount of work that can be obtained from a chemical reaction. Also called Gibbs free-energy function.

nuclear e. The energy given off by a nuclear reaction, especially by fission, fusion, or radioactive deterioration; the energy stored in the formation of an atomic nucleus.

potential e. The energy existing in a particle or system of particles by virtue of its position or state of existence that is not being exerted at the time.

enervation Lack of energy and vigor; lassitude; weakness.

engineering 1. The practical application of the principles of mathematics and the physical sciences. **2.** Work performed by an engineer.

biomedical e. Application of engineering in solving biologic and medical problems.

genetic e. Alteration of genetic material of a living organism to modify heredity or to produce hormones or proteins.

engorged Congested or filled to excess; distended with blood or other fluid.

enkephalin A pentapeptide present in many parts of the brain; believed to be a neurotransmitter.

enol An organic compound containing a hydroxyl group (alcohol) attached to a doubly bonded (ethylenic) carbon atom; the name is derived as an abbreviation of ethyl*ene* alcoh*ol*.

enophthalmos Backward displacement of the eyeball causing it to recede within the orbit.

enostosis A bony growth within a bone.

ensiform Shaped like a sword.

Entamoeba A genus of protozoan parasites.

E. coli A nonpathogenic species found in the intestine. Also called amoeba coli.

E. gingivalis A species occurring in the mouth.

E. histolytica A species that inhabits the intestines of man and causes amebic dysentery; it may also invade the liver.

enteral Within the intestine.

enterectomy Surgical removal of a segment of the intestine.

enteric Relating to the intestines.

enteritis Inflammation of the intestines.

regional e. A chronic recurrent disease, mainly of young adults, caused by inflammation of segments of the small intestine; characterized by abdominal pain, diarrhea, and frequently by fever and weight loss; similar lesions are occasionally found in the large bowel, where the process is referred to as granulomatous colitis; etiology is unknown. Also called regional or terminal ileitis; Crohn's disease.

Enterobacteriaceae A family of gram-negative rod-shaped bacteria (order Eubacteriales) which includes the genus *Escherichia*.

enterobiasis Infestation of the intestines with *Enterobius vermicularis*, a short roundworm commonly called pinworm. Also called pinworm infestation.

Enterobius A genus of nematode worms. Formerly called *Oxyuris*.

E. vermicularis The pinworm, a species that infests the intestines.

enterocele 1. Any hernia of the intestine. **2.** Herniation through the rectouterine pouch (cul-de-sac of Douglas). Also called posterior vaginal, rectovaginal, cul-de-sac, or Douglas' pouch hernia.

enterocleisis Occlusion of the intestinal tract.

omentum e. The operative use of omentum to close an opening in the intestine.

enteroclysis Enema directed into the colon. Also called high enema.

enterococcus Any streptococcus which inhabits the intestinal tract.

enterocolitis Inflammation of the mucous membrane of the small intestine and colon.

pseudomembranous e. An acute form with formation and passage in the feces of membrane-like material; often occurring after prolonged antibiotic therapy.

enterocolostomy Operative creation of an opening between the small intestine and any part of the colon.

enterocyst A cyst of the intestinal wall.

enteroenterostomy Operative connection of any two noncontinuous segments of intestine. Also called enteroanastomosis; intestinal anastomosis.

enterogastrone One of the gastrointestinal hormones released during digestion; it is secreted by the upper intestinal mucosa when a significant amount of gastric contents reaches the upper intestine, and inhibits secretion and movements of the stomach.

enterokinase See enteropeptidase.

enterokinetic Stimulating contraction of the gastrointestinal tract.

enterolith Any concretion or calculus in the intestine.

enterology The branch of medicine concerned with the intestinal tract.

enteron The intestinal tract, especially the small intestine.

enteroparesis Weakness and relaxation of the intestinal walls.

enteropathogenic Causing intestinal disease.

enteropathy Any disease of the intestines.

gluten-induced e See celiac disease.

enteropeptidase An enzyme secreted by the duodenal mucosa that converts trypsinogen (pancreatic secretion) to trypsin (protein-splitting enzyme). Also called enterokinase.

enteropexy Fixation of a portion of the intestine to the abdominal wall.

enteroptosia, enteroptosis Downward displacement of the intestines in the abdominal cavity, as observed sometimes in obese individuals.

enterospasm Intestinal spasm or colic.

enterostenosis Narrowing or stricture of the intestinal lumen.

enterostomy The establishment of an opening into the intestine, temporary or permanent, through the abdominal wall.

enterotomy Incision into the intestine.

enterotoxin A cytotoxin specific for the cells of the mucous membrane of the intestine.

Enterovirus A genus of viruses (family Picornaviridae) that infect the intestinal tract primarily but multiply also in muscles, nerves, and other tissues; incudes viruses causing poliomyelitis, meningitis, gastroenteritis, and viral hepatitis, type A.

enterozoon An intestinal parasite.

enthesitis Irritation of the attachments of muscle or tendons to bone, as in tennis elbow, shin splints, and glass arm of baseball pitchers.

entoderm See endoderm.

entomology The study of insects.

entomophobia Abnormal fear of insects.

entopic Occurring or located in the normal site; opposed to ectopic.

entoptic Located within the eyeball.

entozoon, *pl.* **entozoa** A parasitic animal living in any of the internal organs of its host.

entrapment The act or process of catching in, as if in a trap.

abdominal cutaneous nerve e. syndrome The entrapment of cutaneous nerves when they pass through the abdominal muscles en route to the skin, resulting in neuromuscular compression and pain.

lateral femoral cutaneous nerve e. Compression of the lateral femoral cutaneous nerve in the fascia lata, resulting in a sensory neuropathy (meralgia paresthetica), characterized by pain and numbness over the lateral aspect of the thigh.

median nerve e. Compression of the median nerve at the wrist beneath the transverse carpal

eosinophil

RBCs for size comparison

humerus

lateral epicondyle

medial epicondyle

ephedrine

epicardium

deferent duct

epididymis

testis

stratum corneum
stratum lucidum
stratum granulosum

stratum spinosum

stratum germinativum

epidermis

dermis

ligament, causing pain and numbness in the palmar surface of the hand and the first three fingers (carpal tunnel syndrome).

entropion Inversion or inward displacement of the margin of an eyelid.

entropy **1.** That fraction of energy not available during a chemical reaction for the performance of work, because it has gone to increasing the random motion of the atoms or molecules in a system. **2.** A measure of the ability of a system to undergo spontaneous change.

enucleate **1.** To remove whole, as in shelling out a nut. **2.** To destroy or remove the nucleus.

enucleation The surgical removal of a tumor or of an organ, such as the eyeball, in its entirety, without rupture.

enuresis Involuntary discharge of urine.
   nocturnal e. See bed-wetting.

environment The collection of physical or external conditions affecting the growth and development of organisms.

enzootic Indicating a disease of animals that is indigenous to a specific locality, analogous to an endemic disease among men.

enzymatic Relating to an enzyme.

enzyme A protein secreted by the body that acts as a catalyst by promoting or accelerating a chemical change in other substances while remaining unchanged in the process.
   activating e. An enzyme that activates an amino acid by attaching it to the corresponding transfer ribonucleic acid.
   angiotensin converting e. See dipeptyl carboxypeptidase.
   autolytic e. An enzyme capable of causing autolysis or digestion of the cell in which it was formed.
   digestive e. An enzyme that promotes the hydrolysis of protein, carbohydrate, and fat in the digestive tract prior to absorption.
   induced e. An enzyme produced by the addition of its specific substrate to cells that normally do not metabolize that substrate.
   proteolytic e. An enzyme that acts upon the peptide bonds of proteins and peptides; a protein-splitting or hydrolyzing enzyme. Also called protease.
   restrictive e. Enzyme that acts as a molecular scissors by cutting DNA molecules at specific locations.
   transferring e. An enzyme that catalyzes the transfer of a chemical grouping from one substance to another. Also called transferase.

enzymic Enzymatic.

enzymology The branch of science concerned with the study of enzymes, their structure and function.

enzymolysis The chemical decomposition brought about by an enzyme.

eosin A crystalline product of coal tar, used in solution to stain cells for microscopic study; it imparts a reddish color to the specimen.

eosinoblast A young granular white blood cell (myeloblast) that develops into an eosinophil.

eosinopenia Deficiency of eosinophilic leukocytes in the blood.

eosinophil A cell, especially a white blood cell (eosinophilic leukocyte), that stains easily with eosin dye.

eosinophilia The presence of an abnormally large number of eosinophils in the blood.

eosinophilic Easily stained with eosin dyes. Also called oxyphilic.

eosinophilic endomyocardial disease. See Löffler's disease.

ependyma The lining membrane of the cerebral ventricles and the central canal of the spinal cord.

ependymoma A brain tumor derived from cells of the membrane lining the ventricles (ependyma); occurring most frequently in children and young adults and constituting approximately one to three percent of all intracranial tumors.

ephedrine A sympathomimetic amine obtained from species of *Ephedra* or produced synthetically; it dilates the bronchi and is used in the prevention and treatment of bronchial asthma; it acts, in part, by releasing catecholamines from their storage vesicles.

epicanthus A skin fold extending from the root of the nose to the inner termination of the eyebrow, covering the inner angle (canthus) of the eye; normal in individuals of the Mongolian race; in children under the age of 10 with Down syndrome, a fold is common, but confined to the inner angle. Also called epicanthal fold; plica palpebronasalis.

epicardia The portion of the esophagus from the diaphragm to the stomach.

epicardium The visceral or inner layer of the pericardium that is in contact with the heart.

epicondyle The bony prominence situated above or upon a smooth articular eminence of a long bone.
   lateral e. **1.** Of the femur, a prominence situated above the lateral condyle; it gives attachment to the fibular collateral ligament of the knee-joint; **2.** Of the humerus, a small tuberculated eminence situated at the lower end of the bone; it gives attachment to the radial collateral ligament of the elbow-joint, and to a

tendon common to the origin of the supinator and some of the extensor muscles.
   medial e. **1.** Of the femur, a large convex eminence located above the medial condyle to which the tibial collateral ligament of the knee-joint is attached; **2.** Of the humerus, a large projection situated above and medial to the condyle; it gives attachment to the ulnar collateral ligament of the elbow-joint, to the pronator teres, and to a common tendon of origin of most of the forearm's flexor muscles.

epicondylitis, lateral Pain and tenderness of the tendons near the lateral epicondyle of the humerus; a syndrome affecting the midportion of the upper extremity, usually due to repetitive rotatory motions of the forearm (believed to cause microscopic tears and subsequent chronic tendinitis). Also called tennis elbow.

epicranium The scalp; the structures (muscle, aponeurosis, and skin) covering the skull.

epicrisis A crisis occurring after the first crisis of a disease; a secondary crisis.

epicritic Denoting sensory nerve fibers in the skin and oral mucosa that perceive slight variations of touch and temperature.

epidemic The outbreak and rapid spread of a disease in a community, affecting many people at the same time.

epidemiography A treatise of one or several epidemic diseases.

epidemiologist A person who specializes in epidemiology.

epidemiology The scientific study of epidemics and epidemic diseases, especially of the factors that influence the incidence, distribution, and control of infectious diseases; the study of disease occurrence in human populations.

epidermal Relating to or resembling the epidermis.

epidermatoplasty Skin grafting.

epidermis The outer, thinner layer of the skin, consisting of layers of stratified squamous epithelium; it is devoid of blood vessels and contains a limited distribution of nerve endings. See also skin.

epidermoid **1.** Resembling epidermis. **2.** A tumor containing aberrant epidermal cells.

epidermolysis A loose state of the superficial layer of the skin, often tending to form blisters.

Epidermophyton A genus of fungi causing skin disorders.

epididymectomy Surgical removal of the epididymis.

epididymis A tortuous C-shaped cordlike structure; the first part of the excretory duct of the testis, lying along its posterior surface, in which the sper-after Netter

bolus

epiglottis

trachea

esophagus

thyroid cartilage

epinephrine

OH

epimers

CHO   CHO

H—C—OH   H—C—OH

HO—C—H   HO—C—H

H—C—OH   HO—C—H

H—C—OH   H—C—OH

CH₂OH   CH₂OH

D-glucose   D-galactose

peripheral nerve

epineurium

perineurium

neuron

median **episiotomy** closed by continuous suture

epithelioma

---

matozoa are stored; it consists of a head, a body, and a tail which is continuous with the deferent duct.

epididymitis Inflammation of the epididymis.

epididymo-orchitis Inflammation of both the epididymis and testis.

epididymotomy Surgical incision into the epididymis, usually for relief of tension and pain in epididymitis.

epididymovasostomy The surgical joining of the epididymis and the deferent duct, usually for the purpose of bypassing an obstruction in the deferent duct.

epidural Situated upon or over the dura mater.

epigastrium The upper central area of the abdomen; pit of the stomach.

epigenesis The concept that an organism develops by the new formation of structures, as opposed to the old theory of preformation, i.e., that an organism develops by the growth of structures already existing in miniature in the egg.

epiglottis The leaf-shaped cartilage that covers the aperture of the larynx during the act of swallowing to prevent food from entering the trachea.

epiglottitis Inflammation of the epiglottis; it may cause respiratory obstruction, especially in children.

epilation The removal of hairs with their roots.

epilemma Endoneurium.

epilepsy A chronic neurologic disease, marked by sudden alterations in consciousness and frequently by convulsions.

  focal e. Minor seizures restricted to specific areas of the body. Also called partial epilepsy.

  generalized e. A seizure marked by loss of consciousness and spasms of the trunk and extremities, followed by generalized clonic jerking. Also called grand mal or major epilepsy.

  grand mal e. See generalized epilepsy.

  major e. See generalized epilepsy.

  petit mal e. Brief or mild seizures, lasting from 5 to 30 seconds, characterized by a sudden cessation of activity and blank stare.

  post-traumatic e. Recurring convulsions caused by head injuries.

  psychomotor e. Disorder in which the seizure activity originates in or involves the temporal lobe, producing altered, bizarre activity and behavior. Also called temporal lobe epilepsy.

  sleep e. See narcolepsy.

  temporal lobe e. See psychomotor epilepsy.

epileptic 1. Relating to epilepsy. 2. One who is afflicted with epilepsy.

epileptoid Resembling epilepsy; said of certain convulsions.

epimandibular On the lower jaw.

epimenorrhea Menstruation occurring at excessively short intervals.

epimerase One of a group of enzymes that promote epimeric changes.

epimers Two sugars that differ from one another only in the configuration around a single carbon atom; e.g., glucose and galactose.

epimicroscope Opaque microscope, a microscope with a condenser around the objective; used for observing opaque or translucent specimens.

epimorphosis Regeneration of a cut part of an organism.

epimysium A sheath of connective tissue surrounding individual muscles.

epinephrine 1. Hormone produced by the medulla of the adrenal gland; it stimulates the sympathetic nervous system. 2. A crystalline compound, $C_9H_{13}NO_3$, extracted from the adrenal glands of some mammals or produced synthetically; it produces cardiac stimulation, constriction or dilation of blood vessels, and bronchial relaxation; used as a heart stimulant and in the treatment of bronchial asthma and acute allergic disorders, and as a local vasoconstrictor. Also called adrenaline.

epineural Located upon a neural arch.

epineurial Relating to the connective tissue surrounding a nerve trunk.

epineurium The connective tissue covering of a peripheral nerve.

epipharynx Nasopharynx.

epiphenomenon A symptom occurring during the course of a disease but not necessarily associated with it.

epiphora Persistent overflow of tears onto the cheek, due to obstruction of the tear-conducting passages, eversion of the margin of the lower lid, or excessive secretion of tears.

epiphysiodesis, epiphyseodesis An operation creating a permanent premature closure of an epiphysial plate, resulting in cessation of bone growth.

epiphysiolysis The separation of an epiphysis from the shaft of the bone.

epiphysis, pl. epiphyses The end of a long bone, developed separately, and initially separated from the shaft by cartilage.

  e. cerebri Pineal body; see under body.

epiphysitis Inflammation of an epiphysis.

epiplocele A hernia of the omentum.

epiploectomy Surgical removal of the omentum.

epiploic Relating to the omentum.

epiplopexy See omentopexy.

episclera The loose connective tissue that consti-

tutes the external surface of the sclera and contains a large number of small blood vessels.

episcleritis Inflammation of the connective tissue of the eye between the sclera and the conjunctiva.

episioperineoplasty Reparative surgery of the vulva and perineum.

episioperineorrhaphy Suturing of a lacerated vulva and perineum.

episioplasty Surgical repair of a defect of the vulva.

episiorrhaphy Suturing of a lacerated vulva.

episiotomy Incision of the perineum during childbirth, done to prevent vaginal, vulvar, or perineal tear by controlled enlargement of the vaginal orifice, to shorten the second stage of labor, and to prevent undue pressure on the fetal skull during delivery; the two most commonly used incisions are the mediolateral and median (midline). Also called perineotomy.

episome A class of genetic elements of bacteria that may exist either as autonomous entities, replicating in the host independent of the bacterial chromosome, or as segments of the bacterial chromosome, replicating with it.

epispadias, epispadia A rare congenital defect in the male in which the urethra opens on the dorsal surface of the penis; also a similar defect in the female in which a fissure is present in the upper wall of the urethra.

epispastic Anything that causes blistering.

epispinal On the vertebral column, spinal cord, or any spinelike structure.

episplenitis Inflammation of the capsule of the spleen.

epistasis 1. The film formed on the surface of a bodily discharge such as urine. 2. The nonreciprocal interaction of nonallelic genes in which one suppresses the action of another.

epistaxis See nosebleed.

episternal Situated over or on the sternum. Also called suprasternal.

epistropheus The second cervical vertebra. Also called axis.

epithalamus A small area of the diencephalon consisting of the trigonum habenulae, the pineal body, and the posterior commissure.

epithelial Relating to or composed of epithelium.

epithelialization The final stage in the healing of a surface injury in which epithelium is formed over the denuded area. Also called epithelization.

epithelioid Resembling epithelium.

epithelioma A malignant tumor consisting of epithelial cells and arising mainly in the skin and mucous membrane.

simple squamous epithelium

simple cuboidal epithelium

simple columnar epithelium

basal lamina

ciliated pseudostratified columnar epithelium

columnar cell
goblet cell
intermediate cell
basal cell

strata: skin

disjunctum
corneum
lucidum
granulosum
spinosum — prickle cell
germina-tivum

stratified squamous epithelium

basal cell

transitional epithelium

binucleate dome cell

basal lamina
lamina propria

equivalent measures and weights

US Customary Unit (Avoirdupois)	US Equivalents	Metric Equivalents
LENGTH		
inch	0.083 foot	2.54 centimeters
foot	1/3 yard or 12 inches	0.3048 meters
yard	3 feet or 36 inches	0.9144 meters
CAPACITY		
fluid ounce	8 fluid ounces	29.573 milliliters
pint	16 fluid ounces	0.473 liter
quart	2 pints	0.946 liter
gallon	4 quarts	3.785 liters
WEIGHT		
grain	0.036 dram	64.798 milligrams
dram	27.344 grains	1.772 grams
ounce	16 drams	28.350 grams
pound	16 ounces	453.592 grams

Apothecary Weight Unit	US Customary Equivalents	Metric Equivalents
scruple	20 grains	1.296 grams
dram	60 grains	3.888 grams
ounce	480 grains	31.103 grams

Malherbe's calcifying e. See pilomatrixoma.

epithelium The nonvascular cellular layer that covers the internal and external surfaces of the body.

  germinal e. Specialized peritoneal mesothelium (low cuboidal) that forms a continuous covering over the ovary; it was once thought to give rise to primordial germ cells (oogonia).

epithelization See epithelialization.

epitope The part of the surface of an antigen to which an antibody attaches. Cf. paratope.

epizoic Living as a parasite on the surface of the host's body.

epizoon, *pl.* epizoa An animal parasite living on the exterior of the host's body.

eponychia Infection at the groove of the nail.

eponychium **1.** The fold of skin overlying the root of the nail; its free, cornified margin forms the cuticle. **2.** The horny epidermis at the site of the future nail in the embryo.

eponym The name of a disease, structure, or surgical procedure which includes the name of a person; e.g., Pott's disease.

eponymic Named after a particular person.

epoophoron The vestiges of the mesonephros (wolffian body) consisting of rudimentary tubules located in the mesosalpinx between the ovary and the ovarian tube. Also called pampiniform body; organ of Rosenmüller.

epoxy In chemistry, an oxygen atom bound to two linked carbon atoms.

epulis A tumor of the gums.

  e. gravidarum Tumor of the gums occurring during pregnancy.

equation A mathematical or chemical representation as a linear array of symbols expressing the quality of two things, separated into left and right sides by an equal sign.

  Arrhenius' e. An equation relating chemical reaction rate with temperature.

  Bohr's e. The equation for calculating the volume of the dead space gas in the respiratory tract by measuring the expired air and subtracting it from the alveolar gas volumes.

  Einthoven's e. See law, Einthoven's.

  Hasselbalch's e. See Henderson-Hasselbalch equation.

  Henderson-Hasselbalch e. An equation for determining the pH of a buffer solution such as blood plasma; $pH = pK + \log ([HCO_3^-/CO_2])$. Also called Hasselbalch's equation.

equator bulbi oculi Equator of the eyeball; an imaginary circle around the eyeball at the same distance from both poles.

equicaloric Having the same heat value.

equilibration **1.** The act of bringing about or maintaining equilibrium. **2.** In dentistry, the equalization of pressure.

equilibrium **1.** Condition in which all acting forces cancel each other, resulting in a stable unchanging system. **2.** In chemistry, a stable condition created by two reactions occurring at equal speed in opposite directions. **3.** Mental or emotional stability. **4.** A state of bodily balance.

  Donnan e. The condition that exists when two solutions are separated by a semipermeable membrane (i.e., permeable only to some of the ions of the solutions); the unequal distribution of ions between the two solutions causes an electrical potential between the two sides of the membrane.

  dynamic e. The condition of balance between the varying forces of living processes.

equimolar Containing the same number of moles or having equal molarity.

equimolecular Denoting solutions that contain an equal number of molecules.

equinus Talipes equinus.

equivalence, equivalency **1.** In chemistry, the relative combining powers of a set of atoms or radicals. **2.** Valence.

equivalent **1.** Equal in any way (substance, value, force, etc.). **2.** Having similar or equal effects.

  chemical e. See gram equivalent.

  epileptic e. The occurrence of manifestations such as cough, severe headaches, abdominal pain, etc. instead of a typical seizure, usually observed in psychomotor epileptics.

  gram e. **1.** The weight (usually in grams) of a substance that can combine with, or displace, a unit weight of hydrogen from a compound or its equivalent of another substance. **2.** The atomic or molecular weight in grams of an atom or group of atoms involved in a chemical reaction divided by the number of electrons donated, taken up, or shared by the atom or group of atoms in the course of that reaction. **3.** The weight of a substance contained in one liter of one normal solution. Also called chemical equivalent; equivalent or combining weight.

  migraine e. See under migraine.

  nitrogen e. The nitrogen content of protein.

erbium A soft, malleable, silvery rare earth element; symbol Er, atomic number 68, atomic weight 167.27.

Erb's spastic paraplegia Syphilitic inflammation of the inner coat of the arteries supplying the spinal cord, causing degeneration of the pyramidal tracts.

erectile Able to be erected; relating to vascular tissue, as in the penis, which is capable of filling with blood and becoming somewhat rigid.

erection **1.** The state of erectile tissue when filled with blood. **2.** An erect penis.

erector Something which raises or makes erect; denoting specifically certain muscles that hold up or cause the erection of a body part.

erethism An exaggerated degree of irritability or excitability, either general or in any part of the body, accompanied by mental changes such as instability, memory loss, lack of attention, decrease in intellect, and shyness; may be associated with chronic poisoning.

erg A unit of energy equal to the force capable of moving a weight of one gram a distance of one centimeter.

ergastoplasm The basophilic component of the cytoplasm of certain cells that produce protein substances.

ergocalciferol See vitamin D.

ergodynamograph An instrument used to record the degree of muscular force and the amount of work accompanied by muscular contraction.

ergograph An instrument for recording the work capacity of a muscle.

ergometer Dynamometer.

ergonomics See biotechnology.

ergonomist One who applies his training in the health, behavioral and technologic sciences to the industrial environment for the purpose of reducing stress vectors which cause fatigue, careless workmanship and high labor turnover.

ergosterol A crystalline sterol present in plant and animal tissues, which, under ultraviolet irradiation, is converted to vitamin D_2; derived from ergot, yeast, and other fungi.

ergot **1.** Any fungus (genus *Claviceps*) that attacks cereal plants. **2.** The blackish mass that replaces the grain of rye infected with the fungus; it has vasoconstrictor and oxytocic properties and yields drugs of clinical usefulness.

ergotamine An alkaloid derived from ergot that stimulates smooth muscle, especially of the blood vessels and uterus.

ergotism Poisoning by ergot-infected grain such as rye or from excessive use of medicinal ergot; constriction of the arterioles leads to pain and necrosis of the extremities.

erg-second A unit of work or energy multiplied by time; equal to the amount of energy required to move a weight of one gram a distance of one centimeter in one second.

erogenous, erogenic Producing sexual desire.

erosion **1.** A gradual wearing away. **2.** In dentistry, the progressive loss of tooth substance by a

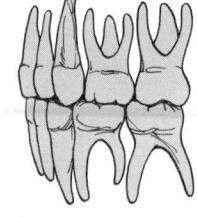

eruption of deciduous teeth

central incisors	6–8 months
lateral incisors	7–9 months
cuspids	16–18 months
first molars	12–14 months
second molars	20–24 months

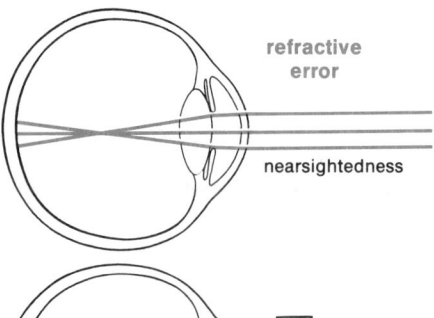

refractive error

nearsightedness

corrected by a lens

eruption of permanent teeth

central incisors	6–8 years
lateral incisors	7–9 years
cuspids	9–12 years
first bicuspids	10–12 years
second bicuspids	10–12 years
first molars	6–7 years
second molars	11–13 years
third molars	17–21 years

erythroblastic island   reticulocyte   red blood cell

maturation of red blood cell precursors

expelling nucleus

erythroblast (normoblast)

section of erythrocyte

erythrocytes

chemical process without the aid of bacteria, producing a hard, polished, smooth depression on the surface of the tooth.

erotic Relating to or tending to arouse sexual desire.

eroticism, erotism 1. Erotic character. **2.** A state of sexual excitement.

erotogenic Producing sexual excitement.

erratic 1. Denoting symptoms that do not follow a usual pattern. **2.** Unconventional.

error, refractive Defect in the refractive system of the eye that prevents light rays from being brought to a focus on the retina.

erubescence A flushing or reddening of the skin; a blush.

eructation The act of belching.

erupt To break or pierce through; said of a tooth.

eruption 1. The act of breaking out, as the appearance of lesions on the skin. **2.** Redness or blemishing of the skin or mucosa as a manifestation of disease. **3.** Cutting of a tooth; the passage of a tooth through the gum.

drug e. The eruption of a skin rash caused by a drug taken internally, generally the result of allergic sensitization.

erysipelas An acute contagious disease caused by *Streptococcus pyogenes*, marked by a circumscribed red eruption on the skin, chills, and fever.

erysipeloid Infection of the hands with the bacillus *Erysipelothrix rhysiopathiae*, marked by red lesions and occurring in persons handling infected fish or meat.

Erysipelothrix A genus of bacteria (family Corynebacteriaceae) containing gram-positive, rod-shaped organisms which have a tendency to form long filaments; parasitic on mammals, birds, and fish.

erysipelotoxin A toxin produced by *Streptococcus pyogenes*, species of bacteria causing erysipelas.

erythema Redness of the skin.

e. chronicum migrans Annular erythema beginning several weeks after the bite of a tick and spreading peripherally with a central clearing; the first lesion of Lyme disease.

e. infectiosum Mild viral infection, most commonly seen in school-aged children, marked by a lacelike skin rash; caused by human parvovirus B19.

e. marginatum A type of erythema multiforme in which the lesions have a disc shape with elevated edges.

e. multiforme An acute inflammatory skin disease, marked by the symmetrical eruption of macules, papules, or vesicles of various shapes presenting a multiform appearance; may be an allergic reaction; severe cases may have a fatal termination; in mild cases (Hebra's disease) the eruption usually recurs.

e. multiforme bullosum A blister-like eruption on the lips, tongue, and mucous membrane of the mouth.

e. multiforme exudativum A rare severe form of erythema multiforme characterized chiefly by eruptive, ulcerative lesions of the skin, oral mucosa, and eyes; frequently the genitalia, lungs, and joints are affected. Also called Stevens-Johnson syndrome.

e. nodosum A skin disease, probably a hypersensitivity reaction, characterized by bright red, painful nodules on the shins and frequently on the anterior thighs and extensor surfaces of the forearms.

e. venenata Erythema due to contact with some sensitizing substance.

toxic e. A diffuse eruption of the skin due to an allergic reaction to a toxic substance.

erythralgia A state of painful redness of the skin.

erythrasma A contagious skin disease caused by the bacterium *Corynebacterium minutissimum*; marked by an eruption of reddish brown patches in the armpits and groin which glow under Wood's light.

erythredema See acrodynia.

erythremia See polycythemia vera.

erythrityl tetranitrate A compound used in the treatment of angina pectoris.

erythroblast A young red blood cell in its immature, nucleated stage.

acidophilic e. See orthochromatic erythroblast.

basophilic e. The second stage in the development of the erythroblast, following the proerythroblast. Also called basophilic normoblast; prorubricyte; early erythroblast.

orthochromatic e. The last stage in the development of the erythroblast in which 80% of the hemoglobin is synthesized. Also called metarubricyte; orthochromatic normoblast; late erythroblast; acidophilic erythroblast.

polychromatophilic e. The third stage in the development of the erythroblast. Also called polychromatic normoblast; rubricyte.

erythroblastemia The presence of nucleated red blood cells (erythroblasts) in the peripheral blood; may be seen in a variety of pathologic conditions.

erythroblastopenia Deficiency in bone marrow of erythroblasts (red blood cells in an early stage of development).

erythroblastosis Excessive number of immature red blood cells (erythroblasts) in the blood.

e. fetalis Erythroblastosis of the fetus and newborn associated with Rh-factor incompatibility between mother and child; often accompanied by enlargement of the spleen and liver. Also called hemolytic disease of the newborn.

erythrochromia A red coloration.

erythroclasis Fragmentation of red blood cells.

erythrocuprein A copper-containing protein present in human red blood cells.

erythrocyanosis Swollen and reddish condition of the limbs upon exposure to cold, but not freezing, temperatures.

erythrocyte A mature red blood cell or corpuscle that transports oxygen to the tissue by means of the hemoglobin it contains; normally it is a yellowish, non-nucleated, biconcave disk, measuring approximately from 7.2 to 8.6 μ in diameter; the thickness at the center is slightly less than 1 μ and at the rim approximately 2 μ; in a normal human adult, 2,500,000 erythrocytes are formed every second; their life span is about 120 days.

crenated e. An erythrocyte possessing a scalloped border.

erythrocythemia Excessive number of red blood cells in the blood. Also called polycythemia.

erythrocytic Relating to a red blood cell.

erythrocytolysin A substance capable of causing dissolution of red blood cells.

erythrocytolysis See hemolysis.

erythrocytometer See hemocytometer.

erythrocytopenia See erythropenia.

erythrocytorrhexis The partial escape of protoplasm from red blood cells, causing changes in the shape of the cells. Also called plasmorrhexis.

erythrocytosis Excessive formation of red blood cells.

erythrocyturia Red blood cells in the urine.

erythroderma A nondescriptive term denoting abnormal redness of the skin, especially over large areas of the body.

erythrodontia Reddish discoloration of the teeth.

erythrogenesis imperfecta Congenital hypoplastic anemia; see under anemia.

erythrogenic 1. Causing a rash. **2.** Producing red blood cells.

erythrogenin An enzymatic factor (renal erythropoietic factor) produced by the kidney which converts a precursor, erythropoietinogen, in plasma to ESF (erythropoiesis-stimulating factor).

erythrogonium, *pl.* **erythrogonia** Denoting tissues from which red blood cells develop.

erythroid Reddish.

erythrokinetics The maintenance of a steady number of circulating red blood cells in the normal individual by the balance achieved between the amount removed from and the amount delivered to

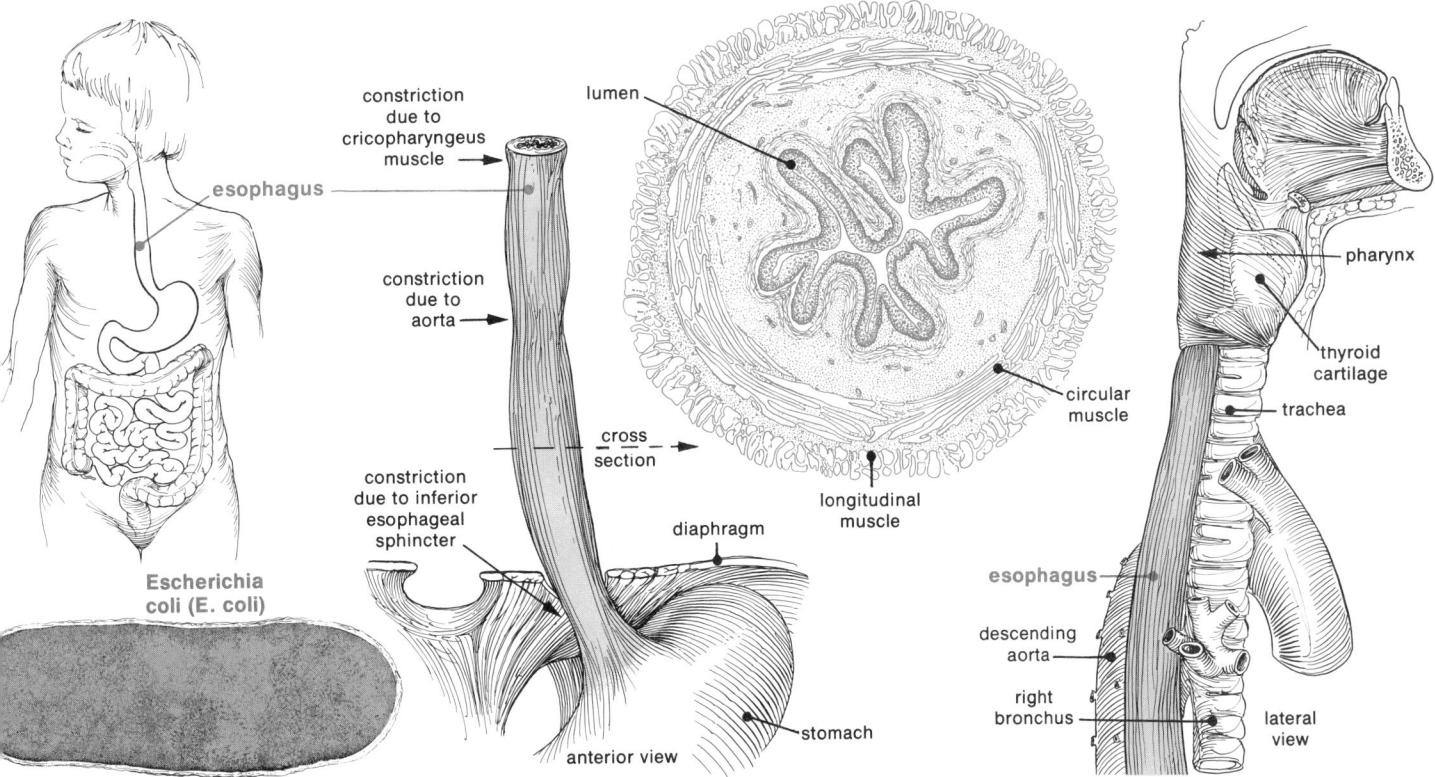

constriction due to cricopharyngeus muscle

esophagus

constriction due to aorta

constriction due to inferior esophageal sphincter

diaphragm

cross section

anterior view

stomach

lumen

circular muscle

longitudinal muscle

pharynx

thyroid cartilage

trachea

esophagus

descending aorta

right bronchus

lateral view

Escherichia coli (E. coli)

the peripheral blood per unit of time.

erythroleukemia Proliferation of immature red and white blood cells.

erythrolysin Hemolysin.

erythromelalgia A circulatory disorder causing a burning sensation of the hands and/or feet, sometimes involving the whole extremity and lasting minutes or hours. Also called erythermalgia.

erythromelia Diffuse atrophy of the skin.

erythromycin An antibiotic substance obtained from a strain of *Streptomyces erythreus*; Ilotycin®.

erythron The total mass of erythropoietic cells and circulating erythrocytes, viewed as a functional, though dispersed, organ.

erythroneocytosis Presence in the peripheral blood of regenerative forms of red blood cells.

erythropenia Deficiency of red blood cells. Also called erythrocytopenia.

erythrophagia Erythrophagocytosis.

erythrophagocytosis The ingestion and digestion of red blood cells by other cells, such as monocytes and polymorphonuclear leukocytes.

erythropia, erythropsia Red vision, the subjective sensation that all objects are covered with a red tint.

erythropoiesis The formation of red blood cells.

erythropoietic Relating to the origin of red blood cells.

erythropoietin Erythropoiesis-stimulating factor (ESF); a hormone produced principally in the kidney which stimulates red blood cell production. Also called erythropoietic factor; hematopoietin.

erythroprosopalgia Burning pain and redness of the face, believed to indicate organic disease of the nervous system.

erythropyknosis Degeneration of red blood cells; which become dark and shrunken (brassy bodies); occurs in malaria.

erythrorrhexis Fragmentation of red blood cells.

erythruria Passing of urine of a red color.

escape The assumption of pacemaker activities by a lower pacemaker when a higher pacemaker defaults or atrioventricular (A-V) conduction fails.

  nodal e. Escape with the A-V node as pacemaker.

  ventricular e. Escape with an ectopic ventricular focus as pacemaker.

eschar A scab or slough.

escharotic Caustic.

Escherichia A genus of bacteria (family Enterobacteriaceae) containing short, gram-negative rods; the motile species are covered with flagella; they ferment glucose and lactose with acid and gas formation, are present in feces, and may cause disease in man.

  E. aurescens A species found in contaminated water supplies and human feces.

  E. coli A motile species normally present in the intestines of humans. Formerly called *Bacillus coli*.

escutcheon A shield-shaped surface, as the pattern of distribution of the pubic hair.

eserine See physostigmine.

  e. salicylate See physostigmine salicylate.

esocataphoria Tendency of the eyes to turn down and in; a combination of esophoria and cataphoria.

esodeviation The inward deviation of one or both eyes in convergent strabismus or in esophoria.

esodic Denoting sensory nerves that conduct impulses toward the brain or spinal cord.

esophagalgia Pain in the esophagus. Also called esophagodynia.

esophageal Of or relating to the esophagus.

esophagectasia, esophagectasis Abnormal dilatation of the esophagus.

esophagectomy Surgical removal of a portion of the esophagus.

esophagitis Inflammation of the esophagus.

  peptic e. See reflux esophagitis.

  reflux e. Diffuse inflammation of the distal esophagus caused by reflux of gastric or duodenal contents through an incompetent lower esophageal sphincter; frequently associated with a hiatal hernia or a duodenal ulcer. Also called peptic esophagitis.

esophagocardioplasty A reparative operation on the esophagus and the cardiac area of the stomach.

esophagocele Protrusion of the mucous membrane of the esophagus through a defect in its muscular layer.

esophagodynia See esophagalgia.

esophagoenterostomy Surgical connection of the esophagus and intestine after excision of the stomach.

esophagogastrectomy Surgical removal of a portion of the lower esophagus and proximal stomach, usually performed for eradicating neoplasms.

esophagogastrostomy The surgical formation of an artificial opening between the esophagus and the stomach.

esophagojejunostomy Surgical union between the esophagus and jejunum.

esophagomalacia Softening of the walls of the esophagus.

esophagomyotomy Incision through the wall of the esophagus.

  Heller e. A longitudinal extramucosal incision on the esophagus, at the level of its junction with the stomach.

esophagoplasty Surgical repair of a defect of the esophagus.

esophagoplication Surgical reduction of a pouch or dilatation in the esophagus by making longitudinal folds on its walls.

esophagoscope An instrument for inspecting the interior of the esophagus.

esophagoscopy Examination of the interior of the esophagus with an esophagoscope.

esophagostenosis Stricture or narrowing of the esophagus.

esophagostomy The surgical formation of an artificial opening into the esophagus.

esophagotomy Incision through the esophagus.

esophagram A roentgenogram of the esophagus.

esophagus The musculomembranous tube extending downward from the pharynx to the cardia of the stomach, a distance of about 25 cm.

esophoria Condition in which the eyes have a tendency to turn inward, manifested when fusion is prevented by covering one eye.

esophoric Relating to esophoria or the tendency of the eyes to deviate inward.

esotropia Convergent strabismus; see under strabismus.

esotropic Relating to convergent strabismus or the inward turning of one eye.

essence 1. The intrinsic properties or qualities of a thing. 2. The fluid extract of a substance that retains its fundamental properties, such as the alcoholic solution of a volatile oil.

essential 1. Necessary. 2. Having no apparent external cause; said of a disease.

ester Any of a group of organic compounds formed by the condensation of an alcohol and carboxylic acid.

esterase Any enzyme that promotes the hydrolysis of an ester.

esthesia The perception of sense impressions.

esthesiogenesis The origin or production of a reaction in a sensory zone.

esthesiography 1. Delineating on the skin the areas of tactile and other forms of sensibility. 2. A description of the mechanism of sensation.

estival, aestival Occurring in the summer.

estivoautumnal Occurring in summer and autumn.

estradiol An estrogenic hormone obtained commercially from the urine of pregnant mares, hog ovaries, and estrone. Also called dihydroxytheelin; dihydroxyestrin.

estriol A white, odorless, estrogenic hormone present in the urine of pregnant mammals. Also called theelol; folliculin hydrate.

estrogens

estrone

estriol

estradiol

ethacrynic acid

ethchlorvynol (tertiary alcohol)

estrus — cycle diagram: proestrus, estrus, metestrus, diestrus

lymphocyte, heterochromatin, euchromatin

eversion of upper eyelid

Walker double evertor

---

estrogen General term for the female sex hormones, responsible for stimulating the development and maintenance of female secondary sex characteristics; formed in the ovary, placenta, testis, adrenal cortex, and some plants; therapeutic uses (with natural or synthetic preparations) include the relief of menopausal symptoms and amelioration of cancer of the prostate gland.

estrone An estrogenic hormone found in the ovary and in the urine of pregnant mammals.

estrus 1. The recurrent period of sexual excitement in the female of animals. Also called heat. 2. In mammals, the cycle of changes in the genital tract produced by ovarian hormones.

ethacrynic acid An unsaturated ketone derivative of aryloxyacetic acid, a potent diuretic; Edecrin®.

ethanol See alcohol (2).

ethchlorvynol A hypnotic and anticonvulsant drug, generally used for inducing sleep in simple insomnia and as a daytime sedative; Placidyl®.

ether 1. Any of a group of organic compounds in which two hydrocarbon groups are linked by an oxygen atom. 2. Term used for the anesthetic diethyl ether.

  diethyl e. An inflammable, volatile liquid, $C_4H_{10}O$, obtained from the distillation of ethyl alcohol and sulfuric acid; used as an anesthetic. Also called ethyl ether.

  ethyl e. See diethyl ether.

  hydrochloric e. See ethyl chloride.

ethereal 1. Relating to, containing, or resembling ether. 2. Evanescent.

etherification The conversion of an alcohol into ether.

etherify To convert into ether.

etherize To produce anesthesia with ether.

ethical 1. Relating to ethics. 2. Being in accord with professionally accepted codes.

ethics Standards of behavior governing an individual or a profession.

ethmoid Resembling a sieve.

ethmoidectomy Surgical removal of the ethmoid cells or of part of the ethmoid bone.

ethmoiditis Inflammation of the ethmoid sinus.

ethmosphenoid Relating to both the ethmoid and sphenoid bones.

ethnopsychiatry The study of varied cultural patterns and their influence on emotional maturation.

ethyl The univalent hydrocarbon radical C_2H_5-.

  e. alcohol See alcohol (2).

  e. chloride A gas at ordinary temperatures, a volatile liquid when compressed; used to produce local anesthesia by superficial freezing. Also called

chloroethane; hydrochloric ether.

ethylcellulose An ethyl ether of cellulose, used as a tablet binder; Ethocel ®.

ethylene A colorless, flammable gas, Ch_2CH_2, somewhat lighter than air; used for inducing general anesthesia. Also called ethene.

  e. dibromide (EDB) Chemical widely used as a fumigant of fruits, soil and grain; identified as a carcinogen.

ethylenediaminetetraacetic acid (EDTA) A heavy-metal antagonist (chelating agent) which forms complexes (chelates) with divalent and trivalent metals; used in the treatment of lead poisoning.

etiocholanolone A metabolite of adrenocortical and testicular hormones excreted in the urine.

etiologic Relating to the causes of disease.

etiology The study of causes, specifically the cause of a disease.

Eubacterium A genus of anaerobic bacteria (family Propionibacteriaceae) containing gram-positive rods; some species may be pathogenic.

eubiotics The science of hygienic living.

eucaryote See eukaryote.

eucholia The normal state of the bile.

euchromatin The lightly stained portion of the cell nucleus containing genetically active DNA. Also called true chromatin.

eugenics The branch of science concerned with the study of the hereditary improvement of man by genetic control.

eugenol Eugenic acid, a light yellow oily liquid obtained from oil of cloves; used in dentistry as an antiseptic and local anesthetic.

euglobulin A simple protein insoluble in pure water, but soluble in saline solutions.

euglycemia Normal level of sugar in the blood.

eugonic Growing rapidly on an artificial medium; applied to cultures of the human tubercle bacillus.

eukaryosis The state of having a true nucleus, as in the higher types of cells.

eukaryote An organism with cells that have nuclear membranes, membrane-bound organelles, and ribosomes and that exhibit mitosis. Also written eucaryote.

eunuch A castrated male, or one whose testes have never developed.

eunuchoid Having the characteristics of a eunuch.

eunuchoidism Condition in which the testes fail to function.

euosmia 1. A pleasant odor. 2. A normal state of the sense of smell.

eupepsia Good digestion.

euphoria 1. A feeling of well-being. 2. In psychiatry, an exaggerated feeling of happiness.

euplasia The normal state of cells or tissues.

euplastic Able to heal readily.

euploidy In genetics, the condition of having the normal full complement of chromosomes; i.e., the chromosome number of a cell is an exact multiple of the haploid number normal for the species from which it originated.

eupnea Normal, easy breathing.

europium A rare earth element; symbol Eu, atomic number 63, atomic weight 151.96.

eustachitis Inflammation of the mucous membrane of the auditory (eustachian) tube.

euthanasia 1. The act of inducing a painless, easy death, as in persons with a painful terminal illness. 2. Painless death.

euthyroidism A normal condition of the thyroid gland.

eutrophia A state of normal nourishment and development.

evacuant 1. Promoting a bowel movement. 2. An agent having such an effect.

evacuate 1. To empty the bowels. 2. To create a vacuum or very low pressure by removing air or any gas from a closed vessel.

evacuation 1. Emptying of the bowels. 2. The waste material discharged from the bowels. 3. The creation of a vacuum.

evagination Protrusion of a part or organ.

evanescent Of short life or duration.

Evans blue A diazo dye injected intravenously to determine blood or plasma volume by the method of dilution (the dye adheres to plasma proteins).

evaporation The change of a liquid into a vapor.

eventration 1. Protrusion of the intestines through an opening in the abdominal wall. 2. Removal of the abdominal organs.

eversion Turning outward, as of a foot, or inside out, as of an eyelid.

evert To turn outward.

evisceration Removal of internal organs.

  e. of the eye Surgical removal of the contents of the eyeball, leaving the sclera intact.

  e. of the orbit Removal of all the contents of the orbit. Also called exenteration.

evolution A continuous and gradual process of change from one state or form to another.

evulsion A pulling out or forcible extraction.

Ewart's sign In large pericardial effusions, bronchial breathing and an area of dullness at the lower angle of the left scapula.

exacerbation Increase in the severity of a disease or any of its symptoms.

examination Any inspection or investigation for the purpose of diagnosis.

  cytologic e. The microscopic examination of cells for the detection of cancer or for the evaluation

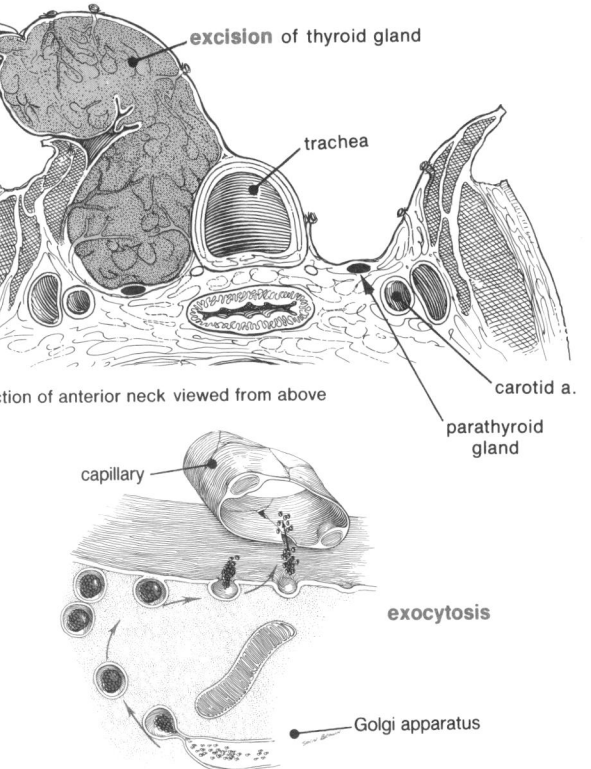

excision of thyroid gland

trachea

section of anterior neck viewed from above

carotid a.

parathyroid gland

capillary

exocytosis

Golgi apparatus

exotoxins produced by some bacteria pathogenic to man

TOXIN	DISEASE	SPECIES	ACTION
tetanospasmin	tetanus	*Clostridium tetani*	spastic hemolytic cardiotoxin
diphtheritic toxin	diphtheria	*Corynebacterium diphtheriae*	necrotizing
α-toxin	pyogenic infection	*Staphylococcus aureus*	necrotizing, hemolytic, leukocidic
whooping cough toxin	whooping cough	*Bordetella pertussis*	necrotizing
neurotoxin	dysentery	*Shigella dysenteriae*	hemorrhagic paralytic
neurotoxin	botulism	*Clostridium botulinum*	paralytic

of hormonal effect; the cells may be obtained by collecting a bodily secretion, such as sputum, urine or vaginal fluid, by scraping a tissue, such as the cervix, or by needle aspiration. Also called Papanicolaou examination.

Papanicolaou e. See cytologic examination.

postmortem e. See autopsy.

examiner, medical 1. A physician whose function is to ascertain the causes of death of those who die suddenly or as a result of violence. **2.** A physician who examines and reports on the physical condition of applicants for life insurance.

exanthem, exanthema 1. Any disease accompanied by a skin eruption. **2.** A skin eruption.

e. subitum An acute febrile disease occurring within the first 3 years of life, most commonly between 6 and 18 months; after 2 to 4 days of fever, the temperature falls and a macular or maculopapular rash appears; caused by human herpesvirus 6 (HH6). Also called roseola infantum.

exanthematous Relating to any disease accompanied by a rash.

excavation 1. A natural bodily cavity or recess. **2.** A cavity resulting from a pathologic process.

atrophic e. An exaggerated depression of the optic disk caused by atrophy of the optic nerve.

glaucomatous e. Glaucomatous cup; see under cup.

physiologic e. Physiologic cup; see under cup.

excavator 1. A spoonlike instrument used to scrape out pathologic tissue. **2.** A dental instrument used to remove carious material from a cavity.

excipient A more or less inert substance used as a diluent or vehicle for a drug.

excise To remove surgically.

excision The surgical removal of a part or organ.

excitability The state of being capable of quick response to a stimulus; the property of muscle tissue by virtue of which it reacts to stimulation by propagation of the impulse.

excitation 1. Stimulation. **2.** In physics, the increase of energy.

excitement The state of being agitated.

excitoglandular Increasing the activity of a gland.

excoriate To scratch or abrade the skin.

excoriation A scratch mark.

neurotic e. Self-inflicted skin lesions by emotionally disturbed persons, usually by the forcible use of fingernails.

excrement Feces.

excrescence Any abnormal outgrowth from the surface.

excreta Discharged natural wastes; excreted material, such as sweat, urine, etc.

excrete To eliminate waste material from the body.

excreter An individual who is a carrier of disease-causing microorganism and who excretes them in the urine or feces.

excretion 1. Process by which the waste products of metabolism or undigested food residues are eliminated from the body. **2.** The product of such a process.

excretory Relating to or used during excretion.

excursion An oscillating or alternating motion from an axis or a mean position.

exenteration Surgical removal of all the contents of a body cavity. See also evisceration.

exercise Physical activity performed to develop or maintain fitness; it may require bodily exertion (active exercise) or effortless motion (passive exercise).

Kegel's e. Repetitive contraction and relaxation of pelvic floor muscles for treatment of urinary stress incontinence.

exergonic Indicating a chemical reaction that is accompanied by a release of free energy, regardless of the form of energy involved.

exflagellation The development of microgametes (male gametes) from microgametocytes (mother cells), as in malaria.

exfoliation 1. The shedding, peeling, or scaling of skin. Also called desquamation. **2.** In dentistry, the casting off of deciduous teeth.

exhalation 1. The act of breathing out. **2.** Exhaled gas or vapor.

exhale 1. To breathe out. **2.** To emit a gas, vapor, etc.

exhaustion 1. Extreme fatigue. **2.** Removal of contents. **3.** Removal of the active ingredients of a drug.

heat e. Condition marked by prostration and weakness caused by prolonged exposure to hot temperatures.

nervous e. Obsolete term for functional neurosis (neurasthenia) or for a mental disorder.

exhibitionism A morbid compulsion to expose the genitalia.

exhumation The process of taking a body out of a place of burial.

exocataphoria A tendency of the eyes to deviate outward and downward.

exocrine 1. A gland that discharges its secretion through a duct. **2.** The secretion of such a gland.

exocytosis Ejection of material from a cell; e.g., ejection of insulin from the beta cells of the pancreas: the membranous sac containing insulin granules migrates to the periphery of the cell; when the sac contacts the cell's plasma membrane, the two fuse;

rupture occurs at the site of fusion and insulin passes out of the cell and into the blood stream via the extracellular space. Also called emiocytosis.

exodeviation The outward deviation of one or both eyes in divergent strabismus or in exophoria.

exodic Denoting nerves that convey impulses toward the periphery.

exodontics The branch of dentistry concerned with the extraction of teeth.

exoenzyme Any enzyme that performs its functions outside of the cell in which it originates, as a digestive enzyme.

exogenous Originating outside the body.

exomphalos See omphalocele.

exonuclease A nuclease (enzyme) that digests or cleaves DNA from the ends of strands (polynucleotide chains).

exopathy Any disease originating from causes outside the body.

exophoria Condition in which an eye has a tendency to turn outward, manifested when fusion is prevented by covering the eye.

exophthalmic Relating to or afflicted with exophthalmos.

exophthalmometer An instrument used to measure the degree of protrusion of the eyeball. Also called proptometer.

exophthalmos Abnormal protrusion of the eyeball.

malignant e. Severe, usually bilateral, protrusion of the eyeballs; occurring mostly in middle age; it may be unresponsive to treatment and can lead to blindness.

exoskeleton 1. The external, supportive covering of certain invertebrates. **2.** Structures, such as hair, nails, feathers, scales, etc., developed from the ectoderm or mesoderm in vertebrates. Also called dermatoskeleton; dermoskeleton.

exosmosis Diffusion from within outward, as from a blood vessel.

exospore A spore produced by budding, as a fungal spore.

exosporium The outer covering of a spore.

exostosis, *pl.* **exostoses** A bony growth on the surface of a bone.

multiple hereditary e. The presence of multiple exostoses in the long bones of children due to a hereditary defect of ossification in cartilage, resulting in severe skeletal deformity and stunting of growth. Also called diaphyseal aclasis.

exoteric Belonging to factors outside the organism.

exothermic, exothermal 1. Releasing heat, as certain chemical reactions. **2.** Relating to the external warmth of the body.

exotoxin A toxin produced and released by bac-

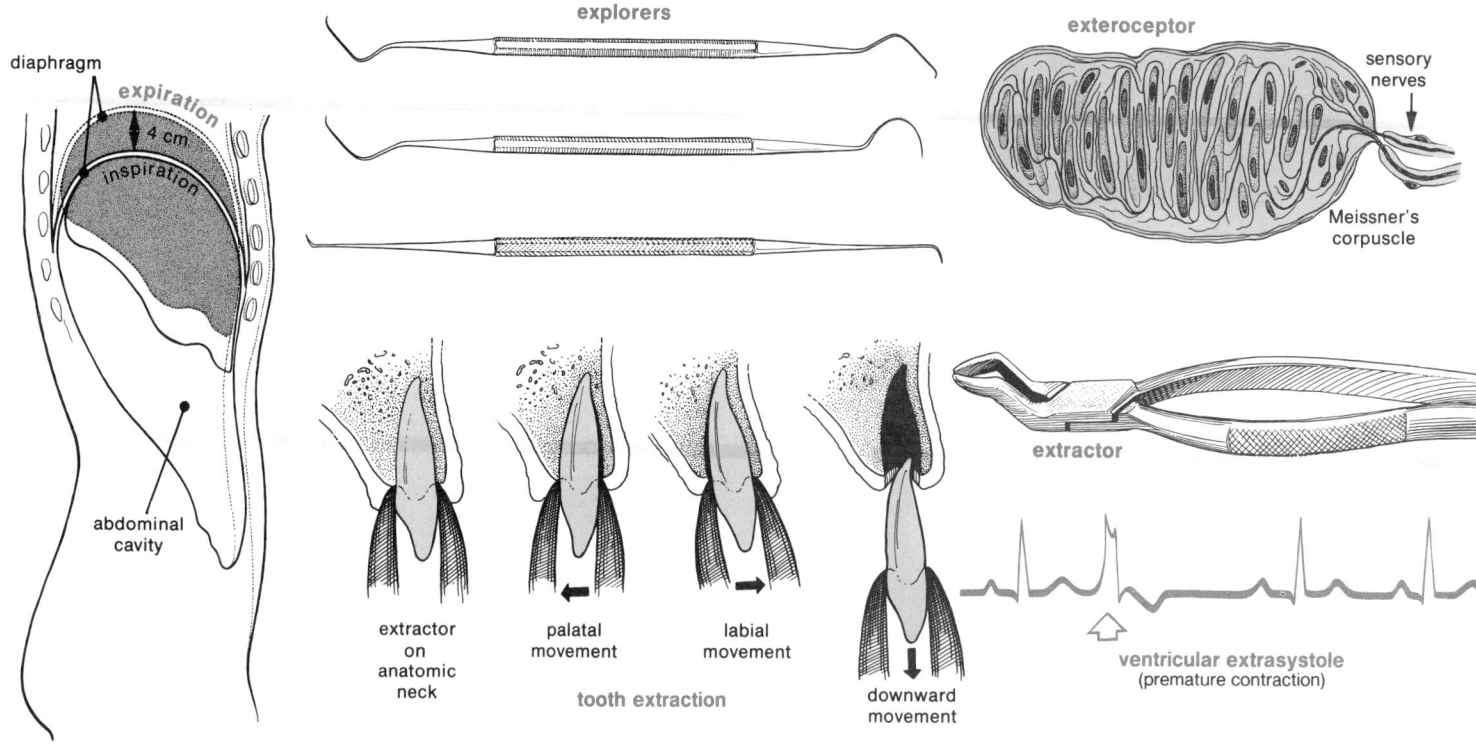

diaphragm

expiration

4 cm

inspiration

abdominal cavity

explorers

exteroceptor

sensory nerves

Meissner's corpuscle

extractor on anatomic neck

palatal movement

labial movement

tooth extraction

downward movement

extractor

ventricular extrasystole
(premature contraction)

terial cells as a normal physiologic process. Also called extracellular toxin.

exotropia Divergent strabismus; see under strabismus.

expansiveness An exaggerated sense of importance.

expectorant 1. Promoting the expulsion of mucus or other material from the air passages. 2. A medicine so acting.

expectoration Mucus or other secretions coughed up from the air passages. Also called sputum.

experiment A test.

 control e. Experiment to check the results of other experiments by keeping the same conditions except for one particular factor.

 double blind e. One in which the control is unknown to the experimenter and the subjects.

expiration 1. The act of breathing out. 2. The act of dying.

expiratory Relating to expiration.

expire 1. To exhale; to breathe out. 2. To die.

explant In tissue culture, to transfer living tissue from the body to another medium.

exploration A surgical, digital, or instrumental examination of tissue as an aid in diagnosis; a diagnostic search or investigation.

explorer A sharp, curved dental probe used to examine teeth.

explosion 1. A sudden, rapid, violent discharge of force from a confined area. 2. A sudden outbreak, as an epidemic or population explosion.

exponent 1. A number or symbol written as a superscript, denoting the number of times a factor is to be involved in a repeated multiplication. 2. One who defines or advocates.

express To squeeze out.

expressivity Strength of the manifestation of a genetic trait in terms of its deviation from the normal.

exsanguinate To drain blood; to make bloodless.

exsiccant 1. Drying; dehydrating; absorbing. 2. A dusting or drying powder.

exsiccate To dry; to remove moisture.

exsiccation The process of removing moisture.

exstrophy Congenital turning inside out of an organ.

 e. of the bladder Malformation in which the interior of the posterior wall of the bladder becomes visible through an opening in the abdominal wall and the anterior bladder wall.

exsufflation Forcible expiration; forced expulsion of the breath by a mechanical apparatus.

extension The act of straightening a limb or the condition of being straightened.

extensor A muscle that, by contracting, straightens a limb.

exteriorize 1. To expose an organ (temporarily or permanently) as a form of therapy or for the purpose of physiologic experimentation. 2. In psychiatry, to direct a patient's interests toward others rather than himself.

extern A nonresident medical student or recent graduate who assists in the care of hospitalized patients.

external Situated on the outside; on the surface.

exteroceptor A sensory nerve ending in the skin or mucous membrane which is affected primarily by the external environment; e.g., Meissner's corpuscle for touch, Krause's end bulb for cold, Ruffini's corpuscle for warmth, Golgi-Mazzoni corpuscle for pressure, and free nerve endings for pain.

extima See adventitia.

extinction 1. In physiology, relating to the point at which a nerve, after responding to a stimulus, becomes completely inexcitable. 2. In psychology, the process by which a stimulus-response bond is broken.

extirpation Complete removal of a part or of a pathologic growth.

extoplasm The outer condensation of the cytoplasm of a cell.

extorsion The act of rotating outward.

extra-articular Outside of a joint.

extracapsular Located or occurring outside of a capsule, as a fracture occurring outside a joint capsule.

extracellular Occurring outside a cell.

extracorpuscular Outside of the blood corpuscles.

extracranial Outside of the skull.

extraction 1. The act of drawing out or removing. 2. The process of preparing an extract.

 breech e. The manual removal of an infant in breech presentation from the uterus.

 tooth e. Removal of a tooth.

extractor An instrument used in drawing out a bodily part; especially forceps for extracting teeth.

extradural Located outside of the dura mater.

extrahepatic Located outside of the liver.

extramedullary Located outside of any medulla.

extraneous Originating outside of the organism, or not belonging to it.

extraocular External to the eye.

extraperitoneal Located outside of the peritoneal cavity.

extrapolate To estimate a value or values beyond the observable range from a known trend of variables; broadly, to estimate or infer from known values.

extrapulmonary Located outside of the lungs.

extrapyramidal Outside of pyramidal tracts; said of descending nerve tracts that are not part of the pyramids of the medulla.

extrapyramidal disease Any disease affecting the extrapyramidal areas of the brain.

extrasensory Not perceptible by the senses, as some forms of perception such as telepathy or clairvoyance. Also called supernatural.

extrasystole A premature contraction of the heart originating at a site other than the usual (ectopic); it may arise from the atrium, the atrioventricular (A-V) node, or the ventricle; the term is loosely applied to all premature contractions, but more correctly limited to interpolated premature contractions.

 atrial e. One due to an irritability of the atria; the early contractions emanate from an impulse in the atria outside of the sinoatrial (S-A) node.

 atrioventricular nodal e. Extrasystole emanating from the atrioventricular (A-V) node and leading to a simultaneous or near simultaneous contraction of atria and ventricles. Also called nodal or A-V nodal extrasystole.

 A-V nodal e. See atrioventricular nodal extrasystole.

 interpolated e. A ventricular extrasystole which, instead of being followed by a compensatory pause, is sandwiched between two consecutive sinus cycles.

 nodal e. See atrioventricular nodal extrasystole.

 supraventricular e. An extrasystole emanating from a center above the ventricles, i.e., atrium or atrioventricular (A-V) node.

 ventricular e. A premature contraction of the ventricles.

extrauterine Located outside of the uterus.

extravasate 1. To escape from a vessel into the tissues. 2. The material that has escaped.

extravasation Escape of fluid from a vessel into the surrounding tissues.

extravascular Outside of the blood vessels or lymphatics.

extraversion See extroversion.

extravert See extrovert.

extremity A limb; an arm or a leg.

extrinsic Originating outside of a part where it is found or on which it acts.

extroversion, extraversion 1. A turning inside out, as of the uterus. 2. A personality trait in which a person's interests lie mainly in the environment and others rather than in himself.

extrovert, extravert A person whose interests lie outside of himself, or who is outwardly directed.

extrude 1. To push out, or reposition distally. 2. In dentistry, to move a tooth into a more occlusal

eye

eyebrow

upper
palpebral
furrow

lateral
canthus

sclera

iris

pupil

lower eyelid

horizontal section
of eyeball
viewed from above

eyeground
(left eye)

vein

artery

upper eyelid:

orbital section

tarsal section

caruncle

medial canthus

eyeball

optic nerve

vitreous chamber

fovea

sclera

choroid

retina

macula

optic
disk

iris

cornea

anterior
chamber

lens

eyelid

tarsal
gland

eyelashes

eyepiece

objective

condenser

light source

position with the teeth of the opposing jaw.

extrusion The process of forcing out of a normal position.

extubation The removal of a tube, specifically, the removal of an intubation tube from the larynx.

exuberant Denoting excessive growth, as of tissue or granulation.

exudate Material gradually discharged and deposited in the tissues or a cavity, usually as a result of inflammation.

exudation The oozing of fluids through the tissues into a cavity or to the surface, usually as a result of inflammation.

exudative Relating to the process of exudation.

exude To ooze; to pass out gradually through the tissues or through an opening.

eye The organ of vision; in humans, it is a nearly spherical body consisting of three concentric coats; the outermost, fibrous, protective coat, made up of

an opaque, white, posterior portion (five-sixths) called the sclera and an anterior transparent part called the cornea; the middle, vascular, nutritive coat, made up (from behind forward) of choroid, ciliary body, and iris; and the innermost, nervous coat called the retina; within, it contains the anterior and posterior chambers, filled with a clear fluid (aqueous humor), the crystalline lens, and the gelatinous vitreous body.

    fixating e. In strabismus, the eye that is directed toward the object of regard.

    pink e. See pinkeye.

    shipyard e. Epidemic keratoconjunctivitis; see under keratoconjunctivitis.

    white of the e. The visible portion of the sclera.

eyeball The globe of the eye.

eyebrow 1. The row of hairs growing between the upper eyelid and the forehead. **2.** The bony ridge over the eye. Also called supercilium.

eyeglasses A pair of ophthalmic lenses mounted on a frame, used as an aid to vision. Also called spectacles; glasses.

eyeground The inner surface of the eye seen through the pupil on ophthalmoscopic examination.

eyelash One of the short hairs growing on the margin of the eyelid. Also called cilium.

eyelid One of two folds (upper and lower) that cover and protect the anterior portion of the eyeball.

eyepiece The lens or system of lenses closest to the eye in an optical instrument such as a microscope, that further magnifies the image formed by the objective lens. Also called ocular lens.

eyestrain Fatigue or discomfort associated with the use of the eyes, due to uncorrected errors of refraction, imbalance of the eye muscles, or prolonged use of the eyes.

eyewash The medicated irrigating solution used in bathing the eyes.

moon face

condylar rods

bite-bow fork

facing

face-bow

jack-screw

first cervical vertebra

articular facets

Ff

fabella Latin meaning little bean; in anatomy, the small sesamoid bone sometimes found in the tendon of the lateral head of the gastrocnemius muscle.

fabrication The feigning of symptoms or illness; the telling of deliberately false statements as if they were true. Also called confabulation.

face The front of the head from the forehead to the chin and from ear to ear.

　hippocratic f. Hippocratic facies; see under facies.

　masklike f. Parkinson's facies; see under facies.

　moon f. The rounded face observed in individuals with Cushing's disease or in hyperadrenocorticalism.

face-bow Instrument used to record the relationship of the jaws to the temporomandibular joint.

facelift See rhytidoplasty.

facet An extremely smooth surface on a bone.

　articular f. A small planar or rounded smooth surface on a bone which articules with another structure.

　costal f. See demifacet.

facetectomy Surgical removal of the facet of a vertebra.

facial 1. Of or relating to the face. 2. The application of cosmetic creams in conjunction with gentle massage of the face.

facies, *pl.* **facies** The outward appearance and expression of the face.

　adenoid f. The open-mouthed expression of children with adenoid growths.

　hippocratic f., f. hippocratica A pinched expression of the face with sunken eyes, hollow cheeks and temples, relaxed lips, and leaden complexion, observed in one dying after an exhausting illness.

　Parkinson's f. Lack of facial expression due to paralysis agitans.

facilitation Reinforcement of the activity of nervous tissue by the introduction of external impulses; an important protective reflex of the spinal cord; e.g., the reflex withdrawal from pain.

facing Plastic or porcelain material used to cover the labial or buccal surface of a dental crown.

faciobrachial Relating to the face and the arms.

faciocervical Relating to the face and neck.

facioplegia Facial palsy; see under palsy.

factitious Artificial; self-induced.

factor (F) 1. An agent or element that contributes to an action, process, or result. 2. A gene. 3. An essential element in a diet, such as a vitamin.

　ABO f.'s See ABO blood group.

　angiogenesis f. Substance, secreted by macrophages, that stimulates growth of new blood vessels; e.g., in cancers and in healing wounds.

　antiberiberi f. Thiamine.

　antihemophilic f. A See factor VIII.

　antihemophilic f. B See factor IX.

　antiheparin f. A glycoprotein released from platelets, following platelet aggregation, which shortens the thrombin clotting time in the presence of heparin. Also called platelet factor 4.

　antinuclear f. (ANF) Antinuclear antibody; see under antibody.

　atrial natriuretic f. (ANF) A peptide (molecular weight 3000-4000 daltons) isolated from the atria of several animal species, including man; when injected, it causes increased excretion of sodium by the kidney; also has vasodilator properties. Also called atriopeptin; auriculin A; cardioinatrin I.

　branching f. An enzyme (transglycosylase) in muscle that cleaves α-1,4 linkages in glycogen or starch, transferring the fragments into α-1,6 linkages and creating branches in the polysaccharide molecules. Also called α-glucan-branching glycosyltransferase; Q or branching enzyme.

　chemotactic f.'s Soluble substances produced by the reaction of antigen with sensitized leukocytes; they induce migration of neutrophils and monocytes from blood vessels into tissues to ingest and destroy potentially dangerous agents, such as bacteria.

　Christmas f. See factor IX.

　citrovorum f. See folinic acid.

　clotting f.'s Various plasma and tissue components involved in the clotting process.

　coronary risk f. Any of several factors that make the likelihood of suffering a coronary occlusion greater than average, including high blood pressure, diabetes mellitus, elevated blood lipids, smoking, and heredity.

　corticotropin-releasing f. (CRF) See corticotropin-releasing hormone, under hormone.

　coupling f.'s Proteins that restore phosphorylating ability to mitochondria that have lost it or have become uncoupled.

　epidermal growth f. Protein substance isolated from submaxillary glands of male mice that, when injected into newborn mice, causes rapid eyelid opening, eruption of teeth, and epidermal growth. Large doses may inhibit these processes.

　extrinsic f. See vitamin B₁₂.

　f. I A protein, present in dissolved form in blood plasma; an important factor in the third stage of blood coagulation during which it is converted to fibrin. Also called fibrinogen.

　f. II A stable glycoprotein of plasma that is important in the second stage of blood coagulation where it is converted to thrombin. Also called prothrombin.

　f. III A lipoprotein complex liberated from injured tissue. Also called thromboplastin.

　f. IV Calcium ions, the presence of which is necessary for many steps of the blood coagulation process.

　f. V A plasma globulin which acts as an accelerator by speeding the conversion of prothrombin to thrombin in the presence of activated factor X; a congenital deficiency of factor V causes parahemophilia. Also known as labile factor; proaccelerin.

　f. VI No longer considered a coagulation factor; formerly applied to serum accelerator globulin, which is activated factor V.

　f. VII A substance that acts as an accelerator in the extrinsic pathway of prothrombin activation; it is not consumed during the clotting of blood and is consequently found in the serum following normal clotting; congenital or neonatal deficiency of factor VII occurs along with hypoprothrombinemia in hemorrhagic disease of the newborn; it is manifested by purpura and bleeding from the mucous membranes. Also called proconvertin; convertin; serum prothrombin conversion accelerator (SPCA); stable factor.

　f. VIII The antihemophilic globulin present in plasma, essential in the first phase of clotting; a deficiency of factor VIII causes the hereditary disease, hemophilia A; transmitted by females as a sex-linked characteristic but causes hemorrhagic difficulties almost exclusively in males. Also called antihemophilic globulin; antihemophilic factor A; antihemolytic factor.

　f. IX A factor essential in the first phase of clotting; a deficiency of factor IX is inherited as a sex-linked recessive trait causing hemophilia B or Christmas disease (after surname of a child in whom this deficiency was first found). Also called Christmas factor; plasma thromboplastin component (PTC); antihemophilic factor B.

　f. X A procoagulant in normal plasma; a factor required for prothrombin conversion in the presence or absence of tissue extract; a deficiency of factor X may be congenital, but it also occurs in hemorrhagic disease of the newborn, liver disease, and deficiency of vitamin K. Also called Stuart-Prower factor.

　f. XI A factor essential in the first phase of clotting; a deficiency of factor XI is most commonly congenital and produces symptoms of mild hemophilia (hemophilia C). Also called plasma thromboplastin antecedent (PTA).

　f. XII A stable factor present in normal blood and serum which initiates the process of blood coagulation when the plasma contacts collagen or a foreign surface; it may be bypassed when absent so that hemostasis occurs normally despite a prolonged coagulation time; deficiency of factor XII is caused by an autosomal recessive gene. Also called Hageman

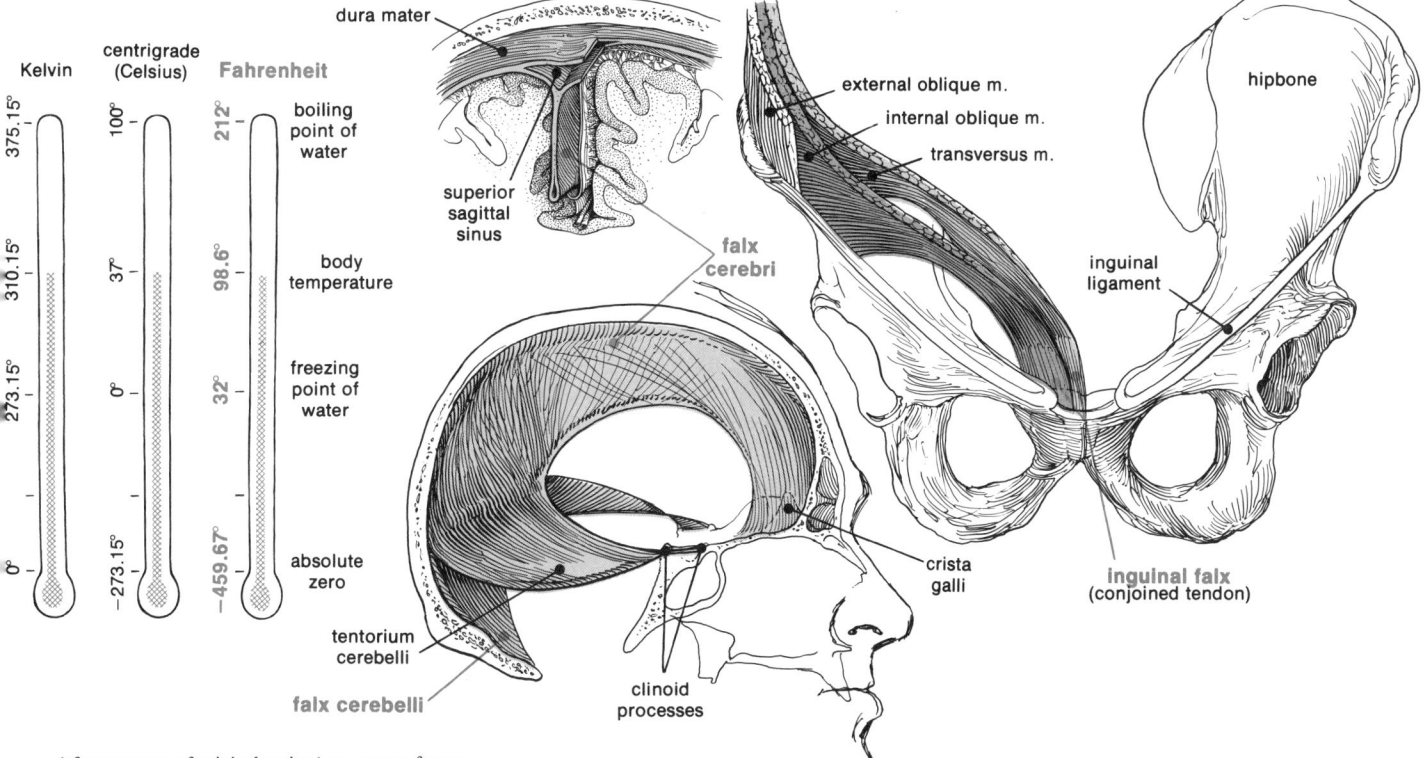

Kelvin — centigrade (Celsius) — Fahrenheit

375.15° — 100° — 212° — boiling point of water
310.15° — 37° — 98.6° — body temperature
273.15° — 0° — 32° — freezing point of water
— — — — — —
0° — −273.15° — −459.67° — absolute zero

dura mater
superior sagittal sinus
falx cerebri
external oblique m.
internal oblique m.
transversus m.
hipbone
inguinal ligament
crista galli
inguinal falx (conjoined tendon)
tentorium cerebelli
falx cerebelli
clinoid processes

(after surname of original patient) or contact factor.

f. XIII A transpeptidase present in normal plasma which cross-links subunits of fibrin monomer to form insoluble fibrin polymer; thrombin catalyzes the conversion of factor XIII into its active form.

follicle-stimulating hormone-releasing f. (FRF; FSH-RF) See follicle-stimulating hormone-releasing hormone, under hormone.

growth hormone-releasing f. (GRF, GH-RF) See growth hormone-releasing hormone, under hormone.

H f. of Lewis Histamine or histamine-like substance present in the deeper layers of the skin, responsible for inflammatory vascular skin reactions.

Hageman See factor XII.

intrinsic f. A mucoprotein produced by the parietal cells of gastric glands essential for absorption of vitamin B_{12} in the ileum; deficiency causes pernicious anemia.

labile f. See factor V.

lopotropic f. Choline.

luteinizing hormone-releasing f. (LRF) See luteinizing hormone-releasing hormone, under hormone.

pellagra-preventing f. (P-PF) Nicotinic acid.

platelet-activating f., platelet-aggregating f. (PAF) Substance released from basophilic leukocytes that induces aggregation of platelets and is involved in immune responses.

platelet derived growth f. (PDGF) A heat-stable polypeptide within the alpha-granules of circulating blood platelets; stimulates fibroblast proliferation and thus helps repair injured cells; normally released only when blood clots; incriminated as a possible link to neoplasia if unregulated.

platelet f. 1 (PF-1) Plasma factor V absorbed on the surface of the platelet.

platelet f. 2 (PF-2) Fibrinogen activator on the surface of the platelet.

platelet f. 3 (PF-3) A lipoprotein of the platelet membrane that reacts with factors VIII and IX to activate factor X; it then participates with factor V and with activated factor X to convert prothrombin to thrombin.

platelet f. 4 (PF-4) See antiheparin factor.

prolactin-inhibiting f. A substance of hypothalamic origin capable of inhibiting the synthesis and release of prolactin by the anterior pituitary gland.

releasing f. (RF) A substance of hypothalamic origin capable of accelerating the rate of excretion of a given hormone by the anterior pituitary gland.

rheumatoid f. (RF) A globulin found in the serum of many individuals with rheumatoid arthritis (70%) and some other conditions; it produces agglutination when added to a suspension of particles coated with pooled human gamma globulin.

secretor f. An inherited factor that permits the secretion of water-soluble forms of A and B-group antigens into saliva and other body fluids.

spreading f. Hyaluronidase.

stable f. See factor VII.

sun-protection f. (SPF) The increased amount of ultraviolet radiation required to produce redness of the skin in the presence of a sunscreen.

thyrotropin-releasing f. (TRF) See thyrotropin-releasing hormone, under hormone.

transfer f. (TF) **1.** A genetic particle in bacterial cells that is transferred from one bacterial cell to another. **2.** A substance, free of nucleic acid and antibody, capable of transferring antigen specific cell-mediated immunity from donor to recipient.

tumor-angiogenesis f. A diffusible factor which is mitogenic to capillary endothelium and stimulates rapid formation of new vessels; secreted by malignant tumors and not found in normal tissue with the exception of the placenta; it has a molecular weight of approximately 100,000 and contains 25% ribonucleic acid.

von Willebrand's f. (VWF) A large glycoprotein polymer that has binding sites for factor VIII.

facultative 1. Relating to a mental faculty. **2.** Capable of adapting to varying environmental conditions; said of certain parasites; opposite of obligate.

faculty 1. An inherent ability. **2.** Any of the powers of the human mind.

fagopyrism, fagopyrismus Poisoning by buckwheat, clover, St. John's wort, etc.

Fahrenheit (F) Denoting a temperature scale that records the freezing point of water at 32° and the boiling point at 212° under normal atmospheric pressure.

failure 1. The condition of being insufficient. **2.** A cessation of normal functioning.

backward heart f. The theory of backward heart failure maintains that congestive heart failure results in engorgement of the veins and raises pressure proximal to the failing heart chambers.

cardiac f. See heart failure (I).

congestive heart f. Abnormal circulatory congestion resulting from heart failure.

forward heart f. The theory of forward heart failure maintains that congestive heart failure results from inadequate cardiac output, resulting in inadequate kidney blood flow and retention of sodium and water.

heart f. 1. Failure of the heart to function effectively as a pump so that it cannot deliver an adequate supply of oxygenated blood to the tissues. Also called myocardial failure; cardiac insufficiency or failure.

2. The resulting clinical syndrome.

high output f. Condition in which the cardiac output, although at normal levels or higher, is inadequate to meet the demands of the body; seen in states such as marked anemia, Paget's disease, and arteriovenous fistulas.

left ventricular f. Heart failure manifested by congestion of the lungs.

low output f. Subnormal cardiac output seen in heart failure, usually due to coronary, hypertensive, or valvular disease.

myocardial f. See heart failure (1).

pacemaker f. Failure of an artificial pacemaker to stimulate the heart muscle.

power f. See pump failure.

pump f. Failure of the heart as a mechanical pump rather than disturbance of the electrical impulse (arrhythmia). Also called power failure.

respiratory f. The failure of the pulmonary system to maintain normal gas tensions of oxygen, carbon dioxide, or both in the arterial circulation.

right ventricular f. Heart failure manifested by distention of the neck veins, edema, and enlargement of the liver.

faint 1. To lose consciousness. **2.** Syncope, generally due to abrupt, usually brief, failure of normal circulation of blood to the brain. **3.** Weak; feeble; lacking strength.

fainting Temporary unconsciousness caused by diminished blood supply to the brain.

falciform, falcate Sickle-shaped.

falling of the womb Prolapse of the uterus.

Fallot's tetralogy See tetralogy of Fallot.

fallout Debris (radioactive material) from the detonation of nuclear weapons that resettles to earth.

local f. Dense radioactive particles propelled into the atmosphere by the explosion; they descend to earth within a day or two near the site of the nuclear explosion.

false-negative Denoting a test result that wrongly indicates that a person does not have the attribute or disease for which the test is conducted.

false-positive Denoting a test result that wrongly indicates that a person has the attribute or disease for which the test is conducted.

falx A sickle-shaped structure.

f. cerebelli The fold of cranial dura mater separating the lateral lobes of the cerebellum.

f. cerebri The fold of cranial dura mater between the cerebral hemispheres.

inguinal f. The united tendons of the abdominal transverse and the internal oblique muscles which insert into the crest of the pubic bone and the pectineal line. Also called conjoined tendon.

familial Affecting several individuals in the same

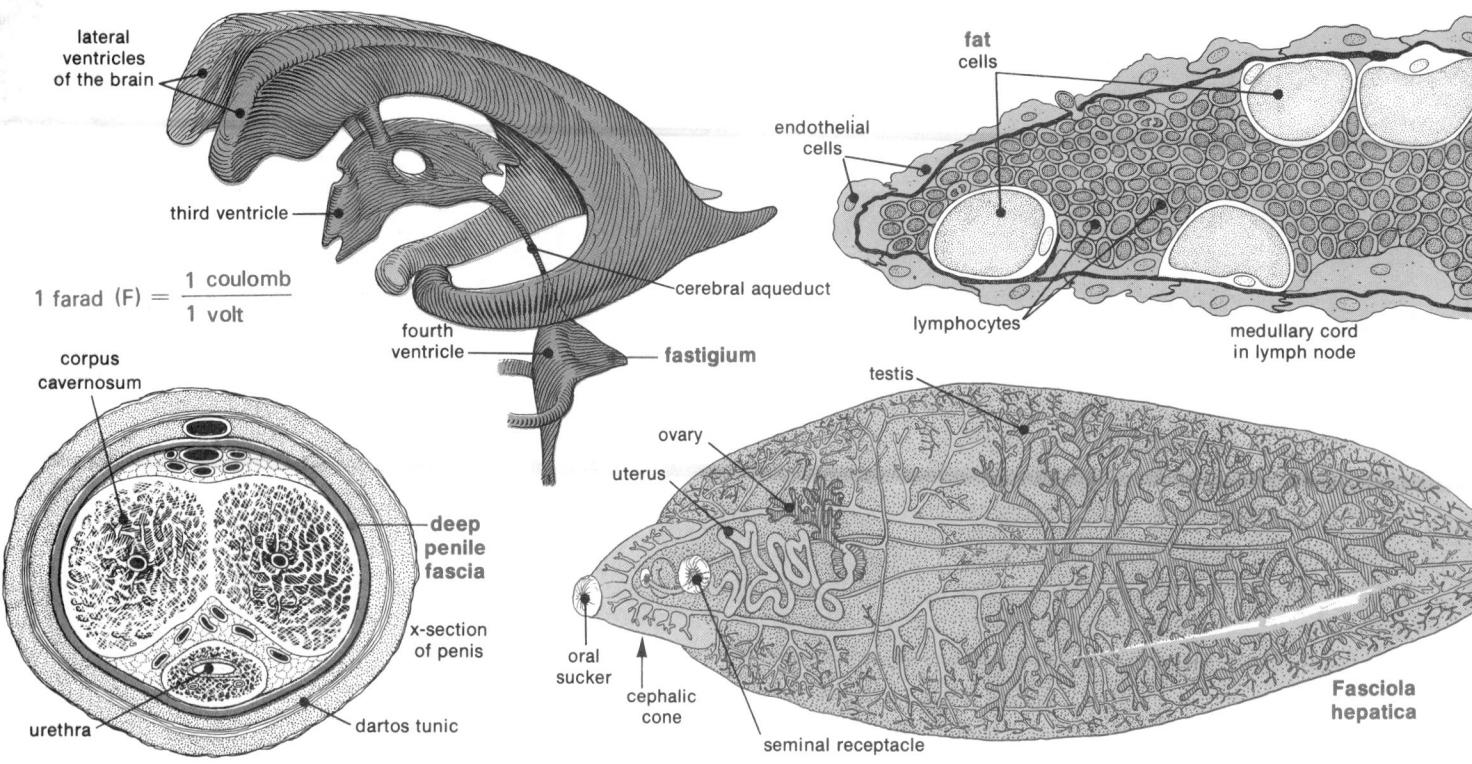

1 farad (F) = $\dfrac{1 \text{ coulomb}}{1 \text{ volt}}$

family; formerly used to denote disorders caused by a recessive gene; distinguished from hereditary.

family In biologic classification, a category ranking above a genus and below an order.

Fanconi's syndrome A functional disturbance of the proximal kidney tubules resulting in glucosuria, generalized aminoaciduria, phosphaturia, and renal tubular acidosis; it may be inherited, e.g., in cystinosis, or acquired as a consequence of numerous causes including drugs, heavy metals, or disease processes such as amyloidosis.

farad (F) A unit of electrical capacity, equal to the capacity of a condenser having a charge of 1 coulomb under an electromotive force of 1 volt.

faraday The amount of electricity required to dissolve or deposit 1 gram equivalent weight of a substance in electrolysis, approximately 9.6494×10^4 coulombs.

faradic Relating to induced electricity.

farcy The cutaneous form of glanders, characterized by ulceration of the skin at the site of inoculation of the bacillus followed by involvement of the lymphatic system.

farinaceous Of the nature of or containing starch.

farsightedness See hyperopia.

fascia, *pl.* **fasciae** A sheet of connective tissue that covers the body under the skin, and envelops the muscles and various organs.

   Buck's f. See deep penile fascia.

   bulbar f. Connective tissue sheath enveloping the eyeball with the exception of the cornea; attached to the sclera at the sclerocorneal junction. Also called Tenon's capsule.

   Camper's f. Superficial fatty layer of the superficial fascia of abdomen and perineum.

   Colle's f. The deep membranous layer of the superficial fascia of the perineum.

   cremasteric f. The part of the fascia of the cremasteric muscle that invests the spermatic cord.

   cribriform f. The part of the superficial fascia of the thigh that covers the saphenous opening.

   deep f. The gray, dense, membranous sheet investing the trunk, neck, limbs, and part of the head; it also covers and holds the muscles and other structures in their proper positions, separating them or joining them for independent or integrated function, respectively.

   deep penile f. A fascial sheath of the penis, derived from the external perineal fascia. Also called Buck's fascia.

   f. clitoridis The dense fibrous tissue that encases the two corpora cavernosa of the clitoris.

   f. lata The broad fascia investing the muscles of the thigh.

   nuchal f. Fascia of dorsal region of neck.

   Scarpa's f. The deep membranous layer of the superficial fascia of the abdomen; it is continuous with the deep layer of the superficial fascia of the perineum (Colle's fascia).

   subcutaneous f. The connective tissue between the skin and the deep fascia, composed of an inner layer and an outer layer that normally contains an accumulation of fat. Also called tela subcutanea; superficial fascia.

   subserous f. The layer of connective tissue located beneath the lining of the body cavities and attaching it to the deep fascia; it also covers and supports the viscera. Also called tela subserosa.

   transversalis f. The fascial lining of the abdominal cavity between the deep or inner surface of the abdominal musculature and the peritoneum.

   triangular f. Reflex inguinal ligament; see under ligament.

fascial Relating to a fascia.

fascicle A small bundle of fibers, as of nerve or muscle fibers.

fascicular Pertaining to a fascicle or arranged in bundles.

fasciculation 1. The formation of small bundles of fibers (fasciculi). 2. Involuntary contraction or twitching of a group of muscle fibers; a coarser form of muscular contraction than fibrillation.

fasciculus, *pl.* **fasciculi** A small bundle of muscle or nerve fibers.

   f. atrioventricularis Atrioventricular bundle; see under bundle.

   inferior longitudinal f. A bundle of association fibers running through the occipital and temporal lobes of the cerebrum.

   medial longitudinal f. A bundle of fibers running under the fourth ventricle from the midbrain to the spinal cord. Also called posterior longitudinal bundle.

   proper fasciculi Ascending and descending association fibers surrounding the gray columns of the spinal cord.

fasciitis Inflammation of fascia.

Fasciola Liver flukes; a genus of Trematoda.

   F. hepatica The liver fluke of sheep and cattle; a species occasionally transmitted to man through the ingestion of uncooked infected liver. Formerly called *Distomum hepaticum.*

fascioliasis Infection with a species of *Fasciola.*

Fasciolopsis A genus of intestinal Trematoda (flukes).

fascioplasty Reparative surgery on a fascia.

fasciorrhaphy Suture of a fascia or an aponeurosis. Also called aponeurorrhaphy.

fasciotomy Surgical incision through a fascia.

fast Resistant to change.

fastigium 1. The peak or highest point of the roof of the fourth ventricle of the brain. 2. The height of a fever or any acute state. Also called maximum.

fat 1. Any of several organic compounds that yield fatty acids and glycerol upon saponification. 2. A mixture of such compounds comprising most of the cell contents of adipose tissue; occurring also in lesser amounts in other animal cells and some plant cells.

   brown f. A lobulated brown mass of tissue composed of cells containing numerous fat globules, found primarily in the interscapular region of the human newborn, hibernating animals, and other mammals. Also called interscapular gland.

   saturated f. Saturated fatty acid; see under acid.

   unsaturated f. Unsaturated fatty acid; see under acid.

fatal Causing death.

fatality Anything resulting in death.

fatigability Condition of becoming easily tired.

fatigue A feeling of exhaustion with decreased efficiency resulting from physical or mental exertion.

   battle f. A severe anxiety state seen in front-line soldiers, characterized by loss of effectiveness, poor judgment, physical complaints, and/or feeling of imminent death.

   flying f. Chronic functional disorder occurring in aviators after prolonged piloting of an aircraft. Also called aeroasthenia.

fatty acid See under acid.

fauces The passage from the oral cavity to the oral pharynx, including the lumen and its boundaries; the aperture by which the mouth communicates with the pharynx.

   anterior pillar of the f. Palatoglossal fold that rises archlike on each side of the posterior limit of the oral cavity.

   posterior pillar of the f. Palatopharyngeal fold just posterior to the palatine tonsil.

faveolus A small depression.

favism Acute hemolytic anemia caused by ingestion of the fava bean or inhalation of the pollen of its flower; seen in individuals of Mediterranean extraction whose red blood cells are deficient in the enzyme glucose 6-phosphate dehydrogenase (not all individuals with this enzyme deficiency are susceptible).

favus A chronic fungus infection, usually of the scalp, caused by *Trichophyton schoenleini.* Also called tinea capitis.

fear A feeling of apprehension or alarm in response to an external source of danger.

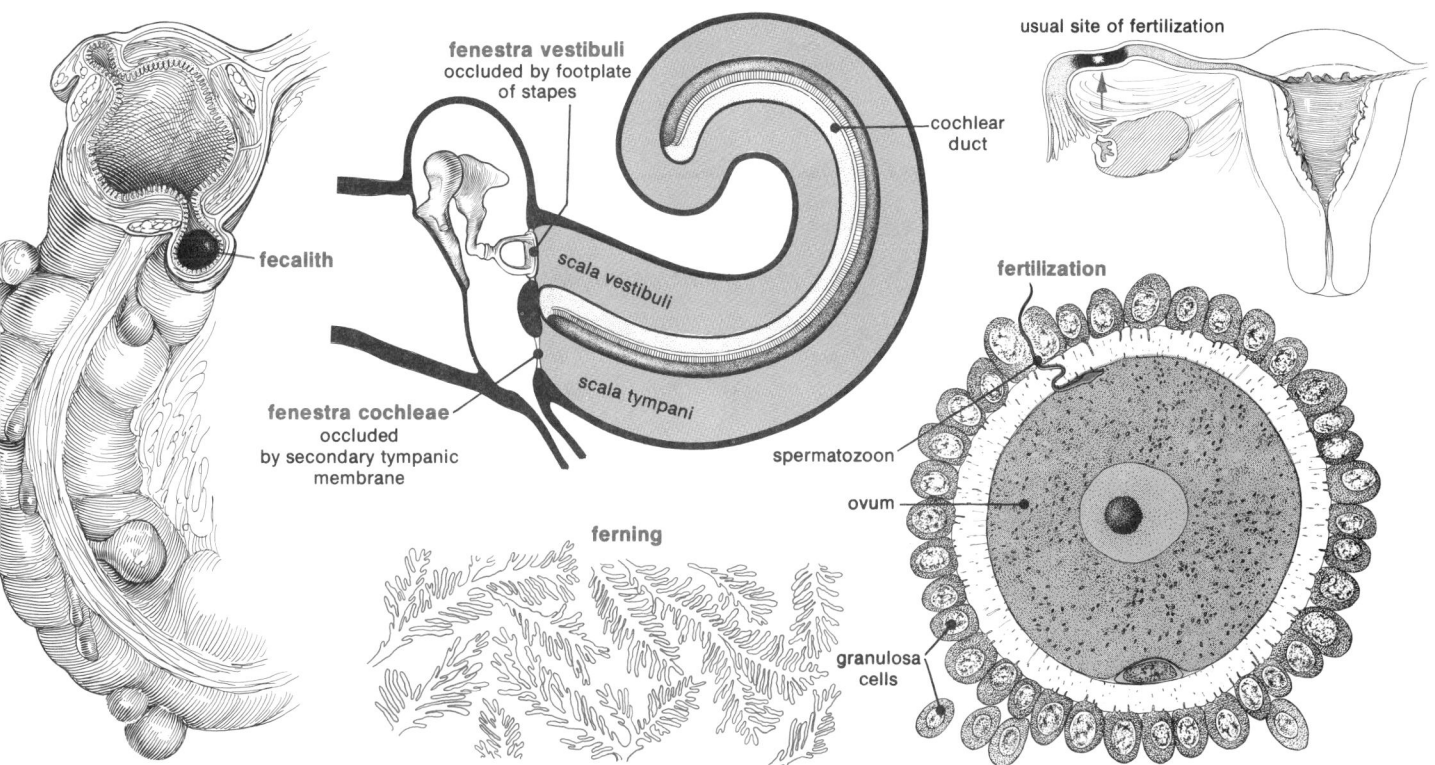

fenestra vestibuli occluded by footplate of stapes

cochlear duct

scala vestibuli

scala tympani

fecalith

fenestra cochleae occluded by secondary tympanic membrane

ferning

usual site of fertilization

fertilization

spermatozoon

ovum

granulosa cells

morbid f. Phobia.

features The outward appearance of the face or any of its parts.

febrifacient 1. Any substance that produces a fever. 2. Causing fever.

febrile Having fever.

fecal Relating to feces.

fecalith A concretion of feces.

fecaluria The passage of fecal matter with the urine in persons with a connecting channel (fistula) between the rectum and the bladder.

feces The waste matter discharged from the bowel.

feculent Fecal; foul.

fecundate To fertilize; to impregnate.

fecundation Fertilization; impregnation.

fecundity Ability to produce offspring abundantly; pronounced fertility.

feeble Infirm; weak; lacking vitality.

feeblemindedness Obsolete term for mental retardation.

feedback 1. The process whereby a portion of a system's output, as of an amplifier, is returned to the input; return of information from the output to the control system so as to modify the nature of the control. 2. The portion of the output so returned. 3. The feeling created by another person's reactions to oneself.

   negative f. A signal or information returning from the output to the control system which results in reduced output.

   positive f. A signal or information returning to the control system from the output which results in increased output.

feeding Administration of nourishment.

   forced f. The administration of liquid food through a lubricated tube which is passed (nasally or orally) into the stomach.

feeling 1. A sensation perceived by the sense of touch. 2. Emotional or affective state or process. 3. A vague belief.

Fehling's reagent See solution, Fehling's.

fellatio Oral penile stimulation.

felon An infection of the distal fat pad at the tip of a finger; manifested by progressive tenderness and throbbing pain.

Felty's syndrome Rheumatoid arthritis, leukopenia, and enlargement of the spleen.

female Relating to or denoting the sex that bears young or produces ova or eggs.

feminine Of or relating to the female sex, or having qualities usually associated with the female.

feminism The possession of feminine characteristics by the male.

feminization The development of female charac-

teristics by the male.

femoral Relating to the femur or to the thigh.

femur The thighbone; the longest and strongest bone in the body; see table of bones.

fenestra, *pl.* **fenestrae** A window-like opening.

   f. cochleae A round opening in the medial wall of the middle ear leading into the cochlea. Also called round window.

   f. vestibuli An oval opening between the middle ear and the vestibule of the internal ear; closed by the footplate of the stapes. Also called oval window.

fenestrated Pierced with one or more small window-like openings.

fenestration 1. The act of perforating. 2. The surgical creation of an opening in the labyrinth of the internal ear to improve hearing in patients afflicted with otosclerosis.

ferment A substance that causes chemical changes in another substance, without itself changing; formerly used interchangeably with enzyme, now applied to a substance that is not removable from the cell that produces it.

ferment To undergo fermentation.

fermentable Capable of undergoing fermentation.

fermentation A chemical decomposition induced in a carbohydrate by a ferment such as yeast, bacterium, or mold.

fermentative Having the ability to cause fermentation.

fermium Radioactive element; symbol Fm, atomic number 100.

ferning The typical palm-leaf pattern formed, upon crystallization, by cervical mucus as a result of electrolyte action on protein; it occurs in the proliferative phase of the menstrual cycle. Also called cervical mucus arborization.

ferric Relating to or containing iron; especially a salt containing iron in its highest valence (3).

ferritin A protein rich in iron (up to 23%) formed by the union of ferric iron with apoferritin; occurs mainly in the liver, spleen, and intestinal mucosa.

ferrocyanide A compound containing the negative ion $Fe(CN)_6^{4-}$.

ferroporphyrin A derivative of ferrous porphyrin in which a central iron atom is linked to the nitrogen atoms of the porphyrin.

ferroprotein A protein containing iron in a prosthetic group.

ferroprotoporphyrin See heme.

ferrous Relating to or containing iron; especially a salt containing iron in its lowest valence (2).

   f. fumarate A reddish orange compound used as a hematinic. Also called iron fumarate.

   f. sulfate. A compound widely used in treating uncomplicated iron deficiency anemia. Also called iron sulfate; green vitriol.

ferruginous Containing iron. Also called chalybeate.

ferrum Latin for iron.

fertile Possessing the capacity to reproduce.

fertility The capacity to initiate or support conception.

fertilization The union of a spermatozoon with an ovum.

   in vitro f. (IVF) Fertilization that occurs outside the body in a glass petri dish.

fervescence An increase of fever.

fester To form pus.

festinant Accelerating; rapid.

festination The involuntary acceleration of walking which occurs when the center of gravity is displaced, as seen in paralysis agitans and some other nervous diseases.

festooning The process of cutting, carving, or grinding material to accommodate the contours of natural tissue, as the cutting of a round copper band in order to fit around a prepared tooth and rest snugly on the gingiva prior to taking an impression.

fetal Relating to a fetus.

fetal alcohol syndrome Congenital mental and growth retardation, heart defects, and defective facial features caused by alcohol consumption by the child's mother during early pregnancy.

feticide The intentional destruction of the embryo or fetus in the uterus. Also called induced abortion.

fetid Having a disagreeable odor.

fetish An object to which excessive attention or reverence is attached; often a source of sexual stimulation or gratification.

fetishism Excessive emotional attachment to an inanimate object or body part which serves as a substitute for a human sexual object.

fetography Roentgenography of the fetus in utero.

fetology The branch of medicine concerned with the fetus and its diseases.

fetometry Estimation of the size of the fetal head prior to delivery.

fetoplacental Relating to the fetus and placenta.

α-fetoprotein (AFP) A protein substance normally found in the fetus, which also has been found in the sera of a large number of individuals with hepatoma.

fetor An offensive odor.

   f. hepaticus An unpleasant odor of the breath of individuals with severe liver disorders.

   f. oris Halitosis.

9 week old fetus 6 cm from crown to rump

fetus at term (38 weeks)

spinal cord

afferent fiber

efferent fibers

fetoscopes

fetoscope Instrument for auscultation of the heart of the fetus. Also called fetal stethoscope.

fetus The developing offspring in the uterus, generally from the second month of pregnancy to birth; during the first two months of development, it is called an embryo.

fever A rise in body temperature above the normal of 98.6°F; usually a temperature of 99.6°F orally or 100°F rectally, or at least 1°F higher than the normal for that individual. Also called pyrexia.

blackwater f. Malarial hemoglobinuria; see under hemoglobinuria.

canicola f. Disease caused by the bacterium *Leptospira canicola;* transmitted to man by contact with infected dog urine.

cat-scratch f. See cat-scratch disease.

Colorado tick f. An acute viral disease (similar to Rocky Mountain spotted fever) transmitted to man by the tick *Dermacentor andersoni;* marked chiefly by fever and leukopenia, but no rash.

desert f. See coccidioidomycosis.

familial Mediterranean f. (FMF) Recurrent attacks of abdominal pain, inflamed peritoneum, fever, and sometimes a rash; the condition is asymptomatic between attacks.

glandular f. Infectious mononucleosis; see under mononucleosis.

Haverhill f. Disorder caused by infection with *Streptobacillus moniliformis;* marked by fever, rash, and arthritis (usually of the large joints and spine), and lasting from two to three weeks; although the disease is caused by the same organism as that causing rat-bite fever, it is not transmitted by a rat's bite.

hay f. A seasonal irritative inflammation of the mucous membranes of the eye and nose, caused by an allergic reaction to various pollens; not actually associated with a rise in body temperature.

hemorrhagic f. Disease of viral origin marked primarily by fever, capillary hemorrhages, and shock. Also called Manchurian or Korean hemorrhagic fever.

icterohemorrhagic f. See Weil's disease.

jungle yellow f. A form of yellow fever transmitted to man by some forest mosquito in the absence of *Aedes aegypti* (the domestic mosquito).

Lassa f. A highly contagious, often fatal, disease marked by fever, chills, muscle aches, rashes, nausea, severe pharyngitis, bleeding gums, and oral ulcerations; caused by the Lassa virus (genus *Arenavirus,* family Arenaviridae); transmitted by a rat (*Mastomys natalensis*).

malignant tertian f. Malarial fever usually occurring every other day. See also malaria.

Mediterranean f. 1. Brucellosis. **2.** Familial Mediterranean fever.

mountain f. Altitude sickness; see under sickness.

Oroya f. The acute form and usually the first stage of bartonellosis, endemic disease of the Peruvian Andes; marked by fever, rheumatic pains, anemia, and albuminuria. See also bartonellosis.

paratyphoid f. An infectious disease with symptoms resembling those of typhoid fever, but milder; caused by strains of *Salmonella.*

pharyngoconjunctival f. Fever, pharyngitis, and acute follicular conjunctivitis caused by a virus usually type 3 adenovirus; conjunctivitis is the chief complaint; it primarily affects children, who acquire it from swimming pools.

pretibial f. A form of leptospirosis first seen at Fort Bragg, North Carolina; marked by mild fever, splenomegaly, and a rash on the anterior surface of the legs. Also called Fort Bragg fever.

puerperal f. Fever occurring after childbirth.

Q f. A bacterial disease resembling influenza, caused by *Coxiella burneti;* marked by headache, fever, and constitutional symptoms; sometimes associated with inflammation of the lungs; usually acquired by inhalation of the agent.

quartan f. Malarial fever in which the paroxysm usually recurs every third day. See also malaria.

quotidian f. Daily fever occurring in quotidian malaria. See also malaria.

rat-bite f. Disease marked by inflammation of the lymph nodes and lymphatic vessels due to infection with *Spirillum minor* or *Streptobacillus moniliformis;* transmitted by the bite of an infected rat or any rodent. Also called headache fever.

recurrent f. Relapsing fever.

relapsing f. An acute infectious bacterial disease marked by alternating periods of fever and apyrexia, each lasting about six days; caused by species of the genus *Borrelia;* transmitted to man by either a louse or a soft tick.

rheumatic f. A disease caused by infection with a β-hemolytic streptococcus; it usually begins with a sore throat and after an interval of several days there is a rapid rise of temperature, prostration, and inflammation of the joints; the heart is often affected.

Rocky Mountain spotted f. An acute infectious bacterial disease marked by fever, bone and muscle pain, headache, and a generalized rash; caused by *Rickettsia rickettsii;* transmitted to man by several varieties of hard ticks. Also called spotted or tick fever; tick typhus.

sandfly f. A viral disease transmitted to man by the fly *Phlebotomus papatassi;* marked by fever, ocular pain, and general malaise, followed by complete recovery. Also called phlebotomus or pappataci fever.

San Joaquin Valley f. See coccidioidomycosis.

scarlet f. An acute infectious disease marked by high fever, sore throat, and a skin rash; caused by β-hemolytic streptococcus. Also called scarlatina.

spotted f. 1. Meningococcal meningitis. **2.** Rocky Mountain spotted fever.

swamp f. 1. A viral disease of horses marked by fever, staggering gait, and progressive anemia. **2.** Malaria.

tertian f. Malarial fever usually occurring every other day. See also malaria.

tick f. 1. Any infectious disease transmitted by the bite of a tick and caused by a protozoan blood parasite. **2.** Rocky Mountain spotted fever.

trench f. A relapsing type of fever caused by *Rochalimaea quintana* and transmitted by infected lice; observed in troops during World War I.

tsutsugamushi f. See tsutsugamushi disease.

typhoid f. An acute infectious disease caused by *Salmonella typhi;* marked by a continued fever that has an insidious start, headache, mental depression, prostration, enlargement of the spleen, a maculopapular rash, and sometimes diarrhea.

typhus f. See typhus.

undulant f. See brucellosis.

West Nile f. Acute illness marked by fever, headache, a papular rash, lymphadenopathy, and leukopenia; caused by a mosquito-borne virus.

yellow f. An acute infectious disease caused by the yellow fever flavivirus (family Togaviridae) and transmitted by *Aedes* mosquitoes; characterized by fever, degeneration of the liver (producing jaundice), and intestinal disturbances. Also called yellow jack; amarilla.

fiber Any slender, threadlike structure.

A f.'s Myelinated fibers of the somatic nervous system having conduction rates from 15 to 100 meters per second.

accelerator f.'s Nerve fibers conveying impulses that increase the force and rapidity of the heartbeat. Also called augmentor fibers.

adrenergic f.'s Nerve fibers that release adrenaline-like substances at the synapse.

afferent f.'s Nerve fibers conveying impulses to a nerve center in the brain or spinal cord.

alpha f.'s Somatic motor or proprioceptive fibers having a conduction rate of 100 meters per second.

association f.'s Nerve fibers connecting different areas of the cerebral cortex in the same hemisphere.

augmentor f.'s See accelerator fibers.

B f.'s Small fibers of the autonomic nervous system having a conduction rate of 3 to 14 meters per second.

beta f.'s Somatic nerve fibers having a conduction rate of 40 meters per second.

C f.'s Unmyelinated nerve fibers of the auto-

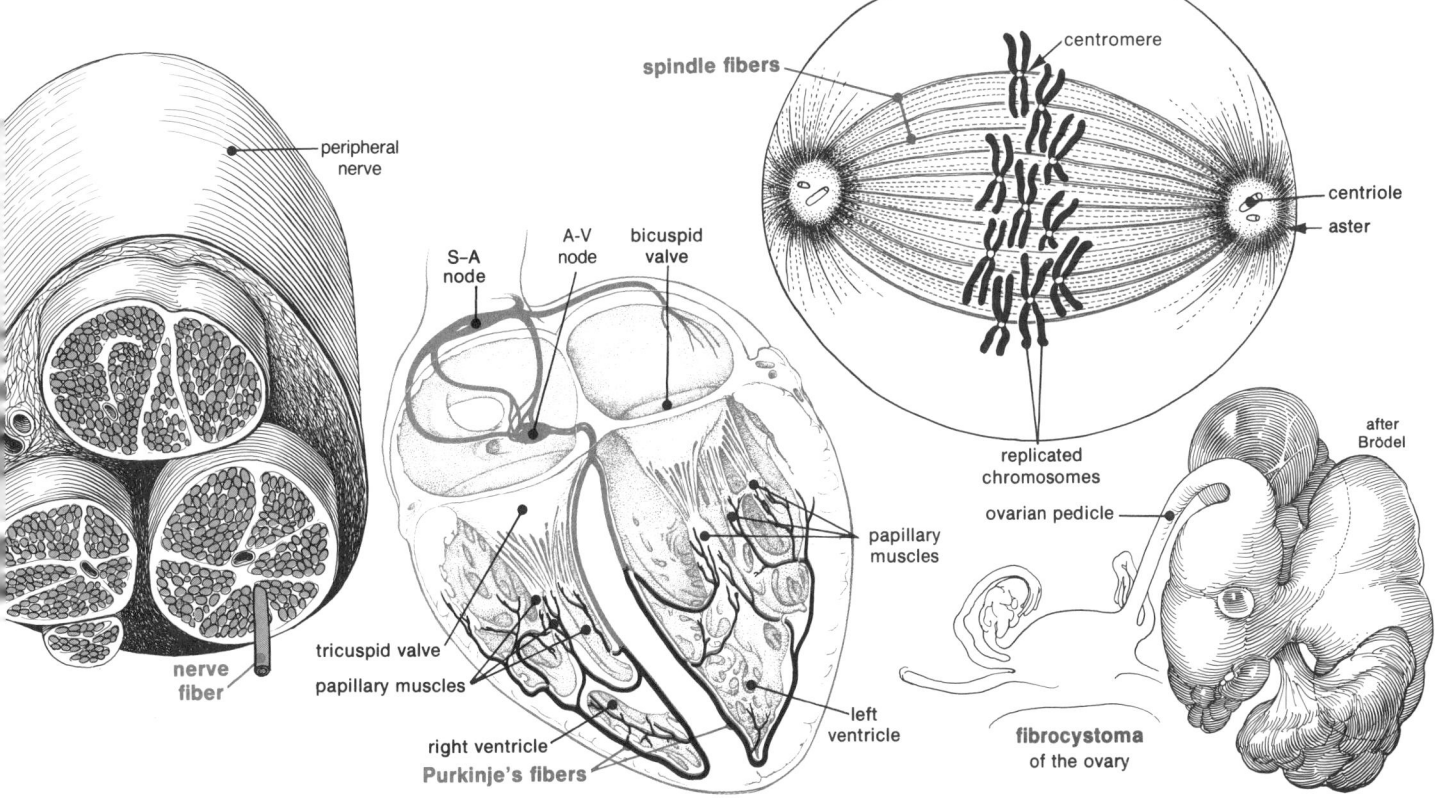

peripheral nerve

spindle fibers

centromere

centriole

aster

nerve fiber

S-A node

A-V node

bicuspid valve

replicated chromosomes

ovarian pedicle

after Brödel

tricuspid valve

papillary muscles

papillary muscles

left ventricle

right ventricle

Purkinje's fibers

fibrocystoma
of the ovary

nomic nervous system having a conduction rate of 2 meters per second.

cholinergic f.'s Nerve fibers that release acetylcholine at the synapse.

collagen f.'s, collagenous f.'s The flexible fibers making up the principal constituent of connective tissue. Also called white fibers.

depressor f.'s Sensory or afferent nerve fibers which, when stimulated, diminish vascular tone and lower blood pressure.

efferent f.'s Nerve fibers that convey impulses from a nerve center in the brain or spinal cord.

elastic f.'s Fibers of elastic properties forming a network in the substance of some connective tissue. Also called yellow fibers.

gamma f.'s Somatic nerve fibers having a conduction rate of 20 meters per second.

Golgi's f.'s (types I and II) Terms given to the axons of Golgi cells, types I and II.

gray f.'s See unmyelinated fibers.

inhibitory f.'s Nerve fibers that slow down the action of an organ.

myelinated f.'s Nerve fibers possessing a myelin sheath.

nerve f. One of the slender units of a nerve trunk; the axon of a nerve cell.

nonmyelinated f.'s Unmyelinated fibers.

pressor f.'s Sensory nerve fibers which, upon stimulation, cause narrowing of blood vessels and rise of blood pressure.

projection f.'s Nerve fibers that connect the cerebral cortex with other areas of the brain.

Purkinje's f.'s Specialized fibers formed of modified heart muscle cells located beneath the endocardium; concerned with the conduction of stimuli from the atria to the ventricles.

Sharpey's f.'s Thick perforating collagenous or fibroelastic bundles that attach periosteum to bone; they are continuations of the periosteal fibers and pierce the bone obliquely or at right angles to its long axis.

spindle f. One of several filaments extending between the poles of a dividing cell, forming together a spindle-shaped structure. Also called traction fiber.

unmyelinated f.'s Nerve fibers lacking a myelin sheath. Also called Remak's or gray fibers.

white f.'s See collagen fibers.

yellow f.'s See elastic fibers.

fiberoptics The transmission of images along a bundle of fine, parallel, flexible rods of plastic or glass.

fiberscope A viewing instrument with very fine, flexible glass rods for light transmission (fiber optics).

fibril A minute, slender fiber or filament.

Ebner's f.'s Slender collagen fibers in the cementum and dentin of a tooth.

fibrillar, fibrillary 1. Relating to a fibril. 2. Relating to twitching of small skeletal or smooth muscles.

fibrillate 1. To be in a state of fibrillation. 2. To become fibrillar. 3. Composed of fibrils.

fibrillation 1. The rapid contractions or quivering of muscular fibrils. 2. The formation of fibrils.

atrial f. The replacement of the normal rhythmic contractions of the cardiac atria by rapid irregular quivers.

ventricular f. Rapid, irregular twitchings that replace the normal contractions of the muscular walls of the ventricles.

fibrilliform Having the general configuration of a fibril.

fibrillogenesis The normal development of minute fibrils in collagenous fibers of connective tissue.

fibrin A fibrous, insoluble protein derived from fibrinogen through the action of thrombin; the basic component of a blood clot.

fibrination 1. The formation of a fibrin. 2. The formation of an abnormally large amount of fibrin; denoting the condition of the blood in certain inflammatory diseases. Also called fibrinosis.

fibrinogen A protein, present in dissolved form in blood plasma, that is converted into a network of delicate filaments (fibrin) by the action of the enzyme thrombin; the blood cells become entangled in the fibrin network, thus producing coagulation. Also called factor I.

fibrinogenopenia Deficiency in the concentration of fibrinogen in the blood.

fibrinoid 1. Resembling fibrin. 2. An acidophilic, homogeneous, refractile material.

fibrinolysin An enzyme that dissolves fibrin in clotted blood.

fibrinolysis The destruction of fibrin in clotted blood by enzyme action, resulting in the dissolution of a clot.

fibrinopurulent Relating to a discharge that contains pus and a large amount of fibrin.

fibrinosis See fibrination (2).

fibrinous Relating to or composed of fibrin.

fibroadenoma A benign tumor derived from glandular epithelium.

fibroadipose Containing both fibrous and fatty elements. Also called fibrofatty.

fibroblast An elongated, flattened, spindle-shaped cell with cytoplasmic processes at each end, having a flat, oval nucleus showing a finely granular chromatin with one or two nucleoli; one of the most common cell types found in growing connective tissue.

fibrocarcinoma See carcinoma, scirrhous.

fibrocartilage A type of cartilage containing collagenic fibers.

fibrochondritis Inflammation of fibrocartilage.

fibrochondroma A benign tumor composed primarily of cartilage and an abundant amount of fibrous tissue.

fibrocyst A lesion consisting of a cyst within a fibrous network.

fibrocystic Marked by the presence of fibrocysts.

fibrocystic disease of breast Benign disease of the female breast marked by one of the three basic morphologic patterns: (a) formation of cysts, (b) overgrowth of stroma and intraductal epithelium, or (c) sclerotic proliferation of gland tissue; there is frequent concurrence of these patterns, with one usually predominating. Also called cystic disease of breast; cystic hyperplasia of breast; chronic cystic mastitis; mammary dysplasia.

fibrocystic disease of pancreas See cystic fibrosis of pancreas.

fibrocystoma A benign tumor characterized by cysts within a conspicuous fibrous stroma.

fibrocyte A resting or quiescent fibroblast.

fibroelastic Made up of collagen and elastic fibers.

fibroelastosis Overgrowth of fibroelastic tissue.

endocardial f. Endomyocardial fibroelastosis.

endomyocardial f. Congenital heart disease characterized by fibroelastic thickening of the mural endocardium, especially of the left ventricle; the rest of the chambers and the valves may also be involved. Also called endocardial sclerosis.

fibroenchondroma A benign tumor located within a bone and composed of mature cartilage and abundant fibrous tissue.

fibroepithelioma A skin tumor composed of fibrous tissue and basal cells of the epidermis; it may be transformed into a basal cell carcinoma. Also called premalignant fibroepithelioma; fibroepithelioma of Pinkus.

fibrofatty See fibroadipose.

fibroid 1. Resembling or containing fibers. 2. Colloquial clinical term for certain types of leiomyoma (a benign tumor), especially those occurring in the uterus.

fibrolipoma A tumor composed predominantly of fat cells but containing abundant fibrous tissue. Also called lipoma fibrosum.

fibroma A benign tumor derived from fibrous connective tissue. Also called fibrocellular tumor.

concentric f. A benign growth that occupies the entire inner wall of the uterus.

f. molluscum gravidarum The occurrence of numerous, small fibrous tumors of the skin, colorless or pigmented, appearing during pregnancy and disappearing as its termination.

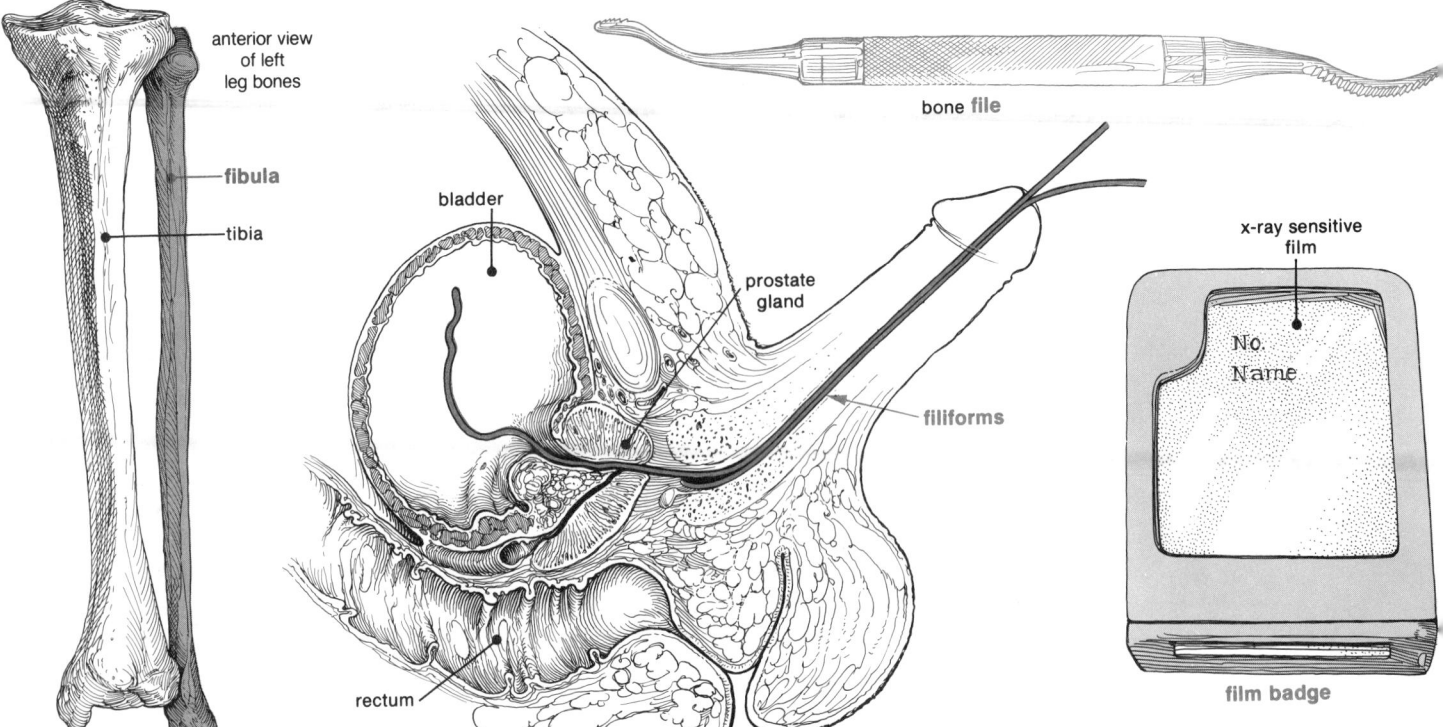

anterior view
of left
leg bones

fibula

tibia

bladder

prostate
gland

filiforms

rectum

bone file

x-ray sensitive
film

No.
Name

film badge

fibromatosis 1. Condition marked by the development of multiple fibromas. 2. Abnormal overdevelopment of fibrous tissue.

fibromuscular Denoting tissues that are both fibrous and muscular.

fibromyoma A benign tumor of smooth muscle origin, containing a relatively small amount of fibrous tissue. Also called leiomyoma.

fibromyositis Chronic inflammation of a muscle with overgrowth of its connective tissue.

fibromyxoma Term formerly used to designate connective tissue tumors that are predominantly fibrous but contain abundant acellular elements.

fibronectin An adhesive glycoprotein present in plasma, where it participates in the phagocytosis of bacteria and other cells, or on the cell surface, where it mediates cellular adhesive interactions.

fibroplasia Abnormal production of fibrous tissue.

  retrolental f. Abnormal increase of fibrous tissue behind the lens of the eye, attributed to exposure of newborn infants, usually premature, to 100% oxygen.

fibroplastic Producing fibrous tissue.

fibrosarcoma A malignant tumor composed of fibrous connective tissue.

fibrosis The formation of fibrous tissue, denoting especially an abnormal degenerative process.

  cystic f. See cystic fibrosis of pancreas.

  endomyocardial f. Thickening of the ventricular myocardium.

  hepatic f. A liver disorder marked by an increase in connective tissue without disturbance of the lobular architecture.

  perimuscular f. Fibrosis involving the renal arteries. Also called subadventitial fibrosis.

  retroperitoneal f. A disorder, usually of unknown etiology, in which an exaggerated fibrocytic response leads to fibrosis involving retroperitoneal structures, particularly the ureters; rarely are the bile ducts involved; the pharmaceutical preparation methysergide has been implicated in some cases as a cause, although the mechanism remains unclear.

  subadventitial f. See perimuscular fibrosis.

fibrositis Inflammatory hyperplasia of fibrous or connective tissue of the muscles.

fibrous Composed of, containing, or resembling fibers of connective tissue.

fibula The lateral and smaller of the two bones of the leg, between the knee and ankle.

fibular Of or relating to the fibula.

fibulocalcaneal Relating to the fibula and the calcaneus.

Fiedler's myocarditis See myocarditis, acute

field A limited area.

  auditory f. The area within which a definite sound is heard.

  magnetic f. The area of space about a magnet in which its magnetic force is perceptible.

  visual f. (F) The area of physical space visible to the eye in a fixed position.

figure Shape; form.

  mitotic f. The appearance of a cell undergoing mitosis.

filament A fine threadlike structure.

filamentous Threadlike; in bacteriology, denoting a colony made up of long, interwoven, threadlike structures.

Filaria Term formerly used for a genus of parasitic threadworms now given other names.

  F. bancrofti Old term for *Wuchereria bancrofti.*

  F. malaya Old term for *Brugia malayi.*

  F. medinensis Old term for *Dracunculus medinensis.*

  F. oculi humani Old term for *Loa Loa.*

filaria, *pl.* **filariae** Any nematode worm of the superfamily Filarioidea.

filariasis A disease caused by the presence of a parasitic threadworm (filaria) in the body; the best known form of filariasis is elephantiasis.

filaricide Any agent that destroys parasitic nematode worms.

filariform Hairlike, as filariae.

Filarioidea A superfamily of true nematode worms that infest man and other vertebrates.

Filaroides A genus of roundworms parasitic in the lungs, bronchi, and trachea of dogs.

file A device used for cutting, smoothing, or grinding.

filial Of or relating to a son or daughter.

filiform 1. Thread-shaped. 2. An extremely slender bougie. 3. In bacteriology, denoting an even, hairlike growth along the line of inoculation in streak or stab cultures.

fillet 1. A thin strip of bandage or tape used for making traction. 2. A band of fibers. Also called lemniscus.

filling Any substance used to fill a space, cavity, or container; e.g., amalgam placed into a tooth cavity to restore the missing portion of the tooth.

  acrylic resin f. A material used for restorations in teeth when esthetic properties are needed.

  combination f. A tooth restoration composed of two or more layers of different materials.

  compound f. A restoration that involves more than one surface of a tooth.

  direct f. A restoration prepared directly in the tooth cavity.

  indirect f. A restoration constructed from an accurate impression of the tooth and then cemented into the tooth cavity.

  overhanging f. A restoration with excessive material at the junction of the filling and the tooth.

  permanent f. A filling intended to be functional for as long a period as possible.

  root canal f. Material placed in the root canal of a tooth to eliminate the space once occupied by the dental pulp.

  silicate f. A restoration of lost tooth structure made with silicate cement, essentially acid-soluble glass.

  temporary f. An interim filling.

  treatment f. A temporary filling for allaying the sensitivity of dentin prior to placing the final restorative material.

  zinc oxide-eugenol f. A temporary filling material, often referred to as ZOE.

film 1. A thin adherent coating on the surface of teeth, consisting chiefly of a mucinous mixture of saliva, microorganisms, and blood and tissue elements. 2. A thin cellulose sheet coated with a light-sensitive emulsion used in taking photographs.

  bite wing f. Dental roentgenographic film with an appendage that is held between the occlusal surface of the teeth.

film badge A small device containing x-ray sensitive film, worn by individuals who are exposed to ionizing radiation, to record the amount of radiation to which they have been exposed; exposure is determined by measuring the degree of darkening of the film.

film fault A defect in an x-ray film due either to physical or chemical causes or to electrical errors in its production.

  fogged f. f. Hazy appearance of a roentgenogram caused by exposure of film to light or stray radiation, subjection to unusual temperatures or chemical actions, or use of outdated film.

film holder A light-tight film container used in extraoral roentgenography.

filopodium, *pl.* **filopodia** A slender process used for locomotion by certain free-living amebae.

filter 1. A porous substance or screen through which liquids or gases are passed in order to separate any suspended material. 2. A device or screen that permits the passage of rays of certain wavelengths only. 3. To pass a substance or rays through such devices.

  Berkefeld f. A filter made of diatomaceous earth through which bacteria do not pass; available in three grades of porosity: W, fine; N, normal; V,

cauda equina of spinal cord

dura mater

filum terminale

filum durae matris spinalis

uterine tube

fimbriae of uterine tube

fingernail

lunula

root of fingernail

fingerprint

longitudinal cerebral fissure

sacral and coccygeal plexuses

coarse.

filterable, filtrable 1. Capable of passing through a filter. 2. Applied to viruses, minute enough to be able to pass through a fine filter.

filtrate Liquid that has passed through a filter.

filtration The process of passing a fluid through a filter employing differential pressure.

filum, *pl.* **fila** Latin for thread; a filamentous or threadlike structure or part.

f. durae matris spinalis Filament of the spinal dura mater; the thin sheath covering the filum terminale and attached to the periosteum of the coccyx; it is continuous above with the dura.

f. radicularia nervorum spinalium Root filament of the spinal nerve emerging from the spinal medulla.

f. terminale The slender fibrous prolongation of the spinal medulla which anchors the spinal cord to the coccyx; it extends from the level of the second lumbar vertebra to the coccyx.

fimbria, *pl.* **fimbriae** 1. Any fringelike structure. 2. See pilus (2).

f. hippocampi A narrow band of white fibers along the medial border of the hippocampus.

fimbriae of uterine tube The numerous irregular fringelike processes on the distal part of the uterine tube.

fimbriate, fimbriated 1. Fringed; having fimbriae. 2. In bacteriology, denoting a colony with slender fringelike projections.

fimbrioplasty A corrective operation on the fringed processes of the uterine tube.

finger One of five digits of the hand.

baseball f. See mallet finger.

drop f. See mallet finger.

clubbed f. Clubbed digit; see under digit.

drumstick f. Clubbed digit; see under digit.

fifth f. The little finger.

first f. The thumb.

fourth f. The ring finger, the thumb being considered the first.

hammer f. See mallet finger.

hippocratic f. Clubbed digit; see under digit.

index f. The second digit, the thumb being considered the first; the finger next to the thumb. Also called forefinger.

mallet f. A finger marked by constant flexion of the distal phalanx; it cannot be actively extended due to detachment of the extensor tendon. Also called baseball, drop, or hammer finger.

middle f. The third finger.

ring f. The fourth finger.

second f. The index finger.

snapping f. See trigger finger.

third f. The middle finger.

trigger f. A finger that locks in a flexed position; it can be extended only with difficulty associated with a snapping or clicking noise; it is due to narrowing of the flexor sheath at the level of the metacarpal neck. Also called snapping finger.

webbed f.'s Congenital abnormality in which two or more fingers are united in various degrees by a fold of skin.

fingeragnosia Loss of ability to recognize the individual fingers of the hand.

finger cot A protective rubber covering for the finger.

fingernail A horny plate on the dorsal surface of the tip of each finger. See also nail.

fingerprint An impression of the configuration of the ridges on the skin surface of the distal phalanx of a finger; usually used as a means of identification; the patterns are sometimes of clinical significance.

Galton's system of classification of f.'s The arch-loop-whorl system of classifying variations in the patterns of the ridges.

first aid Emergency assistance given to the injured or sick before the availability of professional medical care.

fission 1. Division of a cell; form of asexual reproduction. 2. The splitting of an atom in two parts.

fissiparous Reproducing by fission.

fissura, *pl.* **fissurae** Fissure; cleft.

fissuration 1. The condition of being fissured. 2. The formation of a fissure.

fissure A cleft, groove, or slit.

anal f. A painful, difficult to heal slit in the mucous membrane of the anus.

anterior median f. The deep groove in the midline of the anterior aspect of the spinal cord.

auricular f. A groove, between the tympanic and the squamous and mastoid parts of the temporal bone, in which the auricular branch of the vagus nerve is located.

central f. A deep fissure on the lateral surface of each cerebral hemisphere, between the parietal and frontal lobes. Also called central sulcus; fissure of Rolando.

dentate f. Hippocampal fissure.

enamel f. A deep groove on the surface of a tooth resulting from imperfect fusion of adjoining dental lobes.

f.'s of lungs Fissures separating the lobes of the lungs.

f. of Rolando See central fissure.

f. of Sylvius See lateral cerebral fissure.

hippocampal f. A fissure located between the hippocampal convolution and the fascia dentata of

the brain.

horizontal f. of cerebellum A deep cleft encircling the circumference of the cerebellar hemispheres. Also called horizontal sulcus of cerebellum.

inferior orbital f. A groove between the greater wing of the sphenoid and the orbital plate of the maxilla.

lateral cerebral f. A deep fissure separating the frontal, temporal, and parietal lobes of each cerebral hemisphere. Also called fissure of Sylvius.

longitudinal cerebral f. The deep median groove that divides the cerebrum into right and left hemispheres.

superior orbital f. A cleft between the greater and lesser wings of the sphenoid bone. Also called sphenoidal fissure.

transverse cerebral f. A cleft between the corpus callosum and the fornix above and the diencephalon below.

fistula An abnormal passage between two internal organs, or from an organ to the surface of the body; usually designated according to the organs with which it communicates.

anal f. A fistula opening near the anus; it may or may not open into the rectum.

arteriovenous f. An abnormal communication (congenital or traumatic) between an artery and a vein.

branchial f. A congenital defect consisting of a narrow canal on the lateral aspect of the neck in front of the sternocleidomastoid muscle, resulting from incomplete closure of a branchial cleft.

bronchoesophageal f. Passage between a bronchus and the esophagus.

bronchopleural f. A fistula connecting a bronchus and a collection of pus in the pleural cavity.

carotid-cavernous f. Arteriovenous connection formed by rupture of the intracavernous portion of the carotid artery.

colovesical f. A fistula between the colon and the bladder. Also called vesicocolonic fistula.

Eck f. A communication formed by the experimental anastomosing of the vena cava and portal vein with subsequent ligation of the portal vein, for the purpose of shutting off the liver of an experimental animal from its portal circulation.

enterovaginal f. A fistula between the small intestine and the vagina, usually associated with intestinal disease, especially diverticulitis.

gastrocolic f. A fistula between the stomach and the colon.

internal f. Abnormal passage between two internal organs.

pilonidal f. Pilonidal sinus; see under sinus.

rectovaginal f. A fistula between the rectum and the vagina, caused by direct surgical damage, disease of the rectum, or obstetrical injury.

Thiry's f. Artificial fistula made for collecting the intestinal juice of an experimental animal; consisting of an isolated segment of intestine, having one end closed and the other attached to the skin of the abdomen.

Thiry-Vella f. Experimental fistula created by suturing to the skin of the abdomen the two ends of an isolated segment of intestine. Also called Vella's fistula.

tracheoesophageal f. Congenital fistula between the trachea and esophagus.

urachal f., Congenital abnormality which occurs when the lumen of the embryonic allantois (which extends from the navel to the bladder) persists over the entire length, allowing urine to drain from the navel. Also called patent urachus.

urethrovaginal f. A fistula between the urethra and the vagina; may be due to obstetrical injury or may be congenital.

Vella's f. See Thiry-Vella fistula.

vesicocolonic f. See colovesical fistula.

vesicouterine f. A fistula between the bladder and the uterus, usually caused by cancer of the cervix or by surgical injury to the bladder.

vesicovaginal f. A fistula between the bladder and the vagina, often the result of traumatic delivery; almost invariably causes urinary incontinence.

fistulation Formation of a fistula. Also called fistulization.

fistulatome A thin-bladed long knife used for slitting a fistula. Also called syringotome.

fistulatomy See fistulotomy.

fistulectomy Surgical repair of a fistula by the removal of its walls.

fistulization See fistulation.

fistulotomy Surgical incision of a fistula. Also called fistulatomy; syringotomy.

fistulous Relating to or having fistulas.

fitness, physical A state of well being that enables a person to perform his daily work without undue fatigue.

Fitz-Hugh-Curtis syndrome Perihepatitis in women with gonoccocal inflammation of the pelvic organs, resulting from the spread of gonoccoci to the upper abdomen.

fixation 1. The process of making stationary. **2.** In psychiatry, the persistence of immature or earlier patterns of behavior. **3.** In histology, the preservation of tissue elements with minimal alteration of the normal state. **4.** In chemistry, the conversion of a gaseous compound into solid or liquid form. **5.** In ophthalmology, the act of directing the

eye toward an object, causing its image to fall on the fovea.

bifoveal f. Fixation in which the images of the object of regard center simultaneously on the foveae of both eyes, as occurs in normal vision.

binocular f. Bifoveal fixation.

external f. The holding together of a broken bone by means of a plaster cast encircling the injured part or a plaster splint until successful healing occurs.

f. of complement Fixation which occurs when an antigen is allowed to combine with its specific antibody in the presence of complement.

internal f. The use of devices such as metallic pins, screws, wires, or plates, applied directly to the bony fragments to hold them in apposition and alignment.

fixation disparity Condition in which the images of the object of regard do not fall on corresponding retinal points, due to a slight over- or underconvergence of the eyes.

fixative A substance used to preserve histologic specimens.

flaccid Flabby; limp.

flagellantism Erotic stimulation derived from whipping, or being whipped by, a sexual partner.

Flagellata A class of unicellular organisms having one or more whiplike processes (flagella) used for locomotion. Also called Mastigophora.

flagellate A protozoon having one or more flagella.

flagellosis Infection with flagellated protozoa.

flagellum, pl. **flagella** A hairlike protoplasmic structure, present in some microorganisms; it is usually several microns in length and composed of two tightly entwined filaments, each about 100 Å in diameter; it grows out from the basal body in the cytoplasm of the cell and is used for locomotion.

flange 1. A protruding rim or edge. **2.** In dentistry, the part of the denture base which extends from the cervical ends of the teeth to the border of the denture.

buccal f. The portion of the flange of a denture which occupies the vestibule of the mouth adjoining the cheek.

denture f. The nearly vertical extension from the body of a denture into any of the oral vestibules.

labial f. The portion of the flange of a denture which occupies the vestibule of the mouth adjoining the lips.

lingual f. The portion of the flange of a mandibular denture whch occupies the space adjacent to the tongue.

flank The side of the body between the ribs and the pelvis. Also called latus.

flap 1. A flat piece of tissue cut away from the

underlying parts but attached at one end; used to cover a defect in a neighboring part or the sawn end of a bone after amputation. **2.** A characteristic flapping movement of the hands in certain disorders.

bone f. In neurosurgery, a section of the skull attached to muscles and/or other structures which serve as a hinge.

liver f. See asterixis.

pedicle f. A piece of detached tissue (including skin and subcutaneous tissues) in which the attached end or base contains an adequate blood supply.

sliding f. A flap used to either lengthen or shorten a localized area of tissue.

flare Diffuse redness of the skin surrounding an injured point.

flaring of the alae nasi The enlargement of both nostrils during inspiration, due to contraction of the anterior and posterior dilatores naris muscles; a sign of dyspnea since it implies that greater than normal work is required for breathing.

flash 1. A sudden, brief, intense burst of light or heat. **2.** In dentistry, excess material squeezed out of the sections of a mold.

hot f. Sudden sensation of heat through the whole body; a vasomotor symptom of menopause.

flashback The spontaneous and unpredictable reversion of perceptual distortions resulting from having previously taken psychedelic drugs; it can last from several seconds to half an hour.

flashblindness Temporary loss of vision caused by exposure to intense light.

flask 1. A bottle with a narrow neck, used in the laboratory. **2.** A metal case or tube used in investing procedures.

casting f. Refractory flask.

crown f. A small dental flask.

dental f. A metal case in which a sectional gypsum mold is made for the purpose of shaping and curing resinous structures, such as dentures or other resinous restorations.

Dewar f. A glass vessel, often silvered, with two walls; used for maintaining materials at constant temperature or, more usually, at low temperature. Also called vacuum flask.

Erlenmeyer f. A flask with a conical body, broad base, and a narrow neck.

Florence f. A globular long-necked bottle of thin glass used for holding water or other liquid in laboratory work.

refractory f. A metal tube in which a refractory mold is made for casting metal dental restorations or appliances; more commonly known as a casting ring.

vacuum f. See Dewar flask.

volumetric f. A flask calibrated to contain or to

flatfoot

flatworm

(Schistosoma mansoni)

flavin adenine dinucleotide

rat flea
(Xenopsylla cheopis)

normal curve

flexion

sacrum

cephalic flexure

cervical flexure

6 week embryo

caudal flexure

hepatic flexure

splenic flexure

transverse colon

deliver a definite amount of liquid.

flasking In dentistry, the investing of the cast and a wax denture prior to molding the denture-base material into the form of the denture.

flatfoot Condition marked by varying degrees of diminution or depression of the longitudinal arch of the foot, resulting in impairment of its weight-bearing capability; it may be congenital or acquired. Also called pes planus; weak or splay foot.

flatulence Excessive quantities of gas in the stomach and intestines, causing distention.

flatulent Relating to flatulence.

flatus Intestinal gas expelled through the rectum.

flatworm Any member of the phylum Platyhelminthes; e.g., tapeworms and flukes.

flavin Any of various nitrogenous yellow pigments present in numerous plant and animal tissues.

  f. adenine dinucleotide (FAD) A nucleotide containing riboflavin which participates as a coenzyme in oxidation-reduction reactions.

  f. mononucleotide (FMN) A cofactor containing riboflavin in cellular oxidation-reduction systems.

Flavivirus A genus of arthropod-borne viruses (family Togaviridae) that cause diseases such as yellow fever, dengue, and encephalitis. Formerly classified as arbovirus, group B.

Flavobacterium A genus of bacteria; gram-negative rods which, when motile, move by means of flagella located around the mouth opening; they characteristically produce yellow, orange, red, or yellow-brown pigments; some species are pathogenic.

flavoenzyme Any enzyme having a flavin nucleotide as coenzyme.

flavor 1. The distinctive taste of any substance. 2. Inert substance added to a pharmaceutical preparation to give it a pleasing taste.

flea A blood-sucking insect of the genus *Pulex*.

  rat f. A general term for *Pulex fasciatus, Pulex pallidus, Typhlopsylla musculi,* and *Xenopsylla cheopis;* parasitic on the rat and a vector for bubonic plague.

  sand f. See chigoe.

flesh 1. Muscular tissue and other soft tissues of the body excluding the viscera. 2. The meat of animals. 3. Excess tissue; stoutness.

  goose f. Temporary rough appearance of the skin caused by contraction of the arrectores pilorum muscles (erectors of the hair) as a reaction to cold, fear, or other stimuli. Also called goose pimples or bumps.

  proud f. Excessive granulation on the surface of a wound or ulcer.

flex To bend or approximate two parts which are united by a joint.

flexibilitas cerea See cerea flexibilitas.

fleximeter Instrument used to measure the degree of flexion possible in a joint.

flexion 1. The act of bending a limb at a joint so that its proximal and distal parts are brought together; the bending forward of the spine. 2. The condition of being bent.

  palmar f. Flexion at the wrist, causing the hand to be bent toward the anterior surface of the forearm.

  plantar f. Flexion at the ankle joint, causing the foot to be bent downward.

flexor A muscle that flexes a joint; see table of muscles.

flexura Latin for a bend.

flexure A bend.

  caudal f. The bend at the caudal end of the embryo. Also called sacral flexure.

  cephalic f. The bend at the cephalic region of the embryo. Also called cranial flexure.

  cervical f. The bend at the junction of the embryonic brain and spinal cord.

  cranial f. See cephalic flexure.

  hepatic f. The bend between the ascending and transverse colon, near the liver.

  pontine f. A concave flexure dividing the rhombencephalon portion of the embryonic brain into anterior and posterior halves.

  sacral f. See caudal flexure.

  splenic f. The bend between the transverse and descending colon, near the spleen. See also splenic flexure syndrome.

floating Unattached; unduly movable.

floating kidney See under kidney.

floating rib See under rib.

floccillation Aimless plucking at the bedclothes, occurring in delirious patients. Also called carphologia; crocidismus.

flocculation The formation of flaky masses or precipitation in a solution being tested.

flocculent 1. A fluid containing irregularly shaped fluffy particles. 2. In bacteriology, denoting a liquid culture containing small adherent masses of bacteria.

flocculus Latin for small tuft; in anatomy, the small lobule of the posterior lobe of the cerebellum, which adjoins the middle cerebellar peduncle and is continuous with the nodule of the vermis.

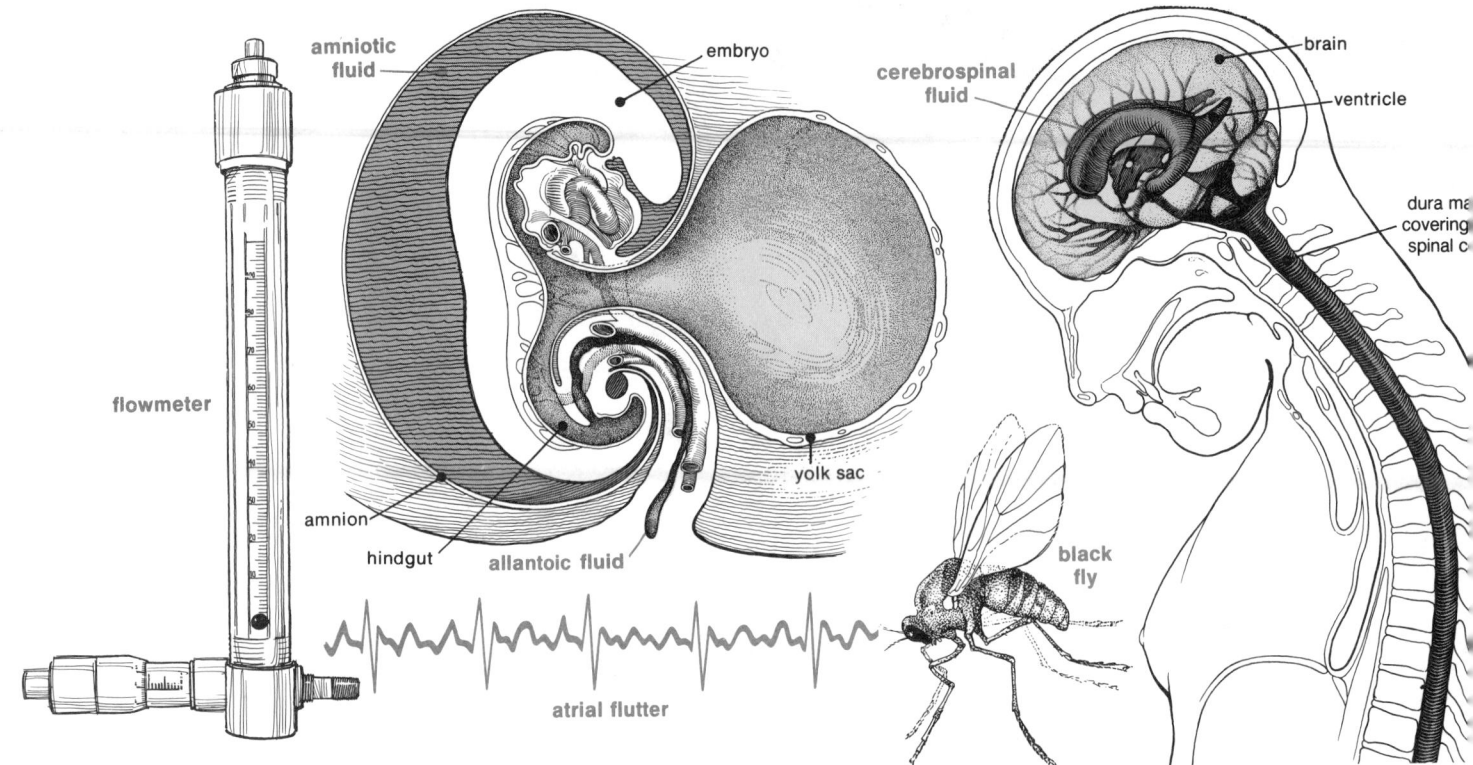

flowmeter

amniotic fluid

embryo

cerebrospinal fluid

brain

ventricle

dura mater covering spinal cord

amnion

hindgut

allantoic fluid

yolk sac

black fly

atrial flutter

---

flood 1. To bleed profusely from the uterus, as after childbirth. 2. Colloquial term for a profuse menstrual flow.

flora Plant life.

　intestinal f. The bacteria in the intestinal contents.

florid 1. Denoting a flushed appearance, as of the skin. 2. Having a bright red color, as of a lesion.

floss 1. To use thread (dental floss) or ribbon (dental tape) to remove particles from spaces between teeth. 2. Dental floss.

flow 1. To circulate; to move freely. 2. Menstrual discharge.

　effective renal plasma f. (ERPF) The amount of plasma passing through the kidneys as measured by clearance of *p*-aminohippurate.

flowers In chemistry, a powdery mineral substance produced by condensation or sublimation.

　f. of zinc Zinc oxide.

flowmeter Device used to measure the flow of liquids in vessels.

floxuridine (5-FUDR) 5-Fluoro-2′-deoxyuridine; a derivative of fluorouracil; used in the treatment of gastrointestinal cancer.

flu A general term given to many brief illnesses presumed to be caused by viruses, mostly the influenza virus; symptoms usually include sudden onset of fever, shivering, headache, muscular aches, and malaise; fever generally lasts three to four days.

fluctuant Having a yielding feel to palpation, suggesting a liquid center.

fluctuate 1. To vary irregularly or change from time to time. 2. To undulate or move in waves.

fluctuation 1. A variation. 2. A wavelike motion produced when a body cavity filled with fluid is palpated.

fluid 1. Any nonsolid substance, either liquid or gas. 2. Flowing.

　allantoic f. The fluid within the allantoic cavity.

　amniotic f. The fluid in the amnion in which the fetus floats.

　cerebrospinal f. (CSF) The fluid filling the ventricles of the brain and the subarachnoid spaces of the brain and spinal cord.

　extracellular f. (ECF) The body fluid outside of the cells, comprised of interstitial fluid, blood, plasma, and lymph; approximately 20% of body weight.

　follicular f. An albuminous fluid secreted by the granulosa (follicular) cells in a developing ovarian follicle; it creates intercellular spaces which eventually give rise to a follicular cavity, the antrum. Also called liquor folliculi.

　infranatant f. The clear liquid that settles on the bottom of a container after separation from an insoluble liquid or solid through the action of gravity or a centrifugal force.

　interstitial f. Fluid lying in the spaces between cells; comprises the major part of extracellular fluid.

　intracellular f. The fluid within the tissue cells, constituting about 40% of the body weight.

　intraocular f. The fluid within the anterior and posterior chambers of the eye.

　seminal f. See semen.

　supernatant f. The clear fluid that settles on top of the contents of a vessel after separating from an insoluble liquid or solid through normal gravity or a centrifugal force.

fluidextract An alcohol solution of a vegetable drug containing one gram of the active principle of the drug in each milliliter.

fluidglycerate A pharmaceutical preparation containing approximately 50% by volume of glycerin and one gram of the active principle of the specific drug in each milliliter.

fluidram, fluidrachm A teaspoonful; ⅛ of a fluid ounce; either of two units of liquid capacity: (a) in the U.S. Customary System, the equivalent of 0.225 cubic inches; (b) in the British Imperial System, the equivalent of 0.2167 cubic inches.

fluke Common name for species of the class Trematoda (flatworms), especially the parasitic variety.

　blood f. Fluke of the genus *Schistosoma*, parasitic in the mesenteric-portal blood stream and the vesical and venous plexuses.

　Chinese liver f. A fluke parasitic in the bile ducts. Also called *Clonorchis sinensis*.

　intestinal f. A large fluke parasitic in the intestines. Also called *Fasciolopsis buski*.

　liver f. See *Fasciola hepatica*.

　lung f. A fluke parasitic in the lungs. Also called *Paragonimus westermani*.

flumina pilorum The lined pattern along which hairs grow on the head and throughout the body. Also called hair streams.

fluocinolone acetonide A fluorinated corticosteroid used topically in the treatment of certain dermatoses.

fluorescein A material used, because of its fluorescence, as a marker, as in immunofluorescent studies and in circulatory studies, particularly of the eye.

　sodium f. An orange-red powder used in solution to detect lesions of the cornea.

fluorescence The ability of certain substances to emit light, to become self-luminous, while exposed to direct light rays from another source, especially ultraviolet rays.

fluoridate To add fluorine salts to a water supply. Also called fluorinate.

fluoridation The addition of fluoride (fluorine compound) to the public water supply to prevent tooth decay.

fluoride A compound containing fluorine.

fluorine A gaseous chemical element of the halogen group; symbol F, atomic number 9, atomic weight 19.

fluorometer A device for detecting and measuring fluorescence. Also called fluorimeter.

fluoroscope A type of x-ray apparatus in which x rays going through part of the body strike upon a fluorescent screen of calcium tungstate, rendering an image on the screen of varying densities of the body.

fluoroscopic Relating to fluoroscopy.

fluoroscopy Direct examination of the inner parts of the body by use of the fluoroscope.

fluorosis Abnormal condition caused by an excessive intake of floride, manifested mainly by mottling of the enamel of the teeth.

fluorouracil (5-FU) 5-Fluorouracil; an antineoplastic drug, $C_4H_3FN_2O_2$, used in the treatment of gastrointestinal cancer and topically for the treatment of multiple premalignant actinic keratoses.

flush 1. To wash with a brief gush of water. 2. Sudden redness of the skin, especially of the face and neck.

　hot f. Sudden redness of the face and neck with a sensation of heat; a vasomotor symptom of menopause.

flutter Rapid vibrations or pulsations.

　atrial f. Extremely rapid but rhythmic contractions of the cardiac atria, usually at a rate of 240 to 300 per min, often producing "sawtooth" waves in the electrocardiogram. Also called auricular flutter.

　auricular f. See atrial flutter.

　diaphragmatic Rapid contractions of all or part of the diaphragm.

　ventricular f. Rapid contractions of the ventricles producing electrocardiographic complexes that have a regular undulating pattern without distinct QRS and T waves.

flutter-fibrillation An electrocardiographic pattern of atrial activity showing both flutter and fibrillation.

flux 1. Excessive discharge of any bodily secretion. 2. Denoting the movement of ions or molecules through a membrane. 3. In dentistry, a substance that increases fluidity of molten metal, thereby promoting fusion; also used to remove oxides from metal surfaces during soldering of dental prostheses.

fly A winged insect of the family Muscidae.

　black f. A small, dark, biting gnat, *Simulium pecuarium* (family Simuliidae); vector of onchocerciasis. Also called buffalo gnat.

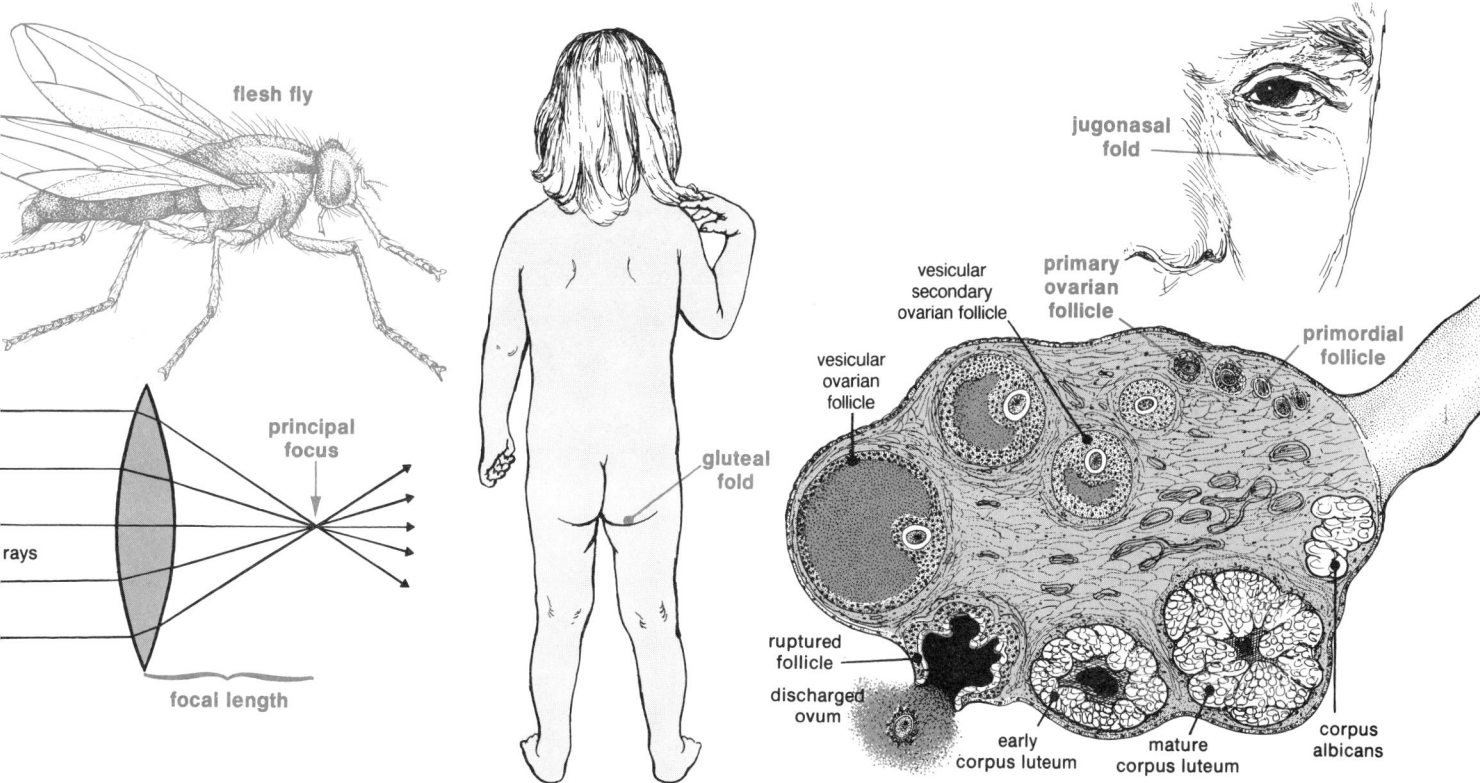

flesh fly

principal focus

rays

focal length

gluteal fold

jugonasal fold

vesicular secondary ovarian follicle

primary ovarian follicle

primordial follicle

vesicular ovarian follicle

ruptured follicle

discharged ovum

early corpus luteum

mature corpus luteum

corpus albicans

flesh f. A fly whose larvae (maggots) develop in putrifying or living tissues.

fruit f. *Drosophila melanogaster,* a fly used extensively in genetic studies.

mangrove f. Species of the genus *Chrysops;* vectors of *Loa loa.*

sand f. A small biting fly of the genus *Phlebotomus;* vectors of leishmaniasis.

Spanish f. See cantharis.

tsetse f. See *Glossina.*

foam 1. Collection of numerous small bubbles on the surface of a liquid. 2. To produce such bubbles.

focal Relating to a focus; localized.

focal glomerulonephritis See under glomerulonephritis.

focal length (f) The distance from a point where the image of a distant object is formed (focal point) to a point in or near the lens.

focal plane The plane at right angles to the optical axis at the focal point.

focal point The point where the light rays coming from a distant object converge after passing through a lens, coming to a focus and forming an image.

foci Plural of focus.

focimeter Instrument used to determine the vergence power of a lens or system of lenses.

focus, *pl.* **foci** 1. The point in an optical system where light rays meet. 2. To adjust a lens system to produce a distinct, clear image. 3. The principal site of a disease.

conjugate foci Two points in an optical system so interrelated that rays originating at one point are focused at the other, and vice versa.

Ghon's f. Ghon's primary lesion; see under lesion.

principal f. The real or virtual axial meeting point of rays passing into a lens parallel to its optical axis.

real f. The point at which convergent light rays meet forming a real image.

virtual f. The point at which the backward extensions of diverging light rays intersect, forming a virtual image.

fog 1. Hazy or dense appearance of a roentgenogram caused by stray radiation, accidental exposure to light, subjection to unusual temperatures or chemical actions, or the use of outdated film. 2. To subject a film to such conditions.

fogging In ophthalmology, the deliberate undercorrection of myopia (nearsightedness) or overcorrection of hyperopia (farsightedness); a procedure used to prevent unconscious accommodation of the eye during the testing for astigmatism.

foil An extremely thin, pliable sheet of metal.

gold f. A foil of pure gold used in dentistry to restore carious or fractured teeth.

platinum f. A foil of pure platinum used in dentistry, because of its high fusing point, as a matrix for soldering procedures and to provide the internal forms of porcelain restorations.

Foix's syndrome See cavernous sinus syndrome.

folate A salt of folic acid.

fold The doubling of a part upon itself.

axillary f. One of the musculocutaneous ridges bounding the armpit anteriorly and posteriorly.

glosso-epiglottic f.'s Three folds of mucous membrane reflected from the base of the tongue onto the epiglottis; the fold in the midline is called the median glosso-epiglottic fold and those to the sides are called the lateral glosso-epiglottic folds.

gluteal f. A fold marking the posterior upper limit of the thigh and the lower limit of the buttock.

jugonasal f. A fold indicating the confluence of the orbicularis oculi and the quadratus labii muscles.

lacrimal f. A fold of mucous membrane in the nasal cavity at the lower end of the nasolacrimal duct; it keeps air from entering the lacrimal sac when the nose is blown.

medial umbilical f. The fold of peritoneum that covers the obliterated umbilical artery as it ascends from the pelvis toward the umbilicus.

median umbilical f. The fold of peritoneum that covers the median umbilical ligament extending from the apex of the urinary bladder to the umbilicus. Also called urachal fold.

neural f. A fold of ectoderm forming the lateral margin of the embryonic neural groove.

rectovesical f. The peritoneal fold that bounds the rectovesical pouch in the male.

salpingopharyngeal f. One of the vertical ridges of mucous membrane extending from the lower portion of the elevation of the auditory tube along the wall of the pharynx on either side.

sublingual f. The fold formed by the mucous membrane of the floor of the mouth, elevated by the sublingual gland and containing its excretory ducts.

transverse f.'s of rectum The three or four crescentric transverse folds in the rectum. Also called rectal valves.

urachal f. See median umbilical fold.

Vater's f. A fold located above the greater papilla of the duodenum.

vocal f. The true vocal cord; it contains the vocal ligament.

foliaceous, foliate Resembling a leaf.

folic acid A constituent of the vitamin B complex; extracted from liver and green leaves, and produced synthetically; deficiency may occur in malnourished individuals, alcoholics, and in malabsorption states and result in a megaloblastic anemia. Also called pteroylglutamic acid.

folic acid antagonist One of a group of compounds that neutralize the action of folic acid; used in the treatment of neoplastic disorders, especially of the hematopoietic system.

folie French for madness or psychosis.

f. à deux Psychosis affecting two closely associated persons in which they share the same delusions. Also called communicated or double insanity.

f. gémellaire Psychosis occurring simultaneously in twins who are not necessarily closely associated at the time.

folinic acid A reduced form of folic acid. Also called citrovorum factor; leucovorin.

folium, *pl.* **folia** A broad thin anatomical structure.

folia of the cerebellum The numerous long parallel infoldings of the cerebellar cortex.

follicle 1. A somewhat spherical mass of cells usually containing a cavity. 2. A small crypt, such as the depression in the skin from which the hair emerges. 3. A small circumscribed body.

atretic ovarian f. A follicle that degenerates before reaching maturity.

graafian f. See vesicular ovarian follicle.

hair f. A saclike invagination of the epidermis from which the root of a hair develops.

lymph f. A small mass of lymphoid tissue, as seen in the mucosa of the gut. Also called lymphatic nodule.

lymphoid f. A collection of proliferating palestaining cells in lymphoid tissue, as in the cortex of lymph nodes.

nabothian f. A cyst resulting from obstruction of a mucous gland of the uterine cervix. Also called nabothian cyst.

ovarian f. The ovum together with its surrounding cells, at any stage of development, located in the cortex of the ovary.

primary ovarian f. A developing follicle in the ovary before the appearance of a fluid-filled antrum; it is composed of a growing primary oocyte and a single or several layers of cuboidal follicular cells surrounded by a sheath of stroma (theca); it usually develops during adolescence.

primordial f. An immature ovarian follicle consisting of the original primordial germ cell, the oogonium, and a thin single layer of squamous (flattened) follicular cells; at birth there are about 400,000 primordial follicles in each ovary; most undergo atresia.

sebaceous f. Oil gland of the skin.

solid secondary ovarian f. A follicle in the ovary in which follicular fluid is gradually accumulating between the follicular (granulosa) cells; it first ap-

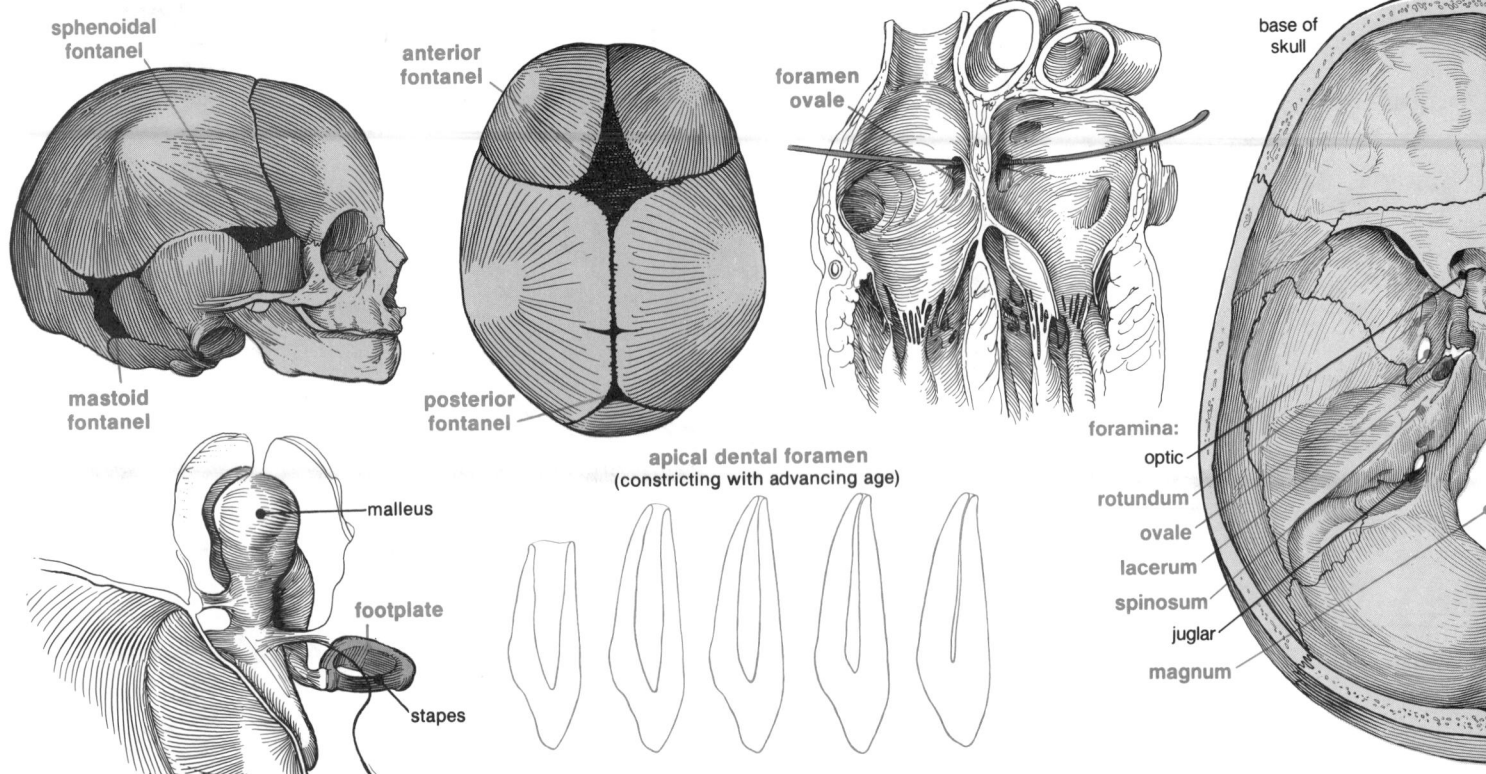

sphenoidal fontanel

anterior fontanel

foramen ovale

base of skull

mastoid fontanel

posterior fontanel

malleus

footplate

stapes

apical dental foramen
(constricting with advancing age)

foramina:

optic

rotundum

ovale

lacerum

spinosum

juglar

magnum

pears during puberty.

thyroid f. The minute components of the thyroid gland in which the thyroid hormone is stored.

vesicular ovarian f. A large mature follicle in the ovary in which the ovum (oocyte) attains full size (about four times that of the primordial germ cell); at this stage of development, the follicle migrates toward the surface of the ovary, causing a preovulatory swelling. Also called graafian follicle.

follicular 1. Having or resembling a follicle or follicles. 2. Growing out of follicles.

folliculitis Inflammation of hair follicles.

f. barbae Tinea barbae.

folliculoma 1. Granulosal cell tumor; see under tumor. 2. Cystic enlargement of a vesicular ovarian (graafian) follicle.

folliculosis Abnormally increased development of lymph follicles.

conjunctival f. A chronic condition, frequently found in children, marked by the presence of multiple tiny lymphatic nodules in the conjunctiva of the lower lids.

folliculus, *pl.* **folliculi** Follicle.

fomentation The therapeutic application of warmth and moisture.

fomes, *pl.* **fomites** Anything (clothing, toys, etc.) capable of transmitting the microorganisms causing a contagious disease.

fontanel, fontanelle Any of the membrane-covered spaces between the incompletely ossified cranial bones of an infant. Commonly called soft spot.

anterior f. A diamond-shaped fontanel located at the junction of the frontal, sagittal, and coronal sutures. Also called frontal or bregmatic fontanel.

anterolateral f. See sphenoidal fontanel.

bregmatic f. See anterior fontanel.

frontal f. See anterior fontanel.

mastoid f. The fontanel on either side at the junction of the mastoid angle of the parietal bone with the mastoid portion of the temporal bone and the occipital bone. Also called posterolateral fontanel.

posterior f. A triangular fontanel at the union of the lambdoid and sagittal sutures. Also called occipital fontanel.

posterolateral f. See mastoid fontanel.

sphenoidal f. An irregularly shaped fontanel located on either side at the junction of the frontal bone with the sphenoidal angle of the parietal bone, the squamous portion of the temporal bone and the greater wing of the sphenoid bone. Also called anterolateral fontanel.

fonticulus Fontanel.

food Nourishment, usually of plant or animal origin. Also called aliment.

convenience f. Food that is partially prepared for cooking so that the time of home preparation is shortened.

conventional f. Common food not subjected to unusual processing.

engineered f. Food made from vegetable or synthetic substances. Also called fabricated food.

enriched f. Food to which vitamins (thiamine, niacin, riboflavin) and iron have been added within specified limits. Also called fortified food.

fabricated f. See engineered food.

formulated f. Imitation of common food, such as an imitation dairy product, or new types of food; blended cereal grains, legumes, roots or tubers, and sources of proteins and calories frequently serve as bases.

fortified f. See enriched food.

food analog Engineered food product designed to look like a traditional food item such as chicken or bacon.

foot The termination of the lower extremity.

athlete's f. See tinea pedis.

ball of the f. The anterior padded portion of the sole of the foot.

burning feet Chronic condition marked by pain and burning sensations, especially in the soles of the feet.

cavus f. See clawfoot.

claw f. See clawfoot.

club f. See clubfoot.

drop f. See footdrop.

flat f. See flatfoot.

Friedreich's f. A foreshortened foot with a high arch and clawed toes, occurring in Friedreich's ataxia.

immersion f. A swollen state of the feet after prolonged immersion in cold water, as after shipwreck.

Madura f. Former name for maduromycosis.

march f. Painful condition of the feet after prolonged stress. Also called Deutschlander's disease.

splay f. See flatfoot.

trench f. Frostbite of the feet after prolonged standing in cold water, snow, or mud; sometimes seen in soldiers on trench duty.

foot and mouth disease A highly infectious disease of cattle, swine, and sheep; when it occurs in man (rarely), it is characterized by fever and a vesicular eruption of the palms, soles, and the oropharyngeal mucosa.

footcandle A unit of illumination on a surface one foot distant from a uniform point source of light of one candela, equal to one lumen per square foot; replaced in the International System of Units by the candela.

footdrop Paralysis or weakness of the dorsiflexor muscles of the foot and ankle causing the foot to fall and the toes to drag on the ground during walking. Also called toe drop.

footplate The base of the smallest ossicle (stapes) of the middle ear which fits in the oval window.

foramen, *pl.* **foramina** A natural opening through a bone or a membranous structure; a short passage.

aortic f. See hiatus, aortic.

apical dental f. The opening at the tip of the root of a tooth through which pass the vessels and nerves supplying the pulp.

carotid f. The inferior opening of the carotid canal giving passage to the internal carotid artery.

epiploic f. The opening connecting the two sacs of the peritoneum, namely the greater sac and the lesser sac (omental bursa). Also called Winslow's foramen.

ethmoidal f. One of two openings (anterior and posterior) in the orbit, giving passage to vessels and nerves.

external auditory f. See meatus, external auditory.

f. cecum The pit on the dorsal surface of the tongue representing the remains of the upper portion of the embryonic thyroglossal duct.

f. lacerum The opening between the apex of the petrous portion of the temporal bone and the body of the sphenoid bone; during life, it is closed with fibrous tissue, giving passage only to the small nerve of the pterygoid canal and a small meningeal branch of the ascending pharyngeal artery. Also called lacerated foramen.

f. of Luschka Lateral aperture of the fourth ventricle; see under aperture.

f. of Magendi Median aperture of the fourth ventricle; see under aperture.

f. magnum The large opening at the base of the skull through which passes the spinal cord. Also called great foramen.

f. of Monro See interventricular foramen.

f. ovale 1. The oval opening between the atria of the fetal heart. 2. A large opening in the great wing of the sphenoid bone, through which pass the third portion of the trigeminal nerve and the small meningeal artery.

f. quadratum See foramen of the vena cava.

f. rotundum An opening located in the great wing of the sphenoid bone, through which passes the maxillary nerve. Also called round foramen.

f. spinosum An opening located in the great wing of the sphenoid bone, transmitting the middle meningeal artery.

f. of the vena cava Opening in the diaphragm

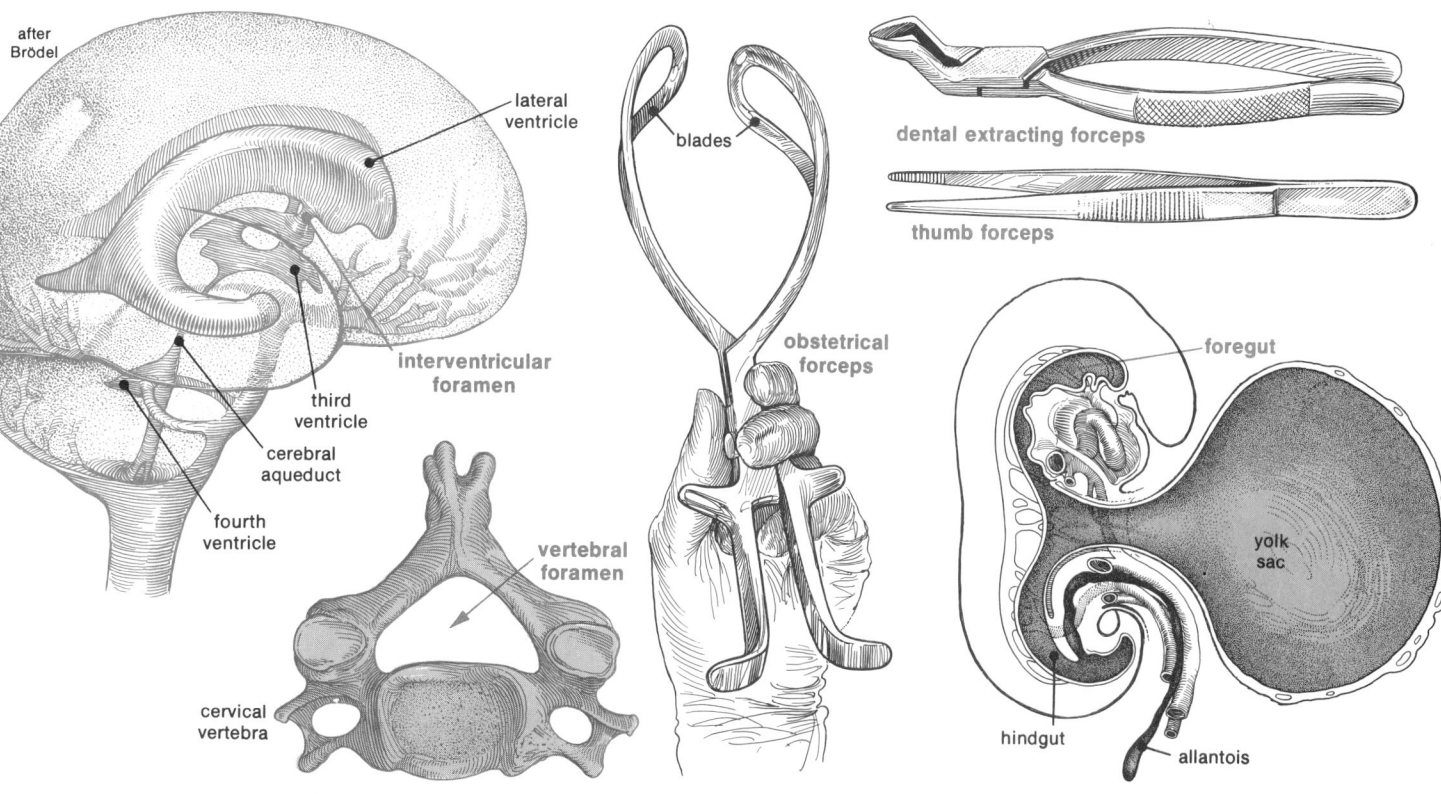

after Brödel

lateral ventricle

blades

dental extracting forceps

thumb forceps

interventricular foramen

third ventricle

cerebral aqueduct

fourth ventricle

obstetrical forceps

foregut

vertebral foramen

cervical vertebra

yolk sac

hindgut

allantois

giving passage to the inferior vena cava. Also called foramen quadratum.

greater sciatic f. A large opening bounded by the sacrum, the greater sciatic notch of the hipbone, and the sacrotuberous and sacrospinous ligaments.

incisal f. The relatively large opening in the midline of the hard palate just behind the central incisors; the opening of the nasopalatine canal.

inferior dental f. See mandibular foramen.

infraorbital f. The external opening of the infraorbital canal, on the anterior aspect of the maxilla.

interatrial f. primum **1.** The temporary opening of the embryonic heart between the right and left atria. Also called ostium primum. **2.** The abnormal persistence of such an opening in the adult heart.

interatrial f., secundum A secondary opening appearing in the embryonic heart between the right and left atria, just prior to the closure of the interatrial foramen primum. Also called ostium secundum.

interventricular f. An oval opening between the third and lateral ventricles of the brain. Also called foramen of Monro.

intervertebral f. One of several openings into the spinal canal formed by adjoining vertebrae.

jugular f. Opening located between the lateral portion of the occipital bone and the petrous portion of the temporal bone.

lesser sciatic f. An opening bounded by the lesser sciatic notch and the sacrotuberous and sacrospinous ligaments.

mandibular f. An opening located in the medial aspect of each ramus of the mandible. Also called inferior dental foramen.

mental f. One of two lateral openings on the body of the lower jaw, usually beneath the second bicuspid tooth. Also called mental canal.

obturator f. The large opening in the hipbone bounded by the pubis and ischium; it is almost completely closed by the obturator membrane except for a small gap (obturator canal) through which the obturator nerve and vessels pass as they leave the pelvis to enter the thigh.

optic f. See canal, optic.

palatine foramina Anterior and posterior openings on either side of the hard palate.

stylomastoid f. An opening on the petrous portion of the temporal bone, between the styloid and mastoid processes; it affords passage to the facial nerve and the stylomastoid artery.

supraorbital f. A canal or groove in the supraorbital margin of the frontal bone which gives passage to the supraorbital nerve and vessels. Also called supraorbital notch.

vertebral f. The space between the arch and the body of a vertebra.

Winslow's f. See epiploic foramen.

foramina Plural of foramen.

Forbes-Albright syndrome Combination of a profuse secretion of milk and absence of the menses, unassociated with recent pregnancy or with acromegaly; believed to be caused by overproduction of prolactin, as in some tumors of the pituitary gland.

force (F) Strength; capacity to produce work or motion, or cause physical change.

electromotive f. (EMF) Force causing the flow of electricity from one point to another, giving rise to an electric current.

f. of mastication Force applied by the muscles during the act of chewing. Also called masticatory force.

masticatory f. See force of mastication.

van der Waals' f.'s The nondescript, attractive forces between atoms or molecules other than electrostatic (ionic), covalent (sharing of electrons), or hydrogen bending (sharing a proton).

forceps An instrument resembling a pair of tongs, used for grasping, compressing, manipulating, or extracting tissue or specific structures.

alligator f. A long, slender forceps with small jaws, the lower of which is stationary.

Allis f. A forceps with serrated jaws for grasping tissues.

bone f. A strong forceps used for grasping and cutting bone.

bulldog f. A forceps for clamping cut blood vessels.

capsule f. A forceps used for extracting the lens in a cataract operation.

chalazion f. A thumb forceps with a flattened plate at the end of one arm and a ring on the other.

dental extracting f. A forceps used for grasping teeth in order to luxate and extract them from the alveolus.

hemostatic f. A forceps with a catch for locking the blades, used for grasping the cut end of a blood vessel to control hemorrhage.

mosquito f. A very small hemostatic forceps.

obstetrical f. A forceps used for grasping and making traction on the fetal head in difficult labor.

rongeur f. A strong biting forceps for gouging away bone.

thumb f. A forceps used by compression with thumb and forefinger for grasping soft tissue; used especially during suturing.

forearm The part of the upper extremity between the elbow and wrist. Also called antebrachium.

forebrain See prosencephalon.

forefinger See finger, index.

forefoot **1.** The front portion of the foot consisting of the toes and metatarsal bones. **2.** One of the front feet of a quadruped animal.

foregut The cephalic portion of the primitive digestive tract in the embryo. Also called headgut.

foremilk A thin, sticky secretion of the breasts occurring a few days before and after childbirth. Also called colostrum.

forensic Relating to or used in legal proceedings.

foreplay Sexual stimulation leading to sexual intercourse.

forepleasure Pleasurable excitement preceding orgasm.

foreskin See prepuce.

forewaters In obstetrics, the part of the amniotic sac that pouches into the cervix in front of the fetal head or presenting part.

form Shape; mold.

accolé f. Appliqué form.

appliqué f. A ring of young species of the malarial parasite *Plasmodium falciparum* which parasitize the marginal portion of red blood cells. Also called accolé form.

convenience f. In dentistry, a form modified beyond the basic to allow access of instrumentation for the preparation of a cavity or the insertion of the restorative material.

L-f. L-phase variant; see under variant.

resistance f. In dentistry, the shape given to the prepared cavity of a tooth to enable the restoration to withstand the stress of mastication.

retention f. In dentistry, the provision made in the prepared cavity of a tooth to prevent displacement of the restoration by lateral forces as well as the stress of mastication.

sickle f. See crescent, malarial.

formaldehyde A colorless, pungent, gaseous aldehyde, CH_2O, used in solution as a disinfectant and preservative.

formalin A 37% aqueous solution of formaldehyde. Also called formol.

formation **1.** The process of giving form or producing. **2.** Something that is formed.

personality f. The development or structure of the components of the personality.

reaction f. The development of conscious attitudes that are the opposite of certain unconscious components of infantile sexuality; e.g., excessive cleanliness as a reaction to anal interests.

reticular f. A collection of intermingled fibers and gray matter in the pons, the anterolateral portion of the medulla oblongata, and the cervical spinal cord. Also called reticular substance.

rouleaux f. The arrangement of red blood cells in groups resembling stacks of coins.

Fischer's projection formula (threose)

left and right groups project in front of plane of projection

top and bottom groups project behind the plane of projection

plane of projection

molecular formula
(methadone)

$C_{21}H_{27}NO$

structural formula
(methadone)

superior fornix
of conjunctiva

eyeball

inferior fornix
of conjunctiva

hypophyseal fossa

cranial
cavity

nasal
cavity

lacrimal
bone

maxillary
bone

lacrimal
fossa

orbit of eye

forme fruste, *pl.* **formes frustes** French expression for a partial or atypical form of a disease.

formic Relating to ants.

    f. acid A colorless caustic liquid, HCOOH, used in solution as an astringent and counterirritant; it occurs naturally in ants and other insects.

formication A paresthesia in which there is an abnormal tactile sensation of ants or other small insects crawling over the skin.

formiminoglutamic acid (FIGlu) An intermediate metabolite of histidine which can appear in the urine of folic acid-deficient individuals.

formula **1.** A symbolic representation of the composition of a chemical substance. **2.** An established group of symbols that express a concept. **3.** A recipe of ingredients in fixed proportion; e.g., a milk mixture for feeding an infant. **4.** A prescription containing directions for the preparation of a medicine.

    Arneth f. A formula that expresses the approximate ratio of polymorphonuclear neutrophils in normal individuals, based on the number of lobes in the nuclei, as follows: 1 lobe, 5%; 2 lobes, 35%; 3 lobes, 41%; 4 lobes, 17%; 5 lobes, 2%.

    Bazett's f. A formula for correcting the observed electrocardiogram $Q - T$ interval for cardiac rate; corrected $Q - T = Q - T \sec/\sqrt{R - R} \sec$.

    Bernhardt's f. A formula for determining the ideal weight, in kilograms, for an adult: the height in cm × the chest circumference in cm ÷ 240.

    DuBois f. Formula for determining the body's surface area from its weight and height; $A = W^{0.425} \times H^{0.725} \times 71.84$.

    Fischer's projection f. A two-dimensional representation of three-dimensional molecules in which the carbon chain is depicted vertically.

    Gorlin f. A formula for calculating the area of the orifice of a cardiac valve, based on the flow across the valve and the mean pressures in the chambers on either side of the valves.

    graphic f. See structural formula.

    Meeh-Dubois f. A formula for determining the body surface area from the height and weight of an individual: $A = W\ 0.425 \times H\ 0.725 \times$ constant 71.84 (A = surface area in cm^2, W = weight in kg, and H = height in cm).

    molecular f. A chemical formula depicting the number of atoms of each element in the molecules of a substance.

    spatial f. See stereochemical formula.

    stereochemical f. A formula depicting a spatial representation of the relative positions of the linked atoms, and the numbers of atoms of each element present in a molecule of a substance.

    structural f. A graphic chemical formula showing

the linkage of the atoms and groups of atoms, as well as their kind and number.

formulary A collection of formulas for the preparation of medicines.

formyl The radical —C(H)O of formic acid.

fornix, *pl.* **fornices** Any arched structure, or the space created by such a structure.

    f. of the cerebrum A harp-shaped, bilateral structure in the brain, composed of two posterior pillars (crura of the fornix), the body, and two anterior pillars (columns of the fornix); it is situated under the corpus callosum and is made up of white fibers arising from the hippocampus and terminating mainly in the mamillary bodies.

    f. of the conjunctiva The space formed by the reflection of the conjunctiva from the upper eyelid to the eyeball (superior fornix) and from the eyeball to the lower eyelid (interior fornix).

    f. of the vagina The space between the vaginal wall and the uterine cervix.

fossa, *pl.* **fossae** A pit or depression.

    acetabular f. A circular, nonarticular depression in the floor of the acetabulum; it lodges a mass of fat.

    amygdaloid f. The hollow between the anterior and posterior pillars of the fauces containing the tonsil.

    axillary f. The armpit.

    coronoid f. The depression on the anterior aspect of the lower end of the humerus where the coronoid process of the ulna rests during full flexion of the forearm.

    cranial f. One of three depressions (anterior, middle, and posterior) on the internal aspect of the base of the skull lodging the cerebrum and cerebellum.

    cubital f. The depression in front of the elbow. Also called bend of the elbow; antecubital space.

    f. ovalis **1.** A depression on the septal wall of the right atrium representing the site of the foramen ovale of the fetal heart. **2.** The saphenous opening in the upper thigh, 38 mm below and lateral to the pubic tubercle, giving passage to the great saphenous vein.

    glenoid f. The depression in the head of the scapula for articulation with the head of the humerus forming the shoulder joint.

    greater supraclavicular f. The triangular depression on each side of the neck above the clavicle, bounded by the lateral border of the sternocleidomastoid muscle, the clavicle, and the omohyoid muscle.

    hyaloid f. The concavity on the anterior aspect of the vitreous body in which the lens of the eye lies. Also called lenticular fossa.

    hypophyseal f. A pit on the sphenoid bone lodging the pituitary gland. Also called pituitary fossa.

    lacrimal f. One located in the medial wall of the orbit, formed by the frontal process of the maxilla and the lacrimal bone; it houses the lacrimal sac.

    lesser supraclavicular f. The space between the two heads of origin of the sternocleidomastoid muscle. Also called Zang's space.

    mandibular f. One of two depressions on the temporal bone that receives the condyle of the lower jaw.

    olecranon f. A depression on the back of the lower end of the humerus in which the olecranon process of the ulna rests when the elbow is extended.

    pituitary f. See hypophyseal fossa.

    popliteal f. The diamond-shaped space situated at the back of the knee.

    pterygoid f. The fossa between the lateral and medial pterygoid plates of the sphenoid bone.

    radial f. A depression on the anterior aspect of the humerus, the site of articulation with the radius.

    submandibular f. See fovea, submandibular.

    tonsillar f. The depression between the palatoglossal and palatopharyngeal arches occupied by the palatine tonsil.

fossette A small deep ulcer of the cornea.

fossula, *pl.* **fossulae** **1.** A small depression. **2.** One of several small depressions on the surface of the cerebrum.

Foster-Kennedy syndrome Ipsilateral optic atrophy with contralateral papilledema or choked disk; most commonly caused by a brain tumor at the base of the frontal lobe. Also called Kennedy's syndrome.

foundation The basis on which something is supported; a base.

    denture f. That portion of the oral structures which supports a denture.

fourchette Tissue connecting posteriorly the labia minora. Also called frenulum labiorum pudendi.

fovea, *pl.* **foveae** A small depression.

    f. centralis An area approximately 1.5 mm in diameter in the macula lutea of the retina; it is the area of greatest visual acuity.

    submandibular f. A pit on the inner surface of the lower jaw on each side which lodges the submandibular gland. Also called submandibular fossa.

foveate, foveated Pitted; having small depressions.

foveation The formation of a pitted scar, as in smallpox.

foveola A minute depression, fovea, or pit.

    f. of the coccyx A small depression or dimple often present in the skin over the tip of the coccyx.

blowout fracture

frontal bone

eyeball

maxillary sinus

comminuted fracture

depressed fracture

closed fracture

open fracture

talus   calcaneus

Pott's fracture

fibula

tibia

medial malleolus

lateral malleolus

calcaneus

ulna

radius

avulsion fracture   Colles' fractures

ulna

radius

transcervical fracture

hipbone

femur

gastric f.   One of the numerous small pits in the gastric mucosa at the bottom of which open the gastric glands.

granular f. of Pacchioni   One of many depressions in the inner surface of the skull, on either side of the superior sagittal sinus groove, in which are lodged the arachnoid granulations (pacchionian bodies).

foveolate   Having minute depressions or pits on the surface.

Fox-Fordyce disease   An uncommon disease of the apocrine glands affecting mainly women from puberty to menopause; characterized by numerous small, follicular, closely aggregated, flesh-colored, intensely pruritic papules in the armpits and on the breasts, pubic area, and perineum; thought to be due to poral closure of the apocrine gland.

foxglove   Any of various plants of the genus *Digitalis* from which the drug digitalis is prepared.

fraction   1. A quotient of two quantities. 2. In chemistry, a component of a substance separated by crystallization or distillation.

blood plasma f.   The separated components of plasma.

ejection f.   A measure of the ability of the left ventricle of the heart to expel blood.

filtration f. (FF)   The fraction of plasma entering the kidney that filters into the renal tubules; glomerular filtration rate/renal plasma flow.

fractionation   The breaking up of a total therapeutic dose of radiation into small fractions of low intensity given over a period of time, usually at daily or alternate daily intervals.

fracture (fx)   The breaking of a bone or cartilage.

articular f.   A fracture involving the joint surface of a bone.

avulsion f.   A breaking off of a small portion of bone at the site of attachment of a tendon or ligament.

basal skull f.   A fracture occurring at the base of the skull.

bimalleolar f.   See Pott's fracture.

blowout f.   A fracture of the floor of the orbit caused by a blow to the eye.

capillary f.   A hairline fracture.

closed f.   A fracture in which the skin is not broken. Also called simple fracture.

Colles' f.   A fracture of the lower end of the radius bone.

comminuted f.   A fracture in which the bone is splintered into several pieces.

compound f.   Former name for open fracture.

depressed f.   A fracture with inward displacement of the skull.

de Quervain's f.   A fracture-dislocation of the wrist; specifically, fracture of the scaphoid (navicular) bone, with dislocation of the lunate bone.

Dupuytren's f.   Fracture of the lower extremity of the fibula or lateral malleolus, with dislocation of the ankle joint.

extracapsular f.   A fracture near but outside of the joint capsule.

fatigue f.   See march fracture.

fissured f.   See linear fracture.

greenstick f.   An incomplete fracture in which one side of the bone is only bent.

impacted f.   A fracture in which one fragment is embedded in the substance of the other and fixed in that position.

incomplete f.   A fracture in which the line of fracture does not include the whole bone.

intracapsular f.   A fracture within a joint capsule.

linear f.   A fracture running parallel with the long axis of the bone. Also called fissured fracture.

longitudinal f.   A fracture in which the direction of the fracture line is along the axis of the bone.

march f.   A fracture of a metatarsal shaft, usually the second or third, caused by stress associated with prolonged weight bearing, as in walking or marching for long periods of time; seen most commonly in army recruits during basic training. Also called fatigue fracture.

oblique f.   A fracture running obliquely to the axis of the bone.

occult f.   A condition in which originally there is no evidence of a fracture, but after three or four weeks an x-ray image shows new bone formation.

open f.   A fracture that is accompanied by an open wound through which the broken bone may protrude. Formerly known as compound fracture.

periosteal f.   A fracture occurring beneath the periosteum, without displacement.

Pott's f.   A fracture-dislocation of the ankle joint; specifically, fracture of the medial malleolus of the tibia, with fracture of the lower extremity of the fibula (lateral malleolus) and dislocation of the ankle joint. Also called bimalleolar fracture.

simple f.   See closed fracture.

spiral f.   A breakage in which the fracture line

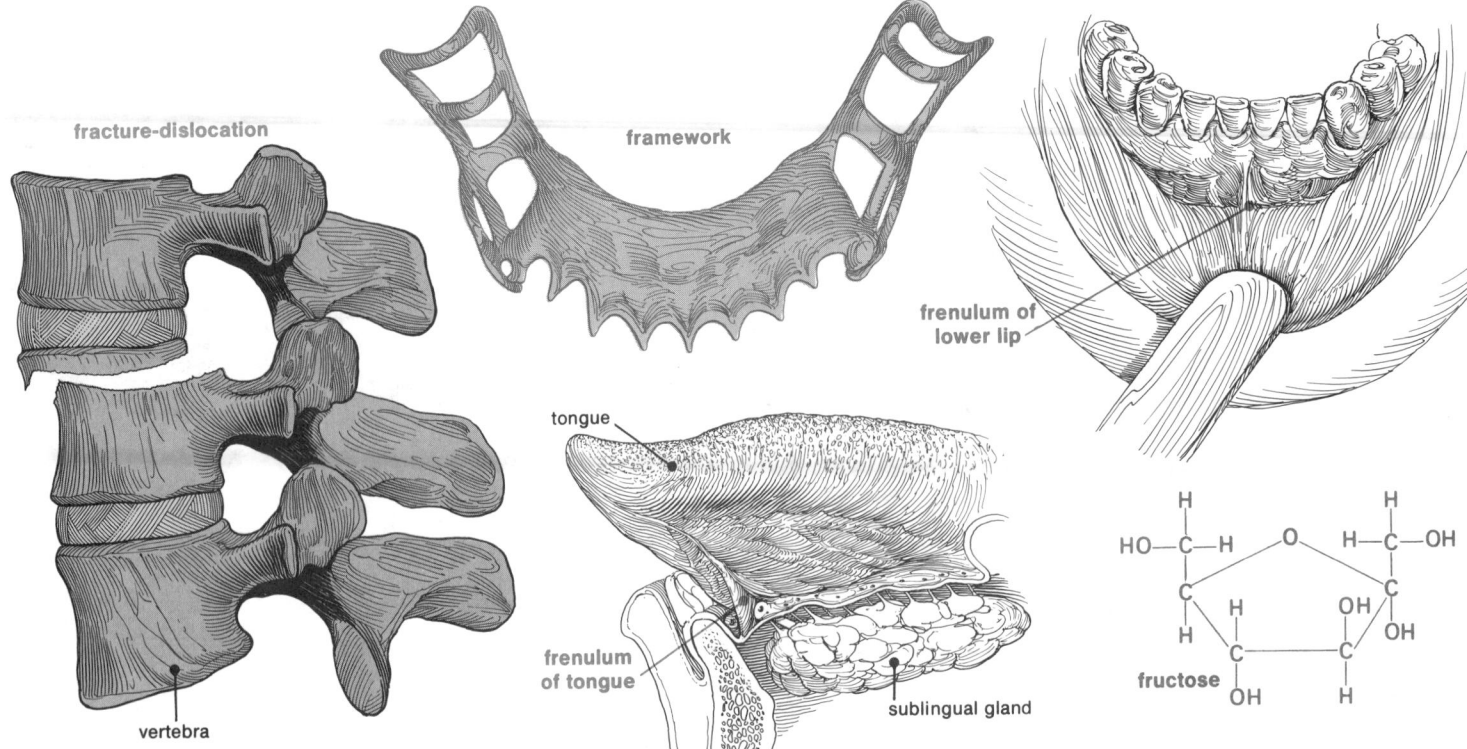

fracture-dislocation

framework

frenulum of
lower lip

tongue

frenulum
of tongue

sublingual gland

fructose

vertebra

runs spirally around the shaft of the bone.

sprain f. Avulsion fracture.

stellate f. A fracture with several break lines radiating from a central point.

strain f. The breaking off by sudden force of a piece of bone attached to a tendon or ligament.

stress f. A fracture occurring at the site of a muscle attachment and caused by sudden, violent, endogenous force; e.g., a closed fracture of the fibula in a runner.

supracondylar f. A fracture in the distal end of the humerus.

transcervical f. A fracture through the neck of the femur.

transcondylar f. A fracture through the condyles of the humerus.

transverse f. A fracture in which the break line runs perpendicular with the axis of the bone.

fracture-dislocation Dislocation and fracture of a bone near its articulation.

fragile X syndrome Inherited defect of the chromosome X causing mental retardation, large testicles, and big ears and chin in males and mild retardation in females.

fragility Brittleness; tendency to break or disintegrate.

erythrocyte f. Tendency of the red blood cells to break down due to mechanical or osmotic factors.

mechanical f. Tendency of the red blood cells to break down when subjected to mechanical trauma.

osmotic f. Tendency of the red blood cells to break down when exposed to increasingly hypotonic saline solutions.

fragment antigen binding (Fab) A segment of the IgG-antibody molecule, derived by papain treatment and reduction, containing one antibody reaction site.

frame A structure designed to immobilize or give support to a part.

Balkan f. An overhead bar supported from the floor or bedposts to suspend a fractured limb. Also called Balkan splint.

Foster f. A reversible bed similar to a Stryker frame.

Stryker f. A device that supports the patient and allows turning without individual motion of parts.

framework 1. Stroma. 2. In dentistry, the skeletal portion of a partial denture around which and to which the remaining portions of the prosthesis are attached.

francium An unstable radioactive metallic element; symbol Fr, atomic number 87, with mass number 223; the heaviest member of the alkali family of elements; the most stable of its isotopes has a half-life of 21 minutes.

freckle A brownish spot on the skin. Also called ephelis.

freeze-drying A method of tissue preparation in which the tissue specimen is instantly frozen and then the ice in the specimen is sublimed away in a high vacuum.

freeze-etching A method of tissue preparation in which the tissue specimen is instantly frozen (−190°C), fragments are splinted away, and then the ice is sublimed away in a vacuum to a depth of about 100 Å; it produces an etching effect especially suitable for the study of the inner surface of plasma membranes.

freezing, gastric Treatment of peptic ulcer by freezing the secretory cells of the stomach for the purpose of reducing or eliminating the production of acid gastric juice.

fremitus A vibration usually produced in the chest and felt on palpation.

pleural f. Vibration produced by the rubbing together of the roughened surfaces of the pleural membranes, as in pleurisy.

tactile f. Vibration felt by the hand when placed on the chest of a person speaking.

vocal f. Vibration in the chest produced by the spoken voice.

frenectomy The surgical removal of a frenum.

frenotomy The dividing of the frenulum of the tongue for the relief of tongue-tie.

frenulum A small fold of mucous membrane that extends from a fixed to a movable part and limits the motion of the movable part.

f. of the clitoris A fold connecting the undersurface of the clitoris with the labia minora.

f. of the lips Either one of the folds extending from the gums to the midline of the upper or lower lips. Also called frenulum labii.

f. of the prepuce A fold that unites the foreskin (prepuce) to the undersurface of the glans penis.

f. of the tongue A fold extending from the midline of the undersurface of the tongue to the floor of the mouth. Also called frenulum linguae.

frenum, *pl.* **frena** A fold of mucous membrane that limits the movement of a part, as the fold passing anteriorly from the gum to the inner surface of the lip.

frequency The number of regular recurrences of a given event.

critical flicker fusion f. Critical fusion frequency.

critical fusion f. The minimal number of intermittent or discontinuous visual stimuli per second that gives rise to a continuous visual sensation obliterating the flicker.

dominant f. The particular frequency appearing most frequently in an electroencephalogram (EEG).

friable Crumbly; easily torn or damaged.

fricative In phonetics, a sound produced by the forcing of breath through a narrow orifice, as the sounds of the letters f, v, s, z.

Friderichsen's syndrome Waterhouse-Friderichsen syndrome.

frigid 1. Very cold. 2. Abnormally lacking the desire for sexual intercourse; said chiefly of women. 3. Unable to achieve orgasm during sexual intercourse.

frigidity A psychologically based inability to respond adequately to a sexual relationship; said chiefly of women.

fringe Fimbria.

fringing Bulbous deformation of the calyx of the kidney and tortuous elongation of the stem sometimes seen in the early stages of tuberculosis of the kidney.

Fröhlich's syndrome Adiposogenital dystrophy; see under dystrophy.

Froin's syndrome Clear yellow color of the lumbar spinal fluid with increased protein content and rapid coagulation, indicating that the communication between the lumbar region and the cerebral ventricles has been cut off; seen in certain organic nervous diseases.

Frommel's syndrome Chiari-Frommel syndrome.

frons Latin for forehead.

frontal Relating to the forehead.

frostbite Local condition of varying degrees of severity caused by freezing of tissues upon exposure to extreme cold temperatures; may lead to gangrene; the fingers, toes, ears, and nose are usually affected Cf. chilblain.

frost, uremic Tiny flakes of urea sometimes seen on the skin of patients with uremia.

fructokinase A liver enzyme that promotes the reaction of ATP (adenosine triphosphate) and D-fructose to form fructose 6-phosphate.

fructosan A polyfructose, such as inulin, present in certain tubers. Also called levan; levulin; levulan.

fructose The sweetest of the simple sugars (monosaccharides) present in honey and fruits; in the body it is formed as one of the two products of sucrose hydrolysis; used intravenously as a nutrient replenisher. Also called fruit sugar; levulose.

fructosemia A rare genetically determined error of carbohydrate metabolism due to a deficiency of fructose-1-phosphate aldolase. Also called hereditary fructose intolerance.

fructosuria The presence of fructose in the urine; disorder of metabolism in which blood fructose levels are excessive and fructose appears in the urine.

frusemide See furosemide.

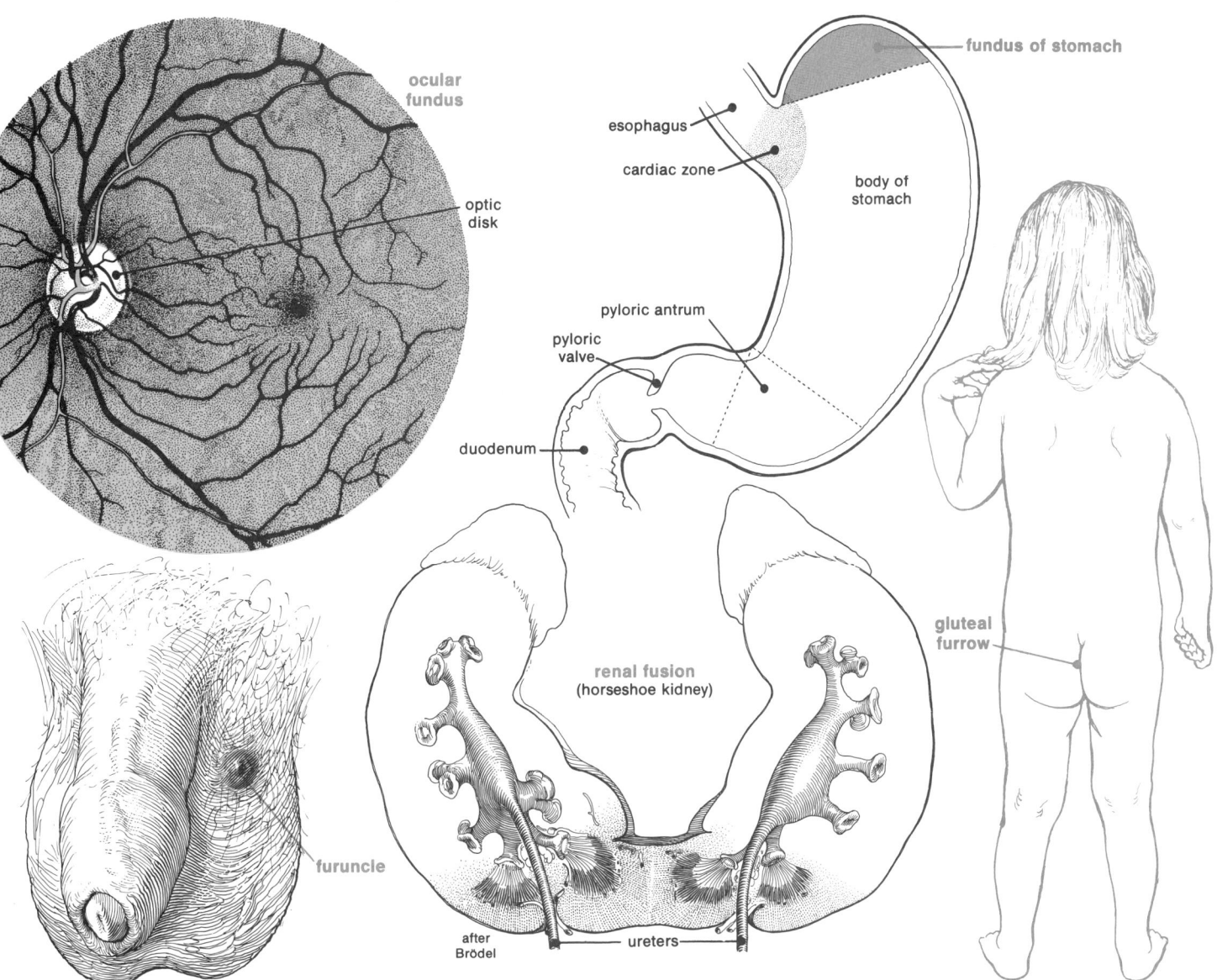

ocular fundus

optic disk

esophagus
cardiac zone
fundus of stomach
body of stomach
pyloric antrum
pyloric valve
duodenum
renal fusion (horseshoe kidney)
gluteal furrow
furuncle
after Brödel
ureters

frustration In psychology, the denial of gratification by reality.

fuchsin Rosaniline monohydrochloride; a bright red dye used in histology and bacteriology.

fugue A form of hysterical loss of memory and actual physical flight from a disturbing environment; when the normal mental state returns, the individual has no recollection of his actions during this period.

fulgurant Sudden, flashing, like lightning; usually said of pain.

fulguration Destruction of tissue by means of a high frequency electric current.

fulminating, fulminant Of sudden, violent onset and rapid course.

fumagillin A crystalline antibiotic used as an amebicide.

fumigation Disinfection by exposure to the fumes of a germicide.

fuming Releasing a visible vapor.

function 1. The natural or special type of activity which is proper for an organ or part. 2. To perform such an action. 3. The general properties of any substance.

fundal Relating to a fundus.

fundiform Sling-shaped.

fundoplication Suturing of the fundus of the stomach, as in the treatment of hiatal hernia.

fundus, *pl.* **fundi** The portion of a hollow organ farthest from, above, or opposite its opening.

f. of the stomach The dome-shaped part of the stomach above its junction with the esophagus.

f. of the uterus The rounded portion of the uterus above the openings of the uterine tubes.

ocular f. The posterior portion of the interior of the eye. See also eyeground.

funduscopy Ophthalmoscopy.

fungal Of or relating to a fungus.

fungate To grow rapidly or to assume a funguslike form.

fungemia Fungal disease disseminated through the blood stream.

Fungi A phylum (subkingdom Thallophyta) that includes saprophytic and parasitic plants, those unable to manufacture their own food because they lack photosynthetic pigments.

fungi Plural of fungus.

fungicide Any substance that destroys fungus.

fungiform Having the shape of a fungus.

fungistat An agent that inhibits the growth of fungi.

fungoid Resembling a fungus.

fungous Of or relating to a fungus.

fungus, *pl.* **fungi** A member of the phylum Fungi (subkingdom Thallophyta) characterized by lack of chlorophyll, asexual reproduction, and parasitic qualities.

funic Of or relating to the umbilical cord.

funicle A small cordlike structure.

funicular 1. Having a cordlike appearance. 2. Relating to the umbilical cord.

funiculitis 1. Inflammation of the spermatic cord. 2. Inflammation of the portion of a spinal nerve located within the intervertebral canal.

funiculus, *pl.* **funiculi** 1. One of the three main divisions or columns of white matter on either side of the spinal cord, called anterior, lateral, and posterior. 2. The spermatic cord. 3. The umbilical cord.

funiform Cordlike.

funis 1. The umbilical cord. 2. A cordlike structure.

funnel A conical vessel with a tube extending from its apex; used for pouring liquids, filtering, etc.

Buchner f. A porcelain funnel consisting of an upper cylindrical portion and a lower conical part, separated by a perforated plate upon which filter paper can be fitted.

furfur, *pl.* **furfures** An epidermal scale.

furfuraceous Scaly; denoting a type of desquamation.

furosemide A powerful diuretic used orally or intravenously. Also called frusemide; Lasix®.

furrow A groove.

digital f. One of the grooves on the palmar surface of the fingers.

gluteal f. The groove between the buttocks.

palpebral f. The groove of the upper eyelid extending from the inner to outer canthi.

furuncle An abscess or pyogenic infection of a sweat gland or hair follicle, usually caused by *Staphylococcus aureus*. Also called boil.

furuncular Relating to or like a furuncle (boil).

furunculoid Like a furuncle (boil).

furunculosis A condition marked by the presence of numerous furuncles (boils).

fuscin The brown pigment of the retina.

fusiform Tapering at both ends.

fusion 1. The process of melting. 2. Joining together by surgery, as of a joint. 3. The integration into one perfect image of the images seen simultaneously by the two eyes. 4. The abnormal union of two adjacent parts.

renal f. The abnormal fusion of the kidneys; named according to either the shape or location; e.g., horseshoe kidney, cake or lump kidney, sigmoid kidney.

spinal f. The fusion of two or more vertebral segments in order to eliminate motion between them.

fusospirochetal Relating to the associated fusiform and spirochetal organisms.

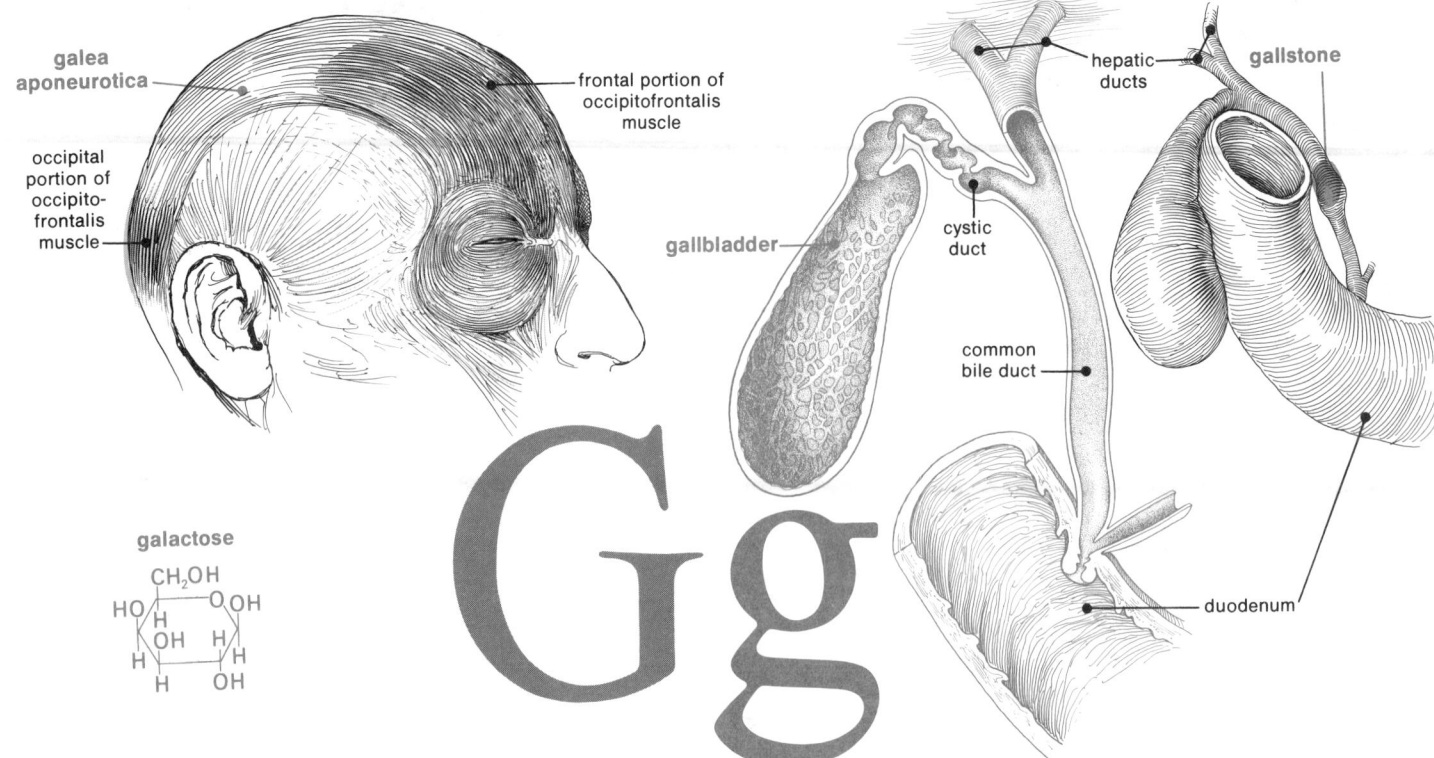

galea aponeurotica

occipital portion of occipitofrontalis muscle

frontal portion of occipitofrontalis muscle

hepatic ducts

gallstone

gallbladder

cystic duct

common bile duct

duodenum

galactose

$$CH_2OH$$

Gg

γ Gamma. For terms beginning with γ, see under specific term.

gadolinium A silvery-white metallic rare-earth element; symbol Gd, atomic number 64, atomic weight 157.25.

gag **1.** To retch; to cause to retch. **2.** An instrument placed between the upper and lower teeth to keep the mouth open during operations on the tongue or throat.

gain **1.** To build up an increase; to acquire. **2.** The ratio of increase of output current, voltage, or power over input; the amplification factor of an electronic circuit.

epinosic g. See secondary gain.

paranosic g. See primary gain.

primary g. The alleviation of anxiety provided by a neurotic illness or symptom. Also called paranosic gain.

secondary g. The additional indirect satisfaction or advantage (e.g., manipulating other people or receiving monetary reward) derived from a neurotic illness or symptom. Also called epinosic gain.

Gaisböck's syndrome Hypertension and polycythemia without splenomegaly, occurring in middle aged white males; the polycythemia is relative, with normal red blood cell mass but decreased plasma volume.

gait A manner of walking or running.

antalgic g. A self-protective limp due to pain.

ataxic g. An unsteady, irregular gait.

cerebellar g. A staggering gait with a tendency to fall, indicative of cerebellar disease; "drunken gait."

festinating g. Festination.

high steppage g. A gait in which the foot is raised high and brought down suddenly, the whole sole striking the ground in a flapping fashion.

tabetic g. A slapping gait characteristic of tabes dorsalis.

galactacrasia Abnormal composition of human milk.

galactagogue An agent that promotes the flow of milk.

galactan Any of several carbohydrates that yield galactose on hydrolysis.

galactic Relating to milk; inducing the flow of milk.

galactoblast One of numerous large, round bodies containing fat droplets, present in colostrum; thought to be a modified leukocyte. Also called colostrum corpuscle.

galactocele A tumor in the breast containing milk; caused by occlusion of a milk duct. Also called lactocele.

galactokinase An enzyme that, in the presence

of ATP (adenosine triphosphate), promotes the phosphorylation of galactose to galactose 1-phosphate.

galactophore A milk duct.

galactophorous Conveying milk.

galactophygous Diminishing or arresting the flow of milk. Also called lactifugal.

galactopoiesis Milk production.

galactopoietic **1.** Relating to the secretion of milk. **2.** Any agent that promotes the secretion of milk.

galactorrhea Excessive discharge of milk from the breasts after the child has been weaned, or unrelated to a recent pregnancy.

galactosamine A crystalline amino derivative of galactose. Also called chondrosamine.

galactosan One of several polysaccharides of galactose. Also called polygalactose.

galactoschesia, galactoschesis Suppression of milk secretion. Also called galactostasia; galactostasis.

galactose A white crystalline simple sugar, $C_6H_{12}O_6$, not found free in food; it is produced in the body by the digestion of lactose (milk sugar) and then converted into glucose for energy.

galactosemia Defect in metabolism of galactose, a nutrient of milk, in which the conversion of galactose to glucose is deficient; the disorder usually becomes evident soon after birth by feeding problems, mental and physical retardation, enlargement of the liver and spleen, and elevated blood and urine galactose levels; can be treated effectively by excluding milk from the diet.

galactosis The formation of milk.

galactostasia, galactostasis See galactoschesia.

galactosuria Presence of galactose in the urine.

galactotherapy Treatment with a milk diet.

galactozymase A starch-hydrolyzing enzyme present in milk.

galea **1.** A helmet-shaped structure. **2.** A form of head bandage.

g. aponeurotica The aponeurosis of the scalp; it covers the upper part of the skull, connecting the frontal and occipital bellies of the occipitofrontal muscle. Also called epicranial aponeurosis.

galeatomy Surgical cutting of the epicranial aponeurosis (galea aponeurotica).

galena See lead sulfide.

galeophobia Morbid fear of cats.

gall **1.** Bile. **2.** An erosion.

gallamine triethiodide A compound used as a skeletal muscle relaxant.

gallbladder A pear-shaped sac which stores bile and is situated under the liver.

hourglass g. Congenital abnormality of the gallbladder in which a septum divides it into two functioning halves.

strawberry g. Gallbladder in which the mucosa is red and congested and dotted with yellowish deposits of cholesterol.

gallium A rare metallic element; symbol Ga, atomic number 31, atomic weight 69.72; liquid near room temperature.

gallium-67 (^{67}Ga) A radionuclide used to detect inflammatory or metastatic lesions.

gallium-68 (^{68}Ga) A positron-emitting isotope of gallium, used in bone scanning to detect metastatic bone lesions; has a 68-minute half-life.

gallon A unit of liquid volume or capacity in the U. S. Customary System, equal to four quarts or 231 cubic inches; it is the equivalent of 3.7853 liters.

gallop A triple or quadruple cadence of heart sounds resembling the canter of a horse, heard on auscultation, due to the addition of a third and/or fourth heart sound. Also called cantering or gallop rhythm.

atrial g. Presystolic gallop sound related to atrial contraction, occurring in late diastole and designated as a fourth heart sound.

presystolic g. Atrial gallop.

protodiastolic g. See ventricular gallop.

summation g. Atrial and ventricular gallop sounds occurring simultaneously.

ventricular g. Third heart sound occurring in early diastole (0.14 to 0.16 seconds after the second heart sound). Also called protodiastolic gallop.

gallstone A stone formed in the gallbladder or a bile duct, thought to be due to a defect in composition of the bile.

cholesterol g. A gray-yellow crystalline translucent stone occurring singly, spherical (when small), or egg-shaped (when large) and reaching a size up to 6 cm in diameter.

silent g. One that does not produce symptoms.

Galton's delta The middle triangular pattern of the lines of a fingerprint.

galvanic **1.** Relating to chemically produced direct current electricity. **2.** Having the effect of an electric shock.

galvanism Direct current electricity, especially when produced by chemical action.

galvanization The application of a direct electric current.

galvanize To stimulate with an electric current.

galvanocautery Cautery with a wire that has been heated with a galvanic current.

galvanocontractility The ability of a muscle to contract under direct current.

galvanofaradization The simultaneous applicaspinal cord

dorsal root ganglion

cochlear nerve

lateral ventricle

spiral ganglia of cochlea

caudate nucleus

claustrum

sympathetic ganglion

lentiform nucleus

insula

ction rain

basal ganglia

amygdaloid nucleus

cochlea

tion of continuous and interrupted electric currents.

galvanometer An instrument for measuring the strength of a current of electricity.

   Einthoven's string g. See string galvanometer.

   string g. A galvanometer designed to record the electrical potentials produced in the heart; the fore-runner of the electrocardiograph. Also called Ein-thoven's string galvanometer.

galvanopalpation The testing of cutaneous nerve responses by means of a weak electric current.

galvanoscope Instrument used for detecting the presence and direction of electric currents.

galvanosurgery Surgical procedure using a direct electric current.

galvanotherapy Treatment of disorders by the application of galvanic current. Also called galvan-otherapeutics.

galvanotonus Tonic muscular response to stim-ulation with an electric current.

gamete One of two sex cells that combines with another in true conjugation to form a zygote, from which a new organism develops.

gametocide Any agent destructive to gametes.

gametocyte A cell from which gametes are pro-duced by division; a spermatocyte or an oocyte.

gametogenesis The production of gametes (ova or spermatozoa).

gametogony, gametogonia Stage in the sexual cycle of protozoa in which gametocytes are formed.

gamma **1.** The third letter of the Greek alphabet, γ; used to indicate the third in a series. **2.** In chemical nomenclature, used to indicate: (a) the third carbon of an aliphatic chain; (b) the location opposite the alpha position in the benzene ring. **3.** Obsolete term for microgram.

gammagram A graphic record of the γ-rays emit-ted by a substance or tissue.

Gammaherpesvirinae Subfamily of viruses (family Herpesviridae) that are specific for either B or T lymphocytes and remain latent in lymphoid tissue. Also called lymphoproliferative virus group.

gammopathy General term for any disorder char-acterized by (a) an abnormal proliferation of anti-body-forming cells and (b) the presence of abnor-mally high levels of immunoglobulins, or any of their constituents, in the plasma and/or the urine; includes disorders such as multiple myeloma, heavy chain disease, and plasma cell leukemia.

   benign monoclonal g. (BMG) A condition marked by the presence of elevated levels of immu-noglobulins (IgG, IgA, or IgM) but, unlike other gammopathies, is asymptomatic and with no appar-ent abnormal proliferation of antibody-forming cells.

   monoclonal g. Gammopathy that involves only

one class and type of immunoglobulin.

   polyclonal g. Gammopathy that involves two or more classes and types of immunoglobulin.

gamogenesis Sexual reproduction.

ganciclovir Agent used in the treatment of cyto-megalovirus (CMV) infections.

ganglia Plural of ganglion.

gangliate, gangliated Having ganglia.

gangliectomy Surgical removal of a ganglion.

gangliform Resembling a ganglion.

ganglioblast An embryonic cell from which gan-glion cells develop.

ganglioma See ganglioneuroma.

ganglion *pl.* **ganglia, ganglions** **1.** A collection of nerve cell bodies located outside of the brain and spinal cord. **2.** A cystic swelling resembling a tumor, occurring on a tendon sheath or joint capsule.

   autonomic g. Any ganglion of the sympathetic and parasympathetic nervous systems.

   basal ganglia Ganglia located within the white matter of each cerebral hemisphere; they serve as important links along various motor pathways of the central nervous system; they include the caudate, lentiform, and amygdaloid nuclei and the claustrum.

   cardiac g. One of several ganglia in the cardiac plexus located between the arch of the aorta and the bifurcation of the pulmonary artery.

   celiac g. One of two large sympathetic ganglia in the upper part of the abdomen on either side of the aorta near the origin of the celiac artery. Also called solar ganglion.

   cervical g. One of three (superior, middle, and inferior) sympathetic ganglia in the neck.

   ciliary g. A parasympathetic ganglion lying be-hind the orbit between the optic nerve and the lateral rectus muscle.

   coccygeal g. An unpaired ganglion of the sym-pathetic trunk located on the anterior aspect of the tip of the coccyx. Also called ganglion impar.

   dorsal root g. A ganglion located on the dorsal root of each spinal nerve containing the cell bodies of the sensory neurons of the nerve. Also called spinal or posterior root ganglion.

   ganglia of glossopharyngeal nerve The two sensory ganglia (superior and inferior) situated on the glossopharyngeal nerve as it passes through the jugular foramen.

   ganglia of sympathetic trunk See paravertebral ganglia.

   g. impar See coccygeal ganglion.

   g. of vagus nerve, inferior A ganglion situated on the vagus nerve a short distance below the jugular foramen, in front of the transverse processes of the first and second cervical vertebrae.

   g. of vagus nerve, superior A ganglion situated

on the vagus nerve as it passes through the jugular foramen at the base of the skull.

   gasserian g. See trigeminal ganglion.

   geniculate g. A ganglion of the facial nerve.

   otic g. A parasympathetic ganglion located just below the foramen ovale medial to the mandibular nerve; its preganglionic fibers are derived from the glossopharyngeal nerve and its postganglionic fibers innervate the parotid gland. Also called Arnold's ganglion.

   parasympathetic ganglia Aggregations of nerve cell bodies of the parasympathetic nervous system; the ciliary, pterygopalatine, otic, and submandibular ganglia of the head and several others located near the organs of the thorax, abdomen, and pelvis.

   paravertebral ganglia Sympathetic ganglia lo-cated at intervals on each sympathetic trunk along the side of the vertebral column; generally there are 3 cervical, 12 thoracic, 4 lumbar, and 4 sacral. Also called ganglia of sympathetic trunk.

   posterior root g. See dorsal root ganglion.

   prevertebral ganglia The sympathetic ganglia situated in front of the vertebral column and form-ing the plexuses of the thorax and abdomen; distin-guished from the paravertebral ganglia, which lie along each side of the vertebral column.

   pterygopalatine g. The largest of the four para-sympathetic ganglia associated with cranial nerves of the head; it is located in the pterygopalatine fossa just posterior to the middle nasal concha; it sends postganglionic parasympathetic fibers to the lacri-mal glands, nose, oral cavity, and the upper-most part of the pharynx. Also called sphenopalatine gan-glion.

   semilunar g. See trigeminal ganglion.

   sphenopalatine g. See pterygopalatine ganglion.

   spinal g. See dorsal root ganglion.

   spiral g. of cochlea The ganglion of bipolar nerve cell bodies located within the modiolus of the internal ear; it sends fibers peripherally to the spiral organ of Corti and centrally to the cochlear nuclei of the brain stem.

   stellate g. A ganglion of the sympathetic trunk containing two components, the inferior cervical and the first thoracic ganglia, which are often fused.

   submandibular g. One of the four parasympa-thetic ganglia associated with cranial nerves of the head; it is located just above the deep part of the submandibular gland; its preganglionic fibers are derived from the facial nerve and its postganglionic fibers innervate the submandibular and sublingual glands.

   sympathetic ganglia Those ganglia of the auto-nomic nervous system that are composed of adre-nergic neurons receiving afferent fibers from pregan-

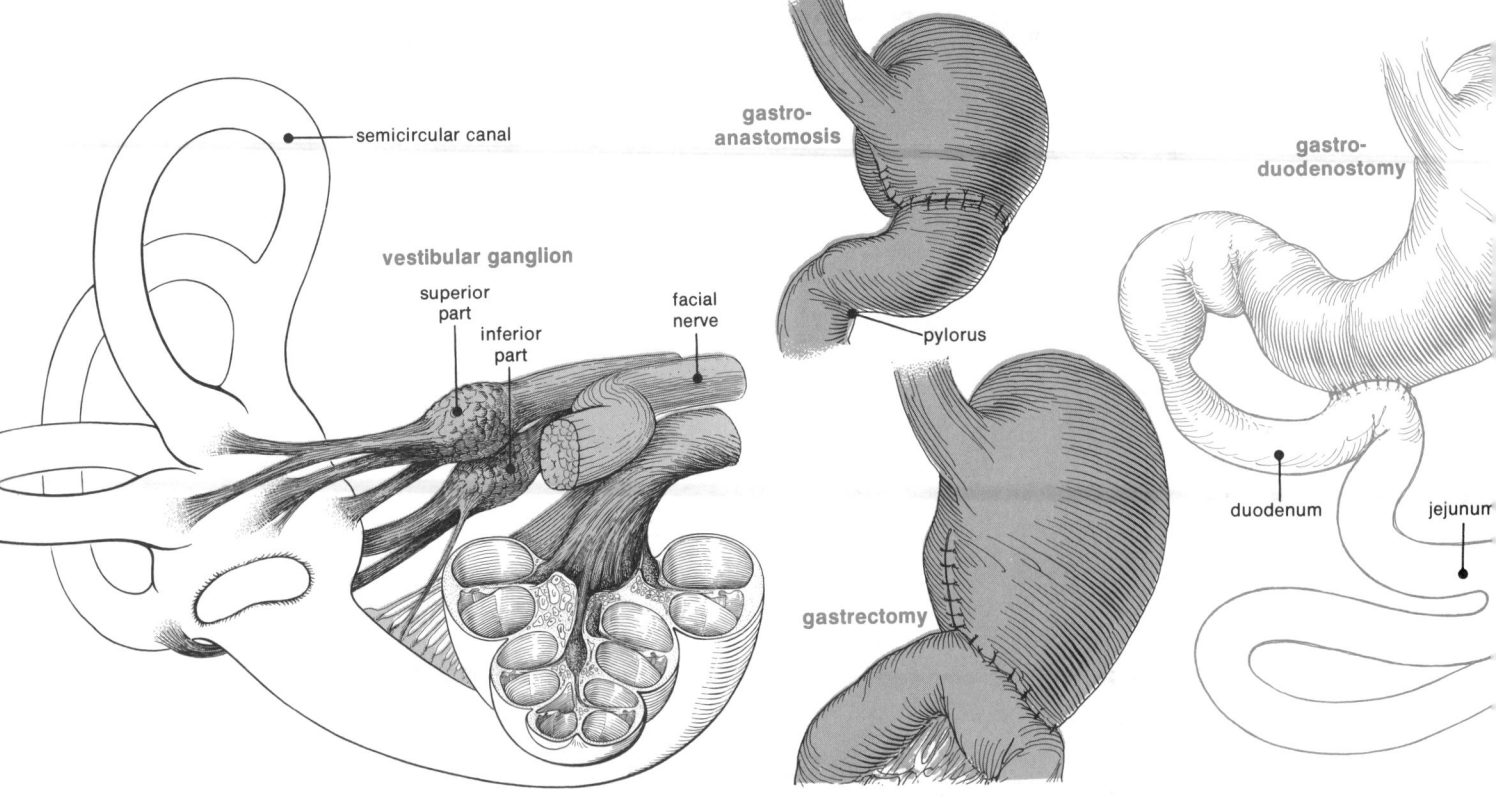

semicircular canal

vestibular ganglion

superior part
inferior part

facial nerve

gastro-anastomosis

gastro-duodenostomy

pylorus

gastrectomy

duodenum

jejunum

glionic visceral motor neurons located in the lateral horn of the thoracic and upper lumbar segments of the spinal cord; classified according to their location as paravertebral and prevertebral ganglia.

    thoracic g. A ganglion on the thoracic portion of the sympathetic system.

    trigeminal g. The large flattened ganglion on the sensory root of the trigeminal nerve, located on the anterior aspect of the petrous portion of the temporal bone. Also called semilunar or gasserian ganglion.

    vestibular g. A collection of bipolar nerve cell bodies forming a swelling of the vestibulocochlear nerve in the internal auditory meatus; it is subdivided into superior and inferior parts. Also called ganglion of Scarpa.

ganglionectomy Surgical removal of a ganglion.

    stellate g. See stellectomy.

ganglioneuroma A small, encapsulated, benign, slow-growing tumor, composed of mature ganglion cells and nerve fibers. Also called ganglioma; neurocytoma.

ganglionic Of or relating to a ganglion, generally a nerve ganglion.

ganglionitis Inflammation of any ganglion.

ganglioplegic Denoting a compound that blocks transmission of impulses (usually for a short period of time) through an autonomic ganglion.

ganglioside A class of sphingoglycolipids present in neural tissue containing *N*-acetylneuraminic acid (NANA).

gangliosidosis Any disease involving an accumulation of specific gangliosides in the nervous system. Also called ganglioside lipidosis.

gangosa Ulceration of the soft and hard palate, nasopharynx, and nose; a sequel to yaws. Also called rhinopharyngitis mutilans.

gangrene Decay of bodily tissue, due to inadequate blood (nutritive) supply; a form of necrosis combined with putrefaction.

    diabetic g. Gangrene due to arteriosclerosis accompanying diabetes.

    dry g. Gangrene not preceded by inflammation. Also called cold or necrotic gangrene; mummification.

    gas g. Gangrene occurring in extensively traumatized and soil-contaminated wounds infected with toxigenic anaerobic *Clostridium;* characterized by the presence of gas in the affected tissue.

    moist g. A soft and moist gangrene due to the action of putrefactive bacteria.

gangrenous Affected with gangrene.

gap An interval or an opening.

    air-bone g. The lag between hearing acuity by air conduction and by bone conduction.

    anion g. The difference between the measured cations and the measured anions in plasma. A simplified formula is: anion gap = [Na] − [HCO₃ + Cl]. The normal range is 8 to 16 mEq/liter.

    auscultatory g. A silent interval sometimes noticed during determination of blood pressure.

    velopharyngeal g. The space behind the palate between the nose and throat.

Gardner's syndrome A hereditary syndrome of polyposis of the rectum and colon, associated with cysts and tumors of skin and bone; transmitted by an autosomal dominant trait; carcinoma of the colon develops in more than 50% of patients by age 40, and colectomy is usually recommended as a prophylactic procedure.

gargle **1.** To rinse the throat and mouth by forcing exhaled air through a liquid held in the mouth while the head is tilted back. **2.** A medicated solution used for rinsing the throat and mouth.

gargoylism See Hurler's syndrome.

gas *pl.* **gases, gasses** **1.** An airlike state of matter distinguished from the solid and liquid states by freely moving molecules capable of great expansion and contraction with changes in pressure and temperature; a vapor. **2.** Gaseous anesthesia.

    inert g. **1.** Any of the gases helium, neon, argon, krypton, xenon, and radon (nitron), which are present in the atmosphere and exhibit no chemical affinity. **2.** Totally unreactive gas, except under extreme conditions.

    laughing g. Nitrous oxide, a mild anesthetic, so called because its inhalation at times causes a hilarious delirium.

    marsh g. See methane.

    mustard g. Dichlorodiethyl sulfide, an oily, volatile substance used in chemical warfare during World War I as a gaseous blistering agent; inhalation of the poison gas may result in chemical bronchopneumonia; progenitor of the so-called nitrogen mustards used in cancer chemotherapy.

    noble g. Inert gas.

    tear g. Any gaseous agent, such as chloroacetophenone (CAP), which irritates the eyes, producing blinding tears.

    water g. An industrial fuel gas produced by passing steam over red-hot coal or coke; consists mainly of hydrogen, hydrocarbons, and carbon monoxide.

gaseous Relating to or of the nature of a gas.

gasiform Gaseous.

gasogenic Gas-producing.

gasometer A calibrated apparatus for measuring volume of gases; generally used for measuring respiration gases.

gasometry The scientific measurement of gases; the determination of the relative proportion of gases

in a mixture.

gastrectomy Surgical removal of part or all of the stomach. Also called gastric resection.

    subtotal g. Excision of a large portion of the stomach.

gastric Of or relating to the stomach.

gastrin One of the gastrointestinal hormones released during digestion; it is secreted by the mucosa of the pyloric region of the stomach upon contact with food; it increases the secretion of hydrochloric acid and, to a lesser degree, of pepsinogen.

gastrinoma A gastrin-producing tumor, usually of the pancreas, associated with the Zollinger-Ellison syndrome.

gastritis Inflammation of the stomach.

    antral g. Condition marked by irregular, concentric narrowing of the stomach. Also called periantritis.

    atrophic g. Chronic inflammation of the stomach with degeneration of the mucous membrane.

    giant hypertrophic g. See Menétrier's disease.

    interstitial g. Gastritis involving the submucosa and muscular coat of the stomach.

    phlegmonous g. Severe inflammation with purulent infiltration of the stomach wall.

    pseudomembranous g. Inflammation of the stomach marked by the formation of a false membrane.

gastroanastomosis Surgical connection of the pyloric and cardiac ends of the stomach. Also called gastrogastrostomy.

gastroblenorrhea Excessive secretion of mucus by the stomach.

gastrocamera A small camera designed to be swallowed, after which the stomach is inflated and photographs are rapidly taken.

gastrocele A hernia of a portion of the stomach.

gastrocnemius See table of muscles.

gastrocolic Relating to the stomach and colon.

gastrocolitis Inflammation of the stomach and colon.

gastrocoloptosis Downward displacement of the stomach and colon.

gastrocolostomy The surgical construction of a passage between the stomach and colon.

Gastrodiscoides hominis A species of trematode worms parasitic in the intestines of swine and man.

gastroduodenal Relating to both the stomach and the duodenum.

gastroduodenoscopy Visualization of the interior of the stomach and duodenum with the aid of a gastroscope.

gastroduodenostomy Surgical creation of an artificial passage between the stomach and duo-

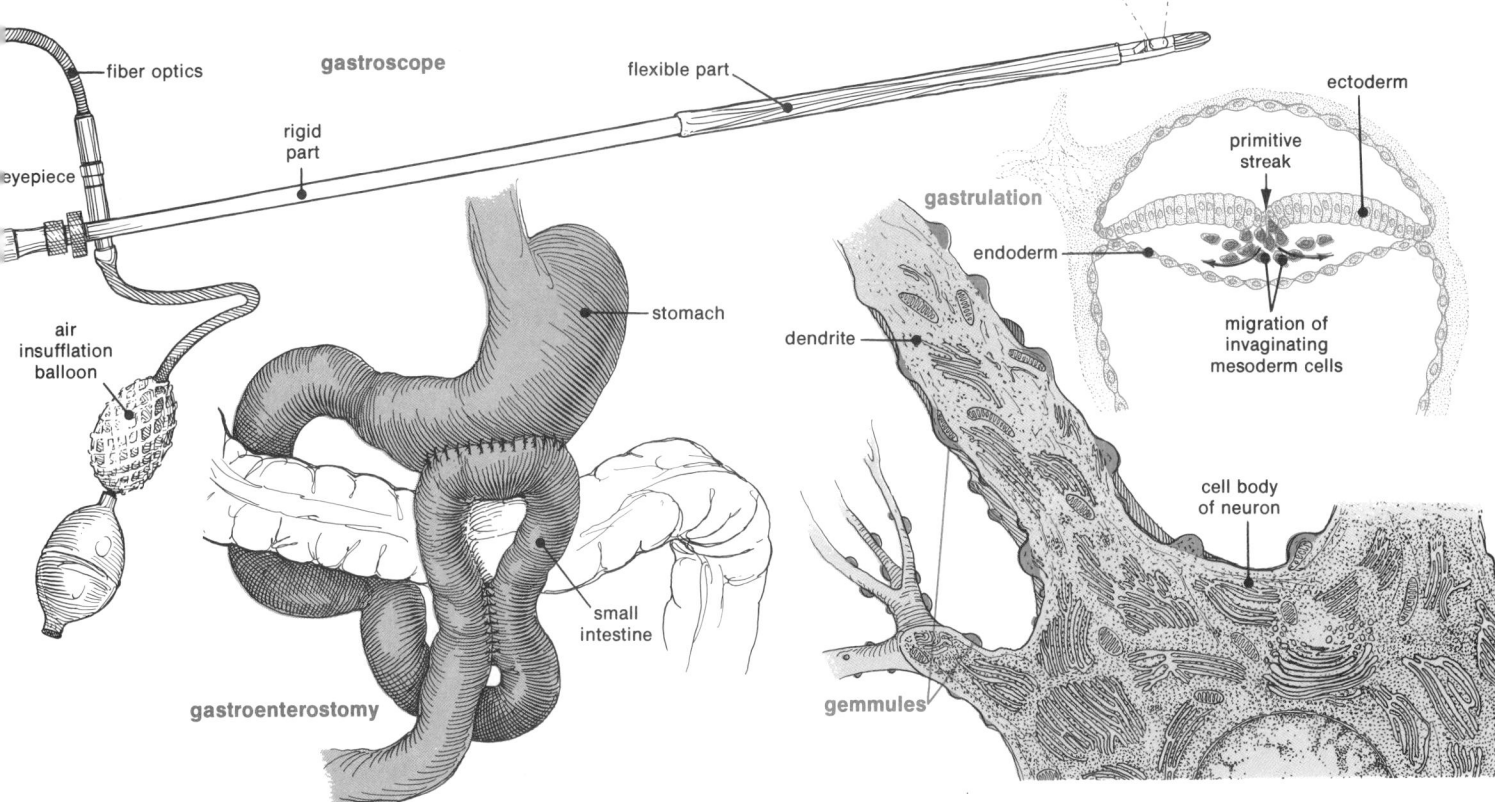

gastroscope

fiber optics

eyepiece

rigid part

flexible part

ectoderm

gastrulation

primitive streak

endoderm

air insufflation balloon

stomach

dendrite

migration of invaginating mesoderm cells

small intestine

cell body of neuron

gastroenterostomy

gemmules

denum.

gastroenteric Relating to the stomach and intestines. Also called gastrointestinal.

gastroenteritis Inflammation of the mucous membrane of the stomach and intestines.

gastroenteroanastomosis A surgical connection between the stomach and any noncontinuous portion of the intestine.

gastroenterologist A specialist in diseases of the stomach and intestines.

gastroenterology The branch of medicine concerned with disorders of the stomach and intestines and also with the esophagus, the liver, and the gallbladder.

gastroenteropathy Any disease of the alimentary canal.

gastroenteroptosis The downward displacement, or prolapse, of the stomach and a portion of the intestine.

gastroenterostomy Surgical creation of a passage between the stomach and the intestine.

gastroenterotomy Surgical incision into the stomach and intestine.

gastroepiploic Relating to the stomach and greater omentum.

gastroesophageal Relating to the stomach and the esophagus.

gastroesophagitis Inflammation of the stomach and esophagus.

gastroesophagostomy Surgical creation of a new opening or connection between the stomach and esophagus.

gastrogastrostomy See gastroanastomosis.

gastrogavage Feeding by way of a gastrostomy (surgical opening through the stomach wall).

gastrogenic Originating in the stomach.

gastrograph An instrument for recording the motions of the stomach.

gastrohepatic Relating to the stomach and the liver.

gastrohydrorrhea Secretion by the stomach of a large quantity of a watery fluid.

gastrointestinal (GI) Relating to the stomach and intestines. Also called gastroenteric.

gastrojejunocolic Relating to the stomach, jejunum, and colon; e.g., a fistula penetrating the three structures.

gastrojejunostomy Surgical creation of an opening or connection between the stomach and jejunum.

gastrolith A calculus in the stomach; a gastric calculus.

gastrolithiasis The presence of one or more calculi in the stomach.

gastrology The scientific study of the stomach

and its diseases; the term gastroenterology is more commonly used.

gastromalacia Softening of the stomach wall.

gastromegaly Abnormal enlargement of the stomach.

gastropathy Any disease of the stomach.

gastropexy Surgical attachment of the stomach to the abdominal wall.

gastrophrenic Relating to the stomach and the diaphragm.

gastroplasty Surgical correction of any defect of the stomach.

gastroplication A surgical procedure to reduce the size of the stomach, usually by suturing a fold along its length.

gastroptosis, gastroptosia Downward displacement of the stomach.

gastropyloric Relating to the stomach as a whole and to the pylorus.

gastrorrhaphy Suture of the stomach.

gastroscope An instrument for viewing the interior of the stomach.

gastroscopy Examination of the interior of the stomach with the gastroscope.

gastrospasm Spasmodic contraction of the stomach.

gastrostenosis Constriction of the stomach.

gastrostomy Surgical construction of a passage into the stomach.

gastrotomy Surgical incision into the stomach.

gastrotropic Having an effect on the stomach.

gastrula An embryo at the stage of development following the blastula when the gastrulation movements occur.

gastrulation The formation of a gastrula; in embryology, the process by which a third germ layer of cells (mesoderm) migrates between the bilaminar disk making it trilaminar (ectoderm, mesoderm, and endoderm); it occurs during the third week of embryonic development.

gather To come to a head; said of a boil when maturing.

gathering 1. The formation of pus in a boil, abscess, etc. 2. Colloquial term for an abscess, boil, etc.

Gaucher's disease A disease characterized by the deposit of glucocerebroside, a glycolipid, in reticuloendothelial cells; manifestations include splenomegaly, hepatomegaly, lymph node enlargement, and bone lesions.

gauge A measuring instrument.

    bite g. A pressure device used in dentistry to determine the biting force. Also called gnathodynamometer.

    Boley g. A caliper-type gauge used in dentistry to obtain measurements necessary for dental pros-

thesis.

    catheter g. A metal plate with perforations of different sizes used to determine the size of catheters.

Gaultheria A genus of plants including the species *Gaultheria procumbens,* commonly known as wintergreen and teaberry; it yields a volatile oil rich in methyl salicylate.

gaunt 1. Very slim and bony. 2. Emaciated.

gauntlet A glovelike bandage protecting the hand and fingers.

gauze A thin, open weave surgical dressing or bandage.

    absorbent g. A bleached cotton gauze of varied thread counts and weight.

    petrolatum g. Absorbent gauze impregnated with white petrolatum.

gavage The passage of nutritive material into the stomach by means of a tube.

Geiger-Müller tube See under tube.

gel 1. The semisolid state of a coagulated colloid. 2. To convert a solution into a gel.

gelate To cause the formation of a gel.

gelatin A colorless, transparent protein derived from the collagen of tissue by boiling in water; used for nutritional purposes and also as a packaging agent for pharmaceuticals.

    zinc g. Jelly containing zinc oxide, gelatin, glycerin, and water; used between layers of bandage as a protective dressing.

gelatinize 1. To convert to gelatin. 2. To become gelatinous.

gelatinoid 1. Like gelatin. 2. Gelatinous.

gelatinous 1. Pertaining to or containing gelatin. 2. Viscous; resembling jelly.

gelation The transformation of a solution to a gel.

gelose In general, any amorphous polysaccharide, such as agar, obtained from red algae and capable of forming a jelly.

gelosis A hard mass in the tissues, especially in a muscle.

gemellology The study of twins and twinning.

geminate Occurring in pairs.

gemma 1. Any budlike structure, such as a tastebud. 2. Any outgrowth or bud that becomes a new organism.

gemmation Asexual reproduction in which a new organism develops as an outgrowth of the parent. Also called budding.

gemmule 1. A bud that develops into a new organism. 2. One of several spherical enlargements sometimes present on the protoplasmic processes (dendrites) of a nerve cell. 3. In Darwin's theory of inheritance, particles transferred from body cells to sex cells.

gender (g) Sex category.

crossing over of genes

loci of genes A, B, a, and b

structural genes

operator gene

regulator gene

mRNA

repressor substance inhibiting function of operator gene

no mRNA, no protein

regulation of protein synthesis

mRNA

mRNA

repressor

inactive repressor

inducer

ribosome

inactivated repressor allows operator gene to function

polypeptides

Mendel's cross for flower colors

parent generation P_1

CC red × cc white

filial generation F_1

Cc red × Cc red

gametes C c C c

possible combination of gametes

filial generation F_2

CC red | Cc red | cC red | cc white

---

gene The hereditary unit occupying a fixed position (locus) in the chromosome; capable of reproducing itself at each cell division and of managing the formation of protein.

allelic g.'s Different genes located in corresponding positions (loci) in a pair of chromosomes and effecting a similar function.

autosomal g. A gene present on any chromosome other than a sex chromosome.

crossing over of g.'s The exchange of material, including genes, between two paired chromosomes during meiosis.

dominant g. A gene that produces a recognizable effect in the organism whether paired with an identical or a dissimilar gene.

hemizygous g. A gene present in a single dose, or without a partner.

holandric g. A gene located on the nonhomologous portion of a Y (male) chromosome. Also called Y-linked gene.

initiator g. One of the regulator genes that codes for the repressor protein which binds to the DNA.

operator g. One of the regulator genes whose function is to activate messenger-RNA production; it is part of the feedback system for determining the rate of enzyme production.

promoter g. One of the regulator genes on which RNA polymerase attaches and catalyzes the synthesis of messenger-RNA.

recessive g. A gene that does not produce a detectable effect in the organism when combined (heterozygous) with a dominant allele.

regulator g. A gene that controls the rate of protein synthesis; it controls the production of a repressor protein which acts on the operator gene.

sex-linked g. A gene located on a sex (X or Y) chromosome.

structural g. A gene that specifies the formation of a particular polypeptide chain.

X-linked g. A gene carried on an X (female) chromosome.

Y-linked g. See holandric gene.

gene dosage The number of times a specific gene is present in the nucleus of a cell.

genera Plural of genus.

generalist A physician who treats a broad range of diseases; a family or general physician.

generalize To become general; said of a primary local lesion that has become widespread or systemic.

generation A stage in the succession of descent of the offspring of plants or animals.

filial g. Offspring resulting from a genetically specified mating: first filial generation (F_1), offspring of the first experimental crossing of animals or plants (parental generation with which the experiment

starts is P_1); second filial generation (F_2), offspring resulting from intercrossing or self-fertilization of F_1 individuals; third, fourth, etc. filial generation (F_3, F_4, etc.), offspring of continued crossing of heterozygotes with continuation of F_2 ratios.

generative Relating to reproduction.

generator 1. A machine for producing electrical energy from some other form of energy. 2. A device that generates vapor, gas, or aerosol from a liquid or solid.

aerosol g. A device for generating airborne suspensions of small particles, usually for inhalation therapy.

asynchronous pulse g. A cardiac pacemaker in which the rate of discharge does not depend on the natural cardiac activity. Also called fixed rate pulse generator.

atrial synchronous pulse g. A ventricular stimulating pacemaker whose rate of discharge is determined by the atrial rate. Also called atrial triggered pulse generator.

atrial triggered pulse g. See atrial synchronous pulse generator.

demand pulse g. See ventricular inhibited pulse generator.

fixed rate pulse g. See asynchronous pulse generator.

pion g. A device that emits a stream of pions (subatomic particles generated by a high-energy accelerator); used experimentally to kill cancer cells.

pulse g. A generator serving as the source for an artificial pacemaker assembly; it generates and discharges electrical impulses to stimulate the heart.

radionuclide g. A receptacle containing a large quantity of a certain radionuclide which decays down to a secondary radionuclide of shorter half-life; the shorter form affords a continuing supply of relatively short-lived radionuclides for laboratory use. Also called "radioactive cow."

standby pulse g. See ventricular inhibited pulse generator.

ventricular inhibited pulse g. A generator that suppresses its electrical output in response to natural ventricular activity but which, in the absence of such cardiac activity, functions as an asynchronous pulse. Also called demand pulse or standby pulse generator.

ventricular synchronous pulse g. A pulse generator that delivers its output synchronously with naturally occurring ventricular activity but which, in the absence of such cardiac activity, functions as an asynchronous pulse. Also called ventricular triggered pulse generator.

ventricular triggered pulse g. See ventricular synchronous pulse generator.

generic 1. Of or relating to a genus. 2. General; relating to an entire group. 3. Used in referring to the non-proprietary name of a drug.

genesial, genesic 1. Pertaining to origin. 2. Pertaining to generation.

genesiology The study of generation and reproduction.

genesis Creation; origin.

genetic 1. Relating to the study of heredity. 2. Inherited. 3. In psychiatry, relating to an earlier period of development in a patient's life in which conflicts or problems originated.

geneticist A scientist who specializes in genetics.

genetics The science of heredity; especially the study of the origin of the characteristics of the individual and hereditary transmission.

medical g. The branch of human genetics concerned with the relationship between heredity and disease.

genetotrophic Denoting inherited nutritional factors, applied especially to certain hereditary deficiency disorders.

genial Of or relating to the chin.

genic Of or relating to the genes.

geniculate, geniculated Shaped like a flexed knee.

geniculum *pl.* **genicula** Latin for small knee; a sharp kneelike bend in a small structure.

g. of facial canal The bend in the facial canal which houses the geniculum of the facial nerve.

g. of facial nerve A kneelike bend of the horizontal portion of the facial nerve at the lateral end of the internal acoustic meatus, above the promontory of the middle ear.

genioglossus See table of muscles.

geniohyoid See table of muscles.

genioplasty Reparative or plastic surgery of the chin. Also called genyplasty.

genital Relating to reproduction.

genitalia The genitals.

genitality In psychoanalysis, a general term denoting the genital constituents of sexuality.

genitals The organs of reproduction.

genitourinary (GU) Relating to the organs of reproduction and the urinary tract. Also called urogenital.

genius 1. Exceptional intellectual and creative abilities. 2. One who possesses such abilities.

genodermatosis A genetically determined disorder of the skin.

genome A complete set of chromosomes (with their genes) from one parent; the total genetic endowment.

genotype The genetic or hereditary constitution of an individual.

genu of corpus callosum

cerebellum

free gingiva

attached gingiva

genu varum

genu valgum

medial view of left elbow joint

humerus

ginglymus

olecranon

radius

ulna

sacrum

ilium

pubis

ischium

pelvic girdle

pubic symphysis

gentamicin sulfate A broad spectrum aminoglycoside antibiotic that inhibits the growth of bacteria; Garamycin®.

gentian Gentian root, the dried roots of the herb *Gentiana lutea*.

gentian violet A compound composed of one or several methyl derivatives of pararosaniline; used as a biological stain, a bactericide in the treatment of minor lesions of the oral mucosa, and a fungicide in the treatment of moniliasis. Also called crystal or methyl violet; methylrosanilin chloride.

genu 1. The knee. 2. Any structure resembling a flexed knee.

   g. of corpus callosum The anterior extremity of the corpus callosum.

   g. recurvatum The backward bending of the knee joint.

   g. valgum A deformity of the leg at the level of the knee, usually bilateral, marked by a lateral angulation of the tibia. Also called knock-knee.

   g. varum A deformity, usually bilateral, in which the leg has an outward curvature at the level of the knee. Also called bowleg.

genus *pl.* **genera** The biologic classification ranking below a family and above a species; a category denoting resemblances in general features but differences in details.

genyplasty See genioplasty.

geophagia, geophagy, geophagism The habit of eating earth, including various forms of clay; a form of pica.

geotrichosis Condition caused by infection with the fungus *Geotrichum*.

Geotrichum A genus of yeastlike fungi, one species of which infects the lungs and bronchi of man.

geriatric Relating to old age.

geriatrics The branch of medicine concerned with old age, its physiology and disease.

germ 1. A pathogenic microbe. 2. An embryonic structure capable of developing into a new organism; a primordium.

   wheat g. The vitamin-rich embryonic or germinating portion of the wheat kernel; used as a cereal or dietary supplement.

germanium A metallic element; symbol Ge, atomic number 32, atomic weight 72.6.

germicidal Destructive to disease-causing microorganisms.

germicide An agent that kills germs or microbes.

germifuge Germicide.

germinal 1. Pertaining to germination. 2. Pertaining to the nature of a germ.

germinoma A tumor arising from germinal tissue, as of the ovaries or testes; e.g., a seminoma.

geroderma Atrophy of the skin.

gerodontics, gerodontology The diagnosis and treatment of dental disorders of the aged.

geromarasmus The atrophy of old age.

gerontal Relating to old age; senile.

gerontology The study of medical and social problems associated with aging.

gerontopia See senopia.

gerontotherapeutics Treatment of diseases of the aged.

gerontoxon See arcus senilis.

gestagen A general term denoting hormones that produce progestational changes in the uterus.

gestalt A unified system of physical, psychological, or symbolic phenomena having properties that cannot be derived solely from its components.

gestation See pregnancy.

Ghon complex Deposits in the peripheral lung field together with calcified hilar nodes; formerly considered pathognomonic of healed primary tuberculosis but may be mimicked by healed primary lesions of histoplasmosis and coccidioidomycosis; the deposits usually go on to calcification.

Ghon focus The primary lesion of pulmonary tuberculosis; that part of the complex which is parenchymal.

ghost, erythrocytic The remaining membranous sac of a red blood cell after the loss of hemoglobin.

Gianotti-Crosti syndrome An acute, papular dermatosis of young children, associated with mild fever and malaise; it generally disappears without treatment within 30 to 70 days. Also called acrodermatitis papulosa infantum.

giantism Gigantism.

Giardia A genus of flagellate protozoa some of which are parasitic in the intestinal tract of man and domestic animals.

   G. lamblia A species with a broad rounded anterior end and a tapered pointed posterior; it has four pairs of flagella, two nuclei, a convex dorsal surface, and a concave ventral surface which forms a functional sucking disc in the anterior half of the body; a common cause of diarrhea and intestinal symptoms in man.

giardiasis Infestation with *Giardia lamblia*.

gibberish Incoherent, rapid talk.

gibbous Humpbacked.

gibbus A hump or kyphos.

GIFT Gamete intra-fallopian transfer; the placing of sperm and unfertilized ova together in a uterine (fallopian) tube to enhance the possibility of fertilization.

gigantism An abnormal condition of excessive growth in height, greatly exceeding the average for the person's race.

gigavolt A billion volts.

gilbert The electromagnetic unit of electromotive force.

Gilbert's disease Familial nonhemolytic jaundice; see under jaundice.

Gilles de la Tourette's disease or **syndrome** See Tourette's disorder.

gingiva (G) The gum; the portion of the oral mucosa which envelops the alveolar process and surrounds the neck of the tooth.

   attached g. The portion of the gingiva that extends from the free gingival groove apically and terminates at the mucogingival junction (where alveolar mucosa begins).

   buccal g. The portion of gingiva facing the cheek.

   free g. The portion of the gingiva that extends from the free gingival groove occlusally, over the free margin of the gingiva, then descends apically into the gingival sulcus and terminates at the epithelial attachment.

   labial g. The portion of gingiva facing the lips.

   lingual g. The portion of gingiva facing the tongue.

gingival Of or pertaining to the gums.

gingivectomy Surgical removal of diseased gingival tissue.

gingivitis Inflammation of the gums.

   necrotizing ulcerative g. A bacterial (fusospirochetal) infection, usually of sudden onset, characterized by tender, bleeding gums with ulcer formation (especially between the teeth), a gray exudate, and fetid breath; most commonly occurring in individuals with poor oral hygiene. Also called Vincent's disease, infection, or stomatitis; trench mouth.

gingivoplasty Surgical contouring of the gingiva.

gingivosis A noninflammatory desquamative condition of the gums.

gingivostomatitis Inflammation of the gums and oral mucosa.

ginglymus A hinge joint which has one concave and one convex articulating surface, as the articulation between the ulna and humerus at the elbow; it allows motion in one plane only.

girdle 1. An encircling band. 2. Any encircling structure or region.

   pectoral g. See shoulder girdle.

   pelvic g. The bony ring formed by the sacrum and the two hipbones.

   shoulder g. A girdle formed by the clavicles (collarbones) scapulas (shoulder blades), and the manubrium part of the sternum (breastbone). Also called pectoral girdle.

girth 1. The measure encircling an animal's body slightly behind the forelegs. 2. Circumference; the distance around anything, particularly the abdomen.

gitalin Extract of *Digitalis purpurea* used in the

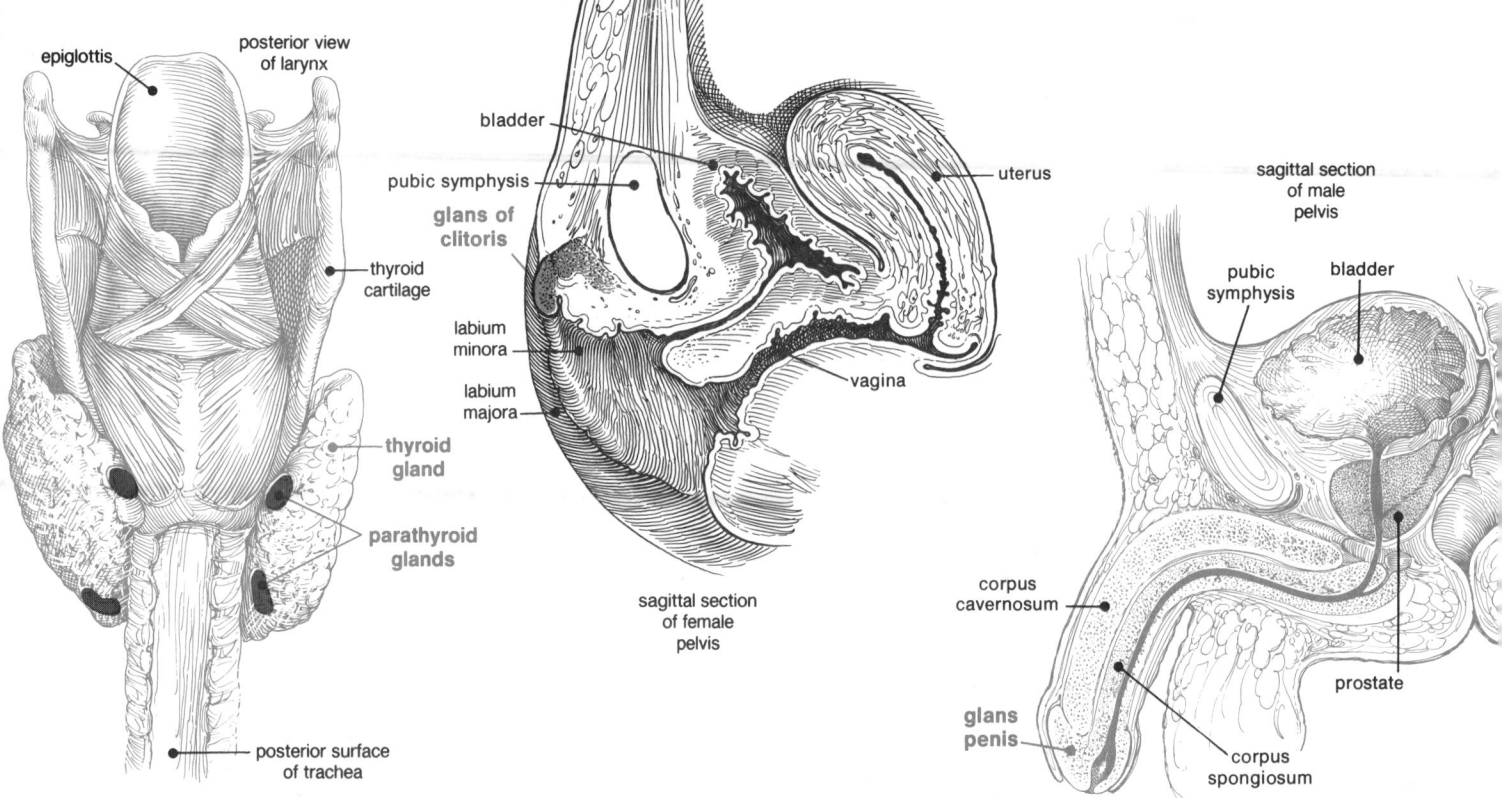

posterior view of larynx

epiglottis

thyroid cartilage

thyroid gland

parathyroid glands

posterior surface of trachea

bladder

pubic symphysis

glans of clitoris

labium minora

labium majora

uterus

vagina

sagittal section of female pelvis

sagittal section of male pelvis

pubic symphysis

bladder

corpus cavernosum

prostate

glans penis

corpus spongiosum

treatment of certain heart diseases. Also called amorphous gitalin; Gitaligin®.

glabella The smooth area of the frontal bone located between the eyebrows, immediately above the root of the nose.

glabrous Hairless; smooth and bare.

gladiolus The body or main portion of the sternum. Also called corpus sterni.

gland (gl) A secreting organ.

  accessory g. A small detached mass of glandular tissue located near a gland or similar structure.

  accessory adrenal g.'s Adrenocortical bodies occurring in areolar tissue around principal glands, or in the spermatic cord, epididymis, and broad ligament of uterus.

  acinous g. A gland made up of one or several saclike structures.

  adrenal g. A flattened, somewhat triangular endocrine gland resting upon the upper end of each kidney; it produces steroid hormones (aldosterone, androgens, glucocorticoids, progestins, and estrogens), epinephrine, and norepinephrine. Also called suprarenal gland.

  apocrine g. A gland producing a secretion which contains part of the secreting cells.

  Bartholin's g. See greater vestibular gland.

  Brunner's g.'s See duodenal glands.

  bulbourethral g.'s Two pea-shaped glands situated dorsal and lateral to the membranous portion of the male urethra; during sexual stimulation, the glands secrete a mucus-like substance into the urethra that serves as a lubricant for the epithelium. Also called Cowper's glands.

  cardiac g.'s The tubular, branched, slightly coiled, mucus-producing glands located in the transition zone between the esophagus and stomach; they also secrete electrolytes.

  compound g. A gland composed of numerous small sacs (acini) whose excretory ducts combine to form larger ones.

  Cowper's g.'s See bulbourethral glands.

  ductless g. A gland with no excretory duct.

  duodenal g.'s Small, branched, compound tubular glands in the submucous layer of the first part of the duodenum; they secrete an alkaline mucoid substance into the crypts of Lieberkühn or directly to the surface between the duodenal villi. Also called Brunner's glands.

  endocrine g. A ductless gland whose secretion (hormone) is absorbed directly into the bloodstream.

  endo-exocrine g. A gland that produces both internal and external secretions, as the pancreas.

  excretory g. Any gland that separates waste material from the blood.

  exocrine g. A gland that discharges its secretion

through a duct onto the internal or external surface of the body; it may be simple or compound.

  gastric g.'s Numerous, straight, sometimes branched, tubular glands in the mucosa of the fundus and body of the stomach (they are absent in the cardiac and pyloric regions); they contain the cells that produce hydrochloric acid and pepsin. Also called fundic glands.

  greater vestibular g. One of two small mucoid secreting glands on either side of the vaginal orifice, in the groove between the hymen and the labium minus; its major function is the production of lubrication of the introitus. Also called Bartholin's gland.

  holocrine g. A gland whose secretion is composed of the disintegrated secreting cell in addition to its accumulated secretion.

  interscapular g. Brown fat; see under fat.

  intestinal g.'s Simple tubular glands in the mucous membrane of the intestines, concerned with the secretion of digestive enzymes and some hormones. Also called crypts of Lieberkühn.

  lacrimal g. A gland that secretes tears; located in the upper lateral portion of the orbit.

  mammary g. A compound milk-producing gland that forms the major part of the female breast; it consists of 15 to 20 lobes, each of which has a separate duct opening at the apex of the nipple; it reaches functional maturity after pregnancy.

  meibomian g. See tarsal gland.

  mixed g. A gland in which some secretory units contain both serous and mucous cells; e.g., the submandibular gland.

  parathyroid g.'s The smallest of the endocrine glands, situated between the dorsal borders of the thyroid gland and its capsule; usually four in number, each the approximate size of an apple seed, they produce parathyroid hormone (parathormone) which regulates the calcium and phosphate metabolism of the body.

  paraurethral g. One of the larger mucous glands located in the lining of the female urethra, just within the orifice. Also called Skene's gland.

  parotid g. A salivary gland located below and in front of each ear.

  pineal g. See body, pineal.

  pituitary g. See hypophysis.

  pyloric g. One of the simple, coiled, mucus-producing tubular glands of the pyloric part of the stomach.

  racemose g. An acinous gland, like the parotid, whose acini are arranged like grapes on a stem.

  sebaceous g. A simple branched holocrine gland in the dermis which usually opens into the distal part of the hair follicle and secretes an oily substance (sebum); some sebaceous glands open di-

rectly onto the skin surface, such as on the vermilion border of the lips.

  seromucous g. A gland whose secretory cells have histochemical and cytologic characteristics that suggest the elaboration of both serous and mucous secretions.

  simple g. A gland consisting of a single system of secretory passages opening into a nonbranching duct; divided into tubular, tubuloalveolar, and alveolar types.

  Skene's g. See paraurethral gland.

  sublingual g. One of two salivary glands in the floor of the mouth with a series of ducts (10 to 30) opening into the mouth at the side of the tongue's frenulum; most of the secretory units are mucus-secreting with serous demilunes.

  submandibular g. One of two predominately serous salivary glands in the upper neck; the main duct opens into the mouth beneath the tongue.

  suprarenal g. See adrenal gland.

  sweat g.'s Coiled tubular glands, located deep in the skin, that secrete a watery solution rich in sodium and chloride (sweat). Also called sudoriferous glands.

  tarsal g. One of numerous sebaceous glands in the eyelids. Also called meibomian gland.

  thymus g. See thymus.

  thyroid g. The largest endocrine gland in man, situated in front of the lower part of the neck, and consisting of right and left lobes, on either side of the trachea, joined by a connecting isthmus; it secretes the iodine-rich hormones thyroxin and triiodothyronine which are concerned with regulating the rate of metabolism; also thought to secrete thyrocalcitonin.

  tubular g. A gland composed of one or more tubules closed at one end.

  urethral g. One of several minute mucous glands located in the lining of the urethra; in the male, also called Littre's glands.

glanders An infectious disease of horses, mules, and donkeys caused by the gram-negative bacillus Pseudomonas mallei; marked by fever and ulcers of the respiratory tract or skin; occasionally transmitted to man; the cutaneous form is called farcy.

glandilemma The enveloping membrane or capsule of a gland.

glandula A small gland.

glandular Of, relating to, or resembling a gland.

glandule A small gland.

glans pl. **glandes** A small glandlike structure.

  g. clitoridis, g. of clitoris A small rounded mass of erectile tissue at the tip of the clitoris.

  g. penis The caplike extension of the corpus spongiosum at the head or tip of the penis.

adrenal glands

left kidney

inferior vena cava

abdominal aorta

ureter

lacrimal gland

lacrimal sac

nasolacrimal duct

mammary gland

bladder

salivary glands

parotid gland

sublingual gland

submandibular gland

prostate

bulbourethral glands

urethra

thyroid cartilage

cornea

iris

lens of the eye

anterior chamber of eye

tarsal gland

thyroid gland

trachea

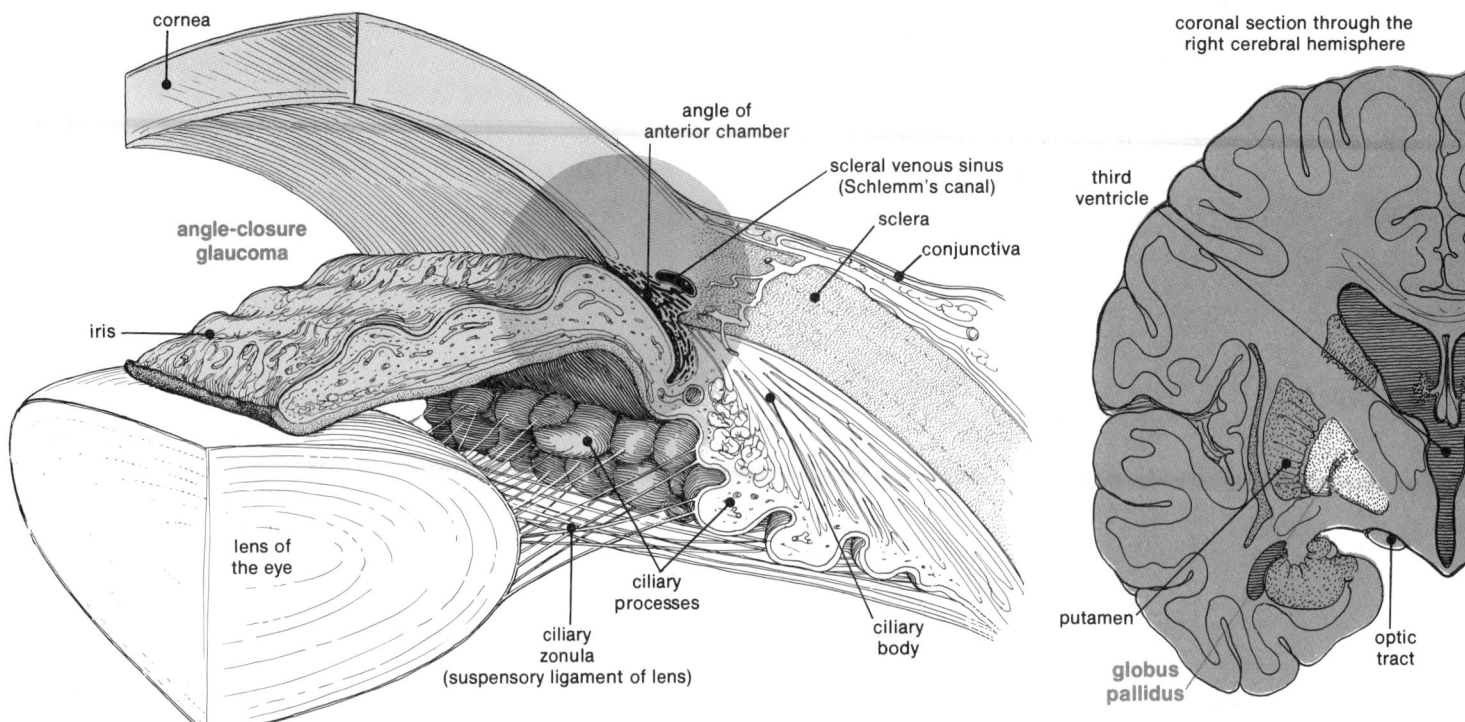

cornea

angle-closure glaucoma

iris

lens of the eye

angle of anterior chamber

scleral venous sinus (Schlemm's canal)

sclera

conjunctiva

ciliary zonula (suspensory ligament of lens)

ciliary processes

ciliary body

coronal section through the right cerebral hemisphere

third ventricle

putamen

globus pallidus

optic tract

Glanzmann's disease See thrombasthenia.

glass Any of a class of transparent or translucent brittle materials composed of silica with oxides of several bases, and considered physically as supercooled liquids instead of true solids.

cover g. A thin piece of glass used to cover an object examined under the microscope.

crown g. Glass having a low dispersion and usually a low index of refraction; a compound of lime, potash, alumina, and silica; used in ophthalmic lenses.

flint g. A heavy, brilliant optical glass having a high dispersion and usually a high index of refraction.

optical g. Glass carefully manufactured to obtain controlled index of refraction and dispersion, purity, transparency, homogeneity, and workability; the two most common types are crown and flint.

quartz g. Crystal made by fusing pure quartz sand; it transmits ultraviolet rays.

Wood's g. A glass containing nickel oxide; used for diagnostic purposes, as in ringworm of the scalp where infected hairs are fluorescent when viewed under light filtered through this glass; also used in conjunction with certain dyes, such as fluorescin, for visualizing abrasions of the cornea.

glasses Eyeglasses.

glaucoma A group of eye diseases characterized by an increase in intraocular pressure, due to restricted outflow of the aqueous humor through the trabecular meshwork and spaces of Fontana in the anterior chamber angle (between the root of the iris and cornea).

acute g. Glaucoma due to an acute obstruction of the anterior chamber angle.

angle-closure g. A chronic form of glaucoma marked by intermittent attacks during which the space between the base of the iris and the cornea at the trabecular meshwork is narrowed. Also called narrow-angle glaucoma.

congenital g. See buphthalmos.

narrow-angle g. See angle-closure glaucoma.

open-angle g. A chronic, slowly progressive glaucoma due to some defect in the trabecular meshwork of the anterior chamber angle resulting in failure of aqueous humor to drain properly.

phacolytic g. Glaucoma occurring as a complication of cataract; fluid from the liquified cortex of the lens seeps into the anterior chamber of the eye, causing swelling of the uvea which obstructs the outflow system and prevents adequate escape of the aqueous humor from the anterior chamber.

secondary g. Increased ocular pressure occurring as a manifestation of another preexisting intraocular disease.

glenohumeral Relating to the glenoid fossa and the humerus.

glenoid Resembling a socket; applied to articular depressions forming the shoulder joint (glenoid fossa) and the articulation of the jaw (glenoid or mandibular fossa).

glia The nonneuronal tissue of the brain and spinal cord. Also called neuroglia.

gliacyte A cell of the non-nervous components of nervous tissue (neuroglia).

gliadin Any of various simple proteins obtained from wheat and rye glutens. Also called glutin.

glial Relating to the non-nervous elements of nervous tissue.

glide, mandibular The side-to-side, protrusive, and intermediate movement of the mandible that occurs when the teeth are in contact.

glioblastoma A general term for malignant forms of neoplasms containing neuroglial cells.

g. multiforme The most malignant of all gliomas (primary brain tumors); a rapidly growing and fatal tumor of the cerebral hemispheres, composed of undifferentiated cells; the most recent term for this tumor is astrocytoma, grade 3 or 4, grade 4 being the most malignant.

glioma Any tumor derived from the various types of cells that make up brain tissue; e.g., astrocytoma, glioblastoma multiforme, medulloblastoma, ependymoma, oligodendroglioma.

gliomatosis Presence within the brain substance of one or several neoplasms originating in the glial cells.

gliomatous Relating to or of the nature of a glioma.

gliosis Tumors of the non-nervous cellular elements of the brain and spinal cord.

gliosome One of several granules occurring in the non-nervous cells of nerve tissue.

globi Brown granular masses sometimes seen in the granulomatous lesions of leprosy.

globin A simple protein constituent of hemoglobin.

globule A minute spherical body, especially a small drop of liquid.

Morgagni's g.'s Minute opaque spheres of fluid beneath the capsule and lens fibers, sometimes seen in cases of cataract. Also called Morgagni's spheres.

globulin Any of a class of simple proteins that are insoluble in water, soluble in saline solutions, and coagulable by heat; found in blood and cerebrospinal fluid; human serum globulin is divided into alpha, beta, and gamma fractions on the basis of electrophoretic mobility.

accelerator g. Factor V.

alpha g., α-g A plasma globulin that has the greatest electrophoretic mobility in neutral or alkaline solutions.

antihemophilic g. (AHG) **1.** See factor VIII. **2.** A sterile preparation of normal human plasma which shortens the clotting time of hemophilic blood; used as an antihemophilic.

antilymphocyte g. (ALG) A preparation of purified globulin obtained after injection of human lymphocytes into animals (usually rabbits or horses) containing antibodies against lymphocytes; used to modify the immune response to allografts, primarily by suppressing cell-mediated immunity in the host.

antithymic g. (ATG) A preparation of purified globulin obtained after injection of human thymic cells into animals (usually rabbits or horses) containing antibodies against thymocytes; used to modify the immune response to allografts primarily by suppressing cell-mediated immunity in the host. Also called antihuman thymocyte globulin; Atgam®.

beta g., β-g A plasma globulin having an electrophoretic mobility intermediate between that of the alpha and gamma globulins.

gamma g., γ-g A blood fraction prepared from plasma, composed of a number of molecular classes and subclasses of immunoglobulins and other nonantibody globulins; used in the prophylaxis of numerous diseases, including measles and hepatitis.

immune serum g. A sterile preparation of globulins containing a number of antibodies normally present in adult human blood; used as an immunizing agent.

thyroxin-binding g. (TBG) An alpha globulin with a strong affinity for thyroxin, thus acting as a carrier of thyroxin in the blood.

globulinuria The presence of globulin in the urine.

globus A globe or ball.

g. hystericus A hysterical sensation of having a lump or ball in the throat.

g. pallidus The inner gray portion of the lentiform nucleus. Also called paleostriatum.

glomangioma Painful, small benign tumor of a glomus body, mainly occurring under the nails of the fingers and toes.

glomerular Of, relating to, or resembling a glomerulus.

glomerulitis Inflammation of the glomeruli of the kidneys.

glomerulonephritis (GN) Kidney disease that is marked by alteration in the structure of the glomeruli; it may be acute, subacute, or chronic.

acute crescentic g. See rapidly progressive glomerulonephritis.

acute g. Disorder occurring primarily in children and sometimes in young adults, most often following streptococcal infections; classical symptoms include fluid retention, periorbital edema, diminished urinary output, dark tea-colored urine, and elevation of the blood pressure; hematuria, red blood cell casts,

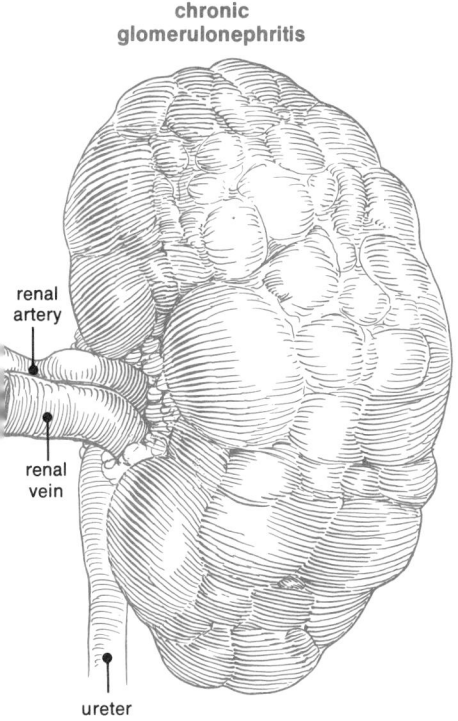

chronic glomerulonephritis

renal artery
renal vein
ureter

Glossina palpalis — a tsetse fly

glucagon

NH₂ — His — Ser — Glu — Gly — Thr — Phe — Thr — Ser — Asp — Tyr — Ser — Lys — Tyr — Leu — Asp — Ser — Arg — Arg — Ala — Gln — Asp — Phe — Val — Gln — Trp — Leu — Met — Asn — Thr — COOH

glomerular (Bowman's) capsule
afferent arteriole
proximal convoluted tubule
glomerulus
efferent arteriole
urinary space

glucose

and proteinuria are characteristic.

chronic g. Glomerulonephritis of insidious onset or occurring as a sequel to acute glomerulonephritis; marked by kidney failure, hypertension, and proteinuria; kidneys become symmetrically shrunken and granular.

diffuse g. Glomerulonephritis involving most of the renal glomeruli.

focal g. A form of glomerulonephritis in which only some of the glomeruli are affected; may be a benign disease or a manifestation of a more serious, progressive disorder, such as lupus erythematosus.

focal embolic g. A complication of subacute bacterial endocarditis.

global g. Complete involvement of the affected glomerulus, as opposed to segmental involvement.

hypocomplementemic persistent g. See membranoproliferative glomerulonephritis.

lobular g. Glomerulonephritis marked by separation of the lobules of glomerular tufts and intralobular hyaline deposits, proteinuria, hematuria, and hypertension; often seen in membranoproliferative glomerulonephritis.

local g. Segmental glomerulonephritis.

membranoproliferative g. A form presenting with symptoms suggesting either acute glomerulonephritis or a nephrotic syndrome with microscopic hematuria; the characteristic lesion is an increase in cellularity of the mesangium, increased lobulation of the tufts, and capillary wall thickening; commonly associated with hypocomplementemia. Also called hypocomplementemic persistent or mesangio-capillary glomerulonephritis.

membranous g. A type marked by thickening of the basement membrane in the glomerular capillaries, causing proteinuria and generalized edema, and often associated with the nephrotic syndrome; a characteristic spiking appearance is found in the basement membrane on microscopy.

mesangiocapillary g. See membranoproliferative glomerulonephritis.

poststreptococcal g. Acute glomerulonephritis.

proliferative g. Acute glomerulonephritis.

rapidly progressive g. A form having an insidious beginning, without a previous episode of streptococcal infection, or possibly an unresolved poststreptococcal nephritis with renal insufficiency leading to death within a few months; characterized by marked crescent formation. Also called crescentic or extracapillary glomerulonephritis.

segmental g. Glomerulonephritis affecting only portions of the glomeruli.

subacute g. A term used variously to describe rapidly progressive glomerulonephritis or a type of glomerulonephritis with nephrotic syndrome and a prolonged course.

glomerulopathy Any disease of the glomeruli.
glomerulosclerosis Fibrosis and degeneration of the structures within the glomeruli of the kidneys.

focal segmental g. A form of progressive renal disease beginning in juxtamedullary capillaries and extending in a centrifugal pattern; usually presents in children or adolescents as a nephrotic syndrome.

intercapillary g. The glomerular lesion present as a complication of diabetes mellitus, associated with proteinuria, edema, and hypertension (Kimmelstiel-Wilson syndrome).

nodular g. A form of diabetic nephropathy in which sclerosis occurs in a peripheral nodular pattern. Also called Kimmelsteil-Wilson lesion.

glomerulus, *pl.* **glomeruli** **1.** A small cluster of nerves or capillaries; when used alone the term refers to a tuft of capillaries at the beginning of each uriniferous tubule in the kidney (malpighian tuft). **2.** The coiled secretory portion of a sweat gland.

glomus A minute globular body composed of anastomoses between small arteries and small veins and having a rich nerve supply.

carotid g. A small neurovascular structure situated on each side of the neck at the bifurcation of the common cartid artery. Also called carotid body.

g. intravagale A collection of chemoreceptor cells on the auricular branch of the vagus nerve; a tumor of this glomus may cause loss of hearing.

g. jugulare A glomus in the adventitia of the jugular bulb.

glossa Latin for tongue.
glossal Of or relating to the tongue.
glossalgia A painful tongue.
glossectomy Amputation of the tongue or of a portion of it.
Glossina A genus of bloodsucking flies, the tsetse flies, which transmit the microorganisms causing African sleeping sickness in humans and domestic animals.
glossitis Inflammation of the tongue.
glossodynia Glossalgia.
glossograph Instrument used to record the movements of the tongue in speaking.
glossolalia Meaningless speech; unintelligible and rapid chatter.
glossopharyngeal Relating to the tongue and pharynx.
glossoplasty Reparative surgery of the tongue.
glossoplegia Paralysis of the tongue. Also called glossolysis.
glossoptosis, glossoptosia Downward displacement of the tongue.
glossorrhaphy Suture of the tongue.
glossospasm Spasmodic contraction of the tongue.
glossotomy Any surgical incision on the tongue.

glossotrichia Hairy tongue.
glottic Relating to either the tongue or the glottis.
glottis The vocal apparatus located in the larynx, consisting of the vocal cords and the opening between them.
glottitis Glossitis.
glucagon A polypeptide hormone, normally produced by α-cells of the islets of Langerhans in the pancreas when the blood sugar level gets too low; it aids in the breakdown of glycogen in the liver, thus elevating the blood sugar concentration.
glucan A polyglucose; e.g., starch amylose, glycogen amylose.
α-glucan-branching glycosyltransferase Branching factor; see under factor.
α-1,4-glucan 4-glucanohydrolase Alpha-1,4-glucan 4-glucanohydrolase; an enzyme which, through a reaction with water, breaks down amylose (a straight chain polysaccharide) to form glucose and maltose; present in plants and obtained in crystalline form from pancreatic juice and saliva. Formerly called α-amylase.
α-1,4-glucan maltohydrolase Alpha-1,4-glucan maltohydrolase; an enzyme which, through a reaction with water, splits amylopectin (a branched polysaccharide) to form maltose; present in soybeans, wheat, barley, and other similar plants. Formerly called β-amylase.
glucocorticoid Any steroid hormone of the adrenal cortex (or synthetic steroid) concerned with gluconeogenesis from amino acids and catabolism of protein; this class of compounds has other activities including anti-inflammatory activity and ability to suppress the synthesis of ACTH and MSH; cortisol is the major naturally occurring hormone of this type in humans.
glucogenic Producing glucose.
glucokinase A specific phosphorylation enzyme for glucose, present in the liver and muscle; it catalyzes the conversion of glucose to glucose-6-phosphate, in which one molecule of adenosine triphosphate (ATP) is used.
glucokinetic Mobilizing glucose in the body, as in the maintenance of sugar level.
gluconeogenesis Formation of glucose from non-carbohydrate sources, such as protein and fat.
glucosamine An amino sugar present in mucopolysaccharides. Also called chitosamine.
glucosan Any anhydride of glucose; a polysaccharide yielding glucose on hydrolysis; e.g., cellulose, glycogen, starch, dextrin.
glucose A dextrorotatory monosaccharide or simple sugar, $C_6H_{12}O_6 \cdot H_2O$, occurring as an odorless, sweet, crystalline powder; present in animal and plant tissue and obtained synthetically from starch; used in medicine as an intravenous nutrient. Also

glutamic acid

$$HOOC—CH_2—CH_2—\underset{\underset{H}{|}}{\overset{\overset{NH_2}{|}}{C}}—COOH$$

glucuronic acid

$$\begin{array}{l}CHO\\HCOH\\HOCH\\HCOH\\HCOH\\COOH\end{array}$$

glycogen

protein molecule consisting of 12 identical bound subunits

model of a glutamine synthetase protein

glutathione

$$\begin{array}{l}COOH\\H_2N—C—H\\CH_2\\CH_2\\C{=}O\\NH\\HS—CH_2—CH\\C{=}O\\NH\\CH_2\\COOH\end{array}$$

glycerol

$$\begin{array}{l}H\\H—C—OH\\H—C—OH\\H—C—OH\\H\end{array}$$

glycine

$$H—\underset{\underset{H}{|}}{\overset{\overset{NH_2}{|}}{C}}—COOH$$

called blood or grape sugar; dextrose.

glucose 6-phosphatase A microsomal enzyme catalyzing the hydrolysis of glucose 6-phosphate to glucose and inorganic phosphate; present in liver, kidney, intestinal mucosa, and endometrium; inherited deficiency of this enzyme is thought to be responsible for the glycogen storage disease known as type 1 glycogenosis or von Gierke's disease.

glucose 6-phosphate dehydrogenase An enzyme that promotes the oxidation of glucose 6-phosphate to 6-phosphogluconolactone.

glucoside One of a variety of substances in nature containing glucose combined by an ether linkage.

glucosuria Presence of glucose in the urine.

glucuronic acid The uronic acid of glucose, $HOOC(CHOH)_4CHO$; it inactivates various substances, e.g., benzoic acid, phenol, and the female sex hormones; the glucuronides so formed are excreted in the urine.

β-glucuronidase An enzyme catalyzing the hydrolysis of various β-D-glucuronides, liberating free glucuronic acid; active in the liver, spleen, endometrium, breasts, adrenal glands, and testes.

glucuronide A glycoside of glucuronic acid.

glue-sniffing The intentional inhalation of fumes from plastic cements, resulting in central nervous system stimulation followed by depression.

glutamic acid An amino acid present in protein; involved in ammonia production in the kidney.

glutamic oxaloacetic transaminase (GOT) See under transaminase.

glutamic pyruvic transaminase (GPT) See under transaminase.

glutamine (Glu) An amino acid found as a constituent of proteins and in free form in blood; it yields glutamic acid and ammonia on hydrolysis.

g. synthetase An enzyme that catalyzes the amination of glutamic acid to glutamine which occurs concurrently with the hydrolysis of ATP to ADP and orthophosphate (P_i).

glutaraldehyde A tissue fixative that causes a fine precipitation of protein, thus permitting sections to be cut without appreciable distortion of structure; universally used as a prefixer in electron microscopy, generally followed by fixation with osmium tetroxide.

glutathione A crystalline tripeptide of glycine, cystine, and glutamic acid that is present in blood and other tissues; it activates certain proteins and takes part in oxidation-reduction processes; the reduced form is abbreviated GSH; in the oxidized form two molecules are linked together and abbreviated GSSG.

gluteal Of or relating to the buttocks.

glutelin One of a number of simple proteins present in the seeds of grain.

gluten A mixture of insoluble plant proteins present in grains such as wheat, rye, oats, and barley; used as an adhesive and as a flour substitute.

glutethimide A compound that is a depressant of the central nervous system; used as a hypnotic; Doriden®.

gluteus, pl. **glutei** Any of the three buttock muscles. See under muscles.

glutin See gliadin.

glutinous Sticky.

glutitis Inflammation of the gluteus muscles of the buttock.

glycemia The presence of sugar in the blood.

glyceraldehyde Compound formed by the oxidation of glycerol. Also called glyceric aldehyde.

glyceridase General term for any of several enzymes that promote the hydrolysis of glycerol esters.

glyceride An ester of glycerol.

glycerin A clear, syrupy, sweet, somewhat colorless liquid, $C_3H_8O_3$, used as a sweetener, a lubricant, and a solvent for drugs. See also glycerol.

glycerol A sweet, syrupy trihydric alcohol, occurring in combination as glycerides and produced by the fermentation of sugar; pharmaceutical preparations are known as glycerin.

glycerose A sugar resulting from the oxidation of glycerin.

glyceryl The trivalent radical, $C_3H_3O_3$, of glycerol. Also called propenyl.

g. guaiacolate $C_{10}H_{14}O_4$; used to promote the ejection of mucus or exudate from the lungs, bronchi, and trachea.

g. nitrate Nitroglycerin.

g. stearate See stearin.

glycine (Gly) The principal amino acid present in sugar cane, $C_2H_5NO_2$; the simplest of the amino acids and one of the first to be isolated from proteins. Also called aminoacetic acid.

glycinuria The presence of glycine in the urine.

glycocalyx A carbohydrate-rich outer fuzz coating on the free surface of certain epithelial cells; it is rich in mucoid components.

glycocholic acid The principal acid of the bile.

glycogen The form in which carbohydrate is stored in the body, especially in the liver and muscles; a highly branched glucosan of high molecular weight; it is broken down as needed to glucose molecules.

glycogenase The enzyme that promotes the breakdown of glycogen to glucose.

glycogenesis The formation of glycogen from glucose or other monosaccharides.

glycogenolysis The breakdown of glycogen to simpler products.

glycogenosis Abnormal accumulation of glycogen in the tissues. Also called glycogen storage disease.

type 1 g. Disorder thought to be caused by deficiency of the enzyme glucose 6-phosphatase, resulting in excessive accumulation of glycogen in the liver and kidneys. Also called von Gierke's disease; glucose 6-phosphatase hepatorenal glycogenosis.

type 2 g. Disease of infancy thought to be caused by deficiency of an enzyme, lysomal α-1,4-glucosidase, resulting in excessive accumulation of glycogen in the heart muscles, liver, and nervous system; associated with marked cardiac enlargement and congestive heart failure usually leading to death within the first year of life. Also called generalized glycogenosis; Pompe's disease.

type 5 g. Disorder attributed to deficiency of muscle glycogen phosphorylase (enzyme that catalyzes the splitting of glycogen to glucose), resulting in accumulation of glycogen in the muscles. Also called McArdle's syndrome; myophosphorylase deficiency glycogenosis.

glycogen storage disease See glycogenosis.

glycogeusia A subjective sweet taste in the mouth.

glycol One of a group of alcohols containing two hydroxyl groups.

glycolysis The energy-producing process in the body, especially in muscles, in which sugar is broken down into lactic acid; since oxygen is not consumed, it is frequently termed anaerobic glycolysis.

glycolytic Causing the hydrolysis or digestion of sugar.

glyconeogenesis The new formation of sugar; the formation of glucose or glycogen from substances other than carbohydrates, such as protein or fat.

glycoprotein Any of several protein-carbohydrate compounds (conjugated proteins); they include the mucins, the mucoids, and the chondroproteins.

glycoside Any of a group of compounds containing a carbohydrate and a noncarbohydrate residue in the same molecule; on hydrolysis they produce sugars and related compounds; found in animal tissues and in many drugs and spices.

glycosphingolipid A ceramide linked to one or more sugars by the terminal OH group.

glycostatic Tending to maintain a constant glycogen level in the tissues.

glycosuria Excretion of sugar in the urine in excess of the normal amount; frequently a sign of diabetes mellitus.

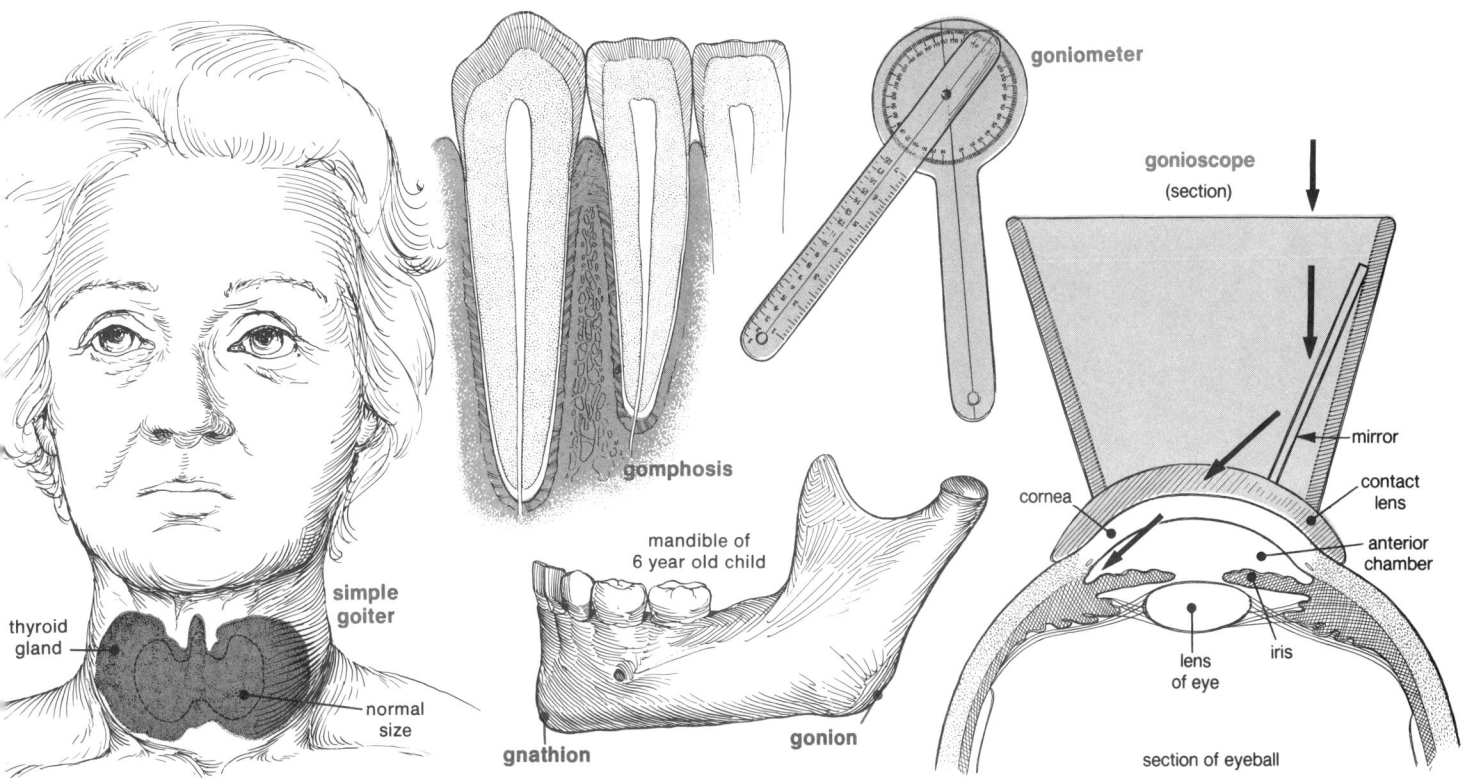

goniometer

gonioscope
(section)

mirror

contact lens

anterior chamber

cornea

lens of eye

iris

section of eyeball

gomphosis

mandible of 6 year old child

gnathion

gonion

thyroid gland

simple goiter

normal size

renal g. Glycosuria occurring with normal blood levels of sugar, due to failure of the renal tubules to reabsorb filtered glucose to the normal degree.

glycyrrhiza The dried roots of *Glycyrrhiza glabra;* used in pharmaceutical preparations. Also called licorice; licorice root.

glycyrrhizic acid A glycoside present in glycyrrhiza which in large amounts produces aldosterone-like effects in the kidney, causing retention of sodium and water and excessive excretion of potassium. Also called glycyrrhizin.

gnat One of several minute, winged, biting insects; a midge.

  buffalo g. *Simulium pecuarium;* a small, biting, black gnat; vector of onchocerciasis. Also called black fly.

gnathalgia See gnathodynia.

gnathic Of or pertaining to the jaw.

gnathion The lowest point of the midline of the mandible; a craniometric point.

gnathitis Inflammation of the jaw.

gnathodynamometer Instrument used in dentistry to measure the biting force of the jaw. Also called bite gauge; occlusometer.

gnathodynia Pain in the jaw. Also called gnathalgia.

gnathoplasty Plastic or reparative surgery of the jaw.

gnathostatics In orthodontic diagnosis, a technique based on relationships between the teeth and certain skull landmarks.

Gnathostoma A genus of parasitic, pathogenic, nematode worms (family Gnathostomatidae). Formerly called *Chiranthus.*

  G. spinigerum A species frequently transmitted to man by ingestion of the larvae in undercooked fish; it causes migratory swelling of the subcutaneous tissues or abscesses in the intestinal wall; the wandering larvae may also invade the eyes and brain.

gnathostomiasis Infection with *Gnathostoma spinigerum.*

gnosis The ability to recognize the nature and significance of objects, based on the reception of sensory stimuli (auditory, visual, or tactile).

gnotobiotic Denoting a laboratory animal that is germ-free or contains only known microorganisms.

goiter Enlargement of the thyroid gland causing a visible swelling in front of the neck.

  adenomatous g. Goiter due to the presence of a benign tumor of glandular tissue (adenoma).

  colloid g. A soft goiter in which the follicles of the gland are distended and filled with colloid.

  cystic g. An enlarged thyroid gland containing one or more cysts.

  exophthalmic g. Disorder caused by excessive production of thyroid hormone; marked by enlargement of the thyroid gland, bulging eyeballs, muscular tremors, rapid pulse rate, and weight loss. Also called Graves' disease.

  parenchymatous g. Uniform enlargement of the thyroid gland due to excessive proliferation of its follicles and epithelium.

  toxic g. A goiter with excessive secretions, causing signs and symptoms of hyperthyroidism.

goitrogen Any agent causing goiter.

gold A soft, deep yellow, corrosion-resistant element; one of the least destructible, and most chemically inert metals known; symbol Au, atomic number 79, atomic weight 196.9.

  white g. A gold alloy with a high palladium content.

gold-198 (^{198}Au) A radioactive isotope of gold; used in colloidal suspension for treating some forms of cancer.

gomphosis A type of fibrous articulation in which a bony process fits into a socket, as of a tooth and its socket.

gonad A sexual gland.

  female g. Ovary.

  male g. Testis.

gonadectomy The surgical removal of an ovary or testis.

gonadoblastoma A benign combined germ-cell and gonadal stromal growth.

gonadogenesis The development of the embryonic gonads.

gonadotropic Influencing the gonads, as the hormones of the anterior pituitary gland which stimulate the ovaries and testes.

gonadotropin A hormone or a substance that stimulates either the ovaries or the testes.

  chorionic g. (CG) Gonadotropin produced by the trophoblastic cells of the chorion; responsible for stimulating ovarian production of estrogen and progesterone during the first trimester of pregnancy.

  human chorionic g. (HCH, hCG) A polypeptide hormone produced by the placenta; its secretion begins soon after implantation of the fertilized ovum (blastocyst); also produced by abnormal chorionic epithelial tissue such as hydatiform moles.

gonalgia Pain in the knee.

gonecystolith A concretion of calculus in a seminal vesicle.

goniometer 1. An instrument for measuring angles. 2. A device used in testing for labyrinthine disease.

gonion The most posterior, inferior, and lateral point of the external mandibular angle.

goniopuncture Operation for congenital glaucoma in which a puncture is made in the trabecular meshwork (at the angle of the anterior chamber) through the corneoscleral junction of the opposite side.

gonioscope A combination of a contact lens and mirror which allows the observer to look directly into the angle of the anterior chamber of the eye.

gonioscopy Examination of the angle of the anterior chamber of the eye by means of a gonioscope.

goniosynechia Adhesion of the iris to the inner surface of the cornea at the angle of the anterior chamber; seen in angle-closure glaucoma.

goniotomy Borkan's operation for congenital glaucoma in which abnormal tissue is removed from the filtration angle of the anterior chamber.

gonococcal Relating to gonococci.

gonococcemia The presence of gonococci in the blood.

gonococcus, *pl.* **gonococci** (GC) The bacterium that causes gonorrhea; an individual organism of the species *Neisseria gonorrhoeae.*

gonocyte A primitive reproductive cell.

gonorrhea (GC) A common contagious disease caused by *Neisseria gonorrhoeae* and transmitted chiefly by sexual intercourse; it is marked by inflammation of the mucous membrane of the genital tract, a purulent discharge, and painful, frequent urination; if untreated it may cause complications such as epididymitis, prostatitis, tenosynovitis, arthritis, and endocarditis; in females it may lead to sterility, and in males to urethral stricture.

  oral g. Gonorrhea of the posterior mouth and pharynx acquired through oral sex.

gonorrheal Relating to gonorrhea.

gonycampsis Any abnormal curvature of the knee.

Goodpasture's syndrome Glomerulonephritis associated with diffuse pulmonary hemorrhage; caused by an antigen directed against the basement membrane of glomerulus capillaries and pulmonary alveoli. Also called hemorrhagic pulmonary-renal syndrome.

gouge 1. A strong chisel with a troughlike blade, usually used for cutting and removing bone. 2. To cut or scoop out in large amounts.

goundou An endemic disease of West Africa marked by egg-shaped swelling of the maxillary bone, on either side of the nose; associated with yaws.

gout A metabolic disorder marked by an excess of uric acid in the blood, by painful inflammation of joints, especially of the big toes, and by deposits of sodium biurate in the cartilages of the affected joints

tophaceous
gout

sclera

iris

caruncle

corneal
graft

bypass
graft

aorta

left coronary
artery

skin
graft

pedicle
graft

heart
(left anterior-
oblique view)

and in the kidney.

   saturnine g.   Gout accompanying lead poisoning.
   secondary g.   Gout occurring as a result of increased nucleoprotein metabolism and uric acid production.
   tophaceous g.   Gout marked by the presence of tophi (deposits of sodium urate) about the joints and cartilaginous areas.
gouty   Resembling or pertaining to gout.
gradient   Rate of change of temperature, pressure, distance, time, or any such variable value.
   concentration g.   A solution with a continuous concentration increase of the solute from top to bottom of the container. Also called density gradient.
   density g.   See concentration gradient.
   mitral g.   The difference in diastolic pressure between the left atrium and left ventricle.
   systolic g.   The difference in pressure during systole between two communicating chambers of the heart.
   ventricular g.   In electrocardiography, the alge-

braic sum of the areas within the QRS complex and the T wave of the electrocardiogram.
grading   A histologic method of providing an estimate of the gravity of a cancerous tumor, based on the degree of cell differentiation and the number of cell divisions within the tumor.
graduate   A laboratory vessel marked off in units of fluid volume.
Graefe's disease   See ophthalmoplegia progressiva.
Graefe's sign, von Graefe's sign   Immobility or lagging of the upper eyelid on downward movement of the eye. Also called lid lag.
graft 1. Any tissue transplanted into a body part. **2.** To insert such a tissue.
   allogeneic g.   A graft derived from a genetically dissimilar individual of the same species. Also called allograft.
   autogenous g.   A graft of tissue derived from the same individual or animal to which it is transplanted. Also called autograft.
   bypass g.   A tubular graft sutured above and

below an occluded arterial segment to circumvent the occlusion and re-establish circulation beyond the occluded site.
   checkerboard g.   See postage stamp graft.
   corneal g.   Donor corneal tissue used in keratoplasty to replace diseased corneal tissue; split thickness (lamellar) and full thickness (penetrating) grafts are the most common types used.
   cutis g.   A piece of skin from which the epidermis and subcutaneous tissue have been removed.
   delayed g.   Grafting postponed until infection has been eliminated.
   double end g.   See pedicle graft.
   full thickness g.   A graft consisting of skin and subcutaneous tissue.
   island g.   See pedicle graft.
   isogeneic g.   See isograft.
   pedicle g.   A stalk of skin and subcutaneous tissue left attached at the donor site until its free end has taken at the recipient site. Also called double end or island graft.
   pinch g.'s   Circular bits of skin a few millimeters

scalp
skull
brain
arachnoid granulations
mitochondrion
matrix granule
platelet formation
multi-lobular nucleus
basophilic granules
megakaryocyte
RBC for size comparison
granulocytes neutrophil
multilobular nucleus
specific granules
bilobular nucleus
eosinophil
basophil

in diameter.

postage stamp g. Multiple, small, thick-split skin graft. Also called checkerboard graft.

prosthetic g. A graft composed of synthetic material; often used in bypass operations of large caliber arteries.

reversed autogenous saphenous vein g. A segment of the patient's own saphenous vein turned inside out prior to insertion to prevent the vein's valves from obstructing the blood flow; used in bypass operations of small caliber vessels, such as coronary arteries.

skin g. A piece of skin removed from one area of the body, or from another person, to cover a denuded area at another site.

split thickness g. A graft consisting of a superficial layer of the dermis.

syngeneic g. See isograft.

tendon g. A piece of tendon used to repair a defect.

thick-split g. A graft consisting of about three quarters of the skin's thickness.

xenogeneic g. A transplant involving two different species, such as the transplantation of a chimpanzee kidney into a human. Also called xenograft.

grafting Transplantation of tissue from one part of the body to another or from one body to another.

grain 1. A minute hard particle. 2. A unit of weight equivalent to 0.0648 gm.

gram (g, gm) A metric unit of mass and weight, equal to one-thousandth of a kilogram and approximately one cubic centimeter of water at its maximum density.

gramicidin A substance produced by the growth of *Bacillus brevis*; used topically to arrest the growth of gram-positive cocci and bacilli.

grammeter A unit of energy equal to the force required to raise a weight of one gram to a height of one meter.

gram-molecule The quantity of a substance that has a weight in grams numerically equal to the molecular weight of the substance; e.g., a gram-molecule of hydrogen weighs two grams. Also called mole; mol.

gram-negative Denoting a microorganism that fails to retain the violet dye used in Gram's stain.

gram-positive Denoting a microorganism that retains the violet dye used in Gram's stain.

grandiose In psychiatry, denoting feeling of great importance; having delusions of grandeur.

grand mal Generalized epilepsy; see under epilepsy.

granular 1. Composed of or resembling granules

or grains. 2. Particles with a strong affinity for stains.

granulase An enzyme capable of splitting starch into dextrins and maltose.

granulation 1. The act or process of dividing substances into small particles or granules; the state of being granular. 2. The formation of small, rounded, fleshy masses on the surface of a healing wound; also, one of these fleshy masses. 3. A granular mass in or on the surface of an organ or membrane, as a mass of lymphoid tissue on the conjunctiva of the eyelids. 4. The formation of crystals by prolonged agitation of a supersaturated solution of a salt.

arachnoid g.'s Small masses of arachnoid projecting into the venous sinuses and on the outer surface of the dura mater, causing, through pressure, the pits on the inner surface of the cranium; they usually appear at the age of seven years and increase in size and number as age advances. Also called pacchionian bodies or granulations.

pacchionian g.'s See arachnoid granulations.

granule 1. A grain or small particle; a minute discrete mass. 2. A small pill, usually sugar coated.

acidophilic g. A granule staining readily with acid dyes such as eosin.

azurophilic g., azure g. A granule that stains readily with azure dye.

basophilic g. A granule staining readily with basic dyes such as azure A.

chromophobe g. A granule that does not stain or stains poorly.

Crooke's g.'s Masses of basophilic material in the basophilic cells of the anterior lobe of the pituitary gland; seen in Cushing's disease or after the administration of ACTH.

matrix g.'s Highly electron-dense intramitochondrial granules, about 500 Å in diameter; thought to be the binding sites for calcium ions.

membrane-coating g. One of several ovoid cytoplasmic granules in the spinous cells of the epidermis about 300 nm in diameter, bound by a double-layered membrane, and filled with lamellae; considered by some to be a specialized epidermal lysosome. Also called keratinosome; lamellated granule.

osmophilic g. A granule that flourishes in the medium of high osmotic pressure.

secretory g.'s Packaged products of synthesized products temporarily stored in secretory cells.

Shuffner's g.'s Fine granules present in red blood cells infected with malarial parasites, particularly *Plasmodium vivax*, giving the cells a dotted or stippled appearance.

zymogen g. One of several granules present in enzyme-secreting cells such as those in a salivary

gland.

granuloblast An embryonic blood cell capable of developing into a granulocyte. Also called myeloblast.

granulocyte A mature granular white blood cell (leukocyte) that develops in the bone marrow from a myeloblast; depending on the specific granules, there are three types: neutrophilic (polymorphonuclear) granulocyte, eosinophilic granulocyte, and basophilic granulocyte.

granulocytopenia Deficiency of granular leukocytes (granulocytes) in the blood. Also called granulopenia.

granulocytopoiesis See granulopoiesis.

granulocytosis The presence of an excessive number of granulocytes in the blood or in the tissues.

granuloma A tumor composed of granulation tissue.

dental g. A mass of chronic inflammatory tissue, usually asymptomatic, occurring at the root of a tooth. Also called periapical granuloma.

eosinophilic g. A relatively benign disorder marked by a single lesion involving one or several bones, beginning in the marrow and gradually eroding the cortex; occurring predominantly in children and young adults.

giant-cell g. A tumor-like mass protruding from the gums (gingiva) believed to be of inflammatory origin.

g. inguinale A chronic disease marked by granulomatous ulcerations in the inguinal region and the genitalia; caused by *Calymmatum granulomatis*.

periapical g. See dental granuloma.

pyogenic g., g. pyogenicum A red, small, benign overgrowth of granulation tissue on the skin or oral mucosa arising as a result of trauma.

swimming pool g. A chronic warty growth, which may ulcerate, arising on abrasions, resulting from infection with *Mycobacterium marinum* in swimming pools, aquariums, or any body of water.

granulomatosis Any disorder marked by the presence of multiple granulomas.

lipoid g., lipid g. See xanthomatosis.

lipophagic intestinal g. See Whipple's disease.

Wegener's g. A rare, often fatal, disease marked by ulceration of the upper respiratory tract progressing to involvement of the lungs, acute necrotizing arteritis, and glomerulonephritis.

granulomatous Resembling a granuloma.

granulopenia See granulocytopenia.

granuloplastic Capable of forming granules.

granulopoiesis The formation of granulocytes. Also called granulocytopoeisis.

granulosis, granulosity A mass of minute gran-

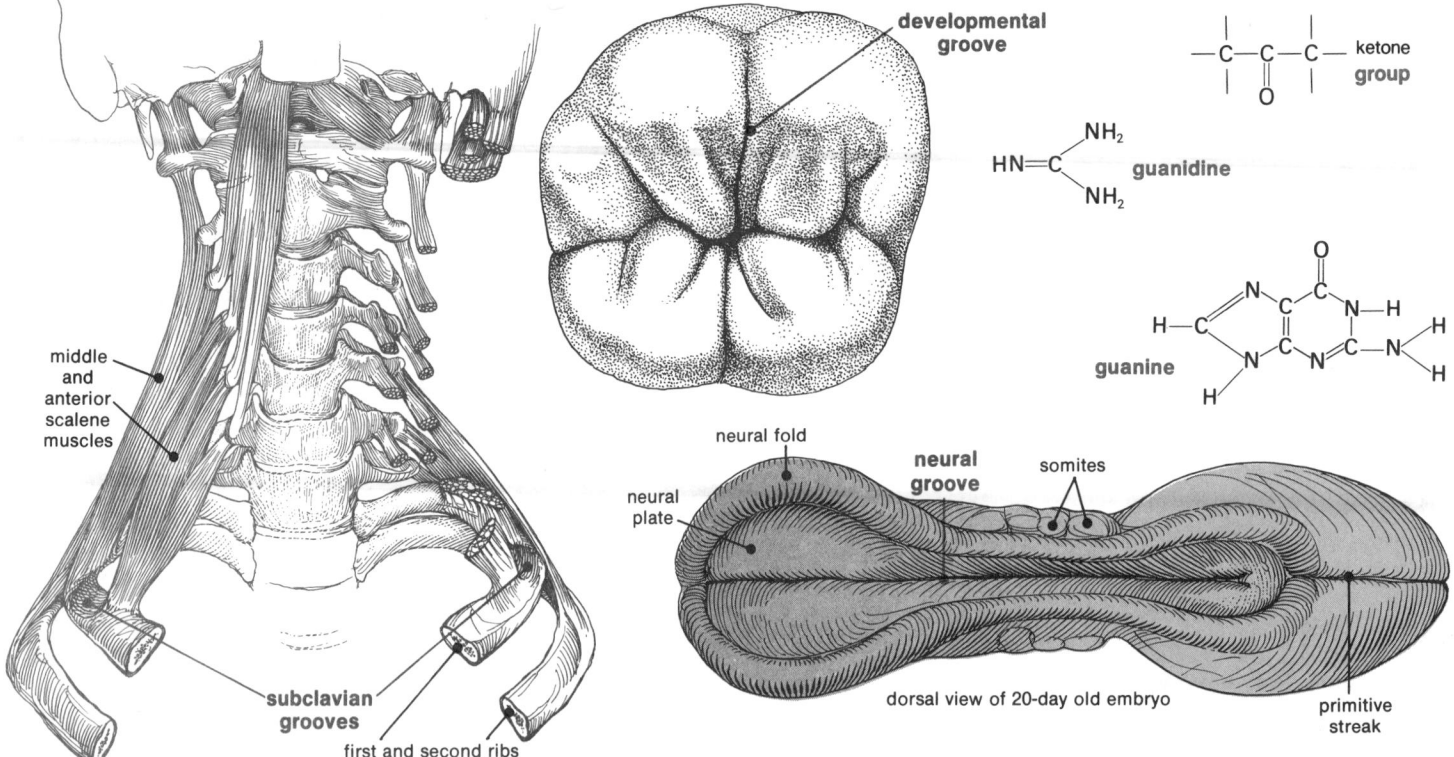

middle and anterior scalene muscles

subclavian grooves

first and second ribs

developmental groove

—C—C—C— ketone group
        ‖
        O

HN=C guanidine
   ⟨NH₂
   ⟨NH₂

guanine

neural fold

neural groove

somites

neural plate

dorsal view of 20-day old embryo

primitive streak

ules.

graph Any pictorial device that displays a relationship of varying values. Also called chart.

graphology The study of handwriting as an aid in analyzing the character of the writer.

graphospasm Writer's cramp; see under cramp.

GRAS Acronym for generally regarded as safe, denoting any safe food additive.

grave Indicating symptoms of an extremely serious or dangerous character. Also called critical.

gravel Numerous minute concretions, usually of uric acid, calcium oxalate, or phosphates, formed in the kidney and bladder.

Grave's disease Exophthalmic goiter; see under goiter.

gravid Pregnant.

gravida A woman who is, or has been, pregnant.

gravidity 1. The pregnant state. **2.** The total number of pregnancies a woman has had, including a current pregnancy.

gravimeter An instrument used to measure the specific gravity of a liquid. Also called hydrometer.

gravimetric Of, determined by, or relating to measurement by weight.

gravity (G) The gravitational force.

  negative g. Gravity in a foot-to-head direction in flying, or in standing on one's head.

  specific g. (sp gr) The ratio of the mass of any substance (usually liquid) compared to the mass of an equal volume of another substance (usually distilled water at 4°C).

Grey Turner's sign Areas of discoloration about the navel and the loins occurring in acute hemorrhagic pancreatitis.

grid 1. A frame of parallel horizontal and vertical lines forming squares of uniform size, used as a reference for plotting curves. **2.** In dentistry, an instrument composed of alternate strips of lead and radiolucent material, placed in apposition to a film to absorb secondary or scattered radiation.

  Wetzel g. A chart for evaluating the growth and physical fitness of young and adolescent children.

grief A state of intense mental anguish normally resulting from the loss of a valued object or person.

griffin claw See hand, griffin-claw.

grinding, selective In dentistry, the modification of occlusal surfaces of teeth with the intent of equalizing occlusal stress or of harmonizing cuspal relations, with the aid of articulator paper or equilibration ribbon.

grinding-in In dentistry, the act of correcting occlusal errors in natural and artificial teeth. Also called equilibrating.

grip 1. Grippe. **2.** Grasp.

  devil's g. Epidemic pleurodynia; see under pleurodynia.

gripe Colic (2); sharp pain in the intestines.

grippe From French *gripper*, to seize; flu-like illness. Also called influenza; grip.

griseofulvin A fungistatic antibiotic derived from a species of *Penicillium*; used systemically in the treatment of superficial fungal infections; Fulvicin-U/F®.

gristle Cartilage.

groin 1. The inguinal region; the region around the crease formed at the junction of the thigh and trunk. **2.** The external genital organs.

Grönblad-Strandberg syndrome An elastic tissue degeneration that involves the retina, gastrointestinal tract, and especially the skin.

groove A narrow, elongated depression.

  carotid g. The groove through the sphenoid bone in which the internal carotid artery lies in its course through the cavernous sinus.

  costal g. A groove in the lower border of the rib, housing the intercostal vessels and nerve.

  developmental g. A groove on the enamel of a tooth, marking the fusion of the lobes of the crown during tooth development.

  neural g. The transitory median dorsal groove in the thickened ectoderm (neural plate) of young embryos; the closure of the groove forms a closed tubular structure with a long caudal portion, the future spinal cord, and a broader cephalic portion, which becomes the brain.

  subclavian g. A shallow groove on the first rib between the anterior and middle scalene muscles through which the subclavian artery and the inferior trunk of the brachial plexus pass.

group 1. A collection of related objects. **2.** In chemistry, a radical.

  characteristic g. A distinctive group of atoms that make one substance different from others.

  Lancefield g.'s Lancefield's classification; see under classification.

  symptom g. 1. Syndrome. **2.** A complex in the electrocardiogram.

growth 1. The progressive development of an organism or any of its parts. **2.** A tumor.

  appositional g. Growth through the addition of layers, typical of rigid structures. Also called growth by accretion.

  differential g. The various growth rates of related tissues, as in embryonic structures, with resulting change in proportions.

  interstitial g. Growth through formation of new tissue throughout the structure, as occurs in soft tissues.

  psychological g. Growth toward self-actualization or personal maturity.

  zero population g. (ZPG) The state of a total population that neither increases nor decreases, oc-

curring when the number of births and immigrants equals the number of deaths and emigrants.

grub The larva of certain insects.

gruel Thin porridge; any semifluid food made of cereal boiled in water.

grunt A deep, guttural sound in the chest; a frequent sign of chest pain implying an acute pneumonic process with pleural involvement; also seen in pulmonary edema and in the respiratory distress syndrome of the neonatal period.

  expiratory g. A laryngeal sound sometimes heard during surgical manipulation of the subdiaphragmatic areas.

gryposis Any abnormal curvature.

guaiacol A colorless, oily liquid, $C_7H_8O_2$, obtained from creosote or made synthetically from pyrocatechin; used chiefly as an expectorant, intestinal disinfectant, and local anesthetic.

guanethidine sulfate A potent antihypertensive drug, thought to interfere with the release of norepinephrine at the sympathetic neuroeffector junction; Ismelin Sulfate®.

guanidine A strong base obtained from the oxidation of guanine; the amidine of aminocarbamic acid, CH_5N_3, considered by some to be one of the factors responsible for part of the uremic syndrome in renal failure.

guanidinemia The presence of guanidine in the blood.

guanidinosuccinic acid A metabolic by-product found in the body in excessive amounts in renal failure and implicated in the clotting abnormality and the neuropathy of the chronic uremic syndrome.

guanine A crystalline purine base.

guanosine 9-β-D-Ribosylguanine; guanine combined with D-ribose.

gubernaculum A guiding cord connecting two structures.

  g. dentis The connective tissue band connecting the permanent tooth follicle to the gingiva.

  g. testis A ligamentous cord extending from the lower end of the fetal testis through the inguinal canal to the floor of the developing scrotum; it guides the descent of the testis from the abdomen into the scrotum.

Guillain-Barré syndrome Acute segmentally demyelinating polyradiculoneuropathy, a disease complex in which the basic mechanism appears to be an immunizing or allergic reaction commonly occurring after a minor febrile illness; inflammatory changes in the spinal cord produce bilateral weakness or paralysis, most commonly beginning in the lower extremities; recovery is usual if respiratory and vasomotor failure do not occur; the classical findings in the spinal fluid are elevated protein concentration without pleocytosis and under normal

guillotine

generally used for resecting the first rib

guinea pig

gynecomastia

precentral gyrus

postcentral gyrus

supramarginal gyrus

angular gyrus

frontal gyri

temporal gyri

pressure. Also called infectious polyneuritis; acute polyradiculitis.

guillotine A surgical cutting instrument with a knifeblade that slides in the grooves of a guide.

guinea pig Any of several small tropical American burrowing rodents of the genus *Cavia*, used extensively for experimental work.

gullet The pharynx and the esophagus; the passage leading from the mouth to the stomach.

gum 1. The dried viscous sap exuded by certain trees and plants; it is water-soluble, noncrystalline, and brittle. **2.** The gingiva.

g. arabic A gummy exudate of various African trees of the genus *Acacia*; used in the preparation of medicinal drugs. Also called acacia.

gumboil Colloquial term for a chronic alveolar abscess that drains itself by perforating the gum. See also abscess, alveolar.

gumma, *pl.* **gummas, gummata** A soft, gummy, infectious tumor that occurs, irregularly, during the third stage of syphilis.

gummatous Relating to or of the nature of a gumma.

gurney A wheeled stretcher or cot for transporting patients, usually within a hospital.

gustation 1. The sense of taste. **2.** The act of tasting.

gustatory Of or relating to the sense of taste.

gut 1. The intestine. **2.** The digestive tube of the embryo.

gutta (gt) Latin for a drop; a volume of liquid considered a unit of measure; equivalent to about 1 minim of water.

gutta-percha A milky latex sap of several tropical trees (family Sapotaceae); used in the manufacture of splints and as a thin waterproof sheet to protect wounds; in dentistry, used for temporary sealing of dressings in cavities and for filling of root canals.

guttate Resembling a drop; said of certain skin lesions.

guttatim Latin for drop by drop.

guttur Latin for throat.

guttural Relating to the throat.

gymnocyte A cell without a limiting membrane.

gymnophobia Morbid fear of the sight of the naked body.

gynandrism A congenital defect marked by overdevelopment of the clitoris and fusion of the labia majora, having the appearance of a penis and scrotum.

gynandromorph An individual with both male and female characteristics.

gynandromorphous Having male and female characteristics.

gynatresia Occlusion of a part of the female genital tract, usually the vagina.

gynecoid Resembling a female.

gynecologic Pertaining to gynecology.

gynecologist A specialist in gynecology.

gynecology The branch of medicine concerned with diseases peculiar to women.

gynecomania Insatiable sexual desire for women.

gynecomastia Excessive development of the male breast.

gynephobia Morbid fear of or aversion to women.

gynopathy Any disease characteristic of women.

gynoplastics Reparative surgery of the female genitalia.

gypsum The dihydrate of calcium sulfate; $CaSO_4 \cdot 2H_2O$, from which plaster of Paris and dental stone are derived.

gyration 1. Revolution about a stationary point. **2.** An arrangement or group of gyri in the brain.

gyri Plural of gyrus.

gyrus A convolution of the brain.

angular g. A convolution arching over the upturned end of the superior temporal sulcus.

cingulate g. A long curved convolution lying above and in front of the corpus callosum; it is continuous posteriorly with the isthmus.

dentate g. A narrow crenated strip of cortex between the fimbria hippocampi and the hippocampal gyrus; it is continued posteriorly, under the splenium of the corpus callosum, as the delicate fasciolar gyrus.

fasciolar g. The transitional band between the dentate gyrus and the indusium griseum (supracallosal gyrus); located near the splenium of the corpus callosum.

frontal gyri The three (superior, middle, and inferior) gyri of the frontal lobe.

hippocampal g. A convolution that lies between the collateral sulcus and the hippocampal sulcus, on the inferior surface of each cerebral hemisphere; posteriorly, it is continuous above the cingulate gyrus through the isthmus and below the lingual gyrus. Also called parahippocampal gyrus.

lingual g. A median occipitotemporal gyrus between the calcarine and collateral sulci.

paraterminal g. A thin sheet of gray matter which covers the undersurface of the rostrum of the corpus callosum.

postcentral g. The anterior convolution of the parietal lobe, bounded in front by the central sulcus (Rolando) and posteriorly by the interparietal sulcus.

precentral g. The posterior convolution of the frontal lobe bounded posteriorly by the central sulcus (Rolando) and anteriorly by the precentral sulcus.

supracallosal g. A thin sheet of gray matter which covers the superior surface of the corpus callosum of the brain. Also called indusium griseum.

supramarginal g. A convolution that arches over the upturned end of the lateral sulcus.

temporal gyri The three convolutions (superior, middle, inferior) on the lateral side of the temporal lobe, inferior to the lateral sulcus.

transverse temporal gyri Two or three convolutions lying transversely on the superior temporal gyrus, mostly in the lateral sulcus.

hallux valgus

varus of
metatarsal

flat, wide
transverse
arch

hallux
valgus

orthopedic head
halter

half-life
decay curve
of radioactive
iodine (¹³¹I)

Percent of activity

100 — 64 mc
75 —
50 — 32 mc
25 — 16 mc
8 mc 4 mc 2 mc 1 mc

1 9 17 25 33 41 49
Days

Hh

habena 1. A restricting band or frenum. 2. A restraining bandage.

habenula The dorsal pedicle of the pineal gland.

habit 1. A constant tendency to perform an act, acquired by frequent repetition of the act. 2. An addiction.

habituation 1. The process of forming a habit; especially the process of becoming addicted to a drug. 2. The method by which the nervous system gradually reduces response to a repeated stimulus.

habitus Physical and constitutional characteristics of a person, especially as related to susceptibility to some disease.

Haemaphysalis A genus of ticks infesting birds and small mammals; vectors of disease.

   H. leporis palustris A species that transmits Rocky Mountain spotted fever and tularemia to rabbits, but not to humans.

Haemodipsus ventricosus The rabbit louse; it transmits the causative agent of tularemia in man.

Haemophilus A genus of bacteria; minute gram-negative, nonmotile, rod-shaped cells, parasitic on media containing blood.

   H. ducreyi A species that is the causative agent of chancroid (soft chancre). Also called Ducrey's bacillus.

   H. influenzae The influenza bacillus; a species found in the respiratory tract; causes acute respiratory infections, acute conjunctivitis, and purulent meningitis in children, rarely in adults. Also called Pfeiffer's, Weeks', or Koch-Weeks bacillus.

   H. parahaemolyticus A species found in the upper respiratory tract; frequently associated with pharyngitis.

haemorrhagia Greek for hemorrhage.

Haemosporidia An order of sporozoa, parasitic in the blood of vertebrates; some of the species cause various diseases.

hafnium Chemical element; symbol Hf, atomic number 72, atomic weight 178.50.

Hageman factor Factor XII.

hagiotherapy 1. Treatment of disease by placing the patient in contact with religious relics, by visiting shrines, or by participating in religious observances.

2. Treatment of disease executed by a holy man.

hair 1. Pilus (1). 2. A long cylindrical filament.

   embryonic h. See lanugo hair.

   ingrown h. Hair that continues to grow but fails to emerge from the pilosebaceous ostium, sometimes causing papules. Also called burrowing hair.

   lanugo h. Soft, fine hair growing on the body of the newborn. Also called embryonic hair.

   tactile h. The whiskers of certain animals.

   taste h. One of the hairlike projections of gustatory cells, formed by the condensation of secretions.

halazone An antibacterial substance used in the sterilization of water supplies.

half-life (HL) The time required for half of the radioactivity originally associated with a radioactive substance to disintegrate (radioactive decay).

   biologic h.-l. ($T_{½}$) 1. The time required for a radioactive isotope within the body to lose half of its activity; this depends both on the natural half-life of the isotope and the rate of excretion from the body. 2. The time it takes for the body to eliminate 50% of a drug.

halide A salt of a halogen (bromide, chlorine, fluorine, or iodine).

halitosis Unpleasant breath; some causes are poor mouth hygiene, infection in the oronasopharyngeal structures, and lung abscess.

halitus 1. Latin for breath. 2. An exhalation; vapor.

hallucal Of or relating to the big toe.

hallucination Perception of objects or events which do not exist.

   hypnagogic h. Vivid sensory, dreamlike experiences occurring during the period between wakefulness and sleep.

hallucinatory 1. Characterized by hallucination. 2. Capable of inducing hallucination.

hallucinogen Any agent that induces hallucinations.

hallucinosis A psychotic state in which an individual is more or less persistently hallucinated; e.g., chronic alcoholic hallucinosis.

hallux *pl.* **halluces** The big toe; the first digit of the foot.

   h. dolorosa A painful condition usually associ-

ated with flatfoot, in which walking causes severe discomfort in the metatarsophalangeal joint of the big toe.

   h. malleus Hammertoe of the big toe.

   h. rigidus Stiff toe; painful flexion of the big toe due to stiffness in the metatarsophalangeal joint.

   h. valgus The most common of the painful conditions of the toes, marked by an abnormal angulation of the big toe toward the other toes of the same foot; the condition is generally attributed to narrow or pointed shoes; predisposing congenital and familial factors may exist. Cf. bunion.

   h. varus An abnormal angulation of the big toe away from the other toes of the same foot.

halo, glaucomatous Colored rings seen around lights by individuals with glaucoma; caused by diffraction of droplets of fluid in the corneal epithelium in the presence of edema of the cornea.

halogen Any of a group of chemically related nonmetallic elements that form similar saltlike compounds in combination with sodium; they include bromine, chlorine, fluorine, iodine, and the radioactive element astatine.

haloid Resembling a halogen.

halophil, halophile A microorganism that thrives in a salty environment.

halothane A liquid hydrocarbon used as a general anesthetic; associated with liver damage in susceptible individuals; Fluothane®.

halter A device for securing the head, particularly for traction.

ham 1. The buttock and back part of the thigh. 2. The popliteal space or poples; the hollow behind the knee.

hamartoblastoma Malignant tumor believed to be derived from a hamartoma.

hamartoma Tumorlike nonmalignant growth composed of cellular elements normally present in that site, but poorly developed.

Hamman-Rich syndrome Progressive interstitial fibrosis of both lungs leading to pulmonary insufficiency, right-sided heart failure, and death; the cause is unknown.

Hamman's sign A rasping sound, synchronous

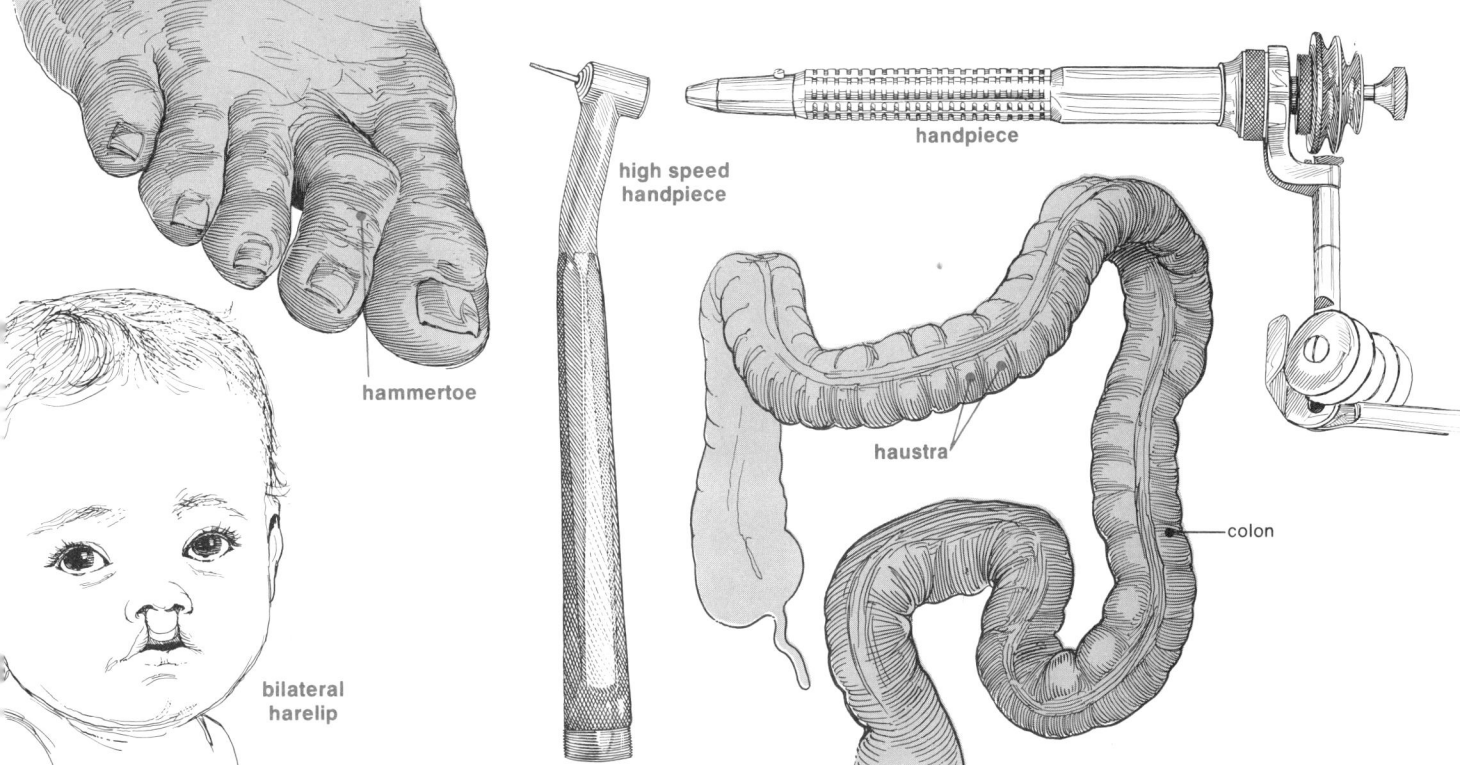

hammertoe

bilateral
harelip

high speed
handpiece

handpiece

haustra

colon

with the heart beat, occurring in pneumomediastinum.

hammer See malleus.

hammertoe A deformed toe in which the second and third phalanges are bent downward.

hamster Any of several ratlike Eurasian rodents (family Cricetidae) extensively used in experimental work.

hamstring Either of two tendons bounding the popliteal space of the knee; the medial or inner one comprises the tendons of the semimembranosus, semitendinosus, gracilis, and sartorius muscles; the lateral or outer one consists of the tendon of the biceps femoris.

hamular Shaped like a hook.

hamulus Any hook-shaped process, as at the end of a bone.

h. lacrimalis The lacrimal hamulus; the hooklike process of the lacrimal bone articulating with the maxilla and forming the upper aperture of the bony nasal duct.

h. laminae spiralis The hooklike termination of the spiral lamina bone of the cochlea.

h. pterygoideus The hooklike process of the sphenoid bone.

hand The terminal part of the upper extremity below the forearm.

accoucheur's h. The characteristic position of the hand produced by spasm in tetany.

griffin-claw h. Permanent extension of the metacarpophalangeal joints. Also called griffin claw; main en griffe.

opera glass h. Deformity of the hand marked by shortening of the fingers and transverse folding of the skin caused by absorption of the phalanges, seen in chronic absorptive arthritis. Also called main en lorgnette.

spade h. The characteristic coarse, thick, square hand of acromegaly or myxedema.

trident h. A hand in which the fingers are short and thick and nearly equal in length, with a deflection (at the second phalangeal joint) of the index and middle fingers toward the radial side and the ring and little fingers toward tne ulnar side, causing the fingers to spread out; characteristic hand of achondroplasia.

H and E stain Abbreviation for hematoxylin and eosin stain; see under stain.

hand-foot-and-mouth disease A highly infectious disease of children characterized by painful ulcerative stomatitis of the tongue, soft palate, and oral mucosa, associated with a vesicular eruption on hands and feet; attributed to type A-16 or A-5 Coxsackie virus.

handpiece In dentistry, the part of a mechanized,

hand-held device that holds rotary instruments such as burs and mandrels during operative procedures; it is connected to a dental engine.

high-speed h. One that operates at rotational speeds in excess of 12,000 revolutions per minute.

ultra high-speed h. One that operates at rotational speeds of 100,000 to 300,000 revolutions per minute.

ultrasonic h. One that vibrates at a frequency of 29,000 cycles per second (above audible range).

water-turbine h. One with a turbine powered by water under great pressure.

Hand-Schüller-Christian syndrome Disorder principally of childhood, occasionally of young adulthood, characterized by exophthalmos (unilateral or bilateral), diabetes insipidus, and destruction of bone (especially of the skull), with tumorlike masses of cholesterol-loaded histiocytes. Also called Schüller-Christian syndrome; Schüller disease.

hangnail A partly detached piece of skin at the base or side of the nail.

Hansen's disease See leprosy.

hapalonychia A state or condition characterized by soft fingernails or toenails; it can be normal or acquired as a result of malnutrition or debility.

haplodont Having peglike, even-surfaced molar teeth.

haploid Referring to the reduced number of chromosomes in the gametes relative to that in the zygotes or in the body cells (diploid); the haploid number is half the diploid number.

haplopia Single, normal vision, distinguished from double vision or diplopia.

haplosis The meiotic reduction of the diploid number of chromosomes to the haploid number.

hapten, haptene Any incomplete antigen which combines specifically with antibody but which does not incite the production of antibody unless attached to a high molecular weight carrier.

haptoglobin A protein present in human blood serum having the ability to combine with hemoglobin; a low level of haptoglobin indicates recent hemolysis.

haptometer Instrument used to determine sensitivity to touch.

haptophore The atom group in the molecule of an antigen or antibody by means of which it becomes attached to a cell or to its corresponding antibody or antigen, respectively.

hard-metal disease A pneumoconiosis attributed to inhalation of a specific industrial dust, especially of tungsten carbide, silicon carbide, or cobalt.

hardness The ability of a material to resist scratching, abrasion, or attrition.

harelip Congenital malformation of the upper lip ranging from a scarlike groove, or a notching of the lip, to a complete cleft extending into the nasal cavity; may be unilateral or bilateral and is frequently accompanied by a cleft palate. Also called cleft lip; cheiloschisis.

harmony, occlusal A contact between upper and lower teeth that is devoid of defects.

harpoon An instrument with a barbed head used to remove small pieces of tissue for microscopic examination.

Hartnup disease A hereditary disorder of amino acid transport, marked by a pellagra-like skin rash upon exposure to sunlight, temporary muscular incoordination, and excretion of excessive amounts of amino acid in the urine. Also called H disease; Hartnup syndrome.

Hartnup syndrome See Hartnup disease.

hasamiyami A fever occurring in Japan in the autumn, caused by a bacterium (*Leptospira autumnalis*).

hashish An intoxicating extract made from the dried flowers of the hemp plant, *Cannabis sativa.* Also written hasheesh.

hatchet An angled cutting hand instrument used in dentistry to remove enamel and dentin.

haunch The region of the upper thigh, buttock, and hip.

haustral Relating to the pouches or sacculations of the colon.

haustration Increase in size of the sacculations of the large intestine.

haustrum *pl.* **haustra** One of the sacculations of the colon.

haversian Term applied to the various osseous structures described by Clopton Havers.

H disease See Hartnup disease.

head 1. The upper or anterior vertebrate extremity, containing the brain and organs of special senses. 2. The proximal extremity of a bone; that which is nearer the axial skeleton. 3. The end of a muscle which is attached to the less movable part of the skeleton. 4. Slang expression denoting one who frequently uses narcotics.

headache Pain or ache in the head. Also called cephalalgia.

blind h. Migraine.

cluster h. A recurrent unilateral headache in the orbitotemporal area; usually of brief duration, often severe, generally occurring in regular intervals of six-week cycles; usually accompanied by stuffiness of the nose and tearing of the eye on the same side as the pain; can be precipitated by the use of histamine, alcohol, or nitroglycerin; more prevalent among males who smoke heavily. Also called histaminic

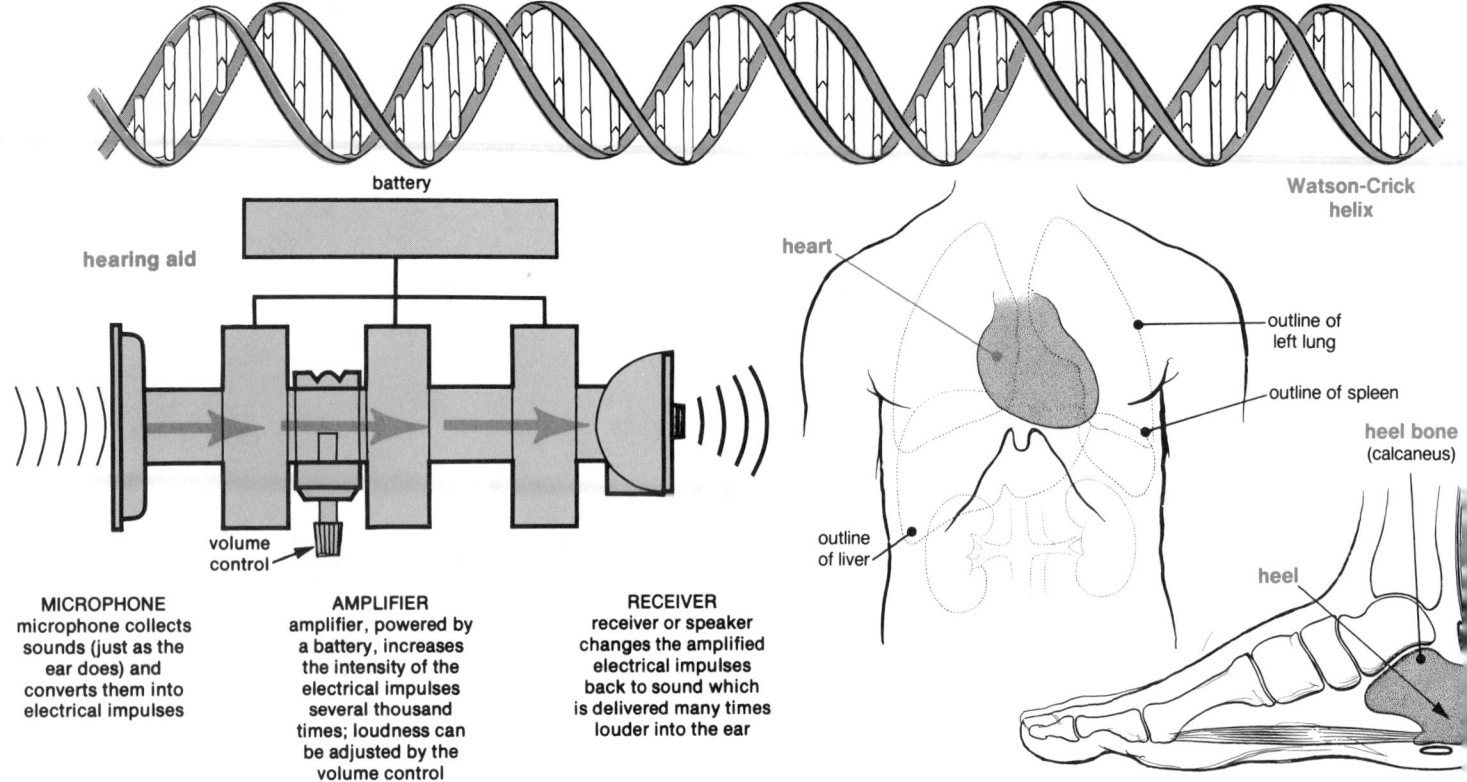

hearing aid

battery

MICROPHONE
microphone collects sounds (just as the ear does) and converts them into electrical impulses

volume control

AMPLIFIER
amplifier, powered by a battery, increases the intensity of the electrical impulses several thousand times; loudness can be adjusted by the volume control

RECEIVER
receiver or speaker changes the amplified electrical impulses back to sound which is delivered many times louder into the ear

heart

outline of left lung

outline of spleen

outline of liver

Watson-Crick helix

heel bone (calcaneus)

heel

---

headache or cephalalgia; Horton's headache.

histaminic h. See cluster headache.

Horton's h. See cluster headache.

migraine h. Migraine.

organic h. Headache caused by disease of the brain or its membranes.

tension h. Headache caused by sustained contraction of skeletal muscle about the scalp, face, and especially the neck.

vascular h. Migraine.

headgear 1. In orthodontics, an apparatus encircling the head or neck which provides anchorage for the attachment of an intraoral appliance. 2. In radiology, a protective device to guard the head from injury by radiation.

heal 1. To close naturally, said of an incision, wound, or ulcer. 2. To restore to health; to cure.

healer One who heals or cures, especially a physician.

healing 1. The process of return to normal health. 2. Denoting an agent that promotes such a process.

health 1. The state of an organism with respect to its physical, mental, and social wellbeing. 2. The state of an organism functioning optimally without disorders of any nature.

community h. See public health.

public h. The organized programs, services, and institutions involved with the prevention of disease and the health needs of the population as a whole. Also called community health.

healthy Of or pertaining to good health.

hear To perceive sound.

hearing The capacity to perceive sound.

color h. A subjective color sensation produced by certain sound waves. Also called pseudochromesthesia.

monaural h. Hearing with only one ear.

hearing aid A small device that amplifies sound; used to compensate for a hearing loss.

hearing loss Reduced auditory sensitivity.

sensorineural h. l. Loss of hearing due to dysfunction of the end organ or nerve fibers or both.

heart The hollow, muscular, four chambered organ that maintains the circulation of the blood by receiving it from the veins and pumping it into the arteries; it lies between the lungs and is enclosed in the pericardium. Also called cor.

artificial h. A device that partially or completely replaces the function of the natural heart.

dextroposition of h. See under dextroposition.

h. failure See under failure.

left h. The left atrium and left ventricle considered together.

right h. The right atrium and right ventricle con-

sidered together.

heartburn Burning sensation in the lower chest and upper central area of the abdomen, caused by irritation of the esophagus; it occurs because of reflux of stomach contents due to an incompetent esophageal sphincter. Also called pyrosis.

heartworm A parasitic nematode worm, *Dirofilaria immitis,* that usually lodges in the right chambers of the heart of dogs; very rarely seen in man.

heat 1. A state characterized by elevation of temperature. 2. A form of energy in transit from a body of higher temperature to another of lower temperature. 3. Estrus.

h. of combustion The quantity of heat released in the complete oxidation of one mole of a substance at constant pressure.

prickly h. A common, noncontagious skin disorder of hot, humid climates; elevated temperatures cause maceration of the skin; leading to blockage of sweat pores, retention of sweat, and formation of tiny vesicular papules that itch and burn. Also called miliaria rubra; heat rash.

heatlabile Susceptible to being destroyed by a rise in temperature.

hebephrenia A type of schizophrenia, usually developing after the onset of puberty, characterized by shallow, inappropriate emotions, unpredictable childish behavior and mannerisms, and delusions.

hectic 1. Relating to the daily fever characteristic of certain diseases such as tuberculosis. 2. Feverish; flushed.

hectogram One hundred grams, the equivalent of 1543.7 grains or 3.527 avoirdupois ounces.

hectoliter One hundred liters, the equivalent of 105.7 quarts.

hedonic Of, relating to, or characterized by pleasure.

hedonics The study of pleasurable and unpleasurable feelings as they relate to behavior.

hedonism A constant pursuit of or devotion to pleasure and avoidance of pain; exhibited in some forms of character disorder.

heel The rounded posterior portion of the foot.

heel bone Calcaneus.

Hegar's sign A compressibility and softening of the lower uterine segment (cervical isthmus) elicited by bimanual examination; a suggestive sign of pregnancy.

helicine Relating to a spiral or helix.

Helicobacter pylori Gram negative, S-shaped spiral bacterium; formerly considered a member of the genus Campylobacter; found in secreting cells of the antral area of the stomach (near the pylorus); responsible for type B chronic gastritis.

helicoid Spiral.

helicotrema The passage at the apex of the cochlea of the internal ear through which the scala vestibuli and scala tympani communicate with one another.

heliopathy Injury from exposure to sunlight.

heliotaxis The tendency of a microorganism to move toward (positive heliotaxis) or away from (negative heliotaxis) a light source.

helium A gaseous element; symbol He, atomic number 2, atomic weight 4.003; present in small amounts in the atmosphere.

helix 1. The folded skin and cartilage forming the margin of the outer ear (auricle). 2. A coiled curve or structure.

alpha- h. The right-handed helical form of many proteins.

DNA h. See Watson-Crick helix.

double h. See Watson-Crick helix.

twin h. See Watson-Crick helix.

Watson-Crick h. A three-dimensional model of the DNA molecule; it consists of a double helix resembling a ladder that has been twisted into a spiral; the sides of the ladder are formed by the deoxyribose-phosphate units and are held together by rungs composed of pairs of bases (adenine and thymine or cytosine and guanine) joined together by hydrogen bonds. Also called DNA, double, or twin helix.

helminth 1. A parasitic intestinal worm, especially the nematode or trematode. 2. A wormlike parasite.

helminthemesis The vomiting of parasitic worms.

helminthiasis The condition of having intestinal worms.

helminthic Of, relating to, or caused by worms, especially parasitic intestinal worms.

helminthoid Resembling a worm.

helminthology The study of worms, especially the parasitic intestinal worms. Also called scolecology.

heloma A corn.

helosis The condition of having horny thickening of the skin, usually on a toe. Also called corns.

helotomy The surgical removal of corns or of calluses.

hemabarometer A device for determining the specific gravity of the blood.

hemacytometer See hemocytometer.

hemacytozoon See hemocytozoon.

hemadsorption Phenomenon in which a substance adheres to the surface of a red blood cell.

hemagglutination Agglutination (clumping) of red blood cells.

hemagglutinin A protein in blood serum that

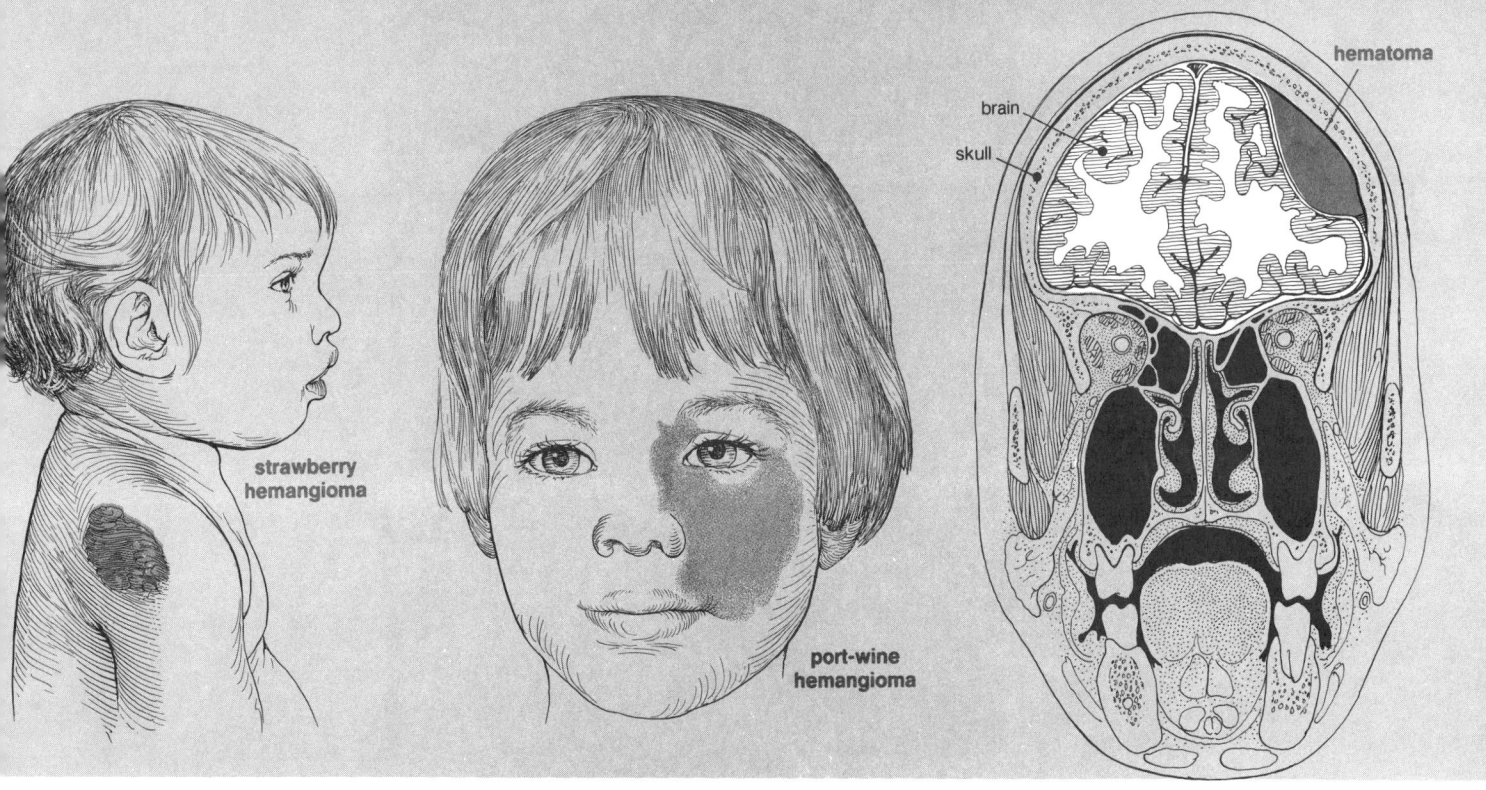

strawberry hemangioma

port-wine hemangioma

hematoma
brain
skull

causes clumping of red blood cells; also present in the surface projections of some viruses.

hemagogue, hemagog Any agent that promotes the flow of blood, particularly during menstruation.

hemal 1. Of or relating to the blood or blood vessels. 2. Relating to or located on the ventral side of the spinal axis where the heart is located; opposed to neural.

hemangiectasia, hemangiectasis Dilation of blood vessels.

hemangioblast An embryonic cell derived from the mesoderm; it develops into cells that give rise to endothelium of blood vessels, to reticuloendothelial elements, and to all types of blood-forming cells.

hemangioblastoma A brain tumor composed of angioblasts. Also called angioblastoma.

hemangioendothelioblastoma A tumor of vascular origin in which the endothelial cells seem to be predominantly immature types.

hemangioendothelioma A tumor derived from blood vessels, composed chiefly of masses of endothelial cells.

hemangioma A benign tumor made up of blood vessels.

   capillary h. A congenital tumor composed of minute, closely packed, thin-walled blood vessels that, for the most part, are of the caliber of capillaries; it varies from bright red to blue and may occur in any tissue or organ; the most common sites are the skin, subcutaneous tissues, and mucous membranes of the oral cavity and lips.

   cavernous h. A tumor containing large blood-filled spaces. Also called cavernous angioma.

   port-wine h. An enlarged red-blue capillary hemangioma that resembles a map, is nonpalpable, and covers large areas of the face and upper trunk. Also called port-wine mark, stain, or nevus; nevus flammeus.

   senile h. A bright red capillary hemangioma varying in size from pinhead to several centimeters in diameter; may be flat or slightly raised; seen in young adults and, most frequently, in elderly individuals. Also called cherry angioma.

   spider h. A dilated arteriole of the skin with radiating capillary branches. Also called arterial spider.

   strawberry h. A bright red raised tumor; present at birth as a pinhead-sized flat lesion that quickly increases in size and becomes elevated and rough; approximately 90% of these hemangiomas disappear without treatment by the ages of 5 to 7. Also called nevus vasculosus.

hemangiomatosis The presence of numerous hemangiomas.

hemangiopericytoma A rare tumor believed to be derived from pericytes (connective tissue cells surrounding capillaries).

hemangiosarcoma A rare malignant tumor composed chiefly of anaplastic cells derived from blood vessels.

hemarthrosis Blood in a joint space, resulting usually in pain, tenderness, and swelling.

hematemesis Vomiting of blood.

hematherm Denoting a warm-blooded animal.

hemathermal Warm-blooded; said of man and certain animals. Also called hemathermous.

hemathermous See hemathermal.

hematic 1. Of, relating to, or contained in blood. 2. A remedy for blood disorders; hematinic.

hematin 1. The hydroxide of heme. 2. Heme.

hematinic Any agent that improves the condition of the blood.

hematinuria The presence of heme in the urine.

hematoblast A primitive blood cell from which develop erythroblasts, lymphoblasts, myeloblasts, and other immature blood cells.

hematocele A swelling caused by the effusion and collection of blood into a cavity of the body, especially under the serous covering of the testis.

hematochezia The passage of bloody stools.

hematocolpometra Accumulation of blood in the uterus and vagina resulting from an imperforate hymen or any other obstruction.

hematocolpos Distention of the vagina with accumulated menstrual blood due to an imperforate hymen.

hematocrit (Hct) 1. The volume percentage of red blood cells in whole blood; in the normal male it constitutes about 45 to 50% of the whole blood volume; in the normal female it constitutes approximately 40 to 45%. Also called packed cell volume. 2. A small centrifuge used to separate the cellular elements of blood from the plasma.

hematocyanin See hemocyanin.

hematocystis Effusion of blood into the urinary bladder.

hematocyte See hemocyte.

hematocytometer Hemocytometer.

hematocytozoon See hemocytozoon.

hematocyturia The presence of red blood cells in the urine. Also called true hematuria.

hematogenesis See hemopoiesis.

hematogenic Hematogenous.

hematogenous 1. Derived from blood. 2. Relating to anything originating in or circulated by the blood.

hematoid 1. Resembling blood. 2. Bloody.

hematoidin Pigment derived from the breakdown of hemoglobin; formed in the tissues as a result of hemorrhage.

hematologist A specialist in the diagnosis and treatment of disorders of blood and blood-forming tissues.

hematology The medical specialty concerned with blood and blood-forming tissues, and the treatment of blood disorders.

hematolysis See hemolysis.

hematoma A localized mass of blood outside of the blood vessels, usually found in a partly clotted state.

   subdural h. Hematoma between the dura and arachnoid membranes of the brain.

hematometra Distention of the uterus with accumulated blood. Also called hemometra.

hematometry Examination of blood to determine (a) the total number, types, and proportions of blood cells; (b) the number or proportion of other formed elements; (c) the percentage of hemoglobin. Also called hemometry.

hematomyelia Effusion of blood into the spinal cord.

hematopathology The branch of medicine concerned with diseases of the blood and blood-forming tissues.

hematopathy See hemopathy.

hematopenia Blood deficiency.

hematopoiesis See hemopoiesis.

hematopoietin See erythropoietin.

hematoporphyrin A dark red substance formed by the decomposition of hemoglobin.

hematosalpinx Distention of a uterine tube with a collection of blood. Also called hemosalpinx.

hematoscope 1. Instrument for determining the number of red blood cells suspended in blood by measuring the dispersion of light. 2. Instrument for determining the percentage of hemoglobin in blood.

hematosepsis Septicemia.

hematospermia Blood in the seminal fluid.

hematostaxis Spontaneous bleeding caused by a blood disease.

hematotrachelos Distention of the uterine cervix, as with accumulated menstrual blood due to an imperforate hymen.

hematoxylin A crystalline compound, extracted from the tropical American tree, logwood; used as a stain in histology and bacteriology; it imparts a bluish tint to the specimen.

hematozoon pl. **hematozoa** Any parasitic protozoan or microorganism that lives in the circulating blood of its host.

hematuria Discharge of red blood cells in the

parietal lobe

frontal lobe

temporal lobe

cerebral hemispheres

occipital lobe

parietal lobe

temporal lobe

lateral and medial views

frontal lobe

hemlock (Conium maculatum)

water hemlock

urine.

heme The nonprotein, iron-containing porphyrin molecule which forms the oxygen-binding element of hemoglobin. Also called ferroprotoporphyrin. Formerly known as hematin.

hemeralopia Defective vision in daylight, with good vision in dim light. Also called day blindness; night sight.

hemialgia Pain on one side of the body only.

hemiamblyopia Reduced vision in one half of the visual field of one or both eyes.

hemianacusia Loss of hearing or deafness in one ear.

hemianalgesia Loss of sensibility to pain on one side of the body.

hemianesthesia Loss of sensibility to touch on one side of the body.

   alternate h. Hemianesthesia affecting one side of the head and the other side of the body and extremities. Also called crossed hemianesthesia.

   crossed h. See alternate hemianesthesia.

hemianopsia Loss of vision in one half of the visual field of one or both eyes.

   bilateral h. Hemianopsia affecting the visual fields of both eyes.

   binasal h. Bilateral hemianopsia affecting the nasal halves of the visual fields of both eyes.

   bitemporal h. Bilateral hemianopsia affecting the temporal halves of the visual fields of both eyes.

   congruous h. Bilateral hemianopsia affecting the nasal half of one visual field and the temporal half of the other, the defects in the two visual fields being identical in size, shape, and location, resulting in a single defect of the binocular field.

   crossed h. Bilateral hemianopsia affecting the upper half of one visual field and the lower half of the other.

   heteronymous h. Bilateral hemianopsia affecting either both temporal halves or both nasal halves of the visual fields.

   homonymous h. Bilateral hemianopsia affecting the nasal half of one visual field and the temporal half of the other.

   incomplete h. Hemianopsia not affecting the entire half of the visual field.

   quadrantic h. See quadrantanopsia.

hemianosmia Loss of the sense of smell on one side only.

hemiatrophy Atrophy confined to one side of an organ or bodily region, as of the face or tongue.

   facial h. Atrophy, usually progressive, affecting the tissues of one side of the face. Also called Romberg's disease or syndrome; facial trophoneurosis.

hemiballism Violent, involuntary movements of the extremities involving one side of the body, due to a lesion in the contralateral subthalamic body. Also called hemiballismus.

hemic Relating to the blood.

hemiblock Blocking of the heart impulse in either of the two main divisions of the bundle of His (atrioventricular bundle).

hemicentrum Either lateral half of the body of a vertebra.

hemichorea Chorea in which the uncontrollable and irregular movements of the muscles are largely confined to one side of the body.

hemicolectomy Removal of part of the colon.

hemicrania Pain on one side of the head.

hemidiaphoresis Sweating on one side of the body.

hemigastrectomy Excision of one half of the stomach, usually of the pyloric end.

α-hemihydrate Alpha-hemihydrate; $(CaSO_4)_2 \cdot H_2O$; gypsum that has been calcined under steam pressure in an autoclave to 130°C; the resulting crystals are somewhat prismatic; used for making casts and models of the oral cavity. Also called dental stone.

β-hemihydrate Beta-hemihydrate; $(CaSO_4)_2 \cdot H_2O$; gypsum that has been calcined in the open air to 110°C; the resulting crystals are irregular in shape; used in the preparation of casts for artificial dentures. Also called dental plaster; plaster of Paris.

hemihypertrophy Congenital overgrowth of one side of the body.

hemikaryon A cell nucleus containing the haploid number of chromosomes.

hemilaminectomy The surgical removal of a portion of the vertebral lamina in order to gain exposure to an underlying nerve root or intervertebral disk; often used to denote unilateral laminectomy.

hemimelia A congenital defect marked by absence of all or part of the distal portion of a limb or limbs.

hemin A crystalline compound, $C_{34}H_{32}N_4O_4FeCl$; the chloride of heme. Also called Teichmann's crystals.

heminephrectomy Surgical excision of part of a kidney.

hemiparesis Muscular weakness or mild paralysis of one side of the body.

hemiplegia Paralysis of one side of the body.

   alternate h. Millard-Gubler syndrome.

hemiplegic One whose body is paralyzed on one side.

Hemiptera A large order of insects that includes the common bedbug.

hemisoantibody (HIID) An antibody that reacts with a surface antigen-determinant on erythrocytes (red blood cells) to cause agglutination of the cells.

hemisphere Half of a symmetrical, spherical object.

   cerebral h. The lateral half of the cerebrum.

hemithorax One side of the chest.

hemizygosity The state of having only one of a pair of genes.

hemizygote An individual or cell having only one of a pair of genes.

hemizygous, hemizygotic Having unpaired genes; said of the male with respect to the X chromosome.

hemlock Any of several poisonous plants (genus *Conium*) capable of producing motor paralysis. More commonly called poison hemlock.

   water h. Probably the most poisonous plant in the United States; the poison is found principally in the roots, which are often mistaken for parsnips.

hemoagglutinin An antibody in serum that causes agglutination of red blood cells (erythrocytes).

hemobilia Bleeding into the biliary passages.

hemochromatosis A disorder of iron metabolism resulting in accumulation of excess iron in the tissues of many organs, especially the skin, liver, and pancreas, leading to fibrosis and functional insufficiency of those organs which are severely involved; the heart and other muscles and endocrine glands are also affected; deposition of iron in the skin causes a bronzed pigmentation; deposits in the pancreas lead to diabetes. Also called iron storage disease; bronze or bronzed diabetes.

hemochrome See hemochromogen.

hemochromogen A substance formed by the union of heme with a nitrogenous compound, as a protein or base. Also called hemochrome.

hemochromometer An apparatus for estimating the percentage of hemoglobin in the blood by comparing the solution of blood with a standard solution of an appropriate compound, such as ammonium picrocarminate.

hemoclasia, hemoclasis Hemolysis or destruction of red blood cells.

hemoconcentration Increase in the concentration or proportion of formed elements in the circulating blood, usually resulting from the loss of plasma from the blood stream. Also called anhydremia.

hemocyanin An oxygen-carrying blue respiratory pigment (chromoprotein) occurring in the blood of lower sea animals (e.g., mollusks) in which copper is an essential component. Also called hematocyanin.

hemocyte Any cell or formed element of the blood; a blood corpuscle; a blood cell. Also called hematocyte.

hemocytoblast A primitive cell derived from the hemohistioblast; the name given to the cell from which granulocytes, red cell precursors, and megakaryocytes are derived.

hemocytometer An instrument used for estimating the blood cell count in a measured volume of blood. Also called hemacytometer; erythrocytometer; globulimeter.

   Thoma-Zeiss h. An apparatus used to count blood cells. Also called Thoma's counting chamber.

hemocytotripsis The destruction of blood cells by mechanical means; e.g., compression between hard surfaces.

hemocytozoon An animal parasite of blood cells. Also called hemacytozoon; hematocytozoon.

hemodialysis Removal of waste materials or poisons from the blood by means of a hemodialyzer (artificial kidney).

hemodialyzer An apparatus used as a substitute for the kidneys to purify the blood in acute or chronic kidney failure and in certain types of poisoning; toxic elements are removed by passing the blood through a semipermeable membrane lying in a bathing solution, then returning it to the body. Commonly called artificial kidney.

hemodilution Increase in the plasma content of the blood with resulting decrease in the concentration of red blood cells.

hemodynamic Of or relating to blood circulation.

hemodynamics The science of the forces connected with the circulation of the blood.

hemofiltration A technique used for purifying the blood by filtering out components of the blood smaller than albumin and replacing a similar quantity of a balanced electrolyte solution; by this process, unwanted solutes such as urea, creatinine and other nitrogenous wastes are removed from the body.

hemoflagellates Flagellated blood parasites.

hemofuscin A brown pigment derived from hemoglobin; sometimes found in urine along with hemosiderin; an indication of increased red blood cell destruction.

hemogenesis See hemopoiesis.

hemoglobin (Hb, Hgb) The oxygen-bearing protein of red blood cells; it is bright red when saturated with oxygen and purple when it is not carrying oxygen.

   fetal h. See hemoglobin F.

   glycated h. A fraction of hemoglobin A to which glucose binds; high concentrations occur in patients with elevated blood sugar levels.

   glycosylated h. See glycated hemoglobin.

   h. A (Hb A) Hemoglobin found in normal adults.

   h. A₂ (Hb A₂) Hemoglobin which is increased in beta-thalassemia; it makes up about 1.5 to 3% of the total hemoglobin concentration in the normal adult.

   h. C A slow-moving abnormal hemoglobin characterized by an amino acid substitution (lysine for glutamic acid at position six of the beta-chains); it reduces the normal plasticity of red blood cells; associated with chronic hemolytic anemia.

   h. F (Hb F) Hemoglobin of a normal fetus; the major hemoglobin component during intrauterine life. Also called fetal hemoglobin.

   h. S (Hb S) Abnormal hemoglobin characterized by an amino acid substitution (valine for glutamic acid at position six of the beta-chain); associated with sickle cell anemia.

   oxygenated h. See oxyhemoglobin.

   reduced h. Hemoglobin present in venous blood, after it has released its oxygen in the tissues.

   sickle cell h. Hemoglobin S.

hemoglobinemia The presence of free hemoglobin in the plasma, resulting from mechanical injury to the red blood cells within the vessels.

hemoglobinometer An apparatus for estimating the amount of hemoglobin in the blood. Also called hemometer.

hemoglobinopathy A hematologic disorder in which the type of hemoglobin within an individual's red blood cells differs qualitatively or quantitatively from that contained in normal red blood cells.

hemoglobinuria The presence of free hemoglobin in the urine, an indication of recent hemolysis of at least moderate severity.

   malarial h. Rare condition caused by malignant tertian malaria. Also called blackwater or remittent fever.

   paroxysmal nocturnal h. Chronic disorder marked primarily by hemolytic anemia, hemoglobinuria (chiefly at night), yellow discoloration of the skin and mucous membranes, and enlargement of the spleen and liver. Also called Marchiafava-Micheli syndrome or anemia.

hemogram A record of the number, proportion, and morphologic features of the cellular elements of blood.

hemohistioblast An undifferentiated mesenchymal cell of the reticulo-endothelial system from which all blood cells are derived; it is probably similar in morphology to other blood blasts. Also called stem cell.

hemolith A concretion in the wall of a blood vessel.

hemolysin 1. An anti-red blood cell antibody which activates complement (C′) to cause destruc-

tion (lysis) of red blood cells. Formerly called amboceptor. **2.** Any substance produced by a living agent and capable of destroying red blood cells by liberating their hemoglobin.

   immune h. Hemolysin made by injecting an animal with red blood cells or whole blood from another species.

hemolysinogen Antigenic substance in red blood cells that stimulates the formation of hemolysin.

hemolysis Liberation of hemoglobin from the red blood cells. Also called erythrocytolysis; hematolysis.

hemolytic Causing disintegration of red blood cells.

hemolytic disease of the newborn See erythroblastosis fetalis.

hemolytic-uremic syndrome A syndrome usually occurring in children, characterized by hemolytic anemia with abnormally shaped erythrocytes, thrombocytopenia, and uremia; minor respiratory or gastrointestinal infection often precedes onset.

hemolyze To cause the liberation of hemoglobin from red blood cells.

hemomanometer An instrument for determining blood pressure. Also called hematomanometer.

hemomediastinum Effusion of blood into the mediastinum. Also called hematomediastinum.

hemometer 1. See hemoglobinometer. **2.** Term occasionally used for hemocytometer.

hemometra See hematometra.

hemometry See hematometry.

hemopathy Any disorder of the blood or blood-forming tissues. Also called hematopathy.

hemoperfusion Passage of the blood over a sorbent (e.g., activated charcoal) in order to remove a toxic substance.

hemopericardium Accumulation of blood in the pericardial sac.

hemoperitoneum Escape of blood into the peritoneal cavity.

hemopexin A serum protein in human plasma, containing 20% carbohydrates; important in binding heme and porphyrins.

hemophagocyte A phagocytic cell that engulfs and destroys red blood cells.

hemophagocytosis The process of engulfment of red blood cells by phagocytic cells.

hemophil, hemophile Denoting microorganisms that thrive in media containing blood.

hemophilia An inherited hemorrhagic disease characterized by a deficiency of factor VIII (antihemophilic factor), causing excessive and sometimes spontaneous bleeding, and inherited as an X-linked recessive trait; although the heterozygous female is

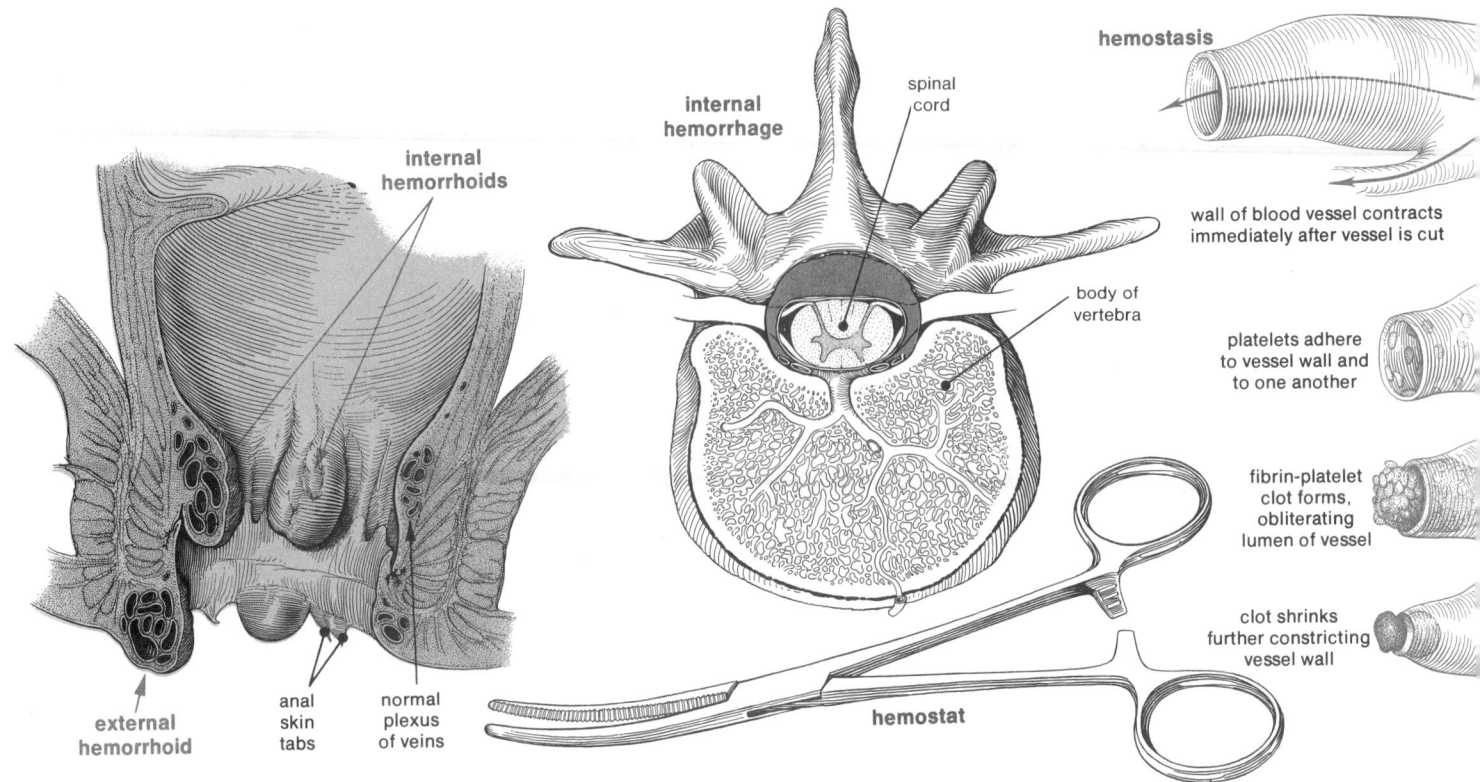

internal hemorrhoids

internal hemorrhage

spinal cord

hemostasis

body of vertebra

wall of blood vessel contracts immediately after vessel is cut

platelets adhere to vessel wall and to one another

fibrin-platelet clot forms, obliterating lumen of vessel

clot shrinks further constricting vessel wall

external hemorrhoid

anal skin tabs

normal plexus of veins

hemostat

the carrier, she is asymptomatic and the disease is manifested only in the affected sons. Also called classic hemophilia; hemophilia A.

h. B A disorder of the blood clotting process caused by hereditary deficiency of factor IX (plasma thromboplastin component). Also called Christmas disease.

hemophiliac An individual afflicted with hemophilia; a bleeder.

hemophilic **1.** Relating to hemophilia. **2.** Thriving in blood or in media with hemoglobin.

Hemophilus See Haemophilus.

hemophobia An abnormal fear of the sight of blood. Also called hematophobia.

hemophthalmia Bleeding into the eyeball.

hemopneumopericardium The presence of blood and air in the membrane enveloping the heart. Also called pneumohemopericardium.

hemopneumothorax Accumulation of air and blood in the pleural cavity.

hemopoiesis The formation of blood cells. Also called hematopoiesis; hematogenesis; hemogenesis.

hemopoietic Relating to the formation of blood cells.

hemoporphyrin The porphyrin component of heme; $C_{34}H_{38}N_4O_6$; the iron-free heme.

hemoprecipitin An antibody that combines with and precipitates soluble antigenic material from erythrocytes; a precipitin specific for blood.

hemoprotein A conjugated compound consisting of a protein linked to heme.

hemopsonin An antibody that combines with red blood cells and renders them susceptible in phagocytosis.

hemoptysis Spitting of blood from lesions in the larynx, trachea, or lower respiratory tract.

hemopyelectasia Dilation of the kidney pelvis with blood and urine.

hemorheology The science of the relation of pressures, flow, volumes, and resistances in blood vessels.

hemorrhage Bleeding, especially profuse.

accidental h. Abruptio placentae.

cerebral h. Bleeding from blood vessels within the brain, usually in the area of the internal capsule.

internal h. Bleeding into an organ or a body cavity.

secondary h. Bleeding that occurs at an interval after an injury or operation.

hemorrhagenic Causing hemorrhage.

hemorrhagic Relating to or characterized by bleeding or hemorrhage.

hemorrhagic disease of the newborn Disorder occurring during the first few days of life,

marked by spontaneous bleeding due to deficiency of procoagulant substances; it is effectively treated with vitamin K.

hemorrhagic pulmonary-renal syndrome See Goodpasture's syndrome.

hemorrhagin Any of a group of toxins that destroy the endothelial cells in capillaries, causing numerous hemorrhages in the tissues; found in certain poisonous substances such as rattlesnake venom, seeds of the castor oil plant, etc.

hemorrhoid A dilated (varicose) vein situated at or near the anus; it is present in about 35% of the population, and occurs usually in persons 25 to 55 years old.

external h. Varicosities of the inferior hemorrhoidal veins situated external to the rectoanal line and covered by skin.

internal h. Varicose enlargement of the superior hemorrhoidal veins situated above the rectoanal line and covered with mucous membrane, causing, at the early stages, intermittent bleeding during or following defecation; the condition may develop in various degrees: (a) the hemorrhoids do not protrude through the anal canal (1st degree); (b) protrusion occurs through the anal canal during defecation, receding spontaneously afterward (2nd degree); (c) protrusion becomes more pronounced, occurring on any extra exertion and receding only by manual reduction (3rd degree); (d) the hemorrhoids are permanently prolapsed (4th degree).

hemorrhoidal **1.** Of or relating to hemorrhoids or piles. **2.** Denoting blood vessels supplying the area of the rectum and anus.

hemorrhoidectomy Surgical removal of hemorrhoids.

hemosalpinx See hematosalpinx.

hemosiderin A granular iron-containing yellow pigment formed during decomposition of hemoglobin; deposits are formed in a variety of tissues when there has been red blood cell breakdown.

hemosiderosis Deposition of hemosiderin (a yellow substance containing iron) in the tissues.

idiopathic pulmonary h. Recurrent hemorrhage of the lungs; cause unknown.

hemospermia See hematospermia.

hemostasis **1.** The arrest of bleeding. Also called hemostasia. **2.** The arrest of the flow of blood through a part or vessel.

hemostat An instrument or an agent that stops bleeding.

hemostatic **1.** Arresting hemorrhage. **2.** Any agent that checks bleeding.

hemostyptic A chemical hemostatic; any chemical agent that stops bleeding by astringent properties.

hemothorax Accumulation of blood in the pleural cavity.

hemotoxic **1.** Causing blood poisoning. **2.** Destructive to blood cells. Also called hematotoxic.

hemotoxin Any toxin that is capable of destroying red blood cells.

hemotympanum Collection of blood in the middle ear.

hemozoon Hematozoon.

hemp A herbaceous plant of the genus *Cannabis.*

henry (H) Unit of electric inductance; may be (a) self-inductance of one circuit, when an increase of current at the rate of 1 amp/sec causes an electromotive force of 1 volt; or (b) mutual inductance of two circuits, when the current of one circuit changing at the rate of 1 amp/sec produces an electromotive force of 1 volt in the other circuit.

hepar Latin for liver.

heparin A mucopolysaccharide acid comprised of D-glucuronic acid and D-glucosamine; found especially in liver and lung tissue; it has the ability to keep blood from clotting and is used chiefly in the prevention and treatment of thrombosis.

heparinize To administer or apply heparin in order to delay the clotting time of blood.

hepatalgia Pain in the liver. Also called hepatodynia.

hepatectomy Surgical removal of a portion of the liver.

hepatic Relating to the liver.

hepatitis Inflammation of the liver.

anicteric h. Hepatitis in which hyperbilirubinemia is mild, serum transaminase levels are elevated, and liver biopsy resembles icteric forms.

cholestatic h., cholangiolitic h. Hepatitis characterized by signs of bile duct obstruction more prominent than the evidence of liver cell necrosis; may be seen occasionally in viral hepatitis or may be drug induced; must be differentiated from extrahepatic obstruction.

chronic aggressive h. Progressive destruction of the liver architecture characterized by piecemeal necrosis and formation of intralobular septa leading eventually to cirrhosis and liver failure; often associated with hyperglobulinemia.

chronic persistent h. Chronic inflammatory infiltration several months after an episode of acute hepatitis with preservation of lobular architecture and little or no fibrosis; symptoms are usually minor; half of the individuals feel well; mild elevation of transaminase may be seen; up to 80% of individuals have hepatitis B antigen present in the serum.

fulminant h. A rapidly progressive form with necrosis of large areas of the liver; usually fatal within

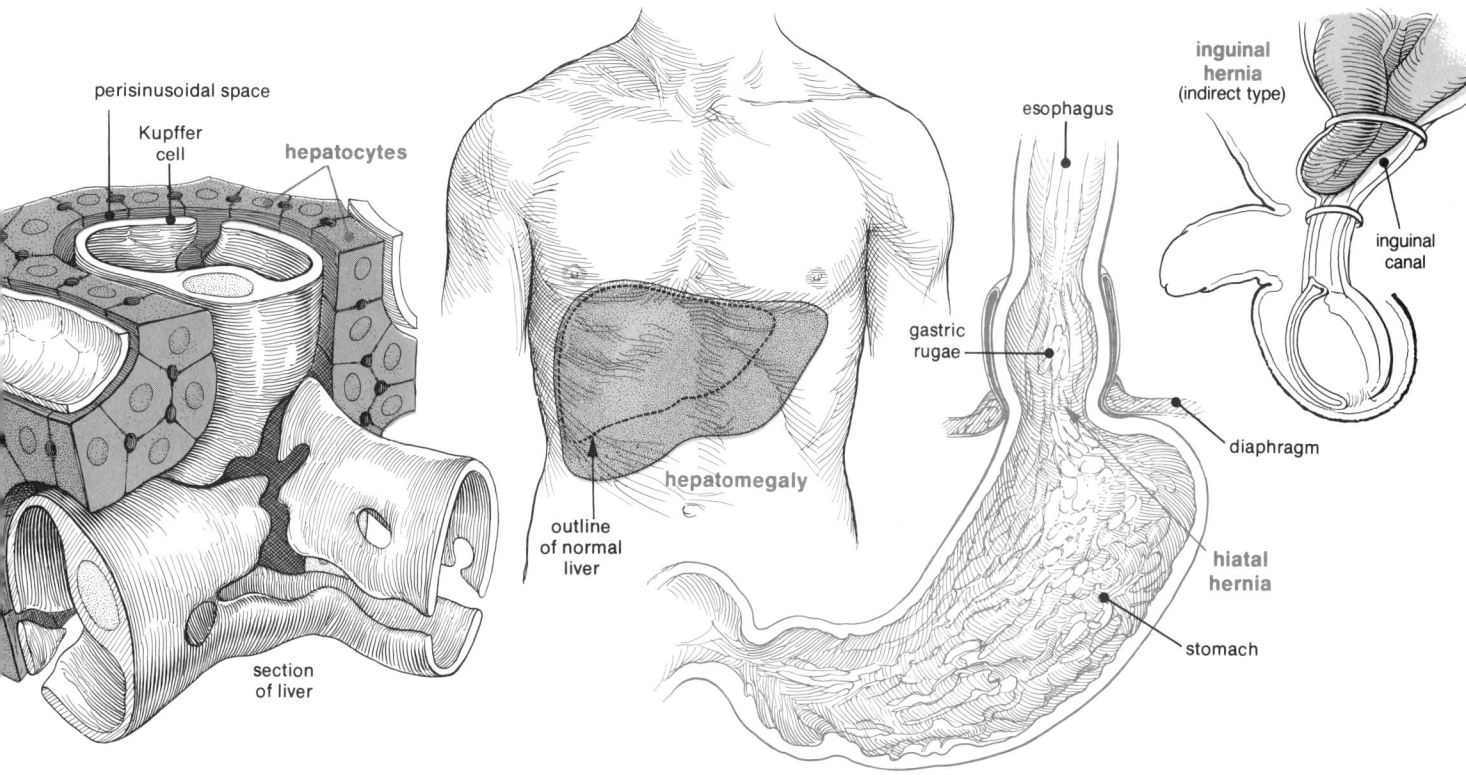

perisinusoidal space

Kupffer cell

hepatocytes

section of liver

inguinal hernia (indirect type)

inguinal canal

esophagus

gastric rugae

diaphragm

hiatal hernia

stomach

hepatomegaly

outline of normal liver

two weeks.

h. A Hepatitis caused by hepatitis A virus (HAV), transmitted by intestinal and oral routes; may occur sporadically or in epidemics. Also called infectious hepatitis.

h. B Hepatitis caused by hepatitis B virus (HBV), spread by transfusion of infected blood, use of contaminated needles, the sexual route, or during childbirth. Also called serum hepatitis.

h. C Hepatitis caused by hepatitis C virus (HCV), transmitted via transfusion of infected blood; often causes chronic hepatitis, leading to cirrhosis. Formerly called transfusion-associated non-A, non-B hepatitis.

h. D Hepatitis caused by hepatitis D virus (HDV), developed only in the presence of hepatitis B virus (HBV); may occur when transfused blood contains both viruses (coinfection), or as an additional infection of a chronic HBV carrier (superinfection).

h. E Self-limited hepatitis (with a high mortality rate in pregnant women) caused by hepatitis E virus (HEV), transmitted via the gastrointestinal route; may occur in waterborne epidemics. Formerly called non-A, non-B hepatitis.

infectious h. See hepatitis A.

non-A, non-B (NANB) h. See hepatitis C and E.

serum h. (SH) See hepatitis B.

viral h. Hepatitis caused by a virus.

hepatization The conversion of loose tissue into a mass resembling liver, as the consolidation of lung tissue in pneumonia.

hepatocyte A parenchymal liver cell.

hepatoduodenostomy Surgical creation of a passage between the hepatic duct and the duodenum.

hepatodynia See hepatalgia.

hepatogenic Formed by or originating in the liver; also called hepatogenous.

hepatogram A radioisotopic scan of the liver.

hepatography 1. The making of a roentgenogram of the liver. 2. A treatise on the liver.

hepatolienography 1. See hepatosplenography. 2. A treatise on the liver and spleen.

hepatolith A calculus in the liver; a biliary calculus.

hepatolithiasis Stones in the liver.

hepatologist A specialist on diseases of the liver.

hepatology Study of the liver and its diseases.

hepatolysin An agent destructive to the parenchymal cells of the liver.

hepatoma Malignant tumor of the liver originating in the parenchymal cells. Also called hepatocellular carcinoma.

hepatomegaly Enlargement of the liver.

hepatonecrosis Death of liver tissue.

hepatopathy Any disease of the liver.

hepatorenal Relating to the liver and kidney.

hepatorenal syndrome Renal failure occurring in the presence of severe disease of the liver or biliary tract, characterized initially by oliguria, marked sodium retention, and a rise in blood urea nitrogen usually out of proportion to the increase in serum creatinine.

hepatorrhaphy The surgical suturing of the liver.

hepatoscan The scanning of the liver after intravenous injection of a radioactive substance that is taken up by the hepatic reticuloendothelial system.

hepatosplenography Roentgenography of the liver and spleen after introduction of a radiopaque medium.

hepatosplenomegaly Enlargement of the liver and the spleen.

hepatotoxic Relating to substances that damage the liver.

hepatotoxin Any agent that destroys the liver cells.

herbivorous Feeding on plants.

hereditary Genetically transmitted from parent to child. Cf. heritable.

heredity 1. The genetic transmission of a specific trait from parent to offspring. 2. The totality of physical and mental traits and potentialities so transmitted to the offspring.

autosomal h. The transmission of a trait by a gene situated on an autosome.

sex-linked h. The transmission of a trait by a gene situated on a sex chromosome.

heredoataxia Friedreich's ataxia; see under ataxia.

heredodegeneration The genetic retrogressive change in cells and tissues.

heredopathia atactica polyneuritiformis See Refsum's syndrome.

heritable Capable of being inherited, such as a trait, provided that it is present in the germ cell of a parent. Cf. hereditary.

hermaphrodism See hermaphroditism.

hermaphrodite An individual who has genital tissues of both sexes.

hermaphroditism, hermaphrodism The presence in the same individual of both ovarian and testicular tissues. Also called intersexuality.

hermetic Completely sealed against the escape or entry of air.

hernia Protrusion of part of an organ through an abnormal opening in the wall that normally contains it.

abdominal h. Hernia protruding through or into any part of the abdominal wall.

acquired h. A hernia resulting from an injury, such as a strain.

concealed h. Hernia not found on inspection or palpation.

congenital h. A hernia that exists at birth, generally umbilical or scrotal.

Cooper's h. Femoral hernia with two sacs, one in the femoral canal and the other passing through a defect in the superficial fascia and appearing immediately beneath the skin.

diaphragmatic h. Passage of a loop of intestine through the diaphragm.

epigastric h. Hernia through the linea alba above the navel.

fascial h. See fatty hernia.

fatty h. Hernia in which a mass of adipose tissue escapes through a gap in a fascia or aponeurosis. Also called pannicular or fascial hernia.

femoral h. Hernia through the femoral canal.

gastroesophageal h. A form of hiatal hernia in which the proximal part of the stomach and adjacent esophagus herniate into the thorax.

hiatal h. hiatus h. (HH) Displacement of the upper part of the stomach into the thorax through the esophageal hiatus of the diaphragm.

incarcerated h. Hernia in which the herniated organ (intestine) is tightly constricted and cannot be returned by manipulation; the flow of intestinal contents is arrested, but the blood circulation is unaffected.

inguinal h. Hernia at the inguinal region; the herniation may pass directly through the abdominal wall (direct inguinal hernia) or through the inguinal canal (indirect inguinal hernia).

irreducible h. Hernia which, as a result of adhesions or for any other reason, cannot be reduced without a surgical operation.

pannicular h. See fatty hernia.

reducible h. Hernia whose contents can be returned to their original position by manipulaton.

sciatic h. A herniation of intestine through the great sacrosciatic foramen.

scrotal h. See scrotocele.

sliding hiatal h., sliding esophageal hiatal h. Hernia in which the junction of the stomach and esophagus moves from time to time or permanently into the thorax through the diaphragm.

spigelian h. An abdominal hernia through the semilunar line.

strangulated h. An incarcerated hernia whose blood supply has been cut off so that the herniated intestine has become, or is likely to become, gangrenous.

umbilical hernia

umbilical cord

hernial sac

newborn

umbilical h. Hernia in which part of the intestine protrudes through the umbilical ring; it usually results from a fascial and muscular defect with failure of the umbilical ring to close.

ventral h. Passage of a loop of intestine through any part of the abdominal wall other than through the inguinal, femoral, or umbilical openings.

herniated Pertaining to any structure protruding through a defect or abnormal opening.

herniation The process of forming an abnormal protrusion.

foraminal h. Protrusion of the cerebellar tonsils through the foramen magnum. Also called tonsillar herniation.

tonsillar h. See foraminal herniation.

herniorrhaphy Surgical repair of a hernia.

heroin A highly addictive narcotic prepared from morphine by acetylation; a white, odorless, bitterish crystalline compound, $C_{21}H_{23}O_5N$. Also called diacetylmorphine.

herpangina An infection of the throat usually caused by a coxsackie virus (coxsackie A); marked by intense swelling of the area, sudden onset of fever, loss of appetite, difficulty in swallowing (dysphagia), and sometimes abdominal pain, nausea, and vomiting; vesiculopapular lesions about 1 to 2 mm in diameter are present around the tonsillar fauces, which soon break down to form grayish-yellow ulcers.

herpes An inflammatory disease of the skin and mucous membrane marked by eruption of a cluster of deep-seated vesicles.

corneal h. Herpes simplex of the cornea characterized by a branch-like ulceration, often occurring in individuals who have had an eruption on the lips or nostrils.

genital h. Sexually transmitted herpes simplex of the genital organs, usually caused by herpesvirus 2 (herpes simplex virus type 2); blisters appear from 2 to 12 days after contact with a person who has active lesions; the ulceration heals spontaneously within two to three weeks; initial infection in a pregnant woman may be transmitted to the fetus through the placenta; if the mother has an active eruption at the time of delivery, the newborn may be infected during its passage through the birth canal. Also called herpes progenitalis; herpes simplex 2; venereal herpes.

h. febrilis Herpes labialis.

h. gestationis Herpes simplex occurring during pregnancy.

h. labialis Herpes simplex of the lips, usually caused by herpesvirus 1. Also called cold sore; fever blister; herpes febrilis.

h. progenitalis Genital herpes.

h. simplex An acute localized eruption of painful blisters, caused by herpesvirus 1 and 2 (herpes simplex virus types 1 and 2); once established, the infection remains in the body and recurs at intervals with complete healing of the eruption between episodes; reappearance may be precipitated by emotional stress, febrile disease, local trauma, or menstruation.

h. simplex 2 Genital herpes.

h. zoster Infection of the ganglia of the posterior roots of the spinal nerves or the fifth cranial nerve by the varicella-zoster virus, which also causes chickenpox; it is marked by a painful eruption of vesicles usually on one side of the body along the course of one or more cutaneous nerves. Also called shingles.

venereal h. Genital herpes.

Herpesviridae A family of viruses (120 to 200 nanometers in diameter) that contain double-stranded DNA and replicate in the cell nucleus; accumulate between inner and outer layers of nuclear membrane and in the cisterna of endoplasmic reticulum; are transported to the cell surface through modified endoplasmic reticulum and may remain latent in their host for the lifetime of the host; comprises three subfamilies: Alphaherpesvirinae (herpes simplex virus group), Betaherpesvirinae (cytomegalovirus group) and Gammherpesvirinae (lymphoproliferative virus group); includes viruses causing herpes, chickenpox, infectious mononucleosis, and cytomegalic inclusion disease. Also called herpesvirus group. See also herpes.

herpesvirus, herpes simplex virus Virus of the subfamily Alphaherpesvirinae (family Herpesviridae) that causes herpes simplex in humans and frequently remain latent in ganglia; occurs in two immunologic types, causing two kinds of infections: **type 1** (primarily nongenital) and **type 2** (primarily genital). See also herpes; Herpesviridae.

herpetiform Resembling herpes.

hertz (Hz) Unit of frequency of a periodic process equivalent to one cycle per second.

heterochromatin The more darkly stained portion of the cell nucleus containing metabolically inactive DNA.

heterochromia Difference in color of a part or parts that are normally alike in color, as of the two irides.

heterecious Having more than one host, i.e., spending different stages of its life cycle on two or more unrelated hosts; e.g., tapeworms.

heteroerotic Relating to sexual feelings that are directed toward another person, as opposed to autoerotic.

heterogametic Having gametes (sex cells) of different types with respect to the sex chromosomes, as in human males.

heterogamy 1. The union of two gametes of different size, structure, and function. 2. Alternation of two kinds of generations, one that reproduces bisexually and another in which the female reproduces without fecundation by the male (parthenogenetic), as in some aphids.

heterogeneity The quality of certain genetic disorders which consist of two or more fundamentally distinct entities; formerly thought to represent single entities.

heterogeneous, heterogenous Composed of dissimilar elements or characteristics; not homogeneous.

heterogenetic, heterogenic Derived from a different species.

heterograft See xenograft.

heterolalia The involuntary uttering of meaningless words instead of those intended. Also called heterophasia; heterophemia.

heterologous 1. Composed of tissues not normal to the area. 2. Xenogeneic.

heterolysis Dissolution or digestion of cells of one species by a lytic agent from a different species.

heteromeric 1. Possessing different chemical composition. 2. Denoting spinal nerve cells that have processes crossing the midline to the opposite side of the spinal cord.

heteromorphism In cytogenetics, a difference in shape or size between homologous chromosomes.

heteronymous 1. Relating to different sides of the two visual fields; e.g., the right side of one field and the left side of the other, both nasal fields or both temporal fields. 2. Having different but correlated names.

heterophasia See heterolalia.

heterophemia See heterolalia.

heterophonia 1. The change of voice in the male at puberty. 2. Any abnormality in the voice.

heterophoria The tendency of the optic axes to deviate toward or away from each other.

heterophthalmia A difference in appearance of the two eyes, as in the coloration of the irides. Also called heterophthalmus.

heterophthalmus See heterophthalmia.

Heterophyes A genus of small sized parasitic flukes.

heterophyiasis Infection with a heterophyid fluke.

heterophyid 1. Relating to flukes of the genus

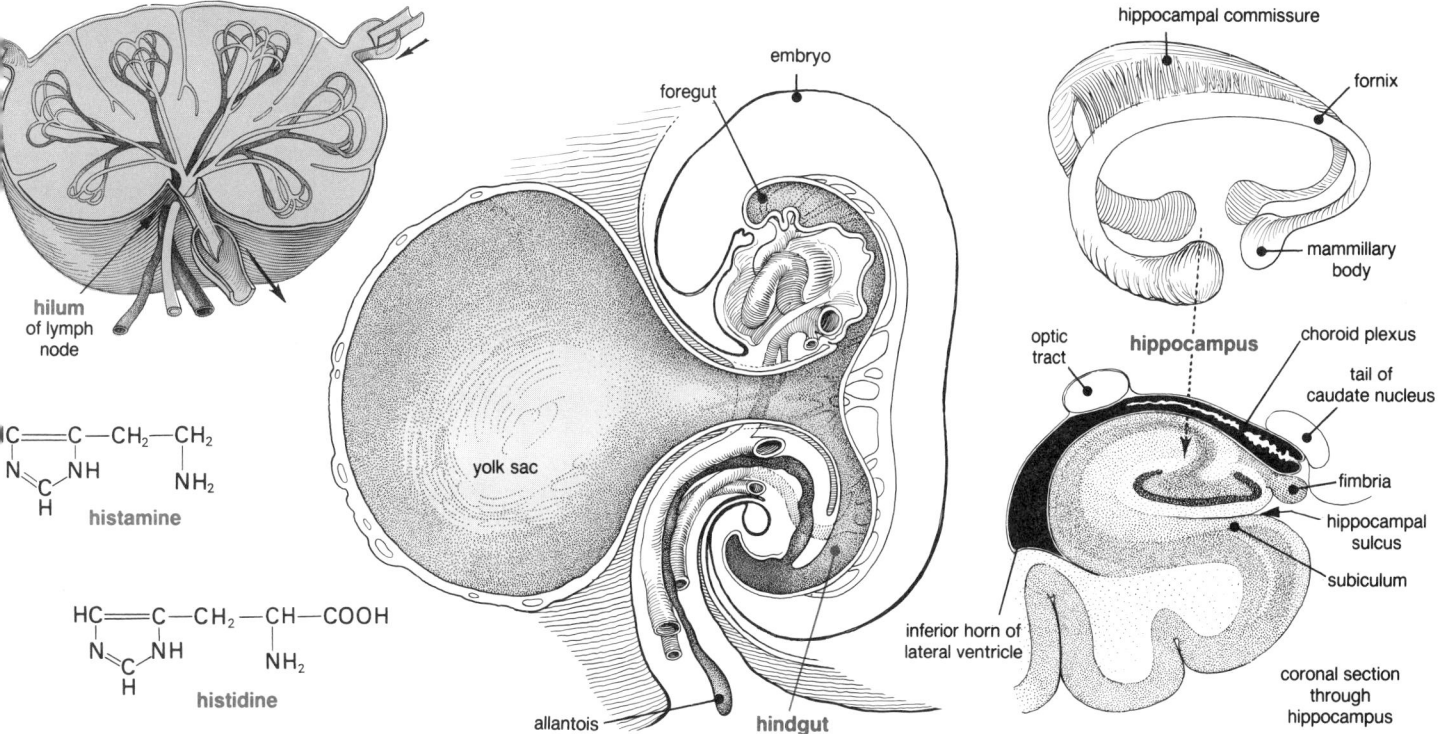

hilum
of lymph node

histamine

histidine

embryo
foregut
yolk sac
allantois
hindgut

hippocampal commissure
fornix
mammillary body
optic tract
hippocampus
choroid plexus
tail of caudate nucleus
fimbria
hippocampal sulcus
subiculum
inferior horn of lateral ventricle
coronal section through hippocampus

Heterophyes (family Heterophilae). **2.** A fluke of the genus *Heterophyes*.

heteroplasia **1.** The presence of tissue elements in an abnormal location; e.g., the growth of bone where normally there should be fibrous connective tissue. **2.** The malposition of a part that is otherwise normal; e.g., the presence of a ureter at the lower pole of a kidney.

heteroplasty **1.** Surgical grafting of tissue donated from another individual. **2.** The replacement of tissue with synthetic material.

heteroploidy The state of an individual or cell with a chromosome number other than the normal diploid number.

heteropsia Unequal vision in the two eyes.

heterosexuality The state of having one's sexual interests directed toward a member of the opposite sex, as opposed to homosexuality.

heterospecific Denoting a graft that is obtained from an individual of a different species. Also called heterologous.

heterotaxia, heterotaxis Abnormal arrangement of bodily organs or parts; anomalous structural arrangement.

heterotaxic Occurring in an abnormal place.

heterotransplant See xenograft.

heterotropia See strabismus.

heterotypic Not typical.

heterozygosity The state of having one or more pairs of dissimilar alleles.

heterozygote A zygote produced by the union of two gametes of different genetic composition.

hexacanth The motile, six-hooked, first-stage larva of a tapeworm. Also called oncosphere.

hexachlorophene A bactericidal agent, $(C_6HCl_3OH)_2CH_2$, used as a local antiseptic.

hexadecanoic acid See palmitic acid.

hexenmilch German for witch's milk; a milky fluid sometimes secreted by the breasts of newborn infants.

hexokinase An enzyme (present in yeast, muscle, and other tissues) that promotes the phosphorylation of glucose and other hexoses to form hexose-6-phosphate.

hexosamine A primary amine derivative of a hexose resulting when NH_2 replaces OH; e.g., glucosamine. Also called amino sugar.

hexosan Any of several polysaccharides that yield a hexose on hydrolysis.

hexose A monosaccharide having six carbon atoms in the molecule; e.g., glucose and fructose.

hexose-1-phosphate   uridylyltransferase An enzyme system that promotes the interconver-

sion of glucose 1-phosphate and galactose 1-phosphate with simultaneous interconversion of UDP glucose and UDP galactose. Also called uridyltransferase.

hexulose A ketohexose, as fructose.

hexylresorcinol A crystalline phenol used as an anthelminthic.

hiatus An opening, aperture, or fissure.

  aortic h. The opening in the diaphragm through which the aorta and thoracic duct pass.

  esophageal h. The opening in the diaphragm through which the esophagus and the two vagus nerves pass.

hibernation The dormant condition or winter sleep in which certain animals pass the cold months.

hiccup A spasm of the diaphragm causing inhalation, followed by sudden closure of the glottis.

hidradenitis Inflammation of a sweat gland.

  h. suppurativa Chronic, relapsing, infectious disease of the apocrine sweat glands; marked by the development of one or more cutaneous pea-sized nodules which undergo softening and suppuration; it occurs most commonly in the genital and perianal regions and in the armpits.

hidradenoma A relatively infrequent benign tumor of sweat gland origin; may be solid or cystic. Also written hydradenoma.

hidroa Hydroa.

hidrocystoma The cystic deformation of sweat glands.

hidropoiesis The formation of sweat.

hidrosis **1.** Excessive perspiration. **2.** Any sweat gland disorder.

high A state of drug induced intoxication, as from a narcotic, alcohol, or hallucinogenic agent.

hilar dance Strong pulsations of the pulmonary arteries seen on fluoroscopic examination in patients with congenital left-to-right shunt.

hilum The point at which nerves and vessels enter and leave an organ. Also called hilus.

hindbrain See rhombencephalon.

hindfoot **1.** The rear portion of the foot consisting of the talus and calcaneus. **2.** One of the back feet of a quadruped animal.

hindgut The caudal part of the embryonic alimentary canal.

hip The lateral area of the body from the waist to the thigh.

  h. pointer Contusion on the iliac crest, or immediately above it.

hipbone A large, flattened, irregularly shaped bone that forms the anterior and lateral walls of the pelvic cavity; consisting of three parts (ilium, ischium, and

pubis). Formerly known as the innominate bone. Also written hip bone.

Hippel-Lindau disease See von Hippel-Lindau disease.

hippocampus One of two curved bands of a very special type of cortex about 5 cm long, on the floor of the inferior horn of the lateral ventricle on each side of the brain.

Hippocrates A Greek physician known as the "Father of Medicine"; his medical science principles were laid down about 400 years before the birth of Christ.

  aphorisms of H. A collection of observations, rules, and brief statements of clinical wisdom found in Books I to III of the hippocratic writings.

hippocratic oath A code of ethical conduct for the medical profession attributed to Hippocrates.

hippus Abnormal, spasmodic, rhythmic contraction and dilation of the pupil.

Hirschsprung's disease Congenital disorder of early infancy characterized by extreme distention of the colon, resulting from absence of ganglion cells of the myenteric plexuses of the rectum and lower colon. Also called congenital megacolon.

hirsute **1.** Hairy. **2.** Of or relating to hair.

hirsutism Excessive hair on cheek, chin, lip, or chest, especially in women.

hirudin An anticoagulant substance secreted by the salivary glands of leeches which prevents coagulation of the blood while the leech is sucking.

histamine A white crystalline amine, $C_5H_9N_3$, occurring in all animal and plant tissue; formed from histidine by decarboxylation and by the action of putrefactive bacteria; its release within the body causes bronchiolar constriction, arteriolar dilatation, increased gastric secretion, and a fall in blood pressure.

histidine α-Amino-β-(4-imidazole)   propionic acid; an amino acid.

histiocyte A large mononuclear phagocyte or macrophage; a tissue cell.

histiocytosis A proliferation of histiocytes.

  h. X The generic name proposed to cover three possibly related entities characterized by histiocytic proliferation of unknown etiology: eosinophilic granuloma, Hand-Schüller-Christian syndrome, and Letterer-Siwe disease.

  nonlipid h. An acute progressive and wasting disease of infants and young children characterized by invasion of the spleen, liver, and bone marrow by proliferating histiocytes, accompanied by generalized involvement of the lymph nodes and enlargement of the spleen and liver; frequently present are

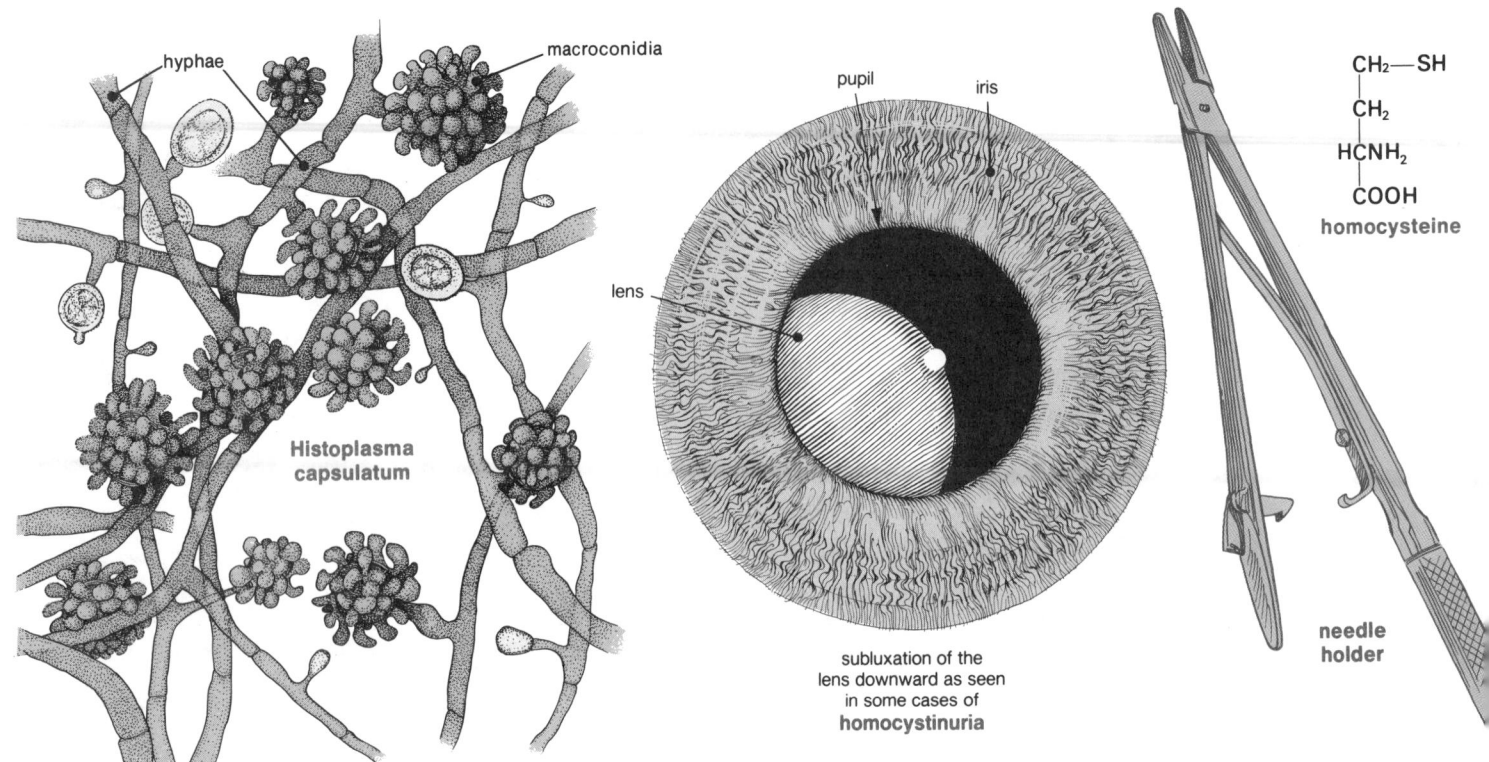

hyphae

macroconidia

Histoplasma
capsulatum

pupil   iris

lens

subluxation of the
lens downward as seen
in some cases of
homocystinuria

CH₂—SH
|
CH₂
|
HCNH₂
|
COOH
homocysteine

**needle
holder**

a purpuric rash, anemia, and chronic inflammation of the middle ear. Also called Letterer-Siwe disease.

histochemistry The chemistry of cell components and tissues.

histocompatibility Ability to accept transplants of tissues from one individual to another; depends on identical genetic constitution of both individuals.

histofluorescence Fluorescence of the tissues produced by exposure to ultraviolet rays after injection of a fluorescent substance.

histogenesis 1. The origin and development of bodily tissues from undifferentiated cells of the embryonic germ layers. **2.** In myology, the development of muscle fibers from primitive cells.

histogram A columnar or bar chart used in descriptive statistics showing the relationship of two factors.

histologic Pertaining to histology.

histologist A specialist in histology.

histology The branch of anatomy dealing with the microscopic structure of tissues. Also called microscopic anatomy; microanatomy.

histolysis The disintegration or breakdown of tissue.

histone Any of several simple water soluble proteins containing a large proportion of basic amino acids; e.g., the globin of hemoglobin.

histopathology The pathology of abnormal or diseased tissue. Also called pathologic histology.

histophysiology The physiology of bodily tissues.

Histoplasma A genus of fungi; some species cause disease in man.

   H. capsulatum Yeastlike fungus occurring in soil; when present in tissue it appears to be encapsulated; the cause of histoplasmosis.

histoplasmin A concentrate of the growth products of the fungus *Histoplasma capsulatum;* used as a dermal reactivity indicator to detect histoplasmosis.

histoplasmosis A fungal disease caused by *Histoplasma capsulatum;* usually asymptomatic but may produce a benign, mild pulmonary illness; it is a frequent cause of pulmonary nodules; the infection may spread throughout the body, and this disseminated form, though uncommon, is quite serious.

hives Eruption of transitory pruritic wheals, often due to hypersensitivity to foods or drugs or to emotional factors.

hoarseness A harsh, rough, grating quality of the voice.

Hodgkin's disease A disease of lymphatic tissue characterized by painless enlargement of the lymph nodes with or without systemic symptoms such as fever, sweats, weight loss, and lassitude; if untreated

the disease may spread to involve the spleen and other organs; treatment and prognosis depend on the clinical staging.

Hoffmann's sign Snapping the nail of the middle finger leads to flexion of thumb and fingers; a sign of a pyramidal tract lesion.

holandric Occurring only in males; denoting a character determined by a gene on the Y chromosome.

holarthritis Inflammation of all or most of the joints.

holder, needle An instrument used for grasping a needle during surgery. Also called needle forceps.

holoblastic Denoting the complete division of the entire ovum into individual blastomeres.

holocrine Wholly secretory; relating to a gland whose secretion is composed of the disintegrated secreting cell in addition to its accumulated secretion, e.g., sebaceous glands.

holodiastolic Relating to or occupying all of diastole from the second heart sound to the succeeding first heart sound.

holoenzyme An enzyme possessing a chemical group that is non-amino acid in nature.

hologram A three-dimensional pattern exposed by holography on a photosensitive surface and then photographically developed.

holography The use of lasers to record on a photographic plate the diffraction pattern of an object from which a three-dimensional image can be constructed.

   acoustic h. A technique for detecting breast cancer by transmitting sound waves through breast tissue.

holosystolic Relating to or occupying all of systole. Also called pansystolic.

Homans' sign Pain in the calf or the back of the knee when the foot is dorsiflexed, suggesting the presence of a deep venous thrombosis in the calf.

homeomorphous Of similar shape.

homeopathist One who practices homeopathy.

homeopathy A system of therapeutics based on the use of small doses of a drug that in large doses is capable of producing symptoms in healthy individuals which are similar to those of the disease being treated.

homeoplasia The formation of new tissue similar to that already existing in, and normal to, the part.

homeostasis A state of physiologic equilibrium in the living body (temperature, blood pressure, chemical content, etc.) under variations in the environment.

homeotherapy Treatment or prevention of a disease with a substance similar to, but not identical

with, the causative agent of the disease; e.g., vaccination.

homicidal Having a tendency to kill.

homicide The killing of a person by another human being.

hominid 1. A member of the family Hominidae. **2.** Relating to the family Hominidae.

Hominidae A family of mammals (order Primates) which includes modern and prehistoric man.

Hominoidea 1. In some classifications, a major division of the order Primates which segregates man from the great apes. **2.** A superfamily (suborder Anthropoidea) which includes the great apes and the fossil hominids.

Homo A genus of the order Primates which includes the extinct and existing species of man.

   H. sapiens The present-day human species.

homoblastic Developing from only one type of tissue.

homocentric Having the same center, as rays originating from one source. Also called concentric.

homocysteine A sulfur-containing amino acid, HSCH₂CH₂CHNH₂COOH.

homocystine A sulfur-containing amino acid (SCH₂CH₂CHNH₂COOH)₂ formed by oxidation of homocysteine.

homocystinuria A genetically determined disorder of metabolism resulting from a deficiency of activity of the enzyme cystathionine synthase; characterized by an elevation of the concentrations of methionine and of homocystine in the blood, homocystine in the urine (not detectable in normal urine), mental retardation, dislocation of the ocular lenses, skeletal abnormalities (dolichostenomelia, genu valgum, osteoporosis), increased stickiness of platelets in the blood, thromboembolic episodes, and abnormality of the palate with crowding of the teeth.

homoeroticism Homosexuality.

homogametic Producing only one kind of germ cell; especially possessing an X chromosome in cell gametes. Also called monogametic.

homogenate A substance that has been homogenized; in biochemistry, tissue that has been reduced to a creamy consistency and that has disintegrated cell structure.

homogeneous Composed of similar elements throughout; of uniform quality.

homogenization The process of making diverse elements homogenous.

homogenize To blend diverse elements into a mixture that is uniform in structure or consistency throughout.

homogenous 1. In biology, correspondence of

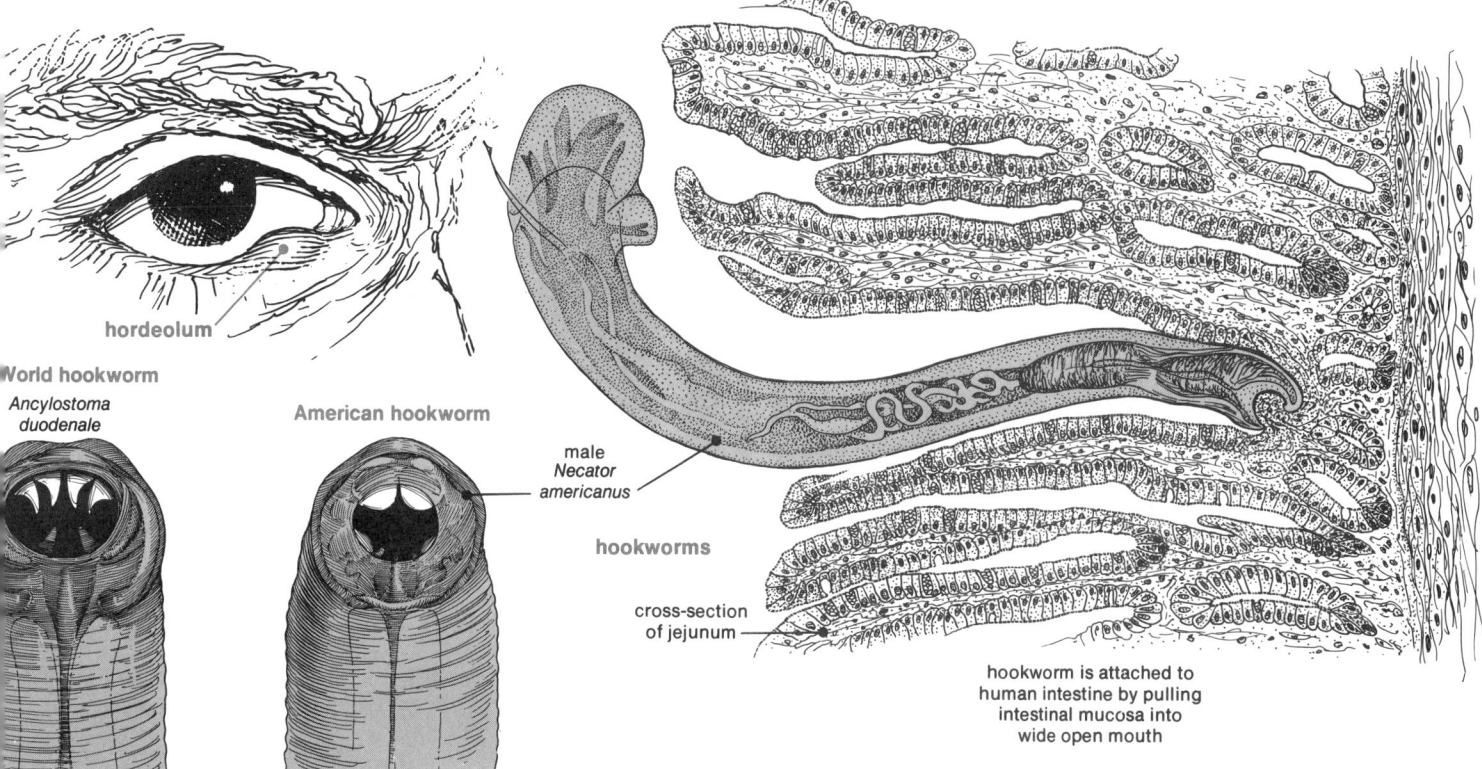

hordeolum

Old World hookworm
Ancylostoma duodenale

American hookworm

male
Necator americanus

hookworms

cross-section
of jejunum

hookworm is attached to
human intestine by pulling
intestinal mucosa into
wide open mouth

parts because of common descent. **2.** Homogeneous.

homogentisate oxygenase An iron-containing enzyme that promotes the cleavage of the benzene ring in homogentistic acid; congenital absence of this enzyme causes alkaptonuria. Also called homogentisase; homogentisic acid oxidase.

homogentisic acid An intermediate in the metabolism of the amino acid tyrosine, excreted in the urine of persons afflicted with alkaptonuria. Also called alkapton.

h. a. oxidase See homogentisate oxygenase.

homogentisuria See alkaptonuria.

homograft Allograft.

homolateral On or relating to the same side. Also called ipsilateral.

homologous Corresponding in structure, position, development, and evolutionary origin, as the wing of a bird, the flipper of a seal, and the arm of man; denoting a homologue.

homologue Any homologous structure; a part or organ similar in structure; position, and origin to another organ. Also written homolog.

homology Correspondence in structure, evolutionary origin, or position.

homolysin Isohemolysin.

homomorphic Denoting structures of similar size and form.

homonomous Denoting parts that are similar in function and structure, as fingers and toes.

homonymous **1.** Relating to the same right or left side of the two visual fields; e.g., the nasal half of one visual field and the temporal half of the other. **2.** Having the same name.

homoplasty Repair of a defect with a graft from another member of the same species.

homopolymer A polymer composed of identical units of a single monomer.

homopolypeptide A peptide chain containing only one type of amino acid residue, as polyglycine, polyalanine, and polyglutamic acid.

homosexual **1.** Relating to or exhibiting homosexuality. **2.** An individual having a sexual interest in or relationship with others of the same sex.

homosexuality Sexual interest or relationship between members of the same sex.

homothermal Having a relatively constant body temperature, more or less independent of the environmental temperature. Also called warm-blooded; homoiothermal; homothermous; homothermic.

homotransplant Allograft.

homotype A part or organ having the same structure or function as another.

homozoic Pertaining to the same animal or the same species of animal.

homozygosis The formation of a zygote by the union of genetically identical gametes.

homozygosity The state of having identical alleles at one or more loci of homologous chromosomes.

homozygote An individual exhibiting homozygosity.

homunculus **1.** The proportional representation of various parts of the body in the motor or sensory areas of the cerebral cortex. **2.** A minute body imagined by 16th and 17th century biologists to be present in the sperm, from which the human body was supposed to be developed.

motor h. One in which the parts of the figure are roughly proportional to the excitable motor cortex associated with evoking movements of the parts; the figure is generally illustrated upside down on the brain, with the lower extremity on the medial surface of the paracentral lobule and with the head near the lateral cerebral fissure.

sensory h. One in which the parts of the figure are proportional to the amount of cortical area associated with sensory innervation density of the body areas, rather than to the size of the area (e.g., the tongue and thumb have a relatively large representation).

honk, systolic A loud, vibratory, often musical heart murmur of relatively clear pitch, usually occurring in late systole; believed to originate in the mitral valve. Also called systolic whoop.

hook A metal instrument with a curved or sharply bent tip, used for traction or fixation of a part.

blunt h. Hook used to make traction upon the groin of a dead infant during a difficult breech presentation.

palate h. Hook used to pull forward the soft palate to facilitate posterior rhinoscopy.

tracheotomy h. A right-angled hook for holding the trachea steady during tracheotomy.

hooklets Small horny residues from *Echinococcus* larval infestation, found in the walls of *Echinococcus* cysts.

hookworm Any parasitic roundworm of the genera *Ancylostoma* and *Necator*.

American h. *Necator americanus.*

Old World h. *Ancylostoma duodenale.*

hora decubitus (h.d.) Latin for at bedtime; used in prescription writing.

hora somni (h.s.) Latin for at hour of sleep; used in prescription writing.

hordeolum A common staphylococcal inflammation of the sebaceous gland of an eyelash, marked by a painful, swollen, erythematous lesion of the external surface of the eyelid. Also called stye.

hormonal Of, relating to, or of the nature of a hormone.

hormone A glandular chemical secretion produced by an organ or part of the body and carried in the bloodstream to another organ or part to stimulate or retard its function; produced by endocrine glands and in the gastrointestinal tract.

adrenocortical h.'s Hormones (steroids) secreted by the human adrenal cortex; the principal ones are cortisol, aldosterone, and corticosterone.

adrenocorticotropic h. (ACTH) A hormone elaborated by the anterior lobe of the pituitary gland which stimulates the adrenal cortex to functional activity. Also called adrenocorticotrophin.

adrenomedullary h.'s Any of the hormones formed by the adrenal medulla; e.g., epinephrine, norepinephrine.

androgenic h. Any of the masculinizing hormones including testosterone, the most potent one.

antidiuretic h. (ADH) One produced by the posterior lobe of the pituitary gland, having a potent antidiuretic action and some vasoconstrictive action on the visceral circulation; it makes the collecting duct of the kidney tubule permeable to water and allows concentration of urine. Also called vasopressin.

corticotropic-releasing h. (CRH) Hormone of hypothalamic origin capable of accelerating pituitary secretion of corticotropin.

follicle-stimulating h. (FSH) A glycoprotein hormone of the anterior lobe of the pituitary gland that stimulates normal cyclic growth of the ovarian follicle in females and stimulates the seminiferous tubules to produce spermatozoa in males.

follicle-stimulating hormone-releasing h. (FSH-RH) A hypothalamic hormone capable of accelerating pituitary secretion of follicle-stimulating hormone.

gastrointestinal h. Any secretion of the gastrointestinal mucosa affecting the timing of various digestive secretions; e.g., secretin.

gonadotropin-releasing h. (GnRH, GRH) A decapeptide secreted by the hypothalamus that stimulates the pituitary gland to produce luteinizing hormone and follicle-stimulating hormone.

growth h. (GH) A hormone secreted by the anterior lobe of the pituitary gland that promotes fat mobilization, inhibits glucose utilization, and affects the rate of skeletal and visceral growth; diabetogenic when present in excess. Also called somatotropin.

interstitial cell stimulating h. (ICSH) An anterior pituitary gland secretion which stimulates testicular interstitial cells to produce androgen; ICSH in the male is identical with luteinizing hormone (LH) in

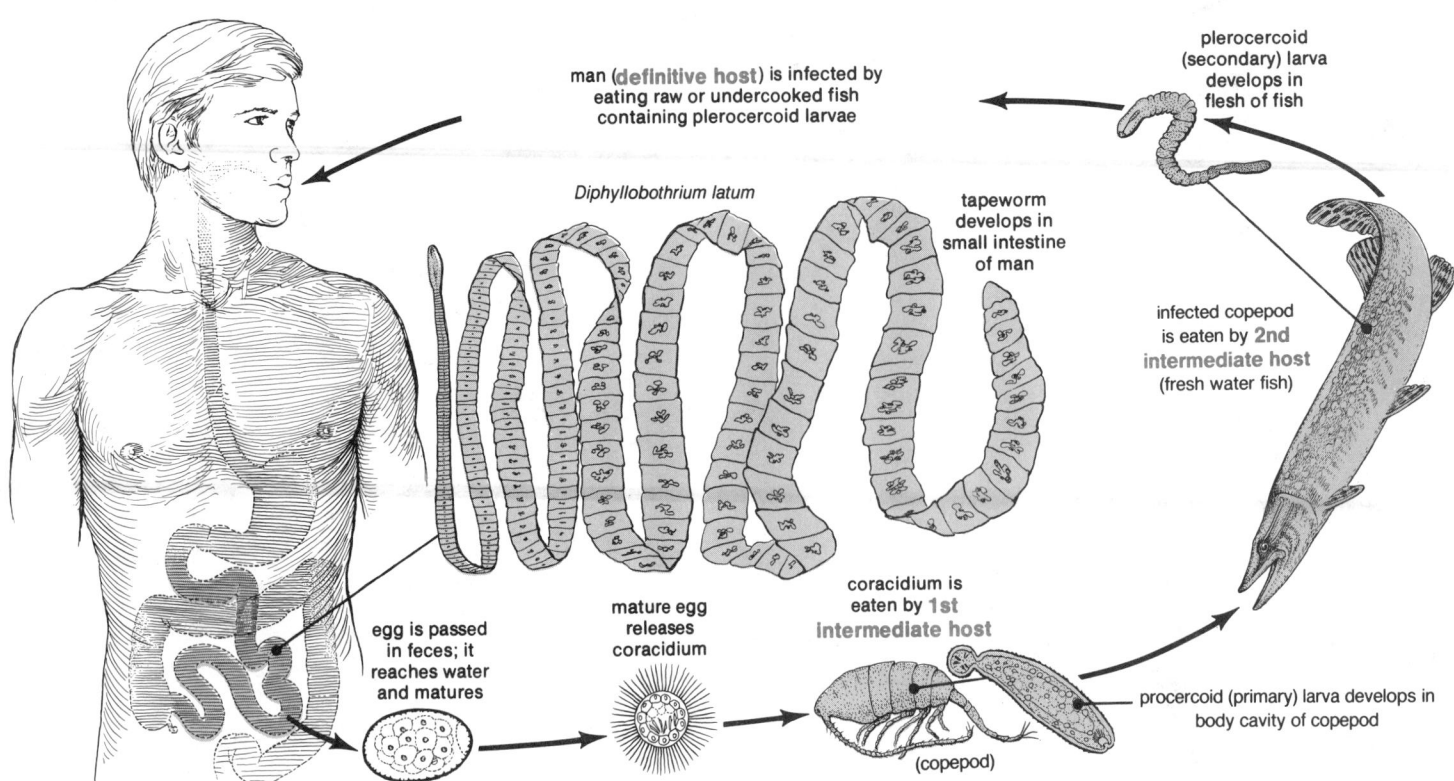

man (definitive host) is infected by eating raw or undercooked fish containing plerocercoid larvae

Diphyllobothrium latum

tapeworm develops in small intestine of man

plerocercoid (secondary) larva develops in flesh of fish

infected copepod is eaten by **2nd intermediate host** (fresh water fish)

egg is passed in feces; it reaches water and matures

mature egg releases coracidium

coracidium is eaten by **1st intermediate host**

procercoid (primary) larva develops in body cavity of copepod

(copepod)

the female, which is essential for ovulation and formation of the corpus luteum in the ovary.

luteinizing h. (LH) A glycoprotein hormone of the anterior pituitary gland that promotes maturation of an ovarian follicle, its secretion of progesterone, its rupture to release the egg, and the conversion of the ruptured follicle into the corpus luteum. Also called lutein-stimulating hormone (LSH).

luteinizing hormone-releasing h. (LH-RH, LRH) Hypothalamic hormone capable of accelerating pituitary secretion of luteinizing hormone.

lutein-stimulating h. (LSH) See luteinizing hormone.

melanocyte-stimulating h. (MSH) A secretion of the middle lobe of the pituitary gland that increases deposition of melanin by the melanocytes.

natriuretic h. A non-peptide substance of less than 500 daltons, isolated from plasma after volume expansion; thought to be released from the brain, it inhibits sodium-potassium ATPase throughout the body and is both natriuretic and vasoconstrictor; possible cause of essential hypertension. Also called endoxin because it binds to digoxin antibodies.

ovarian h.'s Hormones secreted by the human ovary including estradiol, estrone, estriol, and progesterone.

parathyroid h. (PTH) A protein biosynthesized and secreted into the bloodstream by the four parathyroid glands which are located in the neck behind the thyroid gland; it acts on the cells of bone, kidney, and intestinal tract to maintain a constant concentration of calcium in the blood. Also called parathormone.

pituitary growth h. (PGH) The growth hormone of the anterior lobe of the pituitary gland.

placental h. Any of the hormones secreted by the placenta, namely, human chorionic gonadotropin, estrogen, progesterone, and human placental lactogen.

progestational h. Progesterone.

prolactin-releasing h. A hypothalamic hormone that stimulates pituitary secretion of prolactin.

releasing h. (RH) Releasing factor; see under factor.

sex h.'s Estrogens (female sex hormones) and androgens (male sex hormones) formed by ovarian, testicular, and adrenocortical tissues.

somatotrophic h. See growth hormone.

testicular h.'s The hormones elaborated by the human testis, especially testosterone.

thyroid h. A term that commonly refers to thyroxin, but may also include triiodothyronine.

thyroid-stimulating h. (TSH) See thyrotropin.

thyrotrophic h. See thyrotropin.

thyrotropic h. See thyrotropin.

thyrotropin-releasing h. (TRH) A tripeptide hormone from the hypothalamus that stimulates pituitary secretion of thyrotropin.

hormonogenic Denoting any agent that stimulates the production of a hormone.

hormonotherapy Medical treatment with hormones.

horn Any horn-shaped structure or excrescence.

anterior h. of spinal cord The anterior column of the spinal cord as seen in cross sections.

cutaneous h. A horny growth of the skin. Also called warty horn.

posterior h. of spinal cord The posterior column of the spinal cord as seen in cross sections.

pulp h. A prolongation of vital pulp tissue of a tooth directly under a cusp.

hornet Any of several stinging wasps, chiefly of the genera *Vespa* and *Vespula,* having a slender, spindle-shaped body with an elongated waist; they usually construct papier-mâché hives; the antigens responsible for hypersensitivity are present in both the venom sac and body of the insect.

hospice An institution that is organized to provide coordinated multidisciplinary services to dying patients and their families; staff is comprised of professionals in physical, psychological, social, and spiritual care.

hospital An institution whose primary aim is caring for or treating patients.

base h. Hospital located in a large military base for the care of patients received from smaller units near the battle front.

closed h. Hospital in which only members of the attending and consulting staff may admit and treat patients.

day h. Hospital that provides treatment during the day enabling patients to return home at night; it may be a special facility within a large hospital.

evacuation h. A mobile military hospital where patients are taken and cared for until they can be evacuated to a general hospital.

general h. 1. Any large civilian hospital for the care of medical, surgical, and maternity cases. 2. A permanent, large military hospital that receives patients from smaller evacuation hospitals.

maternity h. A hospital for the care of women immediately before, during, and shortly after childbirth and for the care of newborn babies.

mobile Army surgical h. (MASH) See surgical hospital.

proprietary h. A private hospital.

special h. Hospital for the treatment of patients with specific diseases.

surgical h. A mobile military hospital for the immediate care of serious casualties.

host 1. An organism that harbors and provides nourishment for another organism (parasite). **2.** The recipient of an organ or tissue transplant from a donor.

alternate h. Intermediate host.

definitive h. The organism in which a parasite resides during its adult and sexual phase.

intermediate h. The organism in which a parasite resides during its larval or asexual phase.

primary h. The organism in which the mature parasite resides when it has two or more stages of existence in different organisms.

reservoir h. An animal that serves as a host to species of parasites that are also parasitic for man and from which man may be infested either directly through ingestion or indirectly through a carrier, such as a mosquito.

secondary h. Intermediate host.

housefly A common, widely distributed member of the insect order Dipter, *Musca domestica;* it breeds in filth and decaying organic waste, and is a transmitter of numerous disease-causing organisms.

Houssay syndrome Abatement of diabetes mellitus resulting from surgical removal of, or a destructive lesion in, the pituitary gland.

hum, venous A continuous murmur due to altered flow patterns in veins; heard on auscultation over the large veins at the base of the neck when the patient is in a sitting position and looking to the opposite side; commonly heard in association with a goiter.

humectant A substance that helps to retain moisture.

humeral Relating to or located in the proximity of the humerus.

humerus The long bone of the upper arm that extends from the shoulder to the elbow.

humidity Dampness.

absolute h. The amount of water vapor present in the air when saturated at a given temperature, expressed in grains per cubic feet.

relative h. (RH) The percentage of water vapor present in the atmosphere, as compared to the amount necessary to cause saturation at a specific temperature.

humor Any fluid or semifluid occurring normally in the body.

aqueous h. The clear, watery fluid filling the anterior and posterior chambers of the eye.

vitreous h. See body, vitreous.

humulin A biosynthetic human insulin.

hunchback, humpback 1. An abnormally curved spine. Also called kyphosis. **2.** One afflicted with the deformity.

hunger 1. A strong craving for nourishment. **2.** A

islet of Langerhans
in diabetes

beta cell

alpha cell

hyalin

deferent
duct

seminal
vesicle

hydrocephalus

prostate

membrane obstructing
cerebrospinal fluid flow
through cerebral aqueduct

testis

hydrocele

hyaluronic acid
(repeating unit)

COOH   CH₂OH

NHCOCH₃

strong desire for anything.

air h. Dyspnea characterized by deep, labored respiration, as may occur in acidosis.

Hunter's canal See canal, adductor.

Hunter's syndrome A hereditary, X-linked recessive condition characterized by stiff joints, enlargement of the liver and spleen, cardiac involvement, mild retardation, and progressive deafness. Also called mucopolysaccharidosis II.

Huntington's chorea See chorea, hereditary.

Huntington's disease An inherited disorder of the nervous system transmitted by an autosomal dominant gene and marked by degeneration of the basal ganglia and cerebral cortex; manifestations include choreiform movements, intellectual deterioration, and personality changes; onset is usually insidious and occurs in middle life; the disease is often fatal within 5 to 15 years after onset.

Hurler's syndrome An inherited metabolic disorder marked by skeletal deformities, mental retardation, and early death; characterized by an accumulation of an abnormal intracellular material, a deficiency of the enzyme alpha-L-iduronidase, and excretion of chondroitin sulfate B and heparitin sulfate in the urine. Also called mucopolysaccharidosis 1; gargoylism; dysostosis multiplex; lipochondrodystrophy.

hyalin **1.** The homogeneous matrix of hyaline cartilage. **2.** A clear homogeneous substance, occurring in degenerative diseases.

hyaline Glassy or translucent in appearance.

hyaline membrane disease of the newborn (HMD) Condition occurring in premature babies with respiratory distress, marked primarily by the lining of the air spaces of the lungs with an eosinophilic membrane; the symptoms usually appear a few hours after the birth of an apparently healthy infant. See respiratory distress syndrome of the newborn.

hyalitis Inflammation of the vitreous body.

hyaloid Glassy or translucent in appearance.

hyalomere The pale, homogeneous, nonrefractile portion of a blood platelet; found in it are elements of chromatomeres, microtubules, mitochondria, microfilaments, and Golgi vesicles.

hyaluronic acid A mucopolysaccharide present in the form of a gelatinous material in the tissue spaces, thus binding cells together and holding water in the tissues; it has the property of increasing the slipperiness of fluids and of the lubricating and shock absorbing system of joints.

hyaluronidase An enzyme, found in sperm, snake and bee venom, and pathogenic bacteria; it causes the breakdown of hyaluronic acid in the tissue spaces, thus enabling the invading agent to enter cells and tissues. Also called spreading factor.

hybaroxia Oxygen therapy with pressures greater than one atmosphere applied in a room or chamber.

hybrid The offspring (plant or animal) of parents who are genetically dissimilar.

hybridization In somatic cell genetics, the fusing of somatic cells from two different species; may result in hybrid cells (with one fused nucleus) or heterokaryons (with two or more genetically different nuclei); important in mapping of chromosomes.

hybridoma A cell culture composed of fused cells of different kinds, cloned for the purpose of producing antibody of a single specificity.

hydatid **1.** A cystic structure containing the embryo of the *Taenia echinococcus;* a hydatid cyst. **2.** Any structure resembling a cyst.

h. of Morgagni **1.** Testicular appendage. **2.** Vesicular appendage; see under appendage.

hydatid disease See echinococcosis.

hydatidiform Resembling a hydatid.

hydralazine hydrochloride An adrenergic blocking agent that lowers blood pressure by acting directly on arteriolar smooth muscle; it may also increase renal blood flow; Apresoline®.

hydramnios, hydramnion The presence of an excessive quantity of amniotic fluid.

hydrargyrism, hydrargyria Mercury poisoning; see under poisoning.

hydrargyrum Latin for mercury.

hydrarthrosis Collection of fluid in a joint.

hydrase An enzyme that promotes the addition of water, or its removal from a molecule.

hydrate Any compound containing water which is retained in its molecular state.

hydrated Combined with water.

hydration The combination of a substance with water.

hydrencephalocele Hernial protrusion, through a defect in the skull, of brain substance with cerebrospinal fluid. Also called hydrocephalocele; hydroencephalocele.

hydrencephalomeningocele Hernial protrusion of the meninges, brain substance, and cerebrospinal fluid through a defect in the skull.

hydrencephalus Internal hydrocephalus; see hydrocephalus.

hydriatic Applied to the use of water in treating

disease. Also called hydrotherapeutic.

hydride A compound of hydrogen with a more positive element or group, thus assuming a formal negative charge.

hydroa Any vesicular skin eruption.

h. aestivale See hydroa vacciniforme.

h. febrilis See herpes simplex.

h. herpetiforme See dermatitis herpetiformis.

h. puerorum See hydroa vacciniforme.

h. vacciniforme A recurrent form occurring during the summer months. Also called hydroa aestivale or puerorum.

hydroappendix Distention of the vermiform appendix with a serous fluid.

hydroblepharon Edema of the eyelid.

hydrocarbon A compound containing hydrogen and carbon only.

hydrocele Abnormal collection of fluid in any sacculated cavity in the body, especially under the serous covering of the testis or along the spermatic cord.

hernia h. Hydrocele in which the hernial sac is filled with a fluid.

hydrocelectomy Surgical removal of a hydrocele.

hydrocephalic Relating to or afflicted with hydrocephalus.

hydrocephalocele See hydrencephalocele.

hydrocephalus Excessive accumulation of cerebrospinal fluid in the ventricles of the brain (internal hydrocephalus) or in the subarachnoid spaces (external hydrocephalus), causing enlargement of the head and compression of the brain.

communicating h. One in which there is no obstruction between the ventricles.

noncommunicating h., obstructive h. One in which there is an obstruction between the ventricles.

obstructive h. See noncommunicating hydrocephalus.

hydrochloric acid A colorless, compound of hydrogen chloride (HCl); the acid secreted by the stomach to facilitate digestion.

hydrochloride Compound formed by the reaction of hydrochloric acid with an organic base.

hydrochlorothiazide A thiazide compound used as an oral diuretic.

hydrocolloid A gelatinous colloid in unstable equilibrium with its contained water, used in dentistry as an elastic impression material.

irreversible h. A hydrocolloid such as alginate, whose physical condition is changed by an irreversible chemical reaction when mixed with water; used

hydrocortisone (cortisol)

kidney

renal pelvis

measuring specific gravity of a fluid by means of a **hydrometer**

hydronephrosis

hydroureter

ureter

hydromyelia — cross section of spinal cord

uterus

uterine tube

ovary

hydrosalpinx

---

in making diagnostic casts of teeth and partial denture impressions.

reversible h. A hydrocolloid of agar-agar base whose physical state is altered to a liquid by the application of heat and then changed to that of an elastic gel by cooling.

hydrocolpocele, hydrocolpos An accumulation of fluid in the vagina.

hydrocortisone A steroid hormone isolated from the adrenal cortex or produced synthetically; of the naturally occurring adrenal cortical hormones, hydrocortisone is most capable of correcting by itself the effects of adrenalectomy; provides resistance to stresses and maintains a number of enzyme systems. Also called cortisol.

hydrocyanic acid A colorless, volatile, poisonous compound with an almond odor (HCN); used as an insecticide and disinfectant. Also called hydrogen cyanide; prussic acid.

hydrodynamics The branch of physics concerned with fluids in motion and the forces affecting the motion.

hydroencephalocele See hydrencephalocele.

hydrogel A gel having water as its dispersion medium. Cf. hydrosol.

hydrogen A colorless, flammable, gaseous element; the lightest of all known chemical elements; symbol H, atomic number 1, atomic weight 1.0080.

activated h. Hydrogen removed from a compound (donor) by a dehydrogenase.

heavy h. See hydrogen-2.

h. acceptor 1. Hydrogen carrier. 2. A metabolite that transports hydrogen during metabolism.

h. carrier A molecule that carries hydrogen from one substance (oxidant) to another (reductant) or to molecular oxygen to form water (H_2O).

h. cyanide See hydrocyanic acid.

h. donor Substance that gives up hydrogen atoms to another substance.

h. ion The positively charged nucleus of the hydrogen atom, H° or H^+, formed by removal of the electron; it exists in aqueous solution as a hydronium ion, OH_3^+.

h. number A measure of the amount of unsaturated fatty acids in fat, equal to the quantity of hydrogen that 1 g of fat will absorb.

h. sulfide H_2S; a colorless, flammable, poisonous gas with a rotten egg odor; used as a reagent and in chemical manufacturing. Also called sulfuretted hydrogen.

h. transport The transfer of hydrogen from one substance to another; the former is thus oxidized and the latter is reduced.

sulfuretted h. See hydrogen sulfide.

hydrogen-1 (^1H) The hydrogen isotope that makes up about 99 percent of the hydrogen atoms occurring in nature; a mass 1 isotope. Also called protium.

hydrogen-2 (^2H) An isotope of hydrogen having an atomic weight of 2.0141, consisting of one proton and one neutron in the nucleus; a mass 2 isotope. Also called deuterium (D); heavy hydrogen.

hydrogen-3 (^3H) The heaviest of the three isotopes of hydrogen with an atomic mass of 3; weakly radioactive; half-life 12.4 years; a mass 3 isotope, made artificially by bombardment of other species. Also called tritium.

hydrogenation The combination of an unsaturated compound with hydrogen.

hydrokinetics The study of fluids in motion under a force.

hydrolabyrinth Abnormal increase in the amount of endolymph in the labyrinth of the inner ear; thought to be the cause of aural vertigo.

hydrolase An enzyme that promotes the hydrolysis of a compound.

hydrolysate Any product produced by hydrolysis.

protein h. A mixture of amino acids produced by splitting the protein molecule with acid, alkali, or enzyme; used in diets of infants allergic to milk or in special diets for individuals unable to eat ordinary food proteins.

hydrolysis The decomposition or splitting of a compound into simpler substances by the addition of the elements of water; a hydrogen is added to one portion and a hydroxyl group to the other.

hydrolytic Relating to, characterized by, or causing hydrolysis.

hydrolyze To subject to hydrolysis.

hydromassage Massage effected with streams of water.

hydrometer An instrument used to measure the specific gavity of a liquid such as urine. Also called gravimeter.

hydrometra Accumulation of a watery fluid in the uterus.

hydrometrocolpos Accumulation of fluid in the uterus and vagina.

hydrometry The determination of the specific gravity of a fluid.

hydromphalus A cystlike tumor of the umbilicus.

hydromyelia An increase of cerebrospinal fluid in the enlarged central canal of the spinal cord.

hydromyelocele A fluid-filled saclike protrusion of the spinal cord through a spina bifida.

hydronephrosis Distention of the pelvis and calyces of one or both kidneys with urine as a result of obstruction.

hydronium The hydrated hydrogen ion, H_3O^+, as it exists in water. Also called hydronium ion.

hydropenia Condition marked by insufficient content of water in the body.

hydropericardium Abnormal accumulation of serous fluid in the sac around the heart (pericardium).

hydroperitoneum See ascites.

hydrophilia Affinity for water.

hydrophilic, hydrophile Readily absorbing water; opposite of hydrophobic.

hydrophobia See rabies.

hydrophobic 1. Relating to rabies (hydrophobia). 2. Tending to repel water; opposite of hydrophilic.

hydrophthalmos See buphthalmos.

hydropneumopericardium The collection of serous effusion and gas within the pericardial cavity.

hydropneumothorax The presence of both gas and serous fluids in the pleural cavity. Also called pneumohydrothorax.

hydrops Accumulation of clear fluid in bodily tissues or cavities. Also called dropsy.

endolymphatic h. See Ménière's syndrome.

fetal h. Hydrops occurring in the fetus, as in erythroblastosis fetalis.

h. fetalis Fetal hydrops.

hydropyonephrosis The collection of urine and pus in the pelvis and calices of the kidney, usually caused by obstruction of the ureter.

hydrorchis Collection of fluid within the serous covering of the testis.

hydrorrhea Profuse watery secretion.

h. gravidarum Profuse secretion of a clear fluid from the uterus during pregnancy.

hydrosalpinx Accumulation of serous fluid in the uterine tube.

hydrosol A colloid in aqueous solution; a sol in which the dispersing medium is water. Cf. hydrogel.

hydrospirometer A spirometer in which the force of the expired air (air pressure) is indicated by the rise and fall of a column of water.

hydrostatic Relating to the pressures exerted by liquids at rest; opposed to hydrokinetic.

hydrotherapeutic See hydriatic.

hydrotherapy The therapeutic application of water in the treatment of certain diseases.

hydrothermal Relating to hot water.

hydrothorax Noninflammatory accumulation of serous fluid in the pleural cavity.

hydrotropism Growth or movement of an organism toward a moist surface (positive hydrotropism) or away from a moist surface (negative hydrotropism).

hydroureter Abnormal distention of the ureter

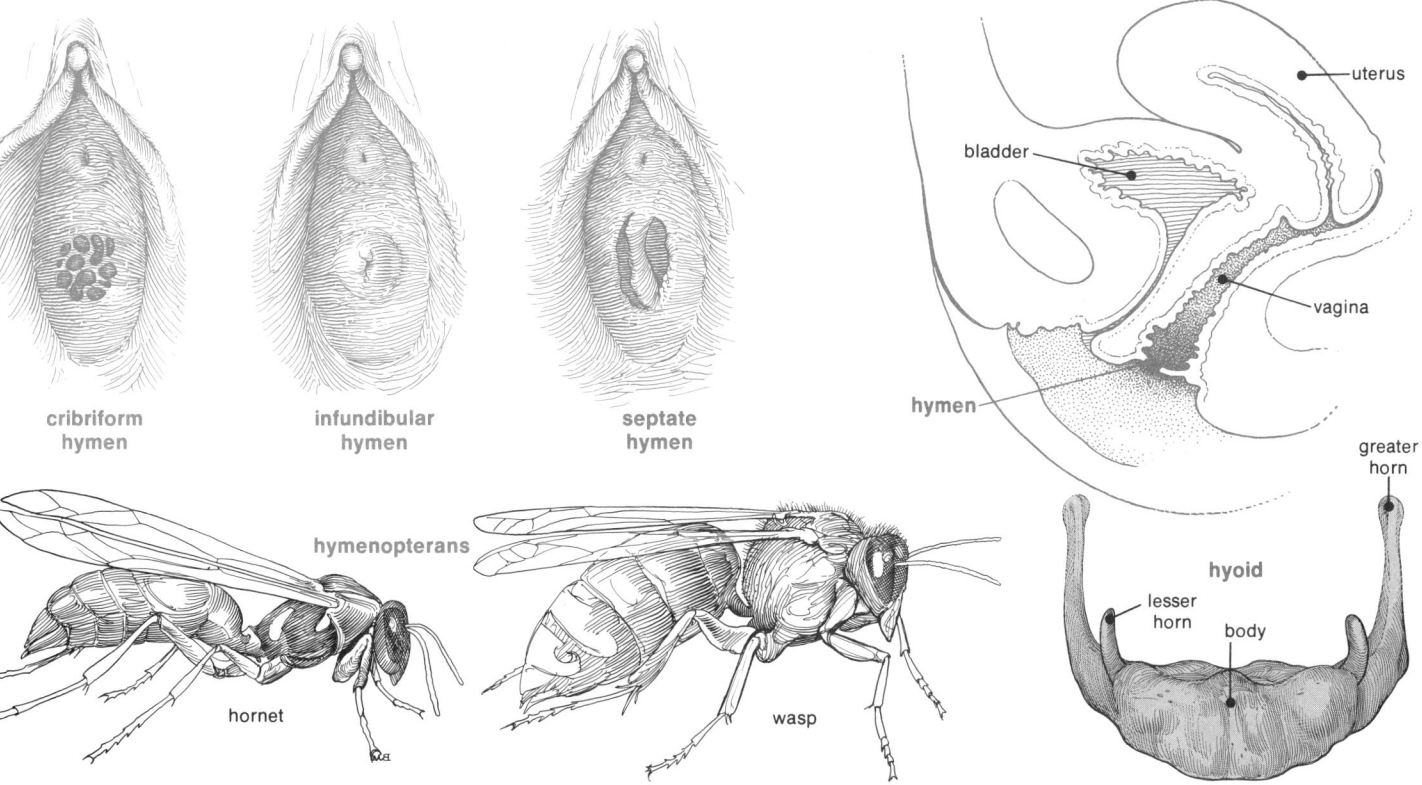

cribriform hymen

infundibular hymen

septate hymen

hymen

bladder

uterus

vagina

hymen

hymenopterans

hornet

wasp

hyoid

greater horn

lesser horn

body

with urine due to obstruction.

hydrous Containing water.

hydroxide Any chemical compound of hydroxyl (OH) with another element or radical.

hydroxyapatite A mineral compound used in chromatography of nucleic acids.

25-hydroxycholecalciferol A product of metabolism of cholecalciferol (vitamin D_3), produced mainly in the liver; by addition of a hydroxy group on the 1 position by the kidney it is converted to 1,25-dihydroxycholecalciferol; thought to be the most active form of vitamin D.

hydroxycortisone Cortisol.

hydroxyl The univalent radical or group OH.

hydroxylysine A basic amino acid found, thus far, only in collagen and gelatin.

hydroxyphenyluria Excretion of tyrosine and phenylalanine in the urine, usually resulting from ascorbic acid deficiency.

hydroxyproline 4-Hydroxy-2-pyrrolidinecarboxylic acid; $C_5H_9NO_3$; a nutritionally nonessential amino acid found among the hydrolysis products of collagen; not found in proteins other than those of connective tissue.

hydroxyprolinemia An inborn error of metabolism characterized by increased blood levels and urinary excretion of free hydroxyproline; associated with severe mental retardation.

5-hydroxytryptamine (5-HT) See serotonin.

o-**hydroxytyramine** See dopamine.

hygiene The science concerned with the methods of achieving or maintaining good health.

  oral h. The proper care of the mouth and teeth for the prevention of disease.

hygienic 1. Of or relating to hygiene. 2. Sanitary clean.

hygienist One who is skilled in the science of health and the prevention of disease.

  dental h. A person trained in the techniques of removing placques from teeth and other preventive treatments.

hygieology 1. The study of hygiene. 2. The sum of all measures for the dissemination and popularization of public health knowledge.

hygroma A bursa or cyst containing fluid.

  subdural h. A collection of fluid beneath the dura mater (subdural space).

hygrometer Any of several devices for measuring the atmospheric moisture.

hygroscopic Readily absorbing moisture.

hymen The membranous fold which partly or completely closes the vaginal orifice in the virgin.

  cribriform h. Hymen with a number of small perforations.

  denticular h. Hymen in which the opening has serrated edges.

  imperforate h. Hymen which completely closes the vaginal orifice.

  infundibuliform h. A protruding hymen with a central opening.

  septate h. Hymen in which the opening is divided by a narrow band of tissue.

hymenal Relating to the hymen.

hymenectomy Excision of the hymen.

Hymenolepis A genus of tapeworms of the class Cestoda.

  H. nana A small tapeworm (7 to 10 mm long) parasitic in rats, mice, and children. Also called dwarf or dwarf mouse tapeworm.

Hymenoptera An order of membrane-winged insects that includes many common stinging members such as the honeybee, yellow jacket, wasp, hornet, and fire ant; the stings are capable of causing severe hypersensitivity reactions and, in some cases, death.

hymenopteran Any of the membrane-winged insects of the order Hymenoptera, including the bees, wasps, and ants.

hymenorrhapy 1. The closing of the vagina by suturing of the hymen. 2. Suture of any membrane.

hymenotomy Surgical incision of the hymen, especially an imperforate hymen.

hyoepiglottic Relating to the hyoid bone and the epiglottis.

hyoglossal Relating to the hyoid bone and the tongue, especially to the hyoglossal muscle from the hyoid bone to the side of the tongue.

hyoid U-shaped, specifically, the horseshoe-shaped bone in the throat between the thyroid cartilage and the root of the tongue.

hyoscyamine A poisonous alkaloid, $C_{17}H_{23}NO_3$, occurring in plants such as belladonna, duboisia, hyoscyamus, and stramonium; isometric with atropine; used as an antispasmodic, analgesic, and sedative. Also called daturine; *l*-tropine tropate.

hypacusis Impairment of hearing; reduction in ability to perceive sound, usually attributable to conductive or neurosensory deficiency in the peripheral organs of hearing. Also called hypoacusis; hypacusia.

hypalgesia Decreased sensitivity to pain.

hypamnios, hypamnion The presence of an abnormally small amount of fluid in the amniotic sac.

hypencephalon The midbrain, pons, and medulla.

hyperabduction syndrome Pain and numbness of the arm and hand occurring after prolonged abduction of the arm, as during sleep, which compresses the axillary vessels and brachial plexus.

hyperacidity An excessive degree of acidity. Also called superacidity.

hyperactivity Excessively increased activity.

hyperactivity syndrome See hyperkinetic syndrome.

hyperacusia, hyperacusis Exaggerated hearing acuteness. Also called auditory hyperesthesia.

hyperadrenocorticism Excessive secretion of adrenocortical hormones.

hyperaldosteronism Condition caused by excessive secretion of aldosterone by the adrenal cortex. Also called aldosteronism.

  primary h. Excessive secretion of aldosterone caused by a tumor of an adrenal gland (aldosteronomal or idiopathic hyperplasia of the zona glomerulosa).

  secondary h. Excessive secretion of aldosterone caused by excess levels of renin and agiotensin; may be seen in cirrhosis, renovascular hypertension, idiopathic edema, etc.

hyperalgesia Excessive sensitiveness to pain.

hyperalimentation Overfeeding for therapeutic purposes.

  parenteral h. The continuous administration of fluids containing nutrients (particularly a solution of amino acids and sugar) into the superior vena cava through a catheter.

hyperbaric Relating to or occurring at pressures greater than atmospheric pressure; e.g., hyperbaric chamber.

hyperbarism Condition resulting from the pressure of ambient gases in excess of that within the body.

hyperbetalipoproteinemia Type II familial hyperlipoproteinemia; see under hyperlipoproteinemia.

hyperbilirubinemia The presence of an abnormally large amount of bilirubin in the blood.

hypercalcemia Abnormally high concentration of calcium in the blood.

  idiopathic h. of infants Persistent hypercalcemia affecting infants, associated with osteosclerosis, renal

Type and prevalence	I RARE	II COMMON	III FAIRLY COMMON	IV COMMON	V UNCOMMON
Appearance of plasma	creamy layer over clear infranatant on standing	clear or only slightly turbid	clear, cloudy, or milky	clear to grossly turbid	creamy layer over turbid infranatant on standing
Cholesterol level	↑	↑	↑	↑	↑
TG level	↑	↑	↑	↑	↑
Signs and symptoms	abdominal pain hepatosplenomegaly lipemia retinalis eruptive xanthomas	tendon xanthomas tuberous xanthomas corneal arcus accelerated atherosclerosis	tendon, tuboeruptive, and planar xanthomas accelerated atherosclerosis	accelerated coronary atherosclerosis abnormal glucose tolerance	abdominal pain hepatosplenomegaly lipemia retinalis eruptive xanthomas abnormal glucose tolerance

insufficiency, and sometimes hypertension.

hypercalciuria Elevated amounts of calcium in the urine, usually a result of hypercalcemia, as in hyperparathyroidism, bone neoplasm, and vitamin D intoxication. Also called hypercalcuria; hypercalcinuria.

  idiopathic h. Condition of elevated amounts of calcium in the urine not explained by hypercalcemia.

hypercapnia, hypercarbia The presence of abnormally high concentration of carbon dioxide in the blood.

hypercementosis Overdevelopment of cementum over the root surface of teeth.

hyperchloremia Abnormal increase of chloride in the blood.

hyperchlorhydria Excessive secretion of gastric juice; may be due to a temporary disturbance of stomach function; chronic hyperchlorhydria may be associated with peptic ulcer.

hypercholesterolemia, hypercholesteremia The presence of an excessive amount of cholesterol in the blood.

hypercholia A condition in which an excessive amount of bile is secreted by the liver.

hyperchromasia Hyperchromatism.

hyperchromatic Overpigmented; having excessive coloration; said especially of a cell which stains more intensely than normal.

hyperchromatism 1. Excessive pigmentation. 2. Degeneration of a cell nucleus which becomes filled with an excessive amount of pigment particles.

hyperchromia 1. Abnormal increase in the hemoglobin content of red blood cells, usually seen in macrocytic cells where the concentration of hemoglobin is normal but the quantity is increased because the cells are larger than normal. 2. Hyperchromatism.

hyperchromic 1. Overpigmented. 2. Relating to an increase in light absorption.

hyperchylia An excessive secretion of gastric juice.

hyperchylomicronemia Type I familial hyperlipoproteinemia; see under hyperlipoproteinemia.

hypercorticoidism, hypercorticism Condition caused by an excess of one or more steroids of the adrenal cortex, or by the administration of large quantities of steroids having glucocorticoid qualities.

hypercryalgesia, hypercryesthesia Excessive sensitivity to cold.

hypercupremia Abnormally high copper content in the blood.

hypercythemia The presence of an abnormally large number of erythrocytes in the circulating blood.

hypercytosis Any condition in which there is an abnormal increase in the number of blood cells, especially of leukocytes.

hyperdipsia Intense thirst.

hyperdistention Extreme distention.

hyperdynamia Extreme muscular activity or restlessness; exaggeration of function.

hyperdynamic Marked by hyperdynamia.

hyperemesis Excessive vomiting.

  h. gravidarum Pernicious vomiting of pregnancy.

hyperemia Excess of blood in an area of the body; congestion.

  active h. Hyperemia caused by increased inflow of arterial blood resulting in dilatation of arterioles and capillaries, as in inflammation.

  collateral h. Increased blood flow through collateral vessels due to an arrest of the flow through the main artery.

  passive h. Hyperemia resulting from an obstruction to the outflow of blood from the affected area.

hyperesthesia Abnormally increased sensitivity to sensory stimuli.

hyperextension Extension of a part of the body beyond the normal limit. Also called superextension.

hyperflexion Flexion of a limb or part beyond the normal limit. Also called overflexion; superflexion.

hypergammaglobulinemia Excess of gamma globulin in the blood.

hypergenitalism Overdeveloped genitalia for age of the individual.

hyperglobulinemia Excess of globulin in the blood.

hyperglycemia Abnormally high concentration of sugar (glucose) in the blood.

hyperglycorrhachia An excessive amount of sugar (glucose) in the cerebrospinal fluid (CSF).

hypergonadism Abnormally increased physiologic activity of the gonads (testes or ovaries), with enhanced secretion of gonadal hormones, marked growth, and precocious sexual development.

hyperhidrosis Excessive perspiration.

hyperhydration See overhydration.

hyperinsulinism 1. Excessive secretion of insulin by the islets of Langerhans, causing the level of sugar in the blood to fall considerably. 2. Insulin shock from excess dosage of insulin.

hyperkalemia An elevated potassium concentration in the blood; it may cause changes in cardiac function leading to cardiac arrest. Also called hyperpotassemia.

hyperkeratosis Overgrowth of the horny layer of the skin.

hyperkinesia, hyperkinesis Abnormally increased muscular activity, as seen in some psychi-

atric disorders, especially in children.

hyperkinetic Of, or relating to, hyperkinesia.

hyperkinetic syndrome Condition marked by excessive energy, emotional instability, and short attention span; may be seen in children with minimal brain dysfunction. Also called hyperactivity syndrome.

hyperlactation Excessive or prolonged secretion of milk.

hyperlipidemia, hyperlipemia The presence of an abnormally large amount of fats in the blood. Also called lipemia; lipidemia.

hyperlipoproteinemia Disorder of fat metabolism marked by high concentrations of lipoproteins in the blood.

  type I familial h. Rare disorder characterized by accumulation of chylomicrons in the blood, proportional to intake of dietary fat; inherited as a recessive trait. Also called hyperchylomicronemia; exogenous hyperlipemia.

  type I h., secondary A form seen in diseases in which there are abnormal circulating globulins, such as multiple myeloma, macroglobulinemia, etc.

  type II familial h. A disorder of autosomal inheritance characterized by increased plasma concentration of low-density (beta) lipoproteins, cholesterol, and phospholipids, with normal levels of triglyceride; associated with xanthomas in the Achilles, patellar, and digital extensor tendons, and susceptibility to atherosclerosis; manifestations are usually detected in infants and young adults. Also called familial hypercholesterolemia; hyperbetalipoproteinemia.

  type III familial h. A rare form, probably inherited as an autosomal recessive trait, characterized by increased plasma levels of abnormal very low-density (pre-beta) lipoproteins and cholesterol, flat, yellowish-orange xanthomas (usually on the palmar and digital creases), glucose intolerance, and premature atherosclerosis; usually detected in young adults. Also called broad-beta disease.

  type IV familial h. A common disorder, usually detected in middle life, probably inherited as an autosomal recessive trait; characterized by increased levels of plasma triglyceride of hepatic origin, contained primarily in very low-density (pre-beta) lipoproteins, and by a predisposition to atherosclerosis. Also called endogenous hyperlipemia; hyperprebetalipoproteinemia.

  type IV h., secondary A form seen in a variety of metabolic disorders including diabetes mellitus, hypothyroidism, and the nephrotic syndrome.

  type V familial h. A rare form with characteristics of both type I and IV, which include increased plasma levels of chylomicrons, very low-density

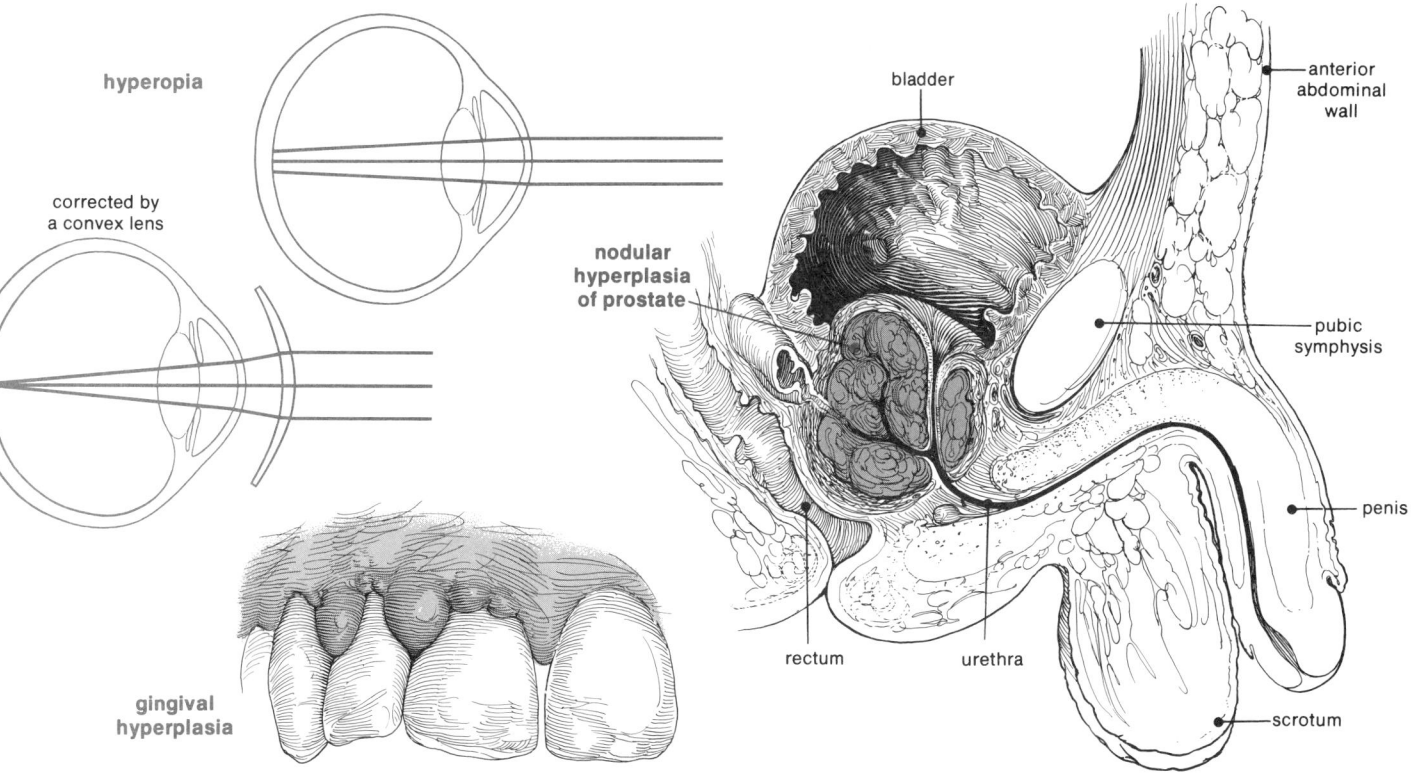

hyperopia

corrected by
a convex lens

gingival
hyperplasia

nodular
hyperplasia
of prostate

bladder

anterior
abdominal
wall

pubic
symphysis

penis

rectum   urethra

scrotum

(pre-beta) lipoproteins, and triglycerides while on ordinary diets, with eruptive xanthomas and recurrent acute pancreatitis; occurs chiefly during adolescence and middle life, probably as an autosomal recessive inheritance. Also called mixed hyperlipemia.

type V h., secondary A form seen in association with any of the diseases capable of producing secondary type IV hyperlipoproteinemia.

hyperlysinemia A hereditary metabolic disorder in which there is an abnormal increase of lysine in the circulating blood; associated with physical and mental retardation, anemia, hypotonia, convulsions, and impaired sexual development; autosomal recessive inheritance.

hyperlysinuria An abnormally high concentration of lysine in the urine.

hypermagnesemia Abnormally large amount of magnesium in the blood.

hypermastia Overdevelopment of the mammary glands.

hypermenorrhea Prolonged or profuse menses. Also called menorrhagia.

hypermetabolism An unusually high metabolic rate; heat production by the body above normal, as in thyrotoxicosis.

hypermetria A manifestation of ataxia characterized by voluntary muscular movement overreaching the intended goal.

hypermetropia (H) See hyperopia.

hypermorph A tall, usually slender person whose standing height is great in proportion to the sitting height, owing to very long legs.

hypermyotonia Marked development of muscular tonicity.

hypermyotrophy Marked development of muscular tissue. Also called muscular hypertrophy.

hypernatremia Abnormally high sodium concentration in the blood.

hypernephroma Renal cell carcinoma; see under carcinoma.

hyperoncotic Denoting an oncotic pressure higher than normal.

hyperonychia Hypertrophy of the nails.

hyperope One afflicted with hyperopia.

hyperopia A condition of the eye in which parallel light rays (rays of light from distant objects) entering the eyeball focus behind the retina, because the eyeball is short or the refractive power of the lens is weak. Also called hypermetropia; farsightedness; far sight.

latent h. (Hl) The portion of the total hyperopia that is not revealed because it is compensated for by the tonicity of the ciliary muscle.

manifest h. (Hm) The portion of the total hyper-

opia that may be measured by the relaxation of accommodation.

total h. (Ht) The sum of the latent and the manifest hyperopia.

hyperorchidism Increased size or functional activity of the testes.

hyperosmia An exaggerated sense of smell.

hyperosmotic Having a greater concentration of osmotically active solutes than another fluid.

hyperostosis 1. Hypertrophy or abnormal growth of bone tissue. 2. Exostosis.

h. frontalis interna Abnormal deposition of bone on the internal surface of the frontal bone.

hyperovarianism Abnormally increased functional activity of the ovaries, usually leading to sexual precocity in young girls.

hyperoxaluria An unusually large amount of oxalic acid or oxalates in the urine; caused by a genetic disorder affecting the metabolism of glyoxylic acid, which forms oxalate rather than glycine; it is one of the common causes of nephrolithiasis and nephrocalcinosis in children.

hyperoxia Excessive amount of oxygen in the tissues.

hyperparathyroidism Excessive secretion of parathyroid hormone.

primary h. Excessive secretion of parathyroid hormone resulting from an adenoma or chief cell or clear cell hyperplasia (80% of cases), or carcinoma (20%); the classic laboratory manifestations are high serum calcium and low serum phosphate.

secondary h. Hyperplasia of the parathyroid glands and increased secretion of parathyroid hormone secondary to abnormal calcium and phosphorus metabolism in chronic renal disease.

hyperpathia Exaggerated response to pain.

hyperpepsia 1. Excessive rapid digestion. 2. Impaired digestion with hyperchlorhydria.

hyperpepsinia Excessive secretion of pepsin in the stomach.

hyperperistalsis Increase in the rate of peristalsis; peristaltic unrest; excessive rapidity of the passage of food through the stomach and intestine.

hyperphagia Overeating.

hyperphoria Tendency of one eye to deviate upward.

hyperphosphatemia Abnormally large amount of phosphates in the blood.

hyperpigmentation Excessive coloration or pigmentation in a tissue or part.

hyperpituitarism Excessive production of growth hormone by the pituitary gland due to a tumor, causing gigantism in children and acromegaly in adults.

hyperplasia The increased size of an organ or part

due to the excessive but regulated increase in the number of its cells. Cf. neoplasm; hypertrophy.

benign prostatic h. See nodular hyperplasia of prostate.

congenital adrenal h. Adrenal hyperplasia with excessive secretion of androgens resulting from enzymatic defects in the biosynthesis of corticosteroids; there are four major types: (a) simple virilizing form; (b) sodium-losing form; (c) hypertensive form; and (d) 3 β-hydroxysteroid dehydrogenase defect, which may produce feminization of male genitalia.

cystic h. of breast See fibrocystic disease of breast.

fibromuscular h. Fibrosis and hyperplasia of the arterial muscular layer, usually involving the renal arteries.

gingival h. Cellular proliferation of the gingiva resulting in swelling.

nodular h. of prostate A common disorder of men over the age of 50, characterized by the formation of large nodules in the prostate which press against the urethra, thus obstructing the flow of urine. Also called benign prostatic hypertrophy or hyperplasia.

hyperplastic Relating to or characterized by hyperplasia.

hyperpnea Abnormally rapid and deep breathing.

hyperpolarization An increase in the positive charges normally present at the surface of a nerve cell membrane.

hyperpotassemia See hyperkalemia.

hyperprebetalipoproteinemia Type IV familial hyperlipoproteinemia; see under hyperlipoproteinemia.

hyperprolactinemia Increased amounts of prolactin in the blood; normal only during lactation; may be caused by certain medications or some pituitary tumors.

hyperprolinemia An inherited metabolic disorder marked by increased proline in the plasma and excretion of proline, hydroxyproline, and glycine.

hyperproteinemia The presence of excessive protein in the blood.

hyperpyretic Relating to high fever. Also called hyperpyrexial.

hyperpyrexia Extremely high fever, usually 105.0°F or more.

hyperpyrexial See hyperpyretic.

hyperreflexia Exaggerated deep tendon reflexes.

hyperresonance An extreme or exaggerated degree of resonance on percussion as heard in pulmonary emphysema.

hypersecretion Excessive secretion.

hypersensitive Overreactive to a stimulus.

hypersensitivity 1. The altered reactivity to a

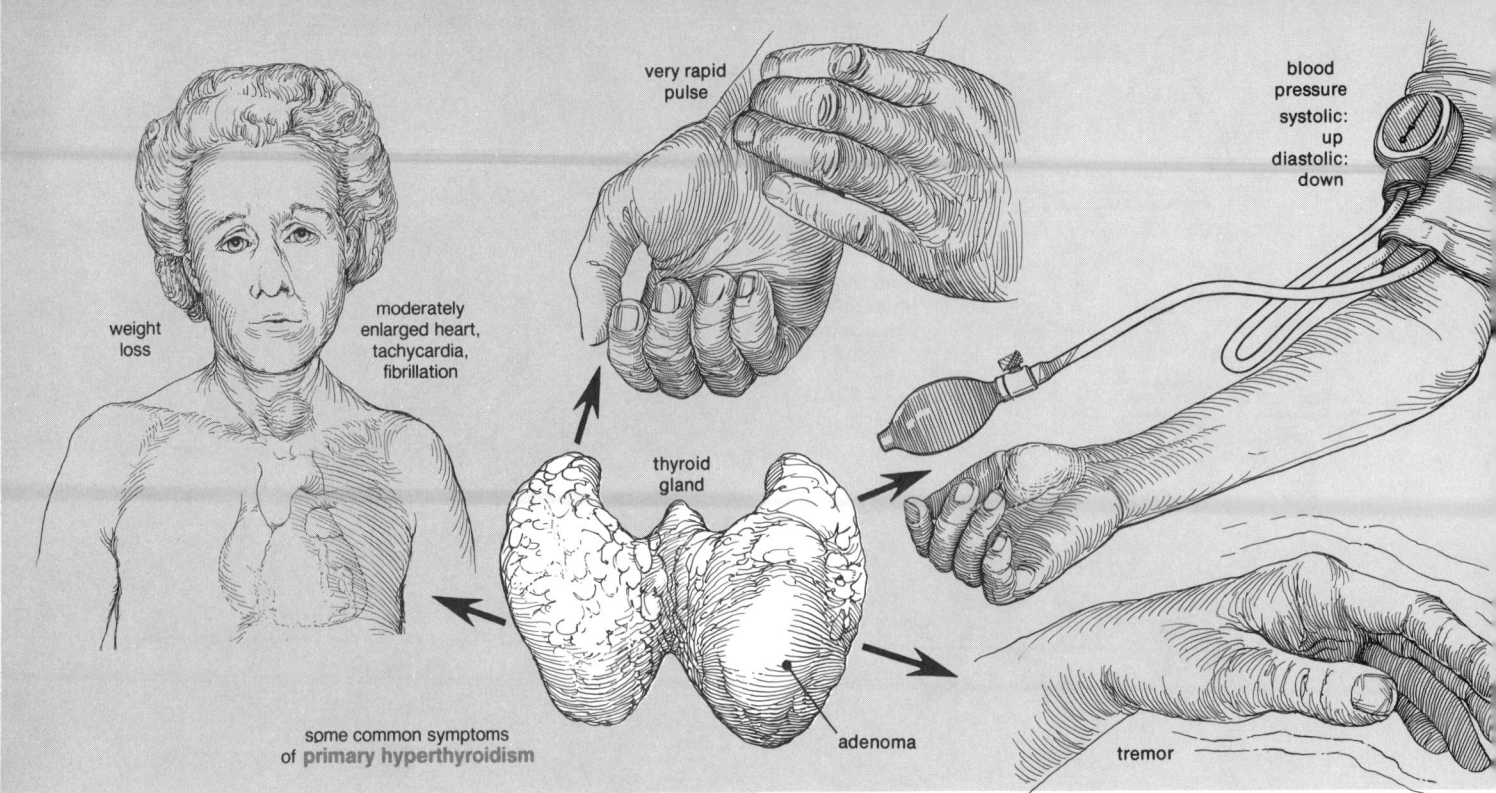

very rapid pulse

blood pressure
systolic: up
diastolic: down

weight loss

moderately enlarged heart, tachycardia, fibrillation

thyroid gland

adenoma

tremor

some common symptoms of **primary hyperthyroidism**

substance, which can result in pathologic reactions upon subsequent exposure to that particular substance. Also called allergy. **2.** Excessive response to a stimulus.

delayed-type h. T-cell mediated immune reactivity to an antigen applied topically or injected subcutaneously; cellular infiltration and swelling are maximal at about 48 hours.

hypersensitization The process of creating an abnormally sensitive state.

hypersialosis Excessive secretion of saliva. Also called hypertyalism.

hypersomatotropism Abnormally increased secretion of pituitary growth hormone.

hypersomia Gigantism.

hypersomnia Abnormal condition in which the individual sleeps for excessive periods of time.

hypersonic Relating to speeds equal to or exceeding five times the speed of sound (speeds less than hypersonic but greater than the speed of sound are called supersonic).

hypersplenism A disorder in which the formed elements of the blood are destroyed by the excessively increased activity of the spleen; it may result in anemia, neutropenia, thrombocytopenia, or a combination of these states.

hypersteatosis Excessive sebaceous secretion.

hypertelorism Abnormally increased distance between paired organs or parts.

ocular h. Congenital malformation marked by enlarged sphenoid bone, causing extreme distance between the eyes. Also called craniofacial dysostosis.

hypertensin See angiotensin.

hypertensinogen See angiotensinogen.

hypertension High arterial blood pressure; in adults, usually defined as pressures exceeding 140/90 mm Hg.

essential h. Hypertension without a known cause.

malignant h. Severe hypertension that causes degenerative changes in the walls of the blood vessels throughout the body; hemorrhages occur in the retina, the kidney, and other areas; cerebral function is altered.

portal h. Increased pressure in the portal venous system; it may result from: intrahepatic causes, such as cirrhosis of the liver; suprahepatic causes, such as heart failure; infrahepatic causes, such as portal vein thrombosis.

pulmonary h. Hypertension in the pulmonary circulation resulting from primary pulmonary changes such as fibrosis of the lung, or from heart diseases such as mitral stenosis.

renal h. Hypertension secondary to kidney disease.

renovascular h. Hypertension due to obstruction of the renal arteries.

hypertensive Marked by or afflicted with high blood pressure.

hyperthecosis Hyperplasia of the theca cells of the vesicular ovarian (graafian) follicles.

hyperthelia The presence of several nipples but only two breasts.

hyperthermia Extremely high body temperature.

hyperthrombinemia The presence of excessive thrombin in the blood.

hyperthymia State of increased emotivity or overactivity.

hyperthyroidism Condition caused by excessive production or ingestion of thyroid hormone; the most common symptoms include weight loss, increased appetite, rapid heart rate, tremor, and fatigue; when exophthalmos is present, the disease is known as exophthalmic goiter.

primary h. A form originating within the thyroid gland.

secondary h. A form caused by abnormal stimulation of the thyroid gland due to a disorder of the pituitary gland.

hypertonia Excessive tension of the muscles or arteries.

hypertonic 1. Having an abnormally increased tension. **2.** Having the greater osmotic pressure of two solutions; frequently, the comparison is to the osmotic concentration of plasma.

hypertonicity The state of being hypertonic.

hypertrichosis, hypertrichiasis A growth of hair in excess of normal for that particular area of the body, e.g., the face in women.

hypertriglyceridemia Excessive concentration of triglyceride in the blood.

familial h. Any one of two heritable forms of the disease: (a) exogenous or fat-induced, occurring after meals of normal or high lipid content; (b) endogenous or carbohydrate-induced, occurring after meals rich in carbohydrates.

hypertrophy The enlargement of an organ or part due to the increase in size of the cells composing it; the overgrowth meets a demand for increased functional activity. Cf. neoplasm; hyperplasia.

adaptive h. Thickening of the walls of a hollow organ, like the urinary bladder, when the outflow is obstructed.

asymmetrical septal h. (ASH) Idiopathic hypertrophic subaortic stenosis; see under stenosis.

compensatory h. of the heart Thickening of the walls of the heart, occurring when a chamber must pump against an increased resistance as in valvular disease or hypertension, thus increasing the power of the heart to maintain the circulation.

concentric h. Thickening of the walls of a hollow organ with little or no change in the size of its cavity; seen in left ventricular hypertrophy associated with essential hypertension or aortic stenosis.

eccentric h. Enlargement of the walls of a hollow organ as well as its cavity; seen in left ventricular hypertrophy of volume overload, as in aortic or mitral regurgitation.

physiologic h. Temporary hypertrophy of an organ to meet the demand of a natural increase in functional activity, as in the female breast during pregnancy and lactation.

ventricular h. Hypertrophy of the muscular wall of either the right (RVH) or the left (LVH) ventricle of the heart.

vicarious h. Hypertrophy of an organ due to dysfunction of another organ of allied activity.

hypertropia Upward deviation of one eye not controllable by fixational efforts; unlike hyperphoria, the condition is continuous.

hyperuricemia Excess of uric acid in the blood.

hyperuricosuria, hyperuricuria Excretion of excessive amounts of uric acid in the urine.

hyperventilation A condition marked by fast deep breathing which tends to remove increased amounts of carbon dioxide from the body and lower the partial pressure of the gas, causing buzzing in the ears, tingling of the lips and fingers, and sometimes fainting. Also called overventilation.

central neural h. A pattern of irregular hyperventilation, usually seen in individuals who have a midbrain lesion and who are comatose.

hyperventilation syndrome A syndrome that is almost always a manifestation of acute anxiety, characterized by difficult, deep, and rapid respiration accompanied by tightness of the chest and a feeling of suffocation; lightheadedness is commonly present and tingling of the hands may appear as a result of marked diminution of carbon dioxide in the blood (hypocapnia), produced by the excessive respiration; it may last half an hour or longer and may recur a few times a day; the attacks may be controlled somewhat by breath-holding or breathing in a paper bag.

hyperviscosity syndrome Visual impairment, neurologic problems, spontaneous bleeding, sluggish blood flow, and organ congestion consequent to increased blood viscosity.

hypervitaminosis Condition caused by ingestion of excessive amounts of a vitamin preparation.

hypervolemia Abnormal increase in the volume of blood, as seen during pregnancy and in some cases of hydatidiform mole.

hypesthesia See hypoesthesia.

hypha *pl.* **hyphae** One of the hairlike structures

hypo-chondrium

hypo-gastrium

hypodactylia

hypo-esophoria

forming the substance of a fungus.

hyphema, hyphemia Collection of blood in the anterior chamber of the eye.

hyphidrosis Diminished or deficient perspiration; abnormally scanty perspiration.

hypnagogic 1. Denoting the transitional state produced by sleep, such as mental images occurring just before sleep. **2.** Inducing sleep. Also called hypnotic.

hypnagogue An agent that induces sleep.

hypnoanalysis Psychoanalysis conducted while the patient is under hypnosis.

hypnogenesis The process of inducing sleep or a hypnotic state.

hypnology The study of sleep or hypnosis.

hypnophobia Abnormal fear of falling asleep.

hypnopompic Relating to the partially conscious state between the stages of sleep and complete awakening.

hypnosis An artificially induced state in which the individual becomes receptive to the hypnotist's suggestions; it may vary in degree from mild suggestibility to a deep sleeplike state with total surgical anesthesia.

hypnotherapy Treatment using hypnosis.

hypnotic 1. Of, involving, or causing hypnosis. **2.** An individual who is hypnotized. **3.** Any agent that induces sleep.

hypnotism 1. The practice of inducing hypnosis. **2.** Hypnosis.

hypnotist One who practices hypnotism.

hypnotize To put into a hypnotic state.

hypo A popular designation for hypodermic injection.

hypoacidity Deficiency of normal acidity. Also called subacidity.

hypoadrenalism Reduced or deficient adrenocortical function.

hypoadrenocorticism Abnormally low secretion of hormones of the adrenal cortex.

hypoadrenocortism Hypoadrenocorticism.

hypoalbuminemia Abnormally low concentration of albumin in the blood.

hypoalimentation Insufficient nourishment.

hypobaric Relating to or occurring at pressures less than atmospheric pressure.

hypobaropathy Condition caused by greatly reduced air pressure and decreased oxygen intake. Also called aviator's, altitude, or mountain sickness; Acosta's disease.

hypocalcemia A marked reduction of calcium in the blood.

hypocalcification Diminished calcification, especially of tooth enamel, producing opaque white spots.

hereditary enamel h. A hereditary defect of tooth enamel development affecting the primary and secondary teeth; it causes a breaking off of the enamel after tooth eruption, exposing the dentin, which gives the teeth a yellow appearance.

hypocapnia Marked diminution in the amount of carbon dioxide in the blood. Also called acapnia.

hypochloremia A marked reduction of chloride in the blood.

hypochlorhydria Abnormally low amount of hydrochloric acid in the gastric juice.

hypochlorite A salt of hypochlorous acid.

hypochlorous acid An unstable acid, HOCl; used as a bleach and disinfectant.

hypocholesterolemia An abnormally small amount of cholesterol in the blood.

hypochondria See hypochondriasis.

hypochondriac An individual afflicted with hypochondriasis.

hypochondriasis The persistent neurotic preoccupation with one's health and fear of presumed diseases that persist despite reassurances; an exaggerated concern over physical health in absence of organic disease. Also called hypochondria.

hypochondrium Any of two lateral regions of the upper zone of the abdomen.

hypochromatic Containing a small amount of pigment, or less than the normal amount for the individual tissue; abnormally deficient pigmentation.

hypochromemia Anemia characterized by an abnormally low color index of the blood.

hypochromia 1. Abnormal decrease in the hemoglobin content of the red blood cells. **2.** Hypochromatism.

hypochromic 1. Having less than the normal amount of pigment. **2.** Relating to a decrease in light absorption.

hypochylia Abnormally low amount of chyle.

hypocorticoidism Hypoadrenocorticism.

hypocupremia Abnormally low concentration of copper in the blood.

hypodactylia The presence of less than the normal number of digits on the hand or foot.

hypoderm See hypodermis.

hypodermic Located in or introduced into the layer beneath the skin; used sometimes to refer not only to the manner of injection, but to the injection per se. Also called subcutaneous.

hypodermis, hypoderm Subcutaneous fascia; see under fascia.

hypodermoclysis The infusion of fluid into the subcutaneous space.

hypodynamia Markedly diminished power.

hypoesophoria Combined downward (hypo-

phoria) and inward (esophoria) deviation of the eyeball.

hypoesthesia Abnormally decreased sensitiveness of the skin. Also called hypesthesia.

hypofibrinogenemia Deficiency of fibrinogen in the blood, usually below 100 mg percent; may occur in amniotic fluid embolism, fetal death, abruptio placentae, and occasionally intra-amniotic instillation of hypertonic saline.

hypofunction Diminished or inadequate functioning of an organ or part.

hypogalactia Insufficient milk production.

hypogammaglobulinemia Lack of gamma globulin in the blood; a deficiency state manifested by recurrent infections; primary forms result from diminished rates of synthesis; secondary forms result from increased catabolism.

hypogastrium The middle region of the lower zone of the abdomen.

hypogenitalism Underdevelopment of the genitalia.

hypogeusia Diminished sensitivity to taste.

hypoglossal Located beneath the tongue.

hypoglottis The undersurface of the tongue.

hypoglycemia A condition marked by lower than normal level of sugar (glucose) in the blood; characterized clinically by sweating, trembling, palpitation, hunger, weakness, and lightheadedness; the symptoms may vary in duration and often disappear rapidly after eating a snack or a sweet, or drinking a glass of milk; may result from excessive production of insulin by the pancreas or excessive administration of insulin to a diabetic.

hypognathous Having an underdeveloped lower jaw.

hypogonadism A condition resulting from deficient secretion of the gonads.

hereditary familial h. See Reifenstein's syndrome.

h. with anosmia A genetic disorder, usually in males, associated with loss of the sense of smell due to failure of develoment of olfactory lobes; X-linked inheritance. Also called Kallmann's syndrome.

testicular h. Condition caused by a decrease of the internal secretion of the testis and marked by the loss of secondary sexual characteristics.

hypohidrosis Abnormally reduced perspiration.

hypokalemia Abnormally low level of potassium in the blood; may result in nephropathy, muscle weakness, gastric atony, paralysis of the muscles of respiration, and arrhythmias. Also called hypopotassemia.

hypokinemia Abnormally reduced cardiac output; reduced circulation rate.

hypokinesia Diminished movement.

bladder

penis

hypospadias

hypophysis
(pituitary gland)

dorsomedial nucleus

para-
ventricular
nucleus

posterior
nucleus

preoptic
nucleus

ventro-
medial
nucleus

Mamillary
body

supra-
optic
nucleus

hypothalamus

optic
chiasma

hypophysis

dura
mater

tuber
cinereum

anterior
lobe

hypothalmo-
hypophysial
tract

posterior
lobe

hypomagnesemia Abnormally low concentration of magnesium in the blood.

hypomania A moderate form of manic activity, usually marked by slightly abnormal elation and overactivity.

hypomastia Abnormal smallness of the breasts.

hypomenorrhea Scanty menstrual flow, possibly with shortening of the duration of the menstrual period.

hypometabolism Reduced metabolism.

hypometria Loss of power of muscular coordination manifested by failure to reach an intended goal; decreased range of voluntary movements.

hypomorph 1. A person who has short legs. 2. In genetics, a mutant gene that acts in the same direction as the normal allele, but at a lower level of effectiveness.

hyponatremia Low concentration of sodium in the blood.

hyponychial Beneath a fingernail or toenail. Also called subungual.

hyponychium The thickened horny zone of the epidermis beneath the free border of the nail.

hypoovarianism Diminished secretion of ovarian hormones.

hypoparathyroidism Condition caused by lack of parathyroid secretion, resulting in reduced plasma calcium level and increased plasma phosphate level.

hypophalangism Congenital absence of a phalanx on a finger or toe.

hypophoria Latent condition in which one eye tends to deviate downward.

hypophosphatasia Lack of alkaline phosphatase in the blood; a rare inherited disorder characterized by rickets and osteomalacia.

hypophosphatemia Deficiency of phosphate in the blood.

hypophyseal, hypophysial Pertaining to the hypophysis (pituitary gland).

hypophysectomize To remove or destroy the hypophysis (pituitary gland).

hypophysectomy Surgical removal of the hypophysis (pituitary gland).

hypophysis A gland of internal secretion situated in the hypophysial fossa of the sphenoid bone, at-

tached to the base of the brain by a short stalk; it consists of two main parts, anterior lobe (adenohypophysis) and posterior lobe (neurohypophysis); its secretions are of vital importance to growth, maturation, and reproduction. Also called pituitary gland or body.

hypopituitarism A condition due to abnormally diminished production of anterior pituitary hormones caused by destruction of the pituitary gland; it leads to atrophy of the thyroid and adrenal glands and the gonads.

hypoplasia Defective or incomplete development of an organ or a part.

hypoplastic Relating to or characterized by hypoplasia.

hypopnea Abnormally shallow breathing.

hypopotassemia See hypokalemia.

hypoproteinemia Abnormally small amounts of protein in the blood.

hypoproteinosis Dietary deficiency of protein.

hypoprothrombinemia Deficiency of prothrombin (blood clotting factor II) in the blood.

hypopyon The presence of pus in the anterior chamber of the eye, secondary to inflammation of the cornea, iris, or ciliary body.

hyporeflexia A condition of weakened reflexes.

hyporeninemia Low levels of the enzyme renin in the blood.

hyporiboflavinosis Disease caused by insufficient intake of riboflavin. Also called ariboflavinosis.

hyposalivation Diminished flow of saliva.

hyposensitivity The condition of less than normal sensitivity; one in which the response to a stimulus is unusually delayed or lessened in degree.

hyposensitization See immunotherapy (3).

hyposensitize To render insensitive, or less sensitive; to reduce sensitivity, usually with reference to allergy (induced sensitivity). Also called desensitize.

hyposmia Reduced sense of smell. Also called hypospheresia.

hypospadia See hypospadias.

hypospadias A congenital defect in the male in which the urethra opens on the undersurface of the penis; it occurs in approximately 1 in 500 births; there is also a similar defect in the female in which

the urethra opens into the vagina. Also called hypospadia.

hypostasis 1. A sediment or deposit. 2. Blood congestion in a part.

hyposthenia A weakened state; decrease or lack of strength.

hyposthenuria Impairment of ability to concentrate the urine.

hypostosis Inadequate development of bone.

hypotaxia Condition marked by imperfect coordination.

hypotelorism Abnormally small distance between two organs or parts such as the eyes.

hypotension Abnormally low blood pressure.

orthostatic h. Hypotension occurring upon arising suddenly from a recumbent position or when standing still. Also called postural hypotension.

postural h. Orthostatic hypotension.

hypotensive Marked by or causing low blood pressure.

hypothalamus A deep-lying part of the brain situated just below the thalamus; it forms the floor and part of the lateral walls of the third ventricle; it includes the mammillary bodies, tuber cinereum, infundibulum, and the optic chiasm; the hypothalamic nuclei are concerned with visceral control, e.g., the regulation of water balance and body temperature.

hypothenar The fleshy portion of the palm of the hand, at its medial side.

hypothermal Relating to a bodily temperature below normal.

hypothermia Abnormally low body temperature, usually below 97°F (36°C).

hypothesis A tentative theory subject to verification.

Lyon h. The concept that in each somatic cell of normal females only one of the two X-chromosomes is active during interphase; as inactivation of the other X-chromosome takes place randomly, females heterozygous for an X-linked mutant gene may show patches of tissue with the phenotype of the mutant gene while the majority of tissue remains normal.

Michaelis-Menten h. The assumption that an in-

hypoxanthine

abdominal hysterectomy (total)

uterus

after Brödel

abdominal skin incision

cutting wall of vagina

frontal / central / temporal / occipital — L R

hypsarrhythmia in an infant with myoclonic spasms

subtotal hysterectomy

cavity of uterus

ovary

uterine tube

total hysterectomy

vagina

labia minora

---

termediate complex is formed between an enzyme and its substrate; it is further assumed that the complex decomposes to yield free enzyme and the reaction products, and that the latter rate determines the over-all rate of substrate-product conversion, i.e., enzyme (E) + substrate (S) ⇌ enzyme + substrate complex (ES) → enzyme + product (P).

sequence h. The concept that the amino acid sequence of a protein is determined by a particular sequence of nucleotides in a definite portion of the DNA of the organism producing the protein.

sliding filament h. The assumption that a contracting muscle shortens because two sets of filaments slide past each other.

Starling's h. The rate of fluid exchange between extracapillary tissue and capillary depends on the hydrostatic and osmotic pressures on both sides of the capillary wall, considering the wall as a semi-permeable membrane.

zwitter h. The supposition that a molecule that behaves as an acid and as a base (ampholytic) yields, in an electrically neutral condition, equal numbers of basic and acid ions, thus becoming an ion (zwitter ion) with an equal number of positive and negative charges.

hypothrombinemia Abnormally small amount of thrombin in the blood, resulting in a tendency to bleed.

hypothyroid 1. Manifested by reduced thyroid function. 2. A person afflicted with hypothyroidism.

hypothyroidism Condition caused by deficient production of thyroid hormone, characterized by a lessened rate of metabolism; clinical features may include cold intolerance, dry skin, hair loss, puffy face, constipation, slow speech, slow heart rate, and retarded mentality; when present at birth it causes cretinism; the severe form is known as myxedema.

hypotonia Lack of muscle tone.

ocular h. Abnormally low tension in the eyeball.

hypotonic 1. Having an abnormally reduced tension. 2. Having the lesser osmotic pressure of two solutions, usually compared to the osmotic concentration of plasma.

hypotoxicity Reduced toxicity.

hypotrichosis Scanty hair on the head and body.

hypotropia Downward deviation of one eye not controllable by fixational efforts; unlike hypophoria, the condition is constant.

hypoventilation Reduced quantity of air entering the lungs.

hypovitaminosis Condition marked by deficiency of one or more essential vitamins.

hypovolemia Markedly diminished blood volume.

hypovolia Reduced water content of a particular compartment.

hypoxanthine A purine present in muscles and other tissues; normally metabolized to uric acid by oxidation, after first being oxidized to xanthine. Also called 6-hydroxypurine.

hypoxemia Abnormally low content of oxygen in the arterial blood. Also called anoxemia.

hypoxia Abnormal reduction of oxygen in body tissues. Also called oxygen deficiency.

hypsarrhythmia Abnormal chaotic encephalogram sometimes observed in infants with spasms.

hysteralgia Pain or discomfort in the uterus.

hysteratresia Pathologic closure of the uterine cavity.

hysterectomy Removal of the uterus.

abdominal h. Removal of the uterus through an incision in the abdominal wall.

cesarean h., caesarean h. Delivery of a baby through an abdominal and uterine incision, followed by removal of the uterus through the abdominal incision.

subtotal h. Removal of the body of the uterus leaving the cervix in place.

total h. Removal of the entire uterus.

vaginal h. Removal of the uterus through the vagina.

hysteresis 1. The failure of coincidence of two associated phenomena, such as the difference between the solidification temperature and the melting temperature of a reversible hydrocolloid. 2. The lag of a magnetic effect behind its cause.

hysteria An illness resulting from emotional conflict, characterized by lack of control over acts and emotions and other mental and physical symptoms not of organic origin; it is derived from the Greek

word for womb, *hystera*, because the illness was originally thought to be caused by disturbances of the uterus.

hysterical Characterized by or pertaining to hysteria.

hysterics Colloquial term for an uncontrollable emotional outburst.

hysterocolposcope Instrument used to inspect the uterine cavity and vagina.

hysterogram An x ray of the uterus utilizing contrast material.

hysterography Roentgenography of the uterine cavity after filling it with radiopaque material.

hysterolith A calculus of the uterus.

hysterometer A graduated sound for measuring the depth of the uterine cavity.

hysteromyoma A benign tumor of the uterine wall.

hysteromyomectomy Surgical removal of a myoma from the uterus.

hysteromyotomy Incision into the muscular wall of the uterus.

hystero-oophorectomy Surgical removal of the uterus and ovaries. Also called hystero-oothectomy.

hysteropexy See ventrofixation of uterus.

hysterorrhaphy See ventrofixation of uterus.

hysterosalpingectomy The surgical removal of the uterus and at least one uterine tube.

hysterosalpingogram A roentgenogram detailing the internal structures of the uterus and uterine (fallopian) tubes.

hysterosalpingography Roentgenography of the uterus and uterine tubes following the injection of a radiopaque material.

hysterosalpingo-oophorectomy Surgical removal of the uterus, uterine tubes, and ovaries. Also called hysterosalpingo-oothecectomy.

hysteroscope A uterine endoscope used for direct visual examination of the cavity of the uterus and cervix.

hysterostomatomy An obstetrical surgical procedure; see Dührssen's incisions, under incision.

hysterotomy Surgical incision of the uterus.

hysterotrachelectomy Surgical removal of the uterine cervix.

idoxuridine

IgG

IgE

light chain

heavy chain

schematic representation of the comparative structures of immunoglobulins

IgA

disulfide bond

IgM

Ii

iatrogenic Caused by a physician; said of an illness unwittingly induced in a patient by the physician's attitude, treatment, or comments.

iatrogeny Abnormal condition caused by a physician.

iatrotechnique Medical and surgical techniques.

ibuprofen A propionic acid derivative having anti-inflammatory properties; an inhibitor of prostaglandin synthetase.

ice Water in a solid state.

Iceland disease Epidemic neuromyasthenia; see under neuromyasthenia.

ichthyoid Fish-shaped.

ichthyosiform Relating to the shape, characteristics, or likeness of ichthyosis.

ichthyosis A disease marked by dry, rough, scaly skin, caused by a congenital defect of the horny layer of the skin; may affect the eyelids, causing loss of the eyelashes, and also affect the eye, causing inflammation of the conjunctiva and keratosis of the cornea. Also called fishskin disease; xeroderma.

ichthyotoxin A toxic substance present in eel serum.

icosanoid See eicosanoid.

ictal Relating to a convulsion.

icteric Relating to or having jaundice.

icterogenic Causing jaundice.

icterus Yellow pigmentation of the skin and/or sclera due to high concentration of bilirubin in the blood. Also called jaundice.

   physiologic i. Physiologic jaundice; see under jaundice.

   scleral i. A yellow pigmentation of the sclera caused by an elevated level of bilirubin in the blood, usually over 2.5 mg per dl.

ictus *pl.* **ictuses** A stroke, beat, or sudden convulsion.

   i. epilepticus An epileptic convulsion.

id **1.** In freudian theory, the part of the personality structure associated with the unconscious instinctive impulses and primitive needs of the individual. **2.** A biologic germ structure, supposed to carry the hereditary qualities. **3.** See reaction, id.

idea A conception existing in the mind as the product of mental activity.

   compulsive i. An inappropriate idea that recurs and persists despite reason.

   fixed i. A loosely used term to describe a compulsive drive, an obsession, or a delusion. Also called idée fixe.

ideal A conception regarded as a standard of perfection.

   ego i. The part of the personality comprising the goals of the self; it usually refers to the emulation of

significant individuals with whom the person has identified.

ideation The formation of ideas or conceptions; indicative of an individual's ability to think.

idée fixe French for fixed idea.

identification A defense mechanism in which a person unconsciously tries to pattern himself after another; distinguished from imitation, which is a conscious process.

identity The role of a person in society and his perception of it.

   ego i. The ego's sense of its own identity.

   gender i. The anatomic-sexual identity of an individual.

   sense of i. A person's sense of his own selfhood.

ideoglandular Eliciting glandular secretions through mental images or thoughts.

ideology The intellectual-moral ideas of reflecting the needs and aspirations of an individual or group.

ideomotion Muscular movements influenced by a dominant idea.

idioagglutinin An agglutinin occurring normally in the blood of a person or an animal.

idiocy Obsolete term for mental retardation; see under retardation.

   amaurotic familial i. Cerebral sphingolipidosis; see under sphingolipidosis.

idiogenesis The origin of an idiopathic disease (one without apparent cause).

idiogram A diagrammatic representation of the chromosomal constitution (karyotype) of an organism.

idioheteroagglutinin An agglutinin occurring normally in the blood of one animal (idioagglutinin), but capable of combining with the antigen of another species.

idioisoagglutinin An agglutinin occurring in the blood of an animal (idioagglutinin) of a certain species, capable of agglutinating the cells from animals of the same species.

idiolysin A lysin occurring naturally in the blood of a person or an animal.

idioneurosis A neurosis originating without an apparent cause.

idionodal Arising in the atrioventricular (A-V) node itself.

idiopathic Denoting a disease of unknown cause.

idiopathic respiratory distress syndrome of the newborn See respiratory distress syndrome of the newborn.

idiophrenic Relating to or originating in the mind or brain exclusively, i.e., neither reflex nor secondary.

idiosyncrasy **1.** A characteristic (physical or be-

havioral) peculiar to an individual. **2.** A susceptibility, peculiar to an individual, to the action of certain drugs or foods.

idiosyncratic Of or relating to an idiosyncracy.

idiot Obsolete term for retardate.

idiot-savant A mentally retarded individual capable of performing certain remarkable mental tasks, such as solving difficult mathematical problems almost instantly, remembering a variety of facts, etc.

idioventricular Relating to the cardiac ventricles alone, as a cardiac rhythm originating from a ventricular focus.

idoxuridine An antiviral agent used locally for the treatment of herpes simplex infection of the eye.

IgA Abbreviation for immunoglobulin A (gamma A globulin); see under immunoglobulin.

IgE Abbreviation for immunoglobulin E (gamma E globulin); see under immunoglobulin.

IgG Abbreviation for immunoglobulin G (gamma G globulin); see under immunoglobulin.

IgM Abbreviation for immunoglobulin M (gamma M globulin); see under immunoglobulin.

ileal Relating to the ileum.

ileitis Inflammation of the ileum.

   backwash i. Inflammation and ulceration of the ileum occurring as an extension of ulcerative colitis.

   regional i. See enteritis, regional.

   terminal i. See enteritis, regional.

ileocecal Relating to the ileum and cecum.

ileocecostomy Surgical connection of the ileum and the cecum.

ileocecum The ileum and cecum taken as a whole.

ileocolic Relating to the ileum and the colon.

ileocolitis Inflammation of the ileum and colon.

ileocolostomy Surgical connection of the ileum and colon.

ileoileostomy Surgical connection of two non-continuous portions of the ileum.

ileojejunitis Inflammation of the ileum and jejunum.

ileostomy Surgical establishment of an opening or fistula into the ileum.

ileotomy Surgical incision of the ileum.

ileotransversostomy Surgical joining of the ileum and transverse colon.

ileum The portion of the small intestine between the jejunum and the cecum; the preferred site for vitamin B_{12} absorption.

ileus Obstruction of the intestines accompanied by severe colicky pain, vomiting, and sometimes fever.

   gallstone i. A mechanical intestinal obstruction caused by impaction of one or more gallstones within the bowel lumen.

Muller-Lyer illusion

(the line on the right appears shorter than the equal line on the left)

Wundt's illusion

optical illusions

(parallel lines do not appear so)

Poggendorf's illusion

(horizontal line appears shorter than the equal vertical line)

retinal image

microscope

virtual image

light

ilium

iliac crest

anterior superior spine

anterior inferior spine

pubis

posterior superior spine

posterior inferior spine

acetabulum

ischium

immobilization of ankle joint with a figure-8 bandage

---

meconium i. Ileus in the newborn due to obstruction caused by excessively thick meconium; frequently the first evidence of cystic fibrosis.

paralytic i. Ileus resulting from paralysis of the intestinal walls.

iliac Relating to the ilium.

iliofemoral Relating to the ilium and the femur.

ilioinguinal Relating to the iliac region and the groin.

iliolumbar Relating to the iliac and the lumbar regions.

iliopectineal Relating to the bones ilium and pubis.

ilium The superior, broad portion of the hipbone which comprises one of the lateral halves of the pelvis.

illness Disease.

functional i. See disorder, functional.

mental i. See disorder, mental.

terminal i. A sickness that ends in death.

illumination 1. The process by which light is made to fall on a surface. 2. In microscopy, the light thrown upon the object to be examined.

critical i. In microscopy, the focusing of the light source directly on the specimen, creating a narrow, intense light beam.

dark-field i. Illumination of a microscopic specimen by a hollow cone of light; the vertically directed light rays are blocked by a black circular shield and the peripheral rays are directed toward the specimen; the object appears bright on a dark background.

direct i. Illumination in which the object is illuminated by a beam of light falling almost perpendicularly upon it. Also called vertical illumination.

vertical i. See direct illumination.

illuminator In a microscope, the source of light which illuminates the specimen to be viewed.

illusion A false perception of reality.

optical i. An erroneous interpretation of a visual sensation.

image 1. A reproduction of the appearance of an object formed by the rays of light emanating or reflected from it. 2. A representation or picture of someone or something not present, formed in the mind from memory.

after-i. Afterimage.

double i. Two images of a single object, as formed perceptually in diplopia.

hypnopompic i. Imagery occurring after the sleeping state and before complete awakening, as when a dream figure persists in waking life.

mental i. Image (2).

mirror i. An image with right and left parts reversed, as the relationship of an object to its image

in a mirror.

real i. An image, formed by converging light rays, which can be seen by inserting a screen, such as a ground glass, into the optical system, or which can be recorded on a photographic plate; the opposite of virtual image.

retinal i. The image formed on the surface of the retina by the refracting system of the eye.

virtual i. An image in which light, originating from a point on the object, and having traversed an optical system, appears to be diverging; it cannot be demonstrated on a screen or photographic plate as in the case of a real image.

image intensifier In radiology, an electronic device for intensification of the fluorscopic image.

imaging Creation of images of body parts.

magnetic resonance i. (MRI) The making of cross-sectional images of body parts by means of nuclear magnetic resonance. The patient is placed in a magnetic field within a cylindrical magnet, which causes the nuclei of the body's hydrogen atoms to line up parallel to each other, like rows of tiny magnets. Radiofrequency pulses are then applied to knock the nuclei out of alignment. As they fall back into alignment, the nuclei produce detectable signals, which are translated into images by computer.

imbibition The absorption of a fluid, as the taking up of water by a gel.

imbrication 1. An overlapping of the free edges of tissue in the closure of a wound or the repair of a defect. 2. A regular overlapping of a surface, as the slight, horizontal, scalelike ridges on the cervical third of the labial surface of some anterior teeth.

imidazole A functional component of histidine.

imide Any compound containing the radical group =NH attached to one bivalent acid radical or two univalent acid radicals.

imino acids Compounds containing both an acid group and an imino group.

imipramine hydrochloride A white crystalline tricyclic substance, soluble in water; used to treat depression; Tofranil®.

immersion The submerging of an object in a liquid.

oil i. In microscopy, the use of a layer of oil between the objective and the specimen.

water i. In microscopy, the use of a layer of water between the objective and the specimen.

immiscible Incapable of being mixed; e.g., oil and water.

immobilization The act of impeding movement.

immobilize To render incapable of being moved; to fix.

immune The state of being secure against harmful effects from pathogenic agents or influences; having immunity.

immune clearance See clearance, immune.

immune complex disease A hypersensitivity reaction marked by deposition of antigen-antibody-complement complexes within tissues, especially vascular endothelium.

immune deficiency syndrome A group of signs and symptoms indicating impairment of one or more of the major functions of the immune system; i.e., protection against infection (defense), preservation of uniformity of a given cell type (homeostasis), or the removal of malignant cells (surveillance).

immunity 1. The physiologic state that enables the body to recognize materials as foreign to itself and to neutralize, eliminate, or metabolize them with or without injury to its own tissues. 2. An inherited, acquired (naturally or artificially), or induced conditioning to a specific pathogen.

acquired i. Immunity acquired after birth.

active i. Immunity acquired as the result of having had a given infectious disease, or by inoculation with a modified form of the causative agent.

adoptive i. Immunity produced by the administration of immune lymphoid cells.

cell-mediated i. (CMI) Specific immune response conducted by antigen-sensitized T lymphocytes. Also called cellular immunity.

congenital i. Immunity present at birth.

humoral i. Immunity in which the involvement of immunoglobulins is predominant.

innate i. Resistance to certain infections that has not been acquired through vaccination or previous infection; included is the species-determined immunity, e.g., resistance of humans to the virus of canine distemper. Also called natural immunity.

local i. Immunity manifested by some organs, tissues, or regions of the body.

natural i. See innate immunity.

passive i. Immunity due to receipt of maternal antibody or injection of antibody.

specific i. Acquired active immunity against a particular disease obtained through vaccination or natural infection.

immunization The act or process by which a person becomes resistant or immune to a harmful agent.

active i. The promotion of antibodies when the injected antigen comes in contact with the plasma cells, reticuloendothelial cells, and large lymphocytes.

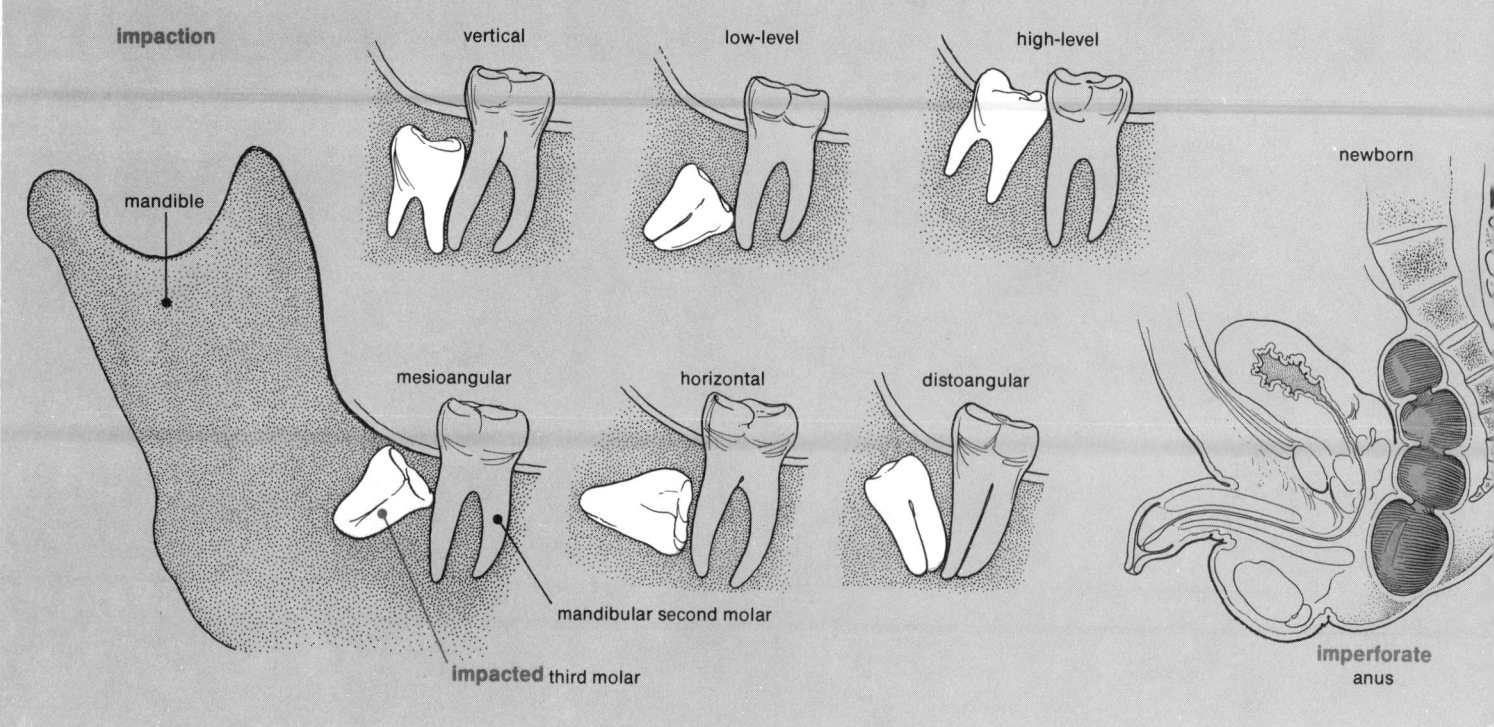

impaction

vertical

low-level

high-level

newborn

mandible

mesioangular

horizontal

distoangular

mandibular second molar

impacted third molar

imperforate
anus

passive i. Transient immunization obtained by injection of serum or gamma globulin from an animal or human already rendered immune.

immunize The process of making an individual resistant or immune to a harmful agent.

immunoagglutination Agglutination brought about by antibody.

immunoassay Technique (e.g., ELISA) for detection of specific protein in body tissue or blood by means of antigen-antibody reactions.

immunochemistry The chemistry of immunologic processes.

immunocompetence Ability to produce antibodies or cell-mediated immunity when exposed to a foreign substance (antigen).

immunocompromised Reduced immune response due to immunosuppressive drugs, radiation, disease, or malnutrition.

immunoconglutinins Conglutinins synthesized in response to antigenic stimulation; these antibodies react with certain antigens masked in molecules of native complement and exposed after the components of complement have been fixed on the antigen-antibody complex.

immunocyte A lymphoid cell capable of reacting with antigen to produce a specific cell product called antibody.

immunocytochemistry Any technique (e.g., the use of fluorescent antibodies) for analyzing cells and tissues to identify particulate antigens.

immunodeficiency Any impairment of immune response.

immunoelectrophoresis (IE) A form of electrophoresis which in addition employs immune precipitation (antigen-antibody reaction). Also called immunophoresis.

immunofluorescence The use of fluorescein-labeled antibodies to identify antigenic material specific for the labeled antibody.

immunogen An antigen which stimulates specific immunity.

immunogenetics The study of all the factors controlling immunologic reactions and the transmission of antigenic specificities from generation to generation.

immunogenic 1. Producing immunity. 2. Relating to an immunogen.

immunoglobulin (Ig) A protein molecule functioning as a specific antibody; it brings about the humoral phase of immunity. Also called immunoprotein.

i. A (IgA) The second most abundant class of immunoglobulins; present in secretions and produced especially by lymphoid tissues in the lining of

the respiratory, gastrointestinal, and urogenital tracts.

i. D (IgD) A class of immunoglobulins present on the surface of lymphocytes, especially of newborns.

i. E (IgE) A reaginic antibody that has ability to attach to the skin and initiate immediate hypersensitivity reactions.

i. G (IgG) The most abundant class of immunoglobulins; present in human serum; they provide immunity to bacteria, viruses, parasites, and fungi that have a blood-borne dissemination.

i. M (IgM) A class of immunoglobulins comprised of the largest immunoglobulins; they are transported across the placenta, play an important role in protecting newborns against infection and agglutinate particular antigens (e.g., bacteria, red blood cells).

monoclonal i.'s Those immunoglobulins derived from a single clone of plasma cells proliferating abnormally and which on electrophoresis of plasma appear as a narrow spike.

immunohematology The branch of hematology concerned with antigen-antibody reactions and their effect on the blood.

immunologist A specialist in immunology.

immunology The study of specific processes by which the host maintains constancy of his internal environment when confronted by substances which are recognized as foreign, whether generated from within the host or introduced from the outside.

immunopathology The study of disorders caused by antigen-antibody reactions.

immunoprophylaxis Prevention of disease through the use of vaccines.

immunoreaction See immune reaction.

immunoscintigraphy The making of a 2-dimensional image of a radiolabeled monoclonal antibody (Mab) that has bound to a preselected antigen at a target tissue. Used to detect specific tumors.

immunoselection Selective death or survival of fetuses of different genotypes depending on immunologic incompatibility with the mother.

immunosuppression The modification of the immune response, in a negative way, so it will have a diminished reaction to a foreign substance.

immunosuppressive 1. Modifying the immune response, in a negative way, so it will have a diminished reaction to a foreign substance. 2. A drug with such a capability.

immunotherapy 1. Passive immunization through the use of serum or gamma globulin which confers temporary protection to one host by the introduction of antibodies actively produced in another. 2. The replacement of immunocompetent tissues, e.g., bone marrow, fetal thymus, or other products, in restoring

immunocompetence to immune deficient individuals. 3. The treatment of allergic respiratory disease by injections of extracts of antigens responsible for the illness. Formerly known as desensitization; hyposensitization.

immunotolerance Immunologic tolerance; see under tolerance.

impact The sudden striking of one body against another.

impact To press firmly together.

impaction Tightly wedged together or firmly lodged so as to be immovable.

ceruminal i. Accumulation of earwax in the external auditory canal.

dental i. Condition in which a tooth is so placed in the alveolus as to be incapable of complete eruption.

impairment Damage resulting from injury or disease.

conduction hearing i. Reduction of hearing ability caused by interference with the conduction of sound to the end organ.

hearing i. Reduction of hearing ability due to either malfunctioning of nerve elements or interference with conduction of sound to the end organ.

mental i. Intellectual defect as manifested by psychologic tests and diminished effectiveness (social and vocational).

impalpable Imperceptible to the touch; unable to be grasped or felt.

impatent Closed.

impedance (Z) A measure of the total opposition to the flow of electric current in an alternating-current circuit.

imperforate Abnormally closed.

impermeable Not allowing the entrance of fluids or particular types of ionic or nonionic substances.

impetigo Contagious skin disease marked by the formation of pustules and caused by staphylococci or streptococci; it occurs mainly in children; the lesions appear as small reddish spots which readily become vesicles and burst, forming a characteristic crust; touching the blisters usually spreads the infection.

impetus In psychoanalysis, the motor constituent of an instinct.

implant 1. To graft. 2. The material grafted.

biocompatible i. An implant of material that permits tissue growth.

cochlear i. A device inserted under the skin adjacent to the ear of persons with total sensory deafness; electrodes of the device leading to the cochlear nerve create sensation of sound.

dental i. Any non-living material placed in a

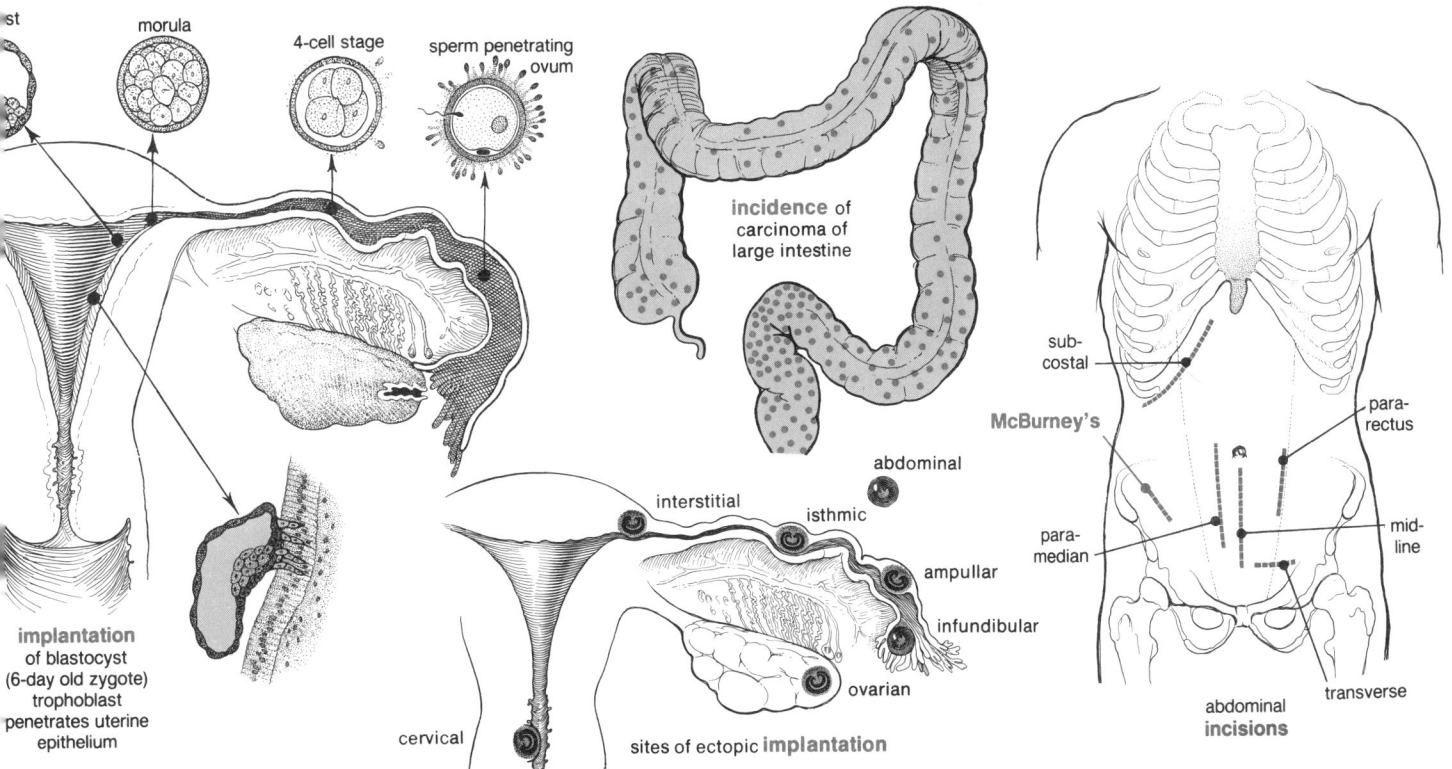

morula
4-cell stage
sperm penetrating ovum

incidence of carcinoma of large intestine

implantation of blastocyst (6-day old zygote) trophoblast penetrates uterine epithelium

cervical

interstitial
isthmic
abdominal
ampullar
infundibular
ovarian
sites of ectopic implantation

sub-costal
McBurney's
para-median
para-rectus
mid-line
transverse
abdominal incisions

dental socket to substitute for a damaged or missing tooth.

intraocular i. Plastic lens inserted in the eye to replace a diseased natural lens removed in a cataract operation.

subdermal contraceptive i. A reversible female contraceptive implanted under the skin; effective for an extended period of time (usually five years); Norplant™.

implantation 1. Tissue grafting. **2.** The embedding of the fertilized ovum.

implant denture substructure A metal framework inserted deeply and in contact with the bone to serve as support for an implant denture superstructure.

implant denture superstructure A denture placed on, and stabilized by, the implant denture substructure.

impotence Lack of power, specifically, lack of copulative power in the male due to failure to achieve adequate erection.

impregnate 1. To render pregnant. **2.** To saturate.

impression An imprint made on a surface by pressure.

complete denture i. An impression of the arch for the purpose of making a complete denture.

dental i. A negative likeness of the teeth or other structures of the oral cavity, made of a setting plastic material which is later filled with plaster of Paris, thus obtaining an exact copy of the structures.

final i. In dentistry, the impression used for making the master cast. Also called secondary impression.

secondary i. See final impression.

imprinting A particular way of learning occurring during early life and marked by rapid acquisition and tendency to forget easily.

impulse 1. A sudden urge to act. **2.** The transference of energy from one neuron to another; a brief action potential in nerve fibers.

cardiac i. The movement of the chest wall produced by cardiac contraction; the point of maximal impulse (PMI) is normally in the fifth intercostal space, on the midclavicular line or somewhat medial.

inactivate To render anything inactive or inert; may be done by using heat or other methods.

inadequacy 1. A state of being deficient. **2.** A failing.

sexual i. Insufficient sexual response (constant or transitory).

inanimate Without life.

inanition Debility resulting from lack of food or defect in assimilation.

inapparent Not apparent; said of certain infections.

inarticulate 1. Not articulate; speechless. **2.** Not joined; not having functional joints.

inattention, selective In psychiatry, failure to pay attention to a part of the perceived situation.

inborn An ambiguous term generally meaning acquired genetically; distinguished from congenital, meaning present at birth.

inbreeding The mating of closely related individuals, occurring naturally or as a deliberate process for the purpose of preserving desirable characters.

incaparina Generic name for a mixture of cereal grains and oilseed meals of a given general range of protein quality, fortified with vitamins and minerals.

incarcerated Confined; held fast, as an irreducible hernia.

incest Sexual intercourse between male and female who are blood-related.

incestuous Relating to or involving incest.

incidence The frequency at which an event occurs, such as the number of cases of a disease.

incident 1. A distinct occurrence or event. **2.** Falling upon, as incident rays.

incipient Beginning to appear; in an initial stage.

incisal Cutting; pertaining to the cutting edges of the anterior teeth.

incise To cut with a knife.

incision A surgical cut into soft tissue.

Dührssen's i.'s Two or three incisions made on the partially dilated uterine cervix to facilitate delivery of the child.

Halsted's i. See operation, Halsted's (1).

McBurney's i. An oblique abdominal incision parallel to the fibers of the external oblique muscle, approximately one inch from the anterior superior iliac spine; used in appendectomy.

incisor Any of the eight front cutting teeth, four in each jaw.

central i. The tooth closest to and on either side of the midsagittal plane of the head, on either jaw.

lateral i. The second tooth, mandibular or maxillary, on either side of the midsagittal plane of the head.

incisura, *pl.* **incisurae** A notch or indention on any structure. Also called incisure.

incisure See incisura.

inclination 1. A trend or disposition toward a particular condition. **2.** The state of being inclined; a leaning or sloping. **3.** In dentistry, the angle of the long axis of a tooth from the perpendicular.

inclusion The act of enclosing or the state of being enclosed.

cell i. Transient substance in a cell that does not participate in the cell's function; e.g., pigmented granules, crystals, lipids.

dental i. A tooth enclosed in bone and unable to erupt.

fetal i. Unequal conjoined twins in which the less developed one is enclosed within the body of the

other.

incoherent Disoriented; confused.

incompatible Incapable of being mixed or used simultaneously without undergoing chemical changes or producing undesirable effects, as two types of blood or certain drugs.

incompetence, incompetency The state of lacking functional ability.

aortic i. Failure of the aortic valve to close tightly, allowing regurgitation of blood into the left ventricle during diastole.

mental i. Legal term denoting defects of intellectual functioning such that comprehension of, or ability to discharge, required duties is inadequate.

mitral i. Defective closure of a mitral valve, allowing regurgitation of blood into the left atrium during systole.

muscular i. Defective action of the papillary muscles of the heart, resulting in imperfect closure of a normal valve.

pulmonary i., pulmonic i. Imperfect closure of a pulmonic valve, allowing regurgitation of blood into the right ventricle during diastole.

pyloric i. A relaxed state of the pylorus, allowing food to pass from the stomach into the intestine before gastric digestion is completed.

tricuspid i. Imperfect closure of a tricuspid valve, allowing regurgitation of blood into the right atrium during systole.

valvular i. Failure of one or more heart valves to close completely.

inconstant 1. Variable; irregular. **2.** In anatomy, denoting a structure that may or may not be present, may have a tendency to change, or is given to change of location.

incontinence 1. Inability to control the passage of urine or feces. **2.** Lack of self-control.

overflow i. Leakage of urine when bladder is over-distended and its sphincters are overcome.

stress i. Involuntary urination occurring during straining, coughing, or sneezing.

urge i. Inability to postpone voiding because the urge to urinate is abrupt and uncontrollable.

incoordination Inability to produce harmonious voluntary muscular movements.

incorporation The act of making something part of oneself, either by eating and digesting food or by taking in and adopting knowledge or the attitudes of another person (especially in psychoanalysis).

incrustation 1. The formation of a scab. **2.** A scab.

incubation 1. The maintenance of optimal conditions of the environment, such as the proper temperature and gas content, for bacterial growth or the development of a premature newborn. **2.** The phase of an infectious disease from the time of introduc-

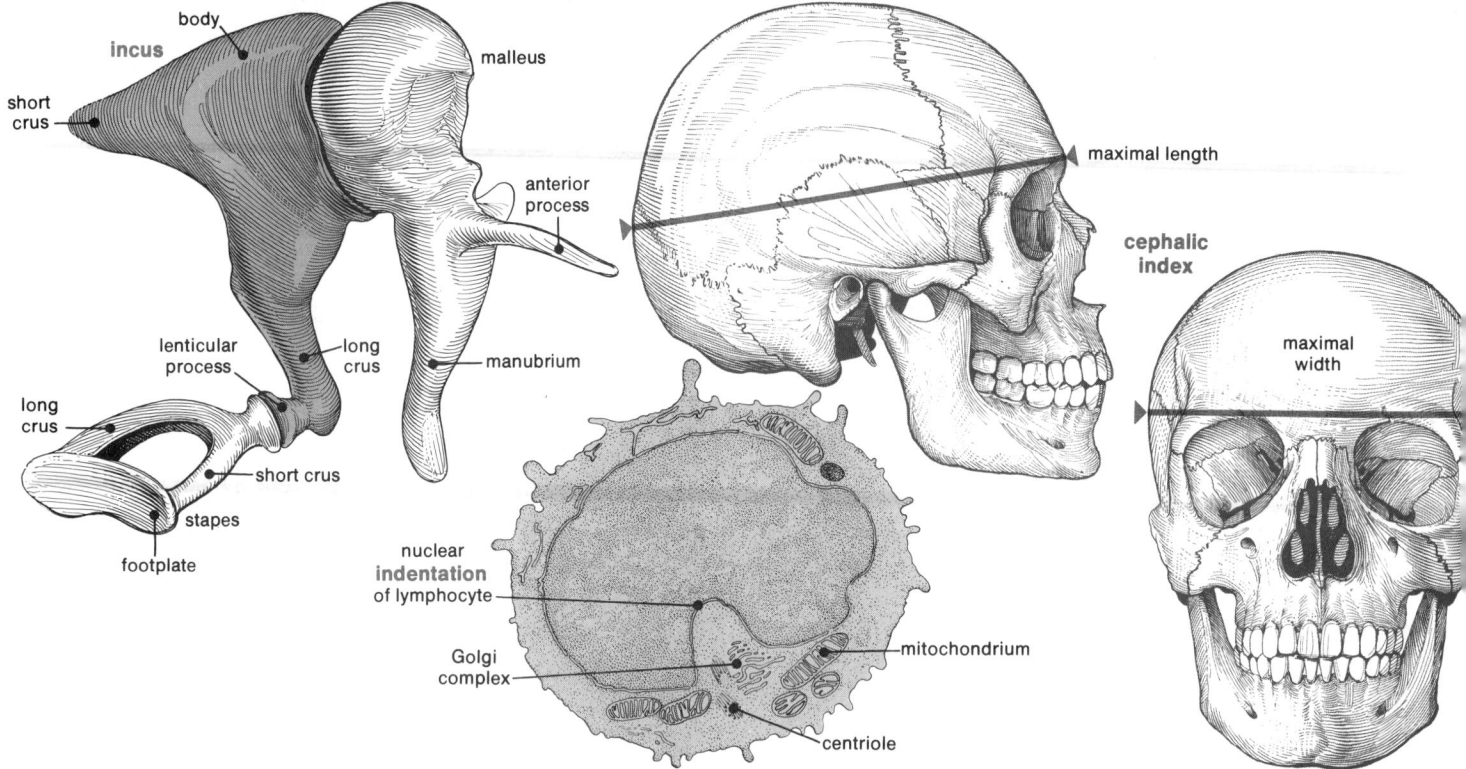

Labels in figure: incus, body, malleus, short crus, anterior process, lenticular process, long crus, manubrium, long crus, short crus, stapes, footplate, maximal length, cephalic index, maximal width, nuclear indentation of lymphocyte, Golgi complex, mitochondrium, centriole

tion to the appearance of the first symptoms.

incubator One of a variety of apparatuses designed to maintain a constant temperature; used to preserve the life of a premature baby, to grow bacterial cultures, etc.

incurable Not curable.

incus The middle of the three auditory ossicles in the middle ear, situated between the malleus and the stapes. Also called anvil.

indentation 1. A deep recess in a boundary; a notch, dent, or impression. 2. The act of indenting or notching.

index, *pl.* **indexes, indices** 1. The forefinger or second digit. 2. A value expressing the ratio of one measurement to another. 3. A mold used to record or maintain the relative position of teeth to one another and/or to a cast. 4. A guide used to reposition teeth, casts, or parts.

  Arneth i. A value obtained by adding the percentages of polymorphonuclear neutrophils with one or two lobes in their nuclei plus one half the percentage of those with three lobes; the normal value is 60%.

  cardiac i. The cardiac output per minute per square meter of body surface.

  cardiothoracic i. The ratio of the maximal transverse diameter of the heart shadow on an x ray to the maximal transverse diameter of the chest, normally less than one half.

  cephalic i. The ratio of the maximal breadth to the maximal length of the head.

  chemotherapeutic i. The ratio of the minimal effective dose of a drug to the maximal tolerated dose.

  color i. (Ci) The ratio of the amount of hemoglobin to the number of red blood cells. Also called blood quotient; globular value.

  icterus i. An index indicating the amount of bilirubin in the blood.

  maturation i. An index used to detect estrogenic activity by indicating the percentage of mature cells exfoliated from the vagina; the action of an estrogen matures vaginal epithelium; therefore, the higher percentage of mature cells exfoliated suggests increased estrogenic activity.

  nasal i. The ratio of the greatest width of the nose to its length.

  orbital i. The ratio of the height of the orbit to its width.

  pelvic-outlet i. Relation of the anteroposterior diameter of the pelvis to the greatest transverse width across the inlet.

  refractive i. (n) The ratio of the speed of light in a medium of reference (vacuum, air, etc.) to the speed of light in a given medium.

  therapeutic i. The ratio of the dose that is fatal to 50 percent of test animals (LD_{50}) to the dose that produces the desired effect in 50 percent of test animals (ED_{50}); used in quantitative comparison of drugs.

  thoracic i. The ratio of the anteroposterior to the transverse diameter of the chest.

  vital i. The ratio of births to deaths in a given population during a given time.

indican 1. A water-soluble glucoside that hydrolyzes to glucose and indoxyl, present in plants yielding the blue dye indigo. 2. Potassium indoxyl sulfate, a product of decomposition of the amino acid tryptophan; formed in the intestines and excreted in the urine.

indicant Serving to indicate, as a symptom that indicates a mode of treatment.

indicanuria The presence of increased indican in the urine; a sign of protein putrefaction mainly in the intestines.

indication Anything that suggests the proper treatment of a disease.

indicator In chemistry, any of various substances (e.g., litmus) that, by means of changing color, indicate the presence, absence, or concentration of a substance, or the degree of completion of a chemical reaction between two or more substances.

indigenous Occurring naturally in an area. Also called native.

indigestible 1. Not capable of being digested. 2. Difficult to digest.

indigestion 1. Discomfort caused by a temporary inability to digest food properly. 2. Failure of digestion.

  nervous i. Indigestion caused by emotional disturbances.

indigo A blue dye obtained from plants of the genus *Indigofera* or produced synthetically.

  i. carmine A blue dye, sodium indigotindisulfonate.

indisposition Malaise.

indium A soft, silvery-white metallic element; symbol In, atomic number 49, atomic weight 114.82.

indium-111 (^{111}In) A gamma-emitting radionuclide used primarily in locating occult abcesses.

individuation The process of forming or becoming a separate person differentiated from the family or community.

indocyanine green A dye used in a variety of blood flow, volume and function studies; most commonly used to measure cardiac output.

indole A normal product of protein decomposition in the large intestine. Also called ketol.

indolent 1. Sluggish. 2. Causing little or no pain.

indolic acids Products of metabolism of the amino acid tryptophan.

indomethacin A nonsteroidal anti-inflammatory compound; an inhibitor of prostaglandin synthetase; used in the treatment of rheumatoid arthritis, osteoarthritis, acute gout, and other musculoskeletal disorders; Indocin®.

induce 1. To bring on or about by stimulation; to cause; to effect. 2. In psychology, to arouse by indirect influence.

inducer A small molecule, usually a substrate of a specific enzyme pathway, capable of combining with the repressor to form an inactive complex that cannot combine with the operator, and as a result permits mRNA synthesis.

inductance (L) A circuit element, typically a conducting coil in which a magnetic field is associated with the circuit when the circuit is carrying current; the unit of induction is the henry (H).

induction Stimulation of the synthesis of an enzyme from amino acids programmed by a structural gene in the presence of a small inducer molecule.

inductor An agent that brings about induction.

inductorium Instrument designed to generate currents of electricity for stimulation of a nerve or a muscle.

indurated Hardened; denoting normally soft tissues that have become abnormally firm.

induration 1. The hardening of a tissue. 2. An abnormally hard spot or area.

  black i. Pigmentation and hardening of lung tissue, as in pneumonia.

  cyanotic i. Induration caused by chronic venous congestion of an organ.

indwelling Denoting a catheter or drainage tube that is fixed and held in position for a period of time.

inebriant Any intoxicating agent; an intoxicant.

inebriation The condition of being intoxicated.

inert 1. Slow to move or act; sluggish. 2. Resisting action. 3. Devoid of chemical activity, as the inert gases. 4. Denoting a compound or drug having no therapeutic action.

inertia 1. Resistance offered by a mass to a change in its position of rest or motion. 2. Denoting inability to move unless stimulated by an external force.

  colonic i. Sluggish muscular activity of the colon.

  uterine i. Absence of effective uterine contractions during labor.

in extremis Latin for at the point of death.

infancy Babyhood; approximately the first two years of life.

infant A child under the age of two years.

  LBW i. An infant with a low birth weight.

  premature i. An infant born after a gestation period of less than the normal length of time; one

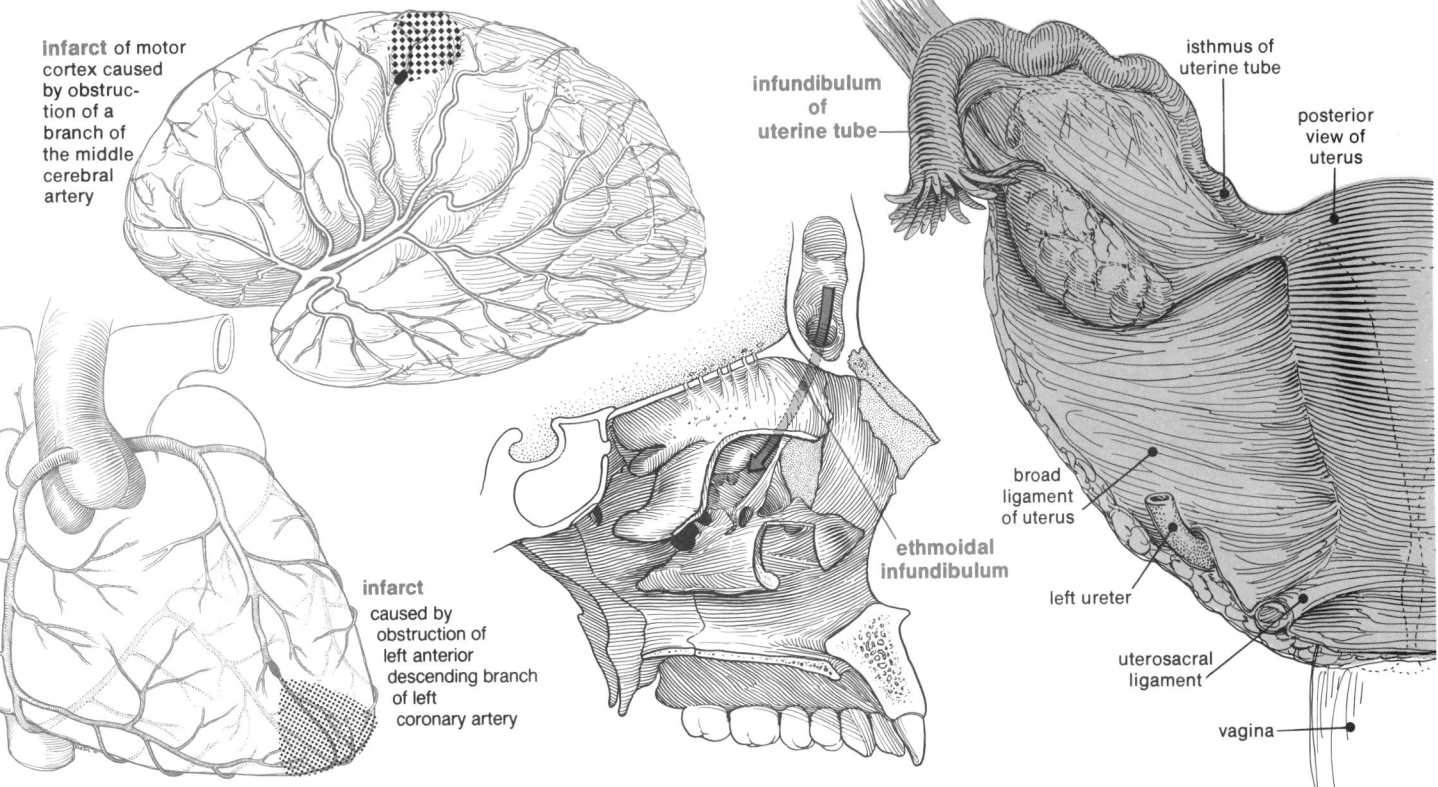

infarct of motor cortex caused by obstruction of a branch of the middle cerebral artery

infarct caused by obstruction of left anterior descending branch of left coronary artery

infundibulum of uterine tube

ethmoidal infundibulum

isthmus of uterine tube

posterior view of uterus

broad ligament of uterus

left ureter

uterosacral ligament

vagina

born before term.

infanticide The killing of an infant.

infantile Relating to an infant.

infantile polycystic disease of kidneys See polycystic disease of kidney.

infantilism Extremely slow development of mind or body, or both.

infarct An area of necrosis in a tissue caused by obstruction in the artery supplying the area.

  anemic i. An infarct caused by the sudden interruption of circulation in the terminal artery. Also called pale infarct.

  hemorrhagic i. An infarct that is red and swollen due to infiltration of blood into the dead area. Also called red infarct.

  lacunar i. A small area (2 to 12 mm) of dead tissue deep in the brain (thalamus, putamen, base of pons, or white matter of cerebral hemisphere), resulting from occlusion or narrowing of the penetrating branches of the anterior cerebral, posterior cerebral, or basilar arteries.

  pale i. See anemic infarct.

  red i. See hemorrhagic infarct.

infarction 1. The formation of an infarction. 2. Infarct.

  myocardial i. Deterioration and/or death of a portion of the heart muscle as a result of deprivation of its blood supply, usually due to occlusion of the artery supplying blood to the area; the occlusion may or may not be due to a thrombus (blood clot).

  pulmonary i. An airless area of lung tissue filled with blood cells as a result of the interruption of the blood supply to the tissues by a clot.

  subendocardial myocardial i. An infarction involving the layer of muscle adjacent to the lining of the heart chambers.

  transmural i. A myocardial infarction thought to involve the whole thickness of the heart muscle, extending through all layers of the myocardium rather than being restricted to the subendocardial region.

infect To contaminate with harmful agents.

infection Invasion of the body by living microorganisms; it may or may not result in an illness.

  clinical i. An infection that has become sufficiently active to give rise to signs and symptoms of a disease (infectious disease).

  focal i. An infection in which the microorganisms remain in a limited area.

  inapparent i. An infection that is not sufficiently active to give rise to recognizable signs and symptoms of disease. Also called subclinical infection.

  latent i. A persistent inapparent infection in which the presence of the organism cannot be detected by currently available methods; it flares up

from time to time under certain conditions; e.g., a herpes simplex infection (cold sore).

  secondary i. An infection occurring in an individual already suffering from a previous infection by another microorganism.

  subclinical i. See inapparent infection.

  terminal i. An acute infection occurring toward the end of another disease (usually chronic) and generally causing death.

infectious Capable of being transmitted or capable of causing infection.

infecundity Inability of a woman to bear children.

inference, statistical In biostatistics, the procedure in which a conclusion is made on the basis of a drawn sample; usually a statistic is computed and, from that, a conclusion is formed about the corresponding parameters.

inferior Located in a lower position in relation to another structure.

infertility The failure to conceive or induce conception, although the potential for reproduction is present.

infest To attack or live on a host as a parasite.

infestation Presence of parasites on the body (e.g., ticks, mites, lice), or in the organs (e.g., worms).

infiltrate 1. To pass into the interstices of a tissue or substance, as a cancer. 2. The material that has infiltrated into the tissue; e.g., a pulmonary infiltrate noted on chest X ray.

infiltration The process of seepage or diffusion into tissue of substances that are not ordinarily present; invasion by cells that are not normal to the location.

  fatty i. Accumulation of fat globules in the cells.

infirm Weak in body due to disease or old age.

infirmary A dispensary for the care of the sick or injured, especially in a school or camp.

infirmity 1. A disabling state of the mind or body. 2. A disease or condition causing bodily debilitation.

inflammation A tissue reaction to irritation, infection, or injury, marked by localized heat, swelling, redness, pain, and sometimes loss of function.

inflammatory Relating to, marked by, resulting from, or causing inflammation.

inflation The act of distending or the state of being distended by a gas or liquid.

inflection, inflexion The act of turning inward, or a state of being turned inward.

influenza A contagious infectious disease caused by an influenza virus (family Orthomyxoviridae); marked by fever, headache, pain in the back and limbs, and inflammation of the respiratory tract; it occurs in epidemics and sometimes pandemics (world epidemics). Also called flu; grippe.

Influenzavirus Genus of viruses (family Orthomyxoviridae) that includes serotypes A and B (prob-

ably C), and several subgroups of strains, classified on the basis of their surface antigens; the cause of respiratory infections of man and other vertebrates; B strains infect primarily man.

infold To fold inward.

infraclavicular Situated below a clavicle (collarbone).

infraclusion Condition in which a tooth fails to erupt. Also called infraocclusion.

infrahyoid Located below the hyoid bone.

inframandibular Below the lower jaw.

infranatant The clear fluid seen after the flotation of particulate matter in a suspension.

infraocclusion See infraclusion.

infraorbital Located beneath or in the floor of the orbit of the eye.

infrapatellar Located below the kneecap (patella), such as a bursa.

infrared The electromagnetic radiation beyond the red end of the spectrum, with wavelengths that are too long (greater than 7700 Å) to be seen by the human eye.

infrascapular Located below the scapula (shoulder blade).

infraspinous Located below a spinous process.

infrasplenic Located below or beneath the spleen.

infrasternal Below the sternum (breastbone).

infratrochlear Located below the pulley (trochlea) of the superior oblique muscle of the eye.

infraumbilical Under the navel.

infundibuliform Shaped like a funnel.

infundibulum Latin for funnel; most commonly refers to the funnel-shaped stalk of the pituitary gland.

  ethmoidal i. The long, curved, funnel-shaped passage connecting the anterior ethmoid cells and the frontal sinus with the nasal cavity.

  i. of uterine tube The lateral, funnel-shaped extremity of the uterine (fallopian) tube.

infusible 1. Resistant to heat. 2. Capable of being infused.

infusion 1. The introduction of a fluid into a vessel. 2. The soaking or steeping of a substance in water in order to extract its soluble parts. 3. The resulting liquid.

ingestion 1. The introduction of food, drink, or medicines into the stomach. 2. Process by which a cell or a unicellular organism takes in foreign material.

inguinal Pertaining to the groin.

inhalant A remedy taken by inhalation.

inhalation The act of breathing in; breathing in of a gas or a medication or a noxious substance.

inhale To draw into the body by breathing; to inspire.

metered
dose
inhaler

Duke
inhaler

insecticides

nicotine

DDT

parathion

inion

inheritance of color blindness

carrier ♀ XX —— XY normal ♂

XX
normal
♀

XX
carrier
♀

XY
color-blind
♂

XY
normal
♂

a possible expression
of the x-linked
recessive trait
for color blindness

inhaler A device that permits medicinal material in vapor form to be inhaled.

inherent Belonging naturally to a person.

inheritance 1. In genetics, the process of genetically transmitting characters from parent to offspring. 2. The characters so transmitted.

  dominant i. See gene, dominant.

  holandric i. Transmission of a character determined by a gene on the Y chromosome, i.e., occurring only in males.

  hologynic i. Transmission of a trait from mother to all daughters but to no sons, i.e., occurring only in females.

  Mendelian i. Mendel's laws; see under law.

  mosaic i. Inheritance characterized by the dominance of paternal influence in one group of cells and the dominance of the maternal in another.

  recessive i. See gene, recessive.

  sex-linked i. X-linkage; see under linkage.

inhibition The restriction or arrest of a function or specific activity.

inhibitor An agent or nerve that represses physiologic activity.

  allosteric i. A substance that decreases enzymatic activity through noncompetitive binding to the enzyme molecule at a site (allosteric site) other than the active site of the enzyme.

inion The most prominent point of the external occipital protuberance of the skull; used as a fixed craniometric point.

initiator A substance, necessary to the process of building certain giant molecules, which helps bring about such reactions and, unlike a catalyst, is altered and may appear in the final product.

inject To drive a fluid into a part.

injectable Any substance that may be injected.

injection 1. The act of forcing or driving a fluid into a part, such as the subcutaneous tissue or a bodily cavity. 2. The fluid injected. 3. The state of being injected. Also called congestion; hyperemia.

  retrograde i. Introduction of a solution into an organ against the normal direction of flow, as injection of a radiopaque solution into the kidney via the ureter.

injector A device for administering injections.

  jet i. A machine that, through high pressure, forces a liquid through a small orifice at high velocity; the liquid is thus able to penetrate the unbroken skin without causing pain.

injure To wound or hurt.

injury A specific bodily damage or wound. Also called trauma.

  blast i. Rupture of lungs or abdominal organs caused by a blast of air, as from explosion of a bomb.

  countercoup i. of brain Injury to the brain at a site opposite to the point of impact.

  repetitive motion i. (RMI) Damage to muscles, nerves, or bones from performing activities for prolonged periods.

  whiplash i. A nonspecific term applied to an injury of the spine, usually at the junction of the fourth and fifth cervical vertebrae, caused by an abrupt jerking motion of the head. Also called hyperextension-hyperflexion injury.

inlay A solid restorative material (gold, fired porcelain, plastic) that is fitted and cemented to a tapered cavity preparation in a tooth.

inlet A passage that leads to a cavity.

innate Present at birth.

innervation The nerve supply of a given area or structure.

innidiation The multiplication of cells in a location where they have been carried by lymph or the blood stream.

innocent Benign; said of a tumor.

innocuous Harmless.

innominate Unnamed.

innominate artery Brachiocephalic trunk; see under trunk.

innominate bone See hipbone.

innominate vein See table of veins.

innoxious Harmless; not injurious.

inoculable 1. Transmissible by inoculation. 2. Susceptible to a disease which is transmissible by inoculation.

inoculate To introduce a virus into the body; to introduce vaccines, immune sera, or other antigenic material into the body in order to prevent, cure, or experiment.

inoculation The introduction of disease-causing microorganisms into the body.

  therapeutic i. The introduction of an antiserum for curative purposes.

inoculum Material containing microorganisms introduced by inoculation.

inoperable That which cannot be operated upon or which cannot be removed by surgery.

inorganic Neither composed of nor derived from organic matter (animal or vegetable); designating compounds that do not contain carbon.

inosculate To make continuous or unite by small openings or anastomoses.

inosine 5'-diphosphate (IDP) A nucleotide which participates in high-energy phosphate transfer.

inositol A substance classified as a member of the vitamin B complex; found in plant and animal tissue. Also called muscle sugar.

inotropic Influencing or affecting muscular contraction.

  negatively i. Weakening the action of muscles.

  positively i. Strengthening the action of muscles.

inotropism The quality of influencing muscular contraction.

inpatient A patient staying overnight in a hospital.

insalivation The mixing of food with saliva in chewing.

insane Relating to insanity, or to one who is of unsound mind.

insanity In law, a mental state in which one is legally nonresponsible or incompetent for some or all purposes. Originally a medical term referring to loss of reason, by the end of the 19th century it came to include diseases of the intellect, the will, or the emotions; since the 1920s, the term has not been used in the United States for medical purposes but continues to have multiple legal meanings, all of which involve some degree of nonresponsibility or incompetence for legal purposes. The law defines different kinds or degrees of insanity (e.g., for making a will, making a business contract, committing criminal acts, or reasonable likelihood of imminent danger to oneself or others); insanity for one act may not necessarily mean insanity for other kinds of acts.

inscription The part of a prescription that stipulates the names and amounts of ingredients to be used by the pharmacist. See also superscription; subscription; signature.

insectarium A place in which living insects are kept and bred for scientific purposes.

insecticide Any agent that kills insects.

insemination 1. Introduction of seminal fluid into the vagina. 2. Fertilization of an ovum.

  artificial i. Deposit of seminal fluid in the vagina by means other than sexual intercourse.

  intrauterine i. The placing of semen within the uterus.

insensible 1. Imperceptible by the senses. 2. Unconscious.

insertion 1. The site of attachment of a muscle to a bone which is more movable than the one from which it originated. 2. The act of introducing or implanting.

insidious Spreading or developing harmfully in a subtle or imperceptible way; applied to certain diseases.

insight 1. The ability to understand the real nature of a situation. 2. Self-understanding.

in situ Latin for in place.

insoluble Not capable of entering into solution.

insomnia Inability to sleep under normal conditions; three varieties are recognized: (a) inability to fall asleep upon retiring; (b) intermittent waking after falling asleep; (c) early awakening.

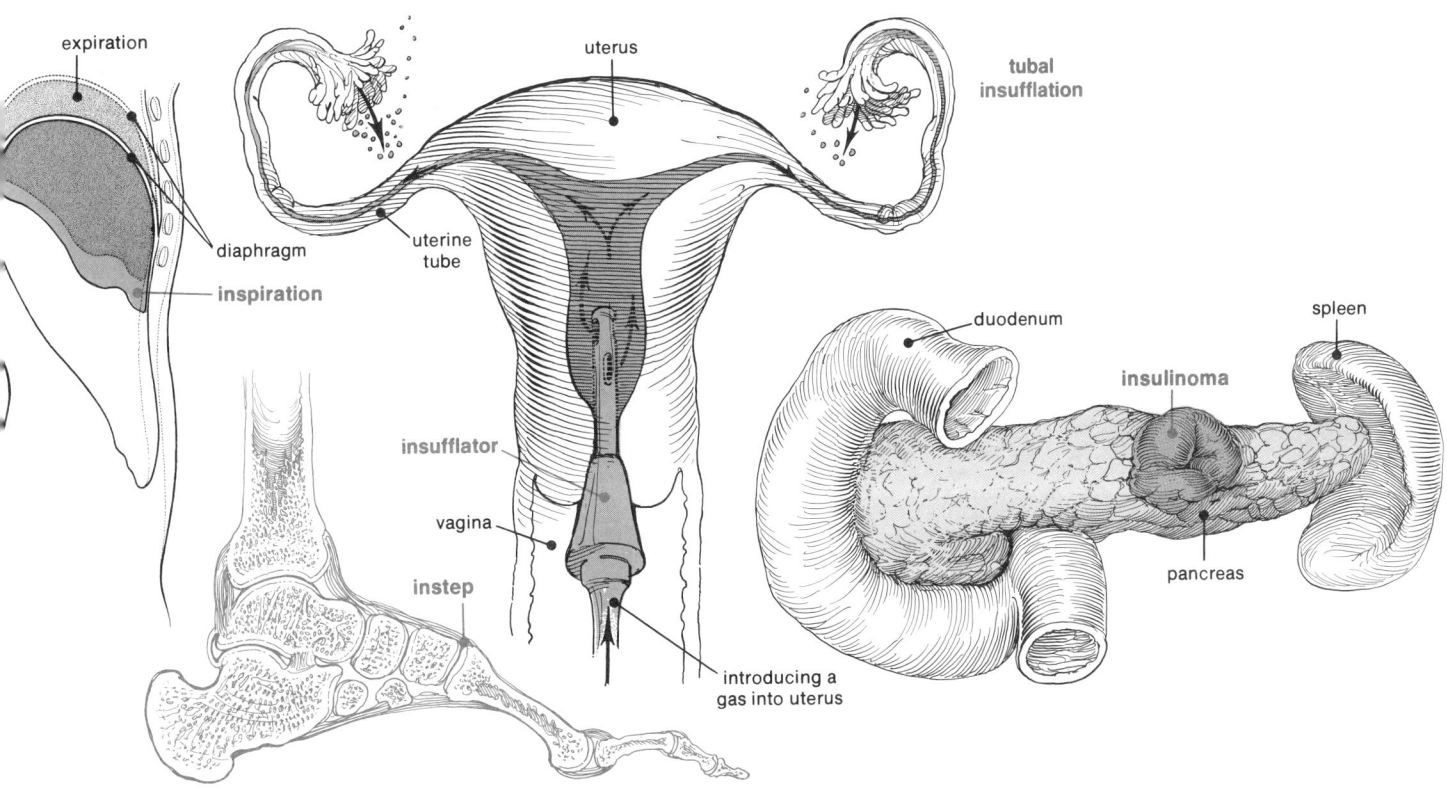

expiration

diaphragm

inspiration

uterus

uterine tube

insufflator

vagina

instep

introducing a gas into uterus

tubal insufflation

duodenum

insulinoma

spleen

pancreas

insomniac A person suffering from insomnia. Inhalation; breathing in.
inspiratory Relating to inhalation.
inspire To inhale; to breathe in.
inspissation The process of thickening as by evaporation of fluid.
inspissator A device used to air-dry fluids.
instep The arched middle part of the dorsum of the human foot.
instillation The gradual, drop by drop, pouring of a liquid.
instinct An inherent drive or tendency to act in a certain way without the aid of reason.
instrumentation The utilization of instruments in the treatment of a patient.
insudate The material passed into vessel walls; from Latin, sweating inward.
insufficiency Inability to perform a normal function; said of an organ or structure.
  adrenal i. See Addison's disease.
  aortic i. Insufficiency of the aortic valve.
  cardiac i. Heart failure; see under failure.
  coronary i. Insufficient blood flow to the cardiac muscle, leading to prolonged pain or discomfort (angina).
  mitral i. Insufficiency of the mitral valve.
  posttraumatic pulmonary i. See adult respiratory distress syndrome.
  pulmonary i. Insufficiency of the pulmonary valve.
  renal i. Defective kidney function, especially a decrease in glomerular filtration manifested by a consequent increase in blood levels of urea and creatinine.
  tricuspid i. Insufficiency of the tricuspid valve.
  valvular i. Failure of a heart valve to close tightly, thus allowing regurgitation of blood; named according to the valve involved, aortic, mitral, pulmonary, or tricuspid.
  venous i. Inadequate drainage of blood from a part, resulting in edema.
insufficiency disease See disease, deficiency.
insufflate **1.** To blow into, as in artificial respiration. **2.** To blow a gas, medicated vapor, powder, or anesthetic into a body cavity.
insufflation The act of blowing a gas, medicated vapor, powder, or anesthetic into a body cavity.
  cranial i. The forcing of air into the ventricles of the brain.
  perirenal i. Injection of air or carbon dioxide in the area around the kidneys for roentgen visualization of the adrenal glands.
  tubal i. The passage of a gas, usually carbon dioxide, into the uterus to determine the patency of the uterine (fallopian) tubes. Also called uterotubal

insufflation.
  uterotubal i. See tubal insufflation.
insufflator An instrument used in insufflation.
insula The central lobe of the cerebrum, lying deeply in the lateral cerebral fissure (fissure of Sylvius). Also called Reil's island; central lobe.
insular Relating to an insula, especially the central lobe of the cerebrum (Reil's island).
insulate To prevent the passage of heat, sound, or electricity from one body or region to another by interposing material with nonconductive properties.
insulation **1.** The act of insulating. **2.** The material used to insulate. **3.** The state of being insulated.
insulator Any nonconductive material used to effect insulation.
insulin A hormone produced in the islets of Langerhans in the pancreas, concerned with the regulation of carbohydrate metabolism by controlling glucose levels in the blood; it is extracted from the pancreas of beef or pork, or produced by bacteria with genetic modification, for use in the treatment of diabetes.
  isophane i. A suspension of insulin, protamine, and zinc; an intermediate-acting preparation. Also called NPH insulin (N denotes a neutral solution; P, the protamine zinc insulin content; H, its origin at Hagedorn's Laboratory).
  lente i. A family of insulin zinc suspensions prepared in three forms: (a) lente, one of intermediate onset and duration of action; (b) semilente, a short-acting preparation; (c) ultralente, a long-acting form.
  protamine zinc i. (PZI) A suspension of insulin, protamine, and zinc chloride; a long-acting preparation.
  regular i. An aqueous solution of the active principle of the islets of Langerhans from beef or pork pancreas, or produced biosynthetically; onset of action after injection is within one hour and duration is up to six hours.
insulinase Enzyme capable of destroying or inactivating insulin.
insulinoma, insuloma An insulin-producing islet cell adenoma of the pancreas.
insulinopenia Decreased or inadequate level of insulin in the blood.
insult An injury or irritation.
integration **1.** The condition of being combined. **2.** The process of bringing all parts together to form a whole, as the building up of living substance by assimilation of nutritive material.
integument A covering or coat, as the skin or the membrane covering an organ. Also called tegument.
intelligence **1.** The faculty of thought, reason, and understanding. **2.** The ability to acquire and apply knowledge.

  abstract i. The ability to acquire and understand abstract ideas and symbols.
  i. quotient (IQ) See under quotient.
  mechanical i. The ability to acquire knowledge and understanding of technical mechanisms.
  social i. Ability to understand and manage social relationships.
intemperance Lack of self-restraint, as in the indulgence of alcoholic beverages.
intensity Degree of activity, tension, strength, etc., usually implying a large measure.
intensive Of or characterized by intensity; applied to an exhaustive and concentrated form of treatment.
intention **1.** A process. **2.** Objective.
  healing by first i. The immediate healing of a wound without suppuration or granulation.
  healing by second i. Healing by the union of two granulating surfaces after some suppuration has taken place.
  healing by third i. Filling of a wound with granulations followed by the formation of scar tissue.
interacinous Between the acini of a gland.
interalveolar Between alveoli.
interarticular Located between two joints or joint surfaces.
interatrial Situated between the atria of the heart.
intercadence The occurrence of an extra pulse beat, between two regular beats.
intercalary Occurring between parts. Also called interpolated; interposed.
intercalate To interpose or insert between others; to interpolate.
interclavicular Located or occurring between the clavicles (collarbones).
intercondylar, intercondylic, intercondyloid Located between two condyles.
intercostal Located or occurring between successive ribs.
intercourse **1.** Interchange between individuals. **2.** Coitus.
intercristal Located between two crests.
intercurrent Occurring during the course of an already existing disease.
interdental Between the teeth.
interdentium The space between two adjacent teeth.
interdigital Between the fingers or toes.
interdigitation **1.** Interlocking of structures by means of finger-like processes. **2.** The processes so interlocked.
interepithelial Situated or passing between epithelial cells.
interface A surface forming a common boundary between two bodies.

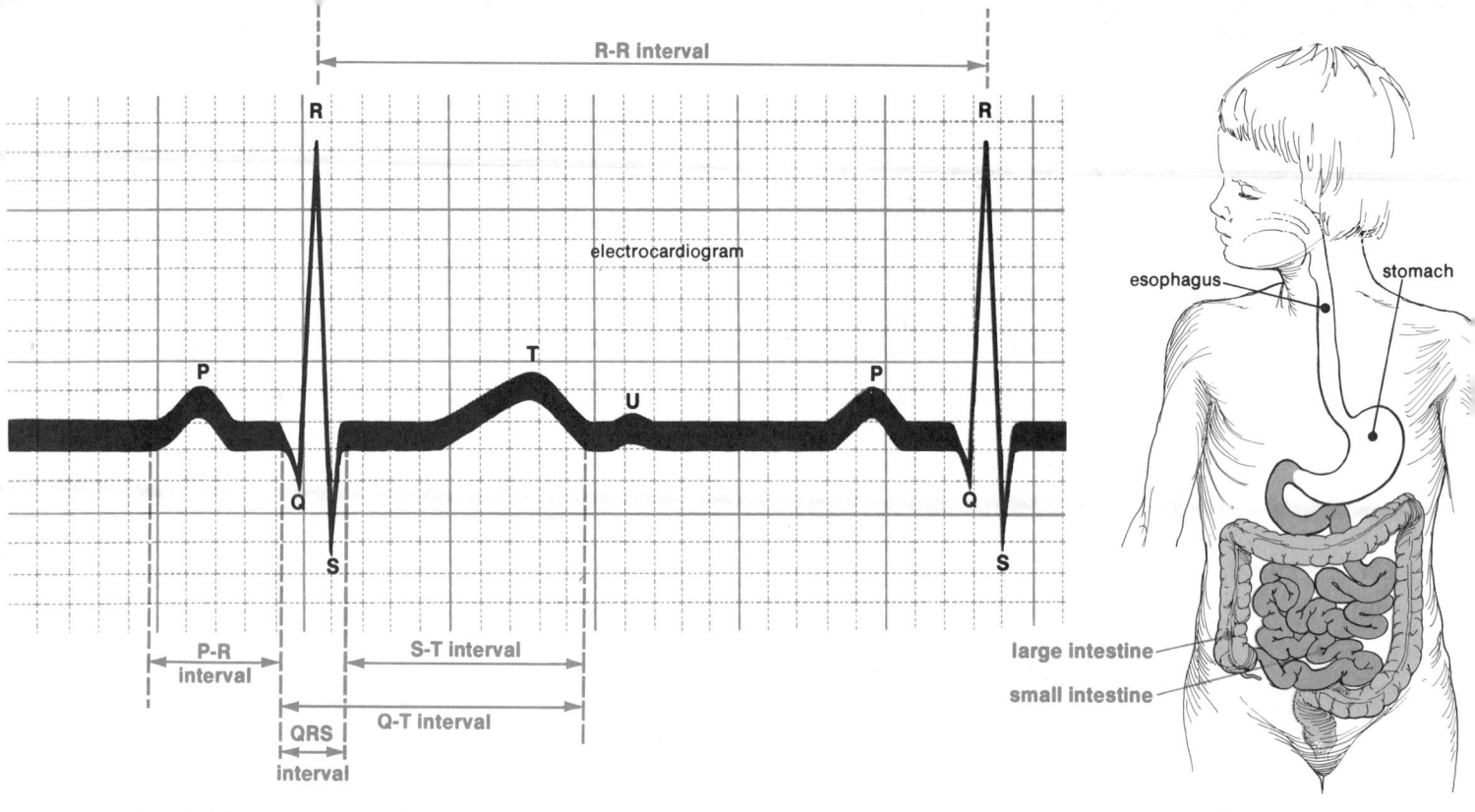

electrocardiogram

R-R interval

P-R interval

QRS interval

S-T interval

Q-T interval

esophagus

stomach

large intestine

small intestine

---

interfacial Relating to an interface.

interference 1. The coming together of waves in various media in such a way that the crests of one series correspond to the hollows of the other; when they cross, they reinforce each other at certain points and neutralize each other at other points. 2. The collision of two waves of excitation in the myocardium, seen in fusion beats. 3. In A-V (atrioventricular) dissociation, the disturbance of the rhythm of the heart ventricles by a conducted impulse from the atria. 4. Superinfection, as occurs when cells are exposed to two viruses.

interferon A protein substance produced by body cells in response to invasion by viruses and other intracellular parasites; it interferes with the synthesis of new virus and is effective against certain protozoal parasitic infections, such as malaria; may also inhibit oncogenic virus growth.

interictal Denoting the interval between convulsions.

interleukin A material which acts as a messenger between leukocytes involved in immunologic or inflammatory responses.

interleukin 1 (IL1) A polypeptide with fever-inducing and lymphocyte-activating properties released by monocyte macrophages; can stimulate production of interleukin 2 by peripheral T lymphocytes. Formerly known as lymphocyte-activating factor.

interleukin 2 (IL2) A glycoprotein that induces proliferation of responsive T lymphocytes; released by certain activated T cells.

interlobar Located between lobes.

interlobular Located between lobules.

intermediate 1. Occurring between two extremes. 2. A substance formed in the course of chemical reactions which then proceeds to participate rapidly in further reactions, so that at any given moment it is present in minute concentrations only.
  metabolic i.'s Substances that appear in the course of the reactions involved in metabolism.

intermediate coronary syndrome Episodes of precordial pain that are too severe or protracted to be called angina, yet are not accompanied by the symptoms of a myocardial infarction. Also called acute coronary insufficiency.

intermenstrual Denoting the interval between two consecutive menstrual periods.

intermittency, intermittence The quality of being recurrent (often at regular intervals); not continuous.

intermuscular Located between muscles.

intern A recent medical school graduate who receives supervised practical training by assisting in the medical and surgical care of patients at a hospi-

tal.

internal Located within or on the inside; away from the surface.

internalization In psychiatry, an unconscious process of taking into one's sense of self aspects of significant persons.

International System of Units (SI) A complete system of units for international scientific and technologic work; based on the metric system to which are added units of time, electric current, temperature, and luminous intensity; the abbreviation SI is from the French equivalent, Système International. See table on page 465.

interneuron An excitatory or inhibitory neuron in the central nervous system which is situated between the primary afferent neuron and the final motor neuron; it usually has a short range of action.

internist A specialist in internal medicine.

internodal Between two nodes; applied to the segment of a nerve fiber between two successive nodes.

internuncial Denoting a connecting agent or part, as a nerve cell connecting two other nerve cells.

interoceptor Any one of the sensory nerve endings which are located in, and receive stimuli from, visceral tissues and blood vessels.

interosseous Connecting or lying between bones.

interphalangeal Positioned between two contiguous phalanges of either the fingers or the toes.

interphase The interval between two successive mitotic divisions; the phase when the cell is not dividing but is actively synthesizing DNA. Formerly called "resting stage."

interplanting In experimental embryology, the transferring of an embryonic part from one embryo to an indifferent evironment in another embryo.

interpretation In psychoanalysis, the process by which the therapist explains to the patient the meaning of a particular aspect of his problems.

interproximal Between adjacent surfaces, as the space between adjacent teeth in the same dental arch.

interradicular Situated between the roots of a tooth.

interscapular Positioned between the scapulae.

interseptal Situated between two septa.

intersex See hermaphrodite.

intersexuality See hermaphroditism.

interspace Space between two similar structures.

interspinal Between the spinous processes of the vertebrae. Also called interspinous.

interstice A minute space in the substances of an organ or tissue.

interstitial Pertaining to or situated in the spaces within a tissue.

interstitium Structures such as fibers, located be-

tween bodily parts, that form a supporting framework of tissue which binds organs together.

intertriginous Characterized by or related to intertrigo.

intertrigo Skin eruption occurring between two adjacent surfaces, as between the scrotum and the thigh.

intertrochanteric Located between the two trochanters of the femur.

interval 1. The lapse of time between two events or between the recurrence of similar episodes of a disease. 2. A distance between two objects. 3. A gap in a continuous process.
  coupling i. The interval between a premature heart beat and the normal beat preceding it.
  lucid i. A period of mental clarity occurring in the course of a mental disorder.
  P-P i. The distance between the same points on two consecutive P waves of the electrocardiogram.
  P-R i. The atrioventricular conduction time, measured from the beginning of the P wave to the beginning of the QRS complex of the electrocardiogram; it includes the time required for atrial depolarization and repolarization plus the normal delay of excitation in the atrioventricular node.
  Q-R i. The interval from the beginning of the QRS complex to the peak of the R wave in the electrocardiogram.
  QRS i. The duration of the QRS complex, representing the measurement of total ventricular depolarization.
  Q-T i. The interval between the onset of the Q wave and the end of the T wave of the electrocardiogram; it measures the duration of electrical systole.
  R-R i. The interval between two consecutive QRS complexes of the electrocardiogram.

intervertebral Between two vertebrae.

intervillous Located among villi.

intestinal Relating to the intestine or bowel.

intestine The portion of the alimentary canal from the stomach to the anus.
  large i. The sacculated portion of the intestine, extending from the ileum to the anus and forming an arch over the convolutions of the small intestines; composed of three parts: cecum, colon, and rectum.
  small i. The convoluted portion of the intestine extending from the stomach to the cecum; divisible into three portions: duodenum, jejunum, and ileum.

intima The inner layer of a blood vessel.

in-toing See pigeon-toe.

intolerance Unfavorable reaction to a substance.
  hereditary fructose i. Metabolic defect due to an autosomal recessive inheritance; marked by a deficiency of fructose 1-phosphate aldolase, causing vomiting and hypoglycemia upon ingestion of fruc-

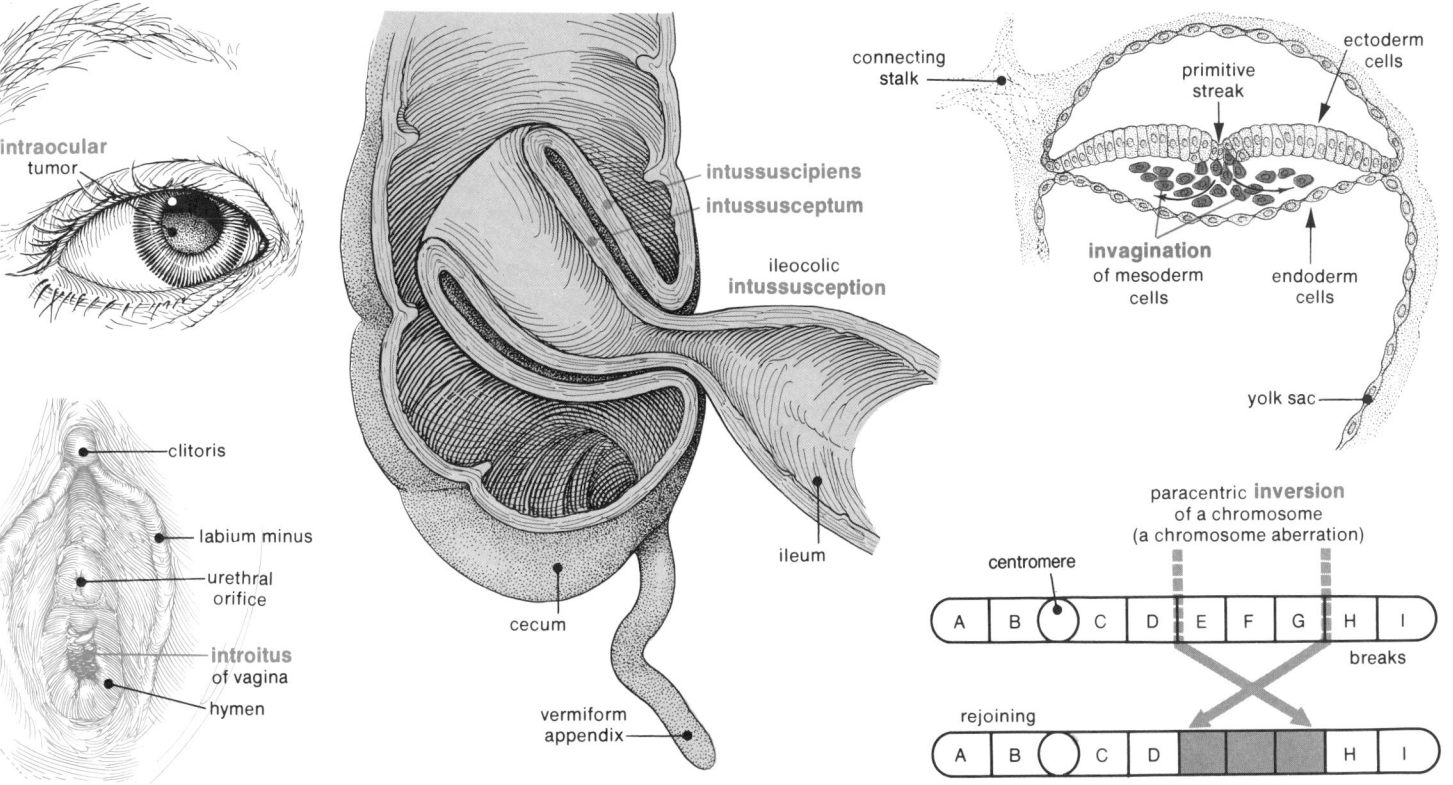

intraocular tumor

clitoris
labium minus
urethral orifice
introitus of vagina
hymen

intussuscipiens
intussusceptum
ileocolic intussusception
ileum
cecum
vermiform appendix

connecting stalk
primitive streak
ectoderm cells
invagination of mesoderm cells
endoderm cells
yolk sac

paracentric inversion of a chromosome (a chromosome aberration)
centromere
| A | B | C | D | E | F | G | H | I |
breaks
rejoining
| A | B | C | D | | | H | I |

tose; repeated ingestion of fructose by infants with this disorder may result in severe disease. Also called fructosemia.

lactose i. Intolerance to lactose due to presence of less than the normal amount of the enzyme lactase; manifested by abdominal cramps and diarrhea upon ingestion of milk and milk products.

intorsion, intortion The real or apparent inward turning of one or both eyes.

intortor A muscle, as an extraocular muscle, that turns a part inward.

intoxicant An intoxicating agent, especially alcohol.

intoxication 1. Poisoning. 2. Acute alcoholism; see under alcoholism.

intra-abdominal Situated within the abdomen.

intra-articular Located within a joint's cavity.

intracapsular Within a capsule, especially the capsule of a joint.

intracardiac Located within the heart.

intracatheter A slender plastic tube inserted into a vein for injection, infusion, or venous pressure monitoring.

intracellular Located or occurring within a cell or cells.

intracerebral Within the cerebrum.

intracostal Situated on the inner surface of a rib or ribs.

intracranial Within the skull.

intractable Resistant to therapy.

intracutaneous Within the layers of the skin.

intradermal Within the dermis (layer of skin).

intradural Situated within the dura mater, the outermost membrane surrounding the brain and spinal cord.

intraepithelial Situated within, or passing through, the epithelial cells.

intrahepatic Located within the liver.

intraluminal Within the lumen of a tubule or tubular structure.

intramedullary Within the bone marrow, the spinal cord, or the medulla oblongata.

intramembranous Between layers of a membrane.

intramolecular Occurring or located within the molecule.

intramural Situated within the wall of an organ or cavity.

intramuscular (I.M., i.m.) Within the substance of a muscle.

intranasal Located or occurring within the nasal cavity.

intraneural Within a nerve.

intraocular Within the eyeball.

intraoral Within the mouth.

intraorbital Within the orbit.

intraosseous Within bone tissue.

intraperitoneal (I.P., i.p.) Within the peritoneal cavity.

intrapsychic Taking place within the mind.

intrapulmonary Within the lungs.

intrarenal Located within the kidney.

intrathecal Within a sheath.

intrathoracic Within the chest cavity.

intrauterine Within the uterus.

intravascular Within the blood or lymphatic vessels.

intravenous Within a vein.

intraventricular Within a ventricle of the heart or brain.

intrinsic Belonging or situated entirely within a part.

introducer Instrument used to introduce a tube into the trachea. Also called intubator.

introitus Entrance into a cavity or hollow organ.

introjection The unconscious symbolic assimilation of a loved or hated object, making it a part of the self.

intromission Insertion; introduction.

introspection Examination of one's own mental processes.

introversion 1. Preoccupation with one's own interests and experiences. 2. The process of turning an organ or part inward.

introvert One whose thoughts are predominantly about himself.

introvert To turn inward.

intubate To introduce a tube into the trachea or the larynx.

intubation 1. Introduction of a tube into any canal. 2. Insertion of a tube into the trachea to allow air to enter the lungs.

intubator See introducer.

intumesce To swell.

intumescence A swelling.

intumescent Enlarging; swelling.

intussuscept To turn inward.

intussusception Condition in which one part of the intestine becomes pushed into the lumen of an adjoining segment; it occurs chiefly at the ilioceal junction, causing acute abdominal symptoms; seen most commonly among children.

intussusceptum The inner or ensheathed segment of intestine in an intussusception.

intussuscipiens The outer portion of intestine surrounding the inner segment in an intussusception.

inulin A fructose polysaccharide found in the roots and underground stems of several plants; used in kidney function tests as a measure of glomerular

filtration rate since it is filtered at the glomerulus, and is neither secreted nor reabsorbed by the tubules.

inunction 1. The rubbing or smearing of a drug, in ointment form, into the skin. 2. Ointment.

in utero Latin for within the uterus.

in vacuo Latin for in a vacuum.

invaginate To turn within or enclose; to ensheathe; to infold one part within another part of the same structure.

invagination Ensheathing or infolding of a part within itself.

invalid A person disabled by a chronic illness or infirmity.

invasion 1. The spread of a malignant tumor to adjacent tissues. 2. The beginning of a disease.

invasive Having a tendency to spread or to invade healthy tissue.

inventory, personality A psychological test for evaluation of personal characteristics; usually a checklist answered by the person about himself.

inversion 1. A turning inside out. 2. Any reversal of the normal relation with other organs. 3. In genetics, a chromosome aberration resulting from fragmentation of a chromosome by two breaks, followed by a turning end for end of the fragment and refusion.

i. of nipple Failure of the nipple to protrude from the breast.

i. of the uterus A turning of the uterus inside out, exposing the lining membrane (endometrium).

invert To turn upside down or inside out.

invertase An enzyme that converts sucrose into glucose and fructose; found in the small intestine. Also called sucrase.

Invertebrata A division of the animal kingdom comprised of animals without spinal columns.

invertebrate An animal that does not have a spinal column.

invertor A muscle that turns a part inward.

invertose A mixture of equal parts of glucose and fructose. Also called invert sugar.

invest To envelop; to cover completely.

investing 1. In dentistry, the process of covering an object, such as a wax pattern of a tooth restoration or a denture, with a refractory investment material before casting or curing. 2. In psychoanalysis, affecting an object with psychic energy or cathexis.

vacuum i. Forming a mold around a pattern in a vacuum in order to avoid trapping air in the investment material.

investment 1. Any material used to invest an object. 2. In psychoanalysis, the affective charge invested in or given to an idea or object.

in vitro In an environment outside of the body, usually in a test tube or other similar artificial envi-

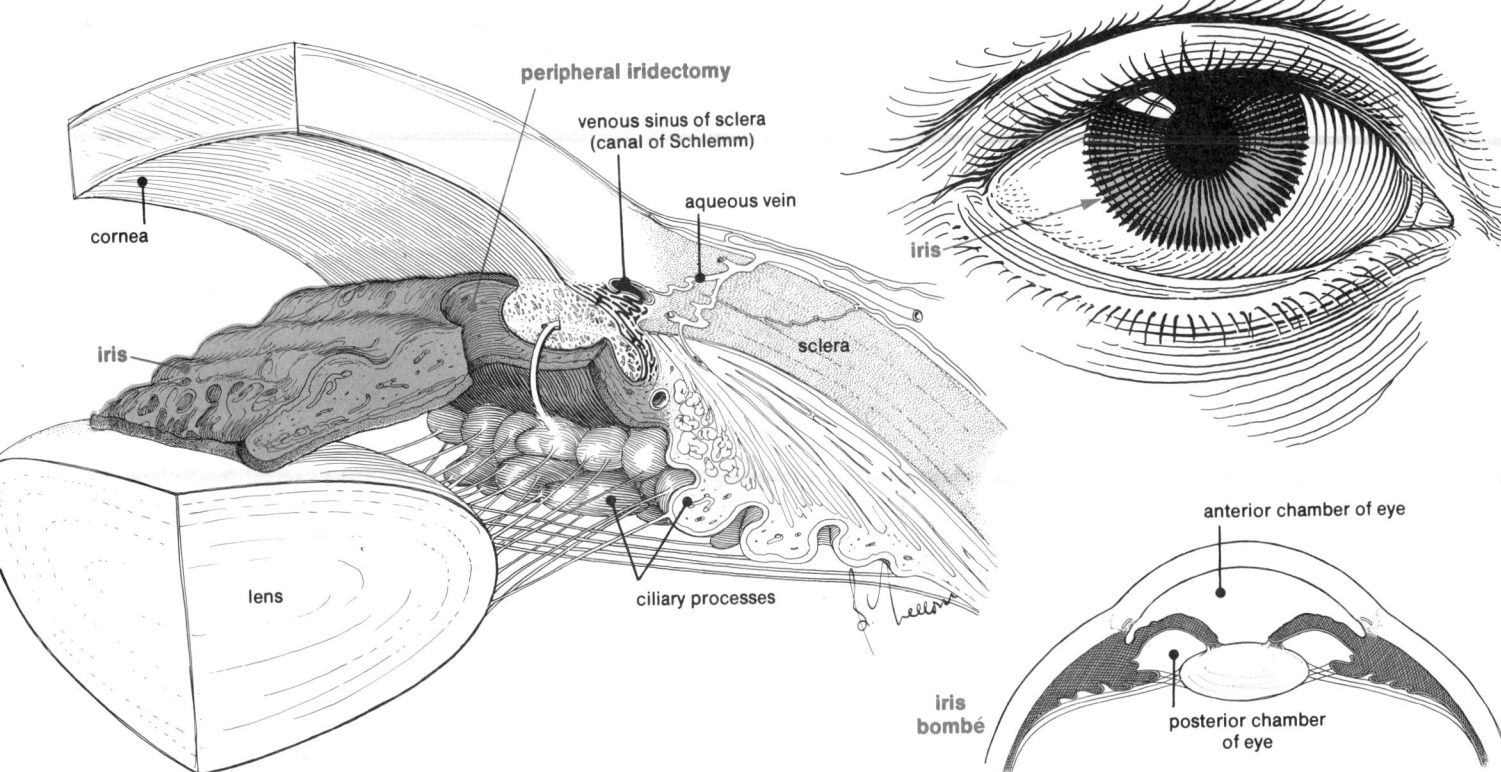

cornea

peripheral iridectomy

venous sinus of sclera (canal of Schlemm)

aqueous vein

iris

sclera

iris

lens

ciliary processes

anterior chamber of eye

iris bombé

posterior chamber of eye

ronment.

in vivo Within the living body.

involucrum An enveloping sheath of new bone, such as that developed around a necrosed bone as a response to infection.

involuntary 1. Performed independently of one's own free will. 2. Not performed willingly.

involution A retrograde process resulting in lessening in the size of a tissue, as the return to normal size of the uterus after childbirth, or the shrinking of organs and tissues in old age.

involutional Relating to involution.

iodate 1. A salt of iodic acid. 2. To iodize.

ioderma Any cutaneous reaction caused by iodine and compounds thereof; lesions may vary from mild acneform to granulomatous.

iodic acid A white or colorless crystalline powder, HIO_3; used as an antiseptic and deodorant.

iodide A compound of iodine with another element, especially with potassium or sodium.

iodimetry See iodometry.

iodine A lustrous, grayish-black, corrosive, nonmetallic element; symbol I, atomic number 53, atomic weight 126.91; used as an antiseptic and in the diagnosis and treatment of thyroid disease; it has no natural isotopes; its most widely used artificial isotopes are ^{131}I and [125]I.

  protein-bound i. (PBI) Thyroid hormone in its circulating form, consisting of one or more of the iodothyronines bound to one or more of the serum proteins. Also called serum protein bound iodine.

[125]**iodine** (^{125}I) Radioisotope used as a label in radioimmunoassay; has a half-life of 60 days.

[131]**iodine** (^{131}I) A beta-emitting radioactive isotope with a half-life of 8.05 days; used to deliver therapeutic doses of radiation to the thyroid gland and to certain types of tumors; it has limited use in imaging the thyroid and adrenal glands.

iodism Poisoning from the prolonged use of iodine or an iodide.

iodize To treat or combine with iodine.

iodochlorhydroxyquin Compound used topically for a variety of skin disorders; also used as an amebicide; Vioform®.

iodoform A lemon-yellow iodine compound used as an antiseptic.

iodohippurate sodium A radiopaque compound used in radiography of the urinary tract.

iodometry The volumetric determination of the amount of iodine in a compound. Also called iodimetry.

iodophilia Affinity for iodine; said of certain cells.

iodopsin A color-sensitive violet pigment composed of a vitamin A derivative and a protein; present in the cones of the retina and important in color vision. Also called visual violet.

ion An atom or group of atoms or molecules having acquired an electric charge by gaining (cations) or losing (anions) electrons.

  dipolar i. An ion that carries both a positive and a negative charge; amino acids are the most notable dipolar ions, containing the positively charged NH_3 group and the negatively charged COO group. Also called zwitterion.

ion exchange Chemical reaction between an insoluble solid and a solution surrounding the solid through which ions of like charge are interchanged; used in the separation of radioactive isotopes and in water softening.

ion exchanger 1. A solid substance used in ion exchange. 2. Apparatus used to effect ion exchange.

ionic Of, containing, or relating to an ion or ions.

ionization Production of ions (electrically charged atoms or molecules) from neutral atoms or molecules; radiation creates ions by dislocating negatively charged electrons from the atoms they impinge upon.

ionize To separate into ions, totally or partially.

ionophore A molecule (e.g., of an antibiotic drug) that increases the permeability of cell membranes (e.g., of bacterial cells).

ion pair Two particles of opposite charge formed during the interaction of radiation and matter.

iontophoresis 1. Term suggested to denote the movement of ions through an electric field. 2. Introduction of the ions of a medication through intact skin by means of an electric current. Also called ion transfer; ionization; ionic medication.

ipecac, ipecacuanha The dried root of *Cephaelis ipecacuanha* or *Cephaelis acuminata*, a shrub of South America; used as an emetic, as an expectorant, and in the treatment of amebic dysentery.

  i. syrup A suspension of ipecac alkaloids that induces vomiting; available without prescription.

ipsilateral Occurring or located on the same side; e.g., symptoms occurring on the same side of a brain lesion.

iridectomy Surgical removal of a portion of the iris.

  peripheral i. Surgical removal of a minute portion of the periphery of the iris, as in the treatment of narrow angle glaucoma.

iridemia Bleeding from the iris.

iridencleisis One of the filtering operations for glaucoma in which a portion of the iris is cut and incarcerated in an incision on the border of the cornea for the purpose of draining the fluid from the anterior and posterior chambers of the eye.

irides Plural of iris.

iridescent Displaying a changeable, colorful, metallic luster.

iridesis Surgical procedure in which a portion of the iris is brought out through an incision in the cornea and fixed with a suture.

iridic Relating to the iris.

iridium A whitish-yellow metallic element, symbol Ir, atomic number 77, atomic weight 192.2; of all chemical elements, it has the greatest resistance to corrosion.

iridization The multicolor halo around a bright light observed by persons afflicted with glaucoma.

iridocapsulitis Inflammation of the iris and the capsule of the lens of the eye.

iridocele Protrusion of a portion of the iris through a defect or wound in the cornea.

iridochoroiditis Inflammation of both the iris and the vascular coat of the eyeball.

iridocoloboma Congenital absence of a portion of the iris.

iridoconstrictor 1. Anything that causes contraction of the pupil, as a nerve or a chemical. 2. The circular muscle fibers of the iris.

iridocyclectomy Surgical removal of the iris and ciliary body.

iridocyclitis Inflammation of the iris and the ciliary body. Also called anterior uveitis.

iridodialysis Separation of a portion of the iris from its attachment to the ciliary body.

iridodilator That which causes dilation of the pupil; denoting the sympathetic ciliary nerve fibers that innervate the pupillary dilator muscle or any chemical that causes constriction of that muscle.

iridodonesis Abnormal trembling of the iris upon movement of the eye, as may occur in partial dislocation (subluxation) of the lens.

iridokeratitis Inflammation of the iris and cornea.

iridokinesia, iridokinesis The movement of the iris resulting in dilation and contraction of the pupil.

iridomalacia Degenerative softening of the iris as a result of disease.

iridoplegia Paralysis of the iris.

iridosclerotomy Incision into the sclera and the margin of the iris.

iridotomy Incision into the iris.

iris, *pl.* **irides** The doughnut-shaped part of the eye, situated between the cornea and the crystalline lens, and separating the anterior and posterior chambers; the contraction of the iris alters the size of the pupil; the amount of pigment in it determines the color of the eye.

  i. bombé A bulging forward of the iris caused by pressure from the aqueous humor in the posterior chamber, which cannot pass to the anterior chamber because of adhesion of the pupillary border of the

erythroblastic island

reticulum cell

reticulocyte

red blood cell

pseudopodlike cytoplasmic extension

ingested nucleus

contracting normoblast expelling nucleus with corona of hemoglobin

normoblast

pronormoblast

maturation of red blood cell precursors

ilium

anterior superior iliac spine

hipbone

acetabulum

spine of ischium

pubis

ischium

obturator foramen

alpha cell (produces glucagon)

delta cell (produces gastrin and somatostatin)

islet of Langerhans

beta cell (produces insulin)

iris to the anterior surface of the lens.

iritic Relating to iritis.

iritis Inflammation of the iris.

iron A metallic element, symbol Fe, atomic number 26, atomic weight 55.85; present in the body as a component of hemoglobin, myoglobin, cytochrome, and the proteins catalase and peroxidase; its role in the body is predominantly concerned with cellular respiration.

iron-59 (^{59}Fe) A radioactive beta-emitter iron isotope with a half-life of 45.1 days; used as a tracer for erythrocyte studies and ferrokinetics.

iron storage disease Accumulation of excess iron in the tissues of many organs, especially the liver and pancreas, leading to fibrosis and functional insufficiency. Also called hemochromatosis.

irradiate To treat with or expose to radiation.

irradiation 1. Exposure to the action of rays. **2.** The condition of having been subjected to radiation. **3.** Therapy by exposure to radiation.

irrational Contrary to reason or to the principles of logic.

irreducible Incapable of being reduced in size or made simpler.

irresponsibility The state of not being responsible.

criminal i. The state of not being responsible for

one's own criminal acts, due to a mental defect or disorder.

irrigate To wash out a wound or bodily cavity with water or a medicated liquid.

irrigation The washing out of a wound or a bodily cavity with a stream of fluid.

irritability 1. Responsiveness to stimuli. **2.** Exaggerated responsiveness to a stimulus.

irritable Capable of reacting, or tending to overreact, to a stimulus.

irritant 1. Causing irritation. **2.** A stimulus.

irritation 1. Incipient inflammation of a bodily part. **2.** The act of eliciting a reaction (normal or exaggerated) in the tissues.

ischemia Lack of blood in an area of the body due to mechanical obstruction or functional constriction of a blood vessel.

myocardial i. Ischemia of the heart muscle, usually due to coronary heart disease.

ischemic Relating to local deficiency of blood.

ischia Plural of ischium.

ischial Relating to the ischium.

ischiodynia Pain in the hip.

ischium, *pl.* **ischia** The lowest of three bones comprising each half of the hipbone; the bone on which the body rests when sitting.

ischuria Suppression or retention of the urine.

island An isolated structure or cluster of cells.

erythroblastic i. One or two central reticulum cells of the bone marrow surrounded by normoblasts at various stages of development; the reticulum cells phagocytize the ejected nuclei of the developing normoblasts just prior to their release into the marrow capillaries as erythrocytes; they also ingest worn out or damaged red blood cells, conserving their iron as ferritin.

i. of Langerhans Islet of Langerhans; see under islet.

Reil's i. See insula.

islet Small island.

i. of Langerhans A cluster of cells in the pancreas that produce insulin. Also called island of Langerhans; pancreatic islet.

isoagglutinin An antibody directed against antigenic sites on the red blood cells of individuals of the same species and causing agglutination of the cells.

isoallele A normal allelic gene that can be distinguished from other normal ones only by the differences in the expression of a dominant trait when paired with another gene in a heterozygous person.

isoantibody An antibody produced by one individual which reacts with antigens of another individual of the same species.

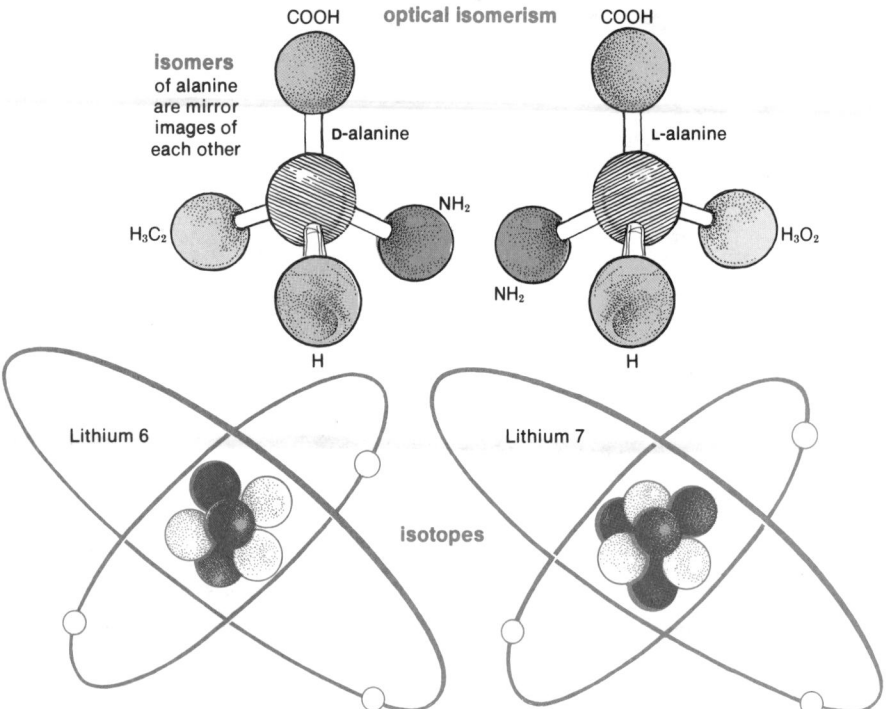

isomers of alanine are mirror images of each other

optical isomerism

D-alanine   L-alanine

isotopes

Lithium 6   Lithium 7

3 electrons, 3 protons, 3 neutrons   3 electrons, 3 protons, 4 neutrons

oleic acid   **geometric isomerism**

cis-2-butane

trans-2-butane

isoantigen An antigen produced by one individual which incites the formation of antibodies in another individual of the same species. Also called homologous antigen; alloantigen.

isobar **1.** Any one of two or more atomic species that have the same atomic weight but not necessarily the same atomic number. **2.** A line on a chart connecting two points of equal barometric pressure at a given time.

isobaric Denoting atoms having the same weight.

isocellular Composed of similar cells.

isochromatic Of uniform or equal color.

isochromosome A chromosome with two identical arms, resulting from transverse rather than longitudinal division of the centromere during meiosis.

isocoria Equal size of the two pupils.

isocortex The non-olfactory, phylogenetically younger part of the cerebral cortex; so called because its cellular and fibrous layers are distributed in a uniform pattern. Also called neocortex; neopallium.

isodynamic Of equal strength.

isoelectric Having an equal number of positive and negative charges; electrically neutral; said of certain molecules.

isoenzyme See isozyme.

isogamete A gamete that has the same size as the one with which it unites.

isogamy Conjugation or fusion of morphologically identical gametes.

isogenic, isogeneic Genetically alike.

isograft A tissue transplant involving two genetically identical or near-identical individuals, such as identical twins or highly inbred animals. Also called syngeneic or isogeneic graft; isotransplant.

isohemagglutinin An antibody that agglutinates blood cells of another individual of the same species; the antibody of blood groups.

isohemolysin A specific antibody from one individual that reacts with antigen in red blood cells of another individual of the same species, resulting in cell destruction. Also called homolysin.

isohemolysis Dissolution of red blood cells caused by reaction between specific antigens present in the cells and antibodies (isohemolysins) from another individual of the same species.

isohydric Having the same pH.

isoimmunization The development of a significant concentration of specific antibody stimulated by the presence of antigens from another individual of the same species, as when fetal cells or other proteins gain access to the maternal circulation, with resulting maternal immunization to the paternal antigens present in the fetal material.

isolate **1.** To separate from a group; to set apart by oneself, as to place an individual in quarantine. **2.** To free or separate (a substance) from a combined form. **3.** In psychoanalysis, to dissociate experiences or memories from the effects pertaining to them, so as to render them a matter of indifference; a defense mechanism against anxiety.

isoleucine An essential amino acid.

isologous Marked by an identical genotype. Also called isoplastic.

isomer One of two or more compounds that have the same percentage composition and molecular weight but different physical or chemical properties due to a different arrangement of the atoms in the molecule.

isomerase A enzyme that catalyzes the conversion of a substance to an isomeric form; e.g., glucosephosphate isomerase.

isomeric Relating to or displaying isomerism.

isomerism The existence of a compound in two or more forms having the same percentage composition and molecular weight but differing in chemical and physical properties, and also in the arrangement of the atoms within the molecule.

  chain i. A form of structural isomerism in which the linkages in the basic chain of carbon atoms vary.

  geometric i. An isomerism in which free rotation about a carbon bond is restricted.

  optical i. Stereoisomerism involving the arrangement of substituents about asymmetric carbon atoms which can rotate the plane of polarized light passing through the substance.

  structural i. Isomerism involving the same atoms in different structural formulas.

isomerization The process in which an isomer is converted into another, as in the action of isomerases.

isometric **1.** Denoting the contraction of a muscle in which its tension is increased without shortening its length; opposed to isotonic. **2.** Of equal dimensions.

isometropia Equality in the refractive state of the two eyes.

isomorphism Similarity of shape or structure.

isoniazid Isonicotinic acid hydrazide (INH); used in the treatment of tuberculosis.

isoplastic See isologous.

isopropyl alcohol A secondary toxic alcohol, $(CH_3)_2CHOH$; used in the preparation of cosmetics and medicines for external use.

isoproterenol sulfate A compound used as an inhalation in the treatment of asthma and emphysema.

isopter A contour line in a visual field representing the area in which the visual acuity is the same as that measured with a specific test target.

isosexual **1.** Relating to characteristics of both sexes in one person. **2.** Denoting the traits of an individual which are characteristic of the sex to which the individual belongs.

isosmotic Having the same osmotic pressure as another fluid.

isospora A genus of coccidia; some species are parasitic in man's intestines and pathogenic.

isosporiasis Infection by *Isospora belli* (genus Isospora) usually causing mild, self-limiting diarrhea except in cases of AIDS, where it causes chronic watery diarrhea and weight loss.

isothenuria Lack of variation in the specific gravity of urine, regardless of amount of fluid intake; inability to concentrate or dilute the urine above or below, respectively, the osmolality of plasma, generally corresponding to a specific gravity of 1.010.

isotherapy Prevention of disease by using the agent that causes the disease, i.e., vaccines.

isothermal Relating to or of the same temperature.

isotonic Of equal tension or osmotic pressure, usually referring to the osmotic concentration of blood plasma.

isotonicity **1.** Equality of tension, as between two muscles. **2.** Equality of osmotic pressure, as between two solutions.

isotope One of two or more chemical elements in which all atoms have the same atomic number but varying atomic weights, due to unequal numbers of neutrons in their nuclei; many are radioactive; designated by the chemical symbol and a superscript number representing the atomic weight, as ^{12}C (isotope of carbon with atomic weight of 12).

  radioactive i. An isotope with an unstable nucleus that emits ionizing radiation in stabilizing itself.

  stable i. An isotope of a chemical element that shows no inclination to undergo radioactive breakdown; a nonradioactive nuclide.

isotoxin A poison in the blood or tissues of an animal that only has toxic effects on other animals of the same species, not on that animal itself.

isotransplant See isograft.

isotropic, isotropous Equal in all directions.

isovalericacidemia A disorder of leucine metabolism characterized by elevated serum isovaleric acid upon protein ingestion or during infectious episodes; associated with recurrent episodes of coma, acidosis, and malodorous sweat; autosomal recessive inheritance.

isovolumic, isovolumetric Equal or unchanged volume; occurring without an associated alteration in volume, as when, in early ventricular systole, the muscle fibers initially increase their tension without

isthmus of external auditory meatus

middle ear chamber

isthmus of auditory tube

bone

cartilage

pinna

tympanic membrane

opening into nasopharynx

hyoid bone

thyrohyoid membrane

thyroid cartilage

isthmus of thyroid gland

trachea

isthmus of uterine tube

fimbria

Progestasert®

Copper 7®

Lippes Loop®

Saf-T-Coil®

posterior aspect of uterus

infundibulum

cervix

IUD's

shortening so that ventricular volume remains unchanged.

isozyme One of a group of enzymes that catalyze the same chemical reaction but have different physical properties. Also called isoenzyme.

isthmus 1. A narrow section of tissue connecting two larger parts. 2. A narrow passage connecting two larger cavities or tubular structures.

  i. of aorta A slight constriction of the aorta between the left subclavian artery and the ligamentum arteriosum.

  i. of auditory tube The narrowest part of the auditory (eustachian) tube, at the junction of the bony and cartilaginous portions.

  i. of cingular lobe The narrow posterior portion of the cingulate gyrus which joins the hippocampal gyrus. Also called isthmus of the limbic lobe.

  i. of external auditory meatus The narrowest portion of the auditory tube near the junction of the bony and cartilaginous parts.

  i. of limbic lobe See isthmus of the cingular lobe.

  i. of nasopharynx The opening between the free edges of the soft palate and the posterior pharyngeal wall.

  i. of oropharynx The constricted aperture by which the mouth is connected with the pharynx;

located at the interval between the two palatoglossal arches.

  i. of prostate The anterior portion of the base of the prostate gland.

  i. of rhombencephalon A marked constriction of the embryonic brain from which the anterior medullary velum is formed; it connects the rhombencephalon with the mesencephalon.

  i. of thyroid The narrow, central portion connecting the two lateral lobes of the thyroid gland.

  i. of urethra The slightly constricted junction of the urethra between the cavernous and membranous portions.

  i. of uterine tube The narrow, medial portion of the uterine tube at its junction with the uterus.

  i. of uterus The elongated constricted part of the uterus between the cervix and the uterine body; it is about 1 cm in length.

  i. Vieussensi The ring or margin of the fossa ovalis.

itch 1. A skin sensation and/or irritation causing a desire to scratch. 2. Common name for scabies.

  barber's i. See tinea barbae.

  swimmer's i. An itchy rash caused by penetration of the skin by the larvae of the worm *Schistosoma mansoni* during immersion in contaminated

fresh water.

iter A passageway leading from one anatomic part to another.

IUD Intrauterine device; see under device.

Ixodes A genus of parasitic ticks (family Ixodidae); transmitters of viral and bacterial diseases to humans and animals.

  I. holocyclus A species prevalent in Australia and South Africa; vector of tick paralysis in sheep, cattle, dogs, and occasionally humans.

  I. pacificus The black-legged tick of California; it infests cattle and deer; may bite humans, causing severe reactions.

  I. persulcatus The vector of Russian spring-summer encephalitis.

  I. ricinus The castor bean tick; it infects cattle, sheep, and wild animals and transmits tularemia, louping ill (infectious encephalomyelitis), and Russian spring-summer encephalitis.

ixodiasis A condition marked by skin lesions and fever caused by ticks, particularly those of the family Ixodidae (hard-bodied ticks).

ixodic Relating to or caused by ticks.

Ixodidae A family of ticks (order Acarina); transmitters of several diseases including tick paralysis. Also called hard ticks.

jimsonweed

Wharton's jelly

umbilical cord

hipbone

ball and socket joint

head of femur

J j

jacket An outer casing, bandage, or garment, especially one extending from the shoulders to the hips.

   Minerva j. A plaster of Paris cast extending from the chin to the hips for immobilization of the lower cervical or upper thoracic spine.

   porcelain j. In dentistry, a porcelain jacket crown.

   strait j. See straightjacket.

jackscrew A device used to approximate or separate teeth or jaw segments.

Jackson's syndrome Paralysis of one side of the tongue, palate, and larynx. Also called syndrome of vago-accessory-hypoglossal paralysis.

jactitation The tossing to and fro of a distressed patient in bed; extreme restlessness.

Jakob-Creutzfeldt disease See Creutzfeldt-Jakob disease.

Jansky-Bielschowsky disease Cerebral sphingolipidosis; see under sphingolipidosis.

Janus green B An azo dye used as a supravital stain for the demonstration of mitochondria.

jargon 1. Language peculiar to a trade, profession, class, etc. 2. Incoherent, meaningless utterance. See also paraphasia.

jaundice Yellow pigmentation of the skin and/or sclera caused by high levels of bilirubin in the blood. Also called icterus.

   familial nonhemolytic j. Jaundice in the absence of liver damage, biliary obstruction, or hemolysis; the unconjugated bilirubin is elevated; believed to be due to an inborn error of metabolism. Also called Gilbert's disease.

   hemolytic j. Jaundice resulting from hemolysis.

   hepatocellular j. A form due to disease of the liver cells.

   obstructive j. Jaundice caused by obstruction of the bile ducts.

   physiologic j. Mild jaundice of the newborn, primarily due to immaturity of the liver. Also called

physiologic icterus.

jaundiced 1. Marked by jaundice. 2. Yellowish.

jaw One of the two bones supporting the teeth; the upper one is the maxilla and the lower one is the mandible.

   lock-j. See trismus.

   lumpy j. See actinomycosis.

jawbone Any bone of the two jaws, especially the mandible.

jejunal Of or relating to the jejunum.

jejunectomy Surgical removal of the jejunum, or a portion of it.

jejunitis Inflammation of the jejunum.

jejunocolostomy Operation in which a communication between the jejunum and the colon is established.

jejunoileitis Inflammation of the jejunum and ileum.

jejunoileostomy Surgical connection between the jejunum and a noncontinuous segment of the ileum.

jejunojejunostomy Surgical joining of two noncontinuous segments of the jejunum.

jejunoplasty Corrective surgery on the jejunum.

jejunostomy The formation of a permanent opening through the abdominal wall into the jejunal part of the small intestine.

jejunotomy Cutting into the jejunum.

jejunum The portion of the small intestine between the duodenum and the ileum; in the adult, it is about 2.5 m in length, with a diameter of approximately 4 cm.

Jellinek's sign Brownish pigmentation of the eyelids, seen in cases of exophthalmic goiter.

jelly A semisolid substance having resilient consistency.

   Wharton's j. The soft, homogenous connective tissue comprising the matrix of the umbilical cord and supporting the umbilical vessels.

jellyfish A free-swimming marine coelenterate

having a gelatinous, umbrella-shaped body and tentacles hanging down into the water; in the tentacles are hairlike structures, called nematocysts, that can be forcibly ejected in order to deposit toxins into the victim's skin; human reaction to stings ranges from skin rashes to death, depending on the species of jellyfish and the sensitivity of the individual; the more sensitive persons experience the symptoms of anaphylactic shock.

Jensen's disease See chorioretinitis.

jerk 1. A sudden abrupt or spasmodic movement. 2. A sudden involuntary muscular contraction following a tap on the muscle or its tendon. Also called muscular reflex or deep tendon reflex.

   ankle j. Calcaneal tendon reflex; see under reflex.

   crossed j. A muscular contraction on one side following a tap on the other side.

   crossed knee j. Movement of one leg when the patellar tendon of the other leg is tapped.

   elbow j. Triceps reflex; see under reflex.

   knee j. Patellar reflex; see under reflex.

jigger Chigoe.

jimsonweed A poisonous plant, *Datura stramonium*, having large funnel-shaped white or purple flowers and prickly fruit. Also called thorn apple.

jitters Extreme nervousness.

joint The point of connection between two or more bones; an articulation.

   amphiarthrodial j. A joint in which the articulating surfaces are united by an articulating disk of fibrocartilage, allowing only slight motion, as between the bodies of the vertebrae. Also called cartilaginous joint; amphiarthrosis.

   ball and socket j. A type of diarthrodial joint in which the globular end of one bone fits into the cuplike cavity of the other, permitting extensive movement in any direction, as seen in the hip and shoulder. Also called spheroidal joint; enarthrosis.

   condyloid j. A type of diarthrodial joint in which the ovoid articular surface of one bone fits into the

amphiarthrodial joint

ribs

costal cartilages

costochondral junctions

dentinoenamel junction

cornea

sclerocorneal junction

sclera

iris

hinge joint (elbow)

elliptical cavity of another, allowing all movements except axial rotation.

diarthrodial j. A joint that permits relatively free movement, characterized by the presence of (a) a layer of cartilage covering the articular surfaces of the bones and (b) a cavity between the bones, the whole being surrounded by a capsule which is lined by synovial membrane. Also called synovial or movable joint; diarthrosis.

gliding j. A type of diarthrodial joint in which the apposed surfaces are more or less flat, permitting a gliding motion, as between the articular processes of the vertebrae. Also called plane joint; arthrodia.

hinge j. A variety of diarthrodial joint which permits only a forward and backward movement, as the hinge of a door; e.g., the interphalangeal joints.

rotary j. A type of diarthrodial joint in which a pivot-like process fits and rotates within a ring which is formed partly of bone and partly of ligaments, as the proximal radioulnar articulation. Also called pivot or trochial joint.

saddle j. A type of synovial joint in which the articular surface of one bone is concave in one direction and convex in a direction at right angles to the first, with the articular surface of the other bone reciprocally convex and concave, as the carpometacarpal joint of the thumb.

spheroidal j. See ball and socket joint.

synarthrodial j. A joint in which two bones are united by fibrous tissue permitting little or no movement between the bones, as the joints between the bones of the skull. Also called fibrous or immovable joint; synarthrosis.

synovial j. See diarthrodial joint.

temporomandibular j. (TMJ) The articulation between the condyle of the mandible and the mandibular fossa and articular tubercle of the temporal bone; divided by a thin oval articular disk into two cavities, each of which is lined by a synovial membrane.

joule **1.** A unit of energy equivalent to that expended when a current of 1 ampere is passed through a resistance of 1 ohm for 1 second. **2.** A unit of energy equivalent to the work done in moving a body 1 meter against a force of 1 newton.

jugal **1.** Connecting. **2.** Relating to the cheek.

jugular **1.** Relating to the neck. **2.** Denoting certain structures in the neck, as a vein.

jugulum The neck or throat.

jugum, *pl.* **juga** A ridge connecting two structures.

juga alveolaria Eminences on the anterior surface of the alveolar processes of the maxilla and mandible, caused by the roots of the incisors and cuspids.

juga cerebralia The cerebral ridges on the internal surface of the cranial bones corresponding to the sulci of the brain. Also called cerebral ridges of cranium.

j. petrosum The eminence of the petrous part of the temporal bone formed by the superior semicircular canal. Also called petrosal ridge.

j. sphenoidale The elevated smooth anterior surface of the body of the sphenoid bone that connects the lesser wings; it forms part of the anterior cranial fossa.

juice A digestive secretion; e.g., gastric juice, pancreatic juice, etc.

junction **1.** A joint or articulation. **2.** The line of union of two parts or surfaces.

cementodentinal j. The surface at which the cementum and dentin of a root of a tooth meet.

cementoenamel j. The line around a tooth where the enamel of its crown and the cementum of its root meet. Also called cervical line.

conjunctivocorneal j. The area of the eye, at the limbus, where the fibrous membrane of the conjunctiva ends and only the epithelium continues centrally to cover the cornea.

costochondral j. The point of articulation between the sternal end of a rib and the lateral end of its cartilage.

dentinoenamel j. The surface at which the dentin and the enamel of the crown of a tooth meet.

esophagogastric j. The junction of the esophagus and the stomach.

gap j. Intercellular space containing channels which connect adjacent cells; seen between certain nerve cells; and in cardiac and smooth muscles.

J j. The point at the end of the QRS complex of the electrocardiogram (principal deflection) and the beginning of the ST segment (segment immediately following the QRS complex). Also called J point.

mucocutaneous j. The area of transition from a mucous membrane to the epidermis.

myoneural j. Neuromuscular junction.

neuromuscular j. The area of contact between the motor nerve and the muscle; the end of the nerve broadens into an endplate that fits into a depression in the skeletal muscle fiber.

sclerocorneal j. The area of the eye, at the limbus, where the sclera and cornea join.

junctura, *pl.* **juncturae** Latin for a joining. Also called articulation.

jurisprudence, medical The application of medical knowledge to legal questions; e.g., in cases of death by poisoning. Also called forensic or legal medicine.

jury-mast An upright bar used in conjunction with a plaster of Paris jacket; used as a head support in cases of diseases of the spine, as in Pott's disease.

juxtaglomerular Near or adjacent to a glomerulus of the kidney.

j. apparatus See under apparatus.

juxtamedullary Referring to that portion of the inner cortex of the kidney adjacent to the medulla, e.g., juxtamedullary glomeruli.

juxtapose To position side by side.

juxtaposition The state of being side by side; the act of placing side by side.

juxtapyloric Located near the pylorus.

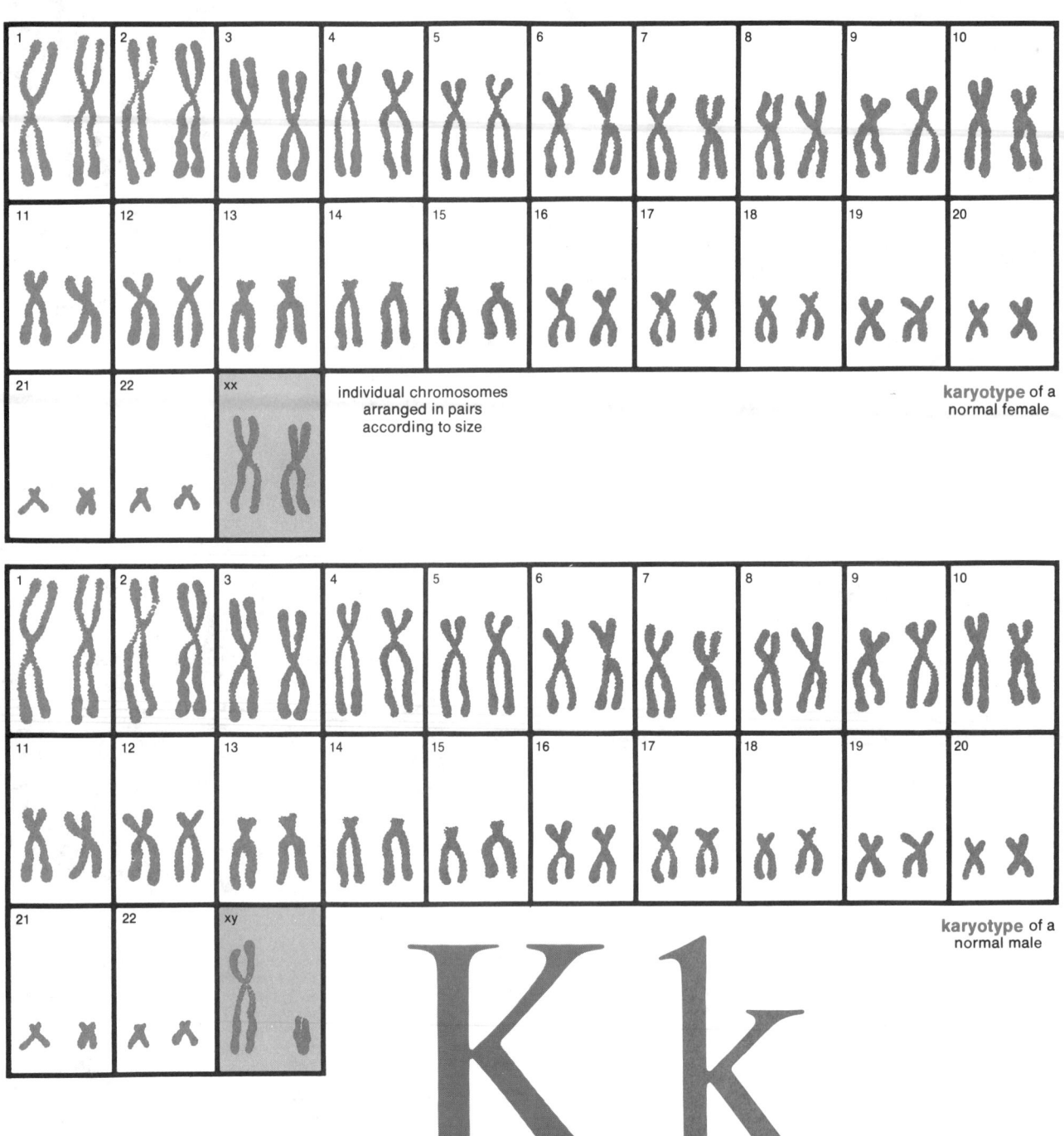

individual chromosomes
arranged in pairs
according to size

karyotype of a
normal female

karyotype of a
normal male

K k

_κ_ Kappa.

kala azar Visceral leishmaniasis; see under leishmaniasis.

kaliopenia Potassium deficiency in the body.

kalium Latin for potassium.

kaliuresis Increased excretion of potassium in the urine. Also called kaluresis.

kaliuretic 1. Relating to kaliuresis. 2. An agent that induces kaliuresis.

kallikrein A peptidase which acts on alpha$_2$ globulins in plasma or in glands to produce kinins.

Kallmann's syndrome Hypogonadism with anosmia; see under hypogonadism.

kaluresis See kaliuresis.

K and k blood groups See Kell blood group.

kaolin A fine, whitish clay used in ceramics and as a demulcent and adsorbent. Also called Fuller's earth; terra alba.

kappa The tenth letter of the Greek alphabet, _κ_; used to denote the tenth in a series.

Kartagener's syndrome Displacement of the viscera to the opposite side of the body (situs inversus) associated with dilation of the bronchial tubes (bronchiectasis) and chronic sinusitis.

karyochrome A nerve cell having a nucleus that stains deeply.

karyocyte A nucleated cell; usually referring to a young nucleated red blood cell (normoblast).

karyogamy Fusion of the nuclei of two cells during cell conjugation.

karyogenesis The formation of a cell nucleus.

karyogram See karyotype.

karyokinesis See mitosis.

karyolobic Having a lobulated nucleus.

karyolymph The clear homogeneous liquid part of a cell nucleus.

karyolysis The destruction or dissolution of the nucleus of a cell.

karyomorphism 1. Development of a cell nucleus. 2. Referring to the nuclear shapes of cells.

karyon The cell nucleus.

karyoplasm The protoplasm of the cell nucleus. Also called nucleoplasm.

karyopyknosis Shrinkage of cell nuclei and condensation of the chromatin.

karyorrhexis Fragmentation of the cell nucleus.

karyosome One of the spherical masses of chromatin resembling a knot in the chromatin network of a resting nucleus during mitosis. Also called net knot; chromatin nucleolus; false nucleolus.

karyotype 1. The chromosome characteristics of an individual or a species. 2. A systematized presentation of individual chromosomes of a single cell, photographed during the metaphase stage of mitosis and arranged in pairs according to size.

karyotyping Analysis of chromosomes.

Kawasaki disease Mucocutaneous lymph node syndrome.

Kell blood group K and k blood groups; red blood cell antigens, specified by the K gene; antibody to the K antigen (anti-K) is the cause of hemolytic disease of the newborn; named after a Mrs. Kell, in whose blood the antibodies were discovered.

keloid A nodular, nonencapsulated, highly hyperplastic mass of scar tissue.

keloidosis The presence of multiple keloids.

keloplasty Surgical removal of a scar or keloid.

Kelvin (K) Relating to the absolute scale of temperature. See scale, absolute.

Kennedy's syndrome See Foster-Kennedy syndrome.

keratalgia Pain in the cornea.

keratectasia Protrusion or bulging of the cornea due to a thinning or weakening of the corneal tissue. Also called kerectasis.

keratoconus

trephine

keratoplasty

donor's eye

graft from donor's eye

cornea of patient's eye

lens

keratoscope

keratome

keratocyte

keratectomy Surgical removal of the superficial layers of the cornea affected by scarring or degeneration, without replacing the excised tissue with a graft.

keratic 1. Horny. 2. Relating to the cornea.

keratin The protein present largely in, and forming the main components of, epidermal structures such as hair, nails, horns, feathers, etc.

   alpha-k. Keratin in its folded form (as in normal hair).

   beta-k. Keratin in its extended form (as in stretched hair).

keratinization The formation of keratin or a horny layer.

keratinize To become horny.

keratinosome Membrane-coating granule; see under granule.

keratinous Relating to or consisting of keratin.

keratitis Inflammation of the cornea. Also called corneitis.

   fascicular k. Superficial corneal ulcer that moves from the periphery to the center of the cornea, carrying with it a narrow band of blood vessels from the conjunctiva; it remains superficial and terminates in a linear opacity; secondary to phlyctenular keratitis.

   herpes simplex k. Herpes simplex infection of the cornea.

   interstitial k. Deep inflammation and vascularization of the cornea involving primarily the middle layer; found chiefly in children and young adults as a late manifestation of congenital syphilis.

   k. sicca A chronic condition of the cornea associated with absence of mucous and lacrimal secretions; usually seen in women at the time of menopause.

   phlyctenular k. Small gray nodules that break down forming a shallow ulcer; usually spreading from the conjunctiva; seen most commonly in the corneal periphery.

keratoacanthoma A rapidly growing benign skin nodule, usually with a central depression, histologically resembling squamous cell carcinoma and occurring chiefly on the face.

keratocele Hernia of the posterior limiting (Descemet's) membrane of the cornea.

keratochromatosis Discoloration of the cornea.

keratoconjunctivitis Inflammation of the cornea and conjunctiva.

   epidemic k. A contagious form caused by a type 8 adenovirus, occurring mainly in persons exposed to dust and trauma in industry. Also called shipyard

eye.

keratoconometer An instrument for determining the degree of keratoconus.

keratoconus A degenerative, noninflammatory, central, conical protrusion of the cornea; usually bilateral; inherited as an autosomal recessive trait. Also called conical cornea.

keratocyte 1. A ruptured or mutilated red blood cell (erythrocyte). 2. One of the flattened cells between the lamellae of the cornea. Also called corneal corpuscle.

keratodermia Thickening of the horny layer of the skin.

   k. blennorrhagica See keratosis blennorrhagica.

   k. palmaris et plantaris Thickening of the skin occurring in symmetrical patches on the palms and soles. Also called keratodermia symmetrica.

   k. symmetrica See keratodermia palmaris et plantaris.

keratogenesis The formation of horny tissue.

keratogenous Causing the production of horny tissue such as nails, feathers, etc.

keratohelcosis Ulceration of the cornea.

keratohemia The presence of blood deposits in the cornea.

keratoid Horny.

keratoiridoscope Instrument used to examine the cornea and the iris.

keratoiritis Inflammation of the cornea and iris.

keratoleptynsis Plastic surgery of the eye; removal of the anterior surface of the cornea and replacement by bulbar conjunctiva.

keratolysis The peeling and shedding of the epidermis.

keratolytic Causing scaling of the epidermis. Also called desquamative.

keratomalacia Dryness, softening, and dissolution of the cornea caused by severe deficiency of vitamin A.

keratome A surgical knife for incising the cornea. Also called keratotome.

keratometer An instrument for measuring the curvature of the cornea.

keratometry The measuring of the anterior curvature of the cornea with a keratometer.

keratomycosis Fungus infection of the cornea.

keratonosus Any disease of the cornea.

keratonyxis Surgical puncture of the cornea, as for needling the lens for soft cataract.

keratopathy A noninflammatory disease of the cornea, distinguished from keratitis.

   calcific band k. Horizontal opacity of the cornea

caused by deposition of calcium salts in its anterior layer; associated with certain inflammatory, metabolic, and degenerative disorders, especially juvenile rheumatoid arthritis.

   climatic k. Corneal degeneration beginning as minute, subepithelial, yellow droplets in the corneal periphery which, as the disorder progresses, extend toward the center, causing blurred vision; seen mainly in persons who spend a great deal of time outdoors; believed to be caused by prolonged exposure to ultraviolet light.

keratoplasty Operation in which the cornea or a portion of it is removed and replaced by healthy corneal tissue (graft). Also called corneal transplantation.

   lamellar k. Procedure in which only the superficial layer of the cornea is removed for the treatment of superficial corneal opacities or recurrent superficial lesions.

   penetrating k. Procedure in which the entire corneal thickness is removed.

keratoprosthesis Plastic corneal implant.

keratorhexis Rupture of the cornea due to a perforating ulcer or to injury. Also written keratorrhexis.

keratoscleritis Inflammation of the cornea and the sclera.

keratoscope Instrument containing a disc of concentric rings used to examine the curvature of the cornea.

keratoscopy Inspection of the anterior surface of the cornea with a keratoscope.

keratose 1. Relating to or marked by keratosis. 2. Horny.

keratosis A circumscribed overgrowth of the horny layer of the epidermis.

   actinic k. See senile keratosis.

   arsenical k. Keratosis resulting from chronic arsenic poisoning.

   k. blennorrhagica Pustules and crusts associated with Reiter's disease. Also called keratodermia blennorrhagica.

   k. pilaris A recurring form of keratosis limited to the hair follicles; most often seen on the upper outer arms and thighs of children and young women.

   seborrheic k. Flat, warty, benign lesions seen in persons after the third decade of life.

   senile k. Premalignant warty lesions occurring on the sun-exposed parts of the aged. Also called actinic keratosis.

keratotome See keratome.

keratotomy Surgical incision through the cornea.

artificial kidney

horseshoe kidney

keraunophobia Abnormal fear of thunder and lightning.

kerectomy Keratectomy.

kerion Suppurative inflammation of the scalp, a complicaton of ringworm; it may simulate a carbuncle, with follicular pustules, exudate, and crusting.

Kerley lines B lines of Kerley; see under line.

kernicterus The neurologic complication of unconjugated hyperbilirubinemia in the infant, causing staining of nuclear masses in the brain and spinal cord by bile pigment, with associated degenerative changes; the clinical signs include spasticity, opisthotonos, twitching, and convulsions.

Kernig's sign Patient's inability to extend his leg completely when lying on his back with his thigh flexed at right angles with his trunk; seen in meningitis.

keroid 1. Resembling the cornea. 2. Horny.

keto acid An acid having the general formula R–CO–COOH.

ketoacidosis Acidosis (diabetic) produced by the presence of an excessive amount of ketone acids in the body.

ketoaciduria Excessive ketonic acids in the urine.

   branched-chain k. See maple syrup urine disease.

ketogenesis The production of ketone bodies (acetone substances).

ketol See indole.

ketone Any of a group of compounds having a carbonyl group (CO) linking to hydrocarbon groups.

ketonemia The presence of ketone bodies in the blood.

ketones Ketone bodies; see under body.

ketonization Conversion into a ketone.

ketonuria The presence of ketone bodies in the urine.

ketose A carbohydrate containing a ketone group in its molecule.

ketosis Abnormally large amounts of ketone (acetone) bodies in the tissues and fluids.

17-ketosteroid A steroid compound with a ketone radical on the seventeenth carbon; a steroid hormone derived from the adrenal gland or gonads; present in excess in the urine in certain tumors of the adrenal cortex; the metabolites of dehydroisoandrosterone are 17-ketosteroids and the metabolites of other steroids, including cortisol and 17-α-OH progesterone, may be oxidized to 17-ketosteroids; normal values in the urine are 6–18 mg/24 hr in the male and 4–13 mg/24 hr in the female.

ketosuccinic acid See oxaloacetic acid.

kick A forceful thrust.

   atrial k. A forceful atrial contraction that tends to improve the performance of the ventricle; usually occurring in aortic stenosis or ischemic heart disease.

Kidd blood group The red blood cell antigens, specified by the Jk gene, that react with the antibodies designated anti-Jk^a and anti-Jk^b; Named after a Mrs. Kidd, in whose blood the antibodies were discovered.

kidney One of two bean-shaped organs, approximately 11 cm long, located in the posterior part of the abdomen, behind the peritoneum, on either side of the spine; it serves to regulate acid-base concentration and water balance in the tissues and to discharge metabolic wastes as urine.

   artificial k. Popular name for hemodialyzer, an apparatus used as a substitute for the kidneys to purify the blood in acute or chronic kidney failure; toxic elements are removed by passing the blood through a semipermeable membrane lying in a bathing solution, then returning it to the body.

   contracted k. A small scarred kidney due to abnormally large amounts of fibrous tissue.

   crush k. Degeneration of renal tubule epithelium following crushing injuries of muscle.

   ectopic k. A permanently abnormally placed kidney; distinguished from a floating kidney.

   floating k. The excessively mobile kidney in nephroptosia; distinguished from ectopic kidney. Also called wandering kidney.

   Goldblatt k. Kidney with impaired arterial blood supply, causing arterial hypertension.

   horseshoe k. Kidney resulting from the fusion of the lower extremities of the two kidneys across the body midline.

   medullary sponge k. Congenital defect marked by cyst formation of the pyramids of the kidney, occasionally associated with dilation of the collecting tubules and formation of stones; often asymptomatic and not generally a cause of renal failure. See also cystic disease of renal medulla.

   polycystic k. A kidney whose substance has been largely replaced by tightly packed cysts of varying sizes resembling a bunch of grapes. See also polycystic disease of kidney.

   wandering k. See floating kidney.

Kikuchi's disease Disease of unknown cause, chiefly affecting young women; marked by unilateral, usually painless, cervical adenopathy. Also called histiocytic necrotizing lymphadenitis.

kilobase (kb) One thousand base pairs in a DNA sequence.

kilocalorie (kcal) Large calorie; see under calorie.

kilogram (kg) One thousand grams or 2.2046

pounds.

kiloliter (kl) One thousand liters, about 1,057 quarts.

kilovolt (kv) A thousand volts.

Kimmelstiel-Wilson disease See Kimmelstiel-Wilson syndrome.

Kimmelstiel-Wilson nodular lesion Nodular glomerulosclerosis; see under glomerulosclerosis.

Kimmelstiel-Wilson syndrome Disorder occurring in patients with diabetes mellitus of several years' duration, marked by hypertension, edema, and proteinuria associated with intercapillary glomerulosclerosis. Also called Kimmelstiel-Wilson disease.

kinanesthesia Loss of ability to perceive sensation of movement.

kinase An enzyme that activates proenzymes or zymogens (inactive enzymes).

kindred An extended group of related persons. Also called family group; clan; tribe.

kinematics The science of motion, particularly of the bodily parts.

kinesalgia Pain occurring during muscular movement.

kinescope Instrument for testing the refraction of the eye; consisting of a disc with a slit, moved across the front of the eye, through which the patient observes a fixed object.

kinesia Motion sickness.

kinesics The study of nonverbal body motion as it relates to communication, as shrugs, waves, etc.

kinesiology The study of muscular movement as it applies to treatment.

kinesitherapy Treatment employing movement. Also called kinetotherapy.

kinesthesia The sense perception of muscular movement by which the individual can estimate the position of his body members.

kinetic Relating to or produced by motion.

kinetics The study of all aspects of motion and forces affecting motion.

   chemical k. The study of the velocities of chemical reactions.

   first-order k. The kinetics characteristic of a reaction whose rate of movement is proportional to the concentration of a single substance.

   zero-order k. The kinetics characteristic of a reaction that proceeds at a constant rate regardless of the concentrations of reactants.

kinetocardiogram Graphic representation of chest wall vibrations caused by heart activity.

kinetocardiograph Apparatus used to make graphic representations of low-frequency move-cortex

interlobular arterioles

arcuate artery

interlobar

kidney

renal artery

papilla of pyramid

ureter

medulla

nephron

arcuate artery

interlobar artery

interlobar vein

collecting duct

filtration membrane of glomerulus

endothelium

basement membrane

podocyte

urinary space

Side View

kidney

ureter

bladder

urethra

adrenal gland

kidneys

Front View

Back View

minor calix

major calix

renal pelvis

ureter

235

articular surface of femur

femur

knee

tibia

fibula

patellar ligament

patella

housemaid's knee

surgeon's kno

clove-hitch knot

granny knot

reef knot

---

ments of the chest wall over the heart area.

kinetochore See centromere.

kinetoplasm 1. The chromophil substance of nerve cells. **2.** The most contractile portion of a cell.

kinetoplast A rod-shaped structure, located at the base of the flagellum of parasitic flagellates; it divides independently prior to the division of the nucleus.

King-Armstrong unit King unit; see under unit.

kinin Any of various small peptides with proinflammatory properties, such as increasing permeability of blood vessels.

kink 1. A bend. **2.** A muscle spasm, usually painful.

kissing disease Infectious mononucleosis; see under mononucleosis.

Klebsiella A genus of coliform bacteria (family Enterobacteriaceae), composed of motile and nonmotile gram-negative microorganisms.

K. pneumoniae The causative agent of Friedländer's pneumonia; normally found in the nose, mouth, and intestinal tract of healthy persons; it causes less than 10 percent of all acute bacterial pneumonias and is frequently present as a secondary invader in the lungs of individuals with chronic pulmonary diseases. Also called Friedländer's bacillus.

kleptomania A morbid compulsion to steal.

Klinefelter's syndrome Common form of genetic disease in males arising from aberrations in sex chromosomes; usually characterized by abnormally long legs, extremely small testes, gynecomastia, eunuchoidism, azoospermia, and a general deficiency of secondary male features such as a deep voice and a beard; syndrome exhibits a classic pattern of 47 XXY karyotype (an extra X chromosome). Also called XXY syndrome; seminiferous tubule dysgenesis.

Klippel-Feil syndrome Congenital defect marked primarily by fusion of one or more cervical vertebrae, resulting in a characteristic short, thick neck with limited movements. Also called cervical fusion syndrome.

knee The articulation between the femur and the tibia.

housemaid's k. Inflammation of the bursa in front of the patella (kneecap), usually due to repeated trauma. Also called prepatellar bursitis.

k. reflex See reflex, patellar.

knock k. See genu valgum.

locked k. Limited motion of the knee due to the presence of loose tissue, such as cartilage, in the joint.

kneecap See patella.

knife A cutting instrument with a sharp blade.

Bard-Parker k. A surgical knife with a disposable blade.

Blair k. A knife with a long sharp blade used to cut skin grafts.

Buck k. A periodontal knife with a spearlike point, used for incising the gums between the teeth.

cautery k. A knife connected to an electric battery that sears tissue while cutting, to control bleeding.

Merrifield k. A gingivectomy knife with a long, narrow, triangular blade.

knitting The union or growing together of the fragments of a broken bone.

knob A protuberance; a nodule.

knock, pericardial Heart sound occurring early during diastole, after the second heart sound but earlier than the normal physiologic third sound; common in patients with constrictive pericarditis. Also called early diastolic sound; third heart sound of constrictive pericarditis.

knot 1. An intertwining of the ends of one or two cords, tapes, sutures, etc., so that they cannot be separated. **2.** A node or circumscribed swelling. **3.** To join the ends.

clove-hitch k. A knot made with two continuous loops around a part.

flat k. See reef knot.

granny k. An insecure double knot in which the two stretches of cord do not pass together under the loop but are separated by it.

reef k. A double knot in which the free ends are parallel to the standing ends of the first knot. Also called flat or square knot.

square k. See reef knot.

surgeon's k. Knot in which the thread is passed twice through the loop of the first knot with a simple knot tied over the first.

knuckle The dorsal part or region around a joint of the finger, especially of the metacarpophalangeal joints of the flexed fingers.

Koch's law Koch's postulates; see under postulate.

Koch-Weeks bacillus See *Haemophilus influenzae*.

koilonychia A rarely seen symptom of iron deficiency anemia in which the nails are concave or spoon-shaped.

koilosternia Funnel chest; see under chest.

kola nut The large caffeine-containing seed of the *Cola acuminata* tree; its extract is used in beverages.

Korsakoff's syndrome Severe impairment of recent memory and inability to learn new informa-

tion, seen in disorders predominantly affecting the hippocampal-mammillary system in the brain, especially thiamine deficiency; confabulation is usually a prominent feature; often associated with Wernicke's disease and called by some the Wernicke-Korsakoff syndrome. Also called Korsakoff's psychosis.

Krabbe's disease A disease of late infancy marked by progressive cerebral demyelination and large globoid phagocytic cells in the white matter of the brain and spinal cord; the development of the infant usually ceases. Also called globoid cell leukodystrophy.

kraurosis vulvae Drying and shriveling of the vagina and vulva accompanied by itchiness and pain.

Krebs' cycle Tricarboxylic acid cycle; see under cycle.

krypton One of the inert gaseous elements found in the atmosphere; symbol Kr, atomic number 36, atomic weight 83.80.

krypton-85 (^{85}Kr) A radioactive form of krypton, used as a tracer, as in studying regional blood flow.

Kufs' disease Cerebral sphingolipidosis; see under sphingolipidosis.

kuru A progressive fatal disease of the central nervous system seen in certain natives of New Guinea; caused by a slow virus. Also called laughing sickness.

Kussmaul's sign Great increase in jugular venous distention and pressure during inspiration; seen in patients with cardiac tamponade.

kwashiorkor A nutritional deficiency syndrome of children due to inadequate intake of proteins relative to the caloric intake; marked by edema, apathy, anorexia, diarrhea, and skin lesions with characteristically low serum protein, especially albumin.

kymograph An instrument for graphically recording pressure variations.

kymoscope Apparatus used to measure pulse waves or the variations in blood pressure.

kynurenic acid A crystalline compound; product of tryptophan metabolism.

kyphos Greek for hump.

kyphoscoliosis Abnormal backward and lateral curvature of the spine; it not only deforms but progressively disables, impairing first lung function and then heart function.

kyphosis Abnormal, rearward increase in the curvature of the thoracic spine. Also called hunchback; humpback.

kyrtorrhachic Relating to curvature of the lumbar spine with the concavity backward.

uterus

cochlea

membranous labyrinth

semi-circular ducts

clitoris

vagina

labium minus

labium majus

labia uteri

L l

lactose

λ   The eleventh letter of the Greek alphabet, lambda.

L+   The lethal plus dose; symbol for a toxin-anti-toxin mixture of diphtheria containing a fatal dose in excess, which will kill an experimental animal in four days.

la belle indifference   Belle indifference.

labia   Plural of labium.

labial   Relating to lips.

labile 1.   Unstable or easily changed, as drugs or preparations that are readily altered when exposed to heat. **2.** In psychiatry, emotionally unstable.

lability   Instability or the condition of being changeable.

labiochorea   Spasm and stiffening of the lips during speech.

labiogingival   Relating to the area of junction of the lips and the gums.

labiograph   Device used to record the movements of the lips in speaking.

labiomental   Relating to the lower lip and the chin.

labionasal   Relating to the lips and nose.

labioplacement   The abnormal position of a tooth toward the lips.

labioplasty   Plastic surgery of the lips. Also called cheiloplasty.

labioversion   Deviation of teeth toward the lips.

labium, *pl.* **labia**   A lip or liplike structure.
  l. majus   One of the two large folds of tissue surrounding the vulva. Commonly called major lip.
  l. minus   One of the two narrow folds within the labia majora. Commonly called minor lip.
  labia uteri   The margin of the vaginal portion of the cervix bounding the opening of the uterus (external os); designated as anterior and posterior labia or lips.

labor   Parturition.
  dry l.   Premature spontaneous breaking of the amniotic sac and escape of most of the fluid that surrounds the fetus, occurring before the onset of uterine contractions.
    first stage of l.   Dilation of the uterine cervix.
    induced l.   Labor brought on by artificial means.
    missed l.   The retention of the (usually dead) fetus for an indefinite period beyond the expected time of delivery.
  precipitate l.   Labor of abnormally short duration, usually lasting three hours or less; frequently a result of abnormally low resistance of the maternal soft structures or abnormally strong contractions of the uterus and abdominal muscles; occurring most frequently in women who have had more than one child.
  premature l.   Labor occurring before term.

prolonged l.   Difficult labor that, for any of several reasons, does not result in vaginal delivery of the child within an 18 to 24 hour period.
  second stage of l.   Stage of childbirth beginning with complete dilation of the cervix and ending with delivery of the baby.
  third stage of l.   Expulsion of the placenta.

laboratory 1. a room or building equipped with scientific equipment for conducting experiments, tests, etc. **2.** A place used for the manufacture of drugs and chemicals.

labrum, *pl.* **labra**   A lip, edge, or liplike structure.

labyrinth 1.   A group of intercommunicating canals. **2.** Internal ear.
  bony l.   A series of cavities in the petrous portion of the temporal bone which houses the membranous labyrinth.
  ethmoid l.   The labyrinth in the lateral part of the ethmoid bone consisting of thin walled cavities or cells. Also called ectethmoid.
  membranous l.   A system of communicating membranous canals, lying within the bony labyrinth.

labyrinthine   Relating to the labyrinth of the internal ear.

labyrinthitis   Inflammation of the labyrinth of the internal ear. Also called otitis interna.

labyrinthotomy   Incision into the labyrinth of the internal ear.

lac, *pl.* **lacta**   Latin for milk; any whitish, milky-looking fluid.

laceration   A wound made by tearing of the tissue.

lacinia   Fringe; fimbria.

lacrimal   Relating to tears.

lacrimation   The secretion, especially excessive, of tears.

lacrimatory   Causing discharge of tears.

lacrimotomy   The operation of incising the lacrimal sac or duct.

lactacidemia   See lacticacidemia.

lactagogue 1.   Any agent that promotes the flow of milk. **2.** Increasing the secretion of milk.

lactalbumin   An albumin of milk.

lactase   An intestinal enzyme that catalyzes the conversion of lactose into glucose and galactose; a sugar splitting enzyme; a deficiency of lactase may lead to gastrointestinal symptoms such as bloating, flatulence, and diarrhea following ingestion of milk and milk products.

lactate 1.   To secrete milk. **2.** Any salt or ester of lactic acid.
  l. dehydrogenase (LDH)   See lactic acid dehydrogenase.

lactation   The production of milk.

lacteal 1.   A lymph vessel that conveys chyle from the small intestine. **2.** Relating to milk.

lactescent 1.   Milky. **2.** Producing a milky fluid, as certain plants and insects.

lactic   Relating to milk.

lactic acid   A colorless syrupy substance formed by the fermentation of milk sugar (lactose); an end product of anaerobic glycolysis in the body.
  l. a. dehydrogenase (LDH)   An enzyme that may be measured in serum for diagnosis of some diseases, e.g., acute myocardial infarction and liver disease. Also called lactate dehydrogenase.

lacticacidemia   The presence of lactic acid in the circulating blood.

lactiferous   Secreting or conveying milk.

lactifugal   See galactophygous.

lactifuge   An agent that arrests the secretion of milk.

lactigenous   Producing milk.

lactin   Lactose.

lactinated   Containing lactose.

Lactobacillus (L)   A genus of rod-shaped, non-motile microorganisms (family Lactobacillacea) that produce lactic acid in the fermentation of carbohydrates, especially in milk.
  L. acidophilus   A species found in the feces of milk-fed infants and individuals on a diet with a high content of milk, lactose, or dextrin.

lactobezoar   A coagulum in the stomach formed by the prolonged ingestion of powdered milk which is mixed with an insufficient amount of water.

lactocele   See galactocele.

lactoflavin 1.   Riboflavin. **2.** Flavin in milk.

lactogen   Any agent that stimulates the production of milk.
  human placental l. (HPL; hPL)   A polypeptide hormone appearing in the serum of pregnant women at about the sixth week of gestation and rising steadily thereafter; it disappears from the blood immediately after delivery; it is produced by the syncytio-trophoblast (in placenta) and is intimately involved in carbohydrate metabolism of both, mother and fetus. Also called chorionic somatomammotropin; chorionic growth hormone.

lactogenic   Inducing milk production.

lactoglobulin   A simple protein found in milk.

lactone   A salt of a hydroxyl acid, formed by the removal of water from the acid.

lactoprotein   Protein normally present in milk.

lactorrhea   Galactorrhea.

lactose   A sugar formed by the mammary glands and constituting about 5 percent of cow's milk; it

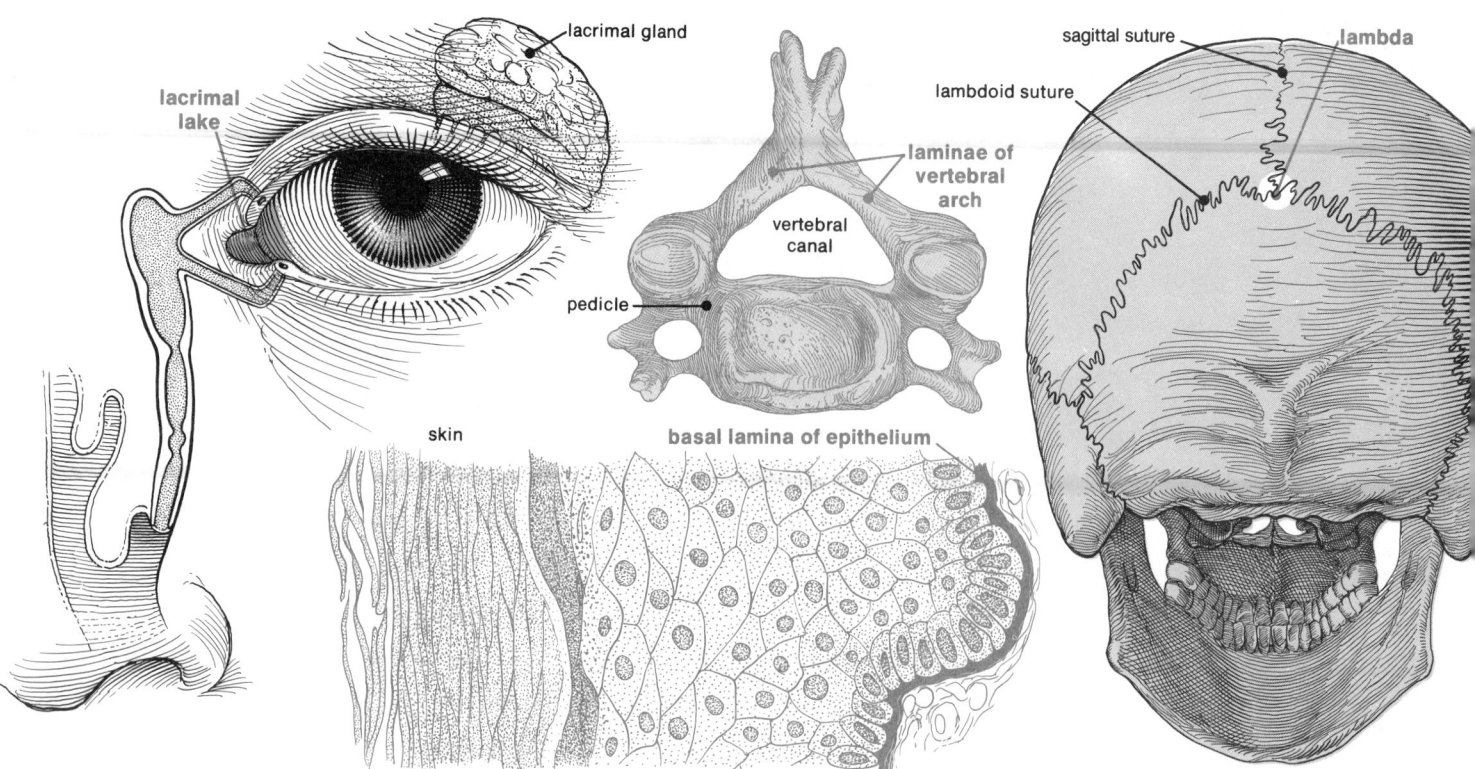

Figure labels: lacrimal gland · lacrimal lake · laminae of vertebral arch · vertebral canal · pedicle · sagittal suture · lambda · lambdoid suture · skin · basal lamina of epithelium

yields glucose and galactose on hydrolysis. Also called milk sugar.

lactosuria The presence of lactose in the urine; occurring sometimes in premature newborn infants.

lactovegetarian One who lives on a diet of vegetables, milk, and milk products.

lactulose Compound used to treat constipation.

lacuna, *pl.* **lacunae** 1. A small cavity. 2. A defect or gap.

   erosion l. A depression in bone caused by resorption of bone tissue by osteocytes. Also called Howship's lacuna.

   Howship's l. See erosion lacuna.

lacus Latin for lake; a small collection of fluid.

   l. lacrimalis Lacrimal lake; see under lake.

Laënnec's cirrhosis See cirrhosis, alcoholic.

lag Lag phase; see under phase.

lagophthalmos, lagophthalmia Condition in which the eyelids cannot be closed completely.

lake 1. A small accumulation of fluid. 2. To cause blood plasma to become red as a result of the release of hemoglobin from the erythrocytes.

   lacrimal l. The area of the conjunctiva, between the medial margins of the eyelids at the inner angle, in which the tears collect after bathing the anterior surface of the eyeball; the caruncle lies in its floor. Also called lacus lacrimalis.

lallation 1. Poor articulation, especially speech sounding like the prattling of a baby; babbling. 2. Defective enunciation of words in which the phoneme "l" is substituted for "r".

lalopathology The study of speech disorders.

lalopathy Any speech defect.

laloplagia Paralysis of muscles involved in the production of speech.

lambda A craniometric point at the junction of the sagittal and lambdoid sutures.

lambdoid Resembling the shape of the Greek letter lambda (λ); denoting the deeply serrated suture in the skull between the occipital bone and the two parietal bones.

lambert (L) Unit of brightness, equal to the uniform brightness of a perfectly diffusing surface emitting or reflecting light at the rate of 1 lumen per square centimeter.

lamella, *pl.* **lamellae** 1. A thin layer or plate, as of bone. 2. A medicated gelatin disc, used under the eyelid in place of solutions.

lamellar 1. Scaly. 2. Relating to lamellae.

lamina, *pl.* **laminae** A thin layer of flat plate, as of muscle or bone.

   anterior elastic l. of cornea Bowman's membrane; see under membrane.

   basal l. of choroid The transparent, inner layer

of the choroid in contact with the pigmented layer of the retina. Also called Bruch's membrane; lamina vitrea.

   basal l. of epithelium A relatively thin layer, about 300 to 1,200 A in thickness, composed of slender filamentous material enmeshed in a mucopolysaccharide matrix; it occurs at the base of epithelial cells where it blends with the reticular lamina to form the basement membrane. Also called boundary membrane; basement lamina.

   basement l. See basal lamina of epithelium.

   choroidocapillary l. The layer of the choroid between the basal lamina and the vascular lamina.

   cribriform l. of ethmoid bone The bony plate that forms part of the roof of the nasal cavity and is transversed by the filaments of the olfactory nerve.

   external cranial l. The outer plate of a cranial bone.

   internal cranial l. The inner plate of a cranial bone.

   interpubic fibrocartilaginous l. The fibrocartilaginous disk uniting the articular surfaces of the pubic bones at the symphysis.

   l. cribrosa sclerae The sievelike portion of the sclera through the holes of which pass the fibers of the optic nerve.

   l. fusca sclerae A layer consisting of a delicate mesh of elastic fibers connecting the sclera and choroid.

   l. vitrea See basal lamina of choroid.

   laminae of vertebral arch Two broad plates directed dorsally and medially from the pedicles of a vertebra; their posterior midline fusion forms the vertebral arch.

   lateral l. of pterygoid process A broad, thin, and everted plate of the pterygoid process of the sphenoid bone; its lateral surface forms part of the medial wall of the infratemporal fossa; its medial surface forms part of the pterygoid fossa.

   medial l. of pterygoid process A narrow, long plate of the pterygoid process of the sphenoid bone that curves laterally at its inferior extremity into a hooklike process, the pterygoid hamulus.

   posterior elastic l. of cornea Descemet's membrane; see under membrane.

   reticular l. A relatively thin layer of reticular and collagenous fibers embedded in a mucopolysaccharide matrix; together with the basal lamina it makes up the basement membrane which holds the basal cells of the epithelium firmly to the underlying connective tissue; it also encloses fat cells, muscle cells, and Schwann cells of peripheral nerves.

   suprachoroidal l. A layer of loose connective tissue forming the external layer of the choroid.

   vascular choroidal l. The layer of the choroid containing the larger blood vessels.

laminar 1. Arranged in layers. 2. Relating to a bony plate.

lamination An arrangement in layers.

laminectomy Surgical removal of the posterior arch of a vertebra.

laminotomy The surgical division of the lamina of a vertebra.

lamp Any device for producing light, heat, or therapeutic radiation.

   annealing l. An alcohol lamp with a soot-free flame used for heating and purifying gold leaf intended as a filling for tooth cavities.

   argon l. A lamp radiating chiefly in the near ultraviolet area around 360 nm; used chiefly in conjunction with fluorescein in fitting of contact lenses.

   Eldridge-Green l. A color perception test lamp containing a single light with color filters mounted in rotating disks.

   Kromayer's l. A U-shaped quartz lamp of mercury vapor that generates ultraviolet rays.

   mignon l. A small electric lamp used in the cystoscope.

   slit-l. See slitlamp.

   ultraviolet l. Lamp that emits rays in the ultraviolet band of the spectrum.

   uviol l. An electric lamp with a globe of uviol glass producing light with a high content of ultraviolet rays; used in phototherapy.

lanatoside A, B, C Digilanid A, B, and C, the three natural glycosides of *Digitalis lanata*.

lance To cut into a part, as into a boil.

lancet A small, pointed, double-edged surgical knife.

lancinating Denoting a piercing or cutting pain.

Landry's paralysis See paralysis, acute ascending.

language The use of vocal sounds in articulate, meaningful patterns, as a form of communication.

   body l. Expression of thoughts and feelings by means of bodily movements.

lanolin Fat obtained from sheep's wool; used in the preparation of ointments.

   anhydrous l. See wool fat.

lanthanum Metallic rare earth element; symbol La, atomic number 57, atomic weight 138.92.

lanuginous Covered with fine, soft, downlike hair (lanugo).

lanugo The fine soft hair covering the body of the newborn.

laparohysterectomy Removal of the uterus through an incision of the abdominal wall.

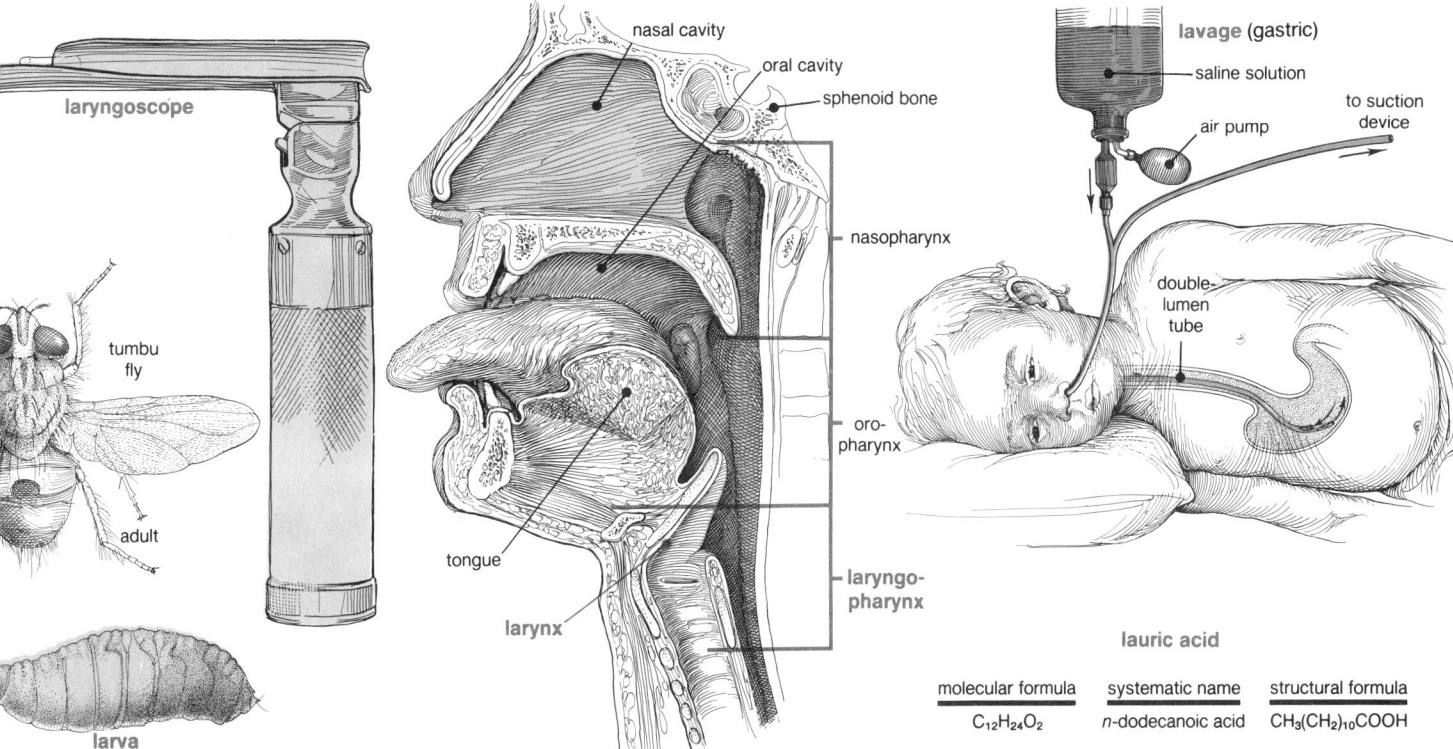

laryngoscope

tumbu fly

adult

larva

nasal cavity

oral cavity

sphenoid bone

nasopharynx

oro-pharynx

laryngo-pharynx

tongue

larynx

lavage (gastric)

saline solution

air pump

to suction device

double-lumen tube

lauric acid

molecular formula	systematic name	structural formula
$C_{12}H_{24}O_2$	n-dodecanoic acid	$CH_3(CH_2)_{10}COOH$

laparohysterotomy Incision of the uterus through an incision of the abdominal wall.

laparoscope Instrument for visualizing the peritoneal cavity.

laparoscopy Visualization of the contents of the abdominal cavity by means of an endoscope. Also called celioscopy.

laparotomy Surgical incision into the flank or through any part of the abdominal wall. Also called celiotomy.

lapsus linguae Latin for a slip of the tongue; usually due to unconscious factors.

larva, pl. **larvae** The wormlike early stage in the development of certain animals, bearing little or no resemblance to the adult form.

larva migrans Larval worms existing for a period of time in the tissues of a host other than the one to which they are adapted.

 cutaneous l. m. A subcutaneous creeping eruption of the skin caused by wandering larvae of *Ancylostoma braziliense* and other domestic animal hookworms; acquired through contact with soil containing contaminated dog or cat feces. Also called creeping eruption.

 visceral l. m. Disease caused by the presence of larvae of *Toxocara canis* (intestinal parasite of dogs) that penetrate the intestinal wall and wander through organs, especially the liver; acquired through consumption of raw vegetables contaminated with eggs of the parasite.

larvicide An agent destructive to larvae.

laryngeal Relating to the larynx.

laryngectome A person who has had the larynx removed.

laryngectomy Removal of the larynx.

laryngismus Spasmodic contraction of the larynx.

 l. stridulus A disease of children marked by sudden attacks of spasm of the larynx, lasting a few seconds, with a crowing noise on inspiration and cyanosis. Also called crowing convulsions; Kopp's asthma; pseudocroup.

laryngitis Inflammation of the larynx.

 acute l. Laryngitis caused by infection or by mechanical irritation; infectious forms are frequently associated with sore throat and cough; characterized by hoarseness that may progress to complete loss of voice.

 atrophic l. A chronic form leading to atrophy of the glands of the mucous membrane, diminished secretions, and formation of crusts.

laryngocele A congenital anomaly of the larynx; a sac formed by the outpocketing of the laryngeal mucosa reaching upward and outward between the true and false vocal cords.

laryngocentesis A small surgical incision or puncture of the larynx.

laryngofissure Surgical incision of the larynx, usually through the midline, for the removal of a tumor. Also called median laryngotomy.

laryngograph Instrument used to make tracings of the movements of the larynx.

laryngology The study of the larynx and treatment of its diseases.

laryngoparalysis Paralysis of the larynx.

laryngopharyngeal Relating to both the larynx and pharynx.

laryngopharyngectomy Removal of both larynx and pharynx.

laryngopharynx The lower portion of the pharynx from the hyoid bone to the esophagus, with which it is continuous. Also called pars laryngea pharyngis. See also pharynx.

laryngoplasty Reparative surgery of the larynx.

laryngoscope Any tubular instrument used in examining the interior of the larynx.

laryngoscopy Examination of the larynx with a laryngoscope.

 indirect l. Examination of the larynx by an instrument giving a reflected view.

laryngospasm A reflex contraction of the laryngeal muscles.

laryngostenosis Stricture or narrowing of the larynx.

laryngostomy Creation of a permanent opening into the larynx.

laryngotome Instrument used to make an incision into the larynx.

laryngotomy Surgical incision into the larynx.

laryngotracheobronchitis Acute inflammation of the upper respiratory passages, occurring as a primary infection or attending a systemic disease such as diphtheria, whooping cough, etc.

larynx The organ of voice production, located at the upper end of the trachea; it is composed of a cartilaginous and muscular frame, lined with mucous membrane, and contains the vocal cords.

lascivia Excessive sexual desire. Also called nymphomania.

Lasègue's sign Pain along the course of the sciatic nerve when the patient, lying on his back, flexes his thigh on his abdomen and then extends his leg at the knee; it indicates disease of the sciatic nerve.

laser Any of several devices that convert light of mixed frequencies into coherent, highly amplified visible radiation; used in surgical and physiological procedures; the term is an acronym for light ampli-

fication by stimulated emission of radiation. Also called optical maser.

laser beam The concentrated, nonspreading (coherent) beam of monochromatic visible light emitted by a laser.

lassitude Weakness or weariness.

latah Nervous disorder marked by imitative behavior and extreme response to suggestion; observed in natives of Malay.

latent Present but not manifest; concealed.

lateral Located on the side; farther from the middle.

laterality A tendency to use either the right or the left parts of the body; right or left dominance of the cerebral cortex.

laterodeviation Displacement to one side.

lateroduction Movement to one side, as of a limb.

lateroflexion Bending to one side.

lateropulsion Involuntary movement toward one side, occurring in certain nervous disorders.

laterotorsion Rotation of the eye around its anteroposterior axis.

lateroversion The displacement of an organ to one side.

lathyrism Disease due to poisoning with some species of peas of the genus *Lathyrus*; neurologic symptoms predominate.

latissimus Broadest; widest.

Latrodectus A genus of highly poisonous spiders. **L. mactans** See black widow.

lattice A regular configuration of ions or molecules in a definite geometric arrangement.

latus, pl. **latera** The side of the body between the ribs and the pelvis. Also called the flank.

laudable Term formerly given to abundant thick pus, thought to indicate the healing of a wound.

laudanum A tincture of opium.

Laurence-Biedl syndrome A recessive hereditary disorder marked by some or all of the following: mental retardation, obesity, polydactyly, hypogonadism, and visual disturbances (retinitis pigmentosa). Also called Laurence-Moon-Biedl or Laurence-Moon-Biedl-Bardet syndrome.

lauric acid A fatty acid present in milk and especially in coconut oil. Also called dodecanoic acid.

Lauth's violet See thionine.

lavage The washing out of a cavity or a hollow organ.

law 1. A principle, rule, or formula expressing a fact based on observed recurrence, order, relationship, or interactions of natural processes or actions. 2. A generalization based on the repetition of events.

 Arrhenius' l. Only those solutions which have

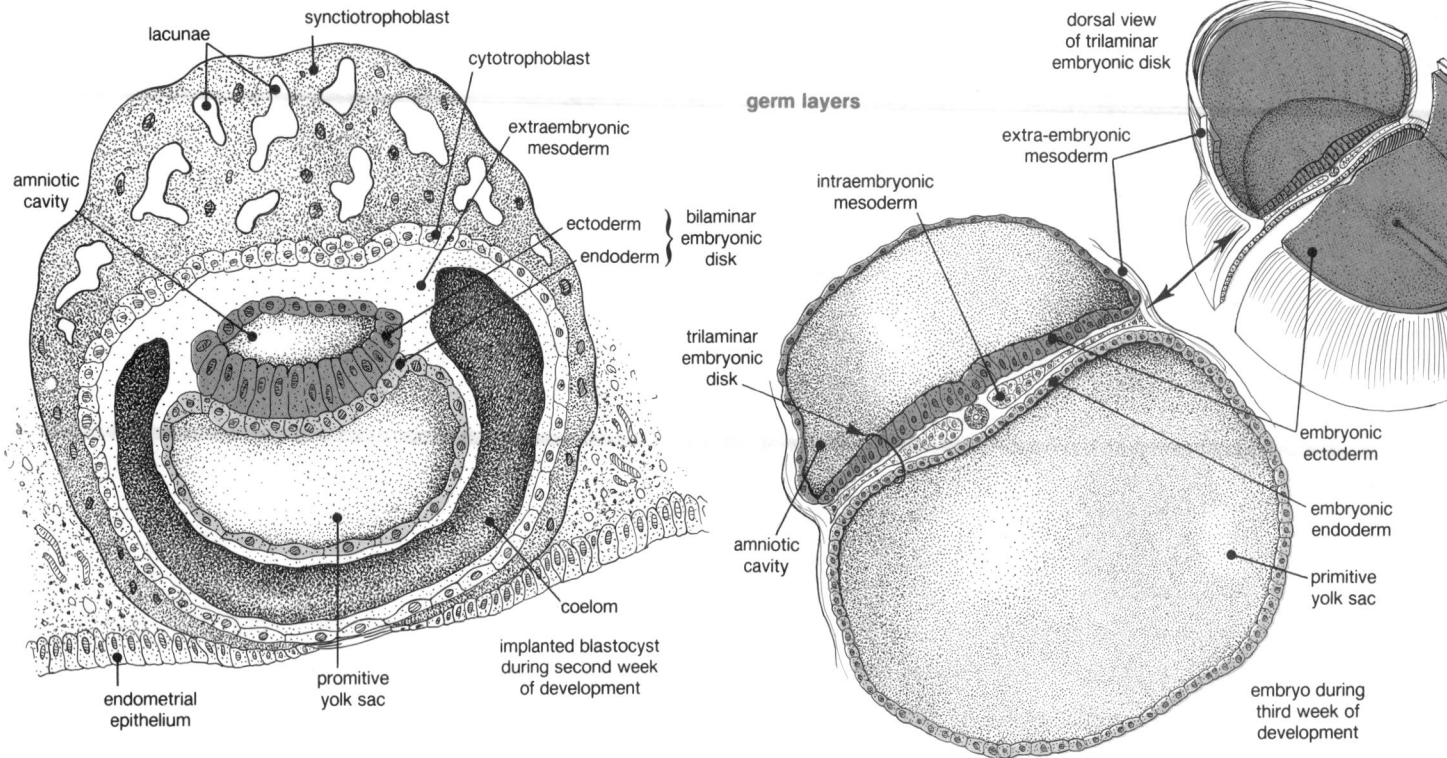

germ layers

lacunae · synctiotrophoblast · cytotrophoblast · extraembryonic mesoderm · amniotic cavity · ectoderm } bilaminar embryonic disk · endoderm } · coelom · promitive yolk sac · endometrial epithelium · implanted blastocyst during second week of development

dorsal view of trilaminar embryonic disk · extra-embryonic mesoderm · intraembryonic mesoderm · trilaminar embryonic disk · amniotic cavity · embryonic ectoderm · embryonic endoderm · primitive yolk sac · embryo during third week of development

---

high osmotic pressures are electrically conductive.

Avogadro's l. Equal volumes of gases contain equal numbers of molecules (pressure and temperature being the same).

Beer's l. The intensity of a light ray is inversely proportional to the depth of liquid through which it is transmitted (the absorption is dependent upon the number of molecules in the ray's path).

Boyle's l. At a fixed temperature, the volume of confined gas varies inversely with the pressure upon it.

Charles' l. All gases expand and contract equally on heating and cooling. Also called Gay-Lussac law.

Courvoisier's l. Obstruction of the common bile duct is more likely to be caused by gallstones when the gallbladder is contracted due to scarring and inflammation; if the gallbladder is enlarged, obstruction is usually due to other causes, such as carcinoma of the head of the pancreas. Also called Courvoisier's sign.

Dalton's l. Each gas in a mixture of gases exerts a pressure proportionate to the percentage of its volume in the mixture as if that were the only gas dissolved. Also called law of partial pressure.

Dalton-Henry l. In dissolving a mixture of gases, a fluid will absorb as much of each gas in the mixture as if that were the only gas dissolved.

Einthoven's l. In electrocardiography, the potential difference in lead II is equal to the sum of the potential differences of leads I and III. Also called Einthoven's equation.

Faraday's l.'s 1. In electrolysis, the amount of an ion liberated by an electric current is proportional to the strength of the current. 2. When the same current is passed through several electrolytes, the amounts of different substances decomposed are proportioned to their chemical equivalents.

Galton's l. While offspring generally tend to resemble their parents, the offspring of parents of extreme types tend to regress toward the mean of the population. Also called law of regression.

Gay-Lussac l. See Charles' law.

Henry's l. The amount of gas which can be dissolved in a liquid solution is proportional to the partial pressure of the gas; when the pressure is doubled, twice as much gas passes into solution.

inverse square l. A law which is especially applied to all point sources of radiation; the intensity of radiation is inversely proportional to the square of the distance.

Laplace's l. The relationship between transmural pressure difference (ΔP), wall tension (T), and diameter (D) related to surface tension in a concave surface: $\Delta P = (4\ T/D)$.

l. of the heart See Starling's law.

l. of independent assortment Mendel's second law.

l. of mass action The speed of a chemical reaction is proportional to the active masses (molar concentration) of the reacting material.

l. of partial pressure See Dalton's law.

l. of refraction For two given media, the sine of the angle of incidence is constantly related to the sine of the angle of refraction.

l. of regression See Galton's law.

l. of segregation Mendel's first law.

l. of universal gravitation See Newton's law.

Mendel's l.'s The principles of heredity summarized in two laws and expressed in modern times as: 1. First law or law of segregation: paired hereditary units (genes) in the offspring (one from each parent) do not mix or alter one another, therefore they are able to separate during the formation of sex cells (gametes) in meiosis and are transmitted independently from generation to generation. 2. Second law or law of independent assortment: the corresponding hereditary units in a pair of gametes unite in the offspring to form new combinations and recombinations according to the laws of chance, provided that the two pairs of genes do not lie on the same chromosome. Also called mendelian laws.

Mendeleeff's l. See periodic law.

mendelian l.'s See Mendel's laws.

Newton's l. All bodies attract each other with a force directly proportional to their masses and inversely proportional to the square of the distance between them. Also called law of universal gravitation.

Ohm's l. The electric current in a circuit is equal to the electromotive force divided by the resistance: amperes = volts/ohms.

Pascal's l. Fluids at rest transmit pressure equally in every direction.

periodic l. The elements when arranged in the order of their atomic weights display a periodic variation of their properties; every element of the series is related in its properties to the eighth element before and after it. Also called Mendeleef's law.

Poiseuille's l. Speed of fluid flowing in a tube is proportional to the cross-sectional area of the tube.

Sherrington's l. Every dorsal spinal nerve root supplies a special area of the skin (dermatome), although the area may be overlapped by fibers from adjacent spinal segments.

Starling's l. The energy liberated by the contracting heart muscle depends on the length of the muscle fibers at the end of diastole; within limits, the stroke volume of the heart is determined by the change in myocardial fiber length associated with ventricular filling in diastole. Also called law of the heart.

van't Hoff's l.'s 1. In stereochemistry, all optically active substances form an unsymmetrical arrangement in space, owing to their having multivalent atoms united to four different atoms or radicals. 2. The osmotic pressure of a substance in a dilute solution is the same that the same substance would exert if present in the state of an ideal gas occupying the same volume as the solution. 3. The velocity of chemical reactions increases between two- and three-fold for each 10°C rise in temperature.

wallerian l. A nerve fiber loses its normal structure and function when continuity with its cell of origin is interrupted. Also called Waller's law.

lawrencium Synthetic transuranic element; symbol Lw, atomic number 103, atomic weight 257.

laxative An agent that stimulates evacuation of a soft formed stool by increasing peristalsis or simply through hydration of the stool; distinguished from a cathartic, which produces a stronger effect.

layer A sheetlike coating, or stratum, covering a surface. Also called stratum; lamina.

bacillary l. The layer of rods and cones of the retina.

choriocapillary l. Choroidocapillary lamina; see under lamina.

conjunctival l. of bulb The mucous membrane investing the anterior surface of the sclera, terminating at the margin of the cornea.

conjunctival l. of eyelids The mucous membrane that lines the posterior surface of the eyelids; it is continuous with the bulbar conjunctiva.

corneal l. The outer layer of the epidermis consisting of several layers of flat keratinized nonnucleated cells.

germ l. Any of three primary layers formed in the early development of the embryo, the ectoderm, endoderm, or mesoderm, that give rise to specific tissues of the body.

l.'s of cerebellar cortex Three distinct layers of the cerebellar cortex that, from the surface inward, are: molecular layer, Purkinje cell layer, and granular layer; the granular layer is adjacent to the cerebellar white matter.

l.'s of cerebral cortex Six not too obvious layers of the cerebral cortex that tend to blend into each other; from the surface inward, they are: molecular layer, outer granular layer, pyramidal cell layer, inner granular layer, ganglionic layer, and the fusiform layer.

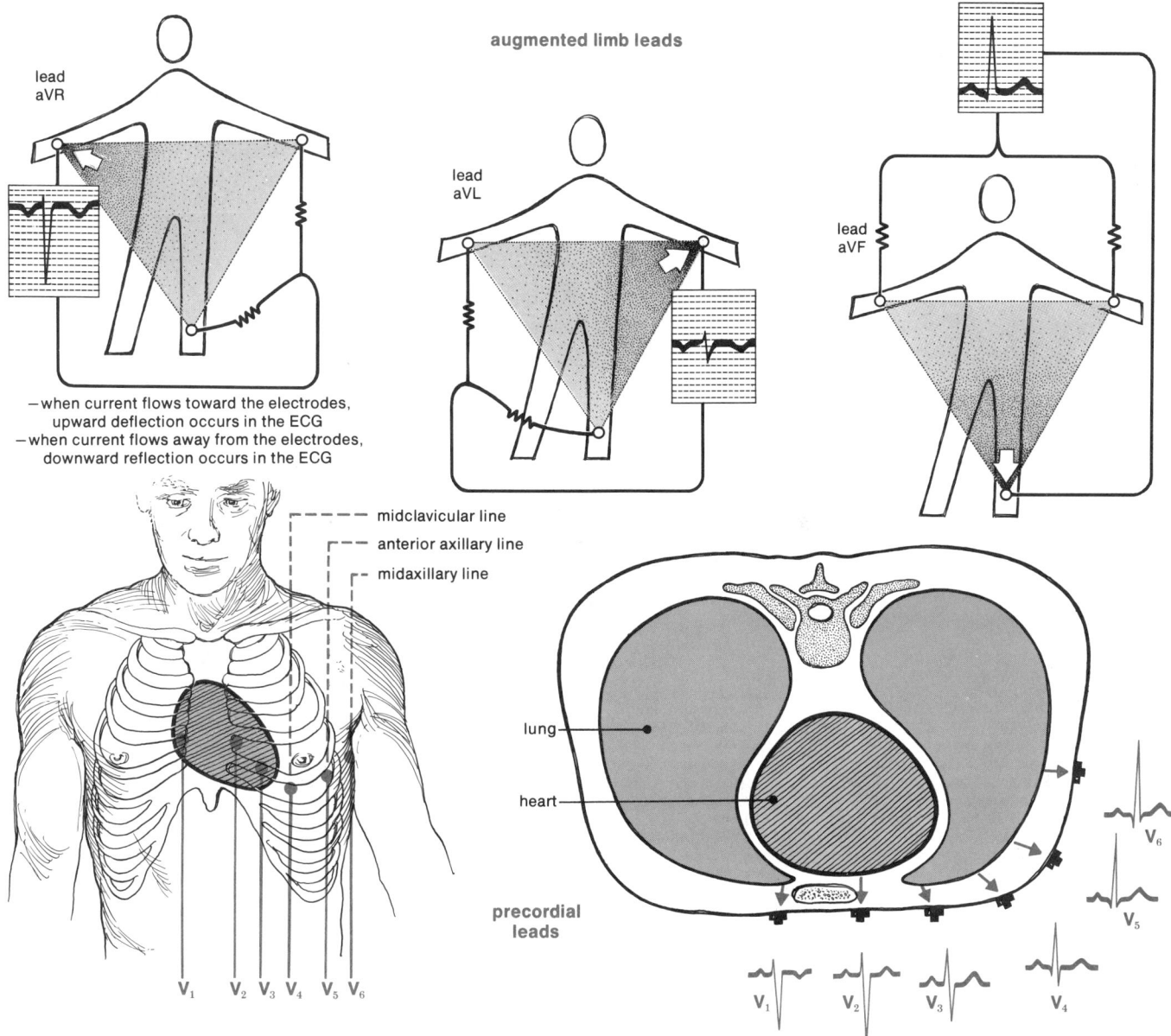

augmented limb leads

lead aVR

−when current flows toward the electrodes, upward deflection occurs in the ECG
−when current flows away from the electrodes, downward reflection occurs in the ECG

lead aVL

lead aVF

midclavicular line
anterior axillary line
midaxillary line

V_1 V_2 V_3 V_4 V_5 V_6

lung

heart

precordial leads

V_6
V_5
V_1 V_2 V_3 V_4

---

l. of rods and cones A layer of the retina between the pigment epithelium and the external limiting membrane, containing the visual receptors (rod and cone cells).

malpighian l. Stratum germinativum; see under stratum.

odontoblastic l. The layer of odontoblast cells lining the pulpal surface of the dentin of teeth.

prickle-cell l. Stratum spinosum; see under stratum.

Purkinje's l. The middle of three layers of the cerebellar cortex consisting of large neuron cell bodies.

subendothelial l. The thin layer of connective tissue situated between the endothelium and elastic lamina in the intima of blood vessels.

layering An arrangement in layers.

leaching The process of washing out soluble matter from a substance by a percolating liquid. Also called lixiviation.

lead A specific array of electric connections (electrodes) used for recording the electric potential created by a functioning organ, as the heart (electrocardiography) or brain (electroencephalography).

augmented limb l. One of three unipolar leads for registering the variations in electric potentials at one point (right arm, aVR; left arm, aVL; or left leg, aVF) with respect to a point which does not vary significantly in electric activity during contraction of the heart; the lead is augmented (increased) by virtue of an electric connection which increases the amplitude; lead aVR records the electric potentials of the right arm with reference to a junction made

by connecting the wires from the left arm and the left leg; lead aVL records the potentials at the left arm in reference to a junction made by connecting the wires from the right arm and the left foot; lead aVF records the potentials at the left foot in reference to a junction made by connecting the wire from the left and right arms.

bipolar l. A lead in which the electrodes detect electric variations at two points and record the difference.

chest l. Precordial lead.

direct l. A lead recorded with the exploring electrode placed directly on the surface of the exposed heart.

esophageal l. An exploring electrode introduced into the lumen of the esophagus in order to improve visualization of atrial deflections on the electrocardiogram (ECG); useful in the recognition of arrhythmias.

indirect l. Standard lead.

intracardiac l. A lead recorded with the exploring electrode placed in one of the heart's chambers, usually by means of cardiac catheterization.

limb l. One of the three bipolar standard leads or one of the three unipolar augmented limb leads (aVR, aVL, aVF).

precordial l. One in which the exploring electrode is on the chest overlying the heart or its vicinity; unipolar chest lead recorded in positions V_1 through V_6 (the V designation denotes that the movable electrode registers the electric potential under the electrode with respect to a V or central terminal connection, which is made by connecting

wires from the right arm, left arm, and left leg; the electric potential of the central terminal connection does not vary significantly throughout the cardiac cycle; as a result, the recordings made with the V connection show the electric variations that are taking place under the movable precordial electrode); position V_1 is at the fourth intercostal space at the right sternal border; V_2 is at the fourth intercostal space at the left sternal border; V_4 is at the left midclavicular line in the fifth intercostal space; V_3 is equidistant between V_2 and V_4; V_5 is the fifth intercostal space in the anterior axillary line; V_6 is at the fifth intercostal space in the left midaxillary line.

standard l. One of the original bipolar limb leads designated I, II, and III; it detects the electric variations at two points and displays the difference; lead I records the potential difference between the right and left arms; lead II records the difference between right arm and left leg; lead III records the difference between left arm and left leg.

unipolar l.'s Leads in which the exploring electrode records the variations in electric potential at one point with reference to a point that does not vary significantly in electric activity during cardiac contraction.

V l. A chest lead with the central terminal as the indifferent electrode.

lead A malleable, bluish-gray, dense metallic element, extracted chiefly from lead sulfide; symbol Pb (plumbum), atomic number 82, atomic weight 207.19.

l. arsenate A poisonous mixture of arsenate of

---

leiomyoma (fibroid)

myometrium

uterine tube

uterine cavity

uterus

uterine cervix

flagellum

lipid body

Leishmanis donovani (amastigote stage)

objective lens

mitochondrion

Golgi apparatus

endoplasmic reticulum

nucleus

kinetoplast

transverse temporal gyrus of brain

medial geniculate body

auditory radiations

nucleus of inferior colliculus

midbrain level

lateral lemniscus

dorsal cochlear nucleus

ventral cochlear nucleus

cochlear nerve

nucleu later lemnisc

med lev

dorsal nucleus of trapezoid body

trapezoid body

internal ear

cochlea

---

soda and acetate of lead, $Pb_3(AsO_4)_2$, used as an insecticide.

l. carbonate A poisonous white powder, $PbCO_3$, used largely in the manufacture of paint.

l. chromate A poisonous lemon-yellow powder, $PbCrO_4$, used as a paint pigment.

l. sulfide (PbS) The natural form in which lead is usually found. Also called galena.

leaflet A structure resembling a small leaf, such as the cusps of a heart valve.

Leber's disease Leber's hereditary optic atrophy; see under atrophy.

lecithin One of a group of phospholipids having a yellowish or brown waxy appearance; found in nerve tissue, egg yolks, and cells (both animal and vegetable).

lecithinase See phospholipase.

lectin A protein found predominantly in seeds, particularly those of the legumes; it binds to specific carbohydrate-containing receptor sites on the red blood cell surface and can cause the cells to agglutinate. Also called plant agglutinin; phytoagglutinin.

leech Any of various annelid worms (class Hirudinea) of which one blood sucking species, *Hirudo medicinalis* (German leech), was used for bleeding patients.

leg The lower limb, especially between the knee and the ankle.

Legg-Calvé-Perthes disease Epiphysial aseptic necrosis; see under necrosis.

Legg-Perthes disease Epiphysial aseptic necrosis; see under necrosis.

Legionella pneumophila A gram-negative, rod-shaped bacterium; the cause of legionnaire's disease.

legionnaire's disease Infectious disease caused by *Legionella pneumophila* (a gram-negative bacillus); symptoms include high fever, headache, abdominal pain and pneumonia; the liver, kidneys and nervous system may also be affected.

legumin A protein found in peas and beans.

leiomyofibroma See leiomyoma.

leiomyoma A benign tumor derived from smooth muscle and containing a relatively small amount of fibrous tissue; may occur anywhere in the body but is most frequently seen in the uterus. Also called fibromyoma; leiomyofibroma; fibroid.

leiomyomatosis The state of having multiple benign tumors of smooth muscle (leiomyomas).

leiomyosarcoma A malignant neoplasm in which smooth (nonstriated) muscle cells proliferate into a fleshy mass.

Leishmania A genus of flagellated parasitic protozoa (family Trypanosomidae) transmitted to humans by the sandfly.

L. braziliensis A species that is the causative agent of mucocutaneous leishmaniasis.

L. donovani A species of intracellular parasite causing visceral leishmaniasis (kala azar).

L. tropica A species that is the cause of cutaneous leishmaniasis.

leishmaniasis, leishmaniosis Infection with a species of *Leishmania*.

cutaneous l. Chronic skin lesions with a tendency to ulcerate produced by *Leishmania tropica*; prevalent in tropical and subtropical areas. Also called oriental sore; Old World leishmaniasis.

mucocutaneous l. Skin lesions often associated with ulcerative lesions of the mucous membranes of the nose, mouth, and pharynx; caused by *Leishmania braziliensis*. Also called American or New World leishmaniasis.

visceral l. A disease characterized by chronic fever, splenomegaly, anemia, leukopenia, and hyperglobulinemia; caused by *Leishmania donovani*; transmitted by the bite of a sandfly. Also called kala azar; tropical splenomegaly.

leishmanid Any lesion that may be infected with a species of the genus *Leishmania*.

lemniscus, *pl.* **lemnisci** A band or bundle of nerve fibers in the central nervous system.

lateral l. The major auditory pathway to the brain stem; it consists of a band of longitudinal ascending fibers that pass through the pons (in the lateral tegmentum) to the level of the midbrain, where most of the fibers terminate in the inferior colliculus with a few projecting directly to the medial geniculate body.

medial l. A bundle of ascending fibers that originates in the nuclei of the lower brain stem and terminates in the ventral posterolateral neuclus of the thalamus.

trigeminal l. A band of fibers in the brain stem passing from the sensory nuclei of the trigeminal nerve to the posterior part of the ventral nucleus of the thalamus.

length (l) Distance between two points.

bond l. The average distance between the nuclei of two atoms linked by a bond.

crown-heel l. (C-H length) The length of an embryo from the top of the head to the heel.

crown-rump l. (C-R length) The length of an embryo from the top of the head to the bottom of the buttocks.

lenitive 1. A soothing agent. 2. Soothing.

lens 1. A transparent object (made of glass, plastic, quartz, etc.) having two polished surfaces of which at least one is curved, usually with a spherical curvature, shaped so that light rays on passing through it are made to diverge or converge. 2. The lens of the eye; the biconvex transparent structure of the eye located between the iris and the vitreous body.

achromatic l. A compound lens that eliminates or reduces chromatic aberration; made of two kinds of glass with different dispersive powers.

acrylic l. A lens made of acrylic material; used to replace a cataractous lens.

aplanatic l. A lens that corrects spherical aberration.

apochromatic l. A lens that corrects both spherical and chromatic aberrations.

bifocal l. Lens having one portion (usually the upper and larger portion) suited for distant vision and the other suited for near vision.

compound l. Optical system having two or more lenses.

concave l. A lens that disperses light rays. Also called minus, diverging, myopic, negative, or reducing lens.

concavoconvex l. Lens having one concave and one convex surface. Also called positive meniscus lens.

contact l. A molded plastic lens that rests directly on the eye in contact with the cornea; used to correct refractive errors.

convex l. A lens that converges or focuses light rays. Also called plus, converging, hyperopic, or magnifying lens.

convexoconcave l. Lens having one convex and one concave surface. Also called negative meniscus lens.

crystalline l. See lens (2).

cylindrical l. (cyl) A lens in which one or both surfaces have the curve of a cylinder, either concave or convex; used to correct astigmatism.

eye l. The lens in an eyepiece which is nearest the eye; it renders light rays from the objective lens parallel prior to entrance into the eye. Also called ocular lens.

field l. The lens nearest the objective lens in an eyepiece; it increases the field of view in a microscopic or telescopic system.

immersion l. The lens in a microscope nearest the object, designed so that it can be lowered into contact with a fluid which is placed on the cover glass.

meniscus l. A crescent-shaped lens; one that is concave on one surface and convex on the other.

minus l. See concave lens.

objective l. The lens in a microscope or telescope

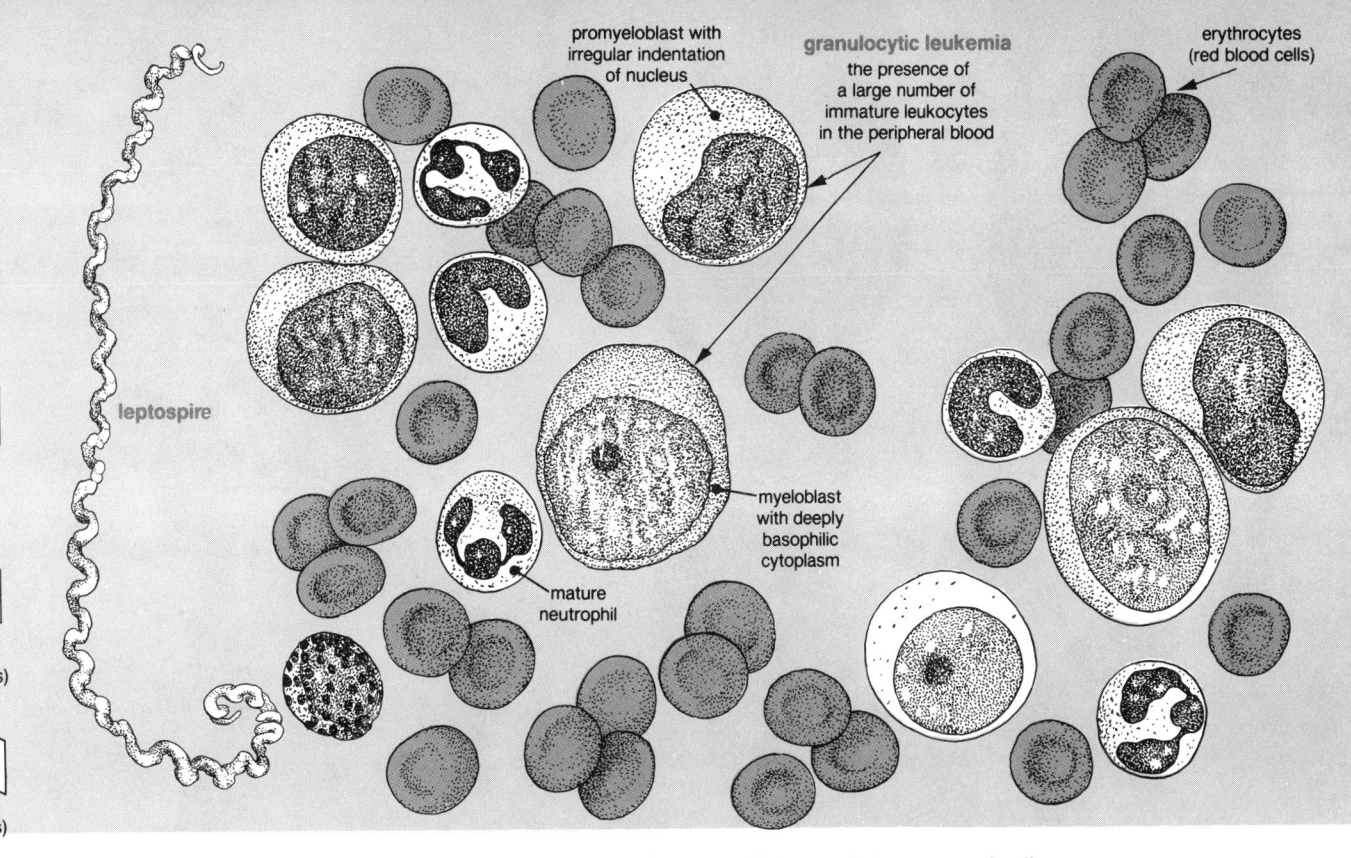

lenses

planoconvex

planoconcave

double convex

convexo-concave
(negative meniscus)

concavo-convex
(positive meniscus)

leptospire

promyeloblast with
irregular indentation
of nucleus

granulocytic leukemia
the presence of
a large number of
immature leukocytes
in the peripheral blood

erythrocytes
(red blood cells)

myeloblast
with deeply
basophilic
cytoplasm

mature
neutrophil

nearest the object; it converges light rays from the field of view.

planoconcave l. A lens that is flat on one surface and concave on the other.

planoconvex l. A lens that is flat on one surface and convex on the other.

plus l. See convex lens.

spherical l. A lens in which all refractive surfaces are spherical.

sphericocylindrical l. A lens in which one surface is spherical and the other is cylindrical.

trifocal l. A lens having three portions with different focal powers serving for distant, intermediate, and near vision.

lensometer An optical instrument used to determine the refractive power, optical center, cylinder axis, and prismatic effect of ophthalmic lenses.

lens system Two or more lenses arranged to work in conjunction with one another in order to accomplish a required function; e.g., microscope, projection lens system.

lenticonus A conical protrusion on either the anterior or posterior surface of the lens of the eye, usually affecting only one eye.

lenticular 1. Relating to a lens. **2.** Shaped like a lentil. Also called lentiform.

lenticulostriate Relating to the lentiform nucleus and the corpus striatum of the brain.

lentiform 1. Lenticular. **2.** Shaped like a lentil.

lentigo, *pl.* **lentigines** A flat, tan or brown spot on the skin which is to be differentiated from a freckle; an early junctional nevus.

leontiasis The lion-like appearance of the face in some cases of advanced leprosy; i.e., ridges and furrows on the forehead and cheeks.

leper An individual afflicted with leprosy.

lepidosis Any scaly eruption of the skin.

lepothrix See trichomycosis axillaris.

lepra Leprosy.

leprid The early skin lesion of leprosy.

leprology The study of leprosy.

leproma The characteristic lesion of the focus of infection with *Microbacterium leprae*.

lepromatous Relating to a leproma.

lepromin Extract made from tissue containing the leprosy bacillus *Mycobacterium leprae,* used in skin tests to determine resistance to leprosy.

leprosarium A special hospital for the care and treatment of those afflicted with leprosy.

leprosery A leper colony.

leprostatic An agent that inhibits the growth of the leprosy bacillus (*Mycobacterium leprae*).

leprosy A chronic infectious disease caused by the bacillus *Mycobacterium leprae* (Hansen's bacillus), which produces granulomatous lesions of the skin, mucous membranes, peripheral nervous system, and bones; it occurs almost exclusively in tropical and subtropical regions and its severity can range from noncontagious and remitting forms to highly contagious malignant forms marked by mutilation. Also called Hansen's disease; elephantiasis graecorum.

leprous Relating to leprosy.

leptocyte A thin red blood cell having a pigmented border surrounding a clear area with a pigmented center.

leptocytosis The presence of leptocytes in the blood, occurring in certain disorders, including thalassemia.

leptodermic Thin-skinned.

leptomeningeal Relating to the pia mater and arachnoid collectively (leptomeninges).

leptomeninx, *pl.* **leptomeninges** The pia-arachnoid.

leptomonad 1. A member of the genus *Leptomonas.* **2.** Former term for promastigote.

Leptospira A genus of spiral, hook-ended spirochetes, bacteria of the order Spirochaetales.

leptospire Any organism belonging to the genus *Leptospira.*

leptospirosis Infection with bacteria of the genus *Leptospira;* the clinical picture may vary from a mild fever to a fulminating, toxic illness with jaundice and renal failure; specific syndromes include aseptic meningitis and pretibial fever, the latter associated with a pretibial eruption and splenomegaly.

leptotene In meiosis, the first stage of prophase in which the chromosomes appear as individual, slender threads, well separated from each other.

Leptotrichia A genus of anaerobic, nonmotile bacteria indigenous to the oral cavity of man.

Leptotrombidium Genus of mites (family Trombiculidae); transmit tsutsugamushi disease.

Leriche's syndrome See aortoiliac occlusive disease.

lesbian 1. A homosexual female. **2.** Relating to lesbianism.

lesbianism Female homosexuality.

Lesch-Nyhan syndrome A disorder of purine metabolism and excess uric acid; clinical features include severe mental retardation and compulsive, self-mutilating behavior; death usually occurs during childhood due to kidney damage.

lesion Any morbid change in the structure or function of tissues due to injury or disease.

coin l. A round shadow the size of a small coin seen in radiographs of the lungs; may indicate tuber-

culosis, cancer, or other diseases.

Ghon's primary l. The primary lesion of pulmonary tuberculosis, appearing in the roentgenogram as a small sharply defined shadow. Also called Ghon's focus.

Janeway l. A small hemorrhagic lesion on the palm or sole, occurring in some cases of bacterial endocarditis.

Kimmelstiel-Wilson nodular l. Nodular glomerulosclerosis; see under glomerulosclerosis.

lethal (L) Deadly.

lethargy A state of drowsiness and sluggishness.

Letterer-Siwe disease Nonlipid histiocytosis; see under histiocytosis.

leucine (Leu) An essential amino acid formed by the hydrolysis of protein; found in many tissues, especially the pancreas and spleen.

leucovorin See folinic acid.

leukapheresis Procedure in which white blood cells are removed from withdrawn blood, which is then retransfused into the patient.

leukemia Disease characterized by the appearance of great numbers of immature and abnormal white blood cells in the bone marrow and often in the spleen and liver; usually these cells appear in the peripheral blood and may also invade other tissues; classified acute or chronic and also on the basis of the dominant type of cell involved (granulocytic, lymphocytic and monocytic); determination of acute or chronic refers in part to the rapidity of its course, but more to the degree of immaturity of the predominant cells.

aleukemic l. A form in which the abnormal cells are present in the blood-forming tissues, but not in the circulating blood; usually associated with decreased total number of normal white blood cells.

basophilic l. A type marked by the presence of great numbers of basophilic leukocytes in the blood and tissues. Also called mast cell leukemia.

embryonal l. See stem cell leukemia.

eosinophilic l. A form in which eosinophilic white cells are present in great numbers in the blood and/or bone marrow.

granulocytic l. A type marked by massive proliferation of myelopoietic cells in bone marrow and large numbers of mature and immature granulocytes in blood and tissues. Also called myelocytic, myelogenic, or myelogenous leukemia.

hairy-cell l. A rare type marked by proliferation of cells covered with hairlike projections.

l. cutis Massive accumulation of leukemic cells in the skin, forming red, brown, or purple nodules which may be localized (usually on the face and

myeloblast
(stem cell of leukocyte series)

promyelocyte

myelocyte

neutrophilic
leukocyte

RBCs for
size comparison

eosinophilic
leukocyte

leukocytopoiesis of
neutrophilic leukocyte

kidney-shaped
nucleus

basophilic
leukocyte

non-segmented
leukocyte (band cell)

segmented
leukocyte
(final stage of
development)

metamyelocyte

neck) throughout the body. Also called lymphoderma perniciosa.

lymphatic l. See lymphocytic leukemia.

lymphoblastic l. Acute lymphocytic leukemia in which the abnormal cells are the large immature forms of cells (lymphoblasts), which make up 50 to 90 percent of the total, with most of the remainder made up of mature lymphocytes.

lymphocytic l. An acute form occurring predominantly in children, characterized by the occurrence of lymphoblasts in the blood-forming tissues (particularly bone marrow, spleen, and lymph nodes); normal bone marrow elements may be replaced by the abnormal cells; a chronic form is usually seen in older people, with rather mature lymphocytes abundantly present in the blood. Also called lymphatic or lymphoid leukemia.

lymphoid l. See lymphocytic leukemia.

mast cell l. See basophilic leukemia.

megakaryocytic l. A rare form characterized by uncontrolled proliferation of megakaryocytes in the bone marrow and the presence of a considerable number in the circulating blood.

monocytic l. A variety in which the predominant abnormal cells are monocytes; in the Naegeli type of monocytic leukemia, the cells are thought to arise from myeloblasts and are associated with neutrophils; in the Schilling type, the latter are not very evident.

myeloblastic l. Leukemia characterized by an increase in myeloblasts which fail to mature (constituting approximately 30 to 60 percent of increased total of white blood cells) and a reduction of the mature forms.

myelocytic l. See granulocytic leukemia.

myelogenic l. See granulocytic leukemia.

myelogenous l. See granulocytic leukemia.

myelomonocytic l. A form of monocytic leukemia in which a moderately large number of monocytes is formed; considered by Naegeli to be a variant of granulocytic leukemia because he believed monocytes to be derived from myeloblasts in bone marrow. Also called Naegeli type of monocytic leukemia.

Naegeli type of monocytic l. Myelomonocytic leukemia.

plasma cell l. An unusual type of leukemia marked by increase of plasma cells and occurring in association with uncontrolled proliferation of plasma cells in bone (multiple myeloma) and in soft tissues (plasmacytoma).

Schilling type of monocytic l. Monocytic leukemia.

stem cell l. An extremely acute and uncommon type in which the abnormal cells are so primitive

and immature that it is impossible to differentiate them, but they are thought to be the precursors of lymphoblasts, myeloblasts, and monoblasts. Also called embryonal leukemia.

subleukemic l. Condition marked by the presence of small numbers of immature cells in the circulating blood; the total count of white blood cells is normal or subnormal.

leukemic Relating to or suffering from leukemia.

leukemogenesis The cause and development of a leukemic disease.

leukemoid Resembling the blood changes of leukemia.

leukoagglutinin Antibody that agglutinates white blood cells.

leukoblast An immature white blood cell.

leukocytactic See leukocytotactic.

leukocytaxia See leukocytotaxia.

leukocyte A white blood cell; any of the colorless cells of the blood; divided into two main groups according to their staining reactions: (a) granular or polymorphonuclear leukocytes, which have readily stainable cytoplasmic granules and lobulated nuclei; they include the neutrophils, eosinophils, and basophils; (b) nongranular leukocytes, which have minute cytoplasmic granules, not detectable with ordinary methods; they include lymphocytes and monocytes.

agranular l.'s See agranulocytes.

basophilic l. A white blood cell containing large coarse granules that stain readily with basic dyes (e.g., methylene blue); it constitutes about 0.5 percent of the total white blood cell count. Also called basophil; mast leukocyte.

eosinophilic l. A granular white blood cell with a bilobed nucleus and numerous, large cytoplasmic granules that stain intensely with acid dyes (e.g., eosin); it constitutes 2 to 5 percent of the total white blood cell count and increases in number during parasitic infestations and allergic states. Also called eosinophil; acidophil; oxyphil.

filamentous polymorphonuclear l. A polymorphonuclear leukocyte whose nuclear segments are united by threadlike filaments of chromatin.

neutrophilic l. A mature granular white blood cell having a nucleus of three to five distinct lobes joined by thin strands of chromatin and having granules that stain with a mixture of acid and basic dyes; it constitutes about 50 to 75 percent of the total white blood cell count; its primary function is ingestion and digestion of particulate matter, especially virulent bacteria. Also called neutrophil; neutrophilic granulocyte.

nonfilamentous polymorphonuclear l. A polymorphonuclear leukocyte whose nuclear segments

are united by wide bands of chromatin.

polymorphonuclear l. (PMN) Common term for any granular leukocyte, especially a neutrophilic leukocyte.

leukocytoblast General term denoting any immature white blood cell.

leukocytogenesis The formation of white blood cells.

leukocytolysin Any agent causing dissolution of white blood cells.

leukocytolysis The dissolution of white blood cells. Also called leukolysis.

leukocytometer A standardized glass slide used to count leukocytes.

leukocytopenia See leukopenia.

leukocytopoiesis The formation of white blood cells.

leukocytosis Abnormal increase in the number of white corpuscles in the blood.

leukocytotactic Relating to leukocytotaxia. Also called leukocytactic; leukotactic.

leukocytotaxia The tendency of white blood cells to move either toward (positive leukocytotaxia) or away from (negative leukocytotaxia) certain microorganisms and substances formed in inflamed tissue. Also called leukocytaxia; leukotaxis.

leukocytotoxin Any agent that causes degeneration of leukocytes.

leukoderma Absence of pigment in the skin. Also called achromia.

acquired l. See vitiligo.

congenital l. See albinism.

leukodystrophy Disease occurring early in life and affecting primarily the white matter of the brain, especially the cerebral hemispheres; thought to be a congenital defect in the formation or maintenance of myelin.

globoid cell l. See Krabbe's disease.

metachromatic l. A progressive disorder of sphingolipid metabolism in which sulfatide accumulates in the tissues; it affects both the central and peripheral nervous systems, causing blindness, deafness, muteness, and quadriplegia; death usually follows a few years from onset; most commonly seen in infants and young children. Also called sulfatide lipidosis.

leukoencephalopathy Leukodystrophy.

leukoerythroblastosis Any anemic condition resulting from lesions in the bone marrow.

leukokoria Any eye condition that causes a white reflection from behind the clear crystalline lens, giving the appearance of a white pupil.

leukolysis See leukocytolysis.

leukoma An opaque white spot on the cornea.

leukomyelitis Inflammation of the white tracts of

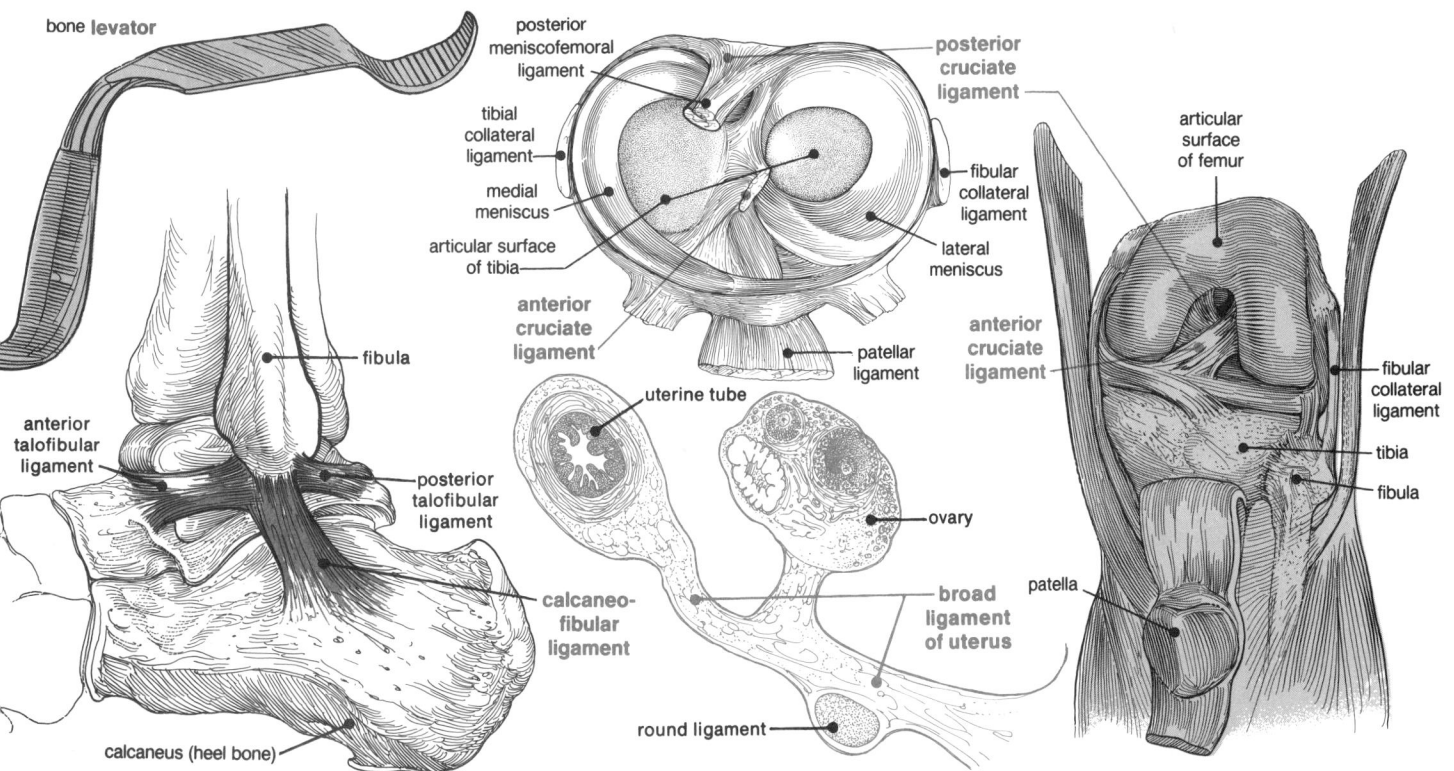

the spinal cord.

leukomyelopathy Any disease that involves the white tracts of the spinal cord.

leukonychia Unduly white nails; especially white spots or patches under the nails.

   l. striata Leukonychia in which the nail plate is marked by horizontal streaks of whiteness.

   l. totalis Leukonychia in which the entire nail is white.

leukopathia, leukopathy Leukoderma.

leukopedesis Movement of white blood cells through the capillary walls into the tissues.

leukopenia Abnormal reduction in the number of white corpuscles in the blood. Also called leukocytopenia.

leukoplakia A disease affecting the mucous membrane of the cheeks, tongue, gums, penis, or vulva, manifested by the formation of white, irregular thickened patches; a chronic inflammatory process, which may ultimately become a squamous cell carcinoma; continued mechanical and chemical irritation is considered the most frequent direct cause. Also called smoker's patch, when the lesion is in the oral cavity.

leukopoiesis The production of white blood cells.

leukoprotease An enzyme, the product of polynuclear leukocytes, formed in an area of inflammation and causing liquefaction of dead tissue.

leukorrhea An abnormal, white, or yellowish discharge from the vagina, containing mucus and pus cells.

leukosis Abnormal proliferation of tissues that form white blood cells.

leukotactic See leukocytotactic.

leukotaxine A crystalline nitrogenous substance prepared from inflammatory exudates and injured degenerating tissue.

leukotaxis See leukocytotaxia.

leukotomy Surgical incision into the white matter of the frontal lobe of the brain.

   prefrontal l. See lobotomy, prefrontal.

   transorbital l. See lobotomy, transorbital.

leukotriene Any 20-carbon unsaturated fatty acid derived from arachidonic acid which contains three alternating double bonds; leukotrienes trigger smooth muscle contraction, as in asthma, and have important roles in the inflammatory response.

levallorphan tartrate White, bitter, crystalline, antianalgesic substance; used in the treatment of narcotics overdose.

levarterenol bitartrate A white, crystalline, sympathomimetic substance that is soluble in water. Also called L-norepinephrine bitartrate.

levator 1. A muscle that raises a part. 2. Surgical instrument used to lift a structure or a depressed

part such as that of a fractured skull.

level A standard.

   hearing l. The measure of hearing ability as read on the hearing loss scale of the audiometer.

   l. of significance The probability that an observed difference is due to some factor or factors other than chance.

   toxic blood l. Level of concentration of a drug in the blood at which toxic symptoms are seen.

levodopa, L-Dopa A crystalline powder, 3-hydroxy-L-tyrosine, used to treat parkinsonism.

levorotatory Denoting the property of certain substances, as levulose, that turn the plane of polarized light counterclockwise.

levulose See fructose.

levulosuria Hereditary fructose intolerance; see under intolerance.

Lewis blood group (Le) Antigens of red cells, saliva, and other body fluids, specified by the Le gene, that react with the antibodies designated anti-Le[a] and anti-Le[b]; named after a Mrs. Lewis in whose blood the antibodies were discovered.

lewisite An oily liquid, $C_2H_2AsCl_3$, used to make a highly poisonous war gas.

libido 1. The emotional energy associated with primitive biologic impulses. 2. In psychoanalysis, the term is applied to the motive force of the sexual instinct.

Libman-Sacks syndrome Nonbacterial verrucous endocarditis associated with lupus erythematosus. Also called atypical verrucous endocarditis.

library, gene A large collection of independently cloned DNA fragments that have been inserted into a vector and theoretically contain at least one copy of each gene of the organism from which the DNA was obtained.

lichen Any eruption of the skin.

   l. planus An eruption of flat, glistening papules with depressed purplish centers.

lichenification Hardening and thickening of the skin resulting from long-continued irritation.

licorice See glycyrrhiza.

lidocaine hydrochloride A widely used local anesthetic; also used in the treatment of cardiac arrhythmias; Xylocaine Hydrochloride®.

lie of the fetus The relation that the long axis of the fetus bears to that of the mother.

   longitudinal l. Relationship in which the long axis of the fetus is roughly parallel to the long axis of the mother, noted in about 99 percent of all labors at term.

   transverse l. Relationship in which the long axis of the fetus is at right angles to that of the mother.

lien Latin for spleen.

lienorenal Splenorenal.

life The state or quality manifested by active metabolism; also called vitality.

life support The act of keeping a person alive.

   advanced l.s. (ALS) Emergency medical care, including the use of drugs, electrical stimulation of the heart and respiratory support, to maintain ventilation and blood circulation.

   basic l.s. (BLS) Emergency treatment that includes basic first aid, cardiopulmonary resuscitation, and treatment of shock.

ligament 1. Any band of fibrous tissue connecting bones. 2. Any membranous fold, sheet, or cordlike structure that holds an organ in position.

   acromioclavicular l. One extending from the acromion process of the scapula to the clavicle.

   alar l. One of two short, rounded cords connecting the second vertebra (axis) to the skull. Also called odontoid or check ligament.

   apical odontoid l. A ligament that extends from the apex of the odontoid process of the axis (second vertebra) to the anterior margin of the foramen magnum.

   arcuate l.'s Two ligaments (lateral and medial) that attach the diaphragm to the first lumbar vertebra and the twelfth rib on either side.

   broad l. of uterus One of two fibrous sheets covered on both sides with peritoneum, extending from the uterus to the lateral pelvic wall, on both sides.

   calcaneofibular l. One extending from the inferolateral side of the lateral malleolus to the lateral side of the calcaneus.

   capsular l. The fibrous membrane of a joint capsule.

   cardinal l. A sheet of subserous fascia embedded in the adipose tissue of the lower uterine cervix and vagina, on either side, extending in close association with the vaginal arteries.

   Cooper's l. 1. See pectineal ligament. 2. See suspensory ligament of breast.

   cricothyroid l. A well defined band of elastic tissue extending from the superior border (midline) of the cricoid cartilage to the inferior border of the thyroid cartilage.

   cruciate l.'s of knee Two ligaments (anterior and posterior) of considerable strength situated in the middle of the knee joint; they cross each other somewhat like the letter X.

   cruciform l. of atlas A cross-shaped ligament consisting of two parts: (a) a thick strong transverse band which arches across the ring of the first vertebra (it retains the dens of the second vertebra in place); (b) a small longitudinal band that divides the ring of the first vertebra into anterior and posterior parts.

   crural l. Inguinal ligament.

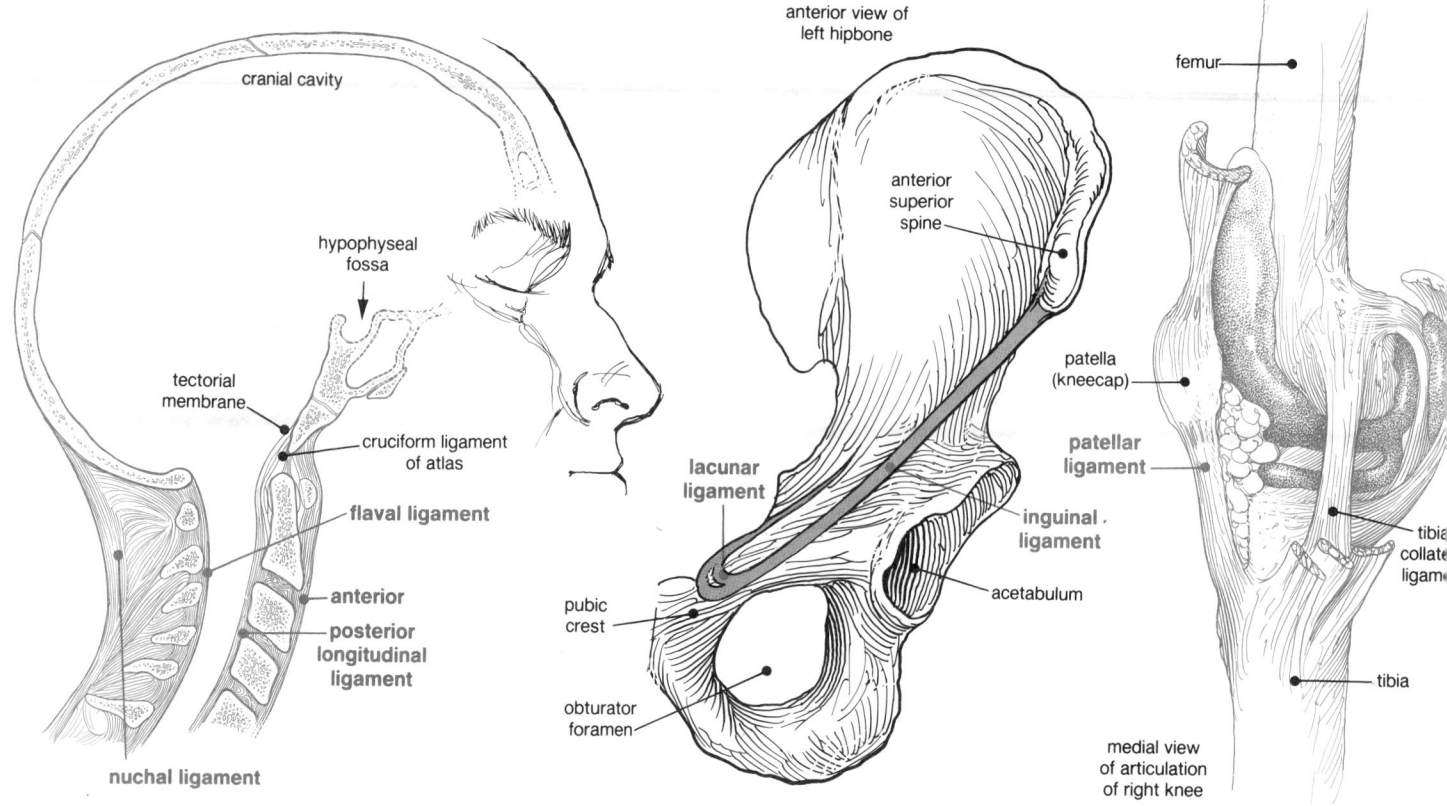

cranial cavity

hypophyseal fossa

tectorial membrane

cruciform ligament of atlas

flaval ligament

anterior

posterior longitudinal ligament

nuchal ligament

anterior view of left hipbone

anterior superior spine

lacunar ligament

pubic crest

obturator foramen

inguinal ligament

acetabulum

femur

patella (kneecap)

patellar ligament

tibial collateral ligament

tibia

medial view of articulation of right knee

deltoid l. The medial reinforcing ligament of the ankle joint.

falciform l. of liver A sickle-shaped ligament composed of two layers of peritoneum that ascends from the navel to the liver; it attaches the liver to the abdominal wall.

fibular collateral l. A strong, round, fibrous cord, situated on the lateral side of the knee joint; it is attached from the lateral condyle of the femur to the lateral side of the head of the fibula. Also called lateral collateral ligament.

flaval l.'s A series of yellow elastic bands that bind together the laminae of adjacent vertebrae from the axis to the first segment of the sacrum; they serve to maintain the upright position.

fundiform l. of penis A fibroelastic tissue that is intimately adherent to the linea alba and the pubic symphysis and is extended on to the dorsum of the penis.

hyoepiglottic l. A short triangular elastic band that unites the epiglottis to the upper part of the hyoid bone.

inguinal l. One extending from the anterior superior spine of the ilium to the tubercle of the pubic bone; it is actually the rolled inferior margin of the aponeurosis of the external oblique muscle. Also called Poupart's or crural ligament.

interfoveolar l. The thickened portion of the transverse fascia that lies medial to the deep inguinal ring, connecting the transverse muscle of the abdomen to the inguinal ligament and pectineal fascia. Also called Hesselbach's ligament.

interspinal l. Short bands of fibrous tissue that interconnect the spinous processes of adjacent vertebrae.

lacunar l.'s A triangular band extending horizontally from the inguinal ligament to the iliopectineal line of the pubis.

longitudinal l., anterior A broad, flat, strong band of fibers which extends along the anterior surface of the vertebral bodies from the axis (second vertebra) to the sacrum; it is thickest in the thoracic area.

longitudinal l., posterior A broad, flat, strong band of fibers in the vertebral canal, extending along the posterior surface from the axis (second vertebra) to the sacrum; it is thickest in the thoracic area.

nuchal l. A broad, somewhat triangular membranous septum in the back of the neck extending from the tips of the cervical spinous processes to the external occipital crest; it forms a septum for attach-ment of muscles on either side of the neck.

ovarian l. A cordlike bundle of fibers between the folds of the broad ligament, joining the uterine end of the ovary to the lateral margin of the uterus, immediately behind the attachment of the uterine tube.

palpebral l., medial Fibrous bands about 4 mm in length that connect the medial ends of the tarsi to the frontal process of the maxilla in front of the nasolacrimal groove.

patellar l. The continuation of the central part of the common tendon of the quadriceps muscle of the thigh (quadriceps femoris) from the patella to the tuberosity of the tibia; it is about 8 cm in length.

pectineal l. A strong aponeurotic band extending from the pectineal line of the pubis to the lacunar ligament with which it is continuous. Also called Cooper's ligament.

periodontal l. Connective tissue fibers that attach a tooth to the bone. Also called periodontal membrane.

Poupart's l. See inguinal ligament.

radial collateral l. A large bundle of fibers that crosses the lateral side of the elbow joint; it is attached above to the lateral epicondyle of the humerus, and below to the annular ligament and neck of the radius.

reflected inguinal l. A small, frequently absent, triangular sheet extending from the medial part of the inguinal ring to the linea alba.

round l. of liver A fibrous cord (the remains of the umbilical vein) extending from the navel to the anterior border of the liver. Also called ligamentum teres hepatis.

round l. of uterus A fibromuscular cord extending from the uterus, on either side, in front and below the uterine tube to the labium majus (usually passing through the inguinal canal).

sacrospinous l. A strong triangular ligament attached by its apex to the spine of the ischium and by its base to the lateral part of the sacrum and the coccyx.

sacrotuberous l. A strong ligament extending from the tuberosity of the ischium to the lateral part of the sacrum and coccyx and to the posterior infe-rior iliac spine.

sphenomandibular l. A flat, thin band which extends from the spine of the sphenoid bone to the lingula of the lower jaw.

stylomandibular l. A condensed band of cervical fascia which extends from the apex of the styloid process to the posterior border of the angle of the lower jaw.

suspensory l. of breast One of numerous fibrous bands distributed between the lobes of the mammary glands, extending from the skin to the deep layer of the superficial fascia. Also called Cooper's ligament.

suspensory l. of lens Ciliary zonula; see under zonula.

suspensory l. of ovary A band of peritoneum arising from the ovary and extending upward over the iliac vessels to become continuous with the peritoneum on the psoas major muscle; it contains the ovarian vessels and nerves.

thyroepiglottic l. An elastic ligament that at-taches the petiole of the epiglottis to the thyroid cartilage.

tibial collateral l. A broad, flat, membranous band, situated toward the medial and posterior part of the knee joint; it is attached from the medial condyle of the femur to the medial condyle and medial surface of the tibia. Also called medial col-lateral ligament.

ulnar collateral l. A thick triangular band of fibers that crosses the medial side of the elbow joint; it is attached above to the medial epicondyle of the humerus, and below to the coronoid process of the ulna (anterior portion) and to the medial margin of the olecranon (posterior portion).

uterosacral l. A fibrous band of subserous fascia extending from the uterine cervix, along the lateral wall of the pelvis, to the sacrum.

vestibular l. of larynx A thin fibrous membrane in the ventricular fold of the larynx that extends from the thyroid cartilage to the arytenoid cartilage. Also called vestibular ligament.

vocal l. The band that extends on either side from the thyroid cartilage to the vocal process of the arytenoid cartilage; it represents the upper border of the conus elasticus of the larynx.

ligamentous Of the nature of a ligament.

ligand An organic molecule attached to a central metal ion by multiple coordination bonds, as oxygen is bound to the central iron atom of hemoglobin.

ligase Enzyme that catalyzes the joining of two molecules coupled with the breakdown of ATP or some other nucleoside triphosphate.

ligate To constrict a blood vessel, a duct, or the pedicle of a tumor by means of a tightly tied thread (ligature).

ligation The tying of a blood vessel.

reater horn hyoid bone

epiglottis

hyoepiglottic ligament

hyoid bone

superior horn thyroid cartilage

thyrohyoid membrane

corniculate cartilage

thyroid cartilage

thyroepiglottic ligament

arytenoid cartilage

vestibular ligament of larynx

vocal ligament

cricoid cartilage

median cricothyroid ligament

posterior wall of trachea

tracheal ring

arytenoid cartilage

vocal muscle

vocal ligament

cricoid cartilage

thyroid cartilage

lateral cricoarytenoid muscle

closed vocal ligaments

posterior cricoarytenoid muscle

open vocal ligaments

uterine tube

ovarian ligament

suspensory ligament of ovary

uterine tube

fimbria

round ligament of uterus

ovary

ovarian ligament

broad ligament

posterior surface of uterus

right ureter

uterosacral ligament

lacrimal sac

lacrimal gland

frontal process of maxilla

lateral palpebral ligament

medial palpebral ligament

left eye

left hipbone (posterior surface)

sacrum

greater sciatic foramen

sacrospinous ligament

lesser sciatic foramen

coccyx

sacrotuberous ligament

obturator foramen

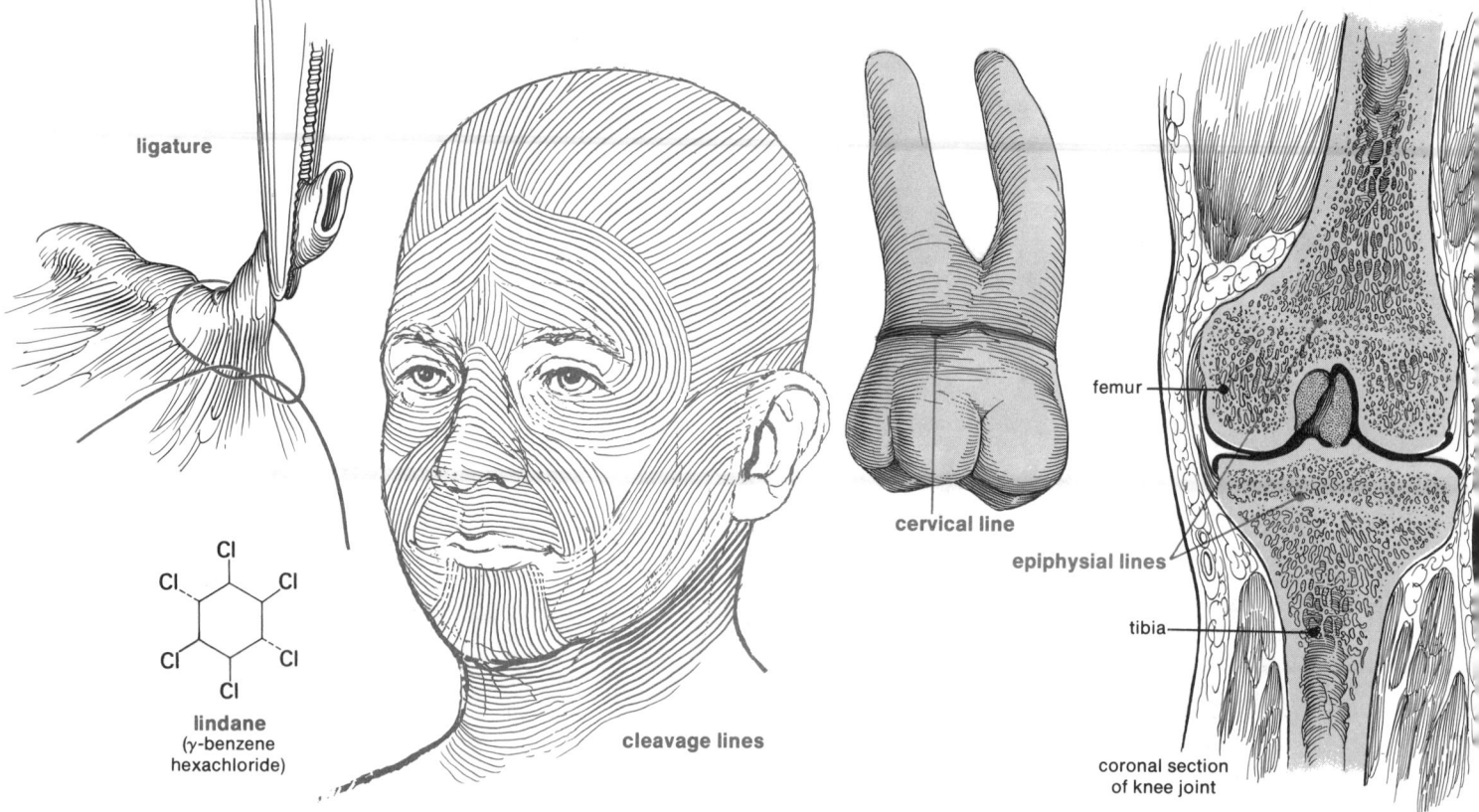

ligature (label, top left)

lindane
(γ-benzene
hexachloride)

cleavage lines

cervical line

femur

epiphysial lines

tibia

coronal section
of knee joint

ligator An instrument used for ligating blood vessels that are generally deep or nearly inaccessible.

ligature A thread used for tying vessels.

light An electromagnetic radiation capable of inducing visual sensation through the eye; radiant energy, approximately between 380 and 760 nm.

axial l. Rays of light parallel to each other and to the axis of an optical system.

coherent l. Electromagnetic radiation in which waves have a continuous relationship among phases.

cold l. 1. Light producing little or no heat, as that by certain luminous insects. **2.** Any visible light essentially devoid of infrared radiation.

diffused l. Light whose rays have no predominant directional component.

infrared l. Infrared rays; see under ray.

Minin l. A lamp that generates violet and ultraviolet light for therapeutic radiation.

polarized l. Light of which the vibrations are all in one plane, transverse to the ray, instead of in all planes.

reflected l. Light whose rays have been bent by a mirror-like surface and which continues to travel in the altered direction.

refracted l. Light whose pathway is altered from its original direction as a result of passing from one transparent medium to another of different density.

transmitted l. Light which passes or has passed through a transparent medium.

ultraviolet l. Ultraviolet rays; see under ray.

Wood's l. A lamp that generates ultraviolet radiation in the region near the visible spectrum; used in diagnosis and treatment of skin diseases, detection of corneal abrasions, and the evaluation of the fit of contact lenses.

lightening The sinking of the fetal head into the pelvic inlet causing the uterus to descend to a lower level and fall forward, thus relieving pressure on the diaphragm and making breathing easier.

Lignac-De Toni-Fanconi syndrome A childhood form of cystinosis; a rare genetic disorder marked by widespread deposits of cystine throughout the body and dysfunction of the renal tubules, associated with vitamin D-resistant rickets, acidosis, dwarfism, glycosuria, and albuminuria.

limb An extremity; an arm or leg.

lower l. The lower extremity that includes the hip, buttock, thigh, leg, and foot.

phantom l. A phenomenon often experienced by amputees in which sensations, sometimes painful, seem to originate in the amputated limb.

upper l. The upper extremity that includes the shoulder, arm, forearm, and hand.

limbic 1. Relating to a limbus or border. **2.**

Relating to the limbic system of the brain, comprising the cortex and related nuclei; thought to control emotional and behavioral patterns.

limbus, *pl.* **limbi** A border.

l. of cornea The highly vascular band at the junction of the cornea and sclera.

lime Calcium oxide, CaO; a white caustic powder used in waste treatment, insecticides, and in several industries. Also called quicklime; unslaked lime; calx.

limen, *pl.* **limina** A threshold; a border; the beginning point; the entrance to a structure.

l. insulae Threshold of the insula (island of Reil) of the brain; a narrow tongue of insular cortex extending ventromedially toward the anterior perforated substance; it receives fibers from the lateral olfactory stria.

l. nasi The threshold of the nose; the curved ridge that forms the superior and posterior boundary between the nasal cavity proper and the vestibule, where the skin is replaced by mucous membrane.

liminal Having the lowest amount of strength necessary to elicit a response; said of a stimulus.

liminometer Instrument to measure a stimulus that has the lowest amount of strength necessary to produce a reflex response.

limp 1. To walk lamely, with a yielding step. **2.** An uneven gait, favoring one leg. **3.** Flaccid.

lincomycin Substance produced by *Streptomyces lincolnensis*; it has antibacterial action against gram-positive organisms.

lindane A drug that repels ticks and kills lice. Also called gamma-benzene hexachloride.

Lindau's disease See von Hippel-Lindau disease.

line 1. A thin, continuous strip, mark, or ridge. **2.** A skin crease; a wrinkle. **3.** An imaginary mark connecting landmarks on the body or passing through them. **4.** A boundary or limit.

absorption l.'s Numerous dark lines in a spectrum due to absorption of specific wavelengths of light by the substance through which it passes.

axillary l. One of three imaginary vertical lines associated with the axilla; the anterior axillary line passes through the anterior fold of the axilla; the posterior passes through the posterior fold; the midaxillary passes through the center of the axilla.

B l.'s of Kerley Horizontal lines in the chest X ray (above the costophrenic angle) of individuals with pulmonary hypertension secondary to mitral stenosis.

blue l. See lead line.

cell l. In tissue culture, cells derived from a primary culture, growing *in vitro* in the first and sub-

sequent subcultures.

cervical l. The line around a tooth marking the junction of the enamel of its crown and the cementum of its root.

cleavage l.'s Definite linear clefts in the skin indicative of the direction of the underlying subcutaneous fibrous connective tissue bundles. Also called Langer's lines.

dentate l. See pectinate line.

epiphysial l. The line of junction of the epiphysis and diaphysis of an adult long bone.

finish l. In the preparation of a dental cavity, the minimal line of demarcation of the wall of the preparation at the cavosurface.

Fleischner l.'s Linear shadows on a chest x-ray, indicating foci of atelectasis.

fulcrum l. An imaginary line of dental appliance rotation. Also called rotational axis.

gingival l. The position of the margin of the gingiva as it extends onto a tooth. Also called gum line.

gluteal l. One of three rough curved lines on the outer surface of the iliac part of the hipbone, designated anterior, posterior, and inferior.

gum l. See gingival line.

Hampton l. In radiography, a line of decreased density surrounding a benign stomach ulcer.

iliopectineal l. An oblique ridge on the surface of the ilium and continued on the pelvis, which forms the lower boundary of the iliac fossa; it separates the true from the false pelvis. Also called linea terminalis.

Langer's l. See cleavage lines.

lead l. A dark bluish area of abnormal pigmentation of the gingival tissues, usually 1 mm from the gingival crest, associated with lead poisoning. Also called blue line.

l. of accommodation The linear extent to which an object can be moved closer to or away from the eye in a given state of refraction without causing noticeable blurriness.

l. of occlusion The alignment of the occluding surface of the teeth in the horizontal plane.

M l. A line formed by the nodular thickenings of the myofilament (myosin) bisecting the H zone of striated muscle myofibrils.

median l. A vertical center line dividing the body surface into right and left parts.

mercurial l. A linear discoloration of the gingival tissues associated with mercury poisoning and seen along the gingival margin; it can be bluish, purplish, or muddy red in coloration.

midaxillary l. An imaginary vertical line passing through the middle of the axilla.

midclavicular
line

anterior
axillary
line

scapular
line

phreno-esophageal
ligament

esophagus

diaphragm

stomach

Z-Z line

basement membrane

sarcolemma

sarcoplasm

xiphoid
process

rectus muscle
of abdomen

myofibril

umbilicus

Z-line

M line

sarcomere

pubic
symphysis

linea alba

actin filament (50Å)

myosin filament (100Å)

anterior abdominal wall

midclavicular l. A vertical line passing through the midpoint of the clavicle on either side; it corresponds closely to a perpendicular line passing through the nipple.

milk l. The line or ridge of thickened epithelium in the embryo, extending from the axillary to the inguinal region, along which the mammary glands are developed.

Muercke's l.'s Parallel, transverse white lines in fingernails and toenails; associated with chronic hypoalbuminemia.

nipple l. A vertical line passing through the nipple on either side.

nuchal l.'s Three lines or ridges (inferior, superior, and highest) on the exterior surface of the occipital bone of the skull.

pectinate l. The line between the rectal mucosa and the skin lining the anus. Also called dentate line.

pectineal l. The line on the superior ramus of the pubic bone from the pubic tubercle to the iliopubic eminence. Also called pecten pubis.

pure l. A strain of animals inbred for many generations, homozygous for certain specific genes. Also called isogenic strain.

scapular l. An imaginary vertical line passing through the lower angle of the scapula on either side.

Schwalbe's annular l. One formed by the peripheral limit of Descemet's membrane of the cornea, indicating the anterior edge of the trabeculae and spaces of Fontana.

simian l. The single flexion crease usually present on the palms of individuals with the Down syndrome.

survey l. 1. A line inscribed on a cast of a tooth by a surveyor scriber; it marks the greatest height of contour in relation to the chosen path of insertion of the restoration. **2.** The line denoting the height of contour of a tooth after the cast has been positioned according to the chosen path of insertion. Also called clasp guideline.

temporal l.'s The two curved lines (inferior and superior) on the outer surface of the parietal bones of the skull.

visual l. An imaginary straight line extending from the object seen to the fovea centralis of the retina. Also called visual axis.

Wagner's l. A narrow line representing the area of preliminary calcification, at the junction of the epiphysis and diaphysis of a long bone.

Z l. One of the transverse septa dividing the myofibrils of skeletal muscle into longitudinally arranged sarcomeres; the region between two Z lines consists of overlapping thick and thin myofilaments. Also called Z band.

zigzag l. See Z-Z line.

Z-Z l. The transition line from esophageal to gastric mucosa; it appears as an irregular dentate or zigzag line. Also called zigzag line.

linea, *pl.* **lineae** A line.

l. alba The narrow portion of the anterior aponeurosis running down the midline of the abdominal wall from the xiphoid process to the pubic symphysis. Also called white line.

l. aspera A longitudinal ridge with two prominent lips, on the posterior surface of the femur. Also called rough line.

l. nigra The dark streak on the abdomen of pregnant women, between the umbilicus and the pubic symphysis.

l. semilunaris The lateral edge of the abdominal rectus muscle; it crosses the costal margin at the tip of the ninth costal cartilage.

l. terminalis Iliopectineal line; see under line.

line breeding A method of breeding designed to perpetuate the desirable traits of an animal by crossbreeding its descendants.

liner A layer of asbestos applied to the inside of a dental casting ring in order to free the investment from the restraint of the ring during heating.

lingua Latin for tongue; denotes any tongue-like anatomic structure.

lingual Pertaining to the tongue.

lingually Toward the tongue.

lingula Any tongue-shaped process.

l. of cerebellum The most anterior tongue-shaped lobule of the superior vermis of the cerebellum.

l. of lung A projection from the upper lobe of the left lung just beneath the cardiac notch.

l. of mandible A projection of bone overlapping the mandibular foramen on the inner surface of the ramus of the mandible; it serves for the attachment of the sphenomandibular ligament.

lingulectomy Surgical removal of the lingular portion of the upper lobe of the left lung.

linguoclusion The displacement of a tooth or group of teeth toward the tongue. Also called lingual occlusion.

linguo-occlusal Relating to the lingual and occlusal surfaces of a posterior tooth; usually denoting the line angle formed by the junction of the two surfaces.

linguopapillitis Small painful ulcers around the papillae on the tongue margins.

linguoversion Malposition of a tooth toward the tongue.

liniment An oily medicinal liquid applied to the

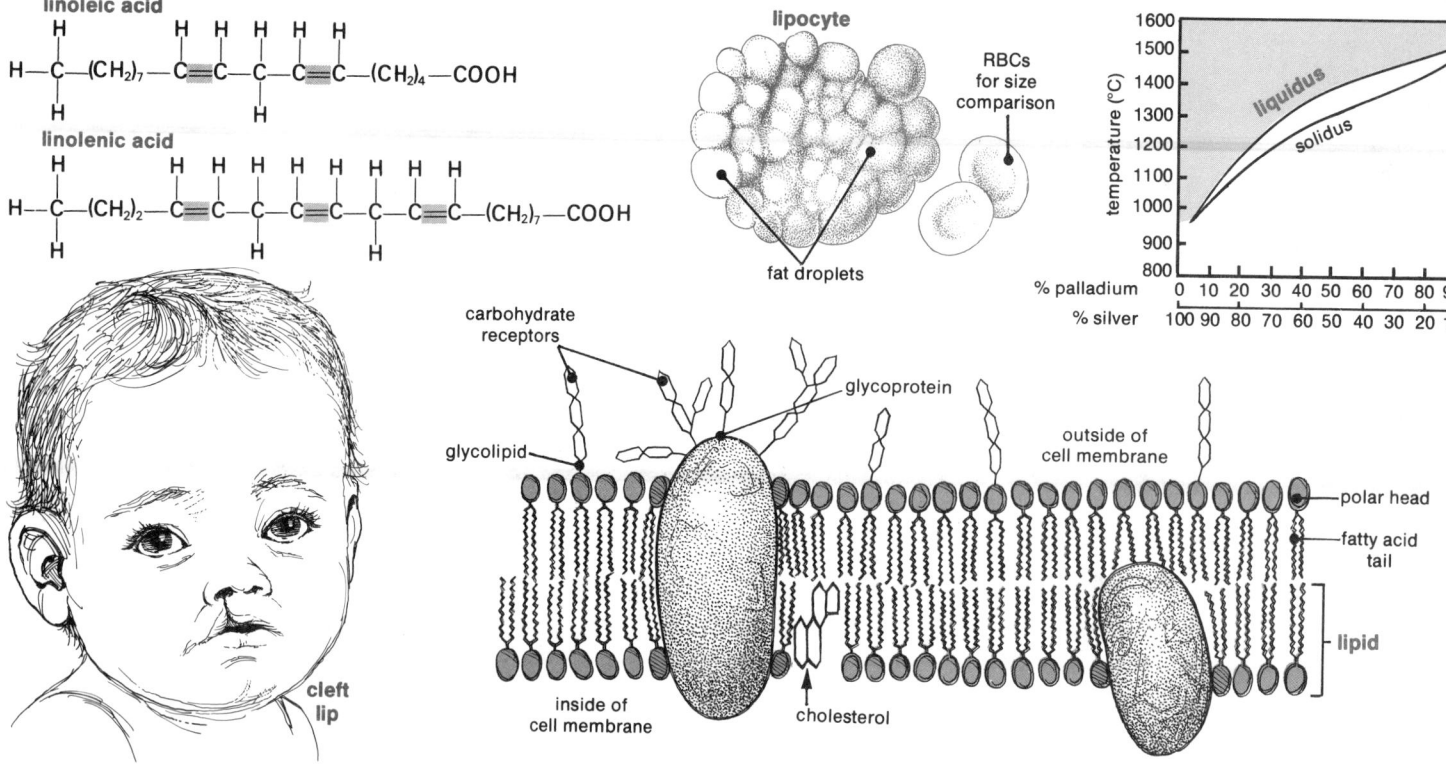

linoleic acid

linolenic acid

lipocyte

RBCs for size comparison

fat droplets

% palladium

% silver

carbohydrate receptors

glycoprotein

glycolipid

outside of cell membrane

polar head

fatty acid tail

lipid

inside of cell membrane

cholesterol

cleft lip

skin by friction as a counterirritant.

linin The fine, threadlike, nonstaining (achromatic) substance of the cell nucleus that interconnects the chromatin granules.

lining In dentistry, a coating applied to the walls of a tooth cavity to protect the pulp from irritation by the restorative filling; most commonly used cements include zinc-oxide eugenol (ZOE), zinc phosphate, and calcium hydroxide.

linitis Inflammation of the cellular tissue of the stomach.

  l. plastica extensive thickening of the stomach wall due to infiltrating scirrhous carcinoma. Also called leather-bottle stomach.

linkage 1. The force that holds together the atoms in a chemical compound, or the symbol used to represent it. 2. The relationship existing between two or more genes in the same chromosome that causes them to remain together from generation to generation.

  sex l. Linkage occurring when a gene that determines a certain trait is carried in a sex (X or Y) chromosome. See also X linkage.

  X l. Sex linkage occurring when a gene that determines a trait is located on the X chromosome; the term sex linkage is often used synonymously with X linkage, but since a Y-linked trait is also sex-linked, the preferred term is X linkage.

linoleic acid A light straw-colored polyunsaturated fatty acid, $C_{18}H_{32}O_2$, that is essential in the human diet; it strengthens capillary walls, lowers serum cholesterol, and prolongs blood clotting time.

linolenic acid A colorless polyunsaturated fatty acid, $C_{18}H_{30}O_2$, that is essential in the human diet.

liothyronine 3,5,3 ′Triiodothyronine.

lip 1. One of the two fleshy folds forming the anterior boundary of the mouth. 2. Any liplike structure.

  cleft l. Congenital malformation of the upper lip ranging from a scarlike groove, or a notching of the lip, to a complete cleft extending into the nasal cavity. Also called harelip.

  double l. An oral anomaly consisting of a fold of excess or redundant tissue on the mucosal side of the lip; the upper lip is involved more than the lower one.

lipase A fat-splitting enzyme present in pancreatic juice, blood, and many tissues.

  lipoprotein l. Enzyme that promotes the breakdown of the triglycerides of chylomicrons to form free fatty acid and glycerol.

lipectomy Surgical removal of adipose tissue, as for certain cases of obesity. Also called adipectomy.

  suction l. See liposuction.

lipedema Chronic swelling of the legs, seen most frequently in middle-aged women.

lipemia See hyperlipidemia.

lipid 1. Generally any fat, oil, or wax, or any derivative of these materials; soluble in organic compounds like alcohol and insoluble in water. 2. Specifically, the fats and fat-like materials which, together with carbohydrates and proteins, constitute the main structural substance in the living cell.

lipidemia See hyperlipidemia.

lipidosis, *pl.* **lipidoses** General term applied to disorders marked by abnormal concentration of lipids in the tissues.

  ganglioside l. See gangliosidosis.

  sulfatide l. Metachromatic leukodystrophy; see under leukodystrophy.

lipoatrophy, lipoatrophia Atrophy of body fat, as the loss of subcutaneous fat after repeated injections of insulin into the same area.

lipocele A hernial sac containing adipose tissue. Also called adipocele.

lipochondrodystrophy See Hurler's syndrome.

lipochrome Any of various naturally occurring fatty pigments such as carotene and lipofuscin.

lipocyte Fat cell; see under cell.

lipodystrophy Defective or faulty metabolism of fat.

lipofibroma A benign tumor composed of fibrous connective tissue and fatty tissue.

lipofuscin A golden brown lipid-containing pigment that represents the indigestible residue of cellular lysosomal activity, associated with normal wear and tear. Sometimes called old age pigment.

lipogenesis The formation of fat.

lipogenic Fat-producing. Also called adipogenic.

lipoid Resembling fat.

lipoidosis The presence of lipid material deposited in various organs.

lipolipoidosis Fatty infiltration of the cells.

lipolysis The splitting up or chemical decomposition of fat.

lipoma A benign tumor composed of mature fat cells. Also called adipose tumor.

  l. fibrosum See fibrolipoma.

lipomatoid Resembling a tumor of fatty tissue.

lipomatosis Deposition of fat, either local or general. Also called liposis.

lipomatous 1. Of the nature of a lipoma. 2. Marked by the presence of a lipoma.

lipophage A fat-absorbing cell.

lipophagic Ingesting or absorbing fat.

lipophil Having affinity for lipids.

lipoprotein A conjugated protein containing fat as the nonprotein substance.

  high-density l. (HDL) A plasma protein of relatively small molecular weight containing propor-

tionally more protein and less cholesterol and triacylglycerides.

  low-density l. (LDL) A plasma protein of relatively large molecular weight containing proportionally less protein and more cholesterol and triacylglycerides.

lipoprotein a [LP(a)] A chemically modified low-density lipoprotein (LDL) by insertion of apolipoprotein a (a glycoprotein).

liposarcoma A rare malignant tumor usually found in the retroperitoneal and mediastinal fat deposits of elderly individuals.

liposis See lipomatosis.

liposuction Removal of fat with a vacuum device.

lipotropic Relating to lipotropy.

lipotropy 1. Prevention of excessive accumulation of fat in the liver. 2. Affinity of basic dyes for fatty tissue.

lipoxygenase Enzyme that promotes oxidation of polyunsaturated fatty acids.

lipping The formation of a liplike border at the articular end of a bone in degenerative bone disease.

lipuria The presence of fat in the urine.

liquefacient An agent that causes a solid to dissolve or become liquid.

liquefaction 1. The act of liquefying. 2. The state of being converted into a liquid form.

liquescent Entering or tending to enter the liquid state.

liquid A substance, neither solid nor gaseous, that exhibits a characteristic readiness to flow, like water.

liquidus The temperature line on a constitution diagram above which the indicated metal element or alloy turns to liquid.

liquor, *pl.* **liquores** 1. A liquid substance. 2. A solution of a nonvolatile substance in water.

Listeria A genus of bacteria (family Corynebacteriaceae) containing small, gram-positive, aerobic rods; found in feces, sewage, and vegetation.

  L. monocytogenes A species causing meningitis, septicemia, abscesses, and local purulent lesions.

listeriosis Infection with bacteria of the genus *Listeria;* commonly occurring in animals, but occasionally transmitted to man, where it may produce a clinical picture resembling infectious mononucleosis or an acute meningitis.

liter (l) A metric unit of capacity equal to a cubic decimeter, or 1000 cubic centimeters; approximately 1.056 liquid quarts.

lithagogue An agent that causes the dislodging or expulsion of a calculus, especially of a urinary calculus.

lithectasy The extraction of a bladder stone through the previously dilated urethra.

lithiasis The formation of stones, especially biliary

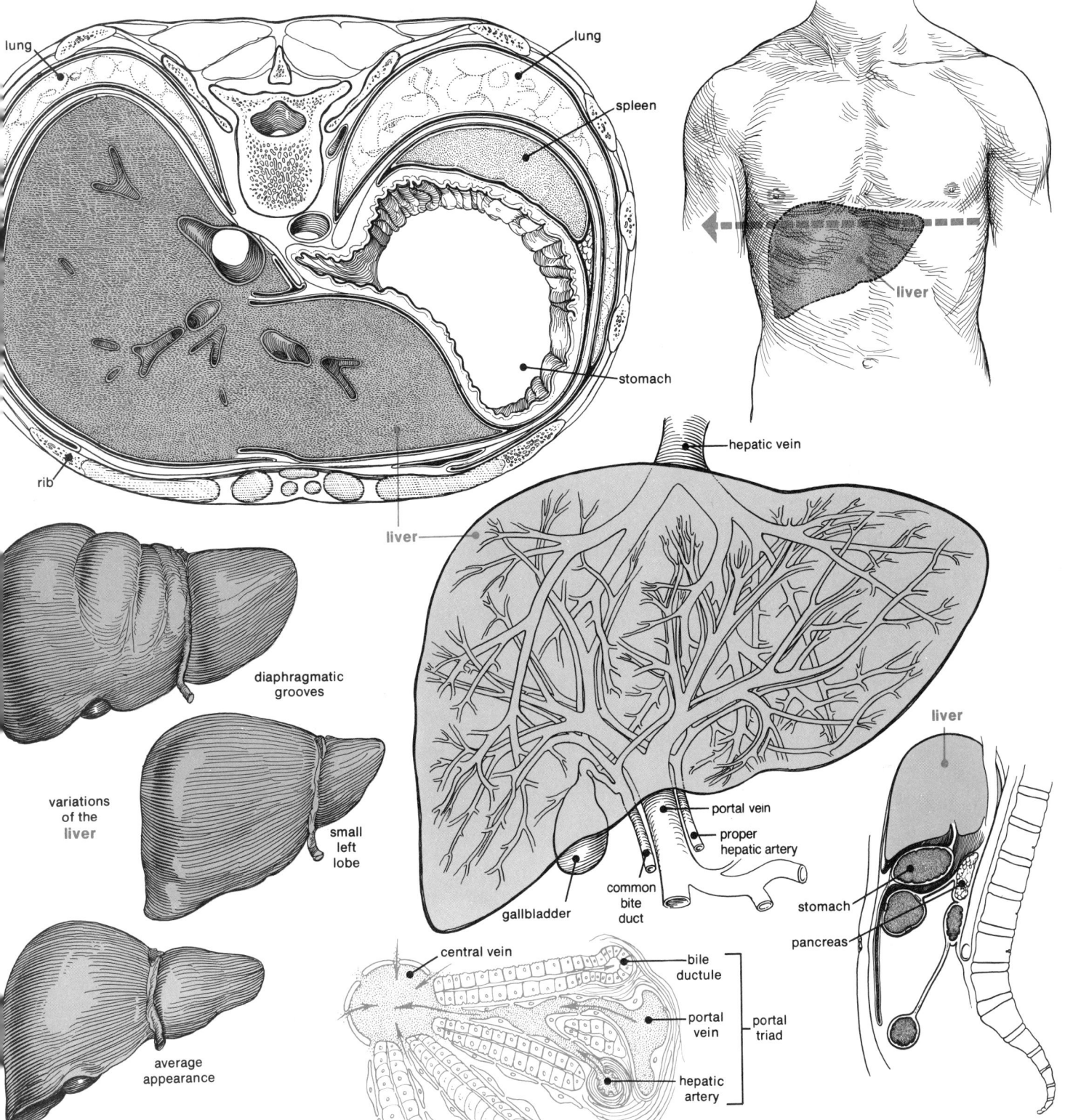

lung

lung

spleen

stomach

hepatic vein

rib

liver

diaphragmatic grooves

variations of the **liver**

small left lobe

average appearance

central vein

bile ductule

portal vein

portal triad

hepatic artery

portal vein

proper hepatic artery

common bile duct

gallbladder

liver

stomach

pancreas

or urinary stones.

lithium A silvery, soft, highly reactive metallic element; symbol Li, atomic number 3, atomic weight 6.939; used in the treatment of mental illness, particularly in manic disorders.

lithocystotomy Removal of stones from the bladder.

lithodialysis The crushing or dissolving of a stone in the bladder.

lithogenic Promoting the formation of stones.

lithogenous Causing the formation of stones.

litholapaxy See lithotripsy.

litholysis Dissolution of stones.

lithometra Calcification of the tissue of the uterus.

lithonephria Stone in the kidney.

lithopedion A retained calcified fetus.

lithotomy Operation for the removal of a stone, especially from the bladder.

lithotresis The boring of holes in a calculus to facilitate its crushing and removal.

lithotripsy The operation of crushing a stone in the urinary bladder by means of a lithotrite and then washing out the fragments through a wide transurethral catheter. Also called litholapaxy.

   extracorporeal shock-wave l. (ESWL) Breaking up of kidney stones by shock waves generated outside the body and focused on the stones electronically; applied mostly to urinary tract but can also be used on gallstones.

lithotrite Instrument for crushing stones in the bladder.

lithous Relating to a calculus or stone.

lithuresis The passage of minute stones or gravel in the urine.

lithuria A condition marked by excess uric (lithic) acid or urates in the urine.

litmus A blue pigment, obtained from *Roccella tinctoria* and other lichens, that turns red with in-

creasing acidity and blue with increasing alkalinity.

litmus paper White paper impregnated with litmus powder and used as a test for acidity and alkalinity; the acid-base pH range is from 4.5 to 8.3.

litter 1. A stretcher for transporting the disabled. 2. A group of animals produced at one birth by a multiparous mammal. Also called brood.

livedo reticularis Circulatory disorder of unknown origin causing constant bluish discoloration on large areas of the extremities.

liver A large, dark red gland that produces and secretes bile, playing an important role in the metabolism of carbohydrates, fats, protein, minerals, and vitamins; located beneath the entire right dome of the diaphragm and approximately one-third of the left dome, it is the largest glandular organ in the body, weighing from 1,200 to 1,600 g in the adult (about $\frac{1}{40}$ the weight of the body); on the basis of the internal distribution of the blood vessels and bile

parietal lobe

occipital lobe

frontal lobe

temporal lobe

lateral and medial aspects of brain

parietal lobe

frontal lobe

cingulate gyrus

occipital lobe

temporal lobe

pyramidal lobe of thyroid gland

left hepatic lobe

medulla

lobule of thymus gland

cortex

septum

lobulated kidney of an infant

right hepatic lobe

Riedel's lobe

ducts, the liver may be divided into nearly equal right and left lobes. Also called hepar.

cirrhotic l. A fibrotic liver associated with alterations of the lobular structure and the presence of regenerative nodules and vascular anastomoses.

fatty l. An enlarged, doughy liver due to fatty degeneration and infiltration (fatty metamorphosis); it may develop as a complication of any disease in which malnutrition, especially protein deficiency, is present; commonly seen in the early stages of alcoholic cirrhosis or in diabetes.

fibrotic l. A liver marked by an increase in connective tissue without disturbance of the lobular architecture.

nutmeg l. A liver presenting a mottled or polymorphic appearance when sectioned.

livid 1. Black and blue. **2.** Denoting a bluish-gray complexion. Also called cyanotic.

lixiviation The process of removing the soluble ingredients from a substance by repeated washing or percolating. Also called leaching.

lixivium The soluble ingredients removed from any substance by leaching. Also called lye.

Loa Congolese for eyeworm; a genus of filarial roundworms.

L. loa The so-called eyeworm, a threadlike round-worm that infests the subcutaneous tissues, causing tumefactions; the worms migrate rapidly and are usually noticed when passing through the conjunctiva across the eyeball or over the bridge of the nose; indigenous to the western part of equatorial Africa.

load 1. The quantity borne or sustained by an organism or a part. **2.** A deviation from normal of any body contents (water, salt, etc.); positive load is more than normal and negative load is less

than normal. **3.** To introduce a defined quantity for some test purpose or to achieve a desired blood level.

lobar Relating to a lobe.

lobate Composed of or divided into lobes; lobed.

lobe 1. A fairly well defined portion of an organ or gland bounded by structural borders such as fissures, sulci, or septa. **2.** A rounded anatomic projecting part, as the fatty lobule of the human ear. **3.** One of the main divisions of the crown of a tooth, formed from a distinct point of calcification.

azygos l. An occasional small triangular lobe on the mediastinal surface at the apex of the right lung, which is delimited by the arch of the azygos vein embedded in the lung substance.

caudate l. A small lobe of the liver situated posteriorly between the inferior vena cava and the fissure for the ligamentum venosum.

ear l. The lower fleshy part of the auricle.

frontal l. The portion of each cerebral hemisphere bounded behind by the central and below by the lateral sulci.

hepatic l. Any of the liver lobes, designated right, left, caudate, and quadrate.

limbic l. A general term that usually denotes the cingulate and parahippocampal gyri along with the olfactory bulb and stalk and the parolfactory and olfactory gyri.

occipital l. The most posterior portion of each cerebral hemisphere, bounded anteriorly by the parieto-occipital sulcus and the line joining it to the preoccipital notch.

olfactory l. A general term that usually denotes the olfactory bulb, tract, and trigone plus the anterior perforated substance.

parietal l. The upper central portion of each cer-

ebral hemisphere between the frontal and occipital lobes, and above the temporal lobe; it is separated from the frontal lobe by the central sulcus.

pyramidal l. of thyroid gland An inconstant, narrow, somewhat cone-shaped lobe of the thyroid gland that arises from the upper border of the isthmus and extends upward; occasionally it arises from the adjacent part of either lobe (most commonly the left), or may be completely detached; sometimes it is attached to the hyoid bone by a fibrous band.

Riedel's l. A tongue-shaped mass of tissue occasionally extending downward from the right lobe of the liver.

quadrate l. A small lobe on the inferior surface of the liver between the gallbladder and the ligamentum teres.

temporal l. A long lobe on the outer side and under surface of each cerebral hemisphere; it is bounded above by the lateral sulcus.

lobectomy Surgical removal of a lobe.

lobelia The dried leaves and tops of *Lobelia inflata*; contains several alkaloids including lobeline, norlobelanine, and isolobelanine.

lobeline A mixture of alkaloids derived from plants of the genus *Lobelia*; it has actions similar to those of nicotine, but less potent.

lobotomy Surgical incision into a lobe.

prefrontal l. A psychosurgical procedure consisting of division of the fibers in the brain connecting the prefrontal and frontal lobes with the thalamus. Also called prefrontal leukotomy.

transorbital l. Lobotomy through the roof of the orbit. Also called transorbital leukotomy.

lobulated Consisting of or divided into lobules.

lobule A small lobe.

lobulet, lobulette A very small lobule or a section

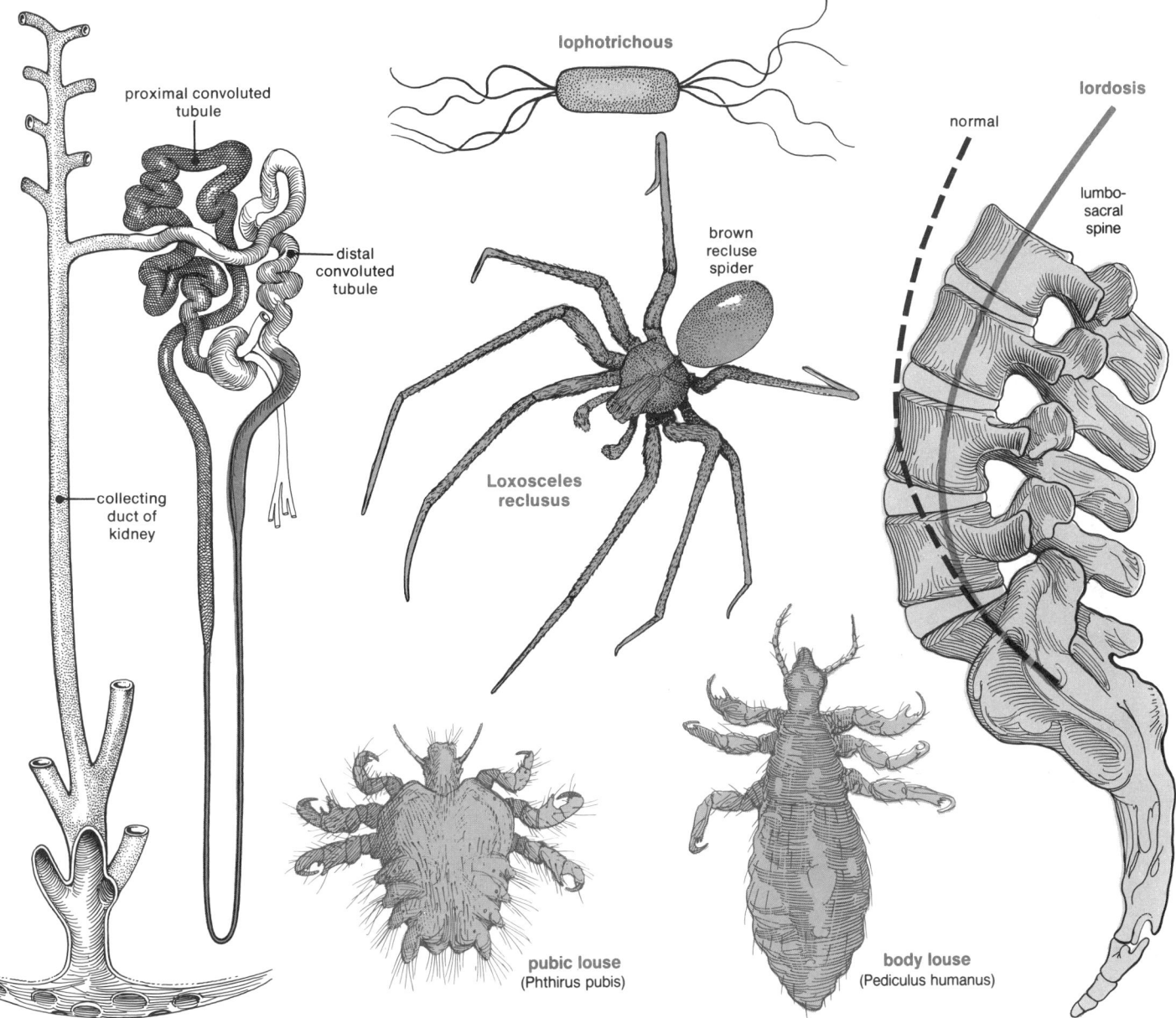

proximal convoluted tubule

distal convoluted tubule

collecting duct of kidney

lophotrichous

brown recluse spider

Loxosceles reclusus

lordosis

normal

lumbo-sacral spine

pubic louse
(Phthirus pubis)

body louse
(Pediculus humanus)

or subdivision of a lobule.

lobulus, *pl.* **lobuli**   Latin for lobule.

lobus, *pl.* **lobi**   Latin for lobe.

local   Confined to a limited area.

localization   1. Restriction of a process to an area. 2. The determination of the site of a morbid process.

localized   Limited to a definite part; generally applied to changes that are restricted or confined to a particular area or part.

localizer   A visual training instrument used in the treatment of amblyopia or anopsia.

lochia   The bloody discharge from the uterus following childbirth.

lochiometra   Retention of blood and mucus (lochia) in the uterus following childbirth.

lochiometritis   Inflammation of the uterus following childbirth.

lochiorrhea   Excessive flow of discharges after childbirth.

lochioschesis   Retention in the vagina of the post-delivery discharges (lochia).

loci   Plural of locus.

lockjaw   1. See tetanus. 2. A symptom of tetanus; see trismus.

loco   A condition affecting cattle who eat loco weed; marked primarily by incoordination and dullness. Also called loco-weed disease.

locomotor   Relating to motion.

loco-weed disease   See loco.

locular   Of or relating to a loculus.

loculate, loculated   Divided into or containing numerous loculi.

loculation   1. A structure or tissue having numerous small cavities. 2. The formation of small cavities or loculi.

loculus, *pl.* **loculi**   A small cavity.

locum tenens   One who temporarily assumes the place of another, e.g., a practitioner assuming someone else's practice during an illness or vacation.

locus, *pl.* **loci**   A place or spot, as the specific site occupied by a gene in a chromosome.

l. ceruleus   A bluish gray area in the floor of the fourth ventricle.

Löffler's disease   An uncommon but distinctive form of disease in which the heart is the organ mainly affected by an eosinophilic arteritis, probably of an allergic type; characterized by progressive congestive heart failure, multiple systemic emboli, and eosinophilia. Also called eosinophilic endomyocardial disease; Loffler's endocarditis.

Löffler's syndrome   Disorder, usually lasting less than a month, marked by transient infiltrates of the lungs, low fever, and increased number of eosinophils in the peripheral blood.

logopathy   Any disorder of speech.

logoplegia   Paralysis of the speech organs.

logorrhea   Excessive, uncontrollable talking.

loin   The part of back and sides of the body between the ribs and the pelvis.

loop   1. A bend in a cord or cordlike structure. 2. A platinum wire attached to a handle at one end and bent into a circle at the other; used to transfer bacterial cultures.

Henle's l.   See nephronic loop.

nephronic l.   The U-shaped portion of the nephronic tubule, between the proximal and distal convoluted portions. Also called Henle's loop or ansa.

lophotrichous   Referring to a bacterial cell with two or more flagella or cilia at one or both poles.

lordoscoliosis   An abnormal backward and lateral curvature of the spine.

lordosis   Abnormally increased forward curvature of the lumbar spine. Also called sway-back.

lordotic   Of, relating to, or characterized by lordosis.

lotion   1. Any of various medicated liquids for external application, especially those containing one or more insoluble substances in suspension. 2. Any of various liquid cosmetic preparations, usually applied to the face and hands.

calamine l.   A preparation of mineral oil with zinc oxide, ferric oxide, glycerin, bentonite magma, and calcium hydroxide solution.

loupe   A small magnifying lens, usually set in an eyepiece.

louse, *pl.* **lice**   1. Any of various small, wingless, flat-bodied, parasitic insects of the orders Anoplura and Mallophaga. 2. Common name for *Pediculus humanus capitis*.

body l.   See *Pediculus humanus corporis*.

crab l.   See *Phthirus pubis*.

head l.   See *Pediculus humanus capitis*.

pubic l.   See *Phthirus pubis*.

Lowe's syndrome   See oculocerebrorenal syndrome.

Loxosceles reclusus   North American brown recluse spider; volume for volume its venom is more potent than a rattlesnake's; its bite is potentially about as lethal as that of the black widow spider.

loxoscelism   A condition resulting from the bite of the North American brown recluse spider, *Loxosceles reclusus*; characterized by gangrenous slough at the affected area, nausea, malaise, fever, hemolysis, and thrombocytopenia.

loxotomy   Surgical amputation by means of an oblique incision through the soft tissue; distinguished from a circular amputation.

lozenge   A medicated disk-shaped tablet for local

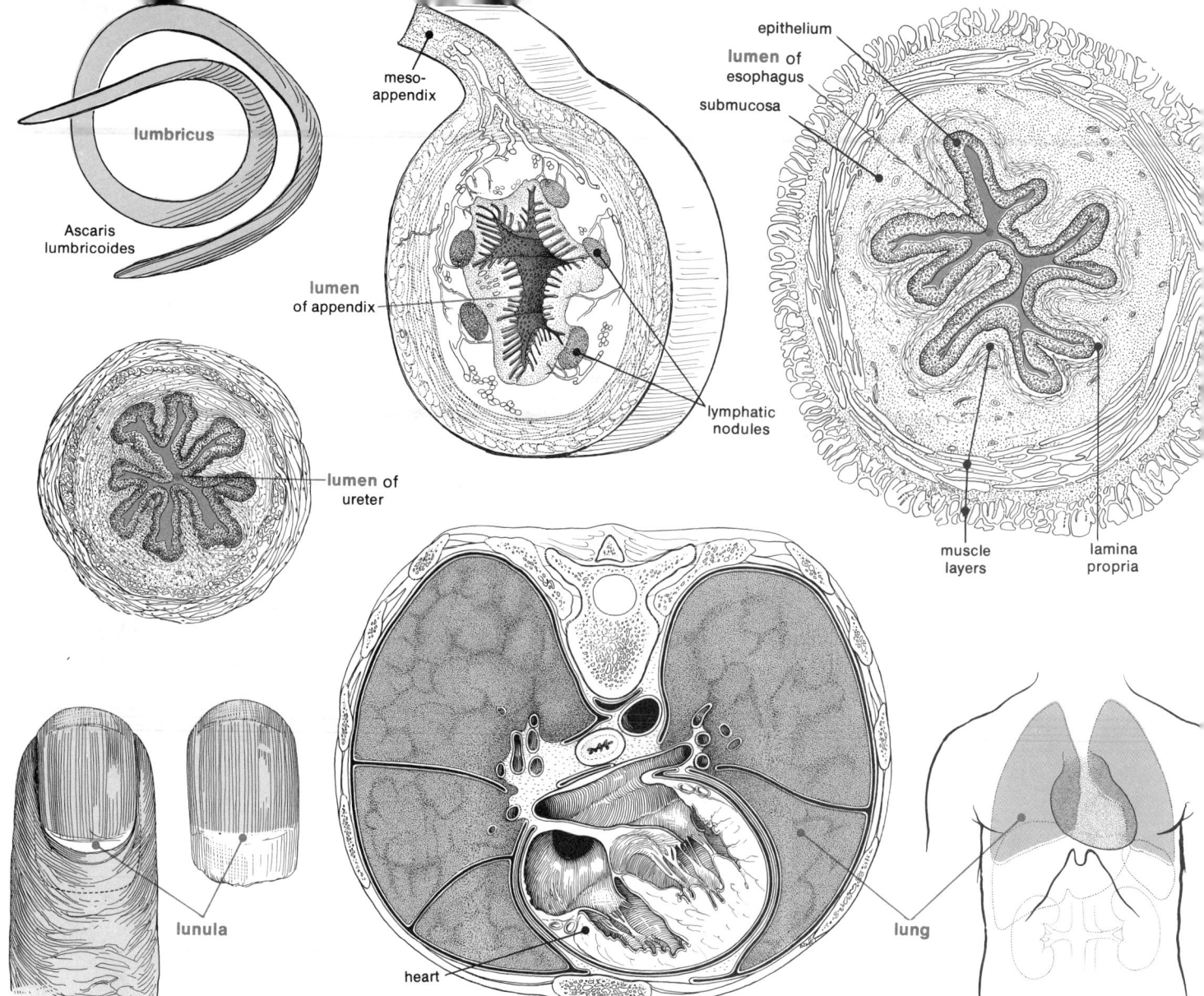

lumbricus

Ascaris lumbricoides

meso-appendix

lumen of appendix

lumen of ureter

lymphatic nodules

epithelium

lumen of esophagus

submucosa

muscle layers

lamina propria

lunula

heart

lung

---

treatment of the mouth or throat. Also called troche.

lubricant Any substance or secretion acting as a surface coating that reduces friction, heat, and wear.

  vaginal l. The transudate-like secretion which appears on the walls of the vagina shortly after the onset of effective sexual stimulation.

lubrication The process of lubricating or making slippery.

lucifugal Avoiding light.

lues Syphilis.

luetic Syphilitic.

lumbago Backache in the lumbar region.

lumbar (l) Relating to the loins.

lumbarization Fusion between the transverse processes of the lowest lumbar and the adjacent sacral vertebrae.

lumbosacral Relating to the lumbar portion of the spine and the sacrum.

lumbrical **1.** Pertaining to or resembling an earthworm. **2.** See table of muscles.

lumbricoid Resembling an earthworm.

lumbricus A worm parasitic in the intestine, *Ascaris lumbricoides*.

lumen **1.** The interior space of a tubular structure, as a blood vessel or the esophagus. **2.** A unit of emitted light; one lumen equals 0.001946 watt.

lumina One of the plural forms of lumen.

luminal Relating to the lumen of a blood vessel, intestine, or other tubular structure.

luminescence The property of giving off light by processes that derive energy from essentially non-thermal sources.

luminiferous Producing, conveying, or transmitting light.

luminophore **1.** Any substance that emits light at room temperature. **2.** An organic radical that produces or increases the property of luminescence of certain organic compounds.

luminous Emitting or reflecting light.

lumirhodopsin An intermediate product in the bleaching process of rhodopsin by the action of light prior to the formation of metarhodopsin and the retinene.

lumpectomy Surgical removal of a hard mass of tissue, especially from the breast.

lunacy Obsolete word for a major mental illness.

lung The paired organ of respiration occupying the chest cavity (together with the heart) and enveloped by the pleura; generally the right lung is slightly larger than the left and is divided into three lobes, while the left has but two; the primary purpose of the lung is the uptake of oxygen and the elimination of carbon dioxide; it is accomplished by the following processes: (a) ventilation (inspired air reaches the alveoli and is distributed evenly to the millions of alveoli in the lungs); (b) diffusion (oxygen and carbon dioxide pass across the alveolar capillary membranes); (c) pulmonary capillary blood flow (flow is distributed evenly to all the ventilated alveoli).

  black l. A form of pneumoconiosis common in coal mines, characterized by heavy deposit of coal dust in the lung; chronic bronchitis and emphysema may be associated with the condition.

  coal miner's l. Black lung.

  farmer's l. An acute reaction or condition due to inhalation of moldy hay dust, usually from handling grains, particularly in threshing; thought to be of allergic origin; the symptoms are distressing dyspnea, cyanosis, and a dry cough. Also called thresher's lung.

  honeycomb l. A lung marked by a spongy or honeycomb appearance from numerous small cysts resulting from diffuse fibrosis and cystic dilation of bronchioles.

  iron l. A popular name for the Drinker respirator; see under respirator.

  miner's l. Black lung.

  rheumatoid l. Infiltrates in the lung associated with rheumatoid arthritis.

  shock l. See adult respiratory distress syndrome.

  thresher's l. See farmer's lung.

  welder's l. Relatively benign form of pneumoconiosis due to deposition of fine metallic particles in the lung; occupational hazard among welders.

  wet l. Accumulation of fluid in the lung as in pulmonary edema.

lungworm Any of various nematode worms parasitic in the air passages of animals.

lunula The pale semicircle at the root of each nail. Also called half moon.

lupoid Resembling lupus.

lupus A general term denoting any of several diseases manifested by characteristic skin lesions; used with a qualifying adjective.

  discoid l. erythematosus A disease confined to the skin, marked by a scaly rash, usually in a butterfly pattern over the nose and cheeks, sometimes extending to the scalp and causing baldness.

  l. pernio Sarcoid lesions of the hands and face, especially the ears and nose, resembling frostbite.

  l. vulgaris Infection of the skin with the bacillus of tuberculosis, causing red-brown nodular lesions most frequently on the face.

  systemic l. erythematosus (SLE) A chronic disease of unknown origin commonly marked by an erythematous rash on the face and other areas exposed to sunlight; it is much more common in

lymphocyte

cytoplasm

nucleus

heterochromatin

euchromatin

villus-like
processes at
cell border

red blood cell
for size comparison

lymphedema

women than men and occurs most often in the third and fourth decades; it involves the vascular and connective tissues of many organs, resulting in a multiplicity of local and systemic manifestations; serologic abnormalities including a false positive VDRL and antinuclear antibodies are manifestations, as well as a positive LE cell test; anti-DNA antibodies appear to be specific for SLE.

luteal Relating to the corpus luteum of the ovary.

lutein The yellow pigment of egg yolks, corpus luteum, and fat cells.

luteinization The formation of luteal tissue; process in which the mature ovarian follicle after discharging the egg, becomes hypertrophied and yellow, thus forming the corpus luteum.

luteinizing See luteogenic.

Lutembacher's syndrome Congenital abnormality of the heart marked by an interatrial defect and mitral stenosis.

luteogenic Inducing the development of corpora lutea. Also called luteinizing.

luteoma An uncommon ovarian tumor believed to be formed in the same way that the lutein cells of the corpus luteum are produced.

luteotrophic, luteotropic Having a stimulating action on the development and function of the corpus luteum.

lutetium A silvery-white rare earth element, symbol Lu, atomic number 71, atomic weight 174.97; the final member of the lanthanide rare earth series; used in nuclear technology.

Lutheran blood group Antigens of red blood cells, specified by the Lu gene, that react with antibodies designated anti-Lu^a and anti-Lu^b; first detected in the serum of an individual who had received many transfusions and who developed antibodies against the erythrocytes of a donor named Lutheran.

lux A unit of illumination, equal to one lumen per square meter.

luxation Dislocation.

lye 1. Sodium or potassium hydroxide. **2.** Lixivium.

lying-in Confinement of a woman during childbirth.

Lyme disease Disorder occurring generally in summer and fall marked by a raised red spot on the skin (erythema chronicum migrans), fever, fatigue, lymph gland swelling and muscle pain; arthritis of a single or several joints develops after several weeks; heart and nerves may be involved; caused by a spirochete transmitted by ticks (genus *Ixodes*).

lymph A transparent or slightly opalescent fluid containing a clear liquid portion, a varying number of white blood cells, chiefly lymphocytes, and a few

red blood cells; it is absorbed from the tissue spaces by the lymphatic capillaries (a system of closed tubes), conveyed, and eventually returned to the bloodstream by the lymphatic vessels, after it flows through a filtering system (lymph nodes).

lymphaden Lymph node; see under node.

lymphadenectasia Enlargement of lymph nodes with excessive lymph.

lymphadenectomy Surgical removal of lymph nodes.

lymphadenia Chronic overgrowth of lymphoid tissue.

lymphadenitis Inflammation of the lymph nodes.

lymphadenography Roentgenographic examination of a lymph node.

lymphadenoma Any tumor made up of lymphoid tissue. See lymphoma.

lymphadenomatosis A condition marked by the presence of numerous enlarged lymph nodes, as in malignant lymphoma.

lymphadenopathy Any disorder of the lymph nodes or lymph vessels.

lymphadenosis Generalized enlargement of the lymph glands and lymphatic tissue of the organs; proliferation of lymphoid tissues.

   benign l. Infectious mononucleosis; see under mononucleosis.

   malignant l. Lymphoma

lymphagogue An agent that increases the formation and flow of lymph.

lymphangiectasia, lymphangiectasis Abnormal dilatation of lymphatic vessels. Also called telangiectasia lymphatica.

lymphangiectomy Surgical excision of a lymphatic vessel.

lymphangioendothelioma A tumor composed of small masses of endothelial cells and aggregations of tubular structures thought to be lymphatic vessels.

lymphangiography Roentgenographic visualization of lymphatic vessels after injection of a contrast medium. Also called lymphography.

lymphangiology See lymphology.

lymphangioma A tumor-like mass of dilated lymphatic vessels.

lymphangitis Inflammation of the lymphatic vessels; a common manifestation of a bacterial infection, usually caused by the hemolytic streptococcus.

lymphatic Relating to lymph, lymph nodes, or lymph vessels.

lymphectasia Dilatation of the lymphatic vessels.

lymphedema Chronic unilateral or bilateral swelling of the extremities caused by obstruction of the lymphatic vessels or disease of the lymph nodes.

lymphoblast An immature cell that is the precursor of the lymphocyte. Also called lymphocytoblast;

immunoblast.

lymphoblastic Relating to lymphoblasts or the production of lymphocytes.

lymphoblastoma A tumor arising in a lymph node or group of nodes, composed mainly of lymphoblasts; a form of malignant lymphoma.

lymphoblastosis Excess of lymphoblasts in the blood.

lymphocele A cystic mass that contains lymph. Also called lymphocyst.

lymphocyte A white blood cell formed in lymphoid tissue and constituting normally from 25 to 33 percent of all white blood cells in adult peripheral blood.

   B l.'s Lymphocytes derived from bone marrow; they interact chiefly with the humoral immune system which involves substances such as antibodies, antigens, and serum complement enzymes in the blood; analogous to the lymphocytes of birds governed by the bursa of Fabricius.

   cytotoxic T l. Lymphocyte that kills target cells (e.g., tumor cells) by releasing a protein (perforin) to perforate the target cell membrane after antibodies have reacted with an antigen on the target cell.

   helper T-l. A subtype of T lymphocytes which stimulate B lymphocytes into producing antibody-forming cells. Also called helper T-cell.

   T l.'s Lymphocytes derived from the thymus; they play a large role in the cellular immune system by responding to antigens and triggering reactions in other cells, such as macrophages.

   virgin l. Inducible cell; see under cell.

lymphocytic Relating to lymphocytes.

lymphocytoblast See lymphoblast.

lymphocytoma A tumor of low grade malignancy, arising in a lymph node or group of nodes; made up chiefly of adult lymphocytes.

lymphocytopenia Marked reduction in the number of lymphocytes in the blood.

lymphocytopoiesis The formation of lymphocytes.

lymphocytosis Excessive number of lymphocytes in the blood.

lymphoderma perniciosa See leukemia cutis.

lymphoepithelioma A malignant tumor derived from the epithelium of the area around the tonsils and nasopharynx, and containing abundant lymphoid tissue.

lymphogenesis The production of lymph.

lymphogenous 1. Originating from lymph. **2.** Producing lymph.

lymphogranuloma venereum (LGV) A chlamydial infection marked by the appearance of a transient ulcer on the genitalia and enlargement of

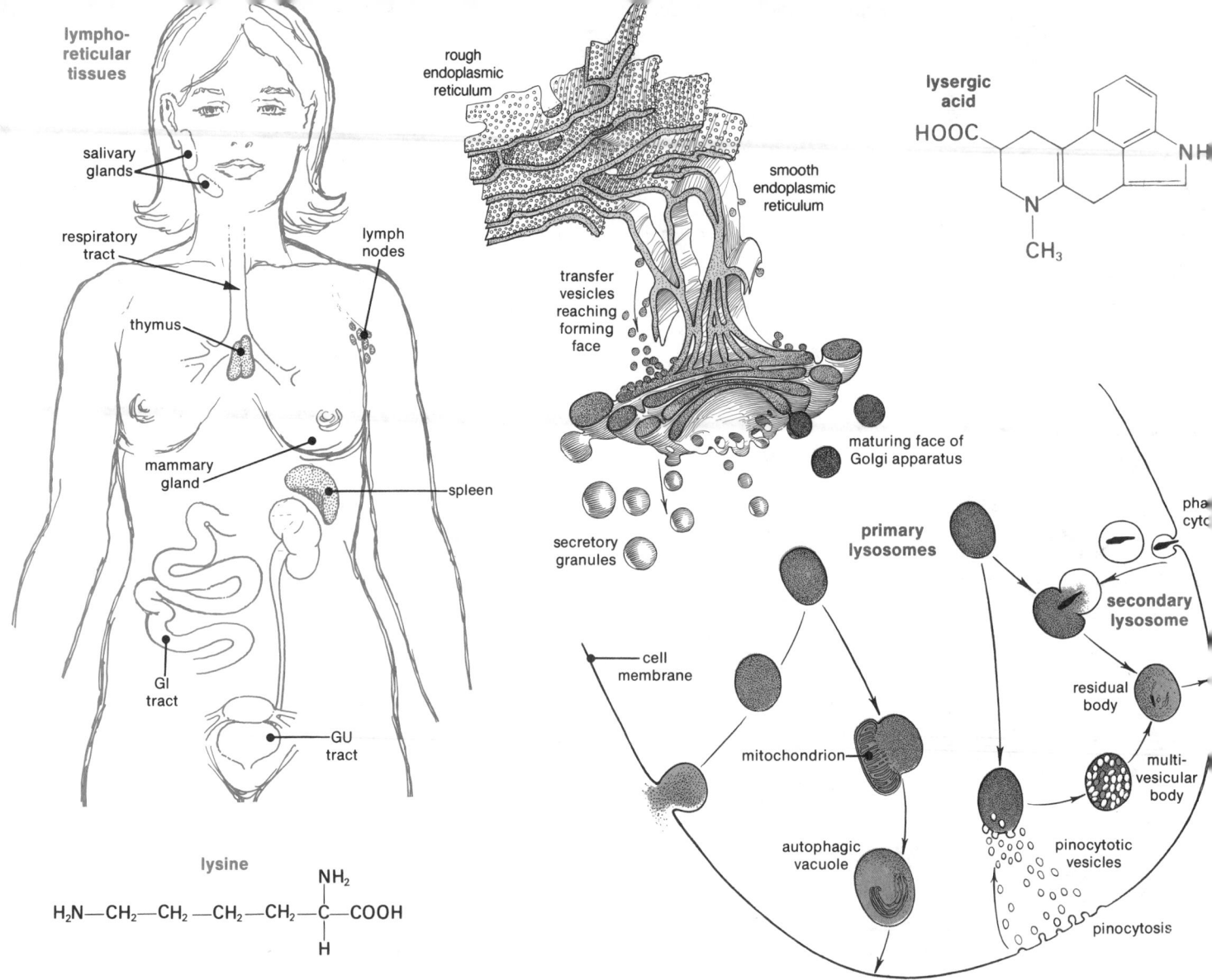

lympho-reticular tissues

salivary glands
respiratory tract
thymus
mammary gland
lymph nodes
spleen
GI tract
GU tract

rough endoplasmic reticulum
smooth endoplasmic reticulum
transfer vesicles reaching forming face
maturing face of Golgi apparatus
secretory granules
cell membrane
primary lysosomes
secondary lysosome
residual body
multi-vesicular body
mitochondrion
autophagic vacuole
pinocytotic vesicles
pinocytosis

lysergic acid
HOOC

lysine
H₂N—CH₂—CH₂—CH₂—CH₂—C—COOH
NH₂
H

the lymph nodes of the groin in the male and the pararectal nodes in the female. Also called tropical bubo; lymphogranuloma inguinale. Formerly called lymphopathia venereum.

lymphography See lymphangiography.

lymphoid Pertaining to or resembling lymph or lymphatic tissue.

lymphoidectomy Surgical excision of lymphoid tissue, such as adenoids.

lymphokine A hormone-like factor produced by sensitized lymphocytes when they come in contact with the antigen to which they were sensitized; acts as an intercellular messenger to regulate immunologic and inflammatory responses.

lymphokinesis 1. Circulation of lymph through the lymphatic vessels and nodes. 2. The movement of endolymph in the membranous labyrinth of the internal ear.

lymphology The science of the lymphatic system comprising lymph, lymphocytes, lymph nodes, and lymph vessels. Also called lymphangiology.

lymphoma Any of a group of malignant diseases originating in the lymphoreticular system, usually in the lymph nodes.

  Burkitt's l. A malignant tumor affecting children of the middle African regions; it involves primarily the jaw and abdominal area. Also called African lymphoma.

  giant follicular l. A malignant tumor of lymphoid tissue characterized by multiple proliferative, follicle-like nodules.

lymphomatosis Any condition characterized by the presence of multiple lymphoid tissue tumors (lymphomas).

lymphopathia venereum Old term for lymphogranuloma venereum.

lymphopathy Any disease of the lymphatic system.

lymphopenia Reduction in the number of lymphocytes in the blood.

lymphopoiesis The formation of lymphocytes.

lymphoreticular Relating to a tissue containing a variety of cell types involved in the elaboration of a cell product when confronted with a substance which is recognized as foreign; the tissue is located within the thymus gland, lymph nodes, spleen, and the lining of the lymphatic and vascular channels, as well as in bodily tracts exposed to the outside.

lymphosarcoma A malignant tumor of lymph nodes composed of lymphoblasts and lymphocytes which enlarges and invades adjacent tissues.

lymphostasis Obstruction of the normal flow of lymph.

lyophil Any substance that easily goes into solution; lyophilic material.

lyophilic Denoting a pronounced affinity between the dispersed particles and the solvent (dispersing medium) of a colloid.

lyophilization 1. The process of freeze-drying; the act of separating a solid substance from solution by freezing the solution and evaporating the ice under vacuum. 2. Process used for preservation of a variety of tissues and bacteria.

lyophilize To separate a solid from solution by rapid freezing and dehydration under vacuum; to freeze-dry.

lyophobic Denoting a lack of affinity between the dispersed particles and the solvent of a colloid.

lyotropic Readily soluble.

lyse To effect lysis (disintegration of cells).

lysergic acid A crystalline compound derived from ergot.

  l. a. diethylamide (LSD) A hallucinogenic drug derived from lysergic acid.

lysin An antibody that destroys cells by dissolving them, as hemolysin and bacteriolysin which destroy

blood cells and bacteria, respectively.

lysine (Lys) One of the essential amino acids; produced by the hydrolysis of casein and other proteins.

lysis 1. Destruction of cells by a specific lysin. 2. The gradual recovery from an acute disease.

lysogen An antigen that stimulates the formation of a specific lysin.

lysogenesis The production of antibodies that cause dissolution of cells and tissues.

lysogeny A form of viral parasitism in which viral DNA becomes incorporated in a cell (bacterial) genome, without destroying the cell, thereby permitting the transmission of the virus to the subsequent generation.

lysokinase An activator agent of the fibrinolytic system, such as streptokinase or staphylokinase, that produces plasma by indirect or multiple-stage action on plasminogen.

lysolecithin A lecithin (phosphatidyl choline) from which the unsaturated fatty acid residue has been removed by partial hydrolysis; it has strong hemolytic properties and is a good detergent and emulsifier of dietary lipid.

lysosome One of the large cytoplasmic particles in a cell containing a powerful digestive juice (hydrolyzing enzyme or lysozyme) capable of breaking down most of the constituents of living matter; it is present in all animal cells, being particularly large and abundant in white blood cells.

  primary l. A lysosome that has not engaged in any digestive activity.

  secondary l. A vacuolated lysosome that is the site of current or previous digestive activity.

lysozyme An antibacterial enzyme naturally present in tear fluid, sweat, saliva, and nasal secretions. Also called mucopeptide glucohydrolase.

lytic Relating to or causing disintegration of cells.

colony

macrodactylia

macrophage

nucleus

macroconidium

Mm

μ The Greek letter mu.

Macaca mulatta The rhesus monkey; a species (genus *Macaca*, family Cercopithecidae) of Southeast Asia that is frequently used as a laboratory animal.

Mace Proprietary name for the lacrimator chloracetophenone, combined with dispersant and a propellant; used in aerosol form as a defensive weapon; disables by means of intense, burning eye pain and respiratory distress.

macerate To soften a solid or a tissue by soaking in a fluid.

maceration **1.** The softening of a tissue or other solid or the separation of its constituents by soaking it in a liquid. **2.** In obstetrics, the softening and disintegration of a fetus remaining in the uterus after its death.

machine A device that accomplishes a specific objective.

  heart-lung m. Any of various machines that make it possible to support the circulation with oxygenated blood while keeping the heart essentially free of blood and permitting surgery within the heart, coronary arteries, and ascending arch of the aorta under direct vision; venous blood ordinarily returning to the right atrium is diverted to an oxygenator (artificial lung) where it takes up oxygen and gives off carbon dioxide; the oxygenated blood is pumped into the individual's arterial system.

  Holtz m. A device for developing high-voltage static electricity by multiplication of an induced charge.

  kidney m. Artificial kidney; see under kidney.

  panoramic rotating m. An x-ray machine capable of radiographing all the teeth and surrounding structures by using a reciprocating motion of the tube and extraoral film.

  Van de Graaf m. An electrostatic machine that produces high potential; used for generating high-voltage x rays.

  Wimshurst's m. A machine capable of converting mechanical energy into electrical energy by electrostatic action.

Macracanthorhynchus hirudinaceus A species of the thorny-headed worms (class Acanthocephala) between 5 and 65 cm in length; a parasite of hogs and, occasionally, of humans.

macrencephaly, macrencephalia Macroencephaly.

macroamylase A form of serum amylase in which the enzyme occurs as a complex joined to a globulin.

macrobrachia Condition of having abnormally long arms.

macrocephalous Having an abnormally large

head.

macrochemistry Chemistry in which the reactions are visible to the naked eye.

macrochilia **1.** Unusually large lips. **2.** A condition of permanently enlarged oral lips, usually due to the presence of distended lymph spaces.

macrochiria A condition of unduly enlarged hands. Also called megalochiria.

macroconidium A large exospore or conidium.

macrocornea See megalocornea.

macrocrania Abnormal general enlargement of the head; distinguished from enlargement of the head in one direction only.

macrocryoglobulinemia The presence of cold precipitating macroglobulins (cold hemagglutinins) in the peripheral blood.

macrocyte A large red blood cell at least 2 μm larger than normal; can be seen in the blood of individuals with pernicious anemia, folic acid deficiency, and other anemias. Also called megalocyte.

macrocythemia See macrocytosis.

macrocytosis A condition in which the red blood cells are larger than normal. Also called macrocythemia.

macrodactylia, macrodactyly A condition in which fingers or toes are abnormally large. Also called dactylomegaly; megalodactylism.

macrodont **1.** An abnormally large tooth. **2.** Denoting a skull with a dental index over 44.

macrodontia The condition of having abnormally large teeth.

macroencephaly Malformation and great increase in size and weight of the brain due partly to proliferation of the glia (nonneuronal tissue); associated with small ventricles, enlargement of the head, and mental retardation.

macrogamete The female of certain unicellular organisms.

macrogametocyte A mother cell producing the females or macrogametes of certain protozoa.

macrogenitosomia Disorder of the adrenal cortex affecting male children, believed by some to originate during prenatal life; characterized by early enlargement of the penis with frequent erections, associated with rapid growth of the skeleton, muscles, body hair, and larynx; ossification of the skeleton occurs prematurely, resulting in abnormally short stature.

macrogingivae Abnormal enlargement of the gums.

macroglia The astrocyte and oligodendrocyte, the two neuroglial elements of ectodermal origin.

macroglobulin Unusually large plasma globulin (protein); molecular weight is often about 1,000,000.

macroglobulinemia A plasma cell dyscrasia; a

disorder marked by excessive production of gamma M globulin; common findings include anemia and bleeding manifestations. Also called primary macroglobulinemia; Waldenström's syndrome.

macroglossia Enlargement of the tongue. Also called megaloglossia.

macrognathia Abnormal largeness of the jaw.

macrogyria A congenital malformation in which the convolutions of the cerebral cortex are larger than normal due to a reduction in the number of sulci.

macrolides A group of antibiotics having molecules made up of large-ring lactones; e.g., erythromycin.

macromastia, macromazia Abnormally large breasts.

macromelia A condition of unduly enlarged limbs; abnormal size of one or more of the extremities. Also called megalomelia.

macromethod A chemical test using ordinary (not minute) quantities.

macromolecule Any molecule composed of several monomers, notably proteins, nucleic acids, polysaccharides, glycoproteins, and glycolipids.

macronucleus **1.** A nucleus that occupies a large area of the cell. **2.** The larger, nonreproductive nucleus in ciliated protozoa.

macroparasite A parasite that is visible to the unaided eye; e.g., a louse.

macropathology Gross anatomic changes caused by disease.

macrophage A large mononuclear cell which ingests degenerated cells and blood tissue; found in large numbers throughout the body, with the greatest accumulation in the spleen, where they remove damaged or aging red blood cells from the circulation; in the brain and spinal cord they are known as microglia; in the blood they are called monocytes.

  alveolar m. A cell that moves about on the alveolar surface of the lung engulfing airborne particles that reach the alveolus; derived from the hematogenous monocyte. Also called dust cell; alveolar phagocyte.

macrophthalmia Abnormal enlargement of the eyeballs.

macroplasia Gigantism.

macropolycyte An extremely large polymorphonuclear neutrophilic leukocyte having a nucleus with numerous segments.

macropsia The condition of seeing objects as larger than their actual sizes. Also called megalopsia.

macrorhinia The condition of having an abnormally large nose.

macroscopic Visible with the naked eye, without need of magnifying equipment.

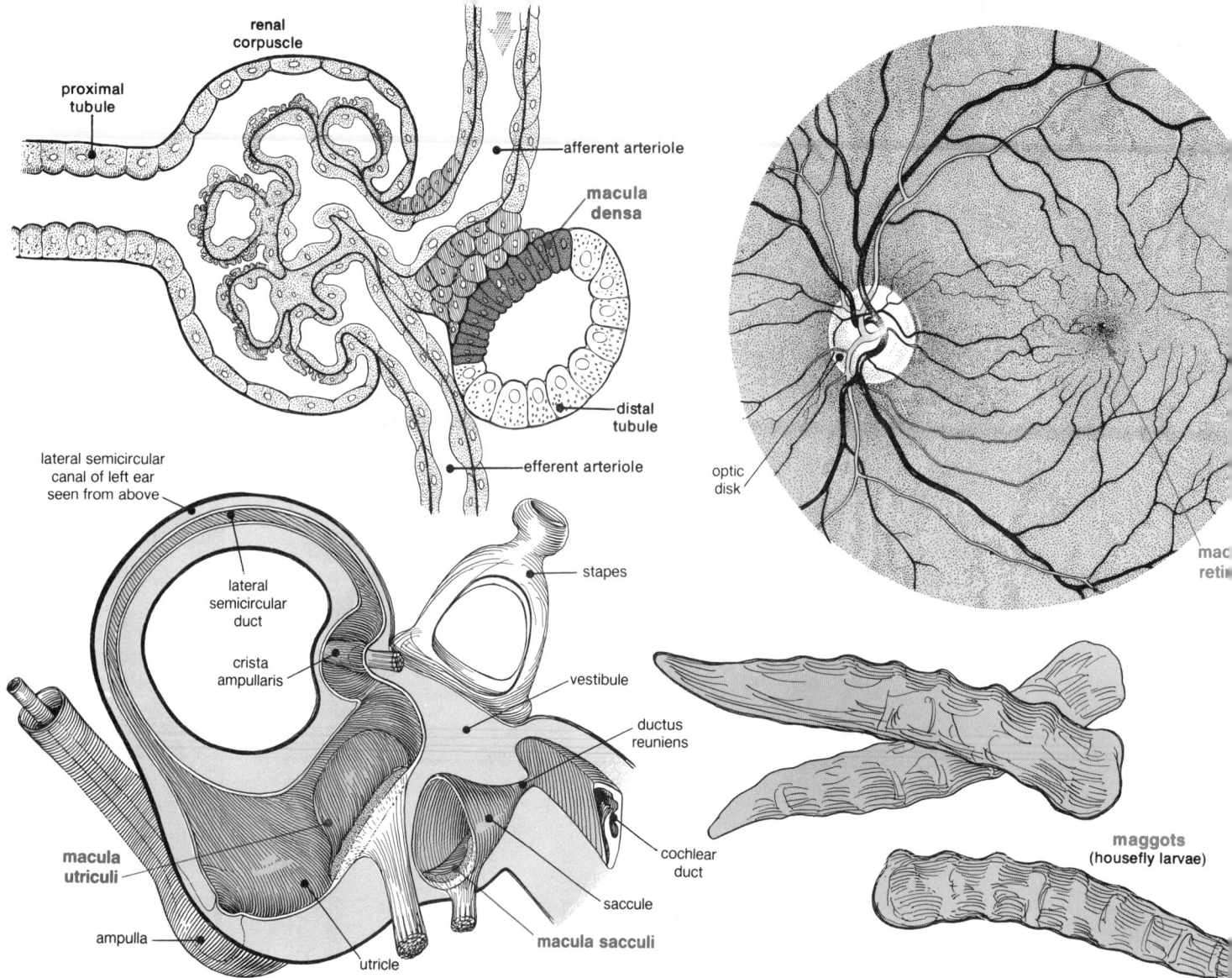

renal corpuscle

proximal tubule

afferent arteriole

macula densa

distal tubule

efferent arteriole

optic disk

mac retin

lateral semicircular canal of left ear seen from above

lateral semicircular duct

crista ampullaris

stapes

vestibule

ductus reuniens

macula utriculi

ampulla

utricle

cochlear duct

saccule

macula sacculi

maggots (housefly larvae)

macrospore See megaspore.

macrostomia Developmental malformation occurring when the embryonic maxillary and mandibular swellings fail to fuse, resulting in extension of the mouth toward the ear; the defect may be bilateral or unilateral.

macrostructure A structure visible with the unaided eye.

macrotia Abnormal largeness of the ears.

macula, *pl.* **maculae** A small area differing in appearance from the surrounding tissue.

  corneal m. A moderately dense whitish opacity of the cornea.

  m. adherens See desmosome.

  m. communis The thickened portion of the medial wall of the auditory vesicle in the embryo; eventually it divides to form the macula sacculi and the macula utriculi.

  m. densa That portion of the distal convoluted tubule of the kidney contacting the wall of the afferent arteriole just before the latter enters the glomerulus; the cells are narrow and slightly taller than those around them; part of the juxtaglomerular apparatus.

  m. lutea See macula retinae.

  m. retinae A small oval yellowish depression on the retina, lateral to and slightly below the optic disk; it contains the fovea centralis. Also called macula lutea; yellow spot.

  m. sacculi The oval neuroepithelial sensory area in the medial wall of the saccule that houses the terminal arborizations of vestibular nerve fibers.

  m. utriculi The neuroepithelial sensory area in the lateral wall of the utricle that houses the terminal arborizations of vestibular nerve fibers.

macular, maculate Of the nature of macules. Also called spotted.

maculation The formation of macules or spots on the skin.

macule A nonelevated, discolored lesion on the skin; a spot on the skin.

maculocerebral Relating to the brain and the macula lutea of the retina.

maculoerythematous Both red and spotted; said of certain lesions.

maculopapular Spotted and elevated.

maculopapule A raised lesion (papule) on a discoloration or spot (macule) on the skin.

maculopathy Any disease of the macula retinae. Also called macular retinopathy.

mad 1. Suffering from a mental disorder. 2. Rabid. 3. Angry.

madarosis Loss of the eyelashes or of the eyebrows.

Madurella A genus of fungi (family Dematiaceae); some species cause maduromycosis.

maduromycosis A chronic disease affecting chiefly the feet, marked by the formation of yellow, white, red, or black granules, draining sinuses, suppuration, and swelling; caused by fungi, especially *Madurella mycetomi.* Formerly called Madura foot after a city in India where it was first observed. Also called mycetoma.

Maffucci's syndrome The combination of multiple cutaneous hemangiomas and dyschondroplasia; the vascular malformations are manifested by extensive birthmarks and dilatation of the veins (phlebectasias) in the form of soft, tender, purple tumors in subcutaneous tissue, lips, and palate; deformities of the hands and feet are usually evident.

maggot A legless, soft-bodied grub that is the larva of various insects of the order Diptera, as the housefly; it develops usually in dead organic matter.

magma A soft inert mass composed of finely divided solids in an aqueous medium; a paste or salve.

magnesia Magnesium oxide.

  citrate of m. See magnesium citrate.

  m. magma See milk of magnesia.

  milk of m. (MOM) An aqueous suspension of magnesium hydroxide; used as a laxative and antacid. Also called magnesia magma.

magnesium A light, moderately hard, metallic element with a silvery luster; symbol Mg, atomic number 12, atomic weight 24.32, valence 2; it is an essential nutritional substance.

  m. carbonate A very light, white powdery compound, $MgCO_3$, used in gastric and intestinal acidity and as a laxative; it is insoluble in water.

  m. citrate A colorless crystalline powder, $Mg_3(C_6H_5O_7)_2 \cdot 14\ H_2O$, used in solution as a laxative. Also called citrate of magnesia.

  m. hydroxide A white powdery compound, $Mg(OH)_2$, practically insoluble in water; used as an antacid and laxative.

  m. oxide A white powdery compound, MgO, insoluble in water; used as an antacid and laxative. Also called magnesia.

  m. sulfate A colorless, crystalline compound, $MgSO_4$, soluble in water; effective cathartic, particularly useful in certain poisonings; the form $MgSO_4 \cdot 7H_2O$ is Epsom salt.

magnetism 1. The property of mutual attraction or repulsion produced by a magnet or by an electric current. 2. The study of magnets and their properties. 3. The force exhibited by a magnetic field.

magneton A unit of measure of the magnetic movement of an atomic or subatomic particle.

magnification An enlargement of an object by an optical element or instrument.

maieusiophobia Abnormal fear of childbirth.

maim To disable, mutilate, or cripple by an injury.

main French for hand.

  m. d'accoucheur Accoucheur's hand; see under hand.

  m. en crochet Permanent flexure of the fourth and fifth fingers, resembling the position of a person's hand while crocheting.

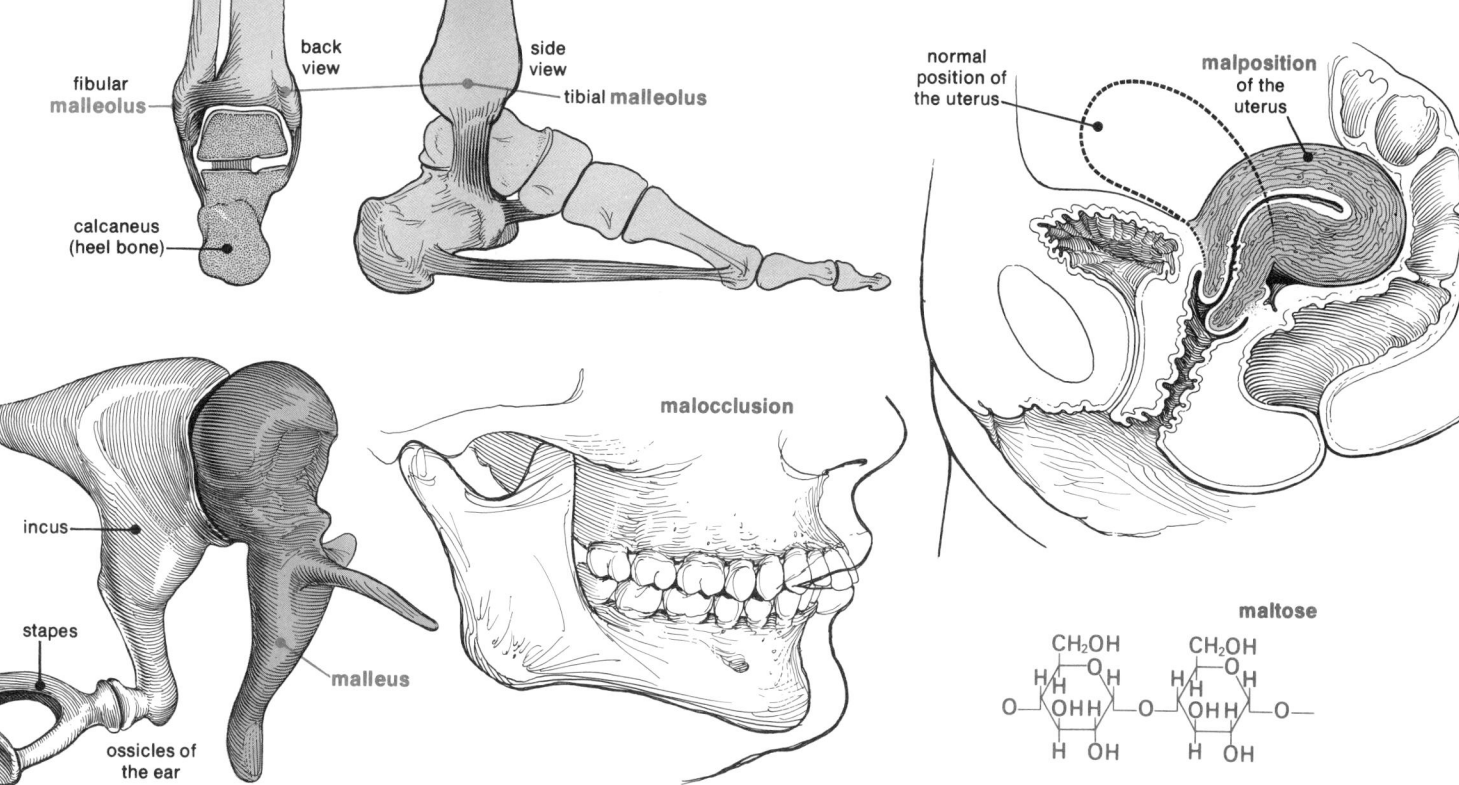

back view

side view

fibular **malleolus**

tibial **malleolus**

calcaneus (heel bone)

normal position of the uterus

malposition of the uterus

malocclusion

incus

stapes

malleus

ossicles of the ear

maltose

CH₂OH ... CH₂OH

m. en griffe Griffin-claw hand; see under hand.

m. en lorgnette Opera glass hand; see under hand.

mainlining Term used by drug addicts denoting intravenous injection of heroin or other drugs.

mainstreaming Placing of a handicapped child into a regular classroom by providing special, but not separate, services and barrier-free education.

Majocchi's disease Annular telangiectatic purpura; see under purpura.

mal French for disease.

grand m. Generalized epilepsy; see under epilepsy.

petit m. Petit mal epilepsy; see under epilepsy.

mala Latin for cheekbone; the cheek.

malabsorption Inadequate or imperfect absorption.

m. syndrome Condition marked by weight loss, weakness, pallor, protuberant abdomen, bleeding tendency and other symptoms and signs, caused by any disease which impairs the absorption of nutrients.

malachite green Green crystalline substance, soluble in water, used as a pH indicator; it changes at pH 1.0 from yellow (acid) to blue-green (alkaline); used also for staining bacteria and as an antiseptic. Also called Victoria green.

malacia Softening of tissues.

malacoplakia See malakoplakia.

maladie French for malady.

m. de Roger See Roger's disease.

malady Illness; disease.

malaise A vague general discomfort or feeling of illness.

malakoplakia The formation of soft, fungus-like growths on the mucous membrane of a hollow organ, especially the urinary bladder. Also written malacoplakia.

malalignment The displacement of a tooth, or teeth, from normal position.

malar Of or relating to the cheek or cheek bone.

malaria An infectious disease caused by any of four species of a protozoan parasite of the genus *Plasmodium*; transmitted by mosquitoes of the genus *Anopheles*; usual symptoms include anemia, fever, and enlargement of the spleen; the typical fever paroxysm has three stages: (a) chills and uncontrollable shaking, (b) high fever, (c) profuse sweating; may occur on alternate days, every third day, or daily, depending on the time required for a new generation of parasites to complete its life cycle in the body. See also *Plasmodium*.

benign tertian m. See vivax malaria.

estivoautumnal m. See falciparum malaria.

falciparum m. A form caused by the most inva-

sive of all malarial parasites, *Plasmodium falciparum*, causing infected blood cells to clump and block capillaries; the paroxysms of fever usually occur every other day but frequently at indefinite intervals; in severe cases cerebral, renal, gastrointestinal, or pulmonary complications may develop. Also called malignant tertian or estivoautumnal malaria.

malariae m. A form caused by *Plasmodium malariae*; the paroxysms of fever usually occur every third day. Also called quartan malaria.

malignant tertian m. See falciparum malaria.

quartan m. See malariae malaria.

quotidian m. A form in which the paroxysms occur daily; usually caused by two groups of *Plasmodium vivax* parasites reproducing alternately every 48 hours may also be caused by a combination of *Plasmodium falciparum* and *Plasmodium vivax* or by two generations of *Plasmodium falciparum*.

relapsing m. A type in which exoerthrocytic forms of the parasite persist after the initial incubation period; if not destroyed, these forms act as a reservoir for repeated clinical episodes due to invasion of the red blood cells.

tertian m. See vivax malaria.

vivax m. A form caused by *Plasmodium vivax* or *Plasmodium ovale*; the paroxysms occur every other day. Also called tertian or benign tertian malaria.

malarial Relating to or caused by malaria.

Malassezia furfur The fungus that causes tinea versicolor; the proper name for *Microsporon furfur*.

malate A salt of malic acid.

malathion Substance used as an insecticide and, in veterinary medicine, against external parasites.

male 1. Designating the sex of an individual containing organs that normally produce spermatozoa; symbol ♂ (the shield and spear zodiac sign for Mars). 2. Masculine.

genetic m. An individual with a male karyotype that normally has one X and one Y chromosome.

malformation A defect or deformity.

congenital m. One evident at birth, either genetic or of environmental origin. Commonly called birth defect.

malfunction Abnormal or inadequate function.

malic acid An intermediate in carbohydrate metabolism; present in unripe apples, cherries, tomatoes, etc.

malignancy The condition of being malignant or resistant to treatment.

malignant Denoting any disease resistant to treatment and of a fatal nature; in the case of a tumor, having the property of uncontrollable growth and dissemination.

malinger To pretend to be ill to avoid work or an unpleasant situation, or for some other type of gain.

malingerer One who pretends to be sick.

malleable Capable of being made into thin sheets; said of certain metals.

malleation A spasmodic movement as of hammering of the hands.

malleolar Relating to one or both prominences on either side of the ankle.

malleolus, *pl.* **malleoli** One of two projections (one on the tibia and one on the fibula) on either side of the ankle joint.

Malleomyces mallei See *Pseudomonas mallei*.

Malleomyces pseudomallei *Pseudomonas pseudomallei*.

malleus The club-shaped and most lateral of the three auditory ossicles in the middle ear chamber, which is firmly attached to the tympanic membrane and articulates with the incus. Sometimes called hammer.

Mallory-Weiss syndrome Lacerations of the lower esophagus with vomiting of blood, usually following protracted, severe, incoordinate vomiting and retching; commonly occurs following excessive alcohol ingestion.

malnutrition Faulty nutrition due to inadequate diet or to a metabolic abnormality; wrong intake of nutrients, i.e., inadequate amounts or the wrong proportions of nutrients.

malocclusion Abnormal contact of opposing teeth (mandibular and maxillary), so as to interfere with the efficient movement of the jaws during mastication.

close bite m. Condition in which the edges of the anterior mandibular teeth extend lingually toward the gums of the opposing teeth when the jaws are closed.

open bite m. A condition marked by the failure of opposing teeth to establish contact when the jaws are closed.

malonyl The bivalent radical of malonic acid.

malpighian body Renal corpuscle; see under corpuscle.

malposition An abnormal or anomalous position of a part or of the body.

malpractice Improper, unskillful, or negligent treatment of an individual by a health practitioner that results in injury.

malpresentation Any position of the baby at the time of birth that differs from the usual face down head first position.

malrotation Failure of all or a portion of the intestines to rotate during embryonic development.

maltase A digestive enzyme that promotes the conversion of maltose into glucose.

maltose $C_{12}H_{22}O_{11}$; a sugar formed by the action of a digestive enzyme on starch; it consists of two

protruded **mandible**

6 years old

adult

mandible

newborn

Mauriceau-Smellie-Veit-Maneuver

glucose moieties. Also called malt sugar.

malum Latin for disease.

malunion Union of a fractured bone in a faulty alignment or position.

mamelon, mammelon One of the three rounded prominences on the cutting edge of an erupting incisor tooth.

mamma, *pl.* **mammae** The mammary gland or breast; rudimentary in the male but containing the milk-producing glands in the female.

mammal A member of the class Mammalia.

Mammalia A class of vertebrates that includes all animals that nourish their young with milk.

mammaplasty Plastic surgery of the breasts. Also called mammoplasty.

   augmentative m. Increase of breast size by insertion of an implant.

   reduction m. Operation to reduce the size of the breasts.

mammary Relating to the breast.

mammectomy See mastectomy.

mammelon See mamelon.

mammilla 1. Nipple. 2. Any nipple-like protuberance.

mammillaplasty Reparative surgery of the nipple. Also called mammilloplasty.

mammillary Relating to or resembling a nipple.

mammillate, mammillated Having nipple-like projections.

mammitis See mastitis.

mammogram A roentgenogram of the mammary gland, usually done for the purpose of detecting cancers.

mammography A soft tissue x-ray technique for visualization of the female breast; used to detect nonpalpable lesions and to identify palpable lesions.

mammoplasty See mammaplasty.

mammotrophic Promoting the development, growth, and function of the mammary gland.

mandelate A salt of mandelic acid.

mandelic acid A crystalline substance, soluble in water; used as a urinary antibacterial agent. Also called phenylglycolic acid.

mandible The horseshoe-shaped bone of the lower jaw which articulates with the skull at the temporomandibular joint; it lodges the lower teeth. Also called jawbone.

mandibular Relating to the lower jaw or mandible.

mandibulectomy Surgical removal of the lower jaw.

mandibulopharyngeal Relating to the mandible and pharynx.

mandragora An herb long known and used in medieval medicine as a sedative, hypnotic, anesthetic, and poison. Also called mandrake.

mandrake See mandragora.

mandrel A shaft on which a working tool is mounted, and by means of which it is rotated.

   disk m. A mandrel designed to hold a polishing disk.

   snap-on m. A mandrel with a split end that supports a rubber polishing cup.

maneuver A procedure or movement requiring skill and dexterity.

   Bracht's m. In obstetrics, maneuver used in breech extraction whereby the breech is allowed to deliver spontaneously up to the umbilicus, then the baby's body is held against the mother's symphysis and moderate suprapubic pressure is applied by an assistant.

   Credé's m.'s Credé's methods; see under method.

   Heimlich m. A maneuver used to dislodge a piece of food stuck in a person's throat and obstructing the airway; standing in back of the victim, the rescuer places both arms around him; he makes a fist with one hand, grasps it with the other hand, and (with the thumb toward the victim) presses his fist sharply upward against the victim's abdomen, between the navel and the rib cage; this causes the diaphragm to elevate and the lungs to compress; the resulting increased air pressure forced through the trachea (windpipe) forces out the food particle.

   Leopold's m.'s In obstetrics, four methods of abdominal palpation to determine position of fetus in the uterus.

   Mauriceau-Smellie-Veit m. In obstetrics, a method of extracting the fetal head in breech presentation when the chin is directed posteriorly; the baby's body straddles the forearm of the operator, the middle finger is introduced into the baby's mouth and applied over the maxilla, and two fingers of the other hand are placed forklike over the fetal shoulder to exert traction.

   Pinard's m. Method of fetal extraction in a frank breech presentation; two fingers are passed along the fetal thigh to the knee to push it away from the midline and flex the leg; the foot is then readily grasped and brought down and out.

   Ritgen's m., modified Delivery of a baby's head by applying forward pressure on the chin through the perineum with one hand while applying pressure on the head with the other hand; the maneuver is performed between contractions and allows for slow delivery of the head.

   Scanzoni's m. Rotation of fetal head with forceps followed by removal and reapplication of instrument for delivery to avoid injury to the maternal soft parts.

   Valsalva m. 1. Forced expiration against the closed glottis to increase pressure within the lungs; **2.** Forced expiration with mouth closed and pinched nose to clear the auditory tube.

manganese A grayish or silvery metallic element; symbol Mn, atomic number 25, atomic weight 54.94; some of its salts are used in medicine.

manganous Denoting a compound containing bivalent manganese.

manganum Manganese.

mange A skin disease of animals caused by burrowing itch mites, usually *Sarcoptes chorioptes;* in man, the disease is called scabies.

mania An emotional disorder characterized by a state of excitement, hyperactivity, and profuse and rapidly changing ideas.

maniac A vague and misleading common term for an emotionally disturbed individual, usually implying violent behavior.

manic Of or relating to mania.

manic-depressive See disorder, bipolar.

manifestation The display of characteristic signs or symptoms of a disease.

   neurotic m. The use of various defense mechanisms, such as depression, conversion, dissociation, etc., in an attempt to resolve emotional conflicts, handicapping the effectiveness of a person in daily living.

   psychophysiologic m. Symptoms which are primarily physical with a partial emotional origin.

   psychotic m. The loss of contact with reality, impairing the ability of the person to function in society, indicating personality disintegration.

manikin, mannikin An anatomic model of the human body used for practicing certain manipulations, as those of obstetrics or dentistry. Also called simulation model.

maniphalanx A bony segment or phalanx of a finger.

manipulation Treatment by the skillful use of the hands, as in reducing a dislocation or changing the position of the fetus.

manna The dried sugary exudate of the ash tree, *Fraxinus ornus;* formerly used as a mild laxative.

mannerism A distinctive characteristic or behavioral trait.

mannitol An alcohol, $C_6H_{14}O_6$, derived from fructose; used in the preparation of dietetic sweets and as an osmotic diuretic.

manometer An instrument for measuring the pressure of gases and liquids.

manometric Relating to a manometer.

Mansonia A genus of mosquitoes in tropical Asia and Africa that transmits microfilaria to man.

manubrium of sternum

manubrium of malleus

malleus
incus
tympanic membrane (eardrum)
stapes

body of sternum
heart
xiphoid process
aorta

enlarged pistillate flower cluster

the source of **marijuana** (Cannabis sativa)

phenotype of **Marfan syndrome** long, thin extremities and digits

port-wine mark

manubrium A structure that resembles a handle; when used alone the term refers to the manubrium of the sternum.

m. of malleus The process of the malleus attached to the inner surface of the tympanic membrane.

m. of sternum The upper portion of the sternum articulating with the clavicles and the first and upper parts of the second costal cartilages on each side.

manus Latin for hand.

m. extensa Backward deviation of the hand.

m. flexa Forward deviation of the hand.

m. valga Deviation of the hand toward the ulnar side.

m. vara Deviation of the hand toward the radial side.

maple syrup urine disease An autosomal recessive inherited disorder marked by deficient oxidative decarboxylation of α-keto acids; the urine has a characteristic maple syrup odor; hypotonia, hypoglycemia, and neurologic manifestations appear within the first week of life. Also called branched-chain ketoaciduria.

mapping In genetics, locating the position and order of gene loci on a chromosome by analyzing the frequency of recombination between the loci.

marantic 1. Marasmic. 2. See under endocarditis.

marasmic Relating to marasmus.

marasmus Gradual, progressive wasting of the body, occurring mainly in young children; caused by protein and calorie depletion.

marble bone disease See osteopetrosis.

Marchiafava-Micheli syndrome, Marchiafava-Micheli anemia Paroxysmal nocturnal hemoglobinuria; see under hemoglobinuria.

Marfan syndrome Disorder inherited as an autosomal dominant trait and marked by defective formation of elastic fibers that affects the skeleton, large arteries, suspensory ligaments of the lens of the eye, tendons, and joint capsules; the affected individuals have abnormally long slender extremities, spidery fingers, high palate, displacement of the lens, lax joints, and aneurysm of the aorta.

margin A border or edge.

ciliary m. of iris The border of the iris attached to the ciliary body.

costal m. The curved lower portion of the thoracic wall, formed by the cartilages of the seventh through tenth ribs.

falciform m. The lower lateral border of the saphenous opening in the deep fascia (fascia lata) in front of the thigh; it lies anterior to the femoral vessels.

free gingival m. The edge of the gum tissue that is not directly attached to the tooth. Also called free gum margin.

free gum m. See free gingival margin.

gingival m. The part of the gum, not attached to the tooth, facing either the lips, cheeks, or tongue.

infraorbital m. The lower border of the orbit.

orbital m. Margin of the ocular orbit bounded by the frontal bone superiorly, the zygomatic bone laterally, the maxilla inferiorly, and the process of the maxilla and frontal bone medially.

pupillary m. of iris The border of the iris forming the edge of the pupil.

right m. of heart The border between the diaphragmatic and sternocostal aspects of the heart.

supraorbital m. The superior edge of the orbit.

margination Adhesion of leukocytes to the interior of capillary walls during early stages of inflammation.

marginoplasty Plastic surgery of the eyelid border.

marijuana, marihuana 1. A tall hemp plant. 2. The dried, chopped leaves, flowers, and stems of the common hemp plant *Cannabis sativa* (family Moraceae); smoked or mixed into food to induce euphoria; the origin of the word is obscure, but may be a composite of the Spanish names Maria and Juana (Mary and Jane).

Marie-Strümpell disease Ankylosing spondylitis; see under spondylitis.

mark A visible impression on a surface; a blemish; a spot.

port-wine m. A congenital discoloration of the skin, usually on the face, varying from pink to purple. Also called port-wine hemangioma.

marker 1. A characteristic or factor by which a cell or molecule can be identified or a disease can be recognized. 2. A general term for any trait that helps to throw light on the genetic nature of a disorder, such as a defect of structure or a deviant enzyme.

marmot A rodent that sometimes carries the plague bacillus and ticks that transmit Rocky Mountain spotted fever. Also called groundhog; woodchuck.

Maroteaux-Lamy syndrome A form of mucopolysaccharidosis characterized by dwarfism, chest deformities, knock knees, stiff joints, corneal clouding, short hands and fingers and excessive dermatan sulfate excretion in the urine; inherited as an autosomal recessive trait. Also called mucopolysaccharidosis VI.

marrow The soft material filling the cavities of the bones. Also called medulla of bone.

red m. The marrow located in the cancellous (spongy) tissue of the ribs, the sternum, and the ends of the long bones; it is concerned with the formation of blood cells.

yellow m. The fatty material located in the center of long bones.

marsupialization Surgical procedure for eradication of a cyst, such as a pilonidal cyst, in which the sac is incised and emptied; its edges are then stitched to the edges of the external incision.

masculine Relating to or marked by the characteristics of the male sex; mannish.

maser A device that converts incident electromagnetic radiation of various frequencies into a beam of highly amplified monochromatic radiation at a

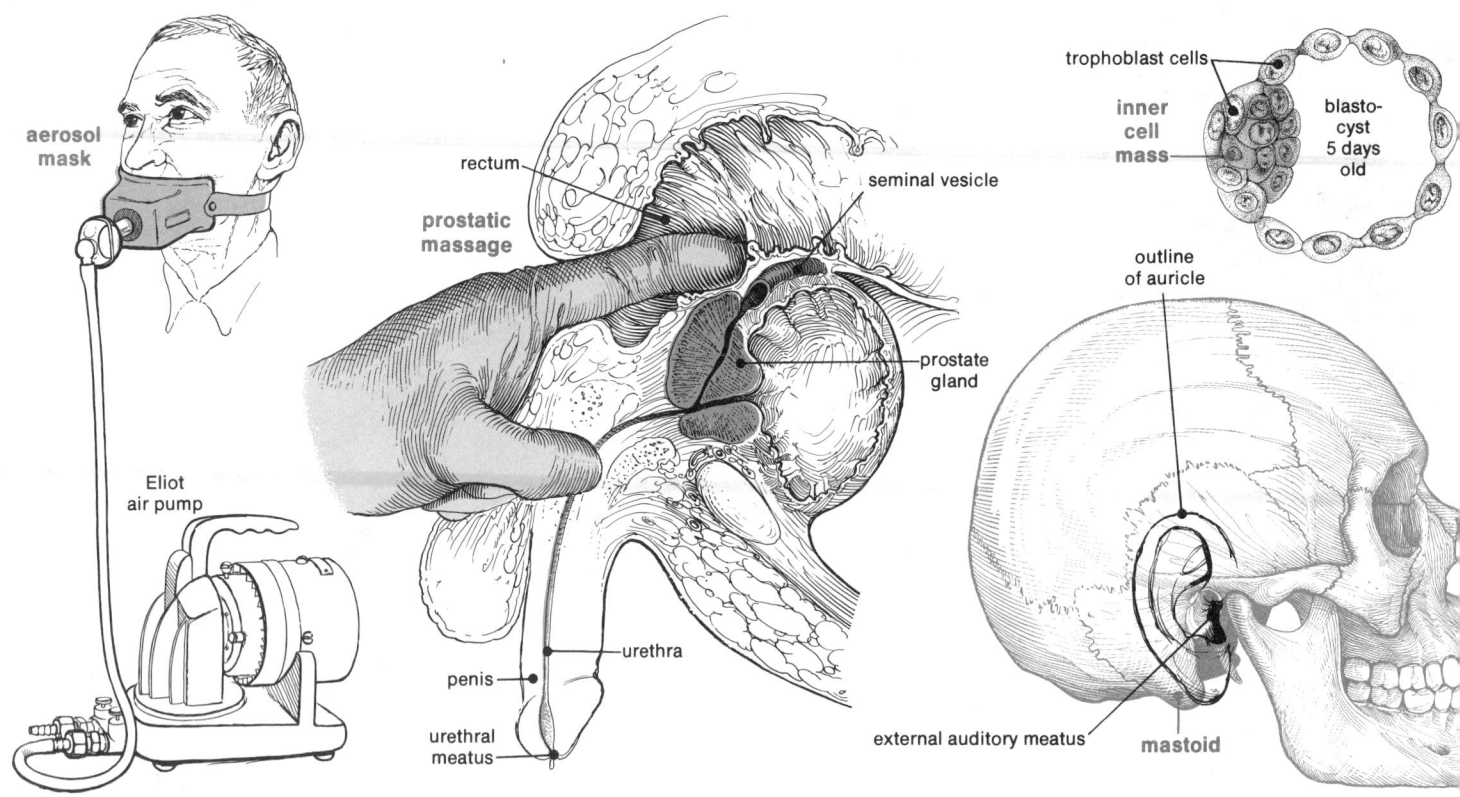

aerosol mask

Eliot air pump

prostatic massage

rectum

seminal vesicle

prostate gland

urethra

penis

urethral meatus

trophoblast cells

inner cell mass

blasto-cyst 5 days old

outline of auricle

external auditory meatus

mastoid

frequency within the microwave region; the term is an acronym for microwave amplification by stimulated emission of radiation.

optical m. See laser.

mask 1. A covering for the face, or a portion of it, for the administration of anesthetics or oxygen, or as an antiseptic measure. 2. An expressionless appearance or a pigmentation of the face characteristic of certain conditions. 3. A facial bandage.

aerosol m. A face mask used in inhalation therapy.

m. of pregnancy See chloasma.

surgical m. A covering for the mouth and nose, made of gauze or plastic material; used by hospital personnel in operating rooms or when caring for patients with communicable diseases or impaired defenses against infection.

masking 1. The introduction of a noise in one ear for the purpose of excluding that ear from a hearing test given to the other ear. 2. The opaque material placed over the metal or any other part of a dental prosthesis.

masochism 1. A form of sexual perversion in which satisfaction depends largely on being subjected to mistreatment or physical pain. 2. The infliction of physical or psychological pain upon oneself to relieve guilt.

masochist 1. The passive partner in the practice of masochism. 2. One who for psychological purposes exposes himself unnecessarily to suffering.

mass 1. A body of coherent material. 2. In pharmacology, a soft pasty mixture of drugs suitable for rolling into pills.

inner cell m. An aggregation of cells that stick together and collect at the embryonic pole of the blastocyst and that give rise to the tissues of the embryo. Also called embryoblast.

lateral m. of atlas The solid parts of the atlas (first vertebra) on either side, articulating above with the occipital condyles of the skull and below with the axis (second vertebra).

massage The rubbing, kneading, tapping, etc. of parts of the body for therapeutic purposes.

cardiac m. The application of manual rhythmic pressure to the ventricles of the heart to restore circulation. Also called open chest massage.

closed chest m. The rhythmic compression of the heart between the sternum and the spine approximately 60 times a minute, in order to restore circulation. Also called external cardiac compression.

gingival m. Stimulation of the gums by rubbing or pressure.

prostatic m. A technique of pressing the prostate gland substance firmly with the pad of the index finger in order to express secretions into the prostatic urethra.

masseter One of the muscles of mastication; its action is to close the jaw. See table of muscles.

massotherapy The therapeutic use of massage.

Mastadenovirus Genus of the family Adenoviridae containing 34 species (types) which infect man, causing respiratory diseases, conjunctivitis, and epidemic keratoconjunctivitis. Also called mammalian adenoviruses.

mastalgia Mastodynia.

mastatrophia, mastatrophy Wasting or atrophy of the breasts.

mastectomy Surgical removal of a breast. Also called mammectomy.

extended radical m. Mastectomy that includes removal of chest muscles, axillary lymph nodes and the internal mammary chain of lymph nodes.

Halsted radical m. Removal of breast, chest muscles, and lymph nodes of axilla.

modified radical m. Removal of breast and axillary lymph nodes, without removal of the pectoral muscles.

total m. Removal of breast only. Also called simple mastectomy.

masthelcosis Ulcers on the breast.

masticate To chew.

mastication The process of chewing food for swallowing.

Mastigophora A subphylum of Protozoa composed of organisms with one or more flagella and a single nucleus; some species are parasitic in man. Trypanosoma and Leishmania are included in this subphylum.

mastitis Inflammation of the breast. Also called mammitis; mastadenitis.

chronic cystic m. See fibrocystic disease of breast.

interstitial m. Inflammation of the connective tissue of the breast.

phlegmonous m. Diffuse inflammation, sometimes accompanied by abscess formation.

plasma cell m. Benign condition characterized chiefly by dilatation and occlusion of mammary ducts with indurated masses of secretion and plasma cells.

mastochondroma A benign breast tumor composed chiefly of cartilaginous tissue.

mastocytogenesis The formation of mast cells.

mastocytoma A nodule resembling a tumor, composed chiefly of mast cells.

mastocytosis See urticaria pigmentosa.

mastodynia Pain in the breast.

mastoid The downward projection of the temporal bone, located behind the ear.

mastoidectomy Removal of the mastoid cells; formerly indicated in the presence of persistent or recurrent mastoiditis and otitis; rarely indicated since the advent of antibiotics.

mastoideocentesis Surgical creation of an opening into the mastoid cells or antrum of the temporal bone.

mastoiditis Inflammation of the mastoid process.

mastoidotomy Surgical opening of the mastoid process of the temporal bone.

mastopathy Any disease of the breast. Also called mazopathy.

mastoplasty See mammoplasty.

mastoptosis Sagging or pendulous breasts.

mastotomy Surgical incision of a breast.

masturbation Self-manipulation of the genital organs to produce sexual excitement.

materia Latin for matter or substance.

m. alba Whitish, loosely adhered deposits on the teeth or dental appliances, composed of mucus, epithelial cells, food debris, and bacteria.

m. medica 1. The science concerned with drugs used in medicine, their origin, preparation, and usage. 2. Any substance used medically.

maternal Relating to or derived from the mother.

maternity 1. The state of being pregnant or a mother. 2. Pertaining to pregnancy.

mating The pairing of male and female for reproduction.

assortative m. Mating that is not random but involves individuals of specific characteristics, which may be similar (positive) or opposite (negative).

random m. Mating without regard to the genetic constitution of the mate. Also called panmixis.

matrilineal Relating to inheritance of traits through the maternal line rather than the paternal.

matrix, *pl.* **matrices** 1. The basic material from which anything (tooth, nail, etc.) develops. 2. The homogeneous intercellular substance of any tissue. 3. A mold in which a cast is made.

matroclinous Inherited through the maternal line; derived from the mother. Cf. patroclinous.

matter 1. Substance. 2. Waste from a living organism.

gray m. See substance, gray.

white m. See substance, white.

maturate To mature.

maturation 1. The process of becoming mature. 2. A stage of cell division in which the number of chromosomes in the sex cells is reduced to one-half the number characteristic of the species. 3. Pus formation.

mature 1. Complete in natural development; ripe;

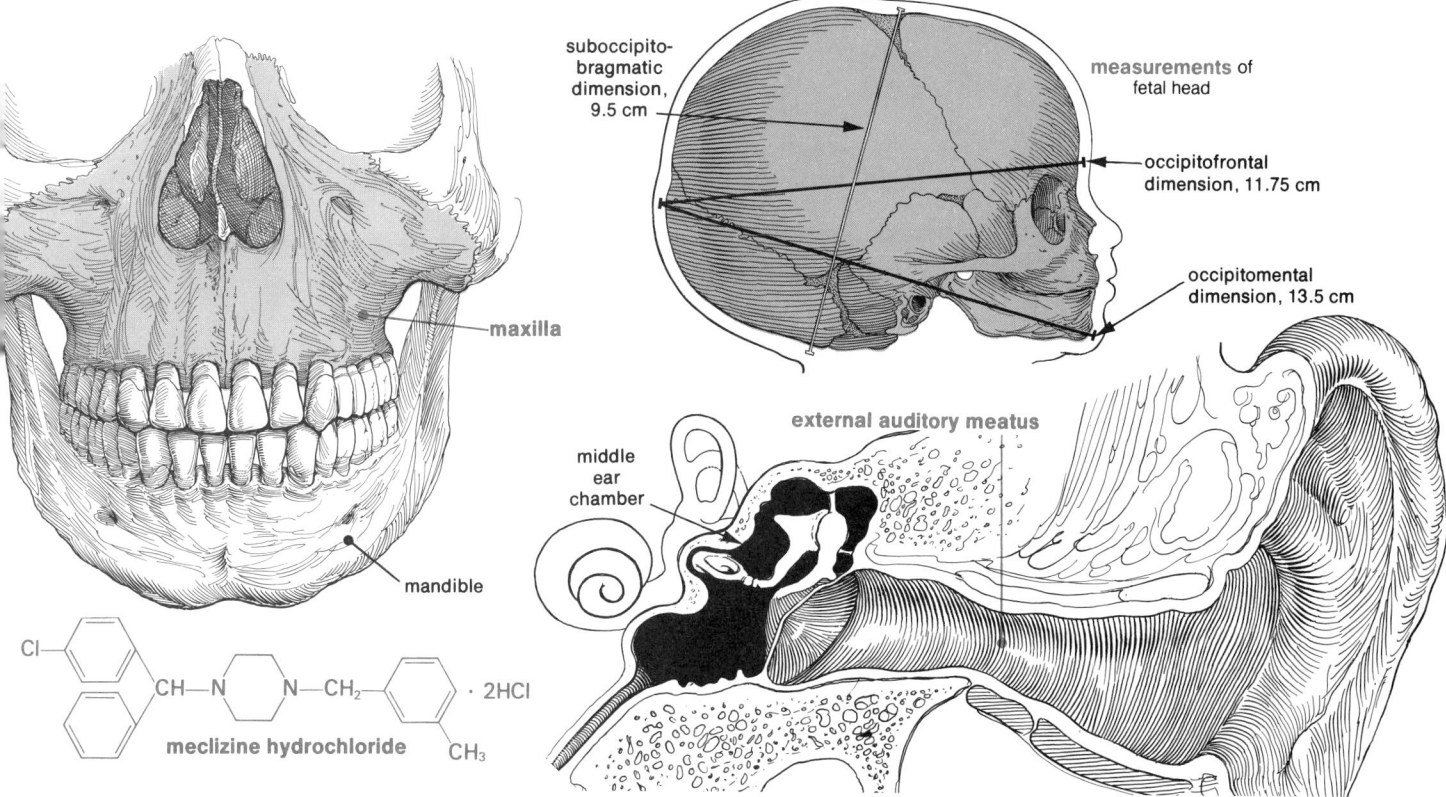

maxilla

mandible

suboccipito-bragmatic dimension, 9.5 cm

measurements of fetal head

occipitofrontal dimension, 11.75 cm

occipitomental dimension, 13.5 cm

external auditory meatus

middle ear chamber

meclizine hydrochloride

e.g., the reproductive cell which has undergone the process of meiosis. **2.** Relating to or marked by full development, either mental or physical. **3.** To achieve full development.

maturity The state of being mature.

Maurer's dots Red-staining granules sometimes seen in the cytoplasm of red blood cells infected with *Plasmodium falciparum.*

maxilla One of a pair of irregularly shaped bones forming the upper jaw; it lodges the upper teeth.

maxillary Relating to the upper jaw (maxilla).

maxillofacial Pertaining to the upper jaw and the face.

maximum 1. The greatest quantity, value, or degree. **2.** The height of a fever or any acute state. Also called fastigium.

glucose transport m. (glucose Tm) The maximum rate at which the kidneys can reabsorb glucose (approximately 300 mg per minute).

tubular m. (Tm) The maximum ability of the renal tubules either to reabsorb or to secrete a given substance.

maze An intricate labyrinth of walled pathways frequently used to study the learning process in experimental animals.

McArdle's syndrome Type 5 glycogenosis; see under glycogenosis.

meal Food.

Boyden m. Meal used to test the evacuation time of the gallbladder; it consists of flour, egg yolks, and milk mixed with sugar or port wine.

test m. Bland food, e.g., toast or crackers and tea, given before analysis of stomach secretions.

mean The numerical average.

arithmetic m. In statistics, the sum of numerical data divided by the number of items.

measle The larva of the tapeworm.

measles An acute contagious viral disease marked by fever, inflammation of the mucous membrane of the respiratory tract, and an eruption of red spots on the skin; the incubation period is usually 10 to 12 days. Also called rubeola.

German m. See rubella.

measly Containing tapeworm larvae.

measure 1. The dimensions, quantity, or capacity of something that can be determined by measuring; e.g., length, area, volume, etc. **2.** The act of determining such dimensions, quantity or capacity. **3.** A device used for measuring; e.g., a graduated container or a marked tape.

measurement The dimensions, quantity, or capacity of something determined by measuring.

measures of central tendency In biostatistics, the tendency of statistical data to group about an

average value.

meatal Relating to a meatus or body opening.

meatometer An instrument for measuring the size of a meatus, as that of the urethra.

meatoscope Instrument for visualization of the urethral meatus.

meatoscopy Examination of the urethral meatus with a meatoscope.

meatotome Knife used in meatotomy.

meatotomy Incision for the enlargement of the urethral opening.

meatus, *pl.* **meatus, meatuses** A body channel or its opening.

external auditory m., external acoustic m. The auditory canal from the concha of the auricle to the tympanic membrane; it is approximately 25 mm in length on its superoposterior wall and 6 mm longer on its anteroinferior wall.

inferior nasal m. The passageway with which the nasolacrimal duct communicates with the nasal cavity below the inferior nasal concha.

internal acoustic m., internal auditory m. A canal through the petrous bone, about 1 cm in length, from the internal acoustic foramen to the medial wall of the vestibule and cochlea; it transmits the labyrinthine blood vessels, the vestibulocochlear nerve, and the motor and sensory roots of the facial nerve.

middle nasal m. The passage from which the anterior ethmoidal cells and the frontal and maxillary sinuses communicate with the nasal cavity below the middle nasal concha.

nasopharyngeal m. The passage in the posterior part of the nasal cavity from the back part of the turbinates to the choanae.

superior nasal m. The passageway with which the posterior ethmoidal cells communicate with the nasal cavity below the superior nasal concha.

urethral m. The external opening of the urethra.

mecapion Device used to measure the output of an x-ray tube in roentgens.

mechanical 1. Produced with the aid of a machine or apparatus. **2.** Automatic.

mechanics The branch of physics dealing with energy and forces acting on bodies (solid, liquid, or gaseous) either in motion or at rest; divided into statics, dynamics, and fluid mechanics.

body m. The study of the action of muscles on the body in motion and at rest.

mechanism 1. An aggregation of parts that interact in order to perform a specific or common function. **2.** The means by which an effect is obtained.

association m. Mental process through which the memory of past experiences may be related to

or compared with present ones.

cough m. A mechanism for the removal of foreign material from the respiratory tract, consisting of a short inspiration, closure of the glottis, forcible expiratory effort, and then release of the glottis with a rush of air at flow rates of usually 3,000 to 4,000 ml/sec.

countercurrent m. A mechanism essential to the production of an osmotically concentrated urine; it involves two basic processes, countercurrent multiplication in the nephronic (Henle's) loop and countercurrent exchange in the medullary blood vessels, the vasa recta.

defense m. A psychic structure, usually unconscious, which serves as a protection against awareness of conflicts or anxiety.

investing m. The structures that surround a tooth and provide retention, including the periodontal membrane, cementum of the tooth, alveolar bone, and gingiva.

pressoreceptive m. Mechanism whereby the pressoreceptive areas (especially the carotid sinuses and aortic arch) react to a stimulus such as a rise in arterial blood pressure.

proprioceptive m. Process by which the body regulates its muscular movements and maintains its equilibrium.

mechanocardiography The use of tracings that represent the mechanical effects of the heart beat.

mechanoreceptor A receptor that responds to the stimulation of mechanical pressure. Also called mechanicoreceptor.

mechlorethamine hydrochloride HN_2; an alkylating agent used in the treatment of Hodgkin's disease; Mustargen Hydrochloride®.

meclizine hydrochloride Preparation used in the prevention and treatment of motion sickness; Bonine®.

mecometer Instrument used to measure the newborn infant.

meconiorrhea The passage of an abnormally large amount of meconium by the newborn infant.

meconium The dark green intestinal contents formed before birth and present in a newborn child.

meconium ileus See ileus, meconium.

media Plural of medium.

mediad Directed toward the midline.

medial Relating to the middle; near the median plane of the body or an organ.

median 1. Situated in the middle, as certain nerves and blood vessels. Also called central. **2.** In statistics, denoting the middle value in a distribution, i.e., the point in a series at which half of the plotted values are on one side and half on the other.

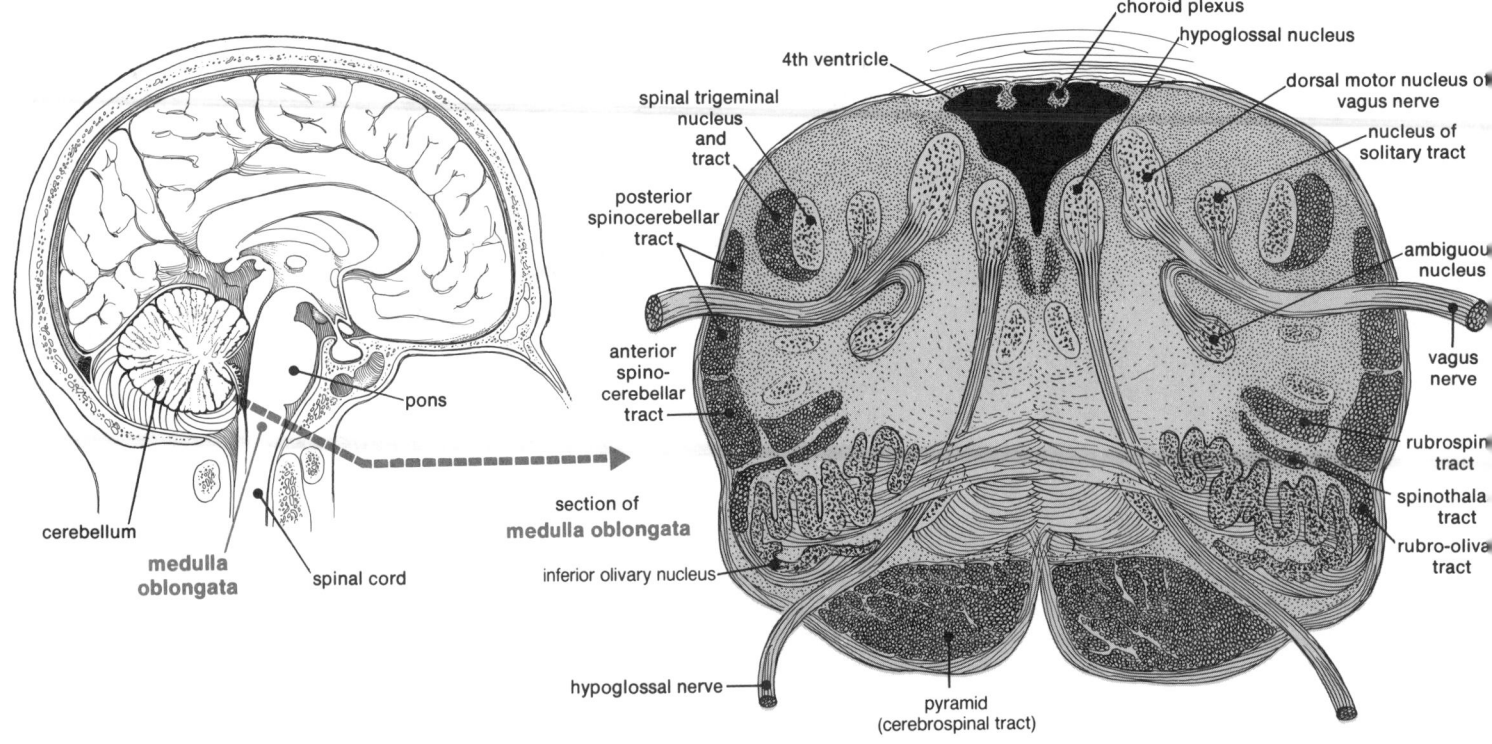

Labels on figure (top diagram, left):
cerebellum · medulla oblongata · pons · spinal cord

Labels on figure (right diagram, section of medulla oblongata):
choroid plexus · hypoglossal nucleus · dorsal motor nucleus of vagus nerve · nucleus of solitary tract · ambiguous nucleus · vagus nerve · rubrospinal tract · spinothalamic tract · rubro-olivary tract · pyramid (cerebrospinal tract) · hypoglossal nerve · inferior olivary nucleus · section of medulla oblongata · anterior spinocerebellar tract · posterior spinocerebellar tract · spinal trigeminal nucleus and tract · 4th ventricle

mediastinal | medulla

mediastinal Of or relating to the mediastinum.
mediastinitis Inflammation of the mediastinum.
mediastinography Roentgenography or x-ray examination of the mediastinum.
mediastinopericarditis Inflammation of the sac enveloping the heart (pericardium) and the tissues and organs between the sternum and vertebral column (mediastinum).
mediastinoscope An instrument for visual inspection of the mediastinum through an incision above the suprasternal notch.
mediastinoscopy Exploration of the mediastinum, under anesthesia, through a transverse suprasternal incision (usually 2 cm above the suprasternal notch); it allows access to the lymph nodes overlying the trachea for surgical biopsy.
mediastinotomy Incision into the mediastinum.
mediastinum, *pl.* **mediastina** 1. The central space in the chest bounded anteriorly by the sternum, posteriorly by the vertebral column, and laterally by the pleural sacs. 2. A septum between two parts of an organ.
  anterior m. The division of the lower mediastinum located in front of the pericardium and behind the body of the sternum; it contains, among other structures, part of the thymus gland, a few lymph nodes, and loose areolar tissue.
  lower m. The part of the mediastinum below the plane that extends from the manubriosternal joint in front to the lower border of the fourth vertebra behind; it is subdivided into anterior, middle, and posterior mediastina.
  middle m. The broadest division of the lower mediastinum; it contains, among other structures, the pericardium and heart and the adjacent parts of the great vessels.
  posterior m. The division of the lower mediastinum located in back of the pericardium and in front of the vertebral column; it contains, among other structures, the esophagus, many lymph nodes, thoracic aorta, thoracic duct, and vagus nerves.
  superior m. The division of the mediastinum above the plane that extends from the manubriosternal joint in front to the lower border of the fourth vertebra behind; it contains, among other structures, the aortic arch with its branches, the brachiocephalic veins and the upper half of the superior vena cava, the vagus, phrenic, cardiac, and left recurrent laryngeal nerves, the trachea, esophagus, thoracic duct, thymus gland, and some lymph nodes.
  upper m. The superior mediastinum.
medicable Potentially curable by drug therapy.
medical 1. Relating to medicine. 2. Medicinal.
medicament A remedy; a healing agent.
medicamentosus Relating to, or caused by, a drug.

medicate 1. To treat disease with a medicinal substance. 2. To impregnate with a medicinal substance.
medicated 1. Permeated with a medicinal substance. 2. Treated medically.
medication 1. A medicine or drug. 2. The act or process of administering remedies.
medicinal Having curative properties.
medicine 1. A drug. 2. The science of diagnosing and treating general diseases or those involving the internal parts of the body, distinguished from surgery.
  clinical m. The study and practice of medicine at the bedside as opposed to theoretical and laboratory investigation.
  community m. The medical specialty dealing with the study and solution of in-depth community health problems.
  family m. The medical specialty dealing with first patient contact, long-term care, and a broad responsibility to all members of a family regardless of age.
  folk m. Treatment of disease in the home with remedies and techniques passed on from generation to generation.
  forensic m. See jurisprudence, medical.
  internal m. The branch of medicine concerned with the nonsurgical aspects of diseases.
  legal m. See jurisprudence, medical.
  nuclear m. The application of nuclear energy in the diagnosis and treatment of disease; e.g., the use of radioisotopes as tracers.
  physical m. See physiatrics.
  preventive m. The study and practice of measures aimed at preventing disease.
  primary m. The care a patient receives during his initial contact with a health practitioner or health-service system; it implies an ongoing responsibility for the patient regardless of the presence or absence of disease and includes that aspect of preventive medicine that can be practiced at the family level.
  proprietary m. A medicinal preparation that is the property of the maker and, by patent or trade mark, is protected against imitation.
  socialized m. The control of medical practice by a branch of the government.
  space m. The branch of medicine concerned with disorders occurring in humans and animals exposed to the conditions of space travel.
  veterinary m. The diagnosis and treatment of the diseases of animals.
medionecrosis Necrosis of the middle layer of an arterial wall.
  m. of the aorta Cystic medial necrosis; see under necrosis.

meditation, transcendental (TM) An exercise of contemplation that induces a temporary hypometabolic state, a sense of well being, and a feeling of complete relaxation; this hypometabolic state is associated with changes in physiologic function including a reduction in oxygen consumption, a decrease in cardiac output, and altered brain wave activity.
medium, *pl.* **media** 1. A means. 2. Any substance through which something is transmitted. 3. Any substance used for the cultivation of bacteria. Also called culture medium.
  clearing m. A substance used in histology to make specimens transparent.
  contrast m. Any substance, e.g., barium, opaque to x rays, used to facilitate visual examination of internal organs. Also called radiopaque medium.
  culture m. Medium (3).
  radiopaque m. See contrast medium.
  rich m. Culture medium containing various kinds of nutrients.
  selective m. Culture medium containing components that limit growth to organisms of a specific type.
  separating m. A substance used in dentistry to coat impressions to facilitate removal of the cast.
MEDLARS (Medical Literature Analysis and Retrieval System) The National Library of Medicine's computerized system of online databases containing citations of the world's biomedical literature; available through a network of centers at universities, medical schools, hospitals, government agencies, and commercial organizations; terminals at these institutions are connected via commercial telephone to the library's computers. To retrieve references, a user types in successive queries until the needed references are identified.
MEDLINE (MEDLARS-online) A segment of MEDLARS; contains references to biomedical journal articles published in the current and two preceding years in the U.S. and foreign countries, and indexed by the National Library of Medicine; coverage of previous periods (from 1966) is provided by backfiles which are searchable online; MEDLINE is updated monthly.
medroxyprogesterone acetate Preparation used in combination with ethynyl estradiol as an oral contraceptive.
medulla Any centrally located soft tissue.
  adrenal m. The inner, reddish-brown portion of the adrenal gland that produces epinephrine and norepinephrine.
  m. oblongata The oblong, caudal portion of the brainstem extending from the lower margin of the pons to, and continuous with, the spinal cord.

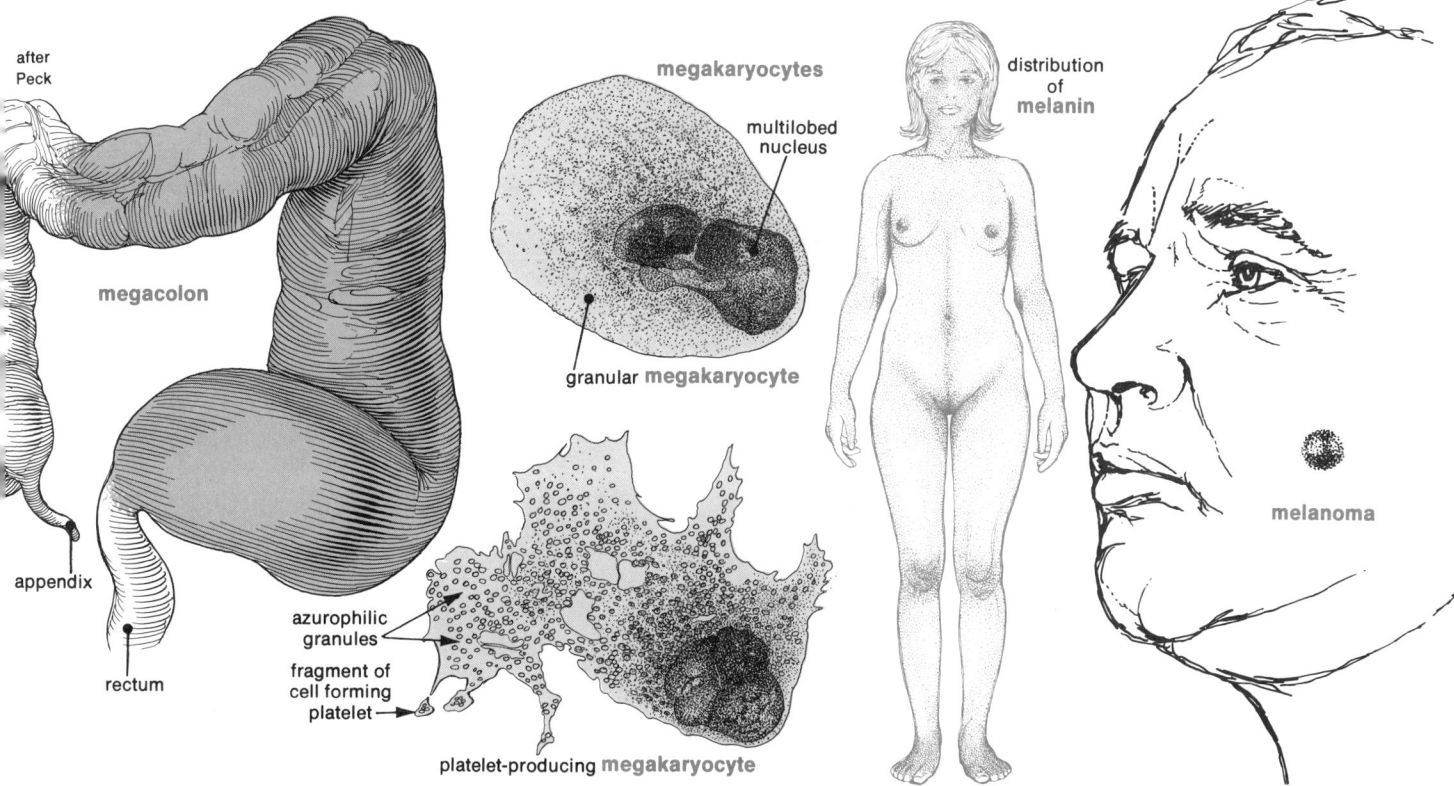

after Peck

megacolon

appendix

rectum

megakaryocytes

multilobed nucleus

granular **megakaryocyte**

azurophilic granules

fragment of cell forming platelet

platelet-producing **megakaryocyte**

distribution of **melanin**

melanoma

m. of bone The soft material filling the cavities of bones, composed of hemopoietic tissue; it produces most of the cells that circulate in the blood. Also called marrow.

m. of kidney The inner, darker portion of the kidney containing the vasa rectae, nephronic (Henle's) loops, and collecting ducts.

m. of ovary The inner part of the ovary composed of loose connective tissue containing lymphatics, nerves, and a mass of large contorted blood vessels.

m. spinalis Spinal cord; see under cord.

medullary Relating to, or resembling, the medulla or marrow.

medullated Containing, or covered with, a soft marrow-like substance.

medullation The formation of marrow or a medullary sheath.

medullization The replacement of bone tissue by marrow, as in rarefying osteosis.

medulloblast An undifferentiated cell of the embryonic neural tube.

medulloblastoma A rapidly growing tumor, usually of the vermis of the cerebellum, composed of undifferentiated preneurogliar cells.

megabladder See megalocystis.

megacolon Abnormally large colon.

congenital m. Megacolon observed in young infants, resulting from absence of ganglion cells of the myenteric plexuses of the rectum and lower colon; the aganglionic area of the intestine is unable to relax during normal peristaltic activity, producing constriction and constipation. Also called Hirschsprung's disease.

idiopathic m. A form having its onset in childhood, characterized chiefly by constipation and distention of colon (sometimes the entire colon) with feces, without constriction or absence of ganglion cells.

toxic m. Marked dilatation of the colon in acute fulminating ulcerative colitis.

megadyne Unit of force, equal to one million dynes.

mega electron volt (mev) One million electron volts.

megaesophagus Abnormal enlargement of the lower esophagus.

megakaryoblast A primitive cell of the megakaryocyte series about 25 to 30 µm in diameter with a large oval or kidney-shaped nucleus and scanty cytoplasm; it develops into a promegakaryocyte before finally differentiating into a megakaryocyte.

megakaryocyte A giant cell with a usually multilobed nucleus, the precursor of platelets; the largest cell in the bone marrow (up to 100 µm in diameter).

megakaryophthisis Deficiency of megakaryocytes in the bone marrow.

megaloblast An embryonic red blood cell of large size, found in the bone marrow in pernicious anemia and folic acid deficiency states.

megalocardia See cardiomegaly.

megalochiria Abnormally large size of the hands. Also called macrochiria.

megalocornea Developmental eye anomaly in which an otherwise normal cornea is abnormally large at birth and continues to grow in diameter; the pressure within the eye remains normal, which distinguishes this condition from buphthalmos. Also called macrocornea.

megalocystis An abnormally enlarged or distended bladder. Also called megabladder.

megalocyte See macrocyte.

megalodactylism See macrodactylia.

megalogastria Abnormally large size of the stomach.

megaloglossia See macroglossia.

megalomania A psychopathologic condition in which the individual has unfounded conviction of his own great importance and power.

megalomelia See macromelia.

megalopenis Abnormally large penis.

megaloureter Excessive dilatation of a ureter in the absence of obstruction.

megarectum Abnormally dilated rectum.

megasigmoid An extremely dilated sigmoid colon.

megaspore The larger of the spores of certain protozoans or heterosporous plants. Also called macrospore.

megavitamin Any quantity of a vitamin far in excess of minimal daily requirement.

megavolt (MV) A unit of electromotive force, equal to one million volts.

megavoltage Electromotive force in the range of 2 to 10 million electron volts (mev); used in radiation therapy.

meglumine N-methylglucamine, a substance used in the preparation of radiopaque compounds.

megohm Unit of electric resistance, equal to 1 million ohms.

meibomianitis, meibomitis Inflammation of the meibomian (tarsal) glands on the inside of the eyelid.

Meig's syndrome The presence of a benign ovarian fibroma associated with the formation of ascites and pleural effusion.

meiosis The special process of cell division during maturation of the sex cells in which two nuclear cell divisions occur in rapid succession, thus forming four gametes, each containing half the number of chromosomes found in the general body cells; when the ovum unites with the sperm in fertilization, the resulting cell then has the normal diploid number of chromosomes (46).

meiotic Relating to meiosis.

mel 1. Honey. 2. A pharmaceutical preparation containing honey as an excipient.

melalgia Pain in the lower extremity.

melancholia Major depression characterized by loss of pleasure in almost all usual activities; symptoms include excessive or inappropriate guilt, psychomotor retardation or agitation, anorexia, and disordered sleep.

mélangeur A glass tube with an enlarged end used to collect and dilute blood specimens.

melanic Having a dark color.

melaniferous Containing any dark pigment.

melanin Black or dark brown pigment found in the skin, hair, and retina.
See melanosis.

melanoameloblastoma Benign tumor of the anterior maxilla, usually occurring in infants; it causes displacement of tooth buds.

melanoblast A cell that when developed to maturity (melanocyte) is capable of producing melanin.

melanocyte Mature pigment cell of the skin that produces melanin.

melanoderma Any abnormal dark pigmentation of the skin predominantly resulting from accumulation of the pigment melanin; usually associated with other conditions.

melanodermatitis Excessive deposit of melanin in an area of dermatitis.

melanogen Substance that may be transformed into melanin.

melanogenemia The presence in the blood of substances that produce melanin.

melanogenesis The formation or production of melanin by living cells.

melanoma A tumor or growth made up of melanin-pigmented cells.

acral lentiginous m. A slow growing type characterized by macular onset and lateral spread within the epidermis; usually occurring on the hands, feet and mucous membranes.

lentigo maligna m. An irregularly shaped, flat patch with various shades of brown, blue, red, white and tan; typically occurring in sun-damaged skin and in older individuals.

malignant m. A malignant neoplasm derived from melanin-producing cells, occurring in the skin of any part of the body. Formerly called melanosarcoma. Also known as melanocarcinoma or simply as melanoma.

nodular m. A deeply invading type that spreads

alveolar epithelium
basal lamina
capillary endothelium
alveolocapillary membrane
air
RBC
lumen of capillary
nucleus

fetal membranes
chorion
allantois
yolk sac
amnion

cell nucleus
microvilli
absorptive cell
basal lamina
reticular lamina
basement membrane

lipid
prote
cell membrane

---

rapidly and vertically, exhibiting a deep black-brown coloration; it occurs anywhere on the skin and mucous membrane.

superficial spreading m. (SSM) A centrifugally expanding type characterized by lateral spread within the epidermis, irregular borders and variable coloration (red, pink, blue, white, brown and black); it occurs most commonly on the legs of women and the chest and back of men.

melanomatosis The presence of numerous melanomas.

melanonychia Black discoloration of the nails.

melanopathy Any disease characterized by black pigmentation of the skin.

melanophage A phagocytic cell that engulfs particles of melanin.

melanophore 1. In human histology and pathology, a pigment cell carrying melanin. 2. In general biology, a cell that produces melanin.

melanoplakia Pigmented patches on the tongue and oral mucosa.

melanoprotein A protein complex with melanin.

melanorrhagia, melanorrhea See melena.

melanosarcoma Malignant melanoma; see under melanoma.

melanosis Abnormal deposits of dark pigment in various organs or tissues. Also called melanism.

melanosome A single melanin-containing organelle that has finished synthesizing melanin.

melanotic Pertaining to melanosis or to a darkened or blackened condition.

melanuria Presence of melanin or other dark pigment in the urine; usually caused by malignant melanoma.

melasma Chloasma.

melatonin A hormone believed to be secreted by the pineal gland.

melena The passage of dark, tarry stools due to blood, usually originating in the upper intestinal tract. Also called melanorrhagia; melenorrhea.

m. spuria Melena in nursing babies in which the blood originates from fissures in the nipples of the mother.

melenemesis Vomiting of dark colored material.

melioidosis Infectious, glanders-like disease of wild rodents of Southeast Asia; caused by the bacillus *Pseudomonas pseudomallei* (*Actinobacillus pseudomallei*); in man it may appear acutely or insidiously and is often associated with fever, cough, purulent sputum, and abscess formation.

melitensis See brucellosis.

melitis Inflammation of the cheek.

melitose See raffinose.

mellitum, *pl.* **mellita** Any pharmaceutical preparation having honey as the excipient.

mellitus Latin for honeyed.

meloplasty, melonoplasty Plastic surgery of the cheek.

melphalen A compound, derivative of nitrogen mustard sometimes used in the management of multiple myeloma.

membrana, *pl.* **membranae** Latin for membrane.

membrane A thin sheet of tissue that covers a surface, envelopes a part, lines a cavity, divides a space, or connects two structures.

abdominal m. Peritoneum.

alveolocapillary m. The blood-air barrier in the lung consisting of the alveolar epithelium, basal lamina, and the capillary endothelium.

anterior limiting m. See Bowman's membrane.

atlantooccipital m. Any of two membranes (anterior and posterior) extending from the border of the foramen magnum to the atlas (first vertebra).

basement m. A thin transparent noncellular layer under the epithelium of mucous membranes and secreting glands.

basilar m. of the cochlear duct Membrane extending from the osseous spiral lamina to the basilar crest of the cochlea; it forms the floor of the cochlear duct and supports the spiral organ of Corti.

Bowman's m. One of the five layers forming the cornea (between the epithelium and the substantia propria), consisting of fine, closely interwoven fibrils. Also called anterior elastic lamina of cornea; anterior limiting membrane.

Bruch's m. Basal lamina of choroid; see under lamina.

cell m. A delicate structure about 90 Å in thickness that encloses the cell, separating the contents of the cell from the surrounding environment; it is comprised of lipids and proteins and regulates the passage of substances into and out of the cell. Also called plasmalemma; unit or plasma membrane.

cricothyroid m. A broad, thin membrane originating from the upper border of the cricoid cartilage, and extending to the vocal process of the arytenoid cartilage and to the thyroid cartilage.

Descemet's m. One of the five layers of the cornea covering the posterior surface of the substantia propria; it is elastic, transparent, homogeneous, and extremely thin. Also called posterior elastic lamina of cornea; posterior limiting membrane.

diphtheritic m. The yellowish-gray, leathery exudate on the mucous membrane of the upper respiratory tract in diphtheria. Also called false membrane.

external limiting m. The third of ten layers of the retina; it has the form of chicken wire, allowing the ample passage of the rod and cone cells.

false m. A tough fibrous exudate on a mucous membrane. Also called pseudomembrane.

fetal m.'s Extraembryonic membranes concerned with the respiration, excretion, nutrition, and protection of the embryo; they include the amnion, chorion, allantois, yolk sac, decidua, and placenta.

glassy m. A prominent basal lamina in the ovary separating the epithelial layer of the follicle from the surrounding connective tissue of the stroma.

glomerular filtration m. The capillary wall of the

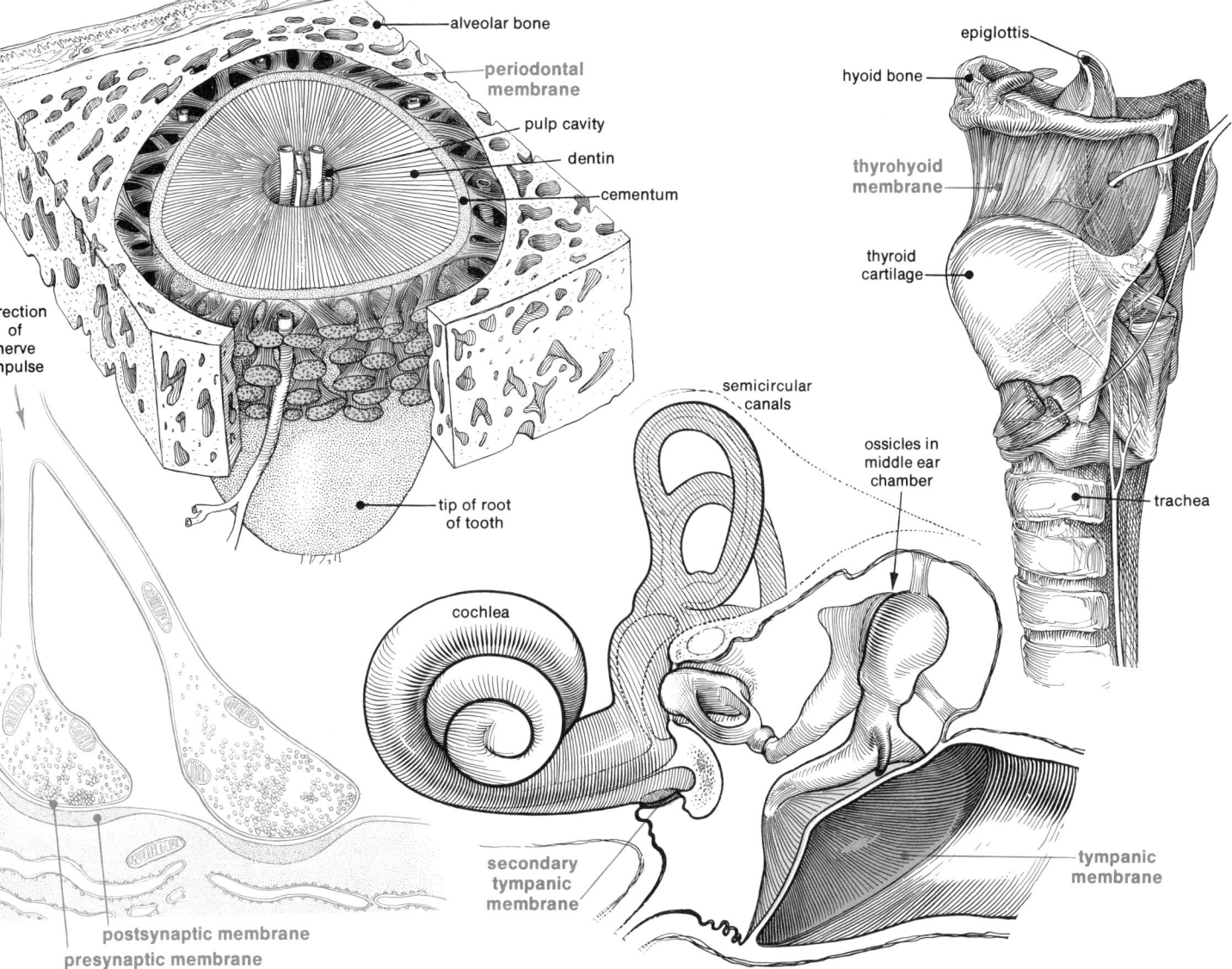

alveolar bone
periodontal membrane
pulp cavity
dentin
cementum

rection of nerve mpulse

tip of root of tooth

postsynaptic membrane
presynaptic membrane

epiglottis
hyoid bone
thyrohyoid membrane
thyroid cartilage

semicircular canals

ossicles in middle ear chamber

trachea

cochlea

secondary tympanic membrane

tympanic membrane

renal corpuscle; it allows ultrafiltration of the blood by delivering the plasma as primary urine to the urinary space within the nephronic (Bowman's) capsule; it does not allow the formed elements of the blood to pass through.

hyaline m.   Basement membrane.

hyaline-like m.   The eosinophilic, homogeneous, transparent membrane lining the alveoli and air passages of newborn (particularly premature) infants afflicted with hyaline membrane disease.

internal limiting m.   The last of ten layers of the retina forming both the inner limit of the retina and the outer boundary of the vitreous.

mucous m.   Membrane lining tubular structures and consisting of epithelium, basement membrane, lamina propria, and lamina muscularis. Also called tunica mucosa.

Nasmyth's m.   An extremely thin membrane covering the enamel of recently erupted teeth; it is soon abraded.

nuclear m. (n.m.)   An ordered membrane interface regulating the exchange of material between the nucleus and cytoplasm of the cell.

obturator m.   Membrane that almost completely closes the obturator foramen of the hipbone; it leaves a small canal for the passage of structures from the pelvis to the thigh.

perineal m.   The inferior layer of fascia of the urogenital diaphragm filling in the gap of the pubic arch of the pelvis.

periodontal m.   Dense white collagenous connective tissue fibers that surround the root of a tooth and attach it to the bone. Also called periodontal ligament.

plasma m.   See cell membrane.

posterior limiting m.   See Descemet's membrane.

postsynaptic m.   The portion of the cell membrane at the site of the synapse, sensitive to neurotransmitter substances. Also called postjunctional membrane.

presynaptic m.   The cell membrane of an axon at the site of the synapse, through which neurotransmitter substances pass into the synaptic cleft. Also called prejunctional membrane.

Reissner's m.   Vestibular membrane of cochlear duct.

secondary tympanic m.   The membrane which closes the round window between the blind end of the scala tympani of the internal ear and the middle ear chamber.

semipermeable m.   A membrane which permits the passage of water and small molecules but prevents the passage of large molecules or colloidal matter.

serous m.   The outermost coat lining the external walls of the body cavities and reflected over the exposed surfaces of protruding organs.

suprapleural m.   A dense, tent-shaped fascial layer attached from the inner part of the first rib and costal cartilage to the transverse process of the seventh cervical vertebra; it helps to close the thoracic inlet.

synaptic m.   The cell membrane of a neuronal ending (presynaptic membrane) in relation to the postsynaptic membrane of the adjacent neuron, usually separated by a 200 Å synaptic cleft.

synovial m.   The connective tissue membrane that lines the cavity of a synovial joint and produces the lubricating fluid.

tectorial m. of cochlear duct   A delicate gelatinous membrane positioned on the spiral organ of Corti of the internal ear.

thyrohyoid m.   A broad fibroelastic sheet that fills in the interval between the hyoid bone and thyroid cartilage.

tympanic m. (TM)   The membrane separating the external acoustic meatus from the middle ear chamber; it is kept tense for better reception of vibrations by the tensor muscle of the tympanum (tensor tympani); during ordinary conversation the tympanic

membrane is displaced only the diameter of a molecule of hydrogen.

undulating m.   An organelle of locomotion of certain flagellate parasites consisting of a finlike extension of the limiting membrane with a wavelike flagellar sheath.

unit m.   See cell membrane.

vestibular m. of cochlear duct   The delicate membrane in the internal ear separating the cochlear duct from the scala vestibuli. Also called Reissner's membrane.

virginal m.   Hymen.

Zinn's m.   The outermost layer of the iris.

membranelle   A minute membrane composed of fused cilia, seen in certain ciliate organisms.

membranocartilaginous   Partly membranous and partly cartilaginous.

membranous   Relating to, or of the nature of, a membrane.

memory   The process of neural mechanism involved in the storage and representation of an experience; the "read-in phase" of learning; the mental faculty of retaining in the subconscious an impression or idea of which the mind has once been conscious.

menacme   The period of menstrual activity in a woman's life.

menadione   A synthetic preparation having vitamin K properties; used in the treatment of hemorrhagic disorders caused by low prothrombin content of blood.

menarche   The first occurrence of the menses.

mendelevium   Radioactive element; symbol Md, atomic number 101.

Menétrièr's disease, Menétrièr's syndrome   A disease of unknown etiology, characterized by huge gastric rugae and pseudopolyps, which may be associated with ulcer-like symptoms, bleeding, or idiopathic hypoproteinemia. Also called giant hypertrophic gastritis.

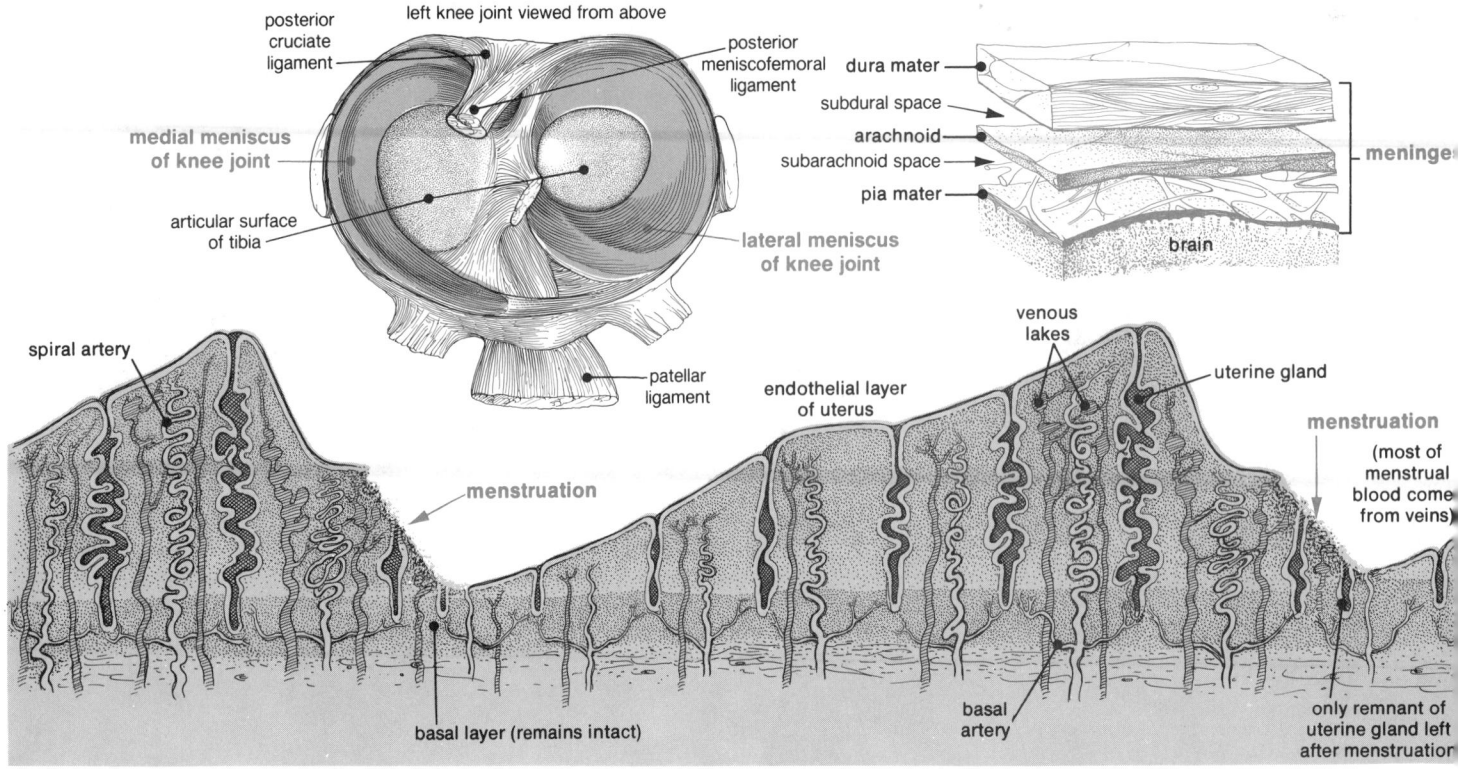

left knee joint viewed from above

posterior cruciate ligament

posterior meniscofemoral ligament

medial meniscus of knee joint

articular surface of tibia

lateral meniscus of knee joint

dura mater
subdural space
arachnoid
subarachnoid space
pia mater

meninges

brain

patellar ligament

spiral artery

venous lakes

uterine gland

endothelial layer of uterus

menstruation

menstruation (most of menstrual blood come from veins)

basal layer (remains intact)

basal artery

only remnant of uterine gland left after menstruation

Ménière's syndrome, Ménière's disease
Paroxysmal labyrinthine vertigo, characterized by recurrent episodes of severe vertigo associated with deafness and tinnitus, due to an unexplained increase in pressures of the endolymph. Also called endolymphatic hydrops; auditory vertigo.

meningeal Relating to the membranes that cover the brain and spinal cord.

meningeorrhaphy Surgical repair of a membrane, especially of those covering the brain and spinal cord (meninges).

meninges Specifically the membranes that cover the brain and spinal cord (pia mater, arachnoid, and dura mater). Also called membranes.

meningioma An intracranial tumor arising from the arachnoid, usually occurring in adults over 30 years of age.

meningism, meningismus Irritation of the brain or spinal cord producing symptoms similar to those of meningitis, but without inflammation of the meninges.

meningitis Inflammation of the meninges (membranes covering the brain and spinal cord); the infection may occur via retrograde thrombophlebitis, via spinal fluid pathways, directly from a local infection, or by the bloodstream.

  bacterial m. One caused by bacteria and generally marked by elevated protein, decrease in cerebrospinal fluid (CSF) sugar, and the presence of polymorphonuclear white blood cells in cloudy CSF.

  cerebrospinal m. Meningococcal meningitis.

  meningococcal m. Inflammation of the coverings of the brain and spinal cord caused by the bacterium *Neisseria meningitidis*. Also called cerebrospinal meningitis; spotted fever.

  viral m. Meningitis caused by a virus and generally marked by lymphocytosis in cerebrospinal fluid (CSF).

meningocele A congenital saclike, skin-covered protrusion of the meninges (membranes of the brain and spinal cord) through a defect in the skull or vertebral column; the most frequent sites are the midoccipital area of the head and the lumbosacral area of the spine.

meningococcemia Presence of meningococci in the blood; may be associated with petechial lesions, cardiovascular collapse, and/or meningitis; the causative agent is the gram-negative coccus *Neisseria meningitidis*.

meningococcus *Neisseria meningitidis*; a microorganism that causes an infectious form of meningitis.

meningocortical Relating to the membranes and the cortex of the brain.

meningocyte A mesenchymal epithelial cell of

the subarachnoid space.

meningoencephalitis Inflammation of the brain and its membranes. Also called encephalomeningitis.

meningoencephalocele Congenital defect consisting of an outpouching of the brain and its coverings (meninges) through a large gap in the skull, usually in the midoccipital area.

meningoencephalomyelitis Inflammation of the brain and spinal cord and their membranes.

meningoencephalopathy Any disease of the brain and its membranes.

meningohydroencephalocele Congenital defect consisting of a saclike protrusion of the brain and its membranes (meninges) containing part of a ventricle filled with cerebrospinal fluid; the outpouching occurs through a large gap in the skull, usually in the midoccipital area.

meningomalacia Softening of the meninges.

meningomyelitis Inflammation of the spinal cord and its membranes, most commonly the arachnoid and pia mater.

meningomyelocele An outpouching of the meninges (membranes covering the brain and spinal cord), containing spinal cord and/or nerve roots, through an abnormal gap in the vertebral column (spina bifida); the protrusion is devoid of a skin cover. Also called myelomeningocele.

meningoradiculitis Inflammation of the meninges and nerve roots.

meningovascular Concerning the meninges and adjacent blood vessels.

meninx, *pl.* meninges A membrane, especially one of the membranes covering the brain and spinal cord.

meniscectomy Surgical removal of an interarticular cartilage, especially from the knee joint.

meniscitis Inflammation of any interarticular cartilage.

meniscocyte Sickle cell; see under cell.

meniscus, *pl.* menisci A crescent-shaped structure, as the fibrocartilage that serves as a cushion between two bones meeting in a joint.

  lateral m. of knee joint A nearly circular, crescent-shaped fibrocartilage attached to the lateral articular surface of the superior end of the tibia.

  medial m. of knee joint A crescent-shaped fibrocartilage attached to the medial articular surface of the superior end of the tibia.

  m. tactus Tactile disk; see under disk.

  temporomandibular m. Articular disk; see under disk.

menolipsis The temporary cessation of menstruation.

menometrorrhagia Abnormal bleeding during

or between menstrual periods.

menopausal Relating to the menopause.

menopause The normal termination of the menses, occurring usually between the ages of 45 and 50; frequent symptoms include hot flushes, headache, vulvar discomfort, painful sexual intercourse, and mental depression; the symptoms correlate with the diminution of ovarian function and hormone production. Commonly known as the "change of life."

  artificial m. Cessation of menstruation by irradiation or surgical removal of ovaries.

  premature m. An abnormally early termination of menstruation.

menorrhagia Excessive or prolonged menstruation; also called hypermenorrhea.

menorrhea 1. Normal menstruation. 2. Menorrhagia.

menoschesis Suppression of the menses.

menostasis, menostasia Amenorrhea.

menothermal Relating to the hot flashes of menopause.

menses Periodic bloody discharge from the uterus. Also called menstruation.

menstrual Relating to the menses.

menstruate To discharge a bloody fluid from the uterus at regular intervals.

menstruation The periodic discharge from the uterus of a normally nonclotting bloody fluid, usually occurring at approximately a four-week interval and lasting from three to five days; in a normal menstrual cycle menstruation is preceded by ovulation. Also called menses.

  anovular m., anovulatory m. Menstrual bleeding not preceded by ovulation.

  vicarious m. Bleeding from sites other than the uterus, occurring at the time when normal menstruation takes place, e.g., bleeding from the nose and other structures of the head.

mensual Monthly.

mensuration Measurement by immediate comparison.

mental 1. Relating to the mind. 2. Relating to the chin.

mental deficiency See retardation, mental.

mentation Mental activity.

menthol Peppermint camphor, an organic compound derived from peppermint oil or prepared synthetically; on the skin or in the respiratory tract (e.g., in cigarette smoke) it provides a sensation of coolness by selective stimulation of nerve endings sensitive to cold.

menton The lowermost point of the median plane of the lower jaw.

mentoplasty Plastic surgery of the chin.

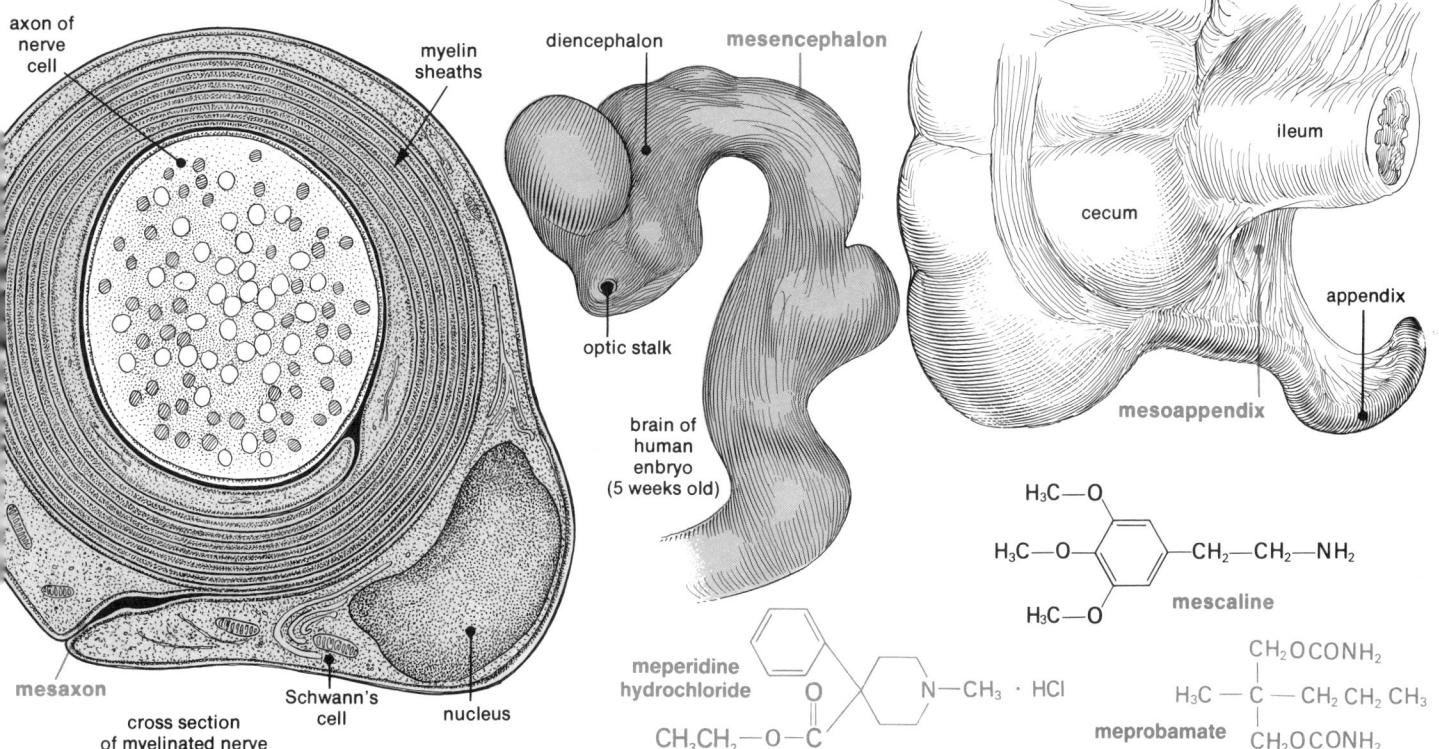

axon of nerve cell

myelin sheaths

mesaxon

cross section of myelinated nerve

Schwann's cell

nucleus

diencephalon

mesencephalon

optic stalk

brain of human enbryo (5 weeks old)

ileum

cecum

appendix

mesoappendix

$$H_3C—O$$
$$H_3C—O \quad CH_2—CH_2—NH_2$$
$$H_3C—O$$

mescaline

meperidine hydrochloride

$$CH_3CH_2—O—C$$ $$N—CH_3 \cdot HCl$$

meprobamate

$$H_3C—C—CH_2 CH_2 CH_3$$
$$CH_2OCONH_2$$
$$CH_2OCONH_2$$

mentum Latin for chin.

meperidine hydrochloride A widely used narcotic and analgesic that may produce addiction; Demerol®.

meprobamate A minor tranquilizer used to allay anxiety; Equanil®; Miltown®.

mepyrapone See metyrapone.

meralgia Pain in the thigh.

  m. paresthetica Burning, tingling, pricking, or numbness of the lateral side of the thigh due to compression of the lateral femoral cutaneous nerve.

meralluride An organic mercurial diuretic.

merbromin A green crystalline compound, used in aqueous solution as a germicide and antiseptic; Mercurochrome®.

mercaptan Any substance containing the radical –SH bound to carbon; analogous to alcohols and phenols but containing sulfur instead of oxygen; the basic ingredient of the polysulfide polymer in rubber-based materials; used in dentistry as an elastic impression compound. Also called thioalcohol; thiol.

2-mercapto-4-hydroxyprimidine See thiouracil.

mercaptopurine A yellow crystalline compound which is an analogue of purine; Purinethol®.

mercurial 1. Relating to mercury. 2. Denoting any pharmaceutical preparation of mercury.

mercurialism Poisoning by mercury or its compounds.

mercuric Denoting a compound containing bivalent mercury.

mercurous Relating to or containing monovalent mercury.

  m. chloride HgCl; compound formerly used as a laxative and intestinal antiseptic. Also called calomel; mercury monochloride; mild mercury chloride.

mercury A heavy, silvery, poisonous metallic element, liquid at room temperature; symbol Hg, atomic number 80, atomic weight 200.59, specific gravity 13.546; used in thermometers, barometers, manometers, vapor lamps, and batteries, and in the preparation of some pharmaceuticals. Also called quicksilver; hydrargyrum.

mercury-197 (^{197}Hg) A radioactive mercury isotope used in brain tumor localization and in the study of renal function.

meridian A line surrounding a spherical body, passing through both poles, or half of such a circle, containing both poles.

  m. of cornea Any line bisecting the cornea through the apex.

  m. of eye Any line surrounding the surface of the eyeball and passing through both poles.

merocrine Denoting secreting cells that remain intact during discharge of the secretory products, as those in the salivary glands.

merotomy Cutting into parts.

merozoite The product of asexual division (schizogeny) of a protozoan in the body of the host; in malaria, one of several small round cells which, on rupture of the red blood cells, reinfect other erythrocytes or liver cells, or form gametocytes (the sexual forms in man, infective for the mosquito).

mesad Toward the middle.

mesal Median.

mesangial Relating to the mesangium.

mesangium The supporting stalk of the glomerulus; a specialized form of connective tissue present in the renal glomerulus (in the center of each lobule); it stabilizes the capillary loops both physically and chemically and consists of a few cells and a small amount of matrix produced by the cells.

mesaortitis Inflammation of the muscular coat of the aorta.

mesarteritis Inflammation of the muscular coat of an artery.

mesaxon A supporting cell membrane that completely encloses the axon, resulting from the fusion of two encircling arms; it generally elongates and encircles the axon like a jelly roll, forming the myelin lamellae.

mescaline A hallucinatory, addictive alkaloid derived from the peyote cactus; also prepared synthetically.

mescalism Addiction to mescaline.

mesencephalon The embryonic midbrain; the second cephalic dilatation of the neural tube that develops into the corpora quadrigemina, the cerebral peduncles, and the cerebral aqueduct (aqueduct of Sylvius).

mesenchyme Embryonic connective tissue consisting of an aggregation of cells in contact with one another by means of long processes, thus forming a loose network; the space between the cells is filled with a ground substance; the mesenchymal cell is multipotential, i.e., it can develop into many kinds of connective tissue.

mesenteric Of or relating to the mesentery.

mesenteritis Inflammation of the mesentery.

mesentery A double layer of peritoneum attaching various organs to the body wall and conveying to them their blood vessels and nerves; commonly used in reference to the peritoneal fold attaching the small intestine to the posterior body wall.

meshwork Network.

mesial Situated in, near, or toward the middle, as toward the middle line or apex of the dental arch.

mesiobuccal Pertaining to the mesial and buccal surfaces of a tooth; usually denoting the line angle

formed by the junction of the two surfaces.

mesiobucco-occlusal Relating to the mesial, buccal, and occlusal surfaces of a posterior tooth; usually denoting the point angle formed by the junction of the three surfaces.

mesiocervical Relating to the mesial surface of the neck of a tooth. Also called mesiogingival.

mesioclusion Malocclusion in which the lower dental arch is anterior to the upper.

mesiodens An accessory tooth located between the two upper incisors.

mesiodistal Denoting the plane of a tooth from its mesial surface across to its distal surface.

mesiolabioincisal Relating to the mesial, labial, and incisal surfaces of an anterior tooth; usually denoting the point angle formed by the junction of the three surfaces.

mesiolingual Relating to the mesial and lingual surfaces of a tooth; usually denoting the line angle formed by the junction of the two surfaces.

mesiolinguoincisal Relating to the mesial, lingual, and incisal surfaces of an anterior tooth; usually denoting the point angle formed by the junction of the three surfaces.

mesiolinguo-occlusal Relating to the mesial, lingual, and occlusal surfaces of a posterior tooth; usually denoting the point angle formed by the junction of the three surfaces.

mesio-occlusal Relating to the mesial and occlusal surfaces of a posterior tooth; usually denoting the line angle formed by the junction of the two surfaces.

mesioversion 1. Position of a tooth closer to the midline than normal. 2. Position of a jaw (upper or lower) anterior to its normal position.

mesmerism Treatment based on the method of Mesmer; thought to be primarily a form of hypnosis.

mesoappendix The mesentery of the appendix; the small, double-layered fold of peritoneum connecting the appendix to the mesentery of the ileum.

mesoblast The mesoderm in its early stage of development; the middle of the three germinal layers of the embryo.

mesoblastic Relating to the mesoblast.

mesobronchitis Inflammation of the middle or muscular layer of the bronchi.

mesocardium, *pl.* **mesocardia** The double layer of mesoderm attaching the embryonic heart to the wall of the pericardial cavity.

mesocecum The mesentery of the cecum; it is frequently absent.

mesocephalic Denoting a skull having a cephalic index between 75 and 80. Also called normocephalic.

mesocolic Relating to the mesocolon.

mesocolon The double layer of peritoneum attaching the colon to the posterior abdominal wall.

mesoderm The middle layer of embryonic cells, between the ectoderm and the endoderm; it gives rise to the dermis, connective tissues, the vascular and urogenital systems, and most skeletal and smooth muscles.

mesoepithelium See mesothelium.

mesogastrium The broad primitive mesentery which encloses the enteric canal (future stomach) in the embryo, and from which the greater omentum is developed. Also called mesogaster.

mesognathic Having a slightly projecting upper jaw with a gnathic index between 98 and 103.

mesognathion The part of the maxilla bearing the lateral incisor tooth.

mesometrium The broad ligament of the uterus below the attachment of the ovary; it extends to the lateral wall of the pelvis.

mesomorph A person having a body build with prominent musculature and heavy bony structure.

meson 1. The median anteroposterior plane of the human body. 2. Subatomic particle with a mass between that of the electron and the proton. Formerly called mesotron.

mesonephroma Rare ovarian tumor believed to be formed from displaced mesonephric tissue.

mesonephros An intermediate excretory organ of the embryo; it is replaced by the more permanent kidney (metanephros) while its duct system is retained in the male as the epididymis and deferent duct. Also called wolffian duct.

mesorchium 1. The fold of peritoneum in the fetus that attaches the developing testis to the mesonephros and holds it in place. 2. A fold of peritoneum in the adult between the testis and epididymis.

mesorectum The short peritoneal fold investing the upper part of the rectum and connecting it to the sacrum.

mesoropter The normal position of the eyes at rest.

mesorrhine Having a nose of moderate width with a nasal index from 47 to 51 on the skull.

mesosalpinx The upper free portion of the broad ligament, above the attachment of the ovary and investing the uterine tube.

mesosigmoid Denoting the portion of peritoneum attaching the sigmoid colon to the posterior abdominal wall.

mesosome A structure present in some bacterial cells, 2,500 to 5,000 Å in diameter, derived from the invagination of the plasma membrane; thought to play a role in the formation of a membrane septum and a crosswall.

mesosternum The body or main portion of the sternum.

mesotendon, mesotendineum The connective tissue fold of synovial membrane extending from a tendon to the wall of its synovial tendon sheath.

mesothelioma A neoplasm composed of cells similar to those forming the lining of the pleura, peritoneum, or pericardium; pleural mesothelioma has been associated with exposure to asbestos.

    m. of genital tract Adenomatoid tumor; see under tumor.

    m. of meninges Meningioma.

mesothelium A single layer of large flattened cells, derived from the mesoderm, which forms the epithelium lining the internal surface of closed body cavities, such as the pericardium, pleura, and peritoneum. Also called mesoepithelium.

mesovarium The short fold of peritoneum attaching the ovary to the posterior wall of the broad ligament.

messenger A conveyor of information.

    second m. Cyclic adenosine monophosphate or cyclic guanosine monophospate; they function as mediators of enzyme action; found on cell membranes.

messenger RNA See under ribonucleic acid.

mestranol Estrogen used in the preparation of certain oral contraceptives.

metabiosis The dependence of an organism upon the pre-existence (and influence on the environment) of another for its development and flourishing.

metabolism A general term applied to the chemical processes taking place in living tissues, necessary for the maintenance of the living organism. See also catabolism; anabolism.

    basal m. The minimum amount of energy required to maintain vital functions in an individual at complete physical and mental rest. Also called basal metabolic rate (BMR).

metabolite Any product of metabolism.

    essential m. The substrate of an essential metabolic reaction.

metacarpophalangeal Relating to the articulations between the metacarpal bones and the phalanges.

metacarpus The five bones of the hand between the carpus and the phalanges.

metacentric Pertaining to a chromosome with the centromere in the middle.

metachromasia 1. The property by which certain cells stain in a color different from the dye with which they are stained. 2. The property through which a single dye stains different tissue elements in different colors.

metachromatic Term applied to cells and dyes exhibiting metachromasia.

metachrosis The ability to change color, possessed by certain animals.

metacresol (m-Cresol) $CH_3C_6H_4$; a local antiseptic.

metacryptozoite A member of a second or subsequent generation of the exoerythrocytic, tissue-dwelling malarial parasite; it develops from the sporozoite, without intervening blood-parasitic generations.

metacyesis Extrauterine pregnancy.

metafemale A female with three X chromosomes and two sets of autosomes, characterized by short stature and a certain degree of obesity; many are mildly retarded. Also called superfemale; trisomy X.

Metagonimus A genus of small flukes which may infect man upon his eating fish containing the larvae.

    M. yokogawai One of the smallest flukes (1.0 to 1.5 mm long) infecting humans; prevalent in the Far East and the Balkan states.

metakinesis The separation of the two chromatids of a chromosome during the anaphase of mitosis.

metal (M) Any of a group of substances that have a characteristic luster, are usually malleable, ductile, and conductors of electricity and heat, and, in chemical reactions, tend to lose electrons.

    alkali-earth m. Alkaline earth; see under earth.

    noble m. Metal that cannot be oxidized by heat alone, nor readily dissolved by acid.

    rare-earth m. Any metallic element of atomic number 57 through 71.

metaldehyde A polymer of acetaldehyde formerly used as an antiseptic.

metalloenzyme An enzyme having a metal ion as an integral part of its active structure.

metallophilia Having an affinity for metal salts; said of certain cells.

metalloporphyrin Compound containing a porphyrin and a metal; e.g., hematin (iron), chlorophyll (magnesium), etc.

metalloprotein A protein containing a more or less tightly bound metal ion or ions; e.g., hemoglobin.

metallotherapy Treatment of disease by the use of metals or metal compounds.

metamale A male with one X chromosome and two Y chromosomes, usually tall and somewhat lean in stature, and often having a tendency toward aggressive behavior. Also called supermale; XYY syndrome.

myeloblast

stages of leukocyte maturation

metamyelocyte

acidophilic cytoplasm

kidney-shaped nucleus

promyelocyte

juvenile neutrophil (band cell)

myelocyte

mature neutrophil (PMN)

cardinal vein

mesonephron in developing embryo

aorta

hindgut

allantois

mesonephric duct

cloaca

metencephalon

myelen-cephalon

metanephric duct

metanephric tissue

metanephros

diencephalon

pontine flexure

telencephalon

methamphetamine hydrochloride

CH₃
|
CH₂—C—H · HCl
|
NH
|
CH₃

model of **methane** molecule

embryonic brain and spinal cord

spinal cord

---

metamere One of a series of homologous body segments.

metamerism The state of having a series of structures arranged in a repetitive pattern.

metamorphosis A change in form and/or function, as the phase in the development of certain insects from larva to adult.

  retrograde m. The gradual degeneration of certain structures through lack of use, as the eyes of certain deep sea-dwelling fish.

metamyelocyte An immature granulocyte; an early stage of a granulocyte derived from a myelocyte; its cytoplasm contains fine specific granules, as well as azurophilic granules, and its nucleus is indented or kidney-shaped.

metanephrine One of the products of catabolism of epinephrine excreted in the urine.

metanephros The permanent kidney in the human fetus, possessing a high degree of excretory function; it is formed caudal to the mesonephros, close to the termination of the cloaca, and develops following the regression of the mesonephros; it is composed of the metanephric duct (primitive ureter) and the metanephrogenic tissue.

metaneutrophil, metaneutrophile Not staining normally with neutral dyes.

metaphase The second stage of cell division by mitosis, during which the chromatids are aligned along the equatorial plane of the cell and attached by spindle fibers to the centromere.

metaphysis The line of junction of the epiphysis with the shaft (diaphysis) of a long bone.

metaplasia The development of adult tissue from cells that normally produce a different type of tissue.

metapsychology A systematic, but usually speculative, attempt to state the underlying general laws of psychology.

metaraminol bitartrate A sympathomimetic compound used to elevate the blood pressure in acute hypotensive conditions.

metarubricyte Orthochromatic normoblast; see under normoblast.

metastable Denoting an intermediate, unstable, or transient state, as of a supersaturated solution or the excited state of an atomic nucleus.

metastasis Transfer of a disease from its primary site to a distant location; metastasis can be accomplished by the transfer of microorganisms or by the transfer of cells as in malignant tumors.

metastasize To pass or spread from one organ or tissue to another.

metatarsal Of or relating to the metatarsus.

metatarsophalangeal Relating to the metatarsus and the bones of the toes.

metatarsus The anterior portion of the foot between the toes and the instep, composed of five bones.

  m. adductus Common deformity in which only the front part of the foot (at the tarsometatarsal joints) is drawn toward the midline; a common cause of the toe-in gait. Also called metatarsus varus.

  m. varus See metatarsus adductus.

metathalamus The part of the thalamencephalon comprising the medial and lateral geniculate bodies.

Metazoa The subkingdom of animals comprised of multicellular individuals in which cells are differentiated into tissues; includes all animals except the protozoa.

metencephalon The portion of the embryonic brain from which develop the pons, cerebellum, and pontine part of the fourth ventricle; together with the myelencephalon it makes up the hindbrain or rhombencephalon.

meteorism Distention of the intestines with gas. Also called tympanites.

meter (M) **1.** Measure of length, equal to 39.37 inches. **2.** A measuring instrument.

  rate m. Device that indicates the magnitude of events averaged over differing time intervals.

  total solids m. A calibrated refractometer used for determining the total solids in a drop of fluid, such as urine or serum.

metestrus, metestrum The period of regression immediately following the period of sexual desire (estrus) in the mating season, prior to diestrus.

methadone A synthetic narcotic compound, used as an analgesic and in the treatment of heroin addiction.

methamphetamine hydrochloride A potent sympathomimetic agent that stimulates the central nervous system and depresses the motility of the digestive tract, thus allaying hunger; taken orally or intravenously by drug abusers; produces strong psychic dependence. Also known by the slang terms meth; speed.

methane An odorless, colorless gas, CH₄; produced by the decomposition of organic matter; it is the smallest and lightest hydrocarbon, and with its next-larger relative, ethane, makes up as much as 90

methantheline bromide

methaqualone

methionine

$$CH_3{-}S{-}CH_2{-}CH_2{-}\overset{\overset{\displaystyle NH_2}{|}}{\underset{\underset{\displaystyle H}{|}}{C}}{-}COOH$$

methoxyflurane

disk sensitivity method (for determining sensitivity of specific microorganisms to multiple antibiotics)

TE – tetracycline
E – erythromycin
S – streptomycin
P – penicillin
B – bacitracin
C – chloramphenicol

multidisk containing a predetermined amount of drug on each segment

---

percent of natural gas. Also called marsh gas.

methanol Methyl alcohol; see under alcohol.

methantheline bromide Drug used in the treatment of peptic ulcer; Banthine;®.

methaqualone A short-acting sedative; Quaalude®.

methemalbumin Compound formed by the combination of heme with plasma albumin; found in the blood of individuals with malarial hemoglobinuria or paroxysmal nocturnal hemoglobinuria.

methemoglobin (MetHb) A dark brown compound sometimes formed in the red blood corpuscles by the action of certain drugs on hemoglobin; equivalent to but chemically different from oxygenated hemoglobin; its oxygen is in firm union with iron and is not available to the tissues.

methemoglobinemia An excessive amount of methemoglobin in the blood.

methenamine $C_6H_{12}N_4$; a urinary antiseptic that acts by releasing formaldehyde in an acid medium; effective against *Escherichia coli*, a common cause of urinary tract infections.

  m. hippurate A compound of methenamine and hippuric acid.

  m. mandelate A compound of methenamine and mandelic acid.

methicillin sodium A semisynthetic penicillin derivative used as an antibiotic in staphylococcal infections resistant to penicillin.

methionine (Met) An organic compound, $C_5H_{11}NO_2S$; one of the protein-derived amino acids, present in proteins such as egg albumin, which on hydrolysis yields about 5% its weight of methionine; it is essential in the diet.

method A set form or mode of procedure, especially a systematic way of performing an examination, test, operation, etc.

  activated sludge m. A method of treating sewage waste by adding 15% bacterially active liquid sludge; it causes the colloidal material of the sewage to coagulate and undergo sedimentation.

  copper-sulfate m. A method for the determination of specific gravity of blood or plasma; solutions of copper sulfate graded in specific gravity by increments of 0.004 are placed in a series of small containers; a drop of blood or plasma is placed into each container; the specific gravity of the copper sulfate solution, in which the drop of blood or plasma remains suspended indefinitely, indicates the specific gravity of the sample.

  Credé's m.'s 1. A method of expressing the placenta in which the body of the uterus is vigorously squeezed in order to produce placental separation; it usually traumatizes the placental site and is not generally recommended. **2.** The application of 1 drop of a 2% solution of silver nitrate onto each eye of the newborn infant to prevent gonococcal conjunctivitis. **3.** Use of manual pressure on the bladder, particularly a paralyzed bladder, to express urine.

  direct m. In dentistry, a technique of fabricating a wax pattern of lost tooth structure directly in the prepared cavity in the tooth; an inlay technique.

  disk sensitivity m. A procedure for determining the relative effectiveness of various antibiotics; small disks of paper are impregnated with known antibiotics and then placed in a Petri dish, on the surface of the medium that was inoculated with the organism being tested; after a period of incubation the lack of growth in areas around the various disks indicates the relative effectiveness of the antibiotics.

  flash m. A method of pasteurizing milk by quickly heating it to a temperature of 178°F, holding it there for a short time, and then reducing it rapidly to 40°F.

  immunofluorescence m.'s Any method in which a fluorescent labeled antibody is used to detect the presence or determine the location of the corresponding antigen.

  indirect m. In dentistry, the fabrication of a wax pattern of lost tooth structure formed on a cast or model that was made from an impression of prepared cavity.

  Kjeldahl m. A method of determining the amount of nitrogen in an organic compound by heating it with strong sulfuric acid in the presence of appropriate catalysts; the nitrogen is thereby converted to ammonia which is distilled off, titrated, and measured, and from this the amount of nitrogen is estimated.

  Lee-White m. A method of determining the coagulation time of venous blood by placing it in tubes of standard bore at body temperature.

  micro-Kjeldahl m. A modified Kjeldahl procedure designed for the analysis of nitrogenous compounds in relatively small quantities, such as 1 or 2 mg.

  Ouchterlony m. Double diffusion, a method of double immunodiffusion using a Petri dish of agar in which antigen and antibody are placed in separate wells cut into the gel; during incubation, both antigen and antibody diffuse from the wells and interact to form precipitins in the agar; as diffusion progresses, concentration gradients are established; distinct bands or lines of precipitate form where diffused specific antigen and antibody meet in optimal proportions; the precipitin reaction is a useful analytic technique for the identification of unknown antibodies or antigens.

  rhythm m. Birth control by avoiding sexual intercourse for several days before and after the approximate day of ovulation.

  Schick's m. A method of producing immunity to diphtheria by the injection of a mixture of toxin and antitoxin of that disease.

  silver cone m. The method in which a prefitted silver cone is placed into the apex of the root canal of a tooth and then sealed.

  Sippy's m. A method of treating peptic ulcer by neutralizing the free acid of the gastric juice with foods (milk and cream especially) administered frequently in small amounts.

  split cast m. A method of indexing dental casts on an articulator to facilitate their removal and replacement on the instrument.

  Westergren m. A method for estimating the sedimentation rate of red blood cells in blood; after mixing 4.5 ml of venous blood with 0.5 ml of 3.8% aqueous solution of sodium citrate, a standard pipet (2-mm bore, 300 mm in length, and graduated at 1-mm intervals from 0 to 200) is filled to the zero mark and kept in an upright position; in 1 hour the fall of the red blood cells is recorded; the average rate for males is 0 to 15 mm and for females, 0 to 20 mm.

  Wintrobe m. A method of determining the sedimentation rate of red cells in blood mixed with an anticoagulant, by the use of the narrow-bore Wintrobe tube; the amount of sedimentation is noted after one hour, then the sample is centrifuged and the measured volume of packed red cells is used to modify the first reading using a standard table; corrected normal value for males is 0 to 10 mm and for females 0 to 20 mm in 1 hour.

methotrexate A folic acid antagonist used in the treatment of choriocarcinoma.

methoxyflurane 2,2-Dichloro-1,1-difluoroethyl methyl ether; a clear, colorless liquid with a fruity odor; nonflammable and nonexplosive in air or oxygen; used as a slow anesthetic; Penthrane®.

methscopolamine bromide A gastrointestinal antispasmodic agent of prolonged action (about eight hours); used chiefly in the treatment of gastrointestinal diseases; Pamine Bromide®.

methyl The radical – CH_3.

  m. chloride CH_3Cl; the hydrochloric acid ester of methyl alcohol; a refrigerant, used in spray form as a local anesthetic. Also called chloromethane.

  m. iodide CH_3I; a somewhat colorless liquid used as a local anesthetic.

  m. methacrylate An acrylic resin; a plastic material.

methyldopa

methylphenidate hydrochloride

methyl salicylate

hydrophyllic heads
hydrophobic tails
micelles
cell membrane
lipids
protein

microaneurysms
retinal capillaries

m. salicylate A colorless liquid, insoluble in water; used as an antipyretic and antiseptic. Also called artificial wintergreen oil.

m. sulfoxide See dimethyl sulfoxide.

methyl orange Sodium salt of helianthin; yellow-orange power used as an indicator with a pH range from 3.2 to 4.4 (yellow at 3.2, pink at 4.4).

methyl red A red compound, $C_{15}H_{15}O_2N_3$, soluble in alcohol; used as an indicator with a pH range of 4.4 to 6 (red at 4.4, yellow at 6).

methyl violet Gentian violet.

methylate **1.** To combine with methyl alcohol or the methyl radical. **2.** A compound of methyl alcohol and a metal.

methylated Combined with or containing methyl alcohol.

methylbenzene See toluene.

methylcellulose A bulk-forming cellulose derivative with laxative properties; available in powder, granules, or capsule forms and used for constipation and occasionally as an appetite depressant in the management of obesity; the synthetic form is used to prolong the duration of contact in ophthalmic drops.

methylcholanthrene A cancer-producing hydrocarbon.

methyldopa A hypotensive drug used in the treatment of hypertension; Aldomet®.

methylene The organic radical CH_2.

methylene blue Methylthionine chloride, an aniline dye which when dissolved in water forms a deep blue liquid; formerly used as a urinary antiseptic; now used in the treatment of methemoglobinemia, as an antidote for cyanide poisoning, and as a staining agent, especially for demonstrating basophilic and metachromatic substances. Also called toluidine blue.

3,4-methylene dioxyamphetamine (MDA) A hallucinogen commonly referred to as the love drug.

methylglucamine diatrizoate An organic compound used as a contrast medium in the making of x-ray transparencies.

methylmalonic aciduria Excretion of excessive amounts of methylmalonic acid in urine.

methylparaben An antifungal preservative; Niapagin®.

methylphenidate hydrochloride A mild central nervous system stimulant similar to amphetamine; used in the management of children with hyperkinetic syndrome and in the treatment of narcolepsy; Ritalin®.

methylprednisolone An anti-inflammatory agent, usually administered orally; a commonly used immune suppressant.

methyltestosterone A methyl derivative of testosterone.

methyl transferase An enzyme that transfers a methyl group from one compound to another. Also called transmethylase.

methyprylon Compound having sedative and hypnotic properties.

methysergide maleate Compound used in the prophylactic treatment of migraine; prolonged use may be associated with retroperitoneal fibrosis; Sansert®.

Metmyoglobin (MetMb) A reddish brown pigment resulting from the oxidation of myoglobin.

metoprolol A beta₁-adrenergic blocking agent.

metopyrone See metyrapone.

Metorchis A genus of flukes; some of its species are found in cats, dogs, and occasionally in man.

metoxenous Heteroecious.

metra Greek for uterus.

metratonia Lack of tone of the uterine wall after childbirth.

metrectomy Hysterectomy.

metria Any inflammatory condition following childbirth.

metric Relating to or based on the meter as a standard of measurement.

metritis Inflammation of the uterus.

metrodynamometer Instrument used to measure the strength of uterine contractions.

metromalacia Abnormal softening of the uterus.

metronoscope Device that exposes printed material at short intervals; used to test and develop reading speed.

metropathia hemorrhagica Excessive, prolonged bleeding from the uterus, associated with cyst formation of the endometrium.

metropathic Related to or caused by disease of the uterus.

metropathy Any disease of the uterus.

metrophlebitis Inflammation of the uterine veins, usually occurring only while bearing a child or immediately thereafter.

metroptosia, metroptosis Prolapse of the uterus.

metrorrhagia Irregular bleeding from the uterus, especially during the intermenstrual period.

metrorrhea Discharge of pus or mucus from the uterus.

metrorrhexis Rupture of the uterus.

metrosalpingitis Inflammation of the uterus and the uterine (fallopian) tubes.

metroscope Instrument for viewing the uterine cavity.

metrostaxis A slight continuous bleeding from

the uterus.

metrostenosis Constriction of the uterine cavity.

metrotomy Hysterotomy.

metyrapone $C_{14}H_{14}N_2O$; 2-methyl-1,2-di-3-pyridyl-1-propanone; an inhibitor of adrenocortical steroid C-11 β hydroxylation; administered orally or intravenously as a diagnostic test to determine the capability of the pituitary gland to increase its production of corticotropin. Also called mepyrapone; metopyrone.

miasm, miasma Noxious vapors, as from a swamp; formerly thought to cause certain diseases such as malaria.

micelle **1.** A formation of approximately 50 to 100 amphipathic molecules arranged spherically, usually with the hydrophobic moiety on the inside and the hydrophilic groups on the outside. **2.** A hypothetical submicroscopic particle thought to be the unit of living matter, capable of growth and division.

Micheli's anemia, Micheli's syndrome Paroxysmal nocturnal hemoglobinuria; see under hemoglobinuria.

microabscess A minute collection of leukocytes in solid tissues; a very small abscess.

microaerophil, microaerophile A microorganism that requires very little free oxygen.

microaerosol A suspension in air of particles between 1 and 10 μm in diameter.

microanalysis Special analytic technique involving quantities weighing 1 mg or less.

microanatomy See histology.

microaneurysm A minute aneurysm of a small vessel as seen in diabetic retinopathy.

microangiography The making of x-ray transparencies of the smallest blood vessels.

microangiopathy Any disorder of the small blood vessels.

thrombotic m. A combination of arteriolar thrombosis and capillary wall thickening resulting in a narrow lumen.

systemic diabetic m. The thickening of capillary basement membranes in many organs.

microbalance A scale designed to weigh minute amounts of materials.

microbe A microorganism; a one-celled animal or plant, especially one that causes disease.

microbial, microbic Relating to a microorganism.

microbicide Anything that destroys microorganisms; a germicide; an antiseptic.

microbiologic Relating to microbiology.

microbiologist A specialist in microbiology.

microbiology The branch of science concerned

micrognathia

microglia

microphthalmos
(left eye)

eyeball

eyepiece

light microscope

phase microscope

filament

condenser

electron microscope

specimen

diffraction plate

objective

objective

specimen

projector

condenser

with the study of microorganisms and their effect on other living organisms.

microbiota A general term denoting both plant and animal organisms that live in streams, as algae and protozoa.

microblast A small nucleated red blood cell.

microbody See peroxisome.

microbrachia Abnormal smallness of the arms.

microcardia Abnormal smallness of the heart.

microcephaly Abnormal smallness of the head.

microchemistry The use of minute amounts (in the range of one milligram) of substances in chemical reactions.

microcirculation Blood circulation in the capillaries, arterioles, and venules.

Micrococcaceae A family of gram-positive spherical or elliptical bacteria which divide in two or three planes, forming pairs, tetrads, or masses of cells; includes some pathogenic species; the type genus is *Micrococcus.*

micrococcus One of several species of bacteria (genus *Micrococcus*) characterized by a spherical shape and occurring singly, in pairs, and (most frequently) in irregular clusters.

microcoria Congenital smallness of the pupil.

microcornea Abnormal smallness of the cornea.

microcoulomb A microunit of electric quantity; one-millionth of a coulomb.

microcurie (μCi) A measure of radioactivity, one-millionth of a curie.

microcyst A tiny cyst, usually undetected by the unaided eye.

microcyte A small red blood cell at least 2 μm smaller than normal; can be seen in the blood of individuals with iron deficiency anemia.

microcytosis, microcythemia Condition in which the red blood cells are abnormally small.

microdactyly Abnormal smallness of the fingers or toes.

microdissection Dissection with the aid of a microscope or enlarging lens.

microdontia, microdentism Abnormal smallness of the teeth.

microelectrode A fine caliber electrode used in physiologic experiments.

microfarad A microunit of electrical capacity; one-millionth of a farad.

microfilament Any of several rodlike structures (4–6 nm in diameter) within cells composed of the proteins actin and myosin; involved in movement of cellular elements within and of the cell itself.

microfilaria The prelarval or embryonic forms of filarial worms.

microgametocyte The mother cell that produces microgametes.

microgamy Conjugation between two young cells in certain protozoans.

microgastria Congenital smallness of the stomach.

microgenia Abnormal smallness of the chin.

microgenitalism Abnormal smallness of the external genital organs.

microglia The smallest neuroglial cells; the macrophages of the brain and spinal cord; they help remove the cellular debris of the central nervous system.

microglossia Abnormal smallness of the tongue.

micrognathia Abnormal smallness of the jaw, especially the lower jaw, usually resulting in a recessive, birdlike profile.

   primary m. See Pierre Robin syndrome.

microgonioscope Instrument used to measure minute angles, as the filtration angle of the anterior chamber of the eye.

microgram (mcg, μg) A unit of weight equivalent to one-millionth of a gram.

microgyria Abnormal narrowness of the convolutions of the brain.

microhm A microunit of electrical resistance equivalent to one-millionth of an ohm.

microincineration The process of heating a tissue section to about 525°C and then observing the mineral ashes under a dark field microscope. Also called spodography.

microincision See micropuncture (2).

microinvasion The earliest stage in the spread of a carcinoma to the adjacent tissues.

microkymatotherapy Treatment of disease with high frequency radiation. Also called microwave therapy.

microliter (μl) One-millionth of a liter.

microlith A minute calculus.

microlithiasis The presence of minute concretions (gravel).

micromanipulation Dissection, teasing, etc. of microscopic structures under the microscope.

micromanipulator An instrument used in the dissection and injection of microscopic specimens and in isolation of single cells.

micromelia The state of having abnormally small limbs.

micrometer (μm) One-millionth of a meter.

micrometer An instrument used to measure microscopic objects.

micromethod Chemical analysis or techniques involving minimal amounts of material or the use of a microscope.

micrometry Measurement with a micrometer.

micromicrogram ($\mu\mu$g) One-millionth of one-millionth (10^{-12}) of a gram. Also called picogram.

micromicron ($\mu\mu$) One millionth of a micron.

micromolar Having a concentration of one millionth of a mole.

micromole (μmole) One-millionth of a mole.

micromyelia Congenital smallness or shortness of the spinal cord.

micron (μ) A unit of length in the metric system equal to one-thousandth of a millimeter.

micronucleus 1. The smallest of the nuclei in a multinuclear cell. 2. The smaller (reproductive) of the two nuclei in ciliates dividing mitotically, the larger being the vegetative nucleus.

micronutrients Essential compounds required by the body only in minute amounts; e.g., vitamins.

microorganic Relating to a microorganism.

microorganism A microscopic animal or plant.

micropathology 1. The microscopic study of disease-caused changes in the tissues. 2. The study of disease caused by microorganisms.

microphage A small neutrophil that leaves the blood stream to phagocytose bacteria and small particles; contrasted with the larger macrophage that characteristically engulfs larger particles.

microphobia Abnormal fear of microorganisms.

microphthalmos, microphthalmia Abnormal smallness of the eyeballs.

micropipette, micropipet Any variously shaped, calibrated glass tubes designed to transfer minute volumes of liquid.

microplasia Arrested growth.

microplethysmography Recording of changes in the size of a bodily part resulting from the flow of blood into and out of it.

micropsia The condition of seeing objects as smaller than their actual sizes.

micropuncture 1. A technique for studying the function of the kidney by placement of a micropipette within a tubule and/or blood vessel of the kidney in order to sample the composition of fluid, measure the pressure, or determine the electric potential at different sites. 2. Destruction of the organelles of a cell by a ruby laser beam. Also called microincision.

microscope An instrument with a combination of lenses used to observe small objects or substances under magnification.

   binocular m. A microscope with two eyepiece tubes, permitting observation with both eyes simultaneously.

   bright field m. A microscope that makes an object visible by passing light through it (transillumination).

   compound m. A microscope having an objective and an eyepiece at opposite ends of an adjustable cylinder.

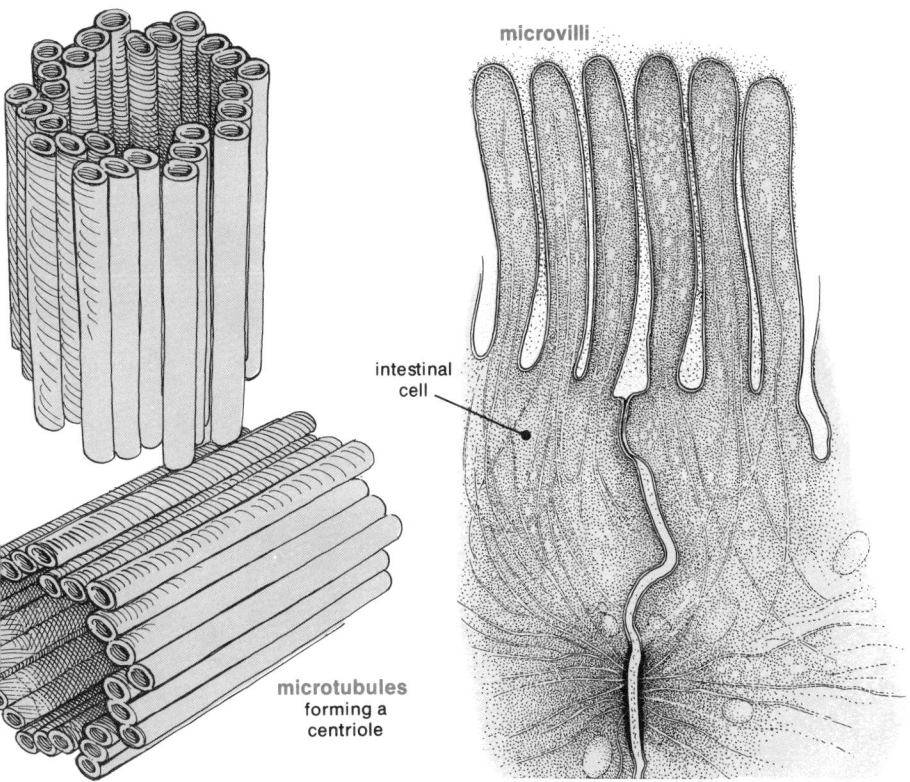

intestinal cell

microvilli

microtubules forming a centriole

	Human	Cow's
protein	2 g	3.5 g
carbohydrate	7 g	5 g
fat	4 g	3.5 g
calcium	25 mg	120 mg
phosphorus	16 mg	95 mg
iron	0.1 mg	0.1 mg
thiamine	17 μg	40 μg
riboflavin	30 μg	150 μg
nicotinic acid	170 μg	80 μg
ascorbic acid	3.5 μg	2.0 μg
vitamin A	170 IU	150 IU
vitamin D	1.0 IU	1.5 IU
calories	70	66

COMPOSITION OF MILK (per 100 g)

dark field m. A microscope that uses a method of illumination by means of which the object structure is made to appear luminous against a dark field.

electron m. (EM) A microscope that uses electrons rather than visible light to irradiate clear, magnified images; capable of magnifying objects having dimensions smaller than the wavelengths of visible light.

interference m. A microscope in which the emerging light is split into two beams which pass through the object and are recombined in the image plane, where transparent and refractile specimen details become visible as intensity differences; useful in the examination of living or unstained cells.

laser m. A microscope in which a laser beam is focused on a microscopic field, causing it to vaporize; the emitted radiation is analyzed by means of a microspectrophotometer.

operating m., surgical m. A microscope used in the operating room for magnifying the surgical field.

phase m., phase contrast m. A microscope that makes use of the relationship between two paths of light: (a) light that enters the microscope objective directly through the specimen and (b) light that enters the objective after being diffracted by the specimens; all points of divergence between these two paths of light reveal a specimen or object whose lack of contrast would make it invisible under other types of illumination.

polarizing m. A microscope especially equipped to polarize light and to examine the alterations of the polarized light by the specimen; useful in the identification of crystals.

scanning electron m. (SEM) A microscope in which the specimen is examined point by point by an electron beam and an image may be viewed on a television screen or photographed.

stereoscopic wide field m. A binocular form of microscope with double objectives, designed to give a three-dimensional view of the specimen; magnifying power is usually limited to about 150 diameters.

x-ray m. A microscope that produces magnified images by recording the differences in the structure's absorption or emission of x-rays.

microscopic 1. Visible only with the aid of a microscope. 2. Relating to the microscope.

microscopy The study of minute objects or organisms by means of a microscope.

microsecond One-millionth of a second; 10^{-6} second.

microsome See ribosome.

microspherocyte A smaller than normal red blood cell having a spherical shape; present in hemolytic diseases.

microspherocytosis Presence in the blood of a large number of small spherical red blood cells (spherocytes); associated with hemolysis.

Microsporum A genus of fungi causing skin infections.

M. audouini Fungus causing ringworm in humans, especially ringworm of the scalp.

microsurgery Surgery aided by stereoscopic magnification that permits precise observation, differentiation, and delicate manipulation of tissues.

microsuture Suture material 40 μm or less in diameter; used in microsurgery.

microsyringe Syringe designed to measure accurately minute amounts of fluid for injection.

microtome An instrument for slicing thin sections of tissue for microscopic examination.

microtomy The slicing of tissue into thin sections with a microtome.

microtonometer Instrument designed to determine the tensions of oxygen and carbon dioxide in arterial blood.

microtubules Long, slender, delicate cylindrical organelles, about 250 Å in diameter, made up of a protein, the amino acid of which resembles the muscle protein actin; they are scattered throughout the cytoplasm of almost every cell type; during cell division they increase greatly in number to form the mitotic spindle; they also form the framework of the basal body and the centriole, and the cores of cilia, flagella, and sperm tails; they play an important role in intracellular movements and in maintaining cell shape.

microvilli Submicroscopic finger-like projections on the surface of the cell membrane which greatly increase the surface area.

microvolt One-millionth of a volt; 10^{-6} volt.

microwave Any electromagnetic radiation having a very short wavelength between 1 mm and 30 cm; wavelengths shorter than 1 mm are in the infrared region, while those above 30 cm are radiowaves. Also called microelectric wave.

micrurgy Manipulative procedures performed on microscopic specimens with the aid of a microscope and often a micromanipulator.

micturate To urinate.

micturition The act of urinating. Also called urination.

midbrain The part of the brain that develops from the embryonic mesencephalon, divided into three parts: the tectum (quadrigeminal plate), the tegmentum (cephalic continuation of the pontine tegmentum), and the crus cerebri (containing massive bundles of cortifugal fibers passing through to the lower brain stem and spinal cord).

middle lobe syndrome A form of chronic ate-

lectasis marked by collapse of the middle lobe of the lung resulting from compression of the bronchus by surrounding lymph nodes, often due to tumor involvement; symptoms include chronic cough, wheezing, recurrent respiratory infections, and chest pains. Also called Brock's syndrome.

midfoot The middle portion of the foot consisting of the navicular, cuboid, and cuneiform bones.

midgut 1. The middle portion of the embryonic digestive tract between the foregut and the hindgut from which the ileum and the jejunum develop. 2. The small intestine.

midmenstrual Occurring midway between two menstrual periods.

midpelvis The area of the pelvis extending from the posterior inferior aspects of the symphysis in a line through the ischial spines to the sacrum, intersecting it at about the second and third vertebrae.

midsection A section or division through the center of an organ or a part.

midwife A woman who attends women at delivery.

midwifery Practical obstetrics.

migraine A recurrent, intense headache, usually confined to one side of the head and associated with nausea, vomiting, and visual disturbances.

migraine equivalent Symptoms produced by a migraine-like mechanism, e.g., transient partial loss of vision, without an associated headache.

migration Passing from one part of the body to another.

Mikulicz's disease Benign bilateral swelling of the lacrimal and salivary glands associated with dryness of the mouth and reduced or absent lacrimation; believed by some clinical investigators to be identical to Sjögren's syndrome.

Mikulicz's syndrome Painless enlargement of the salivary and lacrimal glands, usually bilateral, accompanied by dryness of mouth and decreased lacrimation; thought to be a complication of tuberculosis, leukemia, lymphoma, or sarcoidosis.

miliaria A skin eruption due to retention of sweat in the sweat follicles.

m. rubra Prickly heat; see under heat.

miliary Having nodules of millet seed size (about 2 mm).

miliary tuberculosis See tuberculosis, acute miliary.

milieu French for environment or surroundings.

m. intérieur The internal environment; the fluids bathing the tissue cells of multicellular animals.

milium A minute whitish or yellowish papule on the skin caused by the retention of fatty material (sebum).

milk 1. A white or yellowish liquid secreted by the mammary glands of female mammals for the nour-

275

microscope | **milk**

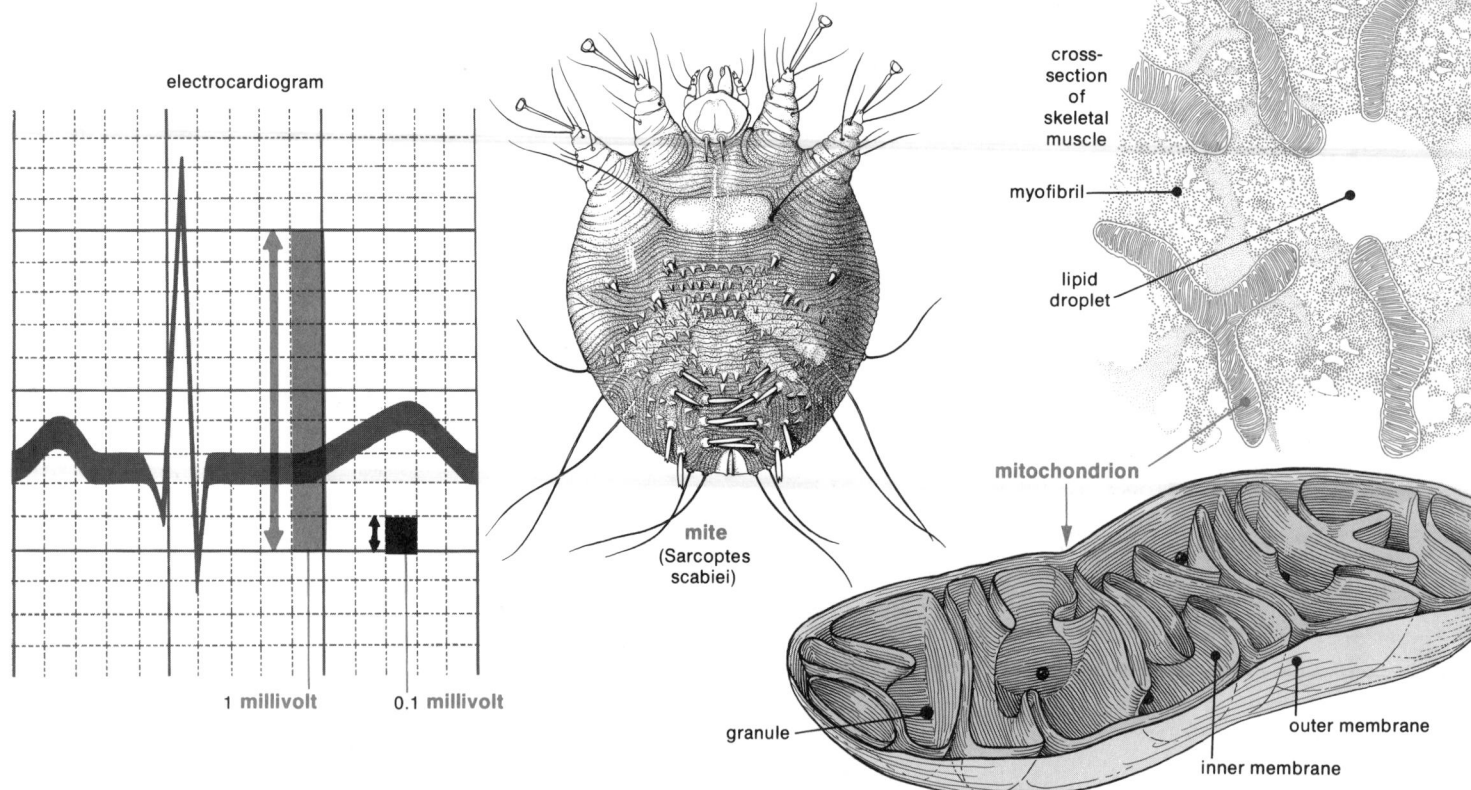

electrocardiogram

1 millivolt   0.1 millivolt

mite
(Sarcoptes
scabiei)

cross-
section
of
skeletal
muscle

myofibril

lipid
droplet

mitochondrion

granule

inner membrane

outer membrane

ishment of the young, containing proteins, sugar, and lipids. **2.** An emulsion or suspension. Formerly called magma. **3.** A milklike liquid.

m. of magnesia See under magnesia.

uterine m. Secretion produced by uterine glands.

witch's m. The milklike fluid sometimes secreted by the breasts of newborn babies of either sex.

milk-alkali syndrome Hypercalcemia without hypercalcuria or hypophosphaturia, induced by the prolonged ingestion of large amounts of milk and soluble alkali, usually as therapy for peptic ulcer; it is reversible in its early stages, but if undetected leads to renal failure. Also called Burnett's syndrome.

milking The removal of the contents of a tubular structure by gently running a finger along its length.

milk leg Colloquial term for a painful swelling of the leg resulting from clotting and inflammation of the great saphenous or femoral veins; occurring sometimes in women after childbirth.

Milkman's syndrome Osteoporosis causing multiple fractures; seen most frequently in postmenopausal women.

milk teeth Deciduous teeth; see under tooth.

Millard-Gubler syndrome Paralysis of facial muscles on one side and of the extremities on the opposite side, produced by a unilateral lesion of the brain stem.

milliampere (ma) One-thousandth of an ampere.

millicurie (mCi) A measure of radioactivity, one-thousandth of a curie.

milliequivalent (mEq) An expression of concentration of substance per liter of solution, calculated by dividing the concentration in milligrams per 100 milliliters by the molecular weight.

milligram (mg) One-thousandth of a gram.

milliliter (ml) One-thousandth of a liter; one cubic centimeter.

millimeter (mm) One-thousandth of a meter.

millimicrogram One-billionth of a gram; preferred term is nanogram (ng).

millimicron (mμ) One-thousandth of a micron; preferred term is nanometer (nm).

millimole (mM) One-thousandth of a mole (gram-molecule).

milling-in The placing of abrasives between the occlusal surfaces of dentures while rubbing them together in the mouth or on the articulator; used to perfect the occlusion.

milliosmole (mOsm) One-thousandth of an osmole; the osmotic pressure exerted by the concentration of a substance in solution; expressed as milligrams per kilogram divided by atomic weight for an ionized substance, or divided by molecular weight for nonionized solutes; normal plasma osmolality is 280 to 300 mOsm/kg.

millirad (mrad) One-thousandth of a rad.

millirem (mrem) One-thousandth of a rem.

milliroentgen (mr) One-thousandth of a roentgen.

millisecond (msec) One-thousandth of a second.

millivolt (mv) One-thousandth of a volt.

Milroy's disease Familial and congenital swelling of subcutaneous tissues (usually confined to the extremities) with large accumulation of lymph.

mimesis State in which one disease presents the symptoms of another. Also called imitation.

mind The totality of conscious and unconscious processes serving to adjust the individual to the demands of the environment. Also called the psyche.

mineral Any naturally occurring homogeneous inorganic substance, having a characteristic crystalline structure and chemical composition.

mineralocorticoid One of the steroids in the adrenal cortex that controls salt metabolism.

minim A unit of fluid measure; in the United States, 1/60 of a fluid dram; about a drop.

minimal brain dysfunction syndrome. A complex of symptoms that involves impairment of some or all of the following functions: learning, language, perception, memory, concentration, and motor; neurologic examination usually yields minor abnormalities if any; diagnosis rests on psychological assessment of cognitive function. See also disability, learning.

minimal change disease A form of nephrotic syndrome in which minimal or no glomerular abnormalities are noted by light microscopy and the major abnormality on electron microscopy is fusion of epithelial foot processes. Also called lipoid nephrosis; idiopathic nephrotic syndrome.

miosis **1.** Reduction in size of the pupil of the eye. **2.** Phase of a disease in which the severity of the symptoms begins to diminish.

miotic Denoting any agent that causes contraction of the pupil.

miracidium, *pl.* **miracidia** A free-swimming ciliated larva of a trematode that penetrates a small intermediate host where it develops into a sporocyst.

mire One of the luminous objects in the ophthalmometer (used to measure the anterior curvature of the cornea).

mirror A polished surface that forms optical images by reflection.

head m. A circular concave mirror attached to a headband; used to illuminate a bodily cavity.

misanthropy Aversion to people.

miscarriage Spontaneous abortion.

miscarry To give birth to a nonviable fetus.

misce (M) Latin for mix; used in prescription writing.

misce et signa Latin for mix and label; used in prescription writing.

miscible Capable of being mixed.

misdiagnosis A wrong diagnosis.

misogyny Hatred of women.

misophobia An abnormal fear of contamination.

mite Any of various minute arachnids that are often parasitic on man and animals; they may infest food and carry disease.

harvest m. See chigger.

hay itch m. See *Pyemotes ventricosus.*

itch m. See *Sarcoptes scabiei.*

northern fowl m. *Ornithonyssus sylviarum.*

mithridatism Immunity to a poison achieved by taking gradually increased doses of it.

miticide An agent that kills mites.

mitochondria, *sing.* **mitochondrion** Compartmentalized, double membrane, self-reproducing organelles present in the cytoplasm of almost all living cells, responsible for generating usable energy by the formation of ATP (adenosine triphosphate); in the average cell there are several hundred mitochondria, each about 15,000 Å in length.

mitogen A substance that stimulates cell mitosis and lymphocyte transformation.

mitogenesis The induction of mitosis in a cell.

mitogenic Causing or inducing cell mitosis.

mitosis Multiplication or division of a cell that results in the formation of two daughter cells normally receiving the same chromosome and deoxyribonucleic acid (DNA) content as that of the original cell. Also called karyokinesis.

mitotic Relating to mitosis or cell division.

mitral Relating to the left atrioventricular valve of the heart.

mitralization In roentgenography, straightening of the left border of the heart shadow with protrusion of the atrial appendage and/or the pulmonary salient.

mittelschmerz Intermenstrual pain, specifically at the time of ovulation.

mixture **1.** An aggregation of two or more substances that are not chemically combined. **2.** A pharmaceutical preparation consisting of an insoluble substance suspended in a liquid by a viscid material such as sugar, glycerol, etc.

binary m. One containing two substances.

Brompton m. A pain relieving mixture of cocaine hydrochloride and morphine hydrochloride given orally to patients who are dying of cancer. Commonly called Brompton cocktail.

explosive m. One capable of instantaneous combustion.

M-mode A diagnostic ultrasound presentation of echo changes in which a B-mode tracing is moved

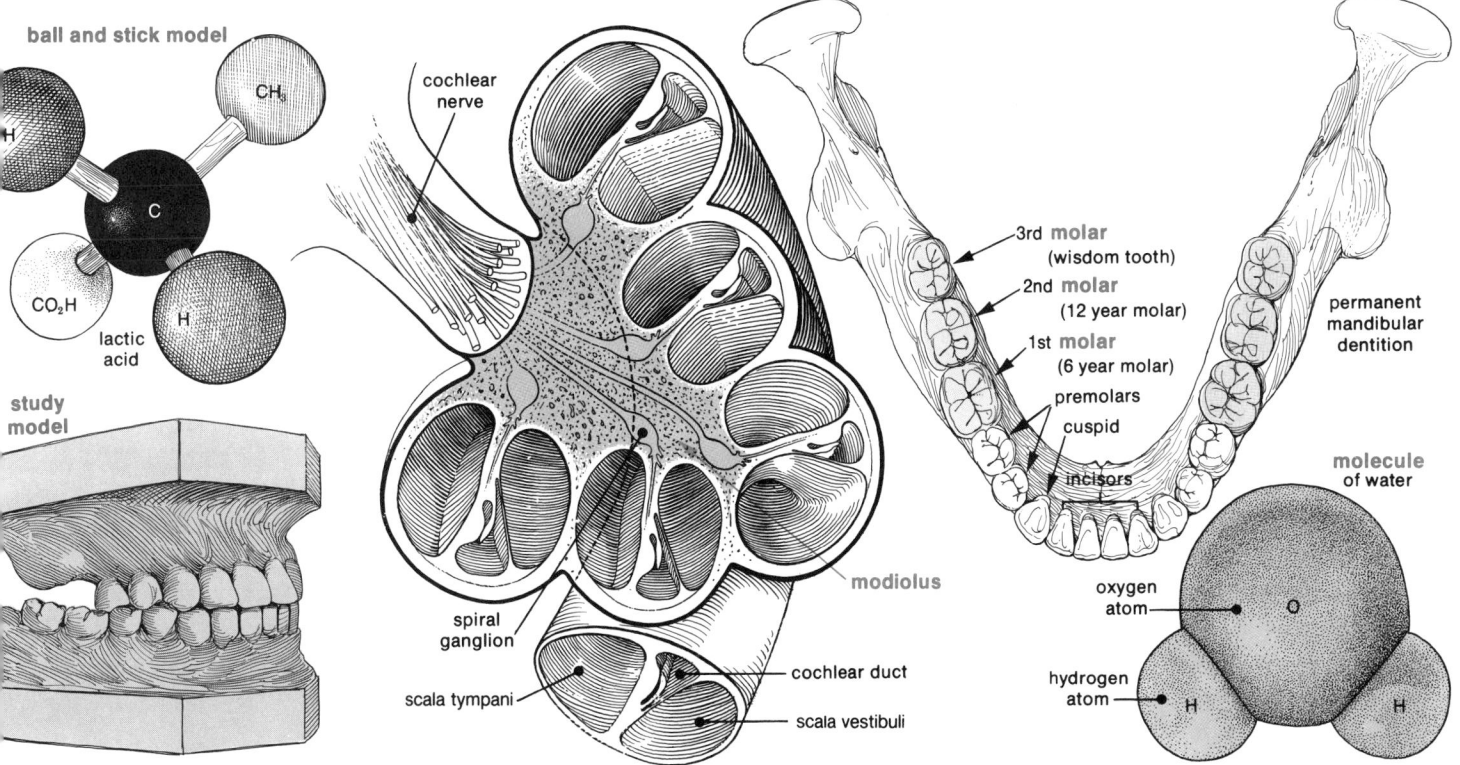

ball and stick model

CH₃

H

C

CO₂H

H

lactic acid

study model

cochlear nerve

modiolus

spiral ganglion

scala tympani

cochlear duct

scala vestibuli

3rd **molar** (wisdom tooth)

2nd **molar** (12 year molar)

1st **molar** (6 year molar)

premolars

cuspid

incisors

permanent mandibular dentition

molecule of water

oxygen atom

hydrogen atom

O

H

H

to indicate the pattern of echo motion (M) as a function of time (T). Also called TM-mode.

mnemonic Relating to or assisting the memory.

mnemonics A system for improving the memory.

MNSs blood group A system of erythrocyte antigens determined by the allelic genes M, N, and S,s; first demonstrated by injecting human blood into rabbits, which developed antibodies against it; originally defined to include antigens to antibodies anti-M and anti-N and later extended to include those reacting to antibodies anti-S and anti-s; the group is primarily used to solve identification problems such as disputed paternity and for genetic linkage population studies.

mobilization 1. Making a part movable. 2. Starting a sequence of physiologic activity.

stapes m. Surgical procedure through which the footplate of the stapes is liberated from adhesions or overlapping bony tissue caused by otosclerosis or middle ear infection.

mobilize To cause stored substances in the body to participate in physiologic activity; to liberate material from storage sites.

Möbius' sign Convergence weakness of the eyes occurring in exophthalmic goiter.

Möbius' syndrome A congenital disorder characterized by bilateral paralysis of both external rectus muscles and face muscles and sometimes associated with other musculoskeletal anomalies or neurologic disorders. Also called congenital facial diplegia; congenital oculofacial paralysis.

modality 1. Any of several forms of therapy; e.g., diathermy. 2. An apparatus used to apply such therapy. 3. Any of the main forms of sensation; e.g., hearing.

mode In statistics, the value occurring most often.

model 1. A three-dimensional shape representing a likeness of some existing structure. Also called replica. 2. In dentistry, positive reproduction of the dentition and adjoining structures. Also called cast.

ball and stick m. A three-dimensional schematic representation of a molecular structure.

disease m. The artificial creation of an abnormality in an experimental animal in order to allow further study of the entity.

study m. A replica of the teeth and adjoining oral structures used as a diagnostic aid. Also called diagnostic cast.

modifier Agent that alters form or character without transforming; e.g., in genetics, a gene which alters the phenotypic effect of another gene.

modiolus The central pillar or column of bone around which the spiral canals of the cochlea turn.

modulation The changes that take place in re-

sponse to changes in the environment, such as the temporary change of osteoblasts into osteocytes and back to osteoblasts in response to altered conditions in the environment.

mogigraphia Writer's cramp; see under cramp.

moiety 1. One of two more or less equal parts. 2. A part or portion of indefinite size.

mol See gram-molecule.

molal Containing one mole of solute per 1,000 grams of solvent. Cf. molar (2).

molality The concentration of a solution expressed as the number of moles of solute per 1,000 kilograms of solvent.

molar (M) 1. A posterior tooth for grinding and pulverizing food. 2. Containing 1 gram-molecular weight (1 mole) of solute per 1,000 milliliters of solution. Cf. molal. 3. Relating to a body of matter; not molecular.

deciduous m. One of 8 posterior teeth in the deciduous (primary) dentition.

first permanent m. Largest permanent tooth in the mouth; first permanent tooth to erupt, usually at the age of 6 years. Also called six-year molar.

impacted m. A molar unable to erupt properly.

permanent m. One of 12 posterior teeth in the permanent (secondary) dentition.

second permanent m. A permanent molar immediately distal to the first molar which usually erupts at the age of 12 years. Also called twelve-year molar.

third permanent m. Last permanent posterior tooth in the mouth which erupts usually between the ages of 17 and 21 years. Also called wisdom tooth.

molarity The concentration of a solution expressed as the number of moles of solute per liter of solution.

mold 1. Any of a group of fungi usually growing on decaying organic matter. 2. A receptacle for shaping any cast material (wax, plastic, etc.). 3. To shape.

mold guide A guide for specifying the shape of artificial teeth.

molding 1. The process of shaping. 2. The change in shape of the fetal head as it passes through the birth canal. Also called configuration.

mole 1. Intrauterine mass. 2. Pigmented cellular nevus; a circumscribed pigmented growth on the skin. 3. Gram-molecule.

hydatid m. See hydatidiform mole.

hydatidiform m. A developmental anomaly of the placenta consisting of a nonmalignant mass of clear vesicles (which resembles a bunch of grapes), formed from cystic swelling of the chorionic villi; the mole may grow to fill the uterus and cause it to

enlarge to the size of a six-month pregnancy; usually there is no embryo present. Also called hydatid mole; hydatid degeneration.

molecular Relating to, or consisting of, molecules.

molecular weight (mol. wt., MW) The sum of the atomic weights of all the atoms making up a molecule; e.g., hydrogen (H) has an atomic weight of one and chlorine (Cl) has an atomic weight of 35.5; thus, a molecule of hydrochloric acid (HCl) has a molecular weight of 36.5.

molecule The smallest unit of a substance (composed of two or more atoms) which can exist in a free state and still retain the chemical properties of the substance.

cyclic m. A molecule that appears in organic compounds, and whose atoms are arranged in a ring or polygon.

molimen, pl. molimina The effort required by a normal physiologic function, especially the menstrual flow.

molluscum A skin disease marked by the presence of soft rounded tumors.

m. contagiosum An infectious disease of the skin, marked by small wartlike lesions containing a substance resembling curds; caused by a virus.

molt To cast off.

molybdate A salt of molybdic acid.

molybdenum Metallic element; symbol Mo, atomic number 42, atomic weight 95.95; it has several isotopes.

molybdic Denoting a salt of trivalent or hexavalent molybdenum.

molybdic acid Any of two acids, H_2MoO_4 (colorless needles), or $H_2MoO_4 \cdot 4H_2O$, a yellow crystalline substance, soluble in ammonia and used as a reagent.

momism The state of being excessively dependent on or subordinate to one's mother or her substitute.

monad 1. A univalent element, radical, or atom. 2. A unicellular organism. 3. The single chromosome formed after the second division in meiosis.

monarthritis Arthritis of one joint.

monarticular Denoting a single joint.

monaural Relating to one ear.

Monday disease The return of symptoms after a weekend away from work, as in the case of an allergic reaction to a substance encountered while at work.

Mondor's disease Inflammation of the subcutaneous veins of the chest and breast, usually extending from the epigastric region to the axilla and occurring in both males and females.

mongolism Down syndrome; congenital defect caused by an abnormal chromosome 21.

SOME DIFFERENTIAL FEATURES OF INFECTIOUS MONONUCLEOSIS

	infectious mononucleosis	infectious hepatitis (hepatitis A)	tonsillitis
usual age	15 to 25 years	15 to 25 years	5 to 20 years
incubation period	30 to 50 days	15 to 45 days	usually 3 to 5 days
fever	irregular; usually about 2 weeks	moderate; disappears when jaundice develops	moderate to high; usually under 5 days
sore throat	marked; whitish-gray exudate	none	constant; yellow or white exudate
adenopathy (enlargement of lymph nodes)	most commonly: anterior and posterior cervical chains; often generalized	minimal; usually cervical	submandibular; anterior cervical
splenomegaly (enlargement of spleen)	approximately 50%	less than 10%	none
hepatomegaly (enlargement of liver)	approximately 10%	over 80%	none

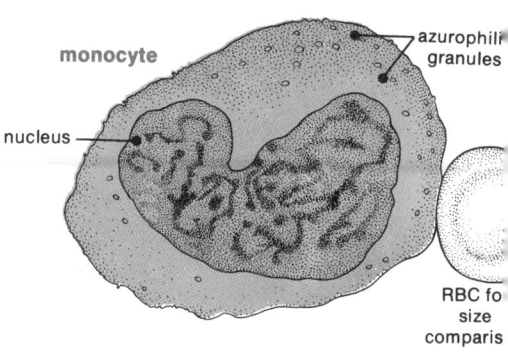

monocyte
azurophilic granules
nucleus
RBC for size comparison

monosaccharide (glyceraldehyde)

morphine

mongoloid, mongolian Having characteristics resembling mongolism (Down syndrome).

monilethrix Beaded hair, an anomalous condition in which the hair shafts exhibit nodosities or points of thickening alternating with normal or constricted girth, giving the appearance of a string of fusiform beads.

Monilia A genus of molds or fungi, commonly known as "fruit molds;" formerly included in this genus was a similar group of organisms now called *Candida*.

moniliasis Infection with any fungi of the genus *Monilia*.

moniliform Shaped like a string of pearls.

monitor, cardiac An electronic device used for observation of each heartbeat of a person.

monitoring Constant observation.
  constant cardiac m. Prolonged observation of the electrocardiogram with the aid of an oscilloscope to detect irregularities in the heart rhythm.

mono Colloquialism for mononucleosis.

monoamine Compound containing only one amine group.
  m. oxidase (MAO) An enzyme that catalyzes the oxidation of a wide variety of physiologic amines to the corresponding aldehydes and NH_3.
  m. oxidase inhibitors (MAOI) Derivatives of hydrazine and hydrazide that inhibit the action of certain enzymes.

monoblast An immature cell of the monocytic series, from 18 to 22 μm in diameter, which has several nucleoli; formed primarily in the spleen and lymphoid tissues.

monochromatic 1. Having one color. **2.** Indicating a spectral color of a single wavelength.

monoclonal Derived from a single clone of cells.

monocrotic Forming a smooth single crest on the downward line of a curve; said of a pulse.

monocular Relating to, having, or used by one eye.

monocyte A large mononuclear white blood cell, generally 15 to 25 μm in diameter, with a round, kidney-shaped, or lobulated nucleus and a cytoplasm that stains a gray-blue color with Wright's stain; it is the largest cell found in normal blood; when it leaves the blood stream, it becomes a macrophage (phagocyte).

monocytopenia Reduction of monocytes in the blood. Also called monocytic leukopenia; monopenia.

monocytosis Abnormal increase in the number of monocytes in the blood; at least 15 or more monocytes per 100 white blood cells.

monodactylism The presence of only one finger on the hand or one toe on the foot.

monogametic See homogametic.

monogenous Produced asexually.

monograph A detailed written account of one particular subject, one class of subjects, or a small area of a special field of learning.

monohybrid A cross between parents that differ in one character.

monoiodotyrosine (MIT) An amino acid formed by the iodination of tyrosine; an initial step in the formation of thyronine.

monokine A hormone-like factor produced by activation of monocytes; acts as an intercellular messenger to regulate immunologic and inflammatory responses.

monolayer A film that consists of a single layer of molecules, formed on a water surface by certain substances, as proteins and fatty acids, in which some atoms are soluble in water while others are insoluble in water.

monomania Pathologic preoccupation with one idea.

monomer A simple molecule of low molecular weight which when repeated in a chain forms a polymer; e.g., ethylene is the monomer of polyethylene.

monomorphic Having but one shape; unchangeable in size and form.

mononeuritis Inflammation or degeneration of a single nerve trunk or some of its branches.
  m. multiplex Neuritis involving single nerves at several distant sites.

mononuclear Uninuclear.

mononucleosis Abnormal increase of mononuclear white blood cells (monocytes) in the blood.
  infectious m. An infectious febrile disease caused by the EB virus (Epstein-Barr virus); marked by fever, sore throat, enlargement of the spleen and lymph nodes, and the presence in the blood of an abnormally large number of atypical lymphocytes that resemble monocytes; the virus can be carried in the mouth and throat of afflicted individuals for several months after the disappearance of clinical illness. Sometimes called glandular fever. Popularly known as mono; kissing disease.

monophasia Disorder in which the individual's vocabulary is limited to a single word or sentence.

monoplegia Paralysis of only one limb or part.

monorchid An individual with only one visible testicle.

monorchism, monorchidism The condition of having or appearing to have only one testicle, the other being absent or undescended.

monosaccharide A carbohydrate which is not further broken down by hydrolysis; a simple sugar.

monosodium glutamate (MSG) See sodium glutamate.

monosome A chromosome without its homologous chromosome.

monosomy Condition in which one chromosome of a pair of homologous chromosomes is missing.

monosubstituted Having only one atom in each molecule replaced.

monotrichous Denoting a unicellular organism having a single flagellum.

monovalent See univalent.

monoxide An oxide containing only one oxygen atom.

monozygotic Denoting identical twins, or twins formed by the division into two of the embryo derived from a single fertilized egg.

mons, *pl.* **montes** In anatomy, a slight prominence or elevation.
  m. pubis The fleshy prominence formed by a pad of fatty tissue over the pubic symphysis in the female.
  m. ureteris A slight prominence on the wall of the bladder at the entrance of the ureter.

mood A prevailing emotional state of mind.

Moraxella A genus of bacteria containing gram-negative, short, rod-shaped cells; aerobic and parasitic; sometimes found on the mucous membranes of man.

morbid Of, pertaining to, or affected by disease; diseased; pathologic.

morbidity 1. The condition of being diseased. **2.** The ratio of disease to the population of a given area.

morbilli Measles.

morbilliform Resembling measles.

Morbillivirus Genus of the family Paramyxoviridae which includes the measles, bovine rinderpest, and canine distemper viruses; all members produce both intranuclear and cytoplasmic inclusion bodies. Also called measles-rinderpest-distemper (MRD) group.

morbillous Relating to measles.

morbus Latin for disease.

mordant A substance used in bacteriology to fix a dye or stain.

morgan (M) The unit of map distance on a chromosome.

morgue A place where the dead are kept pending autopsy and burial.

moribund Dying.

morioplasty Surgical restoration of parts lost through injury or disease.

morphea A skin disease marked by indurated white or yellow lesions surrounded by a violet ring; occurring chiefly on the chest, face, or neck.

morphine An alkaloid compound extracted from

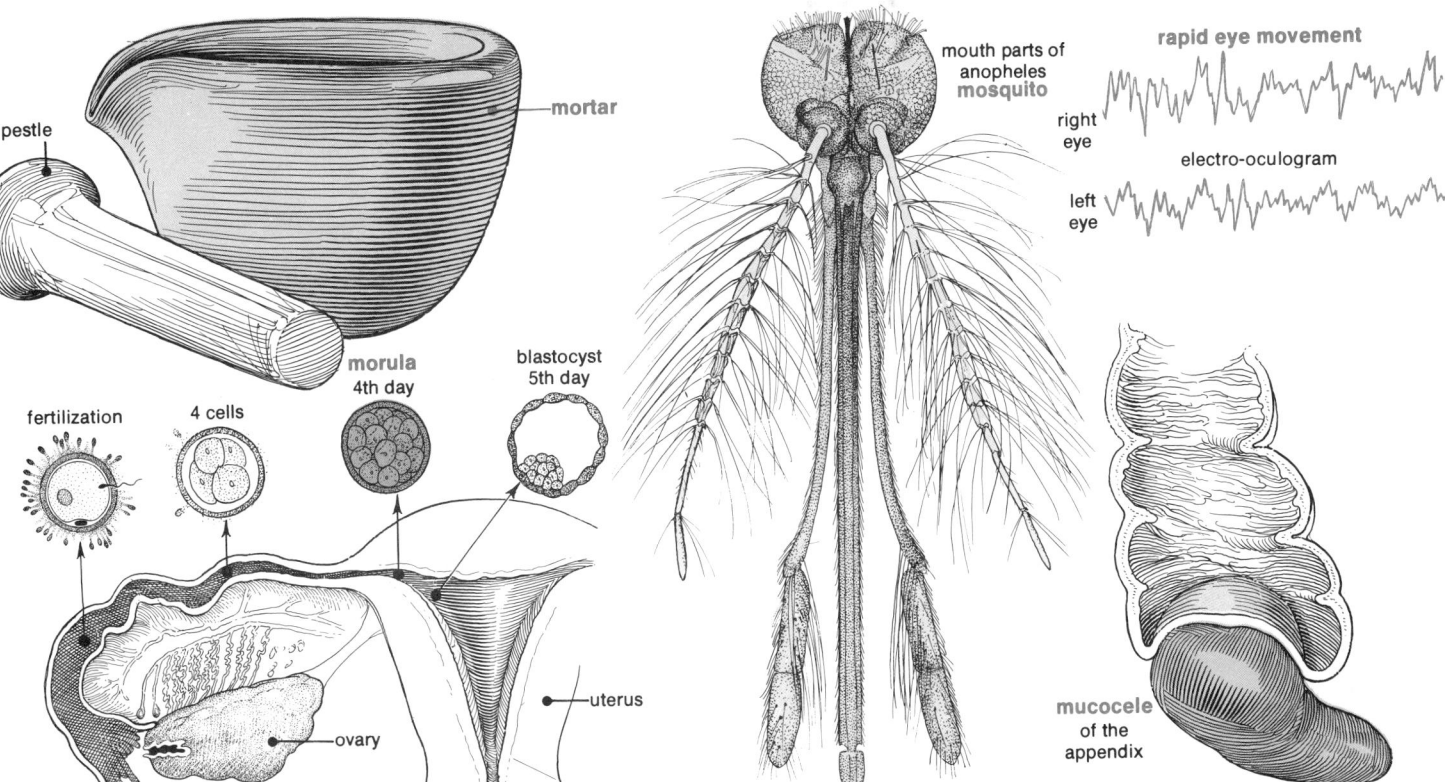

pestle

mortar

morula
4th day

blastocyst
5th day

fertilization

4 cells

ovary

uterus

mouth parts of
anopheles
mosquito

right
eye

rapid eye movement

electro-oculogram

left
eye

mucocele
of the
appendix

opium, used in medicine as an analgesic; prolonged use causes addiction.

morphogenesis The embryonic differentiation of cells leading to the establishment of the characteristic structure and form of the organism or its parts.

morphologic Relating to the structure or form of organisms.

morphology 1. The study of the configuration or structure of living organisms. 2. The form or structure of an organism, exclusively.

Morquio's syndrome A form of mucopolysaccharidosis characterized chiefly by dwarfism, deformed wrist and hands, knock knees, pectus carinatum, osteoporosis, flat vertebrae, and corneal clouding; keratosulfate is excreted in the urine; transmitted as an autosomal recessive trait. Also called mucopolysaccharidosis IV.

mors Latin for death.

mortal 1. Subject to death. 2. Deadly.

mortality 1. The quality of being mortal. 2. The death rate; the whole sum of deaths in a given population or a given time.

mortar A small receptacle in which substances are crushed or pulverized with a pestle.

mortification Gangrene.

mortinatality Natimortality.

mortuary A funeral home where bodies of the deceased are prepared for burial.

morula A cluster of cleaving blastomeres resulting from the early division of the zygote; a stage in the development of the embryo prior to the blastula.

morulation The formation of a morula.

mosaic 1. Resembling inlaid work or a pattern consisting of numerous small pieces. 2. An individual or tissue affected with mosaicism.

mosaicism Genetic condition in which an individual has two or more cell populations differing in genetic composition; the differing cells originate from a single cell type through an error (either genetic mutation or chromosomal aberration) occurring during early cell division of the fertilized egg.

Moschowitz's disease Thrombotic thrombocytopenic purpura; see under purpura.

mosquito Any of various blood-sucking, winged insects (family Culicidae), some species of which are responsible for the transmission of various diseases such as malaria and yellow fever.

mother-surrogate One who replaces an individual's mother in his emotional feelings.

motile Having the capacity to move spontaneously.

motilin A polypeptide hormone of 22 amino acids produced in the mucosa of the lower stomach, duodenum, and upper jejunum; it stimulates motility of the stomach and intestines.

motion 1. Movement. 2. A bowel movement.

motivation An incentive to act or the reason for an attitude.

motor Producing movement; denoting nerves that convey impulses from the nerve centers to the muscles.

m. oculi The oculomotor nerve; the third cranial nerve. See table of nerves.

plastic m. An artificial point of attachment on an amputation stump through which motion is provided to an artificial limb.

mottling 1. A condition marked by spotty coloration. 2. Macular lesions of varying shades or hues.

moulage The making of a mold of a bodily structure, especially for identification, prosthetics, and teaching models.

mount To prepare slides of tissues for microscopic examination.

mounting Dental laboratory procedure in which a maxillary and/or mandibular cast is attached to an articulator.

mouse, *pl.* **mice** Any of numerous small rodents of the genus *Mus*.

cancer-free white m. (CFW) A mouse used in cancer research.

New Zealand black m. (NZB) An inbred strain exhibiting (in the adult form) immune hemolytic anemia and renal disease.

mousepox A viral disease of mice. Also called ectromelia.

mouth The body opening through which an individual takes in food; the upper portion of the digestive tract, including the lips, tongue, teeth, and related parts; the oral cavity.

trench m. Necrotizing ulcerative gingivitis; see under gingivitis.

mouthwash A somewhat antiseptic solution for rinsing the mouth and teeth; it generally contains sodium borate, thymol, potassium bicarbonate, eucalyptol, methyl salicylate, alcohol, glycerin, and water. Also called collutorium.

movement 1. Change of place or position. 2. The act of defecation.

Brownian m. Erratic motion of microscopic particles suspended in a liquid or gas, resulting from collision with molecules in the suspending medium.

ciliary m. Rhythmic motion of the cilia of epithelial cells or protozoa.

circus m. The movement of an excitation wave continuing uninterrupted around a ring of muscle or through the wall of the heart. Also called circus rhythm.

conjugate m. of the eyes Movement of the two eyes in one direction.

passive m. Movement of the body or any of its parts effected by an external force.

rapid eye m.'s (REM) The short, quick movements of the eyes during sleep which last from five to 60 minutes and are associated with dreaming. See under sleep.

saccadic m. A rapid, abrupt movement of the eyes, as occurs in changing fixation from one point to another.

streaming m. The characteristic movement of the protoplasm of certain white cells or unicellular organisms.

moxa 1. A small mass of combustible material placed near the skin or on an acupuncture needle and ignited to produce a counterirritation; used in oriental traditional medicine. 2. A heated button-shaped metal device applied as a cautery.

moxibustion Counterirritation by means of a moxa.

mu 1. The twelfth letter of the Greek alphabet, μ. 2. A micron.

mucid Slimy.

muciferous Secreting or producing mucus.

muciform Resembling mucus.

mucilage In pharmacology, a thick viscous liquid; a water solution of the mucilaginous principles of certain vegetable substances.

mucin A substance secreted by mucous membranes, containing an organic compound (mucopolysaccharide); the main constituent of mucus.

mucinase Any enzyme, such as lysozyme, that acts on mucin.

mucinoid Resembling mucin.

mucinosis A condition in which mucin is present in abnormal amounts.

mucinous Relating to or containing mucin.

mucocele 1. An intrasinus cyst which arises from the mucosal lining. 2. An enlarged cavity that contains mucus. 3. Mucous polyp.

mucocutaneous Relating to both mucous membrane and skin, especially the line of meeting of those tissues as in the nasal, oral, vaginal, and anal orifices.

mucocutaneous lymph node syndrome Condition affecting mainly infants and young children; marked by fever, conjunctivitis, reddening of oral cavity and lips, pharyngitis, and enlargement of lymph nodes of the neck; accompanied by reddening and peeling of the hands and feet; cause is unknown. Also called Kawasaki disease.

mucoenteritis Inflammation of the intestinal mucous membrane. Also called acute catarrhal enteritis.

mucoid 1. Resembling mucus. 2. A mucus-like conjugated protein or polysaccharide of animal origin.

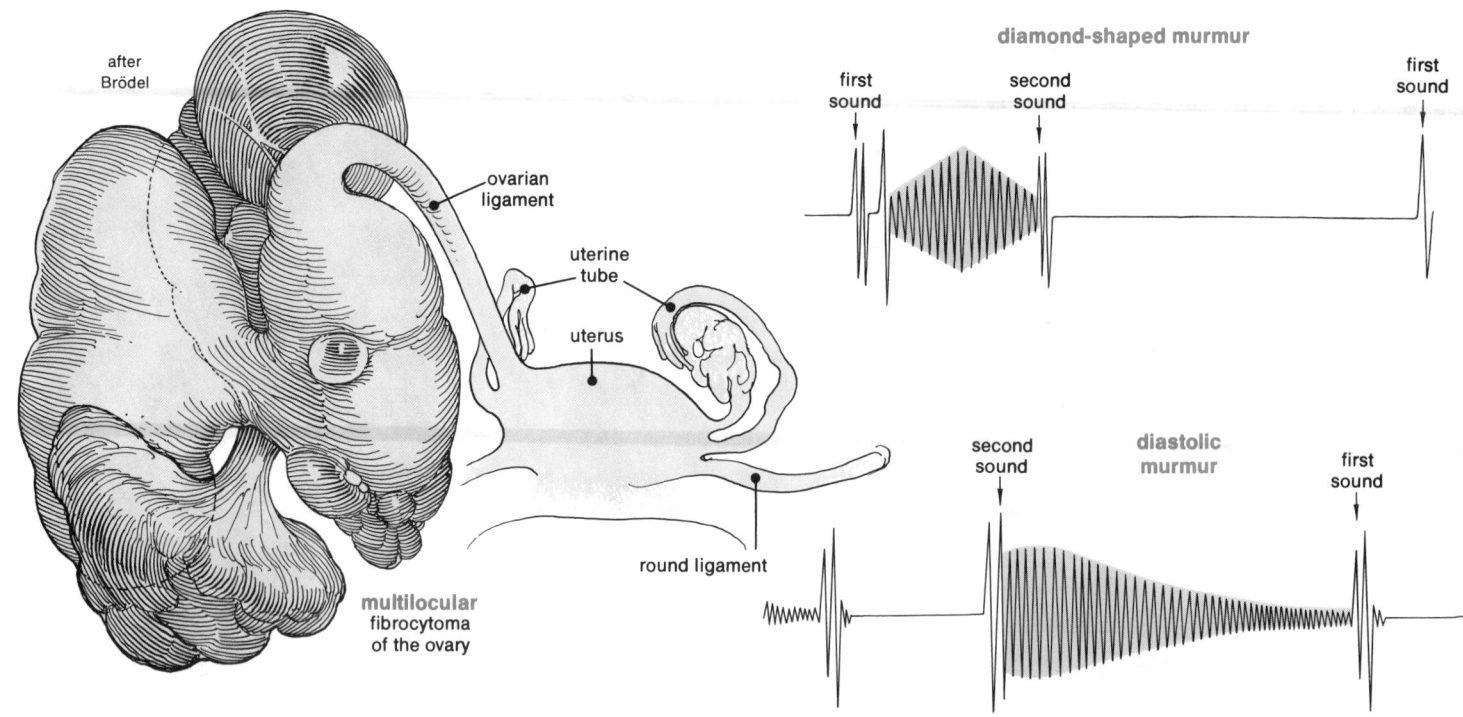

after Brödel

ovarian ligament

uterine tube

uterus

round ligament

multilocular
fibrocytoma
of the ovary

diamond-shaped murmur

first sound

second sound

first sound

second sound

diastolic murmur

first sound

mucolipidosis Any of a group of hereditary disorders transmitted as an autosomal recessive trait; mucopolysaccharides and lipids accumulate in the tissues, but urinary patterns of these substances are normal.

mucolytic Capable of dissolving mucus.

mucomembranous Relating to a mucous membrane.

mucoperiosteum Periosteum with a closely adhered mucous membrane.

mucopolysaccharide Polysaccharide components, such as hyaluronic acid and chondroitin sulfate, attached to a polypeptide component through weak chemical bonding; a ubiquitous macromolecular complex that forms the amorphous component of intercellular material in the body.

mucopolysaccharidosis A group of genetic diseases characterized by defective metabolism of mucopolysaccharides.

    m. I See Hurler's syndrome.

    m. II See Hunter's syndrome.

    m. III See Sanfilippo's syndrome.

    m. IV See Morquio's syndrome.

    m. V Former name for Scheie's syndrome.

    m. VI See Maroteaux-Lamy syndrome.

    m. VII A type caused by beta-glucuronidase deficiency; it resembles a mild form of Hurler's syndrome; transmitted as an autosomal recessive trait.

mucoprotein A group of organic compounds containing proteins and mucopolysaccharides.

mucopurulent Containing mucus and pus.

mucopus Discharge composed of mucus and pus.

Mucoraceae A family of molds (order Mucorales) having a branching, nonsegmented mycelium; some species destroy food products (bread, fruits, and vegetables).

mucormycosis An acute systemic disease characterized primarily by inflammation, necrosis, and suppuration, initially involving the paranasal sinuses, orbit, bronchi, or intestines and spreading to the brain, heart, kidney, or lungs; attributed to fungi of the order Mucorales.

mucosa The inner lining of a cavity, as the lining of the oral cavity.

mucosanguineous Containing mucus and blood; said of a discharge.

mucoserous Relating to or containing serum or plasma and mucus.

mucosin A mucin peculiar to the more tenacious, adhesive variety of mucus, as that of the nasal cavity.

mucous Relating to, resembling, consisting of, or producing mucus.

mucoviscidosis See cystic fibrosis of pancreas.

mucus The slippery, viscous suspension of mucin, desquamated cells, leukocytes, inorganic salt, and water secreted by glands in the mucous membranes; the secretion moistens and protects the membrane.

muliebrity The state of being a woman; any quality characteristic of women; the change of character in the female at puberty.

multangular Having many angles; said of certain bones.

multiarticular Relating to or affecting many joints.

multicellular Composed of numerous cells.

multifactorial Determined by several genetic and nongenetic factors. Cf. polygenic.

multifid Composed of many segments or lobes formed by several clefts.

multifocal Arising from several sites.

multiform Having many forms or shapes.

multigravida A woman who has been pregnant more than once.

multilobular Having many lobules.

multilocular Having several cells or compartments.

multimammae The presence of more than two breasts in the human. Also called polymastia.

multinuclear Having more than one nucleus. Also called polynuclear.

multipara A woman who has completed two or more pregnancies to the stage of viability, regardless of whether the fetuses were live or stillborn.

multiparity The condition of having had two or more children. Also called pluriparity.

multiparous 1. Having borne two or more offspring in separate pregnancies; relating to multipara. 2. Giving birth to two or more children at one birth.

multiple 1. Having more than one part or component. 2. Occurring in several sites at the same time.

multipolar Having more than two poles, as certain nerve cells.

multivalence The property of having the capacity to combine with two or more hydrogen atoms. Also called polyvalence.

multivalent Having the capacity to combine with more than one hydrogen atom, usually more than two. Also called polyvalent.

mummifaction 1. Dry gangrene; see under gangrene. 2. Drying and compression of a dead retained fetus, so that it resembles parchment.

mumps An acute contagious disease caused by an RNA myxovirus, affecting primarily the parotid glands and less often the sublingual and submaxillary glands; characterized by glandular swelling and fever; incubation period is about three weeks; may also involve the pancreas, testes, or central nervous system. Also called epidemic parotitis.

Münchausen's syndrome The fabrication by an itinerant malingerer of a clinically convincing simulation of disease; it may include self-induced fits, faints, anesthesias, hallucinations, or delusions; the individual's history usually shows a long record of hospitalization.

mural Relating to the wall of any cavity.

muramic acid A component of the murein molecule of bacterial cell walls.

muramidase Mucopeptide glucohydrolase, an enzyme that promotes the hydrolysis of muramic acid-containing mucopeptides in bacterial cell walls; e.g., lysozyme.

murein The bag-shaped macromolecule that encases a bacterial cell.

muriatic Hydrochloric.

muriatic acid Hydrochloric acid.

murine Relating to animals of the family Muridae, especially rats and mice.

murmur A relatively prolonged series of auditory vibrations resulting from turbulent blood flow.

    aortic m. Murmur occurring at the aortic orifice.

    Austin-Flint m. A mid-diastolic or presystolic rumble, similar to the murmur of mitral stenosis, which appears to originate at the anterior leaflet of the mitral valve when the normal and abnormal streams of blood enter the left ventricle in cases of aortic incompetence. Also called Flint's murmur.

    cardiac m. Murmur arising in the heart.

    continuous m. Murmur that begins in systole and continues without interruption into all or part of the diastole.

    crescendo m. Murmur that increases in intensity and stops suddenly; the opposite of a decrescendo murmur.

    crescendo-decrescendo m. Murmur that increases to a peak and then decreases. Also called diamond-shaped murmur.

    Cruveilhier-Baumgarten m. Murmur heard on the abdominal wall over collateral veins connecting portal and caval venous systems.

    decrescendo m. Murmur that progressively decreases in intensity; the opposite of a crescendo murmur.

    diamond-shaped m. Named after the shape of its frequency intensity curve. See crescendo-decrescendo murmur.

    diastolic m. Murmur beginning with or after the second heart sound and ending before the first heart sound, i.e., during diastole.

    Duroziez's m. A double murmur heard over the femoral artery in cases of aortic insufficiency.

    dynamic m. Murmur due to a condition other than diseased heart valves, e.g., a flow murmur.

    early diastolic m. Murmur beginning with the second heart sound (at the time of aortic valve

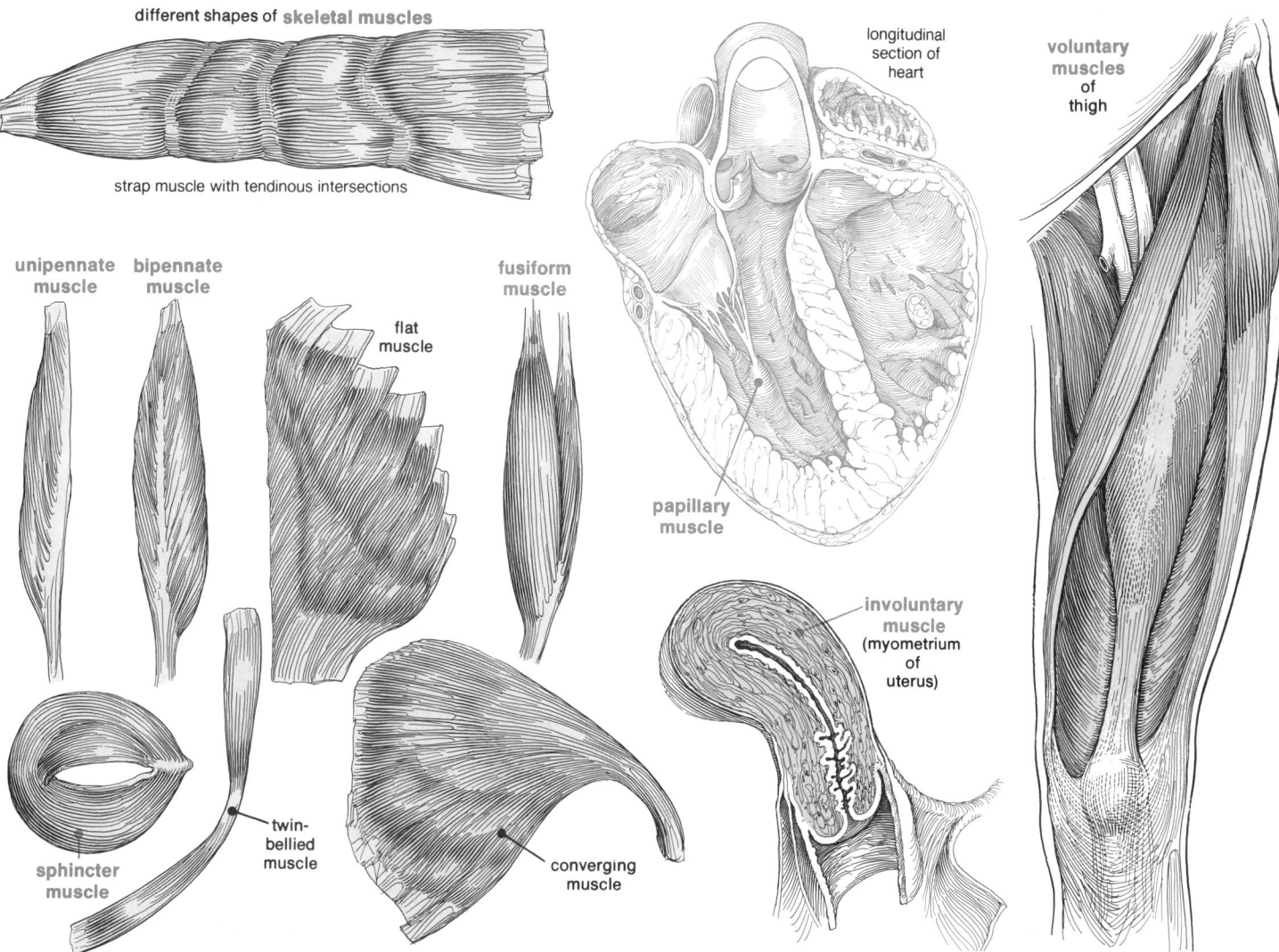

different shapes of **skeletal muscles**

strap muscle with tendinous intersections

unipennate muscle

bipennate muscle

flat muscle

fusiform muscle

longitudinal section of heart

voluntary muscles of thigh

papillary muscle

sphincter muscle

twin-bellied muscle

converging muscle

involuntary muscle (myometrium of uterus)

---

closure); the typical murmur of aortic incompetence.

ejection m. A crescendo-decrescendo murmur occurring when blood is ejected across the aortic or pulmonary valves; the murmur starts with the beginning of ejection; as ejection increases, so does the murmur (crescendo); as ejection decreases, the murmur decreases (decrescendo); it ends before the second heart sound.

extracardiac m. Murmur heard over the heart area but originating from other structures.

Flint's m. Austin-Flint murmur.

functional m. Murmur due to causes other than cardiac disorders. Also called inorganic murmur.

Graham-Steell's m. An early diastolic, high-pitched, usually decrescendo murmur; caused by pulmonary incompetence due to pulmonary hypertension.

hemic m. A cardiac or vascular murmur occurring in anemic individuals without heart disease.

holosystolic m. See pansystolic murmur.

innocent m. Murmur that is not caused by cardiovascular disease.

inorganic m. See functional murmur.

late diastolic m. See presystolic murmur.

machinery m. The continuous murmur typical of patent ductus arteriosus.

mid-diastolic m. Murmur beginning soon, but at a clear interval, after the second heart sound; originating at the atrioventricular valves, usually due either to constriction of the orifices or to abnormal patterns of atrioventricular blood flow.

mitral valve m. A murmur produced at the mitral valve; caused by either constriction of the valve orifice or backward flow of blood through the valve.

musical m. Murmur having a musical quality.

organic m. Murmur caused by organic disease, i.e., a valvular deformity or a septal defect, in contrast to a functional murmur.

pansystolic m. Murmur occupying all of systole, from the first to the second heart sound. Also called holosystolic murmur.

plateau m. Murmur having a relatively constant intensity throughout its duration.

presystolic m. A short, usually crescendo murmur heard during atrial systole, due most often to obstruction of one of the atrioventricular orifices. Also called late diastolic murmur.

pulmonary m., pulmonic m. Murmur heard at the pulmonary orifice of the heart.

regurgitant m. Murmur originating at the valvular orifices of the heart, due to leakage or backward flow of blood.

Roger's m. A loud pansystolic murmur with maximal intensity at the left sternal border caused by a small ventricular septal defect. Also called bruit de Roger.

sea gull m. A musical murmur similar to the cry of a gull.

seesaw m. See to-and-fro murmur.

systolic m. Murmur beginning with or after the first heart sound and ending at or before the second sound, i.e., during systole.

to-and-fro m. Murmurs heard in both systole and diastole. Also called seesaw murmur.

tricuspid m. Murmur originating at the tricuspid orifice.

Musca A genus of flies.

M. domestica See housefly.

muscae volitantes Small spots observed on viewing a bright area which move away when an attempt is made to focus on them; believed to be remnants of embryonic structures in the vitreous body. Also called "flitting flies."

muscarine A poisonous alkaloid present in certain mushrooms, causing inhibition of the heart action and gastrointestinal stimulation.

muscarinic 1. Producing postganglionic parasympathetic stimulation, an effect resembling that of muscarine. **1.** An agent that produces such an effect.

muscle Tissue that serves to produce motion, composed primarily of contractile cells. See table of muscles for individual muscles.

antagonistic m.'s Muscles with opposing actions.

antigravity m.'s Those maintaining the posture characteristic of a given species.

bipennate m. Muscle with a central tendon; e.g., rectus muscle of thigh.

cardiac m. Muscle of the heart (myocardium), composed of striated fibers.

fusiform m. One with a fleshy belly tapering at either extremity. Also called spindle-shaped muscle.

hamstring m.'s Three muscles at the back of the thigh; the biceps muscle of the thigh (biceps femoris), the semitendinous muscle, and the semimembranous muscle; they flex the leg and rotate it medially and laterally at the knee joint, and extend the thigh at the hip joint. Also called posterior femoral muscles.

involuntary m. Muscle that is not under voluntary control; smooth muscle which responds to the autonomic nervous system.

papillary m.'s The fleshy columns in the ventricles of the heart to which the chordae tendinae are attached.

skeletal m. A striated voluntary muscle that is attached to bones.

smooth m. Unstriated, involuntary muscle.

sphincter m. A circular band of muscle; e.g., sphincter muscle of anus.

spindle-shaped m. See fusiform muscle.

strap m. Any flat muscle, especially those of the neck associated with the hyoid bone and thyroid cartilage.

striated m. Skeletal and cardiac muscle in which cross striations occur in the fibers; with the exception of the cardiac muscle, striated muscles are voluntary, as opposed to the smooth muscles under autonomic control.

synergistic m.'s Muscles having a mutually helpful action.

unipennate m. Muscle with a tendon attached along one side; e.g., extensor muscle of little finger.

voluntary m. Muscle whose action is under voluntary control.

transverse head of adductor m. of thumb

oblique head of adductor m. of thumb

short abductor m. of thumb

abductor m. of little finger

palmar view of hand

short flexor m. of great toe

transverse head

oblique head of adductor m. of great toe

plantar view of foot

external obturator m.

hipbor

short adductor m.

great adductor m.

long adductor m.

left femur

MUSCLE	ORIGIN	INSERTION	ACTION
abductor m. of great toe *m. abductor hallucis*	calcaneus, plantar aponeurosis	proximal phalanx of great toe (joined by short flexor muscle of great toe)	abducts and aids in flexion of great toe
abductor of little finger *m. abductor digiti minimi manus*	pisiform bone, tendon of ulnar flexor muscle of wrist	proximal phalanx of fifth digit	abducts little finger
abductor m. of little toe *m. abductor digiti minimi pedis*	lateral tubercle of calcaneus	proximal phalanx of little toe	abducts little toe
abductor m. of thumb, long *m. abductor pollicis longus*	posterior surface of ulna, middle third of radius	first metacarpal bone	abducts thumb and hand
abductor m. of thumb, short *m. abductor pollicis brevis*	flexor retinaculum of hand, scaphoid and trapezium	proximal phalanx of thumb	abducts and aids in flexion of thumb
adductor m., great *m. adductor magnus*	*adductor part:* inferior ramus of pubis, ramus of ischium; *extensor part:* ischial tuberosity	*adductor part:* linea aspera of femur; *extensor part:* adductor tubercle of femur	adducts, flexes, and rotates thigh medially
adductor m., long *m. adductor longus*	pubis, below pubic crest	linea aspera of femur	adducts, flexes, and rotates thigh medially
adductor m., smallest *m. adductor minimus*	the proximal portion of the great adductor muscle when it forms a distinct muscle		
adductor m., short *m. adductor brevis*	pubis, below origin of the long adductor muscle	upper part of linea aspera of femur	adducts, flexes, and rotates thigh laterally
adductor m. of great toe *m. adductor hallucis*	*oblique head:* long plantar ligament; *transverse head:* capsules of metatarsophalangeal joints	proximal phalanx of great toe (joined by flexor muscle of great toe)	*oblique head:* adducts and flexes great toe; *transverse head:* supports transverse arch, adducts great toe
adductor m. of thumb *m. adductor pollicis*	*oblique head:* capitate, second, and third metacarpal bones; *transverse head:* third metacarpal bone	proximal phalanx of thumb	adducts and aids in apposition of thumb
anconeus m. *m. anconeus*	back of lateral epicondyle of humerus	olecranon process, posterior surface of ulna	extends forearm, abducts ulna in pronation of wrist
antitragus m. *m. antitragicus*	outer surface of antitragous of ear	caudate process of helix and anthelix	thought to be vestigial
arrector m.'s of hair *mm. arrectores pilorum*	dermis	hair follicles	elevate hairs of skin
articular m. of elbow *m. articularis cubiti*	posterior distal surface of humerus	posterior aspect of elbow joint capsule	elevates capsule in extension of elbow joint
articular m. of knee *m. articularis genus*	lower part of anterior surface of femur	upper part of synovial membrane of knee joint	elevates capsule of knee joint

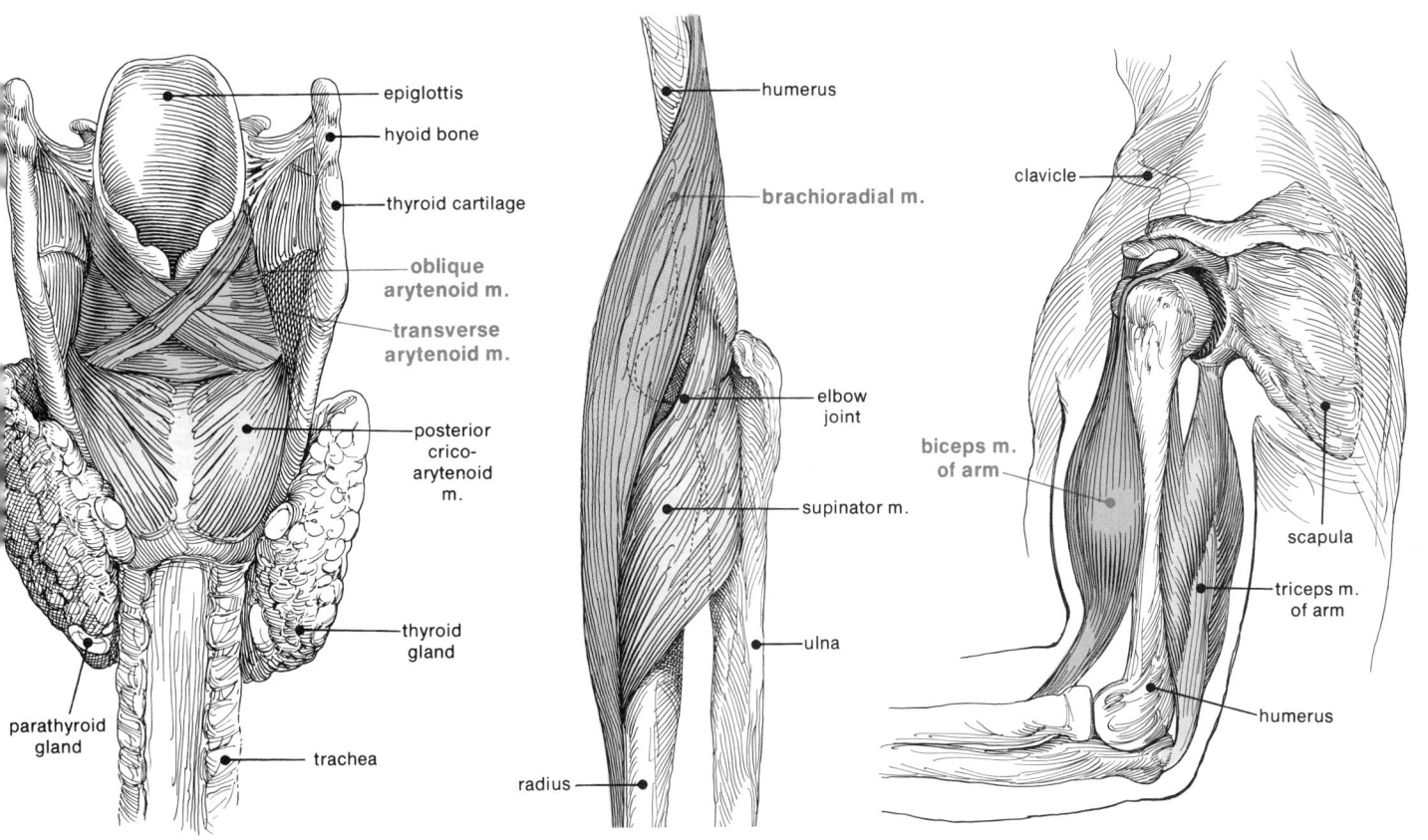

MUSCLE	ORIGIN	INSERTION	ACTION
aryepiglottic m. *m. aryepiglotticus*	apex of arytenoid cartilage	lateral margin of epiglottis	narrows inlet of larynx
arytenoid m., oblique *m. arytenoideus obliquus*	muscular process of arytenoid cartilage	apex of opposite arytenoid cartilage, prolonged as aryepiglottic muscle	approximates arytenoid cartilages
arytenoid m., transverse (only unpaired muscle of the larynx) *m. arytenoideus transversus*	posterior surface of arytenoid cartilage	posterior surface of opposite arytenoid cartilage	approximates arytenoid cartilages; constricts entrance to larynx during swallowing
auricular m., anterior *m. auricularis anterior*	temporal fascia	cartilage of ear	feeble movement of auricle forward
auricular m., posterior *m. auricularis posterior*	mastoid process	cartilage of ear	feeble movement of auricle backward
auricular m., superior *m. auricularis superior*	temporal fascia	cartilage of ear	feeble elevation of auricle
auricular m., transverse *m. auricularis transversus*	upper surface of auricle	circumference of auricle	retracts helix
biceps m. of arm *m. biceps brachii*	*long head*: supraglenoid tubercle of scapula; *short head*: apex of coracoid process	tuberosity of radius	flexes forearm and arm, supinates hand
biceps m. of thigh *m. biceps femoris*	*long head*: ischial tuberosity; *short head*: linea aspera and second supracondylar ridge of femur	head of fibula, lateral condyle of tibia	flexes knee, rotates leg laterally; long head extends thigh
brachial m. *m. brachialis*	anterior surface of distal two-thirds of humerus	coronoid process of ulna	flexes forearm
brachioradial m. *m. brachioradialis*	lateral supracondylar ridge and intermuscular septum of humerus	styloid process of radius	flexes forearm
bronchoesophageal m. *m. bronchoesophageus*	muscle fibers arising from wall of left bronchus	musculature of esophagus	reinforces esophagus
buccinator m. *m. buccinator*	pterygomandibular raphe, alveolar processes of jaws	orbicular muscle (*orbicularis oris*) at angle of mouth	retracts angle of mouth by compressing cheek; accessory muscle of mastication
bulbocavernous m. *m. bulbospongiosus*	*female*: central tendon of perineum; *male*: median raphe over bulb of penis, central tendon of perineum	*female*: dorsum of clitoris, urogenital diaphragm; *male*: corpus cavernosus, root of penis	*female*: compresses vaginal orifice; *male*: compresses urethra

muscle | **muscle**

superior constrictor m. of pharynx

middle constrictor m. of pharynx

inferior constrictor m. of pharynx

esophagus

mandible

buccinator m.

digastric m.

hyoid bone

thyrohyoid m.

thyroid cartilage

cricothyroid m.

trachea

lateral cricoarytenoid m.

posterior cricoarytenoid m.

arytenoid cartilage

cricoid cartilage

vocal ligament

thyroid cartilage

superior view of vocal apparatus

MUSCLE	ORIGIN	INSERTION	ACTION
canine m. *caninus m.*	see levator muscle of angle of mouth		
ceratocricoid m. *m. ceratocricoideus*	muscle fibers arising from posterior cricoarytenoid muscle	inferior horn (cornu) of thyroid cartilage	helps posterior cricoarytenoid muscle separate vocal cords
chin m. *m. mentalis*	incisive fossa of mandible	skin of chin	wrinkles skin of chin
chondroglossus m. *m. chondroglossus*	lesser horn (cornu) of hyoid bone	side of tongue	depresses tongue
ciliary m. *m. ciliaris*	*meridional part*: scleral spur; *circular part*: sphincter of ciliary body	ciliary process	makes lens more convex in accommodation for near vision
coccygeus m. ischiococcygeus m. *m. coccygeus*	ischial spine and sacrospinous ligament	coccyx, lower part of lateral border of sacrum	aids in raising and supporting pelvic floor
constrictor m. of pharynx, inferior *m. constrictor pharyngis inferior*	cricoid and oblique line of thyroid cartilages	median raphe of posterior wall of pharynx	narrows lower part of pharynx in swallowing
constrictor m. of pharynx, middle *m. constrictor pharyngis medius*	stylohyoid ligament and horns of hyoid bone	median raphe of posterior wall of pharynx	narrows pharynx in swallowing
constrictor m. of pharynx, superior *m. constrictor pharyngis superior*	medial pterygoid plate, hamulus, pterygomandibular raphe, mandible	median raphe of posterior wall of pharynx; pharyngeal tubercle of skull	narrows pharynx in swallowing
coracobrachial m. *m. coracobrachialis*	coracoid process of scapula (shoulder blade)	inner side of humerus	flexes, adducts arm
corrugator m. *m. corrugator*	brow ridge of frontal bone	skin of eyebrow	draws eyebrows together, wrinkles forehead
cremaster m. *m. cremaster*	inferior border of internal oblique abdominal muscle	spermatic cord	elevates testis
cricoarytenoid m., lateral *m. cricoarytenoideus lateralis*	upper margin of arch of cricoid cartilage	muscular process of arytenoid cartilage	approximates vocal cords so they meet in midline for phonation
cricoarytenoid m., posterior *m. cricoarytenoideus posterior*	posterior surface of lamina of cricoid cartilage	muscular process of arytenoid cartilage	separates vocal cords, opening the glottis
cricothyroid m. *m. cricothyroideus*	anterior surface of arch of cricoid cartilage	lamina and inferior horn of thyroid cartilage	lengthens, stretches, and tenses vocal cords

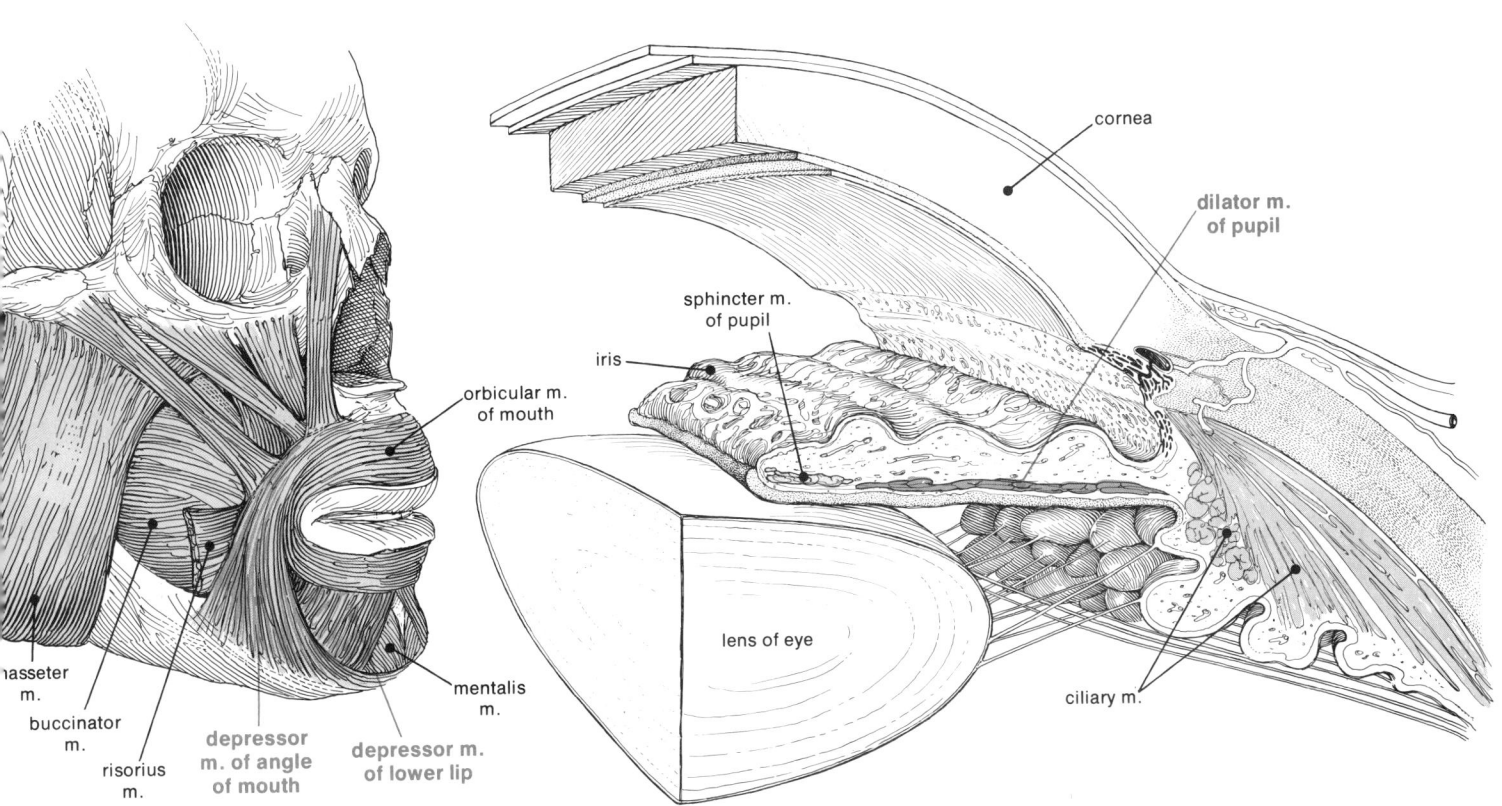

Labels on illustration:

cornea

dilator m. of pupil

sphincter m. of pupil

iris

orbicular m. of mouth

lens of eye

ciliary m.

masseter m.

buccinator m.

risorius m.

depressor m. of angle of mouth

depressor m. of lower lip

mentalis m.

MUSCLE	ORIGIN	INSERTION	ACTION
deltoid m. *m. deltoideus*	lateral third of clavicle, acromion, and spine of scapula	deltoid tuberosity of humerus	abductor of arm; aids in flexion and extension
depressor m., superciliary *m. depressor supercilii*	orbicular fibers of the eye (*orbicularis oculi*)	eyebrow	pulls eyebrow downward
depressor m. of angle of mouth triangular m. *m. depressor anguli oris*	oblique line of mandible	angle of mouth	pulls corner of mouth downward
depression m. of lower lip quadrate m. of lower lip *m. depressor labii inferior*	mandible adjacent to mental foramen	lower lip	draws lower lip downward
depressor m. of nasal septum *m. depressor septi nasi*	incisive fossa of maxilla	ala and septum of nose	widens the nostrils
detrussor m. of urinary bladder *m. detrussor vesicae*	in wall of urinary bladder		empties urinary bladder
detrusor urinae m.	see detrusor muscle of urinary bladder		
diaphragm diaphragmatic m. *diaphragma*	xiphoid process, six lower costal cartilages, four lower ribs, lumbar vertebrae, arcuate ligaments	central tendon of diaphragm	increases capacity of thorax in inspiration (main muscle of inhalation)
diaphragm m., pelvic	composed of the coccygeus and levator ani muscles		forms floor to support pelvic viscera
digastric m. *m. digastricus*	digastric notch at mastoid process	mandible near symphysis	raises hyoid bone and base of tongue, lowers mandible
dilator m. of nose *m. dilator naris*	margin of piriform aperture of maxilla	margin of nostril	widens nostril
dilator m. of pupil *m. dilator pupillae*	circumference of iris	margin of pupil	dilates pupil
epicranial m. *m. epicranius*	the muscular and tendinous layer of the scalp composed of the occipitofrontal and temporoparietal muscles connected by the *galea aponeurotica*		elevates eyebrows, draws scalp forward and backward
erector m. of penis	see ischiocavernous muscle		
erector m. of spine *m. erector spinae*	deep muscle arising from the broad and thick tendon attached to the middle crest of sacrum, spinous processes of lumbar and 11th and 12th thoracic vertebrae, and back part of the iliac crest; it splits in the upper lumbar region into three columns of muscles; iliocostal (lateral division), longissimus (intermediate division), and spinal (medial division)		
extensor m. of fingers *m. extensor digitorum*	lateral epicondyle of humerus	phalanges of digits 2 to 5, via dorsal digital expansion	extends fingers, hand, and forearm
extensor m. of great toe, long *m. extensor hallucis longus*	middle of fibula, interosseous membrane	distal phalanx of great toe	extends great toe, dorsiflexes foot

MUSCLE	ORIGIN	INSERTION	ACTION
extensor m. of great toe, short m. extensor hallucis brevis	dorsal surface of calcaneus	base of proximal phalanx of great toe	dorsiflexes great toe
extensor m. of index finger m. extensor indicis	posterior surface of ulna	extensor expansion of index finger	extends index finger and hand
extensor m. of little finger m. extensor digiti minimi manus	lateral epicondyle of humerus	extensor expansion of little finger	extends little finger
extensor m. of thumb, long m. extensor pollicis longus	middle third of ulna, adjacent interosseous membrane	distal phalanx of thumb	extends distal phalanx of thumb, abducts hand
extensor m. of thumb, short m. extensor pollicis brevis	middle third of radius	proximal phalanx of thumb	extends thumb and abducts hand
extensor m. of toes, long m. extensor digitorum longus pedis	lateral condyle of tibia, upper three-fourths of fibula, interosseous membrane	extensor expansion of lateral toes (by four slips)	extends toes and dorsiflexes foot
extensor m. of toes, short m. extensor digitorum brevis pedis	dorsal surface of calcaneus	extensor tendons of second, third, and fourth toes	extends toes
extensor m. of wrist, radial, long m. extensor carpi radialis longus	lateral supracondylar ridge of humerus	second metacarpal bone	extends and abducts wrist
extensor m. of wrist, radial, short m. extensor carpi radialis brevis	lateral epicondyle of humerus, radial collateral ligament	third metacarpal	extends and abducts wrist
extensor m. of wrist, ulnar m. extensor carpi ulnaris	*humeral head:* lateral epicondyle of humerus; *ulnar head:* posterior border of ulna	fifth metacarpal bone	extends and abducts wrist
fibular m.		see peroneal muscle	
flexor m. of fingers, deep m. flexor digitorum profundus manus	proximal three-fourths of ulna and adjacent interosseous membrane	distal phalanges of fingers	flexes terminal phalanges and hand
flexor m. of fingers, superficial m. flexor digitorum superficialis manus	*humeroulnar head:* medial epicondyle of humerus, coronoid process of ulna; *radial head:* anterior border of radius	middle phalanges of fingers	flexes phalanges, hand, and forearm
flexor m. of great toe, long m. flexor hallucis longus	lower two-thirds of posterior surface of fibula, intermuscular septum	distal phalanx of great toe	flexes great toe and plantarflexes foot

muscle | muscle

posterior
aspect
of leg

long
flexor
m. of
toes

radial
flexor
m. of
wrist

ulnar
flexor
m. of
wrist

after Jones

gastroc-
nemius
m.

short
flexor
m. of
little
finger

ong
exor
. of
reat
oe

ort
xor
of
tle
e

plantar
aspect
of
foot

palmar
aspect
of hand

calcaneus
(heel bone)

posterior
aspect
of leg

MUSCLE	ORIGIN	INSERTION	ACTION
flexor m. of great toe, short *m. flexor hallucis brevis*	cuboid and third cuneiform bones	both sides of proximal phalanx of great toe	flexes great toe
flexor m. of little finger, short *m. flexor digiti minimi brevis manus*	hook of hamate, flexor retinaculum	proximal phalanx of little finger	flexes proximal phalanx of little finger
flexor m. of little toe, short *m. flexor digiti minimi brevis pedis*	base of fifth metatarsal and plantar fascia	lateral surface of proximal phalanx of little toe	flexes little toe
flexor m. of thumb, long *m. flexor pollicis longus*	radius, adjacent interosseous membrane, coronoid process of ulna	distal phalanx of thumb	flexes thumb
flexor m. of thumb, short *m. flexor pollicis brevis*	trapezium, trapezoid, and capitate bones of wrist	proximal phalanx of thumb	flexes thumb
flexor m. of toes, long *m. flexor digitorum longus pedis*	middle half of tibia	distal phalanges of lateral four toes (by four tendons)	flexes second to fifth toes and plantarflexes foot
flexor m. of toes, short *m. flexor digitorum brevis pedis*	calcaneus and plantar fascia	middle phalanges of four lateral toes	flexes four lateral toes
flexor m. of wrist, radial *m. flexor carpi radialis*	medial epicondyle of humerus	bases of second and third metacarpal bones	flexes hand and forearm, aids in pronation and abduction of hand
flexor m. of wrist, ulnar *m. flexor carpi ulnaris*	*humeral head*: medial epicondyle of humerus; *ulnar head*: olecranon and posterior border of ulna	pisiform, hamate, and fifth metacarpal bones	flexes and adducts hand
frontal m.	see occipitofrontal muscle		
gastrocnemius m. *m. gastrocnemius*	*medial head*: popliteal surface of femur, upper part of medial condyle of femur; *lateral head*: lateral condyle of femur	calcaneus via calcaneal tendon (tendo calcaneus) (in common with soleus muscle)	flexes leg and plantarflexes foot
gemellus m., inferior *m. gemellus inferior*	lower margin of lesser sciatic notch	internal obturator tendon	rotates thigh laterally
gemellus m., superior *m. gemellus superior*	upper margin of lesser sciatic notch	internal obturator tendon	rotates thigh laterally
genioglossus m. *m. genioglossus*	mental spine of the mandible	ventral surface of tongue and body of hyoid bone	protrudes, retracts, and depresses tongue, elevates hyoid bone
geniohyoid m. *m. geniohyoideus*	mental spine (genial tubercle) of the mandible	body of hyoid bone	elevates hyoid bone

muscle | muscle

MUSCLE	ORIGIN	INSERTION	ACTION
glossopalatine m.	see palatoglossus muscle		
gluteus maximus m. greatest gluteal m. *m. gluteus maximus*	upper portion of ilium, sacrum and coccyx, sacrotuberous ligament	gluteal tuberosity of femur, iliotibial tract (band of fascia lata)	chief extensor, powerful lateral rotator of thigh
gluteus medius m. middle gluteal m. *m. gluteus medius*	midportion of ilium	greater trochanter and oblique ridge of femur	abducts, rotates thigh medially
gluteus minimus m. least gluteal m. *m. gluteus minimus*	lower portion of ilium	greater trochanter of femur, capsule of hip joint	abducts, rotates thigh medially
gracilis m. *m. gracilis*	lower half of pubis	upper part of tibia	adducts thigh, flexes and rotates leg medially
helix m., smaller *m. helicis minor*	anterior rim of helix	crux of helix	thought to be vestigial
hyoglossus m. hyoglossal m. *m. hyoglossus*	body and greater horn (cornu) of hyoid bone	side of tongue	retracts, depresses tongue
iliac m. *m. iliacus*	iliac fossa, lateral aspect of sacrum	greater psoas tendon, lesser trochanter of femur	flexes thigh
iliococcygeus m. *m. iliococcygeus*	ischial spine and arching tendon over internal obturator muscle	coccyx and perineal body	supports pelvic viscera
iliocostal m. *m. iliocostalis*	the lateral division of erector muscle of spine	inferior borders of angles of last six or seven ribs	extends vertebral column and assists in lateral movements of trunk
iliocostal m. of loins *m. iliocostalis lumborum*	iliac crest and thoracolumbar fascia	transverse processes of lumbar vertebrae, angles of lower six ribs	extends lumbar spine
iliocostal m. of neck *m. iliocostalis cervicis*	upper six ribs	transverse processes of fourth, fifth, and sixth cervical vertebrae	extends cervical vertebral column
iliocostal m. of thorax *m. iliocostalis thoracis*	lower seven ribs, medial to angles of the ribs	angles of upper seven ribs, transverse process of seventh cervical vertebra	keeps thoracic spine erect
iliopsoas m. *m. iliopsoas*	a compound muscle consisting of the iliac and greater psoas muscles, which join to form the iliopsoas tendon		
incisive m.'s of lower lip *mm. incisivi labii inferior*	portion of orbicular muscle of mouth (*orbicularis oris*)	angle of mouth	make vestibule of mouth shallow

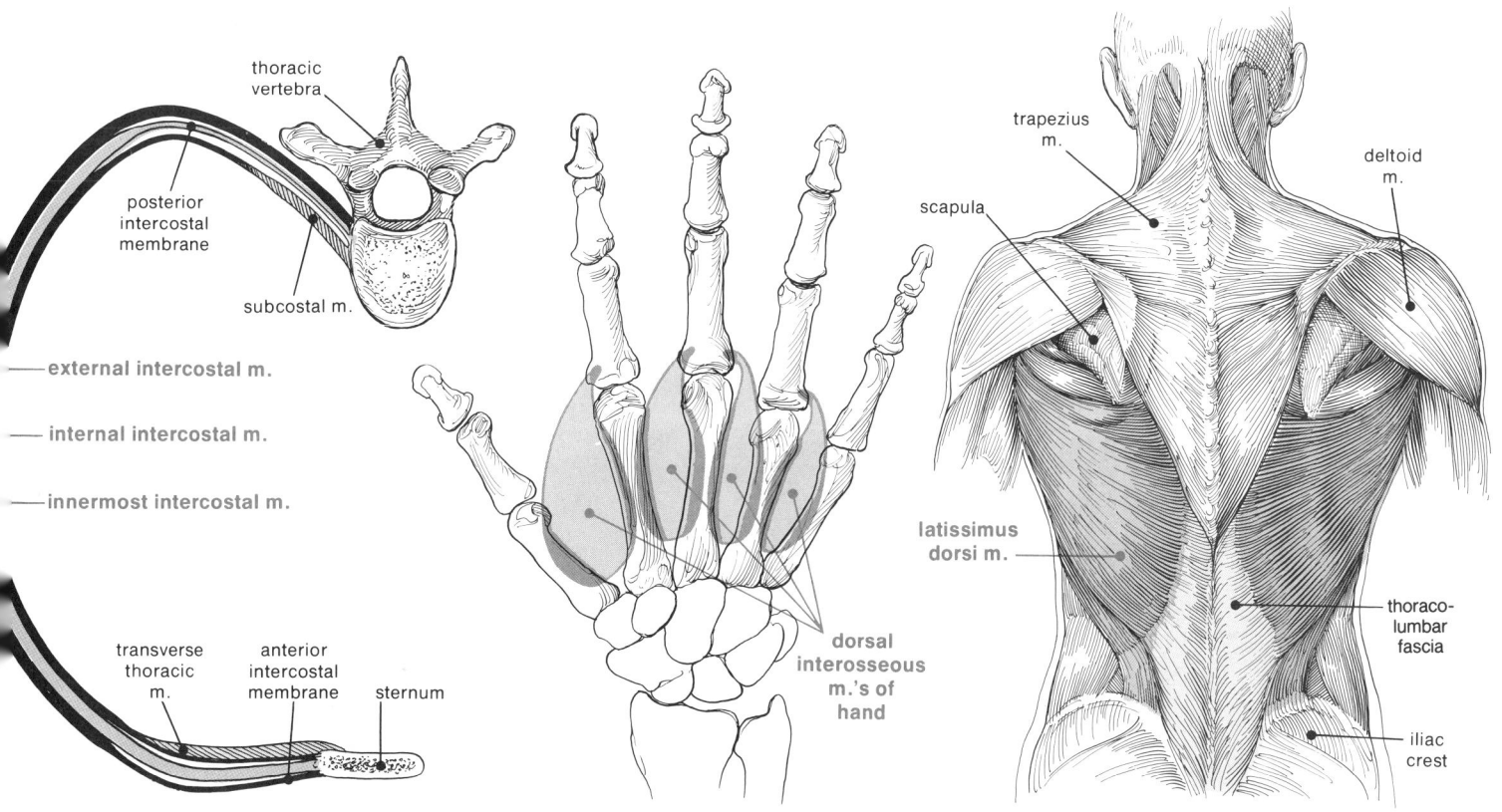

thoracic vertebra

posterior intercostal membrane

subcostal m.

external intercostal m.

internal intercostal m.

innermost intercostal m.

transverse thoracic m.

anterior intercostal membrane

sternum

dorsal interosseous m.'s of hand

trapezius m.

scapula

deltoid m.

latissimus dorsi m.

thoraco-lumbar fascia

iliac crest

MUSCLE	ORIGIN	INSERTION	ACTION
incisive m.'s of upper lip *mm. incisivi labii superior*	portion of orbicular muscle of mouth (*orbicularis oris*)	angle of mouth	make vestibule of mouth shallow
infrahyoid m.'s *mm. infrahyoidei*	the ribbon-like muscles below the hyoid bone including the omohyoid, sternohyoid, sternothyroid, and thyrohyoid muscles		
infraspinous m. *m. infraspinatus*	infraspinous fossa of scapula	midportion of greater tubercle of humerus	rotates arm laterally
intercostal m.'s, external *mm. intercostales externi*	inferior border of rib	superior border of rib below origin	draw ribs together
intercostal m.'s, innermost *mm. intercostales intimi*	superior border of rib	inferior border of rib above origin	draw ribs together
intercostal m.'s, internal *mm. intercostales interni*	superior border of rib	inferior border of rib above origin	draw ribs together
interosseous m.'s, palmar (three in number) *mm. interossei palmares*	medial side of second, lateral side of fourth and fifth metacarpals	base of proximal phalanx in line with its origin	adduct second, fourth, and fifth fingers; aid in extension of fingers
interosseous m.'s, plantar (three in number) *mm. innterossei plantares*	medial side of third, fourth, and fifth metatarsal bones	medial side of proximal phalanges of third, fourth, and fifth toes	adduct three lateral toes toward second toe
interosseous m.'s of foot, dorsal (four in number) *mm. interossei dorsales pedis*	adjacent sides of metatarsal bones	proximal phalanges of both sides of second toe, lateral side of third and fourth toes	abduct lateral toes, move second toe from side to side
interosseous m.'s of hand, dorsal (four in number) *mm. interossei dorsales manus*	adjacent sides of metacarpal bones	extensor tendons of second, third, and fourth fingers	abduct, flex proximal phalanges
interspinal m.'s *mm. interspinales*	superior surface of spinous process of each vertebra	inferior surface of spinous process of vertebra above vertebra of origin	extend vertebral column
intertransverse m.'s *mm. intertransversarii*	extend between transverse processes of adjacent vertebrae		bend vertebral column laterally
ischiocavernous m. *m. ischiocavernosus*	ramus of ischium adjacent to crus of penis or clitoris	crus near pubic symphysis	maintains erection of penis or clitoris
ischiococcygeus m.	see coccygeus muscle		
latissimus dorsi m. *m. latissimus dorsi*	spinous processes of lower six thoracic vertebrae, thoracolumbar fascia, crest of ilium	floor or intertubercular groove of humerus	adducts, extends, and medially rotates arm

muscle | muscle

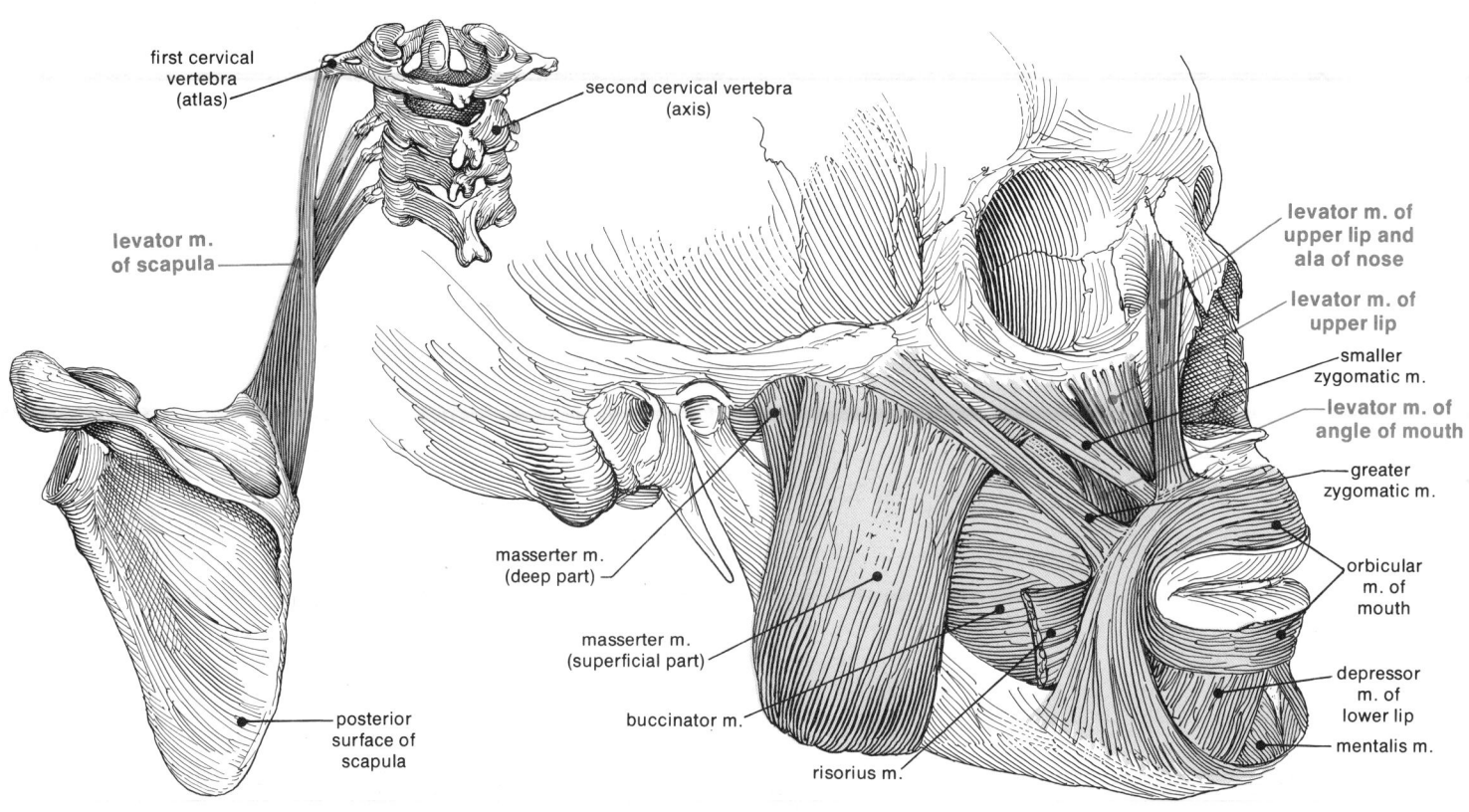

first cervical vertebra (atlas)

second cervical vertebra (axis)

levator m. of scapula

levator m. of upper lip and ala of nose

levator m. of upper lip

smaller zygomatic m.

levator m. of angle of mouth

greater zygomatic m.

masserter m. (deep part)

orbicular m. of mouth

masserter m. (superficial part)

depressor m. of lower lip

buccinator m.

mentalis m.

posterior surface of scapula

risorius m.

MUSCLE	ORIGIN	INSERTION	ACTION
levator ani m. *m. levator ani*	*pubococcygeus m. part*: pubis and pelvic fascia; *puborectal m. part*: pubis; *iliococcygeus m. part*: pelvic surface of ischial spine and pelvic fascia	perineal body, coccyx and anococcygeal raphe	supports pelvic viscera, constricts lower end of rectum and vagina
levator m. of angle of mouth caninus m. canine m. *m. levator anguli oris*	maxilla next to cuspid fossa	corner of mouth	raises angle of mouth
levator m. of soft palate *m. levator veli palatini*	apex of petrous part of temporal bone and cartilaginous part of auditory tube	aponeurosis of soft palate	raises soft palate
levator m. of prostate *m. levator prostatae*	pubic symphysis	fascia of prostate gland	elevates and compresses prostate gland
levator m.'s of ribs *mm. levatores costarum*	transverse processes of seventh cervical and first 11 thoracic vertebrae	angle of rib below	aid in raising ribs
levator m. of scapula *m. levator scapulae*	transverse processes of first four cervical vertebrae	vertebral border of scapula	raises scapula
levator m. of thyroid gland (inconstant muscle) *m. levator glandulae thyroideae*	isthmus or pyramidal lobe of thyroid gland	hyoid bone	stabilizes thyroid gland
levator m. of upper eyelid, *m. levator palpebrae superior*	roof of orbital cavity	skin and tarsal plate of upper eyelid, and superior fornix of conjunctiva	raises upper eyelid
levator m. of upper lip quadrate m. of upper lip *m. levator labii superior*	maxilla and zygomatic bone below level of infraorbital foramen	upper lip and margin of nostril	raises upper lip, dilates nostril
levator m. of upper lip and ala of nose *m. levator labii superior alaeque nasi*	maxilla	skin of upper lip, ala of nose	raises upper lip, dilates nostril (muscle of facial expression)
long m. of head *m. longus capitis*	transverse processes of third to sixth cervical vertebrae	basal part of occipital bone	flexes head
long m. of neck *m. longus colli*	*superior oblique part*: anterior tubercle of transverse processes of third, fourth, and fifth cervical vertebrae;	*superior oblique part*: anterolateral surface of tubercle on anterior arch of first vertebra (atlas);	bends neck forward and slightly rotates cervical portion of vertebral column

longissimus muscle of thorax

mastoid process

longissimus muscle of neck

longissimus muscle of head

scapula

lumbrical muscles of foot

MUSCLE	ORIGIN	INSERTION	ACTION
long m. of neck (cont'd)	*inferior oblique part*: front of bodies of first two or three thoracic vertebrae; *vertical part*: front of bodies of first three thoracic and last three cervical vertebrae	*inferior oblique part*: anterior tubercle of transverse processes of fifth and sixth cervical vertebrae; *vertical part*: front of bodies of second, third, and fourth cervical vertebrae	
longissimus m. of head trachelomastoid m. *m. longissimus capitis*	transverse processes of cervical vertebrae	mastoid process of temporal bone	draws head backward, rotates head
longissimus m. of neck *m. longissimus cervicis*	transverse processes of upper six thoracic vertebrae	transverse processes of second through sixth cervical vertebrae	bends vertebral column backward and laterally
longissimus m. of thorax longissimus dorsi m. *m. longissimus thoracis*	thoracolumbar fascia, transverse processes of lower six thoracic and first two lumbar vertebrae	transverse processes of lumbar and thoracic vertebrae, inferior borders of lower 9 or 10 ribs	bends vertebral column backward and laterally
longitudinal m. of tongue, inferior *m. longitudinalis inferior linguae*	undersurface of tongue at base	tip of tongue	acts to alter shape of tongue
longitudinal m. of tongue, superior *m. longitudinalis superior linguae*	submucosa and septum of tongue	margins of tongue	acts to alter shape of tongue
lumbrical m.'s of foot *mm. lumbricales pedis*	tendons of long flexor muscles of toes	medial side of proximal phalanges and extensor tendon of four lateral toes	flex proximal, extend middle and distal phalanges
lumbical m.'s of hand (four in number) *mm. lumbricales manus*	tendons of deep flexor muscles of fingers	extensor tendons of four lateral fingers	flex proximal, extend middle and distal phalanges
masseter m. *m. masseter*	*superficial part*: zygomatic process and arch; *deep part*: zygomatic arch	*superficial part*: ramus and angle of lower jaw; *deep part*: upper half of ramus, coronoid process of lower jaw	closes mouth, clenches teeth (muscle of mastication)
mentalis m. *m. levator menti*	incisor fossa of mandible	skin of chin	raises and protrudes lower lip
multifidus m. *m. multifidus*	sacrum and transverse processes of lumbar, thoracic, and lower cervical vertebrae	spinous processes of lumbar, thoracic, and lower cervical vertebrae	extends, rotates vertebral column

superior longitudinal m. of tongue

vertical and transverse musculature of tongue

inferior longitudinal m. of tongue

mandible

hyoglossus m.

mylohyoid m.

genioglossus m.

hyoid bone

occipitofrontal m.

frontal part of occipitofrontal m.

occipital part of occipitofrontal m.

inferior oblique m.

superior rectus m.

superior oblique m.

lateral rectus m.

levator m. of upper eyelid

MUSCLE	ORIGIN	INSERTION	ACTION
m. of Treitz	see suspensory muscle of duodenum		
mylohyoid m. *m. mylohyoideus*	mylohyoid line of mandible	median raphe and hyoid bone	elevates floor of mouth and tongue, depresses mandible
nasal m. *m. nasalis*	maxilla adjacent to cuspid and incisor teeth	side of nose above nostril	draws margin of nostril toward septum
oblique m. of abdomen, external *m. obliquus externus abdominis*	external surface of lower eight ribs at costal cartilages	anterior half of crest of ilium, linea alba through rectus sheath, inguinal ligament	flexes and rotates vertebral column, tenses abdominal wall
oblique m. of abdomen, internal *m. obliquus internus abdominis*	iliac crest, thoracolumbar fascia, inguinal ligament	lower three or four costal cartilages, linea alba by conjoint tendon to pubis	flexes and rotates vertebral column, tenses abdominal wall
oblique m. of auricle *m. obliquus auriculae*	eminence of concha	convexity of the helix	thought to be vestigial
oblique m. of eyeball, inferior *m. obliquus inferior bulbi*	floor of orbital cavity at anterior margin	between insertion of superior and lateral recti	rotates eyeball upward and outward
oblique m. of eyeball, superior *m. obliquus superior bulbi*	lesser wing of sphenoid above the optic canal	after passing through a fibrous pulley, reverses direction to insert on sclera deep to superior rectus muscle	rotates eyeball downward and outward
oblique m. of head, inferior *m. obliquus capitis inferior*	spine of second vertebra (axis)	transverse process of first vertebra (atlas)	rotates head
oblique m. of head, superior *m. obliquus capitis superior*	transverse process of first vertebra (atlas)	outer third of inferior curved line of occipital bone	rotates head
obturator m., external *m. obturatorius externus*	external margin of obturator foramen of pelvis, obturator membrane	trochanteric fossa of femur	flexes and rotates thigh laterally
obturator m., internal *m. obturatorius interus*	pelvic surface of hipbone and internal margin of obturator foramen, obturator membrane	greater trochanter of femur	abducts and laterally rotates thigh
occipital m.	see occipitofrontal muscle		
occipitofrontal m. *m. occipitofrontalis*	*frontal part*: epicranial aponeurosis; *occipital part*: highest nuchal line of occipital bone	*frontal part*: skin of eyebrow, root of nose; *occipital part*: epicranial aponeurosis	*frontal part*: elevates eyebrows; *occipital part*: draws scalp backward

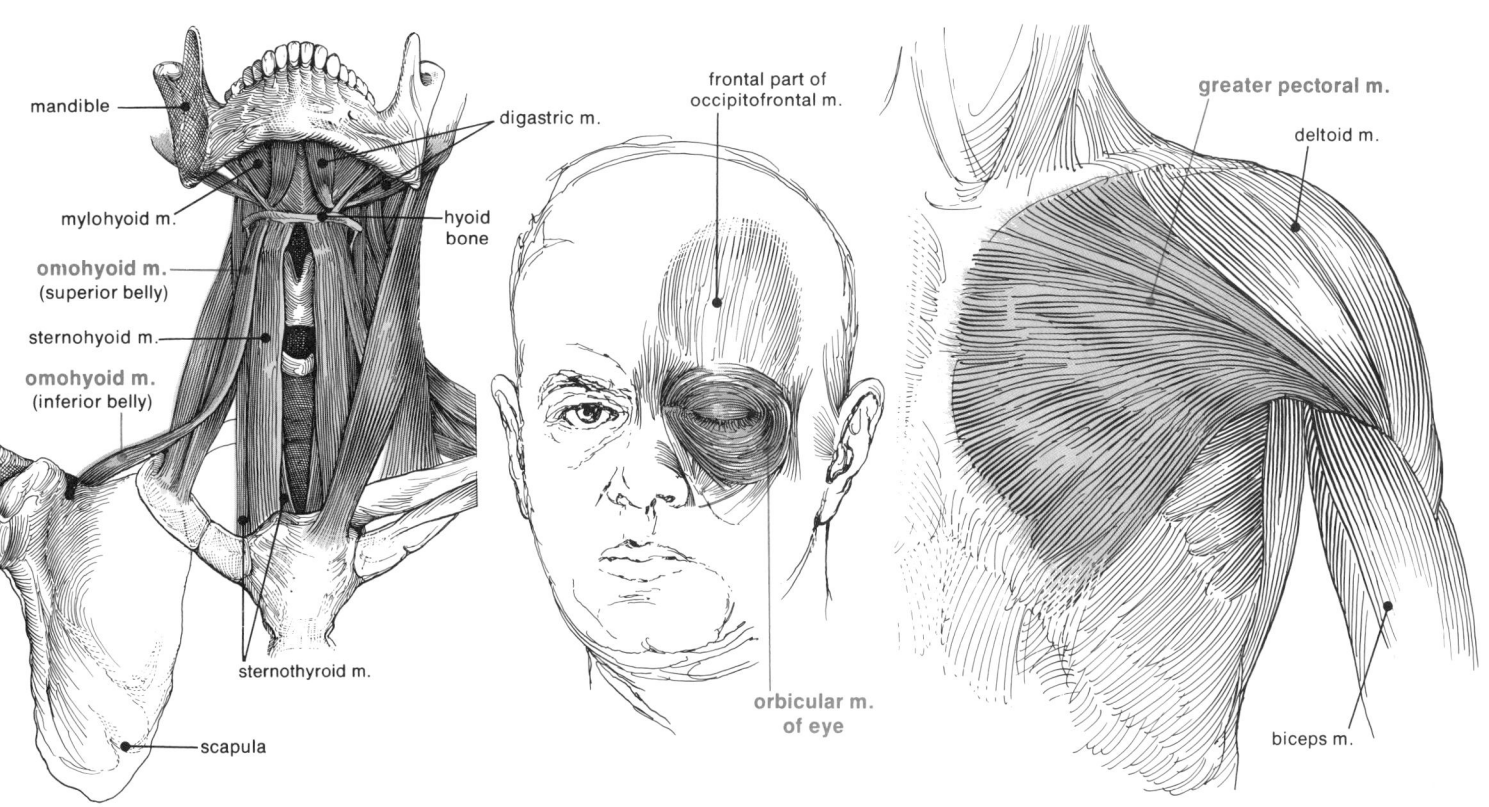

Labels in illustration:
- mandible
- digastric m.
- frontal part of occipitofrontal m.
- greater pectoral m.
- deltoid m.
- mylohyoid m.
- hyoid bone
- omohyoid m. (superior belly)
- sternohyoid m.
- omohyoid m. (inferior belly)
- sternothyroid m.
- orbicular m. of eye
- scapula
- biceps m.

MUSCLE	ORIGIN	INSERTION	ACTION
omohyoid m. *m. omohyoideus*	medial tip of suprascapular notch	lower border, body of hyoid bone	depresses and retracts hyoid bone
opposing m. of little finger *m. opponens digiti minimi manus*	hook of hamate bone, flexor retinaculum	fifth metacarpal	draws fifth metacarpal bone toward palm
opposing m. of thumb *m. opponens pollicis*	tubercle of trapezium, flexor retinaculum	lateral border of first metacarpal bone	draws first metacarpal bone toward palm, opposes thumb
orbicular m. of eye *m. orbicularis oculi*	*orbital part*: frontal process of maxilla, adjacent portion of frontal bone; *palpebral part*: medial palpebral ligament; *lacrimal part*: posterior lacrimal ridge of lacrimal bone	near origin after encircling orbit orbital tubercle of zygomatic bone	closes eyelids, tightens skin of forehead, compresses lacrimal sac
orbicular m. of mouth *m. orbicularis oris*	muscle adjacent to mouth	muscles interlace to encircle mouth	closes and purses lips
orbital m. *m. orbitalis*	bridges inferior orbital groove and sphenomaxillary fissure		thought to be rudimentary; may feebly protrude the eyball
palatoglossus m. glossopalatine m. *m. palatoglossus*	undersurface of soft palate	dorsum and side of tongue	elevates tongue and narrows fauces
palatopharyngeus m. *m. palatopharyngeus*	soft palate	posterior wall of thyroid cartilage and wall of pharynx	elevates pharynx, helps shut nasopharynx, narrows fauces, aids in swallowing
palmar m., long *m. palmaris longus*	medial epicondyle of humerus	flexor retinaculum, palmar aponeurosis	flexes hand
palmar m., short *m. palmaris brevis*	flexor retinaculum	skin of palm	aids in deepening hollow of palm, wrinkles skin of palm
pectinate m.'s *mm. pectinati*	a number of muscular columns projecting from the inner walls of the atria of the heart		contract in systole the atrium of heart
pectineal m. *m. pectineus*	pectineal line of pubis	pectineal line of femur between lesser trochanter and linea aspera	adducts and aids in flexion of thigh
pectoral m., greater *m. pectoralis major*	medial half of clavicle, sternum, and costal cartilages; aponeurosis of external oblique muscle of abdomen; sixth rib	lateral lip of intertubercular groove of humerus	flexes, adducts, and rotates arm medially

muscle | muscle

MUSCLE	ORIGIN	INSERTION	ACTION
pectoral, m., smaller *m. pectoralis minor*	anterior aspect of second through fifth ribs	coracoid process of scapula	draws scapula downward, elevates ribs
pectoralis major m.	see pectoral muscle, greater		
pectoralis minor m.	see pectoral muscle, smaller		
peroneal m., long fibular m., long *m. peroneus longus*	upper aspects of tibia and fibula	first metatarsal bone, first cuneiform bone	aids in plantar flexion and everts foot
peroneal m., short fibular m., short *m. peroneus brevis*	lower two-thirds of fibula	tuberosity of fifth metatarsal bone	aids in plantar flexion of and everts foot
peroneal m., third *m. peroneus tertius*	distal fourth of fibula, interosseous membrane	fascia of fifth metatarsal bone on dorsum of foot	dorsiflexes and everts foot
piriform m. *m. piriformis*	internal aspect of sacrum, sacrotuberous ligament	upper portion of greater trochanter of femur	rotates thigh laterally
plantar m. *m. plantaris*	popliteal groove of lateral condyle of femur	medial side of calcaneal tendon	plantar flexion of foot
platysma m. *m. platysma*	superficial fascia of upper chest	skin over mandible and neck	depresses lower jaw and lower lip, wrinkles skin of neck and upper part of chest
pleuroesophageal m. *m. pleuroesophageus*	muscle fibers from left mediastinal pleura to esophagus		reinforces musculature of esophagus
popliteal m. *m. popliteus*	popliteal groove of lateral condyle of femur	medial two-thirds of popliteal line on posterior surface of tibia	flexes and rotates leg medially
procerus m. *m. procerus*	fascia covering bridge of nose	skin between eyebrows	wrinkles skin over bridge of nose (assists frontal muscle)
pronator m., quadrate *m. pronator quadratus*	distal fourth of shaft of ulna	distal fourth of shaft of radius	pronates forearm
pronator m., round *m. pronator teres*	*humeral part:* medial epicondyle of humerus; *ulnar part:* coronoid of ulna	lateral aspect of radius bone	pronates and flexes forearm
psoas m., greater *m. psoas major*	transverse processes and bodies of lumbar vertebrae	lesser trochanter of femur	flexes and medially rotates thigh
psoas m., smaller *m. psoas minor*	bodies of last thoracic and first lumbar vertebrae	pectineal line of hipbone	flexes vertebral column

lateral pterygoid m.

12th rib

quadrate m.
of loins

iliac
crest

medial
pterygoid m.

superior
constrictor m.

pterygomandibular
raphe

buccinator m.

MUSCLE	ORIGIN	INSERTION	ACTION
pterygoid m., lateral external pterygoid m. *m. pterygoideus lateralis*	lateral pterygoid plate and greater wing of sphenoid	condyle of mandible, capsule of temporomandibular joint	opens and protrudes mandible and moves it side to side
pterygoid m., medial internal pterygoid m. *m. pterygoideus medialis*	maxillary tuberosity and lateral pterygoid plate	medial surface of ramus and angle of mandible	closes and protrudes mandible
pubococcygeus m. *m. pubococcygeus*	pubis and obturator fascia	coccyx and perineal body	supports pelvic floor
puborectal m. *m. puborectalis*	pubis and pubic symphysis	interdigitates to form a sling which passes behind the rectum	holds anal canal at right angle to rectum
pubovaginal m. *m. pubovaginalis*	part of levator ani muscle in the female		
pubovesical m. *m. pubovesicalis*	posterior surface of body of pubis	*female:* around fundus of bladder to front of vagina; *male:* around fundus of bladder to prostate gland	strengthens musculature of urinary bladder
pyramidal m. *m. pyramidalis*	pubis and pubic symphysis	linea alba	tenses abdominal wall
quadrate m. of loins *m. quadratus lumborum*	iliac crest, transverse processes of lumbar vertebrae	12th rib, transverse processes of upper lumbar vertebrae	draws rib cage inferiorly, bends vertebral column laterally
quadrate m. of lower lip *m. quadratus labii inferior*	see depressor muscle of lower lip		
quadrate m. of sole accessory flexor m. *m. quadratus plantae*	calcaneus and plantar fascia	tendons of long flexor muscle of toes (*m. flexor digitorum longus*)	straightens pull of tendon of the long flexor muscle of toes
quadrate m. of thigh *m. quadratus femoris*	proximal part of external border of tuberosity of ischium	proximal part of linea quadrata (line extending vertically and distally from intertrochanteric crest of femur)	rotates thigh laterally
quadrate m. of upper lip *m. quadratus labii superior*	see levator muscle of upper lip		
quadratus lumborum m.	see quadrate muscle of loins		
quadriceps m. of thigh *m. quadriceps femoris*	the large fleshy mass that covers the front and sides of the femur, consisting of the rectus muscle of thigh (*m. rectus femoris*), lateral vastus muscle (*m. vastus lateralis*), medial vastus muscle (*m. vastus medialis*), and intermediate vastus muscle (*m. vastus intermedius*)		great extensor muscle of leg

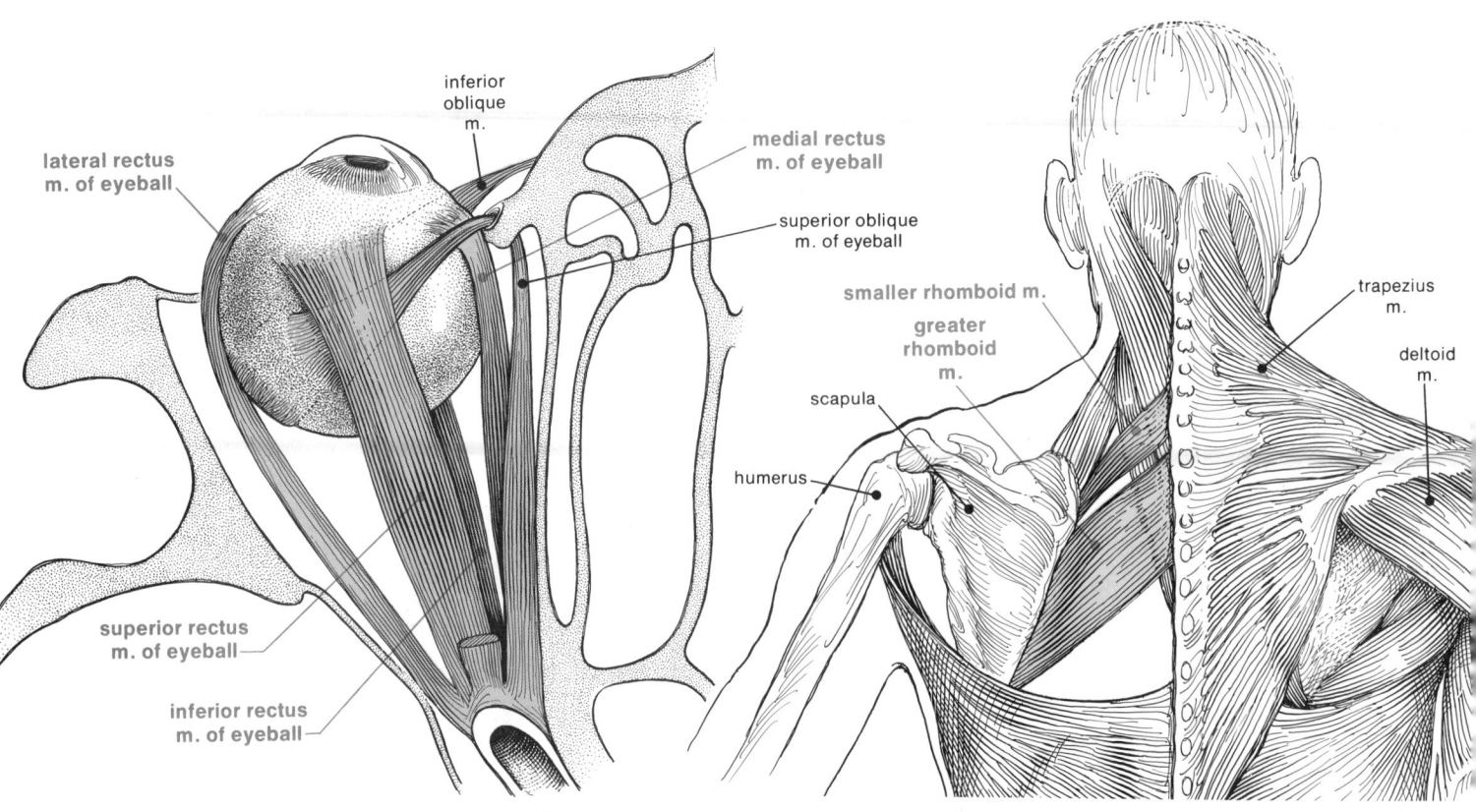

MUSCLE	ORIGIN	INSERTION	ACTION
rectococcygeus m. *m. rectococcygeus*	smooth muscle fibers in the pelvic fascia between the coccyx and rectum		
rectourethral m. *m. rectourethralis*	smooth muscle fibers in the pelvic fascia between the rectum and membranous urethra of male		
rectouterine m. *m. rectouterinus*	bundle of smooth muscle fibers in pelvic fascia between rectum and cervix of uterus		
rectus m. of abdomen *m. rectus abdominis*	pubic crest, pubic symphysis	xiphoid process, fifth to seventh costal cartilages	tenses abdominal wall, draws thorax downward
rectus m. of eyeball, inferior *m. rectus inferior bulbi*	common tendon ring around the optic canal	lower part of sclera just posterior to corneoscleral junction	rotates eyeball downward and somewhat medially
rectus m. of eyeball, lateral *m. rectus lateralis bulbi*	common tendon ring around the optic canal	lateral part of sclera just posterior to corneoscleral junction	rotates eyeball laterally
rectus m. of eyeball, medial *m. rectus medialis bulbi*	common tendon ring around the optic canal	medial part of sclera just posterior to corneoscleral junction	rotates eyeball medially
rectus m. of eyeball, superior *m. rectus superior bulbi*	common tendon ring around the optic canal	top part of sclera just posterior to corneoscleral junction	rotates eyeball upward and somewhat medially
rectus m. of head, anterior *m. rectus capitis anterior*	lateral portion of first vertebra (atlas)	basilar portion of occipital bone	flexes and supports head
rectus m. of head, lateral *m. rectus capitis lateralis*	transverse process of first vertebra (atlas)	jugular process of occipital bone	aids in lateral movements of head, supports head
rectus m. of head, posterior, greater *m. rectus capitis posterior major*	spinous process of second vertebra (axis)	occipital bone	extends head
rectus m. of head, poosterior, smaller *m. rectus capitis posterior minor*	posterior tubercle of first vertebra (atlas)	occipital bone	extends head
rectus m. of thigh *m. rectus of femoris*	anterior inferior iliac spine, rim of acetabulum	base of patella (kneecap)	extends leg and flexes thigh
rhomboid m., greater *m. rhomboideus major*	spinous processes of second through fifth thoracic vertebrae	vertebral margin of scapula	adducts and laterally rotates scapula
rhomboid m., smaller *m. rhomboideus minor*	spinous processes of seventh cervical and first thoracic vertebrae and lower part of nuchal ligament	vertebral margin of scapula above spine	adducts and laterally rotates scapula
risorius m. *m. risorius*	fascia over masseter muscle; platysma muscle	skin at angle of mouth	retracts angle of mouth

muscle | muscle

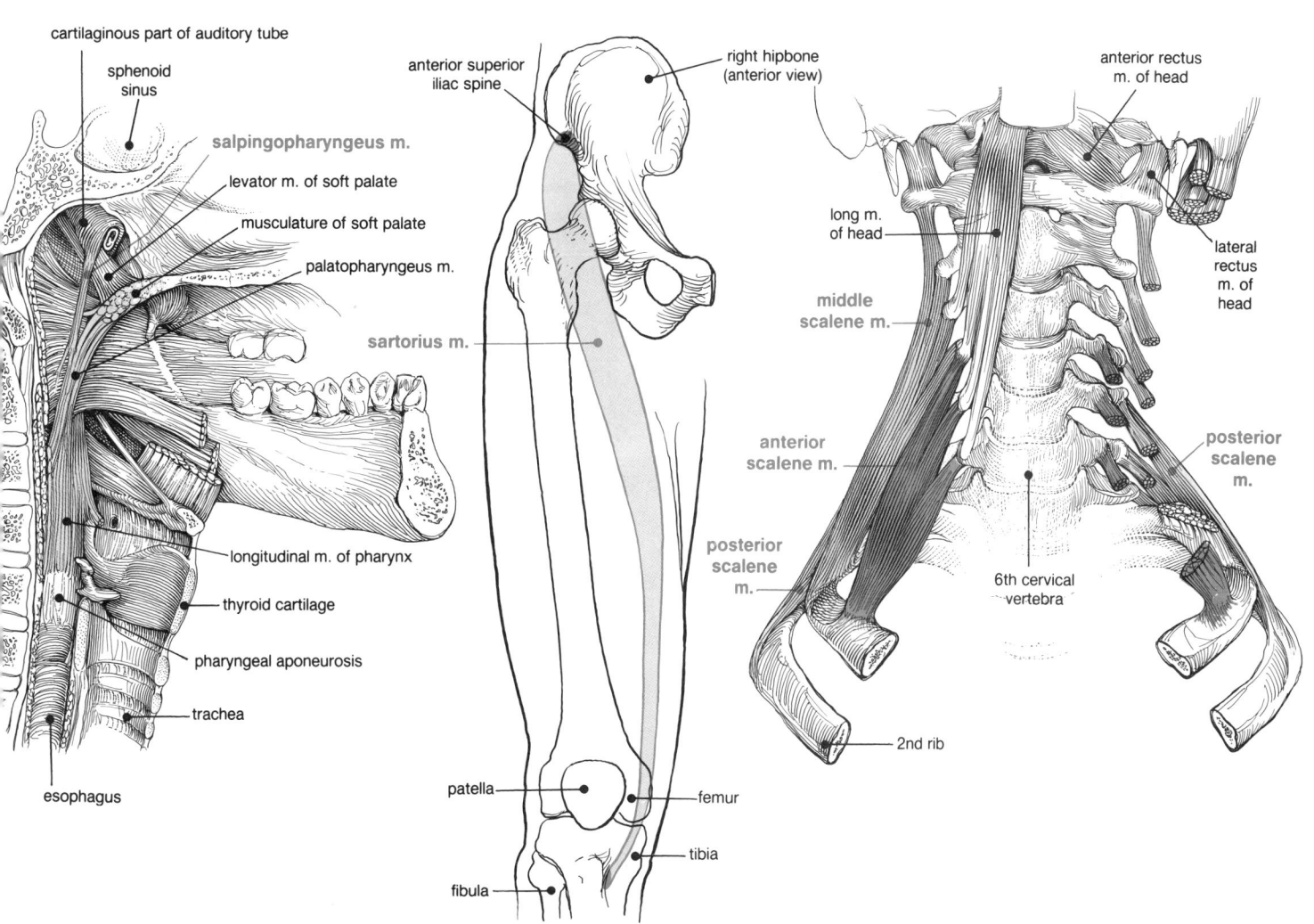

Labels on illustration:

cartilaginous part of auditory tube
sphenoid sinus
salpingopharyngeus m.
levator m. of soft palate
musculature of soft palate
palatopharyngeus m.
longitudinal m. of pharynx
thyroid cartilage
pharyngeal aponeurosis
trachea
esophagus

anterior superior iliac spine
right hipbone (anterior view)
sartorius m.
patella
femur
tibia
fibula

anterior rectus m. of head
long m. of head
lateral rectus m. of head
middle scalene m.
anterior scalene m.
posterior scalene m.
posterior scalene m.
6th cervical vertebra
2nd rib

MUSCLE	ORIGIN	INSERTION	ACTION
rotator m.'s *mm. rotatores*	transverse processes of all vertebrae below second cervical	lamina above vertebra of origin	extend and rotate the vertebral column toward opposite side
sacrococcygeus m., dorsal *m. sacrococcygeus dorsalis*	a muscular or tendinous slip from the dorsal aspect of the sacrum to the coccyx		
sacrococcygeus m., ventral *m. sacrococcygeus ventralis*	a muscular or tendinous slip from the lower sacral vertebrae to the coccyx		
sacrospinal m.	see erector muscle of spine		
salpingopharyngeus m. *m. salpingopharyngeus*	cartilage of auditory (pharyngotympanic) tube	wall of pharynx; thyroid cartilage	elevates pharynx
sartorius m. *m. sartorius*	anterior superior iliac spine	upper medial surface of tibia	flexes thigh and leg
scalene m., anterior *m. scalenus anterior*	transverse processes of third to sixth cervical verebrae	scalene tubercle of first rib	raises first rib, stabilizes or inclines neck to the side
scalene m., middle *m. scalenus medius*	transverse processes of first six cervical vertebrae	upper surface of first and second ribs	raises first rib, stabilizes or inclines neck to the side
scalene m., posterior *m. scalenus posterior*	transverse processes of fifth to seventh cervical vertebrae	outer surface of upper border of second rib	raises second rib, stabilizes or inclines neck to the side
scalene m., smallest *m. scalenus minimus*	occasional extra muscle fibers or slip of posterior scalene muscle		
semimembranous m. *m. semimembranosus*	tuberosity of ischium	medial condyle of tibia	extends thigh, flexes and rotates leg medially
semispinal m. of head *m. semispinalis capitis*	transverse processes of six upper thoracic and four lower cervical vertebrae	occipital bone between superior and inferior nuchal lines	rotates head and draws it backward
semispinal m. of neck *m. semispinalis cervicis*	transverse processes of upper six thoracic vertebrae	spinous processes of second through sixth cervical vertebrae	extends and rotates vertebral column
semispinal m. of thorax *m. semispinalis thoracis*	transverse processes of lower six thoracic vertebrae	spinous processes of upper six thoracic and lower two cervical vertebrae	extends and rotates vertebral column

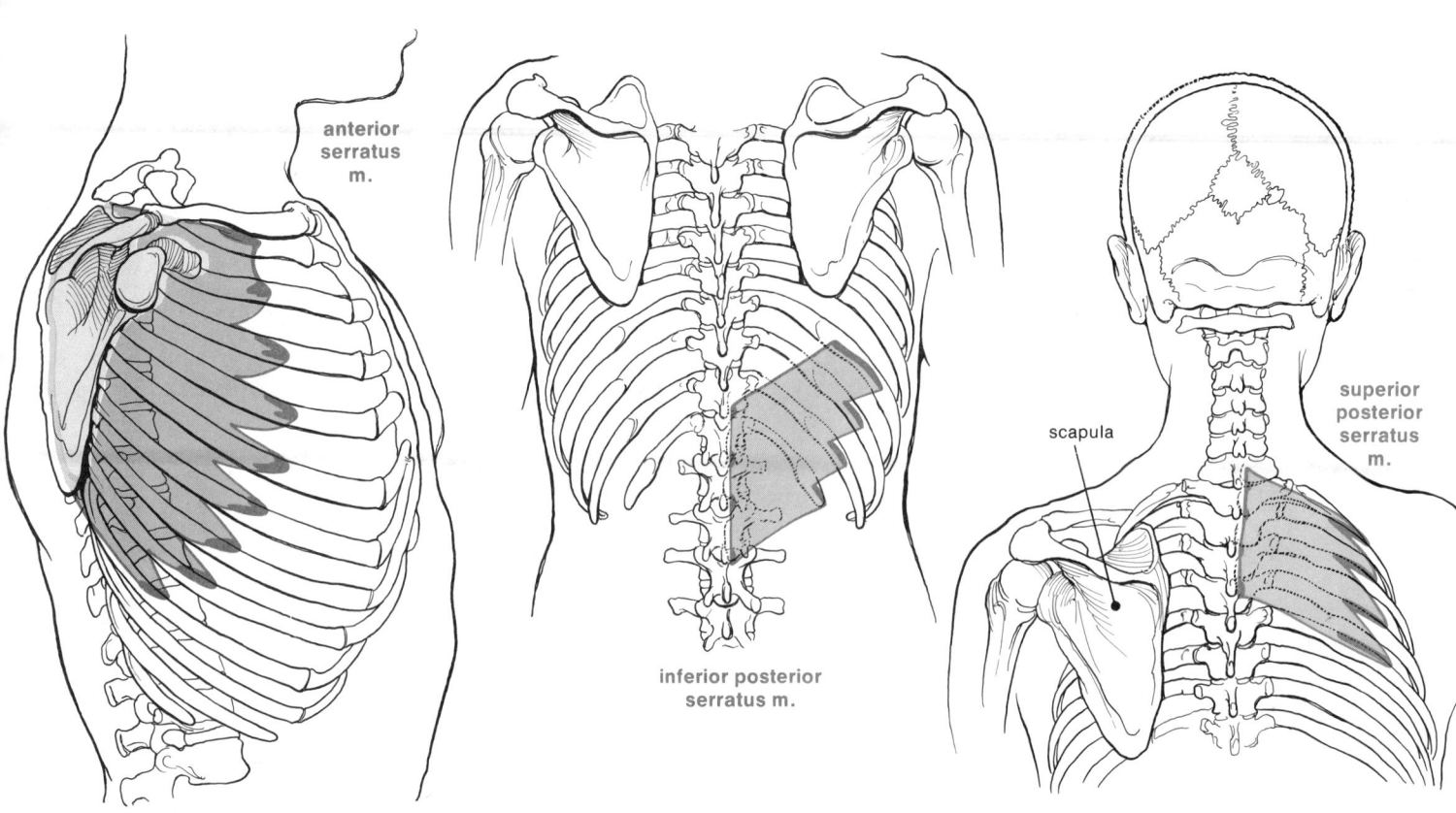

anterior serratus m.

inferior posterior serratus m.

scapula

superior posterior serratus m.

MUSCLE	ORIGIN	INSERTION	ACTION
semitendinous m. *m. semitendinosus*	tuberosity of ischium (in common with biceps muscle of thigh)	upper part of tibia near tibial tuberosity	flexes and rotates leg medially, extends thigh
serratus m., anterior *m. serratus anterior*	lateral surface of eight or nine uppermost ribs	vertebral border of scapula	draws scapula forward and laterally, rotates scapula in raising arm
serratus m., posterior, inferior *m. serratus posterior inferior*	spinous processes of last two thoracic and first two or three lumbar vertebrae, supraspinal ligament	inferior borders of the last four ribs, slightly beyond their angles	draws the ribs outward and downward (counteracting the inward pull of the diaphragm)
serratus m. posterior, superior *m. serratus posterior superior*	caudal part of nuchal ligament, spinous processes of the seventh cervical and first two or three thoracic vertebrae, supraspinal ligament	upper borders of the second, third, fourth, and fifth ribs, slightly beyond their angles	raises the ribs
soleus m. *m. soleus*	upper third of fibula, soleal line of tibia, tendinous arch	calcaneus by calcaneal tendon (*tendo calcaneus*)	plantarflexes foot
sphincter m. of anus, external *m. sphincter ani externus*	tip of coccyx, anococcygeal ligament	central tendon of perineum	closes anus
sphincter m. of anus, internal *m. sphincter ani internus*	muscular ring surrounding approximately 2.5 cm of the anal canal, about 6.0 mm from the orifice of the anus		aids in occlusion of anal aperture and expulsion of feces
sphincter m. of bile duct *m. sphincter choledochus*	a circular muscle around lower part of the bile duct within the wall of the duodenum (part of the sphincter muscle of hepatopancreatic ampulla)		constricts lower part of bile duct
sphincter m. of hepatopancreatic ampulla sphincter of Oddi *m. sphincter ampullae hepatopancreaticae*	circular muscle around terminal part of main pancreatic duct and common bile duct, including the hepatopancreatic ampulla		constricts both lower part of common bile duct and main pancreatic duct
sphincter m. of pupil *m. sphincter pupillae*	circular fibers of iris arranged in a narrow band about 1 mm in width		constricts pupil
sphincter m. of pylorus *m. sphincter pylori*	thick muscular ring at the end of the stomach		acts as valve to close lumen
sphincter m. of urethra external urethral sphincter m. *m. sphincter urethrae*	ramus of pubis	fibers interdigitate around urethra	closes urethra
sphincter m. of urinary bladder *m. sphincter vesicae urinariae*	thick muscular ring toward the lower part of bladder around internal urethral orifice		acts as valve to close internal urethral orifice

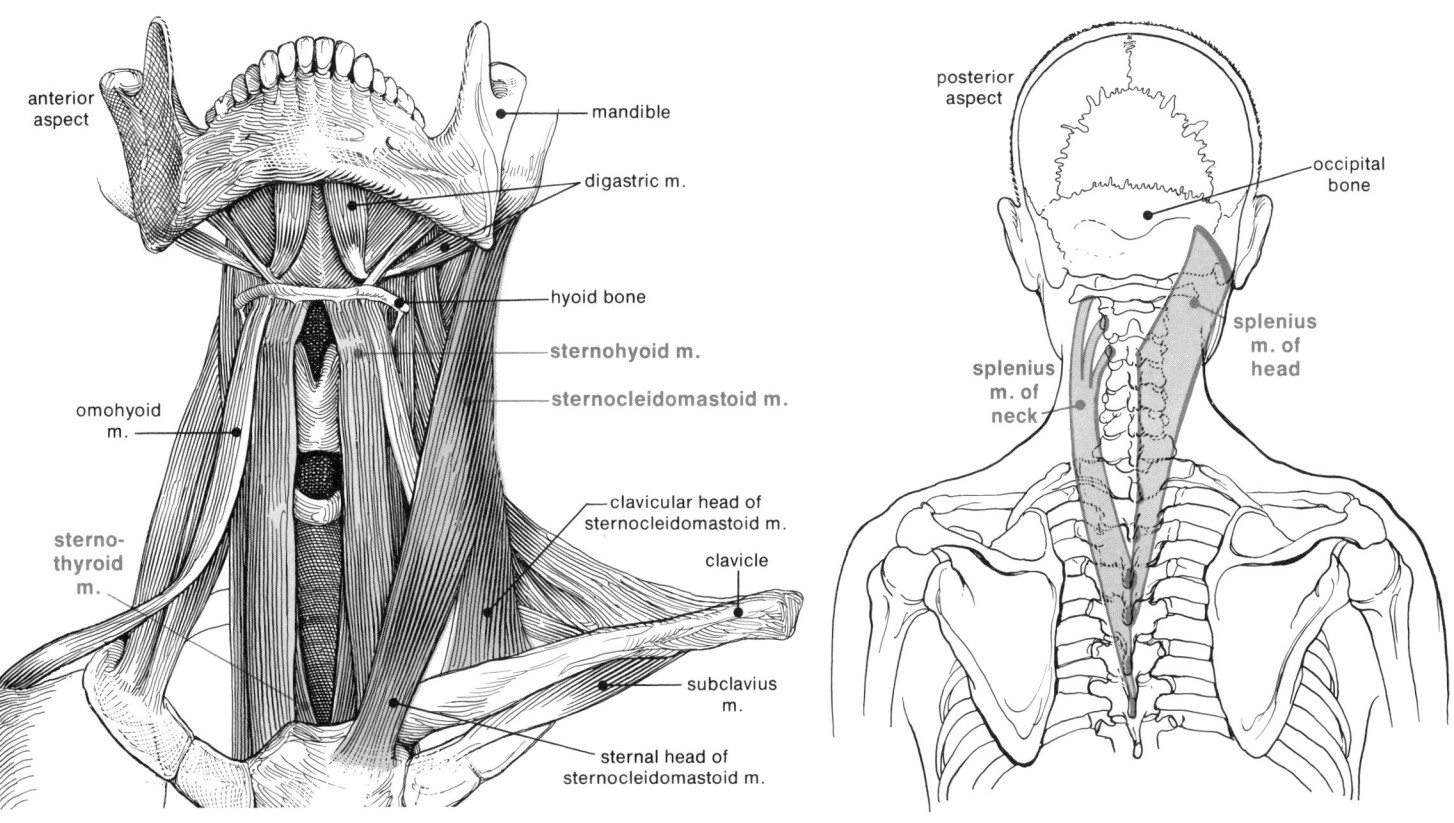

anterior aspect

mandible

digastric m.

hyoid bone

sternohyoid m.

sternocleidomastoid m.

omohyoid m.

clavicular head of sternocleidomastoid m.

clavicle

sterno-thyroid m.

subclavius m.

sternal head of sternocleidomastoid m.

posterior aspect

occipital bone

splenius m. of head

splenius m. of neck

MUSCLE	ORIGIN	INSERTION	ACTION
sphincter m. of vagina *m. sphincter vaginae*	pubic symphysis	interdigitates around and interlaces into vaginal barrel	constricts vaginal orifice
sphincter of Oddi	see sphincter muscle of hepatopancreatic ampulla		
spinal m. of head biventer cervicis m. *m. spinalis capitis*	usually inseparably connected with semispinal muscle of head		
spinal m. of neck *m. spinalis cervicis*	transverse processes of upper six thoracic and seventh cervical vertebrae	spinous processes of second, third, and fourth cervical vertebrae	extends vertebral column
spinal m. of thorax *m. spinalis thoracis*	spinous processes of upper two lumbar and lower two thoraic vertebrae	spinous processes of second through ninth thoracic vertebrae	extends vertebral column
splenius m. of head *m. splenius capitis*	spinous processes of upper thoracic vertebrae	mastoid process and superior nuchal line	inclines and rotates head
splenius m. of neck splenius colli m. *m. splenius cervicis*	nuchal ligament, spinous processes of third to sixth thoracic vertebrae	posterior tubercles of the transverse processes of upper two or three cervical vertebrae	extends head and neck, turns head toward the same side
stapedius m. *m. stapedius*	wall of the conical cavity inside the pyramid of middle ear chamber	posterior surface of neck of stapes	pulls head of stapes posteriorly, tilting the baseplate
sternal m. *m. sternalis*	small superficial muscular band at sternal end of greater pectoral muscle (*m. pectoralis major*), parallel with the margin of sternum		
sternocleidomastoid m. *m. sternocleidomastoideus*	*sternal head:* anterior surface of manubrium; *clavicular head:* medial third of clavicle	mastoid process, superior nuchal line of occipital bone	rotates and extends head, flexes vertebral column
sternocostal m.	see transverse muscle of thorax		
sternohyoid m. *m. sternohyoideus*	medial end of clavicle, posterior surface of manubrium, first costal cartilage	lower border of body of hyoid bone	depresses hyoid bone and larynx
sternothyroid m. *m. sternothyrcideus*	dorsal surface of upper part of sternum and medial edge of first costal cartilage	oblique line on lamina of thyroid cartilage	draws thyroid cartilage downward
styloglossus m. *m. styloglossus*	lower end of styloid process, stylomandibular ligament	*longitudinal part:* side of tongue near dorsal surface; *oblique part:* over hyoglossus muscle	raises and retracts tongue

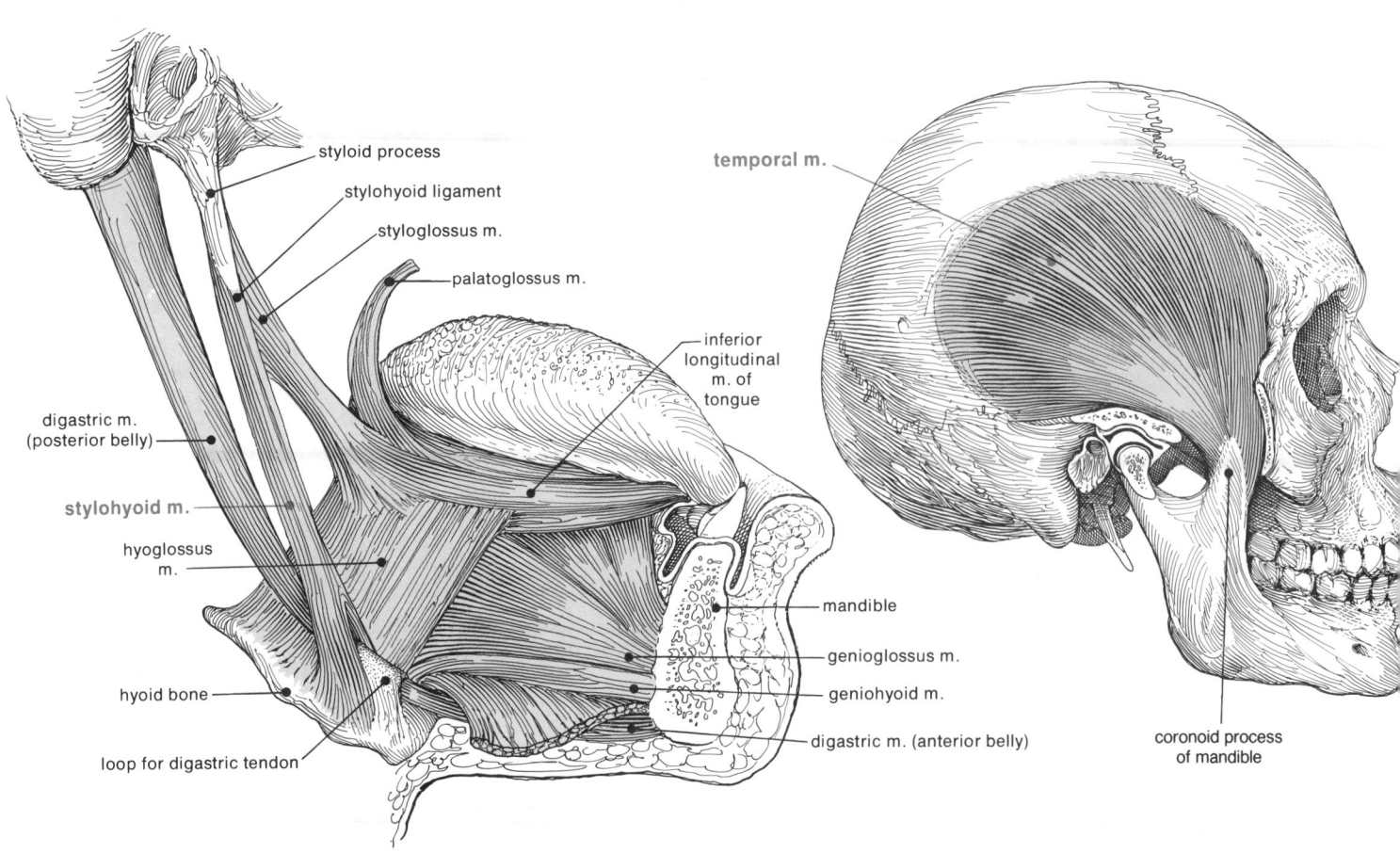

styloid process
stylohyoid ligament
styloglossus m.
palatoglossus m.
inferior longitudinal m. of tongue
temporal m.
digastric m. (posterior belly)
stylohyoid m.
hyoglossus m.
hyoid bone
loop for digastric tendon
mandible
genioglossus m.
geniohyoid m.
digastric m. (anterior belly)
coronoid process of mandible

MUSCLE	ORIGIN	INSERTION	ACTION
stylohyoid m. *m. stylohyoideus*	posterior and lateral surfaces of the styloid process near the base	body of hyoid bone at its junction with the greater horn (cornu)	draws hyoid bone upward and backward
stylopharyngeus m. *m. stylopharyngeus*	root of styloid process	borders of thyroid cartilage, wall of pharynx	elevates and opens pharynx
subclavius m. *m. sbuclavius*	junction of first rib and costal cartilages	lower surface of clavicle	depresses lateral end of clavicle
subcostal m.'s *mm. subcostales*	inner surface of ribs near angle	lower inner surface of second or third rib below rib of origin	draw adjacent ribs together
subscapular m. *m. subscapularis*	subscapular fossa	lesser tubercle of humerus	rotates arm medially
supinator m. *m. supinator*	lateral epicondyle of humerus, supinator crest of ulna	upper third of radius	supinates the forearm
suprahyoid m.'s *mm. suprahyoidei*	the group of muscles attached to the upper part of the hyoid bone including the digastric, stylohyoid, mylohyoid, and geniohyoid muscles		
supraspinous m. *m. supraspinatus*	supraspinous fossa	superior aspect of greater tubercle of humerus	abducts arm
suspensory m. of duodenum ligament of Treitz *m. suspensorius duodeni*	connective tissue around celiac artery and right crus of diaphragm	superior border of duodenojejunal junction, part of ascending duodenum	acts as suspensory ligament of the duodenum
tarsal m., inferior *m. tarsalis superior*	inferior rectus muscle of eyeball	tarsal plate of lower eyelid	widens palpebral fissure
tarsal m., superior lamina profundus m. *m. tarsalis superior*	aponeurosis of levator muscle of upper eyelid	tarsus plate of upper eyelid	raises upper eyelid
temporal m. *m. temporalis*	temporal fossa	coronoid process of mandible	closes mouth, clenches teeth, retracts lower jaw
temporoparietal m. *m. temporoparietalis*	temporal fascia above ear	epicranial aponeurosis	tightens scalp
tensor m. of fascia lata *m. tensor fasciae latae*	iliac crest	iliotibial tract of fascia lata	tenses fascia lata
tensor m. of soft palate *m. tensor veli palatini*	spine of sphenoid, scaphoid fossa of pterygoid process, cartilage and membrane of the auditory tube	midline of aponeurosis of soft palate, wall of auditory tube	elevates palate and opens auditory tube

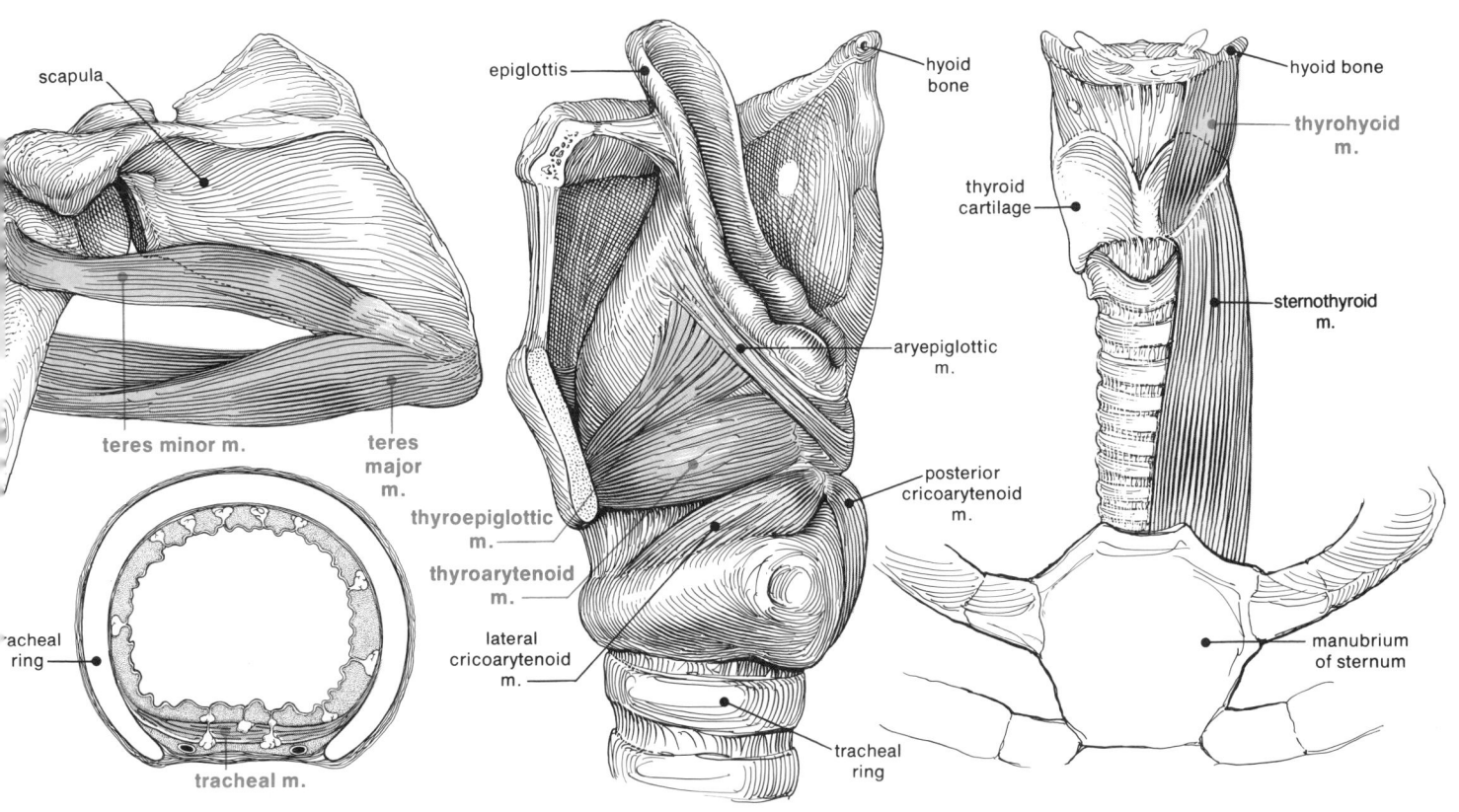

scapula

teres minor m.

teres major m.

epiglottis

hyoid bone

thyroepiglottic m.

thyroarytenoid m.

lateral cricoarytenoid m.

aryepiglottic m.

posterior cricoarytenoid m.

tracheal ring

hyoid bone

thyrohyoid m.

thyroid cartilage

sternothyroid m.

manubrium of sternum

tracheal ring

tracheal m.

MUSCLE	ORIGIN	INSERTION	ACTION
tensor m. of tympanum tensor m. of tympanic membrane (ear drum) *m. tensor tympani*	cartilaginous portion of auditory (eustachian) tube and adjoining part of great wing of sphenoid bone	manubrium of malleus near its root	draws tympanic membrane medially, thus increasing its tension
teres major m. *m. teres major*	inferior axillary border of scapula	crest of lesser tubercle of humerus	adducts and rotates arm medially
teres minor m. *m. teres minor*	axillary border of scapula	inferior aspect of greater tubercle of humerus	rotates arm laterally
thyroarytenoid m. *m. thyroarytneoideus*	inside of thyroid cartilage	base of arytenoid cartilage	aids in closure of laryngeal inlet
thyroepiglottic m. *m. thyroepiglotticus*	inside of thyroid cartilage	margin of epiglottis	depresses the epiglottis
thyrohyoid m. *m. thyrohyoideus*	oblique line of thyroid cartilage	greater horn (*cornu*) of hyoid bone	elevates larynx, depresses hyoid bone
tibial m., anterior *m. tibialis anterior*	upper two-thirds of tibia, interosseous membrane	first metatarsal bone, first cuneiform bone	dorsiflexes and inverts foot
tibial m., posterior *m. tibialis posterior*	interosseous membrane adjoining tibia and fibula	navicular, with slips to three cuneiform bones; cuboid, second, third, and fourth metatarsals	principal inverter of foot, aids in plantar flexion of foot
tracheal m. *m. trachealis*	anastomosing transverse muscular bands connecting the ends of the tracheal rings		
trachelomastoid m.	see longissimus muscle of head		
tragus m. *m. tragicus*	a band of vertical muscular fibers on the outer surface of the tragus of the ear		
transverse m. of abdomen *m. transversus abdominis*	7th–12th costal cartilages, thoracolumbar fascia, iliac crest, inguinal ligament	xiphoid process, linea alba, conjoint tendon to pubis	supports abdominal viscera
transverse m. of auricle *m. transversus auriculae*	see auricular muscle, transverse		
transverse m. of chin *m. transversus menti*	superficial muscular fibers of depressor muscle of angle of mouth (triangular muscle) which turn back and cross to the opposite side below the chin		
transverse m. of nape *m. transversus nuchae*	an occasional muscle passing between the tendons of the trapezius and sternocleidomastoid muscles		
transverse m. of perineum, deep *m. transversus perinei profundus*	inferior ramus of ischium	central tendon of perineum, external anal sphincter	fixes central tendon of perineum

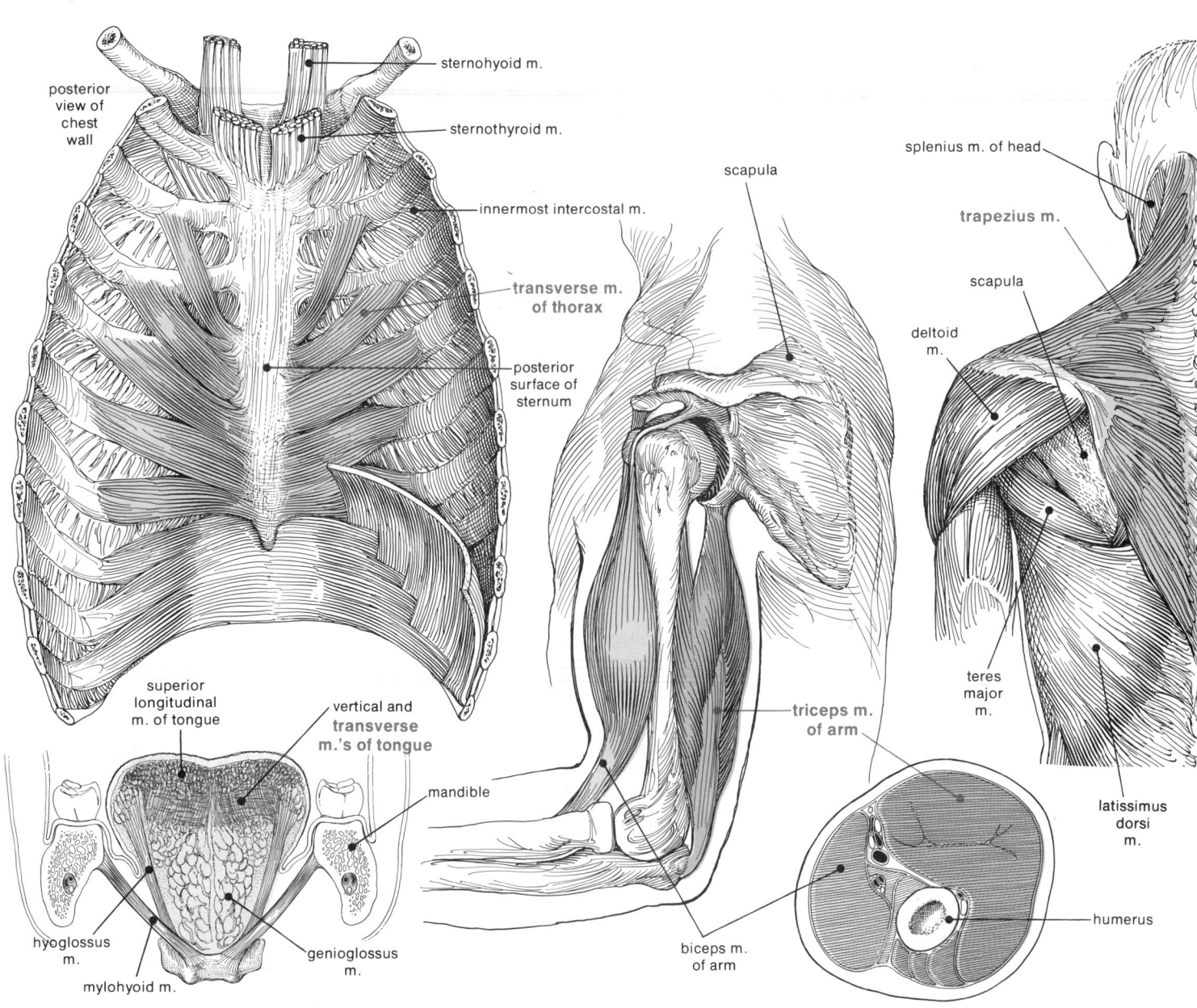

posterior view of chest wall

sternohyoid m.

sternothyroid m.

innermost intercostal m.

transverse m. of thorax

posterior surface of sternum

scapula

splenius m. of head

trapezius m.

scapula

deltoid m.

superior longitudinal m. of tongue

vertical and transverse m.'s of tongue

mandible

triceps m. of arm

teres major m.

hyoglossus m.

mylohyoid m.

genioglossus m.

biceps m. of arm

latissimus dorsi m.

humerus

MUSCLE	ORIGIN	INSERTION	ACTION
transverse m. of perineum, superficial *m. transversus perinei superficialis*	ramus of ischium near tuberosity	central tendon of perineum	supports central tendon of perineum
transverse m. of thorax sternocostal m. *m. transversus thoracis*	xiphoid process, posterior surface of lower part of sternum	second to sixth costal cartilages	narrows chest, draws costal cartilages downward
transverse m. of tongue *m. transversus linguae*	median fibrous septum of tongue	submucous fibrous tissue at sides of tongue	narrows and elongates tongue
trapezius m. *m. trapezius*	superior nuchal line of occipital bone, nuchal ligament, spinous processes of seventh cervical and all thoracic vertebrae	*superior part:* posterior border of lateral third of clavicle; *middle part:* medial margin of acromion, superior lip of posterior border of scapular spine; *inferior part:* tubercle at apex of medial end of scapular spine	elevates shoulder, rotates scapula to raise shoulder in full abduction and flexion of arm, draws scapula backward
triangular m.	see depressor muscle of angle of mouth		
triceps m. of arm *m. triceps brachii*	*long head:* infraglenoid tubercle of scapula; *lateral head:* proximal portion of humerus; *medial head:* distal half of humerus	olecranon process of ulna	extends arm and forearm

muscle | **muscle**

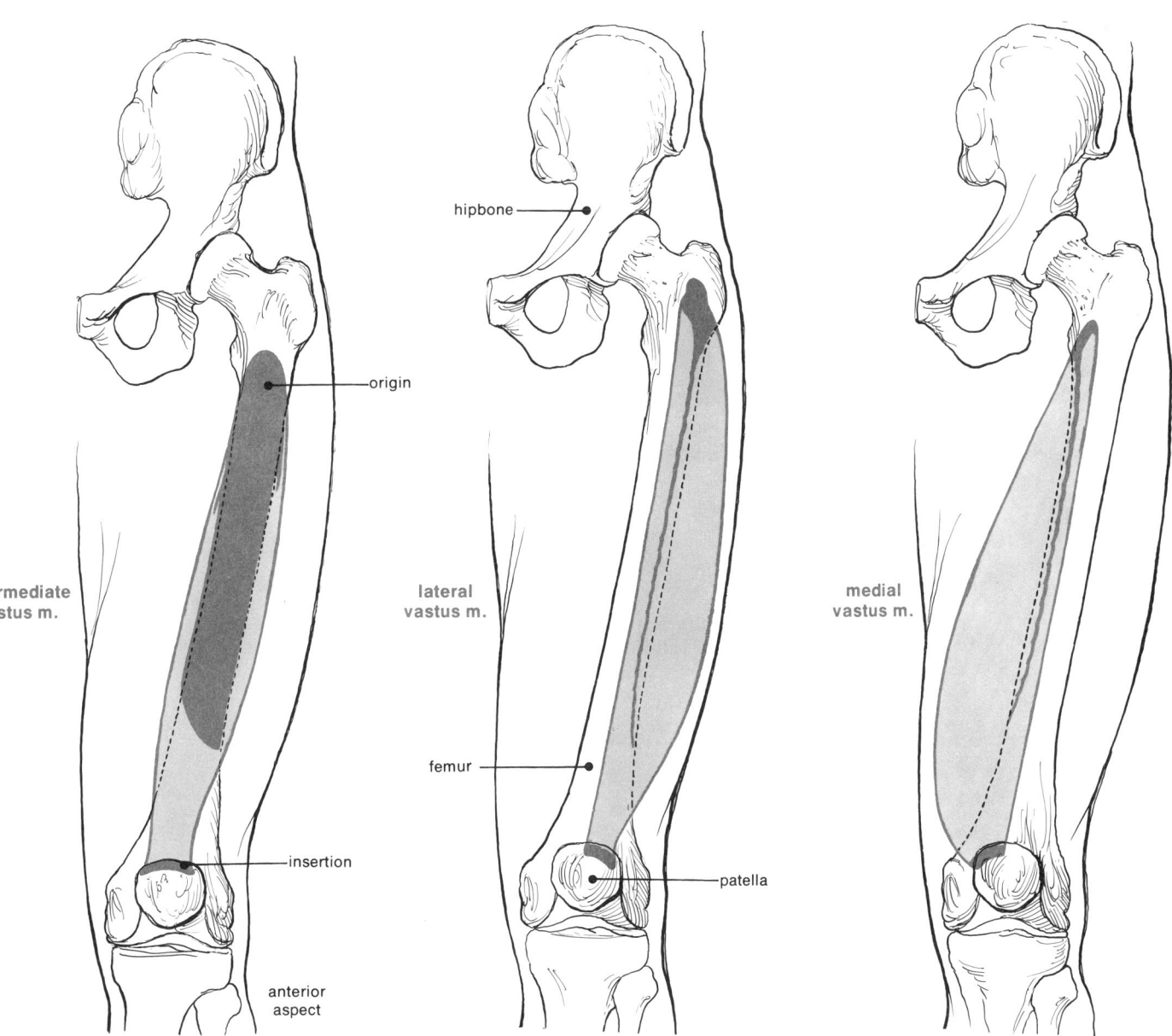

intermediate
vastus m.

origin

insertion

anterior
aspect

hipbone

lateral
vastus m.

femur

patella

medial
vastus m.

MUSCLE	ORIGIN	INSERTION	ACTION
triceps of calf *m. triceps surae*	combined gastrocnemius and soleus muscles; its tendon of insertion is the calcaneal tendon		
uvula m. *m. uvulae*	palatine aponeurosis and posterior nasal spine of palatine bone	mucous membrane of uvula	elevates uvula
vastus m., intermediate *m. vastus intermedius*	anterior and lateral surface of femur	common tendon of quadriceps muscle of thigh, patella	extends leg
vastus m., lateral *m. vastus lateralis*	lateral aspect of femur	common tendon of quadriceps muscle of thigh, patella	extends leg
vastus m., medial *m. vastus medialis*	medial aspect of femur	common tendon of quadriceps muscle of thigh, patella	extends leg
vertical m. of tongue *m. verticalis linguae*	dorsal fascia of tongue	sides and ventral surface of tongue	aids in mastication, swallowing, and speech by altering shape of tongue
vocal m. *m. vocalis*	lamina of thyroid cartilage	vocal process of arytenoid cartilage	adjusts tension of vocal cords
zygomatic m., greater *m. zygomaticus major*	zygomatic arch	angle of mouth	draws upper lip upward
zygomatic m., smaller *m. zygomaticus minor*	malar surface of zygomatic bone	upper lip	aids in forming nasolabial furrow (muscle of facial expression)

muscle | muscle

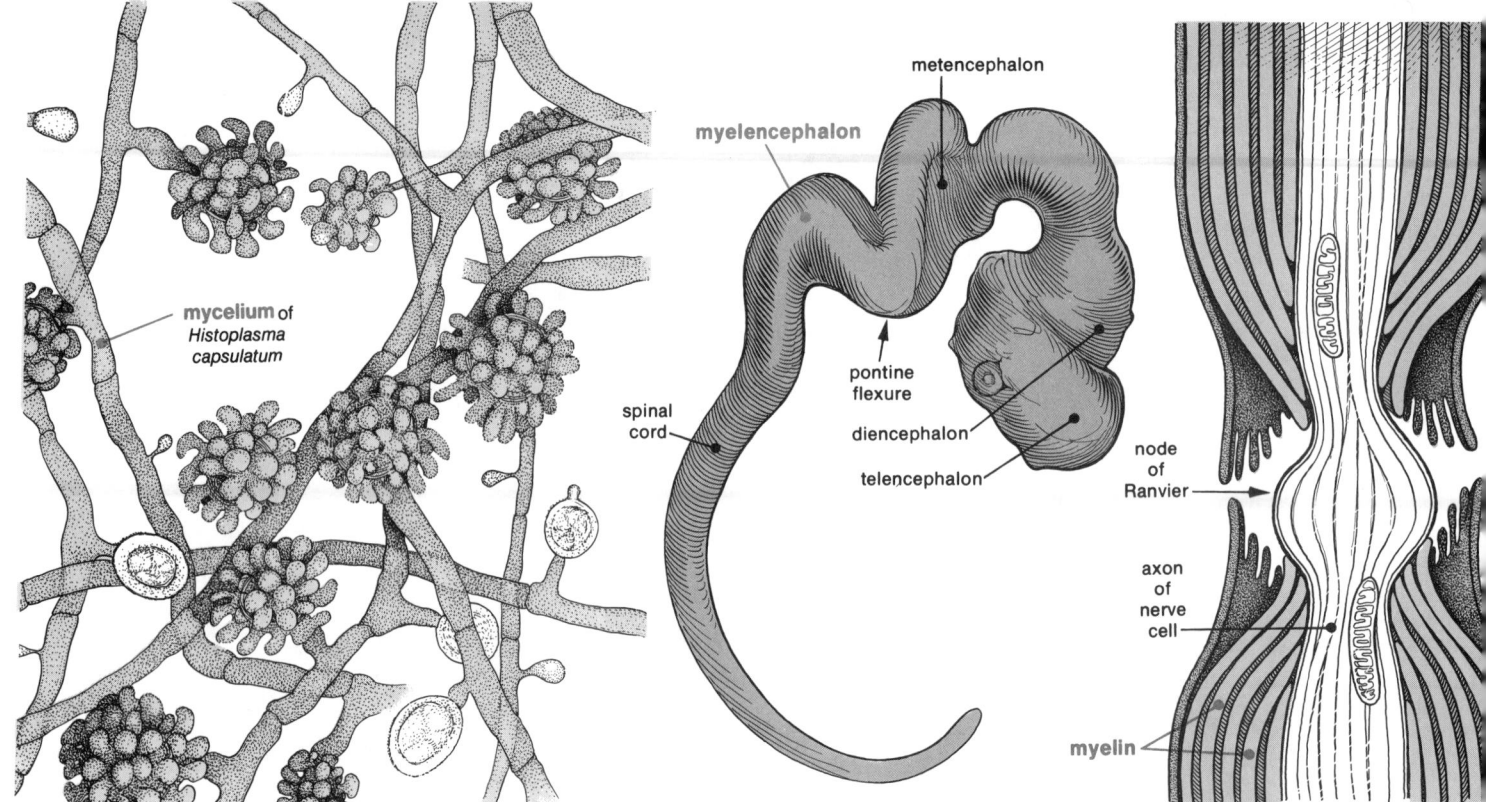

mycelium of *Histoplasma capsulatum*

metencephalon

myelencephalon

spinal cord

pontine flexure

diencephalon

telencephalon

node of Ranvier

axon of nerve cell

myelin

muscle-bound Having overdeveloped muscles which limit movements; usually due to excessive exercise.

muscular 1. Of, or relating to, a muscle or muscles. 2. Provided with well-developed muscles.

muscularis The muscular layer of the wall of a tubular or hollow structure.

muscularize To change into muscle, as the conversion of scar tissue into muscle tissue in a wound of a muscle.

musculature, musculation The system of muscles in the body or a body part.

musculoaponeurotic Relating to muscle and aponeurosis.

musculocutaneous Relating to muscle and skin, as certain nerves that supply both structures.

musculomembranous Relating to or composed of muscular and membranous tissues.

musculoskeletal Relating to the muscles and skeleton.

musculospiral Denoting the distribution of the radial nerve which innervates certain muscles of the arm and forearm and spirals across the back of the humerus.

musculotropic Acting upon muscular tissue.

Musset's sign Rhythmic nodding of the head, occurring in incompetence of the aortic valve.

mutagen Any agent that causes a permanent change in the genetic material (mutation), as radioactive substances, ultraviolet light, etc.

mutagenesis The formation of mutation.

mutagenic Causing mutation.

mutant An organism that differs from the parental strain as a result of having a gene that has undergone structural change.

mutase One of various enzymes that promote the apparent migration of a phosphate group from one hydroxyl group to another of the same molecule.

mutation 1. A permanent, heritable, structural change in a gene. 2. The modified gene.

   point m. One involving minute sections of a chromosome (the purine or pyrimidine bases of a single gene), as seen in sickle cell anemia.

mute A person who is unable to speak.

mutilation 1. Damaging or removing an essential part of the body. 2. The state of being mutilated.

mutism Inability to speak.

mutualism A state in which two dissimilar organisms live together with mutual benefit; a form of symbiosis.

myadenoma A benign tumor derived from glandular epithelial tissue.

myalgia Muscle pain.

myasthenia Weakness of muscle.

   m. gravis A chronic disease characterized by variable degrees of muscular weakness, which may progress to paralysis; it frequently begins in the muscles of the eyes and is often associated with abnormalities of the thymus; the disease attacks the point at which nerve meets muscle, interfering with the normal release of acetylcholine (Ach) and subsequent depolarization of the end plate and excitement of the muscle fiber; may be caused by circulating antibodies to Ach receptors.

myatonia, myatony Absence of muscle tone.

myatrophy See myoatrophy.

mycelial Relating to mycelium; having the filamentous appearance of a mold colony.

mycelium The network of threadlike filaments (hyphae) constituting the body or vegetative portion of a fungus.

mycete A fungus.

mycetism, mycetismus Mushroom poisoning.

mycetogenic, mycetogenetic Caused by fungi.

mycetoma See maduromycosis.

Mycetozoa The slime animals; microscopic animal forms, similar to fungi and often regarded as such.

mycid A secondary lesion occurring in certain mycotic infections.

mycobacteria Microorganisms of the genus *Mycobacterium*.

Mycobacterium A genus (family Mycobacteriaceae) of aerobic gram-positive, acid-fast, nonmotile, rod-shaped bacteria; some of its species are called bacilli.

   M. leprae The causative agent of leprosy. Also called Hansen's bacillus.

   M. tuberculosis The causative agent of tuberculosis in man and animals. Formerly called *Bacillus tuberculosis*.

mycodermomycosis, mycodermatitis A fungal infection of the skin.

mycogastritis Inflammation of the stomach caused by a fungus.

mycologist A specialist in fungi and fungal diseases.

mycology The branch of science concerned with the study of fungi.

Mycoplasma A genus of bacteria lacking a rigid cell wall, having instead a triple-layered membrane (thus occurring in many shapes); the smallest free-living organisms presently known, being intermediate in size between viruses and bacteria; some species are pathogenic.

   M. pneumoniae A species that is one of the main causes of primary atypical pneumonia in man. Also

called Eaton agent.

mycoplasma Any organism of the genus *Mycoplasma*.

   T-m.'s Microorganisms known to inhabit the urinary tracts of a large percentage of individuals; they have the capacity to attach to mammalian cells and to aggregate mucoproteins; so called because they form tiny colonies in agar (about 20 μm in diameter).

mycosis Disease caused by a fungus.

   deep m. See systemic mycosis.

   systemic m. A serious disease, often fatal, caused by various fungi that can invade the subcutaneous tissues and spread throughout the organism. Also called deep mycosis.

mycotic Relating to mycosis or any disease caused by fungi or vegetable microorganisms.

mydriasis Dilatation of the pupil.

mydriatic Any agent that dilates the pupil.

myectomy Surgical removal of a portion of a muscle.

myelencephalon The portion of the embryonic brain from which develop the medulla oblongata and the bulbar part of the fourth ventricle; together with the metencephalon it makes up the hindbrain or rhombencephalon.

myelic 1. Relating to the spinal cord. 2. Relating to bone marrow.

myelin A fatty substance that forms a major component of the sheath that surrounds and insulates the axon of some nerve cells.

myelinated Possessing a myelin sheath.

myelination The formation of a medullary sheath around a nerve fiber.

myelinolysis Demyelination; destruction of the myelin sheath of nerve fibers.

   central pontine m. Demyelination distributed about the midbase of the pons.

myelitis 1. Inflammation of the spinal cord. 2. Inflammation of the bone marrow.

   compression m. A progressive form of myelitis due to pressure on the spinal cord, as from a hemorrhage or tumor.

   concussion m. Inflammation following concussion of the spinal cord.

   disseminated m. Inflammation of several distinct areas of the spinal cord. Also called multiple focal myelitis.

   radiation m. Myelitis caused by excessive exposure to x rays.

   transverse m. Inflammation extending across the whole thickness of the spinal cord.

myeloarchitectonics The study of the arrangement of nerve fibers in the cerebral cortex.

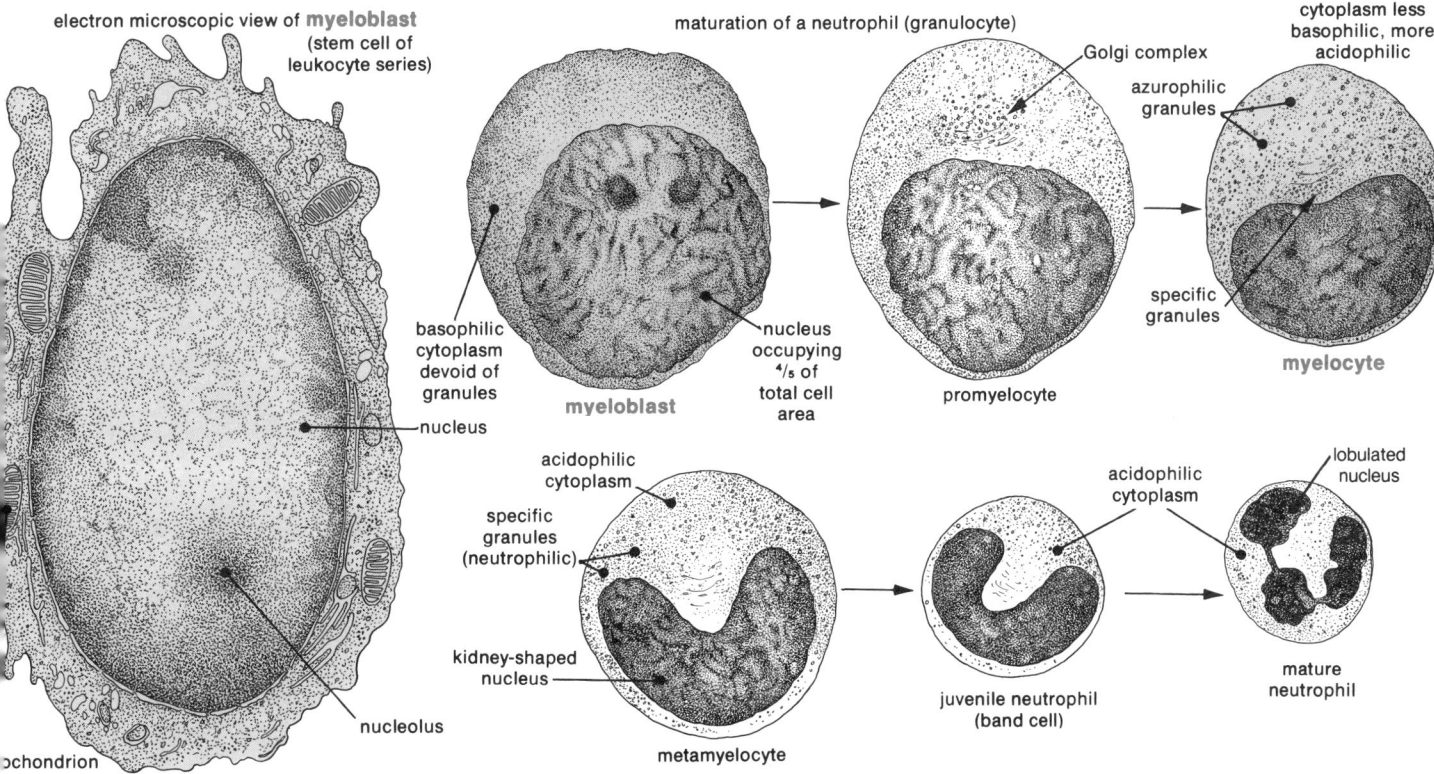

electron microscopic view of **myeloblast**
(stem cell of leukocyte series)

basophilic cytoplasm devoid of granules

nucleus

nucleolus

ochondrion

myeloblast

nucleus occupying ⁴/₅ of total cell area

maturation of a neutrophil (granulocyte)

Golgi complex

promyelocyte

cytoplasm less basophilic, more acidophilic

azurophilic granules

specific granules

myelocyte

acidophilic cytoplasm

specific granules (neutrophilic)

kidney-shaped nucleus

acidophilic cytoplasm

lobulated nucleus

metamyelocyte

juvenile neutrophil (band cell)

mature neutrophil

---

myeloblast A cell in the early stage of development, occurring normally in bone marrow; the first recognizable cell of the granulocytic (myeloid) series; it has a large, oval nucleus that occupies about four-fifths of the cell, usually containing two to five nucleoli; it can differentiate into a neutrophilic, eosinophilic, or basophilic granulocyte. Also called granuloblast.

myeloblastemia The presence of myeloblasts in the blood.

myeloblastoma Malignant tumor composed chiefly of myeloblasts, occurring in certain diseases such as myeloblastic leukemia.

myeloblastosis The presence of a large number of myeloblasts in the blood or tissues, as in acute leukemia.

myelocele Developmental defect in which the vertebral arches are absent, leaving an open groove lined with imperfect spinal cord tissue and through which cerebrospinal fluid drains. Also called rachischisis; spondyloschisis.

myelocyst A cyst originating from a rudimentary medullary canal in the central nervous system.

myelocystic Relating to or of the nature of a myelocyst.

myelocystocele The hernial protrusion of spinal cord substance through a defect in the vertebral column.

myelocyte 1. A young cell of the granulocytic (myeloid) series, developed from the promyelocyte and occurring normally in red bone marrow; its main characteristics are: a cytoplasm containing specific neutrophilic granules, an oval nucleus with the nuclear chromatin appearing as thick strands, and no discernible nucleoli. 2. A nerve cell in the gray matter of the brain or spinal cord.

myelocytosis The increase of myelocytes in the circulating blood above the normal range.

myeloencephalic Relating to the spinal cord and brain.

myeloencephalitis Acute inflammation of the brain and spinal cord. Also called encephalomyelitis.

myelofibrosis A myeloproliferative disorder marked by fibrosis of the bone marrow, associated with abnormal proliferation of blood-forming elements, myeloid metaplasia of the spleen and liver, and anemia. Also called myelosclerosis with myeloid metaplasia; agnogenic myeloid metaplasia; osteomyelofibrotic syndrome; megakaryocytic splenomegaly.

myelogenesis Development of the bone marrow.

myelogenic, myelogenetic Developed in the bone marrow.

myelography Roentgenography of the spinal cord

after introduction of a radiopaque substance into the spinal arachnoid space.

myeloid 1. Relating to, derived from, or of the nature of bone marrow. 2. Of, or relating to, the spinal cord.

myeloma A tumor composed of cell types normally found in bone marrow.

multiple m. Disease characterized by the appearance of scattered malignant tumors in various bones of the body; associated with the production of abnormal globulins and the presence of Bence Jones protein in the urine; the condition occurs mostly in persons in the sixth to eighth decade of life and affects males more often than females. Also called myelomatosis; plasma cell myeloma.

plasma cell m. A general term applied to a number of disorders having in common the proliferation of plasma cells or the formation of abnormal proteins, such as multiple myeloma, soft tissue plasmacytomas, and plasma cell leukemia.

myelomalacia Softening of the spinal cord.

myelomatosis See myeloma, multiple.

myelomeningitis Inflammation of the spinal cord and its membranes.

myelomeningocele See meningomyelocele.

myelon The spinal cord.

myeloneuritis Inflammation of the spinal cord and one or more peripheral nerves.

myelonic Of, or relating to, the spinal cord.

myelopathy Any disease of the spinal cord.

myelophthisis 1. Atrophy or wasting of the spinal cord. 2. Insufficiency of the cell-forming activity of the bone marrow.

myeloplast A leukocyte of the bone marrow.

myelopoiesis The formation of bone marrow or the blood cells derived from it.

myeloproliferative Relating to proliferation of blood-forming elements.

myeloproliferative syndrome A group of disorders characterized by abnormal proliferation of one or more types of bone marrow cells; includes myelofibrosis, polycythemia vera, and idiopathic thrombocytosis.

myeloradiculitis Inflammation of the spinal cord and the roots of the spinal nerves.

myeloradiculodysplasia Congenital abnormal development of the spinal cord and spinal nerve roots.

myeloradiculopathy Disease involving the spinal cord and spinal nerve roots.

myelorrhagia Bleeding into the spinal cord.

myelosarcoma Malignant tumor derived from bone marrow cells.

myeloschisis Cleft spinal cord resulting from fail-

ure of the normal closing of the neural tube.

myelosclerosis Induration of the spinal cord with overdevelopment of the interstitial connective tissue resulting from chronic inflammation. Also called sclerosing myelitis; spinal sclerosis.

myelosis Condition marked by abnormal proliferation of blood-forming cells in bone marrow and other organs.

chronic nonleukemic m. Condition characterized primarily by undue proliferation of elements giving rise to white blood cells, the total count remaining normal; a variant of myelofibrosis.

erythremic m. Disorder marked chiefly by abnormal proliferation of erythroid and myeloid precursors in bone marrow, bizarre red blood cell morphology, anemia, hemorrhagic disorders, and enlargement of the spleen and liver. Also called Di-Guglielmo's syndrome.

myelotomy The cutting of nerve fibers in the spinal cord.

myelotoxic 1. Destructive to bone marrow. 2. Relating to diseased bone marrow.

myelytic Relating to or marked by inflammation of the spinal cord or of the bone marrow.

myenteric Relating to the muscular layer (myenteron) of the intestine.

myenteron The muscular layer of the intestine.

myesthesia Sensation felt within a muscle. Also called muscular sensibility.

myiasis Any infection resulting from infestation of human tissue by fly maggots or flies, usually by deposition of ova by flies in open wounds.

mylohyoid Relating to the posterior portion of the lower jaw and to the hyoid bone.

myoarchitectonic Relating to the structure of muscles.

myoatrophy Wasting away of muscles due to lack of use. Also called myatrophy.

myoblast The embryonic cell which becomes a muscle cell.

myoblastoma Granular cell tumor; see under tumor.

myocardial Pertaining to the heart muscle (myocardium).

myocardiograph An instrument for graphically recording the action of the heart muscle.

myocardiopathy Cardiomyopathy.

primary m. Myocardiopathy of unknown cause.

myocardiorrhaphy Surgical suture of the muscular wall of the heart.

myocarditis Inflammation of the heart muscle.

acute isolated m. An acute form of unknown cause. Also called Fiedler's myocarditis.

Fiedler's m. See acute isolated myocarditis.

Labels in illustration (clockwise from top-left):
endocardium
myograms of myoclonus
peritoneum
myometrium
endometrium
uterus
cervix
vagina
myocardium
epi-cardium
bladder
myoma
uterus
rectum
myopia
nearsightedness
corrected by a concave lens
after Brödel

myocardium The middle and thickest layer of the heart wall composed of specialized striated muscle cells and intervening connective tissue; each cell possesses a central nucleus, a plasma membrane (sarcolemma), and numerous contractile myofibrils that are separated by varying amounts of sarcoplasm.

   infarcted m. Dead heart muscle resulting, usually, from an occluded artery.

myocele Herniation of a muscle.

myocellulitis Inflammation of muscle (myositis) and cellular tissue (cellulitis).

myoclonia Any disorder characterized by twitching or spasmodic contraction of muscles.

myoclonic Marked by myoclonus.

myoclonus A sudden rapid twitch resulting from the sudden contraction of one or more muscle groups.

myocyte A muscle cell.

myodynamometer An instrument used to measure muscular strength.

myodystony A succession of minute contractions during slow relaxation of a muscle following electrical stimulation.

myoedema The localized contraction of a degenerating muscle when struck. Also called mounding.

myoelectric Relating to the electric attributes of muscles.

myoendocarditis Inflammation of the wall and lining of the cardiac cavities.

myoepithelium Tissue composed of contractile epithelial cells that resemble smooth muscle cells.

myofascial syndrome A painful condition of skeletal muscles characterized by the presence of one or more discrete hyperesthetic areas termed trigger points, located within muscles or tendons; when stimulated by pressure, these trigger points produce pain in the area of the patient's symptoms.

myofibril One of the fine longitudinal fibrils present in muscle fiber; each myofibril is divided into a series of repeating units, the sarcomeres, which are the fundamental structural and functional units of contraction.

myofibroma A benign tumor containing fibrous and muscular tissues.

myofibrosis Chronic inflammation of a muscle with excessive formation of connective tissue, resulting in atrophy of the muscular tissue.

myofilaments The microscopic structures that make up the fibrils of striated muscle.

myogen A mixture of proteins, extractable from skeletal muscle with cold water, consisting largely of glycolytic enzymes.

myogenic Of muscular origin.

myoglia A fine network of fibrils formed by muscle cells. Also called muscle cement.

myoglobin An oxygen-transporting protein found in muscle fibers, similar to hemoglobin.

myoglobinuria The presence of myoglobin in the urine, usually after crush injuries or occasionally after very vigorous exercise.

   paroxysmal idiopathic m. See rhabdomyolysis.

myoglobulin (Mb) A globulin present in muscle tissue.

myoglobulinuria Myoglobinuria.

myogram A tracing produced by myography.

myograph An instrument for graphically recording muscular contractions.

myography A technique used to record muscular activity.

myoid Resembling muscle.

myokymia A twitching or tremor of individual fasciculi (bundles of fibers) of a muscle.

myolipoma A benign tumor composed chiefly of adipose and muscle tissues.

myology The branch of science concerned with the study of muscles.

myolysis Disintegration of muscle tissue.

myoma A benign tumor consisting of muscle tissue.

myomalacia Abnormal softening and degeneration of muscular tissue.

myomatectomy Removal of a myoma.

myomatous Resembling a myoma.

myomectomy Surgical removal of a myoma, specifically of a myoma of the uterus.

myometer An apparatus for determining the strength of a muscular contraction.

myometritis Inflammation of the muscular layer of the uterine wall.

myometrium The thick, smooth muscle forming the middle layer of the wall of the uterus.

myon A functional unit consisting of a muscle fiber with its basal membrane, together with the associated blood capillaries and nerves.

myonecrosis Death of muscle tissue.

myoneural Relating to muscle and nerve, as the nerve endings which terminate in muscular tissue.

myopathy Any disease of muscular tissue.

myopericarditis Inflammation of the muscle tissue of the heart and the enveloping membrane (pericardium).

myopia (M, My) A condition of the eye in which light rays entering the eyeball from a distance focus in front of the retina, causing only near objects to be seen in focus. Also called near sight; nearsightedness; shortsightedness.

myopic Relating to or afflicted with myopia.

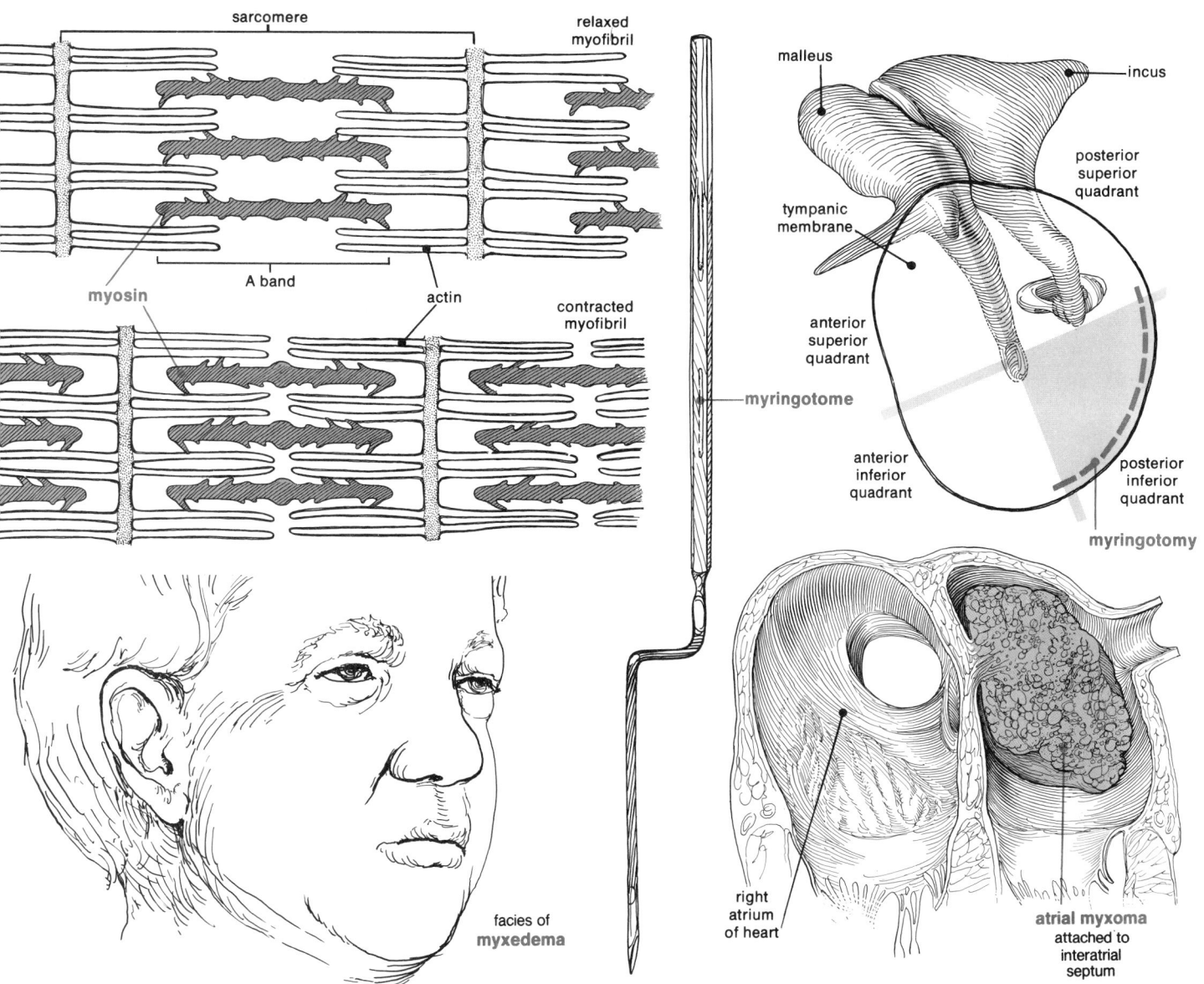

sarcomere

relaxed myofibril

myosin

A band

actin

contracted myofibril

myringotome

malleus

incus

posterior superior quadrant

tympanic membrane

anterior superior quadrant

anterior inferior quadrant

posterior inferior quadrant

myringotomy

facies of **myxedema**

right atrium of heart

atrial myxoma attached to interatrial septum

myoplasm The contractile part of a muscle cell.
myoplasty Surgical repair of a muscle.
myorrhaphy Suture of a muscle wound.
myorrhexis The tearing or rupturing of a muscle.
myosarcoma A general term for a malignant neoplasm or sarcoma derived from muscular tissue.
myosclerosis Chronic inflammation of a muscle with overgrowth of the interstitial connective tissue, resulting in hardening of the muscle.
myosin The thick filaments of polymerized protein molecules in the myofibril which, along with the protein actin, are responsible for muscular contraction; they comprise the dark A bands seen microscopically; called "A" bands because they are anisotropic to polarized light.
myosis Miosis.
myositis Inflammation of a muscle, usually a voluntary muscle.
  m. ossificans Condition in which muscular tissue is replaced by bone; it may be localized following an injury or, rarely, it may be generalized, progressive (beginning in childhood), and due to unknown causes.
myospasm Spasmodic contraction of a muscle or group of muscles.
myotome 1. Knife used in surgery to divide muscle. 2. In embryology, the portion of the mesodermic somite from which skeletal muscle develops.
myotomy 1. Dissection of muscles. 2. Surgical division of a muscle.
myotonia Temporary rigidity of a muscle or group of muscles.
  m. atrophica Disease marked by stiffness and eventual atrophy of the muscles, associated with cataract and slurred speech. Also called myotonic dystrophy; Steinert's disease.

  m. congenita Hereditary disease marked by temporary tonic spasm of certain muscles whenever a voluntary movement is attempted. Also called myotonia hereditaria; Thomsen's disease.
  m. hereditaria See myotonia congenita.
myotonic Characterized by myotonia.
myringectomy Surgical removal of the tympanic membrane (eardrum).
myringitis Inflammation of the tympanic membrane.
myringoplasty A surgical procedure performed to close a perforation of the eardrum acquired through injury or infection. Also called type I tympanoplasty.
myringorupture The tearing or rupturing of the tympanic membrane (eardrum).
myringotome A knife used for puncturing the tympanic membrane.
myringotomy Surgical incision of the tympanic membrane (eardrum) to allow drainage of the middle ear chamber. Also called tympanic paracentesis.
mysophobia Morbid fear of contamination, manifested by constant hand washing.
mythomania An abnormal compulsion to tell lies.
myxadenoma Benign tumor derived from glandular epithelial tissue.
myxedema A severe form of hypothyroidism occurring in juveniles and adults; caused by insufficient circulating thyroid hormone; marked by dry skin, brittle hair, swelling of the face, puffy eyelids, dull expression, and muscle weakness.
  pretibial m. A bulging over the lateral aspect of the lower leg above the lateral malleolus, found in some cases of thyrotoxicosis, usually associated with exophthalmic goiter (Graves' disease).
myxedematous Relating to myxedema.
myxochondrofibrosarcoma A malignant tu-

mor derived from fibrous connective tissue.
myxochondroma A benign tumor composed chiefly of cartilaginous tissue.
myxocyte One of the stellate or polyhedral cells found in mucous tissue.
myxofibroma A benign tumor of connective tissue containing portions that resemble primitive mesenchymal tissue.
myxoid Resembling or containing mucus.
myxolipoma A benign tumor of adipose tissue containing portions that resemble primitive mesenchymal tissue.
myxoma A benign tumor composed of connective tissue embedded in a soft, mucoid matrix. Also called mucoid tumor.
  atrial m. A benign primary tumor arising from the lining of the atria and resembling a polyp; it may cause murmurs which change with shifts in body position or simulate mitral or tricuspid stenosis.
myxomatosis Fatal disease of rabbits marked by the presence of multiple myxomatous growths of the skin and mucous membranes.
myxomycete Fungus or slime mold found in rotting vegetation.
myxoneuroma Tumor resulting from proliferation of Schwann cells in which degenerative changes produce areas that resemble primitive mesenchymal tissue.
myxopoiesis The formation of mucus.
myxosarcoma A malignant tumor derived from connective tissue.
myxospore A spore embedded in a gelatinous mass.
myxovirus Term formerly used for viruses with affinity for mucins, now included in the families Orthomyxoviridae and Paramyxoviridae.

ingrown nail

nail root

eponychium

nail

nail matrix

nail bed

nalidixic acid

nalorphine

naloxone

Nn

nacreous Having a mother-of-pearl luster; iridescent.

nadolol A long-acting β_1- and β_2-adrenergic blocking agent.

nafcillin A semisynthetic penicillin that is not readily destroyed by gastric acids.

nail The flattened, translucent structure on the dorsal surface of the distal end of a finger or toe, composed of several layers of flat, clear cells. Also called unguis.

  hippocratic n. A deformed overhanging fingernail associated with the clubbing of terminal phalanges in certain pulmonary and cardiac conditions.

  ingrown n. A toenail with its edges growing abnormally into the soft tissues. Also called onychocryptosis.

nail bed The portion of tissue to which the nail is firmly adhered.

nail matrix The thick portion of nail bed beneath the nail root from which the nail develops.

nail root The portion of nail which is implanted into a groove of the skin.

nailing The fastening of a fractured bone with a nail.

nail-patella syndrome Hereditary condition characterized by bilateral underdevelopment of the kneecap, deformity and dislocation of the head of the radius, and dystrophy of fingernails.

nalidixic acid An antibacterial preparation effective against infections of the urogenital tract; NegGram®.

nalorphine $C_{19}H_{21}NO_3$; narcotic antagonist used as an antidote to narcotic overdosage; capable of causing withdrawal symptoms in narcotic addicts; Nalline.®

naloxone Narcotic antagonist used in treating respiratory depression suspected of being produced by a narcotic; Narcan®.

name A word that designates and distinguishes one entity from another.

  brand n. See trade name.

  chemical n. A scientific name that indicates a precise chemical structure; e.g., 2-(diphenylmethoxy)-*N*,*N*-dimethylethylamine hydrochloride (Benadryl®). Also called systematic name.

  generic n. Strictly defined, a name that designates a family relationship among drugs, e.g., antihistamine, barbiturate; often used as a synonym for nonproprietary name, e.g., diphenhydramine (Benadryl®).

  nonproprietary n. A name assigned to a drug (by the United States Adopted Name Council) when it is found to have therapeutic value; it indicates the chemical composition of the drug and is not pro-

tected by trademark registration; e.g., diphenhydramine (Benadryl®).

  proprietary n. See trade name.

  semisystematic n., semitrivial n. A name used in the sciences, especially chemistry, composed of two parts, one of which relates to a scientific (systematic) name, the other to a common (trivial) name; e.g., cortisone, derived from cortex and the suffix -one (indicating an aldehyde group).

  systematic n. See chemical name.

  trade n. A name selected by the pharmaceutical company that manufactures and sells the drug; it is registered and protected by a trademark and is usually followed by an encircled superscript R; e.g., Benadryl®. Also called brand or proprietary name.

  trivial n. A common name that tells nothing about the structure of the organism or chemical it designates; e.g., water, caffeine.

nanocephaly Abnormal smallness of the head.

nanocormia Abnormal smallness of the body in relation to the head and extremities.

nanocurie (nCi) A unit of radioactivity equal to one-billionth of a curie; 10^{-9} curie.

nanogram (ng) A unit of weight equal to one-billionth of a gram; 10^{-9} gram.

nanoid Dwarfish.

nanomelia Abnormal smallness of the extremities.

nanomelus Individual characterized by nanomelia.

nanometer (nm) A unit of linear measure equal to one-thousandth of a micron; 10^{-9} meter. Also called millimicron.

nanosecond (nsec) A unit of time equal to one-billionth of a second; 10^{-9} second.

nanosoma, nanosomia Dwarfism.

nanus A dwarf.

nape The back of the neck. Also called nucha.

naphthalene Tar camphor, a crystalline hydrocarbon derived from coal tar, insoluble in water, and soluble in alcohol; used as an insecticide (mothballs) and antiseptic, and in the manufacture of indigo and lampblack.

naphthol A crystalline, antiseptic derivative of naphthalene.

α-naphthol Colorless crystals, soluble in water; used in microscopy. Also written alpha-naphthol.

narcissism Self-love, as opposed to object-love or love of another person; the term is derived from Narcissus, a figure in Greek mythology who fell in love with his own reflected image.

narcolepsy Condition characterized by paroxysmal episodes of sleep lasting from minutes to hours; frequently accompanied by transient muscular

weakness, sleep paralysis, and hallucinations during the period between sleep and wakefulness. Also called paroxysmal sleep; sleep epilepsy.

narcoma See narcosis.

narcomania An uncontrollable craving for narcotics.

narcosis A deep stuporous state produced by certain chemical and physical agents. Also called narcoma.

narcosynthesis Psychotherapeutic treatment conducted with the aid of a partial anesthetic.

narcotherapy Psychotherapy conducted after a state of complete relaxation is induced by injecting a barbiturate drug intravenously (either sodium amytal or sodium pentothal); under this therapy some individuals have a capacity to communicate thoughts previously repressed.

narcotic 1. Producing narcosis. **2.** Generally, any physical or chemical agent that produces narcosis. **3.** A drug intended for the relief of pain that also tends to produce insensibility, stupor, and sleep; with prolonged use it may become addictive.

narcotism Addiction to a habit-forming drug.

narcotize To subject to the influence of a narcotic.

naris, *pl.* **nares** See nostril.

  posterior n. The opening connecting the nasal cavity with the nasopharynx on either side. Also called choana.

nasal Relating to the nose.

nascent Beginning to exist; denoting an atom or element at the moment it is liberated from a compound.

nasion A craniometric point; the midline of the nasofrontal suture.

nasoantral Relating to the nose and the maxillary sinus (antrum).

nasoendoscope An instrument used in examination of the nasal cavity and postnasal space; it possesses a self-contained illumination and magnifying lens which is passed through the anterior naris (nostril).

nasofrontal Of or relating to the nose and the frontal bones.

nasolabial Relating to the nose and lip.

nasolacrimal 1. Relating to the nasal and the lacrimal bones. **2.** Relating to the nose and the structures producing and conveying tears.

naso-oral Concerning the nose and the mouth.

nasopalatine Concerning the nose and the palate.

nasopharyngeal Relating to the nasopharynx.

nasopharyngitis Inflammation of the nasopharynx.

nasopharyngoscope An instrument for visual examination of the nasal passages and the nasopharynx.

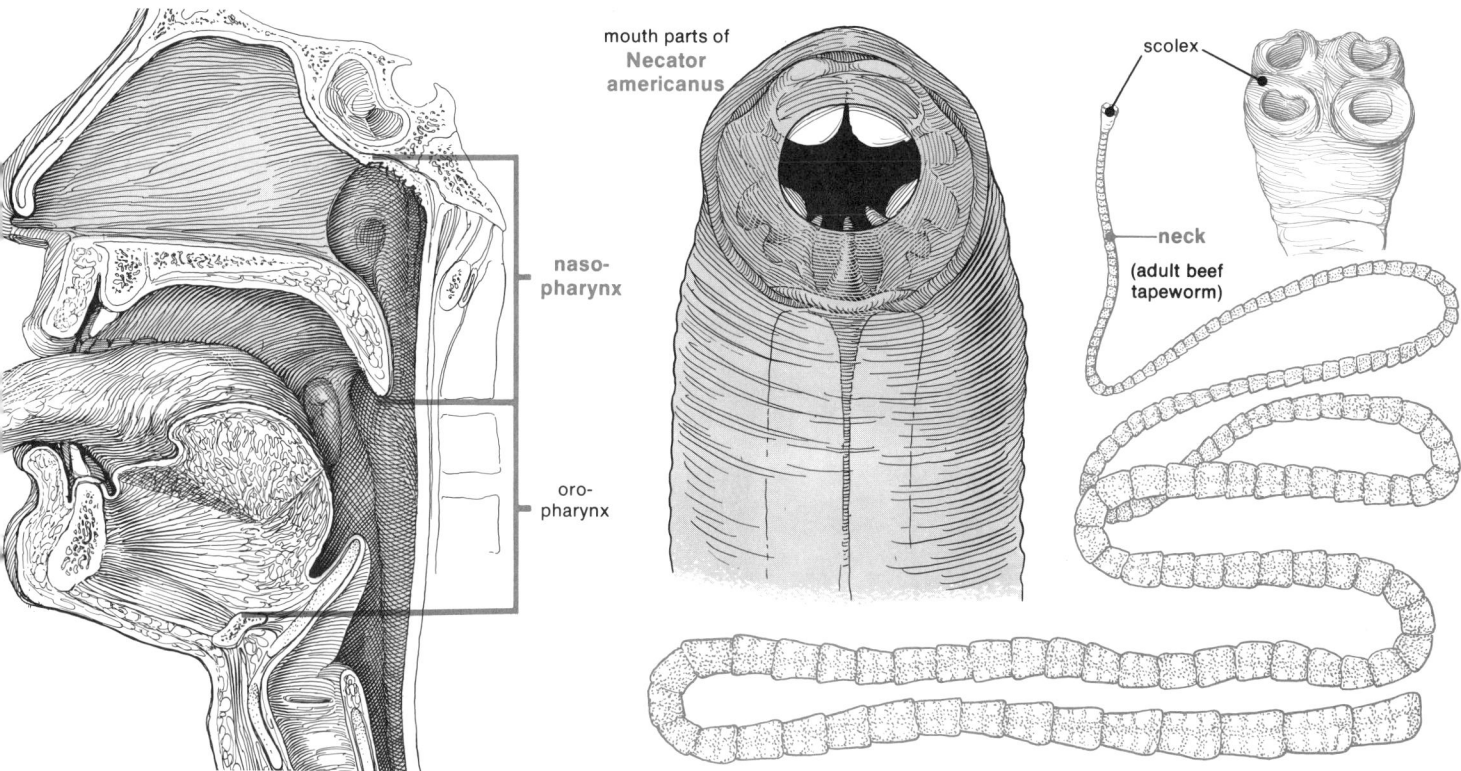

mouth parts of
**Necator
americanus**

naso-
pharynx

oro-
pharynx

scolex

neck

(adult beef
tapeworm)

nasopharynx The uppermost part of the pharynx, located above the level of the soft palate immediately behind the nasal cavity. Also called rhinopharynx; pars nasalis pharyngis.

nasoscope See rhinoscope.

nasoseptal Pertaining to the septum of the cavity of the nose.

nasoseptitis Inflammation of the lining of the nasal septum.

nasosinusitis Inflammation of the lining of the nasal cavity and adjacent sinuses.

nasus Latin for nose.

nasute 1. Having a long or large nose. 2. Possessing a keen sense of smell.

natal Relating to birth.

natality The birth rate.

nates The buttocks.

natiform Shaped like the buttocks.

natimortality The proportion of stillbirths and newborn deaths to the birth rate.

National Formulary (NF) An official publication of the American Pharmaceutical Association which provides authoritative information on drugs.

National Institutes of Health (NIH) An agency of the United States Public Health Service, consisting of eleven health institutes that support integrated programs of research, clinical trials, and demonstrations relating to cause, diagnosis, and treatment of disease.

natrium Latin for sodium (Na).

natriuresis Increased sodium excretion in the urine.

natriuretic 1. Of or relating to the excretion of sodium in the urine. 2. An agent promoting excretion of sodium. 3. Atrial natriuretic factor; see under factor.

naturopath One who practices naturopathy.

naturopathy The treatment of the sick by the exclusive use of physical forces such as sunlight, heat, etc., supplemented with massage and diet.

nausea A feeling of the need to vomit.

n. gravidarum Nausea occurring in pregnant women.

nauseant 1. Nauseating; inducing a feeling of the need to vomit. 2. Any agent that induces nausea.

nauseate To cause a desire to vomit.

nauseous Relating to or causing nausea.

navel The depressed area of the abdominal wall, marking the site of attachment of the umbilical cord to the fetus. Also called umbilicus.

navicular Boat-shaped; see table of bones.

nearsightedness See myopia.

nebula A slight opacity of the cornea.

nebulization The process of converting a liquid

into a fine spray.

nebulize 1. To create a fine spray from a liquid. 2. To medicate through a fine spray.

nebulizer An apparatus for dispersing a liquid in the form of a fine spray.

Necator A genus of hookworms of the class Nematoda.

N. americanus A nematode parasite that produces the human hookworm disease (necatoriasis). Also called American or "New World" hookworm; *Uncinaria americana*.

necatoriasis Human hookworm disease caused by the nematode parasite *Necator americanus*.

neck 1. The part of the body between the head and the trunk. 2. Any relatively constricted portion of a structure or organ. 3. The germinative portion of an adult tapeworm; the region of cestode segmentation behind the scolex. 4. The portion of a tooth between the crown and root.

n. of womb Uterine cervix; see under cervix.

stiff n. See torticollis.

webbed n. A neck with lateral folds extending from the head to the clavicles, giving it a broad, short appearance.

necrobiosis The natural death of tissue with the concurrent replacement thereof.

n. diabeticorum A condition characterized by patchy degeneration of the skin in which fat tissue is extensively involved in the concurrent destructive and reparative process; usually, but not exclusively, associated with diabetes.

necrocytosis The abnormal decomposition and death of cells.

necrogenic Originating in dead matter.

necrology 1. A record of people who have died, especially during a specific period of time. 2. Obituary.

necrolysis Loosening or separation of tissue due to death and decay of cells.

necromania Morbid interest in death or dead bodies.

necroparasite See saprophyte.

necrophile One afflicted with necrophilia.

necrophilia An abnormal fascination with the dead; especially erotic attraction for contact with dead bodies, usually of males with female corpses.

necrophilous Feeding on dead tissue; said of certain bacteria.

necrophobia A morbid fear of death or dead bodies.

necropsy See autopsy.

necroscopy Autopsy.

necrose To cause or undergo irreversible damage, decomposition, and death; said of cells, tissues, and

organs. Also called necrotize.

necrosis Death of tissue within a circumscribed area.

acute tubular n. (ATN) A form of acute renal failure usually caused by a toxic agent or associated with a hypotensive period, especially from shock, sepsis, or trauma; characterized classically by absent or scanty urine followed by gradually increasing flow of dilute urine, often reaching very large amounts.

aseptic n. Necrosis occurring without infection. See also epiphyseal aseptic necrosis.

caseous n. One in which the tissue becomes soft, dry, and cheeselike, as in the lesions of tuberculosis.

central n. Necrosis involving the inner portion of a part, as necrosis in the cells surrounding the central veins of the liver.

coagulation n. Necrosis induced by loss of arterial blood supply to a tissue, leading to denaturation and coagulation of cell protein.

colliquative n. See liquefactive necrosis.

cystic medial n. Accumulation of mucopolysaccharide ground substance between connective tissue fibers of the middle layer of the aorta. Also called medionecrosis of aorta; mucoid medial degeneration.

epiphyseal aseptic n. A form of bone destruction most commonly occurring in the head of the femur (Legg-Perthes disease); also seen in the medial femoral condyle, the humeral head, and the tibial tubercle (Osgood-Schlatter disease); associated with systemic corticosteroid therapy, sickle cell disease, alcoholism, and other disorders. Also called avascular necrosis.

fat n. Death of fatty tissue characterized by the formation of small, white, chalky areas.

liquefactive n. Complete and rapid dissolution of cells (including cell membranes) by enzymes, forming circumscribed areas of softened tissue with a semifluid exudate; characteristic of abscesses and infarcts of the brain. Also called colliquative necrosis.

renal papillary n. Ischemic necrosis of the renal papillae, usually occurring in patients with diabetes and pyelonephritis, in individuals who have habitually ingested large quantities of analgesic medicines, in sickle cell disease, and in the presence of obstructive uropathy and infection. Also called necrotizing papillitis.

necrospermia A condition in which the semen contains a high percentage of nonmotile sperm.

necrotic Relating to dead tissue.

necrotize See necrose.

necrotomy Surgical removal of a dead portion of a bone (sequestrum). Also called necrectomy.

hypodermic **needle**

caudal **needle**

aneurysm **needle**

hemorrhoidal **needle**

Wasserman **needle**

spinal **needle**

acupuncture **needle**

surgical **needles**

weight range.
5 1/2 to 10 pounds
(2.5 to 4.6 kg)
length range:
18 to 22 inches
(45 to 55 cm)

full term **neonate**

---

needle **1.** A slender, pointed implement for stitching or puncturing. **2.** To separate tissues. **3.** To puncture the lens capsule to allow absorption of the lens substance; a surgical procedure for the treatment of soft cataract.

acupuncture n. A fine needle, usually 76.2 to 127.0 mm in length, used to perform acupuncture.

aneurysm n. A needle with a curved blunt end for passing a ligature around a blood vessel.

aspirating n. A long, hollow needle used to withdraw fluid from a cavity.

atraumatic n. An eyeless surgical needle.

biopsy n. A hollow needle used to obtain tissue for microscopic examination.

caudal n. A long, hollow needle used to inject an anesthetic into the epidural space via the sacral hiatus.

exploring n. A grooved needle which is thrust into a tumor or cavity to determine the presence or absence of fluid.

hypodermic n. A hollow needle for injecting fluids beneath the skin.

lumbar puncture n. A needle designed for entering the spinal canal to remove cerebrospinal fluid or to introduce medication.

Menghini n. A needle designed to obtain tissue, especially from the liver, for biopsy; the tissue core is obtained and held in with the aid of suction applied to the end of the needle.

spinal n. A long, hollow needle used to inject an anesthetic into the spinal subarachnoid space.

stop n. A needle with a shoulder permitting insertion to a predetermined depth.

surgical n. Any sewing needle used in a surgical operation.

Vim-Silverman n. One provided with a stylet and tweezer-like cutters used to obtain tissue for biopsy.

needling A surgical technique in which the lens capsule is punctured to permit absorption of a soft cataract.

negative **1.** Absent; nonreactive; not indicative of the presence of a specific abnormal condition, such as a disorder, anomaly, or microorganism. **2.** Denoting a quantity less than zero.

negativism Persistent opposition to suggestions or advice; a symptom of certain psychiatric disorders which also occurs normally in late infancy.

negatron Electron.

Neisseria A genus of bacteria (family Neisseriaceae) composed of small, gram-negative organisms occurring in pairs, each having a coffee-bean shape, flattened at the site of contact with its mate; parasitic (some pathogenic) in man.

N. catarrhalls Nonpathogenic species found in the respiratory tract and saliva.

N. gonorrhoeae Species that causes gonorrhea and ophthalmia neonatorum. Formerly called *Diplococcus gonorrhoeae.*

N. meningitidis Intracellular species that causes meningococcal meningitis.

nemathelminth A member of the phylum Nemathelminthes.

Nemathelminthes A phylum of round worms, including the class Nematoda; characterized by cylindrical bodies with pointed ends.

nematocide An agent that kills roundworms.

nematocyst One of many minute stinging organelles in various marine coelenterates, such as sea nettle, Portuguese man-of-war, and hydra; when stimulated, it ejects a potent venom.

Nematoda A class of round worms of the phylum Nemathelminthes, some species of which are parasitic in man.

nematode Any parasitic worm of the class Nematoda. Also called roundworm.

nematodiasis Infestation with nematode or roundworm parasites.

nematoid **1.** Relating to a nematode worm. **2.** Resembling a thread.

nematology The science that deals with nematode worms.

neoarthrosis See pseudarthrosis.

neoblastic Relating to or originating in new tissue.

neocerebellum The lateral lobes of the cerebellum; so called because it is the last part of the cerebellum to develop.

neocinetic Neokinetic.

neocortex See isocortex.

neocystostomy Surgical procedure whereby a ureter or a segment of the ileum is inserted into the bladder.

neocytosis The presence of immature cells in the blood. Also called skeocytosis.

neodymium A silvery, rare-earth metallic element; symbol Nd, atomic number 60, atomic weight 144.27.

neogenesis New formation of tissue. Also called regeneration.

neokinetic Denoting the area of the cerebral cortex that regulates motor activities.

neolallism Abnormal usage of neologisms.

neologism Any new word or phrase or old word used in a new way; the coining of bizarre neologisms is a common symptom among psychotic individuals.

neomembrane False membrane; see under membrane.

neomorph **1.** New formation; a part or organ that is not evolved from a similar structure in an ancestor. **2.** A mutant gene producing an effect not produced by any nonmutant gene in the same locus.

neomycin An antibacterial substance produced by the metabolism of the bacteria *Streptomyces fradiae.*

neon A rare, inert, gaseous element in the atmosphere; symbol Ne, atomic number 10, atomic weight 20.183.

neonatal Pertaining to the first month of life.

neonate, neonatus A newborn.

neonatologist A specialist in neonatology.

neonatology The study of the newborn; a subspecialty related to obstetrics, pediatrics, and fetal biology.

neopallium See isocortex.

neoplasia The formation and growth of a tumor or new tissue.

neoplasm The abnormal multiplication of cells with the formation of a mass or new growth of tissue; it may be localized (benign) or spreading and invasive (malignant). Also called tumor. Cf. hyperplasia; hypertrophy.

neoplasty **1.** Neoplasia. **2.** Plastic surgery.

neostomy Surgical creation of a new artificial opening.

nephelometer An instrument for measuring the concentration of particles in suspension by means of reflected or transmitted light.

nephelometry The estimation of the number of particles in a suspension with the aid of a nephelometer.

nephrectasia, nephrectasy Dilatation of the pelvis of the kidney.

nephrectomy Surgical removal of a kidney.

nephric Relating to the kidney. Also called renal.

nephridium One of the excretory tubules of invertebrates.

nephritic Afflicted with nephritis.

nephritis Inflammation of the kidneys; a nonspecific term, often used to indicate glomerulonephritis or Bright's disease.

acute n. Acute glomerulonephritis; see under glomerulonephritis.

acute interstitial n. Acute inflammation of the interstitial tissues of the kidney, generally with involvement of the tubules and relative sparing of the glomeruli; commonly caused by reaction to a drug.

Balkan n. A chronic progressive nephritis most commonly seen in Bulgaria, Rumania, and Yugoslavia.

chronic n. Chronic renal disease having a variety of etiologies; the term is most often used to refer to a form of chronic glomerulonephritis.

chronic interstitial n. Fibrotic interstitial tissue accompanied by chronic inflammatory cells;

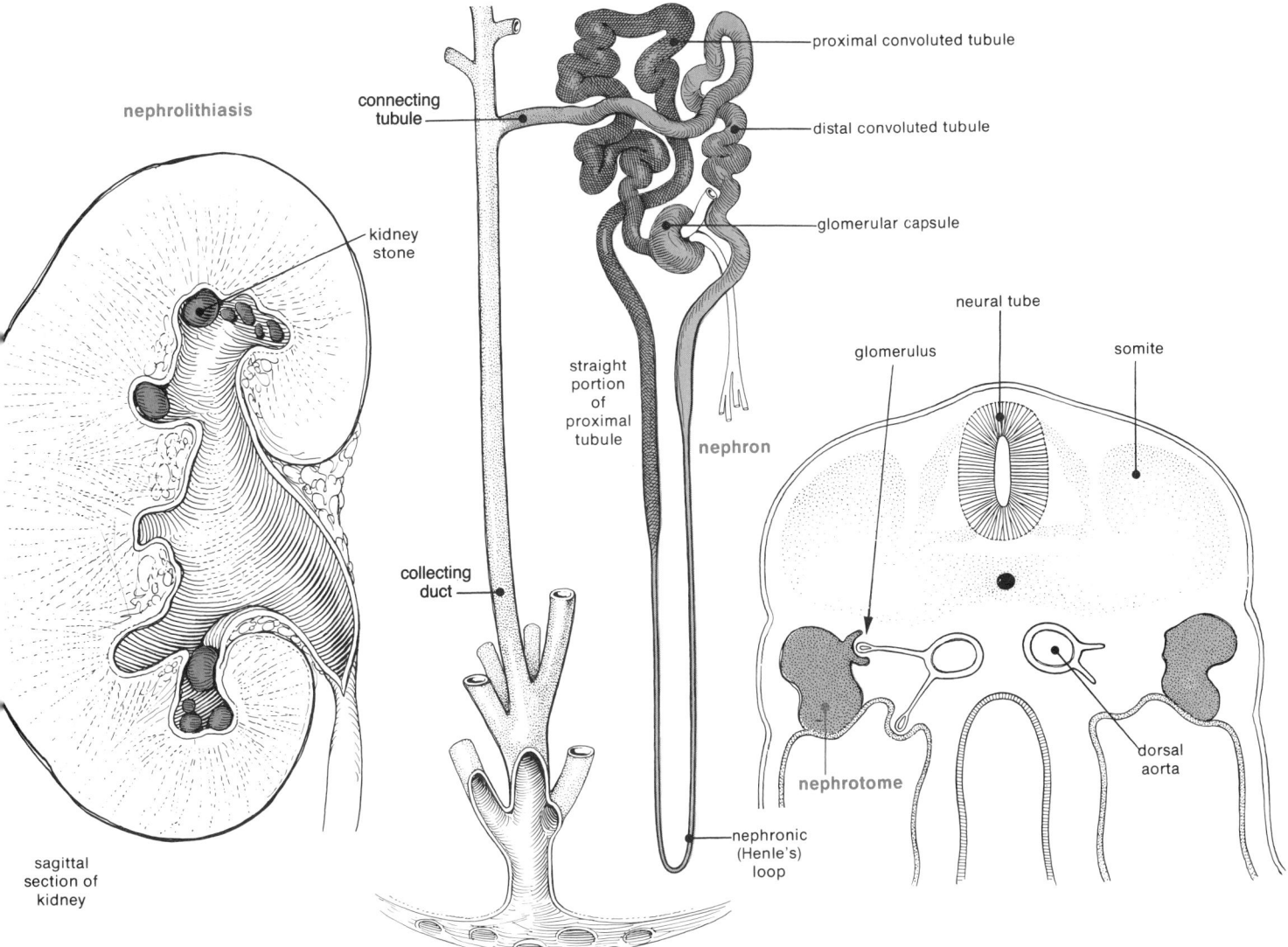

nephrolithiasis

connecting tubule

proximal convoluted tubule

distal convoluted tubule

glomerular capsule

kidney stone

straight portion of proximal tubule

nephron

collecting duct

nephronic (Henle's) loop

sagittal section of kidney

neural tube

glomerulus

somite

nephrotome

dorsal aorta

thought to be caused by many different agents, including chronic drug reaction, heavy metal toxicity, and gout.

hereditary n. Familial renal disease progressing to chronic renal failure; associated with nerve deafness. Also called Alport's syndrome.

IgA n. See under nephropathy.

potassium-losing n. Unusual potassium loss in the urine; may be seen, uncommonly, as a manifestation of renal tubular acidosis and chronic pyelonephritis.

salt-losing n. Tendency of some individuals with chronic renal disease to excrete a high percentage of filtered sodium; most likely to occur with chronic pyelonephritis, polycystic kidneys, analgesic nephropathy, or medullary cystic disease.

nephritogenic Producing nephritis.

nephroblastoma Wilm's tumor; see under tumor.

nephrocalcinosis Condition marked by calcifications scattered throughout the kidneys. Also called renal calcinosis.

nephrogenic, nephrogenetic Originating in the kidney.

nephrogram Roentgenogram of the kidney.

nephrography Roentgenography of the kidney.

nephroid Resembling a kidney.

nephrolith Kidney stone.

nephrolithiasis Condition marked by the presence of stones in the kidney.

nephrolithotomy Cutting through the kidney for the removal of kidney stones.

nephrology The study of the kidney and its diseases.

nephrolysin An antibody that causes specific destruction of kidney cells.

nephromalacia Softening of the kidneys.

nephromere In embryology, a portion of the intermediate mesoderm from which the kidney develops.

nephron The functional unit of the kidney, located mostly within the renal cortex; it consists of the glomerulus and its tubules up to the point where the tubule enters the common collecting duct; the parts include the glomerular (Bowman's) capsule, the proximal convoluted tubules, the straight portion of the proximal tubule (pars recta), the descending and ascending limbs of the nephronic (Henle's) loop, the distal convoluted tubule, and the arched collecting duct.

nephronophthisis Medullary cystic disease of the kidney; see cystic disease of the renal medulla.

nephropathy Any disease of the kidney.

IgA n. Condition marked by deposition of IgA in the central portions of the glomeruli and recurrent excretion of blood in the urine; affects chiefly children and young adults. Also called Berger's disease.

nephropexy Surgical fixation of a displaced kidney.

nephrophthisis 1. Suppurative inflammation with wasting of kidney substance. 2. Tuberculosis of the kidney.

nephroptosia, nephroptosis Downward displacement of a kidney.

nephropyelitis Inflammation of the renal pelvis.

nephropyeloplasty Reparative surgery of the kidney pelvis.

nephropyosis Suppuration of a kidney.

nephrorrhagia Hemorrhage from or into the kidney.

nephrosclerosis Renal impairment secondary to arteriosclerosis or hypertension.

arterial n Atrophy and scarring of the kidney due to arteriosclerotic thickening of the walls of large branches of the renal artery; may cause hypertension. Also called arterionephrosclerosis.

arteriolar n. Renal changes associated with hypertension in which the arterioles thicken and the areas they supply undergo ischemic atrophy and interstitial fibrosis.

malignant n. Rapid deterioration of renal function caused by inflammation of renal arterioles; it accompanies malignant hypertension.

nephrosclerotic Relating to nephrosclerosis.

nephrosis General term denoting diseases of the kidneys which were thought to involve primarily the tubules; noninflammatory disease of the kidneys.

lipoid n. Minimal-change nephrotic syndrome; see under nephrotic syndrome.

lower nephron n. Acute tubular necrosis.

sclerosing n. A condition marked by tubular necrosis, interstitial fibrosis, and sclerosis.

nephrospasia, nephrospasis Floating kidney; see under kidney.

nephrostome, nephrostoma In embryology, one of the ciliated funnels connecting the embryonic uriniferous tubules with the celomic cavity.

nephrostomy The creation of an opening in the kidney pelvis into which a tube is inserted to drain the kidney.

nephrotic Of, relating to, or caused by nephrosis.

nephrotic syndrome Clinical symptom complex caused by various kidney diseases; characterized by generalized edema, low plasma albumin concentration, and severe proteinuria; seen in lipoid nephrosis (minimal-change disease, idiopathic nephrotic syndrome), membranous glomerulonephritis, and varieties of chronic proliferative glomerulonephritis. It also may be secondary to renal involvement by lupus erythematosus, diabetes mellitus, or amyloid; or to a number of drugs, insect bites, etc.

minimal-change n.s. A form of nephrotic syndrome in which the glomeruli appear normal when examined under the light microscope; electron microscopy reveals fused foot processes of the visceral epithelial cells; most commonly seen in children. Also called nil (nothing in light microscopy) disease; idiopathic nephrotic syndrome; lipoid nephrosis.

nephrotome The plate of embryonic mesenchyme of the somites of a vertebrate embryo from

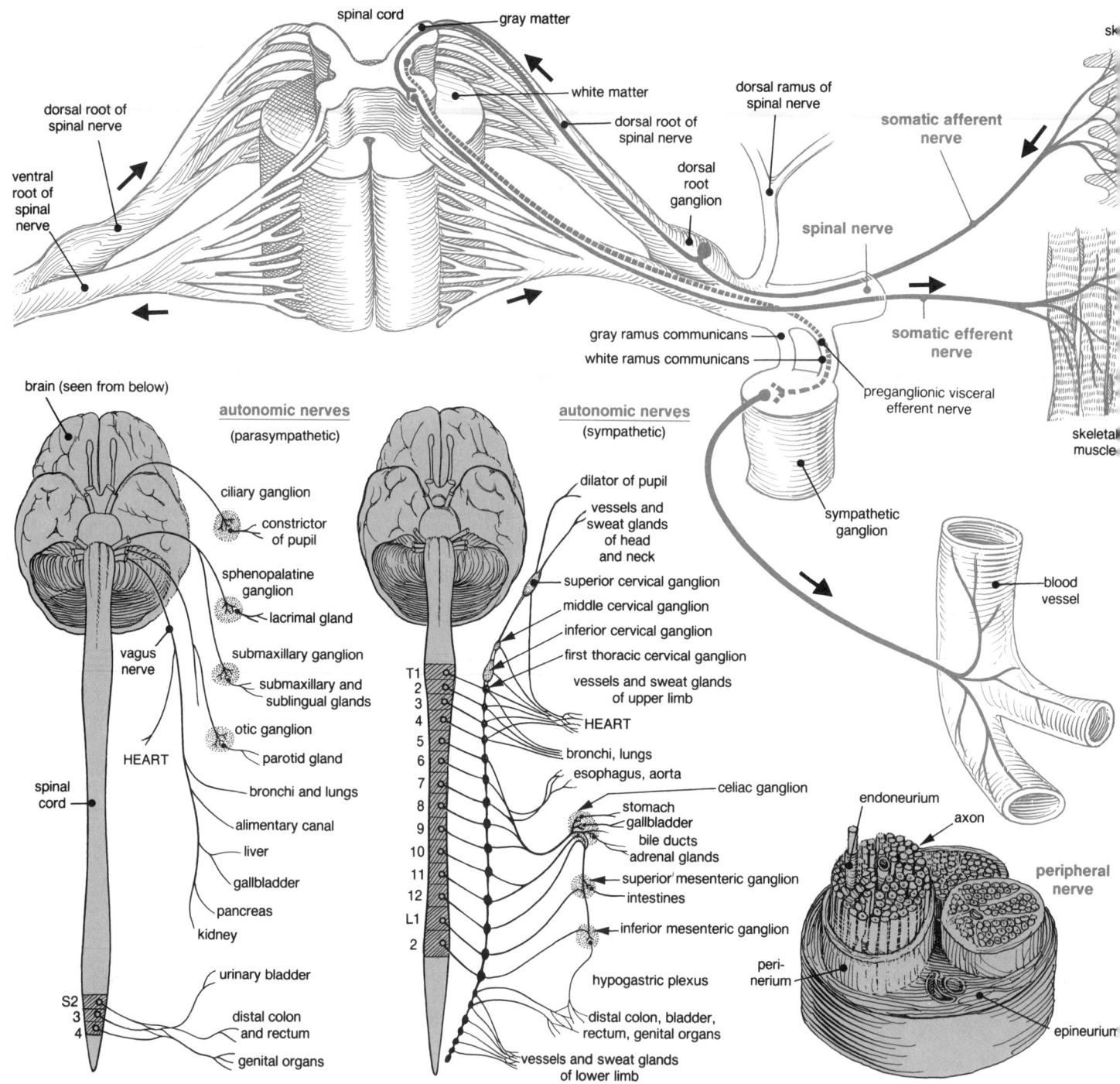

which the kidney tubules develop.

nephrotomogram Sectional x-ray images (tomogram) of the kidney following injection of radiopaque material.

nephrotomography X-ray examination of the kidney by means of tomography.

nephrotomy Incision of the kidney.

nephrotoxic Destructive to the cells of the kidney.

nephrotoxin A particular substance (cytotoxin) that is destructive to kidney cells.

nephrotropic See renotrophic.

nephrotuberculosis Tuberculosis of the kidney.

nephroureterectomy Removal of a kidney with complete or partial removal of its ureter.

neptunium A radioactive metallic element; symbol Np, atomic number 93, atomic weight 237; prepared artificially by the neutron bombardment of uranium atoms.

nerve A cordlike structure of one or more fascicles of nerve tissue that carries impulses (transmissions) from the central nervous system (brain and spinal cord) to the various structures of the body and from the structures to the central nervous system. For specific nerves, see table of nerves.

   accelerator n.'s Nerve fibers arising from the hypothalamus and brain stem which reach the heart

via the cardiac nerves and increase the rate of its beat; they are part of the sympathetic division of the autonomic nervous system.

   afferent n. A nerve that carries an impulse from the periphery to the central nervous system where it is interpreted into the consciousness of sensation; those arising from the skin, muscles, and joints are called somatic afferent nerves; those from the viscera are known as visceral afferent nerves.

   augmentor n.'s Nerves that increase the force as well as the rate of the heart beat.

   autonomic n. A bundle of nerve fibers relating to the activity of cardiac muscle, smooth muscle, and glands; they belong to the autonomic nervous system.

   cranial n.'s Nerves directly connected with the brain. See table of nerves.

   dead n. A misnomer for a functionless tooth pulp.

   depressor n. A nerve that causes depression of a motor center, or one that reduces the function of an organ.

   efferent n. A nerve that conveys impulses from the central nervous system to the periphery; those that terminate at skeletal muscles are called somatic efferent nerves; those that terminate at smooth mus-

cles, cardiac muscles, and gland cells are called visceral efferent (autonomic) nerves.

   inhibitory n. A nerve that carries impulses which diminish functional activity of a structure.

   mixed n. A nerve comprised both of afferent and efferent fibers.

   motor n. Efferent nerve.

   peripheral n.'s The cranial and spinal nerves with their branches; in general, they carry both afferent and efferent fibers.

   pressor n. An afferent nerve which when stimulated excites vasoconstriction, thereby increasing blood pressure.

   sensory n. Afferent nerve.

   somatic n. The afferent (sensory) and efferent (motor) nerves that innervate skeletal muscle and somatic tissue.

   spinal n.'s The thirty-one pairs of nerves directly connected with the spinal cord. See table of nerves.

   vasomotor n. An efferent nerve that can cause blood vessels to dilate (vasodilator nerve) or to constrict (vasoconstrictor nerve).

nervous 1. Relating to nerves. 2. Highstrung; excitable.

nervousness Undue irritability and excitability.

nervus, *pl.* **nervi** Latin for nerve.

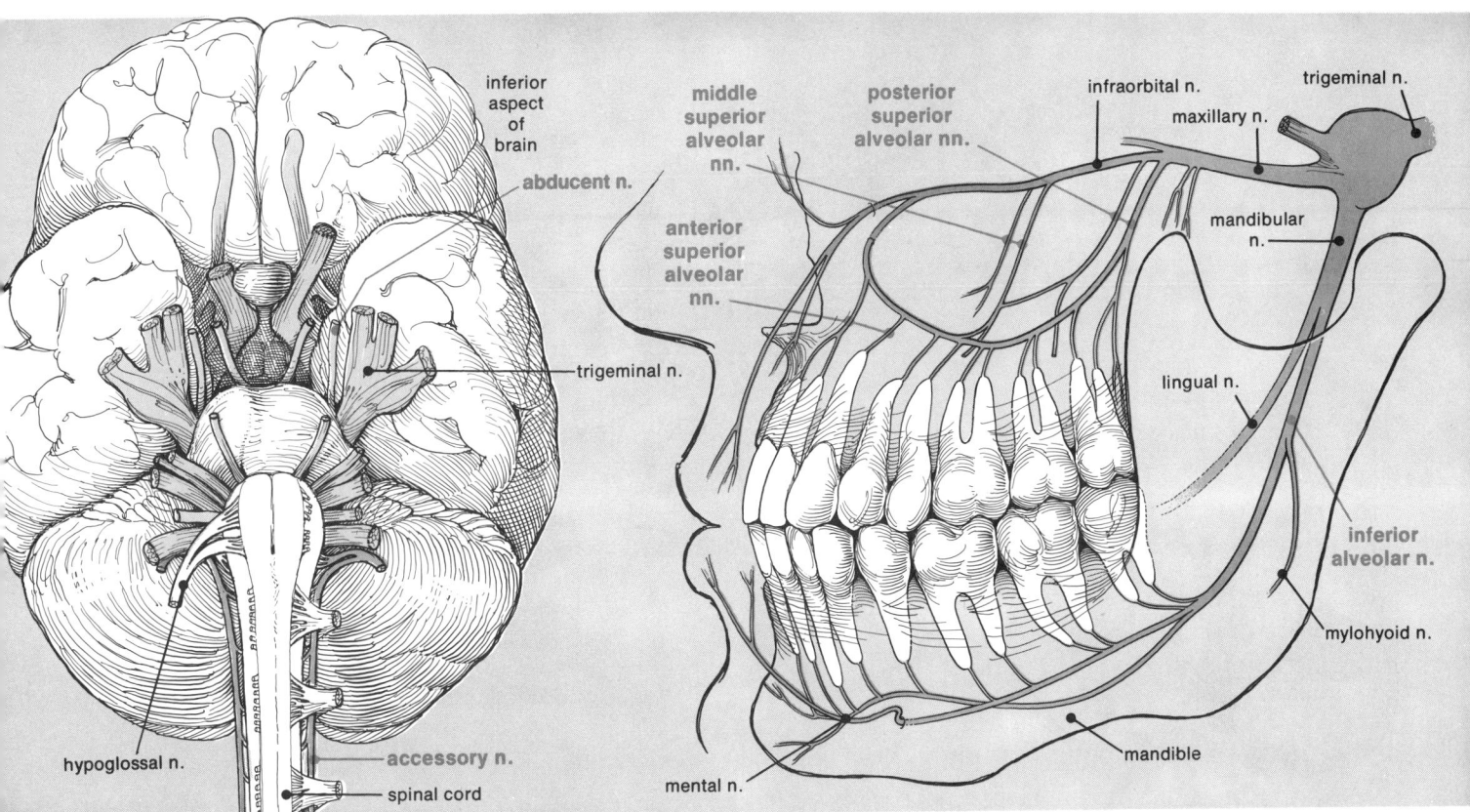

NERVE	ORIGIN	BRANCHES	DISTRIBUTION
abducent n. sixth cranial n. *n. abducens*	brainstem at inferior border of pons	filaments	lateral rectus muscle of eyeball
accessory n. spinal accessory n. eleventh cranial n. *n. accessorius*	*cranial part*: side of medulla oblongata; *spinal part*: first five cervical segments of spinal cord	internal branch external branch	striate muscles of larynx and pharynx sternocleidomastoid and trapezius muscles
acoustic n.	see vestibulocochlear nerve		
acoustic meatus n., external *n. meatus acustici externi*	auriculotemporal n.	filaments	external acoutic meatus
alveolar n.'s, anterior superior anterior superior dental n.'s *nn. alveolares anterior superior*	infraorbital n.	filaments	maxillary sinus, cuspids and incisors, superior dental plexus, floor of nose
alveolar n., inferior inferior dental n. *n. alveolaris inferior*	mandibular n.	mylohyoid, dental, incisive, mental	mylohyoid and anterior belly of digastric muscles, lower teeth, skin of chin, mucous membrane of lower lip
alveolar n., middle superior middle superior dental n. *n. alveolares superior medius*	infraorbital n.	filaments	maxillary sinus, superior dental plexus
alveolar n., posterior superior posterior superior dental n. *n. alveolaris superior posterior*	infraorbital n.	filaments	maxillary sinus, cheek, gums, molar and bicuspid teeth, superior dental plexus
ampullary n., anterior	see ampullary nerve, superior		
ampullary n., lateral *n. ampullaris lateralis*	vestibular n.	filaments	ampulla of lateral semicircular duct
ampullary n., posterior inferior ampullary n. *n. ampullaris posterior*	vestibular n.	filaments	ampulla of posterior semicircular duct
ampullary n., superior anterior ampullary n. *n. ampullaris superior*	vestibular n.	filaments	ampulla of superior semicircular duct
anococcygeal n.'s *nn. anococcygei*	coccygeal plexus	filaments	skin over coccyx
ansa cervicalis ansa hypoglossi *ansa cervicalis*	branch from first cervical uniting with branches from second and third cervical segments of spinal cord	filaments	omohyoid, sternohyoid, and sternothyroid muscles.

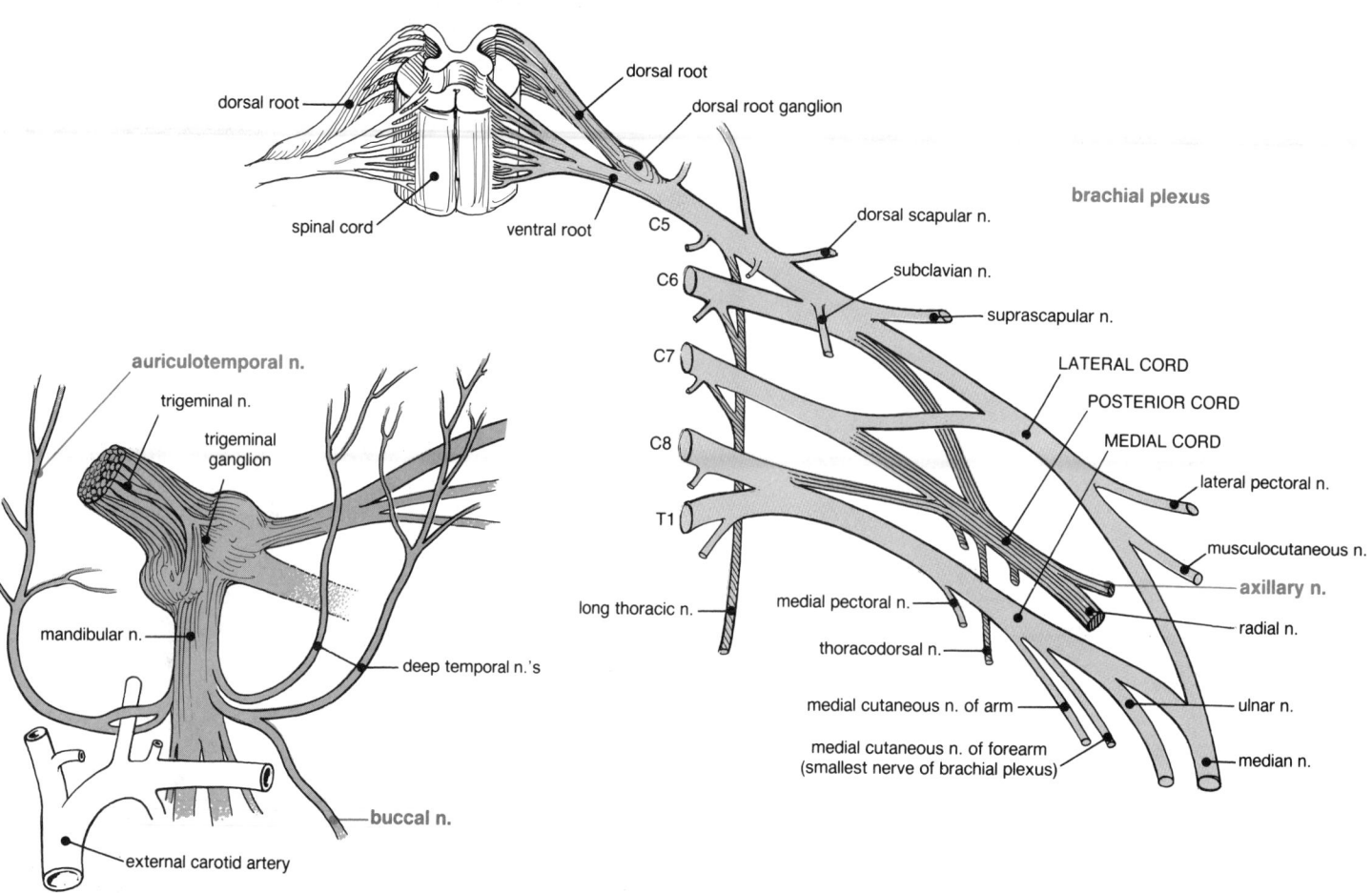

Diagram labels (top):

- dorsal root
- dorsal root
- dorsal root ganglion
- brachial plexus
- spinal cord
- ventral root
- C5
- C6
- dorsal scapular n.
- subclavian n.
- suprascapular n.
- C7
- LATERAL CORD
- POSTERIOR CORD
- C8
- MEDIAL CORD
- lateral pectoral n.
- musculocutaneous n.
- T1
- axillary n.
- long thoracic n.
- medial pectoral n.
- radial n.
- thoracodorsal n.
- medial cutaneous n. of arm
- ulnar n.
- medial cutaneous n. of forearm (smallest nerve of brachial plexus)
- median n.

Diagram labels (left):

- auriculotemporal n.
- trigeminal n.
- trigeminal ganglion
- mandibular n.
- deep temporal n.'s
- buccal n.
- external carotid artery

NERVE	ORIGIN	BRANCHES	DISTRIBUTION
auditory n.	see vestibulocochlear nerve		
auricular n.'s, anterior (usually two in number) *nn. auriculares anterior*	auriculotemporal n.	filaments	skin of anteriosuperior part of external ear, principally helix and tragus
auricular n., great *n. auricularis magnus*	second and third cervical nerves	anterior, posterior	skin about ear, mastoid process and parotid gland
auricular n., posterior *n. auricularis posterior*	facial n.	auricular, occipital	posterior auricular and occipital muscles, skin of external ear
auriculotemporal n. *n. auriculotemporalis*	mandibular division of trigeminal n.	anterior auricular, external, acoustic meatus, articular, parotid, superficial temporal, branches communicating with otic ganglion and facial n.	external meatus and skin of anterior superior part of auricle, temporomandibular joint, parotid gland, skin of temporal region
axillary n. circumflex n. *n. axillaris*	posterior cord of brachial plexus	posterior, anterior	deltoid and teres minor muscles, and neighboring skin
brachial plexus *plexus brachialis*	fifth to eight cervical and first thoracic nerves	*from cervical nerves*: phrenic, muscular, accessory phrenic; *from roots*: dorsal scapular, long thoracic; *from trunks*: subclavius, suprascapular; *from cords*: pectoral, subscapular, thoracodorsal, axillary, medial cutaneous of forearm, medial cutaneous of arm; *terminal nerves*: musculocutaneous, median, ulnar, radial	upper limb
buccal n. buccinator n. long buccal n. *n. buccalis*	mandibular division of trigeminal n.	filaments, branches communicating with buccal branches of facial n.	skin of cheek, mucous membranes of mouth and gums
buccinator n.	see buccal nerve		
cardiac n., inferior cervical *n. cardiacus cervicalis inferior*	inferior cervical ganglion, first thoracic ganglion, stellate ganglion, or ansa subclavia	to cardiac plexus	heart

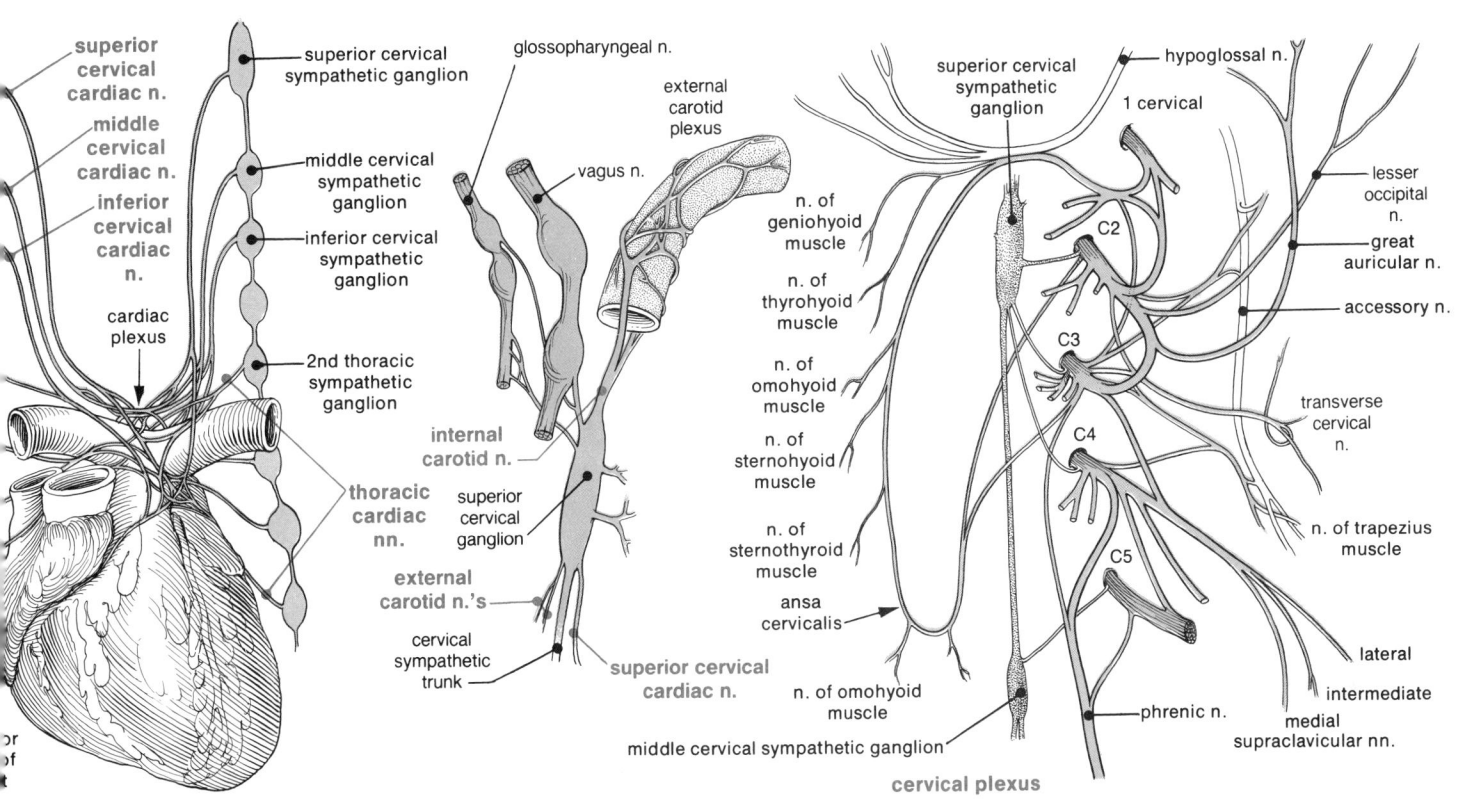

cervical plexus

NERVE	ORIGIN	BRANCHES	DISTRIBUTION
cardiac n., middle cervical great cardiac n. *n. cardiacus cervicalis medius*	middle cervical ganglion	to deep part of cardiac plexus	heart
cardiac n., superior cervical *n. cardiacus cervicalis superior*	lower part of superior cervical ganglion	to cardiac plexus	heart
cardiac n.'s, thoracic *nn. cardiaci thoracici*	second to fifth thoracic ganglion	to cardiac plexus	heart
caroticotympanic n.'s *nn. caroticotympanici*	superior cervical sympathetic ganglion	filaments	middle ear chamber, auditory tube
carotid n.'s, external *nn. carotici externi*	superior cervical ganglion	filaments	external carotid plexus, cranial blood vessels, smooth muscles and glands of head
carotid n., internal *n. caroticus internus*	cephalic end of superior cervical ganglion	medial, lateral	internal carotid plexus, cranial blood vessels, smooth muscle glands of head, cavernous plexus
carotid sinus n. carotid n. *n. caroticus*	glossopharyngeal n. just beyond its emergence from jugular foramen	filaments	carotid sinus, carotid body
cavernous n. of clitoris, greater *n. cavernosus clitoridis major*	uterovaginal plexus	filaments	corpus cavernosum of clitoris
cavernous n.'s of clitoris, lesser *nn. cavernosi clitorides minor*	uterovaginal plexus	filaments	erectile tissue of clitoris
cavernous n. of penis, greater *n. cavernosus penis major*	prostatic plexus	filaments	corpus cavernosum of penis
cavernous n.'s of penis, lesser *nn. cavernosi penis minor*	prostatic plexus	filaments	corpus spongiosum of penis and penile urethra
cervical n.'s (eight pairs of spinal nerves) *nn. cervicales*	cervical segments of spinal cord	filaments	cervical plexus and brachial plexus
cervical plexus *plexus cervicalis*	first to fourth cervical nerves	*cutaneous branches*: lesser occipital, great auricular, anterior cutaneous, supraclavicular; *muscular branches*: anterior and lateral rectae of head, long muscles of head and neck, geniohyoid, thyrohyoid, and omohyoid (superior belly), sternohyoid, and	muscles and skin of neck and upper back; diaphragm

cranial nerves

frontal lobe of cerebrum
hypophysis (pituitary gland)
temporal lobe of cerebrum
olfactory bulb
optic n. (II)
oculomotor n. (III)
abducens n. (VI)
trigeminal n. (V)
trochlear n. (IV)
facial n. (VII)
vestibulocochlear n. (VIII)
glossopharyngeal n. (IX)
vagus n. (X)
accessory n. (XI)
pons
hypoglossal n. (XII)
cerebellum
spinal cord

inferior aspect of brain and brain stem

geniculate ganglion
incus
lesser petrosal n.
n. to tensor tympani
mandibular n.
otic ganglion
chorda tympani n.
tympanic membrane
facial n. (VII)
external carotid artery
maxillary artery
lingual n.

long ciliary nn.
short ciliary nn.
ciliary ganglion
nasociliary n.

NERVE	ORIGIN	BRANCHES	DISTRIBUTION
cervical plexus (cont'd)		omohyoid (inferior belly), phrenic, sternocleidomastoid, trapezius, levator muscle of scapula, middle scalene	
chorda tympani n. *n. chorda tympani*	facial n. (intermediate)	filaments	anterior two-thirds of tongue, submandibular and sublingual glands
ciliary n.'s, long (two or three in number) *nn. ciliares longi*	nasociliary n. as it crosses optic nerve	filaments	iris and cornea
ciliary n.'s, short (6–10 in number) *nn. ciliares breves*	ciliary ganglion from oculomotor n.	filaments	ciliary body, iris, cornea
circumflex n.	see axillary nerve		
clunial n.'s, inferior *nn. clunium inferior*	posterior cutaneous n. of thigh	filaments	skin of lower and lateral gluteal region
clunial n.'s, middle *nn. clunium medii*	first, second, and third sacral nerves	filaments	skin of medial gluteal region
clunial n.'s, superior *nn. clunium superior*	first, second, and third lumbar nerves	filaments	skin of upper gluteal region
coccygeal n. *n. coccygeus*	coccygeal segments of spinal cord	filaments	coccygeal plexus
coccygeal plexus *plexus coccygeus*	fourth and fifth sacral nerves	anococcygeal, filaments	skin of region of the coccyx
cochlear n. n. of hearing *n. cochlearis*	vestibulocochlear n.	filaments	through spiral ganglion of cochlea to spiral organ of Corti of internal ear
common peroneal n.	see peroneal nerve, common		
cranial n.' cerebral n.'s *nn. craniales*	12 pairs of nerves attached to the base of the brain; they include the following: (I) olfactory; (II) optic; (III) oculomotor; (IV) trochlear; (V) trigeminal; (VI) abducent; (VII) facial; (VIII) vestibulocochlear; (IX) glossopharyngeal; (X) vagus; (XI) accessory; (XII) hypoglossal		

osseous labyrinth

semicircular canals of internal ear

anterior view

ampulla

superior vestibular ganglion

inferior vestibular ganglion

vestibular n.

facial n.

cochlear n.

scala tympani

cochlear duct

scala vestibuli

cochlea

spiral ganglion of cochlea

utricle

vestibular nucleus

cochlear n.

vestibulocochlear n.

vestibular n.

cochlear nucleus

saccule

posterior view

cochlear duct

superior ampullary n.

utricular n.

superior saccular n.

greater saccular n.

cochlear n.

cochlear duct

membranous labyrinth

lateral ampullary n.

posterior ampullary n.

ductus reuniens

anterior view

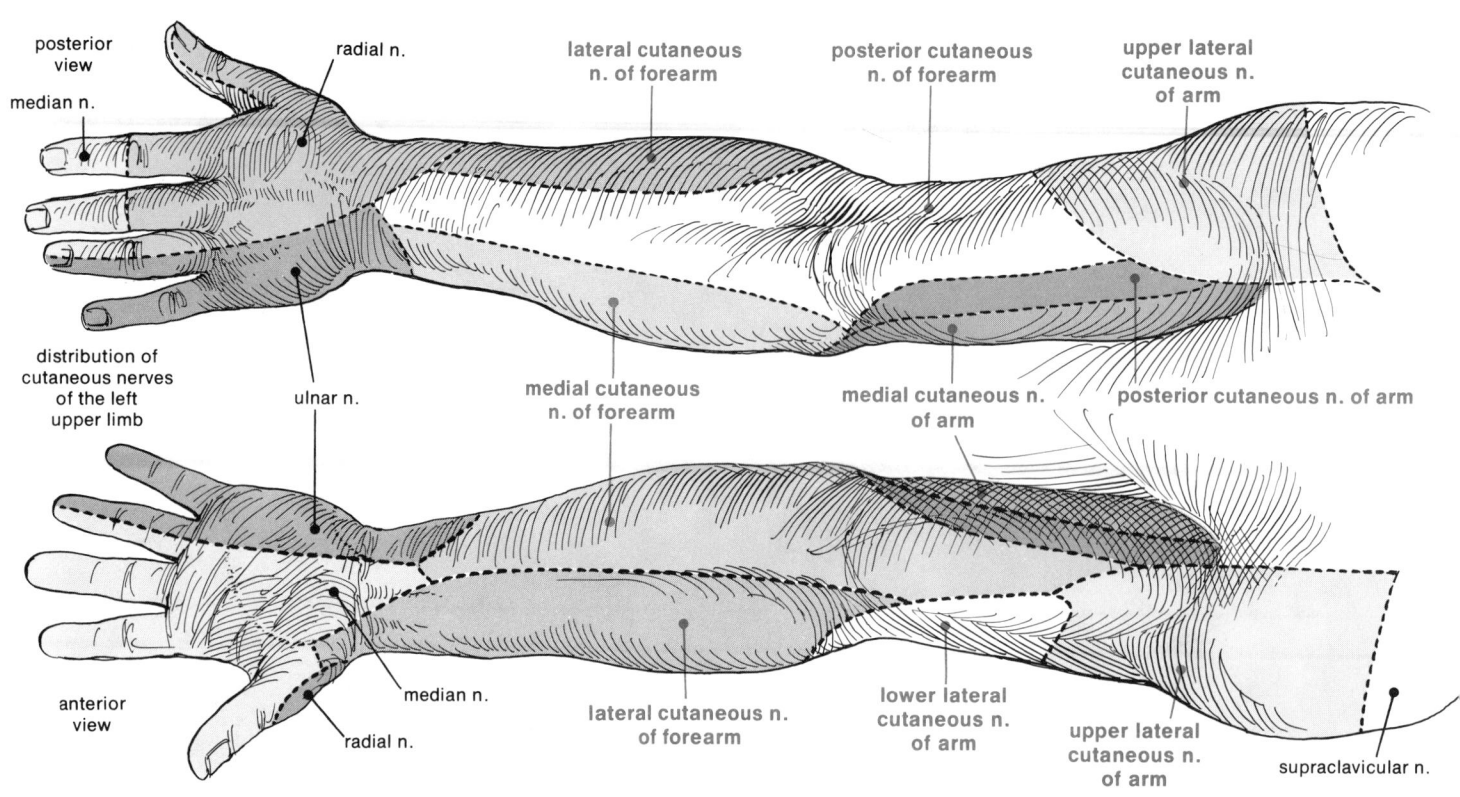

distribution of cutaneous nerves of the left upper limb

posterior view

median n.

radial n.

lateral cutaneous n. of forearm

posterior cutaneous n. of forearm

upper lateral cutaneous n. of arm

ulnar n.

medial cutaneous n. of forearm

medial cutaneous n. of arm

posterior cutaneous n. of arm

anterior view

median n.

radial n.

lateral cutaneous n. of forearm

lower lateral cutaneous n. of arm

upper lateral cutaneous n. of arm

supraclavicular n.

NERVE	ORIGIN	BRANCHES	DISTRIBUTION
cutaneous n. of arm, lower lateral lower lateral brachial cutaneous n. *n. cutaneus brachii lateralis inferior*	radial n.	filaments	skin on lateral aspect of lower part of arm
cutaneous n. of arm, medial medial brachial cutaneous n. *n. cutaneus brachii medialis*	medial cord of brachial plexus	filaments	skin to medial side of arm down to olecranon
cutaneous n. of arm, posterior posterior brachial cutaneous n. *n. cutaneus brachii posterior*	radial n.	filaments	skin on posterior aspect of arm nearly as far as olecranon
cutaneous n. of arm, upper lateral upper lateral brachial cutaneous n. *n. cutaneus brachii lateralis superior*	axillary n.	filaments	skin on lateral aspect of upper part of arm
cutaneous n. of calf, lateral *n. cutaneus surae lateralis*	common peroneal n.	sural, filaments	skin of lateral and posterior aspects of leg
cutaneous n. of calf, medial *n. cutaneus surae medialis*	tibial n.	sural, filaments	skin of medial and posterior aspects of leg
cutaneous n. of foot, intermediate dorsal *n. cutaneus dorsalis intermedius pedis*	superficial peroneal n.	dorsal digital (two)	skin of lateral side of ankle and foot, and adjacent sides of third, fourth, and fifth toes
cutaneous n. of foot, lateral dorsal *n. cutaneus dorsalis lateralis pedis*	sural n.	filaments	skin of dorsolateral part of foot
cutaneous n. of foot, medial dorsal *n. cutaneus dorsalis medialis pedis*	superficial peroneal n.	medial dorsal digital, lateral dorsal digital	skin of medial side of ankle, foot and great toe, skin of adjacent sides of second and third toes
cutaneous n. of forearm, lateral lateral antebrachial cutaneous n. *n. cutaneus antebrachii lateralis*	musculocutaneous n.	anterior, dorsal	skin over radial side of forearm
cutaneous n. of forearm, medial medial antebrachial cutaneous n. *n. cutaneus antebrachii medialis*	medial cord of brachial plexus	filaments, anterior, ulnar	skin over biceps muscle and of ulnar side of forearm
cutaneous n. of forearm, posterior posterior antebrachial cutaneous n. *n. cutaneus antebrachii posterior*	radial n.	proximal, distal	skin on posterior part of lower half of arm and of forearm
cutaneous n. of thigh, lateral external cutaneous n. *n. cutaneus femoris lateralis*	second and third lumbar nerves	anterior, posterior, filaments	skin of lateral and anterior part of thigh
cutaneous n. of thigh, posterior small sciatic n. *n. cutaneus femoris posterior*	first, second, and third sacral nerves	gluteal, perineal, femoral, sural	skin of lower gluteal region, external genitalia, perineum, and posterior aspect of thigh and leg

nerve | nerve

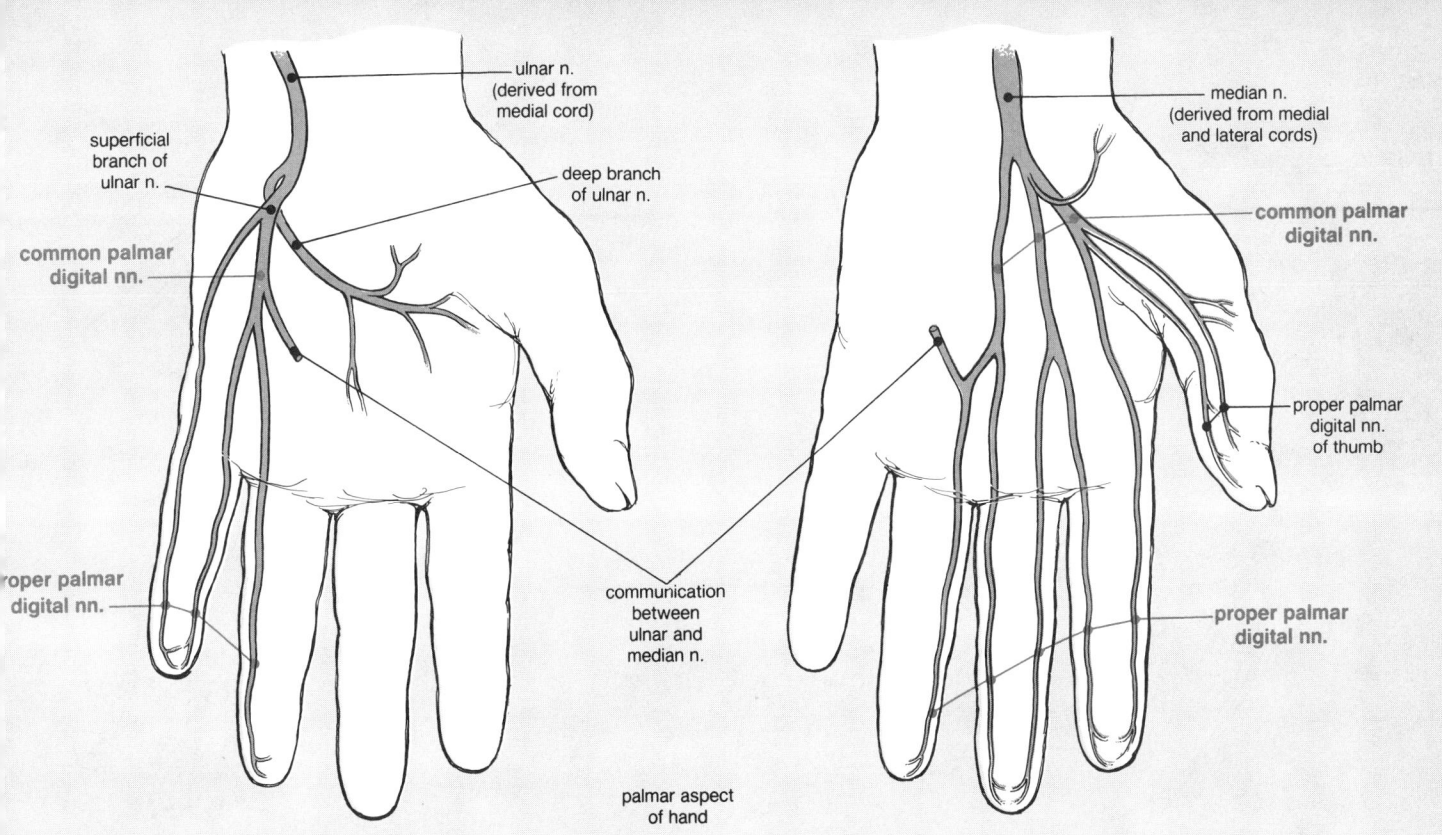

ulnar n.
(derived from
medial cord)

superficial
branch of
ulnar n.

deep branch
of ulnar n.

common palmar
digital nn.

proper palmar
digital nn.

median n.
(derived from medial
and lateral cords)

common palmar
digital nn.

proper palmar
digital nn.
of thumb

communication
between
ulnar and
median n.

proper palmar
digital nn.

palmar aspect
of hand

NERVE	ORIGIN	BRANCHES	DISTRIBUTION
dental n.'s	see alveolar nerves		
digital n.'s, common palmar *nn. digitales palmares communes*	median n. ulnar n.	proper palmar digitals	skin of palmar surface and sides of digits I–IV, first two lumbrical muscles
digital n.'s, proper palmar digital collaterals *nn. digitales palmares proprii*	common palmar digital nerves	filaments	skin of palmar surface and dorsal surface over terminal phalanx of the digits
digital n.'s of foot, dorsal *nn. digitales dorsales pedis*	intermediate dorsal cutaneous n. of foot	filaments	dorsal aspect of toes
digital n.'s of lateral plantar n., common plantar *nn. digitales plantares communes nervi plantaris lateralis*	superficial branch of lateral plantar n.	proper plantar digitals	plantar aspect of lateral toes
digital n.'s of lateral plantar n., proper plantar *nn. digitales plantares proprii nervi plantaris lateralis*	common plantar digital nerves of lateral plantar nerve	filaments	plantar aspect of lateral toes
digital n.'s of lateral side of great toe and medial side of second toe *nn. digitales dorsales hallucis lateralis et digiti secundi medialis*	deep peroneal n.	filaments	adjacent sides of great and second toes
digital n.'s of medial plantar n., common plantar *nn. digitales plantares communes nervi plantaris medialis*	medial plantar n.	proper plantar digitals	plantar aspect of medial toes
digital n.'s of medial plantar n., proper plantar *nn. digitales plantares proprii nervi plantaris medialis*	common plantar	filaments	plantar aspect of medial toes
digital n.'s of radial n., dorsal *nn. digitales dorsales nervi radialis*	superficial branch of radial n.	filaments	skin of dorsum of lateral fingers
digital n.'s of ulnar n., common palmar *nn. digitales palmares communes nervi ulnaris*	superficial branch of palmar branch of ulnar n.	proper palmar digitals	skin of palmar surface of little and ring fingers
digital n.'s of ulnar n., dorsal *nn. digitales dorsales nervi ulnaris*	dorsal branch of ulnar n.	filaments	skin of dorsum of medial fingers
digital n.'s of ulnar, proper palmar *nn. digitales palmares proprii nervi ulnaris*	common palmar digital nerves of ulnar	filaments	palmar surface of little and ring fingers

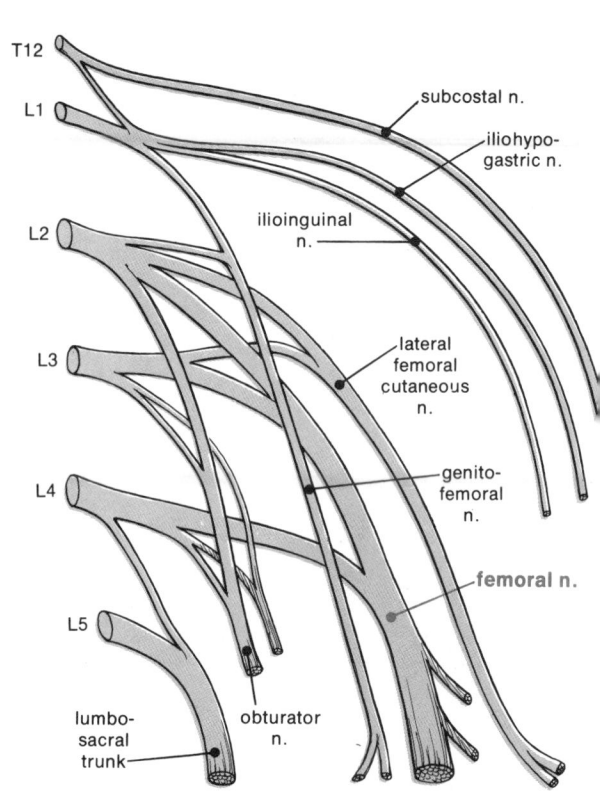

NERVE	ORIGIN	BRANCHES	DISTRIBUTION
dorsal n. of clitoris *n. dorsalis clitoridis*	pudendal n.	filaments	urethra and clitoris
dorsal n. of penis *n. dorsalis penis*	pudendal n.	filaments	urethra and penis
dorsal scapular n.	see scapular nerve, dorsal		
eighth cranial n	see vestibulocochlear nerve		
eleventh cranial n.	see accessory nerve		
ethmoid n., anterior *n. ethmoidalis anterior*	nasociliary n.	internal, external, lateral, and medial nasal	mucous membrane of nasal cavity
ethmoid n., posterior *n. ethmoidalis posterior*	nasociliary n.	filaments	mucous membrane of posterior ethmoidal and sphenoidal sinuses
facial n. seventh cranial n. *n. facialis*	lower border of pons	petrosal, to tympanic plexus, stapedial, chorda tympani, muscular, auricular, temporal, zygomatic, buccal, mandibular, cervical	*motor part*: muscles of facial expression, scalp, external ear, buccinator, platysma, stapedius, stylohyoid, and posterior belly of digastric; *sensory part*: anterior two-thirds of tongue, parts of external acoustic meatus, soft palate, and adjacent pharynx; *parasympathetic part*: secretomotor fibers of submandibular, sublingual, lacrimal, nasal, and palatine glands
femoral n. anterior crural n. *n. femoralis*	second, third, and fourth lumbar nerves	articular, muscular, saphenous, anterior cutaneous	skin of anterior and medial side of leg, hip and knee joint, quadriceps muscle of thigh, pectineal, sartorius, and iliac muscles
fifth cranial n.	see trigeminal nerve		
first cranial n.	see olfactory nerve		
fourth cranial n.	see trochlear nerve		
frontal n. *n. frontalis*	ophthalmic n.	supraorbital, supratrochlear, frontal sinus	conjunctiva, skin of upper eyelid and forehead, corrugator and frontal muscles, scalp, frontal sinus

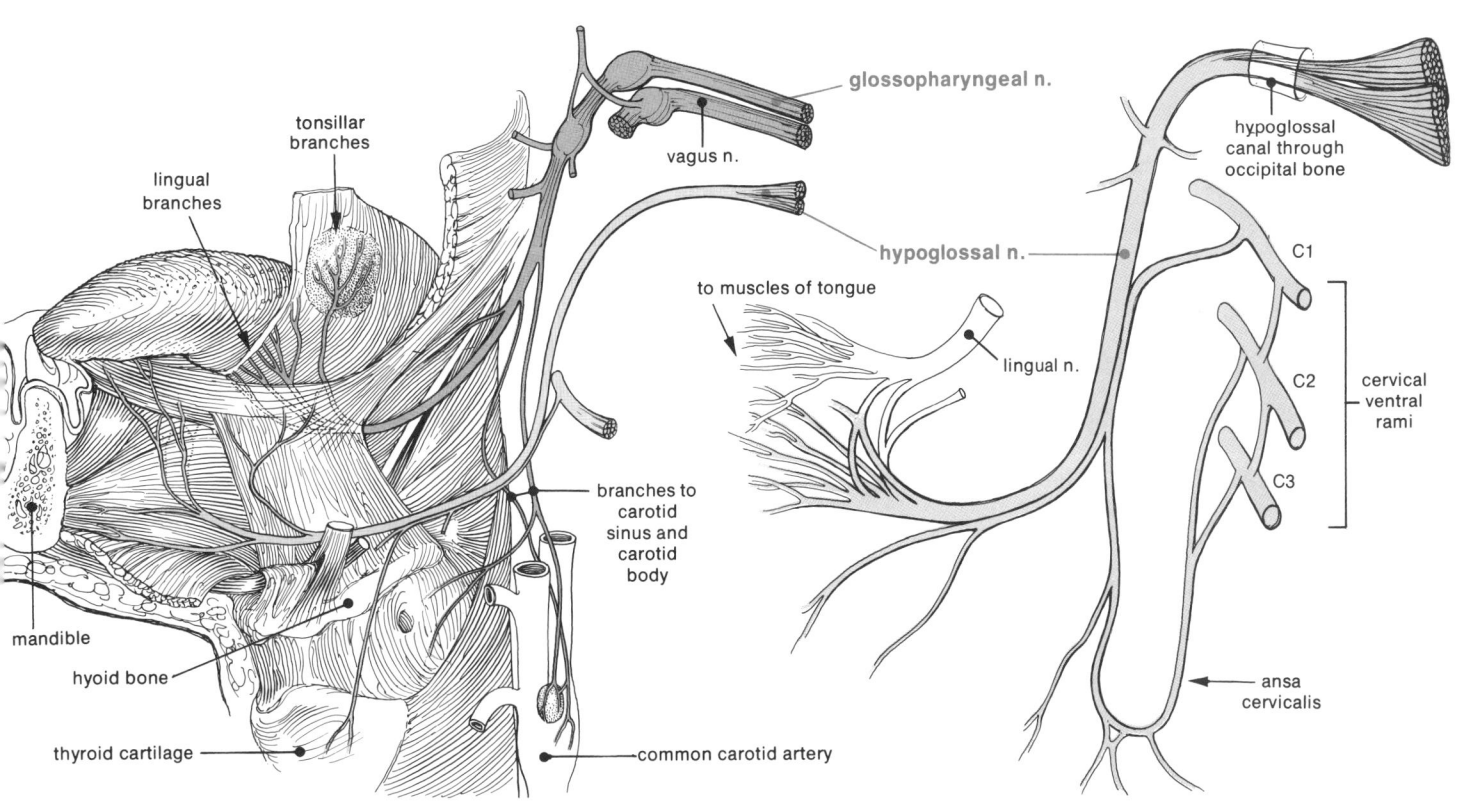

labels on figure:

tonsillar branches

lingual branches

glossopharyngeal n.

vagus n.

hypoglossal canal through occipital bone

hypoglossal n.

C1

to muscles of tongue

lingual n.

cervical ventral rami

C2

C3

branches to carotid sinus and carotid body

mandible

hyoid bone

ansa cervicalis

thyroid cartilage

common carotid artery

NERVE	ORIGIN	BRANCHES	DISTRIBUTION
n. of geniohyoid n. geniohyoideus	first cervical n.	filaments	geniohyoid muscle
genitofemoral n. genitocrural n. n. genitofemoralis	first and second lumbar nerves	genital, femoral	cremaster muscle, skin of scrotum or labium major and adjacent thigh, proximal part of anterior surface of thigh
glossopalatine n.	see intermediate nerve		
glossopharyngeal n. ninth cranial n. n. glossopharyngeus	upper part of medulla oblongata	tympanic, carotid sinus, pharyngeal, stylopharyngeal, tonsillar, lingual	tongue and pharynx, fauces, palatine tonsil, blood pressure receptor of carotid sinus, stylopharyngeus muscle
gluteal n., inferior n. gluteus inferior	fifth lumbar nerve and first and second sacral nerves		gluteus maximus muscle
gluteal n. superior n. gluteus superior	fourth and fifth lumbar nerves and first sacral nerve	superior, inferior, filaments	gluteus minimus and medius muscles, tensor muscle of fascia lata
hemorrhoidal n.	see rectal nerve		
hypogastric n. n. hypogastricus	a single large nerve (or several parallel bundles) which interconnects the superior hypogastric plexus with the inferior hypogastric plexus		
hypoglossal n. twelfth cranial n. n. hypoglossus	series of rootlets between pyramid and olive of medulla oblongata	meningeal, descending hypoglossal, muscular	intrinsic and extrinsic muscles of tongue; dura mater
hypoglossal n., small	see lingual nerve		
iliohypogastric n. n. iliohypogastricus	first lumbar n.	lateral, anterior cutaneous, muscular	abdominal muscles, skin of lower part of abdomen and gluteal region
ilioinguinal n. n. ilioinguinalis	first lumbar n.	anterior scrotal (male), anterior labial (female), muscular, filaments	muscles of abdominal wall, skin of proximal and medial part of thigh, root of penis (male), mons pubis and labium major (female)
infraoccipital n.	see suboccipital nerve		
infraorbital n. n. infraorbitalis	maxillary n.	inferior palpebral, external nasal, superior labial; posterior, middle and anterior superior alveolar	upper teeth, skin of face, mucous membrane of mouth and floor of nasal cavity
infratrochlear n. n. infratrochlearis	nasociliary n.	palpebral	skin of eyelids and side of nose, conjunctiva, lacrimal sac and duct

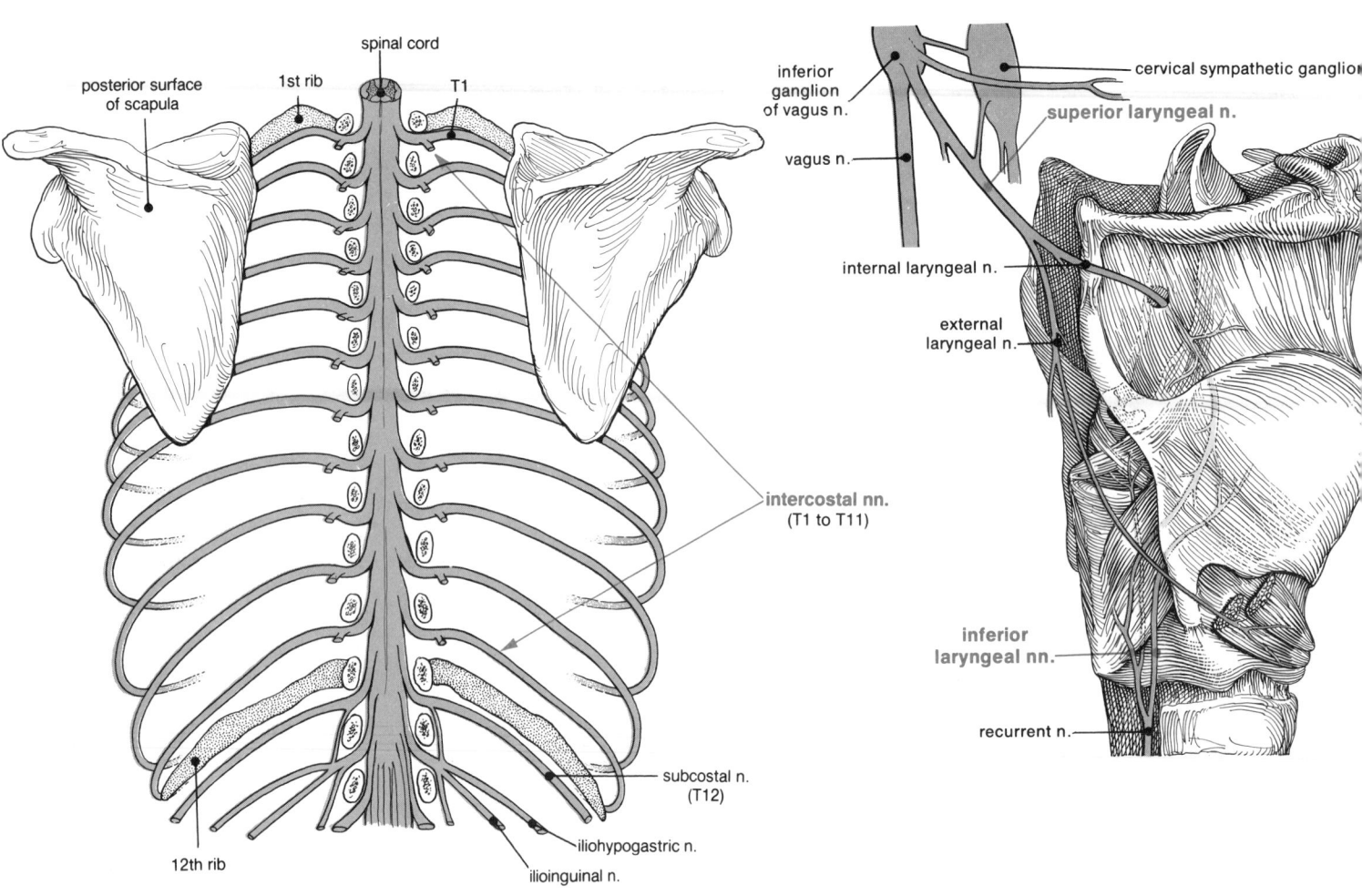

Figure labels (left diagram):
- posterior surface of scapula
- 1st rib
- spinal cord
- T1
- intercostal nn. (T1 to T11)
- subcostal n. (T12)
- iliohypogastric n.
- ilioinguinal n.
- 12th rib

Figure labels (right diagram):
- inferior ganglion of vagus n.
- cervical sympathetic ganglion
- superior laryngeal n.
- vagus n.
- internal laryngeal n.
- external laryngeal n.
- inferior laryngeal nn.
- recurrent n.

NERVE	ORIGIN	BRANCHES	DISTRIBUTION
intercostal n.'s (ventral rami of upper 11 thoracic nerves between ribs) *nn. intercostales*	thoracic segments of spinal cord	lateral cutaneous, anterior cutaneous	first two nerves supply fibers to upper limb and thoracic wall; next four supply thoracic wall; lower five supply thoracic and abdominal walls
intercostobrachial n. *n. intercostobrachialis*	second and frequenty third intercostal n.	filaments	skin of medial and posterior part of arm; axilla
intermediate n. glossopalatine n. n. of Wrisberg *n. intermedius*	brainstem at inferior border of pons	greater petrosal, chorda tympani	taste buds of anterior two-thirds of tongue, glands of soft palate and nose, submandibular and sublingual glands, skin of external acoustic meatus and mastoid process
interosseous n. of forearm, anterior *n. interosseus antebrachii anterior*	median n.	muscular	most of the deep anterior muscles of forearm
interosseous n. of forearm, posterior *n. interosseus antebrachii posterior*	deep branch of radial n.	muscular, articular	wrist and intercarpal joints, deep extensor muscles of forearm, long abductor and extensor muscles of thumb
interosseous n. of leg *n. interosseus cruris*	tibial n.	filaments	ankle joints
jugular n. *n. jugularis*	superior cervical ganglion	filaments	to glossopharyngeal and vagus nerves
labial n.'s, anterior *nn. labiales anterior*	ilioinguinal n.	filaments	skin to anterior labial area of female genitalia
labial n.'s, posterior *nn. labiales posterior*	perineal n.	filaments	skin of posterior portion of labia and vestibule of vagina
lacrimal n. *n. lacrimalis*	ophthalmic n.	superior palpebral, glandular, filaments	lacrimal gland and adjacent conjunctiva, skin of upper eyelid
laryngeal n., inferior *n. laryngeus inferior*	recurrent laryngeal n.	filaments	all intrinsic muscles of larynx except cricothyroid muscle

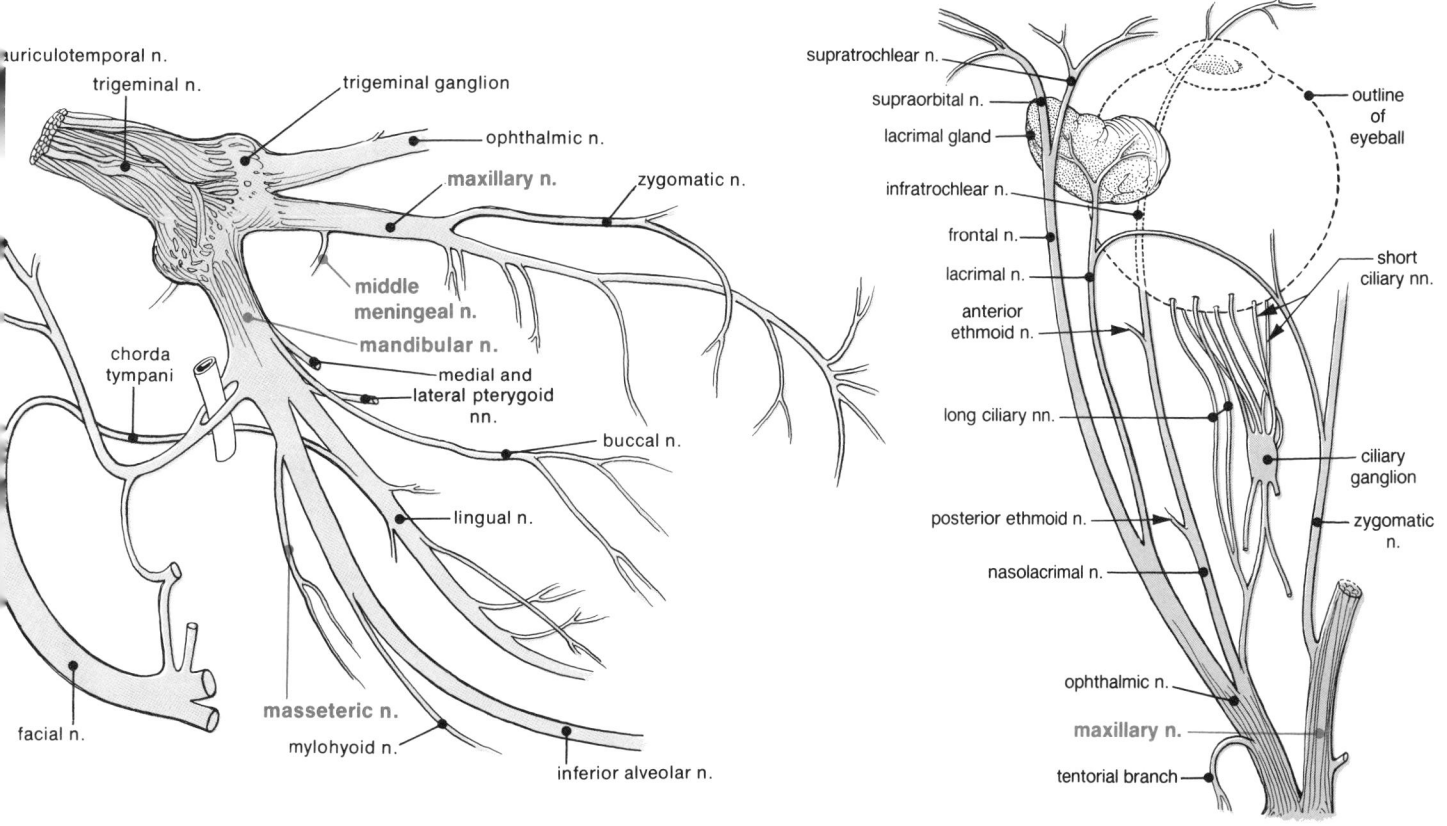

auriculotemporal n.
trigeminal n.
trigeminal ganglion
ophthalmic n.
maxillary n.
zygomatic n.
middle meningeal n.
mandibular n.
medial and lateral pterygoid nn.
buccal n.
lingual n.
chorda tympani
facial n.
masseteric n.
mylohyoid n.
inferior alveolar n.

supratrochlear n.
supraorbital n.
lacrimal gland
infratrochlear n.
frontal n.
lacrimal n.
anterior ethmoid n.
long ciliary nn.
posterior ethmoid n.
nasolacrimal n.
ophthalmic n.
maxillary n.
tentorial branch
outline of eyeball
short ciliary nn.
ciliary ganglion
zygomatic n.

NERVE	ORIGIN	BRANCHES	DISTRIBUTION
laryngeal n., superior *n. laryngeus superior*	vagus n. near the inferior ganglion	external, internal	mucous membrane of larynx and epiglottis; inferior pharyngeal and cricothyroid muscles
laryngeal recurrent n.		see recurrent nerve	
lingual n. small hypoglossal n. *n. lingualis*	mandibular division of trigeminal n.	sublingual, branches communicating with hypoglossal n., chorda tympani, and submandibular ganglion	mucous membranes of anterior two-thirds of tongue, floor of mouth, gums, and sublingual glands
lumbar n.'s (five pairs of spinal nerves) *nn. lumbales*	lumbar segments of spinal cord	ventral, dorsal	lumbar plexus, deep muscles and skin of lower back
mandibular n. inferior maxillary n. *n. mandibularis*	trigeminal ganglion	masseteric, medial pterygoid, lateral pterygoid, deep temporal, buccal, auriculotemporal, lingual, inferior alveolar, meningeal	muscles of mastication, tensor tympani, tensor of palatal velum, anterior belly of digastric, and mylohyoid muscles, mandible, lower teeth and gums, anterior two-thirds of tongue, cheek, lower face, meninges, temporomandibular joint, skin of temporal region, external ear
masseteric n. *n. massetericus*	mandibular n.	filaments	masseter muscle, temporomandibular joint
maxillary n. superior maxillary n. *n. maxillaris*	trigeminal ganglion	middle meningeal, zygomatic, pterygopalatine, infraorbital, superior alveolar, inferior palpebral, external nasal, superior labial	skin of middle part of face, nose, lower eyelid, and upper lip; upper teeth and gums, tonsil and roof of mouth, soft palate, maxillary sinus, mucous membrane of nasopharynx
median n. *n. medianus*	by two roots from medial and lateral cords of brachial plexus	muscular, articular, anterior interosseous, common palmar digitals, proper digital	most of flexor muscles of forearm, short muscles of thumb, lateral lumbricals, skin of hand, hand joints, elbow joint, pulp under nails
meningeal n. *n. meningeus*	vagus	filaments	meninges
meningeal n., middle *n. meningeus medius*	maxillary n.	filaments	meninges, especially dura mater

Labels in the illustration:
- section of midbrain
- crus cerebri
- substantia nigra
- red nucleus
- oculomotor nucleus
- cerebral aqueduct
- oculomotor n.
- medial view of left cerebral hemisphere
- olfactory tract
- olfactory bulb
- olfactor[y]
- nasal cavit[y]
- brain
- olfactory bulb
- olfactory n.
- superior concha
- nasal cavity

NERVE	ORIGIN	BRANCHES	DISTRIBUTION
mental n. *n. mentalis*	inferior alveolar n.	filaments	skin of chin, mucous membrane of lower lip
musculocutaneous n. *n. musculocutaneus*	lateral cord of brachial plexus	muscular, articular, filament, humeral filament, lateral cutaneous n. of forearm	coracobrachialis, brachialis and biceps muscles; skin of lateral side of forearm
musculospiral n.	see radial nerve		
mylohyoid n. *n. mylohyoideus*	inferior alveolar n. just before it enters mandibular foramen	filaments	mylohyoid and anterior belly of digastric muscles
nasal n.'s, external *nn. nasales externi*	infraorbital n.	filaments	skin on side of nose
nasociliary n. nasal n. *n. nasociliaris*	ophthalmic n.	long ciliary, anterior ethmoidal, posterior ethmoidal, infratrochlear, communication with ciliary ganglion	mucous membranes of nasal cavity, anterior ethmoidal and frontal sinuses; iris, cornea, conjunctiva, lacrimal sac, skin of eyelids and side of nose
nasopalatine n. Scarpa's n. *n. nasopalatinus*	pterygopalatine ganglion and maxillary n.	filaments	mucous membrane of hard palate and nasal septum
ninth cranial n	see glossopharyngeal nerve		
obturator n. *n. obturatorius*	second, third, and fourth lumbar nerves	anterior, posterior, filaments	hip and knee joints, skin of medial side of thigh, gracilis muscle, great, long, and short adductor muscles
obturator n., accessory *n. obturatorius accessorius*	third and fourth lumbar nerves	muscular, articular	pectineal muscle, hip joint
n. of obturatur, internal *n. obturatorius internus*	fifth lumbar and first and second sacral nerves	filaments	internal obturator and superior gemellus muscles
occipital n., larger (greater) *n. occipitalis major*	median branch of dorsal division of second cervical n.	muscular, filaments	scalp of top and back of head; semispinal muscle of head
occipital n., smaller (lesser) *n. occipitalis minor*	ventral division of suboccipital n. (from dorsal ramus of C1)	auricular, filaments	skin of side of head and behind ear
occipital n., third least occipital n. *n. occipitalis tertius*	cutaneous part of third cervical n.	filaments	skin of lower part of back of head
oculomotor n. third cranial n. *n. oculomotorius*	midbrain at medial side of cerebral peduncle	superior, inferior	levator muscle of upper eyelid, most intrinsic and extrinsic muscles of eye

geniculate body

optic tract

optic chiasma

optic n.

eyeball

inferior view of brain

field of vision

corpus callosum

medial view of brain

optic n.

optic chiasma

optic tract

geniculate body

visual area

NERVE	ORIGIN	BRANCHES	DISTRIBUTION
olfactory n.'s first cranial n.'s *nn. olfactorii*	olfactory portion of nasal mucosa	filaments	olfactory bulb
ophthalmic n. *n. ophthalmicus*	trigeminal ganglion	tentorial, lacrimal, frontal, nasociliary	dura mater, eyeball, conjunctiva, lacrimal gland, mucous membrane of nose and paranasal sinuses, skin of the forehead, eyelids, and nose
optic n. second cranial n. n. of sight *n. opticus*	ganglionic layer of retina	filaments	lateral geniculate body
palatine n., large anterior palatine n. *n. palatinus anterior*	pterygopalatine ganglion and maxillary n.	posterior inferior nasal, lesser palatine	gums, mucous membrane of hard and soft palates
palatine n.'s, small *nn. palatini medius et posterior*	pterygopalatine ganglion and maxillary n.	filaments	soft palate, uvula, palatine tonsil
palpebral n., inferior *n. palpebralis inferior*	infraorbital n.	filaments	lower eyelid
palpebral n., superior *n. palpebralis superior*	lacrimal n.	filaments	upper eyelid
pectoral n., lateral *n. pectoralis lateralis*	lateral cord of brachial plexus	filaments	greater pectoral muscle
pectoral n., medial *n. pectoralis medialis*	medial cord of brachial plexus	filaments	smaller pectoral muscle and caudal part of greater pectoral muscle
perineal n. *n. perinei*	pudendal n.	superficial (two), deep	urogenital diaphragm, skin of external genitalia, perineal muscles, mucous membrane of urethra
peroneal n., common external popliteal n. peroneal n. *n. peroneus communis*	sciatic n.	articular (three), lateral cutaneous n. of calf, deep peroneal, superficial peroneal	knee joint, skin of posterior and lateral surfaces of leg, short head of biceps muscle of thigh, leg muscles
peroneal n., deep anterior tibial n. *n. peroneus profundus*	common peroneal n.	muscular, articular, lateral terminal, medial terminal	anterior tibial, long extensor of great toe, long extensor of toes, short extensor of toes, third peroneal, ankle joint, tarsal and tarsophalangeal joints of second, third, and fourth toes

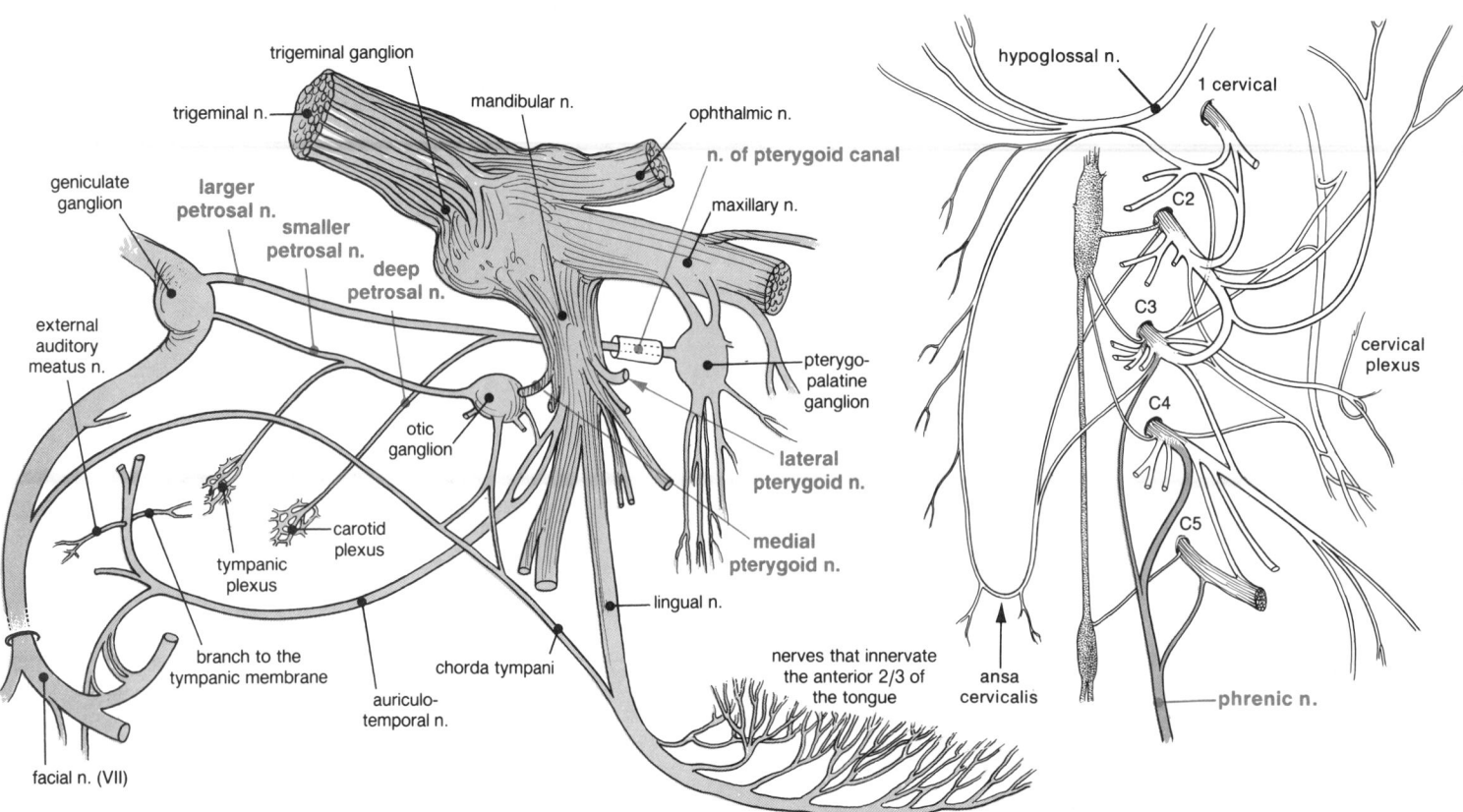

NERVE	ORIGIN	BRANCHES	DISTRIBUTION
peroneal n., superficial musculocutaneous n. *n. peroneus superficialis*	common peroneal n.	muscular, cutaneous filaments, medial dorsal cutaneous, intermediate dorsal cutaneous	long and short peroneal muscles, skin of lower part of leg, skin of medial side of foot, ankle, and side of great toe, skin of adjacent sides of second, third, fourth, and fifth toes
petrosal n., deep *n. petrosus profundus*	internal carotid plexus	joins larger petrosal n. to form n. of the pterygoid canal	glands and blood vessels of the pharynx, nasal cavity, lacrimal gland, and palate
petrosal n., larger (greater) greater superficial petrosal n. *n. petrosus major*	geniculate ganglion of facial n.	joins deep petrosal n. to form n. of pterygoid canal	mucous membrane and glands of palate, nose, lacrimal gland, and nasopharynx
petrosal n., smaller (lesser) lesser superficial petrosal n. *n. petrosus minor*	tympanic n.	ganglionic, filaments	otic ganglion, parotid gland
phrenic n. internal respiratory n. of Bell *n. phrenicus*	third, fourth, and fifth cervical nerves	pleural, pericardial, terminal	diaphragm, pericardium
phrenic n.'s, accessory *nn. phrenici accessorii*	inconstant branch from fifth cervical n. which arises with subclavian n.	joins phrenic n.	diaphragm
n. of piriform *n. piriformis*	second sacral n.	filaments	piriform muscle
plantar n., lateral external plantar n. *n. plantaris lateralis*	tibial n.	muscular, superficial, deep	skin of fifth and lateral half of fourth toes, deep muscles of foot
plantar n., medial internal plantar n. *n. plantaris medialis*	tibial n.	proper plantar digital, common digitals (three), plantar cutaneous, muscular, articular	skin of sole of foot, skin of adjacent sides of great, second, third, and fourth toes, joints of tarsus and metatarsus, short flexor muscle of great toe, lumbrical muscles of foot
pterygoid canal, n. of Vidian n. *n. canalis pterygoidei*	formed by union of larger petrosal and deep petrosal nerves	filaments	glands of nose, palate, and pharynx; pterygopalatine ganglion
pterygoid n., lateral *n. pterygoideus lateralis*	mandibular n.		deep surface of lateral pterygoid muscle
pterygoid n., medial *n. pterygoideus medialis*	mandibular n.	tensor veli palatini, tensor tympani	tensor veli palatini, tensor tympani and medial pterygoid muscles

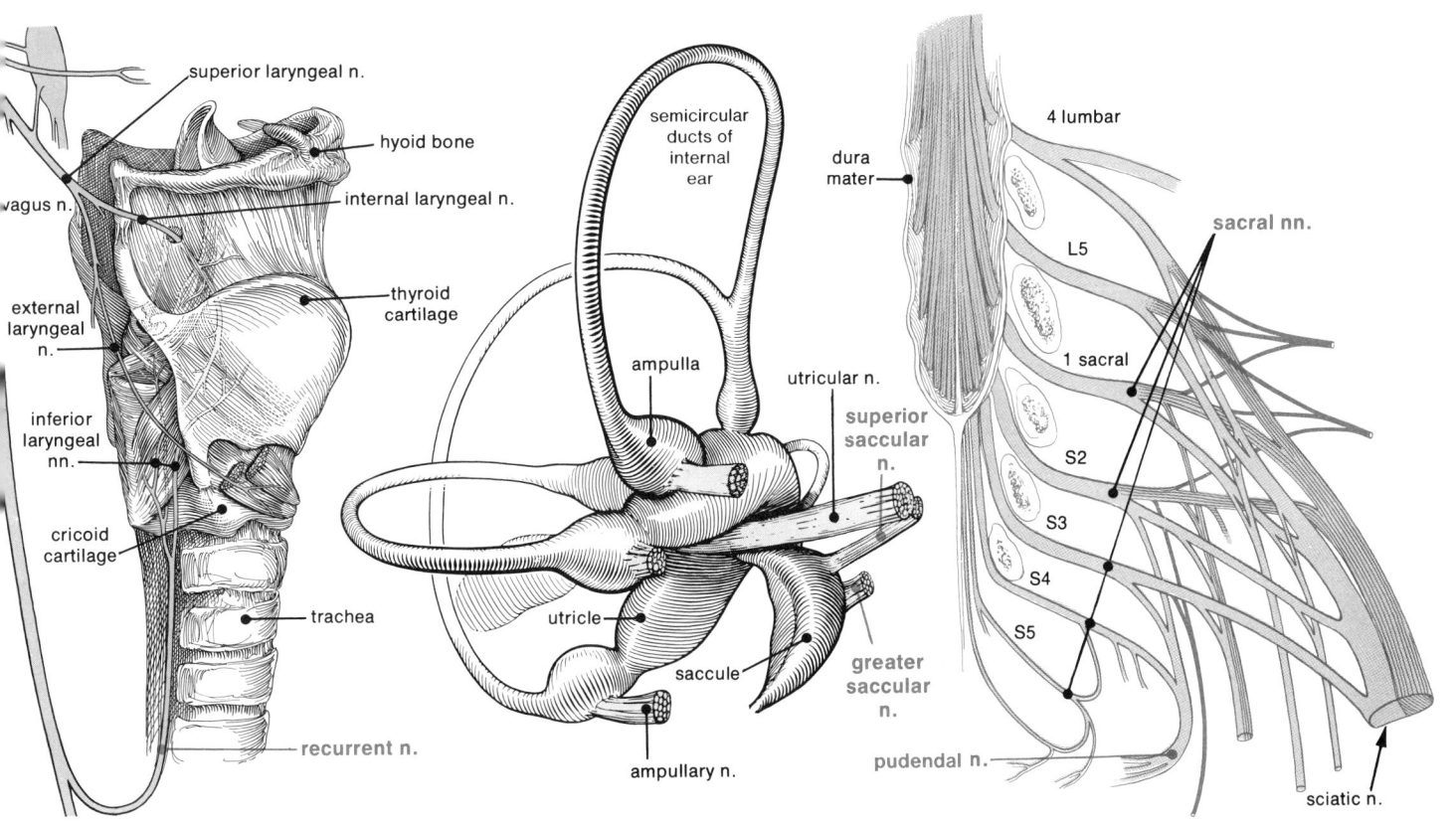

NERVE	ORIGIN	BRANCHES	DISTRIBUTION
pterygopalatine n.'s sphenopalatine n.'s *nn. pterygopalatine* *nn. ganglionares*	maxillary n.	orbital, greater palatine, posterior superior nasal, pharyngeal	mucous membranes of posterior ethmoidal and sphenoidal sinuses, nasal part of pharynx, and hard palate; periosteum of orbit, gums, nasal septum
pudendal n. internal pudic n. *n. pudendus*	second, third, and fourth sacral nerves	inferior rectal, perineal	urogenital diaphragm, skin around anus, skin of scrotum or labium major, external sphincter of anus
n. of quadrate muscle of thigh *n. quadratus femoris*	fourth and fifth lumbar and first sacral nerves	filaments	quadrate muscle of thigh and inferior gemellus muscle
radial n. musculospiral n. *n. radialis*	posterior cord of brachial plexus	muscular, articular, superficial, deep, cutaneous	extensor muscles of arm and forearm, and skin on back of arm, forearm, and hand
rectal n., inferior inferior hemorrhoidal n. *n. rectalis inferior*	pudendal n.	filaments	external sphincter of anus, skin around anus
rectal n., middle *n. rectalis medius*	hypogastric plexus	filaments	rectum
rectal n., superior *n. rectalis superior*	inferior mesenteric	filaments	rectum
recurrent n. recurrent laryngeal n. inferior laryngeal n. *n. recurrens*	vagus n.	pharyngeal, inferior laryngeal, tracheal, esophageal, cardiac	all muscles of larynx except cricothyroid; cardiac plexus, trachea, esophagus
saccular n., greater *n. saccularis major*	vestibular n.	filaments	larger of two nerves that innervate saccule of internal ear
saccular n., superior *n. saccularis superior*	vestibular n.	filaments	smaller of two nerves that innervate saccule of internal ear
sacral n.'s (five pairs of spinal nerves) *nn. sacrales*	sacral segments of spinal cord	dorsal, ventral	deep muscles and skin of lower back, pelvic viscera, sacral plexus
sacral plexus *plexus sacralis*	fourth and fifth lumbar and first, second, and third sacral nerves	internal obturator, superior and inferior gluteals, posterior femoral cutaneous, quadrate muscle of thigh, piriform, sciatic, pudendal	muscle and skin of perineum and lower limb; hip joint

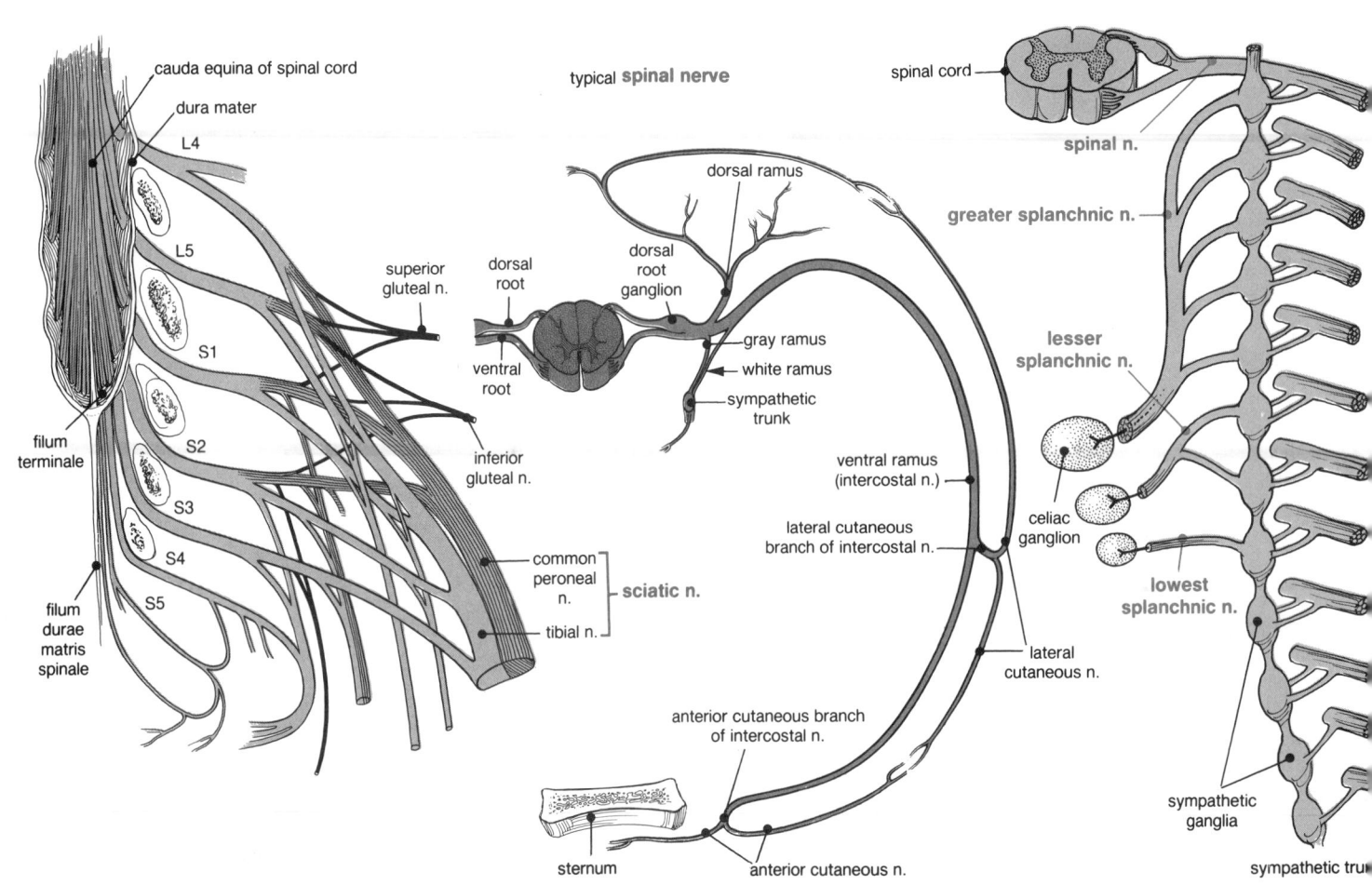

typical spinal nerve

Labels (diagram):
cauda equina of spinal cord
dura mater
L4
L5
S1
S2
S3
S4
S5
filum terminale
filum durae matris spinale
superior gluteal n.
inferior gluteal n.
dorsal root
ventral root
dorsal ramus
dorsal root ganglion
gray ramus
white ramus
sympathetic trunk
common peroneal n.
tibial n.
sciatic n.
ventral ramus (intercostal n.)
lateral cutaneous branch of intercostal n.
lateral cutaneous n.
anterior cutaneous branch of intercostal n.
anterior cutaneous n.
sternum
spinal cord
spinal n.
greater splanchnic n.
lesser splanchnic n.
celiac ganglion
lowest splanchnic n.
sympathetic ganglia
sympathetic trunk

NERVE	ORIGIN	BRANCHES	DISTRIBUTION
saphenus n. *n. saphenus*	femoral n.	infrapatellar, medial crural cutaneous, filaments	skin of medial side of leg and foot, knee joint
scapular n., dorsal posterior scapular n. *n. dorsalis scapulae*	fifth cervical n. near intervertebral foramen	filaments	greater and smaller rhomboid muscle, levator muscle of scapula
sciatic n. (largest nerve in body) great sciatic n. *n. ischiadicus*	fourth and fifth lumbar and first, second, and third sacral nerves	articular, muscular, tibial, common peroneal	skin of foot and most of leg, muscles of leg and foot, all joints of lower limb
sciatic n., small	see cutaneous nerve of thigh, posterior		
scrotal n.'s, anterior *nn. scrotales anterior*	ilioinguinal n.	filaments	skin of anterior scrotal area and root of penis
scrotal n.'s, posterior *nn. scrotales posterior*	perineal n.	filaments	skin of posterior scrotal area
second cranial n.	see optic nerve		
seventh cranial n.	see facial nerve		
sixth cranial n.	see abducent nerve		
spermatic n., external *n. genitalis externi*	genitofemoral	filaments	skin of scrotum and around inguinal ring area
sphenopalatine n.	see pterygopalatine nerve		
spinal n.'s *nn. spinales*	31 pairs of nerves arising from the spinal cord within the vertebral canal, including eight cervical, 12 thoracic, five lumbar, five sacral, and one coccygeal		
splanchnic n., greater *n. splanchnicus major*	fifth (or sixth) to ninth (or 10th) thoracic sympathetic ganglia	filaments	celiac ganglion
splanchnic n., lesser *n. splanchnicus minor*	ninth and 10th thoracic sympathetic ganglia	renal, filaments	aorticorenal ganglion
splanchnic n., lowest least splanchnic n. *n. splanchnicus imus*	last thoracic sympathetic ganglion or lesser splanchnic n.	filaments	renal plexus
splanchnic n.'s, lumbar (two to four in number) *nn. splanchnici lumbales*	lumbar sympathetic trunk at level of first, second, and third lumbar vertebrae	filaments	celiac, mesenteric aortic, and hypogastric plexuses

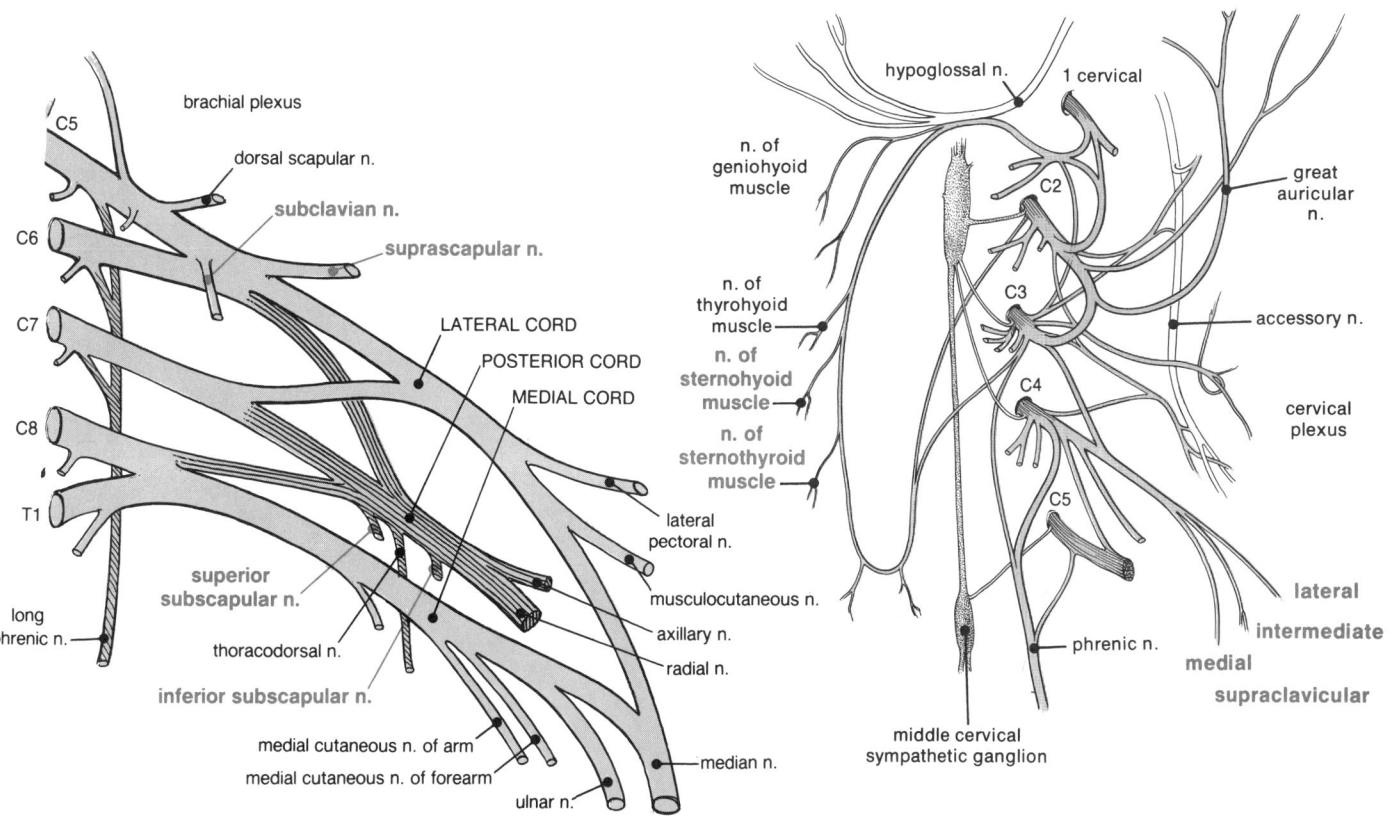

NERVE	ORIGIN	BRANCHES	DISTRIBUTION
splanchnic n.'s, sacral *nn. splanchnici sacrales*	sacral sympathetic ganglion	filaments	inferior hypogastric plexus
splanchnic n.'s, pelvic erigentes n.'s *nn. splanchnici pelvini*	second to fourth sacral nerves	filaments	inferior hypogastric plexus, descending and sigmoid colon, pelvic viscera
n. of stapedius *n. stapedius*	facial n.	filaments	stapedius muscle
n. of sternohyoid *n. sternohyoideus*	convexity of ansa cervicalis	filaments	sternohyoid muscle
n. of sternothyroid *n. sternothyroideus*	convexity of ansa cervicalis	filaments	sternothyroid muscle
subclavian n. *n. subclavius*	superior trunk of brachial plexus	articular, filaments	subclavius muscle, sternoclavicular joint
subcostal n. *n. subcostalis*	12th thoracic n.	filaments	skin of lower abdominal wall and gluteal region; some abdominal muscles
sublingual n. *n. sublingualis*	lingual n.	filaments	sublingual gland and mucous membrane of floor of mouth
suboccipital n. infraoccipital n. *n. suboccipitalis*	first cervical	filaments	deep muscles of back of neck
subscapular n.'s (usually two in number) *nn. subscapulares*	posterior cord of brachial plexus	superior, inferior	subscapular and teres major muscles
supraclavicular n.'s, intermediate middle supraclavicular n.'s *nn. supraclaviculares intermedii*	third and fourth cervical nerves	filaments	skin over pectoral and deltoid muscles
supraclavicular n.'s, lateral posterior supraclavicular n.'s super-acromial n.'s *nn. supraclaviculares laterales*	third and fourth cervical nerves	filaments	skin of upper and dorsal parts of shoulder
supraclavicular n.'s, medial anterior supraclavicular n.'s *nn. supraclaviculares mediales*	third and fourth cervical nerves	filaments	skin of medial infraclavicular region as far as the midline, sternoclavicular joint
supraorbital n. *n. supraorbitalis*	frontal n.	medial, lateral	skin of upper eyelid and forehead, mucosa of frontal sinus, scalp
suprascapular n. *n. suprascapularis*	superior trunk of brachial plexus	supraspinous, infraspinous, articular, filaments	supraspinous and infraspinous muscles, shoulder joint

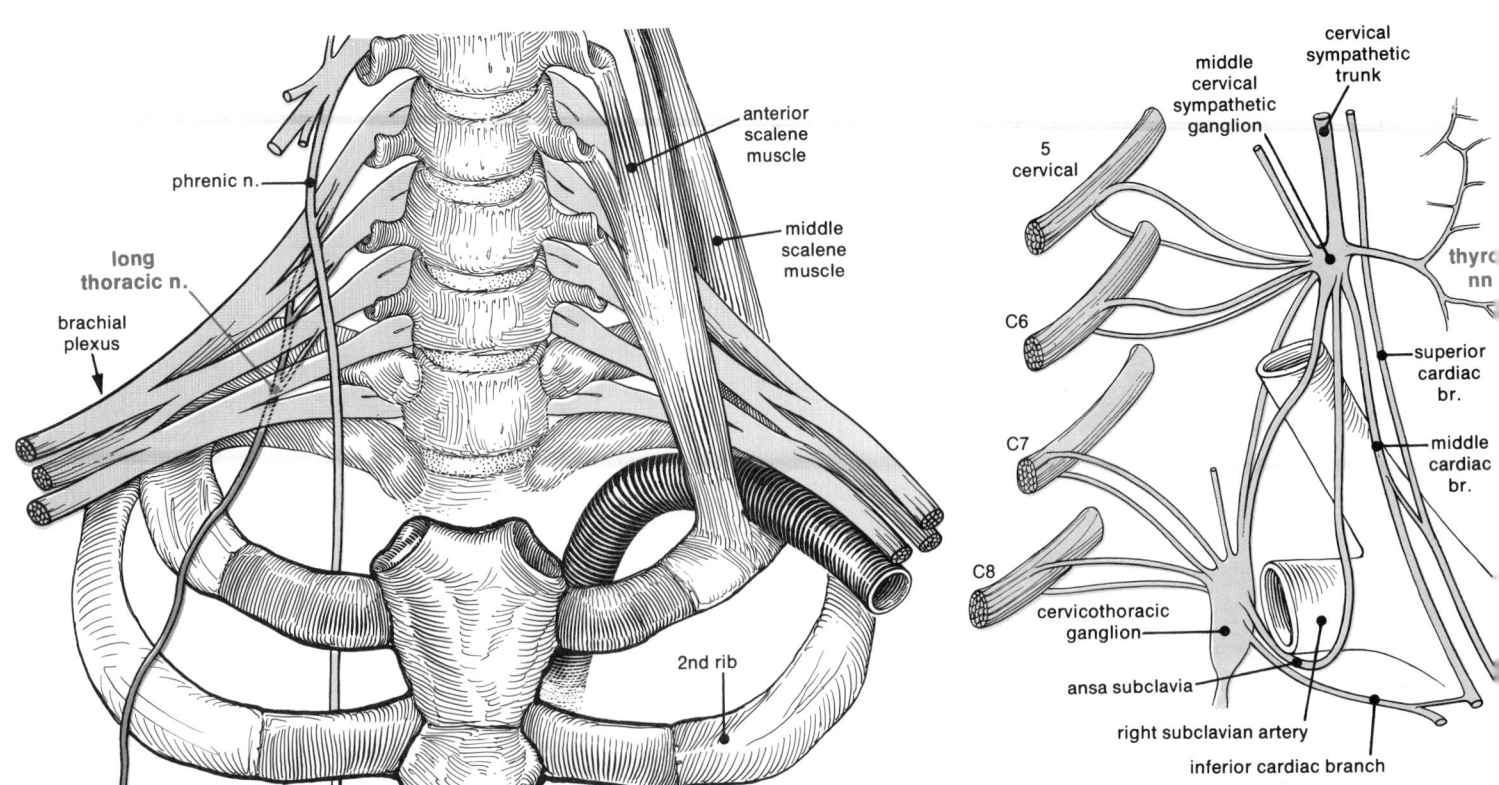

NERVE	ORIGIN	BRANCHES	DISTRIBUTION
supratrochlear n. *n. supratrochlearis*	frontal n.	filaments	conjunctiva, skin of upper eyelid and forehead
sural n. short saphenous n. *n. suralis*	medial and lateral cutaneous nerves of calf	lateral dorsal cutaneous, lateral calcaneal	skin of back of leg and lateral side of foot
temporal n.'s, deep (usually two in number) *nn. temporales profundi*	mandibular division of trigeminal n.	filaments	temporal muscle
n. to tensor tympani *n. tensoris tympani*	medial pterygoid n.	filaments	tensor muscle of tympanum
n. to tensor veli palatini *n. tensoris veli palatini*	medial pterygoid n.	filaments	tensor muscle of palatine velum
tenth cranial n.	see vagus nerve		
tentorial n. *n. tentorii*	ophthalmic n.	filaments	meninges
terminal n. *n. terminalis*	cerebral hemispheres near olfactory trigone	filaments	dura mater, mucous membrane of nasal septum
third cranial n.	see oculomotor nerve		
thoracic n.'s (12 pairs of spinal nerves) *nn. thoracici*	thoracic segments of spinal cord	dorsal, ventral	thoracic and abdominal walls (parietes) and skin of the buttock
thoracic n., long n. of serratus anterior *n. thoracicus longus*	fifth, sixth, and seventh cervical nerves	filaments	all digitations of serratus anterior muscle
thoracoabdominal intercostal n.'s *nn. thoracoabdominales intercostales*	ventral primary divisions of seventh to 11th thoracic nerves beyond the intercostal spaces	filaments	anterior abdominal wall
thoracodorsal n. long subscapular n. n. of latissimus dorsi *n. thoracodorsalis*	posterior cord of brachial plexus	filaments	latissimus dorsi muscle
n. of thyrohyoid *n. thyrohoideus*	first cervical n. traveling with hypoglossal n.	filaments	thyrohyoid muscle
thyroid n.'s *nn. thyroideus*	middle cervical ganglion	filaments	thyroid gland
tibial n. internal popliteal n. *n. tibialis*	sciatic n.	articular, medial calcaneal, medial sural cutaneous, medial and lateral plantar	knee and ankle joints, muscles of posterior leg, plantar muscles of foot

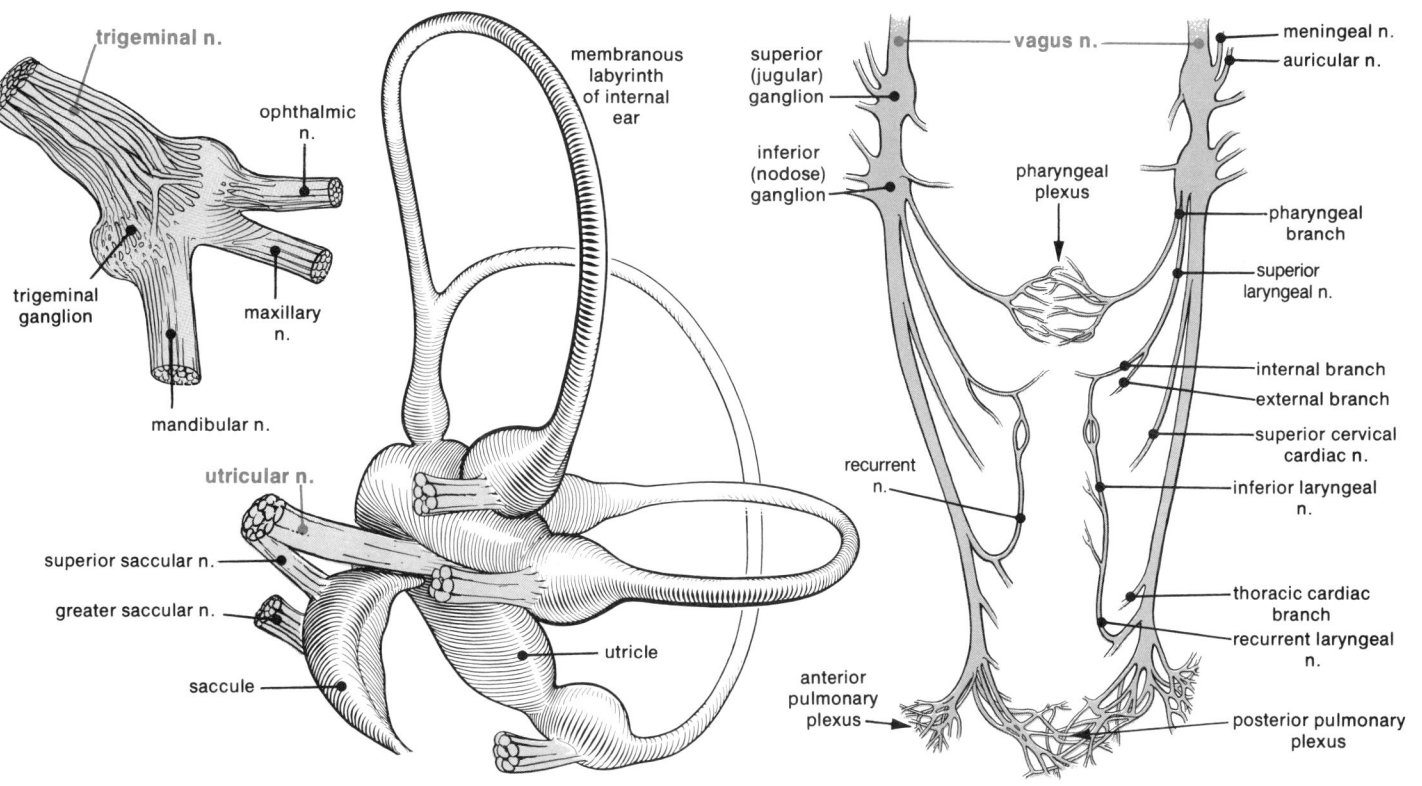

NERVE	ORIGIN	BRANCHES	DISTRIBUTION
tibial n., anterior	see peroneal nerve, deep		
tranverse cervical n. cervical cutaneous n. *n. transversus colli*	second and third cervical nerves	ascending, descending	skin over anterior and lateral parts of neck
trigeminal n. (largest of the cranial nerves) fifth n. trifacial n. *n. trigeminus*	brainstem at inferior surface of pons	two roots (motor and sensory) expand into trigeminal ganglion near apex of petrous portion of temporal bone, from which ophthalmic, maxillary, and mandibular nerves arise	skin of face, muscles of mastication, teeth, mouth, and nasal cavity
trochlear n. (smallest of the cranial nerves) fourth cranial n. *n. trochlearis*	midbrain immediately posterior to the inferior colliculus	filaments	superior oblique muscle of eyeball
twelfth cranial n.	see hypoglossal nerve		
tympanic n. n. of Jacobson *n. tympanicus*	glossopharyngeal n.	lesser petrosal, filaments	middle ear chamber, tympanic membrane, mastoid air cells, auditory tube, parotid gland
ulnar n. cubital n. *n. ulnaris*	medial cord of brachial plexus	articular, muscular, dorsal, palmar (superficial and deep)	intrinsic muscles of hand, elbow, wrist and hand joints, skin of medial side of hand
utricular n. *n. utricularis*	vestibular n.	filaments	utricle of the internal ear
utriculoampullary n. *n. utriculoampullaris*	a division of the vestibular portion of the vestibulocochlear n.; it innervates the macula of the utricle and the ampullae of the anterior and lateral semicircular ducts		
vaginal n.'s *nn. vaginales*	pelvic plexus	filaments	vagina
vagus n. tenth cranial n. pneumogastric n. *n. vagus*	side of medulla oblongata	meningeal, auricular, pharyngeal, superior laryngeal, superior and inferior cardiac, anterior and posterior bronchial, recurrent, esophageal, gastric, hepatic, celiac	dura mater, skin of posterior surface of external ear, voluntary muscles of larynx and pharynx, heart, nonstriated muscles and glands of esophagus, stomach, trachea, bronchi, biliary tract, and intestines, mucous membranes of pharynx, larynx, bronchi, lungs, digestive tract, and kidney

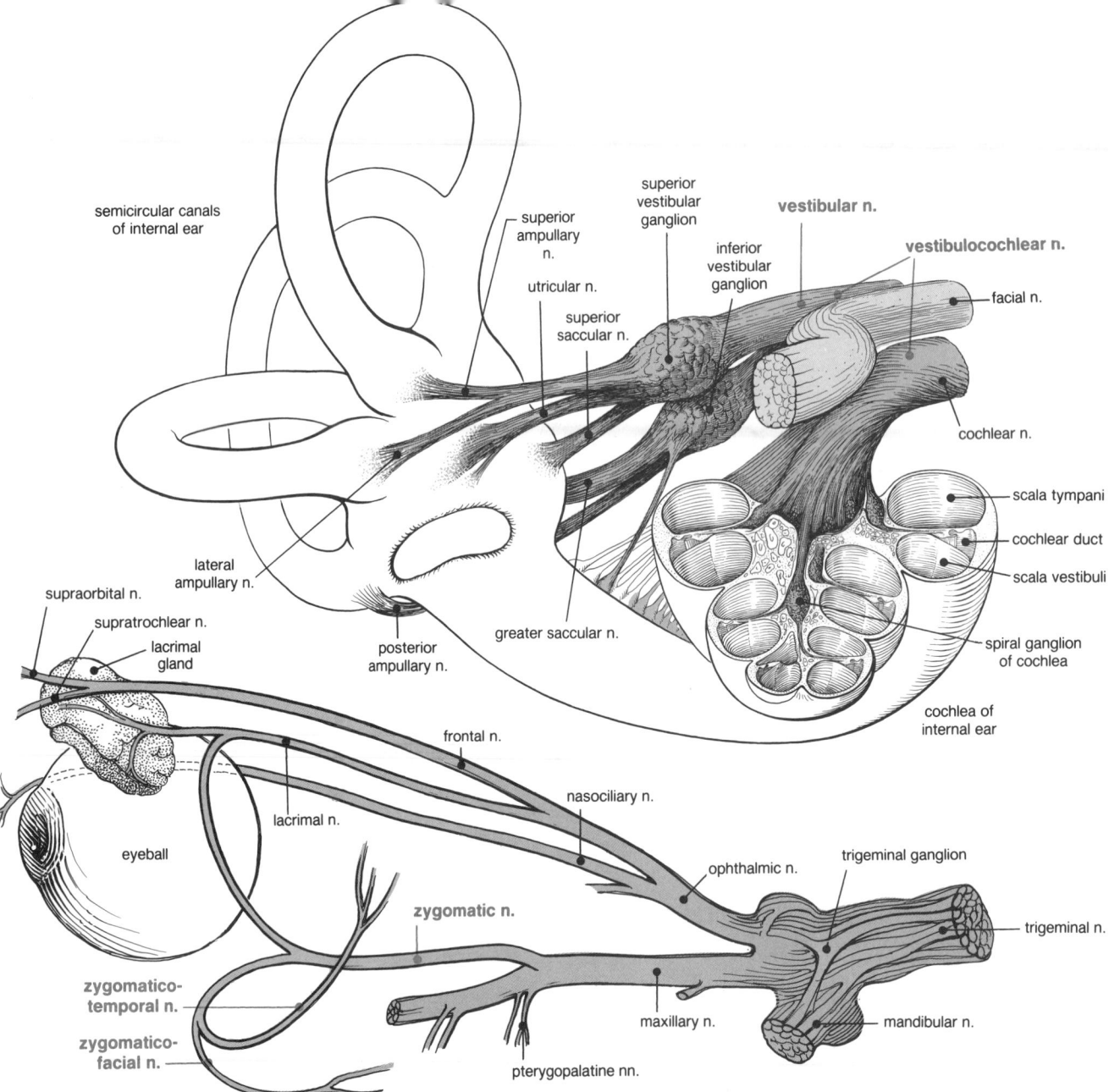

semicircular canals
of internal ear

superior
ampullary
n.

utricular n.

superior
saccular n.

superior
vestibular
ganglion

inferior
vestibular
ganglion

vestibular n.

vestibulocochlear n.

facial n.

cochlear n.

scala tympani

cochlear duct

scala vestibuli

spiral ganglion
of cochlea

cochlea of
internal ear

lateral
ampullary n.

posterior
ampullary n.

greater saccular n.

supraorbital n.

supratrochlear n.

lacrimal
gland

lacrimal n.

eyeball

frontal n.

nasociliary n.

ophthalmic n.

trigeminal ganglion

trigeminal n.

zygomatic n.

maxillary n.

mandibular n.

zygomatico-
temporal n.

zygomatico-
facial n.

pterygopalatine nn.

NERVE	ORIGIN	BRANCHES	DISTRIBUTION
vertebral n. *n. vertebralis*	cervicothoracic ganglion	meningeal, filaments	meninges, joins cervical nerves
vestibular n. n. of equilibration *n. vestibularis*	vestibulocochlear n.	utricular, saccular, ampullary	through vestibular ganglion (ganglion of Scarpa) to maculae of utricle and saccule, and to ampullae of semicircular ducts)
vestibulocochlear n. eighth cranial n. auditory n. acoustic n. otic n. *n. vestibulocochlearis*	brainstem between pons and medulla oblongata formed by union of vestibular and cochlear nerves	vestibular (medial), cochlear (lateral)	receptor organs in membranous labyrinth of internal ear
Vidian n.	see pterygoid canal, nerve of		
vomernasal n. *n. vomernasalis*	present in the nasal septum of the fetus but disappears before birth		
zygomatic n. orbital n. temporomalar n. *n. zygomaticus*	maxillary n.	zygomaticotemporal, zygomaticofacial	skin of temple, skin on prominence of cheek
zygomaticofacial n. *n. zygomaticofacialis*	zygomatic n.	filaments	skin over prominence of cheek
zygomaticotemporal n. *n. zygomaticotemporalis*	zygomatic n.	filaments	skin on side of forehead

node of Ranvier

neurofibrils

axoplasm

axolemma

axon

neurilemma

myelin

processes

oligodendrocyte

neuroglia

gelatinous layer

cilium

microvilli

neuroepithelium

(hair cells of
the utricular
macula of the
internal ear)

cell
body

microglia

protoplasmic
astrocyte

fibrous
astrocyte

nesslerize To treat with Nessler's reagent in order to determine the level of urea nitrogen in the blood and in the urine.

nest A collection of similar cells.
 cell n.'s Small collections of a different type of cell in a tissue.
 epithelial n.'s Small aggregations of neoplastic tissue composed of compressed polygonal cells, frequently seen in squamous cell carcinoma. Also called epithelial pearls; onion bodies.

net Network.

network A structure composed of interlocking filaments. Also called reticulum; rete.
 chromatin n. Basophilic network in the nuclei of many cells, appearing after fixation.
 Purkinje's n. Network of muscle fibers beneath the endocardium of the cardiac ventricles.

neural 1. Relating to the nervous system. **2.** Referring to the dorsal region of an embryo.

neuralgia Severe pain along the course of a nerve.
 trigeminal n. Severe facial pain in the area of the trigeminal nerve. Also called tic douloureux.

neuralgic Relating to neuralgia.

neuranagenesis Regeneration of a nerve.

neurapraxia Injury to a nerve resulting in temporary paralysis.

neurasthenia Condition marked by fatigue, irritability, and poor concentration; originally considered to be due to exhaustion of the nervous system.

neuraxis 1. The central nervous system. **2.** Axon.

neuraxon See axon.

neurectomy Surgical removal of a nerve segment.

neurectopia, neurectopy Abnormal location of a nerve.

neurergic Of or relating to the action of nerves.

neurilemma The thin cytoplasmic membrane of a Schwann cell enwrapping the axon of an unmyelinated nerve fiber and also the myelin layers of a myelinated nerve fiber. Also called sheath of Schwann.

neurilemmitis Inflammation of the neurilemma.

neurilemoma A benign encapsulated tumor originating from a peripheral or sympathetic nerve or from the facial nerve. Also called neurinoma; schwannoma.
 acoustic n. See under neurinoma.
 Antoni type A n. A relatively solid tumor consisting of Schwann cells (arranged in twisting bundles) and reticulum fibers.
 Antoni type B n. A relatively soft tumor consisting of Schwann cells (arranged in a haphazard way), reticulum fibers, and minute cysts.

neurinoma See neurilemoma.
 acoustic n. Benign tumor growing on, and com-

pressing, the vestibulocochlear (VIII cranial) nerve. Also called acoustic neurilemoma.

neuritis Inflammation or degeneration of a nerve.
 intraocular optic n. See papillitis.
 optic n. Neuritis of the optic nerve.
 toxic n. Neuritis resulting from a chemical toxin, as in arsenic or lead poisoning.
 traumatic n. Neuritis following an injury.

neuroanastomosis Surgical union of nerves.

neuroanatomy The branch of anatomy concerned with the study of the nervous system.

neurobiology The integrated study of neuroanatomy and neurophysiology, i.e., of the structure and the normal vital processes of the nervous system.

neurobiotaxis The tendency of nerve cells to move in the direction of the area where most of the impulses originate.

neuroblast An embryonic nerve cell.

neuroblastoma A highly malignant tumor arising most frequently from the medulla of the adrenal gland; it is the most common malignant tumor of childhood and infancy. Also called sympathoblastoma; sympathogonioma.

neurocardiac 1. Relating to the nerve supply of the heart. **2.** Relating to a cardiac neurosis.

neurocele The ventricles of the brain and the central canal of the spinal cord.

neurochemistry The study of the chemical activity of nervous tissues.

neurochoroiditis Inflammation of the optic nerve and the middle, vascular coat of the eye (choroid).

neurocladism Regeneration of a cut nerve by the outgrowth of axonal branches from the proximal stump which grow toward, and make contact with, the distal stump to bridge the gap.

neuroclonic Relating to or marked by nervous spasm.

neurocranium The portion of the skull containing the brain, distinguished from the facial bones.

neurocytoma See ganglioneuroma.

neurodermatitis Localized inflammation of the skin, of nervous or psychological origin.

neurodynamic Relating to nervous energy.

neurodynia Neuralgia.

neuroectoderm In embryology, the part of the ectoderm that gives rise to the neural tube.

neuroendocrine Denoting a relationship between the nervous system and the endocrine glands.

neuroendocrinology The study of the interactions of the nervous system with the endocrine glands.

neuroepithelioma A type of glioma consisting primarily of cells that resemble the precursors of

specialized sensory epithelium or of the brain and spinal cord.

neuroepithelium 1. The specialized epithelium composed of cells that act as receptors of external stimuli, as the hair cells of the internal ear. **2.** The layer of the ectoderm from which the neural tube develops.

neurofibril A nerve fibril; one of numerous aggregates of slender filaments running parallel with one another in the axon and dendrite but crossing and intermingling in the cell body.

neurofibroma A nonmalignant tumor originating in the connective tissues of nerves; it occurs most frequently in the skin, where the nodules are formed.

neurofibromatosis Inherited disorder transmitted as a dominant trait, marked by formation of multiple nerve tumors (neurofibromas).
 n. I A form marked by multiple soft tumors involving nerves of skin and internal organs, light brown (café au lait) spots on the skin, and pigmented (Lisch) nodules in the iris; may be associated with bone cysts and mental impairment. The defective gene is in chromosome 17. Also called Recklinghausen's disease.
 n. II A central, acoustic form marked by tumors in both vestibulocochlear (VIII cranial) nerves. The defective gene is in chromosome 22.

neurogenic, neurogenetic Originating in the nervous system.

neuroglia The nonneuronal tissue of the brain and spinal cord that performs supportive and other ancillary functions; composed of various types of cells collectively called neuroglial cells or glial cells. Also called glia.

neurogliocyte One of the cells composing the supporting, non-nervous portion of the nervous system.

neurogliomatosis The presence of tumors of neuroglial cells in the brain or spinal cord.

neurogliosis 1. Abnormal proliferation of neuroglial cells. **2.** The presence of several gliomas in the brain or spinal cord.

neurogram The hypothesized imprint left on the brain by each mental experience, stimulation of which produces memory. Also called brain residual.

neurohistology Microscopic study of the nervous system.

neurohormone A hormone whose secretion is controlled by the nervous system.

neurohumor An active chemical substance that effects the passage of nerve impulses from one cell to another at the synapse.

neurohypophyseal Relating to the posterior lobe of the pituitary gland. Also written neurohyoptic chiasma

nuclei of hypothalamus

adeno-hypophysis

hypothalamo-hypophyseal tract

neurohypophysis (pars posterior)

posterior hypophyseal vein

inferior hypophyseal artery

axon

dendrite

cell body of neuron

Golgi apparatus

neuron (nerve cell)

neurilemma

axon

axon hillock

gemmules

Nissl bodies

detail of cell body of neuron

---

pophysial.

neurohypophysis   The posterior or nervous lobe of the hypophysis; developed from the floor of the diencephalon.

neuroid   Resembling a nerve.

neurokeratin   **1.** A proteolipid network in the myelin sheath of axons. **2.** The pseudokeratin present in brain tissue.

neurolemma   Neurilemma.

neuroleptic   Any major tranquilizer that acts on the nervous system and has therapeutic effects on psychoses and other types of psychiatric disorders. Also called antipsychotic.

neuroleptic malignant syndrome   Rare, life-threatening reaction to neuroleptic drugs, marked by high fever, rigidity, and coma.

neurologist   A specialist in the nervous system and its diseases.

neurology   The branch of medicine concerned with the nervous system and its diseases.

neurolymph   Cerebrospinal fluid.

neurolysin   An agent that causes destruction of nerve cells. Also called neurotoxin.

neurolysis   **1.** Destruction of nerve tissues. **2.** The removal of adhesions from a nerve.

neuroma   Old term denoting any neoplasm derived from nerve tissue; more specific terms are generally preferred.

   amputation n., traumatic n.   One located at the proximal end of an injured nerve.

neuromalacia   Abnormal softening of nervous tissue.

neuromechanism   That part of the nervous system that controls the function of an organ.

neuromuscular   Relating to nerve and muscle, such as the nerve endings in a muscle, or the interaction of nerve and muscle.

neuromyasthenia   Muscular weakness, especially of emotional origin.

   epidemic n.   An epidemic febrile disorder gener-

ally affecting only adults, marked by stiffness of the neck and back, fever, headache, diarrhea, and localized muscular weakness. Also called Iceland disease; benign myalgic encephalomyelitis.

neuromyelitis   Inflammation of the nerves and spinal cord.

   n. optica   Inflammation of the optic nerves and spinal cord; considered a type of multiple sclerosis. Also called Devic's disease.

neuromyopathy   A disorder of muscle that indicates a disease of the nerve supplying the muscle.

neuromyositis   Nerve inflammation complicated by inflammation of the muscles with which the affected nerve is in relation.

neuron   The basic functional and anatomic unit of the nervous system, concerned with the conduction of impulses; structurally, it is the most complex cell of the body; the human nervous system contains about 28 billion neurons. Also called nerve cell.

   afferent n.   One that conducts impulses toward the spinal cord and brain. Also called sensory neuron.

   bipolar n.   A neuron possessing two separate axons as in the retina, olfactory mucosa, internal ear, and taste buds.

   central n.   A neuron entirely within the spinal cord or brain.

   efferent n.   One that conducts impulses away from the brain and spinal cord. Also called motor neuron.

   internuncial n.   One that connects afferent and efferent neurons. Also called association neuron.

   multipolar n.   A neuron with several short processes (dendrites) and a single long axon.

   pyramidal n.   A multipolar neuron whose cell body lies in the cerebral cortex. Also called pyramidal cell.

   unipolar n.   A neuron having a single process (axon) attached to its cell body.

neuronal   Of or relating to a nerve cell.

neuronic   Relating to a nerve cell.

neuronitis   Inflammation of nerve cells, especially those of the roots of spinal nerves.

neuronophage   A phagocyte that devours injured or diseased nerve cells.

neuronophagia   Destruction of unwanted nerve cells by neuronophages.

neuronyxis   See acupuncture.

neuro-ophthalmology   The branch of ophthalmology concerned with the part of the nervous system related to the eye. Also written neurophthalmology.

neuropapillitis   See papillitis.

neuroparalysis   Paralysis due to disease of the nerve supplying the affected part.

neuropathic   Relating to a disease of the nervous system.

neuropathogenesis   The origin of diseases of the nervous system.

neuropathology   Study of diseases of the nervous system.

neuropathy   Any disease of the nervous system.

   diabetic n.   A complication of diabetes mellitus in which the peripheral nerves and the innervation of the bladder and bowel may be affected.

   peripheral n.   A disorder of the peripheral nerves characterized by motor and sensory changes in the extremities; most commonly associated with alcoholism and/or poor nutrition.

neuropharmacology   Study of drugs that affect the nervous system.

neurophthalmology   See neuro-ophthalmology.

neurophthisis   Wasting of nervous tissue.

neurophysin   A huge endocrine gland molecule produced in nerve cell bodies at the base of the brain and stored in the pituitary gland; this macromolecule with a 92-step chemical sequence is thought to be a transporter of the hormones vasopressin and oxytocin.

neurophysiology   Study of the normal vital proc-

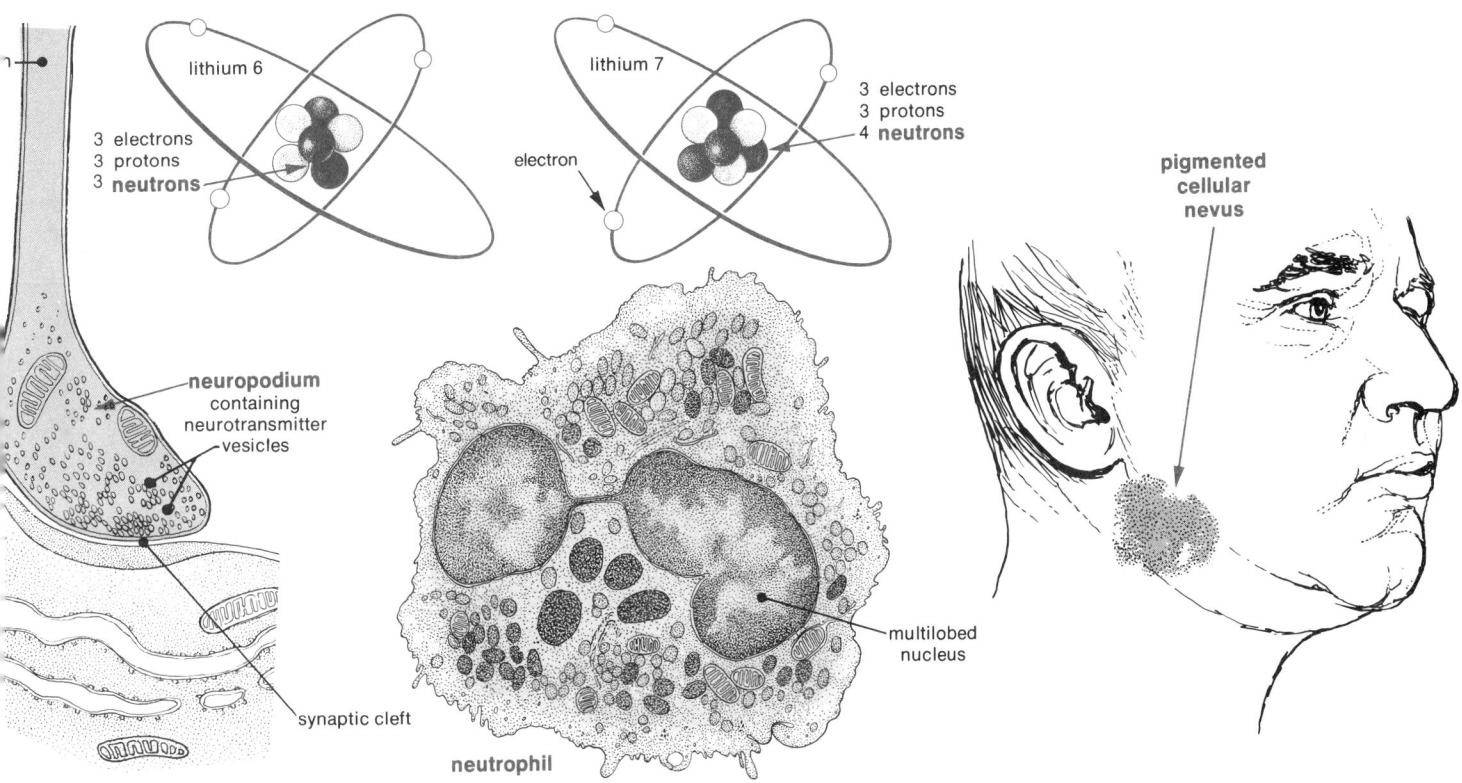

lithium 6
3 electrons
3 protons
3 **neutrons**

lithium 7
3 electrons
3 protons
4 **neutrons**

electron

neuropodium
containing
neurotransmitter
vesicles

synaptic cleft

neutrophil

multilobed
nucleus

**pigmented
cellular
nevus**

esses of the nervous system.

neuropile A dense net of interwoven glia and nerve cells and their processes.

neuroplasm The protoplasm of a nerve cell.

neuroplasty Reparative surgery of the nerves.

neuroplexus A network (plexus) of nerves. See also plexus.

neuropodium, *pl.* **neuropodia** The enlarged, rounded termination of an axon at the site of a synapse.

neuropore The opening at the ends of the neural tube of the developing embryo prior to complete closure around the 20–25 somite stage.

neuropsychiatry The study of both organic and functional diseases of the nervous system.

neuropsychology The study of the relationship between the mind and the nervous system.

neuropsychopathy Functional nervous disease accompanied by mental symptoms.

neuropsychosis Obsolete term; see psychosis.

neuroradiology Study of the nervous system with the aid of x-ray images.

neuroretinitis Inflammation of the head of the optic nerve and adjacent retina.

neurorrhaphy Surgical suturing of the ends of a divided nerve.

neurosarcocleisis Operative removal of the bony canal surrounding a nerve for the relief of neuralgia.

neurosclerosis Hardening of nerves.

neurosecretion Any of several secretory products of nerve cells (e.g., of the neurohypophysis and those of the base of the hypothalamus) that enter the blood stream and act as hormones.

neurosis, *pl.* **neuroses** Emotional maladjustment that may impair thinking and judgment but causes minimal loss of contact with reality.

anxiety n. Neurosis marked by exaggerated uncontrollable anxiety and apprehension of either acute or gradual onset.

battle n. Disorder induced by conditions of warfare. Also called war neurosis. Formerly called shellshock.

cardiac n. Neurosis marked by exaggerated concern with the state of one's heart in the absence of heart disease. Also called cardioneurosis.

obsessive-compulsive n. Disorder marked by the persistent intrusion of unwanted ideas and the compulsion to perform repetitive acts, e.g., repeated hand-washing or touching; anxiety develops when the individual is prevented from performing the ritual.

war n. See battle neurosis.

neuroskeleton The part of the skeleton surrounding the brain and spinal cord.

neurosome 1. One of the minute granules in the protoplasm of a nerve cell. 2. The body of a nerve cell.

neurosplanchnic Relating to the autonomic nervous system.

neurosurgeon A specialist in surgery of the nervous system.

neurosurgery Surgery of the nervous system.

stereotactic n. Neurosurgery involving the use of a mechanically directed probe introduced into the brain through a small hole in the skull; precise topographical coordinates are used to arrive at the desired location.

neurosyphilis Syphilis of the nervous system.

neurotic Relating to or affected with a neurosis.

neurotization Nerve regeneration.

neurotomy Surgical division of a nerve.

neurotonic 1. Stimulating impaired nervous function. 2. An agent having such an effect.

neurotoxin See neurolysin.

neurotransmitter Any substance that aids in transmitting impulses between two nerve cells or between a nerve and a muscle; e.g., acetylcholine.

neurotrophasthenia Condition due to undernourishment and marked by fatigue, poor concentration, and feelings of inadequacy.

neurotropic Having an affinity for nervous tissue; said of certain histologic dyes and microorganisms.

neurula The early vertebrate embryo during the stages when it possesses a neural plate.

neurulation The formation and closure of the neural plate in the early vertebrate embryo.

neutralization 1. The chemical reaction between an acid and a base that yields a salt and water. 2. The process of rendering something ineffective.

neutralize 1. To render ineffective, as in counteracting the effect of a drug or toxin. 2. To make neutral.

neutral red A dye used as an indicator with pH range of 6.8 to 8 (red at 6.8, yellow at 8).

neutrino An uncharged subatomic particle emitted from a radioactive nucleus when a positron is emitted from, or captured by, the nucleus; believed to have zero mass when at rest; it travels at the speed of light and interacts with matter only in the reverse process by which it is produced.

neutrocyte Neutrophil.

neutrocytopenia See neutropenia.

neutron (n) An uncharged subatomic particle existing along with the protons in the nucleus of an atom; slightly heavier than a proton.

neutropenia Abnormally small number of neutrophils in the blood. Also called neutrocytopenia; neutrophilic leukopenia.

neutrophil A mature white blood cell having a nucleus of three to five lobes joined by thin strands of chromatin; the most numerous of the white blood cell population (50 to 75% in normal individuals); its primary function is the ingestion and digestion of particulate matter, especially highly virulent bacteria; after it migrates from the blood stream to a site of infection, it may be called a microphage. Also called neutrophilic or polymorphonuclear leukocyte.

toxic n. A neutrophil having large dark granules (toxic granules) due to severe infection or to a drug reaction.

neutrophilia Increased number of neutrophils in the blood. Also called neutrocytosis; neutrophilic leukocytosis.

nevoid Resembling a nevus.

nevoxanthoendothelioma Single or multiple reddish papules, usually seen in young children. Also called juvenile xanthogranuloma.

nevus, *pl.* **nevi** A benign lesion of the skin; may be pigmented or nonpigmented, flat or elevated, smooth or warty; may become malignant.

blue n. A circumscribed, blue to black nodule beneath the skin, occurring anywhere in the body but most commonly on the dorsum of the hand and foot; chiefly composed of dopa-positive melanocytes (pigment-producing cells) containing a high concentration of melanin pigment; becomes malignant only rarely.

hairy pigmented n. A pigmented cellular nevus (mole) containing hairs.

intradermal n. A nevus occurring in the dermis (layer of the skin deep to the epidermis).

junctional n. A nevus occurring in the area between the dermis and epidermis (layers of the skin).

n. flammeus Port-wine hemangioma; see under hemangioma.

n. vasculosus Strawberry hemangioma; see under hemangioma.

pigmented cellular n. A circumscribed nevus composed of melanocytes (pigment-producing cells) and varying from smooth to rough (depending on the amount of keratin present) and from nonpalpable to nodular. Commonly known as a mole.

port-wine n. Port-wine hemangioma; see under hemangioma.

spider n. See spider, arterial.

systematized n. A widely distributed congenital nevus exhibiting a pattern.

newborn 1. A recently born infant. 2. Just born.

Newcastle disease An acute contagious disease of fowl caused by a paramyxovirus; transmissible to man, causing respiratory and nervous symptoms.

newton (N) A unit of force in the meter-kilogram-second system; the force required to accelerate a amalgam plugger

nicotine

nicotinyl
tartrate

$CH_2O—CO—CHOH—CHOH—COOH$

nicotinic acid

—COOH

NO_2 ... $CH=N—N—C—NH_2$ / H / O

nitrofurazone

5th rib
anterior serratus muscle
pectoralis major muscle
pectoralis minor muscle
external intercostal muscle
internal intercostal muscle
transverse thoracic muscle

costal
cartilage

sternum

costal
cartilage

mammary
gland

lactiferous
sinus

nipple
(mammary papilla)

lactiferous
ducts

---

mass of one kilogram one meter per second per second.

niacin Official designation for nicotinic acid in its role as a vitamin. See nicotinic acid.

niacinamide See nicotinamide.

nib In dentistry, the working part of a condensing instrument corresponding to the blade of a cutting instrument.

niche A small recess or eroded area, especially in the wall of a hollow organ, usually detected by contrast radiography.

nickel A metallic element, symbol Ni, atomic number 28, atomic weight 58.71.

nicking Constriction of a blood vessel of the retina.
 A-V n. Depression of a retinal vein into the tissue of the retina at the point where it is crossed by an artery; usually caused by arteriolar sclerosis. Also called arteriovenous nicking.

nicotinamide White crystalline compound, soluble in water; a B-complex vitamin used to treat pellagra. Also called nicotinic acid amide; niacinamide.

nicotinamide adenine dinucleotide (NAD) One of the coenzymes of the vitamin niacin (nicotinic acid); in association with any of a number of proteins, it acts as an oxidation-reduction catalyst. Formerly called diphosphopyridine nucleotide (DPN). Also called coenzyme I; codehydrogenase I.

nicotinamide adenine dinucleotide phosphate (NADP) A coenzyme that participates in biological oxidation reactions; structurally and functionally similar to NAD. Formerly known as triphosphopyridine nucleotide (TPN). Also called coenzyme II; codehydrogenase II.

nicotine An alkaloid derived from tobacco (*Nicotiana tabacum*); small doses stimulate and large doses depress autonomic ganglia.

nicotinic Resembling nicotine; denoting the action of certain agents on the nervous system.

nicotinic acid An odorless, white crystalline compound, part of the vitamin B complex; used in the prevention and treatment of pellagra. Also called niacin.

nicotinic acid amide See nicotinamide.

nicotinomimetic Simulating the action of nicotine.

nicotinyl tartrate Compound used as a peripheral vasodilator in certain peripheral vascular diseases; Roniacol Tartrate®.

nictitation Winking.

nidation The embedding or implantation of the fluid-filled blastocyst in the lining of the uterus (endometrium); occurs approximately five days after fertilization of the ovum.

nidus 1. A nest. 2. The point of focus of a morbid process. 3. The point of origin or nucleus of a nerve.
 n. avis A cerebellar depression between the biventral lobe and the uvula, which accommodates the cerebellar tonsil.

Niemann-Pick disease A rare form of lipidosis marked by an accumulation of foam cells in the reticuloendothelial system, spleen, liver, kidneys, and pancreas; at a late stage, deposits of sphingomyelin, gangliosides, and cholesterol may be found in the brain and spinal cord; a familial disorder most commonly seen in Jewish infants.

nifedipine A calcium channel-blocking agent used in the treatment of angina pectoris, especially variant angina.

nightmare A dream accompanied by intense anxiety, fear, oppression, and helplessness.

night terror Sleep disorder of children in which the child abruptly awakens agitated and screaming in a semiconscious state.

nihilism In psychiatry, a delusion of nonexistence; it may be total (including the patient and the world as a whole) or selective (referring to a part of the patient or his environment).
 therapeutic n. A disbelief in the value of any type of therapy.

Nikolsky's sign A peculiar vulnerability of the skin in pemphigus vulgaris; the superficial layer of the skin is easily rubbed off with slight friction.

nil disease Lipoid nephrosis; see under nephrosis.

ninhydrin Triketohydrindene hydrate, an important reagent widely used in the analytical determination of amino acids and related substances.

niobium A rare metallic element, symbol Nb, atomic number 41, atomic weight 92.906. Formerly called columbium (Cb).

nipple The conical protuberance at the apex of the mammary gland on which the outlets of the milk ducts are located. Also called mamilla; teat.

nit 1. The egg of a louse. 2. A unit of luminance.

niter See potassium nitrate.

nitrate A salt of nitric acid.

nitric Relating to, derived from, or containing nitrogen.

nitric acid A colorless or yellowish corrosive liquid, HNO_3.

nitric oxide An evanescent vasodilator, possibly the active principle of endothelium-derived relaxing factor.

nitridation Formation of nitrides through the combination with nitrogen.

nitride A compound containing nitrogen and one other element, usually a more electropositive one.

nitrification 1. The conversion of nitrogenous matter into nitrates by the action of bacteria. 2. The treatment of a material with nitrogen or nitrogen compounds.

nitrile, nitril A compound containing trivalent nitrogen (N^{-3}) in a cyanogen group.

nitrite A salt or ester of nitrous acid.

nitritoid Resembling the reaction caused by a nitrite, such as the reaction following the intravenous administration of arsphenamine.

nitrobacteria Bacteria that cause the conversion of nitrogenous matter into nitrites.

nitrofuran Furan derivative containing a nitro group; used as antibacterial agent.

nitrofurazone 5-Nitro-2-furaldehyde semicarbazone; a topical antibacterial agent; Furacin®.

nitrogen A colorless, odorless, gaseous element forming about 47% of the atmosphere by weight; symbol N, atomic number 7, atomic weight 14.008.
 blood urea n. (BUN) A constituent of normal whole blood. See nitrogen; urea.
 n. mustards Toxic compounds similar in composition to mustard gas but with nitrogen replacing sulfur; some have been used to treat neoplastic diseases.
 nonprotein n. (NPN) The nitrogen content of the blood exclusive of the protein bodies; normally urea contains about half of the nonprotein nitrogen in the blood.
 urea n. The portion of nitrogen derived from the urea content of a biologic sample such as blood or urine.

nitrogenous Containing nitrogen.

nitroglycerin A thick, yellow, explosive liquid, used in the production of dynamite; in medicine, the solid form is used as a vasodilator in the treatment of angina. Also called trinitroglycerin.

nitroprusside A salt containing the radical $Fe(CN)_5NO$; e.g., sodium nitroprusside.

nitrosamine Any of various *N*-nitroso derivatives of secondary amines ($R_2N–NO$); some are thought to be carcinogenic; formed naturally from nitrites plus amines; found also in smoke.

nitroso The univalent radical or group –NO, especially when present in organic compounds.

nitrosyl The nitroso radical or group –NO, when attached to an electronegative element such as chlorine.

nitrous Denoting a compound of nitrogen containing the smallest possible number of oxygen atoms.

nitrous oxide A colorless gas of sweet taste, N_2O, used as a mild anesthetic. Also called laughing gas.

nobelium The tenth transuranium element to be discovered; symbol No, atomic number 102, atomic weight 253.

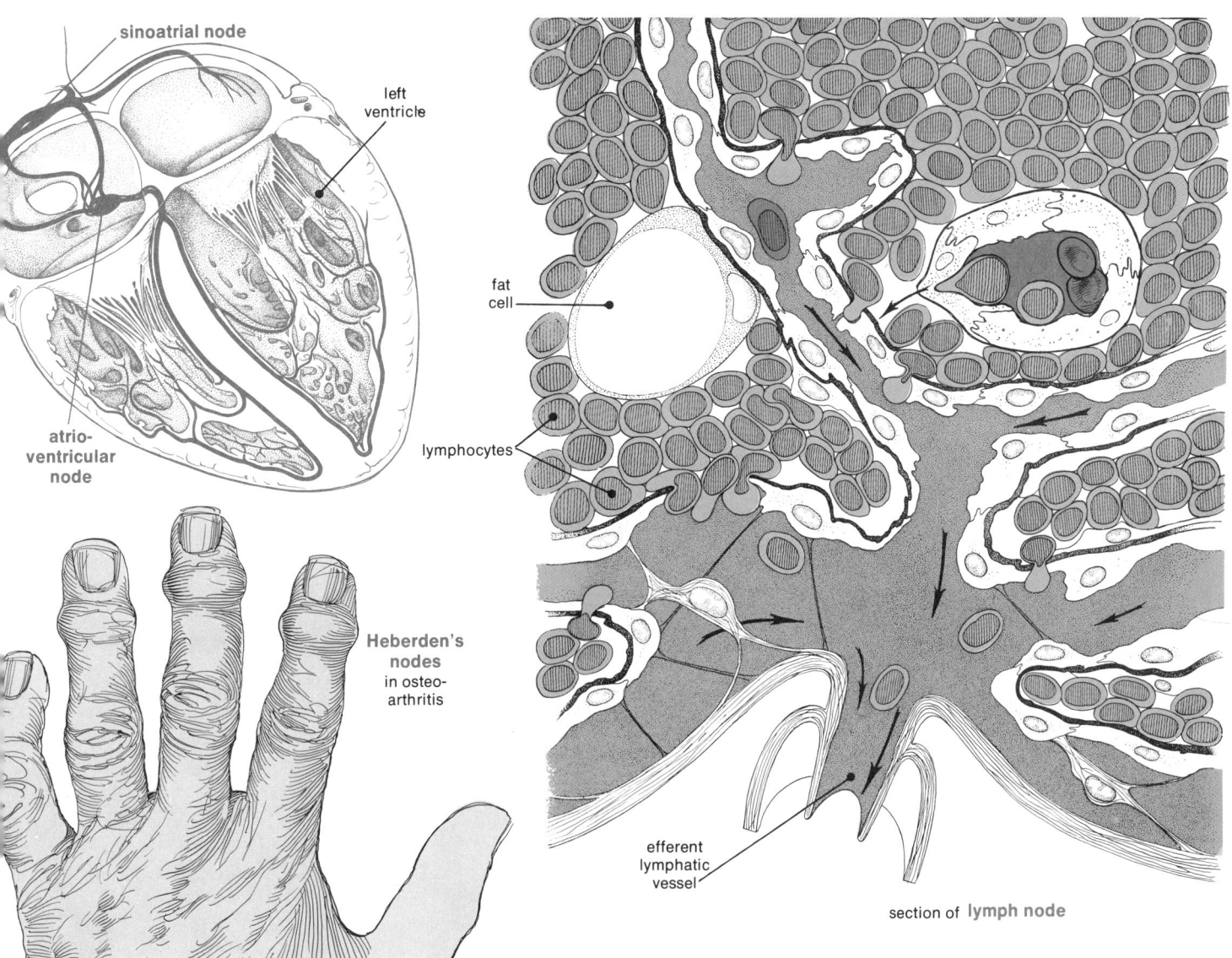

sinoatrial node

left ventricle

atrio-ventricular node

Heberden's nodes in osteo-arthritis

fat cell

lymphocytes

efferent lymphatic vessel

section of lymph node

Nocardia A genus (family Actinomycetes) that in-cludes fungus-like bacteria; the organisms are deli-cate, branching, often beaded, intertwining fila-ments that break into rod-shaped or coccoid forms; they are soil-dwelling and some are pathogenic.

N. asteroides A species isolated from diseases resembling pulmonary tuberculosis and brain ab-scesses.

N. madurae A species that is the causative agent of maduromycosis.

nocardiosis Any of several conditions caused by any species of *Nocardia*.

nociceptor A peripheral nerve organ that receives and transmits painful sensations.

nociperception Perception of painful or inju-rious stimuli.

noctambulism See somnambulism.

noctiphobia An abnormal fear of night and its accompanying darkness and silence.

nocturia Voiding of urine during the night.

node 1. A circumscribed mass of differentiated tis-sue. 2. A swelling.

Aschoff and Tawara's n. Atrioventricular node.

atrioventricular n. A small uncapsulated node made of thin strips of interwoven modified cardiac muscle and situated near the orifice of the coronary sinus; when normally activated by the sinoatrial node, it transmits the impulse, through the Purkinje fibers, to the ventricular muscles, causing practically simultaneous contraction. Also called A-V node.

A-V n. See atrioventricular node.

Bouchard's n. A small, hard nodule located in the proximal interphalangeal joint of a finger in osteoarthritis.

Cloquet's n. The highest of the deep inguinal lymph nodes.

delphian n. A midline node encased in fascia and resting on the thyroid isthmus. Also called prelar-yngeal node.

gouty n. A concretion of sodium biurate gener-ally occurring in the vicinity of joints in certain individuals afflicted with gout.

Heberden's n. A small, hard nodule located in the distal interphalangeal joint of a finger in osteoar-thritis; an enlargement of the tubercle at the articular extremity of the distal phalanx.

Hensen's n. Primitive node.

lymph n. An oval structure located along the course of a lymphatic vessel; its functions are the filtration of foreign matter and the production of lymphocytes; when enlarged, it provides a sign of infection or malignancy.

Osler n. Small, tender, and discolored node usu-ally appearing on the pads of fingers and toes in subacute endocarditis.

primitive n. A local swelling or thickening of ectodermal cells at the cranial end of the primitive streak of the embryo from which a strand of cells grows toward the cranium, between the ectoderm and endoderm in the midline, until it is blocked at the prechordal plate.

Ranvier's n. An interruption or constriction oc-curring at regular intervals (of about 1 mm) in the myelin sheath of a nerve fiber; it is here that a collateral branch may leave the axon; the area be-tween two nodes is occupied by a single Schwann cell.

S-A n. See sinoatrial node.

sentinel n. See signal node.

signal n. An enlarged, palpable, supraclavicular lymph node, usually on the left, that is often the first sign of an abdominal neoplasm. Also called sentinel or Virchow's node.

singer's n. Trachoma of the vocal bands; a small, whitish, beadlike enlargement of the vocal cords, caused by overuse or abuse of the voice, as in prolonged singing, especially of high notes. Also called teacher's node.

sinoatrial n. The mass of interwoven strips of cardiac muscle fibers that normally acts as the pace-maker of the cardiac conduction system; situated in the wall of the right atrium at the upper end of the crista terminalis just at the point of entry of the superior vena cava; receives fibers from both auto-nomic nervous systems and is the part of the heart that originates the heart beat. Also called S-A node.

syphilitic n. A localized swelling of bone resulting from syphilitic periostitis.

teacher's n. Singer's node.

Virchow's n. See signal node.

nodose Having nodes.

nodosity 1. A knotlike swelling. 2. The condition of having nodes.

nodular Relating to or having nodes.

nodulation The presence or the formation of nod-ules.

nodule A small node or closely packed collection of cells appearing distinct from the surrounding tissue.

Aschoff n. See body, Aschoff.

cold n. A thyroid nodule that does not concen-trate an administered dose of radioactive iodine as well as the rest of the gland.

hot n. A thyroid nodule containing a higher con-centration of an administered dose of radioactive iodine than the rest of the gland; usually benign.

juxta-articular n. An inflammatory nodule situ-ated near a joint.

lymphatic n.'s, aggregated Large aggregations of densely packed lymphocytes, present in the sub-mucosa of the intestines, mainly in the ileum and distal jejunum.

lymphatic n.'s, bronchial Small lymph nodes on the larger branches of the bronchi, in the substance of the lungs.

lymphatic n., gastric Solitary mass of lymphoid tissue in the mucous membrane of the stomach.

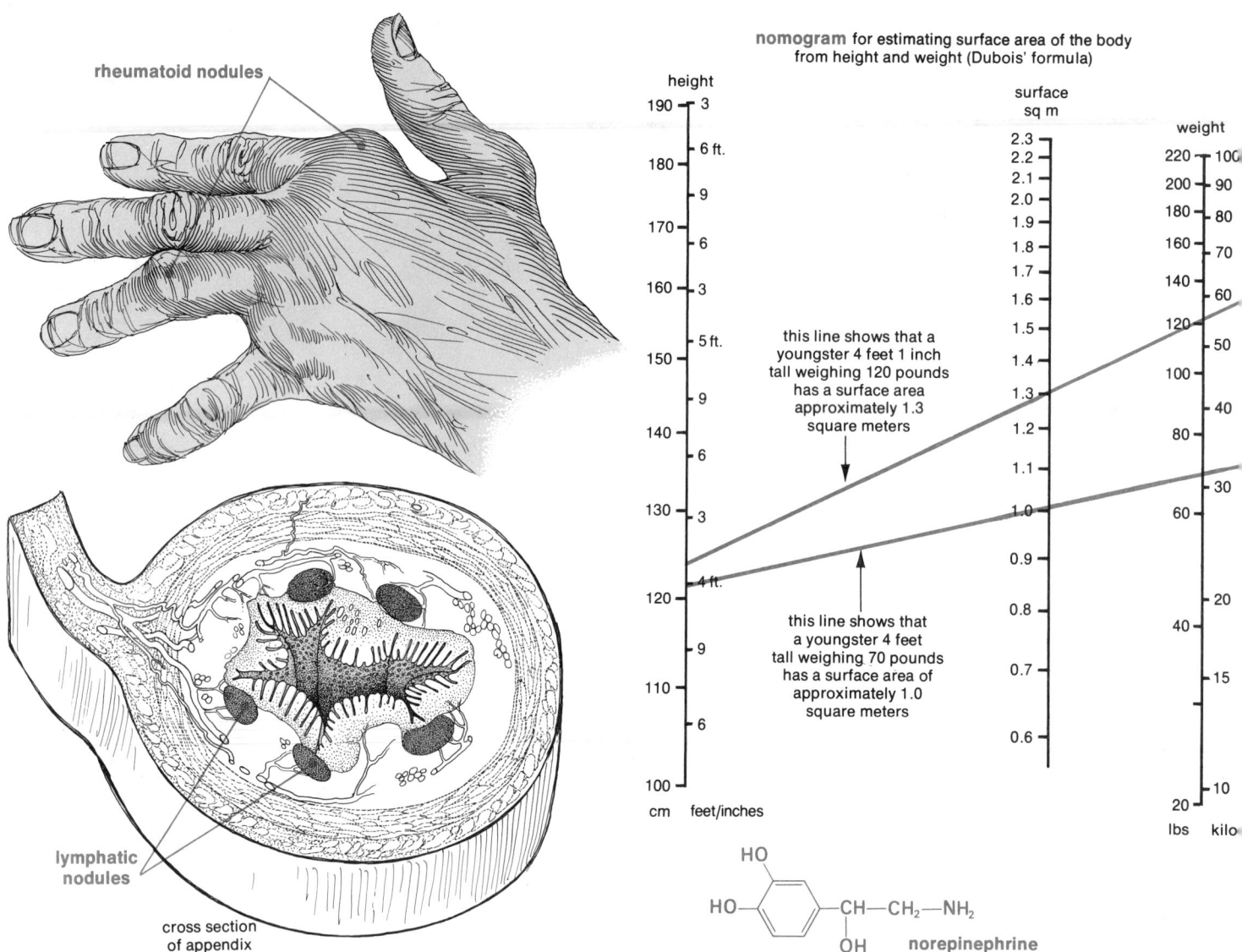

rheumatoid nodules

nomogram for estimating surface area of the body from height and weight (Dubois' formula)

height

surface sq m

weight

this line shows that a youngster 4 feet 1 inch tall weighing 120 pounds has a surface area approximately 1.3 square meters

this line shows that a youngster 4 feet tall weighing 70 pounds has a surface area of approximately 1.0 square meters

cm   feet/inches

lbs   kilo

lymphatic nodules

cross section of appendix

norepinephrine

---

lymphatic n.'s of the vermiform appendix Masses of lymphoid tissue in the submucous coat of the vermiform appendix.

rheumatoid n.'s Round or ovoid masses most commonly occurring subcutaneously over pressure points and near joints, in patients with rheumatoid arthritis.

Schmorl's n. A localized protrusion of the central portion of an intervertebral disk through the cartilage plate and into the spongy bone of the vertebral body.

nodulus, *pl.* **noduli** Latin for nodule.

Noguchia A genus of gram-negative, motile, encapsulated bacteria found in the conjunctiva of man and animals affected by a follicular type of disease.

noma A rapidly destructive gangrenous disease of the mouth; seen in poorly nourished children and debilitated adults. Also called gangrenous stomatitis.

Nomina Anatomica (NA) A system of anatomic terminology prepared by the International Congress of Anatomists.

nomogram, nomograph A graph consisting of three coplanar graduated lines of different variables arranged in such a manner that a straight line connecting two known values on two of the graduated lines intersects the unknown value on the third graduated line; used generally to estimate the surface area of a body on the basis of an individual's height and weight.

nomotopic Located in the normal or usual place.

nonan Recurring every ninth day; said of a fever.

nonapeptide A peptide possessing nine amino acids.

nonchromogens Mycobacteria that either are colorless or produce a light yellow pigment when grown in the presence of light. Also called Group III mycobacteria.

non compos mentis Latin for not having control of the mind; mentally not capable of managing one's

affairs and hence legally not responsible.

nonconductor Anything that does not readily transmit electrical current, light, or heat.

nondisease A disease suspected but not confirmed by further appropriate examinations.

nondisjunction Failure of paired chromosomes to separate at metaphase, so that both chromosomes are received by one daughter cell and none by the other.

nonelectrolyte A substance which, when in solution, does not conduct an electric current.

noninvasive Denoting diagnostic procedures that do not involve the use of instruments that penetrate the skin.

nonmetal Any electronegative element (e.g., iodine and fluorine) which forms oxides that produce acids and, in a solid state, is a poor conductor of heat and electricity.

non-nucleated Without a nucleus.

nonocclusion Condition in which a tooth of one arch fails to contact its opponent of the other arch.

nonparous Never having borne children. Also called nulliparous.

nonpenetrance Failure of a genetic trait to be evident even though the genetic elements that usually produce the trait are present.

nonproprietary See name, nonproprietary.

nonresectable Not capable of being cut off; said of a tumor not suitable for resection.

nonsecretor A person whose body secretions do not contain antigens of the ABO blood group.

nonunion Complication of a bone fracture in which healing stops short of firm union.

nonviable Not capable of living.

Noonan's syndrome Antimongoloid slant of the eyes and low set ears associated with valvular pulmonic stenosis.

noradrenaline See norepinephrine.

norepinephrine (NE) A chemical substance (hor-

mone) that produces constriction of practically all the blood vessels of the body; secreted by the postganglionic endings of the sympathetic nervous system; also produced and stored by the adrenal medulla and released upon stimulation of its sympathetic nerves. Also called levarterenol noradrenaline.

L-norepinephrine bitartrate See levarterenol bitartrate.

norethandrolone $C_{20}H_{30}O_2$; an androgen used in protein anabolism; Nilevar®.

norethindrone A progestational agent used in conjunction with estrogen as an oral contraceptive; Norlutin®.

norethynodrel A steroid structurally similar to progesterone, used in combination with mestranol as an oral contraceptive.

norm An ideal standard or pattern regarded as typical for a specific group.

normal (N) 1. Conformed to an established norm, standard, or pattern. **2.** Perpendicular; a line or plane forming a right angle with another. **3.** In bacteriology, nonimmune; denoting an animal or serum that has not been experimentally exposed to or treated with any microorganism.

normalization 1. The process of making normal. **2.** The process of dispersing fat homogeneously throughout milk after pasteurization.

normal solution See under solution.

normetanephrine A product of norepinephrine catabolism excreted in the urine.

normoblast A young red blood cell in its immature, nucleated stage.

acidophilic n. Orthochromatic normoblast.

basophilic n. The second stage in the development of the normoblast, following the pronormoblast. Also called basophilic or early erythroblast; prorubricyte.

orthochromatic n. The last stage in the development of the normoblast in which 80% of the he-

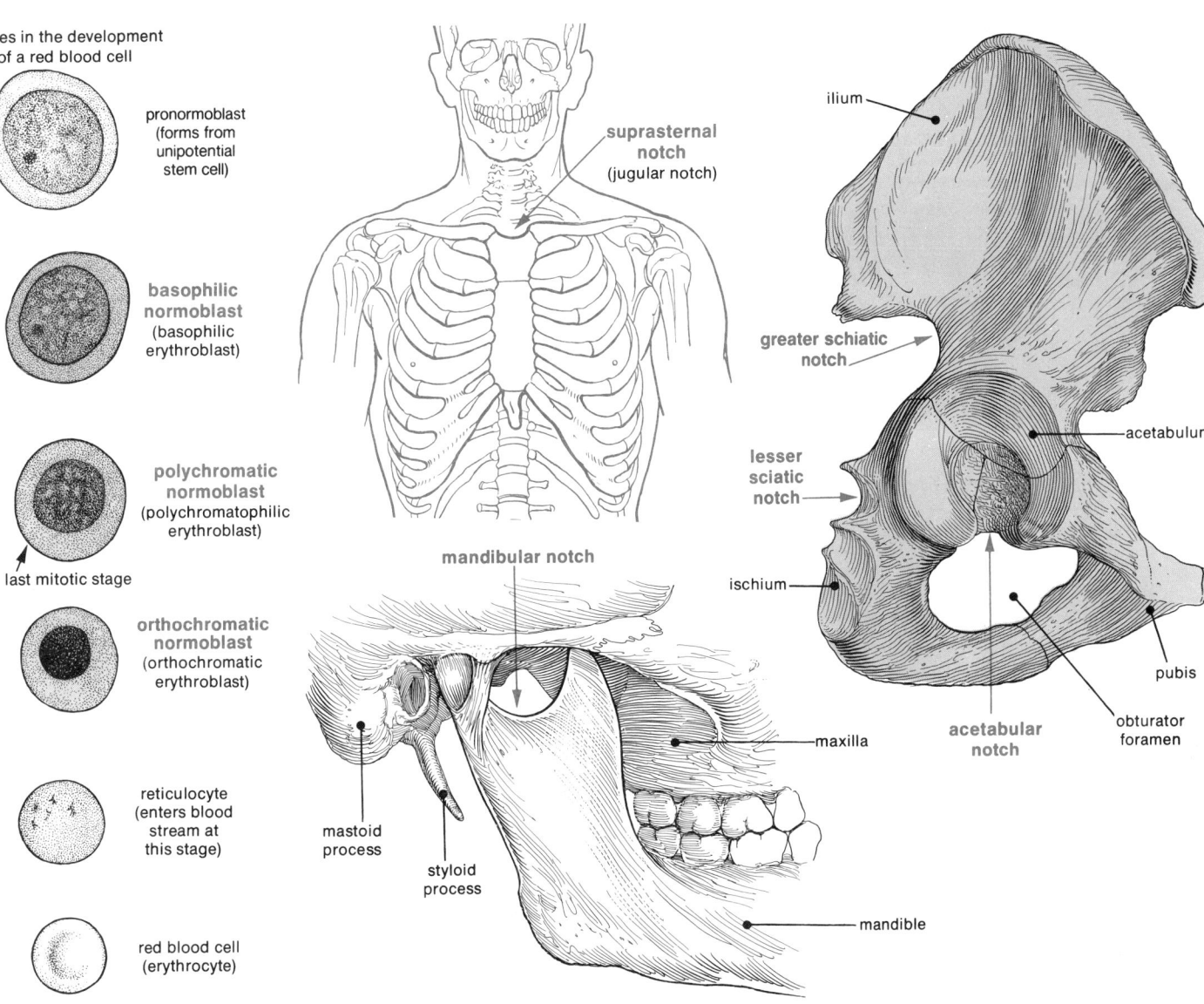

Stages in the development of a red blood cell

pronormoblast (forms from unipotential stem cell)

basophilic normoblast (basophilic erythroblast)

polychromatic normoblast (polychromatophilic erythroblast)

last mitotic stage

orthochromatic normoblast (orthochromatic erythroblast)

reticulocyte (enters blood stream at this stage)

red blood cell (erythrocyte)

suprasternal notch (jugular notch)

mandibular notch

mastoid process

styloid process

maxilla

mandible

ilium

greater schiatic notch

lesser sciatic notch

ischium

acetabulum

acetabular notch

obturator foramen

pubis

moglobin is synthesized. Also called metarubricyte; late or orthochromatic erythroblast; acidophilic normoblast.

    polychromatic n. The third stage in the development of the normoblast. Also called polychromatophilic erythroblast; rubricyte.

normocephalic See mesocephalic.

normochromia Normal color of red blood cells.

normochromic Having normal color; said of red blood cells.

normocyte A red blood cell of normal size.

normoglycemic Having normal glucose concentration in the blood.

normokalemia A normal level of potassium in the blood.

normotensive Denoting a normal arterial blood pressure.

normothermia 1. A normal temperature. **2.** Environmental temperature that does not affect the activity of body cells.

normotonic Having normal muscular tone. Also called eutonic.

normotopia The state of being in the normal location.

normovolemia A normal blood volume.

nose The external organ of the sense of smell and the beginning of the air passages; the midline prominence on the face bearing the nostrils. Also called nasus.

    pug n. A short slightly flattened nose turned up at the end. Also called snub nose.

    saddle n. A nose with a markedly depressed bridge.

nosebleed Bleeding from the nose. Also called epistaxis.

nosepiece A device at the lower end of the microscope body tube for holding two or more readily interchangeable objectives.

nosocomial Of, relating to, or originating in a

hospital.

nosogenesis, nosogeny See pathogenesis.

nosographer One who writes about diseases.

nosography The systematic written description of diseases.

nosology 1. The science concerned with the classification of diseases. **2.** A classification of diseases.

nosomania An unfounded, abnormal fear that one is diseased.

nosomycosis A disease caused by a fungus.

nosoparasite 1. A microorganism occurring in association with, but not causing, a disease. **2.** A pathogenic microorganism living on diseased tissue.

nosophilia An abnormal desire to be sick.

nosophobia An abnormal fear of disease; a dread of having all the symptoms of all the diseases read or heard about.

nosopoietic Pathogenic.

nosotaxy Nosology.

nosotoxin Any toxin associated with a disease.

nostril One of the two external openings of the nose. Also called naris.

nostrum A quack remedy.

notal Of or relating to the back.

notch An indentation or depression.

    acetabular n. A notch in the inferior margin of the acetabulum of the hipbone; it is bridged by the transverse acetabular ligament.

    aortic n. The depression on the sphygmogram caused by the rebound at the closure of the aortic valves.

    cardiac n. A notch in the anterior border of the left lung at the level of the fourth costal cartilage.

    dicrotic n. The depression on the sphygmogram which precedes the dicrotic pulse wave.

    Hutchinson's crescentic n. The somewhat semilunar notch on the incisal edge of upper central incisors in Hutchinson's teeth; seen also occasionally in other anterior teeth.

jugular n. See suprasternal notch.

    mandibular n. The deep semilunar notch between the condyle and coronoid process of the lower jaw (mandible).

    scapular n. A semicircular notch on the superior border of the scapula (shoulder blade), at the base of the coracoid process.

    sciatic n., greater The deep indentation in the posterior border of the hipbone at the junction of the ilium and ischium; it is converted into a foramen by the sacrospinal ligament.

    sciatic n., lesser The notch in the posterior border of the ischium below the ischial spine; it is converted into a foramen by the sacrotuberous and sacrospinal ligaments.

    supraorbital n. A notch or groove (occasionally a foramen) in the superior part of the margin of the orbit through which pass the supraorbital nerve and vessels.

    suprasternal n. The notch between the sternal heads of the two sternocleidomastoid muscles. Also called jugular notch.

    tentorial n. A gap in the tentorium cerebelli, through which the brain stem extends from the posterior into the middle cranial fossa.

    trochlear n. A large concavity on the anterior surface of the olecranon process of the ulna which articulates with the trochlea of the humerus.

    vertebral n. One of two notches above and below the pedicle of a vertebra; the notches of two adjacent vertebrae form an intervertebral foramen.

notochord A supporting rod of cells in the embryo of all chordates; in vertebrates, it is replaced partially or wholly by the skull and vertebral column.

noxa Any harmful agent or influence.

noxious Harmful to health.

nu Thirteenth letter of the Greek alphabet, ν; symbol for kinematic viscosity.

nubile Ready for marriage; said of a sexually ma-coronal section of brain

lateral ventricle

caudate nucleus

insula

lentiform nucleus { putamen, globus pallidus

third ventricle

internal ear

utricle

semicircular ducts

saccule

cochlea

vestibulocochlear nerve

lateral portion
dorsal portion } cochlear nucleus

lumen

nucleus of endothelial cell

vestibular nucleus

cross section of capillary

ture young woman.

nucha The back of the neck.

nuchal Relating to the back of the neck.

nuclear Of or relating to a nucleus.

nuclease An enzyme that promotes the breakdown of nucleic acid into nucleotides.

nucleated Having a nucleus.

nuclei Plural of nucleus.

nucleic acids Chemical compounds, of the utmost biologic importance, contained in all living organisms in the form of deoxyribonucleic acid (DNA) and ribonucleic acid (RNA); they consist mainly of a sugar moiety (pentose or deoxypentose), nitrogenous bases (purines and pyrimidines), and phosphoric acid.

nucleocapsid The protein coat (capsid) of a virus together with its enclosed nucleic acid.

nucleofugal Moving away from a cell nucleus.

nucleogram The data obtained through nucleography.

nucleography A method of observing and recording the chemical composition, structure, size, etc., of a cell nucleus.

nucleohistone A nucleoprotein derived from a histone; a salt between the basic protein and the nucleic acid.

nucleolonema A dense, coarse strand that branches, forming a network within the nucleolus of a cell.

nucleolus, *pl.* **nucleoli** A small, spherical organelle located in the nucleus of a cell; it contains RNA (ribonucleic acid) and protein and is an active center of protein and RNA synthesis, as well as an important center for the formation of ribosomes.

nucleon One of the constituent particles of an atomic nucleus, i.e., a proton or a neutron.

nucleonics The technology and application of nuclear energy.

nucleopetal Moving toward a cell nucleus.

nucleophil, nucleophile The electron donor in a chemical reaction.

nucleoplasm The protoplasm of the cell nucleus, composed mainly of proteins, metabolites, and ions. Also called karyoplasm.

nucleoprotein A nondescript complex of compounds consisting of a simple protein and a nucleic acid; chromosomes and viruses are largely nucleoprotein in nature.

nucleoreticulum Any structural network within the nucleus.

nucleorrhexis The breaking up of a cell nucleus.

nucleosidase An enzyme that promotes the splitting of nucleosides into sugar and purine or pyrimidine base.

nucleoside A purine or pyrimidine base attached to a sugar (pentose, ribose, or deoxyribose).

nucleotidase An enzyme that catalyzes the splitting of a nucleotide into nucleosides and phosphoric acid.

nucleotide One of the compounds into which nucleic acid splits on hydrolysis, consisting of a nitrogenous base (either a purine or a pyrimidine), a sugar (either ribose or deoxyribose), and a phosphate group. Also called mononucleotide.

nucleotidyltransferase Enzymes that transfer nucleotide residues from nucleoside di- or triphosphates into dimer or polymer forms.

nucleotoxin A toxin affecting cell nuclei.

nucleus, *pl.* **nuclei** **1.** The generally oval protoplasmic body in the center of the cell which contains the chromosomes and is surrounded by a nuclear membrane; an essential organelle that controls metabolism, growth, and reproduction. **2.** A localized mass of gray matter, composed of nerve cells, in the brain or spinal cord. **3.** The heavy, central, positively charged portion of the atom (composed of protons and neutrons) which contains the mass of the atom, about which the electrons revolve in orbit. **4.** A central part or mass.

abducens n. A cranial nerve nucleus with fibers directed ventrally to supply the lateral rectus muscle of the eye.

amygdaloid n. An oval mass of gray matter in the anterior portion of the temporal lobe of the cerebrum, near the uncus; it is continuous with the cortex.

anterior horn n. A column of cells extending the entire length of the spinal cord and organized into medial and lateral groups, each with several subdivisions.

caudate n. A long horseshoe-shaped mass of gray matter consisting of an enlarged anterior portion which occupies most of the lateral wall of the anterior horn of the lateral ventricle, a narrower body extending along the floor of the lateral ventricle, and a tapered curved tail which follows the curvature of the inferior horn of the lateral ventricle and enters the temporal lobe, terminating in the amygdaloid complex.

cochlear n. A nucleus located on the surface of the inferior cerebellar peduncle at the junction of the medulla oblongata and the pons; it receives incoming fibers from the bipolar cells in the spiral ganglion of the cochlea.

dentate n. of the cerebellum The largest of the central nuclei of the cerebellum embedded within the hemisphere of the cerebellum; its efferent fibers pass to the brain stem.

diploid n. A cell nucleus containing the diploid or normal double complement of chromosomes.

dorsal motor n. of vagus A nucleus situated in the floor of the fourth ventricle which sends fibers through the medulla oblongata to the vagus and spinal accessory nerves which end in vagal sympathetic plexuses in the chest and abdomen.

dorsomedial n. of hypothalamus The dorsal portion of the two main groups of nerve cell bodies in the tuber cinereum of the hypothalamus; some of their efferent fibers pass to the posterior lobe of the hypophysis (pituitary).

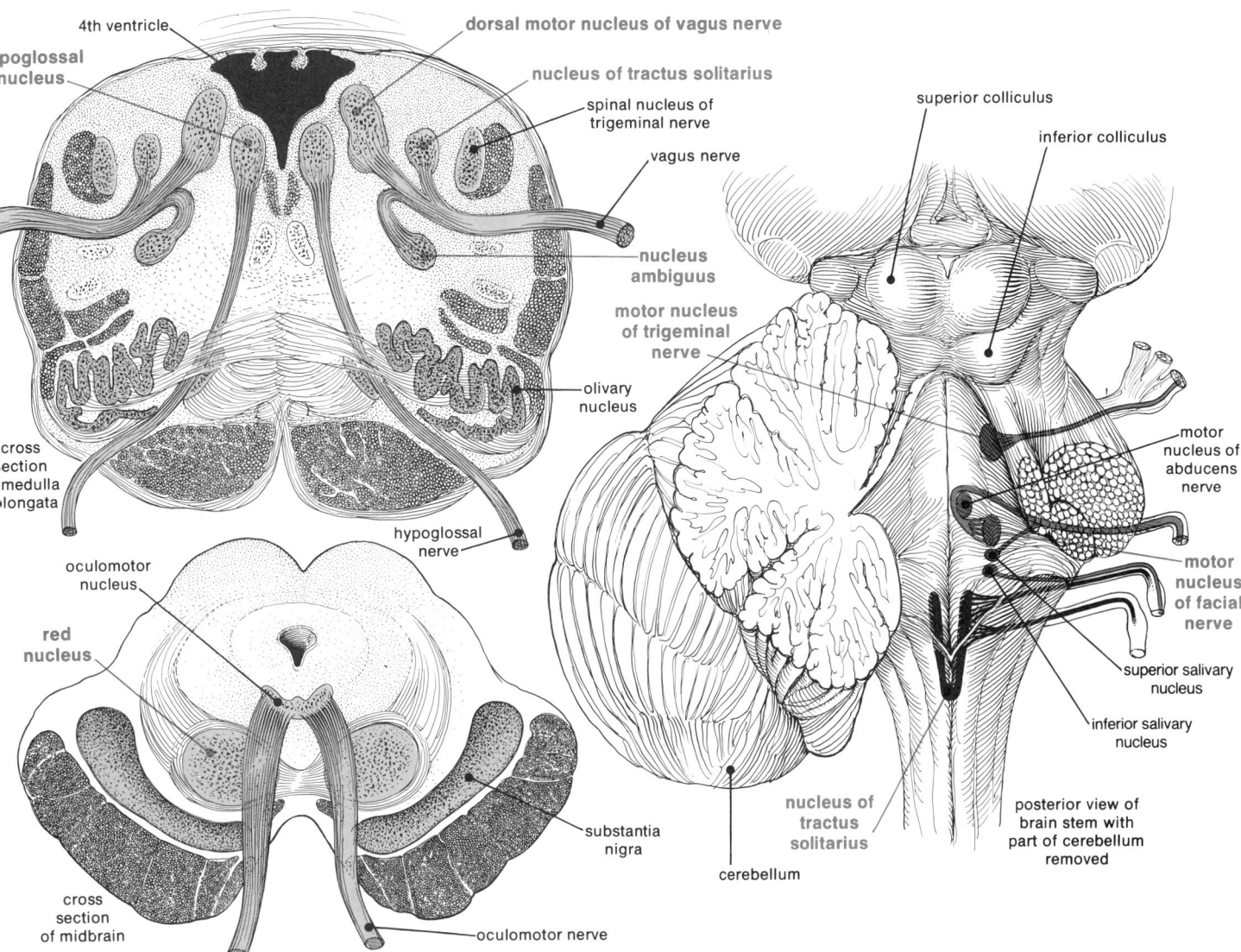

4th ventricle

dorsal motor nucleus of vagus nerve

poglossal nucleus

nucleus of tractus solitarius

spinal nucleus of trigeminal nerve

vagus nerve

nucleus ambiguus

motor nucleus of trigeminal nerve

olivary nucleus

cross ection medulla longata

hypoglossal nerve

oculomotor nucleus

red nucleus

substantia nigra

cross section of midbrain

oculomotor nerve

superior colliculus

inferior colliculus

motor nucleus of abducens nerve

motor nucleus of facial nerve

superior salivary nucleus

inferior salivary nucleus

nucleus of tractus solitarius

cerebellum

posterior view of brain stem with part of cerebellum removed

Edinger-Westphal n. A circumscribed group of nerve cells whose fibers run to the oculomotor nerve and thence to the ciliary ganglion, innervating the intrinsic eye muscles.

hypoglossal n. A cranial nerve nucleus with fibers directed to the lower border of the pyramid to supply the tongue. .

inferior colliculus n. An ovoid cellular mass surrounded by a thin cortex which serves as a relay in transmitting auditory impulses to thalamic levels and is involved in acoustic reflexes.

lenticular n. See lentiform nucleus.

lentiform n. A mass of gray matter the size and shape of a Brazil nut, deeply buried in the white matter of the cerebral hemisphere; a vertical plate of white matter divides the nucleus into a large lateral portion, the putamen, and a smaller medial portion, the globus pallidus. Also called lenticular nucleus.

mesencephalic n. of trigeminal nerve A cranial sensory nerve nucleus which receives fibers from extrinsic eye muscles and muscles of mastication; the mesencephalic root of the trigeminal nerve arises from it.

motor n. of facial nerve A nucleus that gives rise to fibers which innervate the voluntary facial muscles.

motor n. of trigeminal nerve A nucleus from which fibers run laterally with the mandibular nerve to innervate the muscles of mastication.

n. ambiguus A motor nucleus composed of large multipolar cells which send fibers into the glossopharyngeal, vagus, and accessory nerves to supply the pharynx and larynx. Also called ambiguous nucleus.

n. pulposus The central gelatinous part of the intervertebral disk enclosed in several layers of fibrous tissue; it generally becomes fibrocartilaginous in old age.

n. of accessory nerve A cranial nerve nucleus whose fibers form rootlets which join bulbar rootlets

of the spinal accessory nerve to innervate the trapezius and sternocleidomastoid muscles.

n. of tractus solitarius The nucleus of the solitary tract that receives visceral afferent fibers from the facial, glossopharyngeal, and vagus nerves; a slender nucleus extending the entire length of the medulla oblongata.

paraventricular n. of hypothalamus A collection of nerve cells in the anterior part of the hypothalamus on either side of the third ventricle; it gives rise to the paraventriculohypophyseal tract which passes to the posterior lobe of the hypophysis (pituitary gland); related to the autonomic nervous system.

pontine nuclei Groups of nerve cell bodies in the pyramidal tract at the basilar part of the pons, where impulses from the cerebrum to the cerebellum relay.

principal sensory n. of trigeminal nerve A nucleus that receives fibers carrying impulses of touch, pain, and temperature from the head and face.

red n. A large oval nucleus situated in the midbrain, extending from the caudal margin of the superior colliculus to the subthalamic region; it receives fibers mainly from the deep cerebellar nuclei and the cerebral cortex; it is characterized by its pinkish-yellow color, its central position, and its capsule-like covering formed by the fibers of the superior cerebellar peduncle.

salivary nuclei, superior and inferior Scattered nuclei in the dorsolateral reticular formation, just above the pontomedullary junction; the superior sends fibers to the submandibular and sublingual glands via the facial nerve and submandibular ganglion; the inferior sends fibers to the parotid gland via the glossopharyngeal nerve and otic ganglion.

spinal n. of trigeminal nerve A cranial sensory nerve nucleus that receives fibers which mediate pain and temperature for the head and face.

superior colliculus n. A laminated nucleus forming the top half of the tectum (roof of the midbrain)

which serves as a primary relay in transmitting visual impulses.

supraoptic n. of hypothalamus One of two nuclei in the hypothalamus located on either side of the third ventricle near the optic tract; it gives rise to the supraopticohypophyseal tract which passes to the posterior lobe of the hypophysis (pituitary gland).

ventral posterolateral n. (VPL nucleus) A large mass of the thalamus which receives terminal fibers of the spinothalamic tract and medial lemniscus; it projects to the sensory cortex.

ventral posteromedial n. (VPM nucleus) A crescentic mass of the thalamus ventral to the centrum medianum which receives the secondary trigeminal tract; its axons project to the postcentral gyrus for the face.

ventromedial n. of hypothalamus The ventral portion of two main groups of nerve cell bodies in the tuber cinereum of the hypothalamus; thought to be involved in sexual behavior and the control of food intake.

vestibular n. A nucleus located in the floor of the fourth ventricle which receives fibers from the bipolar ganglion cells of the vestibular nerve.

nuclide An atom or a species of atom marked by its particular atomic number and atomic mass (A) or proton number (Z); nuclides with the same proton number are isotopes of a specific element; nuclides with the same atomic mass but different atomic numbers are isobars.

nulligravida A woman who has never been pregnant.

nullipara A woman who has never given birth to children.

nulliparity The condition of not having borne children.

nulliparous Never having borne children.

nullosomic Lacking both members of a single pair of chromosomes.

Periodic Table

Group: I, II, III, IV, V, VI, VII, O

METALS — atomic numbers — NONMETALS

Period	I	II												III	IV	V	VI	VII	O
1	H 1																		He 2
2	Li 3	Be 4												B 5	C 6	N 7	O 8	F 9	Ne 10
3	Na 11	Mg 12												Al 13	Si 14	P 15	S 16	Cl 17	Ar 18
4	K 19	Ca 20	Sc 21	Ti 22	V 23	Cr 24	Mn 25	Fe 26	Co 27	Ni 28	Cu 29	Zn 30		Ga 31	Ge 32	As 33	Se 34	Br 35	Kr 36
5	Rb 37	Sr 38	Y 39	Zr 40	Nb 41	Mo 42	Tc 43	Ru 44	Rh 45	Pd 46	Ag 47	Cd 48		In 49	Sn 50	Sb 51	Te 52	I 53	Xe 54
6	Cs 55	Ba 56	*57-71	Hf 72	Ta 73	W 74	Re 75	Os 76	Ir 77	Pt 78	Au 79	Hg 80		Ti 81	Pb 82	Bi 83	Po 84	At 85	Rn 86
7	Fr 87	Ra 88	**89-103	Rf 104	Ha 105														

* lanthanide elements (rare earth): La 57, Ce 58, Pr 59, Nd 60, Pm 61, Sm 62, Eu 63, Gd 64, Tb 65, Dy 66, Ho 67, Er 68, Tm 69, Yb 70, Lu 71

** actinide elements: Ac 89, Th 90, Pa 91, U 92, Np 93, Pu 94, Am 95, Cm 96, Bk 97, Cf 98, Es 99, Fm 100, Md 101, No 102, Lw 103

---

number (no) One of a series of symbols expressing a specified quantity or a definite value in a fixed order derived by counting.

atomic n. (Z) The number or position of an element in the periodic system; it represents the number of negative electrons outside the atomic nucleus.

Avogadro's n. The number of molecules or particles in one gram mole of any compound; it equals 6.022×10^{23}.

Brinell hardness n. (BHN) A number expressing the hardness of a dental material, derived by measuring the diameter of a dent made by pressing, with the aid of the Brinell tester, a standard carbide ball into the surface of the material under a specified load.

electronic n. The number of electrons in the outermost orbit (valence shell) of an element.

Knoop hardness n. (KHN) A number representing the hardness of material (especially tooth structure and dental materials) determined by the penetration of a diamond indenting tool.

Mach n. (M) A number representing the ratio of the speed of an object to the speed of sound in the same surrounding medium.

mass n. The nearest integer to the number expressing the sum of the protons and neutrons in the atomic nucleus of an isotope; denoted as a prefix superscript, e.g., ^{16}O (oxygen-16).

numbness Insensibility of a part.

nummular 1. Shaped like a small coin; discoid; usually denoting the thick mucous sputum in certain respiratory disorders. 2. Arranged like stacks of coins.

nummulation Formation of disc-shaped masses.

nurse 1. An individual trained to care for the sick, disabled, or enfeebled. 2. To give nourishment from the breast; to suckle. 3. To care for or tend one unable to provide for his own needs.

graduate n. An individual who is a graduate of a school of nursing.

head n. A nurse who is in charge of supervising the nursing staff of a hospital unit.

licensed practical n. (LPN) A practical nurse who is licensed to care for patients but has a range of allowable authority less than that of a registered nurse. Also called licensed vocational nurse (LVN).

practical n. An individual who is trained to provide certain nursing skills but has not graduated from a full nursing school program.

private duty n. A nurse who is not a member of the hospital staff but is privately employed to provide nursing care to an individual patient.

public health n. A graduate nurse who has had special training in the techniques of preventing disease.

registered n. (RN) A graduate nurse who, having passed a state registration examination, is registered and licensed to practice.

scrub n. A nurse who dons a sterile gown and gloves to assist during a surgical procedure.

visiting n. A nurse who provides nursing care to patients in their homes.

wet n. A woman who breast-feeds another woman's child.

nurse-anesthetist A registered nurse who specializes in the administration of anesthetics.

nurse practitioner A registered nurse who is qualified to prescribe and implement nursing care. Also called nurse clinician.

nursing 1. Feeding at the breast. 2. Activities that constitute the duties of a nurse.

nursing home A small private hospital for persons convalescing or people (especially aged persons) who require assistance in caring for and feeding themselves.

nutrient A nourishing component of food.

nutrition The process in which a living organism utilizes food for growth and replacement of tissues through digestion, absorption, assimilation, and excretion.

enteral n. Introduction of nutrients via a tube inserted directly into the stomach or duodenum.

total parenteral n. (TPN) Intravenous infusion of nutrients in place of oral intake.

nutriture The state of the body in regard to nourishment, especially in regard to a specific nutrient, such as protein.

nux Latin for nut.

n. vomica A poisonous nut from *Strychnos nux-vomica*, a tree native to southeastern Asia; it is a source of two alkaloids, strychnine and brucine, and has been used as a bitter tonic, a tincture, and a central nervous system stimulant. Also called strychnos seed; poison nut; Quaker button.

nyctalopia Impaired vision in subdued light, while daylight vision is normal; generally due to vitamin A deficiency; often used incorrectly instead of hemeralopia (day blindness). Also called night blindness; day sight.

nycterohemeral See nyctohemeral.

nyctohemeral Indicating both night and day. Also called nycterohemeral.

nyctophobia Exaggerated and unreasonable fear of darkness.

nymph The wingless stage in the development of certain insects immediately after hatching.

nympholabial Relating to the labia minora and the labia majora.

nymphomania Excessive sexual desire in the female.

nymphomaniac A woman affected with nymphomania.

nymphoncus A swelling or enlargement of one or both labia minora.

nymphotomy Surgical incision of the clitoris or the labia minora.

nystagmic Relating to or affected with a jerky twitching of the eyeball.

nystagmograph Apparatus used to record graphically the movements of the eyeball in nystagmus.

nystagmography The recording of nystagmic movements of the eyes.

nystagmus An involuntary movement of the eyes in either a rotatory, vertical, or horizontal direction; most commonly it is a rhythmic jerking with a fast and slow component, and is described by the direction of the quick component.

nystatin An antibiotic agent obtained from cultures of *Streptomyces noursei;* used in the treatment of monilia infections.

nyxis A puncture.

objectives
housed in nosepiece
of microscope

vertex
sinciput
occiput
newborn skull

occipitomental
dimension

Ω Omega.

obdormition Numbness of a bodily part due to pressure on the sensory nerve.

obelion A craniometric point on the sagittal suture of the skull where it crosses the line joining the two parietal foramina.

obese Very fat; corpulent.

obesity Excessive accumulation of fat in the subcutaneous tissues.

  alimentary o. Simple obesity.

  endogenous o. Obesity attributed to endocrine and metabolic abnormalities.

  exogenous o. Simple obesity.

  morbid o. Obesity that is so severe as to threaten health and limit activities; usually in excess of twice the ideal weight.

  simple o. Obesity that occurs when the caloric intake is greater than the energy expenditure.

obex The small, triangular lamina at the caudal angle of the roof of the fourth ventricle.

obfuscation 1. The process of rendering obscure or indistinct; a darkening. 2. Confusion.

object 1. Anything perceptible through any of the senses. 2. A person or thing that arouses any type of emotion in an observer.

  sex o. A person or thing that arouses sexual feelings in another.

  test o. Device used to determine the defining power of the objective lens of a microscope.

objective The lens or arrangement of lenses in a microscope or other optical system which receives light from the field of view and forms the first image; so named because it is nearest the object.

  immersion o. A high power objective designed to include oil or other liquid instead of air between its front lens and the cover glass.

obligate Capable of surviving in only one environment; said of certain parasites; opposite of facultative.

oblique Having a slanting or sloping direction; deviating from the perpendicular or the horizontal; inclined.

obliquity Former name for a synclitism.

obliquus Latin for oblique.

oblongata Having a long dimension; elongated; oblong.

obmutescence Loss of speech.

obnubilation A confused state of mind.

observerscope A Y-shaped instrument that enables two observers to view simultaneously the interior of a canal or cavity.

obsession A persistently recurring and unwanted idea that cannot be eliminated.

obsessive-compulsive Having an obsessive-

compulsive neurosis. See under neurosis.

obstetric, obstetrical Relating to obstetrics.

obstetrician A physician who specializes in obstetrics.

obstetrics (OB) The branch of medicine concerned principally with the management of pregnancy, labor, and the phenomena following childbirth to complete involution of the uterus.

obstipation Constipation that does not respond to treatment; persistent failure to pass any stool.

obstruction An impedance; a blockage or clogging.

obstruent 1. Causing obstruction. 2. An agent having such an effect.

obtund To diminish pain or touch sensations.

obtundent An agent that dulls perception of pain or touch.

obturation A stoppage or occlusion.

obturator 1. Any structure that closes a bodily opening. 2. A prosthetic device used to close a defect in the hard palate. 3. An instrument used to occlude a hollow cannula during its insertion into the body.

obtusion Dulling of normal sensibility.

occipital Relating to the back of the head. See table of bones.

occipitalization Fusion or ankylosis between the atlas and occipital bone.

occipitoatloid Pertaining to the occipital bone and the first vertebra (atlas); applied to the articulation between the two bones.

occipitobregmatic Pertaining to the occiput and the bregma (a measurement in craniometry).

occipitomental Relating to the back of the head and the chin.

occipitoparietal Relating to the occipital and parietal bones.

occipitotemporal Relating to the occipital and temporal bones.

occiput The lower back of the head.

occlude 1. To close or obstruct. 2. In dentistry, to bring together the upper and lower teeth.

occluder 1. Device placed before an eye to block vision. 2. Device placed on a blood vessel to prevent flow; used in certain physiologic experiments in animals.

occlusal 1. Relating to a closure. 2. In dentistry, relating to the contacting surfaces of teeth or occlusion rims.

occlusion 1. The process of closing or the state of being closed. 2. In dentistry, the contact of the mandibular teeth with the maxillary teeth in any functional relation. 3. In chemistry, the absorption of a gas by a metal.

  abnormal o. Malocclusion.

  afunctional o. Malocclusion that prevents proper mastication.

  centric o. Occlusion in which the upper and lower teeth are together in a normal, relaxed manner, and the mandible is in centric relation to the maxilla.

  coronary o. Impedance of coronary circulation, usually by thrombosis.

  eccentric o. Relating to teeth, any occlusion other than centric occlusion.

  enteromesenteric o. Obstructed blood flow in the wall of the intestine and in the mesentery.

  hepatic vein o. A rare condition characterized by blocking of the hepatic veins, usually by tumor infiltration or by thrombosis of the vessels, causing enlargement of the liver, portal hypertension, and ascites. Also called Budd-Chiari syndrome.

  pathogenic o. An occlusal relationship capable of incurring damage to supporting tissues.

  protrusive o. Protrusion of the lower jaw from centric position.

occlusive Covering; closing.

occlusometer See gnathodynamometer.

occult Hidden, as a concealed hemorrhage.

occupation, prescribed A therapeutic activity recommended by a physician for a particular patient.

ocellus *pl.* **ocelli** A simple eye found in many invertebrates.

ochrodermia Yellow discoloration of the skin.

ochronosis A characteristic brown-black pigmentation of connective tissue occurring in certain metabolic disorders; a result of deposition of homogentisic acid.

ocrylate A tissue adhesive used in surgery.

octamethyl pyrophosphoramide (OMPA) A chemical used as a plant insecticide. Commonly called schradan.

octan Occurring every eighth day; said of certain fevers.

octapeptide A peptide compound of eight amino acid residues, such as the posterior pituitary hormones, oxytocin and vasopressin.

octavalent Having the combining power of eight hydrogen atoms.

ocular 1. Relating to the eye. 2. The eyepiece of a microscope.

ocularist One who designs, constructs, and fits artificial eyes.

oculist Obsolete term for ophthalmologist.

oculocerebrorenal syndrome Hereditary syndrome consisting of congenital cataracts and glaucoma, mental retardation, and reabsorption dysfunction of the kidney tubules leading to proteinuria, glycosuria, aminoaciduria, and inability to con-

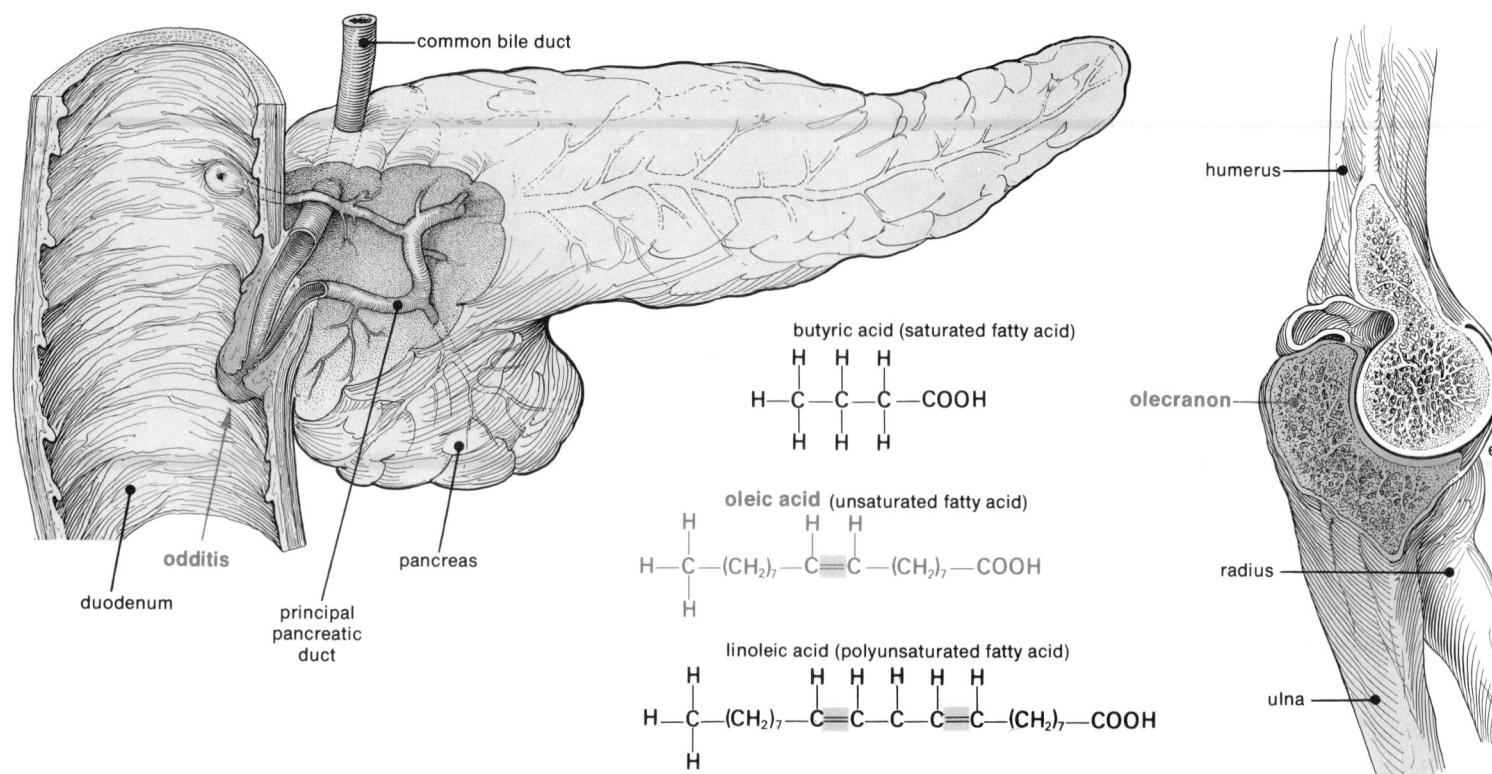

common bile duct

odditis

duodenum

principal pancreatic duct

pancreas

butyric acid (saturated fatty acid)

$$H - \overset{H}{\underset{H}{C}} - \overset{H}{\underset{H}{C}} - \overset{H}{\underset{H}{C}} - COOH$$

oleic acid (unsaturated fatty acid)

$$H - \overset{H}{\underset{H}{C}} - (CH_2)_7 - \overset{H}{C} = \overset{H}{C} - (CH_2)_7 - COOH$$

linoleic acid (polyunsaturated fatty acid)

$$H - \overset{H}{\underset{H}{C}} - (CH_2)_7 - \overset{H}{C} = \overset{H}{C} - \overset{H}{\underset{}{C}} - \overset{H}{C} = \overset{H}{C} - (CH_2)_7 - COOH$$

humerus

olecranon

radius

ulna

centrate and acidify the urine. Also called cerebro-oculorenal dystrophy; Lowe's syndrome.

oculocutaneous Relating to the eyes and the skin.

oculography The graphic recording of eye positions and movements.

oculogyria Rotation of the eyeballs.

oculogyric Relating to or causing rotation of the eyeballs.

oculomotor 1. Relating to or causing movements of the eyeball. 2. Relating to the oculomotor nerve (cranial nerve III).

oculomycosis See ophthalmomycosis.

oculonasal Relating to the eye and the nose.

oculopathy Ophthalmopathy.

oculus *pl.* **oculi** (O) Latin for eye.

  o. dexter (O.D.) Right eye.

  o. sinester (O.S.) Left eye.

  o. uterque (O.U.) The two eyes.

ocutome A miniaturized surgical instrument used in closed vitrectomy to enter the back of the eye through three minute incisions; it consists of three probes: one probe provides light to view the interior of the eye, another cuts and removes tissue, and through the third one a sterile solution is poured in.

odditis Inflammation of the sphincter of the hepatopancreatic duct (sphincter of Oddi), at the junction of the duodenum and common bile duct.

odontectomy The removal of a tooth by the excision of bone around the root before it is extracted.

odontexesis The thorough scaling of teeth.

odontic Of or relating to teeth; dental.

odontoblast A specialized cell in the dental papilla of a developing tooth which produces the matrix that forms the dentin of the tooth; it lines the pulp cavity and may form secondary dentin throughout life.

odontoblastoma 1. Tumor composed chiefly of epithelial and mesenchymal cells that may develop to produce calcified tooth substances. 2. An odontoma in its early stage.

odontocele Alveolodental cyst; see under cyst.

odontoclast A multinucleated cell believed to be involved in the absorption of the roots of primary teeth.

odontogenesis The origin and development of teeth.

  o. imperfecta Developmental defect of teeth; enamel and dentin are thin and pulp cavity is large; affected teeth appear opalescent.

odontogenic Derived from tissues involved in tooth formation; said of certain tumors.

odontogeny Development of teeth.

odontoid Shaped like a tooth, as the odontoid

process of the second cervical vertebra.

odontology Dentistry.

  forensic o. A branch of forensic medicine which applies knowledge of dentistry to civil and criminal problems.

odontolysis Erosion of teeth.

odontoma A tumor developed from tissues involved in tooth formation.

odontopathy Any disease of the teeth.

odontoprisis Grinding of the teeth.

odontorrhagia Profuse bleeding from the socket after extraction of a tooth.

odontoscope A small circular mirror used for inspecting the teeth.

odontotherapy Treatment of diseases of teeth.

odontotomy Cutting into a tooth.

odor An emanation from any substance that stimulates the sense of smell; a smell or a scent.

odoriferous Odorous; giving off an odor.

odorimeter An instrument for determining the intensity of odors.

odorimetry Measurement of relative intensity of odors.

odoriphore See osmophore.

odynacusis Hypersensitivity of the spiral organ of Corti (organ of hearing), so that noises cause actual discomfort; also called painful hearing.

odynometer Instrument used to measure the degree of sensitivity to a painful stimulus. Also called algesiometer.

odynophagia Painful swallowing.

oersted (H) Unit of magnetic intensity, equal to the intensity of a magnetic field exerting a mechanical force of one dyne on a unit magnetic pole.

Oesophagostomum Genus of nematode worms that form nodules in the intestinal wall of ruminants, swine, and man, especially in Africa.

oestrid A two-winged botfly, the larva of which is parasitic in man and animals.

Oestrus A genus of tissue-invading botflies.

official In pharmacology, authorized by or listed in the U.S. Pharmacopeia or the National Formulary.

officinal Kept in stock; available without special preparation; said of pharmaceuticals.

ohm (Ω) A unit of electrical resistance equal to that of any conductor allowing one ampere of current to pass from a one volt potential across its terminals.

ohmmeter An apparatus for direct measurement of the electric resistance (in ohms) of a conductor.

oidiomycetes Common name for a group of fungi that produce arthrospores (reproductive spores) through fragmentation of the mycelium.

oidium *pl.* **oidia** A free, thin-walled hyphal cell

frequently called arthrospore.

oil Any of several substances that are viscous, unctuous, flammable, and not miscible with water but soluble in several organic solvents; classified, according to their origin, as animal, mineral, or vegetable oils.

  castor o. Oil obtained from castor-oil plant seeds (*Ricinus communis*); used as a laxative and externally as an emollient for skin disorders.

  cod liver o. Oil obtained from fresh livers of cod fish; a rich source of vitamins A and D.

  mineral o. Liquid petrolatum, a mixture of liquid hydrocarbons obtained from petroleum. Also called white mineral oil; liquid paraffin.

  o. of vitriol Sulfuric acid.

  o. of wintergreen A fragrant, volatile oil, rich in methyl salicylate, obtained from the macerated leaves of wintergreen.

  peanut o. Oil extracted from peanuts; used as a vehicle in pharmaceutical preparations. Also called arachis oil.

  pine o. The volatile oil (crude turpentine) produced by the destructive distillation of pine wood; used as a deodorant and disinfectant.

  rectified tar o. Oil obtained from pine tar; used in the treatment of certain skin disorders.

  red o. See oleic acid.

  safflower o. Oil from seeds of the safflower, *Carthamus tinctorius,* rich in polyunsaturated fats; used as a dietary supplement and in the manufacture of cosmetics.

  wheat germ o. Oil obtained from the embryo of the wheat kernel; a rich source of vitamin E.

oil red O Oil red O in isopropyl alchol; it stains lipids a cherry red color.

ointment Any of numerous soft, bland, highly viscous preparations used as a vehicle for external medication, as an emollient, or as a cosmetic; a salve.

  benzoic and salicylic acid o. Ointment composed of benzoic acid and salicylic acid in a water-soluble base; used to treat athlete's foot and similar fungus infections. Also called Whitfield's ointment.

  Whitfield's o. Benzoic and salicylic acid oil.

oleate 1. A salt of oleic acid. 2. A pharmaceutical preparation containing an alcohol or metallic base and oleic acid.

olecranon Point of the elbow; the prominent curved process of the ulna forming the tip of the elbow.

olefin An open-chain hydrocarbon having at least one double bond.

oleic Of or relating to oil.

oleic acid A colorless unsaturated fatty acid with

oligodactyly

oligodendroglia

optic nerves

liver

lesser omentum

stomach

pons

transverse colon

greater omentum

mesentery

ileum

neuron in central nervous system

olive

medulla oblongata

spinal cord

a lardlike aroma; a constituent of most of the common fats and oils. Also called red oil.

olein The glyceryl ester of oleic acid; a colorless oily substance occurring in many natural fats and oils; the main constituent of olive oil. Also called triolein.

oleometer Apparatus used to determine the specific gravity of oils.

oleoresin 1. A natural compound of some plants (e.g., pines) containing resin and essential oils. **2.** An extract of a drug.

oleosaccharum, *pl.* **oleosacchara** A homogeneous mixture used in pharmacy that is made by triturating sugar with a small amount of a volatile oil (anise, lemon, etc.). Also called sugar oil.

oleostearate A double salt of the oleic and stearic acids.

oleothorax Therapeutic introduction of oil into the pleural cavity, as in the treatment of pulmonary tuberculosis and other disorders. Also called eleothorax.

oleovitamin A preparation containing an edible oil and a vitamin.

olfactie See olfacty.

olfaction 1. The sense of smell. **2.** The act of smelling.

olfactology The science concerned with the study of the sense of smell.

olfactometer A device for testing the sense of smell.

olfactometry Determination of the degree of acuity of olfactory perception.

olfactory Relating to the sense of smell; denoting the first cranial nerve or olfactory nerve.

olfacty An arbitrary unit of smell, used in olfactometry to determine the strength of a stimulus. Also written olfactie.

oligemia Deficient amount of blood in the body.

olighidria A condition of scanty or diminished perspiration.

oligoamnios See oligohydramnios.

oligocholia Abnormally low secretion of bile.

oligochylia Deficiency of chyle.

oligochymia A lack of chyme.

oligodactyly, oligodactylia Congenital absence of one or more digits of a hand or foot.

oligodendria See oligodendroglia.

oligodendrocyte A cell of the oligodendroglia.

oligodendroglia Non-nervous supportive tissue (neuroglia) surrounding nerve cells and fibers of the central nervous system; composed of small, angular cells (oligodendrocytes) with short, beaded processes and no fibrils; present in both white and gray matter. Also called oligodendria.

oligodendroglioma A relatively slow growing, solid tumor made up of oligodendroglia, usually found in the cerebrum of adults.

oligodipsia Abnormally reduced thirst.

oligodontia Congenital absence of one or more teeth.

oligodynamic Effective in very small quantities.

oligohydramnios Deficient amount of amniotic fluid in the pregnant uterus, sometimes represented by only a few milliliters of a thick viscid fluid. Also called oligoamnios.

oligomenorrhea Reduction in the frequency of menstruation; occurring in intervals between the cycles from 38 days to 3 months.

oligonucleotide A compound made up of a small number of nucleotides (2 to 10).

oligosaccharide A compound made up of a small number of monosaccharide units (2 to 10).

oligospermia, oligospermatism Abnormally low concentration of spermatozoa in the semen.

oligotrichosis See hypotrichosis.

oliguria Abnormally low excretion of urine; arbitrarily defined as less than 400 ml of urine per day for an adult of average size.

olive A smooth prominent oval mass on each side of the medulla oblongata. Also called oliva.

Ollier's syndrome A nonhereditary unilateral disorder marked by the presence of nonossified cartilage in the long bones, resulting in shortening of an extremity. Also called dyschondroplasia; enchondromatosis; hemichondrodysplasia.

ololiuqui A substance present in the seeds of the morning-glory; has been used in ceremonies by Indians of the North American continent to produce altered states of consciousness.

omalgia Pain in the shoulder area.

omega Last letter of the Greek alphabet, Ω.

omental Of or relating to the omentum.

omentectomy Surgical removal of the entire omentum, or of a portion of it.

omentofixation See omentopexy.

omentopexy Suturing of the omentum to the abdominal wall. Also called omentofixation; epiplopexy.

omentorrhaphy Suturing of the omentum.

omentum A peritoneal fold in the abdominal cavity which connects various viscera with each other or with the abdominal wall.

greater o. A prominent double fold of peritoneum descending a variable distance from the greater curvature of the stomach to the front of the small intestine, where turning upon itself (thereby making four layers) it ascends to the top of the transverse colon; it resembles an apron and usually

contains large deposits of fat.

lesser o. The fold of peritoneum extending between the liver and the lesser curvature of the stomach and the beginning of the duodenum; the portion connecting the liver to the stomach is called the hepatogastric ligament, while the portion passing from the liver to the duodenum is named the hepatoduodenal ligament; the right border of the lesser omentum is free, forming the ventral margin of the epiploic foramen.

omni hora (Omn. hor.) Latin for every hour; used in prescription writing.

omnivorous Living on both plant and animal food.

omoclavicular Relating to the shoulder and the clavicle (collarbone).

omohyoid See table of muscles.

omothyroid See table of muscles.

omphalectomy Surgical removal of the navel.

omphalic Umbilical.

omphalitis Inflammation of the navel.

omphalocele Congenital hernia at the umbilicus, either into the umbilical cord, or through a defect of the abdominal wall (omphalocele proper). Also called exomphalos; umbilical eventration; amniotic hernia.

omphalomesenteric Relating to the umbilicus and the mesentery.

omphalophlebitis Inflammation of the umbilical veins.

omphalorrhagia Bleeding from the navel.

omphalorrhea A discharge from the navel.

omphalos, omphalus The navel.

omphalotomy Cutting of the umbilical cord at birth.

omphalotripsy Crushing, instead of cutting, of the umbilical cord after childbirth.

onanism Withdrawal of the penis just prior to ejaculation during sexual intercourse; the term is derived from the story of Onan, son of Judah (Genesis 38:9); commonly used as synonymous with male masturbation. Also called coitus interruptus.

Onchocerca A genus of parasitic worms of the family Onchoceridae (which includes *Wuchereria* and *Loa*); the worms inhabit connective tissues of humans and animals, usually coiled and entangled within firm nodules; two species, *Onchocerca caecutiens* and *Onchocerca volvulus*, can penetrate the skin.

onchocerciasis, oncocerciasis Skin disease caused by infestation with a threadlike work, *Onchocercavolvulus*; marked by irritation of the skin with corneal opacities and skin nodules; transmitted by the bite of infested flies. Also called river blindness; volvulosis.

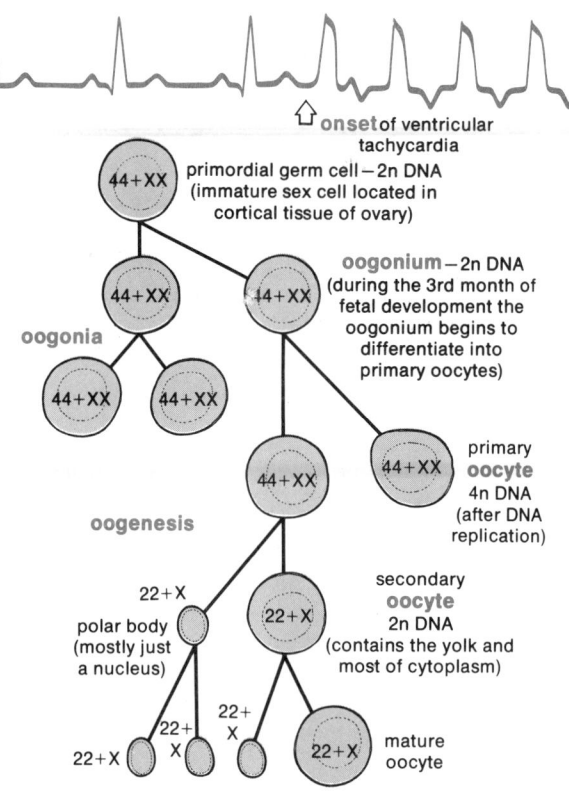

onset of ventricular tachycardia

primordial germ cell – 2n DNA (immature sex cell located in cortical tissue of ovary)

44+XX

oogonia

44+XX   44+XX

oogonium – 2n DNA (during the 3rd month of fetal development the oogonium begins to differentiate into primary oocytes)

44+XX   44+XX

oogenesis

44+XX   44+XX   primary oocyte 4n DNA (after DNA replication)

22+X   polar body (mostly just a nucleus)

22+X

secondary oocyte 2n DNA (contains the yolk and most of cytoplasm)

22+X   22+X

22+X   22+X   mature oocyte

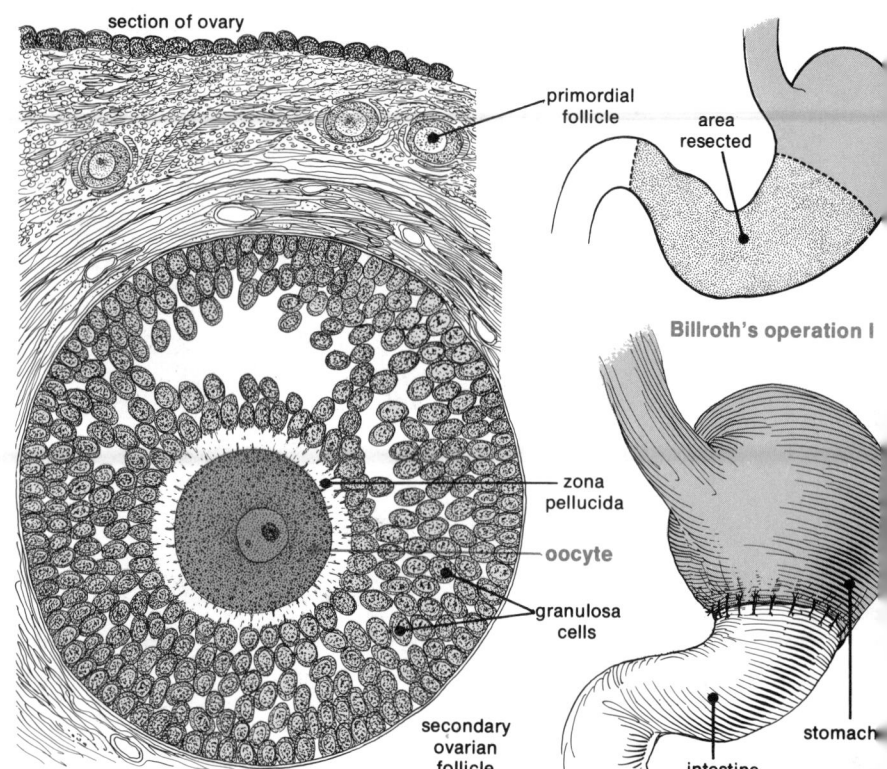

section of ovary

primordial follicle

area resected

Billroth's operation I

zona pellucida

oocyte

granulosa cells

secondary ovarian follicle

intestine

stomach

oncocyte An acidophilic, granular tumor cell.
oncogene Any gene (viral or cellular) implicated in tumor formation.
    retroviral o. A fully tumorigenic version of a cellular proto-oncogene.
oncogenesis The origin of a neoplasm.
oncogenic, oncogenous 1. Causing tumor formation. **2.** Originating from a tumor.
oncolipid A structurally altered fat from a protein molecule found in the blood of many cancer patients.
oncology The scientific study of neoplasms.
oncolysis 1. Destruction of a tumor. **2.** Reduction of any abnormal mass.
oncoma A tumor or a swelling.
oncornavirus Oncovirus.
oncosis Condition characterized by the presence of tumors.
oncosphere See hexacanth.
oncotherapy Treatment of tumors.
oncotic Relating to edema or any swelling. See also pressure, oncotic.
oncotropic Having an affinity for neoplastic cells.
Oncovirinae Subfamily of tumor viruses (family Retroviridae) which, on the basis of morphology and antigenicity, are grouped into types A, B, C, and D; associated with certain malignant diseases. Also called RNA tumor virus or tumor virus group.
oncovirus Any tumor virus (Family Retroviridae, subfamily Oncovirinae). Also called oncornavirus.
oneirology The study of dreams.
oneiroscopy The study of dreams for the purpose of diagnosing a person's mental state. Also called dream analysis.
onlay An extended restoration of a tooth that covers the entire occlusal surface.
onset The start or the beginning.
ontogenesis The biologic development of the individual; distinguished from phylogenesis.
ontogeny Ontogenesis.
onychatrophy, onychatrophia Atrophy or underdevelopment of nails, congenital or acquired.
onychauxis Marked thickening or overgrowth of nails.
onychectomy Surgical removal of a nail or nail bed.
onychia Inflammation of the matrix of a nail.
onychocryptosis Ingrown nail; see under nail.
onychodystrophy Deformity of nails.
onychogryposis Overgrowth of the fingernail or toenail resembling a ram's horn; different factors such as irritation of the nail bed by direct trauma, intermittent pressure, and infection may be possible causes.

onychoid Resembling a fingernail or toenail.
onycholysis Loosening, occasionally with shedding, of the nails.
onychomalacia Abnormal softening of the nails.
onychomycosis Fungus infection, such as ringworm, of the fingernails or toenails.
onychopathy Any disease of the nails. Also called onychosis.
onychophagia, onychophagy Nailbiting.
onychorrhexis Abnormal brittleness of the nails with breakage of the free edge.
onychotillomania A compulsive habit of picking on the cuticles or at the nails.
onychotomy Surgical incision into a fingernail or toenail.
onyx 1. From Greek meaning nail; a fingernail or a toenail. **2.** Collection of pus behind the cornea, resembling a fingernail. Also called hypopyon.
onyxis Ingrown nail.
ooblast A cell from which the ovum develops.
oocyesis Ovarian pregnancy; see under pregnancy.
oocyst The encysted form of a zygote in which the formation of sporozoites (the infectious stage of sporozoans) takes place.
oocyte A cell in the ovary derived from an oogonium that, upon undergoing meiosis, produces an ovum; a primitive egg in the ovary.
oogenesis The formation and development of the egg (ovum). Also called ovigenesis.
oogenetic Relating to oogenesis.
oogenic, oogenous Producing ova.
oogonium One of the cells that form most of the ovarian tissue and serve as a source of oocytes.
ookinesia The movements of the egg during maturation and fertilization.
ookinete A motile zygote; a stage in the life cycle of certain protozoan parasites, e.g., the malarial parasite.
oolemma The cell membrane of the ovum.
oophoralgia Ovarian pain.
oophorectomy Removal of one or both ovaries.
oophoritis Inflammation of one or both ovaries, usually occurring secondary to another infection such as mumps.
oophorocystectomy Surgical removal of an ovarian cyst.
oophorocytosis Formation of a cyst in the ovary.
oophoroma An ovarian tumor.
oophoron The ovary.
oophoropathy Any disease of the ovary.
oophoroplasty Reparative surgery on an ovary.
oophorosalpingectomy Surgical removal of an ovary and its corresponding ovarian duct.

oophorosalpingitis Inflammation of the ovary and uterine tube.
oophorotomy Surgical incision of an ovary.
ooplasm The cytoplasm of an ovum.
ootheca 1. Ovary. **2.** The egg case of certain insects.
ootid One of two cells derived from the maturation division of the secondary oocyte; it corresponds to the spermatid in the male.
ooze 1. Serous discharge or exudate, as from the skin. **2.** To leak out slowly.
opacification The formation of opacities; the process of making opaque.
opacity 1. The state of being opaque. **2.** An area of normally transparent structures of the eye that has lost its transparency and become more or less opaque.
opalescent Exhibiting an iridescence of color resembling an opal; denoting certain bacterial cultures.
opaque 1. Impenetrable or impervious to light rays; not translucent or only slightly so. **2.** Dull; without luster.
opaque media In radiology, contrast substances introduced into a body structure to render it less penetrable, or impenetrable, to x-rays so as to better define parts of the structure.
open Exposed to the air, affording unobstructed entrance; said of a wound.
operable Denoting a pathologic condition that is reasonably expected to be cured by an operation.
operate To perform surgery.
operation Any surgical procedure for remedying a bodily injury, ailment, or dysfunction.
    Abbe-Estlander o. A procedure for correcting a defect on a lip by transferring a full thickness flap from the other lip, using an arterial pedicle to insure survival of the graft.
    Babcock's o. Removal of a varicosed saphenous vein by introducing a sound (usually from the groin to the ankle), fastening the cut vein to it, and drawing it out.
    Billroth's o.'s Operative techniques for removal of part of the stomach: I, removal of the pylorus followed by end-to-end anastomosis of the stomach and duodenum; II, a rarely used procedure consisting of the removal of the pylorus and most of the lesser curvature of the stomach and closure of the cut ends of the stomach and duodenum, followed by a posterior anastomosis of the stomach and jejunum.
    Blalock-Hanlon o. The creation of a large interatrial opening to allow mixing of oxygenated blood; a palliative measure for abnormality of the heart in which the aorta originates from the right ventricle

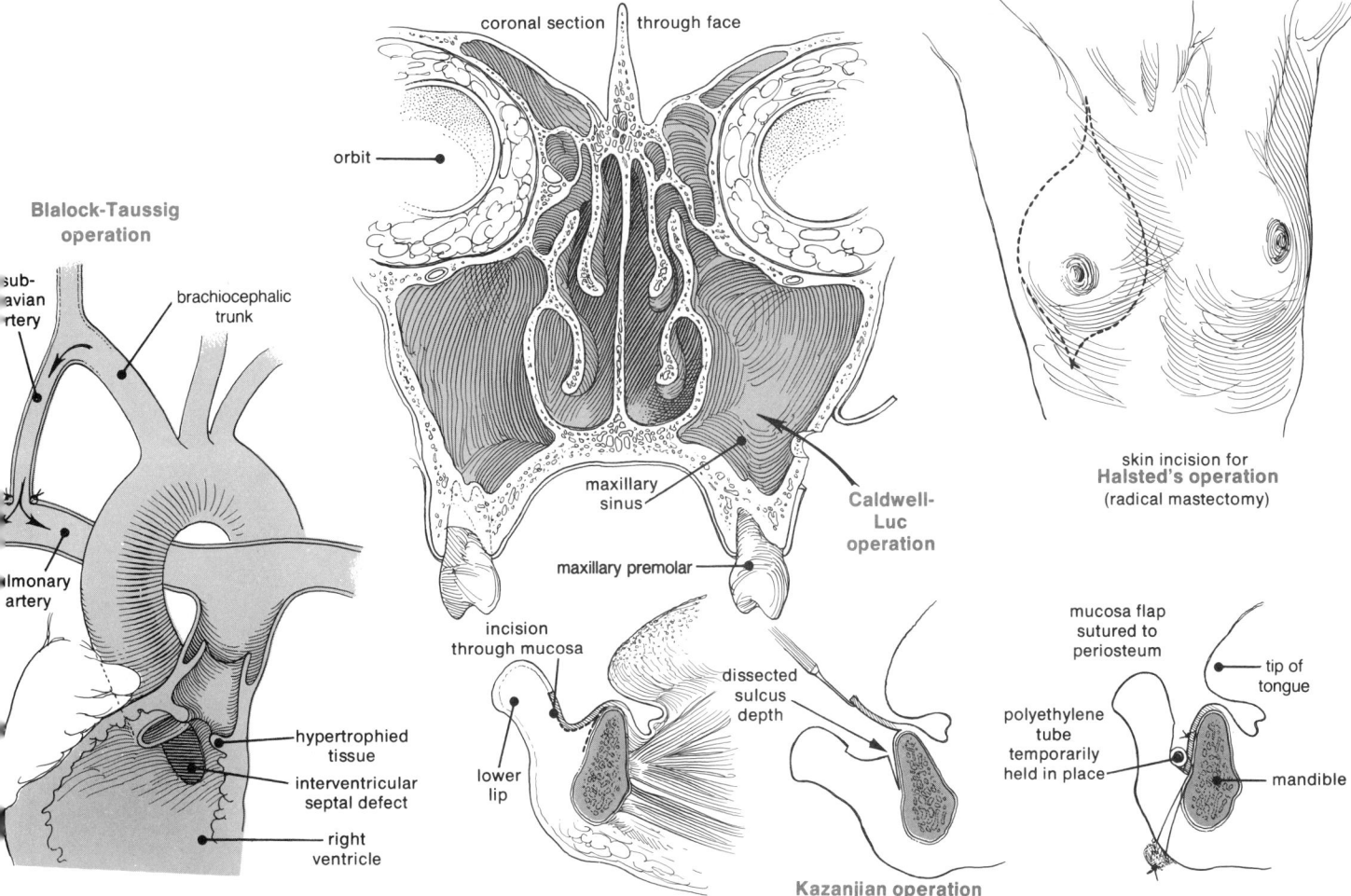

Blalock-Taussig operation

sub-clavian artery

brachiocephalic trunk

orbit

coronal section | through face

maxillary sinus

Caldwell-Luc operation

maxillary premolar

skin incision for **Halsted's operation** (radical mastectomy)

pulmonary artery

incision through mucosa

dissected sulcus depth

mucosa flap sutured to periosteum

tip of tongue

polyethylene tube temporarily held in place

lower lip

mandible

hypertrophied tissue

interventricular septal defect

right ventricle

Kazanjian operation

and the pulmonary artery from the left ventricle.

Blalock-Taussig o. The anastomosing of the brachiocephalic trunk (innominate), a subclavian, or a carotid artery to the pulmonary artery to direct blood from the systemic circulation to the lungs, in cases of congenital pulmonary stenosis with septal defect.

blind o. A procedure in which the surgeon operates by using his sense of touch and knowledge of surgical anatomy without full view of the operative field.

bloodless o. An operation performed with little or no blood loss.

Bricker's o. Diversion of urine disposal from the bladder by connecting the ureter to a pouch of isolated ileum opening onto the abdominal wall.

Caldwell-Luc o. Removal of the contents of a maxillary sinus through an opening on its facial wall above the root of the bicuspid tooth.

debulking o. Removal of a portion of a cancerous tumor that cannot be removed completely.

exploratory o. A procedure used to establish a diagnosis by ascertaining the condition present.

fenestration o. An ear operation in which a sound pathway to the labyrinth is established to take the place of the oval window occluded by otosclerotic stapes fixation; consists of creating a fistula into the osseous labyrinth of the horizontal semicircular canal or promontory and covering the opening with an elastic membrane or skin flap.

flap o. 1. Any procedure involving partial detachment of tissue. **2.** In dental surgery, partial detachment of soft tissue from underlying bone to gain access to the area.

Gillies' o. Reduction of fractures of the zygoma and zygomatic arch through an incision above the hairline.

Halsted's o.'s 1. Removal of a breast for carcinoma along with the greater and smaller pectoral muscles and adjacent lymphatic structures. **2.** Operation for the repair of a direct inguinal hernia.

Hofmeister o. Reestablishment of intestinal continuity after partial removal of the stomach by closure of the lesser curvature side of the stomach and the duodenal stump, followed by anastomosis of the greater curvature side of the stomach and jejunum.

Huggins' o. Removal of testes for cancer of the prostate gland.

Kazanjian o. A surgical procedure for extending the vestibular sulcus of edentulous ridges to increase their height and to improve denture retention.

Manchester o. High amputation of the uterine cervix and suturing together of the broad ligament bases in front of the shortened cervix; devised to relieve first and second degree prolapse of the uterus.

Marshall-Marchetti-Krantz o. An operation for correction of stress incontinence; the tissues on either side of the urethra are sutured together anteriorly, then to the posterior side of pubis and to the rectus muscle.

Naftziger's o.. Removal of the lateral and superior orbital walls for severe malignant exophthalmos.

open o. A procedure in which the surgeon operates with full view of the operative field.

Pott's o. Side-to-side connection between the aorta and the pulmonary artery; a palliative measure for tetralogy of Fallot.

plastic o. An operation intended to restore appearance, function, or lost parts.

radical o. A thorough operation intended to effect a complete cure.

Roux-en-Y o. Procedure in which the jejunum is cut about 15 cm below its origin, the distal end is sutured to the stomach, and the end of the proximal segment is sutured to the side of the jejunum farther down.

stapes mobilization o. Freeing of stapes from overgrowth of bone to restore hearing in individuals with otosclerosis.

Whipple's o. Removal of carcinoma of the head of the pancreas.

operative 1. Relating to an operation. **2.** Active.

operculated Having a caplike cover or operculum, as the eggs of certain parasitic worms.

operculum, *pl.* **opercula 1.** In anatomy, any structure resembling a lid or cover. **2.** The mucus sealing the opening of the endocervical canal of the uterus during pregnancy. **3.** The caplike cover of the eggs of certain parasitic worms. **4.** The attached portion of a retinal detachment. **5.** The tissue covering (partly or completely) an unerupted tooth. **6.**

One of the four gyri of the cerebrum that cover the insula (island of Reil).

o. oculi The eyelid.

operon A cluster of two or more structural genes and an operator gene on a chromosome governing the synthesis of the enzymes of a metabolic pathway.

ophiasis Loss of hair occuring in bands partly or completely encircling the head.

ophidiasis Poisoning by the venom of a snake. Also called ophidism.

ophidic Relating to snakes.

ophidiophobia A morbid fear of snakes.

ophryosis Spasmodic twitching in the area of the eyebrow.

ophthalmalgia Pain in the eyeball.

ophthalmectomy Surgical removal of the eyeball.

ophthalmia Inflammation of the eye.

gonorrheal o. Acute purulent conjunctivitis caused by gonorrheal infection.

o. neonatorum Acute purulent conjunctivitis of the newborn infant acquired during passage through the birth canal when the mother has gonorrhea.

sympathetic o. Bilateral inflammation of the uveal tracts following a perforating wound or retention of a foreign object in one eye, leading to bilateral blindness. Also called metastatic, migratory, or transferred ophthalmia.

ophthalmic Pertaining to the eyeball.

ophthalmitic Relating to inflammation of the eye.

ophthalmoblenorrhea Purulent conjunctivitis.

ophthalmocentesis Surgical puncture of the eye.

ophthalmodiaphanoscope Instrument used to inspect the interior of the eye by means of transmitted light.

ophthalmodonesis A trembling motion of the eyes.

ophthalmodynamometer 1. Instrument for estimating the blood pressure of the retinal vessels. **2.** Instrument for measuring the power of convergence of the eyes, applied to a near point of vision.

ophthalmodynamometry Measurement of the blood pressure in the retinal circulation within the eye by means of an ophthalmodynamometer; used to determine the presence of a stenotic lesion in the

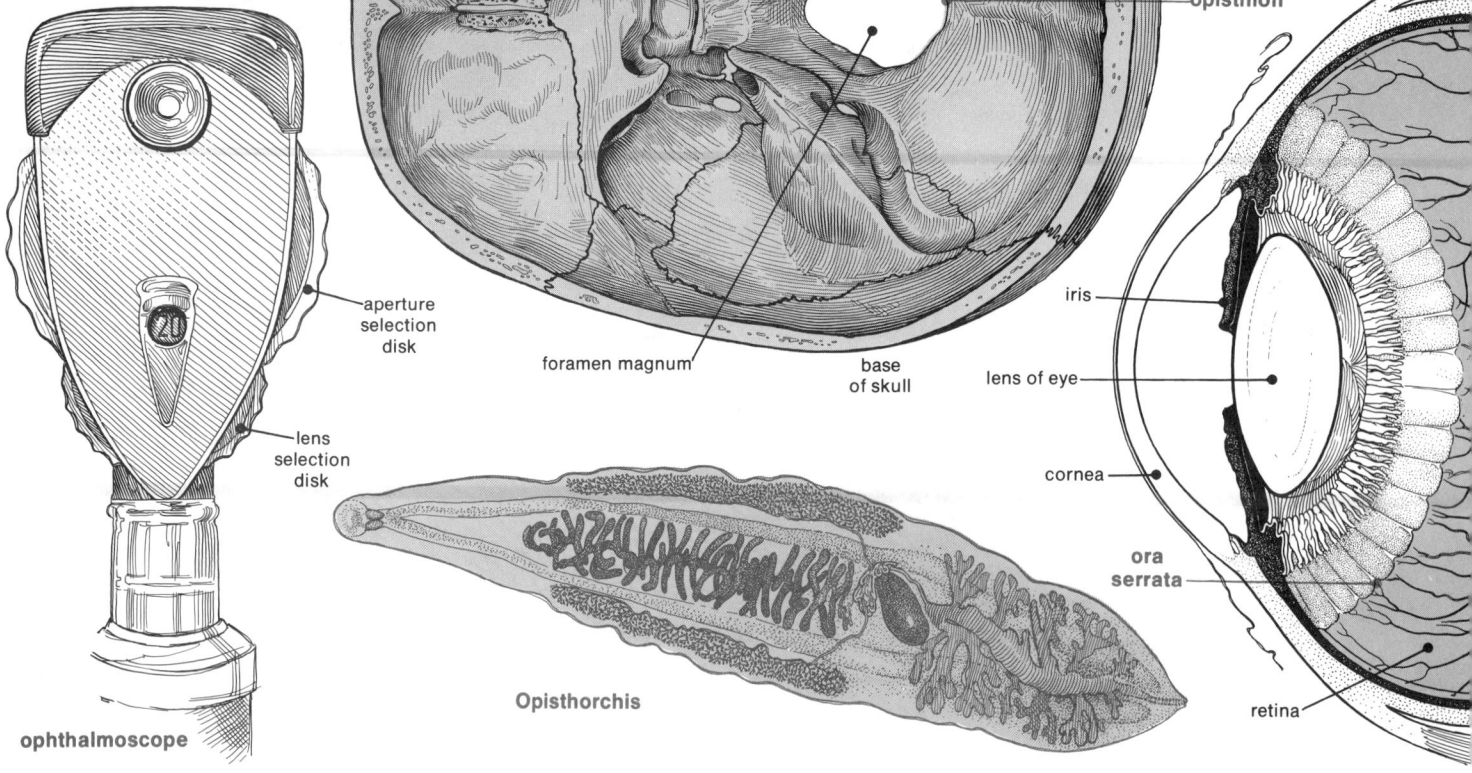

aperture selection disk

foramen magnum

base of skull

lens selection disk

ophthalmoscope

Opisthorchis

opisthion

iris

lens of eye

cornea

ora serrata

retina

carotid artery system.

ophthalmodynia Ophthalmalgia.

ophthalmo-eikonometer Instrument for measuring the ocular disorder, aniseikonia.

ophthalmograph Instrument used to record eye movements during reading.

ophthalmoleukoscope Instrument used to test color perception; it controls color intensities by means of filters to produce a white mixture.

ophthalmologist A physician who specializes in treating diseases and refractive errors of the eye.

ophthalmology The branch of medicine concerned with the eye, its diseases, and refractive errors.

ophthalmomalacia Abnormally low intraocular pressure of the eyeball.

ophthalmometer An instrument for measuring the curvature of the anterior surface of the cornea.

ophthalmometry The measuring of the curvature of the anterior surface of the cornea with the ophthalmometer.

ophthalmomycosis Any disease of the eye or its appendages caused by fungus. Also called oculomycosis.

ophthalmomyiasis Infection of the eye with the larvae of flies. Also called ocular myiasis.

ophthalmomyotomy Surgical division of any of the extrinsic (extraocular) eye muscles.

ophthalmoneuritis Inflammation of the optic nerve.

ophthalmopathy Any disease of the eye.

ophthalmophacometer Instrument used to measure the curvature of the cornea and lens of the eye.

ophthalmoplasty Reparative surgery of the eye.

ophthalmoplegia Paralysis of one or more muscles of the eye.

  external hereditary o. See ophthalmoplegia progressiva.

  o. progressiva Hereditary, progressive paralysis of the external muscles of the eye. Also called external hereditary ophthalmoplegia; Graefe's disease.

ophthalmoplegic 1. Relating to paralysis of the eye muscles. 2. An agent causing such an effect.

ophthalmoptosia, ophthalmoptosis Obsolete terms for exophthalmos.

ophthalmorrhagia Bleeding from the eye.

ophthalmorrhea Abnormal discharge from the eye.

ophthalmorrhexis Rupture of the eyeball.

ophthalmoscope An instrument used in examination of the interior of the eyeball.

ophthalmoscopy Examination of the interior of the eye by means of the ophthalmoscope.

ophthalmotonometer An instrument for determining the tension of the eyeball; used for detection of glaucoma.

ophthalmotonometry Determination of the intraocular tension with the ophthalmotonometer.

ophthalmotonus Intraocular tension; see under tension.

opthalmotrope A model of the two eyes designed to demonstrate the action of the extrinsic eye muscles.

ophthalmoxerosis See xerophthalmia.

opiate Any preparation derived from opium.

opioid Natural or synthetic compounds that have morphine-like pharmacologic activity. Also called narcotic analgesic.

opisthion The middle point on the posterior margin of the foramen magnum of the occipital bone of the skull.

opisthocheilia Receding lips.

opisthocranium The area in the midline of the cranium that protrudes farthest backward.

opisthorchiasis Infection with Asiatic flukes (*Opisthorchis viverrini and felineus*); transmitted through the ingestion of raw or undercooked infested fish.

Opisthorchis A genus of flukes (family Opisthorchiidae) characterized by the presence of testes at the posterior end of the lancet-shaped body; found in the gallbladder or bile ducts of fish-eating mammals, birds, and fish.

  O. felineus The cat liver fluke from Eastern Europe and Asia, measuring from 7 to 12 by 2 to 3 mm; humans are frequently infested by eating raw or undercooked infected fish.

  O. sinensis *Clonorchis sinensis*.

opisthotonos A muscle spasm causing rigidity of the neck and back and arching of the back with convexity forward, as in acute cases of tetanus or meningitis.

opium A bitter, brownish drug prepared from the dried gummy juice of unripe pods of a poppy, *Papaver somniferum*; used as an anesthetic; habitual use causes addiction and excessive use is fatal.

Oppenheim's sign Dorsal extension of the big toe elicited by stroking the medial side of the tibia; seen in pyramidal tract disease.

opponens Opposing; a qualifying addition to the names of several muscles of the hand and foot whose function is to pull the lateral digits across the palm or sole.

opportunistic Denoting a disease, or organisms causing such disease, in people with impaired immune systems or who are undergoing drug therapy.

opsin The protein constituent of the rhodopsin

molecule (a retinal pigment).

opsonin A serum substance naturally present in blood (usually an antibody), which coats particulates, such as bacteria, and renders them susceptible to destruction by phagocytes (phagocytosis).

opsonization The process by which antibody affects antigen so that it is more readily phagocytized.

opsonize To sensitize microorganisms with specific opsonin, thereby rendering them more susceptible to phagocytosis. Also called opsonify.

opsonocytophagic Relating to the increased phagocytic activity of leukocytes in blood containing specific opsonin.

optesthesia The ability to perceive a light stimulus.

optic Pertaining to the eye.

optical Relating to vision.

optical center The point of a lens through which passing light rays suffer no angular deviation.

optician One who makes or sells lenses, eyeglasses, or other optical instruments; a person who adjusts eyeglasses after a prescription furnished by an ophthalmologist or optometrist.

opticociliary Relating to the optic and ciliary nerves.

opticocinerea The gray substance of the optic nerve.

optics The science concerned with the study of light and refracting media, especially of the eye.

optimum Denoting the most suitable or favorable conditions.

optometer Any of several devices used to measure the refractive state of the eye. Also called opsiometer; optimeter.

optometrist An individual who specializes in examining, measuring, and treating visual defects by means of corrective lenses.

optometry The measuring of visual acuity and correction of visual defects by glasses.

optomyometer Instrument used to determine the relative strength of the extrinsic muscles of the eye.

ora, *pl.* **orae** A border.

  o. serrata The serrated margin of the retina, situated in the anterior portion of the eyeball.

orad Toward the mouth.

oral Relating to the mouth.

orality In psychoanalysis, relating to the oral or earliest stage of sexual development.

orange An edible fruit, *Aurantii fructus*; its rind contains numerous oil glands and is used in producing pharmaceutical preparations.

orbicular Circular.

orbiculus ciliaris The dark zone in the eye, within the circumference of the ora serrata.

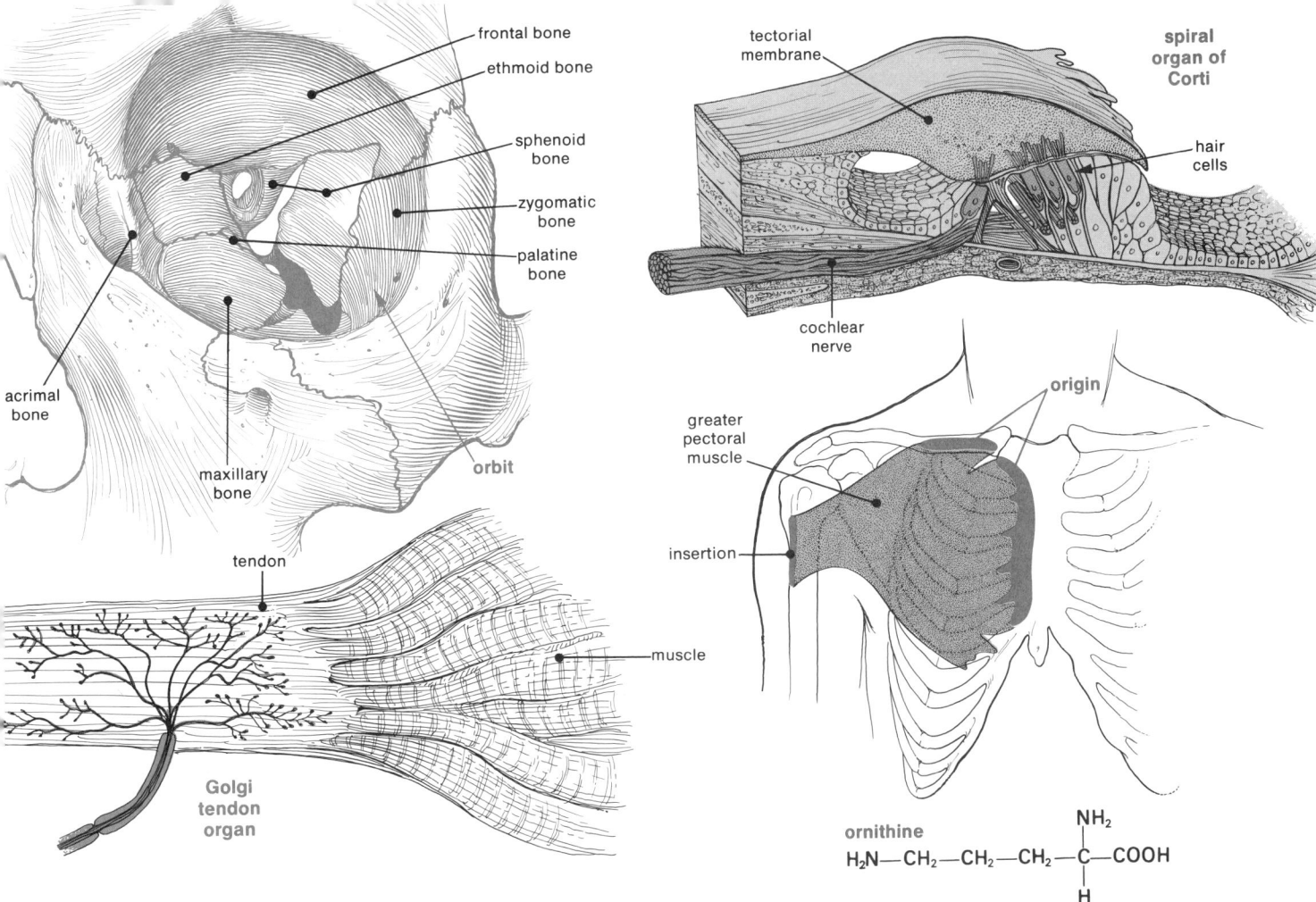

frontal bone
ethmoid bone
sphenoid bone
zygomatic bone
palatine bone
acrimal bone
maxillary bone
orbit

tectorial membrane
spiral organ of Corti
hair cells
cochlear nerve

origin
greater pectoral muscle
insertion

tendon
muscle

Golgi tendon organ

ornithine

$$H_2N—CH_2—CH_2—CH_2—\overset{\overset{\displaystyle NH_2}{|}}{\underset{\underset{\displaystyle H}{|}}{C}}—COOH$$

orbit One of two cavities in the skull which contains the eyeball and its associated structures; it is formed by portions of seven bones: frontal, maxillary, zygomatic, lacrimal, sphenoid, palatine, and ethmoid. Commonly called eye socket.

orbital Relating to the orbit.

orbitography The making of x-ray films of the orbit following injection of a radiopaque substance over the orbit floor; a diagnostic technique used when a blow-out fracture is suspected.

orbitonometer Instrument used to measure the degree of resistance offered by the eyeball when pressed into the socket.

orbitotomy Surgical incision into the orbit.

orcein A purple dye used in cytology.

orchialgia Pain in a testis. Also called orchiodynia; orchidalgia; testalgia.

orchichorea Involuntary twitching of the testis.

orchidorrhaphy See orchiopexy.

orchiectomy, orchidectomy Surgical removal of one or both testes. Also called castration.

orchiepididymitis Inflammation of a testis and epididymis.

orchiocele A tumor of the testis.

orchiodynia See orchialgia.

orchioncus A neoplasm or tumor of the testis.

orchiopathy Any disease of the testes.

orchiopexy Suturing of a testis to the scrotum as in the correction of an undescended testis. Also called orchidorrhaphy; orchiorrhaphy.

orchioplasty Reparative surgery of the testes.

orchiorrhaphy See orchiopexy.

orchioscirrhus Abnormal hardening of the testis.

orchiotomy Surgical incision into a testis.

orchis Greek for testis.

orchitis Inflammation of the testis. Also called testitis.

order A biologic taxonomic category ranking just below class and above family.

orderly An attendant in a hospital ward whose responsibilities do not require professional training.

ordinate The vertical coordinate which, together with a horizontal one (abscissa), forms a frame of reference for the plotting of data.

orexigenic Stimulating the appetite.

orf A viral disease of sheep occasionally transmitted to the skin of man, especially to sheepherders and veterinarians; the chancre-type lesions appear most frequently on the hands and face. Also called ecthyma contagiosum.

organ A differentiated structure of the body that performs some specific function.

  end o. The expanded termination of a nerve fibril as found in muscle tissue, skin, mucous membrane, or glands.

  Golgi tendon o. Special bare nerve ending ramifying about bundles of collagen fibers of tendons, usually at the ends of muscles; the afferent fibers are among the largest fibers in peripheral nerve tissue.

  o. of Corti See spiral organ of Corti.

  o.'s of Zuckerkandl Small masses of chromaffin tissue located along the abdominal aorta; they are most prominent in the fetus.

  sense o. Any organ of special sense, as the eye, and the accessory structures associated with it.

  spiral o. of Corti The sensory receptors for hearing, contained in the cochlear duct of the internal ear. Also called organ of Corti.

  target o. The organ that is stimulated by a hormone.

organelle A specialized cytoplasmic structure of a cell performing a specific function, such as a mitochondrion.

organic 1. Relating to the organs of the body. 2. Relating to living organisms. 3. Organized; structural.

organic brain syndrome (OBS), **organic mental syndrome** (OMS) A syndrome resulting from diffuse or local impairment of brain tissue function, manifested by alteration of orientation, memory, comprehension, and judgment.

  acute o.b.s. Acute confusional state characterized by a sudden onset and a high degree of reversibility.

  chronic o.b.s. Disorder marked by an insidious onset, a progressive course, and a high degree of irreversibility; always due to focal or diffuse brain lesions.

  psychotic o.b.s. Acute or chronic organic brain syndrome associated with psychiatric symptoms.

organism Any living entity, plant or animal.

organization 1. An arrangement of distinct but dependent parts with varied functions that contribute to the whole; the organic structure of an organism. 2. The process of forming into organs.

organizer 1. A group of cells on the dorsal lip of the blastopore that stimulates the differentiation of cells in the embryo. 2. Any group of cells having such an ability.

organoid 1. Resembling an organ. 2. Composed of the cellular elements of an organ.

organoleptic 1. Stimulating an organ of sense. 2. Capable of receiving a sensory stimulus.

organomercurial An organic compound of mercury; some compounds of this type have diuretic properties.

organotropism The predilection of microorganisms and chemicals for certain organs or tissues; e.g., viruses infecting primarily the central nervous tissue.

orgasm The intense sensation experienced at the culmination of sexual intercourse or stimulation of the sex organs; it is accompanied in the male by ejaculation of semen and in the female by involuntary contractions of the vagina.

orientation 1. Awareness of oneself in reference to time, place, and other individuals; the act of finding one's bearings. 2. The relative position of atoms in a compound.

orifice An opening.

origin 1. The site of attachment of a muscle to a bone which is less movable than the one to which it is inserted. 2. The starting point or beginning of a nerve.

ornithine $NH_2(CH_2)_3CHCH_2COOH$; an amino acid formed when urea is removed from arginine; an important intermediate in urea biosynthesis, it possesses one less carbon than its homologue lysine.

Ornithodoros A genus of ticks (family Argasidae) some of which transmit the agents of relapsing fevers.

Ornithonyssus sylviarum A species of mites parasitic on many domestic and wild fowl; they also infest man, producing a pruritic dermatitis. Also called northern fowl mite.

ornithosis An infectious disease of birds occasionally transmitted to man; when transmitted by parrots or other psittacine birds, the disease is known

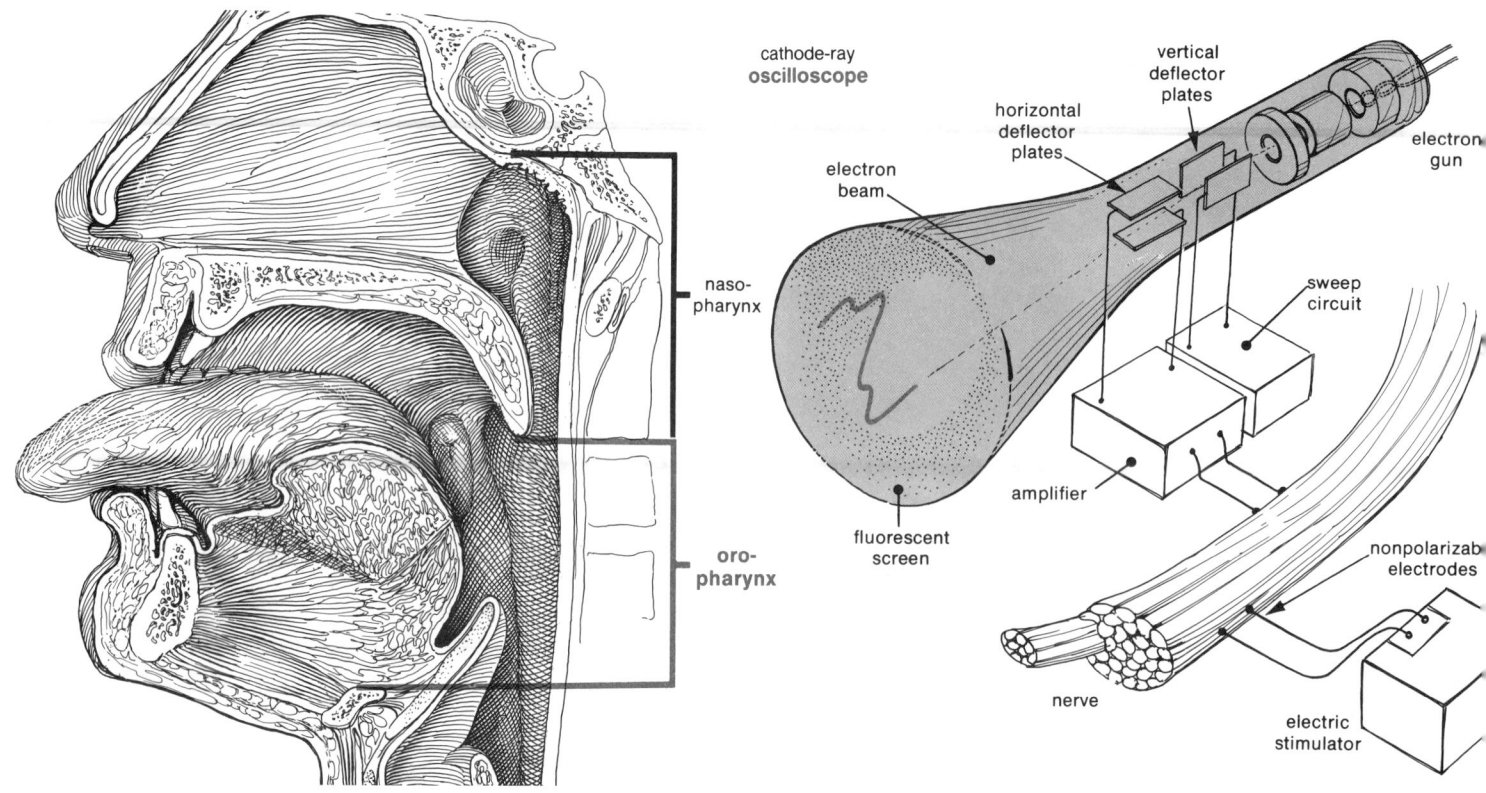

cathode-ray **oscilloscope**

naso-pharynx

oro-pharynx

electron beam

horizontal deflector plates

vertical deflector plates

electron gun

sweep circuit

amplifier

fluorescent screen

nonpolarizab electrodes

nerve

electric stimulator

---

as psittacosis; in man, the disease may cause an influenza-like condition or pneumonia; caused by *Chlamydia psittaci.*

orolingual Relating to the mouth and tongue.

oronasal Relating to the mouth and the nose.

oropharynx The central portion of the pharynx directly behind the oral cavity, extending from the inferior border of the soft palate to the lingual surface of the epiglottis; it contains the palatine tonsils and the posterior faucial pillars.

orotic acid An intermediate in the formation of pyrimidine nucleotides.

orphan Denoting any drug, device, or test that, although useful in some cases, is not manufactured because it is not commercially profitable.

orthetics See orthotics.

orthobiosis Living in a manner that promotes physical and mental health.

orthochromatic Staining the color of the dye used; said of certain cells.

orthocrasia Condition in which the body reacts normally to drugs.

orthodigita Correction of malformed fingers or toes.

orthodontics A specialty of dentistry dealing with correction and prevention of irregularities of the teeth.

orthodontist A dentist who specializes in orthodontics.

orthodromic Conducting impulses along a normal path.

orthogenics The study and treatment of defects (physical and mental).

orthognathic Having straight jaws and a straight profile; having a face with no projection of the lower jaw, one with a gnathic index below 98.

orthograde The erect posture of man; opposed to pronograde.

orthokinetics A method of treatment for hypertrophic osteoarthritis in which a muscular action is transferred from one set of muscles to another in order to protect the affected joint.

orthometer Instrument used to measure the degree of protrusion of the eyeballs.

Orthomyxoviridae A family of viruses, filamentous or spherical (80 to 120 nm in diameter), that contain single-stranded RNA and multiply in cytoplasm; includes all viruses that cause influenza. Also called influenza virus group.

orthopaedics See orthopedics.

orthopedic Relating to orthopedics.

orthopedics The surgically oriented branch of medicine concerned with the preservation and restoration of functions of the skeletal system and associ-

ated structures. Also written orthopaedics.

orthopedist One who practices orthopedics.

orthopercussion Percussion in which the left middle finger is flexed at a right angle and the tip of the finger is placed on the chest wall; the flexed finger is then struck upon the knuckle.

orthophoria Condition in which the visual axes of the two eyes are free from a tendency to deviate.

orthophosphate A salt of phosphoric acid (H_3PO_4).

orthopnea Difficulty in breathing except in an upright position.

orthopneic Relating to or afflicted with orthopnea.

orthopod Slang for orthopedist.

Orthopoxvirus Genus of the subfamily Chordopoxvirinae (family Poxviridae); some viruses included cause smallpox, ectromelia, and vaccinia (cowpox). Also called vaccinia subgroup.

orthopsychiatry The study and treatment of human behavior for the purpose of promoting healthy emotional growth and development.

Orthoptera An order of insects that includes grasshoppers, cockroaches, locusts, etc.

orthoptics The training process or techniques used for the improvement of visual perception and coordination of the two eyes for efficient binocular vision, or for the elimination of strabismus.

orthoptist One who is trained to treat ocular muscle imbalance, as strabismus, by reeducation of visual habits and exercise.

orthoscope An instrument that eliminates the refracting power of the cornea by means of a layer of water in a glass container held in contact with the eye.

orthoscopic 1. Relating to the orthoscope. 2. Having normal vision. 3. Giving a correct and proportioned image.

orthoscopy 1. Examination of the eye with an orthoscope. 2. The state of an optical system that produces images free of distortion.

orthosis Any mechanical device worn on the body to apply force to a part; used in the treatment of physical impairments.

orthostatic Relating to or caused by the upright position.

orthothanasia 1. The science of natural death. 2. The deliberate discontinuance of artificial means of maintaining life.

orthotics The making and fitting of orthopedic appliances. Also called orthetics.

orthotist One who makes and fits orthopedic appliances.

orthotonos, orthotonus Tetanic spasm in which

the head, body, and limbs are fixed rigidly in a straight line.

orthotopic Occuring in the normal position.

orthotropic Growing or extending along a vertical axis.

orthovoltage Medium electromotive force, from 200 to 300 kilovolts; used in radiotherapy.

os, *pl.* **ora** Latin for mouth or orifice, as the os of the cervix.

os, *pl.* **ossa** Latin for bone.

oscheocele Indirect inguinal hernia; see hernia, inguinal.

oscheoplasty Reparative surgery of the scrotum. Also called scrotoplasty.

oscillation 1. A backward and forward movement. 2. A stage of inflammation in which leukocytes accumulate in small vessels, blocking the flow of blood and causing a to-and-fro movement with each cardiac contraction.

oscillogram A graphic record traced by an oscillograph.

oscillograph An apparatus for graphically recording the oscillations of an electric current.

oscillometer An instrument used to measure variations in blood pressure.

oscillopsia A state in which observed objects seem to oscillate.

oscilloscope An electronic instrument that temporarily displays the variations of a fluctuating electrical quantity on the fluorescent screen of a cathode-ray tube.

oscitate To gape; to yawn.

osculum, *pl.* **oscula** A tiny opening.

Osgood-Schlatter disease Epiphysial aseptic necrosis; see under necrosis.

Osiander's sign Pulsation of the vagina in early pregnancy.

Osler's disease Hereditary hemorrhagic telangiectasia; see under telangiectasia.

Osler's sign Small painful swellings in the skin and subcutaneous tissues of the hands and feet occurring in endocarditis.

Osler-Weber-Rendu syndrome Hereditary hemorrhagic telangiectasia; see under telangiectasia.

osmatic Relating to the sense of smell.

osmidrosis Condition marked by a fetid odor of sweat. Also called bromidrosis.

osmiophilic Easily fixed with osmium textroxide.

osmium Metallic element; symbol Os, atomic number 76, atomic weight 190.2.

    o. tetroxide OsO_4; a crystalline compound commonly used as a tissue fixative for electron microscopy; has an irritating odor.

osmoceptor Osmoreceptor.

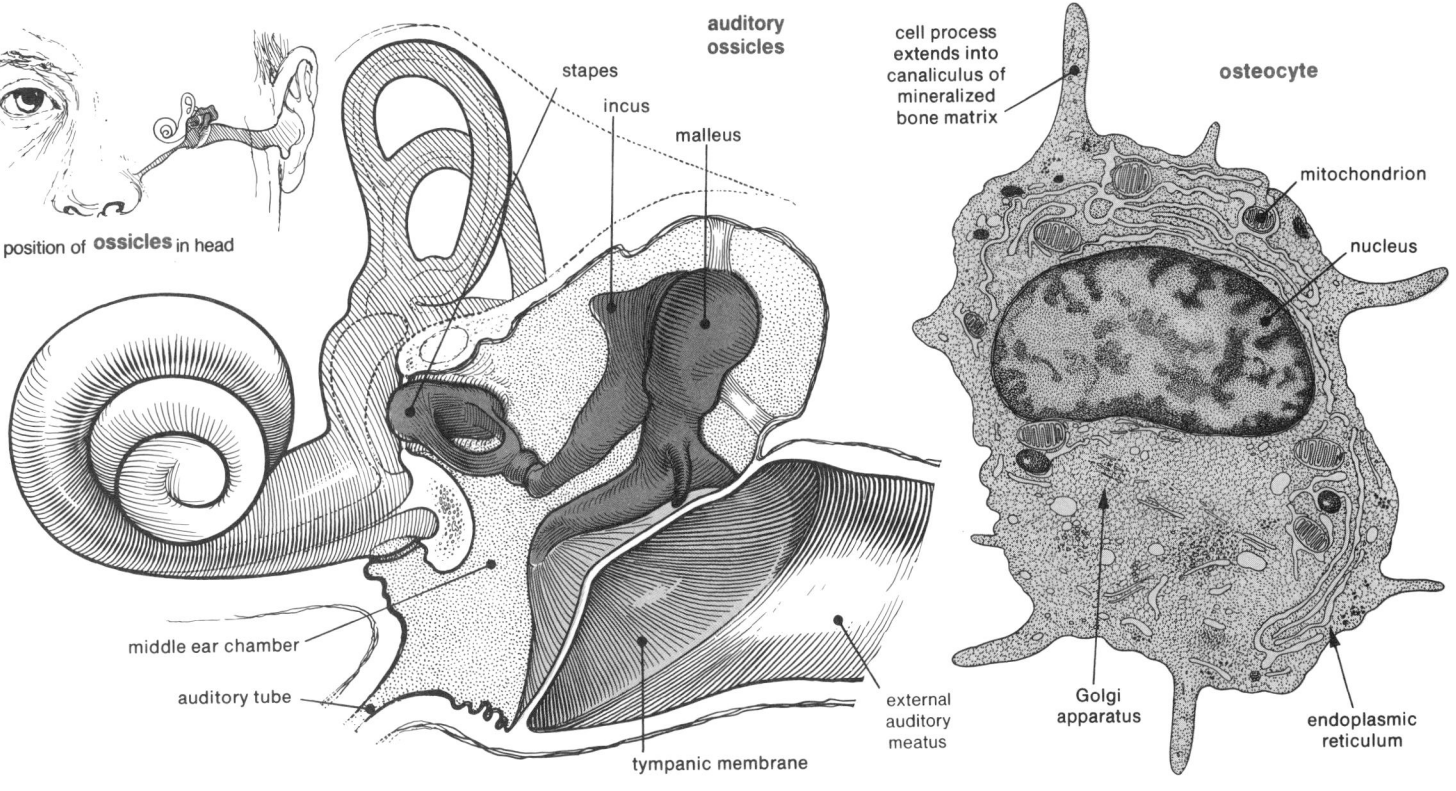

position of **ossicles** in head

auditory ossicles
stapes
incus
malleus

middle ear chamber

auditory tube

tympanic membrane

external auditory meatus

cell process extends into canaliculus of mineralized bone matrix

osteocyte

mitochondrion

nucleus

Golgi apparatus

endoplasmic reticulum

osmol, osmole (Osm.) Molecular weight (MW) in grams of a substance divided by the number of particles one molecule provides when it enters solution; e.g., glucose (MW 180), 1 Osm. $= \dfrac{180 \text{ g};}{1} =$ 180 g; sodium chloride (MW 58.5), 1 Osm. $= \dfrac{58.5 \text{ g}}{2} = 29.75$ g; one osmol provides Avogadro's number (6.023×10^{23}).

osmolality The osmotic concentration of a solution expressed as osmoles of the dissolved substance per kilogram of solvent (water); normal serum osmolality is 280 to 300 mOsm/kg.

osmolar See osmotic.

osmolarity The osmotic concentration of a solution expressed as osmoles of the dissolved substance per liter of solution.

osmometer An instrument for determining osmolality of a liquid, such as urine, by measuring the freezing point depression.

osmometry The measure of concentration of solute per kilogram of water; serum osmolality is normally from 280 to 300 mOsm/kg.

osmophil, osmophilic Thriving in a solution of high osmotic pressure.

osmophore A radical or atomic group whose presence causes the particular odor in a compound. Also called odoriphore; aromatophore.

osmoreceptor 1. A specialized sensory nerve ending in the hypothalamus that responds to increases in the osmotic pressure of the blood by stimulating the secretion of the neurohypophyseal antidiuretic hormone (ADH). **2.** A receptor that responds to the sensation of odors (olfactory stimuli). Also called osmoceptor.

osmoregulatory. 1. Regulating the osmolarity of the blood by acting to alter antidiuretic hormone release. **2.** Influencing osmosis.

osmosis The passage of liquid from a concentrated solution to a diluted one through a semipermeable membrane that separates them.

osmotic Relating to osmosis. Also called osmolar. See also pressure, osmotic.

osseointegration The growing of bone onto an implanted metal device, such as one that serves as a base for a tooth implant.

osseous Bony.

ossicle A small bone.
  auditory o.'s The three bones of the ear: malleus, incus, and stapes which together form a bony chain across the middle ear chamber for the conduction of sound waves from the tympanic membrane (eardrum) to the oval window; they are secured to the walls of the chamber by ligaments.

ossicular Of or relating to an ossicle.

ossiculectomy Surgical removal of one or more ossicles of the middle ear.

ossiculotomy Surgical incision of one of the ossicles of the middle ear or of adhesions that prevent their movements.

ossification The replacement of cartilage by bone.

ossify To change into bone.

ostealgia, ostalgia Pain in a bone.

osteitis Inflammation of bone.
  o. deformans Bone disease of unknown cause, characterized by localized, excessive destruction and repair with associated deformities. Also called Paget's disease.
  o. fibrosa cystica Disease characterized chiefly by softening and resorption of bone and replacement with fibrous tissue; caused by excessive secretion of hormone from the parathyroid glands.

osteoarthritis See degenerative joint disease.

osteoarthropathy Disorder affecting the long bones of the extremities and joints, often accompanied by clubbing of the fingers; almost always associated with disease elsewhere in the body, usually the lungs, pleura, and mediastinum.
  hypertrophic o. Painful swelling and periosteal deposition of new bone in the long bones of the extremities, clubbing of the fingers, and swelling and tenderness of joints; occurs most commonly in association with pulmonary disease, especially pulmonary neoplasm; also seen with cyanotic heart disease, ulcerative colitis, regional enteritis, and liver disorders.
  idiopathic hypertrophic o. Osteoarthropathy that does not occur secondary to any disease. Also called primary osteoarthropathy.

osteoblast A bone-forming cell; it arises from a fibroblast and is responsible for the formation of bone matrix; found on the advancing surface of developing bone.

osteoblastoma A benign tumor derived from primitive bone tissue; occurs most frequently on the spine of young individuals. Also called giant osteoid osteoma.

osteochondritis Inflammation of both bone and its cartilage.

osteochondrodystrophy General term for a group of disorders involving bone and cartilage, including Morquio's syndrome.

osteochondroma A single benign bony outgrowth capped by growing cartilage; most frequently occurring near the end of long bones of individuals between 10 and 25 years of age. Also called solitary osteocartilagenous exostosis.

osteochondromatosis Multiple hereditary ex-

ostosis; see under exostosis.

osteochondrosarcoma A malignant tumor of cartilaginous tissue usually arising from a benign bone tumor.

osteochondrosis Any disorder of the ossification centers in children; characterized by death of tissues in the absence of infection.

osteoclasis, osteoclasia Surgical or manual fracture or refracture of a deformed bone for the purpose of resetting it in a more normal position.

osteoclast A large multinucleated cell which is formed in bone marrow and absorbs bone tissue.

osteoclastoma Giant cell tumor of bone; see under tumor.

osteocranium The fetal cranium after ossification has occurred.

osteocyte One of numerous flattened, nucleated bone cells arising from osteoblasts by modulation; it plays a role in maintaining the constituents of the intercellular matrix at normal levels; each is contained in a space (lacuna) and its processes extend through openings of the lacuna into minute canals within the bone tissue.

osteocytoma Solitary bone cyst; see under cyst.

osteodentin A hard substance, structurally intermediate between dentin and bone, that partially fills the pulp cavity of teeth of the aged.

osteodermia The presence of bony deposits on the skin.

osteodesmosis The conversion of tendons into bone.

osteodynia Ostealgia.

osteodystrophy Defective bone formation.
  renal o. Generalized bone changes consisting of a mixture of osteosclerosis, osteomalacia, osteoporosis, and osteitis fibrosa cystica occurring in children or adults with chronic renal failure.

osteofibroma A benign tumor-like lesion composed chiefly of osseous and fibrous connective tissue.

osteogen The inner layer of periosteum from which new bone is formed.

osteogenesis The formation of bone.
  o. imperfecta A rare disease characterized by bone fragility, blue sclera, and otosclerotic deafness; thought to be transmitted as an autosomal dominant trait.

osteogenic, osteogenetic Relating to bone formation; derived from bone.

osteoid Resembling bone; usually refers to the soft organic part of intercellular bone matrix produced by osteogenic and osteoblast cells.

osteology The study of the structure of bones.

osteolysis Destruction of bone.

section of bone

otoconia

macula of internal ear

gelatinous layer with **otoconia**

hair cell

central canal

osteon (haversian system)

immobilized stapes

otosclerosis

tympanic membrane

osteotomes

middle ear chamber

osteoma A benign tumor composed of bone tissue; it may develop on a bone (homoplastic osteoma) or on other structures (heteroplastic osteoma). Also called osseous tumor.

  dental o. A bony growth projecting from the root of a tooth.

osteomalacia A disease marked by softening of the bones due to faulty calcification; characterized by increased amounts of osteoid or bone matrix which either fails to calcify or does so slowly; similar to rickets in children.

osteomere One of a series of bony structures, such as the vertebrae.

osteometry The branch of anthropology concerned with the relative size of human bones.

osteomyelitis Infection of bone, affecting the metaphyseal regions of the long bones; in the United States 50% of the cases are caused by *Staphyloccus aureus*; salmonella infections are found in individuals with sickle cell disease; spinal lesions are caused commonly by tuberculosis or gram-negative organisms.

osteomyelodysplasia Disease characterized by enlargement of the bone marrow cavities, thinning of the osseous tissue, and associated leukopenia and fever.

osteomyelofibrotic syndrome See myelofibrosis.

osteomyelography X-ray examination of bone marrow.

osteon The basic unit of compact bone structure consisting of a central canal and the concentric bony lamellae around it. Also called haversian system.

osteonecrosis Death of bone tissue, occurring most commonly in the head of the femur, less frequently in the medial femoral condyle, and occasionally in the head of the humerus.

osteopath A practitioner of osteopathy.

osteopathology The study of bone diseases.

osteopathy 1. Disease of bones. 2. A system of medical practice based on the belief that the normal body is capable of making its own remedies against infection; therapeutics is mainly manipulative, although surgical, medicinal, and hygienic methods are used when indicated.

osteopenia Reduced bone mass or density; may or may not be due to deficient bone formation.

osteoperiostitis Inflammation of a bone and its periosteum.

osteopetrosis An uncommon hereditary disorder transmitted as an autosomal recessive trait and characterized principally by overgrowth and denseness of bones and narrowing of the marrow, with resulting anemia, visual disturbances, deafness, and

delayed tooth eruption; seen most frequently in children. Also called Albers-Schönberg or marble bone disease.

osteophlebitis Inflammation of the veins of a bone.

osteophony The conduction of sound by bone.

osteophyte A bony outgrowth.

osteoplasty Plastic surgery of bones, such as bone grafting.

osteoporosis Disease of the bones due to deficiency of bone matrix, occurring most frequently in postmenopausal women.

osteoradionecrosis Death and degeneration of bone tissue caused by radiation.

osteorrhagia Bleeding from bone.

osteorrhaphy Wiring of a broken bone. Also called osteosuture.

osteosarcoma Bone cancer, usually occurring in the shaft at either end of a long bone. Also called osteoma sarcomatosum.

osteosarcomatous Relating to or causing bone cancer.

osteosclerosis Abnormally increased density or hardness of bone.

osteosuture See osteorrhaphy.

osteosynthesis Fastening the ends of a fractured bone.

osteotabes Degeneration of bone marrow.

osteotome A chisel used for cutting bone.

osteotomoclasis, osteotomoclasia Operative procedure for straightening an abnormally curved bone.

osteotomy Cutting a bone, usually with a saw or chisel.

ostial Relating to an orifice or ostium.

ostium A small opening into a hollow structure.

  o. primum Interatrial foramen primum; see under foramen.

  o. secundum Interatrial foramen secundum; see under foramen.

otalgia See earache.

otalgic 1. Relating to earache. 2. Any remedy for an earache.

othelcosis 1. Ulceration of the external ear. 2. Suppuration of the middle ear.

othemorrhea, othemorrhagia Bleeding from the ear.

otic Of or relating to the ear.

otitic Relating to or inflammation of the ear.

otitis Inflammation of the ear.

  chronic suppurative o. media Inflammation of the middle ear attended by a thick mucopurulent discharge from the mucous membrane; the infection may progress to involve the bone.

  o. externa Inflammation of the external auditory canal due to the presence of any of a variety of skin infections.

  o. media Infection of the middle ear, usually secondary to upper respiratory infections, generally transmitted to the middle ear through the auditory tube.

otoantritis Inflammation of the mastoid antrum.

otoblennorrhea Chronic inflammation of the middle ear with perforation of the tympanic membrane (eardrum) and a mucopurulent discharge from the ear.

otocephaly Defect characterized by extreme smallness of the chin and approximation of the ears toward the front of the neck.

otocleisis 1. Closure of the auditory (eustachian) tube. 2. Obstruction of the external auditory canal.

otoconia, *sing.* **otoconium** Granular particles composed of calcium carbonate and protein normally embedded in the gelatinous layer that covers the maculae of the utricle and saccule of the internal ear. Also called otoliths; statoconia.

otodecanoic acid See stearic acid.

otodynia Earache.

otoencephalitis Inflammation of the brain, secondary to inflammation of the middle ear and mastoid cells. Also called otocerebritis.

otoganglion Otic ganglion; see under ganglion.

otolaryngologist A specialist in otolaryngology.

otolaryngology The branch of medicine concerned with the study of the ear and the upper respiratory tract and the treatment of their diseases.

otoliths See otoconia.

otologic Relating to otology.

otologist A specialist in ear diseases.

otology The branch of medicine concerned with diseases of the ear.

otomycosis Fungal infection of the external auditory canal.

otoneuralgia Neuralgic earache.

otopathy Any disease of the ear.

otoplasty Plastic surgery of the auricle of the ear.

otopyorrhea Purulent discharge from the middle ear through a perforated tympanic membrane.

otorhinolaryngology The branch of medicine concerned with the ear, nose, and larynx, and their diseases.

otorhinology Study of the ear and the nose.

otorrhagia Bleeding from the ear.

otorrhea Discharge from the ear.

otosclerosis The formation and overgrowth of new spongy bone in the capsule of the middle ear, which immobilizes the stapes and interferes with the conduction of sound waves, resulting in slow, pro-otoscope

pneumatic otoscope

horizontal overlap

uterine tube

ovarian ligament

uterus

ovary

broad ligament

ureter

ouabain

gressive hearing loss; surgical removal of the stapes and the sclerotic bone covering the oval window and replacement with prosthetic devices frequently restores hearing.

otoscope An instrument for examining the ear.

  pneumatic o. An otoscope that uses alternate positive and negative pressure to observe the degree of flaccidity of the tympanic membrane.

otoscopy Examination of the tympanic membrane with an otoscope.

ototomy 1. Dissection of the ear. 2. Myringotomy.

ototoxic Having a deleterious effect upon the ear.

ototoxicity The capability of having a deleterious or harmful effect upon the ear, especially its neural parts.

ouabain A rapidly acting cardiac glycoside from the seeds of *Stronphanthus gratus*; a constituent of African arrow poison.

ounce 1. An avoirdupois unit of weight equal to 437.5 grains or 16 drams; 1/16th of a pound. 2. An apothecary unit of weight (used in the United States Pharmacopeia) equal to 480 grains or 1.097 avoirdupois ounces.

  fluid o. Either of two units of liquid capacity: 1. In the U.S. Customary System, the equivalent of 1.804 cubic inches or 1/16th of a pint. 2. In the British Imperial System (used in liquid or dry measure), the equivalent of 1.734 cubic inches or 1/20th of a pint.

outlay A graft on the surface of a bone.

outlet 1. A passage or exit. 2. A means of releasing feelings and energies.

  pelvic o. The lower aperture of the pelvis, bounded by the pubic arch, the ischial tuberosities, the sacrotuberous ligaments, and the tip of the coccyx.

outpatient A patient treated in a hospital or clinic without being hospitalized.

output 1. The quantity of a substance produced by or eliminated from the body during a given span of time. 2. The measure of performance by an organ or a system.

  cardiac o. The quantity of blood pumped by the heart per unit of time, usually per minute; the product of stroke volume and cardiac rate.

  minute o. The quantity of blood pumped by the heart during one minute, normally four to five liters at rest in an average sized individual.

  stroke o. The quantity of blood ejected with a single heart beat.

  urinary o. The quantity of urine excreted by the kidneys.

outtoed Foot position in which the toes are turned outward to a marked degree.

ova Plural of ovum.

ovalbumin Albumin from egg whites.

ovalocytosis Inherited disorder in which 25 to 90% of red blood cells have an oval shape. Also called elliptocytosis.

ovaralgia, ovarialgia Pain in an ovary.

ovarian Of or relating to the ovary.

ovariectomy Surgical removal of an ovary.

ovariocentesis Puncture of an ovarian cyst.

ovariocyesis Ovarian pregnancy.

ovariohysterectomy Surgical removal of the ovaries and uterus.

ovariopathy Disease of the ovary.

ovariorrhexis Rupture of an ovary.

ovariosalpingectomy Surgical removal of an ovary and the corresponding uterine tube.

ovariosalpingitis Inflammation of one or both ovaries and uterine tubes.

ovariotomy An incision into an ovary.

ovarium Latin for ovary.

ovary One of the paired sexual glands in which the ova are formed; it produces the hormones progesterone and estrogen.

  polycystic o. A diseased ovary associated with infertility; it contains multiple cysts, is usually enlarged, and is covered with a thick, pearly white capsule; seen in conditions such as Stein-Leventhal syndrome, abnormal bleeding, and virilism. Commonly called large white ovary.

  third o. An accessory ovary.

overbite Vertical overlap; see under overlap.

overclosure A condition in which the mandible rises too far before the teeth make contact, due to modification of tooth shape (through grinding), drifting of teeth, or loss of teeth, resulting in a shortened face length. Also called reduced interarch distance.

overcompensation A type of behavior in which an overwhelming feeling of inadequacy inspires exaggerated correction, e.g., overaggressiveness and the striving for power at all costs.

overdetermination In psychiatry, the multiple causation of a single event, behavior, or emotional symptom.

overdose 1. An excessive dose; too great a dose. 2. To give, prescribe, or take an excessive dose.

  barbiturate o. An overdose of barbiturates causing severe poisoning; a common mode of suicide.

  narcotic o. An excessive dose of a narcotic drug producing the clinical triad of stupor (or coma), respiratory depression, and pinpoint pupils (miosis); treatment generally consists of ventilatory and circulatory care and administration of narcotic antagonists.

overhang An excess of dental filling material beyond the normal tooth contour. Also called gingival margin excess.

overhydration Excess of fluids in the body; may result from the intravenous administration of unduly large amounts of glucose solution. Also called water intoxication; hyperhydration.

overjet, overjut Horizontal overlap; see under overlap.

overlap To extend over; e.g., the suturing of a layer of tissue over another to insure added strength.

  horizontal o. Excessive projection of the upper anterior and/or posterior teeth beyond their antag-

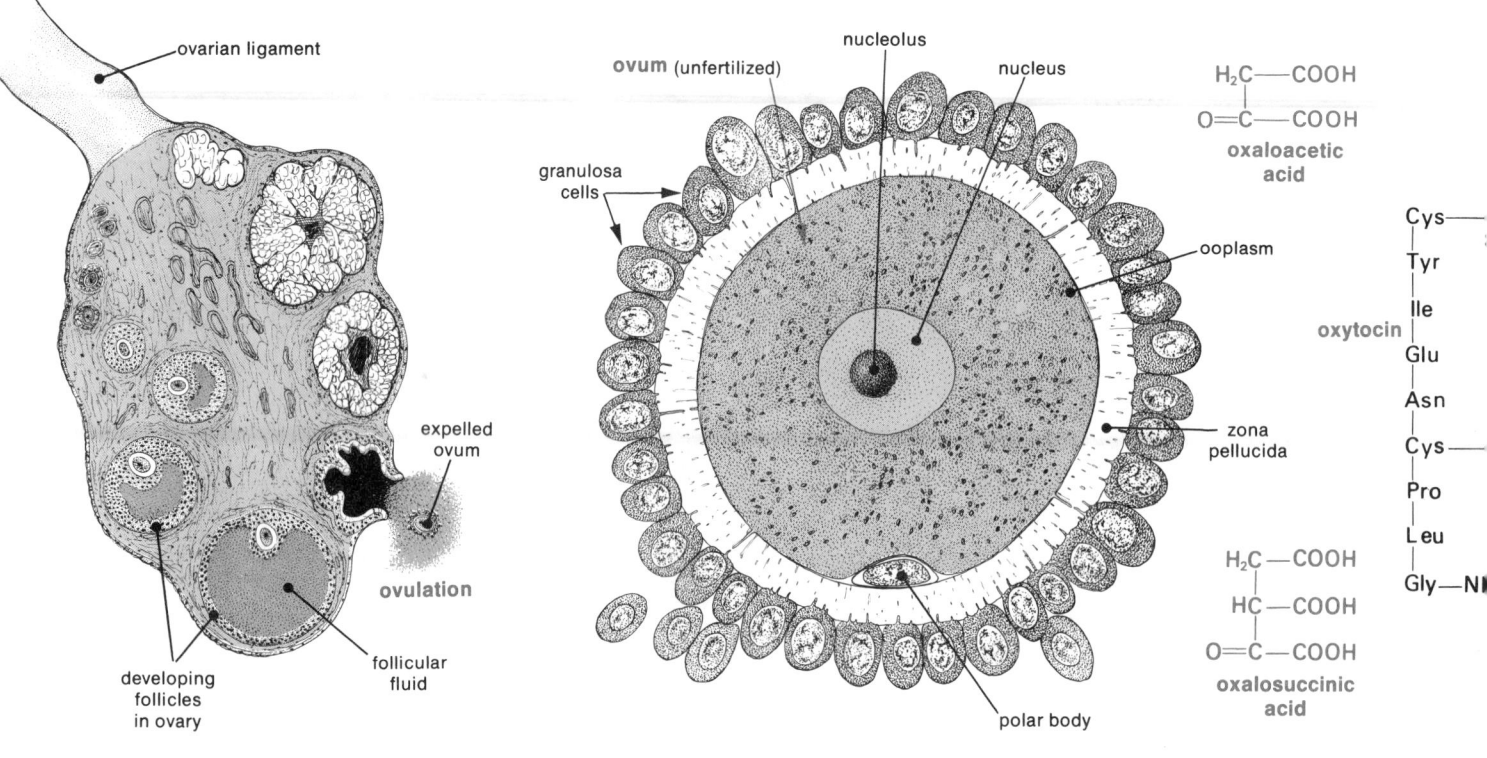

ovarian ligament

ovum (unfertilized)

nucleolus

nucleus

granulosa cells

ooplasm

zona pellucida

expelled ovum

ovulation

developing follicles in ovary

follicular fluid

polar body

$$H_2C—COOH$$
$$O=C—COOH$$
oxaloacetic acid

$$H_2C—COOH$$
$$HC—COOH$$
$$O=C—COOH$$
oxalosuccinic acid

Cys—
Tyr
Ile
oxytocin
Glu
Asn
Cys—
Pro
Leu
Gly—N

---

onists of the lower jaw in a horizontal direction. Also called overjet; overjut; buck teeth.

vertical o. The overlapping of the lower incisors by the upper incisors when the posterior teeth are in normal contact. Also called overbite.

overlay Any condition that is superimposed on an existing one.

emotional o. An emotional disturbance resulting from, or added to, an organic disease.

overnutrition Overeating; excessive caloric intake.

overriding The slipping of one fragment of a broken bone alongside the other.

over the counter (OTC) Denoting a medication not requiring a prescription for purchase.

overventilation See hyperventilation.

ovicidal Causing destruction of the ovum.

oviduct Uterine tube; see under tube.

oviferous Containing or conveying eggs.

ovigenesis See oogenesis.

ovine Relating to sheep.

oviparous Egg-laying; producing eggs that hatch outside the body of the maternal organism. Cf. ovoviviparous; viviparous.

oviposit To lay eggs, especially with the aid of an ovipositor; characteristic of insects.

oviposition The act of laying or depositing eggs; said especially of insects.

ovipositor A specialized tubular structure at the end of the abdomen of many female insects for boring holes to house their eggs.

ovoid Egg-shaped.

ovomucoid Mucoprotein of egg white.

ovotestis A gonad in which both testicular and ovarian tissues are present; a form of hermaphroditism.

ovoviviparous Bearing young that develop from eggs retained within the maternal body, as certain fish, reptiles, and insects.

ovulation The discharge of an ovum from the mature (graafian) follicle of the ovary.

ovule 1. The ovum in the ovarian follicle. 2. Any small egglike structure.

ovulocyclic Denoting any periodic occurrence that is associated with and takes place within the ovulatory cycle; e.g., ovulocyclic porphyria.

ovum, *pl.* ova An egg; the female sexual cell which, when fertilized by union with the male element, develops into a new individual.

oxacillin sodium Preparation used in the treatment of penicillin-resistant staphylococcal infections; Prostaphlin®.

oxalate A salt of oxalic acid.

oxalic acid A compound produced by oxidation of glyoxylate; present in excessive amounts in per-

sons afflicted with primary hyperoxaluria.

oxaloacetic acid An intermediate in the tricarboxylic acid cycle. Also called ketosuccinic acid.

oxalosis Accumulation of calcium oxalate crystals in the kidneys, bones, arteries, and myocardium; a feature of primary hyperoxaluria, usually leading to death by renal failure.

oxalosuccinic acid An intermediate in the tricarboxylic acid cycle.

oxaluria The presence of abnormally large quantities of calcium oxalate in the urine.

oxazepam A benzodiazepine tranquilizer; Serax®.

oxidase One of a group of oxidizing enzymes that promote either the addition of oxygen to a metabolite or the removal of hydrogen or of electrons.

oxidation 1. A chemical reaction in which electrons from one reactant (the reducing agent) are transferred to the other reactant (the oxidizing agent); the atoms in the element losing electrons increase their valence correspondingly. Cf. reduction. 2. The combination of a substance with oxygen.

oxidation-reduction Any chemical reaction in which electrons are transferred from one atom or molecule to another. Also called redox.

oxide A binary compound of oxygen with another element or radical; e.g., mercuric oxide.

acid o. An oxygen compound of nonmetals; e.g., SO_2.

basic o. An oxygen compound of metals; e.g., Al_2O_3.

oxidize To combine or to cause combination with oxygen.

oxidoreductase An enzyme that promotes an oxidation-reduction reaction.

oxime A condensation product of the action of hydroxylamine on a ketone or an aldehyde.

oximeter Instrument used to measure photoelectrically the degree of oxygen saturation in the circulating blood.

oxyacid An acid containing oxygen. Also called oxacid.

oxycellulose Cellulose in which all or most of the glucose residues have been converted to glucuronic acid residues.

oxycephaly Peaked, conical skull.

oxychromatic Staining brightly with eosin and other acid dyes.

oxychromatin Chromatin that stains with acid dyes. Also called oxyphil chromatin.

oxygen An odorless and colorless gas, symbol O, atomic number 8, atomic weight 16; it constitutes about one-fifth of the earth's atmosphere and is essential to animal and plant life.

oxygenase One of several enzymes catalyzing the activation of molecular oxygen and the subsequent incorporation of both atoms of the oxygen molecule into the substrate.

oxygenate To saturate or infuse with oxygen.

oxygenation The combination of hemoglobin with oxygen; provision of oxygen to a tissue or individual.

oxygenator Device for the mechanical oxygenation of venous blood.

oxygenize Oxidize.

oxyhemoglobin (HbO_2) The bright red hemoglobin combined with oxygen, present in arterial blood. Also called oxygenated hemoglobin.

oxylalia Abnormally rapid speech.

oxyphil, oxyphile Eosinophilic leukocyte; see under leukocyte.

oxyphonia Abnormal shrillness of voice.

oxypurine An oxygen-containing purine; e.g., uric acid and xanthine.

17-oxysteroid 17-Ketosteroid.

oxytetracycline Antibiotic produced by *Streptomyces rimosus*; Terramycin®.

oxytocia Rapid childbirth.

oxytocic 1. Relating to rapid childbirth. 2. An agent that hastens the process of childbirth, especially by stimulating contraction of the uterine muscle.

oxytocin A hormone formed in the base of the brain (hypothalamus) and stored in the posterior lobe of the hypophysis (pituitary gland); it stimulates smooth muscle, causing strong contractions of the uterus and ejection of milk from the breast (distinguished from prolactin, which stimulates milk production).

oxyuriasis Infestation with pinworms.

oxyuricide 1. An agent which kills pinworms. 2. Destructive to pinworms.

oxyurid Pinworm.

Oxyuris vermicularis Former name for *Enterobius vermicularis*.

ozena A fetid discharge from the nose in patients with certain forms of chronic rhinitis.

ozone (O_3) A blue, poisonous, gaseous triatomic form of oxygen formed naturally from an electric discharge through oxygen or by exposure of oxygen to ultraviolet radiation; made commercially by passing oxygen over 10,000 volt charged aluminum plates; used chiefly as an antiseptic, disinfectant, and bleaching agent.

ozonometer An apparatus that estimates the amount of ozone in the atmosphere by the use of a series of test papers.

ozostomia Bad breath.

artificial cardiac pacemaker

cephalic vein

axillary vein

catheter electrode at apex of right ventricle of heart

metatarsal pads

synovial membrane

femur

patella

infrapatellar fat-pad

tibia

medial aspect of knee joint

Pp

pablum A precooked food, usually for infants, made from wheat, oat, and corn meals, wheat embryo, alfalfa leaves, brewers' yeast, iron, and salt.

pabulum Any nourishing substance.

pacchionian granulations See granulation, arachnoid.

pacemaker 1. Any bodily structure that serves to establish and maintain a rhythmic pace, as the sinoatrial node of the heart that regulates the heartbeat. 2. A substance whose rate of reaction regulates a series of chain or related reactions.

artificial cardiac p. Any of several usually miniaturized and surgically implanted electronic devices that substitute for the normal cardiac pacemaker and regulate the heartbeat; used in treating individuals with chronic heart block who have (a) episodes of syncope or convulsions owing to ventricular bradycardia, (b) cardiac failure secondary to the bradycardia, and (c) unstable ventricular rhythms associated with the heart block.

brain p. A pacemaker implanted on the surface of the cerebellum that is primarily used to bring intractable epilepsy under control. Also called cerebellar electrical stimulator.

demand p. A pacemaker in which the stimulus is only fired when the ventricular contraction does not occur within a specified period of time; a signal from the heart's previous ventricular depolarization inhibits the pulse generator from firing for an additional second.

ectopic p. Any cardiac pacemaker other than the sinus node.

external p. Artificial pacemaker with electrodes placed externally on the chest wall.

fixed-rate p. An artificial pacemaker that discharges electrical stimuli at a uniform and uninterrupted rate.

shifting p. See wandering pacemaker.

wandering p. Phenomenon in which the point of origin of the heart beat shifts back and forth from one center to another, usually between the sinus and AV nodes. Also called shifting pacemaker.

pachyblepharon Thickening of the border of an eyelid.

pachycephaly, pachycephalia An abnormal thickening of the skull.

pachycholia Abnormal viscousness of the bile.

pachychromatic Having a thick chromatin network.

pachydactyly Abnormal enlargement of the fingers or toes.

pachyderma Abnormally thick skin.

p. laryngis A form of chronic laryngitis, marked by the formation of warty thickening of the epithelium, usually on the vocal cords; it is caused by chronic irritation.

pachydermatocele 1. Congenital looseness of the skin, which hangs in folds. Also called cutis laxa. 2. A large neurofibroma.

pachydermatosis Pachyderma of long duration.

pachydermatous Characterized by pachyderma.

pachydermoperiostosis Inherited condition marked by osteoarthropathy, coarseness of facial features with thickening and oiliness of the skin, excessive sebaceous gland secretion, and enlargement of hands with clubbing of fingers.

pachygyria Abnormally thick convolutions of the cerebral cortex.

pachyleptomeningitis Inflammation of the membranes of the brain and spinal cord.

pachylosis A dry, thickened, scaly state of the skin, especially on the lower extremities.

pachymeningitis Inflammation and thickening of the dura mater.

pachymeningopathy Any disease of the dura mater.

pachymeter Instrument used to measure the thickness of membranes or thin plates.

pachyonychia Excessive thickness of the fingernails or toenails.

p. congenita A congenital deformity characterized by abnormalities of the skin (bullae and papular hyperkeratoses) and mucous membranes (leukokeratoses) and excessively thick nails.

pachyperiostitis Proliferative thickening of the membrane enveloping bones due to inflammation.

pachyperitonitis Inflammation and thickening of the peritoneum.

pachypleuritis Inflammation of the pleura accompanied by thickening of the membrane. Also called productive pleurisy.

pachysalpingitis Chronic interstitial inflammation of the muscular layer of the uterine tube, producing thickening. Also called chronic parenchymatous salpingitis.

pachysomia Abnormal thickening of the soft parts of the body, as in acromegaly.

pachytene The stage of prophase in meiosis in which each paired chromosome separates into its two component sister chromatids, so that each set of homologous chromosome pair becomes a set of four intertwined chromatids called a bivalent.

pack 1. To fill or stuff. 2. To wrap a patient in hot, cold, wet, or dry blankets or sheets. 3. The blankets or sheets so used. 4. In dentistry, the application of a dressing to a surgical site. 5. The dressing so used.

packer Instrument for inserting an absorbent dressing or tampon into a bodily cavity, such as the vagina.

packing The material used to fill a cavity or a wound, such as gauze, sponge, etc.

pad A cushion of soft material.

abdominal p. A large pad used for absorbing discharges from surgical abdominal wounds.

buccal fat-p. An encapsulated mass of fat on the outer side of the cheek situated superficial to the buccinator muscle and pierced by the parotid duct; in infants it is prominent and is called sucking or suctorial pad because it is thought to help prevent the cheeks from being sucked inward while nursing.

fat p. A circumscribed cushion-like mass of fat.

infrapatellar fat-p. A large pad of fat which separates the patellar ligament and part of the patella (kneecap) from the synovial membrane of the knee joint.

ischiorectal fat-p. A pad of fat in the anal region extending upward on both sides of the anus; it contains many fibrous septa that support the anal canal.

metatarsal p. One of various shaped pads worn inside the shoe under the metatarsal bones to shield painful weight-bearing areas from pressure.

Passavant's pad Passavant's ridge; see under ridge.

retropubic fat-p. A large quantity of fat in the U-shaped retropubic space located between the pubic symphysis and the bladder and extending backward on each side of the bladder; it is limited above by the peritoneum.

Paget's disease A bone disease of unknown cause; characterized by localized areas of bone destruction followed by replacement with overdeveloped, light, soft, porous bone and associated with deformities, such as thickening of portions of the skull and bending of weight-bearing bones; Beethoven is believed to have been afflicted with this disease. Also called osteitis deformans.

pagophagia The ingestion of abnormally large quantities of ice.

pain A physical or mental sensation of distress or suffering.

bearing-down p. One accompanying the contractions of the uterus during the second stage of labor.

false p.'s Those resembling true labor pains.

girdle p. A painful sensation encircling the waist like a tight belt, occurring in some diseases of the spinal cord.

growing p.'s Pains in the limbs of children, usually felt at night and resembling rheumatism; attributed to growth, faulty posture, or fatigue.

intermenstrual p. Mild pelvic pain occurring midway between two menstruations, associated with ejection of the ovum from the ovary. Also called

cleft palate (partial) — roof of mouth, nasal cavity

cleft palate (complete) — roof of mouth, cleft of alveolar ridge, nasal cavity, uvula

palate — nasal cavity, uvula, pharynx, oral cavity, tongue, mandible, trachea, esophagus

cerebral palsy (spastic form) — typical positional deformities of the upper and lower extremities

mittelschmerz.

labor p.'s Rhythmic pains of increasing severity, frequency, and duration, caused by contraction of the uterus during childbirth.

phantom limb p. The sensation of pain felt in a limb, although that limb has been amputated.

referred p. Pain felt in an area other than the site of origin, such as the pain near the shoulder associated with biliary disease.

sympathetically maintained p. (SMP) Pain that begins with an injury, grows in severity out of proportion to the injury, and recurs intermittently for months or even years after the injury heals.

pair Two similar, identical, or associated things.

base p. Either of the two pairs of nucleic acid bases (one a purine and the other a pyrimidine), joined by hydrogen bonds, that make up the DNA molecule. Also called nucleotide or nucleoside pair.

pairing Attachment of two homologous chromosomes in a sideward direction, prior to their exchanging of genetic material (crossing over) during meiosis.

palatal Relating to the palate.

palate It consists of a bony anterior part (hard palate) and a soft muscular posterior portion (soft palate). Also called roof of the mouth.

cleft p. Congenitally malformed palate, with a fissure along the midline; may be restricted to the soft and hard palate or extend forward through the dental arch, on either or both sides of the midline; often associated with a cleft lip.

primary p. The embryonic shelf separating the oral and nasal cavities of the early embryo. Also called primitive palate.

secondary p. The embryonic palate that eventually forms the hard palate by fusion of the lateral palatine processes.

palatiform Resembling the palate or roof of the mouth.

palatine Relating to the palate or roof of the mouth.

palatoglossal Relating to the palate and the tongue.

palatograph Instrument for recording the movements of the soft palate during speech and respiration. Also called palate myograph; palatomyograph.

palatopharyngeal Relating to the palate and the pharynx.

palatopharyngoplasty Operative procedure to correct a shortened soft palate (sometimes necessary in plastic repair of a cleft palate).

palatoplasty Reparative surgery of the palate, especially a cleft palate.

palatoplegia Paralysis of the muscles of the soft palate.

palatoschisis Cleft palate.

paleencephalon The phylogenetically older part of the brain that includes all of it except the cerebral cortex and closely related parts.

paleobiology The study of evolution of life from a non-oxygen dominated environment.

paleocerebellum The earlier developed parts of the cerebellum, i.e., vermis and flocculus.

paleocortex The earlier developed parts of the cerebral cortex, i.e., the olfactory cortex.

paleokinetic Denoting the primitive nervous motor mechanism concerned with automatic movements.

paleopathology The study of disease of ancient man as revealed in mummies, bones, and art forms such as paintings, statues, etc.

paleostriatum See globus pallidus.

palilalia See paliphrasia.

palindrome In molecular biology, a length of DNA in which identical (or almost identical) base sequences in the two strands of the double helix run in opposite directions so that the compound reads the same forward or backward (e.g., ACB-BCA).

palindromia Recurrence of a pathologic condition.

palindromic Recurring.

palingenesis The reappearance of ancestral structural features.

paliphrasia The involuntary repetition of phrases in speaking; may be caused by encephalitis. Also called palilalia.

palladium Metallic element resembling platinum; symbol Pd, atomic number 46, atomic weight 106.4.

pallesthesia The perception of vibration, especially through bones. Also called vibratory sensibility.

palliate To mitigate.

palliative 1. Alleviating. 2. A medicine or treatment that affords temporary relief but does not effect a cure.

pallidectomy Surgical removal or destruction of the globus pallidus.

pallidotomy Cutting of nerve fibers from the globus pallidus in the brain for the relief of pathologic involuntary movements.

pallium The cerebral cortex and subadjacent white substance.

pallor Paleness; lack of color.

palm The anterior or inner surface of the hand.

palmar Relating to the palm of the hand.

palmitic acid A saturated fatty acid found in various fats and oils. Also called hexadecanoic acid.

palpable Perceptible by palpation; tangible.

palpate To examine by touching or pressing with the fingers or the palms of the hands.

palpation Examination by touch or pressure of the hand, over an organ or area of the body, as a diagnostic aid.

palpebra, *pl.* **palpebrae** Latin for eyelid.

palpebral Of or relating to the eyelids.

palpitation Rapid or forceful heartbeat, of which the patient is conscious.

palsy Paralysis.

ataxic cerebral p. Cerebral palsy characterized by inability to coordinate voluntary muscular movements.

Bell's p. See facial palsy.

cerebral p. Condition marked by disturbances of voluntary motor function caused by damage to the brain's motor control centers; it is characterized primarily by spastic paralysis or impairment of control or coordination over voluntary muscles and is often accompanied by mental retardation, seizures, and disorders of vision and communication; it may be either congenital or acquired.

dyskinetic cerebral p. Cerebral palsy characterized by uncontrolled and purposeless movements which disappear during sleep.

facial p. Paralysis of the facial muscles on one side, caused by a usually self-limited lesion of the facial (VII) nerve. Also called Bell's palsy.

shaking p. See paralysis agitans.

spastic cerebral p. Cerebral palsy characterized by increased muscle tension and exaggerated reflex activity in an arm and a leg of the same side (hemiplegia) or arms and legs on both sides (tetraplegia or quadriplegia).

trembling p. Paralysis agitans.

paludism Malaria.

panacea A remedy which is supposed to cure all diseases; a cure-all.

panagglutinin An agglutinin that reacts with all human erythrocytes.

panangiitis Inflammation of all layers of a blood vessel.

panarthritis 1. Inflammation of an entire joint. 2. Inflammation of all the body joints.

panatrophy A generalized wasting away of the body.

pancarditis Inflammation of all layers of the heart; i.e., myocarditis, endocarditis, and pericarditis.

Pancoast's syndrome Carcinoma of the apex of the lung or upper mediastinum (Pancoast's tumor) invading the brachial plexus and the cervical sympathetic chain and resulting in pain, weakness, and atrophy of the arm and hand muscles. Also called superior pulmonary sulcus, Ciuffini-Pancoast, or Horner's syndrome.

pancolectomy The removal of the entire colon.

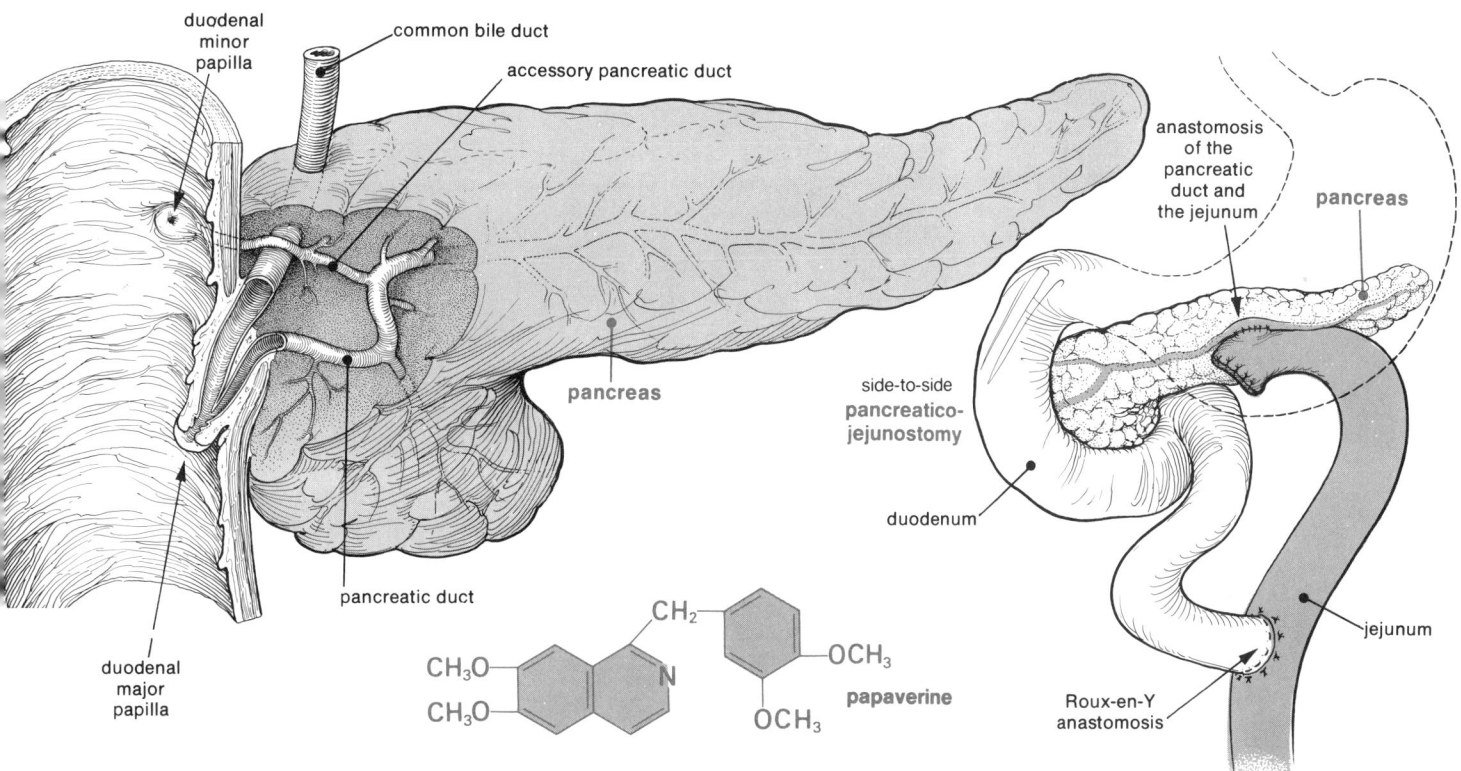

duodenal minor papilla
common bile duct
accessory pancreatic duct
pancreas
duodenal major papilla
pancreatic duct
papaverine

anastomosis of the pancreatic duct and the jejunum
pancreas
side-to-side **pancreatico-jejunostomy**
duodenum
Roux-en-Y anastomosis
jejunum

pancreas A soft gland, 10 to 15 cm long, lying behind the stomach and extending transversely from the concavity of the duodenum to the spleen; it secretes enzymes (amylase, lipase), which aid in digestion of food, into the small intestine; it also produces hormones (glucagon, insulin) which, when taken up by the bloodstream, help regulate carbohydrate metabolism by controlling blood sugar levels.

pancreatectomy Surgical removal of the pancreas.

pancreathelcosis The presence of abscesses of the pancreas.

pancreaticoduodenostomy Surgical joining of the pancreatic duct into the duodenum.

pancreaticogastrostomy The surgical anastomosis of the pancreatic duct to the stomach.

pancreaticojejunostomy Surgical inplantation of the pancreatic duct into the jejunum.

pancreatin A mixture of pancreatic enzymes extracted from hogs or cattle; used as a digestive aid.

pancreatitis Inflammation of the pancreas.

pancreatoduodenectomy Surgical removal of the pancreas and the adjacent portion of the duodenum.

pancreatogenous Originating in the pancreas.

pancreatography The making of x-ray films of the pancreas.

pancreatolith A pancreatic stone. Also called pancreolith.

pancreatolithectomy Surgical removal of pancreatic stones.

pancreatolithiasis Stones in the pancreas.

pancreatolithotomy Incision of the pancreas for the removal of a stone. Also called pancreolithotomy.

pancreatomy See pancreatotomy.

pancreatotomy Incision of the pancreas. Also called pancreatomy.

pancreatropic Exerting an effect on the pancreas.

pancreolith See pancreatolith.

pancreolithotomy See pancreatolithotomy.

pancreozymin A hormone, secreted by the mucosa of the small intestine, that stimulates the secretion of pancreatic enzymes.

pancytopenia Reduction of all the cell components of the blood (red blood cells, white blood cells, and blood platelets).

pandemic Denoting an epidemic that affects the population of a wide geographic area.

panendoscope A cystoscope which offers a wide view of the interior of the urinary bladder.

panendoscopy 1. Endoscopic examination of more than one structure, e.g., of the esophagus, stomach, and duodenum. 2. Visual examination of the interior of the bladder using a panendoscope.

panesthesia The sum of all sensations experienced at one time.

panhypopituitarism Condition characterized by absence of all the recognized anterior pituitary hormones. Also called Simmond's disease.

panhysterectomy Surgical removal of the entire uterus, including the cervix.

panhysterosalpingectomy The removal of the entire uterus and uterine tubes (the ovaries are left intact).

panhysterosalpingo-oophorectomy Removal of the entire uterus, uterine tubes, and ovaries.

panic A sudden, overpowering anxiety and fear.

panmixis Random mating; see under mating.

panniculitis Inflammation of the subcutaneous layer of connective tissue and fat (superficial fascia) of the abdominal wall.

  relapsing febrile nodular nonsuppurative p. See Weber-Christian disease.

panniculus A layer of membranous tissue.

  p. adiposus The subcutaneous layer of connective tissue and fat (superficial fascia).

pannus 1. Superficial infiltration of the cornea with blood vessels; may progress to include a membrane-like granulation tissue; may occur in several degrees of denseness and cover part of or all the cornea; a common complication of trachoma. 2. An inflammatory secretion covering the articular surfaces of affected joints in rheumatoid arthritis and related disorders.

panophthalmia, panophthalmitis Generalized infection and inflammation of the eyeball.

Panorex In dentistry, a radiography machine that rotates the film holder and x-ray tube around the patient's head and shifts the patient to change the axis of rotation of the tube-film assembly relative to his head.

panosteitis, panostitis Inflammation of a bone in its entirety.

panotitis General inflammation of the ear.

pansystolic Occurring throughout systole, from first to second heart sound.

pantothenic acid $HOCH_2-C(CH_3)_2-CHOH-CO-NH-CH_2-CH_2-COOH$; a colorless liquid component of the vitamin B complex, widely distributed in plant and animal tissues, especially the liver; part of coenzyme A.

pap Any soft or semiliquid food, as bread soaked in milk.

papain A proteolytic enzyme obtained from the unripe fruit of the papaya; used as a meat tenderizer and also in medicine as a protein digestant.

papaverine A non-narcotic alkaloid of opium which has vasodilator properties.

paper A thin sheet substance made of the cellulose pulp of wood or other fibrous material; used for writing, filtering, medicating, and testing.

  biuret p. A strip of filter paper dipped in biuret reagent and allowed to dry.

  filter p. Porous unsized paper suitable for filtering solutions.

  litmus p. White blotting paper impregnated with litmus; used as an acid-base indicator; it turns red in a slightly acidic solution and blue in an alkaline one.

paper point In dentistry, a cone of absorbent paper than can be inserted into the entire length of a root canal of a tooth; used to medicate the canal or to absorb fluid.

papilla A small, nipple-like protrusion.

papillary Relating to or resembling a papilla or nipple.

papillectomy Surgical removal of any papilla.

papilledema Swelling of the optic nerve head caused by increased intracranial pressure.

papilliferous Containing papillae.

papilliform Resembling a papilla.

papillitis Inflammation of the optic nerve head. Also called neuropapillitis; intraocular optic neuritis.

  necrotizing p. Renal papillary necrosis; see under necrosis.

papilloadenocystoma A lobulated benign tumor derived from epithelium, characterized by glands or glandlike structures, formation of cysts, and finger-like projections of neoplastic cells enveloping a core of fibrous connective tissue.

papillocarcinoma 1. A malignant tumor originating from a papilloma. 2. A malignant tumor with papillary projections.

papilloma An overgrowth of the papillae of the skin or mucous membrane. Also called papillary tumor; villoma.

  hard p. One derived from squamous epithelium, such as corns or warts.

  villous p. One composed of numerous slender outgrowths, usually found in the bladder, within the mammary gland, or arising from the choroid plexus in the lateral ventricle of the brain.

papillomatosis The development of several papillomas.

papillomatous Resembling a papilloma.

Papillomavirus Genus of viruses (family Papovaviridae), which includes those causing papillomas and warts in humans and animals.

papilloretinitis Inflammation of the optic disk and neighboring parts of the retina. Also called retinopapillitis.

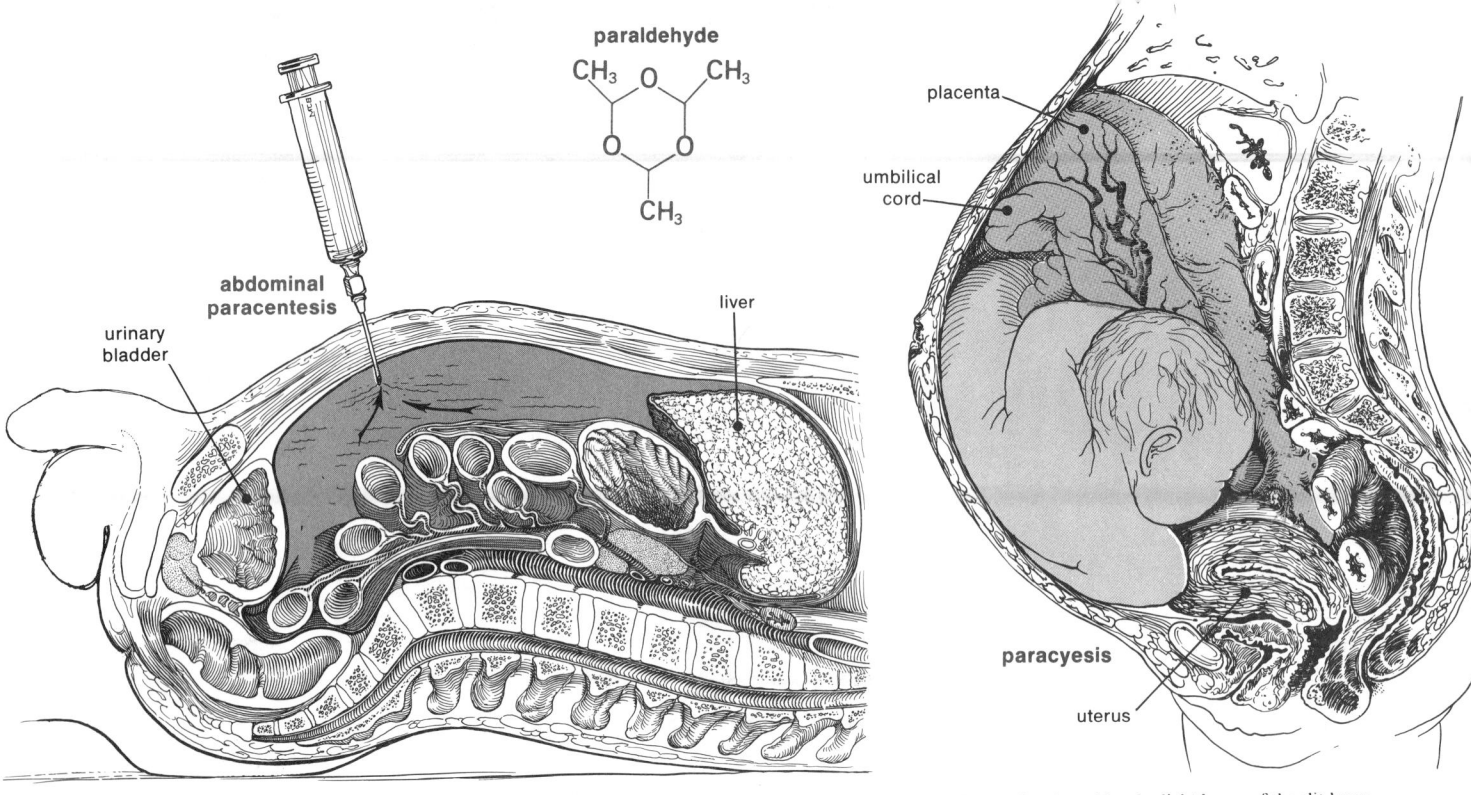

paraldehyde

$$CH_3 \quad O \quad CH_3$$

$$O \quad O$$

$$CH_3$$

abdominal paracentesis

urinary bladder

liver

placenta

umbilical cord

paracyesis

uterus

Papovaviridae Family of viruses (45 to 55 nm in diameter) which contain double-stranded DNA and replicate in nuclei of vertebrate cells; may be transmitted through contact or (mechanically) by arthropods; includes viruses causing warts and papillomas. Also called papovavirus group.

Pap smear See test, Pap.

papula Papule.

papular Relating to papules.

papulation The formation of papules.

papule A superficial solid elevation on the skin, ranging in size up to .1 cm.

papulopustular Denoting an eruption composed of papules (small elevations on the skin) and pustules (elevations on the skin containing pus).

papulosis The occurrence of numerous papules, usually widespread.

papulosquamous Denoting a skin eruption composed of small elevations (papules) and loose scaly lesions.

papulovesicular Having both papules and vesicles.

para Denoting past pregnancies that have reached the period of viability, regardless of whether the child is dead or alive at the time of delivery; the term refers to pregnancies, not fetuses; thus, a woman who gives birth to twins at the end of her first pregnancy is still para I.

parabiosis 1. Union of two organisms, either natural (e.g., conjoined twins) or artificially produced. 2. Temporary loss of conductivity of a nerve.

parablepsia, parablepsis False vision, as in visual illusion or hallucination.

paracasein Compound produced when the enzyme rennin acts upon casein (the protein of milk); it reacts with calcium, resulting in the curdling of milk.

paracentesis The surgical puncture of a cavity for the purpose of removing fluid.

   abdominal p. Paracentesis of the abdomen.

   tympanic p. Incision of the tympanic membrane (eardrum) in order to drain the middle ear chamber. Also called myringotomy.

paracentral Located near a central structure.

parachordal In embryology, located near and anterior to the notochord.

parachromatopsia See dichromatism.

paracoccidioidomycosis A chronic systemic fungal disease caused by a yeastlike fungus (*Paracoccidioides brasiliensis*), characteristically causing gastrointestinal symptoms, painful ulcers of the mouth and nose, and inflammation and suppuration of the lymph nodes of the neck; the infection disseminates to the skin and other organs. Also called South American blastomycosis.

paracolpium Tissues near the vagina.

paracusis 1. Impaired hearing. 2. Auditory hallucination.

paracyesis Extrauterine pregnancy.

paracystic Near the bladder.

paradental Periodontal.

paradidymis A small body made up of a few convoluted tubules attached to the lower part of the spermatic cord above the head of the epididymis; considered to be a remnant of the mesonephros (wolffian body). Also called parepididymis; organ of Giraldès.

paradipsia Abnormal craving for fluids.

paraffin 1. A waxy, somewhat transparent purified mixture of solid hydrocarbons derived from petroleum. Also called paraffin wax. 2. One of the methane or alkane series of saturated aliphatic hydrocarbons having the general formula C_nH_{2n+2}.

paraformaldehyde A water-soluble, white, crystalline polymer of formaldehyde; used in treating various skin disorders.

paraganglia, *sing.* **paraganglion** Collection of chromaffin cells forming globular or ovoid bodies present about the ganglia of the sympathetic chain. Also called chromaffin bodies.

paraganglioma A tumor composed of chromaffin tissue in a paraganglion or the medulla of the adrenal gland. Also called chromaffinoma.

paragene Any extrachromosomal replicating unit or hereditary determinant. Also called plasmid.

parageusia Any abnormality in the sense of taste.

paragglutination Group agglutination; see under agglutination.

paraglobulin A globulin present in blood plasma and lymph.

paragonimiasis Infection with a worm of the genus *Paragonimus*, especially the lung fluke species *Paragonimus westermani*.

Paragonimus A genus of trematode worms that includes the lung worms of man and animals.

parahepatic Located near the liver.

parakeratosis The retention of nuclei in the cells of the stratum corneum of the epithelium, as seen in psoriasis.

parakinesia, parakinesis Any abnormality of motor function.

paralalia Speech defect in which one letter is substituted for another.

paralbumin Albuminous substance usually present in ovarian cysts and ascites.

paraldehyde A polymer of acetaldehyde, $(CH_3CHO)_3$; colorless liquid of pungent odor, used as a hypnotic and sedative.

paralgesia Any abnormal painful sensation.

parallax The apparent displacement of an object caused by a change in the observation position.

parallelepiped, corneal The section of cornea illuminated by the light beam of the slit lamp.

paralysis 1. Loss of voluntary muscular function. 2. Loss of sensation. 3. Loss of any organic function.

   acute ascending p. Paralysis, often fatal, beginning in the lower extremities and ascending rapidly to involve the trunk, arms, and neck. Sometimes called Landry's paralysis.

   ascending p. Paralysis progressing from the periphery to the nerve centers or from the lower limbs upward.

   Brown-Séquard's p. See Brown-Séquard's syndrome.

   congenital oculofacial p. See Möbius' syndrome.

   Duchenne's p. Childhood muscular dystrophy; see under dystrophy.

   Duchenne-Erb p. Paralysis affecting the deltoid, biceps, anterior brachial, and long supinator muscles.

   familial periodic p. Periodic paralysis.

   global p. Paralysis affecting both sides of the body completely.

   hyperkalemic p. Periodic paralysis associated with abnormally high serum potassium concentrations; attacks start in infancy, are frequent, and relatively mild, and last a few minutes to a few hours; autosomal dominant inheritance.

   hypokalemic p. Periodic paralysis in which serum potassium level drops sharply during attacks, which start in late childhood or adolescence, are relatively severe, and last for a day or more; autosomal dominant inheritance.

   infantile p. See poliomyelitis.

   jake p. A form induced by drinking Jamaica ginger (jake). Also called ginger paralysis.

   Landry's p. See acute ascending paralysis.

   p. agitans Parkinson's disease, a disorder characterized, in its fully developed form, by stiffness and slowness of voluntary movement, stooped posture, propulsive gait, rigidity of facial expression, and rhythmic tremor of the limbs; usually has an insidious onset in individuals between 50 and 65 years old; cause is unknown; changes in the melanin-containing nerve cells in the brain stem are regularly observed. Also called shaking palsy.

   periodic p. Recurrent abrupt episodes of paralysis or extreme muscular weakness lasting from a few minutes to a few days, occurring in otherwise healthy individuals.

   postictal p. See Todd's paralysis.

   progressive bulbar p. Progressive paralysis and atrophy of the muscles of the tongue, lips, palate, larynx, and pharynx, due to degeneration of the neurons that innervate them.

   pseudobulbar p. Paralysis of the tongue and lips,

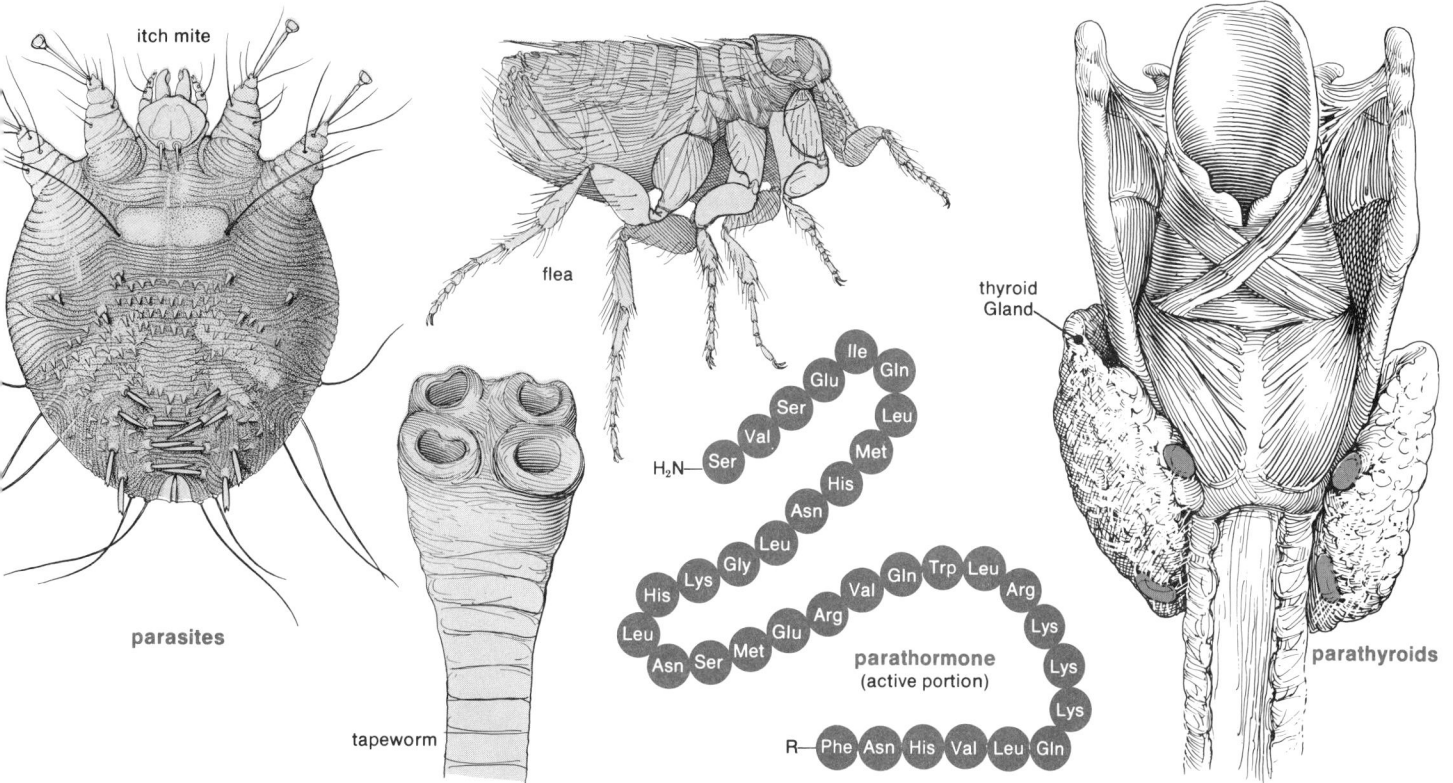

itch mite

flea

parasites

tapeworm

thyroid Gland

parathyroids

Ile
Glu
Gln
Ser
Leu
Val
Met
H₂N—Ser
His
Asn
Leu
Gly
Lys
His
Val
Gln
Trp
Leu
Arg
Leu
Met
Arg
Lys
Asn
Ser
Glu
parathormone
(active portion)
Lys
Lys
Lys
R—Phe
Asn
His
Val
Leu
Gln

resulting in difficulty in speech and swallowing, often accompanied by spasmodic laughter; caused by brain lesions in the upper motor neurons. Also called laughing sickness.

tick p. A rapidly progressive, usually symmetrical paralysis following a tick bite; symptoms include numbness of the extremities, throat, and face, progressing quickly to inability to stand, paralysis of the extremities and trunk, slurred speech, and impaired vision.

Todd's p. Temporary paralysis sometimes occurring after a grand mal epileptic convulsion and usually lasting from several minutes to hours after the seizure. Also called postictal paralysis.

vasomotor p. See vasoparalysis.

paralytic 1. Relating to paralysis. **2.** A person afflicted with paralysis.

paramecium Any of many ciliate protozoans of the genus *Paramecium*, usually slipper-shaped with an oral groove for feeding.

paramedian Near the midline.

paramedic A person trained to provide initial medical care in emergency situations.

paramedical Adjunctive to or relating indirectly to the practice of medicine.

paramenia Any disorder or irregularity of menstruation.

parameter In statistics, a characteristic of the population.

parametritis Inflammation of the connective tissue adjacent to the uterus and the veins and lymphatics contained in it. Also called pelvic cellulitis.

parametrium The connective tissue near the uterine cervix, extending upward along the sides of the uterus, between the two layers of the broad ligaments.

paramyloidosis Accumulation of the protein amyloid in lymph nodes; seen in some chronic nonspecific inflammations.

paramyotonia An atypical form of myotonia; abnormal muscular tonicity and spasms.

Paramyxoviridae Family of viruses that have a variety of shapes but are usually spherical (150 to 300 nm in diameter); contain single-stranded RNA, replicate in cytoplasm, produce cytoplasmic inclusion bodies, and cause cell fusion and hemadsorption; includes viruses causing measles, mumps, and Newcastle disease.

Paramyxovirus Genus of viruses (family Paramyxoviridae), which includes the mumps and Newcastle disease viruses. Also called paramyxovirus group.

paranasal Located near the nose.

paranoia A rare, slowly progressive mental disorder characterized by convincing and logical delu-

sions of persecution and grandeur without any other signs of personality deterioration; some features of true paranoia, such as feelings of persecution, may be found in other psychiatric illnesses.

paranoiac Relating to or suffering from paranoia.

paranoid Resembling paranoia; overly suspicious.

paranuclear Located near the nucleus.

paranucleus An accessory nucleus or a small chromatin body resembling a nucleus, sometimes seen in the cell protoplasm lying just outside of the nucleus.

paraparesis Slight or partial paralysis of both lower limbs.

paraperitoneal Near or alongside the peritoneum.

paraphasia A disturbance of speech marked by substitution of words and disorganized sentence formation; a mild form of aphasia.

literal p. Substitution of words that are similar in sound to the correct one.

verbal p. Substitution of words that are similar in meaning to the correct one.

paraphimosis Tightness of the prepuce or foreskin, which when retracted behind the glans penis cannot be returned to its normal position.

p. palpebrae A turning outward of the margin of an eyelid (usually the upper one) due to spastic contraction of the orbicularis oculi muscle; usually it is of short duration.

paraplegia Paralysis of both legs and lower part of the body.

paraproctitis Inflammation of the tissues surrounding the rectum and anus.

paraprotein An abnormal serum protein, such as a macroglobulin, cryoglobulin, and myeloma protein, characterized by a well defined peak on electrophoresis.

paraproteinemia A disorder marked by the presence of abnormal proteins in the blood as seen in multiple myeloma.

parapsychology The study of extrasensory phenomena.

paraquat A dipyridilium compound used as a herbicide to eradicate marijuana fields and, in farming, to clear fields instead of "plowing under." A small quantity ingested or absorbed through the skin may cause kidney and liver failure and pulmonary insufficiency.

parasalpingitis Inflammation of the tissues surrounding a uterine tube.

parasite Any organism which in its natural habitat feeds and lives on or in a different organism.

parasitic Of, relating to, or characteristic of a parasite.

parasiticide Any agent that destroys parasites.

parasitism 1. The mode of existence between a parasite and its host. **2.** An abnormal condition resulting from infestation with parasites.

parasitize To live as a parasite.

parasitology The scientific study of parasites and parasitism; a branch of microbiology.

parasitosis Infestation with parasites.

paraspadia, paraspadias The presence of a lateral opening into the male urethra.

parasympathetic Relating to the part of the autonomic nervous system concerned with conserving and restoring energy, as by slowing the heart rate.

parasympatholytic Denoting an agent that neutralizes the actions of acetylcholine on structures and smooth muscles innervated by the parasympathetic nerves. Also called anticholinergic; anti-muscarinic; spasmolytic; atropinic; parasympathoparalytic.

parasympathomimetic Producing effects similar to those caused by stimulation of the parasympathetic system.

parasympathoparalytic See parasympatholytic.

parasystole A second automatic cardiac rhythm existing simultaneously with normal sinus rhythm and firing at a regular and uninterrupted rate.

intermittent p. A parasystolic rhythm that is interrupted and subsequently resumes.

parathion A highly poisonous organic phosphate insecticide; an inhibitor of cholinesterase.

parathormone A polypeptide produced and secreted into the bloodstream by the parathyroid glands; its main function is to maintain a constant concentration of calcium in the blood. Also called parathyroid hormone.

parathyroid 1. Located beside the thyroid gland. **2.** A parathyroid gland; see gland, parathyroid.

parathyroidectomy Surgical removal of the parathyroid glands.

parathyrotropic, parathyrotrophic Having an effect on the parathyroid glands.

paratope The region of the surface of an antibody that combines with an antigen. Cf. epitope.

paratrichosis Any disorder affecting hair growth.

paratyphoid Resembling typhoid (fever or bacillus).

paraumbilical Situated near the navel (umbilicus).

paraungual Alongside or near a fingernail or toenail.

paravaginal Near or next to the vagina.

paravertebral Alongside the vertebral column.

parectasia, parectasis Excessive distention of a part or organ.

paregoric An antiperistaltic compound consisting of powdered opium, anise oil, benzoic acid, cam-

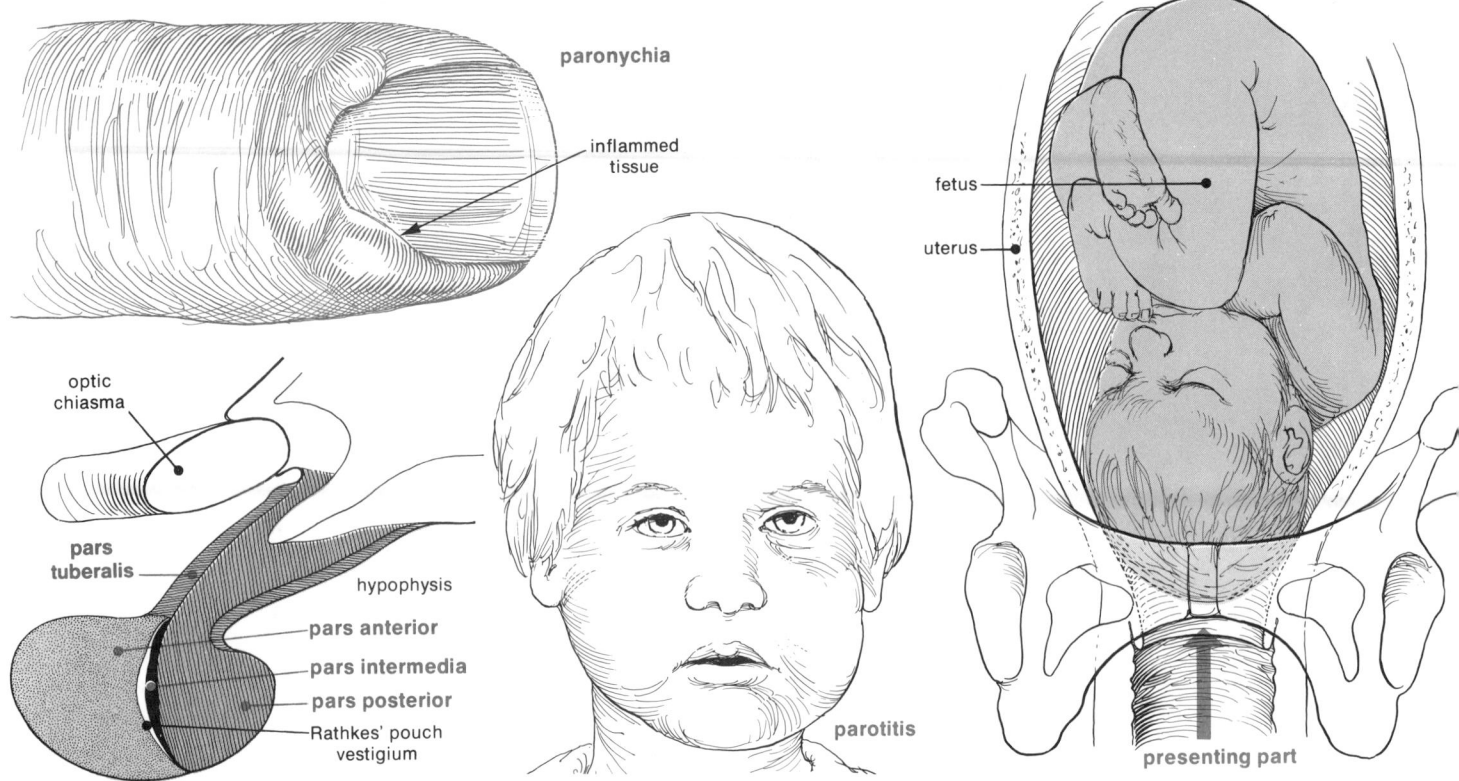

paronychia

inflammed
tissue

optic
chiasma

pars
tuberalis

hypophysis

pars anterior
pars intermedia
pars posterior
Rathkes' pouch
vestigium

parotitis

fetus

uterus

presenting part

phor, and glycerin in diluted alcohol; principally used in relieving abdominal cramps and diarrhea. Also called camphorated opium tincture.

parencephalon Cerebellum.

parenchyma The characteristic tissue of an organ or gland, as distinguished from connective tissue.

parenchymal, parenchymatous Relating to the parenchyma.

parenteral **1.** Situated outside the alimentary tract. **2.** Taken into the body in a way other than through the alimentary canal, as by intravenous or intramuscular injection.

paresis Partial paralysis; weakness.

paresthesia An abnormal sensation, as burning, tingling, or numbness.

paresthetic Characterized by paresthesia.

paretic Relating to or suffering from paresis.

paries, *pl.* **parietes** A wall of a body cavity, as of the chest.

parietal Pertaining to the wall of a cavity.

parieto-occipital Relating to the parietal and occipital bones of the skull or lobes of the cerebrum.

Paris green An insecticide composed of copper acetate and copper meta-arsenite.

parity The state of a woman in respect to having given birth to children.

parkinsonian **1.** Relating to paralysis agitans (Parkinson's disease). **2.** One who suffers from paralysis agitans.

parkinsonism A group of nervous disorders (including paralysis agitans) marked by muscular rigidity, tremors, lack of facial expression, akinesia, and postural abnormalities.

Parkinson's disease See paralysis agitans.

paroniria Terrifying dreams causing sleep disturbance. Also called morbid dreaming.

  p. ambulans Morbid dreaming while sleepwalking.

paronychia Inflammation of the tissues around a nail. Also called whitlow.

paroophoron A group of coiled, vestigial tubules situated in the broad ligament between the epoophoron and the uterus; best seen in the child, the tubules are remnants of the excretory part of the mesonephros or wolffian body.

parosmia Any disorder of the sense of smell, especially a perverted sense of smell as may occur in some cases of schizophrenia, uncinate gyrus lesions, and hysterias.

parotid Situated near the ear, as the parotid salivary gland.

parotidectomy Surgical removal of the parotid gland.

parotitis, parotiditis Inflammation of the parotid gland.

  epidemic p. An acute contagious disease caused

by a virus present in discharges of the nose and in saliva; complications usually involve the ovaries and the testes, sometimes causing sterility in men. Also called mumps.

parous Having borne one or more children.

parovarium The lateral part of the vestigial remains of the mesonephric tubules located in the mesosalpinx between the ovary and the uterine tube.

paroxysm **1.** A sudden onset or recurrence of symptoms of a disease. **2.** A convulsion.

paroxysmal Occurring in or of the nature of paroxysms.

pars, *pl.* **partes** A particular portion of a structure; a part.

  p. abdominalis esophagi The portion of the esophagus between the diaphragm and the stomach.

  p. anterior hypophyseos The anterior lobe of the hypophysis (pituitary gland).

  p. cartilaginea septi nasi The cartilaginous portion of the nasal septum.

  p. flaccida membranae tympani The small, flaccid, somewhat triangular upper part of the tympanic membrane (eardrum). Also called Shrapnell's membrane.

  p. intermedia hypophyseos The intermediate part of the hypophysis, between the posterior and anterior lobes.

  p. membranacea septi nasi The membranous anterior portion of the nasal septum.

  p. membranacea urethrae masculinae The membranous part of the male urethra extending about 1.25 cm from the prostate gland.

  p. muscularis septi interventricularis The muscular portion of the interventricular septum of the heart.

  p. nasalis pharyngis See nasopharynx.

  p. posterior hypophyseos The posterior lobe of the hypophysis (pituitary gland).

  p. prostatica urethra The portion of the male urethra that transverses the prostate gland; it is about 2.5 cm in length.

  p. recta A straight part, e.g., the straight portion of the proximal tubule of the nephron.

  p. tuberalis hypophyseos The part of the anterior lobe of the hypophysis that extends upward and wraps around the infundibular stalk. Also called pars infundibularis.

part A portion.

  presenting p. In obstetrics, the portion of the fetus closest to the birth canal and which is felt through the cervix on vaginal examination; the presenting part determines the presentation.

partes aequales (P.ae.) Latin for equal parts; used in prescription writing.

parthenogenesis Reproduction of organisms in which the female reproduces without fecundation

by the male.

particle **1.** An extremely small part, portion, or division of matter. **2.** One of the minute subdivisions of matter; e.g., an electron.

  alpha p. A positively charged particle ejected from the nucleus of a radioactive atom and consisting of two neutrons and two protons (helium nucleus).

  beta p. An electron, either positively (positron) or negatively (negatron) charged, which is emitted from an atomic nucleus during beta decay of a radionuclide.

  Dane p. A double-shelled particle about 42 nm in diameter; composed of a DNA-containing core (28 nm in diameter) and a lipoprotein outer coat (7 nm thick); has hepatitis B antigen on its surface (HBs Ag) and in its core (HBc Ag).

  elementary p. **1.** The fundamental or simplest unit of matter that so far has defied subdivision. **2.** Platelet. **3.** One of many knoblike repeating units attached to the matrix side of the inner membrane of the mitochondrion; it has a 90 Å spherical head, spaced at approximately 100 Å intervals, and is connected by a 50 Å-long stalklike structure to a baseplate in the membrane itself. Formerly called F_1 particle. Also called elementary transport particle; elementary body.

particulate Relating to, or composed of, fine particles.

parturient **1.** Relating to childbirth. **2.** About to give birth; in labor.

parturifacient **1.** Inducing or accelerating childbirth. **2.** An agent that induces or accelerates childbirth.

parturition The act of giving birth. Also called childbirth.

partus Parturition.

parvicellular Pertaining to or composed of exceptionally small cells.

Parvovirus Genus of DNA viruses (family Parvoviridae) which includes the virus causing erythema infectiosum (fifth disease).

pascal (Pa) The SI unit of pressure; a force of one newton per square meter.

passage **1.** The act of passing. **2.** A channel, duct, pore, opening, or path along which something may pass. **3.** A bowel movement.

Passavant's cushion See ridge, Passavant's.

passive Nonresponsive; submissive; inert; not initiating or participating.

passivity **1.** The inertness exhibited by certain metals under conditions in which chemical activity should take place, due to the formation of a coating of peroxide, oxygen, or salt. **2.** In dentistry, the state of inactivity of the oral structures when a removable partial denture is in place but not used in masticafemur

patella

posterior view

anterior view

tibia   fibula

bladder

patent urachus

hearing centers located in first and second temporal gyri

auditory pathways

medial geniculate body

nucleus of inferior colliculus

superior olive

nucleus of cochlear nerve

auditory radiation

cochlear nerve

cochlea

tion. **3.** Passivism, a passive or submissive attitude or behavior.

paste A soft semisolid substance.

dermatologic p. Pharmaceutical preparation composed of starch, sulfur, dextrin, zinc oxide, or calcium carbonate mixed with glycerin, petrolatum, or soft soap and containing antiseptics for external use.

resorcinol p., mild A bactericidal and fungicidal composed of 10% resorcinol, 25% zinc oxide, 25% starch, and 40% light liquid petrolatum. Also called Lassar's mild resorcin paste.

zinc oxide p. with salicylic acid Mixture of 2% salicylic acid in paste of zinc oxide; used as an antiseptic and soothing agent. Also called Lassar's zinc paste with salicylic acid.

Pasteurella A genus (family Brucellaceae) of round, ellipsoidal, or rod-shaped gram-negative bacteria that usually occur singly.

P. pestis *Yersinia pestis.*

P. tularensis The species causing tularemia in man and rodents.

pasteurellosis Infection with bacteria of the genus *Pasteurella*; it includes hemorrhagic septicemia, tularemia, plague, and pseudotuberculosis.

pasteurization The process of destroying or retarding the growth of bacteria in milk and other liquids, without destroying the flavor of the product, by heating the liquid to a moderate degree (60–70°C) for a sustained period of time (30 minutes) rather than by boiling it quickly.

pasteurize To subject milk or other liquids to pasteurization.

past-pointing See under pointing.

patch A small area or section of a surface differing from or contrasting with the whole.

cotton wool p.'s Coagulated exudates from the retinal capillaries, appearing as white fluffy areas on the retina.

herald p. A solitary large lesion appearing before (sometimes days or weeks) the general eruption of pityriasis rosea.

mucous p. A moist, yellowish lesion on the mucous membrane of the mouth or external genitalia, usually seen in secondary syphilis.

Peyer's p.'s Small whitish masses of lymphoid tissue situated in the mucous and submucous layers of the small intestine.

smoker's p. See leukoplakia.

patella A somewhat flattened triangular bone, embedded in the combined tendons of the extensor muscles of the leg, located at the front of the knee joint; the largest sesamoid bone of the body. Also called kneecap.

patellapexy The surgical fixation of the patella to

the distal end of the femur.

patellar Of, or relating to, the patella.

patellectomy Surgical removal of the patella.

patency The state of being open.

patent 1. Open or exposed. **2.** Apparent.

path The course taken by a nervous impulse.

pathfinder A filiform bougie for passage through a narrow stricture, such as the urethra; it serves as a guide for the introduction of a larger sound or catheter.

pathogen Any microorganism or substance capable of causing disease.

pathogenesis, pathogenesy The origin and development of disease. Also called nosogenesis and nosogeny.

pathogenic, pathogenetic Causing disease.

pathogenicity Disease-producing capability.

pathogenism The relationship between a pathogen and its host.

pathognomonic A special characteristic of a disease; denoting one or more typical symptoms of a disease.

pathologic Pertaining to or caused by disease.

pathologist A specialist in pathology.

speech p. A professional with specialized training in speech pathology.

pathology The branch of medicine concerned with the study of disease in all its aspects (its nature, causes, development, and consequences).

speech p. The study of all aspects of functional and organic speech and language disorders, with particular reference to the underlying cause, evaluation, and treatment.

pathomimesis Imitation of disease, whether intentional or unconscious.

pathoneurosis Abnormal preoccupation with disease.

pathophobia An abnormal fear of disease .

pathophysiology The study of pathologic alteration in bodily function, as distinguished from structural defects.

pathopsychology The study of abnormal psychic processes from the point of view of general psychology.

pathway 1. In neurology, the linked neurons through which an impulse is conducted to the cerebral cortex (afferent pathway), or from the brain to the skeletal musculature (efferent pathways). **2.** The series of metabolic reactions which convert one biochemical substance into another.

direct oxidative p. See pentose phosphate pathways.

Emden-Meyerhof p. In carbohydrate metabolism, the series of anaerobic reactions which convert glucose or glycogen to pyruvate and lactate, releasing

energy in the form of adenosine triphosphate (ATP).

pentose phosphate p. In carbohydrate metabolism, a pathway of hexose oxidation whereby glucose 6-phosphate generates five-carbon sugars; plays major role in production of NADPH for reductive biosyntheses; e.g., of fatty acids. Also called pentose or monophosphate shunt; direct oxidative pathway.

patient (pt) A person who is under medical treatment.

patroclinous Inherited through the paternal line; derived from the father. Cf. matroclinous.

patten A support worn under one shoe to equalize the length of both legs.

pattern 1. An arrangement or design. **2.** In dentistry, a form used to develop a mold from which a restoration is produced, such as an inlay or denture.

early repolarization p. Elevated ST segments with an elevated J-point; often seen in young black males.

juvenile p. Precordial T-wave inversion in the electrocardiogram; a persistent juvenile pattern sometimes seen in healthy adults, especially young Negroes.

wax p. An exact wax model of lost tooth structure which, when invested and burned out, will produce a mold in which a casting may be made.

patulous Freely open; spread widely apart; expanded; patent.

pause 1. Temporary stop. **2.** To suspend activity for a time.

compensatory p. The pause following a premature beat, usually a ventricular extrasystole; the short cycle ending with the premature beat plus the compensatory pause together equal two of the regular cardiac cycles.

sinus p. A spontaneous interruption in the regular sinus rhythm of the heart marked by a long-lasting absence of sinus P waves; thought to result from a high degree of S-A block or sinus arrest.

pearl 1. A small hard mass of mucus found in the sputum in asthma. **2.** A small sphere of thin glass containing a fluid meant to be inhaled after crushing of the sphere in a handkerchief.

enamel p. A spherical nodule of enamel attached to a tooth, usually on the root. Also called enameloma.

Epstein's p. Minute white masses of epithelium seen on the palate of the newborn.

gouty p. Sodium urate concretion, seen on the ear cartilage of individuals with gout.

peau French for skin.

p. d'orange A dimpled appearance of the skin, like that of an orange; seen in some cases of cancer of the breast.

pecten 1. Any anatomic structure resembling a

Labels in figures: glomerular wall, pedicels, endothelium, basement membrane, pore, podocyte, urinary space, Pediculus humanus, peduncle, myxoma, left atrium of heart, intussusceptum, peduncle, tumor, tectum, cerebral aqueduct, substantia nigra, oculomotor nuclei, cerebral peduncle, tegmentum, crus cerebri, red nucleus, oculomotor nerve

comb. **2.** A narrow area in the middle of the anal canal.

pectin A vegetable mucilage found in abundance in certain fruits and roots; a purified form is used in pharmaceutical preparations.

pectinate Comb-shaped.

pectineal Relating to any comb-shaped structure.

pectoral Pertaining to the chest.

pectoralgia Pain in the chest.

pectoralis Relating to the chest.

pectoriloquy Transmission of the voice through the chest wall, audible by use of the stethoscope; indicative of a cavity when present alone; indicative of consolidation when accompanied by bronchophony. Also called pectorophony.

pectorophony See pectoriloquy.

pectus, *pl.* **pectora** The chest; especially the anterior wall.

    p. carinatum Deformity of the anterior chest wall marked by protrusion of the sternum (breastbone); believed to be due to unbalanced or excessive growth of the cartilages. Also called pigeon, chicken, or keel breast.

    p. excavatum Inherited deformity marked by depression of the sternum (breastbone) and rib cartilages; believed to be caused by a short central tendon and muscular imbalance of the diaphragm. Also called funnel chest.

pedal Relating to the feet.

pederasty Anal intercourse, especially between a man and boy.

pediatric Relating to the study and treatment of children's diseases.

pediatrician A physician who specializes in pediatrics.

pediatrics (Ped) The branch of medicine concerned with the care and development of children and the treatment of their diseases.

pedicel The secondary process of a podocyte that helps form the visceral capsule of a renal corpuscle.

Also called foot process or plate.

pedicle **1.** A stem or stalk, as of a tumor. **2.** A tubed or narrow stalk by means of which a skin graft remains attached temporarily to the donor site.

pedicular Relating to lice.

pediculicide Any agent or chemical capable of destroying lice.

pediculosis The state of being infested with lice.

    p. capitis Infestation of the hair of the head with lice.

    p. corporis The presence of lice on the body or clothes; they usually infest the clothes until feeding time.

    p. pubis The presence of lice on the pubic hair or neighboring parts of the body; the infesting louse is usually a species of *Phthirus*, not *Pediculus*; therefore, the condition is more correctly termed phthiriasis pubis.

Pediculus A genus of lice of the family Pediculidae.

    P. humanus The sucking species infesting man and feeding on his blood; a vector of relapsing fever, typhus, and trench fever.

    P. humanus capitis A species that infests the scalp of man and attaches its eggs to hair. Also called head louse.

    P. humanus corporis One that infests the body of man (as distinguished from his head and extremities). Also called body louse.

    P. pubis *Phthirus pubis.*

pediculus, *pl.* **pediculi** **1.** Parasite of the genus *Pediculus*. Also called louse. **2.** Pedicle; stalk.

pedicure **1.** Care and treatment of the feet. **2.** Cosmetic care of the feet, especially of the toenails.

pedigree A diagram setting forth a line of an individual's ancestors. Also called family tree.

pedodontics The branch of dentistry dealing with the preventive care and treatment of children's teeth.

pedodontist A specialist in pedodontics.

pedology A branch of biology and of sociology that studies the behavior and development of children.

pedophilia The engaging in sexual activity with children as a repeatedly preferred or exclusive method by an adult.

peduncle **1.** A large stalklike mass of nerve fibers connecting a suprasegmental structure to other portions of the nervous system. **2.** The narrow part of a structure serving as support or attachment.

    cerebellar p., inferior A bundle of largely afferent nerve fibers on either side of the medulla oblongata, connecting the medulla and spinal cord with the cerebellum. Also called restiform body.

    cerebellar p., middle One of a pair of large bundles of nerve fibers originating in the pontine nuclei and distributed to all parts of the cerebellar cortex. Also called brachium pontis.

    cerebellar p., superior A large bundle of largely efferent nerve fibers extending from each cerebellar hemisphere upward over the pons and reaching the tegmentum of the midbrain, where it decussates; the fibers originate in the dentate and emboliform nuclei and terminate chiefly in the opposite red nucleus and thalamus.

    cerebral p. The part of the midbrain in front of the cerebral aqueduct, composed of the tegmentum (dorsal part) and crus cerebri (ventral part).

    p. of the pineal body The dorsal stalk of the pineal body. Also called habenula.

    thalamic p. The fibers passing between the thalamus and cerebral cortex (subdivided into anterior, posterior, superior, and inferior peduncles).

pedunculate, pedunculated Having a stalk or peduncle.

pedunculotomy Surgical incision of the cerebral peduncle.

peliosis Purpura.

pellagra A condition caused by vitamin (nicotinic acid) deficiency, marked by skin lesions, gastrointesmale **pelvis**

inferior aspect

female **pelvis**

hipbone   sacrum

superior aspect

kidney

renal pelvis (normal capacity 7.5 cc)

pelvimeter

penicillin

S

CH₃

O—NH—C—CH   C—CH₃

C   N   C—OH

area where various penicillins differ

pure crystals of **penicillin**

bladder

ejaculatory duct

urethra

penis

scrotum

---

tinal disturbances, and nervous disorders.

pellagroid   Resembling pellagra.

pellagrous   Relating to pellagra.

pellicle   1. Thin membrane or cuticle. 2. A film on the surface of a liquid. 3. A firm mass formed by some fungi on the surface of a liquid medium.

pelvic   Of, or relating to, a pelvis.

pelvicephalometry   Measurement of the diameters of the fetal head in relation to those of the mother's pelvis.

pelvic inflammatory disease (PID)   Inflammation in the pelvic cavity, especially of the female genital organs.

pelvilithotomy   Pyelolithotomy.

pelvimeter   A caliper-shaped instrument for measuring the diameters and capacity of the pelvis.

pelvimetry   The measurement of the dimensions and capacity of the inlet and the outlet of the pelvis.

   x-ray p.   Pelvimetry performed by application of a grid to roentgenograms of the pelvic bones.

pelviotomy   1. Division of the pubic joint. 2. Incision into the pelvis of the kidney.

pelvis, *pl.* **pelves**   1. A basin-like skeletal structure that supports the spinal column and rests on the lower limbs. 2. A funnel-shaped structure, as the pelvis of the kidney.

   android p.   A female pelvis with characteristics of a male pelvis.

   brim of the p.   The circumference of the plane dividing the major and minor pelves.

   cavity of the minor p.   See cavity, pelvic.

   contracted p.   One in which any of the important diameters is shorter than normal.

   false p.   See major pelvis.

   funnel-shaped p.   One with a normal inlet and a greatly narrowed outlet.

   gynecoid p.   The average female pelvis, having a rounded oval shape.

   inlet of p.   The upper opening of the true pelvis; the space within the pelvic brim.

   major p.   The expanded portion of the pelvis situated above and in front of the pelvic brim. Also called false pelvis.

   minor p.   The portion of the pelvis situated below and behind the pelvic brim. Also called true pelvis.

   renal p.   The funnel-shaped structure, formed by the junction of two tubes (greater calices), into which the urine is discharged from the kidney.

   true p.   See minor pelvis.

pelvisacral   Relating to the pelvis and the sacrum.

pelviscope   An illuminated instrument for examining the interior of the pelvis.

pelvospondylitis   Inflammation of the sacral vertebrae (pelvic portion of spinal column), usually resulting in hardening of the sacroiliac and apophyseal joints.

   p. ossificans   Ankylosing spondylitis; see under spondylitis.

pemphigoid   An eruption of soft blebs resembling those of pemphigus vulgaris.

pemphigus   Any skin disease characterized by severe blistering.

   familial benign chronic p.   A blistering dermatosis; recurrent eruption of vesicles and bullae that become scaling and crusted lesions with vesicular borders, predominantly of the neck, groin, and axillary regions; autosomal dominant inheritance. Also called Hailey-Hailey disease.

   p. erythematosus   See Senear-Usher disease.

   p. foliaceus   A form of pemphigus characterized by widespread leaf-like scaliness and slightly exudative lesions, resembling exfoliative dermatitis; histologically the blisters are high in the epidermis.

   p. vegetans   A form of pemphigus characterized by exuberant overgrowth or vegetations in or about the eroded surfaces left by ruptured blisters. Also called Neumann's disease.

   p. vulgaris   A serious systemic illness of unknown etiology, characterized by an eruption of flaccid vesicles over the entire body, with erosion on the mucous membranes; if left untreated, it is inevitably fatal.

Pendred's syndrome   Congenital deafness and goiter with or without hypothyroidism; inherited as an autosomal recessive trait.

penectomy   Surgical removal of the penis.

penetrance   The frequency with which a heritable trait is manifested in individuals known to carry the gene that causes it.

penetrometer   Device for measuring the penetrating power of a given x-ray beam.

penicillamine   A degradation product of penicillin; a chelating agent used in the treatment of hepatolenticular degeneration (Wilson's disease) and lead poisoning.

penicillin   Any of a family of antibiotic compounds obtained from cultures of the mold *Penicillium notatum* and related species, or produced biosynthetically; it inhibits bacterial cell wall synthesis, resulting in eventual death to the cell when the penicillin-poisoned bacteria outgrows its cell wall.

   benzathine p. G suspension   Aqueous suspension of a salt formed by 1 mol of an ammonium base and 2 mol of penicillin G. Administered intramuscularly, it is very slowly absorbed and provides sustained blood levels of penicillin up to one month. Bicillin®.

   p. V   An oral semisynthetic penicillin which is absorbed from the gastrointestinal tract. Also called phenoxymethyl penicillin.

penicillinase   Enzyme produced by certain bacteria (e.g., some strains of staphylococcus) that render penicillin inactive.

Penicillium   A genus of fungi; a saprophytic mold that yields several antibiotic substances.

   P. notatum   An ascomycete fungus from which penicillin and notatin are derived.

penile   Relating to the penis.

penis   The male organ of copulation and of urinary excretion; composed of three columns of erectile

skin

cauda equina
of spinal cord

interspinal
ligament

spinous
process of
vertebra

dura mater

perforation
of dura mater
with needle

body of
vertebra

**bimanual
percussion**

**sodium
pentobarbital**

tissue, two dorsolateral (corpora cavernosa) and one medial (corpus spongiosum) which contains the urethra and expands at the end forming the glans penis.

pennate Resembling a feather; feathered or winged. Also called penniform; pinnate.

penniform See pennate.

pentabasic Denoting an acid that has five hydrogen atoms replaceable by a metal or radical.

pentamadine Drug used to treat trypanosomiasis, leishmaniasis, and pneumocystis carinii pneumonia (a type often affecting AIDS patients).

pentatomic 1. Denoting a molecule comprised of five atoms. 2. Denoting a compound possessing five atoms in a ring. 3. Denoting a chemical with five replaceable hydrogen atoms. 4. Denoting an alcohol containing five hydroxyl groups.

pentobarbital Short-acting barbiturate, $C_{11}H_{12}$-N_2O_3, generally used for sleep induction; Nembutal®.

    sodium p. The sodium salt of pentobarbital, a short-acting hypnotic that reduces apprehension and produces drowsiness; used for sedation during labor, and prior to surgery and various diagnostic procedures.

pentose Any one of a class of monosaccharides containing five carbon atoms in the molecule (C_5-$H_{10}O_5$); e.g., arabinose, lyxose, ribose, and xylose.

pentosuria The presence of any of the pentoses in the urine.

pepsin An enzyme present in gastric juice; it converts proteins into peptones and proteoses.

pepsinogen The precursor of pepsin, present in the lining of the stomach; an inert substance that is converted into pepsin during digestion by the action of hydrochloric acid.

pepsinogenous Producing pepsin.

pepsinuria The presence of pepsin in the urine.

peptic 1. Of, or relating to, digestion. 2. Relating to pepsin.

peptidase An enzyme that catalyzes the hydrolysis

of peptide bonds of a protein or peptide.

peptide One of various compounds which yield two or more amino acids on hydrolysis; one of the compounds into which the protein molecule is split during digestion.

    C p. A peptide chain in the proinsulin molecule that connects the A chain and B chain; it splits off as residue during conversion of proinsulin to insulin.

    gastric stimulating p. Any peptide that promotes or inhibits secretion from the stomach lining or stimulates gastric motility.

    vasoactive intestinal p. (VIP) A substance found in the intestinal tract, especially the distal small bowel and colon, capable of suppressing acid secretion by the stomach and stimulating secretion in the small intestine and colon; may be responsible for the watery diarrhea syndrome associated with pancreatic islet cell tumor; causes hyperglycemia and hypercalcemia; also found in the brain.

peptize To transform a gel into a sol.

peptolysis The hydrolysis or splitting up of peptones.

peptone Any of various protein derivatives obtained by the action of an enzyme or an acid on a natural protein.

peptonemia The presence of peptone in the blood.

peptonize To convert protein into peptone.

peptonuria The presence of peptones in the urine.

Peptostreptococcus A genus of spherical gram-positive, nonmotile bacteria found normally in the intestinal, respiratory, and female genital tracts, oral cavity, and certain pyogenic infections.

per anum Latin for through the anus.

percept A mental impression of something perceived by the senses that forms an image in the mind.

perception The process of becoming aware of something through any of the senses.

    depth p. The ability to detect by sight the three dimensional quality of objects and their position in space; perception of the third dimension. Also called stereoscopic vision.

    extrasensory p. (ESP) Perception through other than the five senses.

perceptivity The ability or faculty of perception.

perchloride A chloride having the largest possible amount of chlorine.

percolation Extraction of the soluble parts of a solid mixture by passing a liquid solvent slowly through it.

percuss 1. To tap the surface of specific areas of the body to determine the degree of density of the structures beneath by the sound produced. 2. To tap a bodily part as a therapeutic measure.

percussion The act of tapping the body, especially the chest, back, and abdomen, to determine the condition of underlying structures by the sounds produced.

    auscultatory p. Auscultation for the purpose of listening to sounds produced by percussion.

    bimanual p. One in which the finger of one hand taps a finger of the other hand which is placed on the patient.

    palpatory p. Percussion combined with palpation in order to perceive tactile as well as auditory impressions.

percussor 1. A device that sends vibrations through the chest wall to aid in freeing mucus deposits and improve bronchial drainage. 2. A hammer for use in percussion.

percutaneous 1. Having the ability to pass through unbroken skin, as in absorption by inunction. 2. Denoting procedures such as biopsies or intra-venous or intra-arterial catheterizations performed with needle puncture without incision.

perflation The forcing of air into a cavity or canal to expel any contained material.

perforation 1. A small hole or series of holes

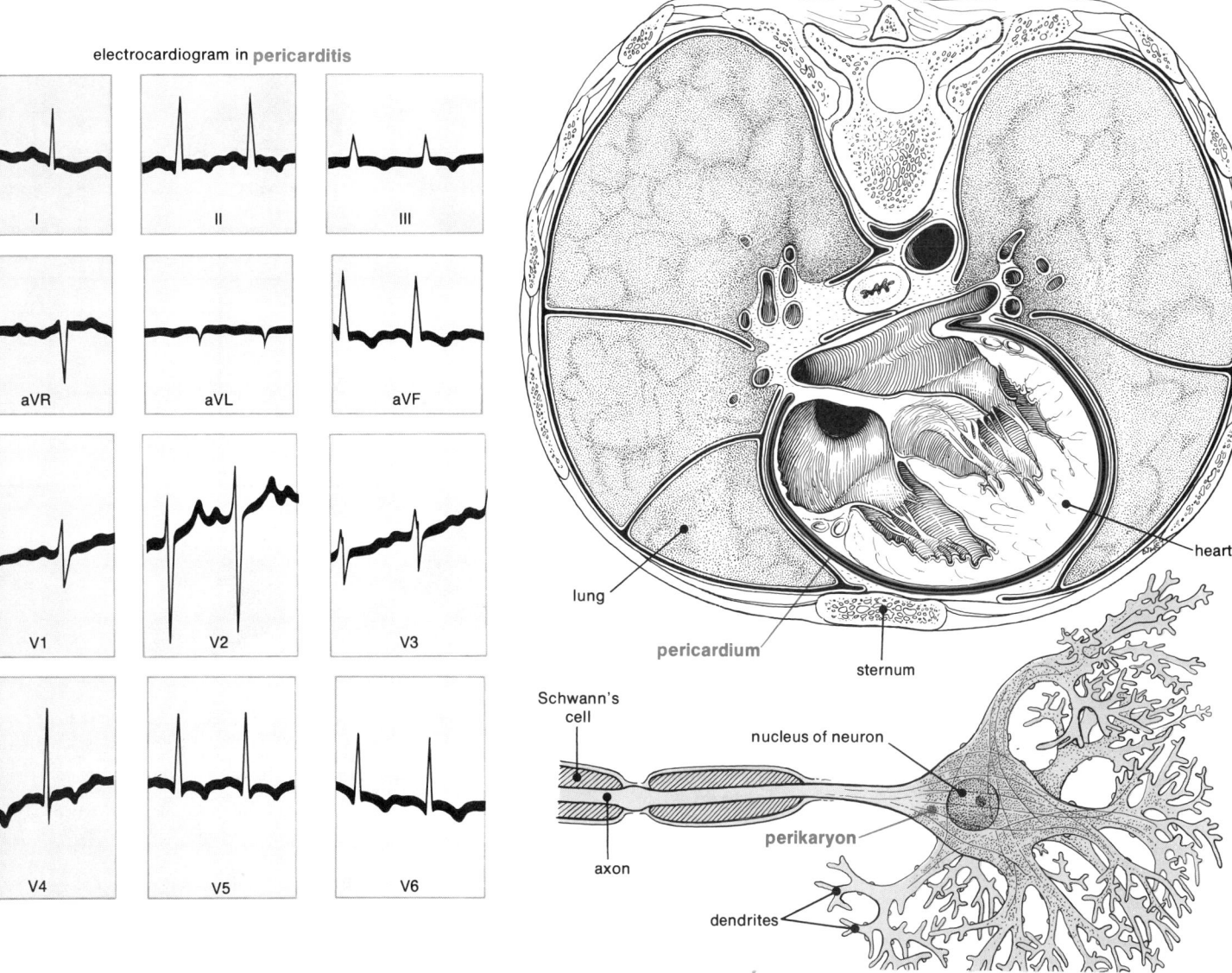

electrocardiogram in **pericarditis**

I

II

III

aVR

aVL

aVF

V1

V2

V3

V4

V5

V6

heart

lung

pericardium

sternum

Schwann's cell

nucleus of neuron

perikaryon

axon

dendrites

through an organ or organelle. **2.** The act of piercing a body part.

perforin A protein present in granules of cytotoxic T lymphocytes; when released, it forms pores in the target cell membrane.

perfusate A fluid that has been poured (a) over a special surface, e.g., a charged plate, or (b) through a tissue or semipermeable membrane.

perfusion The passage of a fluid through the vessels of an organ.

periadenitis Inflammation of the tissues around a gland.

perianal Adjacent to or around the anus. Also called circumanal.

periangitis Inflammation of the tissues surrounding a blood vessel or a lymphatic vessel.

periantritis Antral gastritis; see under gastritis.

periaortic Surrounding or located near the aorta.

periaortitis An inflammatory condition affecting the adventitia of the aorta and the tissues around it.

periapical Relating to the tissues surrounding the tip of a dental root, including the alveolar bone.

periappendicitis Inflammation of the tissues near or surrounding the vermiform appendix.

periarterial Surrounding an artery.

periarteritis Inflammation of the outer coat of an artery.

 p. nodosa See polyarteritis nodosa.

periarthritis Inflammation of the tissues near a joint.

peribronchial Surrounding a bronchus or bronchi.

peribuccal Situated around the mouth.

peribulbar Surrounding any anatomic bulb, especially of the eye and the urethra.

peribursal Situated around a bursa.

pericardectomy See pericardiectomy.

pericardial, pericardiac 1. Situated around the heart. **2.** Of, or relating to, the pericardium.

pericardiocentesis, pericardicentesis Sur-

gical puncture of the membrane covering the heart (pericardium) for the purpose of aspirating a pericardial effusion.

pericardiectomy Surgical removal of a portion of the pericardium. Also called pericardectomy.

pericardiophrenic Relating to the pericardium and the diaphragm.

pericardiorrhaphy The suturing of a wound in the pericardium.

pericardiostomy The making of an opening into the pericardium.

pericardiotomy See pericardotomy.

pericarditis Inflammation of the pericardium.

 adhesive p. The presence of dense fibrous tissue which fixes the pericardium to the heart or to other structures in the chest.

pericardium The thin, double-layered, membranous sac that encloses the heart; the layers are separated by a small amount of fluid which lubricates the constantly rubbing surfaces; the layers fuse as they attach to the great vessels and diaphragm.

pericardotomy Surgical incision of the pericardium. Also called pericardiotomy.

pericecal Surrounding the cecum.

pericellular Surrounding or situated around a cell.

pericementitis Periodontitis.

pericholangitis Inflammation of the tissues around the bile ducts or interlobular bile capillaries.

perichondral Relating to or composed of perichondrium.

perichondritis Inflammation of the perichondrium.

perichondrium A fibrous membrane which covers cartilage except at joint endings, composed of an outer dense irregular connective tissue and an inner layer which is responsible for production of new cartilage.

perichord The sheath covering the notochord.

pericolpitis Inflammation of the tissues surrounding the vagina.

pericoronal Surrounding the crown of a tooth.

pericoronitis Inflammation of the gums around a partially erupted tooth.

pericranial Relating to the fibrous membrane covering the skull.

pericranium The fibrous membrane covering the skull. Also called periosteum of the skull.

pericystic 1. Surrounding the urinary bladder. **2.** Around the gallbladder. **3.** Surrounding a cyst.

pericyte One of the elongated connective tissue cells located around the capillaries.

peridental Periodontal; surrounding a tooth.

peridesmic Surrounding a ligament; relating to the membrane surrounding a ligament (peridesmium).

peridesmitis Inflammation of the connective tissue surrounding a ligament.

peridesmium The connective tissue membrane covering a ligament.

periendothelioma See perithelioma.

periesophageal Surrounding the esophagus.

periesophagitis Inflammation of the tissues around the esophagus.

periganglionic Surrounding a nerve ganglion.

perigastric Surrounding the stomach.

perihepatic Occurring around the liver.

perihepatitis Inflammation of the peritoneum and tissues around the liver; a complication in women with gonococcal inflammation of the pelvic organs, resulting from the spread of gonococci to the upper abdomen. Also called Fitz-Hugh-Curtis syndrome; hepatitis externa.

perikaryon The main cytoplasmic matrix surrounding the nucleus of the cell body of the neuron; it is crowded with granular organelles including neurofibrils, chromidial substance (Nissl bodies), Golgi apparatus, mitochondria, and a centrosome. Also called neuroplasm.

perilymph The fluid contained in the bony labyrinth that surrounds the membranous labyrinth of peristalsis

the internal ear.

perilymphatic 1. Relating to the perilymph. 2. Surrounding a lymphatic vessel.

perimeter 1. An edge or border. 2. A device to determine the extent and characteristics of the visual field.

perimetric 1. Surrounding the uterus. 2. Relating to the measuring of the visual field.

perimetritis Inflammation of the outer coat of the uterus (perimetrium).

perimetrium The serous membrane covering the uterus.

perimetry The determination of the extent of the visual field with the aid of a perimeter, usually for the purpose of diagnosing disturbances in the visual pathways.

perimysial Relating to the perimysium.

perimysium Connective tissue that surrounds the fasciculi (bundles of muscle fibers) and also forms the fibrous septa throughout the muscle.

perinatal Occurring or relating to, immediately before, during, or shortly after birth; applied to the time that usually starts with completion of 20 weeks of gestation and generally ends 28 days after birth.

perinatology A subspecialty concerned with the care of mother and baby during the last stage of pregnancy and early days after birth.

perineal Relating to the perineum.

perineoplasty Reparative surgery of the perineum, as for the correction of a relaxed condition. Sometimes called perineorrhaphy.

perineorrhaphy Suture of the perineum, usually performed for the repair of a laceration occurring during childbirth. See also perineoplasty.

perinephric Surrounding or located about the kidney. Also called perirenal.

perinephrium The connective tissue and fat around the kidney.

perineum 1. The area bounded by the pubis, the coccyx, and the thighs. 2. The area between the external genitalia and the anus.

perineural Surrounding a nerve.

perineuritis Inflammation of the perineurium.

perineurium A layer of connective tissue surrounding and supporting each separate bundle of nerve fibers in a peripheral nerve; it consists of a variable number of layers of squamous epithelial cells.

perinuclear Surrounding or situated near a nucleus.

period 1. An interval of time. 2. An occurrence of menstruation.

 absolute refractory p. 1. The period in the cardiac cycle when the heart muscle does not respond to even a high-intensity stimulus; it corresponds to the contraction phase. 2. The time immediately following the passage of an impulse through a nerve.

 gestation p. Time between conception and parturition; period of pregnancy.

 incubation p. Time between infection with a pathogenic microorganism and appearance of first symptoms.

 latent p. 1. Time elapsed between application of a stimulus and the resulting response. 2. The incubation period of an infectious disease.

 missed p. The failure of menstruation to occur in a month.

 neonatal p. The first 30 days of infant life.

 puerperal p. Time between termination of labor and return of the uterus to its original state (approximately 6 weeks).

 relative refractory p. 1. Time during relaxation of heart muscle in which a stronger than ordinary stimulus is required to elicit a response. 2. Time following the absolute refractory period of a nerve, in which a stronger than ordinary stimulus is necessary to transmit an impulse.

 safe p. The interval during the menstrual cycle when conception is least likely to take place, approximately 10 days after the first day of menstruation and 10 days preceding menstruation.

 vulnerable p. The brief period after contraction of the ventricle when a stimulus applied to it is likely to precipitate fibrillation; occurs approximately at the peak of the T wave on the electrocardiogram.

 Wenckebach p. The progressively lengthened P-R interval in successive cardiac cycles preceding a dropped beat, due to an atrioventricular (A-V) block.

periodic 1. Happening or recurring at regular intervals of time; appearing in cycles, as a disease with regularly recurring symptoms. 2. Intermittent; appearing now and then.

periodic acid A colorless, water-soluble, inorganic acid, $HIO_4 \cdot 2H_2O$, resulting from the action of concentrated hydrochloric acid on iodine.

periodical A journal published at regular intervals.

periodicity 1. Recurrence of a phenomenon at regular intervals of time. 2. Recurrence of similar properties in a group of elements, as seen in the periodic system.

periodontal Surrounding a tooth. Also called peridental.

periodontal disease Any disease of the tissues surrounding and supporting the teeth; there are two principal groups: disease confined to the gingiva (gingivitis) and disease affecting the underlying supporting periodontal tissue (periodontitis).

periodontics The branch of dentistry concerned with the study of the tissues surrounding the teeth and with the treatment of their diseases.

periodontist A specialist in periodontics.

periodontitis A disease of the periodontium manifested by inflammation of the gums, loss of bone tissue around the teeth, degeneration of the periodontal membrane or ligament, and the formation of pockets between the teeth and the surrounding bone. Also called pyorrhea.

periodontium The tissues surrounding and supporting the teeth, including the cementum, periodontal membrane or ligament, alveolar bone, and gingiva (gums). Also called peridentium.

periodontosis A rare condition of unknown cause marked by noninflammatory degeneration of the periodontal tissues, resulting in premature tooth loss.

perioral Situated about the mouth.

periorbita Periosteum lining the interior of the orbit.

periorbital Related to, or situated about, the orbit or periorbita.

periorchitis Inflammation of the tunica vaginalis testis.

periosteal Relating to or of the nature of the periosteum.

periosteoma A tumor surrounding a bone. Also called periostoma.

periosteomyelitis Inflammation of the entire bone and the surrounding periosteum.

periosteotomy, periostotomy The surgical cutting of the periosteum.

periosteum A thick fibrous membrane covering the surface of bones except at points of articulation; it consists, in adults, of two layers: the external layer of dense connective tissue conveying blood vessels and nerves to the bone, and the internal layer of loose connective tissue.

periostitis Inflammation of the periosteum.

periostoma See periosteoma.

periostotomy See periosteotomy.

peripapillary Surrounding the optic disk.

peripheral Pertaining to the outer surface of the body or situated away from the center.

periphery The area of the body away from the center; the outer surface of the body.

periproctitis Inflammation of the tissues situated around the rectum and anus.

perirectal Adjacent to or around the rectum.

perirenal Surrounding the kidney in whole or part. Also called perinephric.

perisplenitis Inflammation of the peritoneum covering the spleen and of the structures surrounding that organ.

peristalsis The alternate contraction and relaxa-

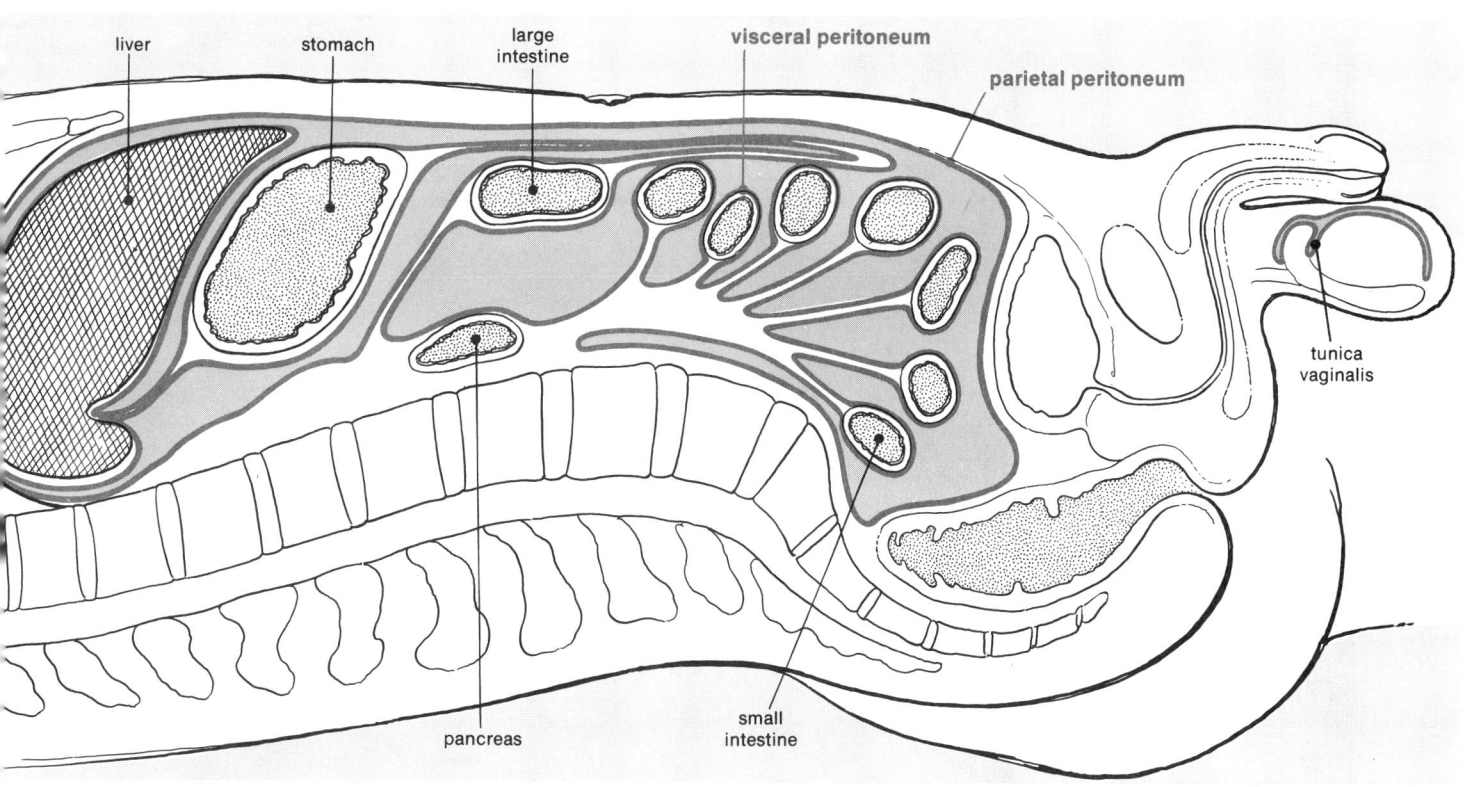

Labels on figure: liver, stomach, large intestine, visceral peritoneum, parietal peritoneum, tunica vaginalis, pancreas, small intestine

tion of the walls of a tubular structure by means of which its contents are moved onward, characteristic of the intestinal tract, ureter, etc.

peristole The ability of the walls of the stomach to contract about its contents following the ingestion of food.

perisynovial Situated around a synovial membrane.

peritectomy See peritomy.

peritendinitis Inflammation of the sheath around a tendon.

perithelioma A tumor which appears to be derived from the tissues surrounding blood vessels (perithelium). Also called periendothelioma.

perithelium Thin layer of connective tissue surrounding the small vessels.

peritomy, peritectomy 1. The cutting of the conjunctiva at the edge of the cornea; a preliminary step in various surgical procedures. 2. Circumcision.

peritoneal Of, or relating to, the peritoneum.

peritoneocentesis Paracentesis or tapping of the peritoneal cavity for the purpose of removing fluid.

peritoneoclysis Irrigation of the peritoneal cavity.

peritoneoscope An illuminated tubular instrument for visual examination of the peritoneum through an abdominal wall incision.

peritoneoscopy Direct inspection of the peritoneal cavity by means of a lighted tubular instrument inserted through the abdominal wall.

peritoneotomy Incision of the peritoneum.

peritoneum The serous membrane lining the walls of the abdominal and pelvic cavities and enclosing the viscera.

   parietal p. The layer of peritoneum lining the walls of the abdominal and pelvic cavities.

   visceral p. The layer of peritoneum investing the abdominal and pelvic organs.

peritonitis Inflammation of the peritoneum, usually attended by abdominal pain, constipation, vomiting, and fever; it may be caused by perforation of the digestive tract, by infection of an organ, such as the appendix, or by a blood-borne infection.

   benign paroxysmal p. Periodic abdominalgia; see under abdominalgia.

peritonize To cover with peritoneum.

peritonsillar Around a tonsil.

peritonsillitis Inflammation affecting the peritonsillar tissues.

peritracheal Situated about the trachea.

peritrichous 1. Relating to cilia or any projections from the surface of a cell. 2. Having flagella uniformly distributed throughout the body; applied to bacteria. 3. Having modified cilia arranged in a spiral fashion around the mouth opening; said of

certain protozoa.

periumbilical Situated around or near the umbilicus. Also called periomphalic.

periungual Around a nail.

periureteral, periureteric Located around one or both ureters.

periureteritis Inflammation of tissues adjacent to the ureter.

periurethritis Inflammation of the tissue around the urethra.

perivascular Around a vessel.

periwinkle Any of several attractive evergreen shrubs or small trees with glossy blue-green leaves and fragrant flowers of the genus *Vinca*, especially *Vinca minor* and *Vinca rosea*; they contain active dimeric alkaloids including vinblastine, vincristine, vinleurosine, and vinrosidine. Also called myrtle.

PERLA Acronym for pupils equal and reactive to light and accommodation.

perlèche A form of oral candidiasis marked by inflammation at the angles of the mouth, with an accumulation of whitish macerated epithelium; it occurs mainly among undernourished children, especially those who have a habit of licking the angles of the mouth.

permanganate Any of the salts of permanganic acid.

permanganic acid An unstable inorganic acid, $HMnO_4$, derived from manganese.

permeability The condition of being permeable.

permeable Being of a substance that allows the passage of another substance. Also called pervious.

permeant Able to penetrate or pass through.

permease A specific protein in the cell membrane of microorganisms that facilitates passage of nutrients, such as sugar, across the membrane in the direction of the concentration gradient.

pernicious Highly destructive; tending to cause death.

pernio See chilblain.

peromelia Severe congenital malformation of the extremities, including absence of a hand or a foot.

peroneal Relating to the fibula or the lateral portion of the leg.

peroneus See table of muscles.

peroral Administered through the mouth.

per os (p.o.) Latin for by mouth.

peroxidase Enzyme found in plant and animal tissues; it causes the decomposition of peroxides which liberate oxygen, thus facilitating oxidation.

peroxide The oxide of a series containing the greatest number of oxygen atoms.

   hydrogen p. Hydrogen dioxide, H_2O_2; an unstable compound, used in solution as an antiseptic, bleaching agent, and oxidizing agent.

peroxisome A membrane bounded organelle (about 0.5 μm in diameter) that contains oxidase and peroxidase; a parenchymal cell contains approximately 200 peroxisomes. Formerly called microbody.

peroxyacetyl nitrate The main pollutant of smog, responsible for the irritation of the eyes and the nose.

per primam, per primam intentionem Latin terms meaning by first intention, a way in which a wound heals; see under intention.

per rectum (p.r.) By way of the rectum.

persalt In chemistry, any salt containing the maximum amount of the acid radical.

per secundum, per secundum intentionem Latin terms meaning by second intention, a way in which a wound heals; see under intention.

perseveration 1. The pathologic, involuntary repetition of a single response to various questions, as seen in organic brain disease. 2. The duration of a mental image.

personality The sum total of an individual's patterns of reaction to his environment.

   borderline p. A personality disorder thought to originate in unsuccessful negotiation of the separation-individuation phase of development; characterized by patterns of unstable and intense interpersonal relationships, identity disturbance, impulsivity, unpredictability of behavior and affect, chronic feelings of emptiness or boredom, intolerance of being alone, and often physically self-damaging acts.

   cyclothymic p. A personality disorder characterized by frequent alternation between moods of elation and depression. Also called affective personality.

   hysterical p. One characterized by dependency, vanity, attention-seeking, and self-centeredness. Also called histrionic personality.

   inadequate p. A personality characterized by inept responses to emotional, social, and intellectual demands.

   multiple p. Condition in which the individual adopts two or more different identities with total intervening amnesia.

   obsessive-compulsive p. Behavior pattern characterized by excessive self-imposed orderliness, rigid adherence to perfectionism, and undue concern with trifles; distinguished from obsessive-compulsive neurosis.

   passive-aggressive p. Character disorder characterized by aggressiveness expressed passively in such ways as procrastination, stubbornness, obstructionism, or intentional inefficiency; this behavior usually indicates hostility that the person does not dare express openly.

pes calcaneus

mortar

pestle

uterus

ring pessary

vagina

Petri dish with growing organisms

pH of some fluids

gastric juice 1.6	urine 5–8	blood plasma 7.4
lemon juice 2.3	saliva 6.5	interstitial fluid 7.4
tomato juice 4.3	cow's milk 6.6	pancreatic juice 7.9

alkaline · neutral · acid

pH 13 12 11 10 9 8 7 6 5 4 3 2

hydrogen ion concentration

---

psychopathic p. An outdated term for sociopathic behavior.

schizoid p. Personality type characterized by avoidance of close or competitive relationships and by a detached reaction to life experiences.

split p. An outdated term for schizophrenia.

perspiration 1. The fluid secreted by the sweat glands, consisting of water, sodium chloride and phosphate, urea, ammonia, creatinine, fats, and other waste products. Also called sweat. 2. The process of sweating.

persuasion In psychiatry, a therapeutic approach directed toward influencing the mind of another by authority, argument, reason, or entreaty.

pertussis An acute respiratory illness of infants and young children usually caused by *Bordetella pertussis*, a gram-negative coccobacillus; in a typical case, the patient manifests paroxysmal coughing with a terminal whoop; a pertussis vaccine is available and is generally administered to infants together with diphtheria and tetanus toxoids. Also called whooping cough.

pervaporation The concentration of a colloidal solution by placing the solution in a bag of semipermeable material and suspending it over a hot plate; only the colloid remains in the bag while the rest of the substances pass through.

perversion A deviation from what is considered normal.

pervert A person who practices perversions, usually sexual.

pervious Being of a substance that is capable of being penetrated. Also called permeable.

pes 1. Latin for foot. 2. Any footlike or basal bodily structure.

p. anserinus 1. The goosefoot-like plexiform branching of the facial nerve in, and in front of, the parotid gland. 2. The combined insertions of the tendons of the sartorius, gracilis, and semitendinosus muscles at the medial border of the tibial tuberosity.

p. calcaneus Foot deformity characterized by dorsiflexion of the foot and prominence of the heel; the weight of the body rests on the heel.

p. cavus See clawfoot.

p. corvinus Crow's foot, the wrinkles radiating from the outer corner (lateral canthus) of the eye, seen in many adults.

p. equinus Foot deformity characterized by plantar flexion; the weight of the body rests on the ball of the foot.

p. planus See flatfoot.

pessary 1. A device used to support a displaced uterus when surgery is contraindicated, or as a contraceptive. 2. A medicated vaginal suppository.

diaphragm p. see diaphragm, contraceptive.

Menge p. a ring pessary with a cross bar and a detachable knob, used when the uterus is markedly prolapsed.

ring p. a ring of plastic, rubber, or metal, used to support the uterus in cases of slight prolapse.

Smith-Hodge p. A pessary used to hold the retroposed uterus in anteposition after it has been brought forward manually.

pesticide Any agent that is used to destroy pests, especially insects, rodents, and fungi.

pestilence An epidemic of a usually deadly disease, especially of the bubonic plague.

pestis Latin for plague.

pestle A club-shaped tool, used for breaking and grinding substances in a mortar.

petechia, *pl.* **petechiae** A small hemorrhage, appearing as a nonraised, purplish-red spot of the skin, nail beds, or mucous membranes.

petiole A slender stalk-like structure; a stem or pedicle. Also called petiolus.

epiglottic p. The pointed lower end of the epiglottic cartilage that is connected by the thyroepiglottic ligament to the back of the thyroid cartilage.

petiolus See petiole.

petit mal See epilepsy, petit mal.

Petri dish A shallow circular container made of glass or plastic with a loose-fitting cover, used for the cultivation of microorganisms. Also called Petri plate.

petrifaction The conversion of an organic substance into stone. Also called fossilization.

petrissage A kneading of the muscles in massage.

petrolatum A pale yellow to amber semisolid mixture of hydrocarbons from petroleum; used as a soothing and lubricant agent and in the preparation of ointments. Also called petroleum jelly; soft paraffin; Vaseline®.

hydrophilic p. A mixture of cholesterol, stearyl alcohol, and white wax.

liquid p. A liquid mixture of hydrocarbons from petroleum; used as an internal lubricant. Also called mineral oil.

white p. White, purified, and deodorized petrolatum.

petrosal Relating to the petrous part of the temporal bone.

petrositis Inflammation of the petrous portion of the temporal bone.

petrous 1. Denoting hardness. 2. Relating to the petrous portion of the temporal bone.

Peutz-Jeghers syndrome, Peutz syndrome A familial disorder characterized chiefly by the presence of numerous polyps in the intestinal tract, especially the jejunum, and dark brown spots on the lips, oral mucosa, and fingers.

peyote, peyotl A small gray-brown cactus, *Lophophora williamsii*, with a carrot-shaped root and a small mushroom-like spineless head ("button"); it has hallucinatory properties.

Peyronie's disease The formation of dense fibrous tissue in the corpus cavernosum of the penis causing painful erection; associated with sclerosis of other parts of the body. Also called fibrous cavernitis.

pH The symbol expressing the degree of alkalinity

---

personality | pH

phagocyte (PMN) — multilobed nucleus, lysosomes (contain acid phosphatase), azurophilic granules, specific granules, mitochondrion, lysosomes

phagocytosis of bacterium — engulfed bacterium, **phagosome**

phalanges of hand — metacarpus, carpus

or acidity of a solution; it denotes the negative logarithm to the base 10 of the hydrogen-ion concentration pH = −log(H+); a solution with pH 7 is neutral; values below 7 indicate a degree of acidity; values above 7 indicate a degree of alkalinity; the normal pH of blood serum is approximately 7.4.

phacitis Inflammation of the eye.

phacoanaphylaxis Introcular inflammation due to hypersensitivity to the protein of the lens of the eye, usually following cataract surgery of one eye.

phacocele Hernia of the lens of the eye, as through a ruptured sclera.

phacocyst Capsule enclosing the lens of the eye.

phacocystectomy Partial removal of the capsule of the lens of the eye.

phacocystitis Inflammation of the capsule of the lens of the eye.

phacoemulsification Removal of a cataractous lens by means of a low frequency ultrasonic needle.

phacoerysis Removal of the lens of the eye by suction.

phacofragmentation The breakup of a cataractous lens of the eye by ultrasonic vibrations.

phacoid Shaped like a lentil.

phacolysis 1. Dissolution of the lens of the eye. 2. Operative procedure to allow dissolution and absorption of the lens.

phacomalacia Softening of the lens of the eye, as may occur in a soft cataract.

phacometachoresis Dislocation of the lens of the eye, either complete or partial.

phacometecesis Displacement of the lens of the eye into the anterior chamber of the eye.

phacoplanesis A free-loating lens of the eye.

phacosclerosis Hardening of the lens of the eye, especially a cataractous lens.

phacoscope An instrument for observing the lens of the eye, especially its changes during accommodation.

phage See bacteriophage.

phagocyte Any cell that ingests bacteria, foreign particles, or other cells.

phagocytic Pertaining to phagocytes or phagocytosis.

phagocytin A basic bactericidal protein found in neutrophils that plays a role in the intracellular destruction of phagocytized gram-negative bacteria.

phagocytize Phagocytose.

phagocytoblast A primitive cell which develops into a phagocyte.

phagocytolysis Destruction of phagocytes.

phagocytose To engulf and digest bacteria and other foreign bodies; denoting the action of phagocytic cells.

phagocytosis A process in which a substance is

engulfed and then held or digested by a cell, as the leukocyte engulfs and destroys pathogens; phagocytosis plays a nutritive and defensive role in cell function.

phagomania A morbid compulsion to eat.

phagosome A compound entity of a phagocytic vesicle combined with a lysosome; formed when a cell ingests a particle by invaginating its cytoplasmic membrane (plasmalemma) and is joined by a lysosome during the process of phagocytosis.

phagotherapy 1. Treatment of infectious disease by a bacteriophage. 2. Treatment by feeding, especially overfeeding.

phagotype In microbiology, a strain of bacteria that differs from other strains of the same species by its vulnerability to the action of a specific virus (bacteriophage).

phalangeal Relating to a phalanx.

phalangectomy 1. Amputation of a finger. 2. Removal of one or more phalanges of a finger or toe.

phalanx, *pl.* **phalanges** Any bone of a finger or toe.

 ungual p. The bone at the end of each digit.

phallectomy Amputation of the penis.

phallic 1. Of, relating to, or resembling a phallus or penis. 2. In psychoanalysis, relating to the penis during the phase of infantile sexuality.

phallicism, phallism Worship of the male genital.

phallocampsis Any curvature of the penis during erection.

phallodynia Pain in the penis.

phalloplasty Reparative surgery of the penis.

phallus Penis.

phanerosis The process of becoming visible.

phantasm The perception of an image; considered a pseudo-hallucination because it is usually recognized as imaginary by the person who sees it.

phantom 1. A teaching model of a bodily part, especially the female pelvis. 2. Something seemingly sensed, but having no physical reality. Also called phantasm; specter.

phantom pain See under pain.

phantosmia The intermittent or persistent odor, pleasant or unpleasant, perceived when no apparent odorant is inhaled.

pharmaceutic, pharmaceutical Relating to pharmacy.

pharmaceutics The branch of science concerned with the preparation and dosage of medicinal products.

pharmacist One who is trained in the preparation and dispensing of drugs. Also called druggist.

pharmacodiagnosis Use of drugs in diagnosis of disease.

pharmacodynamic Relating to the effects of drugs.

pharmacodynamics The study of the effects of drugs on the body and the mechanism of drug action.

pharmacogenetics The branch of biochemical genetics concerned with the genetically determined variations in responses to drugs in man and laboratory animals.

pharmacognosist A practitioner of pharmacognosy.

pharmacognosy, pharmacognostics The branch of pharmacology concerned with the study of medicinal substances in their natural, unprepared, or crude state.

pharmacography A description of drugs in their crude state.

pharmacokinetics The study of the passage of a drug through the body; the extent and rate of absorption, its distribution, localization in tissues, metabolism, and elimination.

pharmacologic Relating to pharmacology.

pharmacologist One who specializes in pharmacology.

pharmacology The branch of science concerned with the unified study of all aspects of the interactions of drugs and their effect on living organisms.

 clinical p. The branch of pharmacology concerned with the effects of drugs on humans.

pharmacomania A morbid impulse to take drugs.

pharmacopedia The total knowledge of crude drugs and medicinal preparations.

pharmacopedics Obsolete term; see pharmacy (1).

pharmacopeia, pharmacopoeia (P) A book containing a list of medicinal drugs, description of their preparation and use, and chemical tests for identifying them and for determining their purity.

pharmacophobia Abnormal fear of taking medicines.

pharmacotherapeutics The administration of drugs in the prevention or treatment of disease and their use in planned alteration of normal function.

pharmacy 1. The preparing and dispensing of medicines. 2. Drugstore.

pharyngalgia Pain in the pharynx. Also called pharyngodynia.

pharyngeal Relating to the pharynx.

pharyngectomy Surgical removal of a portion of the pharynx.

pharyngismus Involuntary convulsive contractions of the pharyngeal muscles. Also called pharyngospasm.

pharyngitis Inflammation of the pharynx.

 fusospirochetal p. Sore throat, foul breath, and

phenacetin

phenformin hydrochloride

phenobarbital

phenolphthalein

phenosulfonphthalein

pharynx

ovarian follicles

ovulation

corpus luteum

luteal phase of menstrual cycle

endometrial layer of uterus

uterine gland

menstrual flow

pharyngeal ulcers covered with a gray film, occasionally accompanied by fever. Also called Vincent's angina; gangrenous pharyngitis.

gangrenous p. See fusospirochetal pharyngitis.

granular p. Pharyngitis with enlargement of the lymphoid follicles of the mucous membrane, which appears granular. Also called clergyman's sore throat.

membranous p. Pharyngitis with a fibrous exudate forming a false membrane.

streptococcal p. Group A streptotoccal respiratory infection, characterized by some or all of the following signs and symptoms: sore red throat, swelling and tenderness of the lymph nodes of the neck, and high fever. Also called hemolytic streptococcal sore throat; strep throat.

pharyngocele Hernial protrusion of the pharyngeal wall into the pharynx.

pharyngodynia Pain in the pharynx. Also called pharyngalgia.

pharyngoesophageal Relating or belonging to the pharynx and the esophagus.

pharyngoglossal Relating to the pharynx and the tongue.

pharyngolaryngeal Relating to both the pharynx and the larynx.

pharyngolaryngitis Inflammation of both the pharynx and the larynx.

pharyngomycosis A fungal invasion of the mucous membrane of the pharynx.

pharyngopalatine Referring to both the pharynx and the palate.

pharyngoplasty Plastic surgery of the pharynx.

pharyngoplegia Paralysis of the muscles of the pharynx.

pharyngorrhinoscopy Visual examination of the nasal portion of the pharynx by means of an instrument (rhinoscope).

pharyngoscleroma A circumscribed area of hard tissue in the mucous membrane of the pharynx.

pharyngoscope An instrument used for inspecting the pharynx.

pharyngoscopy Visual examination of the pharynx.

pharyngospasm The sudden involuntary contraction (spasm) of the pharyngeal muscles. Also called pharyngismus.

pharyngostenosis Constriction of the pharynx.

pharyngotomy Surgical incision of the pharynx.

pharyngotonsillitis Inflammation of the pharynx and tonsils.

pharyngoxerosis Dryness of the mucous membrane of the pharynx.

pharynx A musculomembranous cavity located behind the nasal cavities, mouth, and larynx; it is approximately 12.5 cm long and connects the nose with the larynx and the mouth with the esophagus; the part of the pharynx above the soft palate is the nasopharynx; the portion that lies directly posterior to the mouth is the oropharynx; and the portion behind the larynx and continuous with the esophagus is the laryngopharynx.

phase 1. A stage in a development of cycle. 2. A homogeneous substance (solid, liquid, or gaseous), physically distinct and mechanically separable, present in a heterogeneous chemical system; e.g., the components of an emulsion.

anal p. See stage, anal.

aqueous p. The water portion of a mixture of water and an immiscible liquid.

continuous p. The surrounding or dispersion medium in a heterogeneous mixture. Also called external or dispersion phase.

dispersed p. The insoluble particles in a colloidal solution. Also called internal or enclosed phase.

dispersion p. See continuous phase.

enclosed p. See dispersed phase.

genital p. See stage, genital.

internal p. See dispersed phase.

lag p. The period in the growth of a bacterial culture following inoculation into a medium; there is no increase in cell numbers and very little increase in cell size.

logarithmic p. Period in the development of a bacterial culture in which there is most rapid multiplication.

luteal p. Interval (about 14 days long) of menstrual cycle from formation of corpus luteum to beginning of menstrual flow.

meiotic p. Stage during formation of sexual cells in which the number of chromosomes per cell is halved. Also called reduction phase.

oedipal p. See stage, oedipal.

oral p. See stage, oral.

reduction p. See meiotic phase.

supernormal recovery p. Interval during recovery of heart muscle following excitation, corresponding to the U wave of the electrocardiogram.

phasmid 1. One of a pair of minute lateral postanal chemoreceptors present in roundworms of the class Phasmidia. 2. A roundworm possessing such organs.

phenacetin A bitter compound used as an analgesic and to reduce temperature in fever; when combined in a preparation with aspirin and caffeine, it is commonly known as APC (aspirin, phenacetin, and caffeine). Also called acetophenetidin.

phenanthrene Compound derived from coal; used in the manufacture of dyes and drugs.

phencyclidine (PCP) A hallucinogen that has a pressor effect upon the cardiovascular system. Commonly called angel's dust; peace pill.

phenformin hydrochloride A hypoglycemic agent used alone or in conjunction with sulfonylurea or with insulin in the management of diabetes.

pheniramine maleate An antihistaminic agent.

phenobarbital Phenylethylbarbituric acid, CO-(NHCO)$_2$C(C$_2$H$_5$)(C$_6$H$_5$); used as a sedative and hypnotic. Also called phenobarbitone.

phenobarbitone See phenobarbital.

phenocopy Condition that resembles a genetic disorder but is not inherited; it results from environmental influences.

phenol A caustic crystalline compound, C$_6$H$_5$OH, derived from coal tar; used as an anesthetic and disinfectant. Also called carbolic acid.

phenol red See phenolsulfonphthalein.

phenolphthalein A colorless, crystalline compound, slightly soluble in water; derived from heating phenol with phthalic anhydride in the presence of concentrated sulphuric acid; used as a hydrogen ion indicator (pH 8.2–10.0) and as a cathartic (laxative).

phenolsulfonphthalein (PSP) A dye used by parenteral injection as a test for measuring renal tubular function; also used as an indicator, being yellow at pH 6.8 and red at pH 8.4. Also called phenol red.

phenomenology The study, description, and classification of all possible phenomena in human experience, without attempting to explain or interpret them.

phenomenon, *pl.* **phenomena** An event, manifestation, or fact that is perceptible by the senses.

Arthus p. An inflammatory and, eventually, necrotic lesion produced on the skin of a sensitized animal by the injection of antigen into the skin.

Bell's p. The normal upward turning of the eyes on bilateral closure.

Bordet-Gengou p. The removal of complement from fresh serum, when the serum is incubated with red blood cells or bacteria that have been sensitized with specific lysin.

declamping p. Shock occurring after the removal of clamps from a large blood vessel (e.g., aorta). Also called declamping shock.

déjà vu p. The feeling that an experience, occurring for the first time, has been experienced before.

Donath-Landsteiner p. Destruction of red blood cells occurring when a sample of blood from a person affected with paroxysmal cold hemoglobinuria is cooled to about 5°C and then returned to about 37°C.

escape p. 1. The increase in excretion of sodium and water which occurs after two or three days of

R-on-T phenomenon

phenoxybenzamine hydrochloride

$$OCH_2CH-N-CH_2CH_2Cl \cdot HCl$$
$$CH_3$$

$$NH_2$$
$$CH_2-CH-COOH$$
phenylalanine

$$OH \qquad H$$
$$HO \qquad CH-CH_2-N \qquad \cdot HCl$$
$$CH_3$$
phenylephrine hydrochloride

philtrum

phimosis

narrow opening
of prepuce

glans penis

---

excessive mineralocorticoid activity (endogenous, as in primary aldosteronism, or due to administration of exogenous mineralocorticoid); after the initial phase of sodium and fluid retention there is an "escape" from the sodium-retaining effects and a new equilibrium is established. **2.** After initial constriction, failure of the pupil of an eye to constrict upon repeated and alternate stimulation of both eyes; seen in retrobulbar neuritis.

Goldblatt p. Arterial hypertension caused by partial occlusion of a renal artery. Also called Goldblatt's hypertension.

Gunn's p. Exaggerated opening of the eyes when the mouth is opened and closing of the eyes when the mouth is closed. Also called jaw-winking syndrome.

immune adherence p. The adherence of a cell (platelet, red blood cell, leukocyte, or microorganism), coated with antibody and complement, to normal cells (platelets, etc.), resulting in agglutination. Also called immune adherence.

Pfeiffer's p. Destruction of bacteria when introduced into the peritoneal cavity of an immunized guinea pig, or into that of a normal guinea pig when immune serum is introduced at the same time.

Raynaud's p. Numbness and pallor of the fingers, toes, and/or nose occurring secondary to another disease.

R-on-T p. In electrocardiography, a premature ventricular complex (QRS) interrupting the T wave of the previous beat; predisposes to ventricular tachycardia and/or fibrillation.

Shwartzman p. A reaction elicited when: **1.** Two small subcutaneous doses of endotoxin are given 24 hours apart to an experimental animal; the second injection will cause a localized hemorrhagic necrosis and inflammation of blood vessels. Also called localized Shwartzman phenomenon or reaction. **2.** If the injections are given intravenously, widespread hemorrhages and bilateral necrosis of kidney cortex will occur; the animal dies within 24 hours. Also called generalized Shwartzman phenomenon or reaction.

Wenckebach p. Progressive lengthening of the A-V conduction time (P-R interval) in successive cycles until a beat is dropped.

phenothiazine One of a group of drugs used for antipsychotic effect (e.g., chlorpromazine and promethazine) and for anti-emetic and antihistaminic activity.

phenotype In genetics, the visible appearance of an organism, produced by the interaction of its genetic constitution with the environment.

phenotypic Relating to a phenotype.

phenoxybenzamine hydrochloride An alpha-adrenergic blocking agent that blocks the response of smooth muscle and endocrine glands to the alpha-adrenergic action of epinephrine and norepinephrine; used to treat pheochromocytoma symptoms; Dibenzyline®.

phentolamine An α-adrenergic blocking agent used in the diagnosis of pheochromocytoma; Regitine®.

phenyl The univalent radical of phenol, C_6H_5.

phenylalanine (Phe) An essential amino acid occurring as a constituent of many proteins.

phenylalanine hydroxylase An enzyme that, with NAD (nicotine adenine dinucleotide) as coenzyme, promotes the oxidation of phenylalanine to tyrosine; absence of this enzyme produces phenylketonuria.

phenylbutazone A derivative of pyrazoline, used primarily to relieve pain in musculoskeletal disorders; an anti-inflammatory agent.

phenylephrine hydrochloride A sympathomimetic amine closely related chemically to epinephrine; a powerful vasoconstrictor of sustained action, used as a nasal decongestant, as a mydriatic, and in preventing hypotension during spinal anesthesia; Neo-Synephrine ®.

phenylethylbarbituric acid See phenobarbital.

phenylglycolic acid See mandelic acid.

phenylhydrazine Colorless liquid used in the detection of sugars, aldehydes, and ketones.

phenylketonuria (PKU) Condition in which metabolism of the amino acid phenylalanine (Phe) is deficient, producing increased phenylalanine in the body with resulting nerve and brain cell damage and severe mental retardation; originally known as phenylpyruvic oligophrenia.

phenylpropanolamine hydrochloride Preparation used as a nasal decongestant and bronchodilator.

phenylthiocarbamide See phenylthiourea.

phenylthiourea A substance that is tasteless to those individuals (taste-blind) who are homozygous for an autosomal recessive gene, but tastes bitter to those individuals (tasters) who carry the dominant allele. Also called phenylthiocarbamide.

pheochrome Staining a brownish yellow with chromic salts.

pheochromoblast A young chromaffin (one of the cells forming the medulla of the adrenal gland).

pheochromocyte A chromaffin cell forming the medulla of an adrenal gland, a sympathetic paraganglion, or a pheochromocytoma.

pheochromocytoma A catecholamine-producing tumor of the chromaffin cells of the sympathoadrenal system, usually the adrenal medulla; the symptoms are due to increased secretion of epinephrine and norepinephrine and consist of headache, palpitation, tachycardia, and constant or paroxysmal hypertension of moderate to severe grade.

pheromones Substances secreted externally by an organism that influences the behavior of other organisms of the same species.

phial Vial.

phiala prius agitate (ppa) Latin for shake bottle first.

philtrum The middle vertical groove of the upper lip, below the nose.

phimosis Tightness of the foreskin, so that it cannot be retracted over the glans penis.

phlebalgia Pain originating in a venule or vein.

phlebarteriectasia General dilatation of the veins and arteries.

phlebectasia Dilatation or varicosity of a vein.

phlebectomy Surgical removal of a segment of a vein.

phlebemphraxis Arrest of circulation in a vein by a thrombus. Also called venous thrombosis.

phlebitis Inflammation of a vein.

phleboclysis Injection of medicinal liquids into a vein.

phlebogram A tracing of the venous (usually jugular) pulse made by the phlebograph.

phlebograph A device for recording venous pulsations.

phlebography **1.** The making of phlebograms. **2.** X-ray photography of a vein after intravenous injection with a radiopaque substance. Also called venography.

phlebolith A concretion in a vein resulting from the calcification of an old thrombus. Also called vein stone.

phleboplasty Repair of a vein.

phleborrhagia Bleeding from a vein.

phleborrhaphy Suture of a vein. Also called venisuture.

phleborrhexis Rupture of a vein.

phlebosclerosis Fibrous hardening of the veins, especially the inner coats.

phlebostasis Compression of veins of the extremities for the temporary removal of blood from the circulation. Also called bloodless phlebotomy; venostasis.

phlebothrombosis Clotting of blood within a vein without inflammation of its walls. Cf. thrombophlebitis.

phlebotomize To perform a phlebotomy.

Phlebotomus A genus of bloodsucking sandflies of the family Psychodidae.

P. papatasii The species that is the vector of sandfly fever (phlebotomus or pappataci fever).

phlebotomy Withdrawal of blood from a vein.

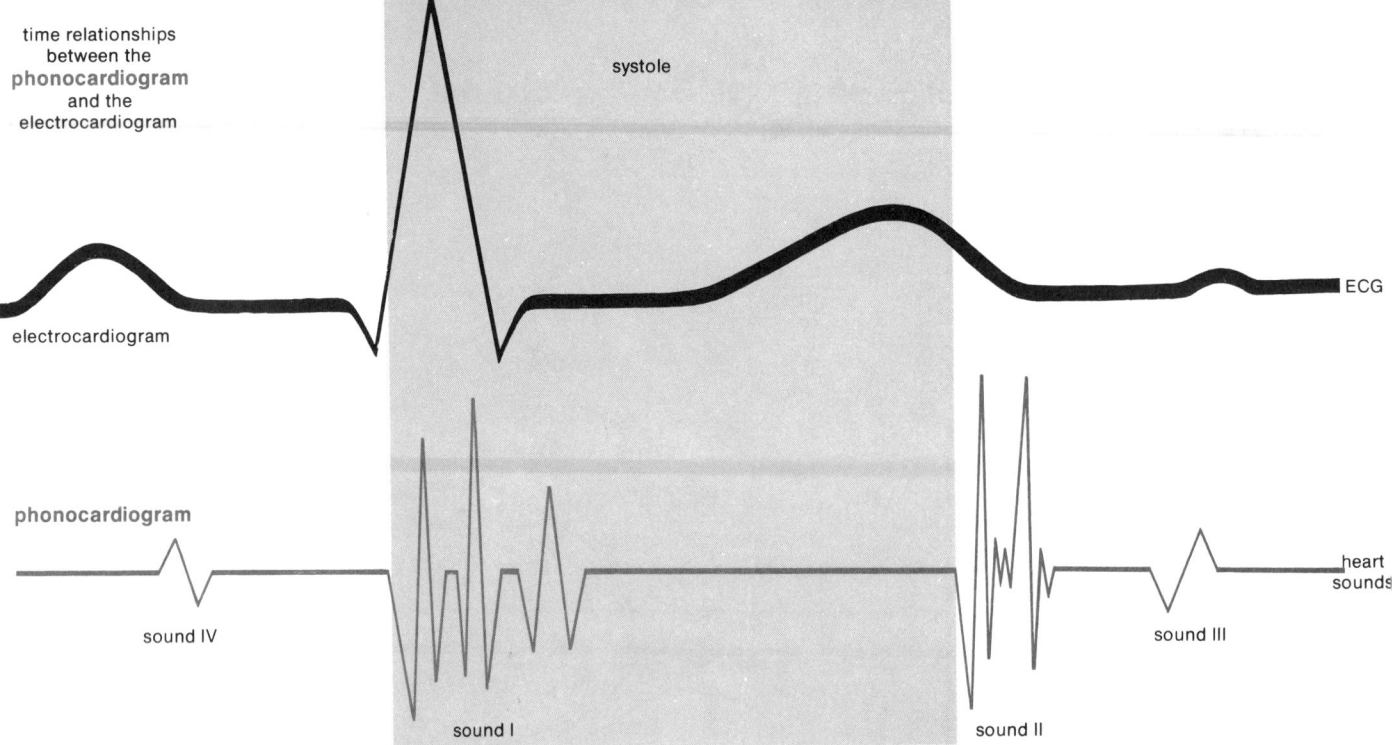

time relationships between the phonocardiogram and the electrocardiogram

systole

electrocardiogram

ECG

phonocardiogram

heart sounds

sound IV

sound I

sound II

sound III

Also called venesection.

phlegm 1. Mucus secreted by the mucosa of the respiratory tract. 2. According to ancient Greek physiology, one of the four humors of the body.

phlegmasia Inflammation.

p. alba dolens Puerperal thrombophlebitis; see under thrombophlebitis.

p. cerulea dolens Severe pain, swelling, and cyanosis of a limb, followed by circulatory collapse and shock, due to thrombosis of the limb.

phlegmatic Apathetic; calm.

phlegmon Acute inflammation of the subcutaneous connective tissue.

phlegmonous Relating to inflammation of subcutaneous tissues.

phlogiston A hypothetical substance of negative mass which, before the discovery of oxygen, was believed to be given off by substances undergoing combustion.

phlorizin Substance extracted from the roots of apple, pear, plum, and cherry trees; injected into experimental animals to produce glycosuria by inhibiting the renal tubular reabsorption of glucose.

phlyctena, *pl.* **phlyctenae** One of several small blisters caused by a burn of the first degree.

phlyctenule A minute red nodular pustule occurring in the conjunctiva or cornea.

phobia Any abnormal, irrational fear.

phobic Relating to abnormal fear.

phobism The state of being affected by a phobia.

phocomelia Gross underdevelopment of extremities, particularly the upper limbs; the hands and feet are attached close to the body, resembling the flippers of a seal.

phocomelus An individual with phocomelia.

phonal Related to the voice.

phonasthenia Difficult or abnormal production of the voice.

phonation The utterance of vocal sounds which are culturally appropriate for human communication.

phonatory Relating to the utterance of vocal sounds.

phonautograph Instrument designed to produce a visible record of a sound.

phoneme The smallest distinctive group of speech sounds in a language.

phonemic Relating to the discrimination of distinctive speech sounds.

phonetic Relating to speech sounds.

phonetics The branch of linguistics concerned with the study of the sounds of speech in all their aspects (their production, combination, and representation by written symbols). Also called phonology.

phoniatrics The study and treatment of speech defects.

phonic Relating to sound or to the voice. Also called phonetic.

phonism A subjective sensation of sound created by, and in addition to, unrelated stimuli, such as light, taste, touch, etc.

phonoangiography The recording and subsequent analysis of sound produced by the blood passing through an artery; useful in determining the extent of narrowing of the lumen by atherosclerosis.

phonocardiogram (PCG) A graphic representation of the heart sounds made with the phonocardiograph.

phonocardiograph An instrument that makes graphic records of the heart sounds.

phonocardiography The recording of the sounds produced by the action of the heart.

phonocatheter A catheter-microphone combination for recording cardiac sounds from within the heart and great vessels.

phono-electrocardioscope A dual-beam oscilloscope that displays both heart sounds and electrocardiographic tracings.

phonogram A symbol representing a sound; e.g., a letter or a syllable in a phonetic alphabet.

phonology The science of speech sounds and their organization into patterns.

phonomassage The application of loud noises in the external auditory canal in order to cause movement of the ear ossicles.

phonometer Apparatus used to measure the intensity and pitch of sounds.

phonopathy Any disease of the organs involved in speech.

phonophore A funnel- or bell-shaped stethoscope.

phonophotography The photographic recording of sound-vibration curves.

phonopneumomassage The application of loud noises and a jet of air into the external auditory canal to produce movement of the ear ossicles.

phonopsia Subjective visual sensations, as of color, induced by the hearing of certain sounds.

phonoreceptor A receptor for sound stimuli.

phonosurgery Surgical procedures upon the larynx, especially the vocal folds, designed for voice preservation, restoration, or enhancement.

phoria The line of direction assumed by one eye in relation to the other eye.

phorometer An instrument for detecting the presence and degree of imbalance of the eye muscles (heterophoria).

phoropter Instrument used to determine the refractive state of the eyes, phorias, amplitude of accommodation, etc.

phose A subjective visual sensation, as of a bright light or color.

phosgene Carbonyl chloride, $COCl_2$; a poisonous gas that condenses to a liquid at temperatures below 8°C.

phosgenic Light-producing.

phosis Any condition that produces subjective visual sensations.

phosphagenic Phosphate-producing.

phosphatase Any of a group of enzymes that promote the hydrolysis of phosphoric esters.

acid p. One active in an acid medium; present in all cells except erythrocytes.

alkaline p. One active in an alkaline medium; found in bone, blood, kidneys, and other tissues.

phosphate A salt or ester of phosphoric acid.

phosphated Containing phosphates.

phosphatic Relating to phosphates.

phosphatidic acid An acid that results from the partial hydrolysis of a phospholipid and that on hydrolysis yields two fatty acid molecules and one molecule each of glycerol and phosphoric acid.

phosphatidylcholine A phospholipid compound resulting from condensation of phosphatidic acid and choline. Also called lecithin.

phosphatidylethanolamine A phospholipid, the product of condensation of phosphatidic acid and ethanolamine. Also called cephalin.

phosphaturia The presence of a high percentage of phosphates in the urine.

phosphene A sensation of light experienced upon pressure on, or electrical stimulation of, the eyeball.

phosphide A compound containing trivalent phosphorus; e.g., sodium phosphide, Na_3P.

phosphine PH_3; a colorless, poisonous gas of characteristic odor. Also called hydrogen phosphide; phosphorated hydrogen.

phosphite A salt of phosphorous acid.

phosphoarginine Compound serving as a store of energy for muscle contraction in invertebrates; it corresponds to phosphocreatine in muscles of vertebrates.

phosphocreatine Creatine phosphate; see under creatine.

phosphodiester A diesterified orthophosphoric acid; $RO-PO_2H-OR-$, as in the nucleic acids.

phosphodiesterase One of a group of enzymes that split phosphodiester bonds, as those between nucleotides.

phosphoenolpyruvic acid A high-energy compound, intermediate in the conversion of glucose to pyruvic acid.

phosphofructokinase An enzyme of the glycolytic pathway that catalyzes the phosphorylation of fructose-6-phosphate to fructose-1,6-diphosphate in

INTERACTION BETWEEN RADIATION AND MATTER

x-ray photon

photoelectric collision

photoelectron (high energy electron)

scattered x-ray (deviated original photon)

photoelectron

ion pair

ion pair

$+ H_3PO_4$

amylose

phosphorolysis

CH_2OH

OPO_3H_2

glucose-1-phosphate

$+$

$n-1$

the presence of ATP and Mg^{++}; it controls the rate of glucose-6-phosphate utilization.

phosphoglucomutase Enzyme that promotes the reaction glucose-6-phosphate $\rightleftharpoons$ glucose-1-phosphate.

phosphokinase See phosphotransferase.

phospholipase Any enzyme that catalyzes the hydrolysis of a phospholipid. Also called lecithinase.

phospholipid A class of waxy or greasy compounds containing phosphoric acid; most of them occur in plant and animal tissues, especially in membranes, such as the myelin sheath of nerve cells and red blood cell membranes; phosphatidylcholine, phosphatidylethanolamine, and sphingomyelin are examples.

phosphoprotein One of a group of conjugated proteins containing a simple protein combined with a phosphorous compound; e.g., casein.

phosphor A substance that glows when stimulated by external radiation; used in the detection of radioactivity.

phosphorated Combined with phosphorus.

phosphorescence 1. The afterglow or continuous emission of light from a substance, without temperature rise, after exposure to light, heat, or electric current; distinguished from fluorescence, in which light is emitted essentially only when the exciting source is present. 2. The faint greenish glow of white phosphorus in the presence of air, due to slow oxidation. 3. The luminescence of certain living organisms such as fire flies.

phosphorescent Having the capacity to glow, especially in the dark.

phosphoribosyltransferase One of a group of enzymes (important in nucleotide biosynthesis) that transfer ribose 5-phosphate from 5-phospho-α-D-ribosyl 1-pyrophosphate to a purine, pyrimidine, or pyridine acceptor.

phosphoric acid H$_3$PO$_4$; colorless crystals that are soluble in water and important as a source of phosphate groups in metabolism; the principal component of silicate and zinc phosphate dental cement liquids.

phosphorism Chronic poisoning with phosphorus.

phosphorized Phosphorated.

phosphorolysis A reaction analogous to hydrolysis in which the elements of phosphoric acid, rather than of water, are added in the course of splitting a bond; the conversion of glycogen to glucose 1-phosphate is an example.

phosphorous 1. Relating to, or containing, phosphorus. 2. Phosphorescent.

phosphorus A poisonous nonmetallic element, symbol P, atomic number 15, atomic weight 30.975;

it occurs in nature always in combined form, as inorganic phosphates in minerals and water and as organic phosphates in all living cells.

phosphorus-32 (^{32}P) A beta-emitting radioactive phosphorus isotope with atomic weight 32 and with a half-life of 14.3 days; used in brain, eye, skin, and stomach tumor localization, as a tracer to study metabolism, and in the treatment of certain osseous and hematopoietic disorders.

phosphorylase An enzyme that triggers the splitting of the glycogen molecule to form glucose.

phosphorylation The addition of phosphate to an organic compound through the action of a phosphorylase.

phosphotransferase An enzyme that catalyzes the transfer of phosphorous-containing groups. Also called phosphokinase.

phosphotungstic acid Green crystals, soluble in water, used as a reagent for alkaloids and for albumin.

phot A unit of illumination equal to one lumen per square centimeter of surface.

photalgia Pain in the eyes caused by light. Also called photodynia.

photesthesia Perception of light.

photic Relating to light.

photism Production of a visual sensation by stimulation of another sense organ.

photoactinic Producing luminous and chemical effects, said of radiation.

photoallergy See photosensitization.

photobiology The study of the effect of light on organisms (plants or animals).

photobiotic Capable of living only in the light.

photocatalyst A substance that brings about a light-stimulated reaction; e.g., chlorophyll.

photoceptor See photoreceptor.

photochemistry The branch of chemistry concerned with chemical changes caused by light.

photochemotherapy Treatment of disease with drugs that react to ultraviolet radiation.

photochromogens Group I mycobacteria, mycobacteria that produce a bright yellow pigment when grown in the presence of light.

photocoagulation Coagulation of protein material in the tissues with the heat generated by an intense, precisely focused beam of light from a carbon arc or laser; used in the treatment of retinal detachment and other intraocular conditions.

photocoagulator Apparatus used in photocoagulation.

    laser p. A laser combined with an ophthalmoscope; used in the treatment of retinal detachment to direct laser beams into selected areas of the detached retina.

photodermatitis 1. Development of skin lesions in areas exposed to sunlight; seen in individuals who have developed a sensitivity to certain drugs; e.g., tetracycline. 2. Any inflammatory skin condition in which light is an important causative factor.

photodisintegration Nuclear deterioration due to absorption of high-energy radiation.

photodynamic Relating to the energy-producing effects of light.

photodynia See photalgia.

photoelectricity Electricity resulting from the action of light.

photoelectrometer Device used to measure concentration of substances in solution by means of a photoelectric cell.

photoelectron An electron which has been set free (ejected from its orbit) by collision with a high energy photon.

photogen A bacterium producing luminescence.

photogenesis The production of light.

photogenic, photogenous Producing light.

photokinesis In biology, movement in response to light.

photoluminescent Having the ability to emit light at room temperature after exposure to radiant energy of a different wavelength.

photolysis Decomposition of a chemical compound by the action of radiant energy, especially light.

photolyte A product of chemical decomposition caused by light.

photomacrography The photographic recording of images of gross specimens at low magnification using photomacro lenses mounted on a camera.

photometer Instrument used to measure the intensity of a light source. Also called illuminometer.

photometry The measurement of the intensity of a light source.

photomicrograph Photograph of an object as viewed through the microscope.

photomicrography The photographic recording of images seen through a microscope.

photon A unit or quantum of energy of a light wave or other electromagnetic wave, regarded as a minute particle of no electric charge and zero mass.

photoperceptive See photoreceptive.

photoperiod The varying length of exposure of a living organism to light.

photoperiodism The physiologic response of living organisms to varying periods of exposure to light (photoperiod).

photophobia Abnormal intolerance or fear of light.

photophobic Relating to abnormal intolerance or fear of light.

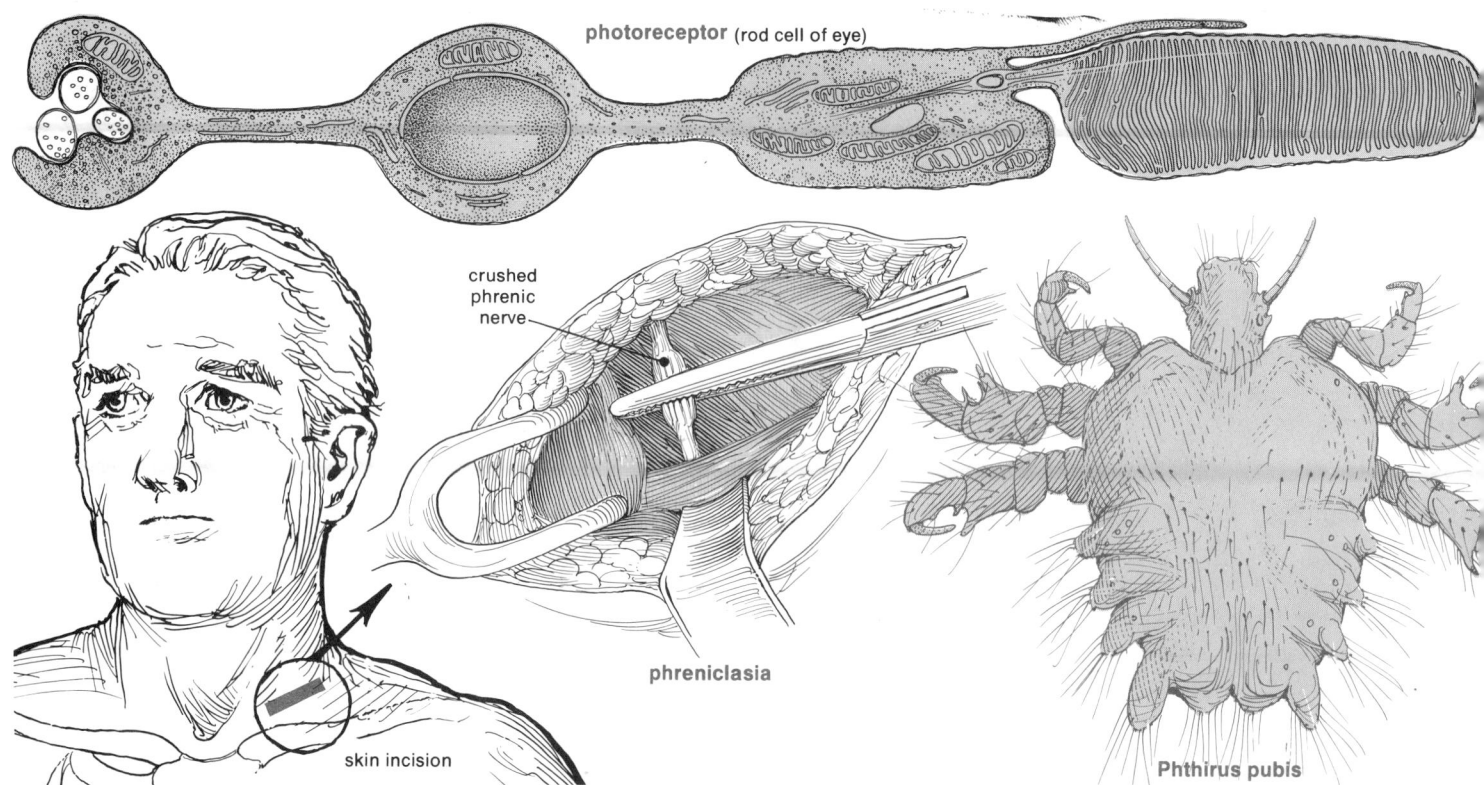

photoreceptor (rod cell of eye)

crushed phrenic nerve

phreniclasia

skin incision

Phthirus pubis

photophthalmia Inflammation of the eyes caused by exposure to intense light, as in snow blindness.

photopsia, photopsy A subjective sensation of flashing light and sparks experienced with certain diseases of the retina, optic nerve, or brain.

photopsin The protein constituent (opsin) of the pigment (iodopsin) in the retinal cones.

photoreactivation The reversal of a photochemical reaction by exposure to light; e.g., reversal of the effect of ultraviolet rays on cells by exposure to visible light rays.

photoreceptive Capable of perceiving light rays. Also called photoperceptive.

photoreceptor A nerve end-organ capable of being stimulated by light, as the rods and cones of the retina. Also called photoceptor.

photoretinitis Inflammation of the retina caused by exposure to intense light.

photoscan A photograph of the distribution and concentration of an internally administered radiopaque substance.

photosensitization Hypersensitization of skin to sunlight or ultraviolet rays; caused by ingestion of certain plants or drugs. Also called photoallergy.

photostable Unchanged upon exposure to light.

photosynthesis The process by which green plants, using chlorophyll and the energy of sunlight, turn carbon dioxide and water into food substance (carbohydrate); molecular oxygen is liberated in the process.

phototaxis, phototaxy Movement of an organism (as a whole) toward or away from a light source. Cf. phototropism.

phototherapy Treatment of disease with light.

photothermal 1. Relating to both light and heat. 2. Relating to heat produced by light.

phototoxic Relating to an injurious effect produced or promoted by overexposure to light, ultraviolet rays, or x rays.

phototropism, phototropy Movement of parts of an organism toward or away from a light source. Cf. phototaxis.

phren 1. Greek for diaphragm. 2. The mind.

phrenectomy See phrenicectomy.

phrenemphraxis See phreniclasia.

phrenic Relating to the diaphragm.

phrenicectomy Surgical removal of a portion of the phrenic nerve. Also called phrenectomy.

phreniclasia Crushing of a portion of the phrenic nerve. Also called phrenemphraxis.

phrenicotomy Division of a phrenic nerve in order to paralyze one-half of the diaphragm.

phrenocolic Relating to the diaphragm and the colon.

phrenogastric Relating to the diaphragm and the stomach.

phrenohepatic Relating to the diaphragm and the liver.

phrenology An obsolete doctrine concerned with the study of mental capacity and traits of character based upon the external configuration of the skull.

phrenoplegia Paralysis of the diaphragm.

phrenosin A cerebroside present in the white matter of the brain. Also called cerebron.

phrenotropic Exerting its foremost effect upon the mind or brain.

phrynoderma A dry eruption of the skin thought to be due to vitamin A deficiency.

phthalein Any of various dyes, such as phenolphthalein, derived from the condensation of phthalic anhydride with the phenols; some are used as indicators and occasionally as purgatives.

phthiriasis Infestation with the species of lice *Phthirus pubis*, more commonly known as crabs.

Phthirus A genus of sucking lice of the order Anoplura.

  P. pubis A parasite of man infesting areas of coarse hair, particularly in the pubic region, but also the hair of the chest, axillae, eyebrows, and eyelashes. Also called pubic or crab louse.

phthisic Relating to or afflicted with phthisis.

phthisiology The study and treatment of pulmonary tuberculosis.

phthisis 1. Tuberculosis. 2. A wasting away of tissue.
  black p., miners' p. Anthracosis.
  marble cutters' p. See calcicosis.
  potters' p. See silicosis.
  stonecutters' p. Pneumoconiosis.

phycomycosis General term for acute and chronic systemic diseases caused by fungi of the class Phycomycetes (Zygomycetes), usually occurring in debilitated individuals.

phylaxis Protection against infection.

phylogenesis The evolutionary development or racial history of the species; distinguished from ontogenesis. Also called phylogeny.

phylogeny See phylogenesis.

phylum One of the first divisions of the animal or vegetable kingdom; below subkingdom and above subphylum.

phyma A small skin tumor.

phymatosis Disorder marked by the presence of small nodules (phymas) in the skin.

physiatrics The branch of medicine concerned with diagnosis and treatment of disease of the neuromusculoskeletal systems with physical elements (heat, cold, water, electricity, etc.) to bring about maximal restoration of physical, physiological, social, and vocational function. Also called physical medicine or rehabilitation.

physiatrist A physician who specializes in physiatrics (physical medicine or rehabilitation).

physic Any medicine, especially a cathartic.

physical Relating to the body.

physician A doctor of medicine; an individual trained and licensed to treat the ill and injured.

physician assistant (P.A.) An individual who has been trained in primary care medicine and is licensed to practice (in the United States) under the supervision of a physician.

physicochemical Relating to both physics and chemistry.

physics The science concerned with the study of matter and energy and the interactions between the two.

physiognomy 1. The art of judging human character and mental qualities from facial features and general bodily carriage. 2. The countenance, especially regarded as an indication of the character.

physiologic, physiological 1. Relating to physiology. 2. Denoting the various normal processes of a living organism.

physiologist A specialist in physiology.

physiology The science concerned with the normal functions and activities of the living organism.

physiotherapy Physical therapy; see under therapy.

physique The structure of the body with reference to its proportions, muscular development, and appearance. Also called biotype.

physohematometra Distention of the uterine cavity with gas and blood.

physostigmine, physostigmin A crystalline compound extracted from the Calabar bean; it is a reversible inhibitor of the cholinesterases and prevents destruction of acetylcholine. Also called eserine.

  p. salicylate Used topically to reduce intraocular tension in glaucoma; also used to overcome excessive cholinergic activity. Also called eserine salicylate.

phytin The mixed magnesium-calcium salt of phytic acid; used as a dietary supplement.

phytoagglutinin See lectin.

phytobezoar An undigested concretion remaining in the stomach over a long period, composed mostly of vegetable fibers, seeds and skins of fruits, and sometimes starch granules and fat globules.

phytohemagglutinin (PHA) An extract derived from the stringbean; originally used as a red blood cell agglutinating reagent; it stimulates human lym-

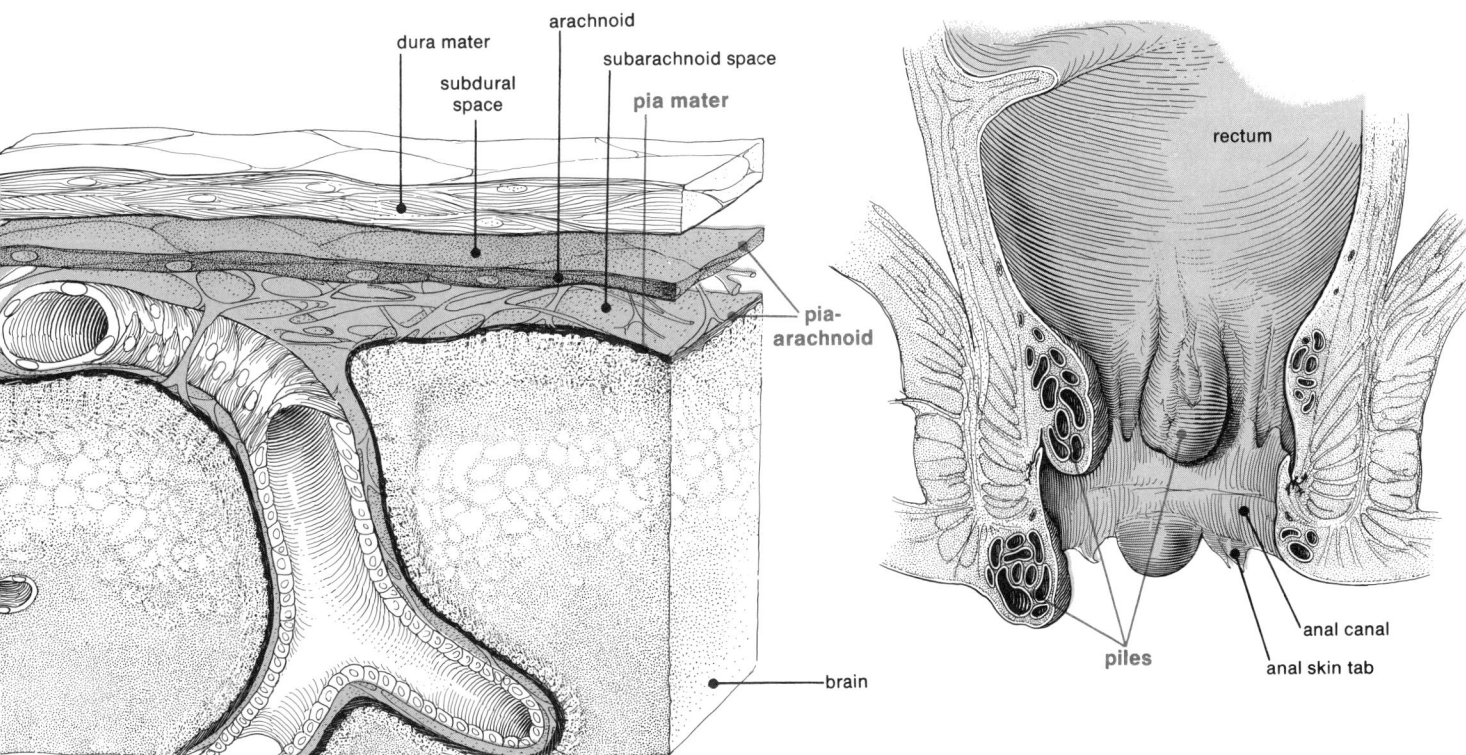

dura mater
subdural space
arachnoid
subarachnoid space
pia mater
pia-arachnoid
brain

rectum
anal canal
piles
anal skin tab

---

phoid cells to divide, replicate their DNA, and transcribe RNA.

phytoid Resembling a plant.

phytol An unsaturated alcoholic fragment obtained on hydrolysis of chlorophyll; an open-chain terpene; used for the synthesis of vitamins E and K₁.

phytopathology The study of plant diseases.

phytotoxic Having a poisonous effect on plant life; inhibiting plant growth.

phytotoxin A toxin produced by certain higher plants.

pia-arachnoid The pia mater and arachnoid as one functional unit.

pial Relating to the pia mater.

pia mater A delicate membrane, innermost of the three membranes enveloping the brain and spinal cord.

pian See yaws.

piarachnoid Pia-arachnoid.

pica Perverted appetite marked by a craving for unnatural food or substances.

pickling In dentistry, the method of removing impurities and oxides from the surface of metals by immersion in acid.

pickwickian syndrome A condition characterized by extreme obesity, breathlessness on exertion, and somnolence; similar to primary alveolar hypoventilation; arterial Pco₂ is elevated; cyanosis, tachycardia, and evidence of heart failure are common; named for the fat boy in Dickens' *Pickwick Papers*.

picogram (pg) A unit of weight equal to one trillionth of a gram (10⁻¹² g). Also called micromicrogram (μμg).

Picornaviridae A large family of viruses that contain single-stranded RNA and multiply in cytoplasm; represents the smallest known viruses (20 to 30 nm in diameter) and includes viruses causing poliomyelitis, meningitis, myocarditis, hepatitis type A, and the common cold. Also called picornavirus group.

picrate A salt of picric acid.

picric acid Crystalline compound used as a reagent and in dyes and antiseptics. Also called trinitrophenol; carbazotic acid.

picrocarmine Solution containing ammonia and picric acid, used to stain tissues in histology.

picroformol Substance containing formalin and picric acid; used as a fixative.

picrotoxin The bitter powder obtained from the fruit of *Anamirta cocculus;* a central nervous system stimulant formerly used as an antidote for barbiturate poisoning.

piebaldness Localized areas of depigmented scalp and hair. Also called albinismus conscriptus.

piedra Spanish for stone; a fungal disease of the hair characterized by formation of numerous small, hard, waxy concretions on extruded hairshafts. Also called trichosporosis.

Pierre Robin syndrome A syndrome characterized by respiratory obstruction in infants with a receding jaw and glossoptosis; frequently accompanied by cleft palate. Also called primary micrognathia; Robin syndrome.

piesesthesia Sensitivity to different degrees of pressure. Also called pressure sense.

piezochemistry The study of the effects of extremely high pressures on chemical reactions.

piezoelectricity Electricity generated by pressure applied to certain crystals.

pigeon-toe The turning in of the feet on walking; may be a physical sign of other disorders such as metatarsus adductus, medial torsion of the tibia, bowlegs, and congenital contraction of the internal rotators of the hip. Also called in-toeing.

pigment 1. Any colored material present in skin, whether deposited in the tissue proper or present in the blood passing through the skin. 2. Any substance that produces a characteristic color in tissue, such as hemoglobin.

hepatogenous p. Bile pigment derived from the destruction of hemoglobin in the liver.

malarial p. Denatured hemoglobin products, in rods or granules within the malarial parasite.

melanotic p. Melanin.

visual p. The photosensitive pigment in the rod and cone cells of the retina that initiates vision by the absorption of light.

pigmentation Coloration by deposition of pigment.

pigmentum nigrum The dark pigment lining the choroid layer of the eye.

piitis Inflammation of the pia mater.

pilar, pilaris, pilary Pertaining to or covered with hair.

pilaster An abnormally prominent linea aspera on the femur, resulting in a backward concavity.

pile 1. A single hemorrhoid. 2. A vertical series of alternate plates of two different metals separated by layers of cloth or paper moistened with a dilute acid solution for producing a current of electricity. Also called voltaic or Volta's pile. 3. A battery consisting of cells similarly constructed.

atomic p. Apparatus containing alternate layers of uranium and graphite in which a chain reaction is initiated and controlled, for the production of heat for power or for the production of plutonium. Also called nuclear reactor; atomic furnace.

sentinel p. A hemorrhoid-like tag at the end of

an anal fissure.

piles Hemorrhoids.

pileus A nipple shield.

p. ventriculi The first portion of the duodenum as seen in an x-ray picture. Also called duodenal cap.

pili Plural of pilus.

pill 1. A small tablet of medicine. 2. An oral contraceptive, commonly referred to as *the pill*.

bread p. A placebo made of bread.

enteric coated p. A pill coated with a substance, such as salol, which prevents its disintegration until it has reached the intestine.

pep p. Colloquialism for an amphetamine or a related pharmaceutical with a pronounced stimulant effect on the central nervous system.

pillar Any vertical anatomic structure somewhat resembling a supporting column.

Corti's p.'s The pillars forming the center and inner walls of the tunnel in the spiral organ of Corti.

p.'s of the fauces, anterior A pair of mucous membrane folds that pass downward from the soft palate to the side of the tongue. Also called glossopalatine arch.

p.'s of the fauces, posterior A pair of mucous membrane folds which pass downward from the posterior margin of the soft palate to the lateral wall of the pharynx. Also called pharyngopalatine arch.

pill-rolling The circular motion of the tips of the thumb and index finger, characteristic of paralysis agitans.

pilocarpine An alkaloid obtained from the leaves of the jaborandi tree; a parasympathomimetic agent used to induce sweating or to increase salivary secretion; also acts topically to contract the pupils and reduce intraocular pressure.

pilocarpus A small genus of shrubs (family Rutaceae) native to the West Indies and tropical America; source of the alkaloid, pilocarpine.

pilocystic Denoting a cyst, usually dermoid, containing hair.

piloerection Erection of hairs.

pilomatrixoma A benign tumor of the growing portion of the hair apparatus. Also called Malherbe's calcifying epithelioma.

pilomotor Relating to muscles or nerves in the skin that control the movement of hairs, as in the formation of goose pimples.

pilonidal Denoting the presence of hairs in a dermoid cyst or ingrown hairs in the deep layers of skin.

pilose Covered with hair.

pilosebaceous Relating to the sebaceous glands that open into the hair follicles.

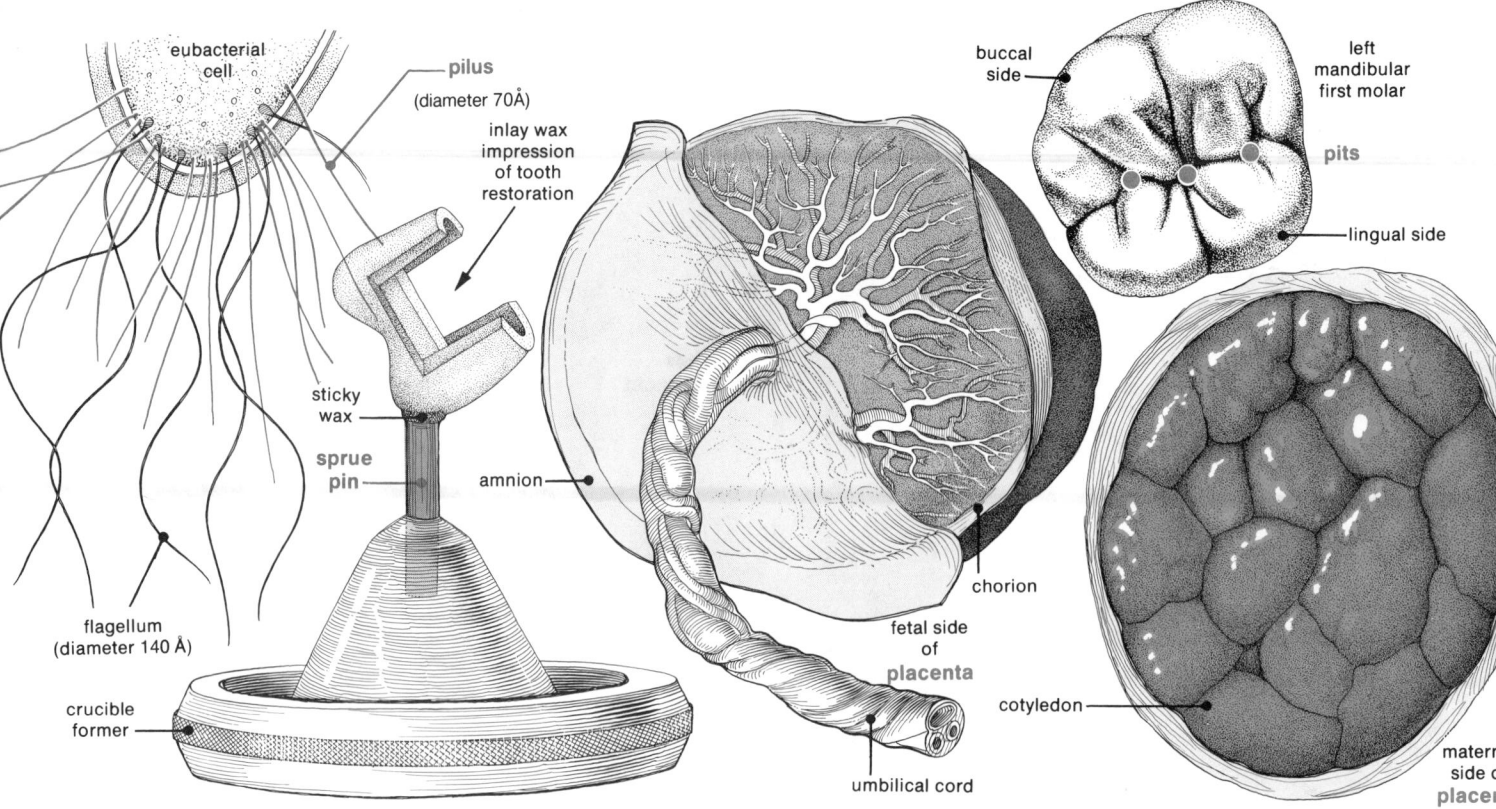

eubacterial cell

pilus (diameter 70Å)

inlay wax impression of tooth restoration

sticky wax

sprue pin

flagellum (diameter 140 Å)

crucible former

amnion

chorion

fetal side of **placenta**

umbilical cord

buccal side

left mandibular first molar

pits

lingual side

cotyledon

matern side o **placen**

pilosis Hirsutism.

pilus, *pl.* **pili 1.** One of the fine hairs covering almost the entire surface of the human body. **2.** A fine, hollow, strawlike filamentous appendage, somewhat analogous to the flagellum, that occurs on some bacteria; it serves to anchor the bacterial cell to the substrate on which it is growing; pili are shorter, straighter, and more numerous than flagella. Also called fimbria.

pimelosis 1. Obesity. **2.** Fatty degeneration.

pi-meson See pion.

pimple A small inflamed swelling of the skin. Also called papule; pustule.

pin A short, straight, cyclindrical piece of metal.

  retention p.'s Small griplike pegs extending from a metal casting into the tooth's dentin.

  sprue p. A short metal pin used to attach a dental wax pattern to the crucible former; it provides the entrance through the investment, permitting the molten metal to flow into the mold.

  Steinman's p. A firm metal pin used for the internal fixation of fractured bones.

pincement In massage, a manipulation in which the skin is gently nipped or pinched.

pineal 1. Shaped like a pine cone. **2.** Relating to the pineal body.

pinealectomy Surgical removal of the pineal body.

pinealocyte One of the cells forming the substance of the pineal body.

pinealoma A relatively rare tumor derived from the pineal gland.

pinguecula A small, slightly raised, yellowish, nonfatty thickening of the conjunctiva of the eye near the sclerocorneal junction, usually on the nasal side.

piniform Pineal (1).

pink disease See acrodynia.

pinkeye Acute contagious inflammation of the conjunctiva.

pin-lay In dentistry, a veneer containing parallel pins for retention.

pinledge In dentistry, vertical parallel pins placed in a tooth or teeth to aid in retention of a restoration.

pinna The projecting portion of the external ear. Also called auricle.

pinocyte A cell that engulfs liquids in a way that resembles the engulfment of solid particles by a phagocyte.

pinocytosis The engulfment of liquid droplets by a cell through minute invaginations formed on the surface, which close to form fluid-filled vacuoles (vesicles); by this process, protein is reabsorbed from the filtrate by tubular cells of the kidney; the phe-nomenon is similar to phagocytosis (the engulfing of solid particles).

pinosome A membrane-bounded vesicle containing pinocytosed fluid.

pint (pt) 1. A unit of liquid measure equal to 16 fluid ounces or 28.875 cubic inches. **2.** A unit of dry measure equal to 33.6 cubic inches.

  imperial p. A British unit of liquid or dry measure equal to 34.659 cubic inches; 20 fluid ounces.

pinta A nonvenereal infection caused by the spirochete *Treponema carateum;* endemic in Mexico, Colombia, Cuba, and the Philippines.

pinworm A nematode worm, *Enterobius vermicularis,* that infests the intestines, especially in children. Also called seat worm (because it may cause pruritus ani); threadworm.

pion A small particle found in the nuclei of atoms; it constitutes the force that holds neutrons and protons together. Also called pi-meson.

piperazine Compound used effectively against the intestinal worms *Ascaris* and *Oxyuris.*

pipette, pipet A calibrated glass tube, open at both ends, used for transferring and/or measuring small quantities of liquids in laboratory work.

  automatic p. An instrument for transferring small amounts of liquid repetitively and automatically.

piriform Pear-shaped.

pisiform Pea-shaped or pea-sized; e.g., one of the carpal bones.

pit 1. Any natural depression on the surface of the body. **2.** A pockmark. **3.** A pointed depression in dental enamel at the junction of two or more developmental grooves, as in the occlusal and buccal surfaces of molars.

pitch One of three important properties of sound (others are intensity and quality) denoting the function of the number of vibrations of sound waves per second; the greater the number of vibrations per unit time, the higher the pitch. Commonly called tone.

pitchblende A brownish-black mineral containing a large proportion of uranium oxide; it is the principal source of radium.

pith 1. The center of a hair. **2.** To pierce the medulla of a laboratory animal, usually by the insertion of a needle or a knife at the base of the skull, to render the animal nonfeeling.

pitocin See oxytocin.

pituicyte The dominant type of cell (fusiform) of the posterior lobe of the pituitary gland.

pituitary 1. Relating to the pituitary gland (hypophysis). **2.** A preparation obtained from either the anterior or posterior lobe of the pituitary gland of domesticated animals; used therapeutically by man.

pityriasis A skin disease marked by fine scaly desquamation.

  p. rosea An eruption of papules of unknown cause usually involving the trunk and the extremities; it begins as an oval patch (herald patch) 6 to 8 cm in diameter, followed in a few days by a generalized eruption which disappears spontaneously in 1 to 2 months; the disorder is benign and exposure to the sun is thought to accelerate clearing; because the lesions may resemble those of secondary syphilis, it is prudent to perform a serologic test for syphilis.

pityroid Scaly.

Pityrosporum A genus of nonpathogenic, yeastlike fungi which produce extremely fine spores and no mycelium; generally found in dandruff and seborrheic dermatitis.

pivot A part about which a related structure rotates or swings.

placebo An inert substance containing no medication but prescribed as medicine, given especially to satisfy a patient; also used in controlled studies to determine the efficacy of drugs.

placenta The organ within the pregnant uterus through which the fetus derives its nourishment; at term it averages one-sixth the weight of the fetus; it is disk-shaped, about 2.5 cm thick, and 17.5 cm in diameter.

  accessory p. A mass of placental tissue distinct from the main placenta.

  fundal p. A placenta that is implanted in the fundus of the uterus.

  p. previa Condition in which the placenta is implanted in the lower segment of the uterus and covers the cervical opening, partly or completely.

  retained p. One that is not expelled after childbirth.

placental Relating to the placenta.

placentascan Determination of the location of the placenta by the use of ultrasound or by means of a scintillation detector after injection of a radioactive substance. Also called placental scan.

placentation The development and organization of the placenta after attachment of the blastocyst to the uterine wall or other structures.

placentitis Inflammation of the placenta; usually limited to the fetal surface, involving especially the zone between the amnion and chorion.

placentography The making of roentgenograms of the placenta following injection of a radiopaque substance.

placode An ectodermal thickening in the early embryo from which a sense organ or a structure

coronal plane

horizontal plane

vertebra

sacrum

coccyx

pelvic plane of inlet

hipbone

pelvic plane of greatest dimension

transpyloric plane

subcostal plane

inter- tubercular plane

inter- spinous plane

right lateral rectus **sagittal plane**

left lateral rectus **sagittal plane**

pelvic plane of midpelvis

pelvic plane of outlet

develops; e.g., lens placode.

pladarosis, pladaroma A soft, wartlike tumor on the eyelid.

plagiocephaly Malformation of the skull in which one side is more developed anteriorly and the other side posteriorly.

plague 1. Acute infectious disease caused by *Yersinia pestis* and marked by high fever, prostration, glandular swelling, or pneumonia; transmitted to humans by fleas that have bitten infected rodents. **2.** Any widespread disease or one causing excessive mortality.

bubonic p. A form marked by buboes (inflammatory enlargement of lymphatic glands).

hemorrhagic p. Bubonic plague in which bleeding may occur into an organ or from the nose and alimentary, respiratory, or urinary tracts.

pneumonic p. A fatal form accompanied by pneumonia with abundant bloodstained sputum.

septicemic p. A variant of bubonic plague leading to death so quickly that localized lesions do not become clinically apparent.

sylvatic p. Bubonic plague in wild animals, especially rodents.

planchet A flat metal disk container on which a radioactive sample is placed while its activity is measured.

plane 1. A flat or level surface. **2.** An imaginary surface formed by extension through any axis or two definite points. **3.** A particular level, as a stage in surgical anesthesia.

bite p. A dental appliance that covers the palate and has an inclined or flat plane at the front border that offers resistance to the upper incisors when they make contact.

coronal p. A vertical plane that passes from side to side at right angles to the sagittal plane, dividing the head into anterior and posterior portions; often used interchangeably with frontal plane.

frontal p. A vertical plane passing at right angles to the sagittal plane, dividing the body into anterior and posterior portions. Cf. coronal plane.

guide p. A plane formed in the occlusal surfaces of occlusion rims to position the lower jaw in centric relation.

horizontal p. The plane extending across the long axis of the body separating an upper portion from the lower part. Also called transverse plane.

intercristal p. A horizontal plane passing through the highest points of the iliac crests; it lies at the level of the fourth lumbar vertebra.

interspinous p. A horizontal plane transecting the body at the level of the anterior superior iliac spine.

intertubercular p. A horizontal plane passing through the tubercles of the iliac crests; it lies at the level of the fifth lumbar vertebra.

median sagittal p. A sagittal plane that passes through the midline.

parasagittal p. Any vertical plane parallel to the sagittal plane.

pelvic p. of greatest dimension The roomiest portion of the pelvic cavity extending from the middle of the posterior surface of the pubic symphysis to the junction of the second and third sacral vertebrae, passing laterally through the ischial bone over the middle of the acetabulum; its anteroposterior diameter is approximately 12.75 cm and its transverse diameter is around 12.5 cm.

pelvic p. of inlet (superior strait) The heart-shaped upper opening of the true pelvis, bounded anteriorly by the upper border of the pubis, laterally by the iliopectineal line, and posteriorly by the sacral promontory.

pelvic p. of midpelvis Plane of least pelvic dimension extending from the lower margin of the pubic symphysis through the ischial spines to the sacrum; the anteroposterior diameter measures approximately 11.5 cm and its transverse diameter is around 10.0 cm.

pelvic p. of outlet (inferior strait) The lower opening of the true pelvis bounded anteriorly by the pubic arch, laterally by the ischial tuberosities, and posteriorly by the tip of the coccyx.

p.'s of reference Planes that serve as a guide for the location of other planes.

sagittal p. A vertical plane extending in an anteroposterior direction.

subcostal p. A horizontal plane passing through the lowest point of the costal margin on each side, generally the inferior border of the tenth costal cartilage.

transpyloric p. A horizontal plane passing through the tips of the ninth costal cartilages; the plane passes through the pylorus, the neck of the pancreas, and the hili of the kidneys.

transverse p. See horizontal plane.

planigraphy Tomography.

planimeter A device that measures the area of any surface by tracing its boundaries with a mechanically coupled pointer.

plano Having a flat surface; said of an afocal lens, i.e., one without refractive power.

planoconcave Flat on one side and curved inward on the other; denoting a lens of that shape.

planoconvex Flat on one side and curved outward on the other; denoting a lens of that shape.

planta, *pl.* **plantae** Latin for the sole of the foot.

plantago Any plant of the genus *Plantago*.

Plantago A large genus of herbs (family Plantaginaceae) comprised chiefly of roadside weeds.

P. psyllium Species producing seeds which are used as a mild laxative. Also called Spanish psyllium; Old World plantain. See also seed, plantago.

plantago seed See under seed.

plantain 1. Any plant of the genus *Plantago*. **2.** A type of banana plant (*Musa paradisiaca*). **3.** The starchy fruit of such a plant, resembling a large banana; a staple food in tropical regions.

plantain seed See under seed.

plantalgia Pain in the sole of the foot.

plantar Relating to the sole of the foot.

plaque A small flat growth.

atherosclerotic p., arteriosclerotic p. A deposit of cholesterol on the intimal surface of the blood vessels.

dental p. A deposit of bacteria and other materials on the surface of a tooth that contributes to tooth decay and to the development of periodontal disease.

neuritic p. A cluster of nerve endings surrounding a core of extracellular amyloid (abnormal complex substance); commonly found in the cerebral cortex of individuals with Alzheimer's disease.

plasma 1. The clear fluid of blood and lymph in which cells are suspended; it also contains dissolved proteins. **2.** Protoplasm.

antihemophilic p. (human) Human plasma in which the antihemophilic components have been preserved; used for the temporary arrest of bleeding in hemophilia.

blood p. The yellow fluid portion of blood devoid of blood cells.

dried p. Preparation consisting of vacuum-dried frozen plasma which contains no added dextrose; it may be preserved at room temperature almost indefinitely, but usually is provided with a five-year expiration date.

fresh-frozen p. (FFP) Preparation made by prompt freezing of liquid plasma and stored at a constant temperature of −18°C or below; usually provided with a five-year expiration date.

liquid p. Preparation made by adding 5% dextrose to normal plasma and preserved at temperatures between 15° and 30°C; usually provided with a two-year expiration date.

plasmablast The precursor of the plasma cell.

plasmacyte Plasma cell; see under cell.

plasmacytoma A solitary tumor made up primarily of plasma cells, usually occurring in the skeleton; almost invariably a precursor of disseminated plasma cell myeloma.

obstetrical measuring plate

mitochondrion

granulomere

hyalomere

oval skull plate

glycogen particles

microtubules (encircling the platelet)

alpha granules

platelet (thrombocyte)

fuzzy coat

smooth interconnected tubules

glycogen particles

plasmacytosis 1. The presence of plasma cells in the blood. 2. Abnormally large percentage of plasma cells in the tissues.

plasma expander Plasma substitute.

plasmalemma Cell membrane; see under membrane.

plasmalogen One of a group of phospholipids present in the brain and muscle.

plasmapheresis A method of obtaining plasma without waste of blood components; blood is drawn, plasma is separated, and the blood cells are returned to the donor suspended in a suitable medium (e.g., Ringer's solution). Also called plasmopheresis.

plasma substitute A solution of a substance such as dextran, administered intravenously as a substitute for plasma; used in hemorrhage and shock.

plasmid See paragene.

plasmin A proteolytic enzyme derived from plasminogen; essential in blood clot dissolution (fibrinolysis).

plasminogen A globulin present in tissues, body fluids, circulating blood, and within clots; the inactive precursor of plasmin.

plasmocyte Plasma cell; see under cell.

Plasmodium A genus of the class Sporozoa; some species cause malaria. See also malaria.

P. **falciform** The parasitic species causing falciparum (malignant tertian) malaria, with fever recurring irregularly every 36 to 48 hours; it invades mature red blood cells that retain normal size and frequently contain basophilic granules and cytoplasmic precipitates (Maurer's dots); reproduction takes place in the visceral capillaries; except in severe fatal cases, only very young forms are seen in peripheral blood; multiple infection of red blood cells is extremely frequent.

P. **malariae** The species causing quartan malaria, with fever recurring every 72 hours; invades mature red blood cells and never fills the cell completely; infected cells occasionally show fine granules (Ziemann's dots).

P. **ovale** A rare parasitic species in man; the cause of ovale (benign tertian) malaria, with fever recurring every 48 hours; infected cells are irregular and fimbriated with abundant acidophilic granules (Schüffner's dots).

P. **vivax** The species causing vivax (benign tertian) malaria, with fever recurring every 48 hours; invades young red blood cells; young forms are ameboid and one-third the size of the cell; mature forms almost fill the distended cell; infected cell appears enlarged, deficient in hemoglobin, and contains acidophilic granules (Schüffner's dots).

plasmodium, *pl.* **plasmodia** A mass of protoplasm with multiple nuclei.

plasmogen Protoplasm.

plasmolysis Process in which the cytoplasm of a bacterial cell shrinks away from the cell wall when the cell is immersed in a hypertonic solution.

plasmopheresis See plasmapheresis.

plasmorrhexis See erythrocytorrhexis.

plaster 1. A white powder, essentially gypsum, which forms a paste when mixed with water and sets to a smooth solid; used for immobilization and impressions of bodily parts. 2. A pastelike material for application to the surface of the body.

adhesive p. A pressure-sensitive, sticky mixture of rubber, resins, and waxes with an absorbent powder filler, spread upon a cotton fabric.

mustard p. A pastelike mixture of powdered mustard seed, flour, and water, spread on cloth and applied to the skin as a poultice; it exerts an emollient, relaxing effect upon the skin and underlying tissues.

p. of Paris Gypsum or calcium sulfate from which water of crystallization has been calcined or expelled by heat in the open air. Also called betahemihydrate.

plastic 1. Capable of being shaped or molded; pliable. 2. In dentistry, a restorative substance that is soft enough to be molded, after which it will harden or set. 3. Any of a large group of synthetic or semisynthetic organic compounds of high molecular weight produced by polymerization. 4. Wellformed.

plasticity The capability of being molded.

plastid A self-replicating organelle in the cytoplasm of plant cells and in some plantlike organisms that serves as a center of special physiologic activities.

plate 1. In anatomy, any flattened, relatively thin structure. 2. In dentistry, an artificial denture, especially the portion to which artificial teeth are anchored. 3. In microbiology, a glass culture container such as the Petri dish. 4. A smooth, flat device of uniform thickness.

axial p. The primitive streak of an embryo.

bone p. A metal bar with perforations for immobilization of fractured bones.

chorionic p. The portion of the chorion that is attached to the uterus at an early stage in the formation of the placenta; the primordium of the chorion frondosum.

epiphysial p. The plate or disk of cartilage between the shaft and the epiphysis of a long bone during its growth.

Ishihara p.'s A series of plates designed as tests for color blindness; they consist of numbers made of primary colored dots printed on a background of many dots of various sizes and in confusing colors; individuals who are color blind are unable to read the numbers.

medullary p. The middle ectodermal thickening in the embryo from which the neural tube develops; the anlage of the central nervous system. Also called neural plate.

motor p. A motor end-plate.

neural p. See medullary plate.

obstetrical measuring p. One for calculating the digital measurements of internal conjugata without a pelvimeter.

occlusal plane p. In dentistry, a metal plate used to establish the occlusal plane of the teeth.

pterygoid p.'s A short, broad lateral plate and a long, narrow medial plate that project inferiorly from the sphenoid bone; the pterygoid fossa lies between them.

platelet A disk-shaped, colorless protoplasmic body, from 2 to 4 μm in diameter (smaller than a red blood cell), derived from a megakaryocyte; a constituent of the blood of mammals; it plays an important role in the process of coagulation: shortly after bleeding begins (before the platelets aggregate to form a plug), a lipoprotein on its surface, platelet factor 3, is activated and reacts with plasma factors to promote prothrombin activation, leading ultimately to the arrest of bleeding (hemostasis); normal level ranges from 150,000 to 300,000 platelets per mm³ of blood.

plateletpheresis The removal of platelets from the drawn blood of a healthy donor, thereby permitting the transfusion of this blood fraction to individuals who have platelet deficiency disorders; the remainder of the blood (white and red blood cells and plasma) is immediately returned to the donor.

plating 1. The planting or streaking of bacteria in a Petri dish or similar container. 2. The application of a metal strip to the fractured ends of a bone to keep them in place. 3. The electrolytic deposition of a metal.

platinum A silver-white metallic element, symbol Pt, atomic number 78, and atomic weight 195.09.

platybasia A developmental deformity in which the floor of the occipital bone of the skull bulges upward, as if pushed by the cervical spine.

platycephalous, platycephalic Having a wide flat head with a vertical cranial index below 70.

platyhelminth Common name for a worm of the phylum Platyhelminthes; any tapeworm or fluke.

Platyhelminthes A phylum of flatworms characleft lung

plexor
(percussion hammer)

pleura

heart

cauda equina
of
spinal cord

lumbosacral
plexus

L4

L5

S1

S2

S3

S4

S5

superior
gluteal
nerve

inferior
gluteal
nerve

sciatic
nerve

posterior
cutaneous
nerve of thigh

terized by bilaterally symmetrical, flat bodies without a true body cavity; some are parasitic, such as tapeworms and flukes.

platyhieric Having a broad sacral bone with an index greater than 100.

platypellic, platypelloid Having a broad, flat pelvis with a pelvic inlet index of less than 90.

platyrrhine 1. Having a broad nose, generally with nostrils directed to the sides. 2. Denoting a skull with a nasal index greater than 53.

platysma See table of muscles.

platyspondylia, platyspondylisis Having broad, flat vertebral bodies.

pledget A small, flattened tuft, usually of cotton or gauze.

pleiotropic In genetics, producing many effects; having several phenotypic expressions.

pleiotropism, pleiotropy Phenomenon in which a single gene is responsible for several distinct and apparently unrelated observable effects, such as a hereditary syndrome.

pleochromatism The property of crystals by which they show different colors when illuminated from different angles.

pleocytosis An increase in the number of leukocytes, especially lymphocytes, in the body; usually the term is applied to an increase in the number of lymphocytes in the spinal fluid.

pleomastia The presence of more than two breasts or nipples.

pleomorphic Occurring in more than one structural form.

pleomorphism 1. The assumption of two or more forms by a single organism during its life cycle. 2. The occurrence of various shapes in the same species.

pleoptics Any type of orthoptic method of treating amblyopia (dimness of vision).

plerocercoid The larval stage of a tapeworm, occurring in an intermediate host.

plesiotherapy See brachytherapy.

plessor See plexor.

plethysmograph Device for measuring variation in size of a part or organ.

plethysmography The recording of the variation in the size of a part produced by changes in the circulation of the blood within it.

plethysmometry Measurement of the fullness of a hollow structure such as a blood vessel.

pleura The serous membrane enveloping the lungs and lining the walls of the chest cavity.

    parietal p. The layer lining the walls of the chest cavity.

    visceral p. The layer covering the lungs.

pleuracotomy Incision into the pleural cavity, as for the introduction of a drainage tube.

pleuralgia Pain in the pleura.

pleurisy Inflammation of the pleura.

pleuritis Pleurisy.

pleurocentesis Puncture and drainage of the pleural cavity.

pleurodynia Pain in the intercostal muscles, usually affecting one side only.

    epidemic p. Acute infectious disease caused by the Coxsackie B virus; characterized chiefly by seizures of chest pain made worse by deep breathing and by movement. Also called devil's grip; benign dry pleurisy; Bornholm disease.

pleurogenic, pleurogenous 1. Originating in the pleura. 2. Originating in a rib.

pleurography Roentgenography of the pleura and lungs.

pleurolith A calculus in the pleural cavity.

pleuropericarditis Inflammation of the membranes enveloping the lungs and the heart.

pleuropulmonary Relating to the pleura and the lungs.

pleurotomy Incision into the pleural cavity.

plexal Relating to a plexus.

plexectomy Surgical removal of a plexus.

plexiform Resembling or forming a network of nerves, veins, or lymphatics.

plexor A small rubber-headed hammer used in percussion. Also called plessor.

plexus, *pl.* **plexuses** or **plexus** A network of nerves, veins, or lymphatics.

    aortic p., abdominal A plexus of nerve fibers around, but mainly in front of, the abdominal aorta which arises from the celiac and superior mesenteric plexuses; below the bifurcation of the aorta, it becomes the superior hypogastric plexus.

    aortic p., thoracic A plexus of nerve fibers around the thoracic aorta formed by filaments from the sympathetic ganglia and vagus nerves.

    Auerbach's p. See myenteric plexus.

    brachial p. A plexus of the ventral primary divisions of the fifth to eighth cervical and the first thoracic nerves; it lies in the lateral part of the neck and extends into the axilla, supplying nerves to the upper limb.

    celiac p. A large plexus of sympathetic nerves and ganglia located in the peritoneal cavity at the level of the first lumbar vertebra; it contains two large ganglionic masses and a dense network of fibers surrounding the roots of the celiac and superior mesenteric arteries; it supplies nerves to the abdominal viscera. Also called solar plexus.

    cervical p. A plexus of the ventral primary divi-

sions of the first four cervical nerves that sends out numerous cutaneous, muscular, and communicating branches.

    choroid p. A vascular proliferation in a cerebral ventricle which regulates the intraventricular pressure by secretion or absorption of cerebrospinal fluid.

    lumbar p. A plexus of the ventral primary divisions of the first three and the larger portion of the fourth lumbar nerves; located ventral to the transverse processes of the lumbar vertebrae.

    lumbosacral p. The combined lumbar, sacral, and pudendal plexuses.

    Meissner's p. See submucosal plexus.

    myenteric p. A network of nerves and ganglia situated between the circular and longitudinal muscular fibers of the esophagus, stomach, and intestines. Also called Auerbach's plexus.

    pampiniform p. A venous plexus in the spermatic cord that drains the testis and empties into the testicular vein.

    pudendal p. Plexus formed from the ventral branches of the second and third sacral nerves and all of the fourth sacral nerve; considered by some to be part of the sacral plexus.

    sacral p. A plexus of the ventral primary divisions of the fourth lumbar to the third sacral nerves; it lies on the posterior wall of the pelvis and supplies the buttocks, perineum, lower extremities, and pelvic viscera.

    solar p. See celiac plexus.

    submucosal p. A plexus of autonomic nerve fibers that ramifies in the submucosal coat of the intestine; it also has ganglia from which nerve fibers pass to the muscles and mucous membrane of the intestine. Also called Meissner's plexus.

    tympanic p. A plexus of nerves on the promontory of the middle ear chamber that supplies the mucous membrane of the middle ear, mastoid air cells, and the auditory tube; it also gives off a small branch to the otic ganglion.

plica, *pl.* **plicae** 1. A fold, as of skin or membrane. 2. A matted state of the hair, resulting from filth and parasites.

    p. circularis One of the transverse folds of mucous membrane of the small intestine. Also called circular fold; valve of Kerckring.

    p. semilunaris conjunctiva The crescent-shaped fold formed by the conjunctiva at the inner angle of the eye.

    p. triangularis A fold of mucous membrane covering the anteroinferior part of the palatine tonsil and projecting from the glossopalatine arch.

plicate Arranged in folds; folded.

plication of small intestine and mesentery

clasp adjusting dental pliers (three prongs)

flat nose dental pliers

angle wire bending dental pliers

amalgam plugger

type I pneumocyte

type II pneumocyte

lamellar bodies

alveolus

basal lamina

endothelium

red blood cell in capillary

---

plication The surgical folding of a muscle or of the wall of a hollow organ.

plicotomy Surgical section of the posterior fold of the tympanic membrane (eardrum).

pliers Any of several tools of varying shapes used in dentistry and orthopedic surgery for bending, cutting, contouring, etc.

ploidy The number of chromosome sets present in a cell nucleus.

plombage The surgical filling of a bodily space with inert material.

plosive Designating a speech sound whose articulation requires retaining the air stream for a moment and then suddenly releasing it.

plug 1. Any mass that occludes a bodily passage or opening. 2. A lumpy mass.

  cervical p. See mucous plug.

  epithelial p. A mass of epithelial cells that temporarily closes the external nares of the fetus.

  mucous p. A plug formed by secretions of mucous glands, especially the mass of cervical mucus secreted by the endocervix which provides a mechanical and antibacterial barrier to the uterine cavity during pregnancy. Also called cervical plug.

plugger An instrument used to compress or condense filling material, such as amalgam, in a tooth cavity.

  root canal p. A fine-tapered instrument with a blunt tip, used for packing dental material, such as gutta percha, into a root canal.

plumbic Relating to lead.

plumbism Lead poisoning; see under poisoning.

plumbum Latin for lead.

Plummer's disease Hyperthyroidism resulting from toxic adenoma of the thyroid gland.

Plummer-Vinson syndrome Postcricoid esophageal web usually seen in middle-aged women with severe iron deficiency and associated with atrophy of the oral and pharyngeal mucosa, inflammation of the lips, spoon-shaped nails, and splenomegaly; symptoms usually include dysphagia, sore tongue, and dry mouth. Also called sideropenic dysphagia; Paterson-Kelly webs.

plumose Feathery.

pluricausal Having two or more causes; applied to a disease that develops in the presence of two or more causative factors.

pluriglandular Denoting several glands. Also called polyglandular.

pluripara Multipara.

pluriparity Multiparity.

pluripotent 1. Capable of affecting more than one organ. 2. Denoting embryonic tissue that may develop in any of several ways.

plutonium A transuranian radioactive element having 15 isotopes with half-lives from 20 minutes to 76 million years; symbol Pu, atomic number 94, atomic weight (chemical scale) 239.11.

P-mitrale A pattern in the electrocardiogram consisting of wide, notched P waves in leads I and II, with flat, inverted P waves in III; occurring in mitral valve disease.

pneuma In ancient Greek philosophy and medicine, (a) a life-giving principle (now identified as oxygen); (b) the soul or spirit of God.

pneumarthrosis Air in a joint.

pneumatic 1. Relating to air. 2. Relating to breathing.

pneumatization The development of air cells or cavities, especially those of the temporal and ethmoid bones.

pneumatocele 1. An air-filled cyst in the lung, characteristic of staphylococcal pneumonia. 2. A swelling of the scrotum with gas. Also called gas tumor. 3. Herniation of lung tissue. Also called pneumonocele.

pneumatograph Pneumograph.

pneumatorrhachis The presence of gas or air in the vertebral column.

pneumaturia The passage of gas through the urethra during urination, usually due to the entrance of air into the bladder from the bowel through a vesicocolic fistula.

pneumoarthrography The making of an x-ray film of a joint after injection of air.

pneumobacillus See *Klebsiella pneumoniae*.

pneumocele Pneumatocele.

pneumocephalus The presence of air within the skull.

pneumocholecystitis Inflammation of the gallbladder with gas-producing organisms.

pneumococcemia The presence of pneumococci in the blood.

pneumococci Collective name for the many serologic types of the bacterium *Streptococcus pneumoniae*, formerly known as *Diplococcus pneumoniae*.

pneumoconiosis, *pl.* **pneumoconioses** Fibrosis of the lungs caused by prolonged inhalation of foreign material, particularly silica, coal, and asbestos, as occurs in coal mining, stone cutting, etc; the main symptoms are chronic dry cough and shortness of breath; specific forms are named according to the offending agent; e.g., silicosis, asbestosis, and anthracosis.

Pneumocystis carinii A parasitic, basophilic microorganism measuring one micrometer or less in diameter, occurring singly or in aggregates within a cystlike structure; the causative agent of pneumocystis carinii pneumonia.

pneumocystosis Pneumocystis carinii pneumonia; see under pneumonia.

pneumocyte, pneumonocyte Any of the alveolar epithelial cells of the lungs.

  granular p. Type II pneumocyte.

  membranous p. Type I pneumocyte.

  type I p. A thin squamous epithelial cell lining the inside of the pulmonary alveolar wall; it has a large attenuated cytoplasm that may extend up to 100 μm. Also called alveolar cell; membranous pneumocyte; respiratory or type I cell.

  type II p. A secretory cuboidal epithelial cell in the niches of the pulmonary alveolar wall; it possesses large, oval lamellar bodies thought to store surfactant, a surface-active phospholipid, which when secreted reduces the surface tension of the alveoli. Also called granular pneumocyte; great alveolar, septal, or type II cell.

pneumodynamics The mechanism of respiration.

pneumoencephalography The making of x-ray films of the brain after replacing the cerebrospinal fluid of the subarachnoid space with a gas.

pneumogram 1. Tracing made by a pneumograph. 2. Roentgenogram following injection of air or gas into a bodily space.

pneumograph An instrument for recording the movements of respiration. Also called pneumonograph; pneumatograph.

pneumography Roentgenography of any air- or gas-filled bodily space.

  retroperitoneal p. Roentgenography following the injection of gas into the retroperitoneal space to increase the contrast between organs (adrenal gland, kidney, etc.) and the surrounding tissues.

pneumohemopericardium See hemopneumopericardium.

pneumohemothorax The presence of gas or air and blood in the thoracic cavity.

pneumohydrometra The presence of gas and fluid in the uterine cavity.

pneumohydrothorax See hydropneumothorax.

pneumolith A calculus or concretion present in the lung.

pneumology Study of the lungs.

pneumolysia, pneumolysis Surgical separation of the pleura from the chest wall in order to allow the lung to collapse.

pneumomediastinum The presence of free air in the mediastinum (the central space of the chest containing all the thoracic organs except the lungs).

pneumomycosis Any disease of the lungs caused

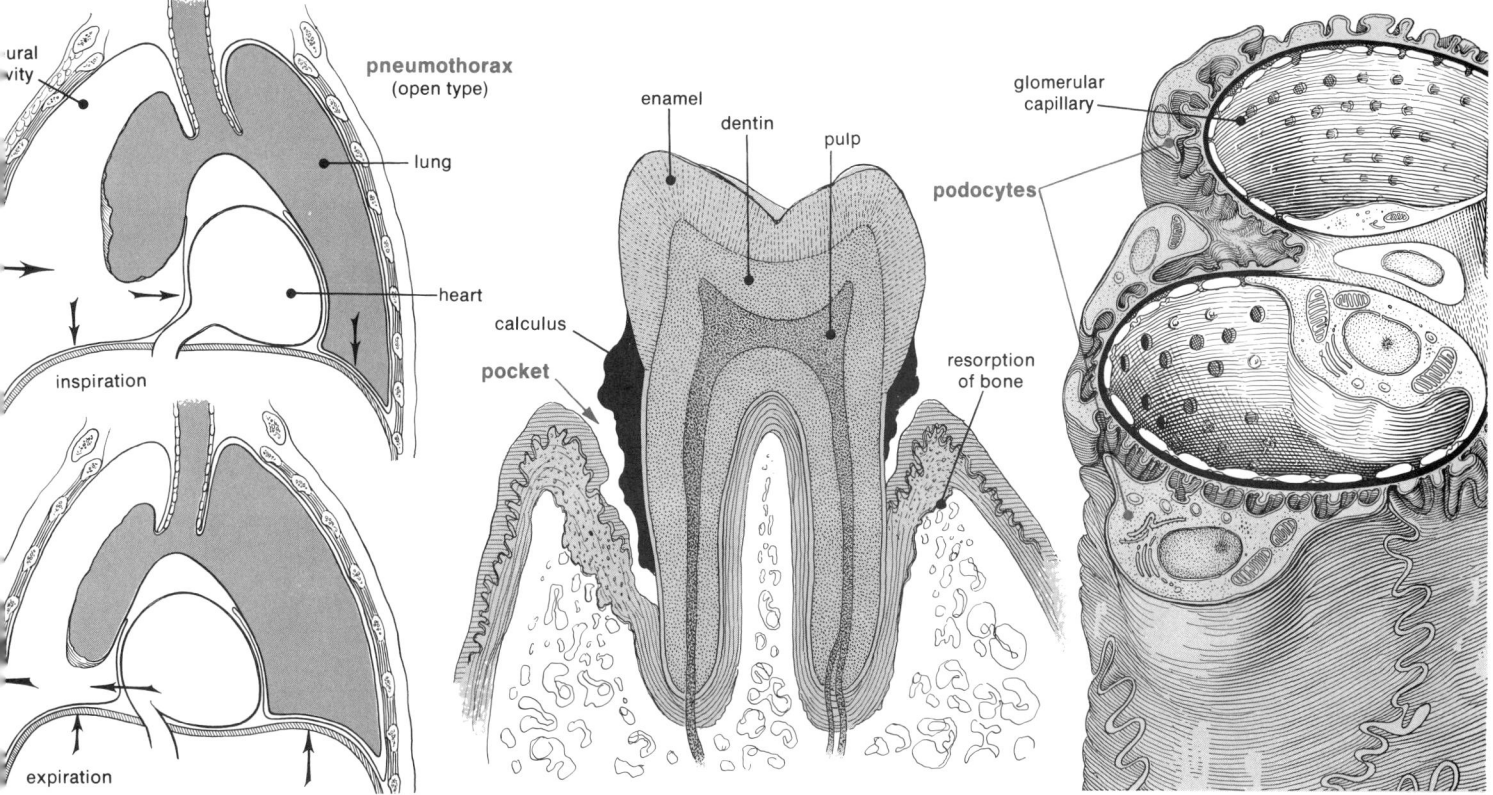

pneumothorax (open type) — lung, heart, inspiration, expiration, pleural cavity

enamel, dentin, pulp, calculus, pocket

glomerular capillary, podocytes, resorption of bone

---

by fungi or bacteria. Also called pneumonomycosis.

pneumonectomy   Surgical removal of a lung or a portion of it. Also called pneumectomy; pulmonectomy.

pneumonia   Inflammation of the lungs, caused by viruses, bacteria, or chemical and physical agents.

   acute p.   Lobar pneumonia.

   aspiration p.   Pneumonia resulting from aspiration of food particles, vomit, water, or infected material from the upper respiratory tract.

   bacterial p.   Disease of sudden onset caused by a variety of bacterial agents (pneumococcus being the most common); high fever, chills, stabbing chest pains, cough, and rusty sputum are typical findings.

   bronchial p.   See bronchopneumonia.

   chemical p.   Pneumonia caused by inhalation of extremely poisonous gas such as phosgene; characterized by edematous and hemorrhagic lungs.

   desquamative interstitial p.   Diffuse proliferation of alveolar lining cells, which desquamate into the air sacs, producing a gradual onset of dyspnea and nonproductive cough, with roentgenographic changes.

   double p.   Lobar pneumonia involving both lungs.

   Eaton agent p.   See mycoplasmal pneumonia.

   Friedländer's p.   A severe form of lobar pneumonia caused by infection with *Klebsiella pneumoniae* (Friedländer's bacillus); marked by much swelling of the affected pulmonary lobe.

   hypostatic p.   Infection occurring in poorly ventilated areas of the lung in the aged or in ill individuals who lie in the same position for long periods of time.

   lipid p., lipoid p.   Condition caused by aspiration of oily or fatty substances. Also called oil pneumonia.

   lobar p.   Acute pneumonia usually caused by a type of pneumococcus bacteria; marked by fever, chest pains, cough, and blood-stained sputum, with inflammation and consolidation of one or more lobes of the lungs.

   Löffler's p.   Löffler's syndrome.

   mycoplasmal p.   A pulmonary inflammation caused by *Mycoplasma pneumoniae* (Eaton agent); marked predominantly by severe cough, tracheal tenderness, pharyngitis with ear involvement, and occasionally blood-specked sputum; it may produce a bronchopneumonia, interstitial, or lobar pneumonia; mild forms are commonly called "walking pneumonia". Also called primary atypical or Eaton agent pneumonia.

   pneumococcal p.   Acute lobar pneumonia caused by the pneumococcus organism.

   pneumocystis carinii p.   An opportunistic, often

---

fatal, lung disease caused by *Pneumocystis carinii* which invade the walls of the alveoli; occurs in premature and debilitated infants during the first three months of life, in individuals receiving immunosuppressive drugs, or in those afflicated with AIDS (acquired immune deficiency syndrome).

   primary atypical p.   See mycoplasmal pneumonia.

   secondary p.   Inflammation of the lungs occurring as a complication of another disease.

   walking p.   See mycoplasmal pneumonia.

   wool-sorter's p.   See anthrax, pulmonary.

   viral p.   Acute systemic disease, caused by a variety of viruses (e.g., adenoviruses), with involvement of the lungs.

pneumonic   1. Of, or relating to, the lungs. **2.** Relating to pneumonia.

pneumonitis   Inflammation of the lungs.

pneumonocele   See pneumatocele (3).

pneumonocyte   See pneumocyte.

pneumonomycosis   See pneumomycosis.

pneumonotomy   Incision into the lungs. Also called pneumotomy.

pneumopericardium   The presence of air in the sac encasing the heart.

pneumoperitoneum   The presence of air or gas in the peritoneal cavity from perforation of a viscus or therapeutic installation.

pneumoperitonitis   Inflammation of the peritoneum with accumulation of air or gas in the peritoneal cavity.

pneumopyothorax   See pyopneumothorax.

pneumoroentgenography   X-ray examination of a bodily part into which air or gas has been injected to provide additional outlines.

pneumorrhachis   The presence of gas in the spinal canal.

pneumorrhagia   Bleeding from or into the lung.

pneumothorax   The presence of air or gas in the pleural cavity.

pneumotomy   See pneumonotomy.

Pneumovirus   Genus of viruses (family Paramyxoviridae), which are intermediate in size between other Paramyxoviridae and the Orthomyxoviridae; includes those causing bronchiolitis and pneumonia in infants. Also called respiratory syncytial virus group.

pock   A pustule caused by an eruptive disease, especially smallpox.

pocket   1. A saclike cavity. **2.** A space between a tooth and the inflamed gum. **3.** To enclose the pedicle of a tumor (after its removal) within the edges of the wound. **4.** A collection of pus.

pockmark   The scar left on the skin after the healing of a smallpox pustule.

---

podagra   Gout of the metatarsophalangeal joint of the big toe.

podagral, podagric, podagrous   Relating to or suffering from gout.

podalgia   Pain in the foot.

podalic   Relating to feet.

podarthritis   Inflammation of the foot joints.

podiatrist   A specialist in podiatry. Also called chiropodist.

podiatry   The study and treatment of foot diseases, injuries, and defects. Also called chiropody.

poditis   An inflammatory disorder of the foot.

podobromidrosis   Perspiration or sweating of the feet with a strong, offensive odor.

podocyte   An epithelial cell of the renal glomerulus which squats upon the glomerular basement membrane, spreading thin cytoplasmic projections over the membrane; the outer surface of the engorged cell projects into the glomerular (Bowman's) space, where it is bathed by the glomerular ultrafiltrate.

pododynamometer   Device for measuring the strength of the foot or leg muscles.

podophyllin   Podophyllum resin; see under resin.

podophyllotoxin   The active principle of podophyllum resin; it has laxative properties.

podophyllum   The rhizome of the mayapple (*Podophyllum peltatum*), used as a bulk-forming laxative.

podophyllum resin   See under resin.

pogonion   The most anterior midpoint of the mandible or chin.

poikilocyte   A red blood cell assuming an abnormal and often bizarre shape; it could be pear-shaped, racquet-shaped, or pessary-shaped; characteristically found in severe hemolytic anemias.

poikilocytosis   The presence in the blood of abnormally shaped red blood cells (poikilocytes). Also called poikilocythemia.

poikiloderma   An atrophic skin condition that has streaks, marks, or patches of a different color or colors.

poikilotherm   An animal having a temperature that varies with the environment.

point   1. A minute spot or area. **2.** The sharp or tapered end of an object. **3.** A specific condition or degree.

   alveolar p.   See prosthion.

   boiling p. (b.p.)   The temperature at which a liquid boils, i.e., at which the vapor pressure of a liquid is equal to the atmospheric pressure.

   contact p.   The small area of the proximal surface of a tooth that touches the adjacent tooth. Also called contact area.

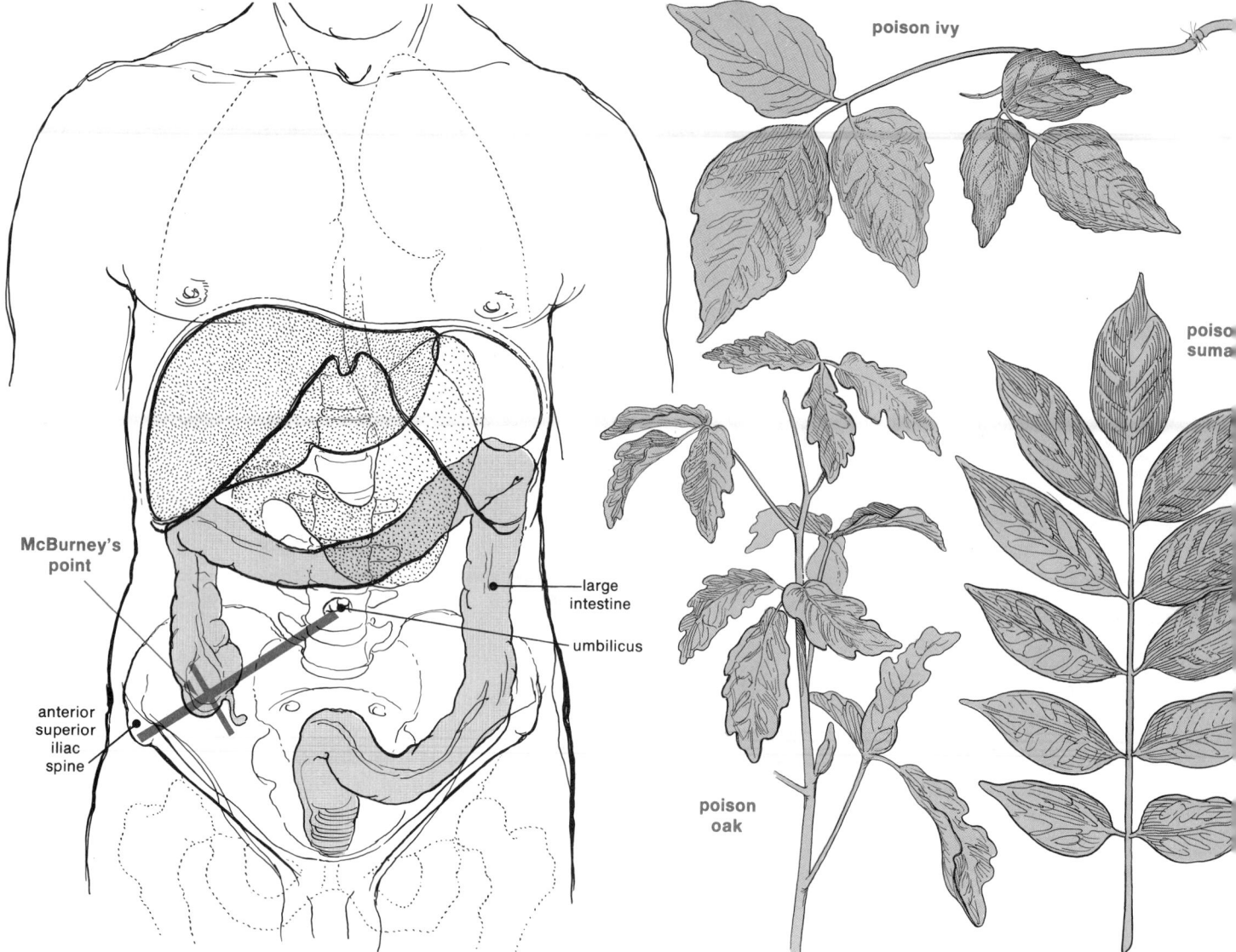

poison ivy

poison sumac

poison oak

McBurney's point

large intestine

umbilicus

anterior superior iliac spine

craniometric p. Any one of many fixed points on the skull used as landmarks in craniometry.

cutoff p. In test interpretation, the value used to separate positive from negative results.

dew p. Temperature at which the moisture of the air condenses.

end p. In volumetric analysis of a solution, the point at which a reaction is completed.

focal p. Point at which light rays meet when deflected by refraction or reflection.

freezing p. The temperature at which a liquid changes to a solid state.

isoelectric p. The pH at which an amphoteric electrolyte, such as an amino acid or protein, is electrically neutral owing to equality of ionization; above or below this pH, it acts as an acid or base, respectively.

J p. The junction between the QRS complex and the ST segment in the electrocardiogram. Also called J junction.

jugal p. The point where the zygomatic arch meets with the frontal process of the zygomatic bone.

McBurney's p. The point located on a line between the anterior superior spine of the right ilium and the umbilicus, about one-third of that distance from the spine; the especially tender point in acute appendicitis.

melting p. (m.p.) The temperature at which a solid changes into a liquid state.

mid-inguinal p. The point on the inguinal ligament halfway between the pubic symphysis and the anterior superior iliac spine.

p. of fixation The retinal point on which an image is formed; in normal vision it is the fovea.

pressure p. 1. A point at which pressure can be exerted to control hemorrhage from an arterial injury. 2. A point on the skin surface which is extremely sensitive to pressure.

trigger p. A spot on the body which, when touched or pressed, initiates pain in adjacent or distant parts.

pointing The process of reaching a point.

p. of an abscess An abscess or boil that is about to open spontaneously.

past p. Incoordination of voluntary movements characterized by inability to place a finger on some designated site (the finger moves past the site).

point source In photometry, the source of light from which light radiates in straight lines in all directions.

poise The unit of dynamic viscosity of a liquid equal to one dyne-second per square centimeter.

poison Any substance that is injurious to health or causes death, either taken internally or applied externally.

p. ivy 1. A shrub or vine that grows abundantly throughout the United States and parts of southern Canada and has smooth, glossy leaflets of three with margins varying from crenate or serrate to deeply lobate; it causes a rash on contact. Also called *Rhus radicans*. 2. The acute, intensely itchy vesicular skin eruption caused by the toxic material (oleoresin) in the sap of the poison ivy plant; the blisters are usually grouped. Also called ivy dermatitis.

p. oak A North American shrub having varied leaflets, often with three to seven subacute lobes resembling oak leaves; it causes a rash on contact; two species exist in the United States: *Rhus toxicodendron* of the Atlantic states and *Rhus diversiloba* of the Pacific states.

p. sumac A swamp shrub that grows in marshy areas of eastern North America and has compound leaves with branches of seven to 13 elongated leaflets; it produces an acutely irritating oil that causes a rash on contact. Also called *Rhus vernix*; poison ash; poison dogwood; poison elder.

"purse" p. Medication carried in the purse for personal use that results in poisoning of the curious child who seeks candy or gum and finds attractive multicolored pills and tablets.

poisoning The condition produced by a poison.

arsenic p. Poisoning caused by ingestion of arsenic-containing compounds, usually insecticides or rodenticides; arsenic reacts with sulfhydryl groups to disrupt vital enzyme systems; symptoms of chronic poisoning include skin changes and peripheral neuropathy; headache and confusion may be seen in both acute and chronic forms.

blood p. A vague colloquial term; see septicemia and bacteremia.

carbon monoxide p. Acute, potentially fatal poisoning with various degrees of severity, caused by inhalation of carbon monoxide; severe headache is usually an early symptom; subsequently, nausea, weakness, and exertional dyspnea develop, and collapse and coma may supervene.

carbon tetrachloride p. Poisoning due to ingestion, inhalation, or absorption of carbon tetrachloride, an industrial solvent; causes hepatic and renal necrosis.

cyanide p. Poisoning caused by inhalation or ingestion of compounds of cyanide; death may occur in minutes; cyanides combine with iron-containing enzymes such as cytochromes and catalase to block energy-releasing metabolism and cause tissue asphyxia; most common sources are fungicides and insecticides.

food p. Poisoning causing acute gastrointestinal illness or neurologic manifestations accompanied by intestinal complaints; resulting from ingestion of foods that (a) have become contaminated with microorganisms, (b) may themselves be poisonous, or (c) may contain harmful chemicals.

heavy metal p. Poisoning caused by such metals as antimony, arsenic, bismuth, cadmium, copper, gold, lead, mercury, silver, and thallium; BAL and EDTA are used to treat many of these disorders.

lead p. Acute or chronic intoxication with lead or its salts, causing gastrointestinal and mental disturbances, anemia, basophilic stippling of red blood

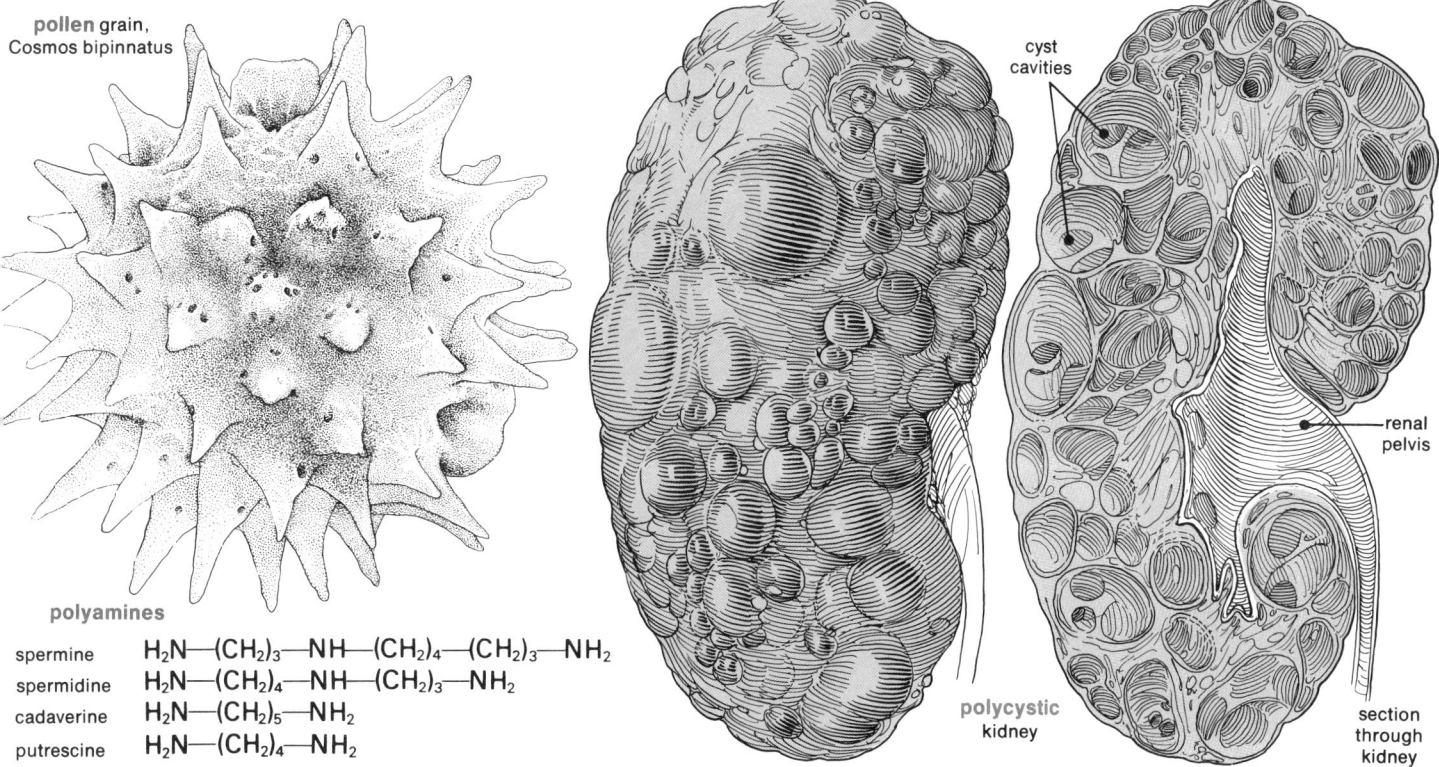

pollen grain, Cosmos bipinnatus

polyamines

$$\text{spermine} \quad H_2N—(CH_2)_3—NH—(CH_2)_4—(CH_2)_3—NH_2$$
$$\text{spermidine} \quad H_2N—(CH_2)_4—NH—(CH_2)_3—NH_2$$
$$\text{cadaverine} \quad H_2N—(CH_2)_5—NH_2$$
$$\text{putrescine} \quad H_2N—(CH_2)_4—NH_2$$

cyst cavities

renal pelvis

polycystic kidney

section through kidney

cells, and a bluish "lead line" on the gums; most commonly seen in young children who eat paint scales; other sources include lead toys, motor fuel, and lead water pipes. Also called plumbism.

mercury p. Poisoning caused by ingestion of soluble mercury salts such as mercuric chloride ($HgCl_2$), producing corrosive damage to the gastrointestinal tract and destruction of the kidney tubules; repeated inhalation of mercury vapor or ingestion of small amounts of mercury salts may lead to chronic mercury poisoning, characterized by mental symptoms, renal damage, and stomatitis.

Salmonella food p. Inflammation of the gastrointestinal tract caused by ingestion of food contaminated with any of several strains of *Salmonella*; symptoms usually appear within 8 to 24 hours and include abdominal pain, nausea, diarrhea, vomiting and fever.

Staphylococcus food p. Inflammation of the intestines caused by a toxin, specific for intestinal mucosa, produced by staphylococci; symptoms appear a few hours after ingestion of contaminated food and include diarrhea and severe vomiting.

polar 1. Relating to poles. 2. Having poles; said of certain nerve cells.

polarimeter Instrument used to determine the amount of polarization of light or the rotation of the plane of polarization.

polarimetry The process of using the polarimeter.

polariscope Instrument used to study the properties of polarized light.

polarity 1. Having two opposite poles. 2. Manifesting two opposite tendencies or attributes.

polarization 1. In optics, the process of altering the transverse wave motion of a light ray, whereby the vibrations of the wave occur in one plane only. 2. In electricity, the deposition of gas in one or both electrodes of an electric cell, whereby the action of the battery is impeded. 3. The development of ions of opposite charges (i.e., differences in potential) in two points of living tissue, as on both sides of a cell membrane.

polarize To induce polarization.

polarizer The part of a polarimeter or polariscope that receives and polarizes the light.

polarography In qualitative or quantitative microanalysis, the recording of the relationship between an increasing current flowing through a solution being analyzed and the increasing voltage used to produce the current.

pole 1. Either end of an axis. 2. Either of two points having opposite physical properties; e.g., terminals of an electric cell or battery.

animal p. The site in the early ovum near the nucleus where most of the protoplasm is concen-

trated, and from which the polar bodies are pinched off. Also called germinal pole.

germinal p. See animal pole.

negative p. Cathode.

positive p. Anode.

vegetal p., vegetative p. The pole of an ovum where the bulk of the yolk is located, opposite to the germinal disk. Also called vitelline pole; antigerminal pole.

vitelline p. See vegetal pole.

polio Colloquial term for poliomyelitis.

poliodystrophy Wasting of the gray substance of the nervous system.

polioencephalitis Inflammation of the gray substance of the brain.

poliomyelitis A highly contagious, infectious disease caused by a poliovirus (genus *Enterovirus*, family Picornaviridae); occurs most commonly in children; in its acute form it involves the spinal cord, causing paralysis, atrophy, and permanent deformity of one or more muscular groups. Also called polio; infantile paralysis.

bulbar p. A form which involves nerve cells in the medulla oblongata and may cause respiratory paralysis and death.

poliomyelopathy Any disease principally affecting the gray matter of the spinal cord and medulla oblongata.

poliovirus The virus (genus *Enterovirus*, family Picornaviridae) causing poliomyelitis in man; serologic types 1, 2, 3, and 4 are recognized.

pollen The powder-like microspores (male fertilizing elements) produced by the authors of flowering plants that are carried by wind or insects and play a major role in the etiology of hay fever and some cases of asthma.

pollenosis, pollinosis Hay fever excited by certain airborne pollens.

pollex The thumb.

pollinosis See pollenosis.

pollutant A substance that contaminates; especially one that contaminates the air, water, or food.

pollute To make impure; to dirty; to contaminate.

pollution The act or process of contaminating, as the discharge of noxious substances into the atmosphere or into a body of water.

polonium A radioactive metallic element; symbol Po, atomic number 84, atomic weight 210; one of the rarest naturally occurring elements, a product of radium disintegration; discovered by Pierre and Marie Curie and named after Mme. Curie's native land, Poland.

polonium-210 (^{210}Po) A 138.4-day alpha-emitter isotope of polonium that is a member of the uranium natural radioactive decay series.

polyacid An acid that yields more than one hydrogen ion per molecule.

polyadenitis Inflammation of several lymph nodes.

poly Polymorphonuclear leukocyte.

polyamine Any of a group of substances, widely distributed in small quantities among living forms, which are essential growth factors for a number of microorganisms, such as *Hemophilus parainfluenzae*; they serve as agents that stabilize membranous structures; putrescine, cadaverine, spermidine, and spermine are polyamines.

polyarteritis Simultaneous inflammation of several arteries.

p. nodosa Polyarteritis with formation of numerous nodules within the walls of the arteries; a collagen vascular disease that may involve a variety of different organ systems, producing renal, gastrointestinal, or nervous system findings. Also called periarteritis nodosa.

polyarthritis Inflammation of several joints.

polybasic An acid that has more than one replaceable hydrogen atom.

polycholia Excessive production and flow of bile.

polychondritis A rare syndrome marked by a widespread inflammatory and degenerative process in cartilaginous structures, such as those in the nose, ear, joints, and tracheobronchial tree; destruction of cartilage leaves deformities, such as saddle nose or floppy ear; death may occur from suffocation due to loss of stability in the tracheobronchial tree.

polychromasia, polychromatia Polychromatophilia.

polychromatic Multicolored; exhibiting many colors.

polychromatophil, polychromatophile 1. A cell or other element that stains readily with both acidic and basic dyes, especially certain red blood cells. 2. A young or degenerating red blood cell that manifests acidic and basic staining affinities.

polychromatophilia 1. Tendency to stain with basic and acid stains. 2. Condition marked by the presence of an excessive number of red blood cells that stain with basic, acid, and neutral dyes.

polyclinic A clinic, dispensary, or hospital that treats any disease or injury.

polycystic Made up of several cysts.

polycystic disease of kidney An inherited kidney disease marked by formation of multiple cysts of varying sizes, resulting in renal parenchymal degeneration and gradual loss of renal function; the adult form of the disease shows autosomal dominant inheritance and uremia appears usually in early or middle adult life; bilateral polycystic kidney disease of infants and children often causes stillbirths or

polyenoic acids

linolenic acid

linoleic acid

adenine
cytosine

polymorph

RBC
for size
comparison

guanine

polynucleotide
(chain of ribonucleic acid)

uracil

supernumerary
mammary
gland

polymastia

milk line

deaths within the first few months of life, is frequently associated with cysts in other organs, and does not follow an autosomal dominant inheritance.

polycystic ovary syndrome Condition of unknown cause characterized by bilaterally enlarged polycystic ovaries, small uterus, menstrual abnormalities, anovulatory infertility (i.e., failure to produce ova), and hirsutism. Also called Stein-Leventhal syndrome.

polycythemia The presence of an abnormally large number of red corpuscles in the blood.

p. vera A disease of unknown cause characterized by hyperplasia of all the cellular elements of the bone marrow and manifested by an increase in the total number of red blood cells in the body, usually accompanied by leukocytosis and thrombocytosis. Also called primary polycythemia; erythremia.

primary p. See polycythemia vera.

relative p. An increase in the number of red blood cells per unit volume of blood due to a decrease in the total plasma of the body.

secondary p. An increase in the total number of red blood cells in the body due to another condition; e.g., the chronic tissue hypoxia of advanced pulmonary disease, high altitude, or the secretion of erythropoietins by certain tumors.

polydactyly Condition marked by the presence of more than ten fingers or toes. Also called polydactylia; polydactylism.

polydipsia Insatiable thirst.

polydysplasia Condition marked by multiple developmental abnormalities of tissues, organs, or systems.

polyene A chemical compound containing many conjugated (alternating) double bonds; e.g., carotenoids.

polyenoic acid A polyunsaturated fatty acid, essential in the diet, with more than one double bond in the carbon chain; e.g., linoleic acid (two double bonds) and linolenic acid (three double bonds).

polyethylene A resin, $(CH_2CH_2)_n$, produced by the polymerization of ethylene under high pressure; a straight-chain paraffin hydrocarbon of high molecular weight.

p. glycol A condensation product of ethylene oxide and water.

polygen A chemical element with two or more valences.

polygene One of a group of genes that, acting together, control a quantitative character, such as height.

polygenic Relating to a quantitative character (e.g., height) dependent on the action of several genes.

polyglandular See pluriglandular.

polygraph An instrument for simultaneously recording changes in such physiologic processes as blood pressure, respiratory motion, and galvanic skin resistance; sometimes used to study emotional reactions, as in lie detection. Also called lie detector.

polyhedral Having many faces.

polyhydramnios An excess volume of amniotic fluid in pregnancy, usually greater than 2,000 ml.

polyhydric Containing more than one hydroxyl group.

polyhypermenorrhea Frequent menstruation accompanied by excessive flow.

polyhypomenorrhea Frequent menstruation accompanied by a scanty flow.

polyleptic Having many relapsing phases; said of a disease.

polylogia Garrulity or talkativeness (often incoherent) caused by a mental disorder.

polymastia The presence of more than two breasts in the human. Also called multimammae.

polymer A complex compound of high molecular weight formed by a chain of simpler molecules; e.g., the combining of many ethylene molecules to form polyethylene.

addition p. A large molecule formed by a chain of smaller molecules (monomers) without the formation of any other product.

condensation p. A large molecule formed by a chain of smaller molecules, involving the elimination of water or some other simple compound.

polymerase Any enzyme that promotes polymerization.

polymerization The chemical joining of similar monomers to form a compound of a high molecular weight.

polymethylmethacrylate The principal base resin employed in making dentures; it is transparent and can be tinted to any shade of translucence; also used as bone cement.

polymicrolipomatosis A condition marked by the presence of a number of small, nodular, fairly discrete masses of lipid (lipomata) in the subcutaneous connective tissue.

polymorph Shortened version of polymorphonuclear leukocyte (PMN).

polymorphic, polymorphous Occurring in many morphologic forms.

polymorphism The occurrence of two or more genetically different classes in the same population; e.g., Rh-positive and Rh-negative humans.

polymorphonuclear Having nuclei of varied shapes, or so deeply lobulated that they appear to be multiple; said of a variety of leukocytes (PMNs).

polymyalgia Pain in several muscles.

p. rheumatica A syndrome of muscular rheumatism in old people, more frequent in men than women, characterized by a markedly elevated erythrocyte sedimentation rate; often associated with cranial arteritis.

polymyositis A painful inflammation of the muscles that may also involve skin and subcutaneous tissue; the muscles most affected are those of the pelvic and shoulder girdles and pharynx; when skin changes are prominent, the disorder is often called dermatomyositis; in 15 to 20 percent of cases there is an associated neoplasm.

polymyxin Any of a group of antibiotic substances derived from strains of the soil bacterium *Bacillus polymixa*; they are polypeptides containing various amino acids and a branched fatty acid, (+)-6-methyloctanoic acid; there are five different types, designated A, B, C, D, and E.

polyneuritis Inflammation of several peripheral nerves at the same time, characterized by widespread sensory and motor disturbances. Also called multiple neuritis.

polyneuropathy A disease in which several peripheral nerves are affected at the same time.

polyneuroradiculitis Inflammation involving nerve roots and peripheral nerves.

polynuclear Containing more than one nucleus. Also called multinuclear.

polynucleotidase A class of enzymes which help to hydrolyze or split up nucleic acids of high molecular weight into their constituent mononucleotide units.

polynucleotide Compound containing several or many nucleotides; a nucleic acid.

polyol General term for an alcohol that contains more than one hydroxyl group in the molecule.

polyopia A condition in which a person perceives more than one image of the same object; multiple vision. Also called polyopsia; polyopy.

p. monophthalmica Condition in which only one eye is affected.

polyorchidism, polyorchism The presence of more than two testes.

polyostotic Affecting several bones.

polyp A general term denoting a growth or mass of tissue that protrudes from a mucous membrane, commonly found in the nose, uterus, rectum, and bladder.

adenomatous p. A benign polyp composed of glandular tissue; may be pedunculated or sessile.

endometrial p. Small benign mass that projects into the cavity of the uterus; composed of tissue from the lining of the uterine cavity (endometrium).

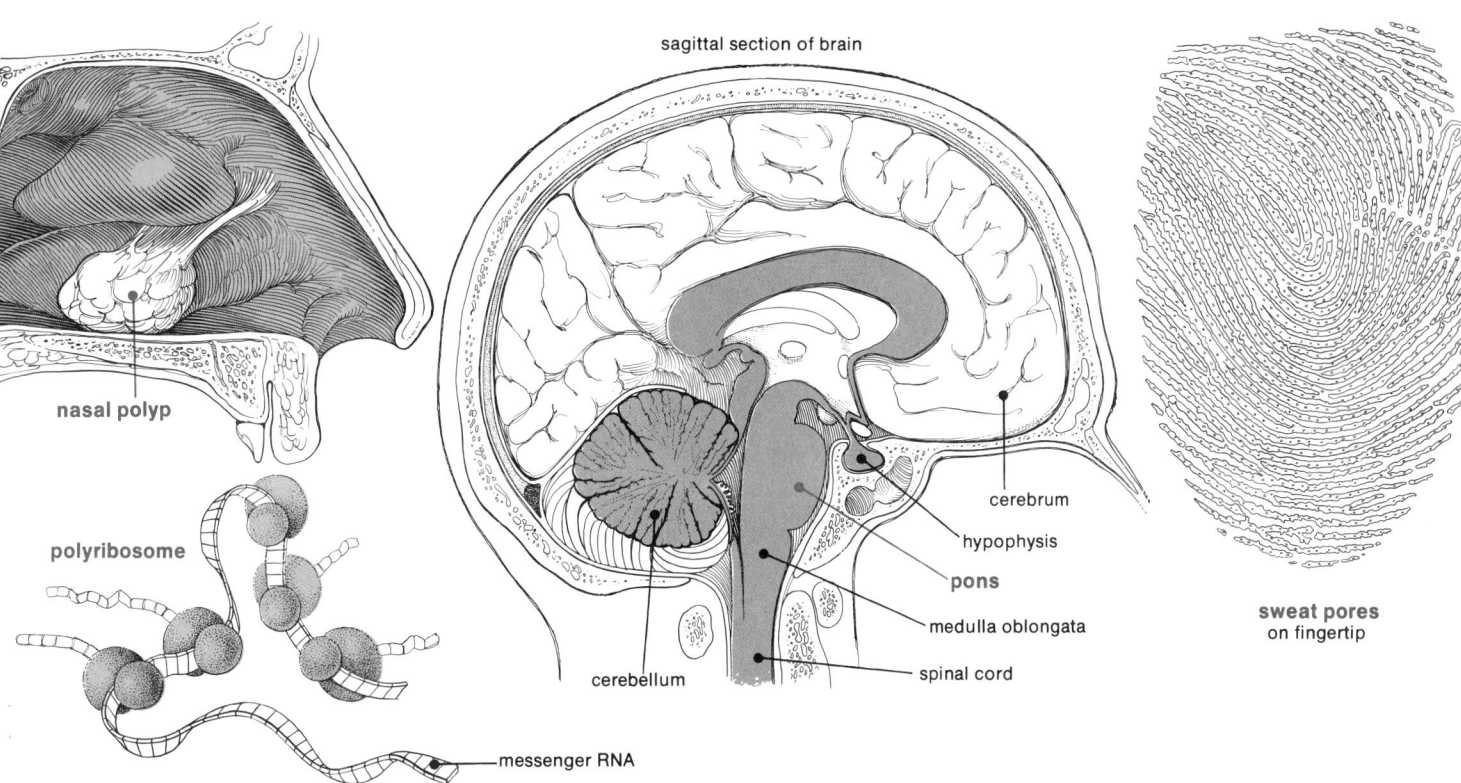

sagittal section of brain

nasal polyp

polyribosome

cerebrum
hypophysis
pons
medulla oblongata
spinal cord
cerebellum
messenger RNA

sweat pores
on fingertip

fleshy p. Polyp composed of smooth muscle tissue.

nasal p. A focal inflammatory swelling of the lining of the nasal cavity or sinuses.

pedunculated p. Polyp that is attached to the mucosa by a slender stalk or pedicle.

sessile p. Polyp that has a broad base.

polypectomy Surgical removal of a polyp.

polypeptide A compound containing two or more amino acids united by peptide linkage; the ribosome is the site of polypeptide synthesis in the cytoplasm.

polypeptidemia The presence of polypeptides in the blood.

polyphagia Morbid or pathological overeating.

polyplast Derived from several structures.

polyplastic Capable of taking many forms.

polyplegia Paralysis of several muscles.

polyploidy The state of having a chromosome number that is a multiple of the normal diploid number, resulting from the replication of chromosome sets without subsequent division of the nucleus; e.g., tetraploid = 92 chromosomes, triploid = 69 chromosomes.

polypoid Having the outward appearance of a polyp.

polyposis The presence of numerous polyps.

polypotome A cutting instrument for excising polyps.

polypous Relating to or characterized by the presence of polyps.

polyribosome A multiple structure composed of two or more ribosomes held together by a molecule of messenger RNA. Also called polysome; ergosome.

polys A colloquial term for polymorphonuclear leukocytes.

polysaccharide A carbohydrate containing a large number of saccharide units, such as starch and glycogen.

polyserositis Inflammation of several serous membranes. Also called multiple serositis.

polysome See polyribosome.

polysomy The state of a cell nucleus in which some but not all of the chromosomes of a set are reduplicated beyond the normal diploid number.

polysorbate 80 Polyoxethylene sorbitan monooleate; a yellow, bitter oil, used as an emulsifier in the preparation of ointments; Tween 80®.

polyspermia Excessive secretion of semen.

polyspermy The entry of more than one sperm into an ovum during fertilization.

polytetrafluoroethylene A waxy synthetic fabric, used for surgical implantation, which resists the clotting of blood upon its surface; Teflon®.

polythelia The presence of more than two nipples.

polytrichia The presence of excessive hair.

polyunsaturated Having two or more unsaturated (double) bonds; said of certain long-chain carbon compounds, especially fats and oils.

polyuria Passage of abnormally large quantity of urine.

polyvalent See multivalent.

polyvinylpyrrolidone (PVP) See povidone.

Pompe's disease Type 2 glycogenosis; see under glycogenosis.

pompholyx A deep eruption of blisters occurring primarily on the hands and feet, accompanied by intense itching. Also called dyshidrosis.

pomphus A blister or a wheal.

pons 1. The part of the brain located between the cerebral peduncle above and the medulla oblongata below. 2. Any bridgelike structure connecting two parts of an organ.

pontic An artificial tooth on a fixed partial denture that replaces the missing natural tooth.

pontile, pontine Relating to a pons, especially of the brain (pons varolii).

pontomedullary Relating to the pons and medulla oblongata of the central nervous system.

pool A collection of blood in a part.

poples The back of the knee.

popliteal Relating to the back of the knee.

porcelain A fine ceramic powder (composed of clay, quartz, and flux) mixed with water to form a paste; used in the manufacture of artificial teeth, inlays, jacket crowns, and dentures.

porcine Relating to pigs.

pore A minute opening on a surface, as of a sweat gland on the skin.

gustatory p. A minute surface opening of a taste bud.

slit p. The linear ultraminute space between the footlike processes (pedicles) of the podocytes that cover the outside of the capillary of the renal corpuscle.

sweat p. The surface opening of a sweat gland.

porencephaly Congenital malformation of the brain characterized by a cystic outpouching of the ventricular system.

porokeratosis A rare skin disease marked by cornification around pores and progressive centrifugal atrophy.

porphin $C_{20}H_{14}N_4$; a fundamental substance that contains four pyrrole-like rings linked by four CH groups or methene bridges in a ring system; the unsubstituted tetrapyrrole nucleus of the porphyrins.

porphobilinogen Organic compound present in large quantities in the urine of individuals with acute or congenital porphyria.

porphyria A disorder of blood pigment metabolism in which there is a marked increase in the formation and excretion of porphyrins.

acute intermittent p. Genetic disorder transmitted as an autosomal dominant trait; marked by neuropsychiatric symptoms, abdominal pain, and dark urine containing excessive amounts of aminolevulinic acid and porphobilinogen; attacks may be induced by certain drugs. Also called porphyria hepatica; acute porphyria.

congenital erythropoietic p. Rare genetic disorder transmitted as an autosomal recessive trait in which excessive porphyrin is produced in the normoblasts of bone marrow; marked by excretion of excessive amounts of porphyrin in the urine, abnormal cutaneous sensitivity to sunlight, hemolytic anemia, and splenomegaly. Also called Gunther's disease.

p. cutanea tarda, symptomatic p. Hereditary disorder expressed only in the presence of liver dysfunction; marked by bullous skin rashes upon exposure to sunlight with scarring and pigmentation of the skin and by excessive porphyrin in the urine.

variegate p. Genetic disorder transmitted as an autosomal dominant trait; marked by light sensitivity, skin fragility, and increased excretion of protoporphyrin and coproporphyrin in feces.

porphyrin Any of various organic compounds present in protoplasm, forming the foundation structure for hemoglobin, chlorophyll, and other respiratory pigments; they are capable of combining with metals such as iron, magnesium, copper, etc. (metalloporphyrins), and with nitrogenous substances.

porphyrinuria, porphyruria Presence of porphyrin in the urine in excess of the normal amount.

porrigo Any disease of the scalp.

porta The point at which vessels, nerves, and excretory ducts enter and leave an organ.

p. hepatis The fissure on the under surface of the liver through which the portal vein, the hepatic artery, and the hepatic ducts pass.

portacaval Relating to the portal vein and the inferior vena cava.

portal Relating to any entrance; specifically, to the porta hepatis.

portio, pl. portiones Latin for part.

portogram An x-ray film of the portal vein.

portography Splenic photography, a roentgenographic technique in which the splenic and portal veins and their tributaries are visualized after injection with a radiopaque material; widely used as a diagnostic and prognostic tool in cirrhosis.

knee-chest position

lithotomy position

Sims' position

porus, *pl.* **pori** Latin for pore; an orifice.
position **1.** The placement of the body in a special way to facilitate specific diagnostic or therapeutic procedures. **2.** The particular arrangement of bodily parts. **3.** In obstetrics, the relationship of a designated point on the presenting part of the fetus to a designated point in the maternal pelvis. **4.** The place occupied. **5.** To place the body in a particular way.

anatomic p. Position in which the body is erect with the arms and hands turned forward.

centric p. The position of the mandible in its most retruded relation to the maxilla; the position in which an individual normally closes his jaws.

eccentric p. Any position of the mandible other than the centric position.

Fowler's p. An inclined position obtained by raising the head of the bed about 50 cm.

frog leg p. Lying on the back with both thighs acutely extended and knees flexed, as seen in infants with scurvy. Also called pithed frog position.

genupectoral p. Knee-chest position.

jackknife p. Position in which the individual is on his back with shoulders elevated and thighs at right angles to the abdomen; used to facilitate urethral instrumentation.

knee-chest p. A prone posture resting on the knees and chest with forearms supporting the head; assumed for rectal examinations.

left lateral recumbent p. Position in which the individual lies on the left side with the right thigh and knee drawn upward; assumed by parturient women. Also called obstetric position.

lithotomy p. The individual lies on his back with buttocks at the end of the examining or operating table, the hips and knees being fully flexed with feet supported by slings or mechanical braces.

obstetric p. See left lateral recumbent position.

occlusal p. The relation of the mandible to the maxilla when the jaws are closed and the teeth are in contact.

orthopneic p. A sitting position with the individual's head and arms resting on an overbed table or on the arms of a chair.

prone p. Lying face down.

recumbent p. A restful position in which the individual is on his back with legs slightly extended and flexed.

Sims' p. Position in which the individual lies on

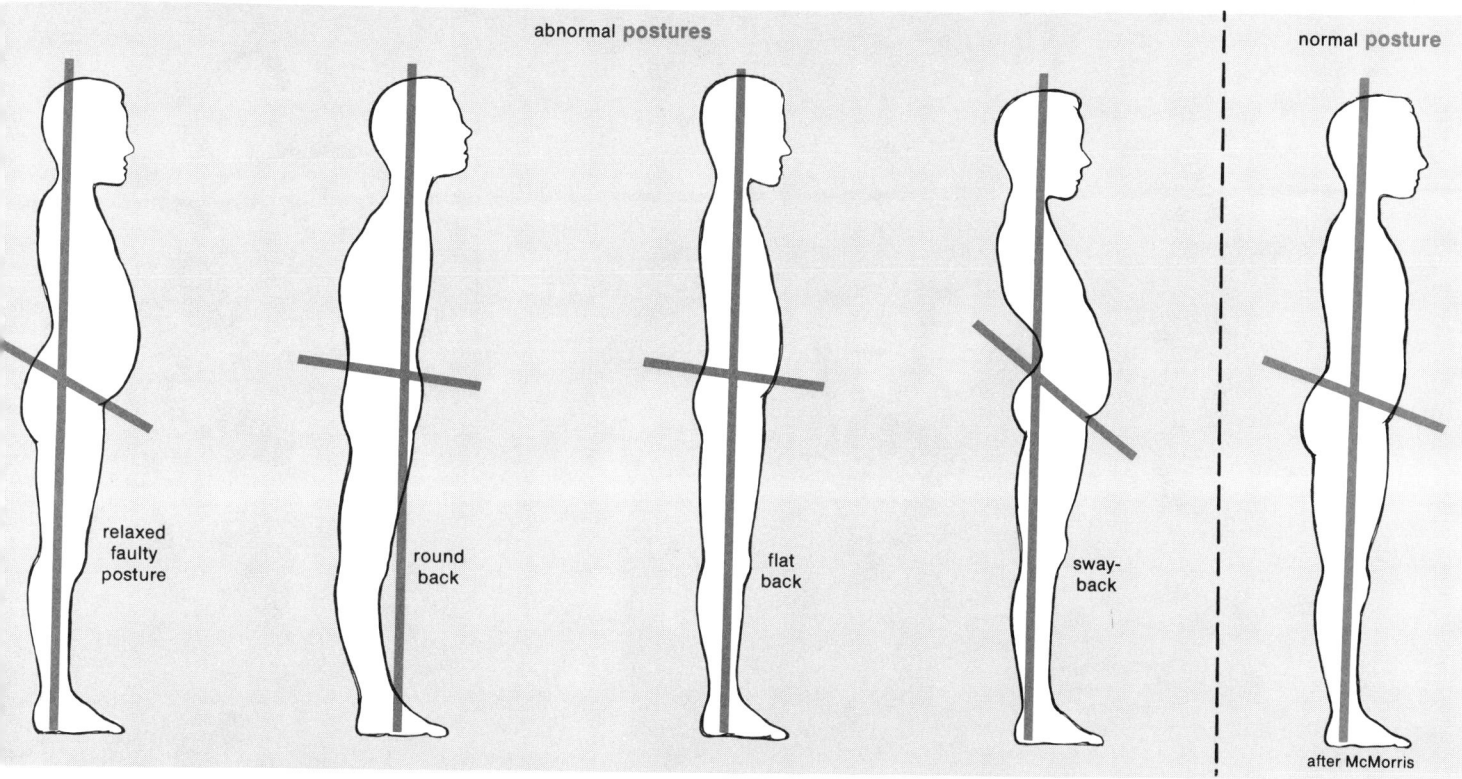

abnormal **postures**　　　　　　　　　　　　　　　　　　　　　　　　　　　　normal **posture**

relaxed
faulty
posture

round
back

flat
back

sway-
back

after McMorris

the left side with the right thigh acutely flexed and the left thigh slightly flexed; the left arm is behind the body; used to facilitate vaginal and rectal examinations, curettement of uterus, intrauterine irrigation after labor, tamponade of vagina, etc.

supine p. Lying on the back.

Trendelenburg's p. Position in which the individual lies on his back on an operating table, inclined at an angle of 45° with the head lower than the rest of the body; the legs and feet hang over the end of the table.

positive 1. Definite; reactive; affirmative; not negative. **2.** Denoting the presence of a particular disorder upon examination. **3.** Having a quantity greater than zero. **4.** Irrefutable.

positron A subatomic particle of the same mass as the electron and of equal but opposite (positive) charge.

postcardiotomy syndrome See postpericardiotomy syndrome.

postcholecystectomy syndrome A group of symptoms suggestive of biliary disease, such as right upper quadrant pain, indigestion, and food intolerance, which persist after removal of the gallbladder (cholecystectomy).

postcibal After meals; after eating.

postcibum (p.c.) Latin for after meals.

postclavicular Situated in back of the clavicle (collarbone).

postclimacteric Following the termination of the reproductive period.

postcoitus The time immediately or soon after coitus (sexual intercourse).

postcommissurotomy syndrome Fever, chest pains, and inflammation of the pericardium and pleura, occurring suddenly, within a few weeks, in patients who have undergone surgery of the heart valves.

postencephalitic Occurring after encephalitis.

posterior 1. Located behind a structure. **2.** Relating to the back or dorsal side of the human body.

posterior inferior cerebellar artery occlusion syndrome Syndrome occurring in occlusion of the posterior inferior cerebellar artery; symptoms include muscular weakness and loss of pain and temperature senses of the face, soft palate, pharynx, and larynx on the same side as the lesion, associated with loss of pain and temperature sensations of the extremities and trunk on the side opposite the lesion. Also called Wallenberg's syndrome.

posteroanterior From the back to the front.

posterolateral Behind and to one side.

posteromedial Behind and to the inner side.

postganglionic Situated behind or distal to a ganglion.

postgastrectomy syndrome See dumping syndrome.

posthioplasty Plastic surgery of the prepuce.

posthitis Inflammation of the prepuce. Also called acrobystitis.

postictal Following a convulsion.

postmaturity Condition in which the fetus remains in the uterus in excess of three weeks after the calculated date of birth.

postmenopausal Relating to the period after the menopause.

postmortem Pertaining to or occurring after death.

postmyocardial infarction syndrome Fever and pericarditis often accompanied by pleuritis occurring a week or more after a myocardial infarction.

postnasal Behind the nasal cavity.

postnatal After birth.

postoperative Occurring after a surgical operation.

postpartum Pertaining to, or occurring after, childbirth.

postpericardiotomy Occurring after surgery that involved cutting through the pericardium (two-layer membrane enveloping the heart).

postpericardiotomy syndrome An unusual complication of heart surgery in which there is a delayed pericardial or pleural reaction characterized by fever, pleuropericarditis, chest pain, and raised erythrocyte sedimentation. Also called postcardiotomy syndrome.

postphlebitic syndrome Chronic swelling of the leg, pain, and dermatitis secondary to stagnation of blood in the veins after phlebitis.

postpolio syndrome Recurrence, 20–30 years later, of weakness and atrophy of muscle groups that had regained function after an attack of poliomyelitis (polio); thought to be due to overuse of motor nerves supplying the muscles rather than a recurrence of the disease.

postprandial After a meal.

postpubertal Of, or occurring during, the period immediately after puberty.

postsynaptic 1. The time immediately following the transmission of an impulse from one neuron to another; occurring right after the crossing of a synapse. **2.** Situated distal to a synapse.

posttraumatic Occurring after an injury or resulting from it.

postulate An unproved assertion.

Koch's p.'s. To prove that a microorganism is the cause of a specific disease, it must be present in all cases of the disease, inoculations of its pure culture must produce the same disease in animals, and from these it must be obtained in pure cultures

and propagated.

posture Way of bearing one's body.

postvaccinal After vaccination.

pot A shortened version of the Mexican Indian word *potaguaya* meaning marijuana.

potable Fit to drink; drinkable.

potassium A soft alkaline metallic element; symbol K (kalium), atomic number 19, atomic weight 39.10; it plays an important physiologic role in muscular contraction, conduction of nerve impulses, enzyme action, and cell membrane function; normal potassium concentration of extracellular fluid is between 3.5 and 5 mEq/liter; normal potassium concentration of intracellular fluid is approximately 150 mEq/liter.

p. chloride A colorless crystalline solid or powder, KCl; used in the treatment of potassium deficiency.

p. iodide A crystalline powder, KI; soluble in water and used medicinally as a source of iodine.

p. nitrate KNO_3; a translucent, crystalline compound. Also called niter; saltpeter.

p. permanaganate A dark purple crystalline compound, $KMnO_4$; used as an antiseptic and deodorizing agent. Also called purple salt.

potassium-42 (^{42}K) An artificial isotope used as a tracer in studies of potassium distribution in body fluid compartments.

potency 1. The quality of being potent; strength. **2.** The comparative expression of drug activity relating to the dose required to produce a specific effect of given intensity as compared to a standard of reference. Cf. selectivity. **3.** Inherent ability for growth and development.

sexual p. Ability of a male to perform sexually.

potent 1. Powerful. **2.** Capable of producing a particular physiologic or chemical effect of strong intensity. **3.** Possessing sexual potency.

potentia Latin for potency.

potential 1. Capable of doing or being, but not yet realized. **2.** The force necessary to drive a unit positive charge from one point in an electrical field to another; the electromotive force that drives a current from one point to another.

action p. The electric current developed in a nerve, muscle, or other excitable tissue during its activity.

dark p. of the eye See resting potential of the eye.

demarcation p. See injury potential.

excitatory postsynaptic p. (EPSP) The change in potential seen in the postsynaptic membrane when an impulse that has an excitatory influence arrives at the synapse; a local change in the direction of depolarization.

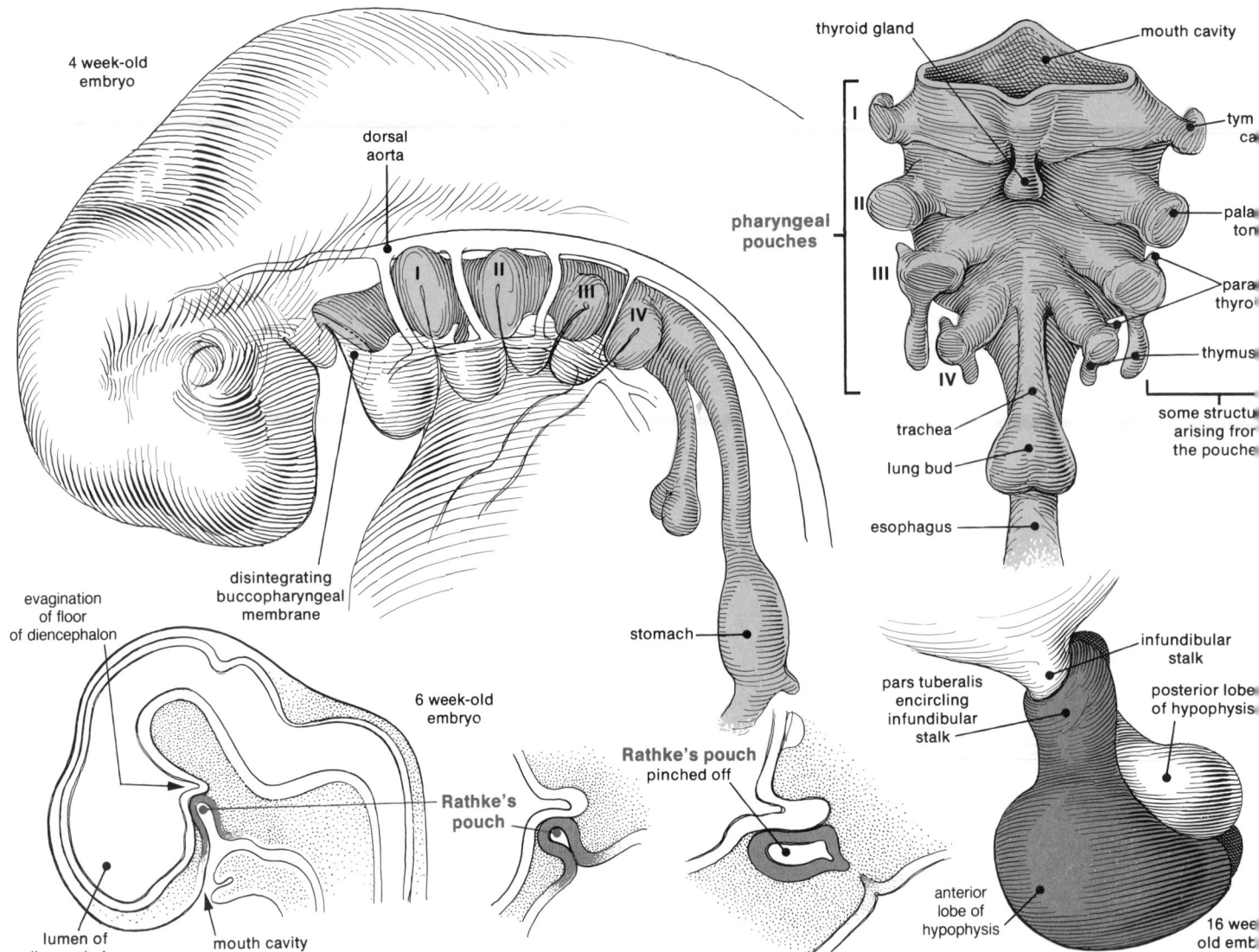

4 week-old embryo

dorsal aorta

disintegrating buccopharyngeal membrane

thyroid gland

mouth cavity

tym ca

pharyngeal pouches

pala ton

para thyro

thymus

trachea

lung bud

esophagus

some structu arising from the pouche

stomach

evagination of floor of diencephalon

6 week-old embryo

Rathke's pouch pinched off

Rathke's pouch

lumen of diencephalon

mouth cavity

pars tuberalis encircling infundibular stalk

infundibular stalk

posterior lobe of hypophysis

anterior lobe of hypophysis

16 wee old emb

inhibitory postsynaptic p. (IPSP) The change in potential seen in the postsynaptic membrane when an impulse that has an inhibitory influence arrives at the synapse; a local change in the direction of hyperpolarization.

injury p. The potential developed between the injured and uninjured parts of a nerve, due to the exposure of the negatively charged inner surface of the polarized membrane at the site of injury. Also called demarcation potential.

membrane p. The difference in potential between the two sides of a cell membrane, especially of nerve or muscle fibers; the outside is positive and the inside negative in the resting state.

oxidation-reduction p. (E_0^+, E^0) The relative potential, in volts, exerted by an inert (nonreacting) metallic electrode in a solution, as measured against that exerted by a normal hydrogen electrode at absolute temperature; the potential difference between an inert electrode and a reversible oxidation-reduction system in which it is submerged. Also called redox potential.

redox p. See oxidation-reduction potential.

resting p. of the eye The direct current potential difference between the anterior pole of the eye (cornea) and the posterior one (retina); usually expressed in millivolts. Also called dark potential of the eye.

visual evoked p. The potential as measured from electroencephalographic recordings taken from the occipital scalp area as the subject fixates a light flashing at ¼-second intervals; the computer averages the response of 100 consecutive flashes.

potentiation The increase in the power of an activity, such as in the force of the contraction of a muscle; the term is frequently used improperly in reference to drug interaction as a synonym of synergism.

potentiometer Instrument for measuring precisely electromotive forces.

potion A large liquid dose, especially of medicine.

Pott's disease Tuberculous spondylitis; see under spondylitis.

pouch A sac or pocket-like space.

Douglas' p. Rectouterine pouch.

Hartmann's p. A dilatation at the neck of the gallbladder.

Heidenhain p. One made for the experimental study of gastric secretions; an isolated part of the stomach, with the nervous supply interrupted, is opened to the outside through the abdominal wall.

Pavlov p. One made for the study of gastric secretions; an isolated part of the stomach, with the nervous supply left intact, is opened to the outside through an opening in the abdominal wall.

pharyngeal p.'s Paired lateral pouches of the embryonic pharynx; each pouch is in close relationship to an aortic arch and is situated opposite a branchial cleft.

Rathke's p. In embryology, the outpocketing of the stomodeum (embryonic mouth) occurring when the embryo is about three weeks old and subsequently forming the anterior (glandular) lobe of the hypophysis. Also called craniobuccal or neurobuccal pouch.

rectouterine p. The pocket-like space between the uterus and the rectum. Also called Douglas' pouch.

rectovesical p. The pouch between the rectum and the bladder in the male.

uterovesical p. The pouch between the bladder and the uterus.

poultice A hot, moist, soft mass of bread meal, linseed, or any other cohesive substance, applied to the skin between two pieces of muslin to soothe, relax, or stimulate an aching or inflamed part of the body.

pound A unit of weight equal to 16 ounces (avoirdupois weight) or 12 ounces (apothecaries' weight).

povidone A synthetic polymer used as a dispersing and suspending medium. Formerly called polyvinylpyrrolidone (PVP).

povidone-iodine Topical antiseptic formed by reacting povidone with iodine.

powder 1. In pharmaceutics, a mixture of dry, fine particles. 2. A single dose of such a powder, enclosed in paper.

Seidlitz p.'s A mild laxative composed of sodium bicarbonate, tartaric acid, and potassium sodium tartrate.

talcum p. A fine, soft toilet powder of perfumed talc.

power 1. The ability or capacity to produce effectively. 2. In optics, the refractive vergence of a lens. 3. Might.

back vertex p. The vergence power of a lens as measured from surface toward eye; standard for measurement of ophthalmic lenses.

focal p. See vergence power.

refractive p. The vergence power of a refracting optical system.

resolving p. A measure of the ability of a lens to image closely spaced objects so that they are recognized as separate objects; calculated by dividing the wavelength of the light used by twice the numerical aperture of the objective.

vergence p. The capability of an optical system to change the vergence of a cylinder of rays. Also called focal power.

pox 1. Any disease characterized by purulent eruptions on the skin. 2. A colloquial term for syphilis.

Poxviridae Family of large ovoid or brick-shaped viruses (300 to 450 nm × 170 to 260 nm) that contain a single molecule of double-stranded DNA and, unlike other DNA-containing viruses, multiply in cytoplasm; classified into two subfamilies of which only one (Chordopoxirinae) contains members infectious to man; includes viruses causing smallpox, vaccinia, and orf. Also called poxvirus group.

poxvirus Any virus of the family Poxviridae.

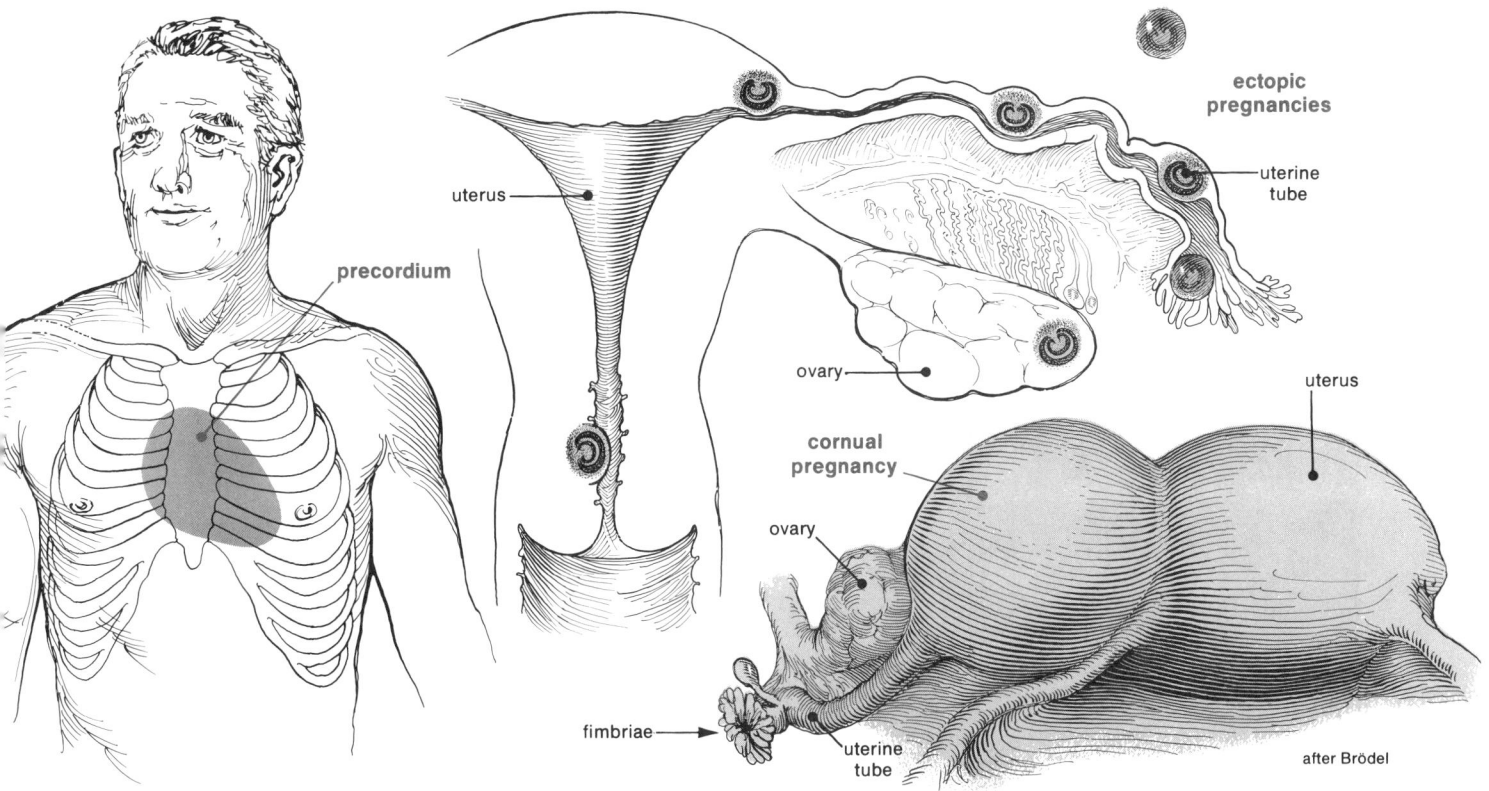

precordium

ectopic
pregnancies

uterus

uterine
tube

ovary

uterus

cornual
pregnancy

ovary

fimbriae

uterine
tube

after Brödel

P-pulmonale In electrocardiography, the P-wave pattern characteristic of cor pulmonale; a tall peaked P wave, usually seen in leads II, III, and AVF.

practice 1. The exercise of a profession or occupation. 2. To engage in, especially as a profession. 3. Collective term for the patients of a physician.

practitioner One who exercises a profession.

pragmatagnosia Loss of the power of recognizing objects formerly known to the individual.

praseodymium A soft, silvery, rare-earth element; symbol Pr, atomic number 59, atomic weight 140.907.

praxiology The study of behavior or conduct.

preagonal, preagonic Preceding the act of dying.

prealbumin A protein constituent of plasma, so named because its mobility is greater than that of albumin (at the alkaline pH values used for electrophoresis).

  thyroxine-binding p. One of the three carrier proteins of thyroxine in plasma.

preanal In front of the anus.

preanesthetic Before anesthesia; a medication administered to facilitate the subsequent induction of general anesthesia.

preauricular Situated in front of the auricle of the ear.

precancerous Subject to malignancy; said of a tumor.

precipitant Anything that causes the chemical separation of a solid from a solution.

precipitate 1. To cause a substance in solution to separate and form a solid deposit. 2. (ppt) The solid deposit thus formed. 3. Occurring abnormally quickly, as a precipitate labor.

precipitation 1. The act of separating a solid held in suspension or solution. 2. The clumping of protein in serum caused by the action of a specific precipitin.

precipitin An antibody that reacts specifically with a soluble antigen to cause a precipitate.

preclinical 1. Occurring before the onset of disease; referring to the stage of a disorder before clinical symptoms can be recognized and diagnosed. 2. Occurring before clinical work; referring to medical training that usually takes place during the first two years.

precocious Characterized by unusually early physical or mental maturity.

precocity Unusually early development, physical or mental.

  sexual p. A complex condition characterized by premature development and maturation of genital organs and secondary sexual characteristics.

precognition Extrasensory perception of an event not yet experienced.

preconscious In psychoanalysis, thoughts and ideas that can be recalled by conscious effort.

preconvulsive Preceding a convulsion.

precordial Relating to the area of the chest over the heart.

precordium The area of the chest wall which corresponds to the location of the heart. Also called antecardium.

precuneus A lobule on the mesial surface of each cerebral hemisphere located between the cuneus and paracentral lobules.

precursor Anything in the course of a process that is the forerunner or precedes a later stage, as a premalignant lesion, or as a physiologically inactive substance that is converted to an active substance, such as a hormone or enzyme.

prediabetes An early stage in the course of diabetes before there is any recognizable impairment of carbohydrate metabolism.

prediastole The interval in the cardiac rhythm cycle just preceding the diastole. Also called late systole.

predigestion Artificial initiation of the digestive process in protein and starch before they are used therapeutically as food.

predispose To render susceptible or liable.

predisposition The state of being predisposed or susceptible to a disease; a special tendency or inclination toward a disease.

prednisolone A synthetic glucocorticoid; white bitter crystals, soluble in water; used as a cortisone substitute.

prednisone A synthetic glucocorticoid; white bitter crystals, insoluble in water; used as a cortisone substitute, as it produces less water retention.

predormitum, predormition The state of waning consciousness that precedes sound sleep.

preeclampsia Disorder of the last trimester of pregnancy marked by hypertension, edema, and proteinuria; most common in first pregnancies.

preemy Informal term for premature infant.

preexcitation Premature activation of the ventricular myocardium by a supraventricular impulse that bypasses the normal A-V conduction pathway; an intrinsic part of the Wolff-Parkinson-White syndrome.

preexcitation syndrome See Wolff-Parkinson-White syndrome.

prefrontal Located in the anterior part of the frontal lobe or region of the brain.

preganglionic Situated before or proximal to a ganglion.

pregnancy The period of time between conception and birth of the child; the normal duration of human pregnancy is about 280 days or 9 calendar months. Also called gestation.

  abdominal p. Development of the impregnated ovum in the abdominal cavity resulting from an early rupture of a tubal pregnancy.

  cervical p. A rare form of ectopic pregnancy resulting from implantation of the fertilized ovum in the lining of the cervix.

  cornual p. Rare ectopic pregnancy, usually occurring in women with a double uterus, in which the fertilized ovum implants in a (usually rudimentary) uterine horn.

  ectopic p. One resulting from implantation of the fertilized ovum in a site other than the normal one in the uterine cavity, i.e., the interstitial portion of the uterine tube and the cervix as well as the ovary, the uterine tube, and the abdminal cavity.

  extrauterine p. Pregnancy occurring outside the cavity of the uterus.

  false p. Spurious pregnancy.

  interstitial p. Pregnancy resulting from implantation of the fertilized ovum in the portion of the uterine tube which pierces the wall of the uterus.

  multiple p. The simultaneous presence of two or more developing fetuses.

  ovarian p. A rare form of ectopic pregnancy in which the impregnated ovum develops in the ovary. Also called oocyesis.

  spurious p. The presence of symptoms of pregnancy without the occurrence of conception, usually occurring in women nearing menopause or in young women with an intense desire to be pregnant. Also called pseudocyesis; false or phantom pregnancy.

  tubal p. Implantation and development of the fertilized ovum in a uterine tube.

pregnane A saturated steroid hydrocarbon, derivative of cholane; a precursor of progesterone and several adrenocortical hormones.

pregnanediol $C_{21}H_{36}O_2$; the main metabolic end product of progesterone; its concentration in the urine is an indicator of corpus luteum function.

pregnanetriol A precursor in the biosynthesis of cortisol.

pregnant Carrying a developing offspring within the body. Also called gravid.

pregnene An unsaturated steroid derivative of pregnane.

prehensile Adapted for grasping.

prehormone An inactive glandular secretion capable of being converted into an active hormone.

preictal Before a convulsion or stroke.

preinfarction syndrome The sudden onset or worsening of angina pectoris prior to myocardial infarction.

preleukemia A defect of cellular differentiation

breech presentation

cephalic
presentation

pelvic
girdle

and maturation that precedes the onset of diagnosable acute leukemia as a primary maturational disturbance.

preload The stretch imposed on the heart muscle due to the ventricular and diastolic volume. Also called venous return.

preluxation Forward dislocation.

premalignant Preceding malignancy. Also called precancerous.

premature Occurring prior to correct or expected time.

prematurity The state of being premature.

premed An abbreviated version for premedical, or premedical student.

premedication A drug or drugs administered prior to a general anesthetic to allay apprehension and produce sedation.

premelanosome All particulate stages in the maturation of melanosomes.

premenarchal Taking place or existing prior to the onset of menstruation.

premenstrual Denoting the time of month prior to the menstrual flow.

premenstrual syndrome (PMS) The occurrence of all or some of the following symptoms during the week before the menstrual flow; lumbar and low abdominal pain, nervous irritability, headache, tenderness of the breasts, and pelvic congestion.

premolar A bicuspid tooth.

premunition Immunity established against a particular microorganism by infection (in a chronic form) with another related organism.

prenaris, *pl.* **prenares** Nostril.

prenatal Prior to birth.

preoperative Prior to an operation.

prepallium The cerebral cortex in front of the central sulcus (fissure of Rolando).

preparation 1. Readiness. 2. A substance, such as medicine, prepared for a particular purpose. 3. The reduction of a natural tooth in order to be able to receive a prosthesis, such as a crown.

cavity p. The removal of caries from a tooth and the establishment of a cavity that is able to receive and retain a restoration.

depot p. A drug whose physical state is altered so that it can be absorbed over an extended period of time; e.g., special microcrystalline suspensions of penicillin.

prepatellar In front of the kneecap (patella).

prepuberty The phase immediately preceding puberty.

prepuce The loose fold of skin that partly or completely covers the glans penis; it is this tissue that is removed by circumcision. Also called foreskin.

p. of clitoris A fold of the labia minora that forms a cap over the clitoris.

preputiotomy Surgical incision of the prepuce (foreskin) of the penis, usually to relieve tightness (phimosis).

prepyloric Located in the stomach, adjacent to the pylorus.

prerenal Located in front of a kidney.

presbycusis Progressive loss of hearing occurring in old age.

presbyopia (Pr) Diminution of accommodation power in the eyes due to advancing age. Commonly known as old sight.

prescribe To recommend a remedy in the treatment of a disorder.

prescription A written instruction by a licensed health science practitioner for the preparation and administration of any remedy, such as medication or corrective lenses.

shotgun p. A drug prescription containing many ingredients, given with the hope that one or more of them may be effective.

presenility 1. Premature old age. 2. Period immediately preceding old age.

present To appear first; said of the part of the fetus that is felt by the examining finger.

presentation The position of the fetus in the uterus during labor with respect to the birth canal.

breech p. Presentation of the pelvic extremity, known as (a) frank breech presentation when the legs of the fetus extend over the anterior surface of its body, (b) full breech presentation when the fetal thighs and legs are flexed, and (c) foot or footling presentation when one or both feet are the presenting parts.

cephalic p. One in which the head is the presenting part, known as (a) vertex presentation when the fetal head is flexed with its chin and thorax in contact, (b) sincipital presentation when the large fontanel is the presenting part, (c) brow presentation when the fetal brow is the presenting part, and (d) face presentation when the face is the presenting part. Also called head presentation.

head p. See cephalic presentation.

placental p. See placenta previa.

shoulder p. Presentation in which the long axis of the fetus lies transversely with the maternal long axis and a shoulder is the presenting part.

preservative 1. A substance added to food products, such as fatty acids, for inhibiting the growth of food-spoiling bacteria. 2. Capable of preserving.

presomite In embryology, before the appearance of somites.

pressor Causing constriction of blood vessels and a rise in blood pressure; said of certain substances and nerve fibers.

pressoreceptor See baroreceptor.

pressure A force applied or acting against resistance.

atmospheric p. The pressure exerted by the atmosphere; approximately 15 pounds per square inch at sea level, capable of supporting a column of mercury 760 millimeters high. Also called standard pressure.

back p. Pressure exerted in the circulatory system resulting from obstruction to flow.

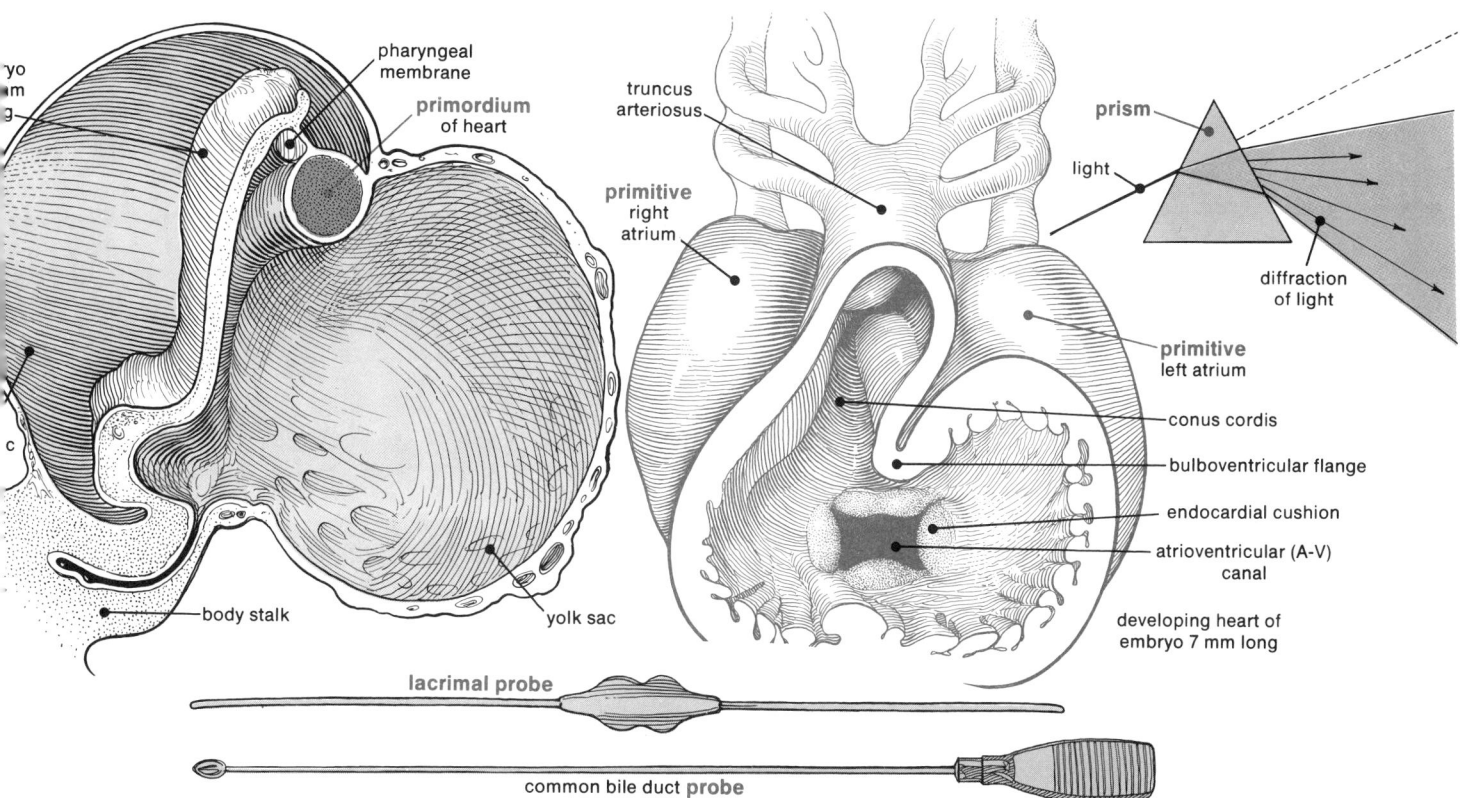

pharyngeal membrane
primordium of heart
truncus arteriosus
primitive right atrium
prism
light
diffraction of light
primitive left atrium
conus cordis
bulboventricular flange
endocardial cushion
atrioventricular (A-V) canal
developing heart of embryo 7 mm long
body stalk
yolk sac
lacrimal probe
common bile duct probe

blood p. The pressure of the circulating blood on the walls of the arteries, primarily maintained by the contraction of the left ventricle, the resistance of the arterioles and capillaries, the elasticity of the arterial walls, and the volume and viscosity of the blood; the maximum or systolic blood pressure occurs at the moment of systole of the left ventricle of the heart; the minimum or diastolic blood pressure occurs during diastole of the ventricle; the upper limits of normal in adults are generally set at 140/90 mm Hg.

central venous p. (CVP) Pressure of blood in the right atrium.

cerebrospinal p. Tension of the cerebrospinal fluid, normally 100 to 150 mm of water (with individual lying on one side).

continuous positive airway p. (CPAP) Respiratory therapy in which pressure within the lung airways is maintained above atmospheric pressure throughout the respiratory cycle.

critical p. The pressure required to condense or liquefy a gas at the critical temperature.

diastolic p. Arterial pressure during diastole; see blood pressure.

effective osmotic p. The portion of the total osmotic pressure of a solution that regulates the tendency of its solvent to pass through a boundary, such as a semipermeable membrane.

hydrostatic p. In a closed fluid system at rest, the pressure exerted at any level by the weight of the fluid above it.

hyperbaric p. Pressure higher than normal atmospheric pressure; used in therapy for shock, carbon dioxide poisoning, clostridial infections, and for some operations.

intracranial p. (ICP) Pressure within the skull.

intraocular p. (IOP) The pressure of the fluid within the eye; (measured by a tonometer, usually in millimeters of mercury).

intrapulmonic p. The pressure of air within the lungs.

negative p. A pressure lower than that of ambient atmosphere.

occlusal p. Any force exerted upon the occlusal surfaces of teeth.

oncotic p. Osmotic pressure exerted by colloids in solution.

osmotic p. Pressure or stress exerted by dissolved substances on a semipermeable membrane that separates a solution from the pure solvent.

partial p. The portion of the total pressure exerted by each component of a gas mixture, expressed in millimeters of mercury (mmHg).

positive end-expiratory p. (PEEP) Technique used in respiratory therapy to increase the amount

of gases remaining in the lungs after expiration by maintaining pressure within the airways.

pulmonary wedge p. See wedge pressure.

pulse p. The difference between the systolic (maximum) and diastolic (minimum) blood pressures within an artery during the cardiac cycle; it normally varies between 30 and 50 mmHg.

systolic p. Arterial pressure during systole; see blood pressure.

vapor p. The pressure exerted by the molecules of a vapor in equilibrium with its solid or liquid phase.

wedge p. (W) Intravascular pressure determined by positioning a catheter in branches of the pulmonary or hepatic venous system; the pressure thus obtained is felt to be a close reflection of pressure at the other end of the capillary bed and helps define the site of increased pressures across either of the two organs.

presynaptic 1. Existing or taking place before the synapse is crossed. 2. Situated proximal to a synapse.

presystole The interval immediately preceding the systole.

pretibial Pertaining to the front of the leg, especially that portion in front of the tibia.

prevalence The number of people with a specific condition in a given population.

preventive Acting to ward off or hinder the occurrence of something such as a disease.

prevertebral In front of a vertebra or of the vertebral column.

prevesical In front of the bladder.

previus Latin for in the way; usually applied to anything that obstructs the birth canal during childbirth. See also placenta previa.

priapism A continuous and pathologic erection of the penis without sexual desire; usually associated with general disorders, especially sickle cell anemia.

primacy The state of being first in importance or occurring first in a sequence.

primaquine phosphate Bitter, orange crystals, soluble in water; used in the treatment of malaria.

primary 1. Being first in a sequence or importance. 2. The simplest or most primitive form.

primate A member of the order Primates.

Primates The highest order of mammals, including man and those animals, such as apes, monkeys, and lemurs, nearest him in physical characteristics; from Latin *primus*, meaning first.

primigravida A woman in her first pregnancy. Also called unigravida.

primipara A woman who has completed one pregnancy to the stage of viability, regardless of whether it was a single or multiple birth, or whether the fetus was live or stillborn.

primaparous Denoting a primipara.

primitive Primary, embryonic.

primordial 1. Relating to the embryonic group of cells that develops into an organ or structure. 2. Formed during the early stage of development.

primordium 1. The earliest cells forming an organ in the embryo. 2. Anlage.

principle 1. A fundamental concept. 2. The essential ingredient characteristic of a drug or chemical compound.

active p. The constituent of a drug to which its physiologic effect is due.

antianemic p. Substance (chiefly found in liver) that stimulates remission of symptoms in pernicious anemia.

Fick p. Principle utilized in measurement of cardiac output and blood flow to some organs.

hematinic p. Vitamin B_{12}.

pleasure p. In psychoanalytic theory, the concept that man instinctively tries to avoid pain and discomfort, and endeavors to obtain gratification and pleasure.

reality p. In psychoanalytic theory, the concept that the pleasure principle is normally modified in personality development by the demands of the external world; e.g., postponement of gratification to a more appropriate time.

Starling p. The principle that the exchange of fluids across capillary membranes is governed by the net difference between the hydrostatic and osmotic pressures.

prion Infectious, viruslike entity highly resistant to inactivation; contains no DNA or RNA.

prism A transparent body, usually made of optical glass or crystalline material, with at least two polished plane faces inclined toward each other from which light is reflected or through which light is refracted.

proarrhythmia Drug-induced worsening of arrhythmia.

probability The ratio of the likelihood of occurrence of a specific event to total events.

proband The member of a family in whom a particular trait is first observed and through whom the rest of the family is brought under observation to study the hereditary characteristics of the trait. Also called propositus and index case. Cf. consultand; relative of interest.

probang A long, slender, flexible rod with a tuft of sponge or some other soft material at the end; used chiefly in removing obstructions from the esophagus or larynx.

probe A slender metal rod with a blunt tip, used to explore bodily cavities or wounds.

lacrimal p. A probe, usually made of silver, that

transverse process · **spinous process** · **scapula** · **acromion** · **coracoid process** · **ribs** · **clavicle** · **incus** · **stapes** · **malleus** · **lenticular process** · **zygomatic process of temporal bone** · **zygomatic process of maxillary bone** · **anterior part of the eye** · **cornea** · **iris** · **mastoid process** · **styloid process** · **condylar process of mandible** · **coronoid process** · **ciliary processes**

can be passed into the upper and lower puncta of the eyelids, through the upper and lower canaliculi, and down the nasolacrimal duct into the nose.

probenecid An agent that enhances the excretion of uric acid by inhibiting its reabsorption by the kidney; also inhibits excretion of penicillin by the kidney; Benemid®.

problem 1. Any situation that presents difficulty or uncertainty. 2. In psychiatry, term often used to denote a person whose behavior deviates from the norm; e.g., problem child; sometimes used in preference to the terms behavior disorder or mental disorder.

proboscis, *pl.* **proboscises** A tubular structure located near the oral cavity of certain insects and worms, often associated with feeding and used as a means of attachment.

procainamide hydrochloride White crystals, soluble in water; a cardiac depressant used in treating ventricular arrhythmias.

procaine hydrochloride A frequently used local anesthetic. $C_{13}H_{20}O_2N_2 \cdot HCl$; Novocaine®.

procaryote Any simple unicellular organism that does not have a nuclear membrane, membrane-bound organelles, and characteristic ribosomes; e.g., bacteria and blue-green algae.

procedure A manner of effecting something.
  cataract operative p. Any of several operations to remove a cataractous lens.

procercoid The larval stage of certain tapeworms, occurring in the intermediate host.

process 1. A marked prominence extending from an anatomic structure, usually for the attachment of muscles and ligaments. 2. A series of actions that attain a result.
  articular p. of vertebra One of the small projections on the upper and lower surfaces of the vertebra, forming the vertebral joint; the surface is coated with hyaline cartilage.

ciliary p.'s Radiating pigmented ridges (from 60 to 80 in number) on the inner surface of the ciliary body of the eye; formed by the inward folding of the various layers of the choroid.

clinoid p. One of three pairs of extensions from the sphenoid bone of the skull.

condylar p. of the mandible The articular process of the ramus of the mandible and the constricted portion (neck) that supports it.

coracoid p. A thick, curved bony projection from the scapula (shoulder blade) overhanging the glenoid fossa; it provides attachment for muscles and ligaments.

dendritic p. See dendrite.

hamulus p. Hamulus.

lenticular p. A right angle extension of the long limb of the incus bone of the middle ear; it articulates with the stapes.

mastoid p. A conical downward projection of the mastoid part of the temporal bone of the skull; situated behind the ear with the apex on a level with the lobe of the auricle; it serves for the attachment of the sternocleidomastoid muscle, the splenius muscle of the head, and the longissimus muscle of the head.

odontoid p. A toothlike process of the second cervical vertebra (axis) that articulates with the first cervical vertebra (atlas).

primary p. A type of thinking characterized by the lack of any sense of time, and the use of allusion, analogy, and symbolic representation. Also called nonlogical thinking.

pterygoid p. A long process extending downward from the junction of the body and great wing of the sphenoid bone on either side; it consists of a medial and lateral plate, the upper parts of which are fused together.

secondary p. A type of thinking controlled by the laws that govern conscious (or preconscious) mental activity.

spinous p. The dorsal projection of the vertebra from the junction of the laminae, forming, with those of other vertebrae, the spine.

styloid p. A slender, pointed projection extending downward and slightly forward from the petrous portion of the temporal bone; it gives attachment to the styloglossus, stylohyoid, and stylopharyngeus muscles, and the stylohyoid and stylomandibular ligaments.

transverse p. A lateral projection present on each side of a vertebra.

trochlear p. A projection from the lateral side of the calcaneus bone of the foot between the tendons of the long and short peroneal muscles.

xiphoid p. The small and pointed process connected with the lower end of the body of the sternum (breastbone); it is cartilaginous in youth, but at its upper part, ossified in the adult.

zygomatic p. of maxillary bone A rough triangular eminence from the maxilla that articulates with the zygomatic bone.

zygomatic p. of temporal bone A long arch projecting from the temporal bone that articulates with the temporal process of the zygomatic bone to form the zygomatic arch.

prochlorperazine A phenothiazine compound used as a tranquilizer and to relieve nausea and vomiting; Compazine®.

prochondral Relating to the stage preceding the development of cartilage.

prochordal Anterior to the notochord.

procidentia Complete prolapse of an organ.

procollagen A precursor of collagen.

proconvertin See factor VII.

procreate To produce offspring.

proctalgia, proctagra Pain in the rectum or in and around the anus. Also called proctodynia.
  p. fuga Acute spasmodic pain of only a few minutes duration in the rectum; occurring in young men usually at night.

proctoscope

progesterone
(corpus luteum
hormone)

scolex

proglottid
(mature segment)

bilobed ovary

uterus

testes

common genital pore

adult beef
tapeworm

prognathism

proctatresia Imperforation of the anus.
proctectasia Dilatation of the anus or rectum.
proctectomy Removal of the rectum.
proctencleisis, proctenclisia Stricture of the anus or rectum.
proctitis Inflammation of the rectum.
proctocele See rectocele.
proctoclysis, proctoclysia Continuous, slow infusion of saline solution into the rectum and colon.
proctocolitis See coloproctitis.
proctocolonoscopy Examination of the rectum and colon.
proctocolpoplasty Surgical closure of a rectovaginal fistula.
proctocystocele Bulging of the bladder into the rectum.
proctocystotomy The incising of the bladder from the rectum.
proctodeum The hollowed ectodermal surface located beneath the tail of the embryo; it rapidly depresses toward the cloaca and comes in contact with the outer surface of the cloacal wall.
proctodynia See proctalgia.
proctologic Of, or relating to, proctology.
proctologist A specialist in proctology.
proctology The branch of medicine concerned with the study of the rectum and anus and the treatment of their diseases.
proctomenia Vicarious menstruation involving the rectum.
proctoparalysis Paralysis of the anus, resulting in fecal incontinence.
proctoperineoplasty Plastic surgery of the anus and perineum. Also called rectoperineorrhaphy.
proctopexy Surgical fixation of a prolapsed rectum by suturing to another part. Also called rectopexy.
proctoplasty Plastic surgery of the anus or rectum. Also called rectoplasty.
proctoplegia Paralysis of the muscles of the rectum and anus.

proctoptosia, proctoptosis Prolapse of the rectum and anus.
proctorrhagia Bloody discharge from the rectum.
proctorrhaphy Suturing of a lacerated rectum or anus.
proctorrhea Mucous discharge from the rectum.
proctoscope Instrument used for inspecting the rectum; a speculum. Also called rectoscope.
proctoscopy Examination of the rectum with a proctoscope.
proctosigmoidectomy Surgical removal of the rectum and sigmoid colon.
proctosigmoiditis Inflammation of the rectum and sigmoid colon.
proctosigmoidoscopy Examination of the interior of the rectum and sigmoid by means of a sigmoidoscope.
proctospasm Spasmodic contraction of the rectum or anus.
proctostat A tube containing radium for insertion through the anus in the treatment of cancer of the rectum.
proctostenosis Abnormal narrowing of the rectum or anus. Also called rectostenosis.
proctostomy The establishment of a permanent opening into the rectum.
proctotomy Surgical incision of the anus or rectum.
proctovalvotomy Incision of rectal valves.
procumbent Lying face down.
prodromal Relating to prodrome.
prodrome An early symptom of a disease, as one seen before the rash of a communicable disease.
product Any substance produced, naturally or artificially.
  cleavage p. Substance resulting from the splitting of large molecules into simpler ones.
  fibrin-fibrinogen degradation p. Any small peptide (X, Y, D, or E) produced by the action of plasmin on fibrinogen and fibrin during the fibrinolytic process.
  fission p. Atomic species resulting from the split-

ting of large atoms.
productive Denoting an inflammatory condition leading to the formation of new tissue.
proencephalon See prosencephalon.
proenzyme The inactive precursor of an enzyme that requires some change to render it active; e.g., profibrolysin. Also called zymogen.
proerythroblast The earliest red blood cell precursor, generally 12 to 19 μm in diameter; characterized by scanty, basophilic cytoplasm without hemoglobin, and a nucleus having fine chromatin. Also called pronormoblast; rubriblast.
proerythrocyte The precursor of a red blood cell; an immature erythrocyte with a nucleus.
profunda, profundus Latin for deep; applied to certain anatomic structures.
progenital On the exposed surface of the external genitalia.
progeria Premature senility of old age.
progestational 1. Conducive to pregnancy. 2. Referring to progesterone.
progesterone A hormone produced in the ovary by the corpus luteum; it stimulates changes in the wall of the uterus in preparation for implantation of the fertilized ovum.
progestin 1. A hormone of the corpus luteum that acts on the lining of the uterus (endometrium). 2. General term for any synthetic drug providing such action.
progestogen An agent that produces effects similar to those of progesterone.
proglossis The tip of the tongue.
proglottid One of the segments of the tapeworm that contains both male and female reproductive organs; in a mature proglottid, ovules are produced and fertilized hermaphroditically.
prognathic See prognathous.
prognathism Abnormal forward projection of the lower jaw.
prognathous Having a projecting lower jaw. Also called prognathic.
prognose To predict the probable course and out-

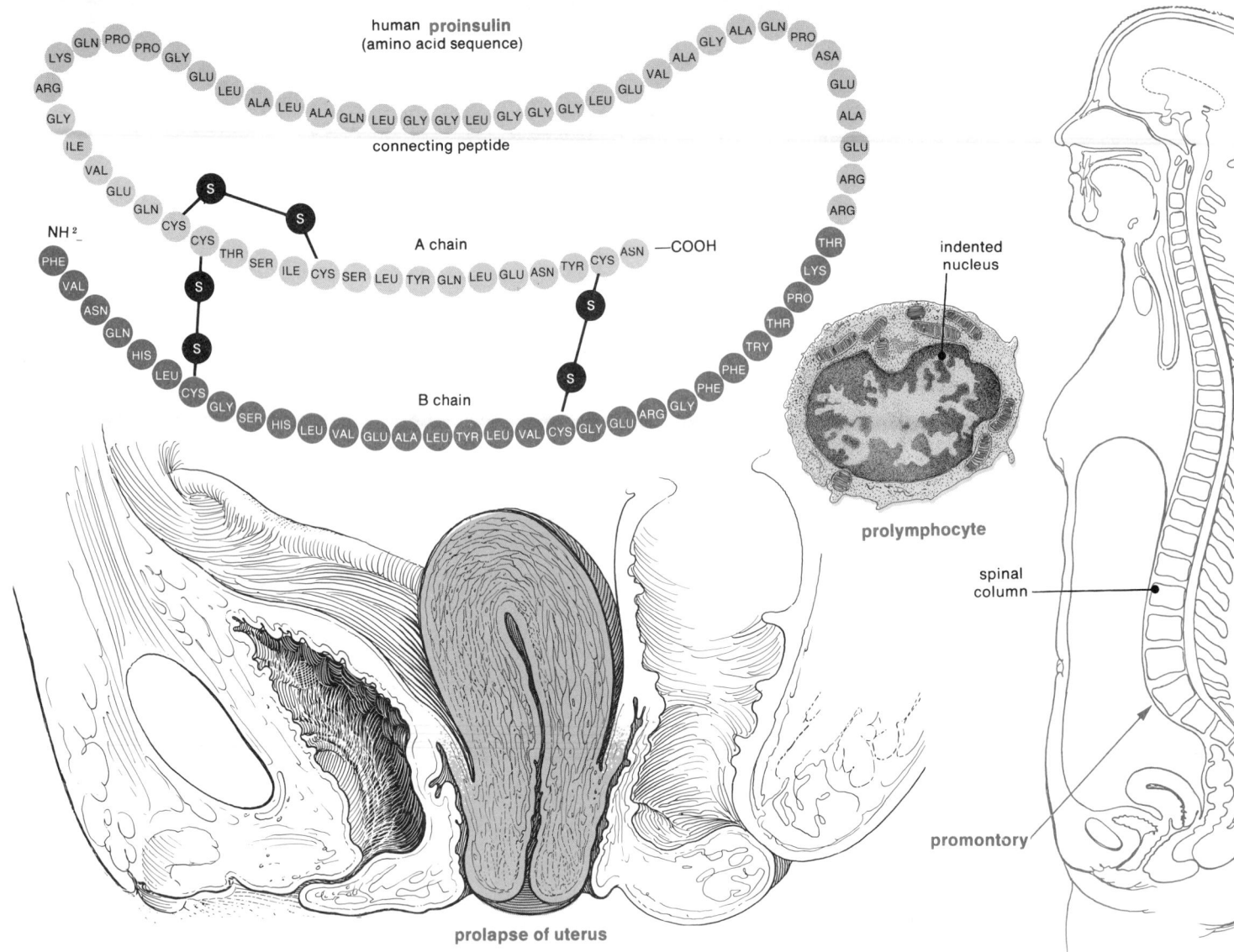

human **proinsulin**
(amino acid sequence)

connecting peptide

A chain

B chain

prolymphocyte

indented
nucleus

spinal
column

promontory

prolapse of uterus

come of a disease. Also called prognosticate.

prognosis A prediction of the outcome of a disease.

prognosticate To give a prognosis. Also called prognose.

program, quality assurance A program designed to insure the quality of patient care within a health facility; peer groups monitor the care given to a patient; necessary changes are brought about through continuing education.

progranulocyte See promyelocyte.

progressive Usually denoting the unfavorable course of a disease, as from bad to worse. Also called advancing.

prohormone Any precursor of a hormone; e.g., proinsulin.

proinsulin A single chain precursor of insulin; formed in the endoplasmic reticulum of the cell and transferred to the Golgi apparatus where the connecting peptide (C-peptide) is removed enzymatically, resulting in the formation of insulin.

projection 1. A prominence. 2. The referring of sensations from the sense organs to the source of the stimulus. 3. The referring to another of one's own unacceptable, repressed attributes. 4. The application of x rays to a bodily part in a particular direction as it relates to the x-ray tube, e.g., anteroposterior (AP), posteroanterior (PA), right anterior oblique (RAO), right posterior oblique (RPO), etc. Also called view.

  Caldwell p. Radiographic projection obtained by placing the face against the cassette and the x-ray tube 15° caudad in a posterior-anterior plane; permits unobstructed viewing of orbital structures.

  Towne p. Radiographic projection obtained by placing the back of the head against the cassette and the x-ray tube 30° caudad in an anterior-posterior plane; permits viewing of occipital bone, foramen magnum, dorsum sellae, and petrous ridges.

prokaryosis A state in which the nuclear sub-

stance of a primitive cell is mixed or is in direct contact with the rest of the protoplasm, due to not having a nuclear envelope.

prolactin A hormone produced by the anterior lobe of the pituitary gland that stimulates milk secretion.

prolactinoma A benign, prolactin-producing pituitary tumor.

prolapse 1. To fall down or slip down. 2. The slipping down of an organ or part from its normal position.

  p. of rectum Protrusion of the inner surface of the rectum through the anus.

  p. of uterus Falling of the uterus into the vagina due to stretching and laxity of its supporting structures.

proliferation Multiplication of similar cells.

prolific 1. Copiously productive. 2. Bearing offspring in great abundance. Also called fertile.

proline (Pro) Amino acid present in collagen.

prolymphocyte A cell midway in maturity between the lymphoblast and the lymphocyte; it has the capacity to divide, and may serve as a reservoir of immunologically uncommitted cells.

promastigote The flagellate stage of a trypanosomatid microorganism. Formerly called leptomonad; leptomonad stage.

promazine hydrochloride Phenothiazine compound used as a tranquilizer and antiemetic; Sparine®.

promegaloblast A large nucleated red blood cell; an early stage in the maturation of the megaloblast.

prometaphase A stage of mitosis, between prophase and metaphase, marked by the disintegration of the nuclear membrane and formation of the spindle.

promethazine hydrochloride An antihistaminic compound used also as an adjuvant with narcotics; Phenergan®.

promethium A radioactive rare-earth element;

symbol Pm; atomic number 61; atomic weight 147 (best-known isotope); half-life 2.6 years; used as a source of beta-rays.

prominence A projection.

  laryngeal p. The projection in front of the neck produced by the thyroid cartilage. Also called Adams's apple.

promontory A projection or elevation.

promoter 1. A substance that increases the activity of a catalyst. 2. The area on DNA in which RNA polymerase binds and initiates transcription.

promyelocyte The developmental stage of a granular leukocyte, between a myeloblast and myelocyte, containing a variable number of large ovoid or irregularly spherical granules; nucleoli are often present. Also called progranulocyte.

pronate To assume, or to be placed in, a prone or face-down position.

pronation The act of lying face downward or of rotating the forearm so that the palm of the hand is turned backward or downward.

prone Lying with the face downward.

pronephros, *pl.* pronephroi The primitive excretory organ of the embryo, consisting of a series of rudimentary tubules; it is replaced by the transitory mesonephros which forms caudally to it.

pronograde The horizontal position of the body of a quadruped; opposed to orthograde.

pronometer An instrument for determining the degree of pronation or supination of the forearm.

pronormoblast The earliest red blood cell precursor, generally 12 to 19 μm in diameter; characterized by scanty, basophilic cytoplasm without hemoglobin, and a nucleus having fine chromatin. Also called proerythroblast; rubriblast.

pronucleus One of two nuclei, or haploid nuclei, undergoing fusion, as of an egg or sperm at the time of fertilization.

proof spirit A mixture of alcohol and water or a beverage containing 50% (100 proof) of ethyl alco-

five member
cyclopentane
ring

20-carbon
carboxylic fatty acid

prostaglandin endoperoxide
(from which all PGs are derived)

hol by volume at 60°F.

pro-opiomelanocortin A precursor molecule, found in many different tissues, capable of yielding a variety of hormones, e.g., ACTH and beta-endorphin.

propagation 1. Reproduction. 2. The continuance of an impulse along a nerve fiber.

propantheline bromide An anticholinergic agent used in treatment of gastrointestinal disorders; Pro-Banthine®.

proparacaine hydrochloride An effective surface anesthetic derived from aminobenzoic acid; used principally in ophthalmology; Ophthaine®.

propenyl The trivalent radical, $C_3H_3O_3$, of glycerol. Also called glyceryl.

properdin A natural euglobulin protein in human blood serum with molecular weight approximately eight times that of gamma globulins; it acts in conjunction with complement and magnesium ions and plays a role in providing immunity from infectious diseases, and possibly in initiating other immune processes.

properitoneal Situated in front of the peritoneum, i.e., between the parietal peritoneum and the abdominal wall.

prophage In lysogenic bacteria, the structure that conveys genetic coding for the creation of a given type of phage and bestows specific hereditary traits on the host. Also called probacteriophage.

prophase The first stage of cell division by mitosis, during which chromatin collects into a chromosomal thread that breaks up into pairs of rod-shaped chromosomes; each chromosome then splits longitudinally into chromatids.

prophylactic 1. Relating to the prevention of disease. 2. An agent that wards off disease. 3. Common name for a condom.

prophylaxis 1. Precautions taken to prevent a disease; preventive treatment. 2. In dentistry, cleaning of the teeth.

propositus, *pl.* **propositi,** *female* **proposita** See proband.

propoxyphene hydrochloride A mild analgesic; Darvon®.

propranolol hydrochloride An adrenergic beta-receptor blocking agent that diminishes the rate and contractile force of the heart, causing a fall in cardiac output and cardiac work; used in the treatment of arrhythmias, angina, and hypertension and for prevention of migraine.

proprioceptor A sensory nerve ending, primarily located within the muscles and tendons, which receives stimuli pertaining to movements and position of the body.

　muscle p. Neuromuscular spindle; see under spindle.

proptometer See exophthalmometer.

proptosis Bulging or protrusion of an organ, as of the eyeball.

propulsion Displacement of the center of gravity producing a tendency to lean forward, seen in persons suffering from paralysis agitans (Parkinson's disease).

propyl The radical of propyl alcohol or propane.

propyl alcohol A clear colorless fluid, CH_3-CH_2CH_2OH, more toxic than ethyl alcohol and widely used as a solvent.

propylene A flammable colorless gas soluble in water; $CH_2 = CHCH_3$.

propylparaben Any of several compounds used as preservatives in a number of pharmaceutical preparations; known to cause contact dermatitis when used in skin creams, lotions, etc.

propylthiouracil Compound used in the treatment of hyperthyroidism.

pro re nata (p.r.n.) Latin for when necessary; used in prescription writing.

prorubricyte Basophilic normoblast; see under normoblast.

prosection An anatomic dissection made specifically for demonstration or for exhibition.

prosector One who prepares or dissects anatomic structures for demonstration.

prosectorium A dissecting room for preparing prosections. Also called anatomy laboratory.

prosencephalon The part of the embryonic brain developed from the most anterior portion of the embryonic neural tube; later it forms the telencephalon and the diencephalon. Also called forebrain; proencephalon.

prosodemic Denoting a disease that is spread from one individual to another; an outbreak of a disease arising in this manner, in contrast to an epidemic.

prosody The variations in the stress and intonation patterns of speech by which different shades of meaning are communicated.

prosopagnosia A form of visual agnosia in which the individual is unable to recognize, or has great difficulty recognizing, familiar faces.

prosoplegia Facial palsy; see under palsy.

prosopotocia Face presentation in childbirth.

prostacyclin See prostaglandin.

prostaglandin (PG) One of a family of hormone-like, lipid-soluble, acidic compounds derived from long-chain polyunsaturated fatty acids; occurring in nearly all tissues (including cerebrospinal fluid), and possessing an intricate array of physiologic actions (e.g., suppression of gastric acid secretions, peripheral vasodilation, increased renal blood flow, and bronchodilation); used for inducing labor and treat-

ing peptic ulcers; other potential uses are in hypertension and asthma; aspirin, indomethacin, phenylbutazone, and other nonsteroidal anti-inflammatory agents prevent prostaglandin synthesis; first found in semen and believed to originate from the prostate, thus the name prostaglandin. PGs are classified by chemical structure, using letters (e.g., PGA, PGB) to designate ring substitution and numerical subscripts (e.g., PGA_1) to denote number of unsaturated bonds. Prostacyclin or PGI_2, a powerful inhibitor of platelet aggregation, appears of importance in maintaining the integrity of blood vessel walls. See also eicosanoids; leukotriene; thromboxane.

prostatalgia Pain in the prostate.

prostate A chestnut-shaped body in the male consisting of glandular and muscular tissue that surrounds the urethra immediately below the bladder; it secretes a milky fluid that is discharged by excretory ducts into the urethra at the time of ejaculation.

prostatectomy Surgical removal of the prostate, or a portion of it.

prostatic Relating to the prostate.

prostatism Any condition caused by hypertrophy or other disease of the prostate; usually refers to symptoms of obstructive uropathy caused by prostatic hypertrophy.

prostatitis Inflammation of the prostate.

prostatocystitis Inflammation of the prostate and the bladder.

prostatocystotomy Incision through the prostate and bladder wall.

prostatolith A stone of the prostate.

prostatolithotomy Incision of prostate for removal of a calculus.

prostatomyomectomy Surgical removal of a myomatous or hypertrophied prostate.

prostatorrhea Abnormal discharge from the prostate.

prostatotomy Incision of the prostate.

prostatovesiculectomy Surgical removal of the prostate and the seminal vesicles.

prostatovesiculitis Inflammation of the prostate and the seminal vesicles.

prosthesis An artificial replacement for a missing or dysfunctional part.

　cleft palate p. Appliance used to correct a congenital structural deficiency in the roof of the mouth.

　dental p. Artificial replacement of one or more teeth and/or related structures.

　discoid valve p. An artificial heart valve consisting of a free disc in an open cage.

　ocular p. An artificial eye.

　penile p. A device implanted within a penis to permit adequate rigidity for coitus; it could be a semirigid rod, or a two-cylinder inflatable device.

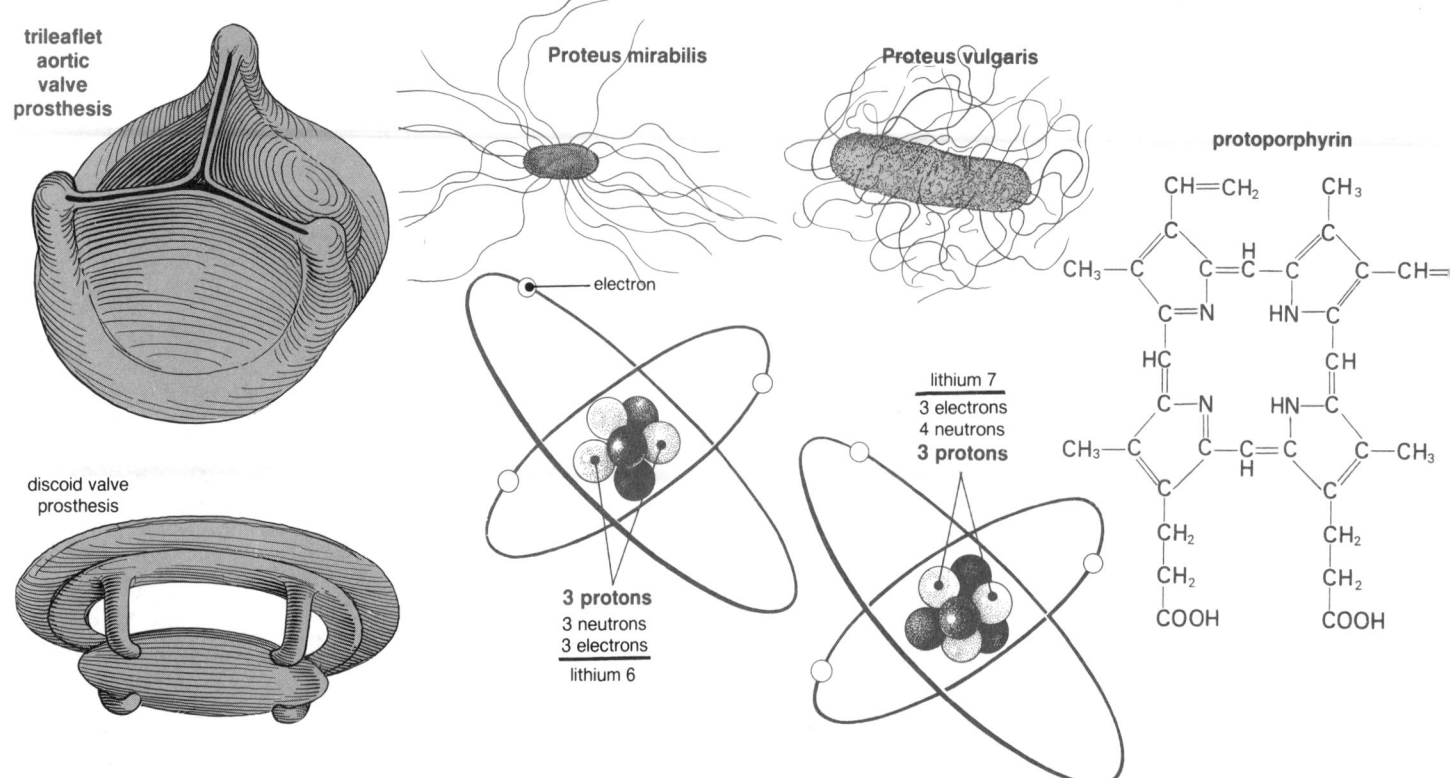

trileaflet aortic valve prosthesis

discoid valve prosthesis

Proteus mirabilis

Proteus vulgaris

electron

lithium 7
3 electrons
4 neutrons
3 protons

3 protons
3 neutrons
3 electrons
lithium 6

protoporphyrin

trileaflet aortic valve p. A one-piece trileaflet artificial heart valve that permits a full central flow pattern similar to that of the normal valve.

prosthetic Relating to an artificial part of the body.

prosthetics The making and adjusting of artificial parts of the body.

dental p. See prosthodontics.

prosthion A craniometric point situated on the maxillary alveolar process that projects most anteriorly in the midline; used in measuring facial depth. Also called alveolar point.

prosthodontics The branch of dentistry pertaining to the restoration and maintenance of oral function by the replacement of missing teeth and associated structures by artificial appliances. Also called dental prosthetics.

prosthodontist A specialist in prosthodontics.

prosthokeratoplasty Reparative surgery of the eye by means of which excised corneal tissue is replaced by a transparent prosthetic implant.

prostration A state of extreme exhaustion.

protactinium A rare radioactive element, symbol Pa, atomic number 91, atomic weight 231; similar to uranium.

protaminase An enzyme of the proteinase class which normally splits up protamines to peptides in the intestine. Also called carboxypeptidase B.

protamine Any of a group of simple, highly basic proteins, rich in arginine and soluble in water; they neutralize the anticoagulant action of heparin.

p. sulfate A heparin antagonist used to neutralize excess amounts of heparin.

protanopia Inability to differentiate red, orange, yellow, and green. Also called red blindness; anerythropsia.

protean Changeable in form; having the capacity to readily assume different shapes or forms. Also called variable.

protease Any enzyme that acts upon the peptide bonds of proteins and peptides; a protein-splitting or hydrolyzing enzyme. Also called proteolytic enzyme.

protection, personal injury In automobile insurance, first party no-fault coverage under which an insurance firm pays, within specified limits, medical, hospital, or funeral costs of the insured, others in his vehicle, or pedestrians hit by him.

protein Any of a group of complex nitrogenous substances of high molecular weight that contain amino acids as their fundamental structural units, are present in the cells of all animals and plants, and function in all phases of chemical and physical activity of the cells.

Alzheimer's disease associated p. (ADAP) A protein found in the brain and spinal fluid of people afflicted with Alzheimer's disease.

Bence Jones p. A protein found in the urine of individuals with multiple myeloma; when the urine is heated, a precipitate forms at 50 to 60°C which dissolves when the temperature is raised to near boiling point. Also called Bence Jones albumin.

conjugated p. Compound formed by the combination of a protein with a nonprotein (prosthetic) group.

C-reactive p. Abnormal protein found in the blood serum of persons in acute stages of inflammatory diseases such as rheumatic fever.

denatured p. One that has undergone a change, so that its characteristic properties are lost.

foreign p. One that differs from those normally found in the blood, lymph, or bodily tissues.

native p. Protein in its natural state.

p. C A protein constituent of blood plasma that prevents coagulation of blood; deficiency of protein C causes recurrent thrombophlebitis.

plasma p.'s Proteins present in blood plasma; e.g., albumin, globulins, fibrinogen.

plasma p. fraction Selected proteins from blood plasma of adult human donors, used as a blood volume supporter.

p. hydrolysate (intravenous) A product of protein hydrolysis used after surgery of the intestinal tract and certain severe illnesses. Also called casein hydrolysate 5%; Amigen®.

p. S A vitamin K-dependent protein of blood plasma needed as a cofactor for the antithrombotic functions of protein C.

simple p. Protein that yields only amino acids upon hydrolysis.

proteinaceous Relating to, or of the nature of a protein.

proteinase Any enzyme that hydrolyzes native protein or polypeptides; e.g., pepsin.

proteinosis Condition marked by an increase in proteins in the tissues, especially abnormal proteins.

pulmonary alveolar p. A chronic progressive disease of the lungs, marked by accumulation of a homogeneous granular substance in the alveoli (air sacs); it affects adults and its cause is unknown.

proteinuria Excretion of protein in the urine in excess of the normal daily amount; an average-size healthy individual normally excretes up to 100 mg of protein per day.

heavy p. Excretion of more than 4 g of protein daily, usually caused by renal disorders that greatly increase glomerular permeability.

orthostatic p. See postural proteinuria.

postural p. Excessive excretion of protein in the urine, usually mild, in healthy adolescents and young adults, occurring when the individual is upright, and disappearing during recumbency. Also called orthostatic proteinuria.

transient p. Proteinuria that may occur with febrile disorders, abdominal crises, heart disease, severe anemia, and emotional stress. Also called intermittent or functional proteinuria.

proteolysis The breaking down (hydrolysis) of proteins into simpler, soluble forms by the action of enzymes, as in digestion.

proteolytic Causing proteolysis.

proteose One of the intermediate products of protein digestion, between a protein and a peptone.

Proteus A genus of gram-negative bacteria, motile only at 25°C; most commonly associated with urinary tract and wound infections; may also be seen in diarrhea and gastroenteritis.

P. mirabilis A species found in putrid meat, effusions, and abscesses; thought to be a cause of gastroenteritis.

P. morganii Species that is a common inhabitant of the gastrointestinal tract; seen in normal and diarrheal stools.

P. vulgaris Species found in putrefying tissues and abscesses; certain strains are agglutinated by typhus serum and therefore are used in diagnosing the disease (Weil-Felix reaction).

prothrombin A plasma protein that is converted into thrombin during the second stage of blood coagulation; an enzymically inactive precursor of thrombin. Formerly called thrombinogen. Also called factor II.

Protista A third kingdom or division of living things comprised of unicellular organisms such as bacteria, protozoa, and many fungi and algae.

protium See hydrogen-1.

protodiastolic Relating to the initial one-third of a cardiac diastole or the period immediately following the second heart sound.

proton (p) The unit of positive electricity; the nucleus of the hydrogen atom; a particle of all other atomic nuclei having a mass of 1.0073 units and a positive charge equal numerically to the negative charge of an electron.

proto-oncogene A cellular gene normally concerned with cell division; may be transformed into a tumor-forming gene (oncogene) if rearranged, mutated, or picked up by a retrovirus.

protoplasm The essential substance of which all living cells, vegetable and animal, are made.

protoporphyria Condition marked by high concentrations of protoporphyrin in red blood cells, plasma, and feces.

protoporphyrin A porphyrin which, linked with iron, forms the heme of hemoglobin and the pros-

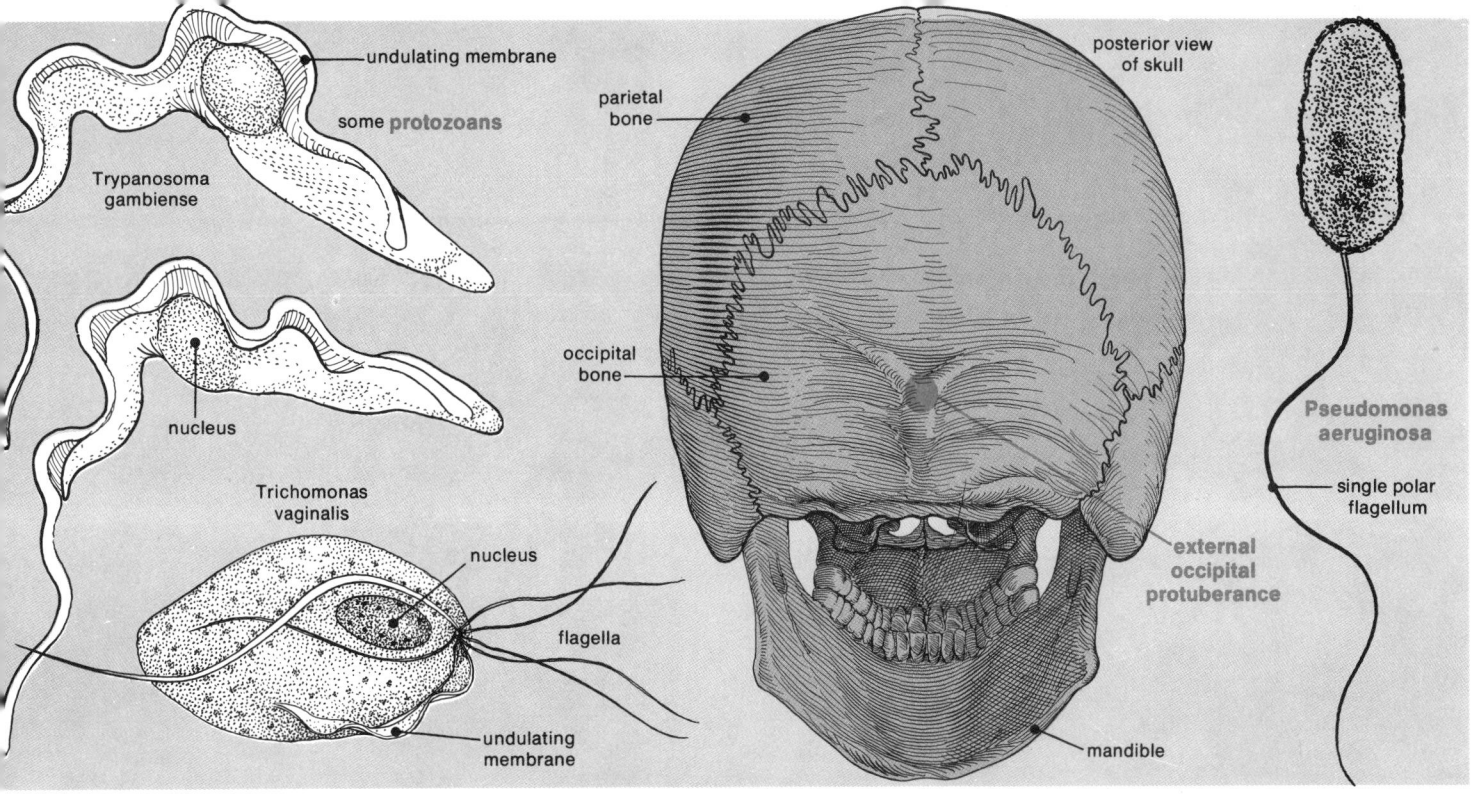

some **protozoans**

Trypanosoma gambiense

undulating membrane

nucleus

Trichomonas vaginalis

nucleus

flagella

undulating membrane

parietal bone

posterior view of skull

occipital bone

external occipital protuberance

mandible

Pseudomonas aeruginosa

single polar flagellum

thetic groups of myoglobin catalase, cytochromes, etc.

prototroph The nutritionally independent, wild-type strain of any organism. Cf. auxotroph.

prototype The primitive or ancestral species from which others develop or to which they conform.

Protozoa A phylum of the animal kingdom which includes all unicellular organisms; members of the subphyla Ciliophora, Mastigophora, Sarcodinia, and Sporozoa are of medical interest.

protozoacide An agent capable of destroying protozoa.

protozoal, protozoan Pertaining to protozoa.

protozoan A unicellular organism, member of the phylum Protozoa. Also called protozoon.

protozoiasis Infestations with protozoans.

protozoology The biological study of the simplest or most primitive forms of animal life (protozoa).

protozoon See protozoan.

protozoophage A cell that ingests protozoa.

protraction In dentistry, condition in which teeth or other maxillary or mandibular structures are located anterior to their normal position.

protractor 1. An instrument for extracting a foreign object, such as a bullet, from a deep wound. 2. A muscle that extends a limb; an extensor muscle.

protrusion In dentistry, position of the mandible forward or laterally forward from the centric position.

protuberance An eminence, projection, or bulge.

external occipital p. A prominence at the center of the outer surface of the occipital bone.

internal occipital p. A prominence at the midpoint of the inner surface of the occipital bone.

mental p. A triangular elevation on the lower portion of the outer surface of the mandible, at the midline, that helps to form the chin.

provirus A virus that has become an integral part of the host cell chromosome and is transmitted from one cell generation to another.

provitamin A substance in certain foods that may be converted into a vitamin; a precursor of a vitamin such as carotene. Also called previtamin.

proximal 1. Nearest the center, midline, point of attachment, or point of origin; opposite of distal. 2. In dentistry, the surface of a tooth, either mesial or distal, which is nearest an adjacent tooth.

proximate Nearest, next; approximate; immediate.

proximoataxia Lack of muscular coordination of the proximal portions of the extremities.

prune The partially dried fruit of the common plum *Prunus domestica*; used as a mild laxative.

prune-belly syndrome Congenital absence of the medial and lower muscles of the abdominal wall, associated with urinary tract abnormalities and un-

descended testicles; males are affected almost exclusively; cause is unknown.

prurient Denoting morbid interest in aberrant matter, especially of a sexual nature.

pruriginous Relating to prurigo.

prurigo An itchy skin eruption of papules.

pruritic Itchy.

pruritus Itching.

p. ani Intense itching at the anus; may be caused by infections, hemorrhoids, or allergy; also, fecal soiling of the perianal skin may play an important role, inducing a chemical dermatosis.

prussiate 1. A salt of hydrocyanic acid; a cyanide. 2. A ferricyanide or ferrocyanide.

prussic acid See hydrocyanic acid.

psammoma A type of meningioma; a benign calcified tumor derived from a connective tissue and occurring along the blood vessels of dura and skull; characterized by the formation of multiple, discrete, concentrically laminated, calcareous bodies (psammoma bodies).

pseudarthrosis A false joint formed on the shaft of a long bone, at the site of a fracture that failed to fuse. Also called neoarthrosis.

pseudesthesia 1. Subjective sensation without an external stimulus. 2. Sensation referred to an absent limb after an amputation. Also called pseudoesthesia.

pseudoallele A gene that behaves as an allele, but occupies a different, closely linked position on a chromosome; it can be separated by crossing over.

pseudoaneurysm Dilatation of an artery resembling an aneurysm.

pseudocoarctation An elongated and tortuous condition of the aortic arch in the area of the ligamentum arteriosum without occlusion of the vessel.

pseudocroup See laryngismus stridulus.

pseudocryptorchism Condition in which the testes occasionally move high into the inguinal canal.

pseudocyst 1. Accumulation of fluid without an enclosing membrane. 2. An aggregation of *Toxoplasma* parasites within a host cell.

pseudodementia Reversible condition, accompanying depression, marked by exaggerated indifference to one's surroundings.

pseudoesthesia See pseudesthesia.

pseudofracture Condition in which new bone tissue and thickening of periosteum is formed at the site of an injury.

pseudoganglion A localized thickening of a nerve trunk simulating a ganglion.

pseudoglaucoma An abnormality of the optic disk resembling glaucoma, due to conditions other than pressure within the eyeball.

pseudogout A disease characterized by calcified deposits in articular cartilage that are free of urate and consist of calcium pyrophosphate crystals; a form of chondrocalcinosis; it leads to goutlike attacks of pain, swelling, stiffness, local warmth, and joint tenderness; the knee is the joint predominantly affected.

pseudohemophilia An acquired condition resembling hemophilia but caused by another disorder.

pseudohemoptysis Spitting of blood from a source other than the lungs or bronchi.

pseudohermaphroditism Condition in which a person is distinctly of one sex but has superficial characteristics of the opposite sex. Commonly, and wrongly, called hermaphroditism.

male p. Condition in which a person has testes but secondary sexual characteristics of both sexes.

female p. Condition in which a person has ovaries but secondary sexual characteristics of both sexes.

pseudohernia A swelling resembling a hernia, caused by inflammation of an inguinal gland or scrotal tissue.

pseudohypha A structure of many fungi which is formed by budding, is composed of a chain of cells, and resembles a hypha.

pseudohypoparathyroidism A genetic disorder resembling hypoparathyroidism in which the primary defect is renal unresponsiveness to parathyroid hormone; usually characterized by short stature, round face, and ectopic calcifications and associated with hyperphosphatemia and hypocalcemia; transmitted as an X-linked dominant trait.

pseudomembrane See membrane, false.

Pseudomonas A genus of gram-negative motile bacteria with polar flagella, occurring in soil, water, sewage, and air.

P. aeruginosa A species found in human feces and skin; it causes blue pus infections of wounds and burns, and may cause infections in other parts of the body through the use of instruments, as in the urinary tract, or in the subarachnoid space through lumbar puncture; some strains produce a blue compound soluble in chloroform (pyocyanin); others produce a greenish compound soluble in water (fluorescin).

P. mallei A species causing glanders in horses, sheep, goats, and man. Also called·glanders bacillus. Formerly called *Actinobacillus mallei*.

P. pseudomallei The species causing melioidosis. Formerly called *Malleomyces pseudomallei*.

pseudomucin A gelatinous substance similar to mucin.

pseudomycelium A group of pseudohyphae.

ameba

pseudopodia

psychopharmaceuticals

CH₃

CH₂CH₂CH₂N

CH₃

Cl

chlorpromazine

imipran

· HCl hydrochl

CH₂CH₂CH₂N(CH₃)₂

CH₂CH₂CH₂NHCH₃

S

· HCl

CF₃

CH₂CH₂CH₂—N   N—CH₃

trifluoperazine
hydrochloride

· HCl   desiprar
        hydrochl

CHCH₂CH₂N

CH₃

CH₃

· HCl   amitript
        hydrochl

CHCH₂CH₂N

CH₃

CH₃

O

· HCl   doxep
        hydrochl

reserpine

CH₃O

N
H

H

H

H

N

O

C

O

O

OCH₃

OCH₃

OCH₃

OCH₃ OCH₃

CH₃

N

O

Cl

N

diazepam
(Valium®)

OH

Cl

N—CH₂CH₂CH₂—C

O

haloperi

pseudomyopia Eye condition resulting from spasm of the ciliary muscle, causing the same focusing defect as myopia.

pseudomyxoma A gelatinous tumor or tumor-like condition resembling a myxoma, but composed of epithelial mucus.

pseudoneoplasm An aggregation of nonneoplastic material that clinically resembles a true neoplasm.

pseudoparalysis Apparent loss of power of voluntary movement.

pseudoparaplegia Apparent loss of power of voluntary movement of the lower extremities.

pseudopodium, *pl.* **pseudopodia** 1. A cytoplasmic process used by certain protozoa (e.g., amebae) for locomotion and feeding. 2. A small cytoplasmic extension from a cell.

pseudopolyp A protruding mass in the colon, composed of edematous mucosa, granulation tissue, or inflamed epithelium; commonly associated with ulcerative colitis.

pseudopregnancy See pregnancy, spurious.

pseudo-pseudohypoparathyroidism Heritable disorder that has the constitutional features of pseudohypoparathyroidism (round face, short stature, obesity, abnormally short hands and feet) but lacks the chemical findings.

pseudopterygium A superficial adhesion of the cornea to the conjunctiva, resulting from injury. Also called scar pterygium.

pseudosmia A sensation of an odor that is not present.

pseudotubercle A nodule resembling a tuberculous granuloma, but not caused by the tubercle bacillus.

pseudotumor The occurrence of symptoms and signs indicating the presence of a tumor in the absence of one, with subsequent spontaneous recovery.

p. cerebri A condition producing signs of increased intracranial pressure suggesting the presence of an intracranial tumor in the absence of any neoplasm. Also called benign intracranial hypertension.

pseudoxanthoma elasticum A condition marked by slightly elevated papules or plaques on the skin that, as yellowish aggregates, resemble but are not xanthomas; the lesions generally appear on the neck, axillae, abdomen, and thighs, and are due to degenerated elastic tissue; so-called angioid streaks occur in the retina; premature arterial degeneration is common and internal hemorrhage occurs in 10% of cases.

Psilocybe mexicana A species of mushrooms (family Agaricaceae) containing the hallucinogenic

substance psilocybin. Commonly known as the Mexican magic mushroom.

psilocybin A hallucinogenic substance obtained from *Psilocybe mexicana.*

psilosis Falling or loss of hair.

psittacosis A disease of birds caused by *Chlamydia psittaci*, transmitted to man by parrots or parakeets through inhalation of infective material; in humans, the disease is characterized by fever, chills, headache, sore throat, and cough. See also ornithosis.

psoas See table of muscles.

psoralen A drug that promotes a sunburn effect on the skin; used in combination with ultraviolet light (PUVA, photochemical therapy) to treat severe cases of psoriasis and vitiligo.

psoriasiform Resembling psoriasis.

psoriasis A chronic skin disease characterized by reddish patches covered with silvery scales, occurring mostly on the knees, elbows, scalp, and trunk.

psoriatic Relating to psoriasis.

psychasthenia Term formerly used for a neurosis characterized by marked anxiety, obsessions, compulsions, phobias, and feelings of inadequacy.

psyche The mind as distinguished from the body.

psychedelic Relating to drugs that cause hallucinations, distortions of perception, and, sometimes, conditions resembling psychosis.

psychiatric Relating to psychiatry.

psychiatrist A specialist in psychiatry.

psychiatry The branch of medicine concerned with the study, diagnosis, and treatment of mental diseases.

social p. The application of psychiatric principles to the solutions of social problems and issues.

psychic 1. Relating to the mind. 2. Relating to extraordinary mental or spiritual processes, such as mental telepathy or extrasensory perception.

psycho Street term for a psychopath.

psychoanalysis 1. Psychotherapy in which a patient is made to recall past experiences, through free association, in order to bring into consciousness repressed experiences causing the emotional problems; originated by Sigmund Freud. 2. A systematic theory of the development and functioning of the human psyche.

psychoanalyst A psychotherapist trained in the techniques of psychoanalytic therapy. Also called analyst.

psychobiology The study of the biology of the mind based on the concept of the individual as a biologic unit whose personality development is dependent on its environmental setting; especially the theory of Adolph Meyer.

psychodiagnosis The use of psychological tests

to determine the causes of abnormal behavior.

psychodrama A method of group psychotherapy in which patients dramatize their emotional problems.

psychodynamics The science of human behavior and its unconscious motivation.

psychodysleptic Any agent that has the capability of producing abnormal mental phenomena, particularly in the perceptual and cognitive spheres.

psychogenesis 1. Development of mental faculties. 2. Production of symptoms by mental factors.

psychogenic, psychogenetic Originating in the mind.

psychogeriatrics The study of old age as it relates to psychological problems and mental illnesses.

psychognosis Diagnosis of mental disorders or psychiatric states.

psychogram A chart depicting the personality traits of an individual. Also called psychograph.

psychokinesis (PK) In parapsychology, the influence on motion, especially of distant inanimate objects, through concentrated directed thought.

psycholagny Sexual excitement and satisfaction from mental imagery.

psychologic Relating to mental processes and behavior.

psychologist One who is trained to perform psychological evaluation, therapy, or research.

psychology The science concerned with the study of the mind in all its aspects, especially as they are manifested in behavior.

psychometry The measuring of mental efficiency, functioning, and potential.

psychomotor Relating to the mental origin of muscular activity, as compulsive movements.

psychoneurosis Emotional and behavioral disorder manifested by anxiety and symptoms such as depression, phobias, compulsions, or obsessions without gross distortion of reality orientation. Currently called neurosis.

psychoneurotic Relating to, or suffering from, a psychoneurosis. Currently called neurotic.

psychopath An individual with a personality disorder, manifested by asocial behavior without accompanying guilt.

psychopathic Relating to mental disease or psychopathy.

psychopathology The pathology of mental disorders; the nature or study of mental disease.

psychopathy Any mental disorder.

psychopharmaceuticals Any of several drugs used in the treatment of emotional disorders.

psychopharmacology The study of the action of drugs on the mind and emotions.

psychophysical Relating to physical stimuli and

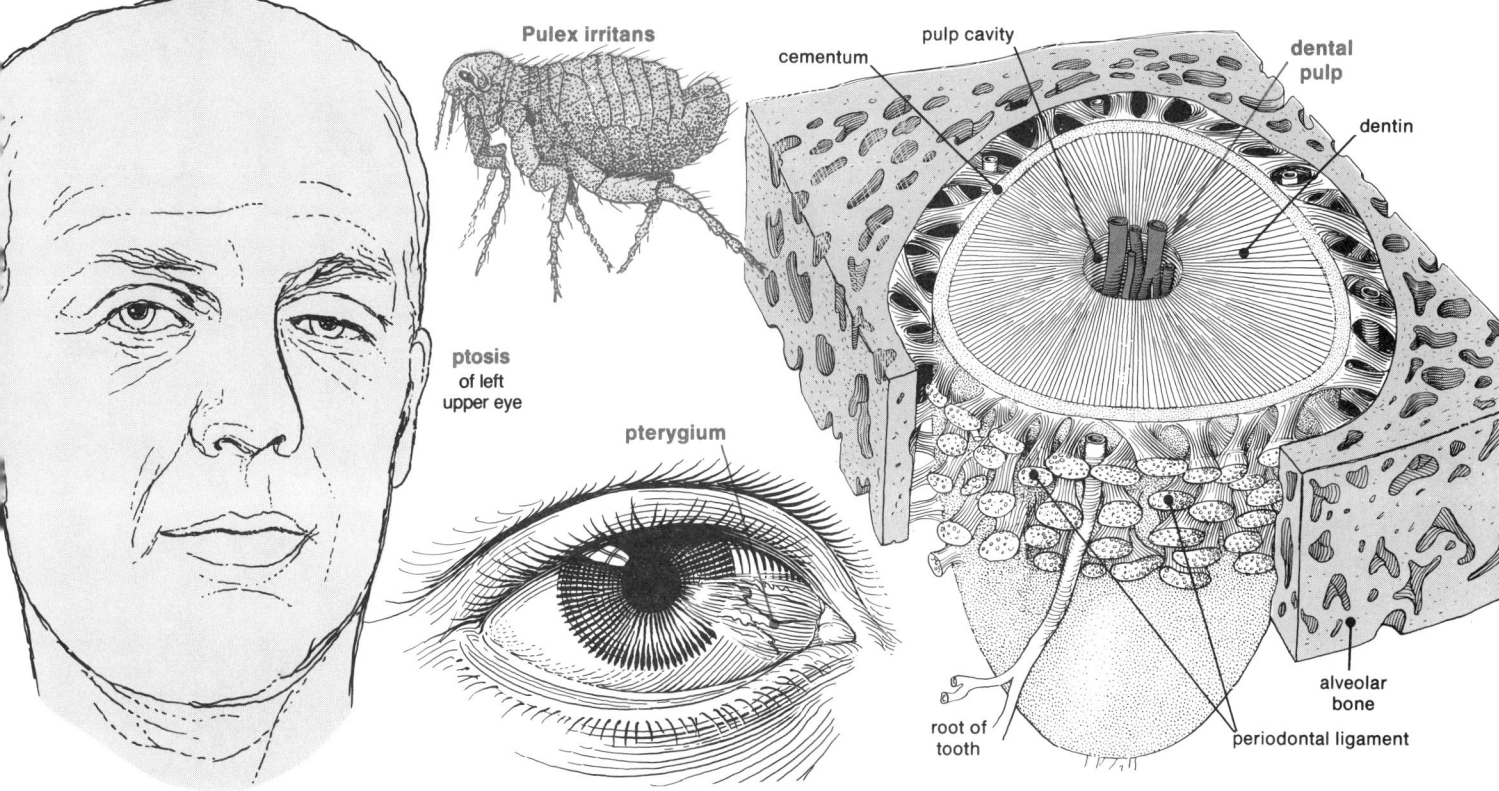

Pulex irritans

cementum

pulp cavity

dental pulp

dentin

ptosis of left upper eye

pterygium

alveolar bone

root of tooth

periodontal ligament

mental responses.

psychophysics The branch of psychology concerned with the relationships between physical stimuli and sensory responses.

psychophysiologic 1. Relating to psychophysiology. 2. Denoting a disease with primarily physical manifestations but emotional causes.

psychophysiology The study of the interaction of psychologic and physiologic processes.

psychoplegia A form of dementia or mental weakness characterized by sudden onset.

psychoplegic 1. Relating to psychoplegia. 2. An agent that dulls mental activity.

psychosensory Of, or relating to, the perception and interpretation of sensory stimuli.

psychosexual Relating to the mental or emotional aspects of sex.

psychosis A severe mental illness of organic and/or emotional origin, marked by loss of contact with reality and frequently by regressive behavior, delusions, or hallucinations. See also insanity.

    Korsakoff's p. See Korsakoff's syndrome.

    manic-depressive p. Conspicuous mood swings from elation to depression.

psychosocial Involving psychological and social factors.

psychosomatic Referring to the influence of the mind over the body; specifically, physical symptoms that have an emotional or mental origin.

psychosomimetic See psychotomimetic.

psychostimulant Any agent that has the capability of increasing the level of an individual's alertness and/or motivation.

psychosurgery Brain surgery for the treatment of mental disorders; e.g., lobotomy.

psychotherapeutic Relating to psychotherapy.

psychotherapist An individual, usually a psychiatrist or a clinical psychologist, trained in psychotherapy.

psychotherapy Treatment of behavioral, emotional, and mental disorders or distress conducted by a variety of psychological methods involving communication between a trained therapist and an individual, couple, family, or group. See under therapy for definitions of various psychotherapeutic approaches.

psychotic Relating to, afflicted with, or caused by a psychosis.

psychotogen An agent that produces psychotic symptoms.

psychotogenic Producing psychosis; said of certain drugs like LSD.

psychotomimetic Producing symptoms that resemble those of a psychosis; said of certain drugs. Also called psychosomimetic.

psychotropic Denoting drugs that affect the mind.

psychrometer Device used to calculate the relative humidity of the atmosphere; it consists of two thermometers, one with a bulb that is kept wet to cause evaporation and the other with a dry bulb.

psychrometry 1. The science of the physical laws that control air and water mixture. 2. Estimation of the relative humidity of the air by means of the psychrometer.

psychrophilic Thriving in cold temperature; said of some bacteria.

psychrophobia 1. Abnormal fear of cold temperatures. 2. Extreme sensitiveness to cold.

psyllium 1. A plant of the genus *Plantago*. 2. Plantago seed; see under seed.

ptarmic An agent that causes sneezing.

pterion A craniometric point on either side of the skull at the junction of the frontal, sphenoid, parietal, and temporal bones.

pteroylglutamic acid See folic acid.

pterygium A horizontal, triangular growth of the bulbar conjunctiva, extending usually from the inner canthus to the border of the cornea or beyond; a slowly advancing lesion, believed to be caused by ultraviolet radiation.

pterygoid Wing-shaped.

pterygopalatine Relating to the pterygoid process of the sphenoid bone and the bony palate.

ptilosis Loss of eyelashes.

ptomaine Vague term denoting a poisonous substance.

    p. poisoning Poisoning attributed to toxic decomposition of ingested food; most of these cases are probably caused by viral or bacterial infection.

ptosed Prolapsed.

ptosis 1. A prolapse or sinking down of an organ. 2. Drooping of an upper eyelid when the eyes are open.

ptotic Relating to ptosis or prolapse.

ptyalin An enzyme present in the saliva, which changes starch into dextrin, maltose, and glucose.

ptyalolith See sialolith.

ptyalolithiasis See sialolithiasis.

ptyalolithotomy See sialolithotomy.

pubarche The beginning of puberty.

puberal, pubertal Relating to the beginning of sexual maturity.

pubertas Puberty.

    p. precox Early arrival of sexual maturity.

puberty The stage of development in which an individual is first capable of reproduction, usually between the ages of 13 and 16 in boys and 12 and 14 in girls.

pubescence The beginning of sexual maturity.

pubescent One who is reaching the age of sexual maturity.

pubic Relating to the pubic bone or area.

pubis, *pl.* **pubes** 1. The pubic bone. 2. The region over the pubic bone. 3. The hair of the pubic region.

pubomadesis Loss or absence of pubic hair.

pubovesical Relating to the pubic bone and the bladder.

pubovesicocervical Relating to the pubic symphysis, bladder, and uterine cervix.

pudendal Relating to the genitals.

pudendum, *pl.* **pudenda** External genitals, especially the female genitals; the vulva.

puericulture The care of the unborn child through attention to the health of the pregnant woman.

puerile 1. Relating to childhood. 2. Childish.

puerilism Second childhood.

puerpera A woman who had just given birth.

puerperal Relating to the first few weeks following childbirth.

puerperalism Any disease state consequent upon childbirth.

puerperium The period from the end of labor to return of the uterus to normal size, usually from 3 to 6 weeks.

Pulex A genus of fleas.

    P. cheopis Former name for the Oriental rat flea species, *Xenopsylla cheopis.*

    P. irritans The species of flea that commonly infects and parasitizes man and various animals; its bite produces itching.

pulicide, pulicicide Any agent that destroys fleas.

pullulation Sprouting; budding.

pulmo, *pl.* **pulmones** Latin for lung.

pulmonary Relating to the lungs.

pulmonectomy See pneumonectomy.

pulmonic Pulmonary.

pulmotor Apparatus used to induce artificial respiration by introducing oxygen into the lungs.

pulp Any soft, moist tissue.

    dental p. The vascular and innervated connective tissue contained in the pulp cavity of the tooth.

pulpal Relating to the pulp or to the pulp cavity of a tooth.

pulpectomy Removal of the pulp tissue from the entire tooth, including the pulp in the root canals.

pulpefaction, pulpifaction The act of reducing to pulp.

pulpitis Inflammation of the pulp of a tooth. Also called odontitis.

pulpless Having a nonfunctioning or dead pulp or one that has been replaced with an inert substance; said of a tooth.

pulpotomy Surgical removal of a portion of the pulp from a tooth, usually the coronal portion.

SYSTOLE DIASTOLE

jugular venous pulse

ECG

dura covering the spinal cord

lumbar puncture

purines

adenine

guanine

pulpy The condition of a solid when it is soft and moist.

pulsate To expand and contract, or beat, rhythmically, as the heart.

pulsatile Throbbing; pulsating.

pulsation 1. The act of pulsating. 2. A single throb, as of the heart.

pulse (p) The rhythmic increase in pressure within a blood vessel produced by the increased volume of blood forced through the vessel with each contraction of the heart.

   alternating p. Pulse with alternating weak and strong beats. Also called pulsus alternans.

   anacrotic p. A pulse (usually palpable in the carotid arteries) in which the ascending limb of the pulse wave has a secondary notch.

   bigeminal p. A pulse in which two beats occur in rapid succession followed by a longer pause; usually produced by a small premature ectopic beat after a normally conducted beat.

   capillary p. See Quincke's pulse.

   Corrigan's p. One characterized by an abrupt rise with rapid collapse. Also called water-hammer pulse.

   coupled p., twice-beating p. A pulse in which two waves are palpated during each cardiac cycle. Also called double beat.

   jugular venous p., jugular p. (JVP) Pulsation observed in a jugular vein.

   paradoxical p. A reduction in the amplitude of the pulse during inspiration, seen in pericardial effusion. Also called pulsus paradoxus.

   plateau p. Pulse with a slowly rising pressure and sustained peak.

   Quincke's p. Alternate pallor and reddening of capillary areas, such as the nail bed; seen in aortic insufficiency. Also called capillary pulse.

   thready p. A small fine pulse.

   trigeminal p. One occurring in groups of three.

   twice-beating p. See coupled pulse.

   venous p. Pulse occurring in the veins.

   water-hammer p. See Corrigan's pulse.

Pulseless disease Progressive inflammation and obliteration of the brachiocephalic trunk, left subclavian, and left common carotid arteries, leading to loss of pulse in the arms and neck among other symptoms. Also called Takayasu's disease. See also aortic arch syndrome.

pulsimeter Instrument used to measure the force and frequency of the pulse.

pulsion A swelling.

pulsus Latin for pulse.

   p. alternans See pulse, alternating.

   p. paradoxus See pulse, paradoxical.

   p. parvus A small pulse.

   p. tardus A pulse with a delayed rise and fall, as seen in aortic stenosis.

pulvinar The angular prominence constituting the posteromedial portion of the thalamus.

pulvis, *pl.* **pulveres** Lain for powder.

pumice A porous volcanic substance; in dentistry, used in powdered form to polish teeth and dentures.

pump An apparatus for transferring a liquid or gas through tubes from or to any part.

   breast p. A suction pump for withdrawing milk from the breast.

   Carrel-Lindbergh p. A perfusion pump by means of which an organ taken out of the body may be kept functioning. Also called Lindbergh pump.

   coronary-sucker p. A pump for aspirating the small quantity of blood that enters the heart while the heart-lung machine is used during open-heart surgery.

   electrolyte p. A process that derives its energy from the metabolic activities of the cell and which can cause a solute to move from an area of relatively low to one of higher chemical potential; e.g., a sodium pump located in renal tubular cells.

   insulin p. Battery-powered pump for infusing a continuous subcutaneous dose of insulin in the management of diabetes mellitus.

   stomach p. A suction pump with a flexible tube for removing the contents of the stomach in an emergency, as in a case of poisoning.

pump-oxygenator A mechanical apparatus that facilitates open heart surgery by temporarily substituting for both the heart (pump) and the lungs (oxygenator).

punch-drunk Suffering from brain dysfunction caused by repeated concussions; characterized by slow body movements, unsteady gait, hesitant speech, and slow intellect; condition seen in some professional boxers.

punctate 1. Marked with minute dots. 2. Material withdrawn by means of a puncture.

punctiform Of the size and shape of a very small point, usually having a diameter of less than one millimeter; used principally to describe minute colonies of bacteria.

punctum, *pl.* **puncta** A point or a spot.

   lacrimal p. The minute opening of the lacrimal duct on the margin of each eyelid at the inner canthus.

puncture 1. To pierce with a pointed instrument. 2. A small hole made with a needle.

   lumbar p. Puncture made into the subarachnoid space between two of the lower lumbar vertebrae to remove cerebrospinal fluid for diagnostic purposes, or to inject an anesthetic solution. Also called spinal puncture; spinal tap.

pupil (p) The circular opening in the center of the iris, through which light enters the eye.

   Argyll-Robertson p. A pupil characterized by the loss of response to light, with retention of a normal response to convergence accommodation.

   fixed p. One that is unresponsive to all stimuli.

pupillary Relating to the pupil.

pupillography The recording of pupillary reactions to light stimuli.

pupillometer An instrument used to measure the diameter of the pupil. Also called coreometer.

pupillometry Measurement of the pupil of the eye. Also called coreometry.

pupillomotor Relating to motor activity affecting the size of the pupil; specifically, denoting the motor nerve fibers supplying the iris.

pupilloplegia Slow or absent response of the pupil to a light stimulus.

pupillostatometer Instrument used to measure the distance between the pupils of the eyes.

pure 1. In genetics, denoting (a) an inherited trait that is transmitted without a break in several generations; (b) an individual who is not a hybrid. 2. Free from contamination.

purebred An animal derived from a line subjected to inbreeding.

purgation Vigorous evacuation of the bowels effected by a cathartic medicine (purgative). Also called catharsis.

purgative See cathartic.

purge 1. To induce evacuation of the bowels. 2. Any agent having such properties.

purine The base of a group of organic compounds (uric acid compounds), known as purines or purine bases; when synthetically produced, it is a colorless crystalline compound; it is not known to exist as such in nature.

purpura Condition in which spontaneous bleeding occurs in the subcutaneous tissues, causing the appearance of purple patches on the skin.

   anaphylactoid p. See Henoch-Schönlein purpura.

   annular telangiectatic p. A form characterized by lesions (usually limited to the lower extremities) appearing as circular pigmented areas with a yellowish necrosed center. Also called Majocchi's disease.

   Henoch-Schönlein p. Purpura, seen especially in children and young adults, associated with gastrointestinal symptoms, joint pains, and hematuria; the appearance of cutaneous lesions (most common on the extremities) is preceded by a pinprick itchy sensation. Also called Schönlein's disease; anaphylactoid purpura.

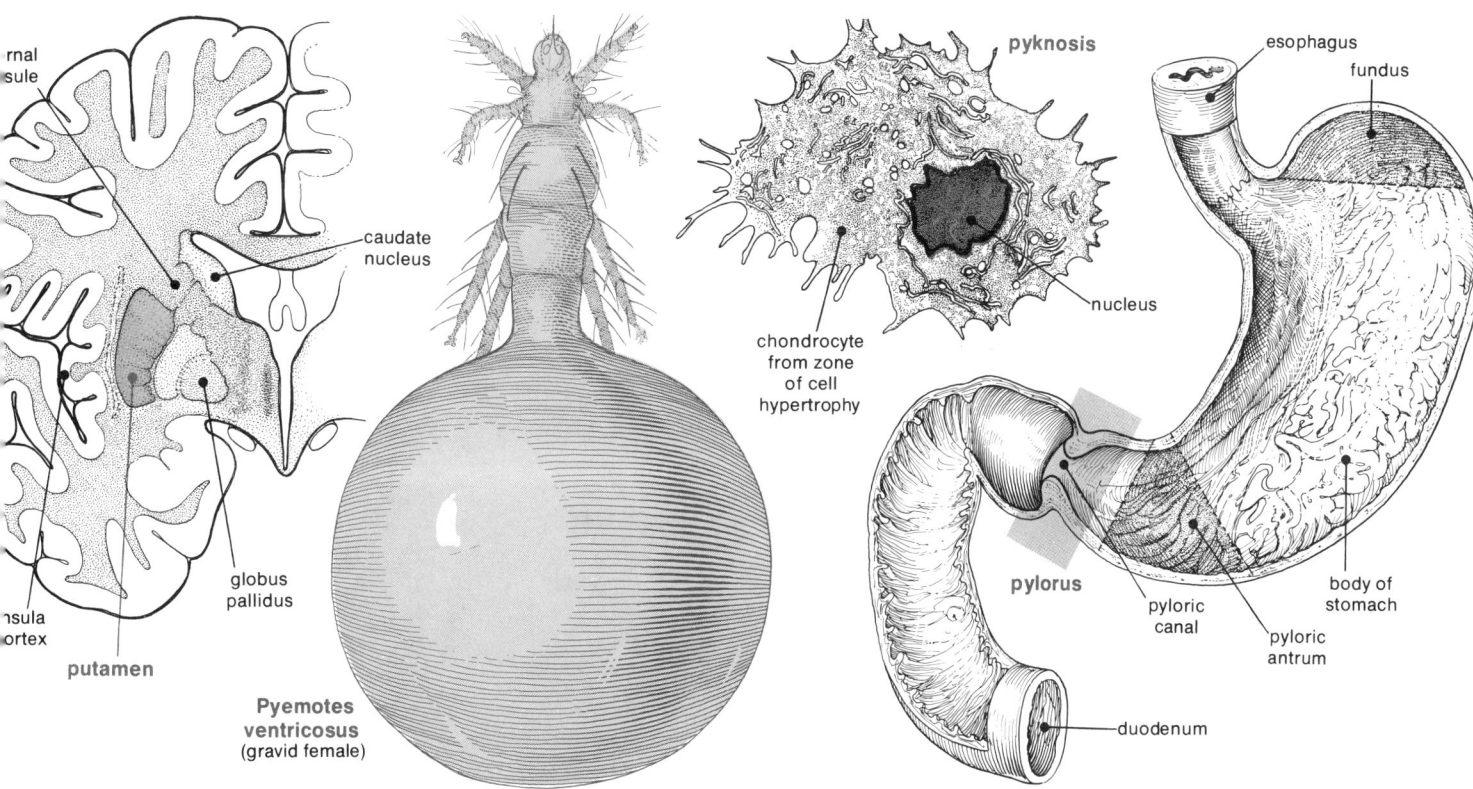

caudate nucleus

globus pallidus

putamen

Pyemotes ventricosus (gravid female)

pyknosis

chondrocyte from zone of cell hypertrophy

nucleus

esophagus

fundus

pylorus

pyloric canal

pyloric antrum

body of stomach

duodenum

idiopathic thrombocytopenic p. (ITP) Purpura over the limbs, upper chest and back unassociated with any systemic disease; may be acute, occurring most commonly in children; bleeding stops after a few days; the chronic form occurs mostly in adult women, with recurring episodes which may last for long periods.

rheumatic p. Purpura associated with acute rheumatic arthritis.

thrombocytopenic p. A form associated with deficiency in platelet count.

thrombotic thrombocytopenic p. (TTP) A severe and frequently fatal form characterized by a low platelet count in the blood and thrombosis in the terminal arterioles and capillaries of many organs; findings may include azotemia, hemolytic anemia, hypertension, and central nervous system symptoms.

purpuric Relating to or afflicted with purpura.

purpuriferous Forming the visual purple or rhodopsin.

purulence, purulency The condition of containing or producing pus.

purulent Containing or producing pus.

pus A thick, viscous, yellowish fluid, product of inflammation, composed chiefly of dead white blood cells (leukocytes) and a thin liquid (liquor puris), and often the microbiologic agent responsible for the inflammation.

cheesy p The thick, nearly solid pus of a tuberculous abscess.

pustular Characterized by pustules.

pustulation The formation or development of pustules.

pustule A small elevation of the skin containing pus.

pustuliform Resembling a pustule.

pustulosis A pustular eruption.

putamen A thick, convex, dark gray mass in the brain between the insular cortex laterally and the globus pallidus and the internal capsule medially.

putrefaction 1. Decomposition of organic matter, especially proteins, by the action of bacteria, resulting in the formation of foul-smelling compounds. 2. Decomposed matter.

putrefactive Relating to or causing the decomposition of organic matter.

putrefy To decompose or decay.

putrescence Rottenness.

putrid Decayed; rotten.

PUVA Acronym for oral administration of psoralen followed by long wavelength ultraviolet light (UVA) for the treatment of psoriasis; a form of photochemotherapy.

pyarthrosis The presence of pus in a joint cavity.

pycnidium, pl. pycnidia A flask-shaped or round spore fruit of various imperfect fungi; it contains conidia.

pyelectasia Dilatation of the renal pelvis.

pyelectomy Surgical removal of the redundant portion of a greatly distended kidney pelvis.

pyelitis See pyelonephritis.

pyelocystitis Inflammation of the kidney pelvis and the bladder.

pyelogram A roentgenogram of the kidney pelvis and the ureter.

pyelography The making of roentgenograms of the ureter and the kidney pelvis.

pyelolithotomy Surgical removal of a stone from the pelvis of the kidney.

pyeloneostomy The division and reimplantation of a ureter for the improvement of kidney drainage.

pyelonephritis Inflammation of the kidney, especially the renal pelvis. Also called pyelitis.

acute p. Active pyogenic infection of the kidney.

chronic p. Disease of the kidney thought to result from scarring from previous bacterial infections.

xanthogranulomatous p. A rare form of chronic pyelonephritis in which the kidney shows xanthogranulomas with lipid-containing foam cells, multinucleated giant cells, lymphocytes, and plasma cells.

pyelonephrolithotomy The removal of kidney stones by combining an incision in the kidney pelvis with one in the cortex.

pyeloplasty Plastic repair of the kidney pelvis either for the purpose of improving drainage or to reduce its size.

pyeloplication Operation to reduce the size of the kidney pelvis when abnormally dilated.

pyeloscopy Fluoroscopic examination of the kidney pelvis after introduction of a radiopaque solution through the ureter or intravenously.

pyelostomy Surgical formation of an opening into the pelvis of the kidney.

pyelotomy Incision into the pelvis of the kidney.

pyeloureterectasis Dilatation of kidney pelvis and ureter.

pyemesis The vomiting of purulent material.

pyemia A form of septicemia in which there is a general secondary infection with formation of multiple abscesses in several areas of the body. Also called metastatic infection.

pyemic Afflicted with pyemia.

Pyemotes ventricosus A small parasite of insect larvae (esp. the grain moth and the wheat grain worm); the young female has an elongated body which becomes greatly distended when gravid; the fertilized eggs are retained in her abdomen where they hatch and become mature mites before they are discharged; the mites may burrow in the epidermis of individuals in contact with grains, straw or hay, causing a skin eruption. Also called hay or grain itch mite.

pyesis Suppuration.

pygmyism Primordial dwarfism; see under dwarfism.

pyknic Having a short, stocky, well rounded body build with ample body cavities.

pyknomorphous Having the stainable elements closely packed; said of a cell.

pyknosis Condensation and shrinking of a cell nucleus; e.g., during maturation of a red blood cell prior to ejection of the nucleus from the cell.

pyla The opening between the third ventricle of the brain and the cerebral aqueduct (aqueduct of Sylvius).

pylemphraxis Obstruction of the portal vein.

phylephlebectasia Dilatation of the portal vein.

pylephlebitis Inflammation of the portal vein or its branches.

pylethrombophlebitis Inflammation and thrombosis of the portal vein.

pylethrombosis Thrombosis of the portal vein or its branches.

pylic Referring to the portal vein.

pylon A temporary artificial leg.

pyloralgia Pain in the pyloric area of the stomach.

pylorectomy Surgical removal of the pylorus.

pyloric Of, or relating to, the pylorus.

pyloric-channel syndrome A syndrome characterized by inflammation of the pylorus and the prepyloric region with muscle hypertrophy and narrowing of the pyloric canal, resulting in pyloric obstruction.

pyloristenosis Stricture of the pylorus.

pyloritis Inflammation of the pyloric area of the stomach.

pylorogastrectomy Surgical removal of the pyloric portion of the stomach.

pyloromyotomy Operative technique for the treatment of congenital pyloric stenosis. Also called Fredet-Ramstedt operation.

pyloroplasty Plastic operation of the pylorus, especially one to enlarge a constricted pylorus; performed sometimes in the treatment of peptic ulcers.

pylorospasm Spasm of the pylorus or the pyloric area of the stomach; in adults, usually associated with nearby duodenal or gastric ulcer or severe gastritis.

pylorotomy Surgical incision of the pylorus.

pylorus The opening between the stomach and duodenum.

pyosalpinx

pyrrole

minor calix

section through kidney

cortex of kidney

arcuate artery

renal pelvis

renal pyramids

pyrimidines

thymine   cytosine   uracil

pyridoxal phosphate

present in RNA   present in DNA

pyocele Distention of a cavity due to accumulation of pus.

pyocephalus The presence of a purulent fluid within the skull.

pyochezia The discharge of pus with the stools.

pyococcus A pus-producing microorganism, as *Streptococcus pyogenes*.

pyocolpos Accumulation of pus in the vagina.

pyocyanic Relating to blue pus or to the bacillus that produces it (*Pseudomonas aeruginosa*).

pyocyanin An antibiotic substance obtained from the bacillus *Pseudomonas aeruginosa*.

pyocyst A pus-containing cyst.

pyoderma, pyodermia Any pus-producing disease of the skin.

   p. gangrenosum An eruption of chronic pustules associated with ulcerative colitis.

pyogen Anything that causes pus formation.

pyogenesis The formation of pus. Also called pyopoiesis.

pyogenic Producing pus.

pyohemothorax The presence of pus and blood in the pleural cavity.

pyoid Resembling pus. Also called puriform.

pyolabyrinthitis Suppurative inflammation of the labyrinth of the internal ear.

pyometra Accumulation of pus in the uterus.

pyometritis Inflammation of the wall of the uterus with accumulation of pus in its cavity.

pyomyositis Condition marked by the formation of single or multiple deep-seated abscesses in voluntary muscles; caused by *Staphylococcus aureus*. Also called tropical pyomyositis.

pyonephrolithiasis The presence of pus and stones in the kidney.

pyonephrosis Distention of the calices and pelvis of the kidney with pus.

pyoovarium Pus in the ovary. Also called ovarian abscess.

pyopericarditis Suppurative inflammation of the pericardium.

pyopericardium Accumulation of pus in the sac enveloping the heart (pericardium).

pyoperitonitis Suppurative inflammation of the peritoneum.

pyophthalmia, pyophthalmitis Suppurative inflammation of the eye, especially the conjunctiva.

pyophysometra An accumulation of gas and pus in the uterine cavity.

pyopneumocholecystitis Distention of an inflamed gallbladder with gas and pus; caused by gas-producing organisms or by the entry of air from the intestine through the biliary tree.

pyopneumopericardium A condition marked by the presence of pus and gas in the membranous sac surrounding the heart (pericardium).

pyopneumoperitoneum A condition marked by the presence of pus and gas in the peritoneal cavity.

pyopneumothorax The presence of pus and air in the pleural cavity. Also called pneumopyothorax.

pyopoiesis The formation of pus. Also called pyogenesis.

pyopoietic Pus-producing.

pyoptysis Spitting of pus.

pyorrhea See periodontitis.

pyosalpingitis Suppurative inflammation of the uterine tube.

pyosalpingo-oophoritis Suppurative inflammation of the uterine tube and the ovary.

pyosalpinx Accumulation of pus in the uterine tube.

pyosis Suppuration.

pyostatic Denoting an agent that arrests the formation of pus.

pyoureter Pus in a ureter.

pyramid Any of numerous anatomic structures that are pyramidal or cone-shaped.

   cerebellar p. The central portion of the inferior vermis of the cerebellum between the uvula and tuber. Also called pyramid of the vermis.

   malpighian p. See renal pyramid.

   p. of light A triangular area on the anterior inferior surface of the tympanic membrane which reflects light brightly; it extends from the umbo to the periphery. Also called cone of light.

   p.'s of the medulla Two anterior and two posterior longitudinal fiber bundles within the medulla oblongata that resemble narrow elongated pyramids.

   p. of thyroid gland Pyramidal lobe of thyroid gland; see under lobe.

   renal p. One of a number of pyramidal masses formed by the medullary substance of the kidney, containing part of the secreting and collecting tubules; the apex projects into the minor calix. Also called malpighian pyramid.

pyramidal Relating to or having the shape of a pyramid; said of certain anatomic structures.

pyretic Feverish.

pyretogenesis The causation of fever.

pyretogenetic Relating to pyretogenesis.

pyretotherapy 1. Treatment of disease by intermittent raising of body temperature. 2. Treatment of fever.

pyrexia Elevation of body temperature above normal. Also called fever.

pyridine A colorless, flammable liquid, C_5H_5N, used in the preparation of vitamins and drugs, as a solvent, and as a denaturant of alcohol.

pyridoxal phosphate A vitamin derivative or coenzyme essential to many reactions of amino acid metabolism, as transamination, decarboxylation, and racemization.

pyridoxine Common name for a group of water-soluble substances of the vitamin B complex, essential in protein metabolism. Also called vitamin B_6.

pyrimethamine An antimalarial agent.

pyrimidine The fundamental substance of several organic bases, some of which are components of nucleic acid.

pyrogallol Pyrogallic acid, $C_6H_3(OH)_3$; used in the treatment of skin disorders, as psoriasis and ringworm.

pyrogen A fever-producing agent.

pyrogenic 1. Producing, or caused by, fever. 2. Produced by or generating heat.

pyroligneous Relating to or obtained from the destructive distillation of wood.

pyrolysis Chemical change produced by heat.

pyromania A morbid desire to set things on fire.

pyrometer An electric thermometer for measuring extremely high temperatures.

pyronin A basic red dye used in histologic stains.

pyrophobia Abnormal fear of fire.

pyrophosphatase Any enzyme that splits a pyrophosphate.

pyrophosphate (PP) A salt of pyrophosphoric acid.

pyrophosphoric acid A water-soluble, crystalline substance, $H_4P_2O_7$, obtained by heating phosphoric acid.

pyrosis A burning sensation in the esophagus caused by the rising of small amounts of acid liquid or gas from the stomach. Also called heartburn. See also water brash.

pyrotic 1. Relating to heartburn. 2. Caustic.

pyrrole A toxic heterocyclic compound possessing an odor suggestive of chloroform; the parent of many biologically important natural compounds such as bile pigments, porphyrins, chlorophyll, etc.

pyruvate A salt or ester of pyruvic acid.

   p. kinase (PK) Enzyme that promotes the transfer of phosphate from phosphoenolpyruvate to ADP, forming ATP and pyruvate; deficiency of pyruvate kinase in red blood cells is the cause of an autosomal recessive hemolytic anemia. Also called phosphoenolpyruvate kinase.

pyruvic acid A colorless liquid, $CH_3COCOOH$, with an odor similar to that of acetic acid; an intermediate product in the metabolism of carbohydrate.

pyrvinium pamoate A deep red, crystalline substance; used in the eradication in pinworms.

pyuria The presence of pus in the urine.

malleus

incus

posterior superior
quadrant

stapes

tympanic
membrane
(eardrum)

anterior
superior
quadrant

manubrium
of
malleus

anterior
inferior
quadrant

posterior
inferior
quadrant

quinacrine

quinidine

quinine

Qq

quack One who fraudulently misrepresents his medical or dental capability to diagnose and treat disease and who generally makes extravagant claims as to the effects achieved by the treatment he offers.

quackery A false claim to medical knowledge and experience in treating the sick.

quadrant (Q) 1. One-quarter of a circle. 2. In anatomy, one of the four sections into which roughly circular areas of the body are divided for descriptive purposes; e.g., the tympanic membrane, the fundus of the eye, the abdomen.

quadrantanopsia Blindness in approximately a quarter of the visual field. Also called quadrantic hemianopsia.

   crossed binasal q. Blindness of the lower nasal quarter of the visual field of one eye and the upper nasal of the other eye.

   crossed temporal q. Blindness of the lower temporal quarter of the visual field of one eye and the upper temporal of the other eye.

   lower heteronymous q. Blindness of either both lower nasal or both lower temporal quarters of the visual fields.

   upper heteronymous q. Blindness of both upper nasal or both upper temporal quarters of the nasal fields.

quadrantectomy Removal of one quarter of an organ, especially a breast, as a treatment for a tumor.

quadrate Having equal sides; square-shaped; four-sided.

quadratus Denoting certain muscles which have a seemingly square shape.

quadribasic Referring to an acid that has four replaceable hydrogen atoms.

quadriceps Having four heads, as some muscles.

quadrigeminal Occurring in a group of four; fourfold, having four parts.

quadripara A woman who has given birth to four children.

quadriplegia Paralysis of all four extremities. Also called tetraplegia.

quadriplegic One whose four limbs are paralyzed.

quadrivalent Having the combining ability of four hydrogen atoms. Also called tetravalent.

quadruplet One of four offspring born at one birth.

quanta Plural of quantum.

quantimeter A device for measuring the quantity of x rays generated by a tube such as a Coolidge tube.

quantitative Involving the measurement of amounts of constituents in a compound.

quantity 1. An indefinite amount. 2. The duration, intensity, and frequency of a speech sound as distinct from its individual quality. 3. The length of time vocal organs remain in specific positions for the production of a particular sound.

quantum, *pl.* **quanta** 1. A unit of radiant energy. 2. A specified amount.

   q. libet (q.l.) Latin for as much as desired.

   q. sufficit (q.s.) Latin for sufficient amount or as much as suffices.

   q. vis (q.v.) Latin for as much as you want; used in prescription writing.

quaque die (q.d.) Latin for every day.

quaque quarta hora (q.q.h.) Latin for every four hours.

quarantine 1. Restriction of freedom of movement of persons who have been exposed to a communicable disease; originally the period of restriction was 40 days. 2. Isolation of a person afflicted with a communicable disease.

quart (qt) 1. A measure of fluid capacity equal to two pints; one-fourth of a gallon; 32 ounces; 0.9468 liter; 57.75 cubic inches. 2. A unit of volume in dry measure equal to 67.2 cubic inches.

   imperial q. A British unit of volume or capacity equal to 1.201 liquid quarts.

quartan Recurring every four days, as a malarial fever; actually, the attack occurs on day one and day four, so that there is really only an interval of two days.

quartile The middle of each half of a set of variables.

quartz A form of silica, used in dentistry as one of three main ingredients of dental porcelain.

quasidominance Direct transmission, from generation to generation, of a recessive trait occurring in inbreeding populations; it results from the mating of a homozygous affected person with a heterozygous carrier of the same recessive gene; the pedigree pattern superficially resembles that of a dominant trait, hence the name.

quater in die (q.i.d.) Latin for four times a day.

quaternary 1. The member of a series that is fourth in order. 2. A chemical compound containing four different elements; e.g., $NaHSO_4$.

Queckenstedt's sign Absence of variation in pressure of the cerebrospinal fluid when the veins of the neck are compressed; indicative of a block in the vertebral canal.

quenching 1. The process of extinguishing or suppressing an energy emission such as heat or an electrical discharge. 2. In liquid scintillation counting, the lowering of the amount of energy recorded from the sample container.

quick A sensitive part, painful to the touch.

quickening The sensation caused by the movement of the fetus within the uterus, felt by the mother for the first time about the fourth or fifth month of pregnancy.

quicksilver See mercury.

quinacrine A bright yellow antimalarial drug with a biologic half-life of 10 days; Atabrine®.

Quincke's sign Quincke's pulse; see under pulse.

quinhydrone A compound of equimolecular quantities of quinone and hydroquinone; $C_6H_4O_2 \cdot C_6H_4(OH)_2$; used in pH determinations.

quinidine An alkaloid from cinchona bark; used to control cardiac arrhythmias.

quinine A white, crystalline, bitter powder, obtained from the bark of the cinchona tree; used in the treatment of malaria. Also called quinina; Jesuit's or Cardinal's bark.

quininism See cinchonism.

quinolones A class of broad spectrum antibiotics used to treat a variety of bacterial infections.

quinquina Cinchona bark from which quinine is extracted.

quinsy Acute suppurative inflammation of the tonsils and surrounding tissue.

quintuplet One of five children born of a single birth.

quod vide (q.v.) Latin for which see; usually placed in parentheses after a cross-reference.

quotidian Recurring every day, as a fever.

quotient The number of times a quantity is contained in another.

   blood q. Color index, see under index.

   intelligence q. (IQ) The ratio of a person's attained score on a standardized test of intelligence to the expected mean score for his age, multiplied by 100.

   respiratory q. (R.Q.) The ratio between the volume of carbon dioxide expired and the volume of oxygen consumed; it varies with the diet, but normally is about 0.82.

medial view of cerebrum

rachiotome

lateral geniculate body

radicular cyst

root of molar

visual cortex

calcarine fissure

eyeball

optic nerve

optic chiasma

optic tract

optic radiation

caries

Rr

rabid Afflicted with rabies.

rabies A viral encephalitis transmitted through saliva of an infected animal; the incubation period varies from 10 days to several months; invariably fatal in man unless preventive treatment is administered. Also called hydrophobia.

racemic **1.** Composed of clustered parts; said of glands. **2.** Denoting a chemical compound composed of equal parts of dextrorotatory and levorotatory substances, therefore incapable of rotating the plane of polarized light.

racemization The chemical conversion of an optically active substance into another that is relatively, or completely, inactive.

racemose Resembling a bunch of grapes.

rachial Spinal.

rachialgia Pain in the spine (vertebral column). Also called spondylalgia.

rachicentesis Lumbar puncture.

rachidian Spinal.

rachiocampsis Spinal curvature.

rachiocentesis Spinal puncture.

rachiodynia Pain in the spinal muscles.

rachiopathy Any disease of the spinal cord. Also called spondylopathy.

rachiotome A surgical bone-cutting instrument for dividing the vertebral laminae.

rachiotomy The operative procedure of cutting into the vertebral column.

rachischisis Developmental defect in which the vertebral arches are absent. Also called myelocele.

rachitic Relating to or affected with rickets.

rachitogenic Producing or causing rickets, as a vitamin D-deficient diet.

rachitome See rachiotome.

rad A unit of radiation exposure expressing the absorbed dose; one rad represents absorption of 100 ergs of energy per gram, and is roughly equivalent to a roentgen.

radarkymography Videotaping of heart motions during fluoroscopy with the aid of an image intensifier; it enables the movements to be calibrated through graphic tracings.

radectomy Removal of a portion or the whole of the root of a tooth.

radial **1.** Relating to a bone in the forearm (radius) or to any radius. **2.** Diverging in various directions from a central point.

radial-immunodiffusion A method of quantifying immunoglobulins; plates of agar impregnated with various antisera to specific immunoglobulins are used as receptacles for the plasma to be tested; as the test sample immunoglobulin diffuses into the agar, a circle of precipitation forms, the diameter of which is proportional to the amount of immuno-

globulin in the test sample.

radiant **1.** Emitting heat or light rays. **2.** A central point from which rays diverge. **3.** Emitted as radiation.

radiate **1.** To expose to radiation. **2.** To emit radiation. **3.** To diverge in all directions from a center.

radiation **1.** The emission and projection of energy (waves or particles) through space. **2.** A bundle of white fibers in the brain.

    background r. The measured radioactivity in a given location, in the absence of a sample.

    Cerenkov r. Light produced when high energy particles travel through a clear liquid at a velocity greater than the speed of light in that liquid.

    corpuscular r. Subatomic particles of specific masses that travel in streams at various speeds; e.g., protons, electrons, neutrons, and alpha or beta particles. Cf. electromagnetic radiation.

    electromagnetic r. Forms of energy that have no mass and travel in waves at the speed of light; they differ in wavelengths (from 10^{17} to 10^{-6} Å), frequency, and photon energy; e.g., x and gamma rays, radio and infrared waves, visible light, and ultraviolet or cosmic radiation. Cf. corpuscular radiation.

    "hard" r. Short wavelength radiation having high energy and the ability to penetrate deeply.

    ionizing r. Electromagnetic radiation (e.g., x rays, gamma rays) or corpuscular radiation (e.g., protons, electrons) capable of producing electrically charged atoms (ions).

    optic r. A band of fibers in the brain passing from the lateral geniculate body of the thalamus to the cortex of the occipital lobe.

    scattered r. The change in direction of the x-ray photon as a result of collision with matter.

    "soft" r. Long wavelength radiation of low penetrability.

radical **1.** A group of atoms that can pass from one compound to another without changing and that forms one of the basic parts of a molecule; in chemical formulas it is enclosed in parentheses. **2.** Carried to the farthest limit in dealing with the root or cause of a disease.

    acid r. A radical formed by an acid by loss of one or more hydrogen ions.

    free r. A chemical group that has unshared electrons available for reaction; e.g., as CH_3.

radiculalgia Neuralgia of the sensory root of a spinal nerve, usually due to an irritation.

radicular Relating to a root, especially a nerve or a tooth root.

radiculectomy Resection of a spinal nerve root.

radiculitis Inflammation of the portion of a spinal nerve root within the dura mater.

radiculomyelopathy Disease of the spinal cord

and nerve roots.

radiculoneuropathy Disease of the spinal nerve roots and nerves.

radiculopathy Disease of the spinal nerve roots.

radioactive Relating to or possessing radioactivity.

radioactivity The property, possessed by certain elements of high atomic weight, of emitting rays and subatomic particles, either through unstable atomic nuclei or as a result of nuclear reaction.

radioautograph See autoradiograph.

radiobiology The branch of science concerned with the effects of radiation on living tissues and with the use of radioactive isotopes.

radiocalcium (^{45}Ca) Radioisotope of calcium, usually used in bone tumor localization and bone metabolism studies.

radiocarbon (^{14}C) Radioactive isotope of carbon.

radiocarpal Relating to the radius and the carpal bones, especially the joint between the radius and the proximal row of carpal bones.

radiochemistry The study of chemical reactions of radioactive elements.

radiocinematography The technique of making motion pictures of the passage of a radiopaque substance through the internal organs as seen on x-ray examination.

radiocurable Susceptible to cure by irradiation; said of some cancer cells.

radiodermatitis Inflammation of the skin caused by excessive exposure to x or gamma rays.

radiodontics The branch of dentistry that specializes in the taking and interpreting of roentgenograms of teeth and related structures.

radioelectrophysiolograph An apparatus by means of which changes in the electrical potential of brain or heart are radiotransmitted and recorded at some other site; the apparatus is carried by the person, who is unrestricted in his movements.

radioelement Any radioactive element.

radioepidermitis Inflammation of the skin caused by exposure to ionizing radiation. Also called radiodermatitis.

radiofrequency A frequency of electromagnetic radiation in the range between audio frequencies and infrared frequencies.

radiogenesis The production of radioactivity.

radiogenic **1.** Producing rays. **2.** Produced by radioactivity.

radiogram Term sometimes used instead of the preferred terms roentgenogram and radiograph.

radiograph The processed photographic film produced in radiography.

    bitewing r. X-ray film adapted to show the crown and cervical third of the roots of both upper and

superior cervical
sympathetic ganglion — hypoglossal nerve

radix superior ansa cervicalis

C1

radix inferior ansa cervicalis

C2

C3

C4

C5

phrenic nerve

radius

radius

ventral ramus of spinal nerve

lateral branch

medial branch

dorsal ramus of spinal nerve

spinal cord

common ragweed

lower teeth and the dental arches.

radiography The development of an image of a bodily part by transmitting radioactive energy (x or gamma rays) through it onto a sensitized film.

radiohumeral Relating to the radius and the humerus.

radioimmunoassay A method of analysis, such as determination of the concentration of substances in blood plasma, through the use of radioactive antibodies.

radioimmunodiffusion The study of antigen-antibody reactions by gel diffusion using radioisotope-labeled antigen or antibody.

radioimmunoelectrophoresis Immunoelectrophoresis using radioisotope-labeled antigen or antibody.

radioiodinated Combined or treated with radioiodine.

radioiodine A radioactive isotope of iodine; about two dozen are known, the most commonly used at present being ^{131}I and ^{125}I.

radioiron A radioactive isotope of iron.

radioisotope An isotope of an element that is naturally or artificially radioactive.

radioligand A radioactive-labeled substance.

radiologist A physician with specific training in radiology.

radiology The science concerned with radiant energy (x rays and radioactive isotopes) and its use for the diagnosis and treatment of disease. Cf. roentgenology.

radiolucency The state of being moderately permeable to x rays or other forms of radiation.

radiometer A device for detecting and measuring radiant energy.

radiomimetic Denoting a chemical that has a destructive effect on tissues which is similar to that of high energy radiation; e.g., sulfur mustards, nitrogen mustards.

radionecrosis Destruction of tissues due to radiation.

radionuclide A radioactive nuclide; a species of nuclide with an unstable nucleus which disintegrates, emitting radiant energy; may be found in a natural state or in a chemical element made radioactive by artificial means.

radiopacity The state of being impenetrable by any form of radiation.

radiopaque Impenetrable by x rays or any form of radiation.

radiopathology The study and treatment of conditions caused by radiation.

radiopelvimetry A radiographic procedure for determining the size and shape of the maternal pelvis, the fetus, and its presenting part.

radiopharmaceutical A radioactive pharmaceutical preparation used for diagnostic or therapeutic purposes.

radio-pharmacy The branch of pharmacy dealing with the preparation and dispensing of radioactive drugs utilizing short-lived radioisotopes.

radioreaction A bodily reaction to radiation, especially of the skin.

radioreceptor A receptor capable of responding to radiant energy, such as light or heat.

radioresistance The relative resistance of cells or organisms to the injurious action of radiation.

radioscopy Examination of internal structures of the body by x rays. Also called roentgenoscopy.

radiosensitivity Relative susceptibility of biologic tissues or substances to the action of radiation. Also called radiosensitiveness.

radiostereoscopy The technique of observing simultaneously two x-ray pictures, taken at slightly different angles, so that the viewed area appears three-dimensional.

radiosurgery Use of radioactive objects such as radium needles or radon seeds in surgical treatment.

radiotherapist A physician who specializes in radiotherapy.

radiotherapy The treatment of disease by any radioactive substance or radiant energy.

radiothermy Therapeutic use of heat from radiant sources.

radiotoxemia Radiation sickness.

radiotransparent Allowing the passage of radiant energy.

radioulnar Relating to the radius and the ulna.

radium A radioactive metallic element that emits alpha, beta, and gamma radiation and a radioactive gas called radon; it has a half-life of 1,590 years; symbol Ra, atomic number 88, atomic weight 226.05; in medicine, it is used in the treatment of some malignancies.

radius, *pl.* **radii** (r) **1.** The smaller of the two bones of the forearm, on the side of the thumb. **2.** A straight line extending from the center to the periphery of a circle.

radix, *pl.* **radices** Latin for root; the beginning or primary portion of a structure, as a nerve at its origin from the spinal cord.

   r. inferior ansae cervicalis. Fibers from the seconds and third cervical nerves that form the inferior root of the cervical loop (ansa cervicalis).

   r. linguae Root of the tongue; the posterior attached part of the tongue.

   r. superior ansa cervicalis Fibers from the first and second cervical nerves that form the superior root of the cervical loop (ansa cervicalis).

radon A colorless gas emanating from radium,

with a half-life of about four days; it is a natural isotope produced during the radioactive decay of radium; symbol Rn, atomic number 86, atomic weight 222. Also called radium emanation.

raffinose $C_{18}H_3O_{16}\cdot5H_2O$; a sugar occurring in cottonseed meal and in sugar beets, composed of D-galactose, D-glucose, and D-fructose. Also called melitose.

rage Intense, violent anger.

   sham r. An outburst of motor activity in an animal whose cerebral hemispheres have been removed, characterized by manifestations of fear and anger on slight provocation and accompanied by struggling, piloerection, dilatation of pupils, and increase in blood pressure.

ragweed A weed of the genus *Ambrosia*, especially the species *A. artemisiifolia* (common ragweed), *A. trifida* (giant ragweed) or *A. psilostachya* (Western ragweed), whose abundant pollen is a hazard to many hay fever sufferers.

rale Abnormal sound heard on auscultation of the chest, originating in the pulmonary airway, and usually indicating disease of the bronchi or lungs.

   atelectatic r. A crackling sound that disappears upon deep breathing or coughing, occurring in persons who tend to breathe superficially; often noted postoperatively.

   coarse r. See rhonchus.

   crepitant r. A fine sound resembling the rubbing of hair between the fingers, produced by a thin secretion in the bronchioles.

   fine r. Short, high-pitched sound originating in the alveoli and terminal bronchi; the sound is simulated by rubbing hair between one's fingers close to the ear.

   medium r. A rale having a pitch that is lower than that of a fine rale.

ramose, ramous Branching.

ramulus A minute terminal branch.

ramus, *pl.* **rami** A branchlike part of a nerve, artery, or vein, especially a primary division.

   dorsal r. of spinal nerve A bundle of nerve fibers given off by a spinal nerve immediately after the union of its dorsal and ventral roots; it innervates the structures of the back.

   r. communicans A bundle of nerve fibers connecting two nerves or a nerve to a ganglion.

   ventral r. of spinal nerve The continuation of a spinal nerve soon after it emerges from the intervertebral foramen, dividing ultimately into the lateral and anterior divisions; it innervates the limbs and the anterolateral parts of the body wall; the major plexuses (cervical, brachial, and lumbosacral) are formed by the ventral rami of spinal nerves.

ranine Pertaining to the undersurface of the

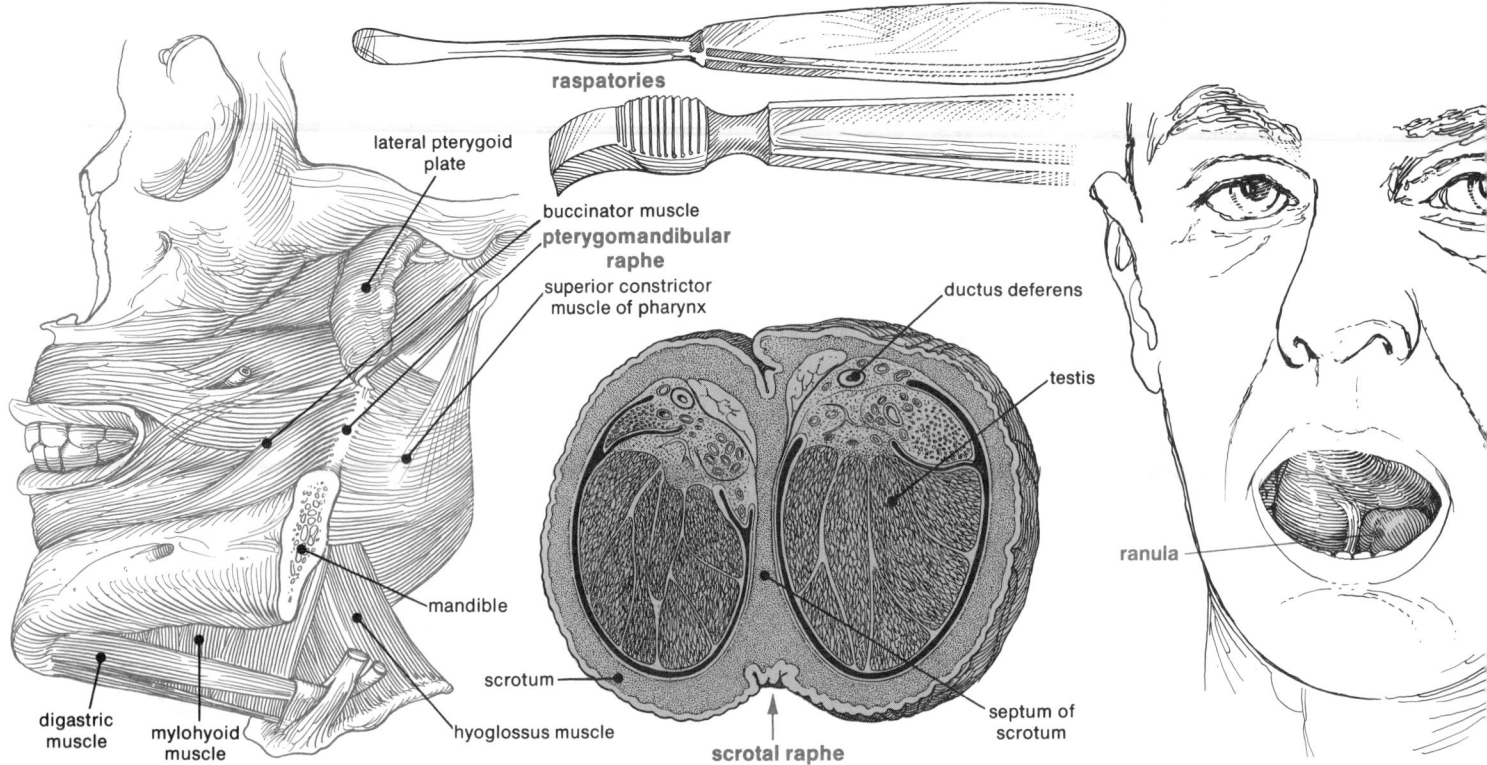

raspatories

lateral pterygoid plate

buccinator muscle

pterygomandibular raphe

superior constrictor muscle of pharynx

ductus deferens

testis

ranula

mandible

scrotum

septum of scrotum

digastric muscle

mylohyoid muscle

hyoglossus muscle

scrotal raphe

tongue.

ranula A cystic tumor occurring on the floor of the mouth or the undersurface of the tongue. Also called sublingual cyst.

rape The criminal act in which an individual forces another individual to submit to sexual intercourse. Also called rape of the first degree.

statutory r. Sexual intercourse with a female under the legal age of consent. Also called rape of the second degree.

raphe A ridge or line marking the union of two similar structures.

pterygomandibular r. A line of interlacing tendinous fibers stretching from the hamulus of the medial pterygoid plate to the inner surface of the mandible at the level of the third molar; the superior pharyngeal constrictor and buccinator muscles attach to it.

r. of medulla oblongata The line between the right and left halves of the medulla oblongata.

scrotal r. A line extending from the anus to the base of the penis; it marks the attachment of the scrotal septum which separates the testes.

raptus Any sudden seizure.

rarefaction The process of becoming less dense.

rarefy To make light, less dense, or less compact.

rash Any eruption of the skin.

heat r. See heat, prickly.

morbilliform r. Condition of the skin resembling the eruption of measles.

nettle r. Urticaria.

raspatory Instrument for scraping bone.

rat Any of various long-tailed rodents of the genus *Rattus*; vectors of human disease.

albino r. White rat used extensively in laboratory experiments.

black r. English black rat, *Rattus rattus*, that harbors the flea, *Zenopsylla cheopis*, responsible for transmitting plague to humans.

brown r. Large brownish-gray rat, *Rattus norvegicus*, with short ears and a smaller than usual tail.

spontaneously hypertensive r. (SHR) A strain of rats prone to develop hypertension without recourse to special diets or hormones; originally developed in Japan; a useful animal in research in hypertension.

Sprague-Dawley r. Genetically similar, inbred strain of rats developed by the Sprague-Dawley Company.

transgenic r. A rat genetically engineered to develop diseases mimicking human disorders.

Wistar r. A white rat extensively used in experimental biology and medicine; strain developed at the Wistar Institute.

rate A quantitative measurement of an event or process in terms of its relationship to some fixed standard; a measured quantity expressed as the ratio of one quantity to another.

basal metabolic r. (BMR) See metabolism, basal.

case r. See morbidity rate.

death r. See mortality rate.

erthrocyte sedimentation r. (ESR) The rate (in millimeters per hour) of settling of red blood cells when anticoagulated blood is allowed to stand under standard conditions in a vertical glass column; the two standard methods commonly used are those of Wintrobe and Westergren (see under method). Also called sedimentation rate.

fetal heart r. (FHR) The number of fetal heart beats per minute, normally ranging from 120 to 140.

glomerular filtration r. (GFR) The volume of plasma filtered through the glomerular capillary membranes of the kidney in one minute.

growth r. Absolute or relative growth increase, expressed in units of time.

infant mortality r. An expression of the relation of the number of deaths in the first year of life to the total number of live births in the same population during the same period of time.

morbidity r. The number of cases of a particular disease occurring in a specified time per given unit of the total population. Also called case rate.

mortality r. The ratio between the number of registered deaths in a specified area and the total population during a given period, usually one year. Also called death rate.

neonatal mortality r. The number of deaths in infants under 28 days of age in a given year per 1000 live births of that year.

perinatal mortality r. The number of deaths in infants less than 7 days of age plus the number of fetal deaths after 28 weeks of gestation in a year per 1000 live births of that year.

pulse r. The number of beats per minute of a peripheral arterial pulse.

respiration r. The rate of breathing; the number of inspirations (breaths) per minute.

sedimentation r. Erythrocyte sedimentation rate.

ratio (r) Proportion; the relation that one thing bears to another in respect to magnitude or quantity. Also called rate.

albumin-globulin r. (A/G r.) The ratio of albumin to globulin in serum plasma, or, in kidney disease, in urine.

body-weight r. Body weight in grams divided by the height in centimeters.

cardiothoracic r. The ratio of the transverse diameter of the heart to the internal diameter of the thoracic cage at its widest point.

extraction r. The fraction of a substance removed from the blood by an organ; A − V/A (A and V being the concentration of the substance in arterial and venous renal plasma, respectively).

lecithin-sphingomyelin r. (L/S r.) The ratio of lecithin to sphingomyelin in amniotic fluid; used to determine the degree of maturity of the fetal lungs and thus predict respiratory problems.

mendelian r. The ratio in which the offspring, or later generations, show the characteristics of their parents, in accordance with genetic principles.

nucleocytoplasmic r. The ratio of the volumes of nucleus and cytoplasm within a given cell; the ratio is generally constant for a particular cell type, and is usually increased in malignant neoplasms.

nucleoplasmic r. See nucleocytoplasmic ratio.

segregation r. Ratio of the various segregating genotypes among offspring.

therapeutic r. The ratio of the maximally tolerated dose of a drug to the minimal effective dose; the higher the ratio the safer the drug.

rational 1. In possession of reasoning qualities; not delirious. **2.** Based on reason.

rationalization The provision of an explanation to justify an act which is governed by factors other than reason.

rauwolfia An alkaloid derived from a number of tropical trees and shrubs of the genus *Rauwolfia*.

r. serpentina The dried root of *Rauwolfia serpentina*; a source of drugs, such as reserpine, with tranquilizing and antihypertensive properties.

ray 1. A straight-line, narrow beam of electromagnetic radiation such as light, heat, or other form of radiation. **2.** A linear anatomic structure.

actinic r. A light ray toward and beyond the violet end of the spectrum, capable of producing chemical changes; photochemically active radiation.

alpha (α) r.'s Fast moving streams of minute alpha particles of matter composed of positively charged composite particles, indistinguishable from helium atom nuclei; derived from radioactive substances.

Becquerel r.'s Alpha, beta, and gamma rays emitted from uranium, radium, and other radioactive substances.

beta (β) r.'s Fast moving streams of negatively charged beta particles of matter, especially of electrons, that have greater penetrative power than the alpha rays derived from radioactive substances.

borderline r.'s Grenz rays.

cathode r.'s A stream of electrons emitted by the negative electrode (cathode) in a vacuum tube (Crookes' tube); their bombardment against the glass wall of the tube or against the anode gives rise to the x rays (roentgen rays).

COMMON MANIFESTATIONS OF ADVERSE REACTIONS TO SOME DRUGS		
Manifestations		Drugs
dermatologic	urticaria (hives)	penicillin aspirin barbiturates sulfonamides
	exfoliative dermatitis (loss of superficial skin layers)	penicillin barbiturates
respiratory	apnea (difficulty in breathing)	local anesthetics
	inflammation of mucous membranes of nose	reserpine
	pulmonary infection	antineoplastic-immuno- suppressive drugs
cardio- vascular	hypotension (fall in blood pressure)	imipramine amitriptyline
	arrhythmia (abnormal rhythm of heart beat)	thyroid hormone sympathomimetic amines
gastro- intestinal	swollen or hairy tongue	tetracycline
	discoloration of dental enamel	tetracycline (in children)
	peptic ulceration hemorrhage	aspirin

cosmic r.'s High energy particles that bombard the earth from outer space.

gamma (γ) r. Electromagnetic radiation emitted from the nucleus of an atom during the radioactive decay process; analogous to the x ray but of shorter wavelength.

grenz r.'s Very soft x rays, greater in length than one Å; closely allied to the ultraviolet rays in their wavelength and in their biologic action upon tissue; used in x-raying soft tissues.

hard r. X ray of short wavelength and great penetrability; produced by a high-voltage tube.

hertzian r.'s Radio waves; see under wave.

incident r. A ray that strikes the surface before reflection.

infrared r.'s Rays having wavelengths greater than 7700 Å, beyond the red end of the spectrum.

medullary r. The center of the renal lobe, which has the shape of a small steep pyramid, consisting of straight ascending or descending limbs of the nephronic loop or collecting tubules.

reflected r. A ray of radiant energy thrown back from a nonabsorbent surface.

roentgen r. See x ray.

soft r. A ray of long wavelength and slight penetrability.

ultraviolet r.'s Rays having wavelengths between 4000 and 40 Å, between the violet end of the visible spectrum and the x-ray region of the electromagnetic spectrum.

vital ultraviolet r.'s Rays of wavelengths between 3200 and 2900 A; necessary for formal growth; they promote calcium metabolism.

x r. 1. An electromagnetic radiation (high energy photon) with a very short wavelength (0.05 to 100 Å), generated at the point of impact of a stream of high-speed cathode electrons on the target of an x-ray tube; x rays, because of their penetrating power, are used to record on film shadows of the varying densities within a portion of the body. Also called roentgen ray. 2. A photograph taken with x rays. Properly termed roentgenogram.

Raynaud's disease Bilateral cyanosis of the digits due to spasmodic contraction of the peripheral arteries, usually precipitated by cold or by emotion.

Raynaud's phenomenon See under phenomenon.

reabsorption The process of reabsorbing or the state of being reabsorbed.

active r. One requiring the expenditure of energy.

passive r. One requiring no energy expenditure; the substances are reabsorbed along a concentration gradient.

tubular r. Selective reabsorption of extracellular fluid in the tubules of the kidney; it helps restore essential components to the body.

reactance (X) Opposition to the flow of an alternating electric current, by passage through a coil of wire or a condenser.

reactant Any substance that takes part in a chemical reaction.

reaction 1. A force produced by and opposing an acting force. 2. Any response to a stimulus. 3. The transformation of molecules into others. 4. The observable color change in, or produced by, indicators or reagents in chemical analysis.

acid r. A positive test indicating the presence of hydrogen ions in a solution; e.g., the reddening of blue litmus.

adverse r. An unexpected, undesirable, and, sometimes, life-threatening response to a therapeutic drug.

alarm r. (AR) The body's response to a sudden exposure to a violent or stressful stimulus.

alkaline r. A positive test indicating the presence of hydroxyl ions in a solution; e.g., the bluing of red litmus.

allergic r. A reaction stimulated by exposure to a substance (allergen) to which the individual has become sensitized.

amphoteric r. The reaction of a substance that is capable of reacting chemically both as an acid and as a base.

anamnestic r. The increased and more rapid production of antibodies upon a second exposure to antigens. Also called secondary response.

antigen-antibody r. The specific binding of antibody with the same type of antigen that activated the formation of the antibody, resulting in precipitation, agglutination, or neutralization of exotoxin.

anxiety r. An uncontrollable apprehension out of proportion to any apparent external cause.

arousal r. Change in the brain wave pattern of an individual when suddenly awakened.

Arthus r. A severe local sensitivity reaction produced at the site of injection of antigen into an animal possessing specific precipitating serum antibodies.

Bence-Jones r. The coagulation of Bence-Jones protein when a urine sample from a patient with Bence-Jones proteinuria is heated, followed by its redissolving on boiling, and coagulation again on cooling.

biuret r. A chemical test used to detect and to quantitate protein.

cell-mediated r. Delayed allergic reaction involving T (thymus-dependent) lymphocytes.

chain r. A series of chemical reactions, each one initiated by the one preceding.

complement fixation r. Reaction occurring when antibody-coated erythrocytes are added to a mixture of a test antigen and a patient's heated serum in the presence of a measured amount of complement; if the patient's serum contains antibody, an antigen-antibody reaction takes place and complement is consumed (fixed); no free complement is left to lyse the sensitized erythrocytes; the reaction is the basis for many serologic tests for infections (e.g., syphilis).

consensual r. Constriction of the pupil of one eye when a light is flashed into the other eye. Also called pupillary reflex; indirect light reflex.

conversion r. Process through which unacceptable unconscious impulses or repressed ideas are converted into bodily symptoms. Also called somatic conversion.

cross r. A reaction occurring between an antibody and an antigen of a type different from, but related to, the one that stimulated the production of the antibody.

cytotoxic r. A reaction that results in damage to or destruction of cells.

delayed r. A late response of the body to an agent to which it is hypersensitive.

dissociative r. A reaction marked by dissociated behavior, such as amnesia, sleepwalking, dream states, etc.

drug r. An adverse reaction arising during the therapeutic administration of a drug; may be immediate (within minutes), accelerated (from one to 72 hours), or late (after three days).

endergonic r. A reaction requiring the expenditure of energy; e.g., certain biologic syntheses.

endothermal r., endothermic r. Chemical reaction in which heat is absorbed.

exergonic r. A reaction that liberates energy, as in certain catabolic processes.

exothermal r., exothermic r. A reaction in which heat is liberated.

false-negative r. An erroneous negative reaction; a negative reaction occurring in the presence of the condition being tested for.

false-positive r. An erroneous positive reaction; a positive reaction occurring in the absence of the condition being tested for.

first-order r. A reaction in which the rate is proportional to the concentration of the substance undergoing chemical change.

Herxheimer's r. See Jarisch-Herxheimer reaction.

id r. A skin eruption occurring in an area of the body other than that of the infection, e.g., on the hands during acute tinea infection of the feet; most commonly follows fungus infections of the feet or the scalp, severe contact dermatitis of the hands,

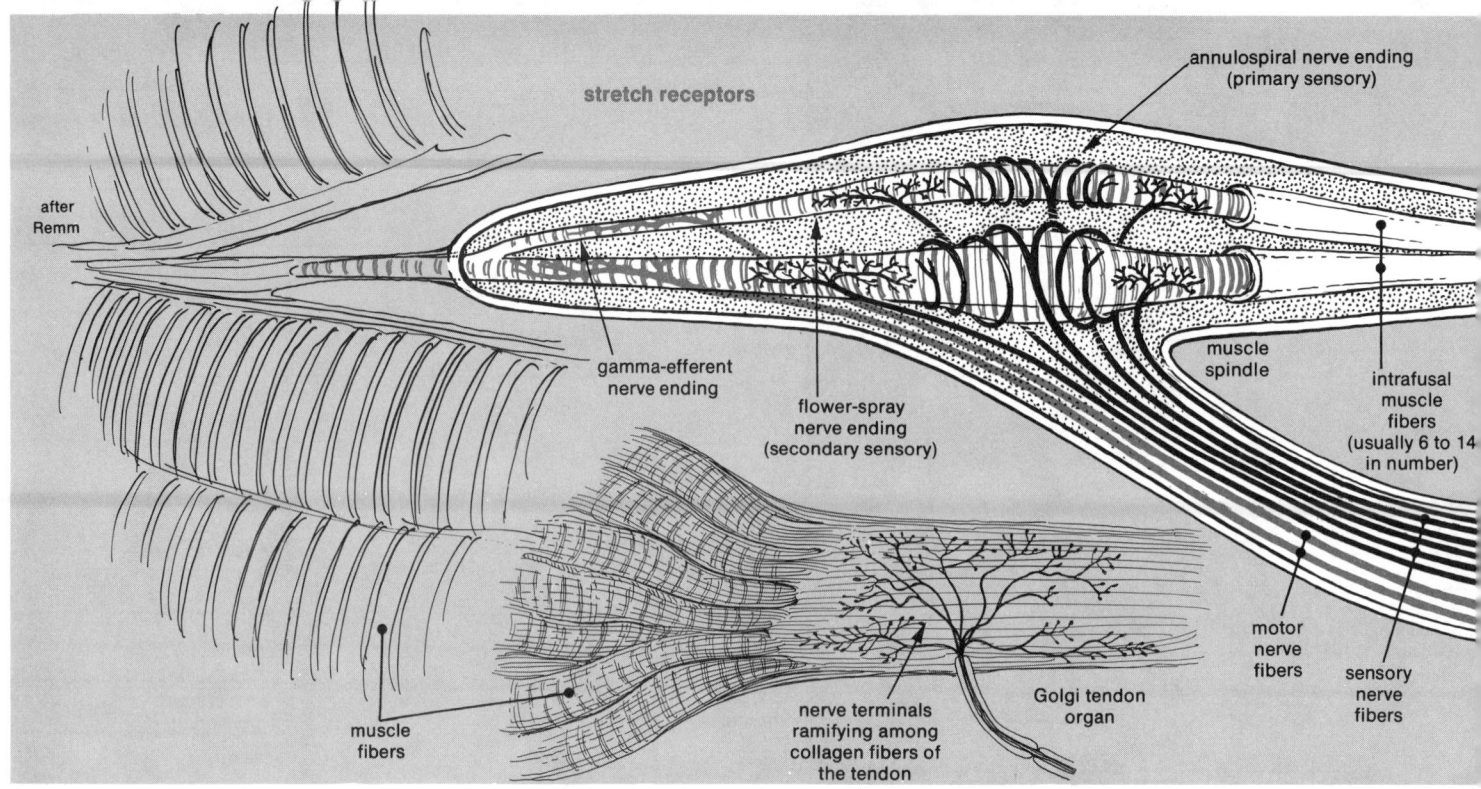

stretch receptors

annulospiral nerve ending (primary sensory)

after Remm

gamma-efferent nerve ending

flower-spray nerve ending (secondary sensory)

muscle spindle

intrafusal muscle fibers (usually 6 to 14 in number)

muscle fibers

nerve terminals ramifying among collagen fibers of the tendon

Golgi tendon organ

motor nerve fibers

sensory nerve fibers

and varicose ulcers; considered to be an allergic reaction.

immune r. 1. The response activated in the lymphoreticular system of vertebrates by the presence of a foreign substance (antigen); the response may be a direct functioning of the cells (e.g., phagocytosis), or the elaboration of a cell product (antibody). 2. The formation of a slight papule without vesicle formation following smallpox vaccination of an immune person.

Jarisch-Herxheimer r. An inflammatory reaction sometimes induced by arsphenamine, mercury, or antibiotics in the treatment of syphilis; believed to be due to rapid release of treponemal antigen. Also called Herxheimer's reaction.

leukemoid r. Condition marked by the presence of increased white blood cells in the blood; similar to, but not associated with, leukemia and occurring in certain conditions, such as infectious diseases and some malignant tumors.

ninhydrin r. The production of violet color by proteins, peptones, peptides, and amino acids having a free carboxyl and an α-amino group, when boiled with ninhydrin.

normal lymphocyte transfer r. (NLT reaction), reaction resulting from the injection of allogeneic lymphocytes into the skin.

nuclear r. A reaction in which an atomic nucleus changes its atomic number (number of protons) or its mass number (number of nucleons), as a result of natural or artificial radioactivity, or through direct nuclear bombardment.

Pandy's r. A qualitative and quantitative test to detect the presence of proteins in the spinal fluid. Also called Pandy's test.

polymerase chain r. (PCR) A method of amplifying a short stretch of DNA; applications include genetic testing, detection of difficult-to-isolate pathogens, mutation analysis, DNA sequencing, diagnosis of disease, and analyzing evolutionary relationships.

Prausnitz-Kustner r. Reaction occurring when blood serum from an allergic person is injected into the skin of a nonallergic individual, followed (48 hours later) by injection of antigens to which the donor is allergic; a wheal appears at the site of injection. Also called Prausnitz-Kustner or P-K test.

quellung r. Neufeld capsular swelling; see under swelling.

Schultz-Charlton r. Blanching of scarlatinal rash at site of intracutaneous injection of scarlatina antiserum. Also called Schultz-Charlton phenomenon.

Schultz-Dale r. Smooth muscle contraction produced in vitro when antigen is applied to the excised muscle of a sensitive animal.

transfusion r. General term for a variety of nonimmune (e.g., hepatitis) and immune complications occurring during or after transfusion of whole blood or blood products; the immune transfusion reaction may be caused by the destruction of the recipient's red blood cells by antibodies present in the blood of either the donor or the recipient or by a reaction to infused white blood cells.

Wassermann r. See test, Wassermann.

Weil-Felix r. The agglutination of *Proteus* X bacteria with blood serum of persons with typhus fever.

wheal-flare r. A skin sensitivity reaction due to histamine, characterized by an edematous elevation and erythematous flare.

white-graft r. A reaction to a tissue graft in which the graft fails to vascularize and is quickly rejected.

Widal's r. Agglutination reaction used in the diagnosis of typhoid.

zero-order r. A reaction that, regardless of the concentration of the reactants, proceeds at a definite rate.

reactivate To restore activity, as in an inactivated immune serum to which normal serum is added.

reactivity The ability to react.

reagent Any substance, added to a solution, that participates in a chemical reaction, especially one employed in chemical analysis for the detection of biologic constituents.

Benedict-Hopkins-Cole r. Magnesium glyoxalate, made by adding a saturated solution of oxalic acid to powdered magnesium; used for testing proteins for the presence of tryptophan.

biuret r. An alkaline solution of copper sulfate.

diazo r. A reagent consisting of two solutions, sodium nitrate and acidified sulfanilic acid; used to bring about diazotization.

Esbach's r. A reagent consisting of a 1% aqueous solution of picric acid mixed with a 2% solution of citric acid; used in estimating the quantity of albumin in urine.

Fehling's r. See solution, Fehling's.

Nessler's r. One used in determining the level of urea nitrogen in the blood and in the urine.

reagin 1. Antibody involved in immediate hypersensitivity reactions; the human IgE antibody. 2. Obsolete term for antibodies detected by the Wassermann test for syphilis.

reality The sum of all things that have an objective existence.

reality testing In psychiatry and psychology, ability to evaluate the outside world and to adequately comprehend one's relationship to it.

reamer A dental instrument used to enlarge root canals.

rebase To replace or add to the base material of a

denture without changing the occlusal relations of the teeth.

rebound 1. In anesthesia, new reflex activity following the withdrawal of a stimulus. 2. Reappearance of a condition often with greater force than originally, after the effect of a therapeutic agent has worn off; e.g., when the effect of a vasoconstrictor (e.g., nosedrops) wears off and there is subsequently increased vasocongestion.

recall 1. The process of summoning back a memory into consciousness; to bring back to awareness; to remember. 2. In psychiatry, the term refers to the recollection of events in the immediate past.

recanalization The process of recanalizing; e.g., the restoration of a lumen in a blood vessel following thrombotic occlusion.

receiver 1. An electronic device capable of receiving incoming electromagnetic signals and converting them to perceptible forms. 2. In chemistry, a vessel attached to a condenser in which the products of distillation are collected.

receptaculum A pouchlike structure.

r. chyli See cisterna chyli.

receptor 1. The sensory end-organ; the small structure in which a sensory nerve fiber terminates; it receives stimuli and converts them into nervous impulses. 2. In pharmacology, a constituent in a cell that combines with a specific drug, resulting in a change of the cell's function; e.g., insulin.

adrenergic r.'s Constituents of effector tissues innervated by adrenergic postganglionic fibers of the sympathetic nervous system.

alpha-adrenergic r.'s Adrenergic receptors that mediate such actions as vasoconstriction, dilation of the iris of the eye, and pilomotor contraction; they are blocked by the action of compounds such as phenoxybenzamine and phentolamine.

beta-adrenergic r.'s Adrenergic receptors that are blocked by action of such compounds as propranolol; beta$_1$-adrenergic receptors are responsible for acceleration of the heart beat and lipolysis; beta$_2$-adrenergic receptors mediate adrenergic bronchodilation.

histamine r.'s Receptors that respond to histamine; vascular dilatation of histamine is mediated by receptors of both H$_1$ and H$_2$ types: (a) H$_1$ receptors that, when stimulated, cause bronchoconstriction and contraction of the intestines; blocked by antihistamines; (b) H$_2$ receptors that, when stimulated, cause gastric secretion; blocked by substances such as cimetidine.

opiate r.'s Specific tissues in the brain, e.g., along the cerebral aqueduct, that have the capacity to combine with morphine or endorphins.

stretch r. One whose function is to detect elon-

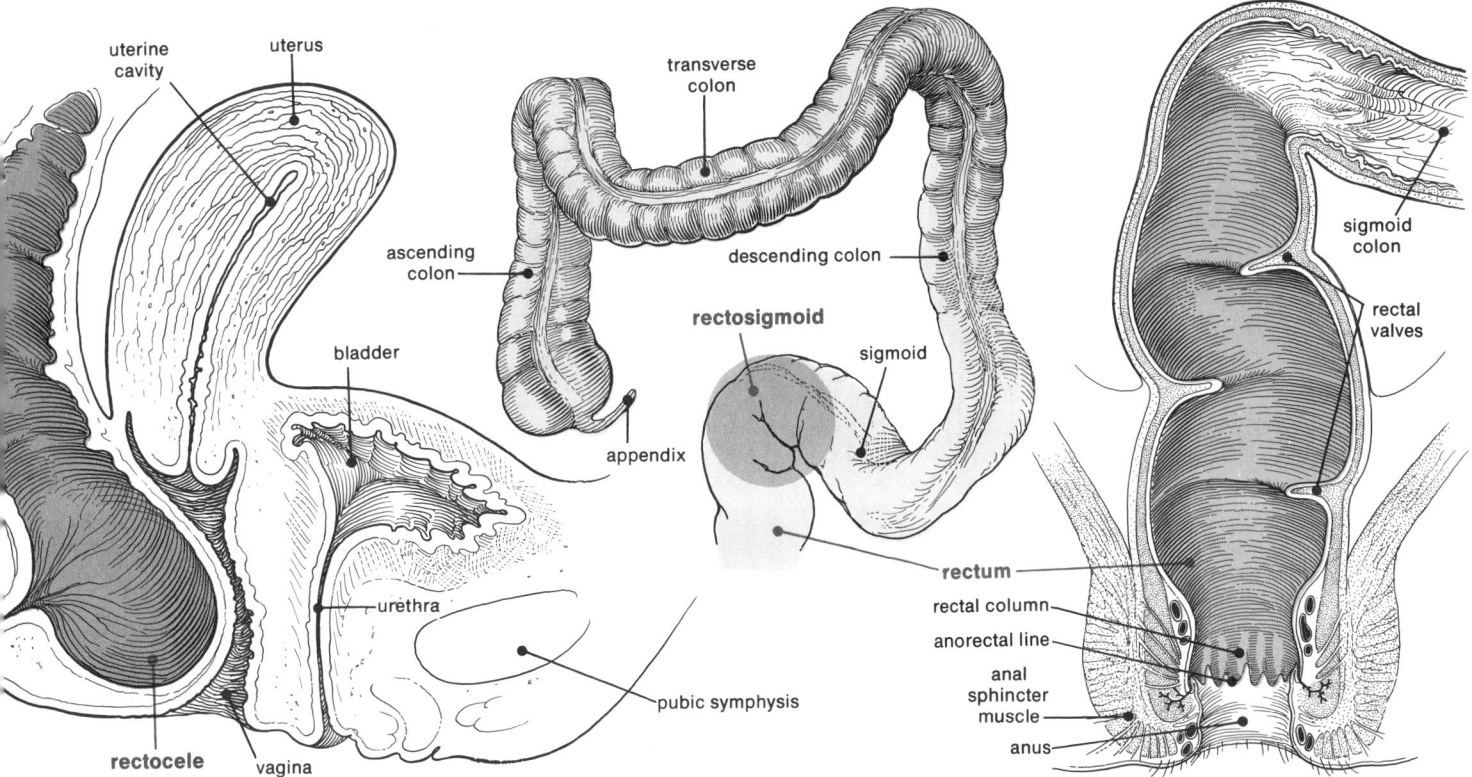

gation; e.g., the muscle spindle and the Golgi tendon organ.

recess A shallow cavity.

    piriform r. A recess in the pharynx on each side of the opening of the larynx.

recession The process of withdrawing.

    gingival r. Displacement of gingiva with resulting added exposure of tooth surface.

    tendon r. Posterior surgical displacement of the insertion of an eye muscle.

recessive 1. Latent; not dominant. 2. In genetics, not expressed unless present in both sets of chromosomes (homozygous).

recidivation Reappearance of a disease, symptom, or pattern of behavior.

recidivism The tendency of an individual to relapse into a previous mode of behavior, especially a tendency to return to criminal or delinquent habits.

recidivist A person who tends to relapse into a previous pattern of bad behavior after rehabilitation; e.g., a habitual criminal.

recipe Latin for take, usually represented by the symbol R_x. **1.** The heading or superscription of a physician's prescription. **2.** The prescription itself.

recipiomotor The recipient of a motor stimulus.

Recklinghausen's disease See neurofibromatosis.

recombinant An organism, chromosome, or DNA that has resulted from the introduction of genetic material from an outside source.

recombination The formation of gene combinations in the offspring that were not present in either parent, caused by the exchange of genes between homologous chromosomes (crossing over).

recon In genetics, the smallest unit of a single DNA nucleotide capable of recombination.

reconduction Retrograde conduction; see under conduction.

reconstitution 1. Restoration to original form, as of a substance previously altered for preservation. 2. Regeneration of a lost bodily part.

record Information preserved in an enduring form.

    interocclusal r. A record of the positional relations of teeth or jaws to each other.

    maxillomandibular r. Maxillomandibular registration, a record of any positional relations of the maxilla to the mandible.

    problem oriented medical r. (POMR) A system of recording medical information about a patient, characterized by a defined universe of information for the data base, a complete up-to-date problem list, and numbered and titled plans and progress notes that preserve the course of action of the physicians and other medical personnel; it is adaptable

for the computer.

    source oriented medical r. The traditional method of recording medical information about a patient as it happens.

record base See baseplate.

recording Preserving, in writing or any other permanent form, the results of a study.

recrement 1. Any secretion, such as saliva or bile, that is reabsorbed after having performed its function. 2. Waste matter.

recrudescence A return of a morbid process after a dormant or inactive period.

recruitment 1. In the testing of hearing, the abnormally rapid increase in loudness experienced by the patient when the sound stimulus is gradually increased. 2. A gradual increase in response to a stimulus which has a constant intensity but prolonged duration.

rectal Relating to the rectum.

rectalgia Proctalgia.

rectify 1. To purify a liquid through redistillation. 2. To transform an alternating current into a direct one. 3. To correct.

rectoabdominal Relating to both the rectum and abdomen, especially a method of examination in which one hand is placed on the abdomen, and one or more fingers of the other hand are inserted into the rectum.

rectocele Prolapse of the rectum into the perineum. Also called proctocele.

rectocolitis See coloproctitis.

rectoperineorrhaphy See proctoperineoplasty.

rectopexy See proctopexy.

rectoplasty See proctoplasty.

rectoscope See proctoscope.

rectosigmoid The portion of the intestinal tract adjacent to the junction of the rectum and the sigmoid colon, on both sides.

rectostenosis See proctostenosis.

rectourethral Relating to both the rectum and the urethra.

rectouterine Relating to both the rectum and the uterus.

rectovaginal Relating to both the rectum and the vagina.

rectovesical Relating to both the rectum and the bladder.

rectum The terminal portion of the intestinal tract extending from the sigmoid colon to the anus.

rectus Straight; describes some muscles which run a straight course, such as the abdominal rectus muscle.

recumbent Lying down; leaning or reclining.

recuperate To recover.

recurrence 1. A return of symptoms, a natural

characteristic of certain diseases, e.g., yellow fever. 2. The return of a morbid state after a period of improvement.

recurrent Returning after abatement or disappearance.

recurvation A backward bending or curving.

Red Cross 1. Red Cross Society; an international organization established for the purpose of caring for the injured and homeless during wartime and natural disasters. 2. The emblem of the Red Cross Society, a red Geneva cross or red Greek cross on a white background; a sign of neutrality.

redia, *pl.* **rediae** The larval stage in the life cycle of a trematode.

redox In chemistry, a coined term meaning a reduction-oxidation reaction state.

reduce 1. To return a part to its normal position; e.g., the ends of a fractured bone. 2. To decrease the valence number of an atom by adding electrons.

reducible Capable of being reduced.

reductant The donor of electrons in an oxidation-reduction reaction.

reductase The reducing enzyme in an oxidation-reduction reaction.

reduction 1. The correction, through surgical or manipulative methods, of a hernia, a fracture, or a dislocation. 2. In chemistry, the removal of oxygen from a substance or the addition of hydrogen; the reverse of oxidation.

reduplication A doubling.

reentry The return of an impulse to an area of heart muscle which it has recently stimulated, as occurs in reciprocal heart rhythms.

refine To purify.

reflect 1. To bend back from a surface, as light or heat rays. 2. To meditate.

reflection 1. The return of light from an optical surface into the same medium from which it came. 2. A bending back.

reflector A surface that reflects light, heat, or sound waves.

reflex 1. An involuntary and immediate response to a stimulus. 2. Turned backward; reflected.

    abdominal r. Contraction of the muscles of the abdominal wall upon stroking of the overlying skin.

    accommodation r. The increase in convexity of the lens of the eye when the eyes are directed from a distant to a near object, in order to bring the image into focus; initiated by an out-of-focus image on the retina.

    Achilles tendon r. Calcaneal tendon reflex.

    acquired r. Conditioned reflex.

    anal r. Contraction of the anal sphincter muscle upon irritation of the perianal area, or upon insertion of a finger into the rectum.

oral
reflex

startle
reflex

eliciting
corneal reflex

ankle r. Calcaneal tendon reflex.

attitudinal r. See statotonic reflex.

Babinski's r. Extension of the large toe with fanning of the small toes upon scratching the sole of the foot. Also called Babinski's sign.

Bainbridge r. Acceleration of the heart beat caused by a rise in pressure in the great veins at the entrance to the right atrium.

biceps r. Flexion of the forearm when the tendon of the biceps is struck.

brachioradial r. Flexion of the forearm upon tapping of the brachioradial muscle at its attachment to the lower end of the radius.

calcaneal tendon r. Contraction of the calf muscles with resulting plantar flexion of the foot on striking of the calcaneal (Achilles) tendon. Also called Achilles tendon reflex; ankle jerk; ankle reflex.

carotid sinus r. See carotid sinus syndrome.

ciliary r. Contraction of the pupils when the gaze is directed from a distant to a near object.

ciliospinal r. See pupillary-skin reflex.

conditioned r. A reflex that is developed through association with, and repetition of, a stimulus. Also called trained reflex.

conjunctival r. Closure of the eyelids upon touching of the conjunctiva with a fine wisp of cotton.

coordinated r. A reflex in which several muscles take part.

corneal r. Blinking induced by touching of the cornea with a fine wisp of cotton while the patient looks in the direction opposite to the approaching cotton.

cremasteric r. Retraction of the testicle upon gently scratching the inner aspect of the upper thigh of the same side.

crossed r. A reflex that causes movement on one side of the body when the opposite side is stimulated.

crossed adductor r. Inward rotation of the leg upon tapping of the sole.

crossed extension r. Response elicited from a newborn infant, indicating spinal cord integrity; placing the child in the supine position, the examiner extends and presses down on one of the child's legs and stimulates the sole of the foot; this causes the free leg to flex, adduct, and then extend.

deep r., deep tendon r. Contraction of a muscle upon tapping of its tendon. Also called tendon reflex.

elbow r. See triceps reflex.

fundus r. The red glow seen in the pupil during inspection of the interior of the eyeball, produced by reflection of light from the choroid.

gag r. Gagging initiated by introduction of a foreign body into the pharynx. Also called pharyngeal reflex.

gastrocolic r. The wavelike contraction of the colon, propelling its contents onward, initiated by introduction of food into the empty stomach.

Gordon r. Extension of the big toe upon firm squeezing of the calf.

grasp r. The immediate grasping of an object placed in the hand; occurring normally only in infants.

Hering-Breuer r. The effects of afferent impulses from the pulmonary vagi in the control of respiration; e.g., deflation of the lungs brings on inspiration.

Hoffmann's r. Flexion of the thumb and fingers when the last joint of the middle finger is quickly flexed and extended.

hung-up r. Prolonged relaxation time of the deep tendon reflexes (particularly the ankle jerks in hypothyroidism).

knee-jerk r. Patellar reflex.

light r. Constriction of the pupil upon light stimulation of the retina.

magnet r. Normal response elicited from a newborn infant; with the baby in the supine position with legs semiflexed, the examiner presses his thumbs against the soles of the child's feet; this causes the child to extend his legs.

micturition r. Any of the reflexes controlling effortless urination and the subconscious ability to retain urine within the bladder. Also called bladder or urinary reflex.

milk-ejection r. The release of milk from the breast upon stimulation of the nipple.

Moro's r. See startle reflex.

myotatic r. Contraction of a muscle in response to a passive stretching force. Also called stretch reflex.

Oppenheim's r. Extension of the toes elicited by pressing down firmly on the shin from the knee to the ankle.

oral r. Normal reflex elicited from a newborn infant; when one corner of his mouth is touched, the bottom lip lowers on the same side and the tongue moves forward and toward the examiner's finger.

orbicularis pulmonary r. Unilateral contraction of the pupil while trying to close the eyelids which are forcibly held open. Also called Westphal's pupillary reflex.

palmomental r. Unilateral twitching of the chin upon scratching of the palm of the hand of the same side. Also called palm-chin reflex.

patellar r. Extension of the leg upon tapping of the patellar tendon while the leg hangs loosely at right angles to the thigh.

patellar-tendon r. Patellar reflex.

pharyngeal r. See gag reflex.

pilomotor r. Formation of goose flesh on lightly touching the skin, or on exposure to cold or emotional stimuli.

plantar r. Flexion of the toes on scratching the sole of the foot. Also called sole reflex.

primitive r.'s Reflexes occurring naturally in the newborn infant; an indication of normal neuromuscular development.

proprioceptive r. Any of various reflexes brought about by stimulation of proprioceptors (labyrinth, carotid sinus, etc.).

pupillary r. Any alteration in the diameter of the pupil.

pupillary-skin r. Dilatation of the pupil upon scratching of the neck. Also called ciliospinal reflex.

quadriceps r. Patellar reflex.

radial r. Flexion of the forearm upon tapping of the end of the radius.

rectal r. Desire to defecate stimulated by accumulation of feces in the rectum.

righting r.'s Reflexes that cause the head and body to resume their normal position in space; initiated by displacement of the body from its normal position.

rooting r. Response elicited from a newborn infant; when the cheek is lightly touched, the infant's head turns in the direction of the touch and his lips purse in preparation for sucking.

startle r. Response of the newborn to loud noises or sudden changes in position; characterized by tensing of muscles, a wide embracing motion of the arms, and extension of the thighs, legs, and fingers, except the thumb and index, which remain in a "C" position. Also called Moro's reflex.

statotonic r. Any of several reflexes stimulated by changes of position of the body in space. Also called attitudinal reflex.

superficial r. Any reflex elicited by stimulation of the skin or mucous membranes.

tendon r. See deep reflex.

trained r. See conditioned reflex.

triceps r. A sudden extension of the forearm on tapping of the triceps tendon at the elbow while the forearm hangs loosely at a right angle to the arm. Also called elbow reflex or jerk.

trunk-incurvation r. Reflex occurring in a newborn infant with normal spinal cord; while the baby is in the prone position, the examiner runs his finger along one side of the spine, causing the child's body to curve in the direction of the stimulus.

tympanic r. Percussion sound heard over a hollow structure.

vagovagal r. A cardiac reflex elicited by irritation of the respiratory tract.

vesical r. The desire to urinate in response to

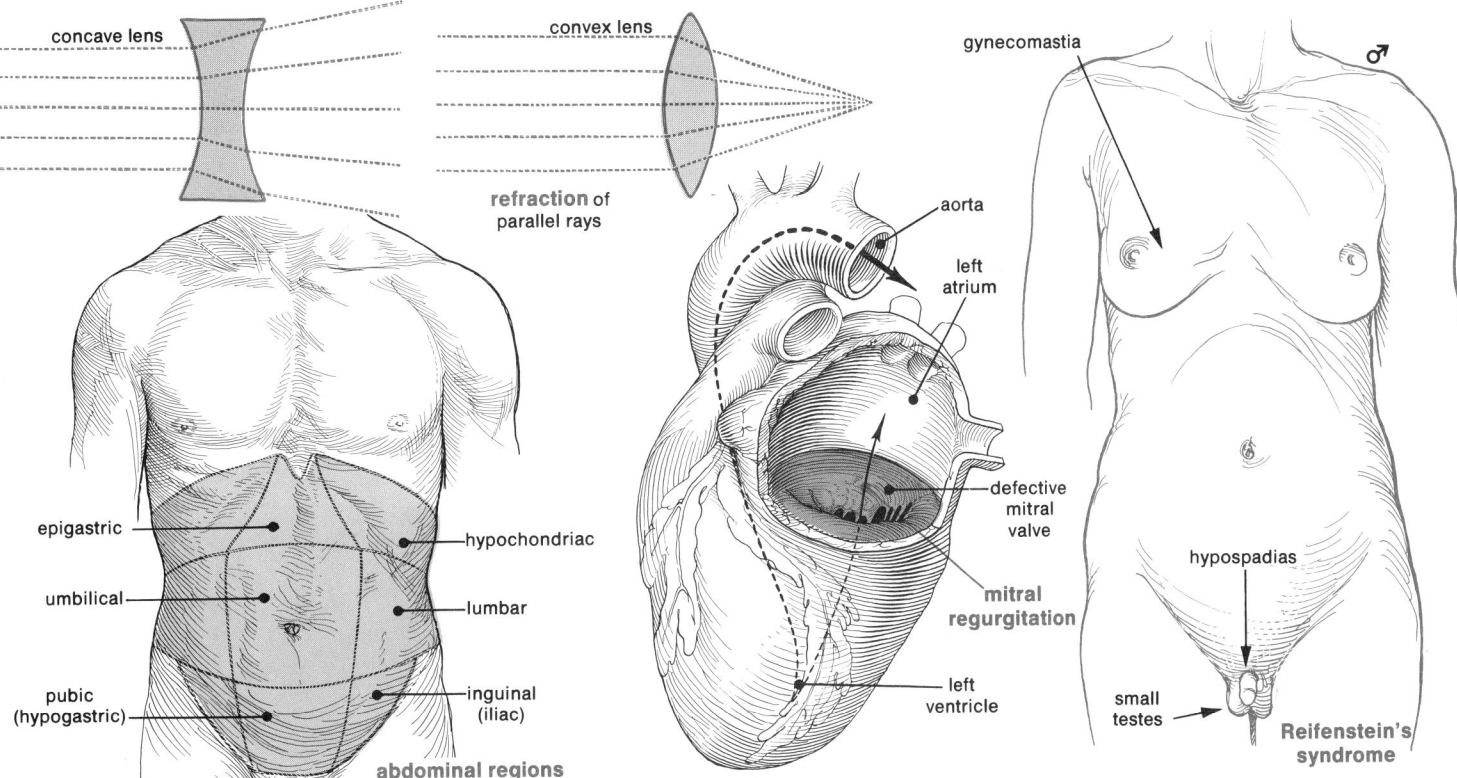

concave lens

convex lens

refraction of parallel rays

gynecomastia

♂

epigastric

hypochondriac

umbilical

lumbar

pubic (hypogastric)

inguinal (iliac)

abdominal regions

aorta

left atrium

defective mitral valve

mitral regurgitation

left ventricle

hypospadias

small testes

Reifenstein's syndrome

pressure within the bladder when full.

Westphal's pupillary r.   See orbicularis pupillary reflex.

reflexograph   An apparatus for graphically recording a reflex.

reflux   Backward flow.

hepatojugular r.   Distention of the jugular veins induced by pressing firmly upon the liver; indicative of congestive heart failure.

vesicoureteral r.   Flow of urine from the bladder back into a ureter during urination.

refract   **1.** To change the direction of a propagating wave, as of light. **2.** To measure the refractive and muscular state of the eyes.

refraction (R)   **1.** The clinical measurement and/ or correction of refractive errors of the eye. **2.** The deflection of a ray of light as a result of passing obliquely from one medium to another of different optical density.

refractive   Relating to refraction.

refractometer   An instrument that measures indices of refraction in translucent substances.

refractory   **1.** Not responsive or readily yielding to treatment. **2.** Not responsive to stimulation, said of a muscle or nerve; immediately after responding to an initial stimulation, it enters a period of functional inactivity during which it does not respond to a second stimulation. **3.** Resisting the action of heat; difficult to melt or work.

refracture   The breaking again of a bone that was improperly set.

refrigerant   An agent that produces a sensation of coolness.

Refsum's syndrome   A rare recessive hereditary disorder marked by cerebellar ataxia, chronic polyneuritis, pigmentary degeneration of the retina, and night blindness; death is commonly due to degenerative heart disease at an early age. Also called heredopathia atactica polyneuritiformis.

refusion   The return of the circulation of blood after its temporary removal from the same individual.

regeneration   **1.** Replacement of a lost or damaged part by the growth of new tissue. **2.** A form of asexual reproduction.

regimen   A systematic procedure or regulation of an activity (exercise, diet) designed to achieve certain ends, usually hygienic or therapeutic in nature.

regio, *pl.* **regiones**   Latin for region.

region   **1.** Any large segment of a bodily surface with more or less definite boundaries. **2.** A bodily part having a special nervous or vascular supply. **3.** A portion of an organ having a special function, as the motor region of the brain.

abdominal r.'s   The nine areas into which the abdomen is divided by four imaginary planes.

registration   In dentistry, a record of jaw relations.

regression   **1.** Abatement of symptoms. **2.** Relapse. **3.** Return to a more primitive or infantile pattern of behavior due to inability to function at a logical adult level (psychological or atavistic regression).

regulation   **1.** A law or rule designed to control details of procedure. **2.** In experimental embryology, the power of a very young embryo to regenerate and continue its development in spite of experimental interference.

regurgitation   A backward flow, as the return of stomach contents.

mitral r.   The back flow of blood from the left ventricle to the left atrium due to a malfunctioning mitral valve (left atrioventricular valve).

rehabilitation   **1.** Restoration of form and function following illness or injury. **2.** Restoration of an individual's capability to achieve the fullest possible life compatible with his abilities and disabilities.

oral r.   The restoration of all lost tooth structure.

physical r.   See physiatrics.

rehalation   Rebreathing of gases previously inhaled; procedure sometimes used in anesthesia.

Reifenstein's syndrome   Familial male pseudohermaphrodism associated with hypospadias, small testes and sterility, absence of beard, short stature, and often gynecomastia; inherited as an X-linked recessive or an autosomal dominant male-limited trait. Also called hereditary familial hypogonadism.

reimplantation   Replacement of a bodily structure to its natural position, as a tooth to the socket from which it was previously removed. Also called replantation.

reinfection   A second infection by the same agent following recovery or during the course of the primary infection.

reinforcement   Added force or strength, such as (a) the increased reflex response when the person performs some mental or physical work while the reflex is being elicited; (b) a structural addition to strengthen a denture.

reinnervation   The restoration of a damaged nerve either by grafting of a live nerve or by spontaneous regrowth of nerve fibers.

reintegration   In psychiatry, the resumption of normal functioning after a mental disorder.

Reiter's syndrome (RS)   A symptom complex consisting of urethritis, conjunctivitis, arthritis, and mucocutaneous lesions; recurrences or chronicity occur in more than one-half of the patients; etiology remains unknown.

rejection   **1.** The term applied to the immunologic response to an incompatible transplanted organ which prevents the graft from being accepted. **2.** Something rejected.

second-set graft r.   Accelerated rejection of a second graft due to immunity developed to a primary graft.

relapse   The return of a disease after apparent recovery or improvement.

relation   The position of one object when considered in association with another.

centric r.   The most posterior position of the mandible from which lateral jaw movements can be made at any given degree of jaw separation.

eccentric r.   Any deviation from the centric relation.

rest r.   The relation of the mandible to the maxilla when the person is resting in an upright position and the jaws are not in contact.

relationship   An association; a kinship.

coefficient of r.   See under coefficient.

object r.   In psychiatry, the emotional bonds existing between one individual and another.

relative biologic effectiveness (RBE)   A measure of the capacity of absorbed doses of various types of radiation (x ray, neutrons, alpha particles, etc.) to produce a specific biologic effect; it may vary with the kind and degree of biologic effect considered, the duration of the exposure, and other factors.

relative of interest   In genetic counseling, anyone who seeks counsel about recurrence of a disease in a family. Cf. proband; consultand.

relax   **1.** To loosen or slacken; to make lax or less tense. **2.** To relieve from tension, effort, or strain.

relaxant   **1.** A drug or therapeutic treatment that produces relaxation by relieving muscular or nervous tension. **2.** Tending to reduce tension or to relax.

relaxation   **1.** Loosening. **2.** The lengthening of muscle fibers.

relaxin   A polypeptide ovarian hormone secreted by the corpus luteum of pregnancy; it relaxes the pubic symphysis and dilates the cervix of some animals during labor; in humans it is thought to inhibit premature contraction of the uterus during pregnancy and to dilate the cervix, thus facilitating delivery of the fetus.

relief   **1.** The lessening of pain or distress, physical or mental; ease from discomfort. **2.** In dentistry, the removal of pressure from a specific area under a denture base.

relieve   **1.** To free wholly or partly from pain, discomfort, anxiety, fear, or the like. **2.** To eliminate bodily waste.

reline   To resurface the tissue side of a denture with new base material in order to make it fit better.

411

native conformation of globular protein chain

unfolded coil

denaturation

renaturation

R

repolarization represented by S-T segment and T wave on electrocardiogram (ECG)

P

Q

S

S-T segment

T wave

U

reserpine

replication of DNA

sugar phosphate backbone

double helix of DNA

original molecule unwinds and strands separate

nucleotides present in cell

two comple molecu form identical the origin

new half-molecules of DNA are formed on old halves

rem Acronym for roentgen-equivalent-man; the amount of ionizing radiation, absorbed by man, that is required to produce a biologic effect equivalent to the absorption of one roentgen of x or γ rays.

remediable Capable of being cured or remedied. Also called curable.

remedial Able to correct a deficiency, especially a reading deficiency.

remedy 1. Something, such as a drug or therapy, that cures, palliates, or prevents disease, or corrects a disorder. 2. To effect a cure.

remembering The neural phenomenon involved in the retrieval of stored information; the "read out phase" of learning; the mental faculty of reviving an impression or idea of which the mind has once been conscious.

remineralization Restoration of mineral elements to the body, especially of calcium salts to bone.

remission A diminution of the severity of a disease or abatement of its symptoms.

remit To temporarily abate in severity without absolutely ceasing; to diminish.

remittent Characterized by alternating periods of abatement and returning of symptoms.

renal Relating to the kidneys. Also called nephric.

renaturation The return of normal characteristic biologic activity to denatured protein, accompanied by the return of its native form. Also called refolding; annealing.

Rendu-Osler-Weber syndrome Hereditary hemorrhagic telangiectasia; see under telangiectasia.

reniform Kidney-shaped.

renin An enzyme formed by the kidney and released into the blood stream; it has an important role in the formation of angiotensin, a potent pressor agent.

rennet A dry extract containing rennin, obtained from the lining of the fourth stomach of the calf; used in curdling milk.

rennin A milk-curdling enzyme obtained from rennet, used in making cheese. Also called chymosin.

renogram, radioactive A graphic record produced by the continuous recording of radioactivity of the kidney after injection of a radiopharmaceutical; an aid in the clinical evaluation of kidney function.

renography Roentgenography of the kidney.

renomegaly Abnormal enlargement of the kidney.

renoprival Resulting from removal of kidneys or absence of kidney function.

renotrophic Affecting the growth of the kidney. Also called nephrotropic.

renotrophin An agent that affects the growth of the kidney.

renovascular Referring to the blood vessels of the kidneys.

reoviruses An RNA group of viruses replicating in the cytoplasm; found in the respiratory and intestinal tracts of man but not yet associated with any disease.

repellent 1. Capable of repelling; tending to repel. 2. Any agent that repels something, especially one that repels insect pests.

repetition compulsion In psychoanalysis, the impulse to reenact earlier experiences.

replantation Replacement of a bodily part to its natural position, as the reinsertion of a dislodged tooth into its original socket; for the soft interior pulp to survive, the tooth should be replanted within about a half-hour; the outer periodontal tissues may survive and reattach after periods of up to six hours. Also called reimplantation.

replication The process of duplicating something; e.g., the repeated formation of the same molecule, as of DNA. Also called autoreproduction.

repolarization A process, immediately following depolarization of the cell, in which the surface of the cell membrane is polarized again by the gradual restoration of the positive charges on the outer and negative charges on the inner surface; for cardiac muscle, graphically shown on the electrocardiogram by the S-T segment and T wave.

repositor An instrument used to replace a prolapsed or dislocated organ, especially the uterus.

repositioning The return of a part to its normal position. Also called reduction.

repression 1. A defense mechanism by which painful experiences are forced into the unconscious sphere; suppression effected unconsciously. 2. The prevention of the formation of an enzyme as programmed by a structural gene in the presence of a small corepressor molecule.

repressor The product of a regulatory gene, capable of combining with a corepressor to form an active complex, or with an inducer to form an inactive complex.

reproduction 1. The process of producing offspring by sexual or asexual means. 2. The act of bringing to mind again a past experience, as a memory.

   asexual r. Reproduction without the union of male and female sex cells.

   sexual r. Reproduction by the union of male and female sex cells.

   somatic r. Reproduction by splitting or budding of cells other than sex cells.

Reptilia A class of cold-blooded, usually egglaying, vertebrates which includes snakes, lizards, turtles, and crocodiles.

repulsion 1. The act of repelling, or the condition of being repelled. 2. Extreme dislike.

reradiation Radiation emanating from a substance as a result of its absorbing radiation.

research Investigation or experimentation.

resect To cut off.

resectable Amenable to surgical removal; capable of being cut off.

resection The surgical removal of a portion of any part.

   transurethral r. of prostate (TURP) Removal of obstructive prostatic tissue with an instrument introduced through the urethra.

resectoscope An instrument for removing prostate gland tissue through the urethra.

reserpine An alkaloid, $C_{33}H_{40}N_2O_9$, isolated from the roots of certain species of *Rauwolfia*; used to reduce blood pressure in hypertension and as a tranquilizer.

reserve Something available, but stored for future use or a special purpose.

   cardiac r. The work which the heart is capable of performing beyond ordinary requirements.

reset To set again, as a broken bone.

resident An individual who is in graduate training to qualify as a specialist in a field of medicine or dentistry.

residual Relating to the quantity remaining or left behind at the end of a process; left over.

residue 1. Material remaining after the completion of an abstractive physical or chemical process. Also called residuum. 2. An amino acid unit in a polypeptide chain.

residuum 1. Residue. 2. That which remains after removal of a part.

   gastric r. The stomach contents during the interdigestive period.

   sporal r. The residual substance after sporulation.

resilience Elasticity.

resin 1. Any of various viscous substances of plant origin, such as amber and rosin, that are usually transparent or translucent; used in synthetic plastics, adhesives, and pharmaceuticals. 2. Any of various polymerized synthetics as polyethylene, epoxies, and silicones, that are used with other components to form plastics. 3. In dentistry, a plastic filling material having good esthetic appearance.

   acrylic r. A thermoplastic resinous material of the various esters of acrylic acid; the principal ingredient of many plastics used in dentistry.

   autopolymer r. A resin which can be polymerized by an activator and a catalyst rather than by the application of heat; it sets at room or body temper-

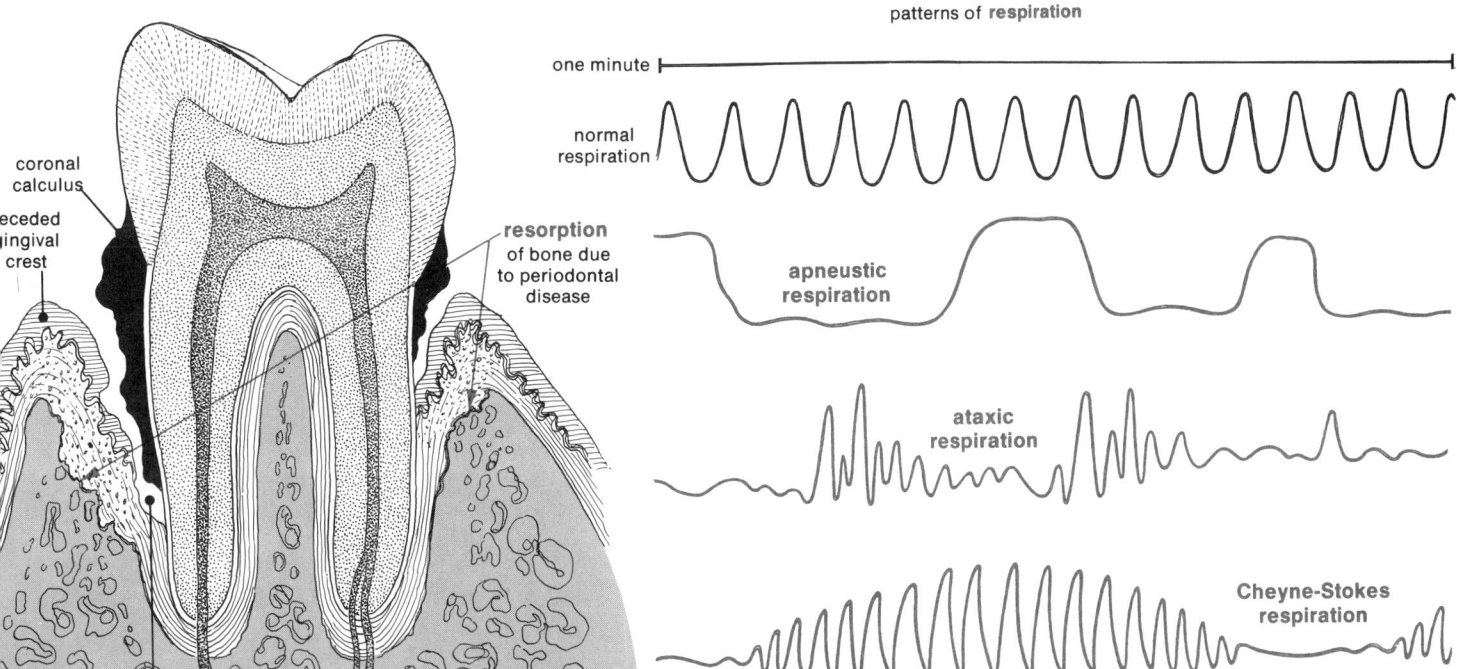

coronal calculus

receded gingival crest

resorption of bone due to periodontal disease

periodontal pocket

patterns of respiration

one minute

normal respiration

apneustic respiration

ataxic respiration

Cheyne-Stokes respiration

ature. Also called cold-curing, quick-curing, or self-curing resin.

cold-curing r. See autopolymer resin.

cholestyramine r. An insoluble chloride salt of a basic anion exchange resin that binds bile acids in the intestine and prevents their reabsorption; the reduced levels of bile acids increase the rate of conversion of cholesterol to bile acids in the liver; used in treatment of hyperlipoproteinemia; Cuemid®; Questran®.

dental r. A synthetic acrylic resin widely used in dentistry.

epoxy r. Any thermosetting resin that is a condensation polymer of epichlorohydrin and bisphenol and forms a tight cross-linked structure that exhibits strong adhesion and chemical resistance; used in surface coatings, adhesives, and as embedding medium for electron microscopy.

ion-exchange r. An insoluble, porous solid material of high molecular weight containing an active electrolyte; it contains either acidic groups (cation-active) or basic groups (anion-active); one type is used to lower the potassium content of the body in the treatment of hyperkalemia.

methyl methacrylate r. A stable, transparent resin of remarkable clarity that is liquid at room temperature and is polymerized by the use of a chemical initiator; widely used in medical and dental appliances.

podophyllum r. A bitter-tasting resin derived from the dried rhizome and root of the May apple (*Podophyllum peltatum*); used as a cathartic and topical caustic.

quick-curing r. See autopolymer resin.

quinine carbacrylic r. A quinine salt of a resin containing about 2% quininium ion; used in testing deficiency of acids in the gastric juice, especially of hydrochloric acid.

self-curing r. See autopolymer resin.

thermoplastic r. A synthetic resin that becomes soft when heated and hard when cooled.

resinous Relating to a resin.

resistance 1. Any force that opposes and/or retards motion. 2. (R) In electricity, the opposition to the passage of electric current. 3. In psychiatry, an individual's psychologic defense against recalling repressed or unpleasant experiences.

drug r. A state of decreased response to drugs that ordinarily inhibit cell growth or cause cell death.

expiratory r. Resistance in the air passages to the flow of air out of the lungs.

peripheral r. See total peripheral resistance.

total peripheral r. The sum of resistance to the flow of blood through the blood vessels; MAP/CO. Also called peripheral resistance.

resolution The termination of a morbid condition such as inflammation or the disappearance of a swelling.

visual r. The ability to perceive two separate adjacent objects as two.

resolve To return to normal after an inflammatory process.

resolvent 1. Causing or capable of causing resolution of a tumor or swelling. 2. Any substance that promotes the dissipation of a pathologic growth or reduces an inflammation. 3. Promoting the separation into constituents.

resonance 1. The sound heard on percussion. 2. In chemistry, the property of a substance whereby two or more structural forms of the substance are simultaneously present.

amphoric r. Sound resembling that produced by blowing over the mouth of an empty bottle.

electron spin r. (ESR) In spectrometry, resonance arising from electron spin, related to the extent of activity of free radicals in an organic reaction.

nuclear magnetic r. (NMR) A measure of the dipole moment of atomic nuclei (i.e., the ratio of the maximum torque applied to the nuclei in a magnetic field to the induction of the field); used in studies of covalent bonds involved in organic reactions; also used for diagnostic imaging. See also imaging.

tympanic r. Percussion sound heard over a hollow structure.

vesicular r. Sound heard on percussion of normal lungs.

vocal r. (VR) Voice sounds heard on auscultation of the chest.

resonator An apparatus designed to create an electric current of very high potential and small volume.

resorcinol A keratolytic compound, $C_6H_4(OH)_2$; in concentrations of 2 to 10%, it is used in treating acne by causing a mild irritation that produces some peeling.

resorption 1. Assimilation of excreted material. 2. Dissolution of tissue by physiologic or pathologic means, as of the gums or of the bones surrounding the teeth.

respirable Fit for breathing.

respiration (r) 1. The physical and chemical processes through which an organism acquires oxygen and releases carbon dioxide. 2. The act of breathing.

abdominal r. Respiration effected mainly by the abdominal muscles. Also called diaphragmatic respiration.

aerobic r. Respiration effected in the presence of air through the consumption of free oxygen.

anaerobic r. Respiration that is carried on in the absence, or near absence, of air, without involving free oxygen.

apneustic r. Breathing characterized by inspiratory spasms of varying duration, often lasting several seconds; seen in persons with lesions of the lower pons.

artificial r. The maintenance of respiratory movements through artificial means.

assisted r. In anesthesia, respiration in which the patient's own respiratory effort initiates the cycle but the volume of air is increased by mechanical means. Also called augmented respiration; assisted breathing.

ataxic r. Gasping, irregular (in rate and depth) breathing; seen in individuals with medullary lesions. Also called Biot's breathing.

Cheyne-Stokes r. A rhythmic increase and decrease in the depth of respiration.

controlled r. In anesthesiology, artificial respiration requiring no effort by the patient; each inspiration is initiated by a timing mechanism of the respirator. Also called controlled ventilation.

diffusion r. Introduction of oxygen into the lungs through a catheter. Also called apneic oxygenation.

external r. The interchange of gases in the lungs. Also called pulmonary respiration.

forced r. Voluntary increase in the rate and depth of breathing.

internal r. Tissue respiration.

Kussmaul r. Respiration marked by deep sighing; characteristic of diabetic acidosis.

mouth-to-mouth r. See under resuscitation.

tissue r. The exchange of gases between tissue cells and blood.

respirator 1. An apparatus used to administer artificial respiration. 2. A screenlike device fitted over the nose and mouth to protect the respiratory passages.

Drinker r. An airtight metal tank designed to enclose the body (except the head) and provide artificial respiration by exerting intermittent negative air pressure on the chest. Commonly known as iron lung.

pressure-controlled r. A respirator that supplies a predetermined pressure to gases during inhalation; the volume of gas delivered varies, depending upon resistance.

volume-controlled r. A respirator that supplies a predetermined volume of gases during inhalation; the pressure needed to move the gases varies, depending upon resistance.

respiratory Of or relating to respiration.

respiratory distress syndrome (RDS) of the newborn A disease of unknown cause characterized by acute difficulty in breathing, cyanosis, easy

orthodontic
retainer

matrix
band

matrix band **retainer**

pronormoblast

orthochromatic
normoblast

basophilic
normoblast

extrusion of
nucleus

reticulocyte

polychromatic
normoblast

erythrocyte

erythropoiesis

collapsibility of alveoli, and loss of pulmonary surfactant; seen most frequently in premature infants,
and those born of diabetic mothers or delivered by
cesarean section. Also called idiopathic respiratory
distress syndrome (IRDS) of the newborn; hyaline
membrane disease of the newborn.

respire   To breathe.

respirometer   Spirometer.

response   A reaction to a specific stimulus.

  autoimmune r.   An immune response in which
the action of an autoantibody is directed to a "self"
antigen; distinguished from autoimmune disease,
with which it may or may not be associated.

  evoked r.   A change in the electrical activity of
the nervous system resulting from an incoming sensory stimulus.

  galvanic skin r.   The change in skin resistance in
response to a stimulus.

  immune r.   A specific response resulting in immunity, which includes an afferent phase during
which responsive cells are primed by antigen, a
central response during which antibodies are
formed, and an efferent response in which immunity
is effected by antibodies.

  triple r.   The three degrees of reaction of the skin
to injury; i.e., a red line, a flare around the red line,
and a wheal surrounded by a flare.

rest   **1.** Repose. **2.** To cease temporarily from any
activity. **3.** A portion of displaced embryonic tissue
that becomes embedded in other structures. **4.** In
dentistry, an extension from a prosthesis that aids
in supporting a restoration.

  adrenal r.   An accessory adrenal gland.

restenosis   Recurrence of stenosis, especially of a
heart valve after corrective surgery of the primary
condition.

restiform   Shaped like a rope, as the ropelike restiform body (inferior peduncle) connecting the cerebellum to the medulla oblongata.

restitution, external rotation   In obstetrics, the
return of the rotated head of the fetus to its natural
relation with the shoulders after its complete emergence from the vulva.

restless legs syndrome   A feeling of creepiness,
twitching, and restlessness deep in the legs, usually
occurring in older individuals after lying down; the
cause is unknown.

restoration   **1.** The process of returning to a
healthy state. **2.** In dentistry, a prosthetic device or
appliance designed to replace lost teeth or oral tissues.

restorative   Tending to renew health.

restraint   In psychiatry, the act of controlling by
physical means an excited or violent patient.

resuscitate   To restore to life after apparent death.

resuscitation   The return to life or consciousness
of one who is apparently dead.

  cardiopulmonary r. (CPR)   Restoration of respiration and cardiac contraction by means of external
assistance (e.g., mouth-to-mouth breathing and external cardiac compression).

  mouth-to-mouth r.   Artificial respiration in which
the operator places his mouth over the patient's
mouth (and nose, if the patient is a small child) and
blows rhythmically at a rate of about 20 cycles per
minute.

resuscitator   An apparatus that forces gas, usually
oxygen, into the lungs to initiate respiration as in
asphyxia.

retainer   **1.** An appliance or device used to maintain teeth in the proper position after orthodontic
treatment. **2.** The part of a fixed denture (dental
bridge) which attaches the prosthesis to the abutment tooth; it may be an inlay, partial-veneer, or a
complete crown. **3.** Any form of device, such as a
clasp, used for the stabilization of a prosthesis.

  continuous bar r.   A metal bar placed in contact
with the lingual surfaces of teeth to aid in stabilizing
the teeth or in retaining a partial denture.

  direct r.   A clasp or attachment placed on a supporting tooth for the purpose of maintaining a removable appliance in position.

  indirect r.   An attachment of a removable partial
denture which assists the direct retainers in preventing displacement of free end denture bases.

retardate   A mentally retarded individual.

retardation   Slowing down of mental and physical
processes, seen in certain forms of severe depression.

  mental r.   Subnormal intellectual functioning,
originating during the individual's developmental
period, often associated with impairment of either
adjustment (social and learning) or maturation, or
both; an IQ score of 69 or below on a standardized
intelligence test.

rete, *pl.* **retia**   A network, as of nerve fibers or
minute blood vessels.

retention   **1.** The act of holding food and drink in
the stomach. **2.** The holding back of body wastes. **3.**
The ability to remember. **4.** Maintaining in position.

  denture r.   The means by which a denture is
maintained in proper position in the mouth.

  direct r.   Retention of a removable partial denture
by means of clasps attached to the anchoring teeth.

  indirect r.   Retention of a removable partial denture by means of an attachment used in conjunction
with a direct retainer.

retention lug   A metal attachment soldered either
to an orthodontic band or an artificial crown to
insure stabilization of a dental prosthesis.

reticular   Netlike; pertaining to a reticulum.

reticulin   A scleroprotein present in the connective
fibers of reticular or lymphatic tissues.

reticulocyte   The youngest red blood cell in the
circulating blood; when it is supravitally stained with
cresyl blue the scattered ribosomes clump together,
giving the cell a reticulated appearance; it constitutes
one percent of the red blood cell population in the
circulating blood.

reticulocytopenia   Diminution of reticulocytes in
the blood.

reticulocytosis   The abnormal increase in the percentage of reticulocytes in the blood.

reticuloendothelial   Relating to the reticuloendothelium, i.e., to tissues having both reticular and
endothelial properties.

reticuloendothelioma   A localized neoplasm derived from reticuloendothelial tissue; e.g., malignant
lymphoma.

reticuloendotheliosis   Abnormal conditions, especially hyperplasia, of the reticuloendothelium in
any of the organs or tissues.

reticuloendothelium   A widely dispersed bodily

preparation for mouth-to-mouth resuscitation

rescuer elevates victim's neck to clear base of tongue from throat and establish patent airway

then he pinches nostrils, grasps jaw with thumb in mouth and fingers under chin, and forcibly draws mandible forward

cardiopulmonary resuscitation (CPR)

heel of one hand is placed over lower half of sternum (3-finger breadth above xiphoid tip) and opposite hand is placed over it

cardiac compressions are performed at a rate of **60** per minute; rescuer breathes into victim's mouth only as pressure is released from sternum

air is puffed into victim to inflate chest (**12** cycles/minute); then rescuer allows victim to breathe out passively

after Netter

heart is intermittently compressed between sternum and vertebral column

depression of sternum (1.5 to 2 inches) compresses cardiac chambers, thus forcing blood into aorta and pulmonary artery; pressure is held for about ¹/₂ second and then released; release of pressure and return of sternum to normal position allows heart chambers to refill with blood

sternum

heart

lung

vertebra

aorta

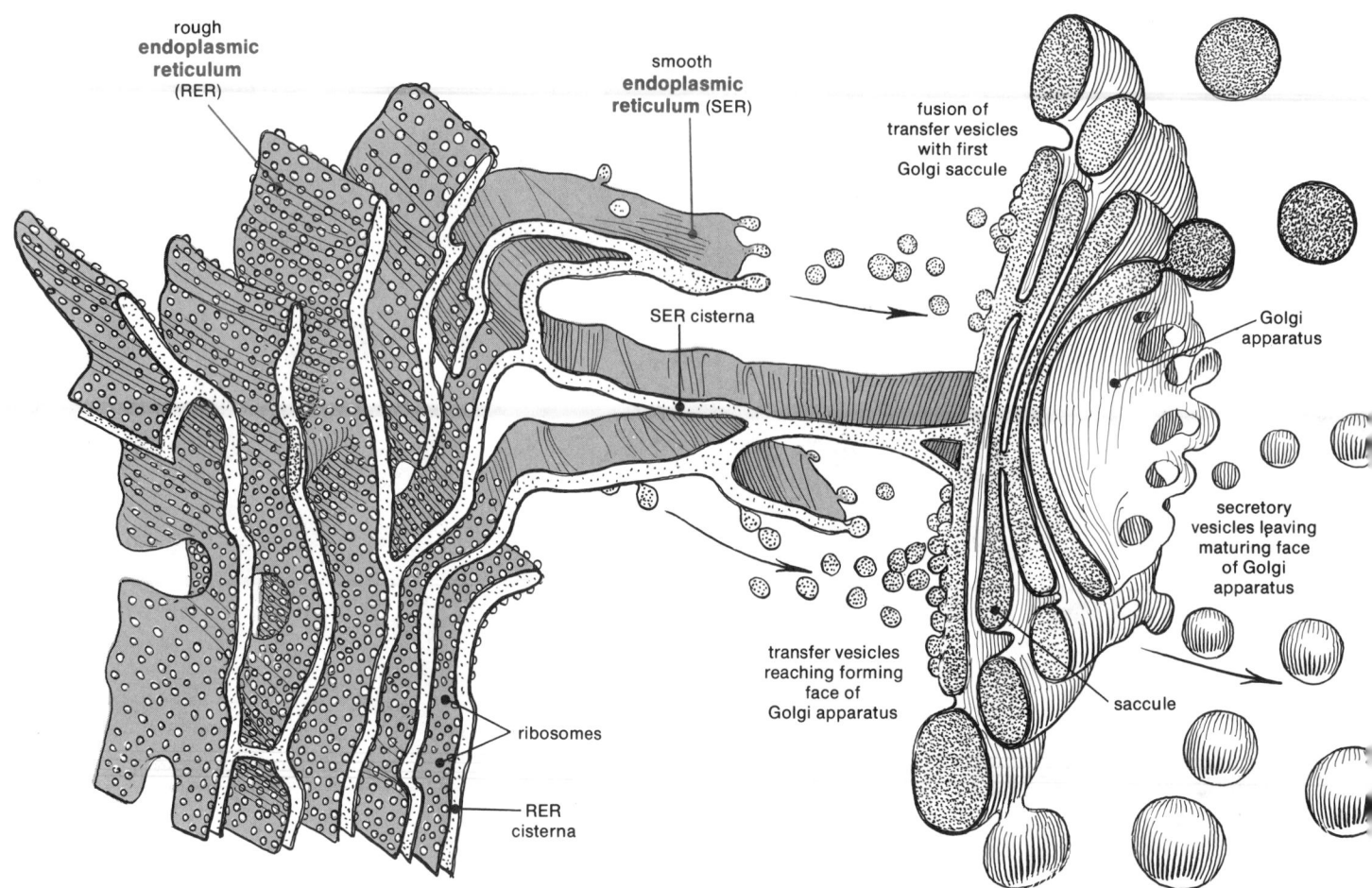

rough **endoplasmic reticulum** (RER)

smooth **endoplasmic reticulum** (SER)

fusion of transfer vesicles with first Golgi saccule

SER cisterna

Golgi apparatus

secretory vesicles leaving maturing face of Golgi apparatus

transfer vesicles reaching forming face of Golgi apparatus

saccule

ribosomes

RER cisterna

system of morphologically varied cells concerned with phagocytosis; present in the thymus, spleen, lymph nodes, etc.

reticulosis A brief term for reticuloendotheliosis.

reticulum A fine network, especially one formed of protoplasmic material within a cell.

endoplasmic r. (ER) An extensive network of fine parallel membranes interspersed throughout the cytoplasm of the cell; it is continuous with the outer portion of the nuclear membrane and with the Golgi apparatus. One possessing ribosomes on its cytoplasmic surface is known as granular or rough endoplasmic reticulum (RER); it receives synthesized material from the ribosomes and isolates it from the rest of the cytoplasm while channeling it to the Golgi apparatus for packaging; differentiated cells engaged in synthesis of protein contain an abundant amount of rough endoplasmic reticulum. One whose surface is free of ribosomes is known as agranular or smooth endoplasmic reticulum (SER); depending on the cell type in which it resides, it can play a role in detoxification of certain drugs, lipid and cholestrol metabolism, production of steroid hormones, etc.

retina The innermost of the three tunics of the eyeball, consisting of an outer pigmented layer and an inner nervous stratum or retina proper which, in turn, is composed of eight microscopic layers, named from within outward as follows: (a) nerve fiber layer, (b) ganglionic layer, (c) inner plexiform layer, (d) inner nuclear layer, (e) outer plexiform layer, (f) outer nuclear layer, (g) layer of rods and cones, (h) pigment layer.

retinaculum, *pl.* **retinacula** A retaining band-like ligament, as seen in the wrist and ankle.

retinal 1. Pertaining to the retina. 2. The aldehyde of retinol present in the visual pigments of the retina; one isomere (11-*cis*-retinal) occurs in rhodopsin in combination with the protein group opsin; another (all-*trans*-retinal) is the yellow pigment resulting from the bleaching of rhodopsin by light. Formerly called retinene; vitamin A₁ aldehyde.

retinene Former name for retinal.

retinitis Inflammation of the retina (the innermost layer of the eyeball).

r. pigmentosa Hereditary degeneration and atrophy of the retina, usually with migration of pigment, causing gradual reduction of peripheral vision; its first symptom, night blindness, is usually seen in children and adolescents.

retinoblastoma A congenital malignant tumor of the retina, composed of embryonic retinal cells; usually observed before the age of four.

retinochoroiditis See chorioretinitis.

retinoic acid Acid derived from oxidation of the alcohol group of retinol (vitamin A) to an aldehyde and carboxyl; used topically to treat acne.

retinoid 1. Resembling a resin. 2. Resembling the retina.

retinoids Compounds derived from retinoic acid; used to treat severe acne and psoriasis.

retinol A 20-carbon alcohol. Also called vitamin A₁.

retinomalacia Degeneration of the retina.

retinopapillitis See papilloretinitis.

retinopathy Any degenerative noninflammatory disease of the retina.

arteriosclerotic r. Changes in the fundus of the eye associated with arteriosclerosis and benign hypertension; vessels show variations in caliber, increased tortuosity, and compression of veins at arteriovenous crossings.

diabetic r. Progressive disease of the blood vessels in the retina, occurring as a complication of diabetes; it may lead to severe visual disability.

hypertensive r. Disease of the blood vessels in the retina occurring as a complication of hypertension; the initial change is narrowing of the arterioles caused by spasm; in later stages hemorrhages and exudates are seen; papilledema may appear in extreme cases associated with hypertensive encephalopathy.

macular r. See maculopathy.

retinopiesis The pressing of a detached retina back into its normal position, as by air, intravitreal silicone, saline, etc.

retinoscope An optical instrument for examining the refractive state of the eye.

retinoscopy Ophthalmologic examination with a

retinoscope to determine the objective measurements of the refractive properties of the eyes. Also called shadow test; skiametry; skiascopy.

retort A closed, long-necked laboratory vessel resembling a flask; used in distillation.

retract 1. To shrink back. 2. To pull back.

retractile Capable of being drawn back.

retraction 1. Drawing back. 2. A shrinking.

gingival r. Retraction of the gums from the tooth surface due to an underlying inflammation.

retractor A surgical instrument used to draw apart the edges of a wound.

retrobulbar 1. Located behind the eyeball. 2. Located posterior to the medulla oblongata.

retrocecal Situated behind or posterior to the cecum.

retrocervical Located behind the uterine cervix.

retrocolic Behind the colon.

retrodisplacement Backward displacement of an organ.

retroflexion The backward bending of an organ.

r. of uterus The backward bending of the body of the uterus while the cervix remains in its normal position.

retrognathia Condition characterized by a retruded position of the lower jaw without diminution of its size.

retrograde Moving backward; retracing original course.

retrogression 1. A return to an earlier or more primitive condition. 2. Degeneration, especially of tissues.

retroillumination The technique of examining transparent or semitransparent tissues, as the cornea, by reflecting light from posteriorly located tissues.

retrolental Located behind the lens of the eye.

retromandibular Located behind the lower jaw.

retroperitoneal Located behind the peritoneum.

retroperitoneum The retroperitoneal space between the parietal peritoneum and the posterior bodily wall.

retropharyngeal Located behind the pharynx.

retroplasia The state of decreased or retrogressive activity in a tissue.

histologic layers of the **retina**

layer of
optic nerve
fibers

yer of
lion cells

r plexiform
layer

r nuclear
layer

plexiform
layer

nuclear
ayer

of rods
cones

ment
yer

macula lutea

retinaculum

**retroflexion
of uterus**

bladder

posterior
surface
of the
body

adrenal
gland
(retroperitoneal)

peritoneum

kidney
(retroperitoneal)

Richardson abdominal **retractor**

Shuman dental **retractor**

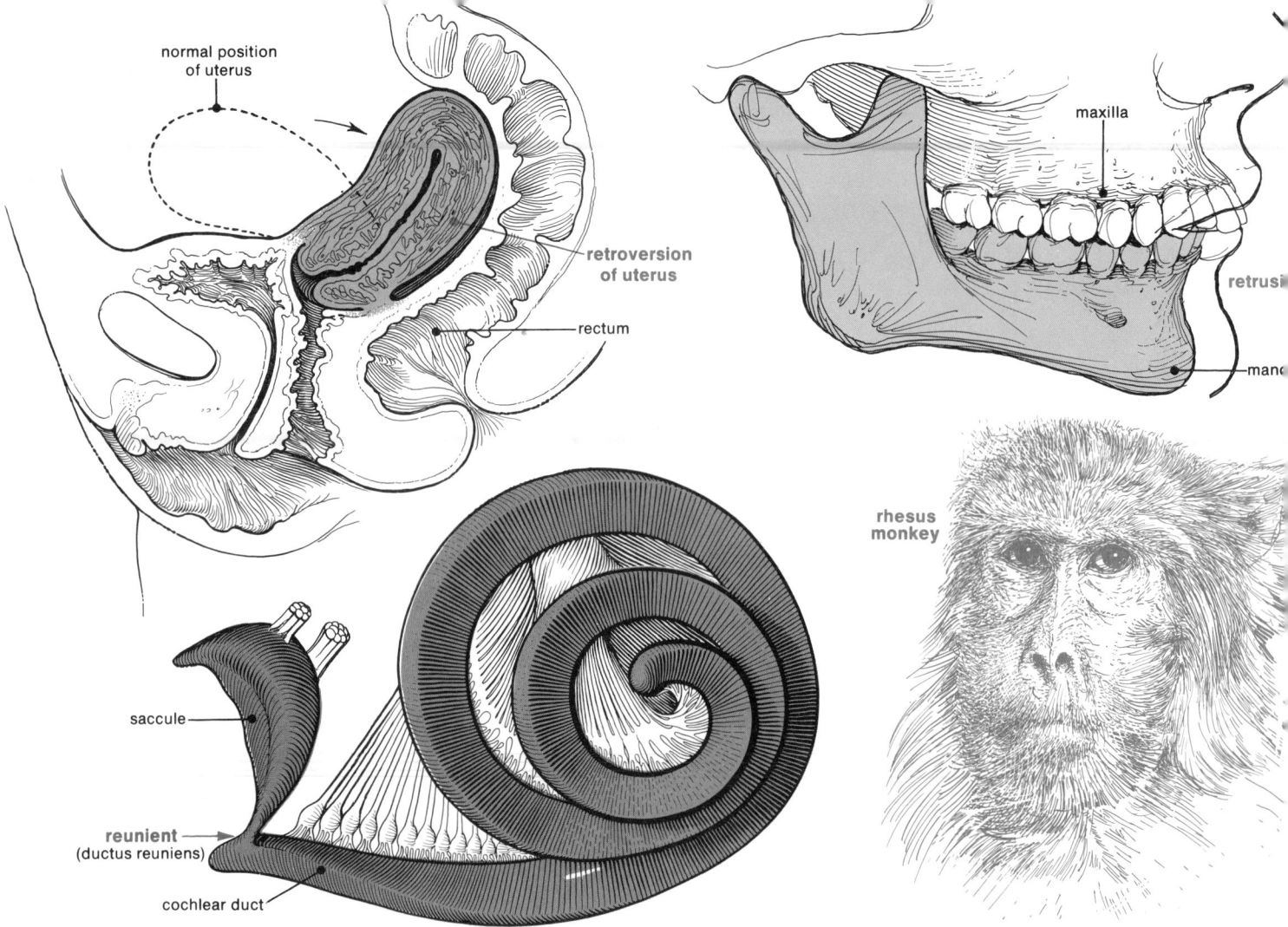

normal position of uterus

retroversion of uterus

rectum

maxilla

retrus...

man...

rhesus monkey

saccule

reunient (ductus reuniens)

cochlear duct

retroposition Backward displacement of an organ without retroflexion or retroversion.

retropulsion An involuntary walking or falling backward.

retrospondylolisthesis Posterior displacement of a vertebra, bringing it out of alignment with the other vertebrae.

retrosternal Situated behind the sternum (breastbone).

retrouterine Situated behind the uterus.

retroversion The backward tilting of an entire organ.

  r. of uterus The leaning backward of the uterus with the cervix pointing forward.

retroverted Inclined backward.

Retroviridae Family of viruses (100 nm in diameter) that have RNA-dependent DNA polymerases (reverse transcriptases); included are the tumor viruses. Also called RNA tumor viruses.

retrovirus Any virus of the family Retroviridae. Retroviruses are named for their ability to convert RNA into DNA and thus use genetic material of the cells they infect to make the proteins they need to survive, causing several diseases in the process. Retroviruses include the cancer-causing virus HTLV (human T-cell leukemia/lymphoma virus) and HIV (human immunodeficiency virus), the cause of AIDS (acquired immune deficiency syndrome); these viruses have a tropism for T4 (helper) lymphocytes and contain a Mg++ dependent reverse transcriptase.

retrusion The backward displacement of the lower jaw.

reunient Connecting; denoting the ductus reuniens which connects the saccule to the cochlear duct in the internal ear.

revascularization The reestablishment of blood supply to a part of the body by blood vessel grafting, or by development of collateral channels.

reversal A turning in the opposite direction.

  sex r. The apparent change to the opposite sex, as in certain pseudohermaphroditic individuals.

reversible Capable of returning to the original form or state.

reversion 1. Reverse mutation; the restoration in a mutant gene of its ability to produce a functional protein. 2. The appearance in an individual of a characteristic that has been absent for several generations.

Reye's syndrome An acute and frequently fatal childhood syndrome marked by encephalopathy, hepatitis, and fatty accumulations in the viscera; usually starts as a mild illness with respiratory and gastrointestinal symptoms of a few days' duration, terminating in rapid brain swelling, hepatomegaly, convulsions, and coma.

Rhabditis A genus of small phasmid nematode worms; some are parasitic in man.

rhabdoid Rod-shaped.

rhabdomyolysis An acute, fulminating, potentially fatal disease of skeletal muscle, characterized by disintegration of skeletal muscle accompanied by excretion of myoglobulin in the urine. Also called paroxysmal idiopathic myoglobulinuria.

rhabdomyoma A benign tumor or neoplasm of striated muscle elements.

rhabdomyosarcoma A malignant tumor derived from skeletal muscle.

Rhabdoviridae Family of relatively large bullet-shaped or rod-shaped viruses that contain single-stranded RNA and replicate in cytoplasm; includes viruses causing rabies. Also called bullet-shaped virus group.

rhagades Cracks or fissures in the skin, especially around bodily openings; seen in congenital syphilis and in vitamin deficiencies.

rhagadiform Denoting the shape of a fissure.

rhe The absolute unit of fluidity; the reciprocal of the unit of viscosity.

rhenium A rare, silvery-white metallic element with a melting point exceeded only by tungsten and carbon; symbol Re, atomic number 75, atomic weight 186.2.

rheobase The minimal strength of an electric stimulus required to excite a tissue if allowed to flow through it for an adequate time.

rheoencephalography The measurement of blood flow in the brain.

rheology The study of the deformation and flow of liquids and semisolids; e.g., the flow of blood through the heart.

rheometer 1. A device for measuring the velocity of viscous liquids, such as blood. 2. A galvanometer.

rheometry The measurement of blood flow.

rheostat An appliance for regulating the current entering an electric circuit; it basically consists of a continuously variable electrical resistor.

rheotaxis The movement of an organism in response to the direction of fluid flow.

  negative r. Rheotaxis in which the organism moves in the same direction as that of fluid flow.

  positive r. Rheotaxis in which the organism moves in the opposite direction from that of fluid flow.

rhesus monkey A light brownish monkey, *Macaca mulata*, of India and China; used in medical research.

rheum Any watery discharge from the nose or eyes.

rheumatic Relating to or afflicted with rheumatism.

rheumatic heart disease (RHD) A manifestation of rheumatic fever consisting of inflammatory changes (carditis) and/or damaged heart valves.

rheumatid An eruption sometimes accompanying rheumatism.

rheumatism A general term applied to various diseases that cause pain in the muscles, joints, and fibrous tissues.

rheumatoid 1. Resembling rheumatism. 2. Associated with rheumatoid arthritis.

rheumatology The study of the diagnosis and treatment of rheumatic conditions.

rhexis The rupture of a vessel or an organ.

rhinal Relating to the nose.

rhinalgia Pain in the nose.

rhinedema Edema or swelling of the nasal mucous membrane.

rhinencephalon The region of the forebrain involved with the function of olfaction (smell), con-

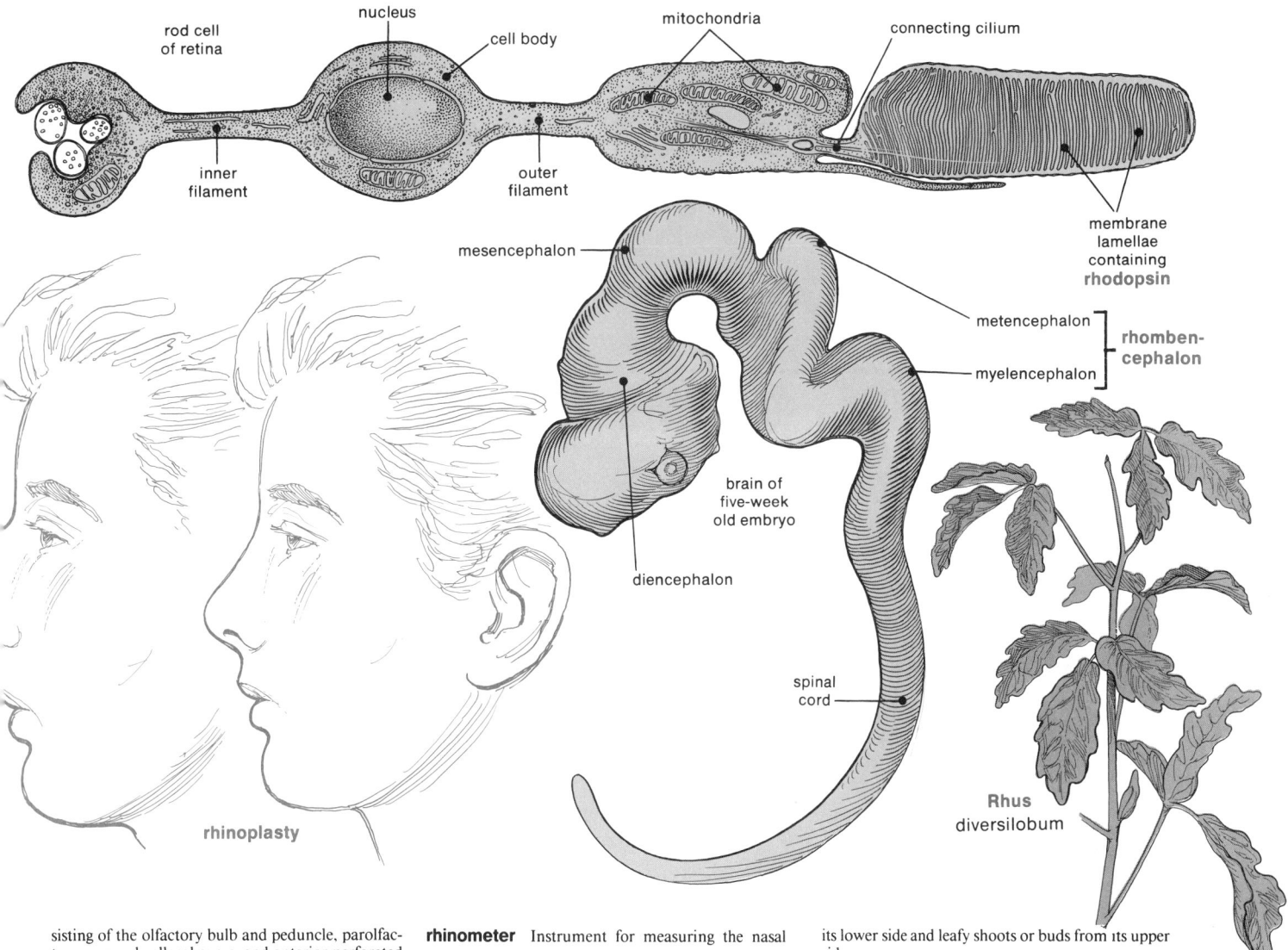

rod cell of retina · nucleus · cell body · mitochondria · connecting cilium · inner filament · outer filament · membrane lamellae containing **rhodopsin** · mesencephalon · metencephalon · myelencephalon · **rhomben-cephalon** · brain of five-week old embryo · diencephalon · spinal cord · **rhinoplasty** · **Rhus diversilobum**

sisting of the olfactory bulb and peduncle, parolfactory area, subcallosal gyrus, and anterior perforated substance.

rhineurynter A dilatable bag that is inflated after insertion into a nostril to arrest a profuse nosebleed (epistaxis).

rhinion A craniometric point; the lower end of the suture between the nasal bones.

rhinitis Inflammation of the mucous membrane of the nose accompanied by excessive mucus discharge.

acute r. Self-limiting rhinitis accompanied by headache, general malaise and, frequently, fever; caused by a rhinovirus. Also called head cold.

allergic r. Pale boggy swelling of nasal mucosa associated with sneezing and watery discharge due to hypersensitivity to foreign substances such as pollens, dust, etc.

atrophic r. Chronic rhinitis causing thinning of the mucous membrane; often associated with crusts and foul-smelling discharge.

hypertrophic r. Chronic rhinitis causing permanent thickening of the mucous membrane.

vasomotor r. Rhinitis without infection.

rhinoantritis Inflammation of the mucous membrane of the nasal cavity and maxillary sinuses.

rhinocanthectomy Surgical incision of the inner canthus of the eye. Also called rhinommectomy.

rhinochiloplasty Reparative surgery of the nose and lip.

rhinocleisis Nasal passageway obstruction.

rhinodacryolith A concretion in the nasolacrimal duct.

rhinogenous Originating in the nose.

rhinokyphosis A deformity of the nose characterized by an abnormal hump in the ridge.

rhinolalia Nasal speech due to disease or defect of the nasal passages.

rhinolith A stone in the nasal cavity formed in layers, usually around a foreign body.

rhinolithiasis The presence of calculi in the nose.

rhinology The study of the nose and its diseases.

rhinomanometer Instrument for determining the amount of nasal obstruction.

rhinometer Instrument for measuring the nasal passages.

rhinomycosis Fungus infection of the mucous membrane of the nose.

rhinopathy Disease of the nose.

rhinopharyngitis Inflammation of the mucous membrane of the nasopharynx.

r. mutilans See gangosa.

rhinopharynx See nasopharynx.

rhinophyma Acne rosacea of the nose, causing the skin to become coarsened, purplish, and thickened with nodulation and pitted scars.

rhinoplasty 1. Plastic surgery of the nose. 2. Surgical reconstruction of the nose with tissue taken from another site.

rhinorrhagia Nosebleed.

rhinorrhaphy Operation for the relief of epicanthus, in which a piece of skin is removed from the bridge of the nose and the edges of the wound are sutured together.

rhinorrhea A profuse, watery nasal discharge.

rhinosalpingitis Inflammation of the nasal mucosa and the lining of the auditory (eustachian) tube.

rhinoscleroma Chronic disease involving the nose and upper respiratory tract, marked by the formation of hard nodules, sometimes leading to deformity.

rhinoscope An instrument for inspection of the nasal cavity; a speculum. Also called nasoscope.

rhinoscopy Visual examination of the nasal cavity with a rhinoscope.

median r. Inspection of the nasal cavity and the openings of the ethmoid cells and sphenoidal sinus with a long nasal speculum.

rhinostenosis Abnormal narrowing of the nasal passage; nasal obstruction.

rhinotomy Operative incision of the nose.

Rhinovirus Genus of viruses (family Picornaviridae) that includes those causing the common cold in humans and foot-and-mouth disease in cattle; over 100 antigenic types have been identified.

rhizome A horizontal rootlike stem, growing under or along the ground, which gives off roots from

its lower side and leafy shoots or buds from its upper side.

rhizomeningomyelitis Inflammation of the nerve roots, the meninges, and the spinal cord. Also called radiculomeningomyelitis.

rhizoplast A fine fibril connecting the flagellum to the nucleus of certain flagellate organisms.

Rhizopoda A subclass of protozoa of the class Sarcodina, characterized by having rootlike pseudopodia.

rhizotomy Surgical division of a posterior spinal nerve root for the relief of pain. Also called radicotomy; radiculotomy.

rhodium A hard metallic element of the platinum group; symbol Rh, atomic number 45, atomic weight 102.91.

rhodopsin A purplish red, light-sensitive pigment found in the membrane of the outer segments of the rod-shaped photoreceptor cells of the retina; composed of a vitamin A derivative (11-*cis*-retinal) and a protein group (opsin); when light is absorbed by rhodopsin, it is transformed and separated into all-*trans*-retinal and opsin, but regenerates in the dark (the all-*trans*-retinal reverts back to 11-*cis*-retinal, which combines with opsin to form rhodopsin); this unique property makes possible the transformation of light energy into visual perception. Also called visual purple.

rhombencephalon The embryonic hindbrain; the third cephalic dilatation of the neural tube which divides into the metencephalon (anterior portion), which later forms the pons and cerebellum, and the myelencephalon (posterior portion), which develops into the medulla oblongata.

rhombocele The terminal expansion of the central canal of the spinal cord in the lumbar region. Also called rhomboidal sinus.

rhomboid Resembling a rhomb or parallelogram with unequal adjacent sides; somewhat kite-shaped.

rhonchus, *pl.* rhonchi A loud rale or snoring sound produced in the bronchial tubes or the trachea. Also called coarse rale.

Rhus A genus of plants (family Anacardiaceae),

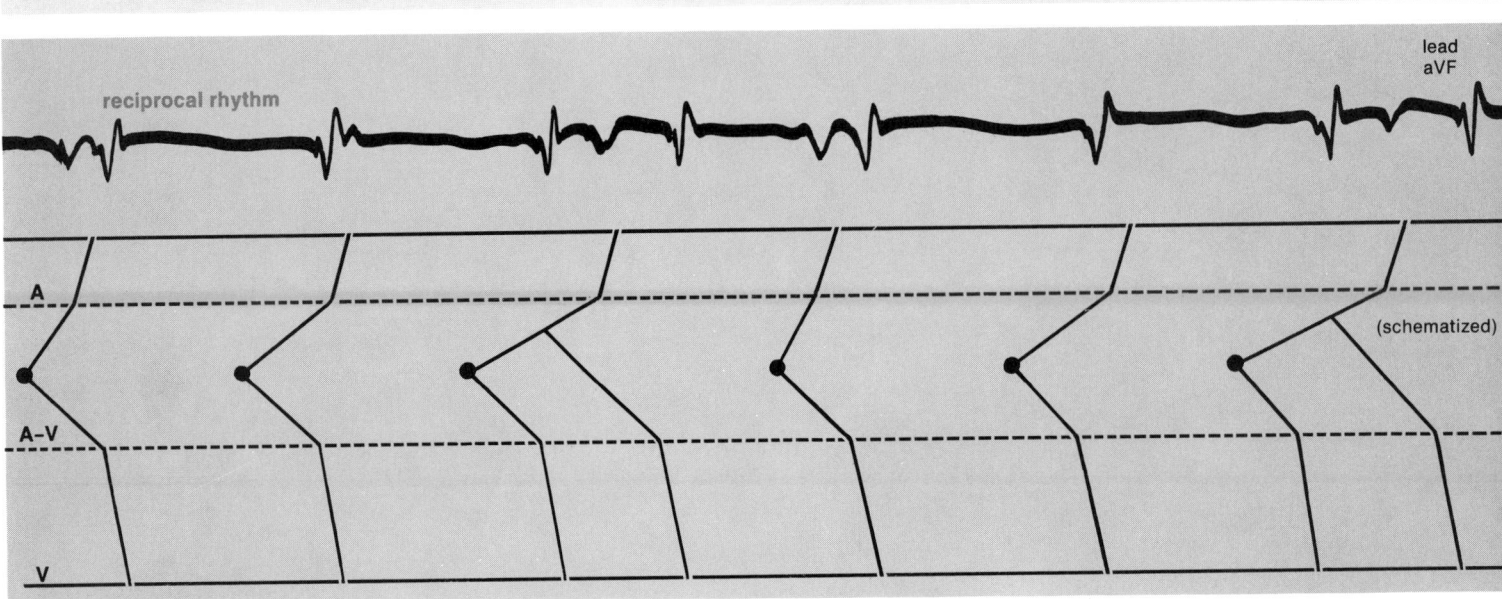

agonal rhythm

reciprocal rhythm

lead aVF

(schematized)

A

A-V

V

various species of which produce pruritic skin lesions on contact; the irritating ingredient is urushiol, a catechol contained in the sap.

R. diversiloba See poison oak.

R. radicans See poison ivy (1).

R. vernix See poison sumac.

rhythm The pattern of recurrence of a biologic cycle; e.g., the heart beat and sexual cycle.

agonal r. A rhythm appearing in the electrocardiogram as wide distorted ventricular complexes, often seen in dying patients.

alpha (α) r. See wave, alpha.

A-V nodal r. A heart rhythm originating in the atrioventricular (A-V) node; resulting from anything that suppresses sinus node activity, or from anything that enhances A-V node automaticity. Also called nodal rhythm and junctional rhythm.

beta (β) r. See wave, beta.

bigeminal r. Heart rhythm in which every beat is followed by a weak premature beat and then a pause, so that the beats appear coupled. Also called coupling.

cantering r. See gallop.

circus r. See movement, circus.

coronary nodal r. Term, not uniformly accepted, for rhythm appearing in the electrocardiogram with normal upright P waves in leads I and II with a short P-R interval. Occasionally called short P-R interval.

coronary sinus r. A heart rhythm appearing in the electrocardiogram with inverted P waves in inferior leads with a normal P-R interval; thought to originate in the coronary sinus.

delta (δ) r. See wave, delta (1).

ectopic r. Heart rhythm originating from any focus other than the sinus node.

gallop r. See gallop.

idionodal r. A slow independent heart rhythm arising in the atrioventricular (A-V) junction and controlling only the ventricles.

idioventricular r. A slow independent heart rhythm arising in an ectopic center in the ventricles and controlling only the ventricles.

junctional r. See A-V nodal rhythm.

nodal r. See A-V nodal rhythm.

quadruple r. A quadruple cadence of the heart sounds, not heard in normal hearts.

reciprocal r. Phenomenon in which the impulse arises in the A-V junction and travels both downward to the ventricles and upward to the atria; before reaching the atria, it is reflected and descends to reactivate the ventricles. Also called reciprocal beating.

reciprocating r. A variation of the reciprocal rhythm in which the impulse circulates around the A-V junction and gives off two daughter impulses,

one to the atria and one to the ventricles.

sinus r. The normal heart rhythm originating in the sinoatrial node.

theta (θ) r. See wave, theta.

trigeminal r. One in which the heart beats are grouped in three; either two premature beats follow each normal beat, or two normal beats are followed by a premature beat. Also called trigeminy.

triple r. A triple cadence to the heart sounds, generally caused by the presence of a third (diastolic) or fourth (presystolic) heart sound or gallop in addition to the usual first and second heart sounds.

rhythm method See under method.

rhytidectomy See rhytidoplasty.

rhytidoplasty A face lift; surgical elimination of wrinkles from the face; the excess skin is removed so that the remaining skin may be tightened, thus smoothing out the wrinkles. Also called rhytidectomy.

rhytidosis 1. Premature wrinkling of the face. 2. Wrinkling of the cornea.

rib One of a series of long, thin, rather elastic, curved bones which articulates posteriorly with a thoracic vertebra and extends anteriorly toward the sternum; normally there are 12 on each side.

cervical r. An extra rib similar to, but independent of, the first dorsal rib; usually attached to the seventh cervical vertebra.

false r. One of the five lower pairs of ribs that is not directly connected anteriorly, through the costal cartilage, to the sternum. Also called vertebrochondral rib.

floating r. One of the two lower pairs of false ribs that is free at the anterior end. Also called vertebral rib.

true r. One of the seven upper pairs of ribs that is connected anteriorly, through the costal cartilage, to the sternum.

riboflavin A yellow, crystalline pigment present in milk, egg yolk, and fresh meat, and produced synthetically; it acts as coenzyme for hydrogen transfer in reactions catalyzed by flavoproteins. Also called vitamin B₂. Formerly called vitamin G.

ribonuclease (RNase, RNAase) An enzyme responsible for the breakdown of ribonucleic acid.

ribonucleic acid (RNA) Any of a family of polynucleotides, component of all living cells, especially the cytoplasm and nucleolus, that are characterized by their constituent sugar (d-ribose) and single stranded molecules.

messenger RNA (mRNA) An RNA fraction with a base ratio that corresponds to the DNA of the same organism; it carries information from DNA to the protein-forming areas of the cell. Also called template RNA.

ribosomal RNA (rRNA) The RNA ribosomes and polysomes.

soluble RNA (sRNA) Transfer RNA.

template RNA See messenger RNA.

transfer RNA (tRNA) An RNA molecule that transfers an amino acid to a growing polypeptide chain; the smallest biologically active nucleic acid known, present in cells in at least 20 varieties. Also called soluble RNA.

ribonucleoprotein (RNP) A complex macromolecule containing ribonucleic acid (RNA) and protein.

ribonucleoside A nucleoside in which the sugar component is ribose; e.g., adenosine, cytidine, guanosine, and uridine.

ribonucleotide A compound consisting of a purine or pyrimidine base bonded to the sugar component ribose, which in turn is esterified with a phosphate group; the most common ribonucleotides are adenylic, guanylic, cytidylic, and uridylic acids.

ribose A five-carbon sugar present in ribonucleic acid (RNA); an aldopentose.

riboside A glycoside that, on hydrolysis, yields ribose.

ribosome One of the minute granules free in the cytoplasm or attached to the endoplasmic reticulum of a cell, containing a high concentration of RNA; it plays an important role in protein synthesis, ranges in size from 100 to 150 Å in diameter, and is assembled from two subunits produced in the nucleolus. Also called microsome.

ribosuria Excessive excretion of ribose in the urine; seen in muscular dystrophy.

ribosyl The radical formed from ribose, C₅H₉O₄.

riboviruses RNA viruses; see under virus.

rib-spreader A surgical instrument for widening and maintaining space between ribs, facilitating intrathoracic operations.

ricin A highly toxic protein occurring in the castor-oil bean; used as a biochemical reagent.

rickets A disease of infants and young children caused by deficiency of vitamin D, resulting in defective bone growth. Also called rachitis.

renal r. A form of rickets occurring in children due to chronic disease of the kidneys.

vitamin D-resistant r. A severe form of rickets that is not relieved by the administration of vitamin D; it is caused by a congenital defect of the kidneys; the disease is seen most frequently in males.

Rickettsia A genus of gram-negative, pathogenic, intracellular parasitic bacteria that are transmitted to humans through the bites of infected fleas, ticks, mites, and lice.

R. akari A species that is the causative agent of rickettsialpox; transmitted to humans by a mite that

riboflavin

two common **ribonucleosides**

ribose component

adenosine

cytidine

sternum

clavicle

scapula

true ribs

false ribs

floating ribs

costal cartilages

rough endoplastic reticulum

ribose

ribosome

small subunit

large subunit

ribosomes

molar

triangular
ridge

marginal
ridge

lymphoid
ring

ringworm

tracheal
rings

cross section
of
tracheal ring

infests mice.

R. mooseri   A species that is the causative agent of murine (endemic or flea-borne) typhus; transmitted to man by the rat flea. Also called *Rickettsia typhi*.

R. prowazekii   Species causing epidemic typhus and Brill-Zinsser disease (carrier or latent type of typhus); transmitted by lice.

R. rickettsii   A species which is the causative agent of Rocky Mountain spotted fever; transmitted through the bites of infected ticks.

R. tsutsugamushi   Species causing tsutsugamushi disease (scrub typhus); transmitted by mites.

R. typhi   See *Rickettsia mooseri*.

rickettsialpox   An acute, mite-borne disease of several days' duration, characterized by an initial cutaneous lesion followed by a rash, fever, backache, and headache; caused by *Rickettsia akari*.

rickettsiosis   Any disease due to a species of *Rickettsia*, such as Rocky Mountain spotted fever, epidemic typhus, endemic typhus, scrub typhus, rickettsialpox, and Q fever.

ridge   A linear elevation or projection on a bone or a tooth.

alveolar r.   The bony ridge of the jaw that contains the sockets (alveoli) in which the roots of the teeth are held.

dental r.   Any linear elevation on the surface of a tooth forming the border of a cusp or the margin of a crown.

incisal r.   The cutting portion of the crown of an anterior tooth.

labial r.   One of three smooth, vertical ridges on the labial surface of an anterior tooth.

lateral supracondylar r.   A curved ridge on the lateral surface of the humerus to which two of the dorsal muscles of the forearm attach.

lingual r.   A vertical ridge extending from the cingulum on the lingual surface of an anterior tooth; on the cuspid it may be confluent with the cusp tip.

marginal r.   The rounded border of the enamel of a tooth that forms the proximal margin of the occlusal surface of an anterior tooth.

medial supracondylar r.   A curved ridge on the medial surface of the humerus to which two of the muscles of the arm attach.

oblique r.   A variable ridge, formed by the union of two triangular ridges, which crosses obliquely the occlusal surface of a maxillary molar.

palatine r.   One of four or six transverse ridges on the anterior portion of the hard palate.

Passavant's r.   The prominence formed in the posterior wall of the pharynx by the contraction of the superior constrictor muscle during the act of swallowing. Also called Passavant's bar or cushion.

supraorbital r.   The curved elevation of the frontal bone forming the upper border of the orbit.

transverse r.   A ridge, formed by the union of two triangular ridges, which crosses transversely the occlusal surface of a posterior tooth.

triangular r.   The ridge that runs from the tip of the cusp toward the central part of the occlusal surface of a posterior tooth.

rigidity   **1.** Stiffness; immobility; the quality of being rigid or inflexible. **2.** In psychiatry, an individual's excessive resistance to change.

anatomic r.   Rigidity of the uterine cervix in labor without any pathologic infiltration.

cerebellar r.   Stiffness of the body and limbs due to an injury or lesion of the veins of the cerebellum.

clasp-knife r.   See spasticity, clasp-knife.

cogwheel r.   Rigidity of a muscle which, when passively stretched, gives way to a series of small jerks, as seen in Parkinson's disease.

decerebrate r.   Rigid extension of the extremities of an experimental animal following transsection of the brain between the red nucleus and the vestibular nuclei; lesions of the upper part of the brain stem produces similar effects in humans.

lead-pipe r.   The diffuse tonic contraction of muscles as seen in paralysis agitans.

mydriatic r.   A tonic pupil, usually large, that responds very slowly, if at all, to light and accommodation.

pathologic r.   Rigidity of the uterine cervix in labor, due to fibrosis, cancer, or other diseases.

postmortem r.   Rigor mortis.

rigor   **1.** Rigidity; stiffness. **2.** A chill.

r. mortis   Stiffness of the body occurring from one to seven hours after death and lasting from one to six days; caused by coagulation of the muscle plasma.

Riley-Day syndrome   Familial dysautonomia; see under dysautonomia.

rim   The outer edge, border, or margin, generally circular in form.

bite r.   See occlusion rim.

occlusion r.   Occluding surface built on denture bases for recording maxillomandibular relation and for arranging teeth. Also called record or bite rim.

record r.   See occlusion rim.

rima   A slit or elongated opening.

r. glottidis   The opening between the true vocal cords.

r. oris   The longitudinal aperture of the mouth.

r. palpebrarum   The slit between the lids of the closed eye.

ring   **1.** A circular or oval object with a vacant center. **2.** In anatomy, any circular band surrounding an opening. **3.** In chemistry, a group of atoms bound in a manner graphically representable as a circle.

benzene r.   The hexagonal ring arrangement of carbon and hydrogen atoms in the benzene molecule. Also called benzene nucleus.

casting r.   A metal ring or tube in which a mold is made for casting metal tooth restorations or dental appliances. Also called refractory flask.

inguinal r.   One of two (superficial or subcutaneous and deep or abdominal) openings of the inguinal canal through which pass the spermatic cord in males or round ligament in females. See also anulus inguinalis profundus and superficialis.

Kayser-Fleischer r.   A brownish pigmented ring, about one to three millimeters wide, in the periphery of the cornea; seen in Wilson's disease.

lower esophageal r.   Annular fibrous narrowing of the esophagus occurring 1 to 4 cm above the hiatus (diaphragmatic opening); may be asymptomatic or may cause attacks of difficult swallowing precipitated by hasty swallowing of improperly chewed solid foods; may also be asymptomatic. Also called Schatzki's ring.

lymphoid r.   A mass of lymphoid tissue, encircling the entrance to the pharynx, that includes the palatine, pharyngeal, and lingual tonsils and the small lymph follicles on the posterior oropharyngeal wall. Also called Waldeyer's ring.

signet r.   An early trophozoite of the malaria parasite (plasmodium), appearing as a small hyaline disc with a nucleus on one side.

teething r.   A ring, usually of hard rubber or plastic, designed for a teething baby to bite on.

tonsillar r.   Lymphoid ring.

tracheal r.   One of the cartilages forming the trachea. Also called tracheal cartilage.

umbilical r.   The opening in the linea alba of the fetus through which the umbilical vessels pass.

Waldeyer's r.   See lymphoid ring.

ringworm   A superficial infectious condition of the skin marked primarily by ring-shaped or oval itchy lesions; caused by any of a number of fungi, chiefly of the genera *Trichophyton*, *Microsporum*, and *Epidermophyton*.

risk   The possibility of harm. Also called hazard.

ristocetin   Antibiotic produced by *Nocardia lurida*; used against staphylococcic and enterococcic infections.

risus   A laugh.

r. caninus, r. sardonicus   A peculiar grin caused by spasm of the facial muscles, occurring in tetanus. Also called sardonic grin.

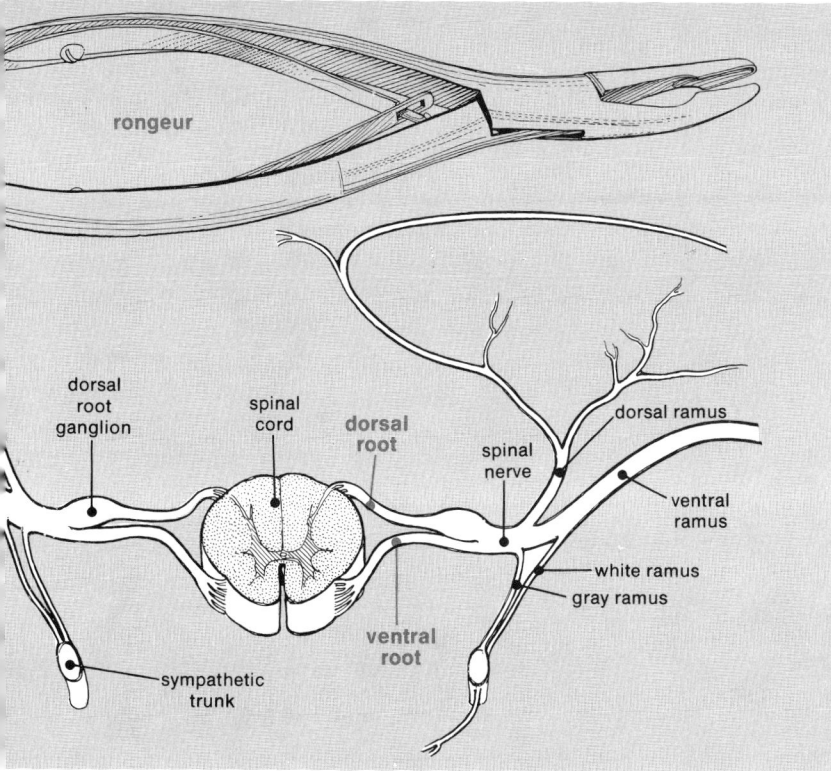

rongeur

dorsal root ganglion · spinal cord · **dorsal root** · dorsal ramus · spinal nerve · ventral ramus · white ramus · gray ramus · **ventral root** · sympathetic trunk

MANDIBULAR TEETH	LENGTH OF ROOT OF TOOTH	LENGTH OF CROWN OF TOOTH
central incisor	12.5 mm	9.0 mm
lateral incisor	13.0 mm	9.5 mm
cuspid	16.0 mm	11.0 mm
first bicuspid	14.0 mm	8.5 mm
second bicuspid	14.5 mm	8.5 mm
first molar	14.0 mm	6.0 mm
second molar	13.0 mm	7.5 mm
third molar	11.5 mm	7.0 mm
MAXILLARY TEETH		
central incisor	13.0 mm	10.5 mm
lateral incisor	12.0 mm	9.0 mm
cuspid	17.0 mm	10.0 mm
first bicuspid	14.0 mm	8.5 mm
second bicuspid	14.0 mm	8.5 mm
first molar	12.5 mm	7.5 mm
second molar	11.5 mm	7.0 mm
third molar	10.5 mm	6.5 mm

Ritter's disease See dermatitis exfoliativa infantum.

ritual In psychiatry, any psychomotor behavior or activity performed compulsively and repeatedly to relieve or forestall anxiety; seen in obsessive-compulsive neurosis.

riziform Resembling rice grains.

Robin syndrome See Pierre Robin Syndrome.

Rocher's sign See drawer sign.

rod 1. Any slender, cylindrical structure or formation. 2. One of the cells forming, with the cones, the layer of rods and cones of the retina.

rodenticide An agent lethal to rodents.

roentgen (R) Primary unit of x-ray dosage, equal to the quantity of ionizing radiation that can produce one electrostatic unit of electricity in one cubic centimeter of dry air at 0°C and standard atmospheric pressure.

roentgen-equivalent-man (rem) The amount of ionizing radiation absorbed by a human that is required to produce a biologic effect equivalent to the absorption of one roentgen of x or gamma rays; the dose is determined by multiplying the dose in rads (units of radiation exposure expressing the absorbed dose) by the appropriate RBE (relative biologic effectiveness); maximum permissible doses (MPD) used as a guideline for occupational exposure are as follows: gonads, red bone marrow, and whole body, 5 rems in a year; skin, thyroid, and bone, 30 rems in a year; hands and forearms, 75 rems in a year; all other organs, 15 rems in a year.

roentgen-equivalent-physical (rep) The amount of ionizing radiation which, upon absorption by living tissue, produces an energy gain per gram of tissue equivalent to that produced by one roentgen of x rays or gamma rays.

roentgenism 1. Any disorder caused by x-ray radiation. 2. The use of x rays in the treatment of disease.

roentgenkymograph Apparatus for graphically recording the movements of the heart and great vessels on a single x-ray film.

roentgenogram A processed photographic film on which an image is produced by x rays striking a sensitized film after their passage through a portion of the body. Loosely called an x ray.

  cephalometric r. X-ray picture of the skull, including the mandible, for purpose of taking measurements.

roentgenography Radiography with the use of x rays.

  body section r. Sectional roentgenography in which a single layer of a part of the body is put into focus. Also called tomography.

  mucosal relief r. Roentgenography of the lining of the rectum, made after a barium enema has been evacuated and the rectum has been distended with air; the small amount of barium remaining on the intestinal wall reveals fine details. Also called air contrast study.

  spot-film r. The making of several localized x-ray pictures during a fluoroscopic examination.

roentgenologist A specialist in the use of x rays in the diagnosis and treatment of disease. Cf. radiologist.

roentgenology The study of x rays as applied to diagnosis and treatment of disease. Cf. radiology.

roentgenometry Measurement of (a) the therapeutic dosage of x rays; (b) the penetrating power of x rays.

roentgenoscopy Examination of any bodily part by visualization of images cast upon a roentgenoscope, fluoroscope, or fluorescent screen by a beam of x rays, following introduction of a radiopaque material. Also called radioscopy.

Roger's disease Congenital heart anomaly consisting of a small defect of the interventricular septum. Also called maladie de Roger.

role 1. The pattern of social behavior that an individual develops, influenced by what others expect or demand of him. 2. A part played by an individual in relation to a group.

role-playing A method of treating emotional conflicts by having the subject assume various roles.

Romberg's disease Facial hemiatrophy; see under hemiatrophy.

Romberg's sign Swaying and loss of balance when standing with feet together and eyes closed; indicates a loss of proprioceptive control; occurs in disease of the posterior columns of the spinal cord.

Romberg's syndrome Facial hemiatrophy; see under hemiatrophy.

rongeur Instrument used to cut bone.

roof A top covering structure.

  r. of fourth ventricle The upper structure of the fourth ventricle of the brain; formed by the superior and inferior medullary vela and by the epithelial lining, the tela choroidea. Also called tegmen ventriculi quarti.

  r. of mouth The bony and muscular partition between the nasal and oral cavities. Also called palate.

room An area in a building surrounded by walls.

  anechoic r. A room that is devoid of echo; used in acoustical testing.

  delivery r. A hospital room to which women in labor are taken for delivery.

  emergency r. (ER) An area in a hospital where immediate attention is given by trained personnel to individuals brought in with sudden and unexpected medical problems, such as acute illness, trauma, etc. Also called accident ward.

  operating r. (OR) A hospital facility in which surgical procedures are performed.

  predelivery r. A hospital room in which a woman is placed during the first stage of labor. Also called labor room.

  recovery r. (RR) A hospital room provided for the immediate care of postoperative patients.

rooming-in The practice of allowing a newborn to stay in the mother's hospital room, in a crib, instead of the nursery during the hospital stay.

root 1. The embedded part of a structure, as of a tooth, hair, or nail. 2. The origin of a structure; e.g., the proximal end of a nerve.

  anatomic r. The root of a tooth extending from the cervical line to its apical extremity and contained in the bony socket of the jaw.

  anterior r.'s See ventral roots.

  clinical r. The portion of the tooth below the gingival crevice.

  dorsal r.'s The nerve roots that carry impulses from bodily parts to the back of the spinal cord; they are attached along the dorsal lateral sulcus of the cord by six to eight rootlets. Also called sensory or posterior roots.

  motor r.'s See ventral roots.

  posterior r.'s See dorsal roots.

  r. of aorta The origin of the ascending aorta from the left ventricle.

  r. of hair The part of hair embedded in the hair follicle.

  r. of lung All the structures entering or emerging at the hilus of the lung, forming a pedicle.

  r. of nail The proximal end of the nail, embedded under a fold of skin.

  r. of penis The proximal attached part of the penis, including the two crura of the corpora cavernosa and the bulb.

  r. of tooth The part of the tooth below the neck which is normally embedded in the alveolar process and covered with cementum.

  sensory r.'s See dorsal roots.

  ventral r.'s The nerve roots which carry impulses from the anterior part of the spinal cord out to muscles and other structures; they are attached along the ventral lateral sulcus in two or three irregular rows of rootlets. Also called motor or anterior roots.

rosacea Chronic inflammatory disorder superficially resembling acne; occurring most often in middle-aged individuals; characterized by papules, pustules, and dilation of capillaries on the cheeks and

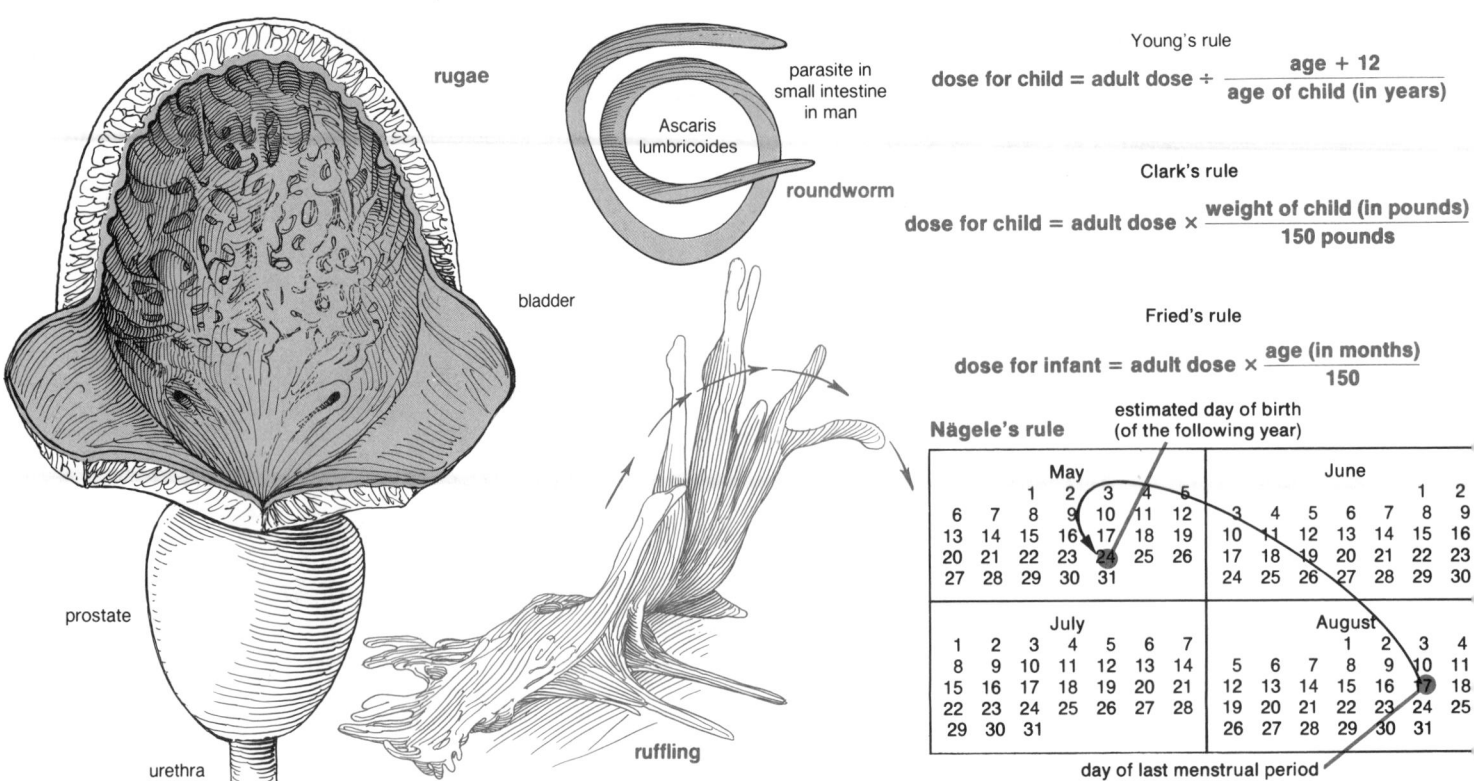

rugae

parasite in small intestine in man

Ascaris lumbricoides

roundworm

bladder

prostate

urethra

ruffling

Young's rule
$$\text{dose for child} = \text{adult dose} \div \frac{\text{age} + 12}{\text{age of child (in years)}}$$

Clark's rule
$$\text{dose for child} = \text{adult dose} \times \frac{\text{weight of child (in pounds)}}{150 \text{ pounds}}$$

Fried's rule
$$\text{dose for infant} = \text{adult dose} \times \frac{\text{age (in months)}}{150}$$

Nägele's rule

estimated day of birth (of the following year)

	May								June					
		1	2	3	4	5						1	2
6	7	8	9	10	11	12	3	4	5	6	7	8	9
13	14	15	16	17	18	19	10	11	12	13	14	15	16
20	21	22	23	24	25	26	17	18	19	20	21	22	23
27	28	29	30	31			24	25	26	27	28	29	30

	July								August					
1	2	3	4	5	6	7				1	2	3	4
8	9	10	11	12	13	14	5	6	7	8	9	10	11
15	16	17	18	19	20	21	12	13	14	15	16	17	18
22	23	24	25	26	27	28	19	20	21	22	23	24	25
29	30	31					26	27	28	29	30	31	

day of last menstrual period

---

nose, and sometimes the forehead and chin. Also called acne rosacea.

rosanilin Red needle-like crystals, soluble in water; a component of the stain fuchsin.

rosary An arrangement resembling a string of beads.

rachitic r. A row of nodules at the junction of the ribs with their cartilages, sometimes seen in rachitic children. Also called rachitic beads.

Rosenbach's sign 1. Fine tremor of gently closed eyelids, occurring in exophthalmic goiter. 2. Loss of abdominal reflexes seen in cases of acute inflammation of the abdominal organs.

roseola A reddish rash.

r. infantum Exanthem subitum.

rosette A spherical group of fine red vacuoles surrounding the cytocentrum of a monocyte.

rostellum The anterior, hook-bearing portion of a tapeworm.

rostral, rostrad 1. Directed toward the front end of the body. 2. Relating to any beaklike structure.

rostrum Any beak-shaped structure.

rot 1. To decay. 2. The process of decomposition.

rotameter A flow-rate meter used to measure gases during administration of anesthesia.

rotation 1. Motion around an internal axis. 2. In obstetrics, the turning of the fetal head or any presenting part, whereby it is accommodated to the birth canal.

rotator A muscle that rotates a part, as one of several muscles that rotate the vertebral column.

Rotavirus Genus of wheel-shaped RNA viruses (family Rotaviridae) including the human gastroenteritis virus; the most important cause of severe dehydrating diarrhea, vomiting, and low-grade fever in children under 3 years of age.

Rothmund's syndrome A hereditary syndrome, probably transmitted as an autosomal recessive trait, characterized by juvenile cataracts, saddle nose, premature graying and loss of hair, and wasting of muscles. Also called Rothmund-Thomson or congenital poikiloderma-juvenile cataract syndrome.

rouge A fine red powder of iron oxide; used as a final polishing agent for dental restorations made of gold and precious metal alloys.

rough Denoting the granular surface of certain bacterial colonies.

roughage Indigestible material in the diet (coarse vegetable fibers and cellulose) that serves to stimulate peristalsis.

roughing The grinding of lenses with a coarse abrasive.

roundworm A member of the phylum Nemathelminthes.

rub 1. To apply pressure and friction on a surface. 2. Friction encountered in moving a structure against another.

friction r. The auscultatory sound produced by the rubbing together of two serous surfaces roughened by an inflammatory exudate. Also called friction sound.

pericardial r. A friction or scraping sound produced by the rubbing together of inflamed pericardial surfaces during each heart beat.

pleuritic r. A grating sound produced by the rubbing together of the inflamed surfaces of the costal and visceral pleurae.

rubber-dam See dam.

rubedo Temporary redness of the skin.

rubefacient Causing redness and irritation of the skin.

rubella A contagious exanthematous disease of short duration, caused by a virus and capable of causing congenital defects in infants born of mothers who acquire the disease during the first three months of pregnancy; the incubation period is usually two to three weeks. Also called German measles.

rubeola See measles.

rubeosis Redness.

r. iridis The formation of numerous new blood vessels on the anterior surface of the iris; most frequently associated with diabetes; occasionally seen in other conditions.

rubescent Reddening.

rubidium Chemical element; symbol Rb, atomic number 37, atomic weight 85.48.

Rubivirus A genus of viruses (family Togaviridae) which, unlike other members of Togaviridae, are not transmitted by arthropods; man is the only vertebrate host; includes the rubella (German measles) virus.

rubor Latin for redness.

rubriblast See pronormoblast.

rubricyte Polychromatic normoblast; see under normoblast.

rubrospinal Relating to the red nucleus and the spinal cord.

rudiment An incompletely developed structure.

rudimentary Incompletely developed.

Ruffini's corpuscle Ruffini's nerve ending; see under ending.

ruffling The method by which a cell moves (perambulates) across a surface; characterized by the extension of thin, veil-like folds (ruffles) sprouting upward, extending out like an arm, and then dropping to the surface; when this "arm" adheres to the surface the cell flows into it as if it were pulling itself along.

ruga, pl. rugae A fold or wrinkle.

gastric r. One of the folds in the lining of the stomach.

r. palatina One of several transverse ridges on the anterior portion of the palate.

r. of vagina One of several transverse folds of the vaginal mucosa.

rugal Wrinkled; creased; corrugated.

rugitus Intestinal rumbling.

rugose Marked by rugae or ridges; wrinkled.

rugosity 1. The state of having folds or ridges. 2. A fold or ridge (ruga).

rule A guide.

American Law Institute r. A 1962 American rule stating, ". . . a person is not responsible for criminal conduct if at the time of such conduct as a result of mental disease or defect he lacks substantial capacity either to appreciate the wrongfulness of his conduct or to conform his conduct to the requirements of law."

Durham r. A 1954 American test of criminal responsibility stating, ". . . an accused is not criminally responsible if his unlawful act was the product of mental disease or mental defect." This test was repudiated in 1966 (Brawner vs. U.S.) by the court that originated it.

M'Naghten r., McNaughton r. A British test of criminal responsibility stating, ". . . it must be shown that, at the time of committing the act, the accused was acting under such defect of reason from a diseased mind as not to know the nature and quality of the act or if he knew this, that he did not know that what he was doing was wrong."

Nägele's r. Estimation of the day of birth by counting back three months from the first day of the last menstrual period and adding seven days.

ruminant Any of various hoofed, usually horned, animals (cattle, goats, etc.) that have a stomach with four compartments and that regurgitate and chew partially digested food (cud).

rumination 1. The process of chewing cud. 2. The recurring of thoughts.

rump Buttocks or gluteal region.

rupture 1. Hernia. 2. The bursting or tearing of a part.

rut A period of sexual desire in the males of certain species of mammals; corresponds to heat or estrus in the female.

ruthenium A rare, brittle, metallic element; symbol Ru, atomic number 44, atomic weight 101.1.

rutherford Unit of radioactivity, equal to the amount of radioactive material that undergoes one million disintegrations per second.

rypophobia A morbid fear of dirt.

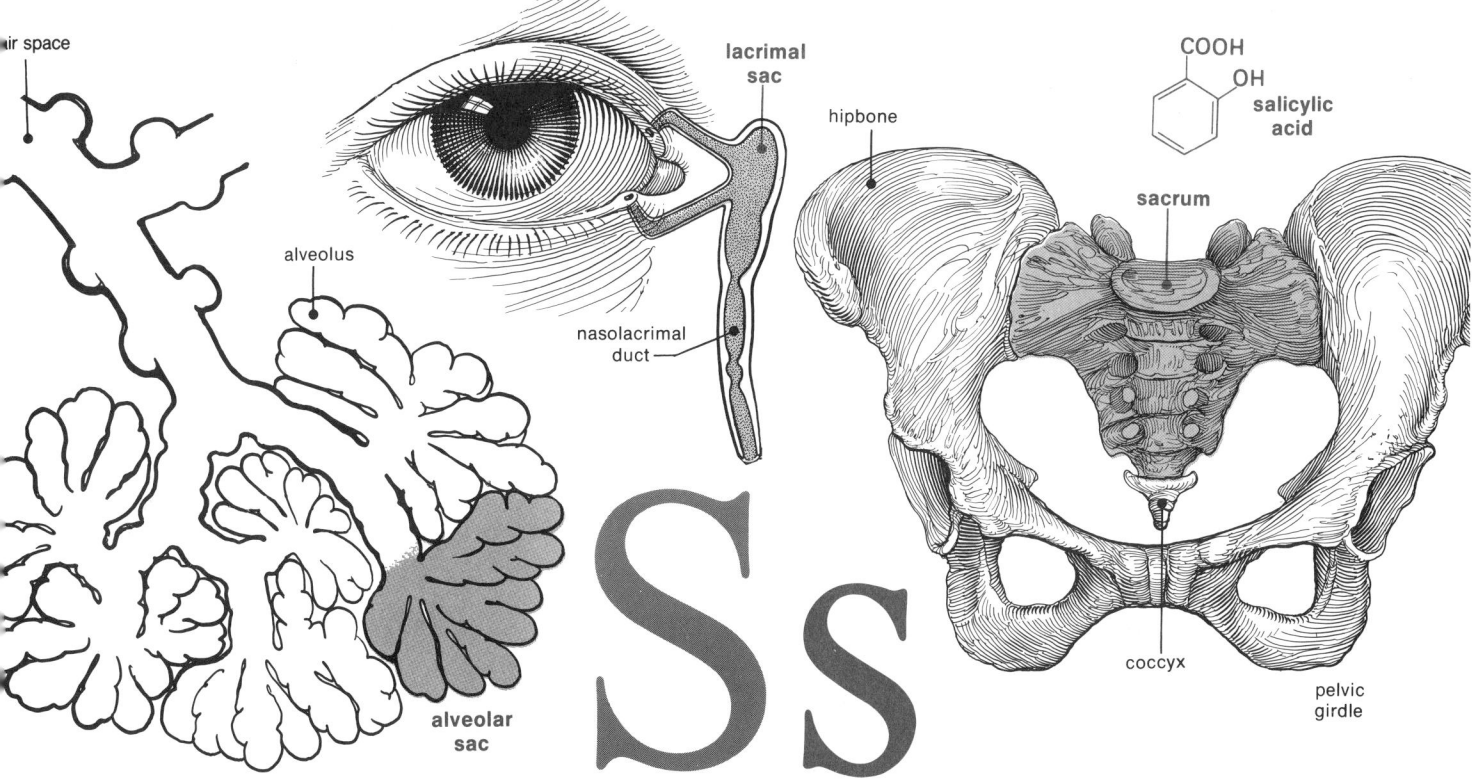

air space

alveolar
sac

alveolus

lacrimal
sac

nasolacrimal
duct

hipbone

COOH

OH

salicylic
acid

sacrum

coccyx

pelvic
girdle

S s

sabulous Sandy; gritty.

sac A bag or pouchlike anatomic structure.

  abdominal s. The part of the embryonic coelom that develops into the abdominal cavity.

  air s. See alveolar sac.

  allantoic s. The dilated distal part of the allantois.

  alveolar s. A cluster of alveoli in the lungs sharing a common central air space. Also called air sac.

  aneurysmal s. The dilated wall of an artery in a saccular aneurysm.

  dental s. The fibrous layer of mesenchyme surrounding a developing tooth.

  endolymphatic s. The blind extremity of the endolymphatic duct of the inner ear.

  greater s. of peritoneum The main part of the peritoneal cavity; it extends across the whole breadth of the abdomen, and from the diaphragm to the pelvis.

  heart s. Pericardium.

  hernial s. The peritoneal envelope of a hernia.

  lacrimal s. The slightly dilated upper part of the nasolacrimal duct situated in the lacrimal fossa. Also called tear sac.

  lesser s. of the peritoneum The smaller part of the peritoneal cavity; a diverticulum of the greater sac of the peritoneum, situated behind the lesser omentum; it extends upward as far as the diaphragm, extends downward between the layers of the greater omentum, and opens through the epiploic foramen. Also called omental bursa.

  omental s. A recess of the lesser sac of the peritoneum situated between the layers of the greater omentum.

  pleural s. A closed sac enveloping each lung, composed of a double-layered membrane (pleura).

  synovial s. A closed sac formed by the synovial membrane; it contains a thick, viscous, lubricating fluid (similar to the white of an egg) that facilitates movement of joints.

  tear s. See lacrimal sac.

  vitelline s. See yolk sac.

saccadic Quick; jerky; sudden; said of certain movements of the eye.

saccate Pouched.

saccharate A salt of saccharic acid.

saccharated Sweetened; sugary.

saccharic Relating to sugar.

  s. acid A white crystalline compound obtained by oxidation of glucose or its derivatives.

saccharide Any of a series of compounds containing carbon, hydrogen, and oxygen in which the ratio of hydrogen to oxygen is 2:1.

sacchariferous Containing or producing sugar.

saccharimeter A device for measuring the amount of sugar in a solution.

saccharin A white crystalline powder, C_6H_4-$COSO_2NH$; used as a sugar substitute.

saccharine Sweet.

saccharometabolism Utilization of sugar by the tissues.

Saccharomyces A genus of yeast fungi, some species of which ferment sugar.

  S. cerevisiae The beer, wine, and bread yeast. Also called brewer's, baker's, or wine yeast.

saccharose See sucrose.

saccharum Latin for sucrose.

saccharuria Glycosuria.

sacciform Baglike.

saccular Resembling a bag.

sacculated Formed of or divided into a series of pouches.

sacculation The presence or the formation of sacs.

saccule, sacculus 1. A small sac. 2. The smaller of the two sacs of the membranous labyrinth in the vestibule of the internal ear.

saccus, *pl.* **sacci** Latin for sac.

sacrad Toward the sacrum.

sacral Relating to the sacrum.

sacralgia Pain in the sacral area. Also called sacrodynia.

sacralization A bony anomaly in which one or both (usually both) transverse processes of the fifth lumbar vertebra are wing-shaped and long, and articulate with the sacrum or ilium, or both.

sacrectomy Surgical removal of a portion of the sacrum.

sacrococcygeal Relating to both the sacrum and coccyx.

sacroiliac Relating to the sacrum and the ilium, as the sacroiliac joint.

sacrosciatic Relating to the sacrum and ischium.

sacrospinal Relating to the sacrum and spine.

sacrovertebral Relating to the sacrum and the vertebrae.

sacrum A slightly curved, triangular bone comprised of five fused vertebrae, wedged dorsally between the two hip bones, and forming the posterior section of the pelvis.

saddle Denture base; see under base.

sadism The existence of destructive-aggressive attitudes in an individual; i.e., the person derives pleasure from inflicting physical or psychological pain on others, in both social and sexual relationships.

sadist One who practices sadism.

sadomasochism The simultaneous existence of destructive-aggressive and self-destructive-passive attitudes in an individual, in both social and sexual relationships.

safflower *Carthamus tinctorius*, a plant having seeds from which safflower oil is extracted.

safranin O A red basic dye used in biologic stains.

safranophile Staining readily with safranin.

sagittal In an anteroposterior direction.

sal, *pl.* **sales** Latin for salt.

salicin A glucoside obtained from the bark of willow and poplar trees; used as a bitter tonic.

salicylamide A white, crystalline compound having analgesic properties.

salicylate A salt of salicylic acid.

  methyl s. Oil of wintergreen.

salicylazosulfapyridine A sulfonamide used in the treatment of ulcerative colitis.

salicylic acid $C_7H_6O_3$; a white crystalline powder derived from phenol; used externally for the local treatment of corns and warts.

salicylism Poisoning by salicylic acid or its salts.

salicyluric acid $C_9H_9NO_4$; an acid found in the urine after administration of salicylic acid or some of its derivatives.

salient Projecting; protruding.

salify To convert into a salt.

salimeter Instrument used to determine the concentration of saline solutions.

saline Relating to or containing salt.

saliva The fluid mixture of secretions from the parotid, sublingual, and submandibular glands and the mucous glands of the oral cavity; it contains an enzyme (ptyalin) which partially digests carbohydrates.

salivant 1. Increasing the flow of saliva. 2. An agent having such an effect.

salivary Relating to saliva.

salivary gland virus disease See cytomegalic inclusion disease.

salivate To produce excessive secretion of saliva.

salivation 1. The secretion of saliva. 2. Excessive flow of saliva. Also called sialorrhea.

Salmonella A genus of gram-negative, rod-shaped, motile bacteria, some species of which cause acute intestinal inflammation.

  S. typhi Species that is the causative agent of typhoid fever. Formerly called *Salmonella typhosa*. Also called typhoid bacillus.

  S. typhimurium Species causing food poisoning in man.

  S. typhosa Former name for *Salmonella typhi*.

salmonellosis Infection with bacteria of the genus *Salmonella*, usually marked by severe diarrhea.

salpingectomy Surgical removal of a uterine tube. Also called tubectomy.

salpingemphraxis Obstruction of a uterine or an auditory tube.

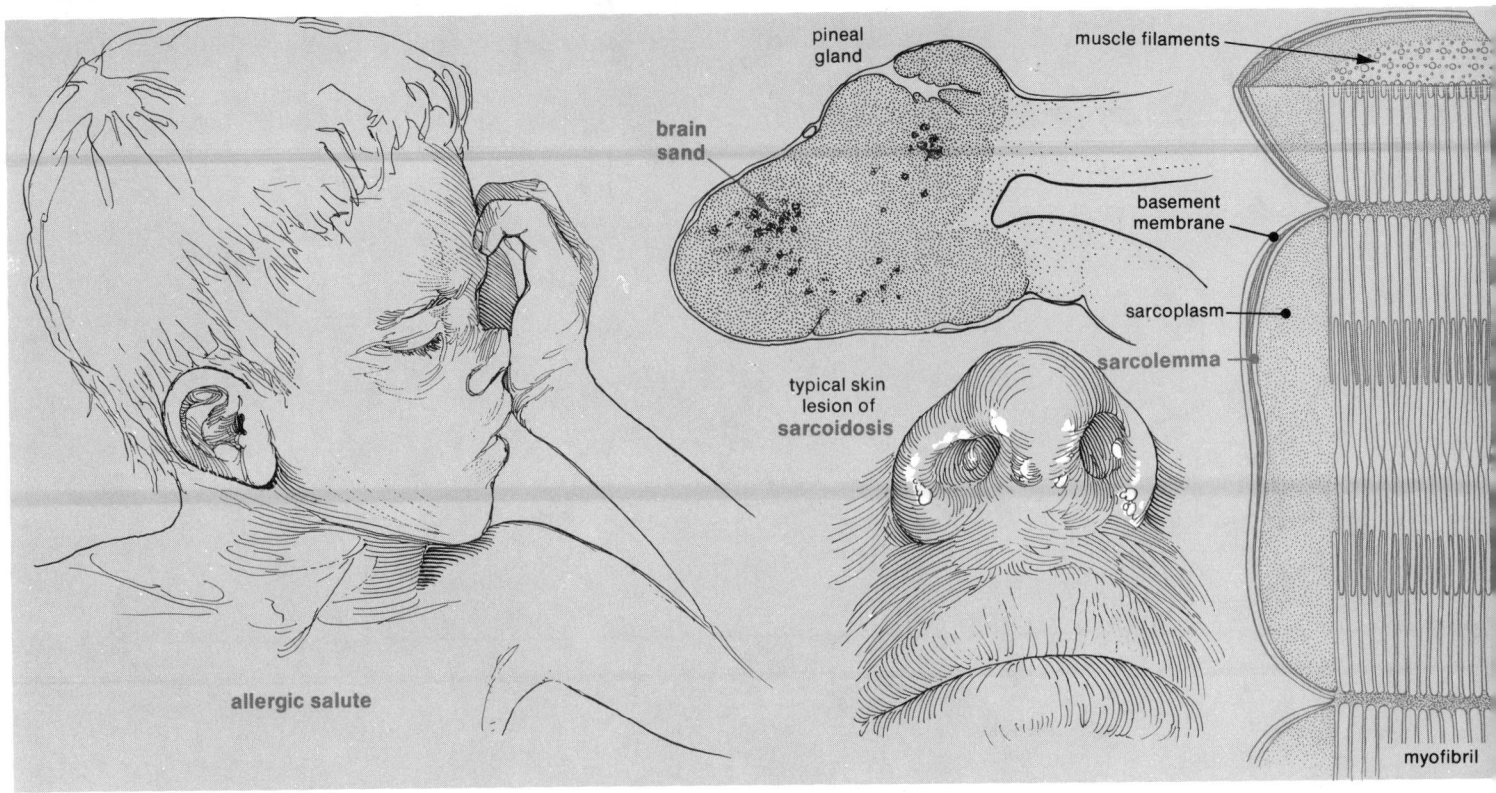

pineal gland

brain sand

muscle filaments

basement membrane

sarcoplasm

sarcolemma

typical skin lesion of **sarcoidosis**

allergic salute

myofibril

salpingian Relating to the uterine (fallopian) or to the auditory (eustachian) tubes.
salpingitis Inflammation of the uterine tube.
salpingocele Hernia of a uterine (fallopian) tube.
salpingocyesis Tubal pregnancy; see under pregnancy.
salpingography Radiography of a uterine tube after the injection of a radiopaque compound.
salpingolysis The release of adhesions about a uterine (fallopian) tube or its fringed end.
salpingo-oophorectomy Surgical removal of an ovary and its corresponding uterine (fallopian) tube.
salpingo-oophoritis Inflammation of a uterine tube and ovary. Also called salpingo-oothecitis.
salpingo-oothecitis See salpingo-oophoritis.
salpingoperitonitis Inflammation of a uterine (fallopian) tube and adjacent peritoneum.
salpingopharyngeal Relating to the auditory tube and the pharynx.
salpingoplasty Reparative operation on a uterine tube.
salpingorrhaphy Stitching of a uterine (fallopian) tube.
salpingostomy The making of an artificial opening in a uterine tube when the fringed end of the tube is occluded; an operative treatment for sterility.
salpingotomy Surgical incision into a uterine tube.
salpinx A tube; especially, the uterine (fallopian) tube or the auditory (eustachian) tube.
salt 1. Compound produced by the reaction between an acid and a base in which all or part of the hydrogen ions of the acid are replaced by one or more radicals of the base. 2. Table salt (sodium chloride).
  acid s. A salt containing unreplaced hydrogen atoms from the acid; e.g., $NaHSO_4$.
  basic s. A salt containing unreplaced hydroxyl radicals from the base; e.g., $Bi(OH)Cl_2$.
  binary s. A salt containing only two elements.
  effervescent s. One of several preparations containing sodium bicarbonate, tartaric and citric acids, and an active salt; when mixed with water, the acids break up the sodium bicarbonate, releasing the carbonic acid gas.
  Epsom s. See magnesium sulfate.
  iodized s. Table salt containing one part sodium or potassium iodide to 10,000 parts sodium chloride.
  smelling s. A preparation of ammonium carbonate with any of several aromatic oils, sniffed as a restorative.
salt-abrasion Technique of superficially rubbing away the skin with salt to a uniform depth; used to remove tatoos.
saltation Leaping, as in certain nervous disorders.

salting out The separation of a protein from its solution by the addition of a neutral salt such as sodium chloride.
saltpeter See potassium nitrate.
salubrious Healthful.
saluresis Excretion of sodium in the urine.
saluretic Promoting excretion of sodium.
salutary Healthful.
salute, allergic Rubbing of the tip of the nose in a characteristic transverse or upward motion, commonly seen in children afflicted with allergic rhinitis.
salve 1. An ointment. 2. Anything that soothes or heals. 3. To dress with salve; to soothe.
samarium A rare earth element; symbol Sm, atomic number 62, atomic weight 150.35.
sample 1. A representative segment of the whole. 2. In biostatistics, the portion of the population being studied. 3. A specimen.
  random s. One made in such a way that all group members have equal chances of selection.
sampling Selection and examination of a sample.
  chorionic villus s. (CVS) Sampling of placental tissue of an 8–12 week old fetus to detect chromosomal defects.
sanative, sanatory Curative.
sanatorium Institution for treating long term illnesses, such as tuberculosis and mental disorders.
sand Granules of disintegrated rock.
  brain s. Minute crystals, mainly composed of calcium carbonate, present in the pineal body. Also called acervulus.
sandfly A tiny, long-legged fly (genus *Phlebotomus* or *Lutzomyia*); vector of leishmaniasis.
sane Relating to sanity or to one who is of sound mind.
Sanfilippo syndrome A form of mucopolysaccharidosis characterized by severe mental retardation and excretion of heparan sulfate in the urine; skeleton may be normal or exhibit slight dwarfism; inherited as an autosomal recessive trait. Also called mucopolysaccharidosis III.
sanguiferous Conveying blood.
sanguineous Relating to or containing blood.
sanguinolent Blood-tinged.
sanguinopurulent Denoting a discharge or matter containing blood and pus.
sanguis Latin for blood.
sanguivorous Blood-sucking, as certain animals.
saniopurulent Denoting a blood-tinged discharge with pus.
sanioserous Denoting a blood-tinged serum.
sanitarium A health resort. Cf. sanatorium.
sanitary Relating to or conducive to health.
sanitation Application of measures to create environmental conditions conducive to health.

sanity 1. Soundness of mind. 2. In a legal sense, the state of a person's mind whereby he is legally responsible for his actions and their consequences.
santonin The bitter principle of santonica (dried flower heads of the plant *Artemicia cina*); sometimes used to effect expulsion of roundworms.
saphenectomy Surgical removal of a saphenous vein.
saphenous 1. Relating to either of two large superficial veins of the leg (saphena) that carry blood from the toes upward. 2. Denoting various structures in the leg.
saponaceous Soapy; resembling soap.
saponification The formation of a soap by the hydrolytic action of an alkali upon fat.
saponify To convert fat into soap.
saponin Any of a group of vegetable substances possessing the property of making suds.
sapphism Lesbianism.
saprogen An organism that causes decay of organic matter.
saprogenic Causing decay.
saprogenous Resulting from decay.
saprophilous Thriving on decaying matter.
saprophyte A plant, such as a bacterium or fungus, that lives on dead or decaying organic matter. Also called necroparasite.
saprophytic Relating to a saprophyte; deriving nourishment from dead organic matter.
saprozoic Thriving in decaying organic material; said of certain protozoa.
sarcocele A fleshy tumor of the testis.
sarcoid 1. Sarcoidosis. 2. Resembling flesh.
sarcoidosis Multiple benign nodular lesions involving any tissue of the body, especially the lungs; a systemic granulomatous disease of undetermined etiology. Also called Boeck's sarcoid.
sarcolemma The delicate plasma membrane that invests every striated muscle fiber.
sarcoma A malignant tumor composed of connective tissue.
  Ewing's s. A rapidly growing malignant tumor arising from medullary tissue within a single bone, usually the long bones; occurring most frequently in individuals between the ages of 10 and 25 years; symptoms include fever, pain, and leukocytosis. Also called Ewing's tumor; diffuse endothelioma of bone.
  Kaposi's s. Malignant skin tumor occurring on multiple sites, especially lower extremities; spreads to lymph nodes and internal organs; initial lesions are small red papules which enlarge and fuse to form purple to brown spongy nodules; usually a slowly progressive disease, its course is much more agressive when associated with AIDS.

satellite

centric
nosome

scabies

Gigli
wire
saw

scalers

	absolute scale (Kelvin)	Celsius scale (centigrade)	Fahrenheit scale
boiling point of water	373.15	100	212
body temperature	310.15	37	98.6
freezing point of water	273.15	0	32
absolute zero	0	273.16	-459.67

scala tympani
scala media
scala vestibuli

cochlea
of internal
ear

Rous s.   A sarcoma-like growth of fowl; shown in 1910 by Peyton Rous to be caused by a virus.

sarcomatoid   Resembling a sarcoma.

sarcomatous   Pertaining to or of the nature of sarcoma.

sarcomere   One of a series of repeated segments of a muscle fibril that comprises the fundamental units of contraction; the area between two Z lines, composed of overlapping thick and thin myofilaments.

sarcoplasm   The interfibrillary cytoplasm of a muscle fiber; the substance in which the muscle fibrils are embedded.

sarcopoietic   Forming muscle.

Sarcoptes scabiei   The species of itch mite that causes the parasitic skin disorder scabies; the fertilized female tunnels intradermally and deposits eggs and excreta; the male mites generally do not burrow, but remain on the surface of the skin searching for unfertilized females.

sarcosome   A mitochondrion of muscle; in cardiac muscle, sarcosomes are large, numerous, and usually aligned in columns between the myofibrils.

sarcostosis   Ossification of muscle tissue.

sarcotubules   A system of membranous tubules surrounding each fibril of striated muscle.

sardonic grin   See risus caninus.

satellite   In genetics, a small globoid chromatin mass attached to the end of the chromosome by a slender secondary constriction; in man, usually associated with the short arm of an acrocentric chromosome.

satellitosis   Phenomenon in which interstitial brain cells of a certain type (oligodendroglia), normally found as satellites about nerve cells, increase in number about a damaged nerve cell.

saturate   1. To impregnate completely.   2. To neutralize.

saturated   Denoting a solution in which the addi-

tion of any more of a solute will cause precipitation.

saturnine   Relating to lead.

saturnism   Lead poisoning.

satyriasis   Excessive sexual desire in the male.

sauriasis   Severe ichthyosis. Also called lizard skin.

saw   A cutting instrument with a serrated edge, used to cut bone.

   Gigli wire s.   A wire with saw teeth.

   Stryker s.   A saw designed for cutting hard material such as bone or plastic casts.

scab   1. The crust formed on the surface of an ulcer or a superficial wound, composed of dried pus, lymph, or blood.   2. To develop a scab.

scabicide   An agent destructive to itch mites.

scabies   A contagious, parasitic skin disorder caused by the mite *Sarcoptes scabiei*; the female mite excavates tunnels in the superficial layers of the skin and deposits eggs and irritating excreta, causing red lesions, itching, and swelling of the skin surface along the elevated tracts; the most common sites of entry are between the fingers, the hands, and wrists; the infection can persist for months or years in untreated individuals, hence the colloquial term seven-year itch. Also called sarcoptic acariasis.

scabrites   Rough, scaly skin.

scala   One of the spiral canals of the cochlea.

   s. media   Cochlear duct; see under duct.

   s. tympani   The spiral canal of the cochlea located below the spiral lamina. Also called tympanic canal.

   s. vestibuli   The spiral canal of the cochlea located above the spiral lamina. Also called vestibular canal.

scald   1. To burn with a hot liquid or vapor.   2. The lesion produced in such a manner.   3. Any crusty lesion of the scalp.

scale   1. A small thin piece of epithelium shed from the skin.   2. To shed such material.   3. In dentistry, to scrape tartar off the teeth.   4. A system of

marks at regular intervals serving as a standard of measurement.   5. An instrument having such marks.

   absolute s.   A temperature scale with its zero point at absolute zero (approximately −273.16°C). Also called Kelvin scale.

   Celsius s.   A temperature scale in which 0° represents the freezing point of water and 100° its boiling point, at sea level; the normal human body temperature is recorded at 37°; named after Anders Celsius, the Swedish astronomer who invented it. Also called centigrade scale.

   centigrade s.   One having 100 equal units between two standard points; e.g., the Celsius scale.

   Fahrenheit s.   Temperature scale that records the freezing point of water at 32°, the boiling point of water at 212°, and the normal human body temperature at 98.6° under standard atmospheric pressure; named after the German physicist Gabriel D. Fahrenheit.

   Kelvin s.   See absolute scale.

scalene   Having sides of unequal length; said of a triangle or a muscle of such proportions.

scalenectomy   Surgical removal of a scalene muscle, or a portion of it.

scalenus-anticus syndrome   Pain in the shoulder, often radiating to the arm and back of the neck, caused by compression of nerves and vessels between the first thoracic rib and a hypertonic anterior scalene (scalene anticus) muscle.

scaler   An instrument designed to be used in removing deposits, especially tartar, from the teeth.

scaling   Removal of calculus from the exposed surfaces of the teeth and the area under the margin of the gums by use of special instruments called scalers.

scalp   The skin covering the cranium.

scalpel   A thin surgical knife, usually with a removable blade.

scalpriform   Resembling a chisel.

scaly   1. Flaking.   2. Covered with scales or flakes.

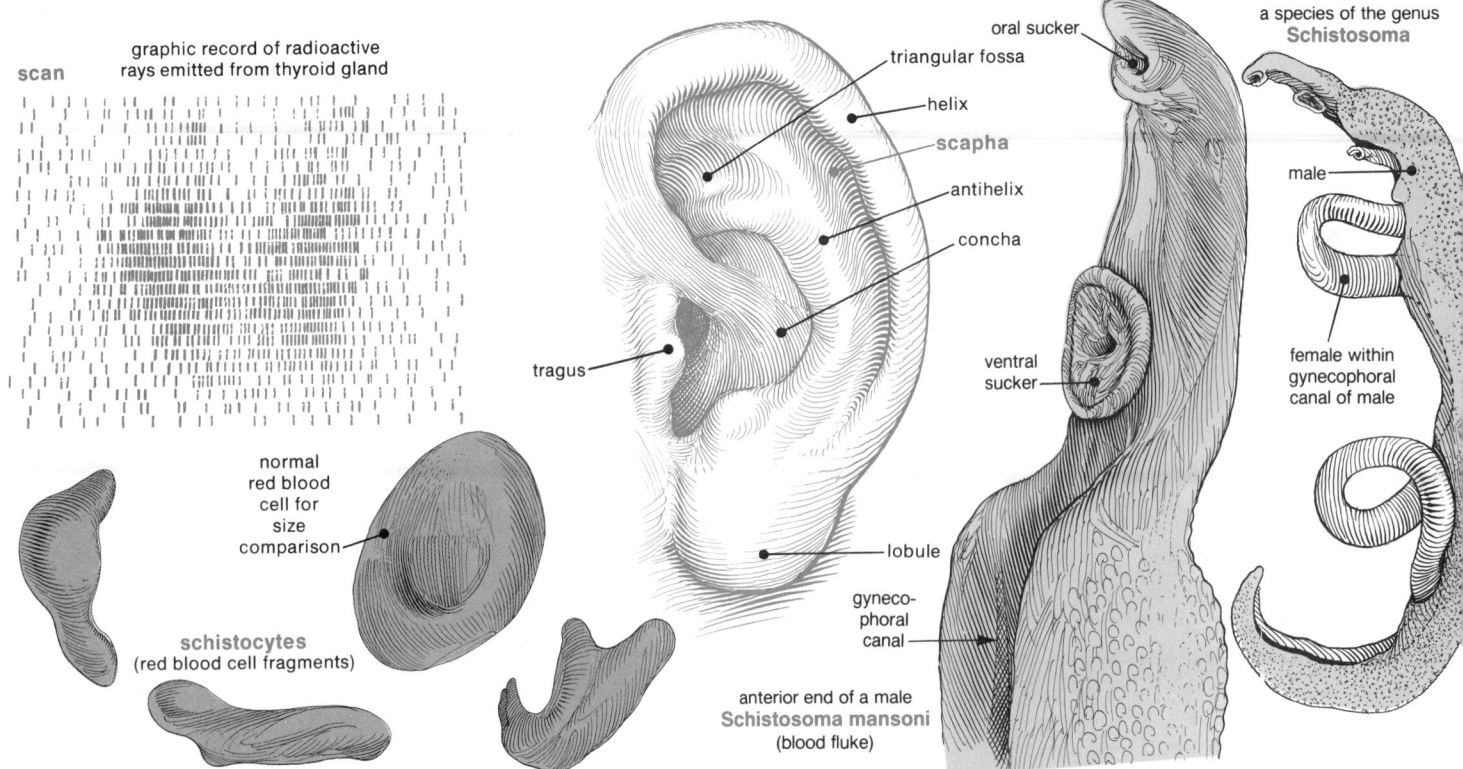

scan

graphic record of radioactive
rays emitted from thyroid gland

normal
red blood
cell for
size
comparison

schistocytes
(red blood cell fragments)

triangular fossa

helix

scapha

antihelix

concha

tragus

lobule

gyneco-
phoral
canal

anterior end of a male
Schistosoma mansoni
(blood fluke)

oral sucker

a species of the genus
Schistosoma

male

female within
gynecophoral
canal of male

ventral
sucker

scan **1.** A graphic record of the distribution of a specific radioactive element within an organ. **2.** To obtain a record of the distribution of radioactivity within an organ.

   brain s. One of the essential methods of cerebro-spinal diagnosis; it entails injection or inhalation of radioisotopes and production of pictures by radiation detectors. Also called radioisotopic brain scan.

    radioisotopic brain s. See brain scan.

scandium A light, silvery-white metallic element that reacts rapidly with acids; symbol Sc, atomic number 21, atomic weight 44.956; present in the earth's crust in a concentration of about five parts per million.

scanner **1.** Apparatus used to determine radioactivity distribution within an organ; it consists of a sensitive, collimated detector that is mechanically coupled to a recorder. **2.** Any device that scans a region point by point in a continuous systematic manner.

   CT s. A machine for performing computed tomography. Also called CAT scanner.

scanning The procedure of making a radioactivity scan.

   bone s. A sensitive technique of scanning bone for detecting lesions; a valuable aid in the diagnosis, treatment, and prognosis of a variety of benign and malignant skeletal disorders.

scapha The long longitudinal depression or furrow between the helix and the antihelix of the auricle.

scaphocephalic Characterized by scaphocephalism.

scaphocephalism A deformity in which the skull is abnormally long and narrow (high vertex, bulging forehead, lateral flattening, and increased anteroposterior diameter), due to the premature closure of the sagittal suture.

scaphocephaly Scaphocephalism.

scaphoid Boat-shaped; sunken; hollowed.

scapula Either of two large, flat, triangular bones overlying the upper portion of the ribs, and forming the back of the shoulder; articulates with the clavicle and the humerus. Also called shoulder blade.

scapular Of or relating to the scapula (shoulder blade).

scar The fibrous tissue formed during the healing of a wound. Also called cicatrix.

scarification The making of several superficial scratches on the skin, as when vaccinating.

scarlatina An acute infectious disease caused by a beta-hemolytic streptococcus. Also called scarlet fever.

scarlatiniform Resembling scarlatina; said of a rash.

scatology **1.** The scientific study and analysis of the feces. **2.** In psychiatry, the study of disorders manifesting excessive concern with excrement.

scatoma An inspissated fecal mass in the colon or rectum resembling, on palpation, an abdominal tumor.

scatophagy Eating of feces or filth. Also called rhypophagy.

scatoscopy Examination or inspection of the feces for diagnostic purposes.

scattering The change in direction or dispersal of a beam of particles or radiation as a result of physical interaction, as the dispersal of electrons by the specimen in the electron microscope.

Schamberg's disease Progressive pigmentary dermatosis, a benign chronic disorder marked by repeated crops of petechiae on feet and legs, especially in men; associated microscopically with capillary dilatation, diapedesis, and hemosiderosis.

Scheie's syndrome A type of mucopolysaccharidosis considered to be a variant of Hurler's syndrome; characterized by progressive corneal clouding, stiff joints, hirsutism, aortic valvular disease, and excretion of dermatan sulfate and heparan sulfate in the urine; inherited as an autosomal recessive trait. Also called mucopolysaccharidosis I S and, formerly, mucopolysaccharoidosis V.

schema An arrangement or plan.

Schilder's disease See encephalitis periaxialis diffusa.

Schilling's hemogram A differential blood count in which the polymorphonuclear leukocytes are separated into four groups according to the number and arrangement of nuclear segments in the cells. Also called Schilling's blood count; Schilling's index.

schistocelia Congenital furrow of the abdominal wall.

schistocystis Fissure or exstrophy of the bladder; a congenital gap in the anterior wall of the bladder and the abdominal wall in front of it, with the posterior wall of the bladder presenting through the opening.

schistocyte, schizocyte A fragment of a red blood cell; it can assume a variety of sizes and shapes.

schistocytosis The occurrence of many red blood fragments (schistocytes) in the blood.

schistoglossia Congenital cleft of the tongue.

Schistosoma A genus of blood flukes (class Trematoda); some species are parasitic in man, causing debilitating illnesses over wide geographical areas of the world; parasites penetrate the skin of persons who come in contact with infested waters.

   S. haematobium Species found in the Middle East, large areas of Africa, and small areas of India; invertebrate host is a snail of the genus *Bulinus*; adult worms live exclusively in humans, within the veins of the bladder, causing symptoms of the urinary tract and, to a lesser degree, of the intestines.

   S. japonicum Species found in the Far East; invertebrate host is a snail of the genus *Oncomelania*; adult worm inhabits rodents, domestic animals, and humans; in humans, it lives within the venules of the small intestine and, because of the large number of eggs it deposits, causes the most serious of blood fluke diseases, with intestinal, hepatic, and pulmonary symptoms.

   S. mansoni Species found mainly in northeastern Brazil and the Caribbean islands; invertebrate host is a snail of the genus *Biomphalaria*; main definitive host is man, within veins of the large intestine; disease is similar to that caused by *Schistosoma japonicum* but milder.

schistosome A member of the genus *Schistosoma*.

schistosomiasis Infestation with schistosomes (blood flukes); involves mainly the intestinal tract, liver, or bladder. Also called bilharziasis; bilharziosis.

schizogony A stage in the asexual cycle of the malarial parasite occurring in the red blood cells of man. Also called multiple fission.

schizoid See under personality.

Schizomycetes A class of microorganisms containing all bacteria.

schizont The adult asexual form of the malarial parasite in man, following the trophozoite, with two or more divisions of its nucleus; it eventually divides, producing merozoites.

schizophasia The disordered, incomprehensible speech of the schizophrenic individual. Also referred to as "water-salad" speech.

schizophrenia A category of severe emotional disorders marked by disturbances of thinking including misinterpretation of reality and sometimes delusions and hallucinations; there are associated changes in mood and behavior, particularly withdrawal from people. Formerly called dementia precox.

schizophrenic Relating to or afflicted with schizophrenia.

schizotrichia A splitting of hairs at their ends. Also called scissura pilorum.

Schlemm's canal Scleral venous sinus; see under sinus.

Schmidt's syndrome **1.** Primary hypothyroidism and adrenal insufficiency; organ-specific antibodies against the adrenal gland and thyroid gland may be present; diabetes mellitus may also be pres-

Kelly angular scissors

bandage scissors

crown and collar scissors

scoleces of tapeworms

Dibothriocephalus latus (fish tapeworm)

sucking groove

globular scolex

rostellum with double row of hooks

four muscular suckers

scolex (head)

Taenia solium (pork tapeworm)

neck

Taenia saginata (beef tapeworm)

lateral curvature of spine

scoliosis

asymmetry of the thoracic cage (rib hump)

ent. **2.** Unilateral paralysis of a vocal cord, the palate, and the trapezius and sternocleidomastoid muscles.

Schönlein's disease Henoch-Schönlein purpura; see under purpura.

Schüffner's dots The dots or stipples appearing in red blood cells infected with malarial parasites (especially *Plasmodium vivax*), due to accumulation of granules. Also called Schüffner's granules.

Schüller disease See Hand-Schüller-Christian syndrome.

schwannoma See neurilemoma.

granular cell s. See tumor, granular cell.

sciatic Relating to the hip or ischium, or to any structure in its vicinity, as the sciatic nerve.

sciatica Any condition characterized by pain along the course of the sciatic nerve; usually a neuritis and generally caused by mechanical compression or irritation of the fifth lumbar spinal root.

scinticisternography A test for diagnosing hydrocephalus and for studying the dynamics of cerebrospinal fluid movement, by use of a radioactive tracer.

scintigraphy Injection of a radioactive substance and determination of its distribution in the tissues with the aid of a scintiscanner.

scintillation A flash of light produced in a chemical crystal by absorption of an ionizing photon; the minuscule flash of light seen on a fluorescent screen results from the spontaneous emission of charged alpha particles across the sensitized surface.

scintillator Scintillation counter; see under counter.

scintiphotography The recording on photographic film of the distribution of an internally administered radioactive substance.

scintiscan A graphic pattern recorded on paper of pulses derived from a radioactive isotope, revealing its concentration in a specific organ or tissue; it serves to outline the tissue or organ or its actively metabolizing portion.

scintiscanner A directional scintillation counter that automatically scans a region of the body to record the concentration of a gamma-ray-emitting isotope in tissue.

scirrhous Relating to a scirrhus; hard.

scirrhus A hard cancerous tumor composed chiefly of fibrous connective tissue.

scissors A double-bladed cutting instrument.

sclera The tough, white membranous tunic, outermost of three, which covers all of the eyeball except the anterior portion, which is occupied by the cornea.

scleradenitis Inflammatory hardening of a gland.

scleral Of or pertaining to the sclera.

sclerectasia Bulging of the sclera.

sclerectomy Surgical removal of a small portion of the sclera, as for the treatment of glaucoma.

scleredema Disease of unknown cause marked by induration and swelling of the skin and subcutaneous tissues.

sclerema Hardening of the skin and underlying tissues.

scleritis Inflammation of the sclera.

annular s. Anterior scleritis that extends around the limbus of the cornea (ring-shaped).

anterior s. Scleritis of the anterior part of the eyeball where the sclera adjoins the limbus of the cornea.

brawny s. Annular scleritis involving the episcleral tissue of the peripheral part of the cornea.

herpetic s. Herpes zoster involving the sclera.

posterior s. Inflammation of the posterior sclera and Tenon's capsule; may also involve the underlying choroid and retina.

pyogenic s. Scleritis caused by a bacterial embolus lodged in a scleral vessel, resulting in an abscess.

sclerochoroidal Relating to both the sclera and choroid, the outer and middle layers of the eyeball.

scleroconjunctival Relating to the sclera and the conjunctiva.

sclerocornea The sclera and cornea considered as a unit.

sclerodactyly Scleroderma affecting the fingers or toes.

scleroderma Progressive thickening and hardening of the skin.

sclerodermatitis, sclerodermitis Inflammation thickening and hardening of the skin.

sclerogenous Producing a hard tissue or substance; causing sclerosis. Also called sclerogenic.

scleroiritis Inflammation of the sclera and iris.

scleroma A circumscribed area of hard or granulation tissue in the skin or mucous membrane.

scleromalacia Extreme thinning of the sclera, occurring in patients with rheumatoid arthritis.

scleronychia Excessively hardened and thickened condition of the nails.

sclero-oophoritis Inflammatory hardening of the ovary. Also called sclero-oothecitis.

sclero-oothecitis See sclero-oophoritis.

sclerophthalmia Rare congenital condition in which scleral tissue encroaches on the cornea, with only a small central area remaining clear.

scleroplasty Reparative surgery of the sclera.

scleroprotein A hard fibrous protein resembling albumin. Also called albuminoid.

sclerose To harden or to become sclerotic.

sclerosis Hardening of tissues due to proliferation

of connective tissue, usually originating in chronic inflammation.

amyotrophic lateral s. A disease characterized by degeneration of the lateral motor tracts of the spinal cord, causing progressive muscular atrophy and exaggerated reflexes.

arterial s. See arteriosclerosis.

endocardial s. Endomyocardial fibroelastosis; see under fibroelastosis.

medical calcific s. Mönckeberg's arteriosclerosis; see under arteriosclerosis.

multiple s. (MS) Disease of the brain and spinal cord affecting mostly young adults and characterized by loss of the fatty sheaths (myelin) that surround nerve fibers; its name is derived from the plaques or patches of scarred (sclerosed) nervous fibers that dot the central nervous system; symptoms vary with distribution of the sclerotic patches, but the most frequently seen are weakness, incoordination, scanning (halting, monosyllabic) speech, involuntary oscillation of the eyeballs (nystagmus), and coarse tremors.

tuberous s. A familial disease marked by progressive mental deterioration, epileptic convulsions, and sometimes sebaceous adenomas of the skin.

sclerostomy Operative creation of a fistulous opening in the sclera, as for the relief of glaucoma.

sclerotherapy Injection of a chemical into a vein to obliterate its lumen; a method of treating varicose veins.

sclerotic **1.** Relating to or characterized by sclerosis. **2.** Of or relating to the sclera or outer layer of the eyeball.

sclerotome In embryology, the cells that break off from the somite, surround the notochord and spinal cord, later differentiate into cartilage, and eventually form the vertebrae.

sclerotomy Surgical incision of the sclera.

sclerous Hardened; indurated; calloused; leatherlike; scarred.

scoleces Plural of scolex.

scolecology See helminthology.

scolex, *pl.* **scoleces** The head of a tapeworm by which it attaches to the mucosa of the small intestine; it is connected by a short and narrow neck to a large number of proglottids (segments).

scoliosis A rotary lateral curvature of the spine.

congenital s. Scoliosis resulting from malformation of the spine or chest.

idiopathic s. Scoliosis of unknown cause.

myopathic s. Scoliosis due to weakness of the spinal muscles.

neuromuscular s. Scoliosis caused by any of various diseases affecting the motor nerve cells.

osteopathic s. Lateral curvature resulting from

Criteria	Score		
	0	1	2
skin color	pale blue	pink body blue extremities	all pink
heart rate	absent	<100	>100
respiratory effort	absent	irregular; slow	good; crying
muscle tone	limp	some flexion of extremities	active
reflex response to nose catheter	limp	grimace	sneeze; cough

scrotum — body of epididymis — septum of scrotum — testis

scorpion

immature goblet cell — build-up of mucin — greatly distended mature cell — goblet cell secretion — epithelial cells

pathologic conditions of the vertebrae, such as tuberculosis, rickets, osteomalacia, and tumors.

static s. Scoliosis due to difference in the length of the legs.

scoliotic Relating to or afflicted with scoliosis.

scopolamine A nonbarbiturate hypnotic alkaloid found in the leaves and seeds of *Hyoscyamus niger* (henbane), *Scopola carniolica*, *Atropa belladonna*, and other solanaceous plants; used to prevent motion sickness; in toxic doses, it can cause excitation, hallucinations, delirium, and other peculiar mental effects; because of its amnestic qualities, it is used with morphine to produce "twilight sleep"; formerly used extensively in obstetrics.

scorbutus See scurvy.

score An evaluative record, usually expressed numerically.

Apgar s. Evaluation of the general condition of a newborn soon after birth; numerical values are assigned to the status of skin color, heart rate, respiratory effort, muscle tone, and reflex irritability; a score of ten denotes a newborn in excellent condition.

scorpion A member of the order Scorpionida having a segmented body and an erectile tail which possesses a venomous sting.

scotochromogens Group II mycobacteria that produce a yellow pigment when grown in the dark and an orange pigment in the presence of light.

scotoma 1. An abnormal blind spot; an area in the visual field in which vision is absent or greatly diminished. 2. In psychiatry, a figurative blind spot in an individual's psychologic awareness characterized by an absence of insight into or inability to grasp a mental problem.

scotomatous Relating to an area of absent or depressed vision (scotoma) in the visual field.

scotometer Instrument used to plot and measure an isolated area of absent or depressed vision (scotoma) in the visual field.

scotopic 1. Relating to vision that is adapted to low levels of illumination. 2. Denoting the low levels of illumination to which the eye's sensitivity to light becomes greatly increased when it is dark-adapted.

scrapie 1. A disease-causing viroid that may represent a missing link between viruses and genes, and may be an agent of extrachromosomal inheritance. 2. A contagious disease of sheep and goats, manifested by various nervous symptoms and usually leading to death.

screen 1. A thin sheet of any material used as a shield. 2. To make a fluoroscopic examination.

fluorescent s. One coated with calcium tungstate crystals, used in the fluoroscope; activation

produces images on screen.

tangent s. A large, usually black screen used in the clinical measurement of the central field of vision.

screening 1. The process of examining large groups of people for a given disease. 2. Survey of a specimen for a variety of substances; e.g., a narcotic screen of a urine sample.

genetic s. Any method of identifying individuals in a given population at high risk of having, or transmitting, a specific genetic disorder.

scrofula Tuberculous inflammation of lymph nodes of the neck in children, caused by *Mycobacterium bovis*; relatively rare in the United States as a result of elimination of tuberculous cattle and pasteurization of milk. Also called cervical adenitis.

scrotal Of or relating to the scrotum.

scrotectomy Surgical removal of part of the scrotum.

scrotitis Inflammation of the scrotum.

scrotocele A complete inguinal hernia which rests in the scrotum. Also called scrotal hernia.

scrotoplasty See oscheoplasty.

scrotum The two-layered sac enclosing the testes and lower part of spermatic cords; composed of skin, muscles, and fascia, and divided on its surface into two portions by a ridge (raphe).

scruff Nape.

scruple A unit of apothecary weight equal to 20 grains or one-third of a dram.

scurvy A nutritional deficiency disease resulting from a lack of vitamin C (ascorbic acid), characterized by spongy, swollen, and bleeding gums, hemorrhages, and extreme weakness. Also called scorbutus.

scute A thin lamina or plate, as the thin bony plate separating the upper part of the middle ear from the mastoid cells.

scybalum An abnormally hard mass of feces in the intestine.

Scyphozoa A class of marine animals (phylum Coelenterata) that includes the jellyfishes.

seal 1. To effect an airtight closure. 2. Any agent used to prevent seepage of air or moisture.

seasickness Nausea, pallor, sweating, and vomiting provoked by the motion of a vessel at sea.

sebaceous Relating to or secreting fatty material (sebum).

seborrhea See dermatitis, seborrheic.

sebum The secretion of a sebaceous gland.

secobarbital A short-acting, fast-onset sedative and hypnotic; Seconal®.

secondary 1. Sequential to something considered primary; e.g., secondary syphilis, a stage of syphilis that must be preceded by the primary stage.

2. Sequential to anything; not primary; e.g., secondary infection, an infection which is superimposed upon an existing condition.

secreta Secretions.

secretagogue, secretogogue 1. A substance that promotes secretion, as of the stomach. 2. Stimulating secretion.

secrete To produce cell products and deliver them into the blood or bodily cavity either through a duct or by direct diffusion.

secretin An intestinal hormone released primarily by the mucosa of the duodenum during digestion; it stimulates the secretion of water and bicarbonate by the pancreas.

secretion 1. The production of a substance by a cell or a gland. 2. The substance produced.

secretogogue See secretagogue.

secretomotor, secretomotory Stimulating secretion; said of certain nerves.

secretor A person whose saliva and other body fluids contain water-soluble forms of the ABO blood group antigens.

secretory Relating to secretion.

sectile Capable of being cut.

section 1. The act of cutting. 2. One of several component segments of a structure. 3. A thin slice of tissue suitable for examination under the microscope. 4. A cut surface.

cesarean s. (CS) Incision through the walls of the abdomen and uterus for delivery of the fetus.

coronal s. A section parallel to the coronal suture of the skull, at right angles to the saggital section.

cross s. A section at right angles to the long axis.

sagittal s. An anteroposterior section which divides the body in more or less equal right and left parts.

serial s. One of several consecutive histologic sections of a structure (e.g., spinal cord) for the purpose of microscopic examination.

secundigravida A woman who has been pregnant twice.

secundines The placenta, umbilical cord, and membranes expelled from the uterus after the birth of the child. Also called the afterbirth.

secundipara A woman who has given birth twice. Also called bipara.

sedate 1. To bring under the influence of a sedative. 2. To administer a sedative to an individual.

sedation The reduction of anxiety or stress by the administration of a sedative drug.

sedative Any agent that slows down nervous activity.

sediment The insoluble material that settles to the bottom of a liquid. Also called hypostasis (that which rises to the surface is called epistasis).

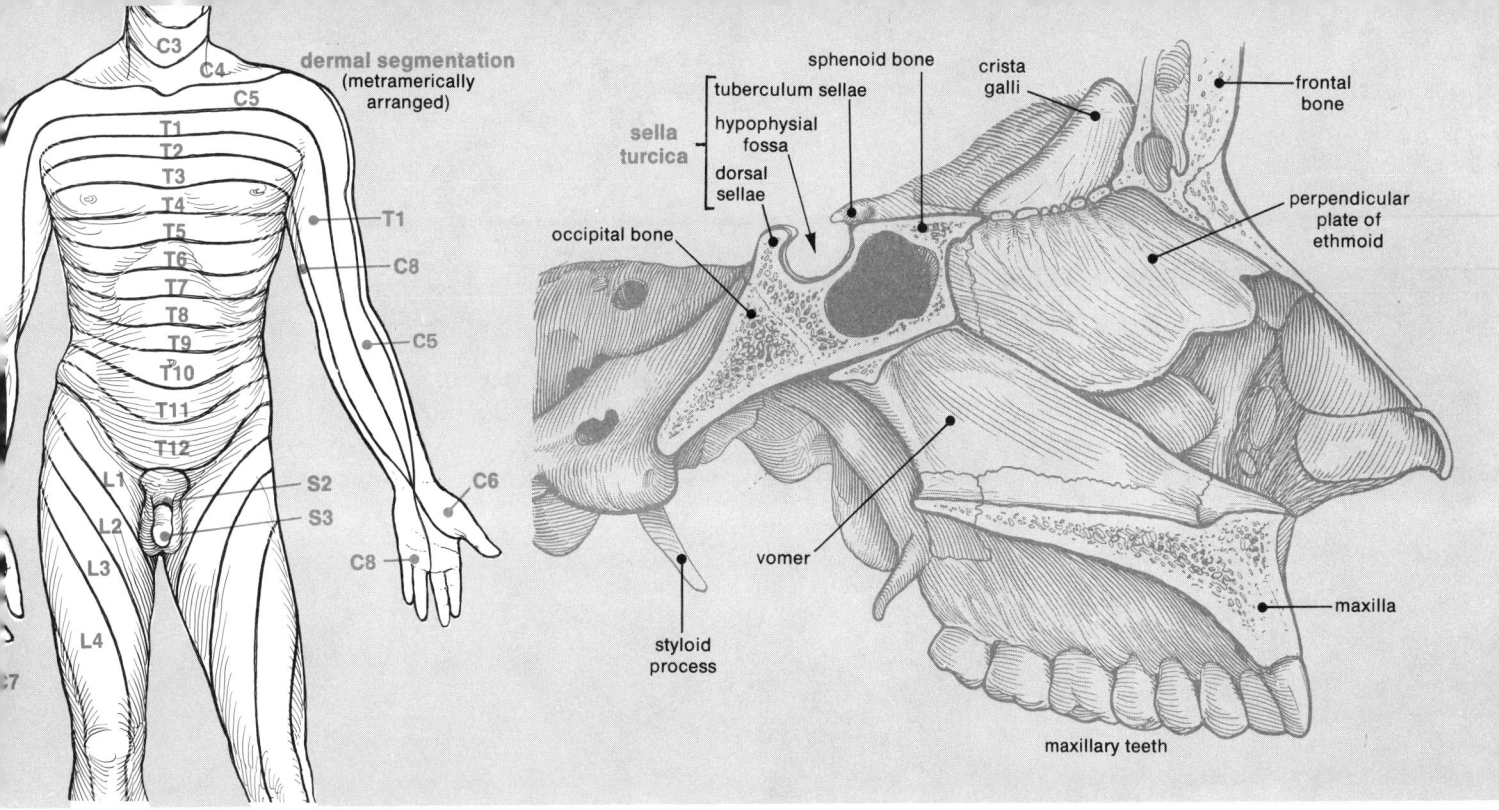

dermal segmentation (metramerically arranged)

C3 C4 C5 T1 T2 T3 T4 T5 T6 T7 T8 T9 T10 T11 T12 L1 L2 L3 L4

T1 C8 C5 C6 C8 S2 S3

sella turcica — tuberculum sellae, hypophysial fossa, dorsal sellae

sphenoid bone
crista galli
frontal bone
perpendicular plate of ethmoid
occipital bone
vomer
styloid process
maxilla
maxillary teeth

urinary s. The solid matter that sinks to the bottom after urine has been allowed to stand for some time or has been centrifuged; microscopic examination of urine is usually performed on sediment resuspended in a few drops of the supernatant urine.

sedimentation The formation of a deposit of insoluble materials at the bottom of a liquid.

sedimenator Centrifuge.

seed The fertilized ovule of a plant.

plantago s.'s The seeds of the herb *Plantago psyllium,* which, when moist, swell and become gelatinous; used as a mild laxative in the treatment of simple constipation.

segment 1. One of the parts into which a structure can be divided. **2.** A differentiated subdivision of an organism or part, as a metamere.

anonymous DNA s. A piece of DNA of unknown gene content that has been localized to a chromosome.

segmentation 1. The process of becoming divided into similar parts. **2.** Cleavage, as of the fertilized ovum.

cutaneous s. See dermal segmentation.

dermal s. The division of the skin into segments (dermatomes) according to the different nervous innervation of each segment. Also called cutaneous segmentation.

segregation In meiosis, the separating of two alleles of a pair of allelic genes so that they can pass to different gametes.

seizure An attack; the sudden onset of a disease or symptoms, especially of epilepsy.

jacksonian s. A form of epilepsy with involuntary clonic motion or sensation.

selection In population genetics, the biologic process that results in preventing some individuals from surviving and in allowing others to do so, with the result that the frequency of particular genes in the population is altered.

artificial s. The purposeful interference by man with natural selection to produce organisms with a desired trait; e.g., breeding of specific strains of cows for the abundant production of milk.

natural s. The biologic process that causes survival and reproduction of those organisms best adjusted to the conditions under which they live.

sexual s. A form of natural selection through which male and female members of a species are attracted by certain traits, thus ensuring the passing of those traits to subsequent generations.

selectivity In pharmacology, a comparative measure of the tendency of one drug to produce several effects; the relationship between the desired and undesired effects of a drug. Cf. potency (2).

selenium An element; symbol Se, atomic number

34, atomic weight 78.96; it resembles sulfur.

self A person's awareness of his own being.

self-abuse Masturbation.

self-accusation Condemning oneself to misery, often because of some trivial error; a psychiatric symptom seen frequently in the depressive phase of manic-depressive psychosis.

self-analysis See autoanalysis.

self-digestion See autodigestion.

self-hypnosis See autohypnosis.

self-infection See autoinfection.

self-limited Denoting a disease that runs a definite course in a specific time, limited by its own characteristics rather than external factors.

self-poisoning 1. Autointoxication. **2.** The intentional or accidental taking of a substance that causes illness or death, especially by chemical means.

sella turcica A depression with two prominences (anterior and posterior) on the upper surface of the sphenoid bone at the base of the skull, resembling a Turkish saddle and housing the pituitary gland.

semeiography See semiography.

semeiology See symptomatology (1).

semelincident Occurring only once; said of certain diseases.

semen A viscous whitish secretion of the male reproductive organs; composed chiefly of sperm, fructose-rich secretions from the seminal vesicles, and secretion from the prostate gland (sperm usually comprises about 10% of the semen). Also called seminal fluid.

semenuria The discharge of seminal fluid with the passage of urine. Also called seminuria; spermaturia.

semicoma A state of impaired responses to stimuli which is not profound and from which a person can be aroused.

semicomatose In a state of unconsciousness or stupor from which one can be aroused.

semiconscious Partly conscious; half-conscious.

semiflexion The position of an extremity midway between extension and flexion.

semilunar Shaped like a half-moon. Also called crescentic.

semimembranous Consisting partly of membrane or fascia.

seminal Of or relating to the semen.

semination Insemination.

seminiferous Conveying semen.

seminoma A malignant testicular neoplasm made up of large cells resembling spermatogonia; it usually metastasizes to paraortic lymph nodes. Also called dysgerminoma of the testis.

ovarian s. See dysgerminoma.

seminuria See semenuria.

semiography A description of the symptoms of a disease. Also written semeiography.

semiology See symptomatology (1).

semipenniform Shaped like a feather on only one side; said of certain muscles.

semipermeable Of, or relating to, a membrane that allows some molecules in a solution to pass through but not others.

semiprone About three-quarters prone, between the midposition and pronation.

semis (ss, s) Latin for half; in prescriptions, it follows the sign indicating the measure.

semisulcus A slight groove on the edge of a structure which, when united with a similar groove of an adjoining structure, forms a complete sulcus.

semisupination A position midway between supination and pronation.

semisupine Lying in semisupination.

semisynthetic Made from chemical reactions in which a naturally occurring substance was used as a starting material.

semitendinous Partly tendinous, as the semitendinous muscle.

Senear-Usher disease or **syndrome** An eruption of scaling macules and blisters resembling both lupus erythematosus and pemphigus vulgaris; occurs on the scalp, face, and trunk. Also called pemphigus erythematosus.

senescence The process of aging or growing old.

senescent Aging; growing old.

senile 1. Characteristic of or resulting from old age. **2.** Exhibiting mental deterioration with old age.

senilism Premature old age or senility, as in progeria.

senility 1. The condition of being senile. **2.** The physical and mental changes associated with old age.

senna The dried leaves of the plants *Cassia acutifolia* or *Cassia angustifolia*; a laxative.

senopia The unaided improvement of near vision in the aged; usually a sign of incipient cataract. Also called second sight; gerontopia.

sensate 1. To perceive through a sense, especially the sense of touch. **2.** One who is so able; referring to a patient who regains sensation after partial paralysis.

sensation The conscious perception of a stimulus acting on any of the organs of sense.

sense 1. The power of perceiving any stimulus. **2.** Any of the special functions of sight, hearing, touch, taste, or smell.

sensibility The capability of perceiving sensations.

sensibile 1. Perceptible by the senses. **2.** Able to feel.

sensimeter An instrument for measuring degrees of cutaneous sensation, as in anesthetized areas.

ascending aorta
section of heart
nasal septum
perpendicular plate of ethmoid bone
septal cartilage
septum secundum
septum primum
right atrium
lef atri
vomer
nasal cartilage
LV
palatine bone
maxilla
scrotum
RV
interventricular septum
septulum of testis
section of heart of developing fetus
septum of scrotum
cross-section of testes

sensitive 1. A state of increased capacity to respond specifically to an antigen or hapten. 2. Responsive to external stimulation. 3. Easily irritated or altered by the action of some agents. 4. Susceptible, as to the action of an antibiotic.

sensitivity 1. The state of being sensitive; often implying a keen perception of, or responsiveness to, a stimulus. 2. Applied to a screening test: The proportion of persons who truly have a disease in a screened population, and who are identified as such by the screening test.

disk s. A measurement of the susceptibility of a bacterial species to a variety of antibiotics placed on the culture medium in the form of disks; the sensitivity is measured by the area of inhibition of growth produced by the antibiotic disk.

sensitization The process of increasing the reactivity of a subject, usually to specific antibodies or immune cells.

sensitize To render sensitive; to increase the specific reactivity of a subject to an agent.

sensorimotor Both sensory and motor; said of certain nerves.

sensorium In psychiatry, the state of mental clarity and consciousness at a given time.

sensory Relating to sensation; said of a nerve.

separator 1. Instrument used to separate two teeth, so as to gain access to adjacent surfaces. 2. A substance applied to a surface to prevent other material from adhering to that surface.

Sephadex Proprietary name for gel particles composed of cross-linked dextrans; used as molecular sieves in gel filtration.

sepsis Presence in the blood of pus-forming microorganisms or their toxins.

septa Plural of septum.

septal Of, or relating to, a septum.

septate Divided into compartments by a septum.

septation The formation of thin dividing walls or septa.

septectomy Surgical removal of part of the nasal septum.

septic Relating to sepsis.

septicemia Systemic disease caused by the presence of pathogenic microorganisms in the body.

septivalent Having a valency of seven.

septomarginal Relating to the margin of a partition or septum.

septonasal Relating to the nasal septum.

septotome An instrument for incising the nasal septum.

septotomy Surgical incision of a septum.

septulum, *pl.* **septula** Latin for a minute partition or septum.

septum, *pl.* **septa** A thin wall dividing two bodily cavities or masses of soft tissue.

interalveolar s. One of the bony partitions between the tooth sockets.

interatrial s. The partition between the atria of the heart.

interventricular s. The musculomembranous wall dividing the ventricles of the heart. Also called ventricular septum.

nasal s. The thin wall dividing the nasal cavities, composed posteriorly of bone and anteriorly of cartilage.

rectovaginal s. The thin layer of fascia separating the vagina from the anterior wall of the rectum.

s. lucidum See septum pellucidum.

s. of scrotum The layer of fascia dividing the scrotum into two completely separate sacs, each containing a testis.

s. pellucidum A thin triangular partition between the anterior portions of lateral ventricles of the brain; it is composed of the two laminae and is attached to the undersurface and reflected portion of the corpus callosum and to the fornix. Also called septum lucidum.

s. primum In embryology, the sickle-shaped partition that initiates the division of the single atrial cavity of the embryonic heart into right and left chambers.

s. secundum The sickle-shaped partition appearing on the roof of the right atrium of the embryonic heart, adjacent to the septum primum; it never closes completely; its unclosed area forms the foramen ovale.

sequel, sequela, *pl.* **sequels, sequelae** Any abnormal condition following and caused by another disease.

sequencer, protein An instrument that sequentially removes amino acids from the parent protein chain in order to determine the composition and structure of the protein.

sequester 1. To undergo sequestration. 2. To detach, separate, or isolate.

sequestration 1. The formation of a sequestrum. 2. The isolation of a person with a contagious disease. 3. An increase in the quantity of blood within the blood vessels, occurring physiologically or produced artificially.

bronchopulmonary s. Congenital anomaly marked by the presence of an independent mass of lung tissue having its own bronchial branch and artery (a branch from the thoracic aorta).

sequestrectomy The surgical removal of a dead bone fragment that has become separated from the surrounding healthy bone.

sequestrum A piece of dead bone that has become separated from the surrounding healthy bone

tissue.

sera Plural of serum.

series A group of related events, objects, or compounds, arranged systematically.

aromatic s. Compounds derived from benzene.

erythrocytic s. The group of cells in various stages of development that ultimately form red blood cells.

fatty s. The series of saturated open-chain hydrocarbons, denoted by the suffix *-ane* (methane, ethane, propane, etc.). Also called methane or paraffin series.

granulocytic s. The cells in various stages of development, culminating in the formation of granulocytes.

homologous s. A succession of organic compounds, each one differing from the preceding one by a radical or atomic group such as CH_2.

lymphocytic s. Cells in different stages of development leading to the formation of mature lymphocytes.

serine (Ser) A nonessential amino acid; one of the hydrolysis products of proteins.

seriograph Instrument for taking a series of six to eight radiographic exposures; used in radiography of the cerebral blood vessels.

seriscission Division of soft tissue, as the pedicle of a tumor, by a silk ligature.

seroconversion A change in immunologic reactivity of the serum from negative to positive for a particular antibody; most commonly refers to one of the serologic tests for syphilis.

serocystic Composed of, or relating to, cysts containing serous fluid.

serodiagnosis Diagnosis by means of reactions tested in the blood stream. Also called orthodiagnosis.

seroenteritis Inflammation of the serous or peritoneal coat of the intestine.

serofibrinous Containing serum and fibrin; said of a discharge or exudate.

serofibrous Relating to both a serous membrane and a fibrous tissue.

seroimmunity Passive immunity; see under immunity.

serologic Relating to serology.

serology 1. The study of serum, especially with respect to immunity phenomena. 2. Commonly used to refer to a serologic test for syphilis.

seroma A tumor-like mass formed by the collection of serum in the tissues, usually in a wound site.

seromembranous Relating to a serous membrane.

seromucous Composed of serum and a mucinous material.

serotonin

$NH_2-CH_2-CH_2-C$ ... OH (serotonin chemical structure)

serrefine

composition of **serum**

PO₄⁼ SO₄⁼ → $PO_4^= SO_4^=$

protein
nonprotein organic anion
CO_2
Cl^-
Na^+
Mg^{++}
Ca^{++}
K^+

sesamoid

bones of hand

musculo-cutaneous nerve
median nerve
radial nerve
ulnar nerve
lateral portion of **axillary sheath**

orthopedic plaster **shears**

---

seropurulent Containing serum and pus; said of a discharge.

seropus Serum mixed with pus.

serosa Any smooth membrane, such as that covering the intestines, composed of a mesothelial layer and a layer of connective tissue.

serosanguinous Containing serum and blood; said of an exudate or discharge.

seroserous Relating to two or more serous membranes.

serositis Inflammation of a serous membrane.
multiple s. See polyserositis.

serosynovitis Inflammation of the synovial membrane of a joint with effusion of serum.

serotonin 5-Hydroxytryptamine; $C_{10}H_{12}N_2O$; a stimulant of smooth muscle contraction; occurs predominantly in the gastrointestinal mucosa, in small amounts in blood platelets, and in the brain; also found in carcinoid tumors.

serotype A taxonomic subdivision of bacteria based on the antigenic characteristics of the microorganisms.

serous Relating to, resembling, secreting, or containing serum.

serovaccination Combination of injection of serum to produce passive immunity and vaccination to produce active immunity.

serpiginous Creeping; denoting an ulcer or skin lesion that heals at one margin while spreading on the opposite side.

serpigo 1. Ringworm. 2. Herpes. 3. Any creeping eruption.

Serratia Genus of motile gram-negative, rod-shaped bacteria (family Enterobacteriaceae) which thrive in decaying organic matter and produce a characteristic red pigment.
S. marcesscens Species found in soil, water, and food; occasionally found in pathologic specimens in which the red pigment produced suggests erroneously the presence of blood; e.g., in sputum; a cause of hospital acquired infection, especially in patients with impaired immunity.

serrate, serrated Notched.

serration 1. The state of having a sawlike edge. 2. A series of toothlike projections.

serrefine A fine clamp; a small surgical spring forceps, usually used for clamping blood vessels.

serrulate, serrulated Having small notches.

serum, *pl.* **serums, sera** 1. The clear fluid of blood, devoid of fibrinogen and cells. 2. Loosely used term denoting serum that contains antitoxins, used for therapeutic or laboratory diagnostic purposes.
anticomplementary s. A serum that destroys complement.

antilymphocyte s. (ALS) A serum used to inhibit rejection of grafts or organ transplants.

antitoxic s. One containing antibodies to the toxins of a disease-causing microorganism.

blood s. The clear, fluid portion of blood that is left after fibrinogen (a protein) and the cellular elements of blood are removed by coagulation; distinguished from plasma, which is the cell-free liquid portion of uncoagulated blood.

convalescent s. Blood serum from a person recovering from an infectious disease.

polyvalent s. A serum containing antibodies against more than one strain of a microorganism.

truth s. A name for certain chemicals (sodium amobarbital and sodium thiopental) administered intravenously to facilitate questioning of an individual who is unwilling or unable to answer queries; a misnomer since the subject's revelations elicited under the influence of the drug are not necessarily factually true.

serum sickness Generalized allergic reaction to a foreign serum or to a drug; characterized by fever, skin rash, enlarged lymph nodes, and painful joints.

servomechanism 1. An automatic control device used to maintain the operation of a mechanical system. 2. A self-regulatory biologic process.

sesamoid Resembling a grain of sesame; denoting a small bone that is embedded in a tendon or in a joint capsule; it is found mainly in the hands and feet; the patella (kneecap) is the largest such bone in the body.

sessile Attached by a broad base rather than by a peduncle; applied to certain polyps.

set 1. To put into a position that will restore function; said of a fractured bone. 2. Denoting plastic material after it has hardened or jelled.

seta A short bristle-like hair or structure.

setaceous 1. Having bristles or setae. 2. Resembling a bristle.

setting Hardening, as of plaster of Paris.

setup The arrangement of artificial teeth on a trial denture base, preliminary to construction of an appliance.

sex The classification of organisms as male or female by means of their reproductive characteristics.
chromosomal s. An individual's sex determined by the presence or absence of the Y chromosome in the spermatozoon at the time of its union with the ovum.

genetic s. Chromosomal sex.

morphologic s. Sex determined by the morphology of the external genitalia.

sex-influence The occurrence of autosomal traits predominantly in one sex, either male or female.

sexivalent Having the combining power of six

hydrogen atoms.

sex limitation The occurrence of autosomal traits in one sex only, either male or female.

sex linkage See under linkage.

sex-linked Determined by a gene that is carried on the X chromosome; said of a trait; often used synonymously with X-linked, but as a Y-linked trait is also sex-linked, the preferred term is X-linked.

sexology The study of the sexes and their relationship.

sextan Denoting a malarial paroxysm recurring every sixth day.

sexual 1. Relating to or endowed with sex. 2. Causing erotic desires.

sexuality The state of having sexual characteristics, experiences, and behaviors.
infantile s. In psychoanalysis, the capacity of the infant and child to have experiences of a sexual nature.

Sézary syndrome Erythroderma associated with infiltration of the skin by atypical cells, believed to be of T-lymphocyte origin, which spill into the blood.

shadow-casting A method of increasing the visibility of ultramicroscopic specimens under the microscope by coating them with a film of carbon, platinum, or chromium.

shaft The rodlike portion of a structure, such as that of a long bone.

shakes 1. Colloquial term for severe chills, especially those of malarial fever. 2. A popular name for the tremor associated with withdrawal from acute alcoholism.

shank The anterior part of the human leg, from the knee to the ankle.

shears Large double-bladed cutting instrument, similar to a pair of scissors.

sheath An enveloping structure.
axillary s. A tubular, fibrous membrane encasing the large vessels and nerves of the arm (axillary artery and vein and brachial plexus); located between the clavicle (collarbone) and the first rib.

carotid s. A tubular sheath enclosing the carotid artery, internal jugular vein, and vagus nerve; extends from the base of the skull to the first rib and sternum (breastbone).

femoral s. A funnel-shaped sheath located in the groin below the inguinal ligament and divided into three compartments by two vertical partitions; the lateral compartment contains the femoral artery, the middle one contains the femoral vein, and the medial one (femoral canal) contains lymphatic vessels and a lymph node. Also called crural sheath.

Henle's s. See endoneurium.

medullary s. Myelin sheath.

cross section of axon of nerve cell

myelin sheath (jelly-roll configuration)

Schwann cell

nucleus

nipple shield

breast shield

superior vena cava

right atrium

septal defect

right ventricle

section of heart

left atrium

left-to-right shunt

myelin s. The multiple-layered covering of many of the axons of both central and peripheral nerves; composed of lipid and protein molecules, and serving mainly to increase the velocity of conduction of nerve impulses.

s.'s of optic nerve The three sheaths (dura, arachnoid, and pia) surrounding the optic nerve; continuous with the membranes of the brain.

s. of Schwann See neurilemma.

synovial tendon s. A double-layered sheath forming a closed sac; one layer surrounds the tunnel through which the tendon passes, the other covers the surface of the tendon; serves to facilitate the gliding of tendons through fibrous and bony tunnels.

Sheehan's disease or **syndrome** Hypopituitarism due to postpartum pituitary necrosis, usually following hemorrhage and shock during delivery; results in failure to lactate, absence of menstrual function, loss of hair, cold intolerance, atrophy of sex organs, and wrinkling of the skin; a specific form of panhypopituitarism.

sheet, draw A folded sheet placed under the buttocks of a bedridden patient, with its long axis across the bed, to facilitate its removal without lifting the patient.

shelf A structure in the body resembling a shelf.

rectal s. A shelf occurring in the rectum due to infiltration by neoplasm or inflammation. Also called Blumer's shelf.

shield 1. A means of protection, such as a lead rubber apron or sheet used to protect an individual from radiation. 2. A dense substance that encloses radioisotopes in order to reduce the amount of radiation that escapes into the area. 3. To protect from radiation or other toxic agents.

breast s. A rubber cap or dome, used to protect inflamed or irritated nipples from contact with clothing.

Buller's s. A watchglass in a frame of adhesive tape secured over the unaffected eye to protect it from the infected eye.

embryonic s. A swelling of the embryonic blastoderm within which the primitive streak appears.

eye s. A protective covering for the eye.

nipple s. A round glass or plastic plate with a short central projecting tube to which a rubber nipple is attached; used over sore nipples during nursing so that the pressure from the infant's mouth is attenuated by the resistance of the rubber nipple.

shift A change.

axis s. See deviation, axis.

Doppler s. The magnitude of the frequency change with the velocity of motion in the Doppler effect.

s. to the left Increased percentage of young neu-

trophils in the blood.

threshold s. A deviation in decibels from an individual's previous audiogram, indicating loss of hearing.

Shigella A genus of nonmotile, gram-negative bacteria (family Enterobacteriaceae) that is the principal cause of human dysentery; divided into four major groups (A, B, C, and D) and subdivided serologically into different types.

S. dysenteriae Group A species, a particularly virulent form that causes dysentery in man; found in the excreta of infected individuals or convalescent carriers.

S. flexneri Group B species, one of the commonest causes of dysentery epidemics and sometimes of infantile gastroenteritis.

S. sonnei Group D species, a cause of mild dysentery in man and summer diarrheal disorders in children.

shigellosis Acute infection of the bowel caused by *Shigella* organisms, often occurring in epidemic patterns; characterized by frequent passage of stools containing blood, pus, and mucus and accompanied by cramps, tenesmus, and fever.

shin The anterior portion of the leg below the knee.

shin splints Irritation or inflammation of the extensor muscles of the lower lateral area of the legs caused by an unusually great adduction of the legs and aggravated by overexercise.

shinbone See tibia.

shingles See herpes zoster.

shiver To shudder or shake, especially from a chill produced by fever-induced decreased skin temperature.

shock A severe physiologic reaction to bodily trauma characterized by pale clammy skin, diminished blood pressure, weak rapid pulse, and sometimes unconsciousness.

anaphylactic s. Violent reactions, sometimes accompanied by a rash, following injection of a foreign protein to which the individual has been previously sensitized.

cardiogenic s. Shock due to the sudden reduction of the cardiac output, as in myocardial infarction.

counter s. See countershock.

deferred s., delayed s. Shock occurring a number of hours after the injury.

electric s. The effects of the passage of an electric current through any part of the body.

endotoxin s., endotoxic s. Septic shock caused by toxins produced and released by bacteria.

histamine s. Shock produced by the injection of histamine.

hypovolemic s. Shock produced by reduction of

blood volume, as in hemorrhage.

insulin s. Shock resulting from a sudden reduction of blood sugar caused by an overdose of insulin.

irreversible s. Shock that does not respond to any form of treatment.

neurogenic s. Shock due to the action of the nervous system immediately after injury.

primary s. Shock appearing immediately after a severe injury, mainly due to anxiety, pain, etc.

septic s. Shock due to severe infection, particularly with gram-negative bacilli.

spinal s. Loss of spinal reflexes after injury to the spinal cord, manifested in the muscles innervated by the nerves situated below the injury.

shoe An outer covering for the human foot having a durable sole and heel.

Scarpa's s. A metal brace that prevents plantar extension of the foot beyond a right angle; used in treating talipes equinus.

short bowel syndrome Condition that occurs following removal of an extensive segment of small intestine, characterized by intractable diarrhea with impaired absorption of fats and other nutrients.

shortsightedness See myopia.

shoshin The acute fulminating form of cardiovascular beriberi. See also beriberi.

shoulder The region where arm and trunk meet.

shoulder blade See scapula.

shoulder-hand syndrome Pain and stiffness of the shoulder and hand, sometimes with late atrophy of hand muscles; usually associated with neck or upper arm injuries or with myocardial infarction; thought to be a reflex sympathetic dystrophy.

show The discharge from the vagina of blood-stained mucus indicating the onset of labor; it is caused by the expulsion of the mucus plug that has filled the cervical canal during pregnancy.

shunt 1. To bypass or divert. 2. A passage between two natural channels; may be congenital, as a defect between the two atria of the heart, or a surgical anastomosis to divert blood from one part of the body to another or to divert intestinal contents from one portion of the intestinal tract to another.

left-to-right s. Diversion of blood from the left to the right side of the heart (through a septal defect) or from the systemic to the pulmonary circulation (through a patent ductus arteriosus).

LeVeen peritoneovenous s. A device to restore ascitic fluid to the circulation; plastic tubing, equipped with a valve, is inserted into the peritoneal cavity, tunneled under the skin and connected to a large vein in the neck. The Denver variation of the LeVeen shunt has a valved chamber that is manually compressible.

metabolic s. Catabolism of a substance by an

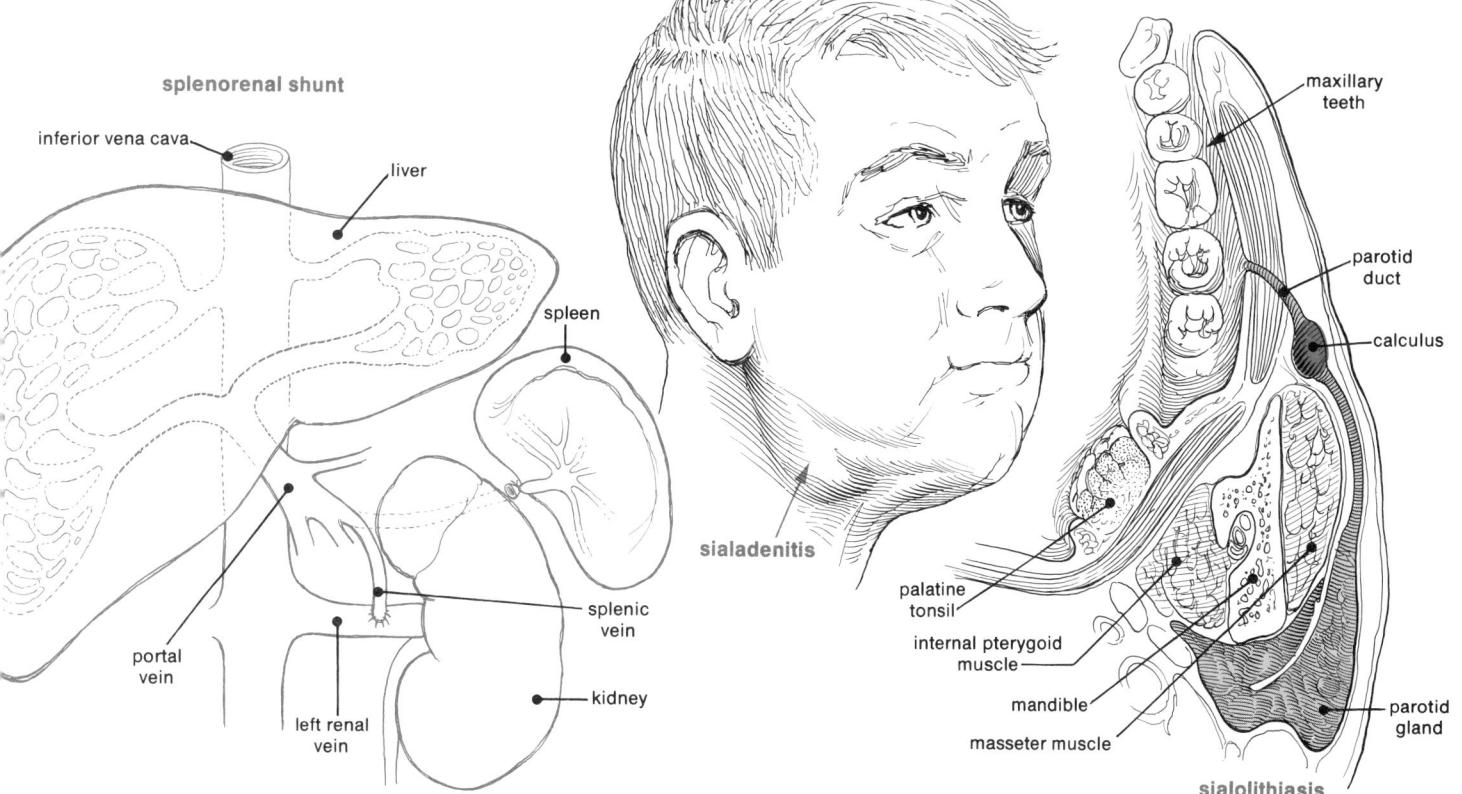

splenorenal shunt

inferior vena cava

liver

spleen

splenic vein

portal vein

left renal vein

kidney

sialadenitis

maxillary teeth

parotid duct

calculus

palatine tonsil

internal pterygoid muscle

mandible

masseter muscle

parotid gland

sialolithiasis

alternate pathway.

monophosphate s. See pathway, pentose phosphate.

pentose s. See pathway, pentose phosphate.

portacaval s. Any communication between the portal vein and the systemic veins; surgical anastomosis between the portal and caval veins.

reversed s. See right-to-left shunt.

right-to-left s. The passage of unoxygenated venous blood from the right heart into the arterial circulation without passing through the lungs. Also called reversed shunt.

splenorenal s. Surgical anastomosis between the splenic vein and the left renal vein.

Shy-Drager syndrome A rare condition, resembling parkinsonism, characterized by tremors, muscular wasting, atrophy of the iris, ocular palsies, and ortho-static hypotension.

sialadenitis Inflammation of a salivary gland.

sialadenotropic Influencing the activity of salivary glands.

sialaporia Deficient secretion of saliva.

sialectasis Dilatation of a salivary duct.

sialic Salivary.

sialic acids A group of naturally occurring derivatives of a 9-carbon, 3-deoxy-5-amino sugar acid; present in bacteria and in animal tissue as constituents of lipids, polysaccharides, and mucoproteins.

sialism, sialismus Sialorrhea.

sialoadenectomy Surgical removal of a salivary gland.

sialoadenitis Sialadenitis.

sialoadenotomy Incision of a salivary gland.

sialoangiectasis 1. Condition in which a salivary duct is vastly dilated by stagnated saliva, usually resulting from an obstructive stone or ductal constriction. 2. Dilatation of salivary ducts, usually by means of bougies.

sialoangiitis Inflammation of a salivary duct.

sialodochitis Inflammation of the duct of a salivary gland.

sialodochoplasty Repair of a salivary duct.

sialogenous Producing saliva.

sialogogue An agent that promotes the secretion of saliva.

sialogram A roentgenogram of one or more salivary ducts, produced by sialography. Also called sialograph.

sialograph See sialogram.

sialography Roentgenographic examination of the salivary glands and ducts after the injection of radiopaque material into the ducts; an invaluable technique for determining the presence and location of an obstruction in the ducts and the condition of the salivary acini.

sialolith A salivary calculus. Also called ptyalolith.

sialolithiasis Presence of a calculus in the salivary gland or duct. Also called ptyalolithiasis.

sialolithotomy Surgical incision of a salivary duct or gland for the removal of a calculus. Also called ptyalolithotomy.

sialorrhea An excessive flow of saliva for any reason, including teething, mental retardation, ill-fitting dental appliances, mercurialism, periodontic disease, and acute inflammation of the mouth. Also called salivation.

sialoschesis Suppression of the secretion of saliva. Also called dry mouth.

sialosis Salivation (1).

sialostenosis Stricture or stenosis of a salivary duct.

sialosyrinx 1. A salivary fistula. 2. A syringe for cleansing the salivary ducts. 3. A salivary duct drainage tube.

sibilant Hissing or whistling; said of a rale.

sibilus A hissing or whistling sound heard on auscultation.

sibling One of two or more children having one, but especially both, parents in common.

sibship Relationship between children of the same parents; occasionally used to denote all blood relatives.

siccant Drying.

sicca syndrome See Sjögren's syndrome.

siccolabile Destroyed by drying.

siccostabile Not destroyed by drying.

siccus Latin for dry.

sick 1. Ill. 2. Nauseated. 3. Mentally disturbed.

sickle cell disease See anemia, sickle cell. See also sickle cell trait, under trait.

sickle cell C disease Hemolytic anemia present in patients who are heterozygous for hemoglobin S and C.

sickle form See crescent, malarial.

sicklemia Outmoded term, formerly used to denote any sickle cell disorder.

sickling The production of sickle-shaped blood cells.

sickness Disease.

African sleeping s. Disease of the central nervous system caused by protozoans of the genus *Trypanosoma*, transmitted by several species of tsetse flies (genus *Glossina*). Also called African trypanosomiasis.

air s. Motion sickness occurring during travel in aircraft flying at low altitude where the atmosphere is most turbulent.

altitude s. Condition marked by giddiness, headache, difficult rapid breathing on exertion, insomnia, and nausea; experienced by some unacclimatized

individuals within a few hours after exposure to high altitude. Also called mountain sickness.

car s. Motion sickness brought about by riding in an automobile or on a train.

decompression s. See caisson disease.

morning s. Nausea and/or vomiting sometimes occurring during early pregnancy.

motion s. A group of symptoms such as pallor, sweating, excessive salivation, nausea, and frequently vomiting, occurring in persons riding in airplanes, automobiles, ships, or trains and occasionally in children riding on playground equipment; caused by stimulation of the semicircular canals and/or certain psychic factors.

mountain s. See altitude sickness.

radiation s. Illness caused by excessive exposure to ionizing radiation; massive exposure usually causes symptoms occurring in four stages: (a) nausea, vomiting, and sometimes diarrhea and weakness; (b) a period of relative well being; (c) fever, loss of appetite, nausea, abdominal distention, bloody diarrhea, and loss of hair (death usually occurs during this stage); (d) those who survive experience temporary sterility and eventually develop cataracts.

sea s. Seasickness.

serum s. An immune response following injection of a foreign serum, marked by fever, skin eruptions, edema, and painful joints.

sleeping s. African sleeping sickness.

sick-sinus syndrome (SSS) A syndrome caused by failure of the sinus node to maintain normal rhythmicity; characterized by chaotic atrial activity with continual changes in P wave contour, bradycardia interspersed with multiple and recurring ectopic beats, and by runs of atrial or nodal tachycardia. Also called sick sinus node.

side effect See under effect.

sideroblast An immature red blood cell containing granules of iron.

siderocyte A red blood cell having iron-containing granules.

sideroderma Brownish discoloration of the skin of the legs caused by accumulation of hemosiderin deposits.

siderofibrosis Abnormal formation of fibrous tissue associated with multiple small deposits of iron.

sideropenia Iron deficiency, especially in the blood and bone marrow.

siderophil A cell or tissue that has an affinity for iron.

siderophilin See transferrin.

siderosis 1. Pneumoconiosis due to inhalation of iron dust. 2. Deposit of iron dust or particles in a tissue.

s. bulbi Rusty discoloration of the eyeball caused

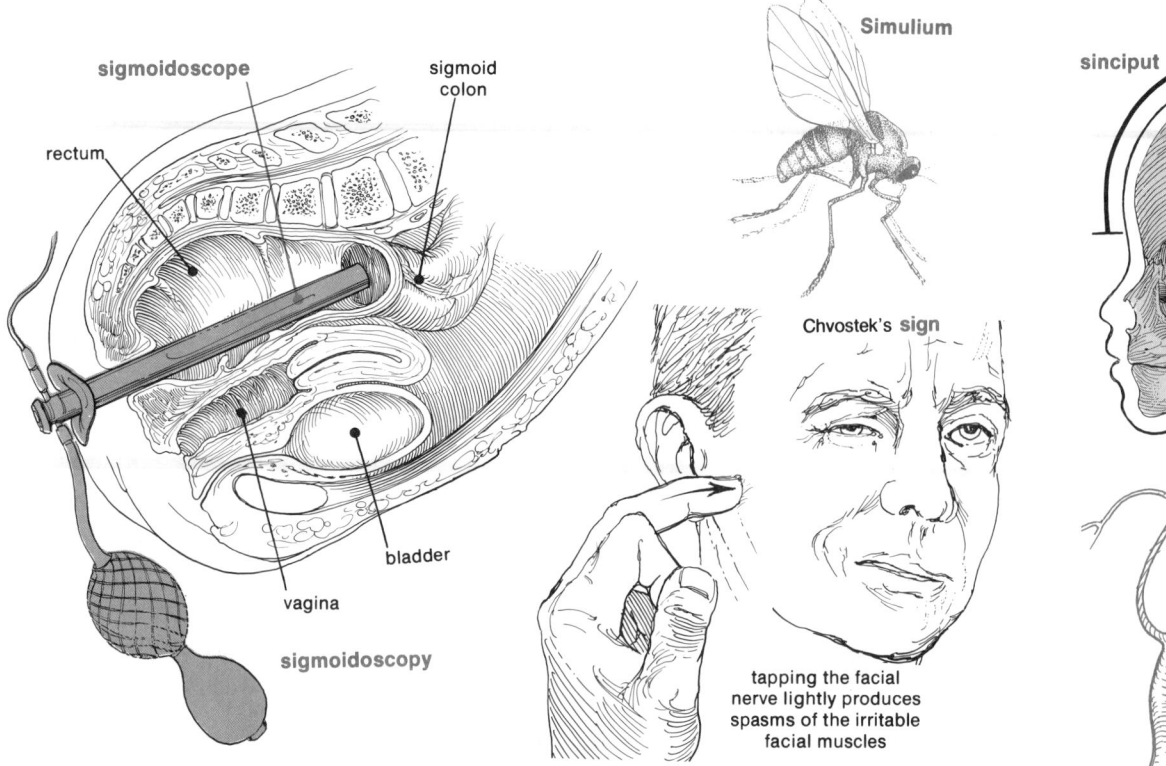

sigmoidoscope   sigmoid colon

rectum

bladder

vagina

sigmoidoscopy

Simulium

Chvostek's sign

tapping the facial
nerve lightly produces
spasms of the irritable
facial muscles

sinciput

newborn
skull

aortic
sinus

coron
arte

by the prolonged presence of an iron foreign body in the eye.

sigh 1. A deep audible inspiration and expiration made involuntarily under the influence of some emotion or an anesthetic. **2.** To emit such a sound.

sight The ability to see.

    day s. See nyctalopia.

    far s. See hyperopia.

    near s. See myopia.

    night s. See hemeralopia.

    old s. See presbyopia.

    second s. See senopia.

sigmatism Inability to pronounce sibilant (s, sh) sounds correctly.

sigmoid Having the shape of the letter S.

sigmoidectomy Surgical removal of part of the sigmoid colon; excision of the sigmoid flexure.

sigmoidopexy Suturing of the sigmoid colon to the abdominal wall for the correction of a prolapsed rectum.

sigmoidoscope An instrument for inspecting the interior of the sigmoid colon.

sigmoidoscopy Inspection of the interior of the sigmoid colon by means of an instrument (sigmoidoscope).

sigmoidotomy Surgical incision of the sigmoid colon.

sign 1. Any objective evidence indicative of disease, perceptible to the examiner, as compared to subjective sensations (symptoms) of the patient. For individual signs, see specific names. **2.** An indication of continued existence.

    vital s.'s (VS) Breathing, heart beat, and blood pressure; the signs of life.

signa (Sig. or S.) Latin for write, or set a mark upon; used in prescriptions to introduce the signature.

signature The part of a pharmaceutical prescription containing instruction to the patient for the use of the medication. Also called transcription. See also superscription, inscription, and subscription.

significant In statistics, anything that is probably not the result of chance.

silica Silicon dioxide, SiO_2; a white or colorless crystalline compound; one of the three major ingredients of dental porcelain.

silicate A salt of silicic acid.

silicic acid Generally, any acid containing silicon.

silicious Resembling, relating to, or containing silica.

silicon A nonmetallic element abundantly present in the earth's crust in silica and silicates; symbol Si, atomic number 14, atomic weight 28.09.

silicone Any of a group of semiorganic polymers marked by physiochemical inertness and a high degree of water repellence and lubricity; used in prosthetic replacement of bodily parts, protective coatings, and adhesives.

silicosis Fibrosis of the lungs caused by prolonged inhalation of silica dust (stone dust, SiO_2); a pneumoconiosis. Also called stone mason's disease; potters' phthisis.

silicotuberculosis Silicosis associated with tuberculosis.

silk The fine lustrous fiber produced by the silkworm to make its cocoon.

    surgical s. Thread made from the cocoon fiber of the mulberry silkworm; used as suture material in surgical operations.

silver A lustrous white, malleable, ductile metallic element; symbol Ag (from the Latin *argentum*), atomic number 47, atomic weight 107.87.

    s. nitrate A caustic colorless crystalline compound, $AgNO_3$, which becomes grayish black when exposed to light; used in solution as an antiseptic in the eyes of the newborn.

Simmond's disease See panhypopituitarism.

simulation 1. Imitation; said of a disease or symptom that resembles or mimics another. **2.** A feigning or pretending. Also called malingering.

simulator A device designed to produce effects simulating or approximating actual conditions.

    patient s. A functional replica of a bodily part.

    space s. A hermetically sealed chamber with human or animal subjects at ground level, used to study some of the physiologic effects of space traveling.

Simulium A genus of biting black gnats (family Simuliidae), some species of which transmit onchocerciasis.

sincipital Relating to the forehead and upper part of the head.

sinciput 1. The upper anterior part of the head from the forehead to the crown. **2.** The top of the skull where the sagittal and coronal sutures meet. Also called bregma.

sine (s, ŝ) Latin for without; used in prescription writing.

sine (sin) A trigonometric ratio between parts of a triangle; in a right triangle, it is the side opposite an acute angle divided by the side opposite the right angle (hypotenuse); graphed with two coordinates, the values produce a sinusoid or sine curve with the equation $y = \sin x$.

sinew A tendon.

singlet A single member, as a single microtubule in the middle of a cilium.

singultation Hiccupping.

singultus A hiccup.

sinister (s) Latin for left.

sinistral 1. Of or relating to the left side. **2.** Left-handed.

sinistrality Left-handedness.

sinistrocardia Displacement of the heart toward the left, beyond its normal position.

sinistrocerebral Relating to the left hemisphere of the brain.

sinistrocular 1. Having better vision in the left eye. **2.** Relating to dominance of the left eye.

sinistropedal Using the left foot in preference to the right.

sinoatrial, sinoauricular (S-A) Relating to the sinus venosus and the right atrium of the heart; especially the sinus (S-A) node.

sinus 1. A mucus-lined, air-filled cavity in one of the cranial bones which communicates with the nasal cavity. **2.** A dilated channel for the passage of blood or lymph which lacks the coats of an ordinary vessel; applied especially to those of the dura; e.g., cavernous sinus. **3.** An abnormal fistula or tract.

    aortic s. Any of the three slight dilatations of the aorta between each semilunar valve and the wall of the aorta. Also called sinus of Valsalva.

    carotid s. A slight dilatation of the most proximal part of the internal carotid artery containing in its wall pressoreceptors which, when stimulated by changes in blood pressure, cause slowing of the heart, vasodilation, and a fall in blood pressure. Also called carotid bulb.

    cavernous s. A paired, irregularly shaped venous sinus in the dura mater on each side of the body of the sphenoid bone in the middle cranial fossa; it drains the superior ophthalmic vein, superficial middle cerebral vein, and sphenoparietal sinus; it empties by way of the petrosal sinuses into the transverse sinus and internal jugular vein.

    cerebral s.'s See dura mater sinuses.

    circular s. 1. A venous ring around the hypophysis (pituitary gland) formed by the anterior and posterior intercavernous sinuses communicating with the cavernous sinus. Also called Ridley's sinus. **2.** The venous sinus at the periphery of the placenta. **3.** The scleral venous sinus of the eye.

    coronary s. The short venous sinus receiving most of the veins of the heart, situated in the posterior part of the coronary sulcus between the left atrium and the ventricle; it opens into the right atrium between the inferior vena cava and the atrioventricular orifice.

    dermal s. A congenital sinus tract lined with skin and usually extending from the skin to the spinal canal.

    dura mater s.'s The venous sinuses in the dura mater; e.g., cavernous, superior sagittal, and transverse. Also called cerebral sinuses.

nasal cavity

ethmoid sinuses

cavernous sinus

sphenoid sinus

superior sagittal sinus

inferior sagittal sinus

straight sinus

transverse sinus

occipital sinus

sigmoid sinus

great cerebral vein

cerebrum

urachal sinus

bladder

sagittal section of newborn

epididymal s. A narrow slitlike recess between the upper part of the testis and the overlying epididymis; formed by the invagination of the tunica vaginalis.

ethmoid s. Any of the air cells of the ethmoid bone.

frontal s. One of the paired sinuses in the lower part of the frontal bone; it communicates by way of the nasofrontal duct (infundibulum) with the nasal cavity of the same side.

jugular s.'s Two slight dilatations of the internal jugular vein; a superior one located at its origin near the base of the skull and an inferior one near its termination, just before it unites with the subclavian vein.

lactiferous duct s. The spindle-shaped dilated portion of the lactiferous duct of the mammary gland, just before it enters the nipple.

lymphatic s. Irregular, tortuous channels of a lymph node through which a continuous flow of lymph passes on its way to the efferent lymphatic vessels.

marginal s. of placenta A discontinuous, circumferential venous sinus at the margin of the placenta.

maxillary s. A mucus-lined air cavity in the body of the maxilla on either side, communicating with the middle meatus of the nasal cavity.

occipital s. The smallest of the sinuses of the dura mater, usually unpaired, that drains the area of the foramen magnum, ascends along the attached margin of the falx cerebelli, and terminates in the confluence of the sinuses near the internal occipital protuberance.

omphalomesenteric duct s. A sinus caused by persistent patency of the distal part of the embryonic omphalomesenteric (vitelline) duct.

paranasal s. Any of the mucus-lined air sinuses (frontal, ethmoid, sphenoid, maxillary) in the bones of the face which open into the nasal cavity.

petrosal s., inferior A paired venous sinus passing along in the groove of the petro-occipital fissure connecting the cavernous sinus with the beginning of the internal jugular vein.

petrosal s., superior A paired venous sinus passing along the attached margin of the tentorium cerebelli connecting the cavernous sinus with the transverse sinus.

pilonidal s. A congenital sinus in the sacral region, leading to the exterior; often containing a tuft of hair and prone to suppuration.

piriform s. Piriform recess; see under recess.

prostatic s. The sinus or recess on either side of the urethral crest in the prostatic part of the urethra.

rhomboidal s. A dilatation of the central canal of the spinal cord in the lumbar region. Also called rhombocele.

Rokitansky-Aschoff s. One of a number of small evaginations of the gallbladder extending through the lamina propria and muscular layer; may be seen in chronic cholecystitis.

sagittal s., inferior An unpaired venous sinus in the lower margin of the cerebral falx, running parallel to the superior sagittal sinus and emptying into the upper end of the straight sinus.

sagittal s., superior An unpaired venous sinus in the sagittal groove of the cranium, beginning near the crista galli and extending backward to empty into the confluence of the sinuses near the internal occipital protuberance; it is invaginated by arachnoid granulations.

scleral venous s. The ringlike sinus in the corneoscleral junction of the eye; it serves as a flow drainage for the excess aqueous humor of the anterior chamber of the eye. Also called venous sinus of the sclera; Schlemm's canal.

sigmoid s. The S-shaped continuation of the transverse sinus on either side, situated along the posterior surface of the petrous portion of the temporal bone to the jugular foramen where it joins the jugular vein.

s. of Valsalva See aortic sinus.

s. rectus Straight sinus.

s. venosus The common venous chamber of the embryonic heart into which the cardinal, vitelline, and umbilical veins drain.

sphenoid s. One of the paired, asymmetrical, mucus-lined sinuses situated in the body of the sphenoid bone; it opens into the nasal cavity, of which it forms part of the roof.

sphenoparietal s. A small dural venous sinus along the lesser wing of the sphenoid bone; it empties into the cavernous sinus.

splenic s.'s Dilated venous sinusoids, lined with reticuloendothelial cells, that connect splenic capillaries with collecting venules and serve to convey blood through the spleen.

straight s. A triangular venous sinus formed by the union of the great cerebral vein and the inferior sagittal sinus; it receives the cerebellar veins before draining into the transverse sinus.

tonsillar s. Tonsillar fossa; see under fossa.

transverse s. Either of two (right and left) large venous sinuses of the dura mater lying along the attached margin of the tentorium cerebelli; the right one is frequently the direct continuation of the superior sagittal sinus; the left, of the straight sinus; at their origin in the confluence, they communicate with each other; they drain via the sigmoid sinuses to the internal jugular veins.

urachal s. Congenital abnormality that occurs when the lumen of either end of the embryonic allantois (which extends from the navel to the bladder) fails to close.

urogenital s. In embryology, an elongated sac formed by the division of the cloaca below the entrance of the genital ducts; it develops into the lower part of the bladder in both sexes, the vestibule in the female, and most of the urethra in the male.

venous s. of sclera See scleral venous sinus.

endothelial cells

perisinusoidal space

liver cells (hepatocytes)

Kupffer cells forming **sinusoids**

dip slide

skull

cytologic smear

vaginal smear

uterus

vagina

snare

sinusitis Inflammation of the mucous membrane of a sinus, especially of a paranasal sinus.
   frontal s. Infection in the frontal sinuses.
sinus node syndrome A syndrome of reduced sinoatrial (S-A) nodal automaticity; often precedes the development of the sick-sinus syndrome.
sinusoid 1. Like a sinus. 2. An irregular blood channel formed by anastomosing blood vessels; present in certain organs, such as the liver and spleen.
siphon 1. A U-shaped tube, used to transfer liquids or in draining wounds. 2. The act of transferring a fluid by means of a siphon.
   carotid s. The U-shaped bend of the intracranial portion of the internal carotid artery alongside the sella turcica.
Sipple syndrome A familial syndrome consisting of pheochromocytoma and medullary thyroid carcinoma with occasional parathyroid carcinoma.
site A location.
   active s. The area of an enzyme molecule that binds the substrate (substance that undergoes chemical change) and activates the reaction.
   allosteric s. The part of an enzyme molecule that binds an effector (substance that does not undergo chemical change but either inhibits or accelerates the enzymatic reaction). Also called regulatory site.
sitosterol Any of several widely occurring plant sterols, or a mixture of such sterols.
situs Position or location; especially normal location.
   s. inversus Congenital anomaly in which internal organs are located on the side of the body opposite to their normal location.
Sjogren's syndrome Disorder of unknown cause marked chiefly by atrophic changes of the lacrimal and salivary glands, leading to scanty lacrimal and salivary secretions with dryness of the eyes and mouth (keratoconjunctivitis sicca and xerostomia), and rheumatoid arthritis; rheumatoid factor is usually present and other abnormal antibodies are common in the patient's serum. Also called sicca syndrome.
skatole A crystalline compound formed in the intestine as a result of protein decomposition.
skein A length of coiled thread; said mainly of the coiled chromatin seen in the prophase stage of mitosis.
skeletal Relating to the skeleton.
skeletogenous Giving rise to bone formation.
skeleton The internal framework of vertebrates, composed of bones and cartilages and supporting the soft tissues.
skeneitis, skenitis Inflammation of Skene's glands of the female urethra.

skeocytosis See neocytosis.
skin The membranous covering of the body; the human skin is an integument composed of a thin outer layer (epidermis) and a thicker, deeper, connective tissue layer (dermis).
skin popping Slang expression denoting the injection of a narcotic drug intradermally; often results in ulcerations.
skull The framework of the head composed of the bones encasing the brain and the bones of the face. Also called cranium.
sleep A natural, periodically recurring state of rest in which consciousness is temporarily interrupted.
   non-rapid eye movement s. The dreamless period of sleep during which breathing is slow and deep, heart rate and blood pressure are low and regular, and brain waves are slow and of high voltage. Also called NREM sleep.
   paroxysmal s. See narcolepsy.
   rapid eye movement s. Phenomenon occurring at regular intervals during the dreaming phase of sleep, in which both eyes move rapidly and in unison under the closed eyelids; thought to represent the activated state of sleep, in which activity levels of many functions approach those occurring during wakefulness. Also called REM sleep.
   REM s. See rapid eye movement sleep.
   twilight s. State in which, although pain is felt, the memory of it is abolished, induced by injection of a mixture of morphine and scopolamine.
sleep apnea syndrome Clinical manifestations resulting from recurring periods of cessation of breathing during sleep; symptoms include morning headaches, daytime sleepiness, personality changes, and sexual impotence.
sleeplessness Insomnia.
sleeptalking Talking while asleep or while in a condition resembling sleep. Also called somniloquism.
sleepwalking Walking while asleep. Also called somnambulism.
slide A glass plate for mounting specimens to be examined under the microscope.
   dip s. A special plastic slide capable of holding an even thickness of culture medium on a molded grid; used to quantify the bacterial population of urine.
sling A band suspended from the neck, serving as a supporting bandage for an injured arm or hand.
slit A long, narrow opening, entrance, or cleft.
   vulvar s. The cleft between the labia majora.
slitlamp An instrument that projects obliquely a thin beam of intense light for illuminating any transparent structure, such as the cornea, by sections; usually used in examination of the eye through a

magnifying apparatus.
slough A mass of dead tissue separated from, or partially attached to, a living structure.
sludge A muddy sediment.
smallpox A severe contagious viral disease with an incubation period of 12 days; at the onset symptoms are headache, fever, abdominal and muscular pain, and vomiting; after three or four days, symptoms lessen and the eruptive stage occurs, with papules developing into vesicles and pustules throughout the body, especially on the face, hands, and feet; the trunk and legs are last affected; the lesions in any area are all in the same stage of development; after about three weeks, scabs form and upon falling leave permanent markings on the skin (pock marks). Also called variola.
smear A substance or preparation spread thinly on a slide for microscopic examination.
   buccal s. A smear obtained by scraping the inside of the cheek.
   cervical s. One obtained from the uterine cervix.
   cytologic s. A smear made by spreading the specimen onto a glass slide, then fixing it and staining it. Also called cytosmear.
   Pap s., Papanicolaou s. See test, Papanicolaou.
smegma The material that collects under the foreskin of the penis, consisting of sebaceous secretions of preputial glands mixed with desquamated epithelial cells.
smell 1. To perceive the scent of a substance by means of the olfactory apparatus. 2. To emit an odor.
smog A fog made heavier and darker by industrial gases, motor vehicle exhaust fumes, or smoke.
snap A sharp sound.
   closing s. The accentuated first sound of the heart occurring during closure of the abnormal mitral valve in mitral stenosis.
   opening s. A highpitched click heard during diastole; caused by opening of the abnormal mitral valve in mitral stenosis.
snare A surgical instrument with a wire loop which is tightened about the pedicle of a tumor polyp, etc., in order to sever it; also used to remove an intrauterine device.
sneeze The forceful, involuntary expulsion of air through the nose and mouth.
snore 1. To breathe through the mouth and nose with a rattling noise produced by vibration of the soft palate. 2. The noise produced while snoring.
snorting Slang expression denoting the inhalation of a narcotic drug, especially heroin or cocaine.
snuff 1. To inhale forcibly through the nose; to sniff. 2. Finely pulverized tobacco which is inhaled through the nostrils or applied to the gums. 3. Any

tooth socket

periodontal membrane

sole of newborn

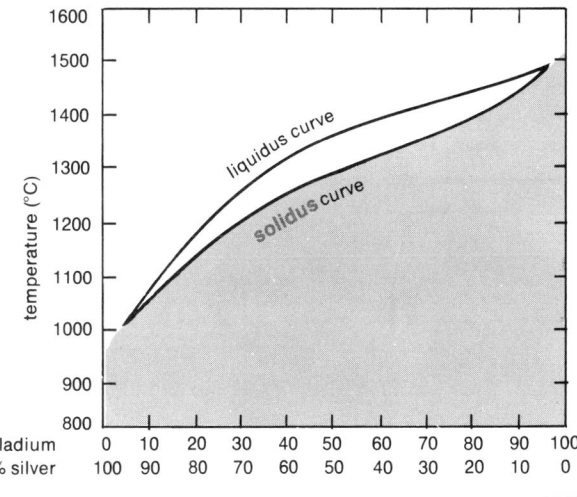

% palladium
% silver

COMPOSITION AND MELTING RANGES OF DENTAL GOLD **SOLDERS**

Solder no.	Gold %	Silver %	Copper %	Zinc %	Tin %	Melting range °F	Melting range °C
A	65.4	15.4	12.4	3.9	3.1	1375–1445	745–785
B	66.1	12.4	16.4	3.4	2.0	1385–1480	750–805
C	65.0	16.3	13.1	3.9	1.7	1410–1470	765–800
D	72.9	12.1	10.0	3.0	2.0	1390–1535	755–835
E	80.9	8.1	6.8	2.1	2.0	1375–1595	745–870

medicated powdery substance which is inhaled through the nose.

snuffbox, anatomic A somewhat triangular depression formed on the radial aspect of the wrist when the thumb is extended and abducted.

snuffles Noisy breathing due to obstructed nasal passages; when occurring in the newborn, it is usually caused by congenital syphilis.

soap A cleansing agent; a salt formed by fatty acids with potassium or sodium.

　insoluble s. A salt formed by fatty acids and metals other than sodium or potassium; insoluble in water and without detergent properties.

soapstone A relatively soft stone having a soapy feel and composed mainly of talc and chlorite.

social psychiatry The application of psychiatric principles to the solutions of social problems and issues.

socioacusis Denoting a hearing loss caused by a noisy environment.

sociomedical Pertaining to the interrelations of the practice of medicine and social welfare.

sociopath An individual with a behavior disorder marked by disregard for societal rules, immaturity, difficulty in postponing gratification, poor impulse control, and little ability to consider the consequences of his actions.

socket A cavity into which another part fits, as the socket of the eye or of a joint.

　dry s. A condition sometimes occurring after extraction of a tooth in which the blood clot in the socket disintegrates, leading to exposure of the bone and secondary infection.

　eye s. See orbit.

　tooth s. The cavity in the jaw in which a tooth is embedded. Also called alveolus.

soda General term commonly used to designate sodium bicarbonate, sodium carbonate, and sodium hydroxide.

sodium A soft, silvery-white metallic element; symbol Na, atomic number 11, atomic weight 22.99.

　s. benzoate A white, crystalline, odorless powder, C_6H_5COONa; used as a food preservative and in the manufacture of pharmaceuticals. Also called benzoate of soda.

　s. bicarbonate A white crystalline compound with a slight alkaline taste, $NaHCO_3$; used medicinally as a gastric antacid. Also called baking soda; bicarbonate of soda.

　s. bisulfite White, water-soluble crystals, $NaHSO_3$; used as a preservative, a disinfectant, and an antioxidant in certain injections.

　s. borate A colorless crystalline compound, $Na_2B_4O_7 \cdot 10\ H_2O$; used in dentistry as a retardant and in the manufacture of pharmaceuticals and detergents. Also called borax.

　s. carbonate 1. A white powdery compound, Na_2CO_3; used as a reagent and in water treatment. **2.** Any of several hydrated forms, such as $Na_2CO_3 \cdot 10H_2O$ (washing or sal soda).

　s. chloride A crystalline compound, $NaCl$; used medicinally in solution. Also called table or common salt.

　s. citrate A white, water-soluble, granular powder, $Na_3C_6H_5O_7 \cdot 2H_2O$; used as a blood anticoagulant.

　s. cyclamate A water-soluble powder, used as an artificial sweetener.

　s. diatrizoate A radiopaque, water-soluble powder, an organic compound of iodine, $C_{11}H_8O_4 \cdot N_2I_3Na \cdot 4H_2O$; used in excretory radiography of the urinary tract.

　s. glutamate A white crystalline compound used in cooking to enhance flavor. Also called monosodium glutamate (MSG).

　s. hydroxide Alkaline, water-soluble compound, $NaOH$; used in the chemical and pharmaceutical industries. Also called caustic soda; lye.

　s. iodide White crystalline powder, NaI; used as a source of iodine.

　s. levothyroxine The sodium salt of the natural isomer of thyroxin; used in the treatment of thyroid deficiency conditions.

　s. liothyronine The sodium salt of L-triiodothyronine; used in the treatment of thyroid deficiency.

　s. nitrate White crystalline compound, $NaNO_3$; formerly used to treat dysentery. Also called Chile saltpeter; soda niter.

　s. pentothal See thiopental sodium.

　s. perborate A white odorless compound, $NaBO_2H_2O_2 \cdot 3H_2O$; used as an antiseptic.

　s. peroxide A white or yellowish powder, Na_2O_2; used in the manufacture of pharmaceuticals.

　s. phosphate A crystalline, water-soluble sodium salt of phosphoric acid, $Na_2HPO_4 \cdot H_2O$; used as a laxative.

　s. salicylate White scales, soluble in water, formerly used in the treatment of rheumatic fever.

　s. thiosulfate A crystalline compound, $Na_2S_2O_3 \cdot 5H_2O$; used as an antidote in cyanide poisoning, to prevent ringworm infection, and as a photographic fixing agent. Also called hypo; hyposulfite.

sodium group The alkali metals: lithium, sodium, potassium, rubidium, and cesium.

sodoku Rat-bite fever; see under fever.

sodomy Sexual practice in which the penis is introduced into the anus or mouth of another person.

softening The process of becoming soft. Also called malacia.

　gray s. A stage in softening of the brain in which absorption of fat occurs, following yellow softening.

　hemorrhagic s. Red softening.

　red s. Softening of the brain with bleeding into the necrotic tissue.

　white s. Softening of the brain caused by obstruction of blood supply.

　yellow s. Late stage in softening of the brain in which fatty degeneration takes place.

sol A colloidal dispersion of a solid in a liquid.

Solanaceae A family of herbs, shrubs, and trees, including several poisonous species and some that are used medicinally.

solanaceous Relating to the family Solanaceae.

solation In chemistry, the conversion of a gel into a sol, as the melting of gelatin.

solder A fusible alloy of metals used to join metallic parts when applied in the melted state to the solid metal.

soldering The joining of metals by the fusion of intermediate alloys which are of a lower melting point than that of the components to be connected.

sole The plantar surface (undersurface) of the foot.

solid 1. Of definite shape; not liquid or gaseous. **2.** Compact; firm; without gaps.

solidus The temperature line on a constitution diagram below which the indicated metal element or alloy is in a solid state.

solubility 1. The property of being soluble. **2.** The degree to which a substance possesses the property of being soluble.

soluble Capable of being dissolved.

solute The substance dissolved in a solution.

solution (sol) 1. A homogeneous substance formed by the mixture of a gaseous, liquid, or solid substance (solute) with a liquid or a noncrystalline solid (solvent), and from which the dissolved substance can be recovered. **2.** The process of making such a mixture.

　alcoholic s. A solution in which alcohol is used as the solvent.

　Benedict's s. A water solution of sodium citrate, sodium carbonate, and copper sulfate; used to detect the presence of reducing substances in the urine.

　Burrow's s. A solution of aluminum acetate.

　C3 s. One used for perfusion of tissues before freezing.

　Collins s. See C3 solution.

　Dakin's s. A mixture of hypochlorite and perborate of sodium with hypochlorous and boric acids; an antiseptic. Also called Dakin's modified solution.

　gram-molecular s. Molar solution.

　hyperbaric s. A solution possessing a higher specific gravity than a standard of reference; e.g., in spinal anesthesia, one having a specific gravity higher than that of the cerebrospinal fluid (CSF),

SELECTED SOLVENTS

Name	Molecular weight	Melting point °C	Boiling point °C
water	18.02	0.0	100.0
methanol	32.04	−97.7	64.7
acetaldehyde	44.05	−123.0	20.4
ethanol	46.07	−114.1	78.3
acetone	58.05	−94.7	56.3
acetic acid	60.05	16.7	117.9
cyclopentane	70.13	−93.8	49.3
benzene	78.12	5.5	80.1
hexane	86.17	−95.3	68.7
pyruvic acid	88.06	13.6	165.0
toluene	92.14	−94.9	110.6
phenol	94.12	40.9	181.8
caprylic acid	144.22	16.5	239.9
engenol	164.20	9.2	255.0
oleic acid	282.47	13.4	360.0

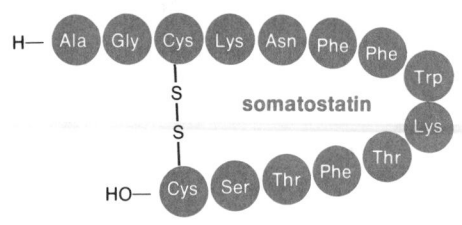

somatostatin

MOLECULAR WEIGHT OF SOME PROTEINS

ribonuclease	14,000
somatotropin (growth hormone)	21,500
carboxypeptidase	34,000
pepsin	35,500
serum albumin	66,500
catalase	250,000
fibrinogen	330,000
urease	480,000
thyroglobulin	660,000

thereby producing anesthesia below the level of injection due to its downward migration.

hypertonic s. A solution possessing a higher osmotic pressure than a standard of reference; e.g., a solution of sodium chloride having a higher osmotic pressure than that of blood; often denoting a solution which, when surrounding a cell, causes a flow of water to leave the cell through the semipermeable cell membrane.

hypobaric s. A solution possessing a lower specific gravity than a standard of reference; e.g., in spinal anesthesia, one having a specific gravity lower than that of the cerebrospinal fluid (CSF), thereby producing anesthesia above the level of injection due to its upward migration.

hypotonic s. A solution possessing a lower specific gravity than a standard of reference; e.g., a solution of sodium chloride having a lower osmotic pressure than that of blood; often denoting a solution which, when surrounding a cell, causes a flow of water to enter the cell through the semipermeable cell membrane.

iodine s. A solution containing approximately 2% iodine and 2½% sodium iodide in water; generally applied to superficial lacerations to prevent bacterial infections.

iodine s., strong A solution containing iodine 5 g, potassium iodide 10 g, and enough distilled water to make 100 ml; used as a source of iodine. Also called Lugol's solution.

isotonic sodium chloride s. A solution of sodium chloride with the same osmotic pressure as plasma; 0.9% sodium chloride. Also called physiologic salt solution.

lactated Ringer's s. A solution containing sodium chloride 600 mg, sodium lactate 310 mg, calcium chloride 20 mg, and potassium chloride 30 mg in 100 ml of boiled distilled water; the ionic concentration of the solution is 130 mEq sodium, 4 mEq potassium, 4 mEq calcium, 111 mEq chloride, and 27 mEq lactate.

Locke-Ringer s. A solution containing sodium chloride 9 g, calcium chloride 0.24 g, potassium chloride 0.42 g, and magnesium chloride 0.2 g, with sodium bicarbonate 0.5 g, glucose 0.5 g, and water to make one liter; used for physiologic and pharmacologic experiments.

Locke's s. A solution consisting of sodium chloride 0.9 g, calcium chloride 0.024 g, potassium chloride 0.042 g, with sodium bicarbonate 0.01 to 0.03 g, glucose 0.1 g, and distilled water to make 100 ml; used for irrigation of tissues during laboratory experiments.

Lugol's s. See iodine solution, strong.

molal s. A solution in which one-gram molecular weight of the solute is dissolved in enough solvent to make one liter.

molar s. A solution in which one-gram molecular weight of the solute is dissolved in one liter of the solvent.

normal s. A solution that contains one gram equivalent weight of the dissolved substance in each liter of solution.

ophthalmic s. A sterile solution for application into the eye, containing a preservative and having an osmotic pressure and pH similar to that of normal tears.

ophthalmic irrigating s. See eyewash.

phsyiologic salt s. See isotonic sodium chloride solution.

pickling s. An acid solution used to remove oxide and other impurities from dental casts; commonly made from one part of concentrated hydrochloric acid and one part water.

Ringer's s. A solution containing sodium chloride 8.6 g, potassium chloride 0.3 g, and calcium chloride 0.33 g in one liter of boiled distilled water; the ionic concentration of the solution is 147 mEq sodium, 4 mEq potassium, 5 mEq calcium and 156 mEq chloride; used locally for burns and wounds. Also called Ringer's mixture.

saline s. A solution of any salt, especially of sodium chloride. Commonly known as saline.

saturated s. A solution containing the maximum amount of solute that a given amount of solvent can dissolve.

sclerosing s. A solution that causes formations of fibrous tissue; used in oral surgery to arrest bleeding, cauterize ulcers, etc.

Shohl's s. A solution containing citric acid 140 g, sodium citrate 90 g, and enough water to make one liter.

standard s. A solution of known concentration, used as a basis of comparison.

supersaturated s. A solution containing a greater amount of the solute than a given amount of solvent would dissolve at ordinary temperatures.

test s. Standard solution of specific substances, used in analysis.

Tyrode's s. One containing sodium chloride 8 g, potassium chloride 0.2 g, calcium chloride 0.2 g, and magnesium chloride 0.1 g, with sodium biphosphate 0.05 g, sodium bicarbonate 1 g, glucose 1 g, and water to make one liter; used in irrigation of the peritoneal cavity and in laboratory work.

volumetric s. (V.S.) A standard solution containing a specific quantity of a substance (usually 1, ½, or 1 mg mole) dissolved in one liter of water.

Ziehl's s. A staining solution for microorganisms such as the tubercle bacillus; contains basic fuchsin, ethyl alcohol, phenol, and distilled water. Also called carbolfuchsin.

solvate A compound formed by the loose combination of a solvent (the dissolving substance) and a solute (the substance dissolved).

solve (solv) Latin for dissolve.

solvent Capable of dissolving another substance. Also called dissolvent.

soma 1. An organism as a whole, exclusive of its germ cells. 2. The body, distinguished from the mind. 3. The body of a nerve cell.

somatesthesia Bodily awareness. Also called somesthesia.

somatic 1. Of, or pertaining to, the body. 2. Parietal; relating to the wall of the body cavity.

somatization The unconscious conversion of anxiety into physical symptoms.

somatogenic Of bodily origin; originating in the body cells.

somatology The study of the human body in relation to form and function.

somatomammatropin See lactogen, human placental.

somatomedin A peptide present in plasma, formed in the liver and probably in the kidney; able to stimulate synthesis of protein, DNA, and RNA, and the uptake of sulfate; mediates the effect of growth hormone (somatotropin) on cartilage. Also called sulfation factor.

somatometry Measurement of the body.

somatoplasm The totality of protoplasm of all cells (except germ cells) that make up the body.

somatopsychic Relating to the relationship of the body and mind; denoting the effects of the body on the mind.

somatopsychosis An emotional disorder associated with visceral disease.

somatosexual Relating to both physical and sexual characteristics; usually refers to physical manifestations of sexual development.

somatostatin A peptide found in the central nervous system, stomach, small intestine, and islets of Langerhans; it inhibits the release of growth hormone, insulin, and glucagon; it may act as a neurotransmitter in the central nervous system. Also called somatotropin release-inhibiting factor.

somatotherapy Treatment directed toward physical ailments, as opposed to psychiatric treatments.

somatotonia Personality type marked by dominance of vigorous muscular activity and assertiveness.

somatotropic, somatotrophic Having a stimulating effect on body growth or an influence on the body.

somatotropin (STH) A hormone secreted by the

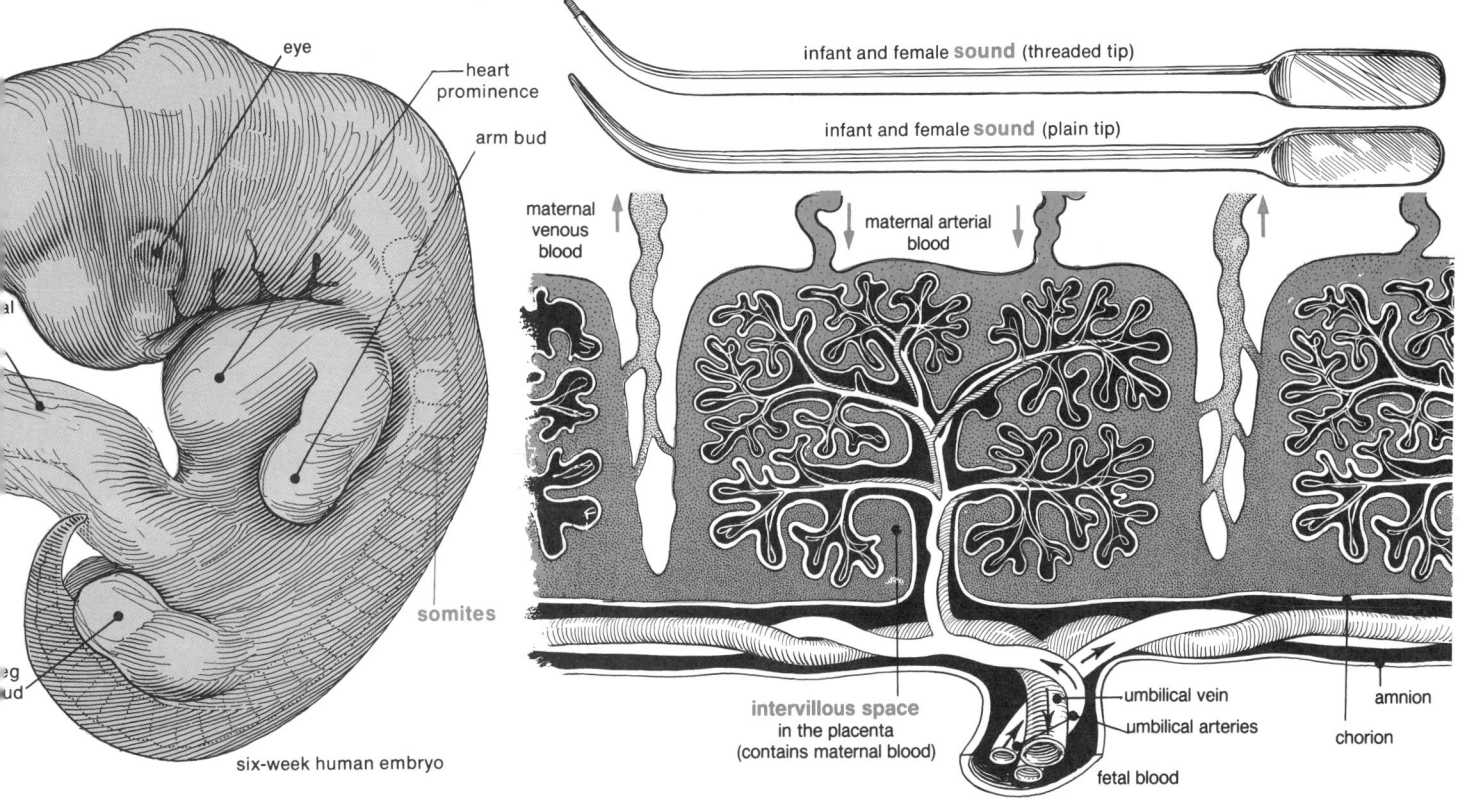

eye

heart prominence

arm bud

somites

six-week human embryo

infant and female **sound** (threaded tip)

infant and female **sound** (plain tip)

maternal venous blood

maternal arterial blood

intervillous space in the placenta (contains maternal blood)

umbilical vein

umbilical arteries

amnion

chorion

fetal blood

anterior lobe of the pituitary gland which affects the rate of skeletal growth and gain in body weight. Also called growth hormone.

somatotype A classification of individuals based on physical characteristics of the body. Also called biotype; physique; body build.

somesthesia See somatesthesia.

somite One of paired, segmented blocks of epithelioid cells on either side of the neural tube of the embryo, which in later stages of development give rise to connective tissue, bone, muscle, and the dermis and subcutaneous tissue of the skin; the size of the embryo may be expressed in the number of somites; usually 42 to 44 develop in man.

somnambulism Walking while asleep without any recollection upon awakening; applied also to some states of hypnosis. Also called sleepwalking; noctambulism.

somnambulist One who walks in his sleep.

somniloquism, somniloquence Talking while asleep or in a condition resembling sleep. Also called sleeptalking.

somniloquist A person who talks in his sleep.

somnolence, somnolency Drowsiness; sleepiness.

somnolent Drowsy.

somnus Latin for sleep.

sone A subjective unit of loudness; the intensity of sound of a pure tone of 1000 cycles per second at 40 decibels above an individual's threshold of audibility.

sonic 1. Of or pertaining to audible sound. 2. Relating to the speed of sound in air (approximately 740 mph at sea level).

sonography See ultrasonography.

sopor Unusually profound sleep. Also called stupor.

soporific Producing sleep.

soporose, soporous Comatose.

sorbefacient Facilitating absorption.

sorbitan A general term for esters of sorbitol.

sorbitan polyoxyalkalene A compound from which the nonionic emulsifying compounds with the trademark Tween are derived.

sorbitol A sweet crystalline substance occurring in mountain ash fruits and made synthetically by reduction of glucose; used in the preparation of ascorbic acid and as a laxative, working by an osmotic effect. Also called D-glucitol.

sordes Foul brown or blackish crust formed about the lips and teeth of patients with some forms of prolonged low grade fever.

sore Any open skin lesion.

bed s. Decubitus ulcer; see under ulcer.

canker s. Aphthous stomatitis; see under sto-

matitis.

cold s. A lesion occurring singly or in clusters, usually on the lips, usually caused by herpesvirus 1; it often accompanies a fever, common cold, or exposure to the sun. Also called fever blister. See also herpes labialis.

hard s. See chancre.

oriental s. Cutaneous leishmaniasis; see under leishmaniasis.

pressure s. Decubitus ulcer; see under ulcer.

soft s. See chancroid.

souffle A soft blowing sound heard on auscultation.

fetal s. A blowing, whistling sound synchronous with the fetal heart beat, heard during late pregnancy; caused by blood rushing through the umbilical arteries when the umbilical cord is subject to torsion, tension, or pressure. Also called funic or umbilical souffle.

mammary s. A blowing murmur heard at the medial border of the breast during late pregnancy and lactation; attributed to a change of dynamics in blood flow through the internal thoracic (mammary) artery.

placental s. Uterine souffle.

splenic s. A soft blowing sound heard over the spleen in malaria.

umbilical s. Fetal souffle.

uterine s. A soft, blowing sound synchronous with the maternal heart beat, heard during late pregnancy; caused by blood flowing through engorged uterine vessels; also may be heard in nonpregnant women with large myomatous tumors of the uterus or enlarged ovaries.

sound 1. A noise. 2. A cylindrical, usually curved metal instrument used for exploring bodily cavities or for dilating a canal such as the urethra. 3. Healthy.

friction s. A grating sound heard on auscultation, produced by the rubbing of two inflamed surfaces. Also called friction rub.

heart s.'s Sounds heard on auscultation over the area of the heart: first heart sound (S_1) is caused by closure of the atrioventricular valves (mitral and tricuspid); second heart sound (S_2) results from closure of the semilunar valves (aortic and pulmonic); third heart sound (S_3) is audible sometimes during rapid filling of the ventricles; fourth heart sound (S_4) coincides with atrial contraction. The presence of a third or fourth heart sound generally indicates an abnormality. Also called cardiac sounds.

soya The seed of the soybean plant.

soybean 1. A leguminous, climbing Asiatic plant, *Glycine soya* or *Glycine hispida*. 2. The seed of this plant, rich in protein and low in starch content;

given to individuals who are allergic to cow's milk.

space Any bodily area or volume between specified boundaries; a delimited three-dimensional area.

antecubital s. Cubital fossa; see under fossa.

arachnoid s. Subarachnoid space.

Bowman's s. The space or sac between the parietal and visceral epithelial of the renal corpuscle; it receives the filtrate of the blood from the glomerular vessels. Also called glomerular or urinary space.

corneal s.'s The interlamellar spaces of the cornea; very small spaces between the lamellae of the corneal stroma which contain tissue fluid.

dead s. 1. A space or cavity left after improper closure of a surgical or other wound. 2. The portion of the respiratory tract from the nostrils to the terminal bronchioles where no gaseous interchange can take place. Also called anatomic dead space.

epidural s. The space between the spinal dura mater and the periosteum of the vertebrae; it contains loose areolar tissue and a plexus of veins.

epitympanic s. The upper portion of the middle ear cavity above the tympanic membrane; it contains the head of the malleus and the body of the incus.

free-way s. Interocclusal distance; see under distance.

glomerular s. See Bowman's space.

intercostal s. (I.C.S., I.S.) The space or interval between two adjacent ribs; the breadth is greater between the upper ribs and ventrally.

interpleural s. The space in the middle of the chest between the two pleurae.

interproximal s. The space between adjacent teeth in a dental arch.

interradicular s. The space between the roots of a multirooted tooth, occupied by bony septum and the periodontal membrane.

intervillous s. The space in the placenta in which maternal blood bathes chorionic villi, thus allowing exchange of materials between the fetal and maternal circulation; it is bounded by the chorion on the fetal side and the decidua basalis on the maternal side.

medullary s. The central cavity and the cellular intervals between the trabeculae of marrow-containing bone.

palmar s. A large fascial space in the hand, divided by a fibrous septum into the middle palmar space (toward the little finger) and the thenar space (toward the thumb).

pharyngeal s. The area within the pharynx.

physiologic dead s. The portion of the respiratory passage, at the end of inspiration, which is filled with air that has not mixed with alveolar air.

pleural s. The potential space between the pari-

dura mater   arachnoid
**subdural
space**   **subarachnoid
space**

pia mater

brain

spasm of the
bronchial
musculature

plaster-dental stone **spatula**

dental cement **spatulas**

**Frenzel
spectacles**

Ayre wooden spatula

etal and visceral layers of the pleura. Also called cavum pleurae.

  retroperitoneal s. The space between the parietal peritoneum and the structures of the posterior abdominal wall.

  retropubic s. The extraperitoneal area of loose connective tissue separating the bladder from the pubis and anterior abdominal wall. Also called Retzius' space.

  Retzius' s. See retropubic space.

  s. 's of Fontana The spaces of the trabecular tissue that connect the anterior chamber of the eye to the venous sinus of the sclera (Schlemm's canal); involved with drainage of the aqueous humor.

  subarachnoid s. The space or interval between the arachnoid and the pia mater; it is filled with a delicate meshwork of fibrous trabeculae and contains cerebrospinal fluid.

  subdural s. The narrow space between the dura mater and the arachnoid; it contains only a small amount of fluid sufficient to moisten the opposing surfaces of the two membranes.

  subphrenic s. The space between the diaphragm and the organs immediately below it.

  subpodocytic s.'s Spaces beneath the cell body of the podocyte and its trabeculae; they contain numerous fine foot processes (pedicels) that support the trabeculae on the basement membrane of glomerular capillaries.

  Traube's s. A space on the left side of the chest about 7.6 cm wide, bounded on the right by the sternum, above by the oblique line from the cartilage of the sixth rib to the ninth rib, and below by the inferior border of the rib cage.

  urinary s. See Bowman's space.

  Zang's s. Lesser supraclavicular fossa; see under fossa.

  zonular s. The circumlental space between the equator of the lens of the eye and the ciliary processes; it contains aqueous humor.

space maintainer A dental appliance, either fixed or removable, used to preserve the space created by the premature loss of a tooth.

space obtainer An orthodontic appliance that slowly increases space between teeth.

spallation 1. A nuclear reaction in which nuclei eject a number of protons and alpha particles when bombarded by high energy particles. 2. The process of breaking up or splintering into small fragments; applied to the breaking off of the coating from a catheter.

span A full extent or reach.

  auditory s. The number of words, letters, or digits that can be repeated after hearing them once; used to test immediate memory.

sparganosis Infection with spargana.

sparganum The intramuscular parasitic larva of tapeworms of the genus *Spirometra*.

spargosis Excessive distention, especially of the breasts with milk.

spasm An involuntary, sudden, violent contraction of a muscle or a group of muscles.

  carpopedal s. A spasm of the feet and hands occurring in tetany and other disorders.

  clonic s. A spasm characterized by alternate rigidity and relaxation of the muscles.

  intention s. A spasm occurring when voluntary movements are attempted.

  nictitating s. Involuntary winking.

  tonic s. A spasm in which the muscular contraction is persistent.

  vasomotor s. Spasm of small arteries.

spasmodic Relating to or characterized by spasm.

spasmogenic Causing spasms.

spasmolysis The arrest or elimination of spasm.

spasmolytic A drug that reduces spasm. Also called antispasmodic.

spastic Convulsive.

spasticity Increased tone or rigidity of a muscle.

  clasp-knife s. Spasticity of the extensor muscles induced by passive flexion of a joint which suddenly gives way on exertion of further pressure, allowing the joint to be easily flexed; the rigidity is due to an exaggeration of the stretch reflex. Also called clasp-knife rigidity.

spatula 1. A thin, flat, blunt, blade-shaped instrument used especially for spreading or mixing substances such as dental impression materials. 2. A device used for scraping tissue for biopsy.

  Ayre wooden s. A spatula generally used for taking a smear from the cervix or fornix of the uterus.

  Roux s. A small steel spatula for transferring bits of infected material to culture tubes.

spatulate 1. Shaped like a spatula, or having a flat blunt end. 2. To mix substances by forced compression with a spatula.

spatulation The manipulation of two or more substances with a spatula in order to mix them into a homogeneous mass; usually done by repeatedly and forcefully smoothing out the mass on the side of a mixing bowl or on a flat surface.

spay To remove the ovaries of an animal.

specialist One who confines his interest to one branch of knowledge, as a physician who confines his practice to the treatment of a specific group of patients (e.g., of children, a pediatrician) or of diseases (e.g., of urogenital tract, a urologist).

specialize To channel one's training or practice to a specific branch of health science.

species 1. A toxonomic classification of organisms, ranking after a genus and before a variety, that bear a close resemblance to one another and are capable of interbreeding; a subdivision of a genus. 2. A variety or type of pharmaceutical preparation consisting of a mixture of crushed, but not pulverized, dried leaves used in making decoctions.

species-specific Affecting a particular species in a characteristic manner; term applied to a drug or a virus.

specific 1. Relating to a species. 2. Relating to one disease only. 3. A remedy intended for one particular disease.

specificity 1. The state of being specific, having a fixed affinity, as the antigen-antibody relation. 2. Applied to a screening test: The proportion of persons who are truly free of a disease in a screened population, and who are identified as such by the test.

specimen A small part or sample of any substance, as tissue, blood, or urine, obtained for analysis and diagnosis.

spectacles Eyeglasses.

  crutch s. Spectacles with a ptosis crutch attachment (little offsets of smooth metal which engage below the upper eyelid to keep it raised above the pupil). Also called Masselon's spectacles.

  Frenzel s. Plano spectacles with built-in illumination and 20-diopter lenses for the purpose of dazzling the eyes and preventing their fixation on an external object; used in a darkened room to observe and record nystagmus.

  half-glass s. See pantoscopic spectacles.

  Masselon's s. See crutch spectacles.

  pantoscopic s. Eyeglasses used for reading in which the top halves of the lenses are removed so as not to affect distant vision. Also called clerical or half-glass spectacles.

  stenopaic s. Spectacles having, in place of lenses, opaque disks with narrow slits or circular perforations allowing a minimum amount of light to enter.

spectrochemistry The study and analysis of chemical substances by the use of light waves (spectroscopy); the study of the spectra of substances.

spectrocolorimeter An instrument used to detect color blindness for one color through the use of a light source from a selected wavelength.

spectrogram 1. A machine that translates sounds into a pattern on paper. 2. A photograph, graph, or map of a spectrum.

spectograph A spectroscope specifically designed for photographic recording of a spectrum.

spectrometer An instrument designed to break up light from a source into its constituent wavelengths and to indicate wavelength on its calibrated

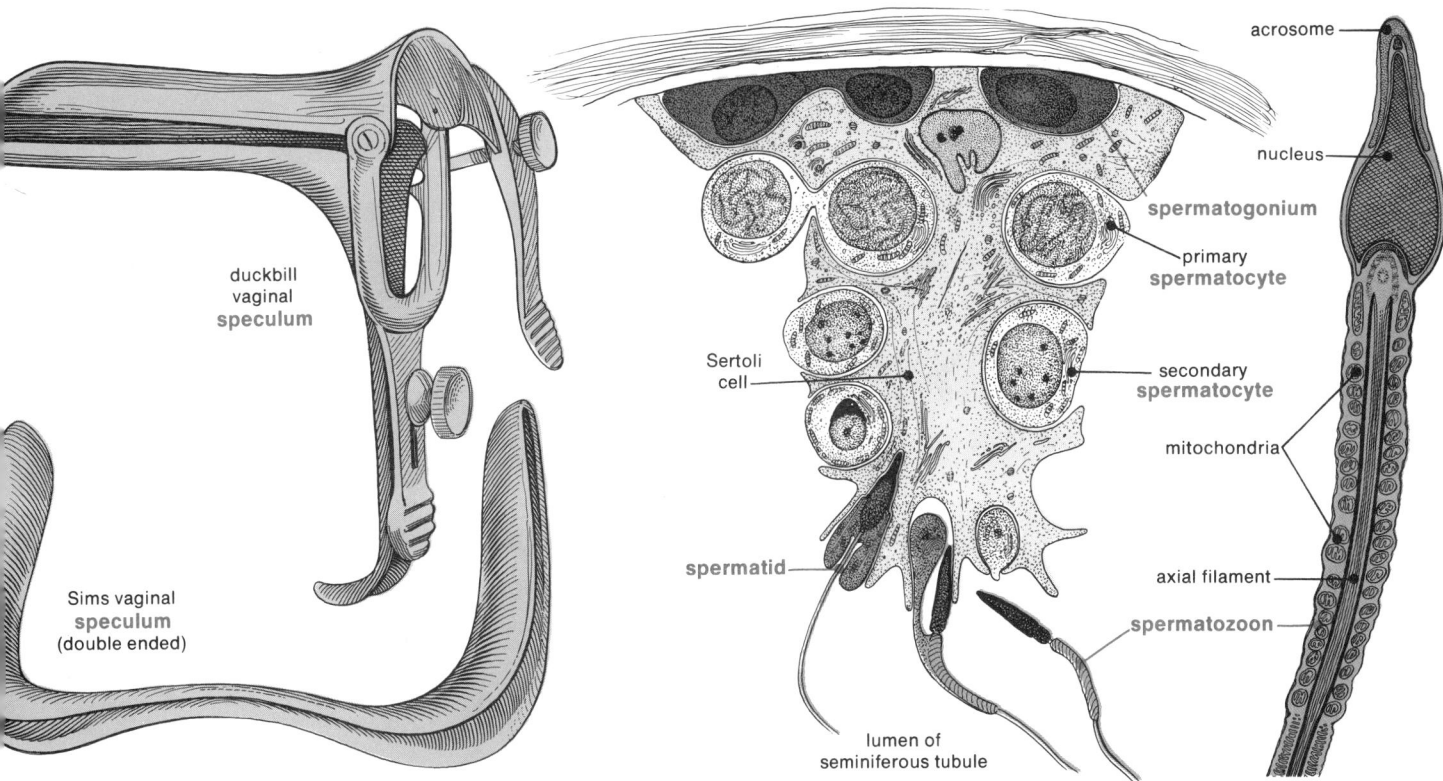

duckbill vaginal **speculum**

Sims vaginal **speculum** (double ended)

acrosome

nucleus

spermatogonium

primary **spermatocyte**

Sertoli cell

secondary **spermatocyte**

mitochondria

spermatid

axial filament

spermatozoon

lumen of seminiferous tubule

---

scale.

nuclear magnetic resonance s. One that makes it possible to observe the magnetic properties of atoms in a molecule and provide information which describes their spatial relationships and movements.

spectrometry Measuring of the wavelengths of rays of a spectrum with the spectrometer.

spectrophotofluorimetry The photometric measurement and analysis of the intensity and quality of fluorescence spectra.

spectrophotometer An optical instrument for measuring photometrically the intensity of any particular wavelength range absorbed by a colored solution.

spectropolarimeter An instrument for measuring optical rotation of different wavelengths of light passing through a solution or translucent solid; a combined spectroscope and polariscope.

spectroscope Any one of several forms of optical instruments used for dispersion of light and visual observation of the resulting spectrum.

spectroscopy The experimental observation and study of optical spectra.

spectrum 1. An orderly distribution of radiant energy presented when white light is dispersed into its constituent colors by passing through a prism or a diffraction grating; the colors, arranged according to the increasing frequency of molecular vibration or decreasing wavelength, are red, orange, yellow, green, blue, indigo, and violet. **2.** A range of activity of pathogenic microorganisms affected by an antibiotic or antibacterial agent.

antibacterial s. Spectrum (2).

s. of disease The complete range of manifestations of a disease.

speculum An instrument used to dilate and hold open the orifice of a body cavity or canal to facilitate the inspection of its interior.

speech The production of articulate sounds to convey ideas.

esophageal s. Speech produced by swallowing air and regurgitating it; used by an individual who has had his larynx removed.

scanning s. Slow speech with pauses between syllables.

staccato s. Jerky, abrupt speech in which each syllable is pronounced separately.

telegraphic s. Sparse speech usually consisting mainly of nouns, important adjectives, and transitive verbs, omitting articles, prepositions, and conjunctions; seen in certain types of aphasia.

speed Slang name for methamphetamine hydrochloride.

sperm 1. A mature reproductive cell of the male. **2.** Semen.

spermatic Relating to the sperm.

One of the four cells resulting from the division of a spermatocyte; it develops into a spermatozoon without further division.

spermatoblast See spermatogonium.

spermatocele An intrascrotal, painless cyst containing sperm, usually less than 1 cm in diameter and occurring just above and posterior to the testis; caused by obstruction of the sperm-transporting tubules. Also called spermatocyst.

spermatocide Any agent that destroys spermatozoa. Also called spermicide.

spermatocyst 1. Seminal vesicle; see under vesicle. **2.** See spermatocele.

spermatocystectomy Removal of the seminal vesicles.

spermatocyte A cell originating from the division of a spermatogonium which in turn divides into four spermatids.

spermatogenesis The formation of spermatozoa.

spermatogenetic Relating to spermatogenesis.

spermatogenic, spermatogenous Producing sperm.

spermatogonium, spermatogone An undifferentiated young cell located close to the basement membrane of the seminiferous tubules which either gives rise to new spermatogonia (type A) or differentiates to a more developed primary spermatocyte (type B), which eventually becomes a sperm. Also called spermatoblast.

spermatoid Resembling semen.

spermatolysin A specific lysin of spermatozoa formed in the female body following exposure to spermatozoa.

spermatolysis Destruction and dissolution of the spermatozoa.

spermatorrhea Abnormal involuntary discharge of semen without orgasm.

spermatoschesis Suppression of seminal discharge; nonsecretion of semen.

spermatotoxin Spermotoxin.

spermatozoa Plural of spermatozoon.

spermatozoon, *pl.* **spermatozoa** The male sexual cell produced in the testes; a nucleated cell with a thin motile tail by means of which it migrates up the female reproductive passages where fertilization takes place.

spermaturia See semenuria.

spermiation The release of spermatozoa from the seminiferous epithelium.

spermicide See spermatocide.

spermiogenesis The phase of spermatogenesis in which spermatids develop into spermatozoa.

spermolith A stone in the deferent (spermatic)

duct.

spermotoxin A cytotoxic antibody destructive to spermatozoa. Also called spermatotoxin.

sphacelate To become gangrenous.

sphaceloderma Gangrene of the skin.

sphenion A craniometric point located at the tip of the sphenoid angle of the parietal bone.

sphenoid Wedge-shaped; denoting a large wedge-shaped bone at the base of the skull.

sphenoiditis Inflammation of the sphenoid sinus.

sphenoidostomy Removal of a portion of the anterior wall of the sphenoid sinus.

sphenoidotomy Incision into the sphenoid sinus.

sphenopalatine Relating to the sphenoid and palatine bones.

sphenorbital Relating to the sphenoid bone and the orbit.

sphenosquamosal Relating to the sphenoid bone and the thin portion of the temporal bone.

sphere A ball-shaped structure; a globular body.

attraction s. See astrosphere.

Morgagni's s.'s Morgagni's globules; see under globule.

spherocyte A red blood cell that appears spherical in the living state and has a diameter of less than 6 μm; it has a greater than normal density of hemoglobin and a decreased surface-to-volume ratio; characteristic of hereditary spherocytosis and certain other hemolytic anemias.

spherocytosis The presence of red blood cells that are more spherical than biconcave, as in hemolytic anemia. Also called congenital spherocytic anemia.

spherule 1. A small sphere. **2.** A minute, thick-walled, spherical structure containing many fungal spores; characteristic of the parasitic phase of *Coccidioides immitis*.

rod s. The miniature terminal part of the retinal rod cell that forms synaptic relationships with the processes of bipolar cells and horizontal cells of the retina.

sphincter 1. Any circular muscle that, when contracted, closes a natural body opening. **2.** A portion of a tubular structure that functions as a sphincter.

external anal s. A two-layered flat band of muscular fibers, elliptical in shape, surrounding the anal orifice.

ileocecal s. Ileocecal valve; see under valve.

internal anal s. A muscular ring surrounding about 2.5 cm of the anal canal; in contact with, but separate from, the external anal sphincter.

lower esophageal s. (LES) A high pressure zone in the distal portion of the esophagus where resting pressure is usually higher than pressure in the fundus of the stomach; acts as a barrier preventing the reflux

cerebroside

sphingolipids

sphingomyelin

sphingosine

sphygmo-
manometer

brown
recluse
spider
(Loxosceles reclusus)

spina
bifida

of gastric contents; cannot be identified anatomically but its pressure can be measured and demonstrated; normally it straddles the diaphragm extending 1–3 cm below to 1–2 cm above the diaphragmatic hiatus.

pupillary s. A narrow circular band of muscle fibers, about 1 mm in width, in the pupillary margin of the iris.

vesicular s. A thickening of the middle circular layer of the muscular fibers of the bladder, surrounding the internal urethral opening.

sphincteralgia Pain in a sphincter muscle, especially of the anus.

sphincteritis Inflammation of a sphincter, particularly the sphincter of the hepatopancreatic duct.

sphincterotomy Surgical division of a sphincter muscle.

sphingolipid A group of lipids containing in their structure a long-chain, aliphatic base; e.g., ceramide, cerebroside, sphingomyelin, ganglioside; found primarily in tissues of the central nervous system.

sphingolipidosis General term for a number of disorders marked by abnormal metabolism of sphingolipids.

cerebral s. Any of a group of inherited diseases caused by a disturbance of metabolism resulting in increased lipids in the brain and characterized by progressive decrease in vision leading to complete blindness (usually within two years), severe mental deterioration, retinal atrophy, convulsions, and paralysis; there are four types of the disorder: infantile (Tay-Sachs disease), early juvenile (Jansky-Bielschowsky disease), late juvenile (Spielmeyer-Vogt or Batten-Mayou disease), and adult (Kufs' disease). Also called cerebromacular degeneration. Formerly called amaurotic familial idiocy.

sphingomyelin One of a group of phospholipids present in large quantities in brain and nerve tissue; on hydrolysis, it yields a fatty acid, phosphoric acid, choline, and the amino alcohol sphingosine.

sphingosine A complex amino alcohol; a constituent of cerebrosides.

sphygmic Relating to the pulse.

sphygmogram A curve representing the arterial pulse, made with a sphygomograph.

sphygmograph Instrument used to make a graphic representation (curve) of the arterial pulse.

sphygmography **1.** The graphic recording of the arterial pulse by means of the sphygmograph. **2.** A treatise on the pulse.

sphygmoid Resembling the pulse.

sphygmomanometer An instrument for measuring arterial blood pressure.

sphygmometer Sphygmomanometer.

sphygmopalpation Feeling or "taking" the pulse; palpation of the pulse.

sphygmophone An instrument for rendering audible the vibrations of each individual beat of the pulse.

sphygmoscope Instrument used to render the pulse beat visible.

spica A plaster cast resembling a figure 8, used to immobilize the trunk and an extremity; e.g., shoulder spica; its name is derived from the overlapping turns that give it the appearance of an ear of barley.

spicule A small needle-shaped structure.

spider **1.** Any of numerous arachnids having four pairs of legs, usually eight eyes, a body divided into a cephalothorax and an abdomen, and a complex of web-spinning spinnerets that produce silk; some venomous spiders are the black widow (*Latrodectus mactans*), brown recluse (*Loxosceles reclusus*), Chilean brown (*Loxosceles laeta*), and red-legged widow (*Latrodectus bishopi*). **2.** Exhibiting a pattern suggestive of a spider or a spider's web.

arterial s. A dilated arteriole in the skin, with radiating capillary branches resembling the legs of a spider; characteristic of parenchymatous liver disorder, but also seen in pregnancy and at times in normal individuals. Also called spider nevus; spider

hemangioma; nevus arachnoideus.

Spielmeyer-Vogt disease Cerebral sphingolipidosis; see under sphingolipidosis.

spike A brief electrical cerebral activity of 3 to 25 milliseconds' duration that is recorded on the electroencephalogram as a rising and falling vertical line.

spillway The labial, buccal, and lingual embrasures or passageways through which food escapes from the occlusal surfaces of teeth during chewing.

spina, *pl.* **spinae** **1.** The spine. **2.** Any sharp projection.

s. bifida Congenital defect in which part of the vertebral column is absent; it allows the spinal membranes and sometimes the spinal cord to protrude.

s. bifida occulta Spina bifida without protrusion of the spinal cord or its membranes. Also called cryptomerorachischisis.

spinal **1.** Relating to a spine. **2.** Relating to the vertebral column.

spinal column See column, vertebral.

spinal cord See under cord.

spinal curvature See under curvature.

spindle Any spindle-shaped or fusiform anatomic structure.

mitotic s. The fusiform figure characteristic of a dividing cell formed by protoplasmic fibers extending between the two asters, along which the chromosomes are distributed.

muscle s. Neuromuscular spindle.

neuromuscular s. Small bundle of delicate muscular fibers (intrafusal fibers) invested by a capsule within which the sensory nerve fibers terminate; they vary in length from 0.8 to 5 mm and have a fusiform appearance. Also called muscle proprioceptor.

neurotendinous s. An enclosed capsule containing a number of enlarged tendon fasciculi (intrafusal fasciculi) around which the sensory nerve fibers terminate; chiefly found near the junctions of tendons and muscles. Also called Golgi tendon organ.

spine **1.** A short projection of bone. **2.** Vertebral

Labels in figures: nasal bone, anterior nasal spine, maxilla, mandible, normal spirogram, spirometer, spirochetes, vertebra, spleen, lung, stomach, liver

column; see under column.

anterior nasal s. The anterior projection of the anterior crest of the maxilla.

cervical s. The seven cervical vertebrae considered as a whole.

iliac s. One of the four spines of the ilium.

ischial s. A spine situated on the posterior aspect of the ischium near the posteroinferior border of the acetabulum.

lumbar s. The five lumbar vertebrae considered as a whole.

mental s. One of two spines located on the internal surface of the mandible, near the lower part of the midline.

neural s. The middle spinous process of a typical vertebra.

thoracic s. The twelve thoracic vertebrae considered as a whole.

spinnbarkeit The ability to form a thread; designates the stringy cervical mucus of decreased or low viscosity which, when smeared on a slide, dries in a fernlike pattern and is indicative of ovulation in some women. Also written spinnbarkheit.

spinobulbar Relating to the spine and the medulla oblongata.

spiradenoma A benign tumor or overdevelopment of sweat glands.

spiral Circling around a fixed center; coiled.

Curschmann's s.'s Coiled masses of mucus sometimes found in the sputum in bronchial asthma.

spirillosis Any disease caused by bacteria of the family Spirillaceae.

Spirillum A genus (family Spirillaceae) of flagellated spiral or corkscrew-shaped bacteria which are found in water and putrid infusions.

spirit 1. An alcohol solution of a volatile substance. 2. Archaic term denoting any liquid produced by distillation. 3. Used in the plural, an alcoholic beverage.

pyroxylic s. Methyl alcohol; see under alcohol.

Spirochaeta A genus of nonflagellated microorganisms with a slender wavy shape; found in sewage and stagnant water.

spirochete Any organism of the genus *Spirochaeta*.

spirochetosis Any infection caused by a spirochete, such as syphilis.

spirogram The tracing made by a spirometer.

spirograph A device for graphically recording the depth and rapidity of respiratory movements.

spirometer Device for measuring the rate and volume of breathing; it records the volume of air and the time used to complete both inspiration and expiration.

spironolactone A drug that acts directly on the renal tubules to block the action of aldosterone, producing sodium loss with potassium retention; used to minimize the hypokalemia induced by the thiazides or other potassium-losing diuretics; Aldactone®.

spissated Thickened by evaporation or absorption of fluid.

spit 1. To expectorate. 2. Saliva.

spittle Saliva.

splanchnectopia Malposition of any of the abdominal organs.

splanchnic Pertaining to the viscera.

splanchnicectomy Surgical resection of a portion of the greater splanchnic nerve, usually performed along with a sympathectomy for treating essential hypertension.

splanchnicotomy Surgical transection of a splanchnic nerve or nerves; a surgical procedure tried in the treatment of arterial hypertension.

splanchnocele 1. Hernia of an abdominal organ. 2. The embryonic body cavity.

splanchnomegaly Abnormal largeness of abdominal organs.

splayfoot See flatfoot.

spleen A large vascular lymphatic organ situated in the abdominal cavity on the left side below the diaphragm; it is the sole lymphatic tissue specialized to filter blood; it removes effete or worn out cells from the circulatory system, converts hemoglobin to bilirubin, and releases iron into the blood for reuse. Also called lien.

accessory s. A mass of splenic tissue sometimes present in one of the peritoneal folds.

sago s. A spleen containing deposits of amyloid.

splenectomy Surgical removal of the spleen.

spleneolus Accessory spleen.

splenic Relating to the spleen.

splenic flexure syndrome Painful discomfort in the upper left abdomen which may radiate to the area over the heart and to the left shoulder; believed to be due to distention or spasmodic contraction of the colon.

splenitis Inflammation of the spleen.

splenium A bodily structure resembling a bandaged part.

s. of corpus callosum The round, thick, posterior part of the corpus callosum of the brain.

splenocele 1. Hernial protrusion of the spleen. 2. A splenic tumor.

splenocolic Relating or belonging to the spleen and colon, as the peritoneal fold connecting the organs.

splenocyte A large mononuclear white blood cell of the spleen which is phagocytic; a splenic macrophage.

splenogram A roentgenogram of the spleen.

splenogranulomatosis A granulomatous condition of the spleen with enlargement of the organ and thickening of the capsule.

splenography Roentgenography of the spleen following injection of radiopaque material into it.

splenohepatomegaly Abnormal enlargement of the spleen and the liver.

splenolysis Destruction (lysis) of spleen tissue.

airplane splint

cervical splint

clavicular splint

Frejka's splint

splenomalacia Pathologic softening of the spleen.

splenomegaly Enlargement of the spleen. Also called splenomegalia; megalosplenia.

  chronic congestive s. Disorder usually following hypertension of the portal vein, marked by splenic enlargement, anemia, and occasional gastrointestinal bleeding; leukopenia and thrombocytopenia may develop in some cases. Also called Banti's syndrome; splenic anemia.

  tropical s. Visceral leishmaniasis; see under leishmaniasis.

splenonephric See splenorenal.

splenopancreatic Relating or belonging to the spleen and the pancreas.

splenopathy Any disease or disorder of the spleen.

splenophrenic Relating to the spleen and the diaphragm.

splenoportogram X-ray image of the splenic and portal veins obtained after injection of radiopaque material into the spleen.

splenoptosis Abnormal mobility of the spleen resulting in downward displacement.

splenorenal Relating to the spleen and the kidney. Also called splenonephric.

splenorrhagia Bleeding from a ruptured spleen.

splenosis The presence of numerous nodules composed of splenic tissue throughout the peritoneal cavity.

splenotomy Incision into the spleen.

splenotoxin A cytotoxin that has a particular affinity for the cells of the spleen.

splint A device used to immobilize, support, and correct injured, displaced, or deformed structures.

  acrylic s. A splint covering only the labial and lingual (outside and inside) surfaces of teeth and connected around the last molar by continuous acrylic material or a wire; used only to anchor fractured jaws of children with deciduous teeth.

  acrylic resin bite-guard s. An appliance used to eliminate movement of teeth.

  airplane s. A splint designed to hold the arm in abduction at shoulder level.

  Balkan s. See frame, Balkan.

  cast cap s. A one-piece metal appliance, cemented over the crowns of teeth to immobilize the fragments of a fractured jaw.

  cervical s. A splint for supporting the head, thus taking some pressure off the cervical area.

  Cramer's s. A flexible splint resembling a ladder, consisting of two parallel wires connected with a series of fine wires.

  Denis Browne s. A splint used to correct clubfoot, consisting of two padded metal plates which are securely fastened to the infant's feet and connected by a metal crossbar.

  Frejka's s. A pillow splint used to correct dislocations of the hip in infants under the age of 12 months.

  Hodgen's s. A splint designed for a fractured femur, essentially used to apply balanced traction.

  open-cap s. A cast cap splint that does not cover the occlusal surface of teeth.

  palatal s. A splint applied to the palate and fastened to the upper teeth by clasps or wires; used to hold tissue flaps in place for 48 hours after removal of a maxillary bony growth (torus) from the hard palate; thereafter the splint is worn as a removable bandage until the wound heals.

  plaster s. A splint made of gauze impregnated with plaster of Paris.

  Thomas' s. A splint used to immobilize the leg, consisting of an iron ring that fits on the upper thigh (near the groin) connected to a continuous iron bar that has a W shape at the opposite end.

  treatment s. Temporary artificial tooth or teeth (restoration) that protect and hold in position the teeth adjacent to the space while the fixed partial denture is being constructed.

splinting 1. The application of a rigid device to a limb to prevent motion of a dislocated joint or the ends of a fractured bone. 2. In dentistry, the linking of two or more teeth with a fixed restoration. 3. Protection against pain by reducing motion of the painful part; e.g., the shallow breathing and fixed position assumed by a patient to reduce pain in his chest.

splitting In chemistry, the conversion of a complex substance into two or more simpler products.

spodogenous Resulting from accumulation of waste material in an organ.

spodophagous Denoting one who eats body wastes.

spondylarthritis Inflammation of one or more intervertebral articulations.

spondylitis Inflammation of one or more vertebrae.

  ankylosing s. Ossification of the ligaments of the spine with involvement of the hips and shoulders. Also called Strümpell-Marie arthritis; Marie-Strümpell disease; rheumatoid spondylitis.

  tuberculous s. Tuberculosis of the spine. Also called Pott's disease.

spondylolisthesis Forward slippage of one vertebra over another, usually of a lumbar vertebra on the vertebra below it, or upon the sacrum. Also called spondyloptosis.

spondylolysis Breaking down or destruction of a vertebra.

spondylopathy Any disorder of the vertebrae. Also called rachiopathy.

spondyloptosis See spondylolisthesis.

spondylopyosis Suppurative inflammation of the body of a vertebra.

spondyloschisis Congenital fissure of the vertebral column. Also called myelocele.

spondylosis Abnormal immobility and fixation of a vertebral joint.

ocular fundus

wax pattern of dental restoration

sprue pin

sprue-former

calcaneal spur

cut-out in insole of heel for added comfort

macula lutea

blind spot (optic disk)

modified shoe for calcaneal spur

squalene

sponge 1. The light fibrous skeleton of certain aquatic animals used as an absorbent. 2. A folded piece of gauze or cotton.

absorbable gelatin s. A sterile, absorbable, water-insoluble gelatin-based sponge, used in surgery to control bleeding.

spongiform Resembling a sponge.

spongioblast An embryonic cell of the supportive (non-neuronal) component of the central nervous system.

spongioblastoma Tumor composed mainly of spongioblasts.

spongiocyte 1. A cell of the supportive tissue of the central nervous system. 2. One of the vacuolated cells situated in the cortex of the adrenal gland.

spongiositis Inflammation of the corpus spongiosum of the penis.

spontaneous Arising without appararent cause.

spoon 1. An implement consisting of a small, shallow, oval bowl on a handle. 2. A slang expression for a measure of pure heroin, about 1/16 ounce.

cataract s. An instrument used for removing a cataractous lens from the eye.

sharp s. A sharp-edged spoon used for scraping away granulations, carious bone, or other diseased tissue.

sporadic 1. Occurring infrequently or at irregular intervals. 2. Not widespread.

sporangia Plural of sporangium.

sporangiophore A fungal structure that bears one or more sporangia.

sporangium, *pl.* **sporangia** A capsule or encystment within a plant in which spores are produced.

spore A primitive, thick walled, usually unicellular reproductive cell that is capable of giving rise to a new plant.

sporicide A substance that destroys spores.

sporidium The spore stage of a protozoan organism.

sporoblast An early stage in the development of a sporocyst, from which sporozoites later develop.

sporocyst A stage in the life cycle of many protozoa in which two or more parasites are enclosed within a common wall.

sporogenesis The production of spores.

sporogony A sexual cycle of certain protozoans in which spores are produced as a result of sexual fusion of gametes prior to multiple fission.

sporont A sexually mature protozoan parasite.

sporotrichosis A fungal disease usually affecting cutaneous, subcutaneous, and lymphatic tissues; caused by *Sporotrichum schenkii*.

Sporotrichum A genus of cigar-shaped parasitic fungi.

S. schenkii A species that is the cause of sporotrichosis in man and animals.

Sporozoa A class of the phylum Protozoa which includes parasitic organisms that reproduce by spores.

sporozoan A member of the class Sporozoa.

sporozoite The infectious stage in the life cycle of sporozoan organisms; one of the minute elongated bodies formed by division of the encysted zygote (oocyst); in malaria, forms of the plasmodium organism are concentrated in the salivary glands of mosquitoes and transferred to man in the act of feeding.

sporozoon Sporozoan.

sporulate To produce spores.

sporulation Reproduction by spores.

sporule A minute spore.

spot 1. A small area of discoloration. 2. To discharge a small amount of blood from the vagina.

blind s. The area in the eye, insensitive to light, where the optic nerve leaves the retina. Also called optic disk.

cafe au lait s.'s Hyperpigmented light brown patches on the skin, as seen in neurofibromatosis.

cherry red s. See Tay's cherry red spot.

cotton-wool s. See patch, cotton-wool.

Koplik's s.'s One of the signs of measles; minute bluish white lesions surrounded by a bright ring on the mucous membrane of the cheeks, occurring about two days before the appearance of the skin rash.

liver s.'s See chloasma.

mongolian s. A type of blue nevus of infants, appearing as a dark blue-to-brown spot 2 to 15 cm in diameter over the sacrum; usually disappears in childhood.

rose s.'s Pinkish spots on the abdomen, seen in the early stages of typhoid fever.

Roth's s.'s Round white spots sometimes seen in the retina of patients with bacterial endocarditis.

soft s. See fontanel.

Tay's cherry red s. The cherry red spot in the macular area of the retina, seen in patients with Tay-Sachs disease.

yellow s. See macula retinae.

sprain Injury to a joint in which only the soft tissues are affected.

spray 1. A jet of liquid droplets. 2. To sprinkle.

sprue 1. A malabsorptive disorder. See celiac disease. 2. In dentistry, the wax or metal used to form the opening through which a material such as gold or resin is poured into a mold to make a casting; also the waste piece of material that fills the opening.

nontropical s. See celiac disease.

tropical s. Disease occurring in certain tropical

areas, characterized by abnormal small bowel structure and malabsorption; unlike celiac disease, it is not associated with gluten intolerance but is caused by vitamin deficiencies and/or bacterial contamination of the intestines; it responds to treatment with folic acid, sometimes supplemented by antibiotics. Cf. celiac disease.

sprue-former In dentistry, the cone-shaped base to which the sprue pin is anchored while the wax pattern is being invested.

spur A spinelike projection from a bone or a horny outgrowth from the skin.

calcaneal s. A bony outgrowth from the plantar surface of the calcaneus (heel bone) which often causes pain when walking. Also called heel spur.

heel s. See calcaneal spur.

sputum, *pl.* **sputa** Expectorated matter from the air passages. Also called expectoration.

squalene An unsaturated terpene hydrocarbon found in shark liver oil and an intermediate in the biosynthesis of cholesterol; present in small amounts in blood plasma.

squama, *pl.* **squamae** 1. A thin plate of bone. 2. A scalelike structure.

squamomastoid Relating to the squamous and mastoid portions of the temporal bone.

squamopetrosal Relating to the squamous and petrous parts of the temporal bone.

squamosa The scalelike portion (squama) of the temporal bone.

squamous 1. Scaly; covered with scales. 2. Resembling scales.

squint Strabismus.

S₁S₂S₃ syndrome Prominent S waves in the three standard limb leads with a small R' deflection in V_1 and a normal QRS interval; most commonly seen in young adults without heart disease, but may also be seen in right ventricular hypertrophy, and occasionally with acute myocardial infarction.

stab To pierce or wound with a pointed instrument or weapon.

stabile 1. Stable; unchangeable; fixed; immobile; unaffected, as certain constituents of serum which are unaffected by ordinary degrees of heat, etc. 2. Resistant to chemical change.

stability 1. The condition of being resistant to change in the presence of forces. 2. The ability of a denture to resist displacement by functional forces.

dimensional s. The property of a material to retain its shape.

emotional s. Character of a person not given to marked mood swings or labile emotions.

stabilizer 1. An instrument employed in an x-ray unit to render constant the milliamperage output of the x ray. 2. Any substance used to maintain the

Stain	demonstrates	Stain	demonstrates	Stain	demonstrates
acid stain acid-fast stain	pancreatic alpha cells acid-free bacteria	hematoxylin and eosin stain	cytoplasm and nuclei of cells muscle fibers collagen	silver and gold impregnation stain	reticular fibers collagenous connective tiss Golgi apparatus neurofibrils
alcian blue stain	mucoproteins	Janus-green stain	mitochondria	Sudan stain	lipids myelin
aldehyde fuchsin	elastic fibers basement membranes beta cells of islets of Langerhans neuro secretion mast cell granules thyrotrophs	Mallory's stain	collagen reticular fibers elastic fibers nuclei neuroglia	Toluidine blue stain	nucleic and cytoplasmic ribonucleic acid cartilage matrix mast cell granules basophilic granules Nissl bodies
		Nissl stain	cell bodies of neuron dendrites of neuron	van Gieson's stain	connective tissue
azan stain	nuclei of cells muscle fibers collagen	oil red O stain	lipids	von Kossa's stain	calcium salts in bone
basic stain	nuclei of cells	orcein stain	elastic fibers	Weigert's stain	elastic fibers nerve fibers
Best's carmine stain	glycogen	osmic acid stain	lipids myelin Golgi apparatus	Wright's stain	bone marrow erythrocytes eosinophils basophils neutrophils malarial parasites
brilliant cresyl blue stain	platelets reticulocytes	periodic acid-Schiff stain	glycoproteins glycogen basement membranes granules in some pituitary cells		
Feulgen nuclear reaction stain	chromatin	picric acid and carmine stain	collagenous fibers epithelium muscle fibers	Ziehl-Neelsen stain	tubercle bacilli
Giemsa stain	blood, spleen, and bone marrow certain protozoan parasites	potassium dichromate stain	catecholamine granules of the adrenal medulla and paraganglionic cells		
Golgi stain	nerve tissue				

equilibrium or velocity of a chemical reaction.

stable   Denoting a balanced condition, resisting alteration.

staff   **1.** The personnel who have a specific responsibility and authority in a hospital. **2.** A grooved probe or sound used for guiding the scalpel, as in a lithotomy. Also called guide. **3.** A pole, rod, or stick, especially when used as a symbol.

house s.   The resident or junior physicians and surgeons of a hospital.

stage   **1.** A phase in the course of a disease or the life cycle of an organism. **2.** The platform of a microscope on which the slide is placed for viewing.

anal s.   Stage in infantile psychosexual development during which interest is focused on elimination and retention of feces. Also called anal phase.

exoerythrocytic s.   Stage in the life cycle of the malarial parasite (*Plasmodium*) outside of the red blood cells of the host.

incubation s.   Stage in the course of a disease prior to the appearance of symptoms.

mechanical s.   Device attached to, or built into, the stage of a microscope which permits moving of the specimen slide while holding it in the plane of focus.

Oedipal s.   Stage in psychosexual development following the phallic stage in which the child has an erotic attachment to the parent of the opposite sex. Also called Oedipal phase.

oral s.   Stage of infantile psychosexual development (from birth to approximately 12 months); divided into oral erotic, associated with the pleasurable sensation of sucking, and oral sadistic, related to aggressive biting. Also called oral phase.

phallic s.   Stage in psychosexual development (usually between the ages of 3 and 6) during which the child becomes aware of his/her genital sexuality.

prodromal s.   Incubation stage.

psychosexual s.'s   Stages of development of infantile sexuality, especially in psychoanalytic theory (oral, anal, phallic, Oedipal).

resting s.   The period in the life of a cell when no mitotic changes occur. Properly called interphase.

separation-individuation s.   Stage in personality (around 18 months) when the child begins to develop his/her own sense of self as an autonomous person.

symbiotic s.   Earliest stage in personality development during which the child just barely sees itself as separate from its environment and perceives the self and parent (usually mother) as a single omnipotent being.

s.'s of labor   See under labor.

staging   A clinical method of providing an estimate of the gravity of a cancerous tumor, based on the size of the primary tumor and the extent of local and distant spread.

TNM (tumor-node-metastasis) s.   A system that assigns to higher stages those tumors that are larger, more invasive, or metastatic.

stain   **1.** Any dye used to render cells and tissues visible for microscopic study. **2.** To impart color to cells and tissues for microscopic examination. **3.** A superficial discoloration of the skin.

acid s.   A dye salt whose acid radical combines with the basic components of cells; it stains mainly the protoplasm.

acid-fast s.   Procedure for staining acid-free bacteria (those retaining Ziehl's solution even when decolorized with acid alcohol); after decolorization, a contrasting second stain (counterstain) is applied; the acid-fast cells remain red; others take the color of the counterstain.

aldehyde fuchsin s.   A stain containing potassium permanganate, sulfuric acid, sodium bisulfate, fuchsin, and paraldehyde; used to demonstrate elastic fibers, beta cells of islets of Langerhans, and basement membranes.

basic s.   A dye salt whose basic radical combines with the acidic components of cells; it stains mainly the nuclei.

contrast s.   A stain used to stain a portion of tissue which is unaffected by a previously used dye of another color.

differential s.   A stain used to differentiate between kinds of bacteria that are morphologically indistinguishable although of different species.

Giemsa s.   A stain consisting of azur-II-eosin, azur II, glycerin, and methanol; used for blood cells, Negri bodies, and certain protozoan parasites.

Golgi s.   A heavy metal stain used to enhance the cytoarchitectural appearance of nervous tissue; usually the metal (silver or gold) becomes impregnated along the membranes or within neurons or neuroglia.

Gram's s.   Method used to classify bacteria, based on the ability of the organisms to retain a basic dye (crystal violet); those retaining the violet stain are gram positive and those that do not retain it are gram negative.

H & E s.   Hematoxylin and eosin stain.

hematoxylin and eosin s.   Method of tissue staining employed in numerous variations; consists mainly of the use of a water solution of hematoxylin and eosin; it stains cytoplasm pink and nuclei blue.

Janus-green B s.   A supravital stain used to demonstrate mitochondria.

Mallory's aniline blue s.   One suitable for demonstrating connective tissue and secretion granules.

metachromatic s.   A stain that produces different colors in varied cell elements.

Nissl s.   A method for staining neuronal cell bodies and proximal dendrites; based on the ability of the cell to take up basic aniline dyes, such as cresyl-fast violet, thionine, or toluidine blue.

oil red O s.   Oil red O in isopropyl alcohol; it stains lipid a cherry red color.

orcein s.   A natural dye used to demonstrate elastic fibers and membranes.

osmic acid s.   Aqueous solution of osmic acid (OsO_4) used in electron microscopy as a fixative and stain.

Papanicolaou s.   One employed on smears of body secretions to detect the presence of malignancy; consists generally of aqueous hematoxylin with multiple counterstaining dyes in ethyl alcohol.

periodic acid-Schiff s.   (PAS) A tissue stain for demonstration of polysaccharides and mucopolysaccharides of epithelial mucins, basement membranes, and connective tissue.

port-wine s.   A capillary hemangioma varying in color from pink to purple. Also called port-wine hemangioma.

potassium dichromate s.   A stain used to demonstrate catecholamine granules of the adrenal medulla and paraganglionic cells.

silver and gold impregnation s.   Solutions of silver and gold compounds used to demonstrate reticular fibers, collagenous connective tissue, Golgi apparatus, and neurofibrils.

Sudan s.'s   Oil-soluble compounds used for demonstrating lipids.

supravital s.   A relatively nontoxic dye such as neutral red; used to study living cells.

tumor s.   In radioscopy, a dense area in an x-ray film indicating accumulation of contrast material in abnormal distorted blood vessels, thought to represent a tumor.

vital s.   A dye introduced into a living organism.

von Kossa's s.   A silver nitrate stain for calcium salts in bone.

Weigert s.   A stain that stains nerve fiber tracts blue to black.

Wright's s.   A stain commonly used for the demonstration of blood cells; consists of both acid (eosin) and basic (methylene blue, methylene azure, and methylene violet) dyes; also used to stain malarial parasites.

Ziehl-Neelsen s.   Stain used in the identification of tubercle bacilli.

staining   **1.** The coloration of a microscopic specimen with a dye to improve the visibility of certain parts. **2.** In dentistry, modification of the color of teeth.

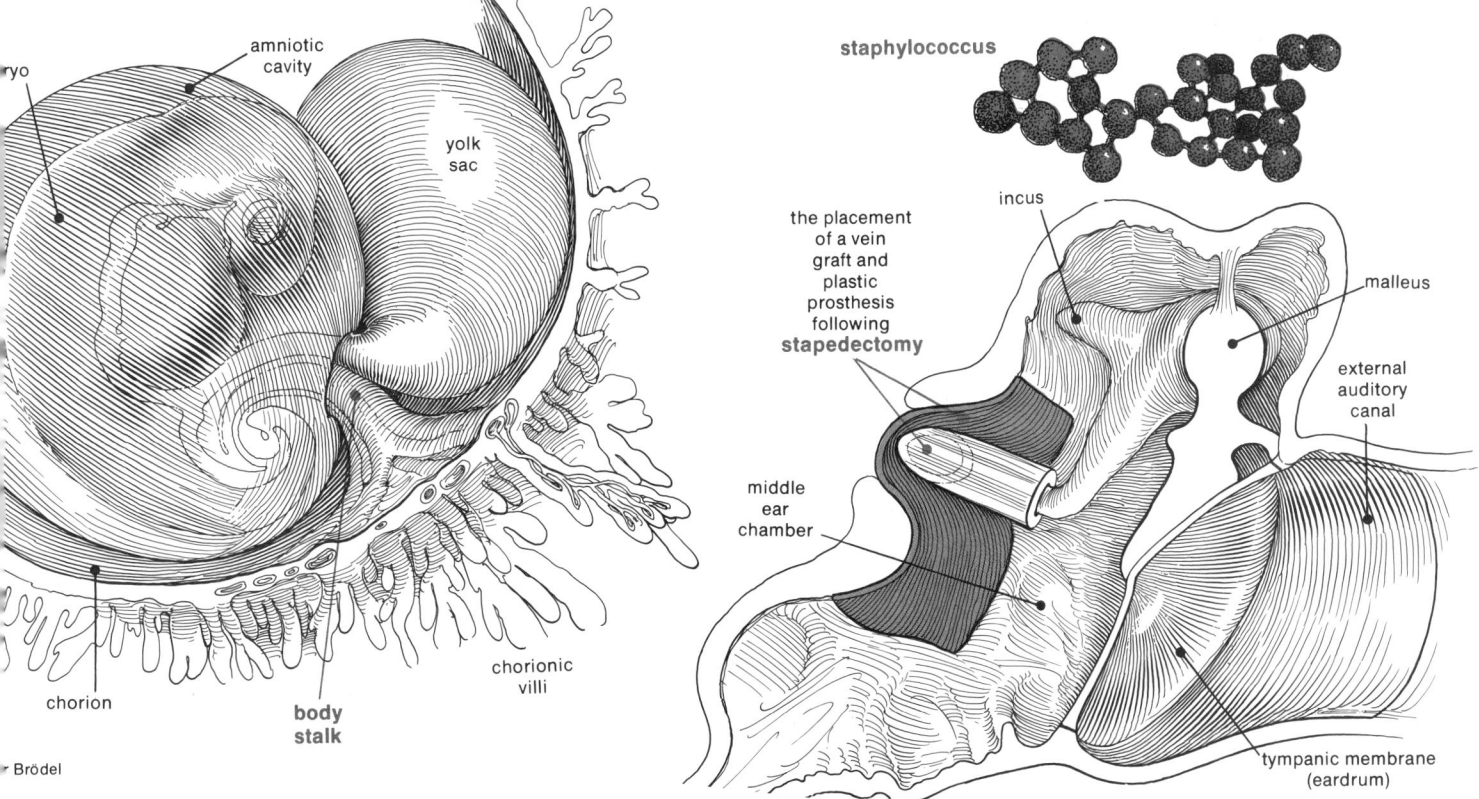

amniotic cavity

yolk sac

ryo

chorion

body stalk

chorionic villi

Brödel

staphylococcus

the placement of a vein graft and plastic prosthesis following **stapedectomy**

incus

malleus

external auditory canal

middle ear chamber

tympanic membrane (eardrum)

negative s. Process of suspending bacteria in an opaque medium (e.g., India ink) that fails to penetrate the organism, thus providing contrast.

simple s. Staining with one dye only.

stalagmometer Device used to obtain and measure drops from a liquid at definite intervals with a view to calculating the surface tension of the liquid.

stalk A slender or elongated connection with a structure or organ.

allantoic s. A narrow connection between the urogenital sinus and the allantoic sac.

body s. A bridge of mesenchymal mass connecting the caudal end of the young embryo to the inner face of the chorionic vesicle.

optic s. A slender structure connecting the optic vesicle to the forebrain in the early embryo.

yolk s. Omphalomesenteric duct; see under duct.

stammering A faltering manner of speaking marked by involuntary pauses and syllabic repetitions; distinguished from stuttering.

stanch To arrest bleeding. Also called staunch.

standard An established rule of comparison for qualitative or quantitative value.

standardization 1. The formulation of standards for any preparation or procedure. 2. Making anything fit a standard.

stannic Relating to or containing tin with valence four.

stannous Relating to or containing tin with valence two.

stannum Latin for tin.

stapedectomy Surgical removal of the stapes from the middle ear chamber.

stapedial Relating to the stapes of the middle ear.

stapediotenotomy Surgical division of the stapedius muscle of the middle ear.

stapediovestibular Relating to both the stapes and the vestibule of the ear.

stapedius A minute muscle in the middle ear. See table of muscles.

stapes The smallest and innermost of the three ossicles of the middle ear; it articulates by its head with the incus, and its base (footplate) is inserted and attached to the margin of the oval window; the smallest bone of the human body. Also called stirrup.

staphylectomy Surgical removal of the uvula.

staphyline Resembling a bunch of grapes.

staphylion A craniometric landmark; the midpoint of the posterior edge of the hard palate.

staphylococcal Relating to or caused by staphylococci.

staphylococcemia The presence of staphylococci in the blood.

staphylococcus, *pl.* **staphylococci** Any organism of the genus *Staphylococcus.*

Staphylococcus A genus (family Micrococcaceae) of gram-positive, nonmotile, usually pathogenic bacteria which tend to aggregate in irregular grapelike clusters.

S. aureus A species containing the pigmented, coagulase-positive variety which causes boils, carbuncles, abscesses, and other suppurative inflammations.

S. epidermidis A species containing the nonpigmented, mannitol- and coagulase-negative nonpathogenic variety which causes stitch abscesses; normally present on skin.

staphyloderma Pus-forming skin disorder caused by staphylococci.

staphylolysin 1. A substance elaborated by a staphylococcus that causes destruction of red blood cells and liberation of hemoglobin. 2. An antibody causing dissolution of staphylococci.

staphyloma Protrusion of the cornea or sclera; usually lined with uveal tissue.

staphyloplasty Surgical repair of the uvula and/or the soft palate.

staphyloptosia, staphyloptosis Relaxation or lengthening of the uvula.

starch 1. A carbohydrate with the general formula $(C_6H_{10}O_5)_n$; exists abundantly in the vegetable kingdom and is converted into dextrins and glucose by amylase enzyme action in saliva and pancreatic juice. 2. A substance consisting of granules separated from the mature grain of *Zea mays* (Indian corn); used in pharmaceuticals and as a dusting powder.

stare To look intently with a steady, often wide-eyed, unblinking gaze.

postbasic s. An odd expression of the eyes marked by downward rolling of the eyeballs and retraction of the upper eyelids; seen in persons with posterior basic meningitis.

starvation The condition of suffering from prolonged lack of food.

stasis Stoppage of the flow of a fluid, especially of the blood.

state A condition.

anxiety s. Anxiety neurosis; see under neurosis.

carrier s. The condition of harboring pathogenic microorganisms without being affected by them.

central excitatory s. A condition of hyperexcitability of nerve cells produced by the storing up of subthreshold stimuli in a reflex center of the spinal cord.

convulsive s. Spasmodic jerking of the extremities and trunk with varying degrees of unconsciousness.

dreamy s. A semiconscious condition associated with an attack of epilepsy.

paranoid s. Psychotic disorder in which the primary abormality consists of a delusion, usually of persecution or grandeur.

refractory s. The reduced excitability of a nerve following a response to previous stimulation.

standard s. The pure and stable form of an element at 1.0 pressure and 25°C temperature.

steady s. Dynamic equilibrium.

twilight s. Condition of impaired consciousness in which a person may perform elaborate purposeful acts and have no recollection of them afterward.

statim (stat) Latin for at once, immediately; used in prescription writing.

statistics A collection of organized numerical data.

vital s. A collection of data pertaining to human birth, health, disease, and death.

statoconia See otoconia.

stature The natural height of a person.

status State; condition.

s. choleraicus The stage of shock and collapse in cholera, marked by cold skin, weak pulse, and lethargy.

s. epilepticus A series of epileptic attacks in rapid succession.

s. thymicolymphaticus Enlargement of the thymus and lymph nodes; formerly believed to cause crib death of infants.

staunch See stanch.

steal Diversion of blood from a vascular area to one deprived of circulation.

subclavian s. See subclavian steal syndrome.

steapsin A fat-splitting enzyme in pancreatic juice. Also called pancreatic lipase.

stearate A salt of stearic acid.

stearic acid A common fatty acid made by the hydrolysis of fats; used in pharmaceutical preparations. Also called octadecanoic acid.

steatocryptosis Dysfunction of sebaceous glands.

steatocystoma A sebaceous cyst.

s. multiplex See steatomatosis.

steatogenous 1. Causing fat degeneration. 2. Producing any disease of the sebaceous glands.

steatolysis The hydrolysis or emulsion of fat preparatory to absorption.

steatoma 1. A tumor composed chiefly of fatty tissue. 2. A sebaceous cyst.

steatomatosis A condition characterized by the presence of numerous sebaceous cysts, often widespread. Also called steatocystoma multiplex.

steatonecrosis A histologic abnormality seen almost exclusively in the liver of an alcoholic patient; marked by the presence of Mallory bodies (coagu-

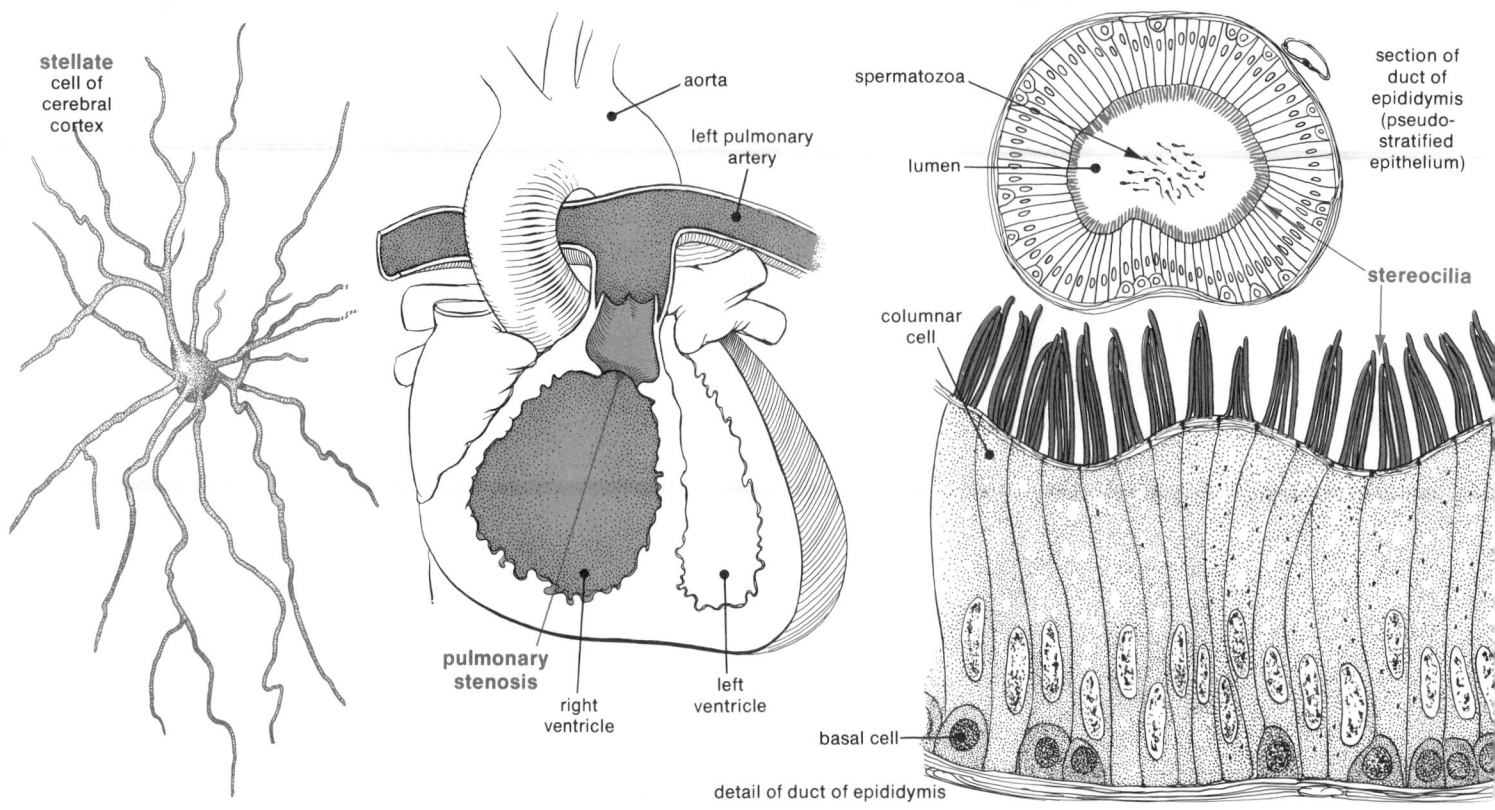

stellate cell of cerebral cortex

aorta

left pulmonary artery

pulmonary stenosis

right ventricle

left ventricle

spermatozoa

section of duct of epididymis (pseudo-stratified epithelium)

lumen

stereocilia

columnar cell

basal cell

detail of duct of epididymis

lated, hyalinized cytoplasm that forms a coarse, acidophilic network around the nucleus of liver cells), usually in association with fatty changes.

steatopathy Disorder of the sebaceous glands.

steatopygia, steatopyga Excessively fat buttocks.

steatorrhea Excessive amount of fat in the feces, a manifestation of the malabsorption syndrome.

steatosis 1. Fatty degeneration. 2. Any disease of the sebaceous glands.

stegnosis 1. Stoppage of secretions or excretions. 2. Constriction.

Stein-Leventhal syndrome Condition characterized primarily by menstrual abnormalities, enlarged cystic ovaries, and infertility. Also called polycystic ovary syndrome.

stellate Having the shape of a star.

stellectomy Excision of the stellate ganglion; usually performed for the relief of intractable pain. Also called stellate ganglionectomy.

Stellwag's sign Infrequent and incomplete blinking; seen in exophthalmic goiter.

stem cell renewal A residual population of cells that retain the ability to divide.

stenion The craniometric point located at each end of the shortest transverse diameter of the skull in the temporal region.

stenochoria Constriction of a duct or orifice.

stenopeic Having a narrow opening.

stenosed Constricted.

stenosis Abnormal constriction of a channel or orifice.

 aortic s. Pathologic constriction of the orifice between the aorta and the left ventricle of the heart.

 congenital pyloric s. See hypertrophic pyloric stenosis.

 hypertrophic pyloric s. Overdevelopment of the pyloric sphincter muscle causing narrowing of the pyloric orifice and projectile vomiting, occurring in the second or third week of life. Also called congenital pyloric stenosis.

 idiopathic hypertrophic subaortic s. (IHSS) Disease of the heart muscle marked by disproportionate hypertrophy of the interventricular septum and left ventricular wall which sometimes causes obstruction to the left outflow tract. Also called asymmetric septal hypertrophy (ASH).

 infundibular pulmonic s. Obstruction of the infundibulum (outflow tract) of the right ventricle of the heart, usually caused by either or both of two conditions; (a) a fibrous ring just below the pulmonic valve; (b) hypertrophy of heart muscle surrounding the infundibulum.

 mitral s. Narrowing of the opening between the left atrium and the left ventricle.

 pulmonary s. Constriction of the orifice between the pulmonary artery and the right ventricle.

 pyloric s. Constriction of the pyloric orifice of the stomach.

 subaortic s., subvalvular s. Obstruction of the outflow tract of the left ventricle of the heart; caused by either a fibrous band or muscular hypertrophy just below the aortic valve.

 tricuspid s. Narrowing of the tricuspid orifice of the heart.

stenostenosis Constriction of the parotid duct.

stenostomia A narrow state of the oral cavity.

stenothermal Capable of withstanding only slight changes in temperature.

stenothorax An abnormally narrow chest.

stenotic Narrowed abnormally; affected with stenosis.

stent 1. A mold for holding a skin graft in place. 2. A device for supporting tubular structures that are being anastomosed.

steppage High steppage gait; see under gait.

stercobilin A brown pigment present in the feces, derived from bile.

stercolith A fecal concretion.

stercoraceous Fecal; relating to feces.

stere A metric unit of volume equal to one kiloliter or 1,000 liters (nearly one cubic meter).

stereoanesthesia See astereognosis.

stereoarthrolysis Surgical creation of a movable joint.

stereocampimeter Instrument used to examine the central visual field of each eye separately while both eyes fixate similar targets.

stereochemistry The branch of chemistry concerned with the spatial arrangement of atoms in a compound.

stereocilia Unusually long, slender, nonmotile microvilli, found primarily in parts of the male reproductive tract; thought to aid in secretion and absorption.

stereocinefluorography Motion picture photography of x-ray images obtained by stereoscopic fluoroscopy, producing three-dimensional visualization.

stereognosis The recognition of objects through the sense of touch.

stereoisomer One of two compounds which contain the same chemical structure but which have different optical properties because the atoms in each have different spatial positions.

stereoisomerism Isomerism in which two compounds have the same structural formula but the atoms are linked in a different order.

stereology A study of the three-dimensional aspects of morphology, especially ultrastructure.

stereo-orthopter A visual training instrument used to correct strabismus.

stereopsis Visual depth perception produced by slight disparateness of images, i.e., when images fall on slightly disparate points of the retina.

stereoroentgenography The taking of an x-ray picture from two slightly different positions to produce a three-dimensional effect.

stereoscope Instrument that permits two different portions of the same picture (or two photographs of different views of the same object) to be viewed by the two eyes at the same time, resulting in a three-dimensional perception.

stereospecific Denoting enzymes or synthetic organic reactions that act only with a given molecule or with a limited class of molecules.

stereotaxis 1. The localization of the three-dimensional arrangement of body structures by means of coordinate landmarks. 2. The movement of an organism toward, or away from, a rigid surface with which it comes in contact; applied to the organism as a whole.

stereotaxy A method of inserting an electrode into a specific area of the brain by means of a stereotaxic apparatus; used to destroy nuclear masses and fiber tracts within the brain.

stereotropism The movement of parts of an organism toward (positive stereotropism) or away from (negative stereotropism) a solid body with which it comes in contact.

stereotypy The persistent mechanical repetition of certain movements or speech; common in schizophrenia.

 oral s. See verbigeration.

steric Relating to stereochemistry.

sterile 1. Incapable of reproducing. 2. Free from bacteria or other microorganisms. Also called aseptic.

sterility Absence or nonfunctioning of the organs of reproduction.

sterilization 1. A treatment that deprives living organisms of the ability to reproduce. 2. The process of destroying or removing all living microorganisms.

sterilizer An apparatus for rendering anything germ-free.

sternal Of or relating to the sternum (breastbone).

sternalgia 1. Pain in the sternum or sternal area. Also called sternodynia. 2. Angina pectoris.

sternoclavicular Relating to the sternum and the clavicle.

sternocleidal Relating to the sternum and the clavicle.

sternocleidomastoid Relating to the sternum, clavicle, and mastoid process; denoting the muscle that has its origin and insertion on these structures.

steroid

three fused cyclohexane rings plus

a terminal cyclopentane ring

stilbestrol

esophagus
cardiac incisure
fundus
lesser curvature
pyloric canal
pyloric sphincter
pyloric antrum
body
stomach
greater curvature
duodenum

hourglass stomach

sternocostal   Relating to the sternum and the ribs.
sternodynia   See sternalgia.
sternotomy   Cutting through the sternum.
sternum   A long, flat bone forming the middle part of the anterior wall of the thoracic cage, articulating with the clavicles and the costal cartilages of the first seven pairs of ribs. Also called breastbone.
steroid   1. One of a family of chemical substances characterized by four interlocking rings of carbon atoms; included are the adrenal steroids, corticosteroids, the male and female sex hormones, and the D vitamins; cholesterol is one of the main building blocks for the other steroids; examples include aldosterone, androsterone, cholecalciferol, cholesterol, cortisol, cortisone, estradiol, estriol, progesterone, and testosterone. 2. A shortened form for an adrenal corticosteroid or a synthetic compound with similar actions.
   anabolic s.   Any of a group of synthetic drugs with protein-building properties; they promote muscle recovery after injury and help strengthen bones. Adverse effects include acne, liver and adrenal gland damage, and infertility.
steroidogenesis   The natural production of steroids.
steroid withdrawal syndrome   Weakness, nausea, fever, malaise, and slight hypotension experienced by persons upon withdrawal of steroid therapy to which they have been subjected for prolonged periods.
sterol   One of a group of unsaturated solid alcohols, a subdivision of the steroids, present in all animal and plant tissue except bacteria; the best known member of the group is cholesterol.
stertor   A snoring sound produced in breathing.
stertorous   Characterized by snoring.
stethograph   Apparatus used for recording the respiratory movements of the chest.
stethoscope   An instrument used for listening to sounds produced within the body, especially respiratory and vascular sounds; originally designed by René Laënnec.
Stevens-Johnson syndrome   Erythema multiforme exudativum; see under erythema.
stibialism   Poisoning with antimony.
stiff-man syndrome   A chronic disorder of unknown cause marked by fluctuating muscular rigidity and spasm which progresses to generalized stiffness involving the extremities, neck, and trunk; associated with severe muscle pains and disability, dysphagia, and weight loss.
stigma, *pl.* **stigmata**   1. Visible evidence characteristic of a disease (spot, blemish, symptom, sign, etc.). 2. The pigmented eyespot of certain protozoa.
stilbestrol   A colorless crystalline compound derived from stilbene; formerly used as an estrogen in humans and as a fattener for livestock; now thought to have carcinogenic properties. Also called diethylstilbestrol.
stillbirth   Death of the fetus while in the uterus.
stillborn   Born dead.
stilus   A pencil-shaped medicinal preparation for external application.
stimulant   Anything that accelerates organic activity.
stimulation   1. The process of exciting the body, or a part, to increased functional activity. 2. The state of being stimulated.
   photic s.   The use of a flickering light to alter the pattern of the electroencephalogram.
stimulator   An agent that increases functional activity.
   cerebellar electrical s.   Brain pacemaker; see under pacemaker.
   long-acting thyroid s.   (LATS) Substance found in the blood of hyperthyroid patients, not elaborated in the pituitary gland, and having a prolonged stimulatory action on the thyroid gland.
stimulus, *pl.* **stimuli**   1. Anything causing a response. 2. A stimulant; an agent or action that elicits a physiologic or psychologic activity.
   conditioned s.   (CS) A stimulus which prior to the procedure does not evoke the specific reflex or response under study.
   unconditioned s.   (UCS) A stimulus which normally evokes the particular response under study.
sting   1. To pierce the skin with a sharp-pointed organ or part, such as the ovipositor of a wasp, and deposit venom. 2. The sharp transitory pain produced by stinging.
stippling   In histology, the staining of basophilic granules in a cell protoplasm when exposed to the action of a basic stain.
   Ziemann's s.   Fine spots sometimes seen in red blood cells of persons with quartan malaria.
stirrup   See stapes.
stitch   1. A suture. 2. A sudden, short sharp pain. 3. The act of suturing.
stoichiometry   The study of the combining proportions (by weight and volume) of elements participating in a chemical reaction.
Stokes-Adams syndrome   See Adams-Stokes syndrome.
stoma   1. Any small opening. 2. The mouth or an artificial opening between two cavities or channels or between any cavity or tube and the exterior.
stomach   The enlarged, saclike portion of the digestive tract, between the esophagus and the small intestine, in which ingested food is acted on by the enzymes and hydrochloric acid of gastric juice, and then released spasmodically into the duodenum by gastric peristalsis; the stomach is entirely covered with peritoneum and normally has a capacity of about one quart.
   hourglass s.   One with a stricture at the midpoint.
   leather-bottle s.   See linitis plastica.
stomachache   Pain in the stomach or abdomen.
stomal   Pertaining to a stoma or small aperture.
stomatalgia   Pain in the mouth, occurring in varying degrees of severity as a result of injury or disease. Also called stomatodynia.
stomatic   Relating to (a) the mouth; (b) an artificial opening.
stomatitis   Inflammation of the mucous membrane of the mouth.
   angular s.   Superficial fissuring and inflammation at the angles of the mouth.
   aphthous s.   A chronically recurrent disease marked by the appearance of small, painful, single or multiple ulcers on the mucous membrane of the mouth. Also called canker; canker sore; ulcerative stomatitis.
   gangrenous s.   See noma.
   herpetic s.   A recurrent infection of the oral mucosa, caused by the herpes simplex virus, with painful vesicle and ulcer formation.
   ulcerative s.   See aphthous sore.
   Vincent's s.   Necrotizing ulcerative gingivitis; see under gingivitis.
stomatocyte   Red blood cell in which the central area appears as a slit rather than a biconcave circular area.
stomatodynia   See stomatalgia.
stomatology   The study of the structures, functions, and diseases of the mouth.
stomatomalacia   Abnormal softening of structures in the mouth.
stomatomycosis   Fungal disease of the mouth.
stomatopathy   Any disorder of the oral cavity.
stomatorrhagia   Bleeding from any structure in the mouth.
stomodeum   A midline invagination or depression of the ectoderm of the embryo between the maxillary and mandibular processes which later develops into the mouth cavity.
stone   An abnormal concretion usually composed of mineral salts and formed most frequently in the cavities of the body which serve as reservoirs for fluids. Also called calculus.
   bladder s.   A stone lodged in the bladder; it may be either formed in the bladder or passed from the kidney or ureter. Also called vesical calculus.
   chalk s.   See tophus.
   dental s.   Gypsum that has been calcined under

normal
well
balanced
foot

normal
transverse arch

normal longitudinal arch

development of foot **strain**

deltoid
ligament
strain

head of talus
is depressed

talus
slides
medially

flattened transverse arch

navicular bone drops

heel everts
into valgus
position

plantar fascia **strain**

diverge
strabism

kidney
stones

steam pressure to 130°C; used for making casts and models of the oral cavity. Also called α-hemihydrate.
  gallbladder s. Gallstone.
  kidney s. Stone in the kidney, most commonly made up of calcium oxalate, uric acid, or calcium phosphate. Also called renal calculus.
  pulp s. The collection of calcified material in the pulp chamber of a tooth or a projection into the chamber from the cavity wall. Also called pulp nodule; denticle.
  tear s. A stone located in the lacrimal apparatus (tear-forming and tear-conducting structures). Also called dacryolith.
  womb s. A calcified myoma of the uterus.
stool **1.** A bowel movement. **2.** Feces.
  tarry s. Bloody stool, especially one in which blood can be grossly recognized.
stopcock A valve that stops or regulates the flow of a liquid through a tube or pipe.
storm, thyroid Thyrotoxic crisis; see under crisis.
strabismal, strabismic Relating to or afflicted with strabismus.
strabismometer Instrument used to measure the angle of strabismus.
strabismus A visual disorder in which one eye cannot focus with the other. Also called heterotropia.
  convergent s. Strabismus in which the eye deviates inward, toward the nose. Also called cross-eye; internal strabismus; esotropia.
  divergent s. Strabismus in which the eye deviates outward. Also called wall-eye; external strabismus; exotropia.
strabotomy Division of one or more of the ocular muscles or their tendons in treatment of strabismus.
straight back syndrome Loss of the physiologic dorsal kyphosis of the thoracic spine; this may result in the leftward shift of the heart or a "pancake" appearance; the close proximity of the outflow structures to the anterior chest wall results in an easily heard innocent systolic murmur.
straightjacket A longsleeved garment used to restrain a violent patient by securing the arms tightly against the body.

strain **1.** Tearing or stretching of a muscle or its tendon. Cf. sprain. **2.** To injure a part by misuse or excessive effort. **3.** The injury resulting from such activity. **4.** A group of microorganisms, such as bacteria, made up of descendants of a single isolation in pure culture. **5.** An inherited trait. **6.** A measure of the deformation produced on a structure by an external force; used in reference to the elastic property of solids.
  S s. The strain of pneumococcus that has a slime capsule and causes pneumonia.
strait A narrow space or passageway.
  inferior pelvic s. Pelvic plane of outlet; see under plane.
  superior pelvic s. Pelvic plane of inlet; see under plane.
strait jacket See straightjacket.
stramonium The dried leaves of jimsonweed (*Datura stramonium*), formerly used in the treatment of asthma.
strangle To suffocate by compressing the trachea so as to prevent respiration; to choke.
strangulation **1.** Constriction of the air passages that interferes with or terminates normal breathing. **2.** Compression that cuts off the blood supply to a part, specifically to a loop of intestine.
strangury Difficult, slow, painful urination.
strap **1.** A strip of adhesive plaster. **2.** To bind with adhesive plaster.
stratified Arranged in layers.
stratiform Arranged in a series of superimposed layers.
stratum, *pl.* **strata** A layer, especially of differentiated tissue comprising one of several associated layers.
  horizontal strata Portion of dorsal horn of gray matter of spinal cord. Formerly called zona spongiosa.
  malpighian s. Stratum germinativum.
  s. bacillare retinae The neuroepithelial layer of rods and cones of the retina.
  s. basale The deepest (basal) layer of the endometrium (mucosa of the uterus) which undergoes only minimal changes during the menstrual cycle;

the portion of the endometrium which is not sloughed off during menstruation; it contains the narrow terminal portion of the uterine glands.
  s. basale epidermidis The deepest (basal) layer of the epidermis consisting of columnar or high cuboidal cells arranged in a single row and resting on a thin basement membrane; usually contains granules of melanin pigment.
  s. compactum The innermost layer of the endometrium (mucosa of the uterus) containing the necks of the uterine glands and a rather compact layer of interglandular tissue.
  s. corneum The outermost horny keratinized layer of the epidermis, composed of flattened, dehydrated, nonnucleated epithelial cells; it is very thick in the palms and soles. Also called corneum.
  s. cylindricum Stratum basale epidermidis.
  s. functionale The thick part of the lining of the uterus (endometrium) which is sloughed off during menstruation; it consists of a compact layer and a spongy layer.
  s. germinativum The growing part of the epidermis containing several rows of cells undergoing mitosis; composed of a basal layer (stratum basale) and a spiny layer (stratum spinosum). Also called malpighian layer.
  s. granulosum epidermidis The layer of epidermis between the stratum spinosum and the stratum lucidum composed of a few rows of flattened rhombic cells with their long axis parallel with the skin; thought to represent the transitional stage in the formation of soft keratin; the cells contain conspicuous granules of keratohyalin.
  s. granulosum ovarii The epithelial layer of granulosa (follicular) cells in the developing ovarian follicle, located between the zona pellucida surrounding the ovum and the glassy membrane.
  s. lucidum A narrow homogeneous layer of the epidermis between the stratum corneum and the stratum granulosum; it consists of a few rows of flattened clear cells containing a refractile substance (eleidin); nuclei and cell boundaries are not visible.
  s. pigmenti retinae The outer pigmented layer of the retina.

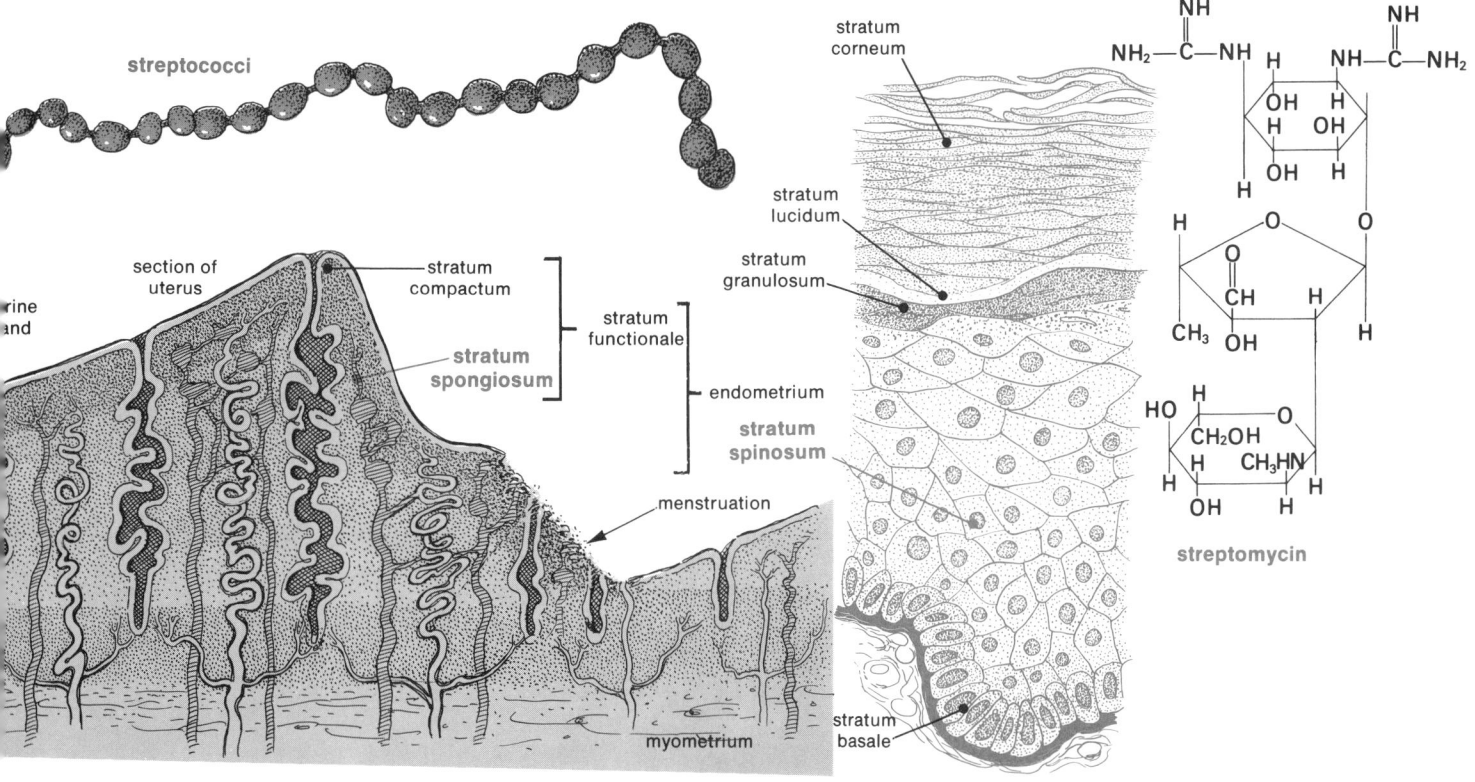

streptococci

stratum corneum

stratum lucidum

stratum granulosum

section of uterus

stratum compactum

stratum functionale

stratum spongiosum

endometrium

stratum spinosum

menstruation

stratum basale

myometrium

streptomycin

s. spinosum The thick layer of the epidermis between the stratum basale and stratum granulosum, composed of irregular polyhedral cells with short cytoplasmic spines which may contain melanin; mitosis is frequent in this layer. Also called prickle-cell layer.

s. spongiosum The middle of three layers of the lining of the uterus (endometrium) containing the tortuous and dilated glands and a small amount of interglandular tissue; the layer is discharged at each menstrual flow and at the termination of pregnancy.

streak A striation, line, or furrow.

angioid s.'s Brownish-red pigmented lines in the fundus of the eye, radiating from the disk and situated beneath the retinal vessels, due to degeneration of the lamina vitrea of the choroid; may be seen in pseudoxanthoma elasticum, osteitis deformans, and sickle-cell anemia.

germinal s. Primitive streak.

Knapp's s.'s Pigmented streaks resembling blood vessels, seen occasionally in the retina following hemorrhage. Also called Knapp's striae.

medullary s. The embryonic neural groove, the closure of which forms the primordium of the brain and spinal cord.

primitive s. A midline narrow groove, with slightly bulging regions on either side, situated on the caudal end of the embryonic disk; site from which the mesodermal cells migrate from the surface to form the middle germ layer; clearly visible in a 15- to 16-day embryo and provides the earliest evidence of the cephalocaudal axis.

strephosymbolia A perception disorder, occurring mainly in children, in which certain letters or words are seen reversed, as if in a mirror.

strepitus A sound heard on auscultation.

Streptobacillus A genus (family Bacteriodiaceae) of bacteria containing gram-negative rods; some species are pathogenic.

streptococcal Relating to or caused by streptococcus.

streptococcemia The presence of streptococci in the blood.

streptococci Plural of streptococcus.

streptococcosis Any infection with streptococci.

Streptococcus A genus of gram-positive, round or ovoid bacteria (family Streptococcaceae), pathogenic and/or nonpathogenic in man, occurring in pairs or chains; medically classified according to their hemolytic activity on blood agar as alpha-hemolytic streptococci, which produce a zone of incomplete hemolysis and green discoloration adjacent to the colony; beta-hemolytic streptococci, which produce a clear zone of hemolysis around the colony; and gamma-streptococci, which produce no

hemolysis. Beta-hemolytic forms are classified into groups (A, B, C, etc.) according to the carbohydrate found in the cell wall; group A strains are pathogenic for humans; they are further subdivided by Arabic numerals into types based on the cell wall protein.

S. fecalis An enterococcus normally found in the intestinal tract; a cause of subacute bacterial endocarditis.

S. pneumoniae A rarely spherical species that causes lobar pneumonia and other acute pus-forming conditions such as middle ear infections and meningitis. Formerly called *Diplococcus pneumoniae*.

S. pyogenes A species that is the cause of several acute pyogenic (pus-forming) infections in man, such as scarlet fever, erysipelas, and sore throat.

S. salivarius Species found in saliva and throughout the intestinal tract; generally nonpathogenic but has been implicated in contributing to the formation of dental caries.

streptococcus, *pl.* **streptococci** Any member of the genus *Streptococcus*.

streptodermatitis Inflammation of the skin caused by streptococci.

streptodornase Enzyme produced by hemolytic streptococci, capable of causing liquefaction of purulent exudates.

streptokinase Enzyme present in hemolytic streptococci, capable of dissolving fibrin; used to dissolve blood clots and fibrinous adhesions.

streptolysin A hemolysin produced by streptococci.

Streptomyces A genus of bacteria (family Streptomycetacea) present in the soil; antibiotics have been obtained from cultures of some species.

S. antibioticus Species that yields actinomycin.

S. fradiae Species that yields neomycin.

S. griseus Species that yields streptomycin.

streptomycete A member of the genus *Streptomyces*.

streptomycin An antibiotic obtained from cultures of *Streptomyces griseus*; white granules or powder soluble in water, acid alcohol, and methyl alcohol; active against the tubercle bacillus, many gram-negative bacteria, and some gram-positive bacteria; excessive dosage leads to damage to the eighth cranial (vestibulocochlear) nerve, usually affecting the vestibular part first.

streptotrichosis Infection with bacteria of the genus formerly called *Streptothrix* but now classified in other genera, e.g., *Actinomyces*, *Nocardia*, *Streptobacillus*.

stress 1. The internal force of a body generated to resist an external force that tends to deform it. 2. In dentistry, pressure against the teeth and their

attachments exceeding that produced by normal function. 3. Abnormal conditions that tend to disrupt normal functions of the body or mind. 4. An emotionally disrupting influence.

stressbreaker An attachment in a removable partial denture that relieves the anchoring teeth of all or part of the pressure during mastication.

stretcher A canvas stretched over a frame, used to transport disabled or dead persons. Also called litter.

stria, *pl.* **striae** A thin stripe or band, especially one of several that are more or less parallel.

s. atrophica One of several glistening white bands in the skin of the abdomen, breasts, buttocks, and thighs, caused by overstretching and weakening of the elastic tissues; associated with pregnancy, obesity, rapid growth during puberty, Cushing's syndrome, and other conditions.

striate, striated Marked by striae; striped.

striation 1. A stria. 2. The state of having stria.

stricture An abnormal narrowing of a tubular structure.

strident Harsh, shrill, or grating, as certain sounds heard on auscultation.

stridor A harsh, shrill respiratory sound, as in acute laryngeal obstruction.

stridulous Having a harsh, shrill sound.

strip 1. To remove the contents of a tubular structure by gently running a finger along the structure; to milk. 2. To excise a varicose vein of the leg with a stripper. 3. Any narrow piece.

abrasive s. A piece of linen with an abrasive material bonded to one side; used to shape and polish proximal surfaces of artificial teeth.

lightning s. A metal strip with abrasive on one side; used to remove rough or improper points of contact between artificial teeth.

stripe A streak.

Mees' s.'s White stripes on fingernails occurring in arsenic poisoning.

stripper An instrument for the removal of a diseased vein; generally consists of a cable with a disk or cup at one end and a guide tip at the other.

strobila, *pl.* **strobilae** The linear collection of segments comprising the body of a tapeworm.

strobiloid Resembling the segmented body of a tapeworm.

strobolaryngoscope A type of stroboscope used to observe in detail the vibratory motion of the vocal cords.

stroboscope 1. An instrument used to observe moving objects by making them appear stationary through intermittently interrupted illumination. 2. An electronic instrument that produces brief pulses of light at controllable frequency, used to alter electrical activity of the cerebral cortex.

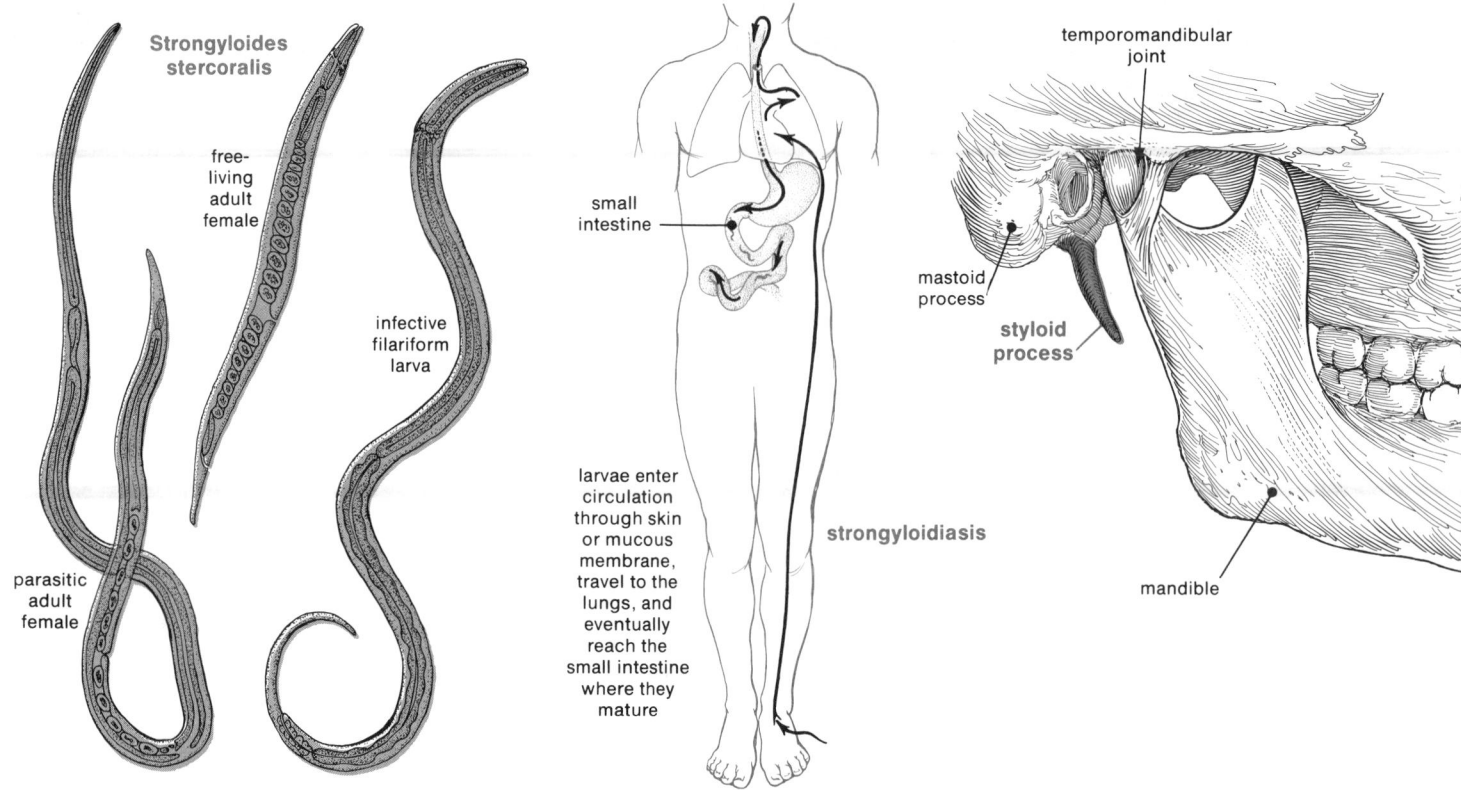

Strongyloides stercoralis
free-living adult female
infective filariform larva
parasitic adult female

small intestine

larvae enter circulation through skin or mucous membrane, travel to the lungs, and eventually reach the small intestine where they mature

strongyloidiasis

temporomandibular joint
mastoid process
styloid process
mandible

stroke **1.** Occlusion or rupture of a blood vessel in the brain. Also called cerebrovascular or cerebral vascular accident. **2.** Any sudden, severe attack or seizure.

heat s. Condition caused by excessive exposure to high temperatures, marked by high fever, dry skin, and in severe cases, coma.

paralytic s. Sudden paralysis caused by injury to the brain.

stroma The framework of an organ, usually composed of connective tissue, which supports the functional elements or cells.

stromuhr Instrument used to measure the amount of blood flowing per unit of time through a blood vessel.

Strongyloides A genus (class Nematoda) of intestinal parasites of herbivorous animals and man.

S. stercoralis A species that is the causative agent of strongyloidiasis of man.

strongyloidiasis, strongyloidosis Parasitic infection caused by a nematode, *Strongyloides stercoralis*; the threadlike worms enter the body through the skin or mucous membrane of the mouth, travel to the lungs, and eventually reach the small intestine where the female lays her eggs.

strontium A soft, easily oxidized metallic element similar to calcium in chemical properties; symbol Sr, atomic number 38, atomic weight 87.62.

s. 90 A radioactive isotope which emits a high energy beta particle and has a half-life of 28 years; a product of atom bomb blasts that constitutes an important fallout hazard, since it is incorporated into bone tissue upon absorption.

Strophanthus A genus of African vines of the family Apocynaceae.

S. gratus Species containing ouabain, a cardiac glycoside.

S. kombe A species containing strophanthin, a cardiac glycoside.

structure The configuration of the component parts of an entity.

brush heap s. The fibrils in a gel or hydrocolloid impression material.

denture-supporting s. The tissues, teeth, and/or residual ridges that serve as support for removable dentures (partial or complete).

fine s. See ultrastructure.

struma Goiter

Hashimoto's s. Lymphocytic thyroiditis; see under thyroiditis.

s. lymphomatosa Lymphocytic thyroiditis; see under thyroiditis.

Riedel's s. See thyroiditis, Riedel's.

strumitis Inflammation of the thyroid gland accompanied by swelling.

strychnine An extremely poisonous alkaloid, derived from seeds of *Strychnos nux-vomica* and possessing an intensely bitter taste; occasionally used as a stimulant for the central nervous system.

strychninism A toxic condition resulting from excessive use of strychnine. Also called chronic strychnine poisoning.

Strychnos A genus of tropical trees or shrubs (family Loganiaceae) that yield the alkaloids strychnine, curare, ignatia, and brucine.

study The pursuit and acquisition of information.

bioavailability s. See bioequivalence study.

bioequivalence s. The comparison of two or more different formulations of the same parent drug, one of which is an acceptable standard. Also called bioavailability study.

blind s. A study in which the patient is not aware of the type of medication being administered.

case control s. Epidemiological study that begins with identification of persons with the disease of interest, and a comparison (control) group of people without the disease; the relationship of a particulate attribute (e.g., sex, age, race) to the disease is examined by comparing the frequency with which the attribute appears in both groups. Also called case comparison, case history, or case referent study.

double blind s. A study in which neither the patient nor the individual in contact with the patient is cognizant of the type of medication being administered in order to obviate bias of observation.

longitudinal s. A study of a defined cohort (group of individuals having a statistical factor in common) over a protracted period of time, in contrast to a cross-sectional study examining a cohort at a particular time.

stump **1.** The extremity of a limb left after amputation. **2.** The pedicle remaining after removal of the tumor that was attached to it.

stun To daze, stupefy, or render senseless, as by a blow or other force.

stupe A hot compress applied externally as a counterirritant; prepared by wringing out a cloth of hot water; a medicament is usually added to the water or directly to the cloth.

stupefacient **1.** Causing stupor. **2.** Any agent that causes stupor, as a narcotic.

stupefaction The act of inducing stupor or narcosis.

stupefy To make senseless; to induce a stupor.

stupor A state of semiconsciousness.

stuporous In a semiconscious state.

Sturge-Weber syndrome An uncommon congenital condition marked by localized atrophy and calcification of the cerebral cortex, and an ipsilateral port-wine hemangioma on the face; often associated with mental retardation; attributed to faulty development of certain mesodermal and ectodermal elements.

stuttering A speech disorder characterized by involuntary spasmodic hesitation and repetition of sounds.

St. Vitus' dance Acute chorea; see under chorea.

stye, sty See hordeolum.

stylet, stylette, style A wire inserted into the lumen of a flexible catheter in order to stiffen it during passage.

styliform Having the shape of a peg. Also called styloid.

styloglossus Relating to the styloid process of the temporal bone and the tongue; the term is given to certain structures, as a muscle extending between the tongue and the process.

styloid Shaped like a peg; denoting certain bony processes. Also called styliform.

stylomastoid Relating to the styloid and mastoid processes of the temporal bone.

stylostixis Acupuncture.

stylus A sharply pointed instrument used in drawing or as the marking instrument on certain recorders.

stype A tampon; a plug or pledget of absorbent material.

stypsis **1.** The action of an astringent or hemostatic agent. **2.** The application of an astringent.

styptic An agent that contracts the tissues; an astringent.

subacromial Situated beneath the acromion process.

subacute Denoting the intensity of a disease, somewhat between acute and chronic.

subalimentation Insufficient nourishment.

subarachnoid Beneath the arachnoid membrane of the brain or spinal cord.

subarcuate Slightly bowed.

subareolar Beneath the areola, particularly of the nipple.

subatomic Relating to the components of the atom.

subaural Below the ear.

subcapsular Situated beneath a capsule.

subcarbonate Any basic carbonate such as bismuth subcarbonate; a complex of a base and its carbonate.

subcartilaginous **1.** Beneath a cartilage. **2.** Partly cartilaginous.

subchondral Beneath or just under the cartilages of the ribs.

subclavian **1.** Situated beneath the clavicle. **2.** Relating to the subclavian artery.

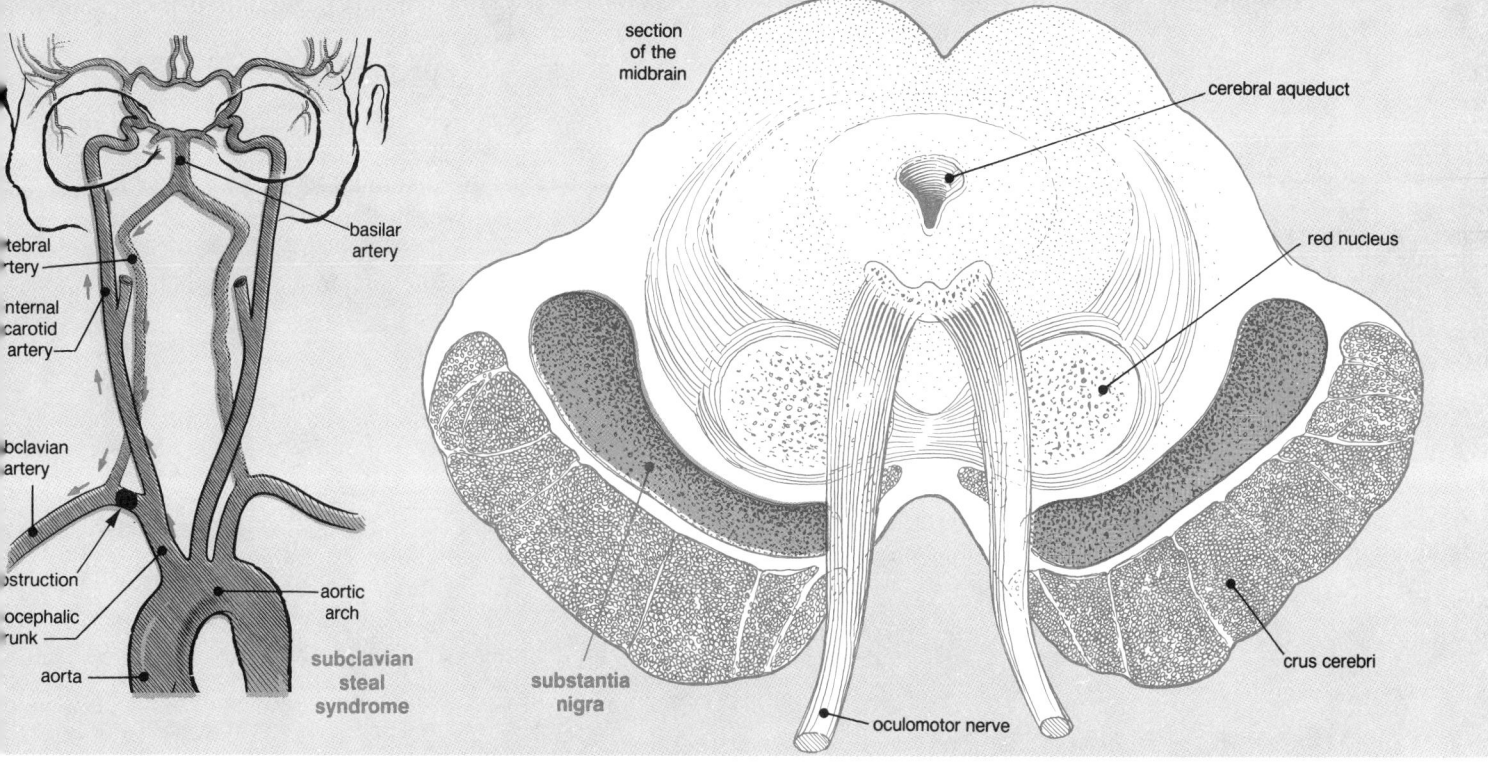

section of the midbrain

cerebral aqueduct

red nucleus

crus cerebri

oculomotor nerve

substantia nigra

subclavian steal syndrome

vertebral artery

internal carotid artery

subclavian artery

obstruction

brachiocephalic trunk

aorta

aortic arch

basilar artery

subclavian steal syndrome Reduced blood supply of the brain stem caused by obstruction of the subclavian artery proximal to the origin of the vertebral artery; blood flow through the vertebral artery is reversed and diverted from the brainstem to the arm, thus the subclavian "steals" cerebral blood.

subclavicular Situated beneath the clavicle (collarbone).

subclinical Denoting the phase of a disease prior to the manifestation of symptoms.

subconjunctival Under the conjunctiva of the eye.

subconscious 1. Less than fully conscious. 2. In psychology, not fully in conscious awareness but easily accessible; distinguished from unconscious, which implies inaccessibility to awareness.

subcorneal Beneath or just under the stratum corneum of the skin.

subcortex The portion of an organ immediately below the cortex, especially below the cerebral cortex.

subcostal Beneath the ribs.

subcranial Below the skull.

subculture A secondary culture of microorganisms, derived by inoculation from the primary culture.

subcutaneous Located beneath the skin. Also called hypodermic.

subcuticular Below the epidermis.

subcutis The loose fibrous tissue directly below the skin. Also called tela subcutanea.

subdermic Subcutaneous.

subdiaphragmatic Located beneath the diaphragm. Also called subphrenic.

subdural Located beneath the dura mater.

subendocardial Under the endocardium.

subfamily A taxonomic category between a family and a tribe.

subfertility Less than normal ability, in either the male or the female, to accomplish fertilization.

subgenus A taxonomic classification ranking between a genus and a species.

subgingival At a level below the gingival margin.

subglottic Situated or occurring beneath the glottic opening between the vocal cords.

subhepatic Situated below the liver.

subintimal Under the intima (of a vessel).

subinvolution Failure of an organ to return to its normal size, as when the uterus remains abnormally large after childbirth.

subjacent Situated beneath or below.

subject 1. A person or animal under treatment or experimentation. 2. A cadaver used for dissection.

subjective Perceived by the patient only and not

by the examiner; e.g., the symptom of pain or a sense of fatigue or malaise.

sublation Detachment of a bodily part.

sublethal Slightly less than lethal.

sublimate 1. To convert a solid into a gas and back into a solid without passing through the liquid stage. 2. A substance that has been subjected to sublimation. 3. In psychoanalysis, to divert consciously unacceptable, instinctive drives into personally and socially acceptable channels; an unconscious process.

sublimation 1. The conversion of a solid directly into vapor and then back into the solid state without passing through the intermediate liquid stage. 2. The unconscious process of changing instinctive impulses which may be socially unacceptable into personally and socially acceptable channels.

subliminal Below the level of sensory perception.

sublimis Latin for superficial.

sublingual Located beneath the tongue.

subluxation Partial dislocation.

s. of lens Incomplete dislocation of the lens of the eye.

submandibular Situated below the lower jaw.

submaxillary Located beneath the upper jaw.

submental Situated beneath the chin.

submicroscopic Too small to be seen through an ordinary light microscope.

submucosa The layer of tissue located beneath the mucous membrane.

subnormal Less than normal.

suboccipital Situated below the occipital bone or the back of the head (occiput).

suborbital Located beneath the orbit.

suborder A taxonomic classification ranking between an order and a family.

suboxide An oxide of an element (e.g., carbon suboxide) containing the smallest proportion of oxygen. Cf. protoxide.

subphylum A taxonomic classification ranking between a phylum and a class.

subscapular Located beneath or below the scapula (shoulder blade).

subscleral Beneath the sclera.

subscription The part of a pharmaceutical prescription that contains directions to the pharmacist for the compounding of ingredients, or dispensing of medication, in a form suitable for use by the patient; it indicates the class of preparation (e.g., capsules) and the number of doses (e.g., 20). See also superscription, inscription, and signature.

subserous Located beneath a serous membrane.

substage An attachment to a microscope, situated beneath the stage, by means of which accessories (mirror, diaphragm, condenser, or prism) are

held in place.

substance Matter; material.

gray s. The gray portion of the brain and spinal cord composed of cell bodies. Also called substantia grisea; gray matter.

reticular s. 1. A mass of filaments seen in immature red blood cells after vital staining. Also called alpha substance; filar mass. 2. See formation, reticular.

Rolando's s. Substantia gelatinosa of Rolando.

slow-reacting s. (SRS SRS-A) Substance (possibly a leukotriene) released in anaphylactic shock, formed through the interaction of antigen with sensitized cells; produces a slow prolonged contraction of smooth muscle.

specific capsular s. A polysaccharide present in the capsule of many bacteria, believed to have a role in the transport of nutrients and protection against noxious agents. Also called specific soluble substance.

specific soluble s. (SSS) See specific capsular substance.

s. P A polypeptide found in the brain (concentrated in the substantia nigra) and elsewhere; a sensory transmitter that mediates pain perception; may also serve as a neurohormone.

white s. The white portion of the brain and spinal cord consisting of nerve fibers. Also called substantia alba; white matter.

substantia Latin for substance.

s. adamantina Tooth enamel.

s. alba See substance, white.

s. eburnea The dentin of teeth.

s. gelatinosa of Rolando A mass of translucent gelatinous tissue, containing small nerve cells, on the posterior gray column of the spinal cord; appearing in cross-section as a crescentic cap over the horn.

s. grisea See substance, gray.

s. nigra A layer of gray substance in the cerebral peduncles containing deeply pigmented nerve cells; it extends from the upper border of the pons into the subthalamic region; on cross-section it appears crescentic. Also called black substance; intercalatum.

substernal Situated beneath the sternum (breastbone).

substitution 1. In chemistry, the replacement of one or more atoms of one element by those of another. 2. An unconscious mechanism by which an unacceptable goal or emotion is replaced by a more acceptable one.

substrate Any substance upon which an enzyme or ferment acts.

substratum Any layer of tissue located beneath

succinyl coenzyme A

COOH
CH₂
CH₂
O=C
CoA

sucrose

(structural chemical diagrams)

lateral view of cerebrum

superior frontal sulcus
inferior frontal sulcus
superior frontal gyrus
middle frontal gyrus
inferior frontal gyrus
anterior branch
ascending branch
posterior branch of lateral sulcus
precentral sulcus
central sulcus
postcentral sulcus
intraparietal sulcus
parie occip sulc
inferior temporal sulcus
superior temporal sulcus
lateral occipital sulcus

---

another layer.

substructure A structure or a dental appliance that is partly beneath the surface.

subthalamic 1. Situated beneath the thalamus. **2.** Relating to the subthalamus.

subthalamus The portion of the diencephalon lying immediately beneath the thalamus, between the tegmentum of the midbrain and the dorsal thalamus.

subungual Beneath the nail of a toe or finger. Also called hyponychial.

subunit A secondary unit or part of a more comprehensive unit.

suburethral Located beneath the urethra.

subvirile Characterized by deficient potency or masculine vigor; lacking in virility.

subvitrinal Beneath the vitreous body.

subvolution The operative procedure of turning over a flap of mucous membrane to prevent adhesion.

succagogue 1. Stimulating glandular secretion. **2.** An agent having such property.

succedaneum A substitute, as the permanent teeth that replace the deciduous teeth, or a drug with properties similar to those of another.

succenturiate Supplemental; accessory.

succinate A salt of succinic acid.

succinic acid An intermediate in the metabolism of tricarboxylic acid.

succinylcholine chloride Choline chloride succinate, a muscle-relaxant drug used as an anesthetic.

succinyl coenzyme A (succinyl-CoA) The condensation product of succinic acid and coenzyme A.

succorrhea An excessive flow of a digestive fluid, such as saliva or gastric juice.

succus, *pl.* **succi 1.** Juice. **2.** The fluid component of tissues. **3.** A fluid secretion, especially of the digestive tract.
s. entericus Intestinal juice.

succussion The act of shaking the body as a diagnostic procedure; a splashing sound is produced in the presence of fluid and air in a body cavity.

suck 1. To draw fluid into the mouth. **2.** To draw fluid into a tube by establishing a partial vacuum.

sucrase See invertase.

sucrose A disaccharide, $C_{12}H_{22}O_{11}$, which on hydrolysis yields glucose and fructose (monosaccharides); obtained chiefly from sugar cane, sugar beet, and maple; used as a sweetener and preservative. Also called cane sugar; saccharose.

suction The process of aspirating or sucking.

sudamen, *pl.* **sudamina** A minute vesicle formed by retention of sweat.

Sudan Name given to a series of histologic dyes.

See under stain.

sudanophilia Affinity for Sudan stain.

sudation Sweating.

sudden infant death syndrome (SIDS) The sudden death of a baby caused by a disease which can be neither predicted nor prevented and that displays no specific symptoms; it is a major cause of death in infants after the first month of life. Also called crib death.

Sudeck's atrophy See Sudeck's syndrome.

Sudeck's syndrome Bone atrophy usually of the hands, wrists, or feet following minor injuries; associated with painful swelling of the overlying soft tissue; thought to be due to abnormal vasomotor regulation. Also called Sudeck's atrophy.

sudomotor Stimulating sweat glands.

sudor Perspiration.

sudoral Relating to perspiration.

sudoresis Profuse perspiration.

sudoriferous Producing or carrying perspiration.

sudorific Causing perspiration. Also called diaphoretic; sudoriferous.

sudoriparous Producing perspiration.

suet The fat within the abdomen or around the kidneys of sheep and cattle.
prepared s. Purified suet from sheep, used in pharmaceutical ointments.

suffocate To impede respiration; to choke.

suffusion 1. Pouring of a fluid over the body. **2.** Flushing of the skin. **3.** Extravasation or spreading of a bodily fluid, such as blood, into surrounding tissues.

sugar A type of carbohydrate having a sweet taste.
amino s. A sugar containing an amino group; e.g., glucosamine. Also called hexosamine.
blood s. Glucose.
brain s. Galactose.
cane s. See sucrose.
deoxy s. A sugar that contains fewer atoms of oxygen than of carbon; e.g., deoxyribose.
fruit s. See fructose.
grape s. Glucose.
hexose s. A simple sugar having six carbon atoms per molecule.
invert s. A mixture of equal parts of glucose and fructose, used in solution as a parenteral nutrient. Also called invertose.
malt s. See maltose.
milk s. See lactose.
pentose s. A sugar having five carbon atoms per molecule.

suggestion 1. In psychiatry, the technique by which a therapist induces an idea or attitude that is adopted by the patient without questioning. **2.** Any idea or attitude so induced.

suicide 1. The act of taking one's own life voluntarily and intentionally. **2.** One who commits such an act.

suicidology The study of the nature, causes, and control of suicide.

suit An outer garment designed to be worn under particular environmental conditions.
antiblackout s. Anti-G suit.
anti-G s. A flight garment worn by pilots to increase their ability to withstand the effects of high acceleration (gravitational force or G) by exerting pressure on parts of the body below the chest; bladders (balloons) in the suit expand to apply external pressure to the abdomen and lower extremities during positive G maneuvers in flight, thereby preventing the pooling of blood in those areas.
G-s. Anti-G suit.

sulcate, sulcated Furrowed.

sulculus, *pl.* **sulculi** A small groove.

sulcus, *pl.* **sulci** A groove or furrow.
alveololabial s. The oral sulcus between the anterior alveolar bone and the lips.
alveololingual s. The sulcus at the floor of the mouth between the mandibular alveolar bone and the tongue.
arterial sulci Grooves on the interior surface of the skull which house the meningeal arteries. Also called arterial grooves.
calcarine s. A deep arched fissure on the medial surface of the occipital lobe; it divides the cuneus from the lingual gyrus. Also called calcarine fissure.
central s. A deep sulcus between the parietal and frontal lobes of the brain. Also called central fissure.
cingulate s. A sulcus on the medial surface of each cerebral hemisphere from the front of the corpus callosum to a point just behind the central sulcus.
collateral s. A long sagittal sulcus on the inferior surface of each cerebral hemisphere; it separates the fusiform gyrus from the hippocampal and lingual gyri.
coronary s. A sulcus encircling the external surface of the heart between the atria and ventricles, and occupied by arterial and venous vessels. Also called atrioventricular groove.
dorsal lateral s. A shallow longitudinal sulcus on either side of the dorsal median sulcus of the spinal cord; it marks the line of entrance of the posterior nerve roots.
dorsal median s. A shallow sulcus in the median line of the posterior surface of the spinal cord.
gingival s. The shallow space or groove between the free gingiva and the surface of a tooth.
horizontal s. of cerebellum Horizontal fissure of cerebellum; see under fissure.

substructure | sulcus

456

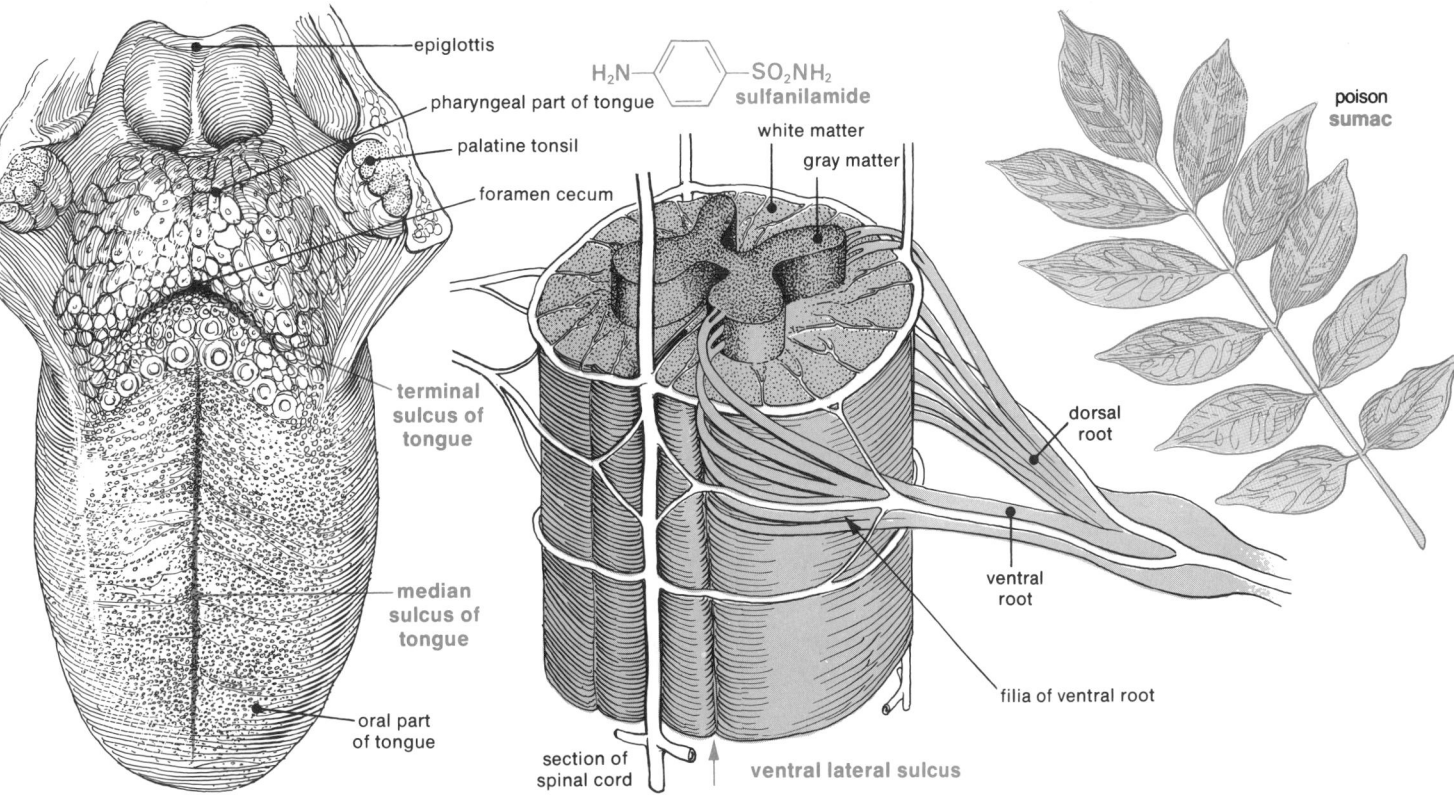

epiglottis
pharyngeal part of tongue
palatine tonsil
foramen cecum
terminal sulcus of tongue
median sulcus of tongue
oral part of tongue

H_2N —⟨ ⟩— SO_2NH_2 sulfanilamide

white matter
gray matter

poison sumac

dorsal root

ventral root

filia of ventral root

section of spinal cord

ventral lateral sulcus

median s. of tongue A slight, median, longitudinal depression running forward on the dorsal surface of the tongue from the foramen cecum; it divides the tongue into symmetrical halves.

occlusal s. A sulcus on the occlusal surface of a tooth.

parietooccipital s. A sulcus on the medial surface of the occipital region of each cerebral hemisphere extending upward from the calcarine sulcus; it separates the occipital lobe from the parietal lobe.

postcentral s. A sulcus on the lateral surface of the parietal lobe of the cerebrum; it separates the postcentral gyrus from the remainder of the parietal lobe.

precentral s. An interrupted sulcus on the lateral surface of the frontal lobe, anterior and somewhat parallel to the central sulcus.

terminal s. of tongue A shallow V-shaped groove on the tongue running laterally and forward from the foramen cecum; it marks the separation between the oral and pharyngeal parts of the tongue. Also called sulcus terminalis.

ventral lateral s. An indistinct sulcus on either side of the ventral median fissure of the spinal cord, marking the line of exit of the ventral nerve roots.

sulfa Denoting any of the sulfa drugs chemically similar to sulfonamide, such as sulfisoxazole and sulfadiazine.

sulfanilamide A potent antibacterial crystalline compound, $C_6H_8N_2SO_2$; first of the sulfonamides discovered and used in the treatment of bacterial infections.

sulfate A salt of sulfuric acid; a compound containing the group SO_4.

sulfhemoglobin A compound derived from the action of hydrogen sulfide on hemoglobin. Also called sulfmethemoglobin.

sulfhemoglobinemia Condition marked by persistent cyanosis, caused by the presence of sulfhemoglobin in the blood.

sulfide A compound of bivalent sulfur with a metal.

sulfisoxazole A sulfonamide (sulfa drug) used chiefly in the treatment of bacterial infections of the urinary tract; Gantrisin®.

sulfite A salt of sulfurous acid.

sulfmethemoglobin Compound formed by the combination of sulfide with the ferric ion of methemoglobin.

sulfobromophthalein sodium (BSP) A crystalline powder, soluble in water and used in testing liver function; Bromsulphalein®.

sulfonamides General term for a group of antibacterial drugs containing the sulfanilamide group; commonly known as sulfa drugs.

sulfonate 1. A salt of sulfonic acid. 2. To treat with sulfonic acid.

sulfone Any of various compounds containing the radical SO_2 and carbon.

sulfonic acid Any of various acids containing one or more sulfonic groups (—SO_3H).

sulfonylurea compounds Derivative compounds of isopropylthiodiazylsulfanilamide; because of their hypoglycemic action, they are used in the treatment of certain cases of diabetes mellitus. Also called sulfonylureas.

sulfosalicylic acid A soluble solid, $C_6H_3(OH)\cdot(COOH)\cdot SO_3H$, used as a reagent for albumin and ferric ion.

sulfur A pale yellow nonmetallic element, symbol S, atomic number 16, atomic weight 32.06; used in the preparation of pharmaceuticals and insecticides.

sulfur-35 (^{35}S) A radioactive sulfur isotope; a beta emitter with a half-life of 87.1 days; used as a tracer in studying protein systems, since it can be taken up by proteins by way of the sulfur-containing amino acids.

sulfuric Containing sulfur, especially with valence 6.

sulfuric acid A heavy, oily, highly corrosive liquid, H_2SO_4. Also called oil of vitriol.

sulfurize To combine with sulfur.

sulfurous 1. Containing or derived from sulfur; denoting compounds of sulfur with a low valence (+4). 2. Having the characteristics of sulfur.

sulfurous acid A solution of sulfur dioxide, H_2SO_3; used as a disinfectant and bleaching agent.

sumac Any of various plant species of the genus *Rhus;* some cause an acute itching lesion shortly after contact. Also written shumac.

   swamp s. See poison sumac.

sumat (sum) Latin for let him take; used in prescription writing.

sumendum (sum) Latin for to be taken; used in prescription writing.

summation 1. Totality. 2. The quality of two or more drugs whereby their combined effects are equal to the sum of their individual effects.

   s. of stimuli Muscular or neural effects produced by the frequent repetition of slight stimuli, one of which alone might not excite a response.

sunburn An inflammation or blistering of the skin caused by excessive exposure to ultraviolet rays of the sun.

sunstroke A state of extreme prostration and collapse caused by prolonged exposure to intense sunlight.

superacidity An excess of acid beyond the normal; particularly increased acidity of the gastric juice. Also called hyperacidity.

superacute Extremely acute; said of a disease.

superalimentation The therapeutic administration of nutrients in excess of the patient's nutritional requirements for the treatment of certain wasting diseases.

superalkalinity Excessive alkalinity beyond the normal. Also called hyperalkalescence.

superciliary Relating to or located in the area of the eyebrow.

supercilium Eyebrow.

superego In psychoanalytical theory, the part of the personality structure associated with ethics and standards formed during the individual's early life through identification with important persons, particularly his parents; the conscience.

superexcitation Excessive stimulation.

superfamily A taxonomic category between an order and a family.

superfatted Containing additional fat; said of certain soaps.

superfecundation The impregnation of two or more ova, liberated at the same ovulation, by successive coital acts.

superfemale Nonscientific term for metafemale.

superficial 1. On, near, or affecting the surface, as a wound. 2. Shallow, not thorough.

superinfection Appearance of a new infectious agent complicating an infection already under treatment.

superior Above; higher.

superior cerebellar artery syndrome Syndrome occurring in occlusion of the superior cerebellar artery; consists of loss of pain and temperature sensations on the side of the face and body opposite to that of the lesion, with incoordination in executing skilled movements.

superior mesenteric artery syndrome Obstruction of the superior mesenteric artery, marked by vomiting, pain, and extreme abdominal distention.

superior vena cava syndrome Edema of the face, neck, and/or upper arms caused by obstruction of the superior vena cava, usually by lung cancer or lymphoma invading the mediastinum.

supermale Nonscientific term for metamale.

supernatant Floating on a surface; denoting the liquid floating above a precipitate.

supernumerary 1. Accessory. 2. Exceeding a normal or fixed number.

supersaturate To add a substance beyond saturation.

superscription The part of the pharmaceutical prescription that directs the pharmacist to take the drugs listed to prepare the medication; indicated by the symbol ℞ (from the Latin term *recipe*, take). See also inscription; subscription; signature.

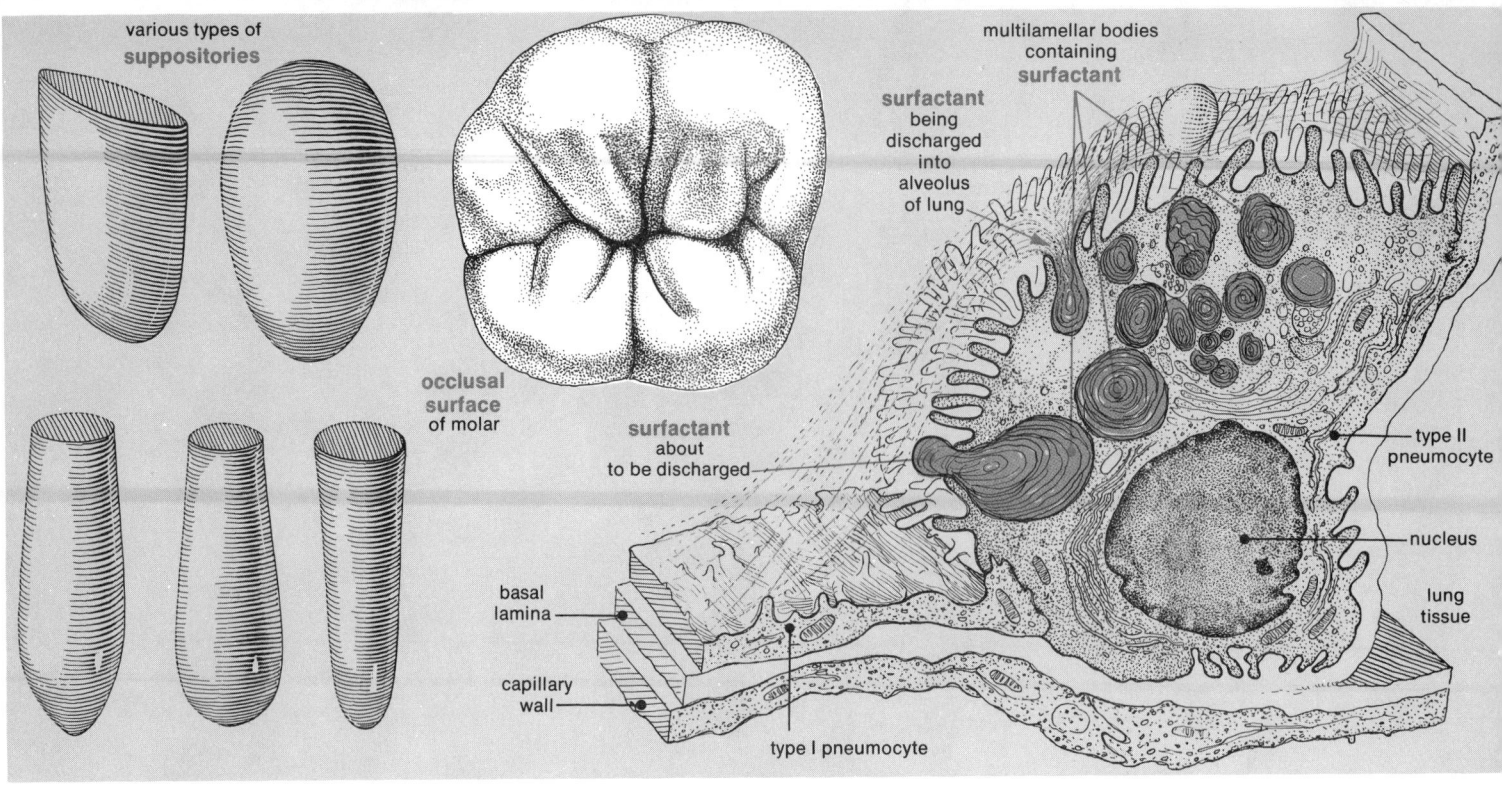

various types of **suppositories**

occlusal surface of molar

surfactant about to be discharged

surfactant being discharged into alveolus of lung

multilamellar bodies containing **surfactant**

type II pneumocyte

nucleus

lung tissue

basal lamina

capillary wall

type I pneumocyte

supersonic 1. Having a frequency above the level of audibility of the human ear. 2. Of or relating to speeds greater than the speed of sound in air.

supervoltage A very high electromotive force, from 10 to 50 million electron volts; used in radiation therapy.

supination 1. The act of lying on the back. 2. Rotation of the forearm so that the palm of the hand is turned forward or upward.

supinator A muscle that supinates the forearm.

supine Lying on the back.

support A device for holding a part in position.

suppository A solid medication designed for introduction into and dissolving within a body cavity other than the mouth.

suppression 1. In psychoanalysis, the conscious exclusion from awareness of painful memories or feelings; distinguished from repression, which is unconscious. 2. The cessation of a secretion; contrasted with retention, in which secretion occurs without discharge from the body.

suppuration The production and discharge of pus.

suppurative Pus-forming.

supra-anal Situated above the anus.

suprabuccal Above the cheek.

suprachoroid The outer layer of the vascular (choroid) coat of the eye, consisting chiefly of pigmented, loose, connective tissue.

supraclavicular Located above a clavicle (collarbone).

supracondylar, supracondyloid Situated above a condyle.

supracostal Located above or over the ribs.

supradiaphragmatic Located above the diaphragm.

supraduction In vertical divergence testing, upward movement of one eye when an ophthalmic prism is placed base down before it.

suprahepatic Located above the liver.

suprahyoid Located above the hyoid bone.

suprainguinal Located above the groin.

supraliminal Above the threshold of sensory perception.

supralumbar Located above the lumbar region.

supramandibular Located above the mandible (lower jaw).

supramental Above the chin.

supranuclear Situated above a nucleus.

supraorbital Located above the orbit.

suprapubic Located above the pubic arch.

suprarenal 1. Situated above or over the kidney. 2. Pertaining to the adrenal (suprarenal) gland.

suprascapular Situated above or in the upper part of the scapula (shoulder blade).

suprasellar Above the sella turcica of the sphenoid bone.

supraspinal Located above or over a spine or spinal column.

supraspinatus syndrome Pain and tenderness over the supraspinatus tendon upon abduction of the arm.

supraspinous Situated above a spine, especially those of the vertebrae.

suprasternal Located above the sternum (breastbone).

supratympanic Above the middle ear.

supraventricular Above the ventricles.

supravergence The upward movement of one eye while the other remains stationary. Also called sursumvergence.

supraversion 1. Condition in which a tooth is abnormally elongated. 2. The upward movement of both eyes. Also called sursumversion.

sura Latin for the calf of the leg.

surface The outer boundary of an object.

buccal s. The surface of premolars and molars facing the cheek.

distal s. 1. The surface of a structure that is farther from a point of reference. 2. The surface of a tooth most distant from the median line.

dorsal s. 1. The surface of a structure that is directed toward the back of the human body. 2. The back of the human body.

facial s. The combined buccal and labial surfaces of anterior teeth.

incisal s. The cutting surface of incisors and cuspids.

labial s. The surface of incisors and cuspids facing the lips.

lingual s. The surface of a tooth facing the tongue.

mesial s. The proximal surface of a tooth facing the median line.

occlusal s. The grinding surface of a posterior tooth which comes in contact with one in the opposite jaw during occlusion.

proximal s. 1. A surface that is nearer to a point of reference. 2. The surface of a tooth that faces an adjoining tooth in the same dental arch.

ventral s. 1. The anterior or abdominal surface of the human body. 2. The surface of a structure that is directed toward the anterior side of the human body.

surface-active Altering the surface of a liquid, usually by reducing the surface tension.

surfactant A surface-active lipoprotein that normally serves to decrease the surface tension of fluids within the alveoli (air sacs) of the lungs; permits pulmonary tissues to expand during inspiration and prevents alveoli from collapsing and sticking together after each breath; in the fetus, it is largely produced after the 35th week of gestation.

surgeon A health practitioner who specializes in surgery.

dental s. A dentist.

house s. A resident training in surgery in a hospital who acts under the orders of the attending surgeon.

oral s. A dental specialist concerned with the diagnosis and the surgical and adjunctive treatment of diseases, injuries, and defects of the jaws and associated structures.

Surgeon General The chief medical officer in the United States Army, Air Force, or Public Health Service; although the chief medical officer in the Navy is referred to as the Surgeon General, he is more properly called the Chief of the Bureau of Medicine and Surgery.

surgery The treatment of disease, injury, or deformity by means of manual and instrumental operations.

laser s. The use of laser beams (e.g., carbon dioxide, argon, excimer) for thermal cutting, vaporizing, coagulation, or destruction of tissues.

open heart s. Surgical correction of defects of the heart's interior through direct visualization.

oral s. The branch of dentistry dealing with the surgical treatment of disorders of the oral cavity.

orthopedic s. The branch of surgery specializing in the treatment of injuries and deformities of bones and chronic joint diseases.

plastic s. Surgery for the repair of physical defects or for the replacement of tissues lost through injury.

surrogate 1. A person who substitutes for another. 2. In psychiatry, refers to a person who replaces a parent in the feelings of the patient.

surveying In dentistry, studying the relative position of teeth and associated structures before designing a removable partial denture, in order to select a path of insertion and removal that will encounter the least interference.

susceptibility 1. The condition or quality of being sensitive or predisposed, as to a familial disease. 2. The state of lacking bodily resistance to disease.

susceptible 1. Capable of being influenced or affected. 2. Unresistant or not immune to an infectious disease.

suscitate To stimulate; to excite; to arouse to increased activity.

suspension 1. The hanging of a bodily part from a support in order to subject it to traction. 2. A noncolloidal dispersion of solid particles in a liquid.

suspensory 1. A structure, such as a ligament or

blanket suture button suture cobbler suture continuous suture Connell's suture

after Jones

Cushing suture interrupted suture Halstead suture Lembert suture purse-string suture

muscle, that aids in keeping an organ or part in place. **2.** A support for a dependent bodily part, such as a pouch attached to a body belt that provides support for the scrotum (used to relieve discomfort from such conditions as orchitis, varicocele, or epididymitis, or from scrotal surgery).

sustentacular Supporting.

sustentaculum A supporting structure.

s. lienis The phrenicocolic ligament that supports the left flexure of the colon, and upon which rests the base of the spleen (lien).

s. tali A process that projects medially from the anterior end of the calcaneus and that serves to support the head of the talus bone of the foot.

Sutton-Rendu-Osler-Weber syndrome See telangiectasia, hereditary hemorrhagic.

sutura A type of immovable fibrous articulation occurring only between the bones of the skull. Also called cranial suture.

suture 1. Stitch or stitches used in surgery to unite two surfaces. **2.** To apply a surgical stitch. **3.** The material used. **4.** An immovable joint uniting the bones of the skull. Also called sutura.

absorbable s. A sterile strand obtained from tissues of healthy animals that is capable of being gradually absorbed by living tissue; it may be treated to alter its absorbability, may be impregnated with antimicrobial substances, and may be treated with coloring materials.

blanket s. A continuous self-locking stitch. Also called lock-stitch suture.

button s. One in which the ends of the strand are passed through the eyes of a button and then tied.

catgut s. An absorbable suture obtained from

the small intestine of sheep.

cobbler s. A suture made with a needle at each end of the strand.

continuous s. A suture running the length of the wound with only two anchoring knots, at the beginning and at the end.

Connell's s. Continuous suture in which the apposing edges are inverted.

cranial s. A junction between the bones of the skull. Also called sutura.

Cushing s. A continuous inverting suture passed through the seromuscular layers of the gastrointestinal tract.

Halsted s. Interrupted inverting stitch, parallel to the wound and tied on one side.

interrupted s. A single stitch inverted and tied separately.

inverting s. A suture that turns in the apposing surfaces.

Lembert s. An inverting suture, either continuous or interrupted, used to join two segments of intestine without entering the lumen.

lock-stitch s. See blanket suture.

mattress s. A suture that may be parallel to the wound (interrupted and continuous) or at right angles (interrupted on-end or vertical) and is inserted deep into the tissues.

nonabsorbable s. A suture that is not absorbed by living tissues, i.e., silk, cotton, plastic, and alloy steel wire.

purse-string s. A continuous, circular inverting suture.

subcuticular s. Continuous suture inserted so as to approximate the tissues immediately under the

skin, without penetrating the skin.

tension s. Large simple or mattress interrupted stitch used to prevent undue stress.

uninterrupted s. A continuous suture.

Svedberg (S) Unit of sedimentation, proportional to the rate of sedimentation of a molecule in a given centrifugal field; a sedimentation constant of 1×10^{-13} sec.

swab A small ball of cotton or gauze wrapped around the end of a stick or wire; used for cleansing, for applying medication, or for obtaining samples of material for bacteriologic examination.

swallow To pass a substance from the mouth via the throat and the esophagus into the stomach; to perform deglutition.

swarming Denoting the progressive spreading of motile bacteria, especially *Proteus* species, over the surface of the colony or solid culture medium.

sway-back See lordosis.

sweat 1. Perspiration. **2.** To perspire.

sweetbread The thymus or pancreas of a calf used for food.

swelling An enlargement that may be inflammatory or noninflammatory; like fever, it is not a disease in itself, but rather a sign of an underlying disorder.

Neufeld capsular s. Swelling and opacity of the capsule of pneumococci when exposed to specific immune serum. Also called quellung reaction.

sycoma 1. A pendulous growth. **2.** A large soft wart.

sycosiform Latin for resembling the form of a fig; resembling sycosis.

sycosis Disease involving the hair follicles of the

Chemical Symbols

Sb	antimony	N	nitrogen
As	arsenic	Os	osmium
Ba	barium	O	oxygen
Bi	bismuth	Pb	palladium
Br	bromine	P	phosphorus
Cd	cadmium	Pt	platinum
Ca	calcium	Pu	plutonium
C	carbon	K	potassium
Cl	chlorine	Ra	radium
Cr	chromium	Rn	radon
Co	cobalt	Se	selenium
Cu	copper	Si	silicone
F	fluorine	Ag	silver
Au	gold	Na	sodium
He	helium	Sr	strontium
H	hydrogen	S	sulfur
I	iodine	Sn	tin
Fe	iron	W	tungsten
Pb	lead	U	uranium
Mg	magnesium	Xe	xenon
Mn	manganese	Y	yttrium
Hg	mercury	Zn	zinc

Symbols Used in Genetics

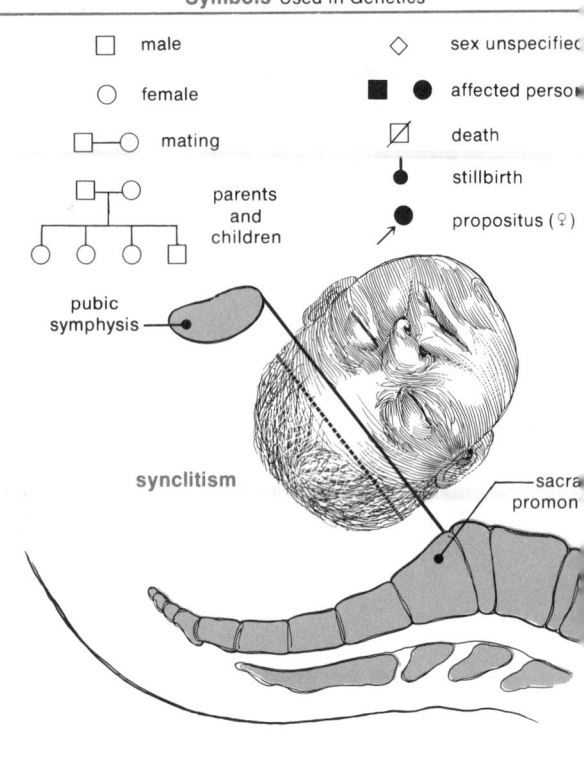

beard, marked by pustules and crusting of the skin.

symbiont One of the organisms associated with another in a symbiotic relationship. Also called symbiote; symbion.

symbiosis 1. The living together in intimate association of two dissimilar organisms. 2. In psychiatry, the relationship of two disturbed individuals who become dependent on each other.

symbiote See symbiont.

symblepharon Adhesion of the eyelid to the eyeball.

symblepharopterygium Adhesion of the eyelid to the eyeball through a cicatricial band resembling a pterygium.

symbol 1. A mark or character representing a substance, quality, quantity, or relation. 2. Something that represents something else.

chemical s. A symbol (letter or combination of letters) representing an atom or molecule of an element.

phallic s. In psychoanalysis, any slender, upright, pointed object representing, in disguise, a penis (phallus).

symbolization An unconscious mental process whereby one object or idea stands for another through some aspect that both have in common.

symmetry Exact correspondence of constituent parts on opposite sides of a dividing plane or about an axis.

sympathectomy, sympathetectomy Surgical removal of a portion of a sympathetic nerve or of a sympathetic ganglion.

chemical s. Interruption of a sympathetic nervous pathway by means of a chemical.

sympathetic 1. Denoting the thoracolumbar autonomic nervous system. 2. Of or expressing sympathy.

sympathicotripsy Crushing of a ganglion of the sympathetic nervous system.

sympathicotropic Having an influence upon the sympathetic nervous system.

sympathoadrenal Relating to the sympathetic nervous system and the hormones of the medulla of the adrenal gland, epinephrine and norepinephrine, which produce effects similar to those produced by sympathetic stimulation.

sympathoblast One of the primitive undifferentiated cells that migrate from the embryonic neural crest and give rise to sympathetic ganglion cells and to the adrenal medulla.

sympathoblastoma See neuroblastoma.

sympathogonia The primitive ectodermal stem cells that migrate down from the neural crest to form the medulla of the adrenal (suprarenal) glands during embryologic development.

sympathogonioma See neuroblastoma.

sympatholytic Inhibiting the activity of the sympathetic nervous system. Also called sympathoparalytic.

sympathomimetic Producing effects similar to those caused by stimulation of the sympathetic nervous system.

sympathoparalytic See sympatholytic.

sympathy 1. Expression of compassion or sorrow for another's grief. 2. The capacity for understanding the feelings of another person.

symphyseal Relating to a symphysis.

symphysiorrhaphy Fastening of a divided symphysis.

symphysiotomy, symphyseotomy Division of the pubic symphysis, by means of a wire saw, to facilitate delivery.

symphysis 1. A type of articulation in which two bones are united by fibrocartilage, as the pubis. 2. In pathology, the abnormal fusion of two surfaces.

symport The simultaneous transport of two compounds across a cell membrane in the same direction by a common carrier mechanism.

symptom Any manifestation of illness consciously experienced by a patient. For individual symptoms, see specific names.

symptomatic Relating to a symptom.

symptomatology 1. The group of symptoms of a disease. 2. The study of the symptoms of a disease, their causes, and the information they furnish. Also called semiology; semeiology.

synalgia Pain felt in an area other than the site of its origin.

synapse The site of communication between two nerve cells; a synaptic gap exists through which a nerve impulse must pass to be transmitted from one nerve cell to another; this is accomplished by release of a transmitter substance.

axodendritic s. The junction of the axon of a nerve cell with a dendrite of another nerve cell.

axosomatic s. The junction of the axon of a nerve cell with the cell body of another.

synapsis Process during the prophase stage of meiosis in which homologous chromosomes pair off and unite.

synaptic Relating to a synapse.

synarthrosis A joint in which two bones are united by fibrous tissue permitting little or no movement between the bones. Also called synarthrodial joint.

syncanthus Adhesion of the eyeball to orbital structures.

synchondrosis The union of two bones by cartilage, in some instances replaced by bone before adulthood, as in the skull of the newborn or the union of the manubrium with the body of the sternum (breastbone).

synchronia 1. Synchronism. 2. The formation and development of tissues at the normal time.

synchronism The simultaneous occurrence of two or more events.

synchrotron An accelerator for generating high speed electrons or protons around a fixed circular path by a radio-frequency potential.

synchysis Condition of the eye marked by liquefaction of the vitreous body.

s. scintillans The presence of numerous minute, glistening particles floating in a liquefied vitreous body, occurring secondarily to degenerative disease of the eye.

synclitism A condition in which the planes of the fetal head and the maternal pelvis are parallel; the fetal head presents into the pelvis with the sagittal sutures midway between the maternal pubic symphysis and sacral promontory. Also called parallelism.

syncopal Relating to fainting.

syncope A brief loss of consciousness; a faint.

syncytiotrophoblast The peripheral trophoblast, developed as a thick layer of syncytium from the single-layered trophoblast, which penetrates maternal tissues to attach the blastocyst to the uterus; eventually covers each chorionic villus and opens channels to maternal blood vessels.

syncytium A mass of protoplasm with many nuclei, seemingly resulting from the merging of several cells.

syndactily, syndactilism Partial or total webbing or fusion of two or more fingers or toes.

syndesmitis Inflammation of a ligament.

syndesmectomy Excision of a section of a ligament.

syndesmopexy Operative fixation of a dislocation by reconstruction of the ligaments of the joint.

syndesmoplasty Reparative surgery of a ligament.

syndesmorrhaphy Surgical suture or repair of a ligament.

syndesmosis A type of fibrous articulation in which the fibrous tissue between the bones forms a membrane or ligament, as the tibiofibular articulation or the union of the footplate of the stapes to the oval window of the internal ear.

syndrome A set of signs and symptoms that appear together with reasonable consistency. For individual syndromes, see specific names.

syndrome of inappropriate secretion of antidiuretic hormone (SIADH) Persistent high levels of antidiuretic hormone, expanded extracellular volume, and low concentration of plasma sodium; osmolality of urine is greater than that of plasma despite low plasma osmolality.

synechia, *pl.* **synechiae** Any adhesions; espe-

DISEASE	APPEARANCE	MUCIN CLOT VISCOSITY	LEUKOCYTES PER ML (% polymorphonuclear leukocytes)	OTHER FEATURES
normal	clear, straw-colored	good	<200 (<25%)	sugar is 90% of serum level

ROUP I   NONINFLAMMATORY

osteoarthritis	clear, straw-colored	good	100–1,000 (<25%)	
traumatic arthritis	clear to bloody	good	1,000 (<25%)	red blood cells may be present

ROUP II   INFLAMMATORY—IMMUNOLOGICAL

systemic lupus erythematosus	clear to slightly cloudy	good to fair	2,000–5,000 (10–15%)	low complement + LE prep
rheumatoid arthritis	cloudy, light yellow	poor	8,000–20,000 (60–75%)	low complement, slightly low sugar
Reiter's syndrome	cloudy	poor	10,000–40,000 (60–90%)	high complement

ROUP III   INFLAMMATORY—CRYSTALLINE

gout	cloudy	poor	10,000–20,000 (60–95%)	sodium urate crystals (negatively birefringent)
pseudogout	cloudy	fair to poor	5,000–40,000 (60–95%)	calcium pyro-phosphate crystals (weakly positive birefringent)

ROUP IV   INFLAMMATORY—INFECTIOUS

acute bacterial arthritis	cloudy, gray	poor	50,000+ (98%)	low sugar (less than 2/3 plasma level)
tuberculous arthritis	cloudy, yellow or gray	poor	25,000 (50–90%)	low sugar (less than 1/2 plasma level)

cially adhesion of the iris to the cornea or to the lens of the eye.

synechiotomy   Division of the adhesions in synechia.

synectenterotomy   Separation of intestinal adhesions.

syneresis   The shrinking or contraction of gels upon prolonged standing, causing the solid components to become more concentrated and droplets of the liquid medium to form on the surface; e.g., the shrinkage of blood clots, agar culture media, custards, etc.

synergism, synergy   1. Cooperation in action, as the coordinated action of two or more substances or organs to produce an effect of which each is individually incapable. 2. In pharmacology, the quality of two drugs whereby their combined effects are greater than the algebraic sum of their individual effects.

synergist   Anything, such as a drug or muscle, that acts in conjunction with another toward a common purpose.

synesthesia   Condition in which, in addition to the normal sensation, a stimulus produces another unrelated sensation.

synesthesialgia   Condition in which a stimulus, in addition to exciting the normal sensation, produces pain somewhere else.

syngamy   Conjugation or union of the nuclei of two gametes in fertilization to produce a zygote nucleus.

syngeneic   Relating to genetically identical (isogenic) or near-identical mammals (identical twins or highly inbred animals).

syngenesis   Sexual reproduction.

synkaryon   The nucleus formed when the nuclei of two cells fuse during fertilization.

synkinesis   Involuntary motion of one part when another part is moved.

synoptophore   A modified stereoscope used in training individuals afflicted with ocular muscle imbalance.

synorchidism, synorchism   Congenital fusion of the testes.

synostosis   The fusion of adjacent bones, normally separate, by means of osseous tissue.

synovectomy   Surgical removal of a portion or all of a diseased synovial membrane of a joint.

synovia   The clear, thick, lubricating fluid in a joint, bursa, or tendon sheath; it is secreted by the membrane lining the cavity or tendon sheath (synovial membrane).

synovial   Relating to, containing, or secreting synovia.

synovianalysis   The microscopic examination, crystal identification, and cell count of joint fluid (synovia); five categories can be distinguished: (a) normal, (b) noninflammatory, (c) inflammatory-immunologic, (d) inflammatory-crystalline, and (e) inflammatory-infectious.

synovin   Mucinous substance found in synovia.

synovioma   Tumor of synovial origin.

synovitis   Inflammation of the membranes lining a joint (synovial membranes).

synteny   In genetics, the association of genes that have loci on the same chromosome.

synthermal   Of the same temperature.

synthesis   A building up; especially the formation of a compound by the combination of simpler compounds or elements.

synthesize   To combine so as to produce a complex compound from simpler compounds; to form

central canal

cavitation of spinal cord

gray matter

white matter

syringomyelia

cross-section of spinal cord

tuberculin syringe

disposable syringe and needle

insulin syringe

control syringe

Luer-Lok syringe

syringe for irrigation and aspiration

aspiration biopsy syringe

spinous process of vertebra

syringo-myelocele

protrusion of spinal cord through defect in vertebral column

central canal of spinal cord

---

by synthesis.

synthetase Trivial name for a ligase.

synthetic Made by synthesis.

syntonic In balance.

syntrophism Enhanced growth of a strain of bacteria resulting from admixture with or nearness of another strain.

syntrophoblast See syncytiotrophoblast.

syntrophus Any congenital disease.

syphilid Any of the skin lesions of syphilis. Also called syphiloderma.

syphilis An infectious venereal disease caused by *Treponema pallidum*, transmitted through sexual intercourse or any direct contact; the first symptoms develop after an incubation period of 12 to 20 days.

　congenital s. Syphilis present at birth.

　late latent s. A form of the disease in which there is serologic or historic evidence of syphilis of more than four years' duration; it is not detectable by physical examination, by examination of the cerebrospinal fluid, or by roentgenographic examination of the heart and aorta.

　latent s. A phase of syphilis following the primary infection in which the organisms disappear from the skin and blood, and the foci of infection are beyond diagnostic reach; if evidence of infection is present in the cerebrospinal fluid the stage is designated as asymptomatic neurosyphilis.

　primary s. The first stage of the disease, beginning with the appearance on the genitalia, and sometimes the oral cavity, of a small ulcer which develops into a chancre.

　secondary s. The second stage of syphilis, beginning after healing of the initial chancre (between 6 and 12 weeks after its appearance) and lasting indefinitely; it is marked by infectious, copper-colored skin eruptions, mucous patches, fever, and other constitutional symptoms.

　tertiary s. The final, noninfectious stage of the disease, beginning after a lapse of several months or

years; marked by the development throughout the body of masses of granulomatous tissue (gummas); serious disorders of the nervous and vascular systems may occur.

syphilitic Relating to or suffering from syphilis.

syphilogenesis Origin of syphilis.

syphiloid Resembling or characteristic of syphilis.

syphilology The medical study pertaining to the nature and treatment of syphilis.

syphiloma A gumma; a syphilitic tumor.

syphilophobia An unwarranted fear of acquiring syphilis.

syringadenoma A benign sweat gland tumor. Also called syringoadenoma.

syringadenosus Relating to sweat glands.

syringe A device used for injecting or withdrawing fluids.

　fountain s. An apparatus consisting of a reservoir for holding water or special solutions, to the bottom of which is attached a tube with a nozzle at the end; used for enemas and vaginal irrigations (douches).

　hypodermic s. A syringe for the introduction of liquid remedies through a hypodermic needle into subcutaneous tissues.

syringitis Inflammation of a bodily tube, such as the uterine tube.

syringoadenoma See syringadenoma.

syringobulbia The presence of abnormal cavities in the brainstem.

syringocystoma Cystic tumor of a hair follicle.

syringoma A benign neoplasm of the tubular portion of a sweat gland.

syringomyelia A disease marked by the presence of cavities in the gray matter adjacent to the central canal of the spinal cord, causing loss of the senses of pain and temperature with retention of the sense of touch; in advanced cases, it often causes paralysis of the extremities and scoliosis of the lumbar spine.

syringomyelitis Inflammation of the spinal cord with formation of cavities in its substance.

syringomyelocele Protrusion of the spinal cord, with the central canal greatly distended with cerebrospinal fluid, through an abnormal gap in the vertebral column.

syringotomy See fistulotomy.

syrinx A cavity in the brain or spinal cord caused by disease.

syrup In pharmacy, a solution of sugar in water used as a vehicle for active ingredients.

syssarcosis A muscular articulation; the union of bones by muscular tissue, as in the connection between the hyoid bone and the mandible (lower jaw).

system 1. A functionally related group of parts or organs. 2. An organized set of interrelated ideas, procedures, techniques, etc.

　ascending reticular activating s. The upward neural projections of the reticular formation and thalamus which are responsible for normal wakefulness and alertness.

　autonomic nervous s. The division of the nervous system that innervates the striated muscles of the heart and the smooth muscles and glands of the body; it is divided into the sympathetic (thoracolumbar) system and the parasympathetic (craniosacral) system.

　cardiovascular s. (CVS) The heart and blood vessels.

　centimeter-gram-second s. (CGS) A system of metric units in which the basic units of length, mass, and time are the centimeter, gram, and second.

　central nervous s. (CNS) The brain and spinal cord.

　digestive s. The alimentary canal from the mouth to the anus and the associated glands.

　endocrine s. Collectively, all the ductless glands.

　extrapyramidal s. A functional system of tracts in the brain which controls and coordinates motor activities, especially postural, static, and supportive.

　female reproductive s. The genital organs in the

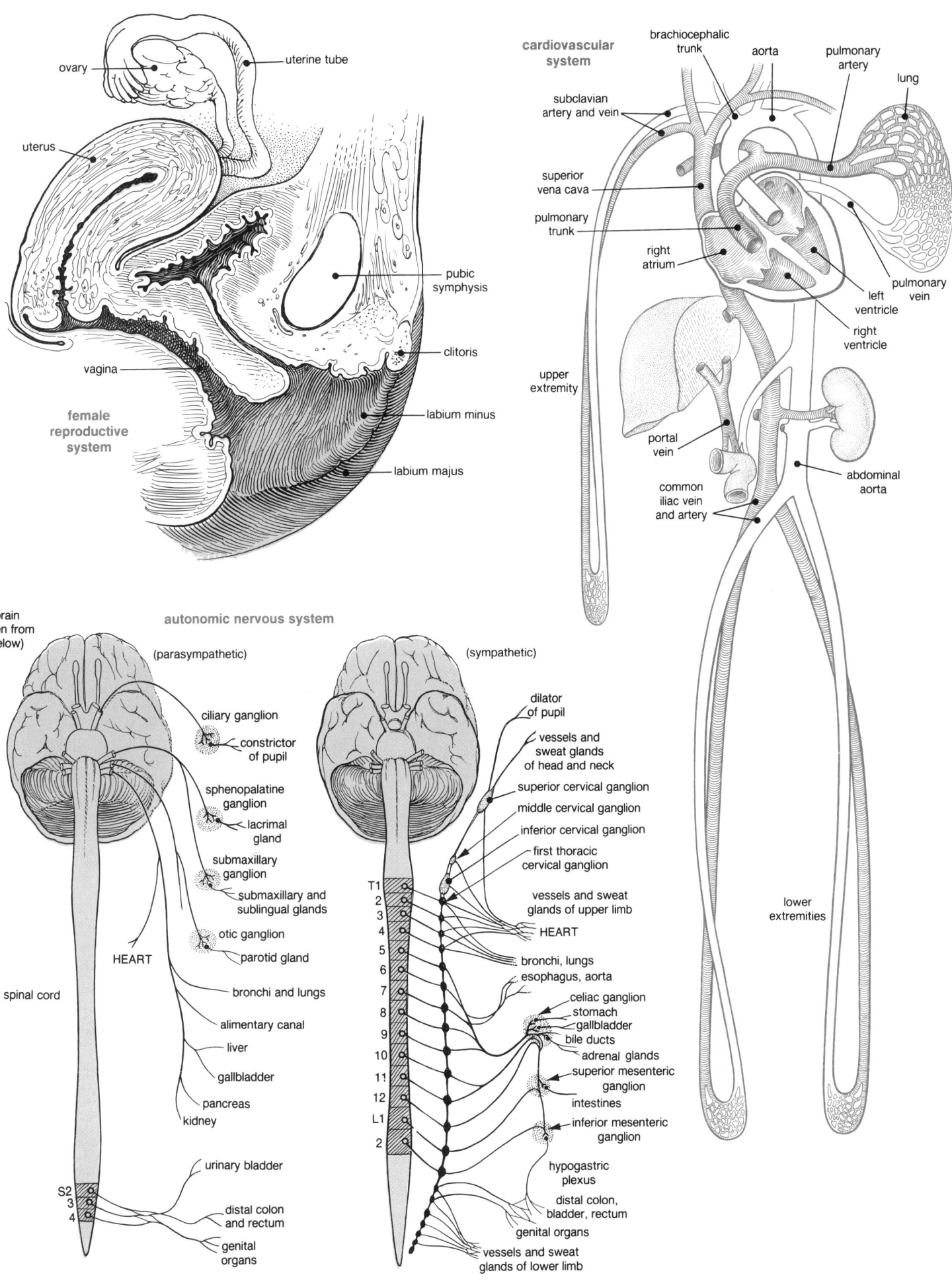

ovary

uterine tube

uterus

pubic
symphysis

vagina

clitoris

**female
reproductive
system**

labium minus

labium majus

**cardiovascular
system**

brachiocephalic
trunk

aorta

pulmonary
artery

lung

subclavian
artery and vein

superior
vena cava

pulmonary
trunk

right
atrium

pulmonary
vein

left
ventricle

right
ventricle

upper
extremity

portal
vein

common
iliac vein
and artery

abdominal
aorta

lower
extremities

brain
(seen from
below)

autonomic nervous system

(parasympathetic)

ciliary ganglion

constrictor
of pupil

sphenopalatine
ganglion

lacrimal
gland

submaxillary
ganglion

submaxillary and
sublingual glands

otic ganglion

HEART

parotid gland

spinal cord

bronchi and lungs

alimentary canal

liver

gallbladder

pancreas

kidney

urinary bladder

S2
3
4

distal colon
and rectum

genital
organs

(sympathetic)

dilator
of pupil

vessels and
sweat glands
of head and neck

superior cervical ganglion

middle cervical ganglion

inferior cervical ganglion

first thoracic
cervical ganglion

vessels and sweat
glands of upper limb

HEART

bronchi, lungs

esophagus, aorta

celiac ganglion

stomach

gallbladder

bile ducts

adrenal glands

superior mesenteric
ganglion

intestines

inferior mesenteric
ganglion

hypogastric
plexus

distal colon,
bladder, rectum

genital organs

vessels and sweat
glands of lower limb

T1
2
3
4
5
6
7
8
9
10
11
12
L1
2

463

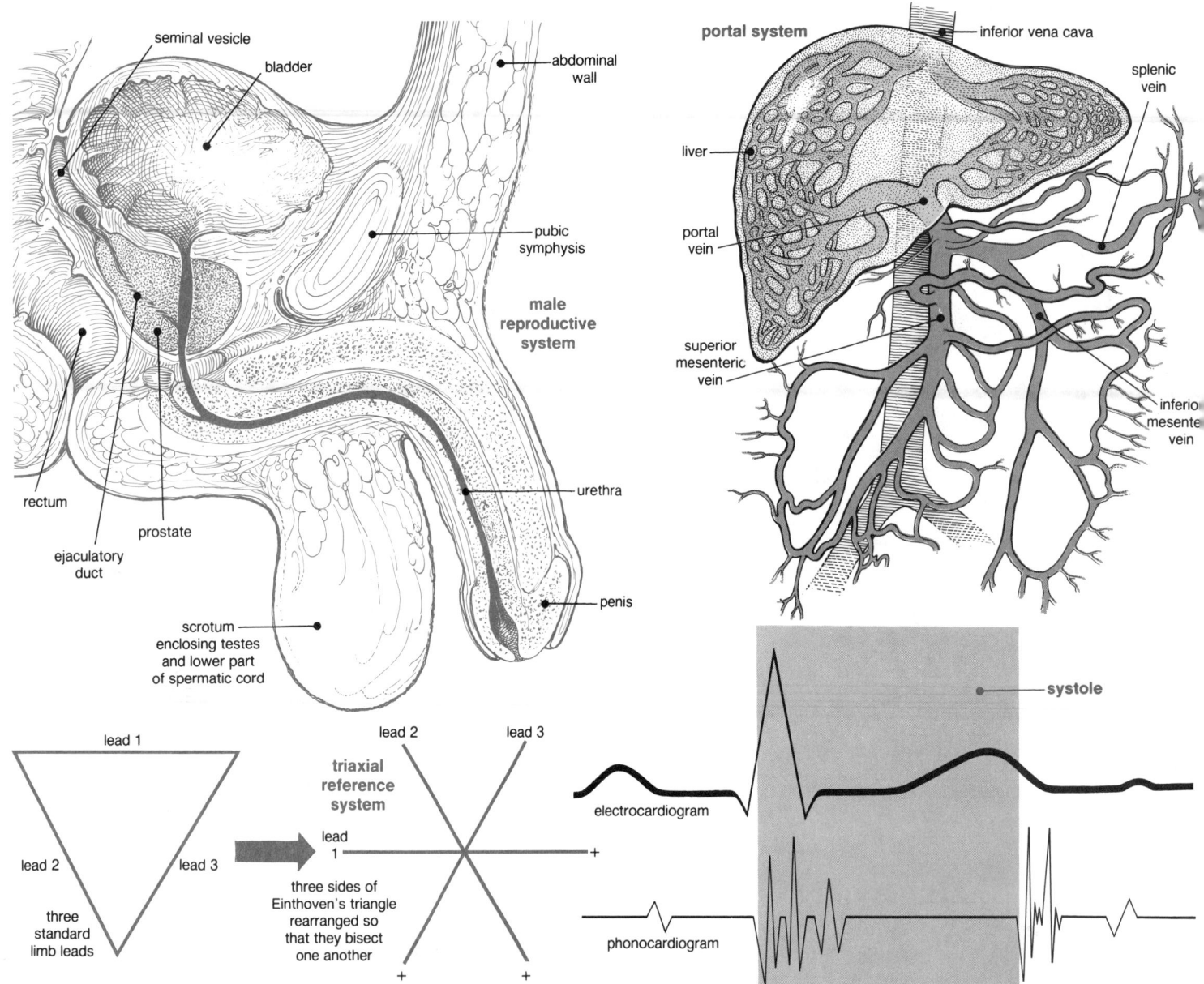

female, consisting of the ovaries, uterine tubes, uterus, vagina, and external genitalia.

   genitourinary s. The reproductive organs, kidneys, and urinary tract considered as a whole. Also called urogenital system.

   haversian s. See osteon.

   hematopoietic s. The blood-producing organs.

   heterogeneous s. A combination of matter containing two or more distinct components that have definite boundaries; e.g., a suspension or an emulsion.

   international s. of units A system of units for the basic quantities of length, mass, time, electric current, temperature, luminous intensity, and amount of substance; the corresponding units are: meter, kilogram, second, ampere, kelvin, candela, and mole. In all languages it is abbreviated SI.

   limbic s. Term loosely applied to the part of the nervous system that controls autonomic functions and the emotions.

   lymphatic s. The lymphatic vessels, nodes, tonsils, spleen, thymus, and lymphoid or adenoid tissue.

   lymphoreticular s. In immunology, a collection of cellular elements strategically distributed throughout the body; they can be activated by a variety of influences which are recognized as foreign by the host.

   male reproductive s. The genital organs in the male, consisting of the testes, excretory ducts, seminal vesicles, prostate gland, and penis.

   metric s. A system of measures and weights based upon the meter and the gram, respectively.

   muscular s. The muscles of the body collectively.

   nervous s. The brain and spinal cord (central

nervous system), the cranial and spinal nerves (peripheral nervous system), and the autonomic nervous system.

   neuromuscular s. The nerves and the muscles which the nerves supply.

   oculomotor s. The part of the nervous system that controls eye movements.

   oxidation-reduction s. A system in which the reversible oxidation-reduction reaction can take place; e.g., the enzyme systems of living cells.

   parasympathetic nervous s. A division of the autonomic nervous system.

   peripheral nervous s. (PNS) The nervous system that connects the central nervous system (CNS) to the rest of the body.

   portal s. The arrangement of vessels and capillaries in the liver; the portal vein and its branches.

   Purkinje s. The system of modified muscle fibers in the heart concerned with conduction of impulses.

   respiratory s. The air passages, lungs, and the muscles of respiration.

   reticular activating s. (RAS) A portion of the central cephalic brain stem which controls wakefulness, arousal from sleep, and focusing of attention.

   reticuloendothelial s. (RES) The phagocytic cells present in the bone marrow, spleen, and liver, where they free the blood or lymph of foreign matter.

   sympathetic nervous s. A division of the autonomic nervous system.

   triaxial reference s. In electrocardiography, the figure resulting from rearranging the sides of the Einthoven triangle (which represent the three standard limb leads) so that they bisect one another.

   urogenital s. See genitourinary system.

   vascular s. The blood vessels.

   vertebral-basilar s. The system composed of the two vertebral arteries as they join to form the basilar artery and their immediate branches.

systematic Relating to a system or arranged in accordance with a system.

systematization Formulation or arrangement of ideas in orderly sequence, according to a system.

systematized Denotes widespread pathology that has a significant pattern rather than haphazard distribution.

systemic Relating to or affecting the entire body.

systole The rhythmic and synchronous contraction of the muscles of the heart chambers.

   atrial s., auricular s. Atrial contraction giving impetus to the blood flowing from the atria into the ventricles; it has a duration of about 0.1 sec.

   ventricular s. Ventricular contraction immediately following atrial systole; it is divided into two phases: (a) isometric contraction, which occurs when the ventricular pressure firmly closes the atrioventricular valves, and (b) the period of ejection, occurring when the pressure in the ventricles overcomes the diastolic pressure of the aorta and pulmonary trunk and the aortic and pulmonic valves open, forcefully ejecting the ventricular blood; in an individual with a heart rate of 70 beats per minute, the ejection period lasts 0.3 sec.

systolic Relating to or resulting from ventricular systole.

systremma A cramp in the muscles of the leg, chiefly of the bellies of the gastrocnemius and soleus muscles; may be associated with swimmer's cramp or a charleyhorse.

INTERNATIONAL SYSTEM OF UNITS (SI)

Quantity	Name	Symbol
base units:		
length	meter	m
mass	kilogram	kg
time	second	s
electric current	ampere	A
thermodynamic temperature	kelvin	K
amount of substance	mole	mol
luminous intensity	candela	cd
supplementary units:		
plane angle	radian	rad
solid angle	steradian	sr

PREFIXES AND THEIR SYMBOLS USED TO DESIGNATE DECIMAL MULTIPLES AND SUBMULTIPLES

Prefix	Symbol	Factor
tera	T	10^{12} =
giga	G	10^{9} = 1 000 000 000
mega	M	10^{6} = 1 000 000
kilo	k	10^{3} = 1 000
hecto	h	10^{2} = 100
deka	da	10^{1} = 10
deci	d	10^{-1} = 0.1
centi	c	10^{-2} = 0.01
milli	m	10^{-3} = 0.001
micro	μ	10^{-6} = 0.000001
nano	n	10^{-9} = 0.000000001
pico	p	10^{-12} = 0.000000000001
femto	f	10^{-15} = 0.000000000000001
atto	a	10^{-18} = 0.000000000000000001

EXAMPLES OF SI DERIVED UNITS EXPRESSED IN TERMS OF BASE UNITS

Quantity	SI unit	Unit Symbol
area	square meter	m^2
volume	cubic meter	m^3
speed, velocity	meter per second	m/s
acceleration	meter per second squared	m/s^2
wave number	1 per meter	m^{-1}
density, mass density	kilogram per cubic meter	kg/m^3
current density	ampere per square meter	A/m^2
magnetic field strength	ampere per meter	A/m
concentration (of amount of substance)	mole per cubic meter	mol/m^3
specific volume	cubic meter per kilogram	m^3/kg
luminance	candela per square meter	cd/m^2

SI DERIVED UNITS WITH SPECIAL NAMES

Quantity	Name	Symbol	Expression in terms of other units
frequency	hertz	Hz	s^{-1}
force	newton	N	$kg \cdot m/s^2$
pressure, stress	pascal	Pa	N/m^2
energy, work, quantity of heat	joule	J	N·m
power, radiant flux	watt	W	J/s
quantity of electricity, electric charge	coulomb	C	A·s
electric potential, potential difference, electromotive force	volt	V	W/A
capacitance	farad	F	C/V
electric resistance	ohm	Ω	V/A
conductance	siemens	S	A/V
magnetic flux	weber	Wb	V·
magnetic flux density	tesla	T	Wb/m^2
inductance	henry	H	Wb/A
luminous flux	lumen	lm	cd·sr
illuminance	lux	lx	lm/m^2
activity (of a radionuclide)	becquerel	Bq	s^{-1}
absorbed dose	gray	Gy	J/kg

RECOMMENDED UNITS

Quantity	Symbol	Dimension	Unit	Unit symbol	Recommended sub-units	Not recommended units
Length	l	L	meter	m	mm, μm, nm	cm, μ, u, mμ, mu, A
Area	A	L^2	square meter	m^2	mm^2, μm^2	cm^2, μ^2
Volume	V	L^3	cubic meter / liter	m^3 / l	dm^3, cm^3, mm^3, μm^3 / ml, μl, nl, pl, fl	cc, ccm, μ^3, u^3 / L, λ, ul, $\mu\mu$l, uul
Mass	m	M	kilogram	kg	g, mg, μg, ng, pg	Kg, gr, γ, ug, mμg, mug, $\gamma\gamma$, $\mu\mu$g, uug
Number	N	I	one	1	10^9, 10^6, 10^3, 10^{-3}	all other factors
Amount of substance	n	N	mol	mol	mmol, μmol, nmol	M, eq, val, g-mol, mM, meq, mval, μM μeq, μval, nM, neq, nval
Mass concentration		L^{-3} m	kilogram per liter	kg/l	g/l, mg/l, μg/l, ng/l	g/ml, %, g%, % (w/v), g/100 ml, g/dl, ‰, ‰, ‰ (w/v), mg%, mg% (w/v), mg/100 ml, mg/dl, ppm, ppm (w/v), μg%, μg% (w/v), μg/100 ml, μ/dl, γ%, ppb, ppb (w/v), $\mu\mu$g/ml, uug/ml
Substance concentration	c	L^{-3} N	mol per liter	mol/l	mmol/l, μmol/l, nmol/l	M, eq/l, val/l, N, n, mM, meq/l, mval/l, μM, uM, μeq/l, nM, neq/l
Molality	m	M^{-1} N	mol per kilogram	mol/kg	mmol/kg, μmol/kg	m, mmol/g, μmol/mg, mm, μm, mm

Tt

periodic table

METALS NONMETALS

Group	I	II													III	IV	V	VI	VII	O
Period																				
1	H 1																			He 2
2	Li 3	Be 4													B 5	C 6	N 7	O 8	F 9	Ne 10
3	Na 11	Mg 12													Al 13	Si 14	P 15	S 16	Cl 17	Ar 18
4	K 19	Ca 20	Sc 21	Ti 22	V 23	Cr 24	Mn 25	Fe 26	Co 27	Ni 28	Cu 29	Zn 30			Ga 31	Ge 32	As 33	Se 34	Br 35	Kr 36
5	Rb 37	Sr 38	Y 39	Zr 40	Nb 41	Mo 42	Tc 43	Ru 44	Rh 45	Pd 46	Ag 47	Cd 48			In 49	Sn 50	Sb 51	Te 52	I 53	Xe 54
6	Cs 55	Ba 56	*57-71	Hf 72	Ta 73	W 74	Re 75	Os 76	Ir 77	Pt 78	Au 79	Hg 80			Ti 81	Pb 82	Bi 83	Po 84	At 85	Rn 86
7	Fr 87	Ra 88	**89-103	Rf 104	Ha 105															

*	lanthanide elements (rare earth)	La 57	Ce 58	Pr 59	Nd 60	Pm 61	Sm 62	Eu 63	Gd 64	Tb 65	Dy 66	Ho 67	Er 68	Tm 69	Yb 70	Lu 71
**	actinide elements	Ac 89	Th 90	Pa 91	U 92	Np 93	Pu 94	Am 95	Cm 96	Bk 97	Cf 98	Es 99	Fm 100	Md 101	No 102	Lw 103

T-1824 Evans blue.

Tabanus A genus of biting flies, some species of which transmit anthrax, infectious equine anemia, and other diseases. Commonly called horseflies; gadflies; breezeflies.

tabefaction Atrophy or wasting of the body.

tabes Progressive wasting away.

t. dorsalis A late manifestation of syphilis characterized by sclerosis of the sensory nerve roots and the posterior columns of the spinal cord; the usual symptoms are: shooting pains, muscular incoordination and atrophy, and functional disturbance of certain organs. Also called locomotor ataxia.

tabescent Wasting away progressively.

tabetic Afflicted with tabes.

tabetiform Resembling tabes dorsalis.

table 1. An orderly arrangement of written, typed, or printed data. 2. A flat layer, as one of the two laminae, separated by the diploë, into which the cranial bones are divided. 3. An article of furniture having a flat horizontal surface.

Aub-DuBois t. Table of rates of basal metabolism in calories per square meter of body surface per hour for all age groups.

examining t. Table on which the patient lies during a medical examination.

operating t. Table on which a patient is placed during a surgical procedure.

periodic t. An arrangement of chemical elements listed according to their atomic number; it demonstrates the recurrence of similar properties after certain intervals.

tilt t. One with a top that tilts so that the patient lying on it can be brought toward an erect position.

Reuss' color t.'s Diagrams in which colored letters are superimposed on colored backgrounds as a test for colorblindness.

vitreous t. The inner table of the cranial bones; it is denser than the outer table.

tablespoon (tbsp) A large spoon used as a measure in the dosage of liquid medicines; equivalent to 15 milliliters, 4 liquid drams, one-half fluid ounce, or 3 teaspoons.

tablet A small disc containing measured amounts of medicinal substances.

buccal t. Tablet placed between the cheek and the gum where it dissolves quickly, permitting the medicinal substance to be absorbed through the mucosa.

compressed t. Tablet prepared by compressing granulated medicinal substances under several hundred kilograms of pressure per square centimeter.

enteric coated t. Tablet coated with material that does not disintegrate in stomach fluids; the medication is released in the intestines.

hypodermic t. A small water-soluble tablet, intended to be dissolved in the barrel of a hypodermic syringe prior to injection.

sublingual t. Tablet placed under the tongue to permit absorption of the medicinal ingredients through the mucosa.

taboparesis Condition marked by symptoms of tabes dorsalis and general paresis.

tabular 1. Arranged as a table or list. 2. Having a flat surface.

tache A minute spot or blemish.

t. noir The crust-covered lesion produced by the bite of a tick.

tachistesthesia Perception of a flicker of light.

tachistoscope Instrument that projects a slide for a brief period of time; used in experimental optics to measure the speed of conscious visual perception.

tachogram The graphic record made by tachography.

tachography The recording of the rate of arterial blood flow.

tachyarrhythmia Heart rhythm with over 100 beats per minute.

tachycardia An abnormally fast heart beat. Also called tachyrhythmia.

paroxysmal atrial t. (PAT) Sudden onset of rapid heart action originating in the atria.

paroxysmal atrial t. with block PAT with a block in transmission of some of the beats from the atria to the ventricles so that the ventricular rate is less than the atrial.

tachycardiac Relating to, or afflicted with, tachycardia.

tachycrotic Relating to a rapid pulse.

tachykinin One of a group of structurally related peptides involved in blood vessel dilation, smooth muscle contraction, stimulation of saliva secretion, and neurotransmission of painful stimuli.

tachylalia Tachylogia.

tachylogia Rapid speech.

tachyphagia Abnormally rapid eating; bolting of food.

tachyphrasia Tachylogia.

tachyphylaxis Rapid production of immune tolerance, as by repeated injections of small doses of a substance.

tachypnea Abnormally rapid, shallow breathing.

tachyrhythmia See tachycardia.

tachysterol A sterol produced by ultraviolet irradiation of ergosterol.

tachysystole Tachycardia.

tactile Relating to the sense of touch.

taction 1. An act of touching; a contact. 2. The sense of touch.

tactometer Instrument used to determine the condition of the sense of touch.

tactor A sensory (tactile) end-organ.

tactus Latin for touch; the sense of touch.

Taenia A genus of tapeworms (family Taeniidae).

T. echinococcus *Echinococcus granulosus.*

T. saginata The common tapeworm transmitted to man by the ingestion of infected beef; the larvae exist in the muscles and organs of cattle; the adults, measuring from 5 to 10 m in length, are found in the human small intestine, attached to the mucosa by means of muscular suckers on the scolex (head). Also called beef tapeworm.

T. solium A species whose larval state exists in the muscles of the hog; the adult forms are found in the human intestine, to which they gain access by the ingestion of insufficiently cooked infested pork. Also called pork tapeworm; armed tapeworm because of the double row of hooks present on its head.

tag 1. To introduce a radioactive isotope to a substance. 2. The radioactive material so used. 3. A small outgrowth of flaplike appendage. 4. To add an

anal skin tags

talipes calcaneus

talipes valgus

talipes varus

adult tapeworm

scolex of tapeworm

easily identifiable marker, such as a radioactive isotope.

anal skin t. A polypoid projection in the anus.

skin t. A small flesh-colored to brown polypoid growth. Also called fibroepithelial papilloma.

tagged Said of a compound to which a radioactive isotope has been added. Also called labeled.

Takayasu's syndrome Pulseless disease occurring mostly in young females. See also pulseless disease; aortic arch syndrome.

take A successful grafting procedure.

talalgia Discomfort or pain in the heel or ankle.

talc, talcum A fine-grained hydrous magnesium silicate, having a soft texture; used in face and talcum powder, and in cosmetic and pharmaceutical preparations.

talcosis Disorder of the lungs produced by inhalation of talc.

taliped 1. A person who is afflicted with a clubfoot. 2. Clubfooted.

talipes General term that denotes a deformity involving the ankle and foot.

t. calcaneovalgus A relatively common congenital disorder in which the ankle joint is dorsiflexed and the foot is everted; believed to be caused by the position of the fetus in the uterus; the opposite of clubfoot (talipes equinovarus).

t. calcaneus Fixed dorsiflexion of the foot, causing the weight of the body to rest on the heel.

t. equinovarus See clubfoot.

t. equinus Fixed plantar extension of the foot, causing the weight of the body to rest on the ball of the foot; the ankle joint is plantar flexed.

t. valgus Outward turning of the foot, causing only the inner side of the sole to touch the ground; accompanied by flattening of the longitudinal arch.

t. varus Deformity considered to be an incomplete form of clubfoot (talipes equinovarus); characterized by a turning inward of the foot, causing only the outer part of the sole to touch the ground; accompanied by increased height of the longitudinal arch.

talocalcaneal Pertaining to the talus and calcaneus bones of the foot; denoting the joint between those bones and the ligaments attaching them.

talocrural Relating to the ankle joint.

talonavicular Relating to the talus and the navicular bone.

talus The large bone articulating with the tibia and fibula to form the ankle joint. Also called astragalus; ankle bone.

tambour A drum-shaped apparatus used to transmit and register slight movements.

tampon A plug of any absorbent material placed in a canal or cavity to control hemorrhage or absorb secretions.

tamponade The use of a tampon as a surgical aid. Also called tamponage.

cardiac t. Compression of the heart due to accumulation of blood in the pericardium, as in rupture of the heart or after penetrating wounds.

Tangier disease An inherited disorder of lipid metabolism marked by deficiency of high density lipoproteins, deposition of cholesterol esters in foam cells, enlargement of liver, spleen, and lymph nodes, enlarged orange-colored tonsils, and corneal opacity; the disease was named after Tangier Island, a geographically isolated community located in the Virginia part of the Chesapeake Bay, where the disease was first discovered.

tangle A twisted interwoven mass.

neurofibrillary t. An accumulation of paired helical filaments within a cell body; commonly seen in areas of the cerebral cortex of individuals with Alzheimer's disease.

tannate A salt of tannic acid.

tannic acid A lustrous brownish-yellow amorphous, powdered, or spongy mass, $C_{76}H_{52}O_{46}$, extracted from the bark and fruit of various plants; used as an astringent and styptic, and occasionally in treating diarrhea; toxic to the liver. Also called tannin.

tannin See tannic acid.

tantalum A metallic noncorrosive element; symbol Ta, atomic number 73, atomic weight 180.95; used in surgery as a skull plate, a wire mesh in the abdominal wall, etc.

tantrum Unprovoked fit of bad temper; unreasoning anger that may be accompanied by violent acts or gestures.

tap 1. To deliver a quick, gentle blow or blows, as when eliciting a tendon reflex. 2. To strike lightly but audibly. 3. To withdraw fluid from a bodily cavity.

spinal t. Lumbar puncture; see under puncture.

tapetum 1. The portions of the corpus callosum that border the posterior horns (laterally) of the lateral ventricles of the brain. 2. The outer and posterior part of the choroid (the vascular layer of the eyeball).

tapeworm Any of several ribbonlike worms (class Cestoda) that infest the intestines of vertebrates, including man; its body consists of a head or scolex with hooks for attachment to the intestinal wall and a series of segments or proglottids (from four to several thousand) containing the reproductive organs.

beef t. See *Taenia saginata.*

fish t. See *Diphyllobothrium latum.*

dwarf t., dwarf mouse t. See *Hymenolepis nana.*

pork t. See *Taenia solium.*

tapinocephalic Characterized by a flattened skull.

tapinocephaly Deformity in which the skull is flattened.

tapotement Tapping with the side of the hand; a massage movement.

tar A dark, semisolid substance obtained from the destructive distillation of various organic materials, as wood or coal.

coal t. Tar obtained from bituminous coal; used in the preparation of certain drugs and dyes.

pine t. A dark, viscous syrup produced by the destructive distillation of pine wood; it contains resins, turpentine, and oils and is used as a disinfectant and antiseptic in the treatment of skin disorders such as eczema. Also called wood tar; liquid pitch.

tarantula Any of several large, hairy, dark spiders (family Theraphosidae) capable of inflicting a painful but not significantly poisonous bite.

black t. *Sericopelma communis,* a large black tarantula of Panama, whose bite is poisonous although the effect is localized.

tardive Term applied to the characteristic lesion of a disease that is late in appearing. Also called late; tardy.

tare In chemistry, (a) the weight of an empty container; (b) a weight used to counterbalance the weight of the container holding the substance being weighed.

target An object of fixation or observation used in vision training or testing.

tarsadenitis Inflammation of the borders of the eyelids and of the meibomian glands.

tarsal 1. Relating to the small bones forming the instep of the foot. 2. Relating to the border of an eyelid.

tarsectomy 1. Surgical removal of the tarsus of the foot, or part of it. 2. Surgical removal of the margin of an eyelid, or part of it.

tarsitis 1. Inflammation of the margin of the eyelid. Also called marginal blepharitis. 2. Inflammation of the tarsus of the foot.

tarsoclasia, tarsoclasis Surgical fracture of the tarsus, as for the correction of clubfoot.

tarsomalacia Softening of the tarsal cartilage of an eyelid.

tarsometatarsal Relating to the tarsus and metatarsus.

tarsophyma A tarsal tumor.

tarsoplasty Plastic surgery of the eyelid. Also called blepharoplasty.

tarsorrhaphy A surgical procedure to close or to reduce the length of the palpebral fissure by suturing the upper and lower eyelids.

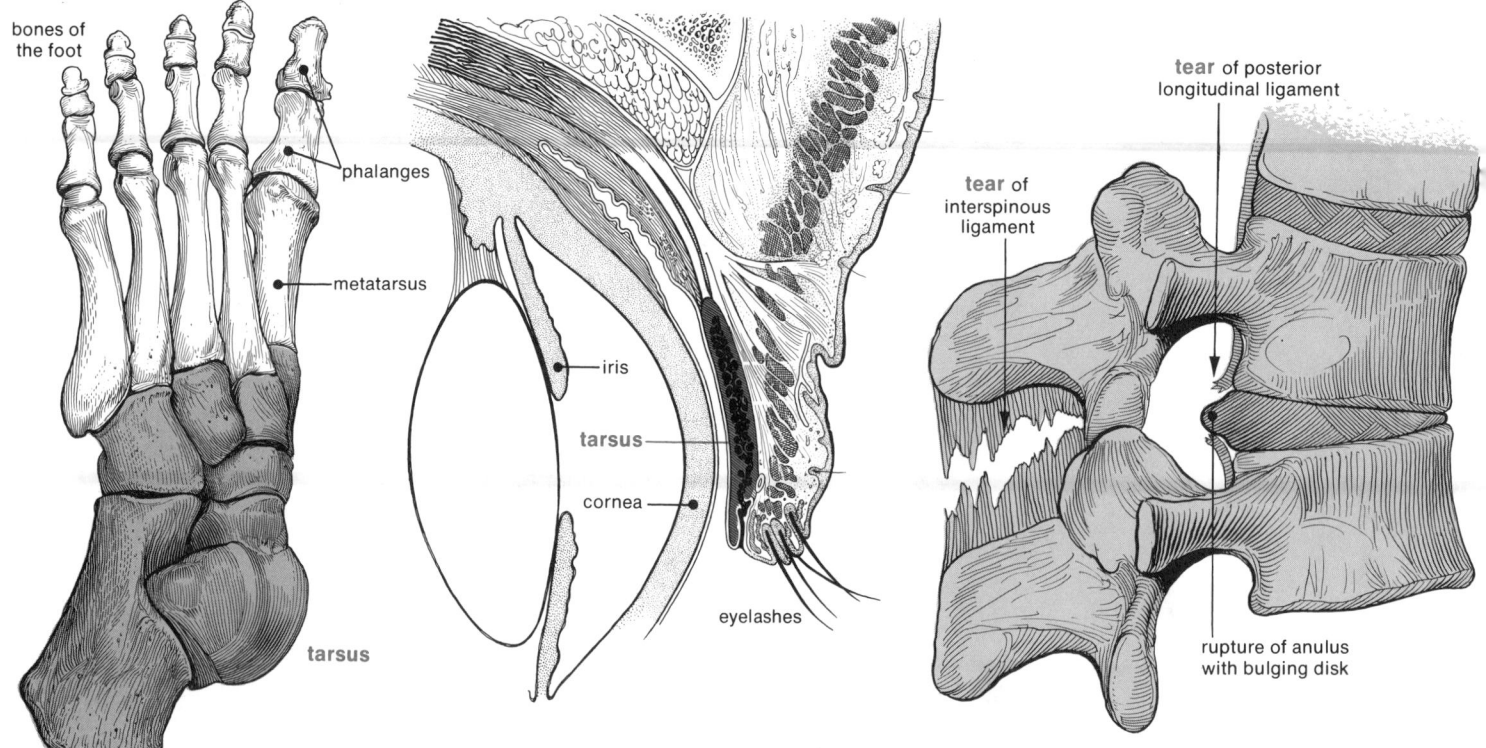

bones of the foot

phalanges

metatarsus

tarsus

iris

tarsus

cornea

eyelashes

tear of posterior longitudinal ligament

tear of interspinous ligament

rupture of anulus with bulging disk

tarsotomy Surgical incision of the eyelid.

tarsus, *pl.* **tarsi** 1. The part of the foot between the leg and the metatarsus formed by seven small bones. 2. The fibrous tissue that strengthens and shapes the edge of the eyelid.

tartar A hard yellow to brown deposit on the teeth, usually most heavily accumulated on the teeth nearest the salivary duct openings. Also called dental calculus.

tartaric acid A soluble white powder, a laxative and refrigerant, used in preparing Seidlitz powders and effervescing tablets.

tartrate A salt of tartaric acid.

tartrated Containing tartar or tartaric acid.

taste 1. The special sense that distinguishes the different flavors of substances that come in contact with the taste buds in the mouth. 2. To perceive such sensations.

taste bud See bud, taste.

tattoo A permanent design made on the skin by ingraining an indelible pigment through punctures.

taurine Water-soluble, colorless crystals produced by the decomposition of taurocholic acid.

taurocholate A salt of taurocholic acid.

taurocholic acid A bile acid; a compound of cholic acid and taurine; also called cholytaurine.

taurodontism Abnormal development of the molars of either or both primary or secondary dentition; the teeth have short roots, long crowns, and large pulp cavities.

Taussig-Bing syndrome Congenital malformation of the heart in which the aorta arises from the right ventricle (instead of the left) and the pulmonary artery arises from both ventricles, anterior to the aorta; a ventricular septal defect is also present.

tautomerism Phenomenon in which a chemical compound exists in a state of equilibrium between two isomeric forms and is able to react according to either. Also called dynamic allotropy.

taxis 1. Correction of a dislocation or reduction of a hernia by gentle pressure. 2. The reaction of certain organisms to a stimulus, i.e., motion away from or toward the stimulus, or arrangement in a particular position relating to the stimulus; used with a prefix indicating the type of stimulus; e.g., chemotaxis, electrotaxis, etc.

taxon, *pl.* **taxa** A category in a systematic classification; e.g., genus, species.

taxonomy The classification of living organisms into categories (taxa).

Tay-Sachs disease Cerebral sphingolipidosis; see under sphingolipidosis.

tear 1. The clear saline liquid secreted by the lacrimal gland, serving to keep the cornea and conjunctiva moist and to facilitate movement of the eyelid. 2. The act of secreting tears.

tear 1. To pull apart or divide forcefully. 2. To wound by lacerating.

tease To separate gently with a fine instrument, as the minute components of a tissue.

teaspoon (tsp) A small spoon used as a measure in the dosage of fluid medicines, equivalent to 5 ml.

teat A nipple or breast.

technetium A radioactive element, symbol Tc, atomic number 43, atomic weight 99.

technetium-99M (⁹⁹mTc) A radioisotope with a half-life of 6 hours suitable for clinical and research purposes; used in the preparation of radiopharmaceuticals and as a radiotracer in determining blood flow and for tumor localization.

technical 1. Relating to technique. 2. Specialized.

technician A person who has a high school diploma or an Associate Degree and who has been trained in the performance of special technical procedures.

dental laboratory t. A person trained in the making of dental appliances, such as dentures, crown and bridge work, restorations, and orthodontic appliances.

histologic t. One trained in processing body tissues that have been removed from the body for microscopic examination (such as fixing, embedding, sectioning, mounting, and staining).

medical laboratory t. A person who has an Associate Degree with special training in medical laboratory techniques (such as physical, chemical, and microscopic analysis of body fluids and tissues) and who works under appropriate supervision, such as that of a certified medical technologist. Cf. medical technologist.

radiation therapy t. One who assists the radiologist in treatment of disease by exposing specific areas of the patient's body to prescribed doses of x-ray or other forms of ionizing radiation.

x-ray t. A person trained to make x-ray films of a bodily part. Also called radiologic technologist.

technique The systematic procedure by which a surgical operation, scientific experiment, or any complex act is accomplished.

fluorescent antibody t. An immunofluorescent technique used for detecting antigen in tissue sections by either: (a) *direct method,* in which immunoglobulin (antibody) treated with a fluorescent dye is added to the tissue, specific antigen in the tissue (e.g., microbe) combines with the fluorescent antibody, and the resulting antigen-antibody complex is then detected through fluorescence microscopy; or (b) *indirect method,* in which unlabeled immunoglobulin (antibody) is added to tissue, specific antigen in the tissue combines with the antibody resulting in an antigen-antibody complex), fluorescein-conjugated anti-immunoglobulin antibody is added, and the resulting triple complex is then located by fluorescence microscopy.

flush t. One used to determine the systolic blood pressure in infants.

hydro-flow t. In dentistry, a method of cavity preparation in which the tooth being prepared is kept under a stream of water.

invasive t. Technique in which the skin of the patient is punctured or incised.

non-invasive t. Technique in which the skin of the patient is not punctured or incised.

Ouchterlony t. A double diffusion method for performing a precipitin test.

Shouldice t. A technique for repairing direct and indirect inguinal hernias.

technologist An individual who is a graduate of a four-year college with special training in a particular field and who is certified in that field.

medical t. (M.T.) One who performs or supervises test procedures in the clinical laboratory, including the fields of serology, immunology, chemistry, blood typing, hematology, parasitology, microbiology, urinalysis, and histochemistry. Cf. medical technician.

nuclear medicine t. A certified medical technologist or a registered nurse who has been trained in the use of radioactive materials for diagnostic purposes.

pharmaceutical laboratory t. Certified medical technologist in industry who analyzes and tests medications for strength and purity.

tectiform Shaped like a roof.

tectonic Relating to plastic surgery or grafting.

tectorial Relating to, or forming, a cover or roof.

tectorium Any rooflike structure.

tectum Any anatomic covering or roofing structure, especially the roofplate of the midbrain; it is dorsal to the cerebral aqueduct and includes the superior and inferior colliculi, their brachii, and the tectal lamina.

teething The eruption of the primary or baby teeth into the oral cavity.

tegmen A structure that covers or roofs over a part.

t. tympani Roof of the middle ear chamber formed by the thin plate of the petrous part of the temporal bone; it separates the middle ear chamber from the middle cranial fossa.

t. ventriculi quarti Roof of fourth ventricle; see under roof.

tegmentum The larger dorsal portion of the brain stem.

tegument See integument.

tela, *pl.* **telae** A thin, delicate, weblike membrane.

telangiectasia
dilatation of small blood vessels

tenaculum

tenia mesocolica

tenia omentalis

tenia libera

meso-colon

colon

NORMAL RECTAL BODY temperatures

Species	°F (±1°F)	°C (±0.5°C)
mouse	97	36
man	98.6	37.0
cat	101.5	38.5
dog	102	39
chicken	106.2	41.5

telangiectasia, telangiectasis Dilatation of a group of capillaries.

  hereditary hemorrhagic t. Telangiectasia in the skin and mucous membranes, usually appearing after puberty; transmitted as a simple dominant trait. Also called Rendu-Osler-Weber disease; Sutton-Rendu-Osler-Weber syndrome.

telangiectatic Afflicted with telangiectasia.

telangioma A tumor made up of dilated capillaries or arterioles.

telediagnosis Diagnosis of disease in a patient located at some distance from the physician by evaluation of data transmitted to a receiving station.

telelectrocardiogram An electrocardiogram recorded at some distance from the patient. Also called telecardiogram.

telelectrocardiograph An apparatus for the transmission and remote reception of electrocardiograph signals. Also called telecardiograph.

telemetry The science and technology of remote sensing for monitoring living systems by use of radio transmitters placed in or on animal or human subjects; such parameters as blood pressure, heart rate, etc., may be monitored in this way.

  cardiac t. Transmission of electrical signals from the heart to a receiving location where the electrocardiogram is displayed for monitoring.

telencephalon The portion of the embryonic brain from which develop the cerebral hemispheres, the lateral ventricles, the anterior part of the third ventricle, and the olfactory lobes; together with the diencephalon it makes up the prosencephalon.

teleneuron A nerve ending.

teleology Doctrine according to which all biologic events are directed toward some final purpose.

telepathy The phenomenon of communication of thought from one individual to another without the aid of physical means; since the means of extrasensory thought transference is unknown, it is generally not accepted as scientifically valid.

telereceptor An organ that perceives sense stimuli from a distance; e.g., the eye.

teletherapy Radiotherapeutic treatment with an external radiation source many centimeters from the patient.

tellurium A lustrous semimetallic element; symbol Te, atomic number 52, atomic weight 127.6.

telocentric Denoting a chromosome with its centromere at the end.

telodendron The terminal branching of an axon.

telogen The resting or final phase of a hair cycle; the period of time before a hair is shed.

telomere One of the two ends of a chromosome.

telophase The last stage of cell division by mitosis, beginning when the chromatids reach the poles

of the cell and the nuclear membranes enclose each new set of chromosomes to complete the separation of two daughter cells.

temperament The unique natural predispositions of an individual that influence his manner of thinking, behaving, and reacting.

temperature (t) **1.** Intensity of heat as measured in any of several arbitrary scales. **2.** A feverish condition.

  absolute t. (T) Temperature measured on an absolute scale.

  critical t. Temperature above which a gas cannot be reduced to liquid form.

  effective t. A comfort index that takes into consideration the temperature, movement, and moisture content of the air.

  normal t. The temperature of a normal person at rest (usually about 98.6°F or 37°C oral).

temper-tantrum A habit disorder, seen principally among emotionally immature children, characterized by screaming and kicking.

template **1.** The macromolecular mold for the synthesis of another macromolecule. **2.** In dentistry, a curved or flat plate used as an aid in setting teeth. Also called pattern.

  wax t. A wax impression of the occlusion of the teeth.

temple The lateral region on either side of the forehead above the zygomatic arch.

tempolabile Unstable over a period of time or changed or destroyed by time; said of a serum.

temporal Relating to the side of the head or temple.

temporomandibular Relating to the temporal bone and mandible, as the articulation of the lower jaw (temporomandibular joint, TMJ).

temporo-occipital Relating to the temporal and occipital bones of the skull.

tempostabile, tempostable Not altered by the passage of time; said of certain chemicals.

tenacious Sticky; adhesive.

tenacity The state of being adhesive or cohesive.

tenaculum A hooked surgical instrument for grasping and holding parts, such as the divided end of a blood vessel during an operation.

tenalgia Pain in a tendon. Also called tenontodynia; tenodynia.

tender Painful on pressure; sensitive.

tenderness Abnormal sensitivity to pressure or contact.

  rebound t. Pain felt when pressure is released suddenly; in the abdomen it is characteristic of peritonitis.

tendinitis Inflammation of a tendon. Also called tenontitis; tenonitis; tendonitis.

tendinoplasty See tenoplasty.

tendinous Relating to or of the nature of a tendon.

tendolysis The removal of adhesions from a tendon. Also called tenolysis.

tendon A fibrous band that attaches a muscle to a bone.

  Achilles t. See calcaneal tendon.

  calcaneal t. The large common tendon that attaches the gastrocnemius and soleus muscles to the calcaneus (heel bone). Also called Achilles tendon; tendo calcaneus.

  conjoined t. The fused tendons of the transversus abdominis and internal oblique muscles; it inserts onto the crest of the pubic bone and the pectineal line. Also called inguinal falx; conjoint tendon.

tendonitis See tendinitis.

tendoplasty See tenoplasty.

tendotomy See tenotomy.

tenectomy Surgical removal of part of a tendon.

tenesmic Relating to or afflicted with tenesmus.

tenesmus A painful, ineffectual straining to defecate or urinate.

tenia, *pl.* **teniae** **1.** Any narrow bandlike anatomic structure. **2.** The line of attachment of a choroid plexus. **3.** Any flatworm of the genus *Taenia*.

  t. coli Any of three thickened bands of longitudinal muscular fibers about 6 mm broad, on the wall of the colon.

  t. libera The tenia coli almost midway between the tenia mesocolica and tenia omentalis. Also called free band.

  t. mesocolica The tenia coli situated along the attachment of the mesocolon to the colon.

  t. omentalis The tenia coli of the transverse colon situated along the site of attachment of the greater omentum.

  t. thalami The tenia, or line of attachment, of the choroid plexus that runs along the dorsomedial border of the thalamus; the lateral ventricles lie above it and the third ventricle lies below it. Also called tenia of the thalamus; tenia of the third ventricle.

teniacide Any agent that destroys tapeworms.

teniafuge An agent for expelling tapeworms.

tenial **1.** Relating to a tapeworm. **2.** Relating to a band of tissue (tenia).

teniasis Infestation with tapeworms in the intestine.

tenioid **1.** Resembling a ribbon. **2.** Resembling a tapeworm.

tenodesis The transferring of the proximal end of a tendon to another site.

tenolysis See tendolysis.

tenonectomy Surgical procedure for shortening a tendon in which a segment of the tendon is removed

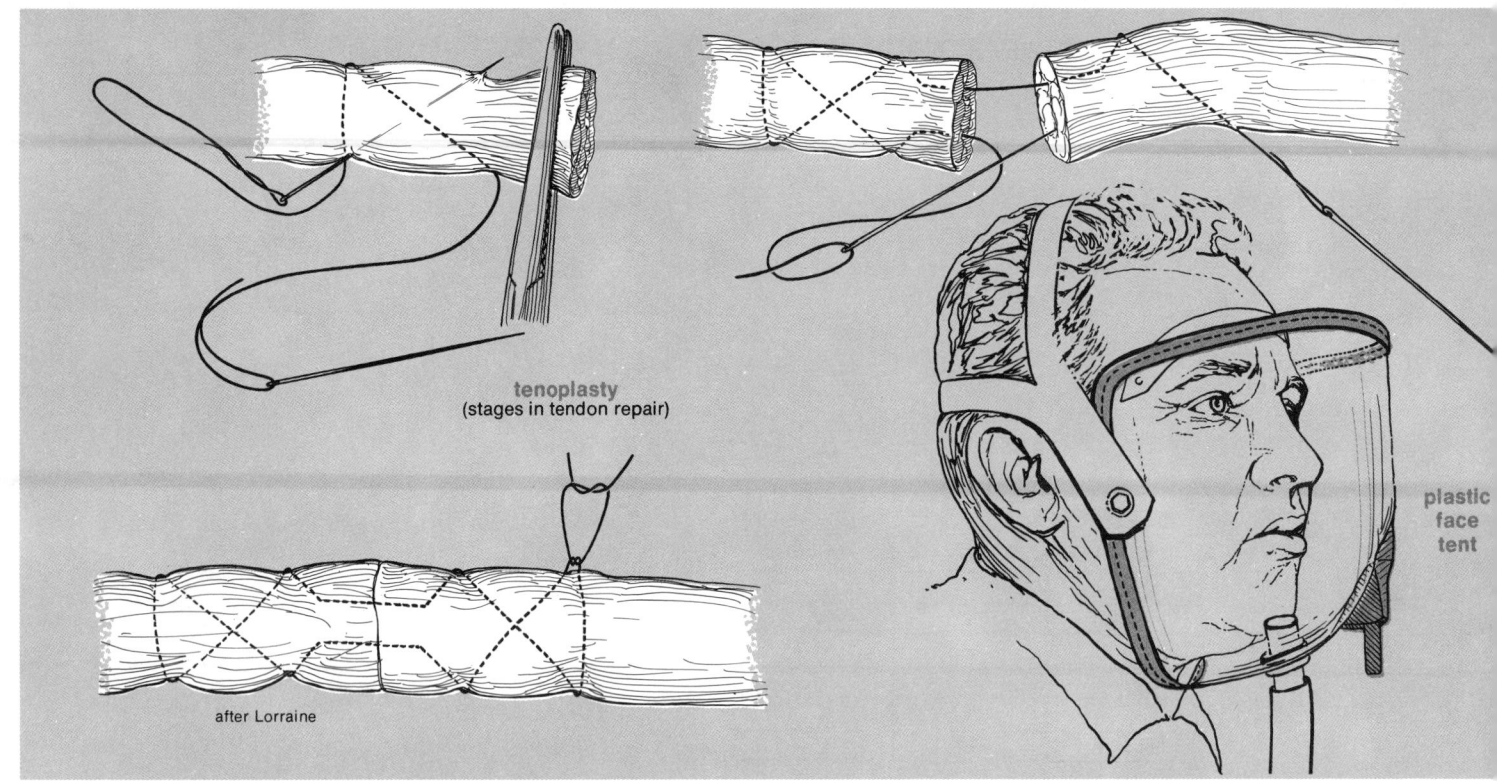

tenoplasty
(stages in tendon repair)

after Lorraine

plastic
face
tent

and the two remaining ends are joined.

tenontitis See tendinitis.

tenophyte A growth of cartilaginous or bony tissue attached to a tendon.

tenoplasty Reparative surgery of the tendons. Also called tendinoplasty; tendoplasty; tenontoplasty.

tenorrhaphy The suturing of a divided tendon.

tenosynovectomy Surgical removal of a tendon sheath.

tenosynovitis Inflammation of a tendon sheath. Also called tenovaginitis.

tenotomy The cutting of a tendon for corrective measures, as for clubfoot or strasbismus. Also called tendotomy.

tenovaginitis See tenosynovitis.

tension (T) 1. The act of stretching or the condition of being taut or strained **2.** A force tending to produce extension or expansion, as of a liquid or gas, when a confining force is removed. **3.** Emotional or mental strain.

arterial t. The pressure produced on the wall of an artery by the blood current at the peak of a pulse wave.

interfacial surface t. The resistance to separation offered by the film of liquid between two well adapted surfaces, as that of the thin film of saliva between a denture base and the tissues.

intraocular t. (Tn) Pressure within the eyeball.

premenstrual t. Temporary condition marked by irritability, nervousness, and/or headache, occurring during the week prior to menstruation and disappearing after the onset of the menstrual flow.

surface t. The force that tends to pull together the molecules of a liquid surface when in contact with another substance.

tensor A muscle that makes a part tense or firm.

tent 1. A covering of canvas or plastic placed over a patient's bed for the administration of inhaled medications or oxygen. **2.** An expandable plug placed in an orifice to keep it open.

oxygen t. Tent placed over a patient's bed into which oxygen is conducted.

plastic face t. One placed over a patient's face to facilitate the administration of gaseous medications.

steam t. Tent in which steam is provided.

tentorial Of, or relating to, the tentorium.

tentorium A membranous partition.

t. cerebelli A fold of dura mater separating the cerebellum and the posterior part of the cerebrum.

tephromalacia Condition marked by softening of the gray substance of the brain and spinal cord.

ter Latin for three times.

t. die sumendum (t.d.s.) Latin for to be taken three times a day; used in prescription writing.

t. in die (t.i.d.) Three times a day; used in prescription writing.

teratocarcinoma 1. A malignant tumor composed of several types of tissues, usually occurring in the testis. **2.** A malignant epithelial tumor originating in a teratoma.

teratogen Any environmental or chemical agent that causes abnormal development of the fetus.

teratogenesis, teratogeny The origin of congenital malformations.

teratogenic Causing physical abnormalities.

teratoid Resembling a malformed fetus.

teratology The subspecialty of developmental anatomy that deals with abnormal development. Also called desmorphology.

teratoma A tumor composed of multiple tissues, including tissues not normally found in the organ in which it arises; occurs most frequently in the ovary, where it is usually benign and forms dermoid cysts; also occurs in the testis, where is it usually malignant, and, uncommonly, in other sites.

teratomatous Relating to, or having, the characteristics of a teratoma.

teratophobia Morbid fear of giving birth to a grossly deformed baby.

terbium A metallic element; symbol Tb, atomic number 65, atomic weight 158.93.

teres Round and elongated, such as certain ligaments and muscles.

term A definite or limited period of time.

at t. At the normal time; at the end of a normal pregnancy or gestation period.

terminal 1. Relating to the end. **2.** Relating to, situated at, or forming the extremity of any structure. **3.** The part of an electric circuit at which an electric connection is generally made.

ternary Composed of three, as a molecule containing three different types of atoms.

tertian Recurring every third day, as a type of malarial fever; the attack actually occurs on day one and day three, so that there is really only an interval of one day.

tertigravida A woman who has been pregnant three times.

tertipara A person who has borne three children.

test 1. An examination. **2.** A means to determine the presence and quantity of a substance. **3.** To perform such functions. **4.** A substance used in a test.

achievement t. A standardized test used to evaluate acquired learning in specific subjects.

acoustic impedance t. A test that assesses the integrity and function of the middle ear, especially transmission characteristics, by measuring the reflected sound waves (acoustic impedance) at the tympanic membrane.

ACTH stimulation t. Test for adrenal cortex function; limited or nonexistent increase of plasma cortisol after administration of ACTH indicates adrenal cortex insufficiency.

Adson's t. A test for the detection of thoracic outlet syndrome; the patient sits with the palm of the hands on his knees, chin held high, head turned toward the side to be examined; if on deep inspiration the radial pulse disappears, it indicates temporary occlusion of the subclavian artery.

alkali denaturation t. Test to determine the concentration of fetal hemoglobin.

antiglobulin t. See Coombs' test.

aptitude t. A test that measures a person's skills, interests, talents and abilities; useful in vocational counseling.

association t. A method for examining the content of the mind, whereby the subject is required to respond as quickly as possible to a given stimulus word with the first word that comes to mind. Also called word association test.

Bárány's caloric t. Test for vestibular function of the ear; reduced or absent response (e.g., nystagmus or past pointing) after irrigation of external auditory canal with hot or cold water indicates vestibular disease.

Bender-Gestalt t. A test of visual motor function in which the subject is asked to copy nine standard designs; its chief application is to determine organic brain dysfunction in both children and adults and level of development of visual motor function in children; secondarily used to assess personality variables. Also called Bender visual-motor Gestalt test.

benzidine t. Test to detect the presence of blood; a portion of the suspected sample is added to benzidine reagent (benzidine, glacial acetic acid, and hydrogen peroxide); a blue color develops in the presence of blood.

Bernstein t. Test to establish that a pain under the breastbone is due to reflux esophagitis; a weak hydrochloric acid solution is instilled into the lower esophagus; pain disappears when the acid solution is replaced by saline solution.

Binet t., Stanford-Binet t. Test used to determine the mental age of a child; it consists of a series of questions standardized according to the mental capacity of normal children at different ages.

biuret t. Test used to determine the presence of proteins in body fluids; the sample is mixed with alkaline copper sulfate; a violet-pinkish color indicates a positive result.

blood urea clearance t. See urea clearance test.

individual supine, limb elevated to 65°; veins emptied by gravity, tourniquet applied to thigh tight enough to constrict superficial but not deep veins

individual stands erect; if varices remain empty for 20 seconds, the valves in communicating veins are competent

on removal of tourniquet, veins fill rapidly from above indicating incompetence of valves in great saphenous vein

if veins fill rapidly with tourniquet in place, there is incompetence of valves in communicating veins, including the small saphenous vein

Brodie-Trendelenburg test

a rabbit is immunized with whole serum, gamma globulin or complement

anti serum

anti-human protein antibodies (e.g., antigamma globulin, anticomplement)

direct Coombs' test (direct antiglobulin test)

test samples of red blood cells

red blood cells sensitized with incomplete antibodies or complements result in agglutination of cells

POSITIVE

NEGATIVE

nonsensitized red blood cells do not agglutinate

Brodie-Trendelenburg t. Test for determining the presence of incompetent valves in the communicating veins between the superficial and deep vessels in patients with varicose veins; tourniquet is applied around the thigh with the individual in the recumbent position; if the valves are incompetent, they allow the varicosities to fill rapidly when the person assumes an erect position.

CAGE t. A screening test for alcoholism. The patient is asked if he (she) ever Cut down on drinking; felt Annoyed by criticisms about drinking; had Guilty feelings about drinking; had an Eye opener in the morning.

capillary fragility t. A tourniquet test to determine weakness of the capillary walls; a circle 2.5 cm in diameter is drawn on the inner aspect of the forearm 4 cm below the crease of the elbow, and a blood pressure cuff is inflated above the elbow (not to exceed

100 mm Hg) for 5 minutes; the petechiae (minute hemorrhagic spots) formed within the circle are counted; a number over 20 is abnormal. Also called Rumpel-Leede test.

complement-fixation t. A widely used test to detect the presence of antibodies in serum; based on the fact that antibodies, when combined with their specific antigens, are able to fix or remove complement (thus making it undetectable in a subsequent test).

Coombs' t. (CT) An agglutination test designed to detect the presence on cells of serum proteins (commonly functionally univalent antibodies) not usually identifiable by simple in vitro agglutination techniques; two methods may be used: direct (test for antibody on cells) or indirect (test for antibody in serum); also called antiglobulin test. See also direct and indirect Coombs' tests.

cross-agglutination t. One of several tests used in blood typing; red blood cells from a donor of an unknown blood type are mixed with sera of known blood types.

cytotoxicity t., cytoxicity t. One used in testing for compatibility for organ transplant; living cells are mixed with antibody and complement; if antibody to a cell-bound antigen is present, cell death will occur in the presence of complement.

dexamethasone suppression t. 1 mg of dexamethasone suppresses cortisol secretion in normal persons but not in those with Cushing's syndrome.

Dick t. Intracutaneous test to detect susceptibility to scarlet fever.

direct Coombs' t. Test for detecting sensitized red blood cells in erythroblastosis fetalis and acquired hemolytic anemia; a sample of the patient's red blood cells is washed with saline and mixed with

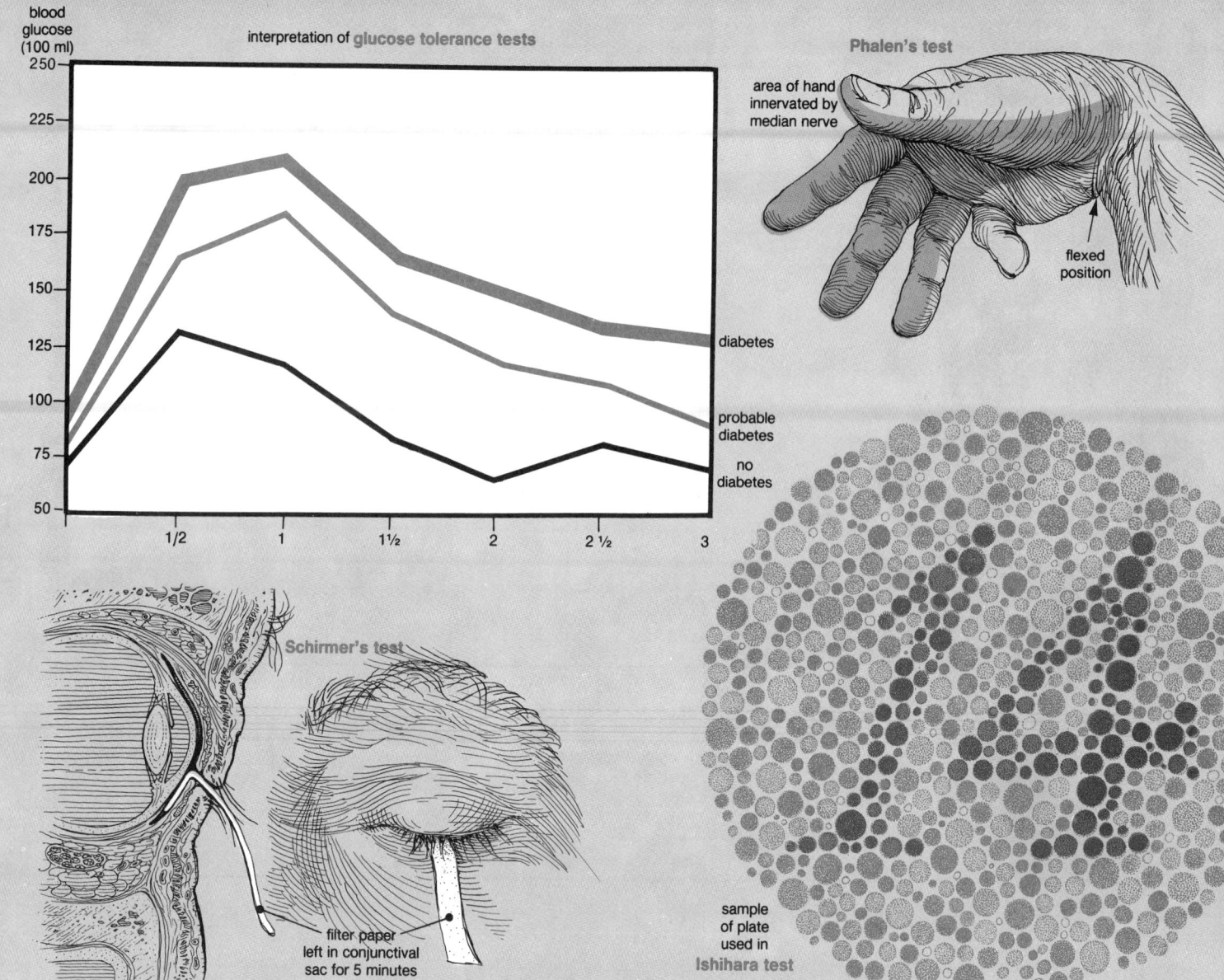

blood glucose (100 ml)

interpretation of glucose tolerance tests

Phalen's test

area of hand innervated by median nerve

flexed position

diabetes

probable diabetes

no diabetes

Schirmer's test

filter paper left in conjunctival sac for 5 minutes

sample of plate used in Ishihara test

Coombs' antihuman globulin, then centrifuged; agglutination indicates a positive test.

double-blind t. Test in which neither the person giving the test nor the one receiving it knows whether the drug used is active or inert.

draw-a-person t. In psychology, (a) a method of determining a child's level of intellectual development based upon the complexity of the subject's "best" drawing of a human figure; also called Goodenough test; (b) a projective personality test requiring the subject to draw a person. Also called Machover test.

Ellsworth-Howard t. The measuring of urinary phosphate after intravenous administration of parathyroid extract for the diagnosis of pseudohypoparathyroidism; an increase in urinary phosphate is seen in hypoparathyroidism but not in pseudohypoparathyroidism (however, exceptions may occur).

ferric chloride t. Test for detecting phenylketonuria, which is indicated when a urine sample turns blue-green by addition of ferric chloride.

finger-nose t. Test of ability to coordinate voluntary movement of the arm; the person is asked to slowly touch the end of his nose with the tip of his extended index finger.

fluorescent treponemal antibody-absorption t. (FTA-ABS t.) A specific test for syphilis using a suspension of *Treponema pallidum* (Nichols strain).

fragility t. One that measures the osmotic fragility of red blood cells; cells are placed in a series of test tubes with saline of decreasing concentrations ranging from 0.85 to 0.10%; the red cells absorb water, swell to a spheroid shape, and rupture; in normal cells hemolysis begins at concentrations of 0.45 to

0.39%; and complete hemolysis occurs at 0.33 to 0.30%.

galactose tolerance t. A liver function test that measures the ability of the liver to convert galactose to glycogen; after ingestion of 40 g of galactose, excretion of not more than 3 g in urine after 5 hours is considered normal.

glucose tolerance t. (GTT) Test for diabetes based on the response to a glucose load; in the oral glucose tolerance test (OGTT), 100 g of glucose are ingested after an overnight fast; normally, blood sugar rises quickly, then falls to normal within 2 hours; in diabetes mellitus, the increase is greater and the return to normal is abnormally prolonged; additional information can be obtained if plasma insulin levels are measured simultaneously; in patients with gastrointestinal disease, a smaller dose of glucose (usually 25 g) may be given intravenously to avoid difficulty in interpretation due to abnormal absorption.

guaiac t. Test for detection of blood; specimen is mixed with glacial acetic acid and gum guadiac solution; blood is present if a blue color develops upon addition of hydrogen peroxide.

Hickey-Hare t. Test for diabetes insipidus; hypertonic saline is infused intravenously after establishment of water diuresis; test is positive when antidiuresis is not produced; when the posterior pituitary is normal, the hypertoxicity causes release of antidiuretic hormones, which concentrates the urine.

histamine t. **1.** A test for determining the absence of gastric acidity; histamine phosphate is injected subcutaneously to stimulate secretion of gastric juice. **2.** A provocative test for pheochromocytoma; histamine phosphate is injected intravenously; nor-

mally there is a prompt, slight fall in blood pressure, but if a lesion is present, a marked rise in blood pressure follows immediately after the fall.

immunologic pregnancy t. Test utilizing latex particles coated with human chorionic gonadotropin (HCG) as antigen, anti-HCG serum, and urine to be tested; if the latex particles do not clump, the woman is pregnant. Also called agglutination inhibition test for pregnancy.

indirect Coombs' t. Test used in crossmatching of blood and transfusion reaction studies; the patient's serum is incubated with a suspension of donor red blood cells; after a washing with saline, Coombs' serum is added; clumping indicates that the cells had been coated or sensitized by antibodies present in the patient's serum.

intelligence t. Any test designed to measure the mental capacity of the subject.

Ishihara t. A test for detection of color blindness, based on the ability to see patterns in a series of multicolored plates or cards (Ishihara plates).

Kolmer's t. **1.** A complement-fixation test for certain bacterial diseases. **2.** A modified Wassermann test for syphilis.

Kveim t. Test for detection of sarcoidosis; a dose of ground sarcoid lymph nodes, tested for sterility and preserved in phenol, is injected intradermally; a papule appears; biopsy of the papule in a positive test shows giant cell formation.

latex t. Test for rheumatoid arthritis; minute spherical particles of latex in suspension are coated with antigen and incubated with the patient's serum; when rheumatoid factor is present in the serum, clumping of the latex particles occurs. Also called latex agglutination or latex fixation test.

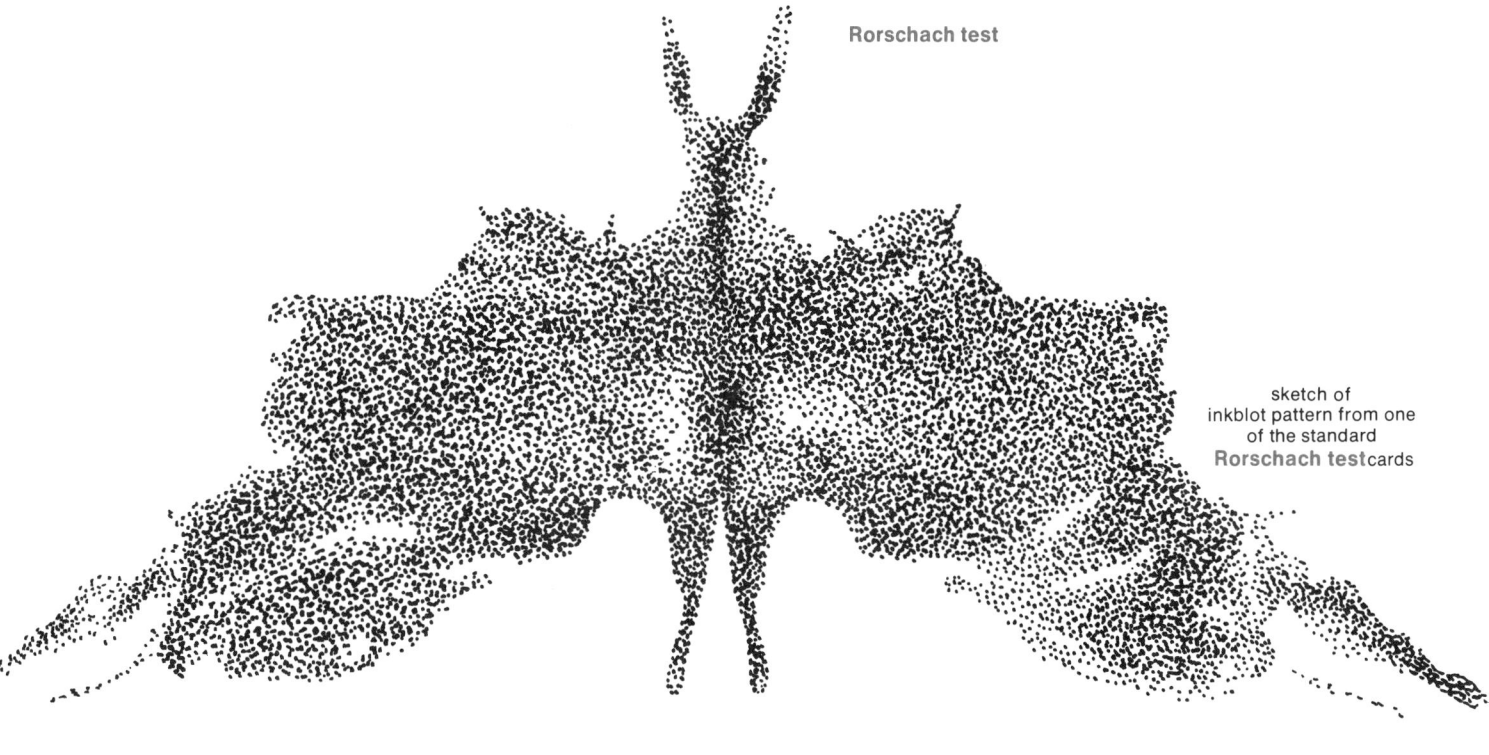

Rorschach test

sketch of
inkblot pattern from one
of the standard
Rorschach test cards

LE cell t. A test for systemic lupus erythematosus; polymorphonuclear leukocytes engulf nuclear material from damaged white blood cells, forming LE cells, in blood or serum samples from patients with the disease.

lepromin t. Test for leprosy; a lepromin injection produces a papule in tuberculoid leprosy; no such reaction occurs in lepromatous leprosy.

Mantoux t. A tuberculin test in which a derivative of tuberculin, such as purified protein derivative (PPD), is injected intracutaneously; considered positive if redness and induration of 10 mm diameter occur.

migration inhibition t. In vitro test for delayed type sensitivity (cell mediated); when specific antigen is present, peritoneal exudate cells (macrophages) from a sensitized animal do not migrate from a chamber in the manner typical of those from a normal animal.

Minnesota multiphasic personality inventory t. (MMPI) Psychological test in the form of a questionnaire composed of 550 true-false statements; answers are scored by codes, standardized on different diagnostic groups and personality types.

mixed lymphocyte culture t., MLC t. Test to measure a person's ability to accept a tissue transplant; lymphocytes from donor and recipient are mixed in culture, whereupon the degree of incompatibility is measured by estimating the number of cells that have undergone transformation and mitosis, or by the amount of radioactive isotope-labeled thymidine that was incorporated.

nitroblue tetrazolium (NBT) **t.** Test of neutrophil capacity to kill bacteria; normally, phagocytosis of bacterial cells is accompanied by NBT reduction to a blue formazan pigment; absence of NBT reduction indicates neutrophil defects.

nitroprusside t. Test to detect cystine in the urine; sodium cyanide is first added to the urine sample, then nitroprusside; a red-purple color develops if the cyanide has reduced to cysteine any cystine that was present in the urine.

Pap t., Papanicolao t., Procedure in which cells from body secretions are fixed and stained and examined microscopically for abnormal cells; used in the detection of cancer (especially of the female genital tract, but also of the respiratory, urinary and gastrointestinal tracts) and for the evaluation of the hormonal state. Also called Pap smear; Pap smear test.

partial thromboplastin time t. A one-stage clotting test for detection of plasma factor deficiencies.

patch t. A test for allergic sensitivity made by placing filter paper or gauze saturated with a suspected allergen against the skin (usually on the forearm) under a small patch; on removal of the patch the reaction of the skin is observed; a positive reaction is indicated by reddening at the site; also used for tuberculin testing.

paternity t. A medicolegal test based upon genetic interpretation of blood groups of mother, child, and alleged father for the purpose of excluding the possibility of paternity.

Paul-Bunnell t. A test to determine the presence of heterophil antibodies in the circulating blood; an elevated titer is found in infectious mononucleosis.

Phalen's t. A test for determining median nerve compression in the carpal tunnel of the wrist; the wrists are placed in a flexed position; if there is median nerve compression, paresthesias of the fingers usually occur after several seconds; most normal individuals develop paresthesias after a few minutes of acute wrist flexion.

phenotolamine t. Test for pheochromocytoma in patients with sustained hypertension; administration of phentolamine produces a sustained fall in blood pressure in the presence of pheochromocytoma.

postprandial blood sugar t. A test utilizing a sample of blood drawn, usually two hours after the ingestion of a 100-gram carbohydrate meal, for the diagnosis of diabetes mellitus.

precipitin t. Any test in which a positive result is indicated by the formation of a precipitate. Also called precipitation test.

pregnancy t. Any test for pregnancy (e.g., Aschheim-Zondek test, immunologic pregnancy test).

prostate-specific antigen t., PSA t. Blood test for detection of prostatic cancer; it measures serum concentrations of a protein (antigen) produced exclusively by prostate epithelial cells; levels of up to 4 micrograms/liter are generally considered normal.

protein-bound iodine t. (PBI t.) A test formerly used for assessment of thyroid function.

prothrombin t. Test that determines the amount of thrombin present in plasma, based on the clotting time of blood; used to measure blood coagulability and as a guide to anticoagulation with coumarin and related drugs.

provocative t. A test for pheochromocytoma performed on patients with normal blood pressure; the presence of pheochromocytoma causes a sudden rise in blood pressure immediately following the administration of histamine, tyramine, or glucagon.

PSA t. See prostate-specific antigen test.

psychological t. Any test dealing with mental phenomena.

pulp t. See vitality test.

Queckenstedt-Stookey t. When the jugular vein is compressed in a healthy person, there is rapid increase in the pressure of the cerebrospinal fluid (CSF), and an equally rapid return to normal when pressure is released; when there is a block in the vertebral canal, compression of the jugular vein causes little or no increase in pressure.

radioactive iodine uptake t. A test of thyroid function; ^{131}I-iodine is given orally; 24 hours later the amount present in the thyroid gland is measured against normal values.

radioallergosorbent t. (RAST) Test for detection of IgE-bound allergens causing tissue hypersensitivity; antigen is fixed in an insoluble medium, serum from the patient is added, and then a radiolabeled anti-gammaglobulin; if antibody to the allergen is present in the serum, it complexes to the allergen.

rapid plasma reagin t., RPR t. A test for syphilis using unheated serum and a standard antigen containing charcoal particles.

Rinne's t. Hearing test that compares bone conduction with air conduction by alternately holding a vibrating tuning fork in contact with the skull and in the air near the auditory orifice; in normal hearing, the vibrations are heard twice as long by air as by bone conduction; in conductive hearing loss, the ratio varies in favor of bone conduction.

Rorschach t. Projective psychological test for evaluating conscious and unconscious personality traits and emotional conflicts through the individual's associations to a set of inkblot patterns.

Rumpel-Leede T. Capillary fragility test.

Sabin-Feldman dye t. One used to diagnose toxoplasmosis; heat-inactivated serum from the patient (in the presence of a nonspecific serum factor) kills *Toxoplasma* organisms; methylene blue fails to stain damaged organisms.

Schick t. A test to measure immunity to diphtheria; diphtheria toxin (one-fiftieth of a guinea pig median lethal dose) is injected intracutaneously; if the person does not have sufficient antitoxin to neutralize the dose of toxin, an inflammation appears at the site of injection, usually within 48 hours.

Schiller's t. A test for early squamous cell carcinoma of the cervix; the cervix is coated with an aqueous iodine solution; a normal cervix turns brown; a cancerous cervix turns yellowish-white.

Schirmer's t. Test to measure the production of tears with a strip of filter paper.

scratch t. See skin test.

screening t. One devised to separate individuals or objects according to a fixed characteristic or property.

secretin t. Test for excretory function of the pancreas; secretion of pancreatic enzymes is stimulated for analysis by intravenous injection of the hormone secretin.

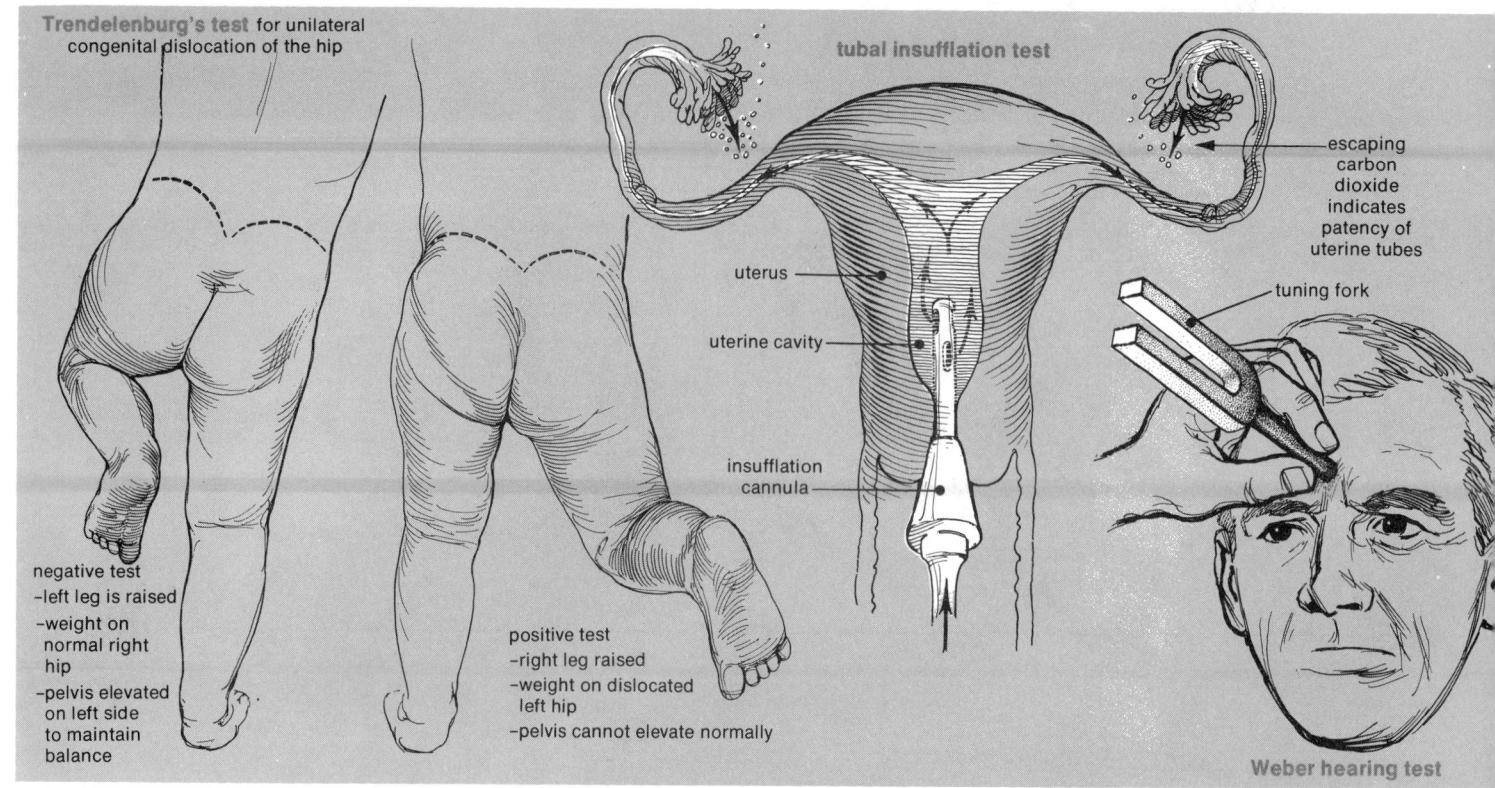

Trendelenburg's test for unilateral congenital dislocation of the hip

tubal insufflation test

escaping carbon dioxide indicates patency of uterine tubes

uterus

uterine cavity

insufflation cannula

tuning fork

negative test
-left leg is raised
-weight on normal right hip
-pelvis elevated on left side to maintain balance

positive test
-right leg raised
-weight on dislocated left hip
-pelvis cannot elevate normally

Weber hearing test

---

seroigic t. Any test using serum.

serologic t. for syphilis (STS) Any test for serum antibodies indicative of *Treponema pallidum* presence; may detect antitreponemal antibodies (treponemal test) or substances derived from host tissues (nontreponemal test).

sickle cell t. When blood is mixed with sodium bisulfite, red blood cells containing the abnormal sickle hemoglobin (Hb S) assume a crescentic or elongated shape.

skin t. Any test for allergy or infectious disease in which the allergen or an extract of a disease-causing organism is injected intracutaneously or applied to the skin by means of a patch. Also called scratch test.

skinfold t. Measurement of skinfolds with special constant tension calipers to determine the degree of obesity.

string t. Any of various tests to determine the approximate site of bleeding from the upper gastrointestinal tract, using a white string which is passed into the duodenum or beyond; the string is removed and checked along its length for blood; the blood-stained portion indicates the site of hemorrhage.

sweat t. Test for diagnosis of cystic fibrosis of the pancreas; high concentration of sodium chloride in the sweat is suggestive of the disease.

thematic apperception t. (TAT) Psychological test in which the subject is asked to tell stories about ambiguous pictures that may be interpreted in different ways according to the patient's personality.

three-glass t. Test for locating the site of inflammation of the male urinary tract; the patient urinates into three glass containers; the contents of each container reveal the approximate site; the urine in the first container has washings from the anterior urethra, that in the second from the bladder; after prostatic massage, the third has cells from the prostate, seminal vesicles and posterior urethra.

thromboplastin generation t. (TGT) A coagulation test based on the principle of mixing reagents; if thromboplastin formation is deficient, recombination of reagents determines which of the ingredients is defective.

tilt t. (1) Test to measure predilection for fainting (syncope); excretion of urinary epinephrine and norepinephrine is measured during three consecutive intervals with the patient first in a horizontal and then in a nearly vertical position; a marked increase in the second period indicates a positive test. (2) A rise in pulse or drop in blood pressure as a patient is moved from the supine toward the upright position indicating a loss of extracellular fluid, as during hemorrhage or dehydration.

tine t. Test for skin sensitivity performed by pressing tines previously impregnated with antigens into the skin; used for tuberculin testing.

Töpfer's t. Quantitative test for free hydrochloric acid in the gastric contents, by means of the indicator *p*-dimethylaminoazobenzene (0.5% alcoholic solution).

Trendelenburg's t. Test for unilateral congenital dislocation of the hip; when weight is borne on the normal side of the hip, the opposite side of the pelvis is elevated to maintain balance (negative test); when weight is borne on the dislocated side, the opposite side of the pelvis cannot be elevated normally (positive test).

treponemal immobilization t. (TPI) Test for syphilis; serum from a syphilitic patient (in the presence of complement) immobilizes the actively motile *Treponema pallidum* obtained from testes of a syphilitic rabbit (antigen).

triiodothyronine uptake t. (T_3 t.) An in vitro measurement using the patient's serum and radioactive triiodothyronine to determine the concentration of thyroxin-binding globulin present.

tubal insufflation t. Insufflation of the uterus with carbon dioxide to determine patency of the uterine (fallopian) tubes; if patent, the escape of gas into the abdominal cavity is heard over the lower abdomen. Also called Rubin test.

tuberculin t. Any test for tuberculosis in which tuberculin or its protein derivative is introduced into the skin by means of a patch (patch test), multiple punctures (tine test), or injection (Mantoux test).

two-glass t. Test for determining whether infection is located in the urethra or higher in the urinary tract; the patient collects his urine in two glasses; first glass contains urine which has washed out cells originating from the urethra, especially the anterior portion; the second contains urine characteristic of bladder urine.

Tzanck t. Microscopic examination of fluid from vesicles or blisters to identify characteristic cells of certain vesicular diseases, such as herpes and pemphigus.

van den Bergh's t. A test used to determine bilirubin in body fluids.

vanillylmandelic acid t. Test for tumors, such as neuroblastomas, by measuring vanillylmandelic acid levels in a 24-hour urine specimen. Also called VMA test.

VDRL t. Flocculation test for syphilis developed by the Venereal Disease Research Laboratory of the United States Public Health Service.

vitality t. A test that measures the response of the dental pulp to various stimuli (thermal, electrical, or mechanical); it determines whether a pulp is alive, diseased, or dead. Also called pulp test.

vitamin A absorption t. A gastrointestinal absorption test; blood specimen is obtained after a fasting period; the subject ingests 200,000 units of vitamin A in oil; serum vitamin A level normally should rise to twice fasting level in 3 to 5 hours.

VMA t. See vanillylmandelic acid test.

Wassermann t. A complement-fixation test used in the diagnosis of syphilis; the antigen is a cardiolipin diphosphatidylglycerol. Also called Wassermann reaction.

Watson-Schwartz t. A test for diagnosing acute intermittent porphyria, based on the formation of red coloration upon addition of Ehrlich's reagent to a urine specimen.

Weber hearing t. The application of a vibrating tuning fork to the midline of the forehead, bridge of the nose, and against the chin, for audiologic assessment; if the individual hears the tone in the middle of his head, he may have either normal hearing or deafness equal on both sides; if there is nerve deafness on one side, the tone will be heard better on the other side; when asymmetric conductive deafness is present, the tone is heard better in the poor ear.

D-xylose absorption t. A test of gastrointestinal absorption; after fasting for 8 hours, an individual drinks 10 ml per kg body weight of a 5% solution of D-xylose and then abstains from eating or drinking until the test is completed; all urine voided during the following 5 hours is pooled; blood samples are taken just prior to ingestion of the solution and at 1 and 2 hours later; normally, 16 to 33% of the ingested xylose is excreted within 5 hours; the serum xylose reaches a level between 25 and 40 mg/100 ml after 1 hour and is maintained at this level for another 60 minutes.

testa An outer shell.

testalgia Testicular pain. Also called orchialgia.

testcross A way of determining an unknown genotype by crossing it with a homozygous recessive.

testes Plural of testis.

testicle See testis.

testicular Of, or relating to, the testes.

testicular feminization syndrome Familial male pseudohermaphroditism marked by female external genitalia with a short vaginal pouch and absent uterus, undescended or labial testes, and absent or sparse pubic and axillary hair; the karyotype is XY, but there is a lack of end organ response to testosterone.

---

test | testicular

474

ampulla of deferent duct

deferent duct

ejaculatory duct

seminal vesicle

prostate

urethra

testes

epididymis

CH₃ OH

CH₃

O

testosterone
the male hormone, obtained directly from the testis, has a double bond in the first ring

CH₃

OH

9

8

7

10a

6a

6

H₃C CH₃ O

5

4

3

C₅H₁₁

tetrahydrocannabinol

spasm of hand in **tetany**

testis, *pl.* **testes** One of the two egg-shaped glands which produce spermatozoa, normally situated in the scrotum. Also called testicle.

   descent of the t. The gradual change of location of the testis, in the fetus and infant, from the abdominal cavity to the scrotum.

   undescended t., retained t. A testis that fails to descend into the scrotum, but remains in the abdominal cavity or inguinal canal.

testitis See orchitis.

testosterone A hormone produced by the testes, responsible for the development and maintenance of secondary sexual characteristics; the most potent of the naturally produced androgens, it is produced in the Leydig's cells under control of luteinizing (interstitial cell-stimulating) hormone.

test types Letters or figures printed on a card, used to test visual acuity.

   Jaeger's t. t. Words and phrases printed in ordinary printer's type of varying sizes, used to test near vision.

   Snellen's t. t. Block letters of varying sizes printed on a white card; used to test visual acuity.

tetanic Relating to tetanus or tetany.

tetaniform Resembling tetanus.

tetanize To produce a sustained contraction of a muscle by the application of numerous stimuli in rapid succession.

tetanode The quiet period between the muscle spasms in tetanus.

tetanoid 1. Resembling tetanus. 2. Resembling tetany.

tetanolysin A hemolysin produced by the tetanus bacillus (*Clostridium tetani*).

tetanospasmin The neurotoxin produced by *Clostridium tetani*, the causative agent of tetanus; it interferes with neuromuscular transmission by inhibiting the release of acetylcholine from nerve terminals; sites of action include: the motor end plates in skeletal muscles, spinal cord, brain, and sympathetic nervous system.

tetanotoxin A filtrate of a culture of *Clostridium tetani* (the tetanus bacillus) containing the toxins tetanospasmin and tetanolysin.

tetanus 1. An acute infectious disease caused by the toxin of *Clostridium tetani*, which affects the central nervous system, and marked by painful muscular contraction, most commonly beginning in the jaws (trismus) and neck muscles; it results from deposition of spores of *Clostridium tetani* in an area of injury, often minor, where the devitalized tissue permits growth; its incubation period is from three days to four weeks or longer; in generalized tetanus, the mortality rate approximates 50 percent; severity is related to the rapidity of onset of symptoms. Also

called lockjaw. 2. Sustained or prolonged contraction of a muscle.

   local t. Tetanus that affects only the muscles of the immediate area of the wound.

   t. neonatorum A form of tetanus affecting newborn infants due to infection through the open end of the umbilical cord.

tetany A disorder marked by intermittent muscle spasms, usually beginning with sharp flexion of the wrists and ankles, and progressing to involve other muscles and produce convulsions; it occurs as a result of hypocalcemia, alkalosis, or hypokalemia.

   hyperventilation t. Tetany caused by reduction of carbon dioxide in the blood, as in prolonged forced breathing.

   latent t. Tetany which is made apparent only by certain stimulating procedures.

   neonatal t. A relatively continuous hypertonicity of muscles in newborn infants.

tetartanopsia Loss of vision in homonymous quadrants of the visual fields of both eyes; e.g., the lower nasal quadrant of one eye and lower temporal quadrant of the other eye.

tetracaine hydrochloride A white crystalline compound used as a local or spinal anesthetic.

tetrachloride A compound possessing 4 atoms of chlorine per molecule.

tetracycline A yellow crystalline compound produced synthetically or from certain species of *Streptomyces*; a broad spectrum antibiotic.

tetrad 1. A set of four related things. 2. In chemistry, an element that has the combining power of four. 3. A group of four chromatids (chromosomal elements) that were formed during meiosis.

tetradactyl Having only four fingers or toes.

tetraethylammonium chloride Compound of ammonium having a ganglionic blocking action of short duration.

tetrahydrocannabinol (THC) The chief active ingredient in marijuana; it has no accepted medical use.

3,5,3′,5′-tetraiodothyronine (T₄) See thyroxin.

tetralogy Any series of four related elements, such as four concurrent defects.

   t. of Fallot A form of cyanotic congenital heart disease; the four abnormalities that constitute the deformity are pulmonic stenosis (usually infundibular), right ventricular hypertrophy, ventricular septal defect, and overriding of the aorta; thought to be due to a single embryologic error whereby the conus septum is located in an abnormally anterior position.

tetraplegia Paralysis of the four extremities. Also called quadriplegia.

tetraploid A cell with four haploid sets of chro-

mosomes in its nucleus.

tetravalent See quadrivalent.

tetrose A four-carbon sugar; a monosaccharide containing four carbon atoms; e.g., threose and erythrose.

thalamic Relating to the thalamus.

thalamic syndrome Hemianesthesia, hemichorea, central pain, and hemiparesis caused by arterial occlusion. Also called Dejerine-Roussy syndrome.

thalamocortical Relating to the thalamus and the cerebral cortex.

thalamolenticular Relating to the thalamus and the lentiform nucleus of the brain.

thalamomammillary Relating to the thalamus and the mammillary bodies of the brain.

thalamotegmental Relating to the tegmentum of the brain stem and the thalamus.

thalamotomy Operative destruction of a portion of the thalamus.

thalamus, *pl.* **thalami** An ovoid gray mass about 4 cm in length, located on either side of the third ventricle of the cerebrum, which primarily serves as a relay center for sensory impulses in the cerebral cortex; it is also an important structure for the perception of some types of sensation.

thalassemia A genetically transmitted type of hemolytic anemia; caused by a decreased rate of synthesis of one of the polypeptide chains in the globin portion of hemoglobin; the different forms are classified according to the polypeptide chain involved, i.e., alpha, beta, or gamma; in the presence of one normal gene and one thalassemia gene (the heterozygote state), clinical findings are generally mild and the condition is termed thalassemia trait or thalassemia minor; the homozygous state produces thalassemia major, generally a severe illness characterized by the appearance, in early childhood, of anemia, hepatosplenomegaly, jaundice, and growth retardation.

   A₂ t. Beta thalassemia.

   alpha t. A form in which there is a decrease in the rate of synthesis of the alpha polypeptide chain of hemoglobin; the homozygous form is incompatible with life.

   beta t. Thalassemia characterized by a decrease in the rate of synthesis of the beta polypeptide chain of hemoglobin; if the defect is only in the beta chain, levels of hemoglobin A₂ are increased even in the heterozygous form. Also called Cooley's or Mediterranean anemia.

   F t. A form of thalassemia in which heterozygotes show high levels of fetal hemoglobin and normal levels of A₂ hemoglobin; both beta and gamma polypeptide chains are affected.

thalidomide A sedative and hypnotic drug,

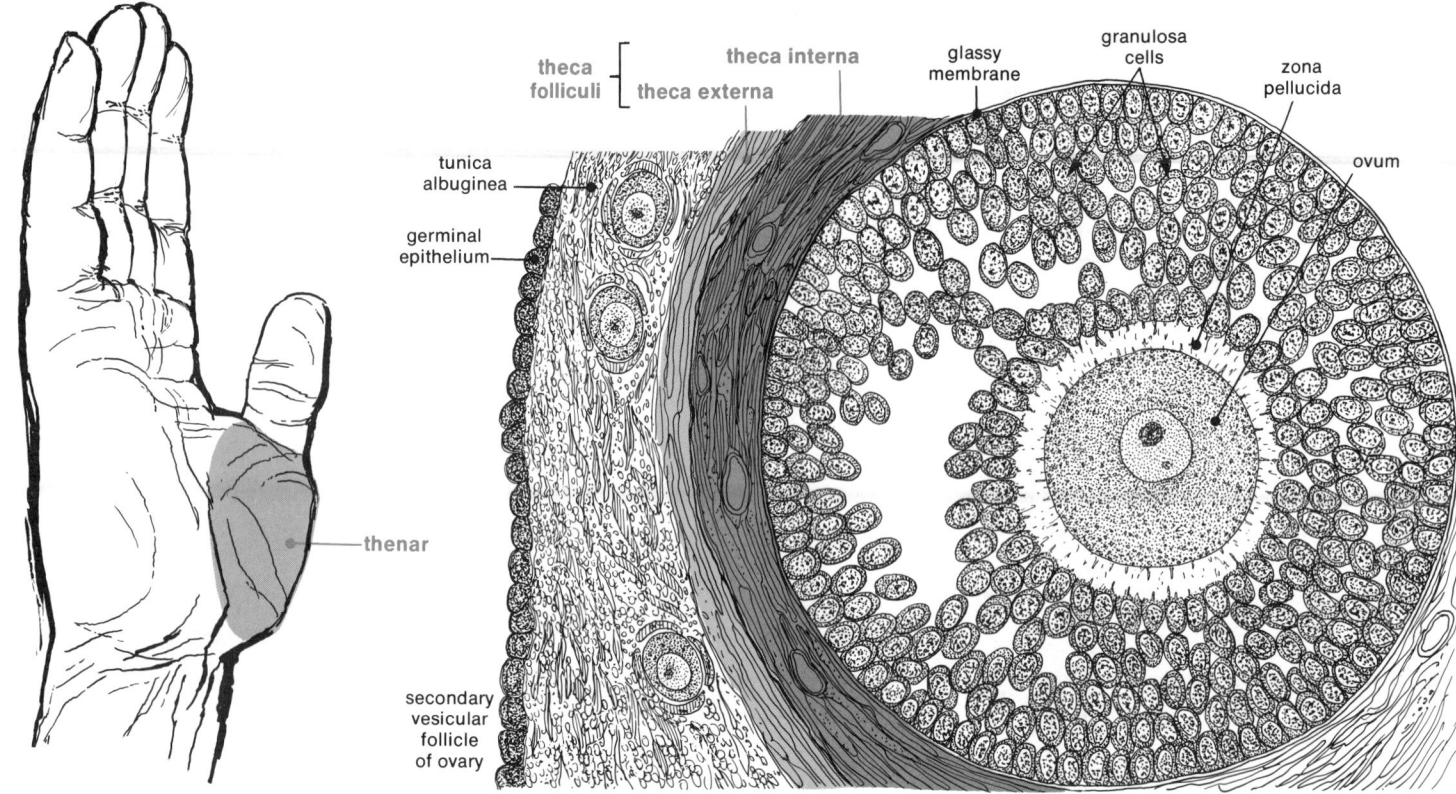

theca folliculi [theca interna / theca externa]
theca interna
glassy membrane
granulosa cells
zona pellucida
ovum
tunica albuginea
germinal epithelium
thenar
secondary vesicular follicle of ovary

$C_{13}H_{10}N_2O_4$; when taken by pregnant women, it has been associated with abnormalities of the fetus' limbs.

thallium A rare metallic element, symbol Tl, atomic number 81, atomic weight 204.37; the lightest known element with naturally radioactive isotopes; used in scintillation scanning.

thallospore An organ of reproduction derived directly from the thallus or vegetative portion of certain fungi and algae.

thallotoxicosis Poisoning resulting from the intake (accidental or purposeful) of thallium salts (widely used as pesticides); clinical features include ptosis, ataxia, tremors, paresthesias, and a toxic encephalopathy.

thallus The vegetative plant body of certain fungi and algae, which is not differentiated into root, stem, and leaf.

thanatoid 1. Resembling death. **2.** Deadly.

thanatology The study of death in all its aspects.

thanatophobia Extreme fear of death.

thanatopsia, thanatopsy Autopsy.

theca, *pl.* **thecae** A sheath, such as the one covering a tendon or a vesicular ovarian follicle.

t. **externa** The outer fibrous part of the theca folliculi; it is poorly vascularized.

t. **folliculi** An envelope of concentrically arranged hypertrophied stromal cells surrounding the vesicular ovarian follicle.

t. **interna** The inner secretory part of the theca folliculi; it is permeated by a rich capillary network.

thecitis Inflammation of a tendon sheath.

thecoma A functional ovarian neoplasm, composed of spindle-shaped cells (predominantly theca lutein cells with bands of collagen), that produces considerable quantities of feminizing endocrine substances; it generally causes irregularities in the menstrual cycle, breast enlargement, and occasionally increased libido. Also called theca lutein cell or theca cell tumor.

thelarche The beginning of breast development at puberty.

theleplasty Mammillaplasty.

thelerethism Erection of the nipple.

thelitis Inflammation of the nipple.

thelorrhagia Hemorrhage or bleeding from the nipple.

thenar The fleshy mass of the palm at the base of the thumb.

theophylline Drug used to treat bronchial asthma.

theorem A proven proposition.

theory A hypothetical concept given credibility by working experimentation but lacking absolute proof.

clonal selection t. Theory according to which certain predestined antibody-producing cells, when exposed to the host's own tissues during fetal life, were deleted or destroyed; thus there would be no "antiself" clones or colonies of cells to react against one's own tissues.

germ layer t. The concept that the embryo develops three primary germ layers (ectoderm, mesoderm, and endoderm) and that each layer gives rise to specific tissues and organs.

gestalt t. Theory claiming that mental phenomena are total configurations and cannot be analyzed into their component parts.

Lamarckian t. The theory that acquired characteristics may be transmitted.

Planck's t. See quantum theory.

quantum t. Theory that atoms emit and absorb energy discontinuously, in finite discrete amounts (quanta) in individual acts of emission and absorption, rather than in a continuous fashion. Also called Planck's theory.

reentry t. Theory that extrasystoles are caused by reentry of the sinus impulse into the ectopic focus.

van't Hoff's t. The theory that substances in dilute solutions obey the gas laws.

Young-Helmholtz t. The theory that the perception of colors depends on three sets of receptors in the retina; for red, green, and violet.

therapeutic Curative or healing.

t. **blood level** See under level.

therapeutics The aspect of medicine concerned with the treatment of disease.

therapist A specialist in the conduction of therapy, as in speech therapy, physical therapy, etc.

rehabilitation t. A member of the health-care team (i.e., physical, occupational, and recreational therapists) engaged in restoring the injured, the disabled, and the physically or mentally sick to their rightful place in society.

therapy The treatment of disease or disability.

anticoagulant t. The use of drugs that prevent or arrest formation of blood clots in the cardiovascular system.

behavior modification t. See behavior modification.

cognitive t. Psychotherapeutic treatment that aims to alter a patient's distorted thinking process; based on the belief that the way a person perceives the world determines his feelings and behavior.

electroshock t. (EST) **electroconvulsive t.** (ECT) A form of shock treatment for mental illness (especially depressive reactions) in which an electric current is used to produce unconsciousness and/or convulsions.

extracorporeal shock-wave t. See lithotripsy, extracorporeal shock-wave.

gene t. Introduction of one or more specific genes into the cells of an organism for correction of a specific defect.

gestalt t. Psychotherapeutic treatment concerned with developing the human potential through a growth process involving the whole person as he experiences and interacts with the environment.

hyperbaric oxygen t. The use of oxygen in a compression chamber at a prevailing pressure greater than one atmosphere.

inhalation t. Administration of gases, steam, or vaporized medications through inhalation.

interpersonal t. (IPT) Psychotherapeutic treatment that focuses on interpersonal behavior rather than intrapsychic phenomena, aiming to change the way the patient thinks, feels, and acts in current problematic relationships.

occupational t. (O.T.) An adjunctive method of treatment for the sick or injured through purposeful and healthy activity.

oxygen t. Treatment with oxygen inhalation.

parenteral t. Administration of medications through routes other than the alimentary canal, i.e., intramuscular or intravenous.

physical t. The use of physical agents (heat, massage, electricity, and exercise) to restore bodily functions; also called physiotherapy.

play t. A method of psychotherapy for treating emotional disorders of children in which the child's play with toys, pictures, drawings, etc. is used as a communication medium between the child and the therapist.

psychoanalytical t. See psychoanalysis.

psychodynamic t. Psychotherapeutic treatment that focuses on intrapsychic conflict, aiming to help the patient gain insight into both conscious and unconscious factors affecting thoughts, feelings and behavior.

replacement t. Administration of natural body products, or synthetic substitutes, to compensate for a deficiency.

roentgen t. Treatment with x rays.

shock t. See treatment, shock.

specific t. Administration of medication that has a selective action upon the course of a disease.

speech t. The application of special techniques to correct speech disabilities.

therm Any of the following units of quantity of heat: a small calorie; a large calorie; 1,000 large calories; 100,000 British thermal units.

thermal Relating to heat.

thermalgesia Extreme sensitivity to heat.

thermanalgesia See thermoanesthesia.

thermatology The study of heat as applied to the treatment of disease.

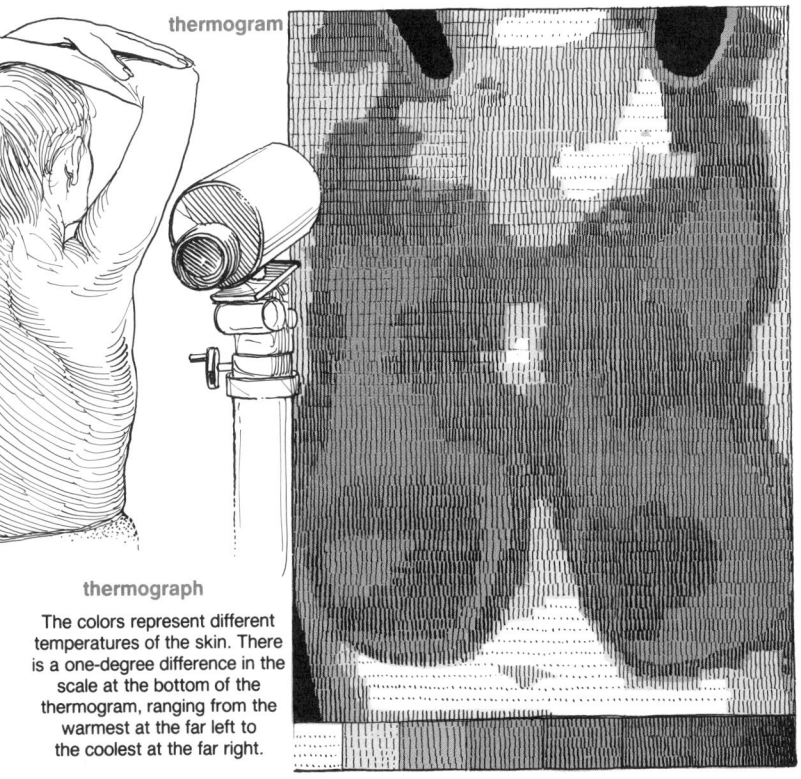

thermogram

thermograph

The colors represent different temperatures of the skin. There is a one-degree difference in the scale at the bottom of the thermogram, ranging from the warmest at the far left to the coolest at the far right.

thiamine

thiopental sodium

thiouracil

thermoreceptor

Krause's end bulb

thermelometer An electric thermometer.

thermoanesthesia Inability to distinguish between heat and cold or to feel variations in temperature. Also called ardanesthesia; thermanalgesia.

thermocautery The destruction of tissue (cauterization) by means of a heated wire. Also called thermoelectric cautery.

thermochemistry The branch of chemistry concerned with the relationship of heat and chemical reactions.

thermochrose The property of heat rays which enables them to be reflected, refracted, and absorbed.

thermocoagulation Coagulation effected by the application of heat.

thermocouple Device used to measure slight variations in temperature. Also called thermopile.

thermodiffusion Diffusion of a gas or a liquid through heat; the rise in temperature increases the molecular motion.

thermodilution Reduction in temperature of a liquid occurring when it is added to a colder liquid; the volume of the latter liquid can be calculated from the degree of rise in its temperature; the principle is employed to measure the volume or the rate of flow through a chamber; e.g., ventricular volume, cardiac output, or renal blood flow.

thermodynamics The branch of physics concerned with heat and its conversion to other forms of energy.

thermoesthesia The ability to perceive changes in temperature. Also called thermesthesia.

thermogenesis The production of heat in the body; a physiologic process.

thermogram A colored photograph displaying the surface temperatures of the body; produced by infrared sensing devices.

thermograph A thermometer that records variations in temperature.

thermography A process for measuring temperature by photographically recording infrared radiations emanating from the body's surface; it can aid in diagnosing underlying pathology by indicating thermal variations.

thermohyperesthesia Extreme sensitivity to variations in temperature.

thermohypesthesia Diminished sensitivity to temperature fluctuations. Also called thermohypoesthesia.

thermoinhibitory Preventing or arresting the production of heat.

thermolabile Susceptible to alteration or destruction by heat.

thermolysis 1. The loss of body heat. 2. The chemical decomposition of compounds by heat.

thermomassage The use of heat and massage in physical therapy.

thermometer A device for measuring temperature, usually consisting of a graduated, sealed, glass vacuum tube with a bulb at its lower extremity and containing a liquid, generally mercury (sometimes alcohol), that rises in the tube when expanded by increase in temperature.

  digital t. An electronic thermometer that reads and/or numerically prints out the temperature.

  electronic t. Thermometer that measures and/or electronically records temperature.

thermometry Measurement of temperature by direct contact.

thermophile, thermophil An organism which grows best at warm temperatures, usually from 40° to 70°C.

thermophore An appliance for (a) applying heat to a bodily part; (b) maintaining the temperature of the mask during ether inhalation.

thermoplacentography Determination of the placental location by recording the increased temperature (due to large amounts of blood) with the thermograph.

thermoplastic A type of material which can be made soft by heating and which rehardens upon cooling (without chemical change).

thermoplegia Heat stroke; see under stroke.

thermoreceptor A special nerve-ending (receptor) that is sensitive to change in temperature.

thermoregulation The regulation of heat. Also called temperature control.

thermoset A material which becomes rigid or hardened by a chemical reaction involving heat.

thermostable, thermostabile Not changed or destroyed by moderate heat.

thermotaxis 1. Movement of an organism toward (positive thermotaxis) or away from (negative thermotaxis) a heat source. 2. The adjustment of the body to temperature changes.

thermotherapy The use of heat as an aid in the treatment of disease.

thesaurosis, thesaurismosis Abnormal or excessive storage in the body, or in particular organs, of phosphatides, fats, heavy metals, or other material.

thesis An essay containing results of original research written by a candidate for an academic degree.

thiaminase A thiamine-splitting enzyme.

thiamine, thiamin A vitamin of the B-complex, present in yeast, meat, and the bran coat of grains; essential in carbohydrate metabolism; lack of thiamine causes beriberi. Also called vitamin B_1.

  t. pyrophosphate The diphosphoric ester of thia-

mine; a coenzyme which is a cofactor in decarboxylation. Also called cocarboxylase.

thiazides A shortened term for the class of diuretics called benzothiadiazides; widely used in treating both edema and hypertension.

thigh The portion of the upper leg between the knee and the hip.

  driver's t. Inflammation of the sciatic nerve due to prolonged pressure on the nerve, as from the continued use of the accelerator pedal in long distance driving of an automobile.

thighbone The femur; see table of bones.

thigmesthesia Sensitiveness to touch. Also called tactile sensibility.

thigmotaxis The response of animal or plant protoplasm to contact with a solid body.

thioguanine An antineoplastic agent used in the treatment of some types of leukemia.

thiol 1. The univalent radical —SH. 2. Any substance containing the radical —SH bound to carbon. Also called mercaptan.

thionine A greenish-black powder giving a violet color in solution; often used to stain the Nissl substance of nerve cells. Also called Lauth's violet.

thiopental sodium A rapid-acting, potent barbiturate capable of inducing anesthesia within 30 to 60 seconds after being administered intravenously or rectally. Also called sodium pentothal; Pentothal Sodium®.

thiosemicarbazone One of several compounds containing the radical –N–NH–C(S)–NH₂, having an inhibitory effect on tuberculous infections.

thiosulfate A salt of thiosulfuric acid.

thiosulfuric acid A highly unstable acid, $H_2S_2O_3$, which decomposes readily to sulfur and sulfurous acid.

thiotepa A white crystalline compound $C_6H_{12}N_3PS$; an alkylating agent used as a palliative medication in malignant diseases.

thiouracil A compound that inhibits the formation of thyroid hormones. Also called 2-mercapto-4-hydroxypyrimidine.

thiourea An antithyroid substance of the thiocarbamide group.

thirst A desire to drink, often associated with an uncomfortable sensation of dryness in the mouth and pharynx.

  excessive t. Polydipsia.

Thoma's counting chamber Thoma-Zeiss hemocytometer; see under hemocytometer.

thoracectomy Resection of part of a rib.

thoracentesis The removal of fluid from the chest cavity by puncture. Also called thoracocentesis.

thoracic Relating to the thorax or chest.

thromboangiitis obliterans

- partially occluded lumen
- organizing thrombus
- microabscess (inflammatory process in the thrombus)

artery of medium size

sphenoid sinus

nasal cavity

nasopharynx

uvula

throat

tongue

epiglottis

esophagus

trachea

CHO glyceraldehyde
HCOH
CH₂OH

CHO
HCOH
HCOH
CH₂OH
erythrose

CHO
HOCH
HCOH
CH₂OH
threose

thrombocytes

COOH
H₂N—C—H
H—C—OH
CH₃
threonine

---

thoracicoabdominal, thoracoabdominal Relating to the thorax and the abdomen.

thoracicoacromial See acromiothoracic.

thoracic outlet syndrome Abnormal sensations of fingers (numbness, burning, etc.) attributed to compression of the brachial plexus; similar symptoms also may be caused by cervical disk or carpal tunnel syndromes.

thoracoabdominal See thoracicoabdominal.

thoracocentesis See thoracentesis.

thoracolumbar Relating to the thoracic and lumbar regions of the spine.

thoracomyodynia Pain in the muscles of the chest.

thoracopathy Any disease of the chest.

thoracoplasty Plastic surgery or repair of defects of the chest.

thoracopneumoplasty Reparative surgery of the lung and chest.

thoracoscopy Visual examination of the pleural cavity by means of an endoscope.

thoracostomy The surgical creation of an opening into the chest wall.

thoracotomy Surgical incision on the chest wall.

thorax The upper part of the body between the neck and the diaphragm; it contains the chief organs of the circulatory and respiratory systems. Also called chest.

thorium A radioactive metallic element; symbol Th, atomic number 90, atomic weight 232.038.

threadworm See pinworm.

threonine (Thr) An amino acid present in most proteins; essential to the diet of man and other mammals.

threose A monosaccharide containing four carbon atoms; C₄H₈O₄; one of the two aldoses, the other being erythrose.

threshold The point where a stimulus just begins to produce a sensation; the intensity below which a mental or physical stimulus cannot be perceived.

absolute t. The stimulus of least strength which will cause a response. Also called stimulus test.

auditory t. The intensity of the lowest perceptible sound.

galvanic t. Rheobase.

radiologic t. The level of radiation dose below which there may not be permanent injury to the body.

renal t. The level at which the kidney can no longer reabsorb all of a substance (sugar, ketones, etc.) presented, and some of it appears in the urine.

stimulus t. See absolute threshold.

t. of consciousness The lowest gradient of sensation that can be perceived.

thrill A tremor or vibration associated with a vascular or cardiac murmur and discerned by palpation.

throat 1. The back part of the mouth extending to the beginning of the esophagus; generally the area from the nasopharynx to the larynx. 2. The front of the neck.

sore t. A throat condition characterized by discomfort, especially when swallowing, due to inflammation of the fauces, pharynx, tonsils, or larynx.

strep t. Streptococcal pharyngitis; see under pharyngitis.

throb 1. To pulsate. 2. A pulsation.

throe A severe pang or seizure of pain, as experienced during childbirth.

thrombasthenia Abnormality of the blood platelets in which they lack factors that are effective in blood coagulation. Also called Glanzmann's disease.

thrombectomy Surgical removal of a thrombus (blood clot).

thrombelastograph Device for recording elastic variations of a thrombus during the process of coagulation.

thrombi Plural of thrombus.

thrombin An enzyme in the blood derived from factor II (prothrombin) that converts fibrinogen into fibrin, thus producing a blood clot.

thrombinogen Factor II (prothrombin).

thromboangiitis Inflammation of the wall of a blood vessel with clot formation.

t. obliterans Disorder of the medium-sized arteries and veins, especially of the lower extremities; marked by inflammation of the wall of the vessel and surrounding connective tissue, resulting in tissue ischemia and gangrene. Also called Buerger's disease.

thromboblast The giant cell precursor of the blood platelet (thrombocyte). More commonly called megakaryocyte.

thrombocytasthenia A disorder of platelet function characterized by abnormal adhesion and/or aggregation; congenital varieties are known, and acquired forms are seen, especially in uremia.

thrombocyte A blood platelet.

thrombocythemia A rare disorder of middle adult life, marked by abnormal proliferation of megakaryocytes with increase in circulating platelets; bleeding, thromboembolic diathesis, splenomegaly, and leukocytosis are frequently present.

thrombocytopathy General term denoting any disorder involving faulty function of blood platelets. Also called thrombopathia.

thrombocytopenia Abnormally small number of platelets in the blood. Also called thrombopenia.

thrombocytosis Increase in the number of platelets in the blood.

thromboembolectomy The removal of an embolism which obstructs the flow of blood through a vessel.

thromboembolism Embolism (obstruction) in a blood vessel caused by a dislodged thrombus (clot).

thromboendarterectomy The surgical removal of an obstructing blood clot together with the inner lining of the obstructed artery.

thrombogenic 1. Producing thrombosis or coagulation of the blood. 2. Relating to factor II (prothrombin).

thrombolysis The dissolving of a clot. Also called thromboclasis.

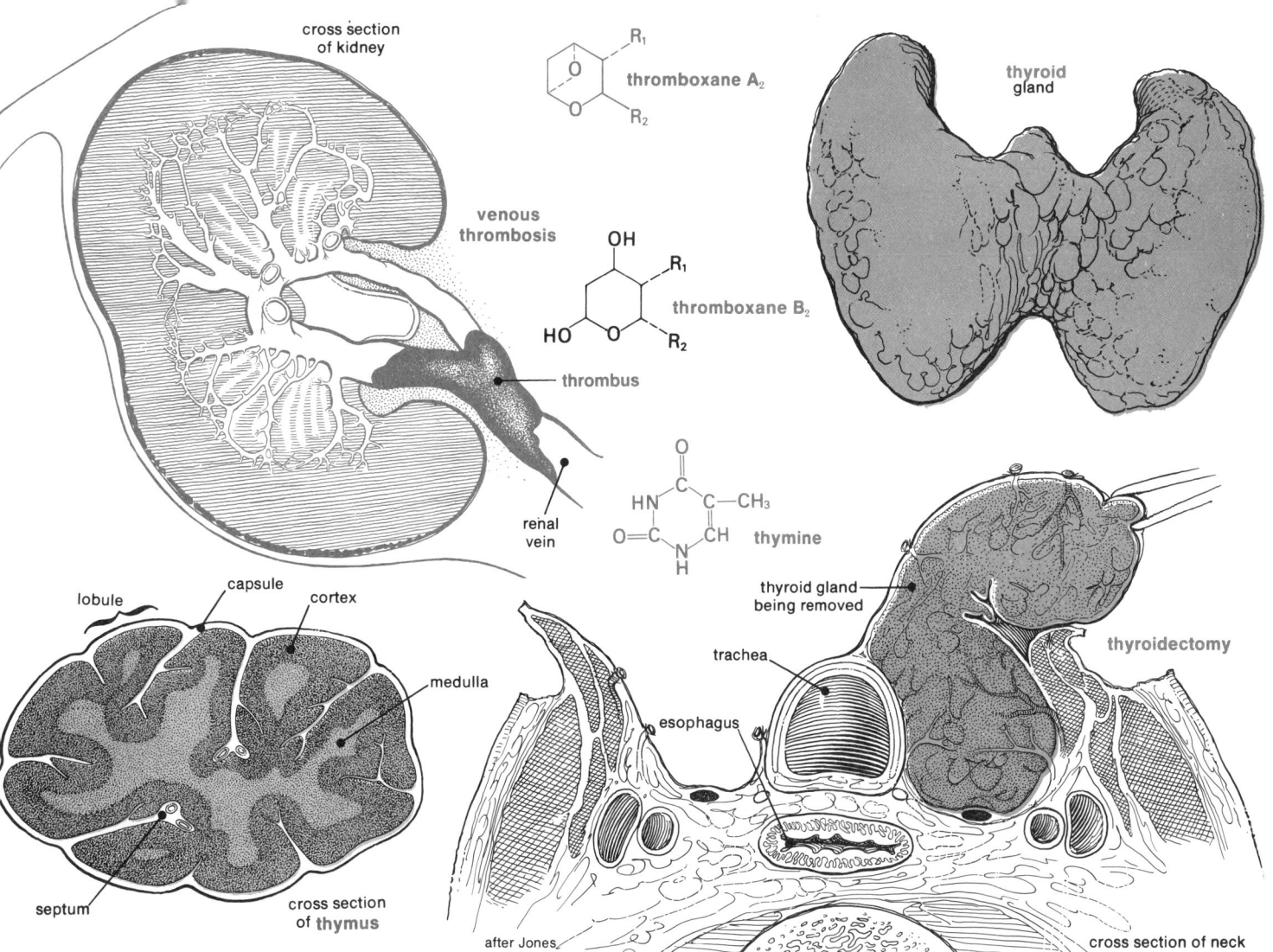

cross section of kidney

thromboxane A₂

venous thrombosis

thromboxane B₂

thrombus

renal vein

thymine

thyroid gland

thyroid gland being removed

thyroidectomy

trachea

esophagus

lobule capsule cortex

medulla

septum

cross section of thymus

after Jones

cross section of neck

thrombopathia See thrombocytopathy.
thrombopenia See thrombocytopenia.
thrombophlebitis Inflammation of the walls of a vein associated with formation of a thrombus (blood clot).
  puerperal t. Thrombophlebitis of the great saphenous or femoral veins, causing a sudden painful swelling of the leg; it usually occurs in women with a low-grade infection of the birth canal after delivery; also called phlegmasia alba dolens and milk leg.
thromboplastin A protein complex that initiates the clotting of blood. Also called factor III.
  plasma t. A complete thromboplastin capable of converting factor II (prothrombin) to thrombin directly.
  tissue t. An incomplete thromboplastin requiring the presence of factor V, factor VII, and factor X in order to convert prothrombin to thrombin.
thrombopoiesis 1. The formation of a blood clot. 2. The formation of blood platelets.
thrombosis The formation or presence of a blood clot.
  cerebral t. Obstruction of a blood vessel of the brain by a thrombus; one of the causes of stroke.
  coronary t. The presence of a blood clot in an artery that supplies the heart muscle; a cause of heart attack.
  venous t. Arrest of circulation in a vein by a blood clot. Also called phlebemphraxis.
thromboxane A compound isolated from blood platelets (thrombocytes); it contains an oxane ring and is related to the prostaglandins; thromboxane exists in two forms; A₂ and B₂; the A₂ form appears to be much more potent than prostaglandin in some important biologic activities, such as smooth muscle contraction and platelet aggregation.
thrombus A blood clot, usually one located at the point of its formation, in a blood vessel or a chamber of the heart.
thrush Infection of the mouth with *Candida albicans;* marked by the appearance of white patches in the oral mucosa, which later become shallow ulcers; seen most commonly in infants or in patients receiving antibiotics or immunosuppressive drugs.
thulium A metallic element of the lanthanide series, symbol Tm, atomic number 69, atomic weight 168.94.
thumb The first digit on the radial side of the hand, apposable to each of the other four digits.
  gamekeeper's t. A subluxation of the metacarpophalangeal joint of the thumb.
  tennis t. Tendonitis accompanied by calcification in the tendon of the long flexor muscle of the thumb due to activities in which the thumb is subject to great pressure and strain, as in tennis playing.
thumbprinting A sign of submucosal edema of the bowel wall; the colon appears in the x-ray image as having a series of smooth depressions; seen in such disorders as Crohn's disease and ischemia.
thumb sign When making a fist over the thumb, the thumb extends clearly beyond the ulnar margin of the hand, as seen in individuals with the Marfan syndrome.
thymectomy Surgical removal of the thymus.
thymic Relating to the thymus.
thymidine A condensation product of thymine with deoxyribose; a nucleoside in DNA.
thymidylic acid A constituent of DNA.
thymine One of the pyrimidine bases which is commonly found in deoxyribonucleic acid (DNA).
thymitis Inflammation of the thymus.
thymocyte A lymphocyte that originates in the thymus.
thymogenic 1. Originating in the thymus. 2. Of hysterical origin.
thymokinetic Stimulating the thymus.
thymoma A tumor of the anterior mediastinum arising from the thymus; associated with a variety of diseases, including myasthenia gravis, agammaglobulinemia, and hematologic abnormalities; it may undergo malignant change.
thymopathy 1. Any disease of the thymus. 2. Any mental disorder.
thymosin An immunologically active thymic fraction of low molecular weight; believed to develop immunologic competency in T lymphocytes (thymus-dependent lymphocytes).
thymus 1. A ductless glandlike lymphoid structure located just behind the top of the sternum; it appears to be the master organ in immunogenesis in the young and is believed by some to monitor the total lymphoid system throughout life; it consists of two lobes surrounded by a thin capsule of connective tissue; it grows quickly until the age of 3 years, after which it grows very slowly until the age of about 13, at which time it begins to decrease in size; in old age, very little thymic tissue remains, having been replaced by fat and connective tissue. 2. One of the organs of cattle called sweetbread.
thyroaplasia Congenital defects associated with faulty thyroid functioning.
thyroarytenoid Relating to both the thyroid and arytenoid cartilages.
thyrocalcitonin See calcitonin.
thyrocricotomy Tracheostomy performed in extreme emergency conditions whereby the neck opening is made through the most superficial portion of the respiratory tract, the cricothyroid membrane. See also tracheostomy.
thyroglobulin A protein produced and stored in the thyroid gland; a prohormone (precursor of hormone), which on hydrolysis yields iodinated tyrosines and thyroxin.
thyroglossal Relating to the thyroid cartilage and the tongue.
thyrohyoid Relating to the thyroid cartilage and the hyoid bone.
thyroid 1. Pertaining to the thyroid gland; see under gland. 2. Resembling a shield. 3. A pharmaceutical preparation derived from the thyroid gland of certain domestic animals; used in the treatment of hypothyroid states.
thyroidectomy Removal of the thyroid gland.

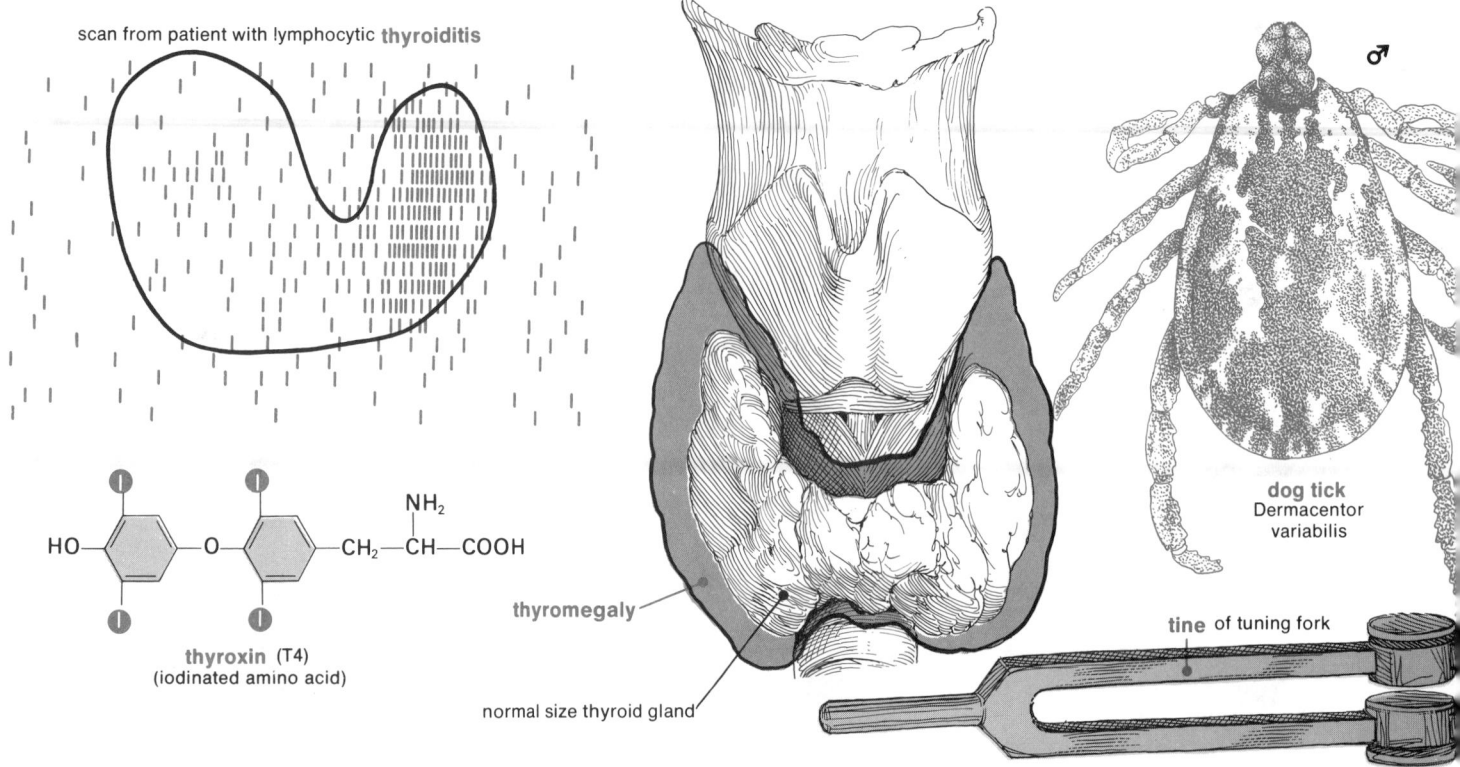

scan from patient with lymphocytic **thyroiditis**

thyroxin (T4)
(iodinated amino acid)

thyromegaly

normal size thyroid gland

dog tick
Dermacentor
variabilis

tine of tuning fork

♂

thyroiditis Inflammation of the thyroid gland.
  de Quervain's t. See subacute thyroiditis.
  granulomatous t. See subacute thyroiditis.
  Hashimoto's t. See lymphocytic thyroiditis.
  lymphocytic t. A form of chronic thyroiditis in which the thyroid gland is massively infiltrated with lymphoid and fibrous tissues causing destruction of the gland substance, goiter formation, and thyroid hormone insufficiency; thought to be an autoimmune disease; it occurs 20 times more frequently in women than in men, usually between the ages of 30 to 50. Also called Hashimoto's thyroiditis; Hashimoto's struma.
  Riedel's t. A rare chronic condition in which the thyroid gland and adjacent structures are replaced by dense fibrotic tissue.
  subacute t. Inflammation of the thyroid gland following viral infection, usually of the upper respiratory tract. Also called de Quervain's or granulomatous thyroiditis.
thyromegaly Abnormal enlargement of the thyroid gland.
thyronine An amino acid present in proteins only as iodinated derivatives (iodothyronines).
thyroparathyroidectomy Surgical removal of the thyroid and parathyroid glands.
thyropathy Disease of the thyroid gland.
thyroprival Caused by removal of the thyroid gland or the arrest of its function.
thyroprotein 1. Thyroglobulin. 2. Preparation made by iodinating protein (such as casein), having a physiologic action similar to that of thyroxin.
thyrotomy 1. Surgical division or cutting of the thyroid cartilage. 2. Operative cutting of the thyroid gland.
thyrotoxicosis Toxic condition caused by an excess of thyroid hormone.
thyrotropic, thyrotrophic Stimulating the thyroid gland.
thyrotropin Hormone of the anterior hypophysis (pituitary) that stimulates the growth and function of the thyroid gland. Also called thyrotropic or thyroid-stimulating hormone.
thyroxin, thyroxine (T₄) An active iodine-containing hormone, produced normally in the thyroid gland, that aids in regulating metabolism; produced synthetically or extracted from the thyroid gland in crystalline form for treatment of thyroid disorders such as hypothyroidism, cretinism, and myxedema. Also called tetraiodothyronine.
tibia The larger and medial of the two bones of the leg between the knee and the ankle. Commonly called shinbone.
tibiofibular Relating to both the tibia and fibula.

tic An involuntary, brief, and recurrent twitching of a group of muscles, most commonly involving the face, neck, and shoulders.
  t. douloureux Spasmodic facial neuralgia, marked by piercing pain of short duration along the trigeminal nerve. Also called trigeminal neuralgia.
tick A mite of the families Ixodidae (hard shell ticks) and Argasidae (soft shell ticks), some of which are parasitic and the carriers of disease-causing microorganisms.
  dog t. *Dermacentor variabilis*, a hard shell tick that can transmit Rocky Mountain spotted fever; found on the East Coast of the United States; usually in mountainous, heavily wooded, or sagebrush areas. Also called the American dog tick.
  Rocky Mountain wood t. *Dermacentor andersoni*, a hard shell, reddish-brown tick of the Western United States; most important vector of Rocky Mountain spotted fever; also conveys tularemia, Colorado tick fever, and Q fever, and is a cause of tick paralysis.
tickle 1. To feel a tingling or restless sensation. 2. To excite the surface nerves by repeated light stimulation of the skin. Also called titillate.
tide An alternate rise and fall; a lapse of time.
  alkaline t. Alkalinity of the urine following ingestion of food; a consequence of secretion of gastric juice. Also called alkaline wave.
Tietze's syndrome Pain and tenderness of the chest at the junction of ribs with cartilage; the pain may mimic that of coronary artery disease. Also called costochondral junction syndrome; costal chondritis.
timbre The characteristic quality of a sound whereby one may distinguish between two sounds of equal pitch and loudness.
time A degree or measure of duration.
  bleeding t. The duration of bleeding (normally from 1 to 3 minutes) from a small puncture made on the skin.
  circulation t. Time required for blood to flow once through a given circuit of the circulatory system.
  clot retraction t. Time required for a blood clot to become firm and separated from the sides of the tube containing it; about 50 percent retraction is considered normal.
  clotting t. Coagulation time.
  coagulation t. Time required for blood to clot in a test tube.
  doubling t. In microbiology, the time needed for a population of cells to double in number. Also called division or generation time.
  partial thromboplastin t. See test, partial thromboplastin.

  prothrombin t. Time required for a clot to form when calcium and a preparation of thromboplastin (e.g., brain tissue) are added to plasma.
  reaction t. Time elapsed between application of a stimulus and an observable response.
  recognition t. Time elapsed between the application of a stimulus and the recognition of its nature.
  survival t. 1. Interval between the completion or institution of a procedure and death. 2. The life span of cells.
tin A malleable, silvery metallic element; symbol Sn (stannum), atomic number 50, atomic weight 118.69; a member of the subgroup containing carbon, silicon, germanium, and lead.
tinctorial Relating to staining.
tinctura (tinct, tr) Latin for tincture; used in prescription writing.
tincture An alcohol or hydroalcohol solution of nonvolatile animal or vegetable drugs or chemical substances, prepared usually by a percolation or maceration process; the strength is usually 1 to 2 parts by weight of the dry drug to 10 parts by volume of the tincture, i.e., 1 to 2 g per 10 ml.
  alcoholic t. One made with undiluted alcohol.
  belladonna t. An anticholinergic, antispasmodic, alcoholic preparation containing between 27 and 33 mg of alkaloids of belladonna leaf to 100 ml of tincture.
  iodine t. A simple 2% solution of iodine with 2.5% sodium iodide in water and 44 to 50% alcohol; used as an antinfective on the skin (iodine solution is generally preferred to the tincture as an antiseptic).
  opium t. A tincture containing 10 mg of morphine per ml; used for the symptomatic treatment of diarrhea.
  opium t, camphorated See paregoric.
tine, *pl.* **tines** 1. One of a set of slender prongs on a tuning fork. 2. An instrument used for introducing an antigen, such as tuberculin, into the skin.
tinea A superficial infectious condition of the skin caused by fungi belonging chiefly to the genera *Trichophyton*, *Microsporum*, and *Epidermophyton*; the fungi live on the dead horny layer of the skin and produce an enzyme that enables them to digest keratin, thus disintegrating hair, nails, and the kertanized cells of the skin. Also called ringworm.
  t. barbae Tinea of the beard area; the lesions are dark red and dotted with perifollicular abscesses; it is prevalent in the United States, particularly in cattle-raising regions, where the usual causative organisms are *Trichophyton mentagrophytes* and *Trichophyton verrucosum*. Also called barber's itch; tinea of the beard.
  t. capitis Infection of the scalp and hair caused

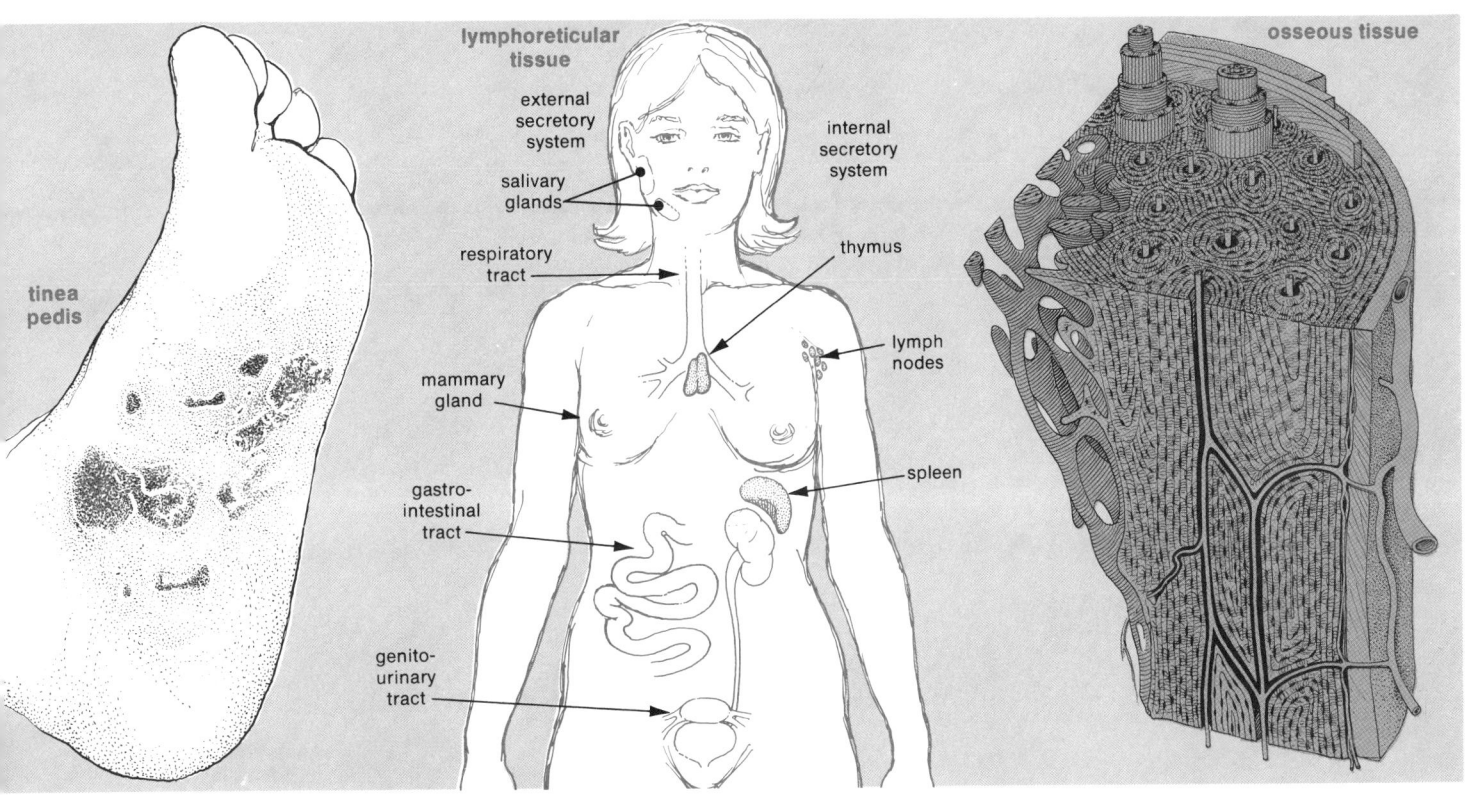

tinea pedis

lymphoreticular tissue

external secretory system

salivary glands

respiratory tract

mammary gland

gastro-intestinal tract

genito-urinary tract

internal secretory system

thymus

lymph nodes

spleen

osseous tissue

by species of *Microsporum* and *Trichophyton,* producing patches of round balding areas; likely sources of infection are hair clippers, theater seats, and domestic animals. Also called tinea of the scalp; scalp ringworm.

t. corporis A highly contagious form most commonly seen in children; caused by many species of *Microsporum* and *Trichophyton* and transmitted through contact with kittens, puppies, and other children; the typical lesion is round or oval, with a scaly center that usually tends to heal; the periphery of the lesion is an advancing circle of vesicles and papules. Also called tinea of the smooth skin; ringworm of the smooth skin; tinea circinata.

t. cruris Tinea involving the groin, perineum, and perianal region; most frequently caused by *Epidermophyton floccosum.* Also called tinea of the groin; eczema marginatum; epidermophytosis cruris.

t. pedis A common infection of the feet; the acute form, caused by *Trichophyton mentagrophytes,* is characterized by blisters on the soles and sides of the foot and/or between the toes; the chronic form is caused by *Trichophyton rubrum* and the lesions are dry and scaly. Also called athlete's foot; tinea of the feet; ringworm of the feet.

t. sycosis Tinea barbae.

t. unguium Infection of the nails, especially the toenails, usually caused by *Trichophyton mentagrophytes, Trichophyton rubrum,* and *Epidermophyton floccosum.* Also called tinea of the nails; onychomycosis trichophytina.

t. versicolor A mild, superficial infection of the skin, usually of the trunk, appearing as tan, irregularly shaped, scaly patches; caused by *Malassezia furfur.*

tinfoil An extremely thin, pliable sheet of tin; a base metal foil used in dentistry as a separating material, as between a cast and denture-base material during flasking and curing procedures.

t. substitute An alginate solution that serves as a separating medium.

tingle To have a peculiar pricking or stinging sensation, as from an emotional shock or striking a nerve, such as the "funny bone" sensation.

tinkle A metallic sound sometimes heard on auscultation over large pulmonary cavities, e.g., pneumothorax, or over a distended loop of bowel as in an ileus.

tinnitus Noises in the ear, such as ringing, buzzing, roaring, etc.

tintometer An apparatus containing a standard color scale for determining by comparison the relative proportion of coloring matter in a fluid, such as blood.

tissue A mass of similar cells and the substances that surround them.

adipose t. Connective tissue composed of fat cells clumped together and surrounded by reticular fibers.

areolar t. A type of connective tissue composed of loosely woven collagenous bundles and elastic fibers with comparatively wide interspaces that are filled with a mucopolysaccharide ground substance.

bone t. See osseous tissue.

cancellous t. A honeycomb arrangement of bone cells as seen in the center of some bones such as the clavicle, vertebrae, the end of long bones, etc.

cartilaginous t. Connective tissue with a solid, elastic matrix which may or may not have fibers embedded in it.

chondrogenic t. A connective tissue forming the inner layer of perichondrium, concerned with the formation of cartilagenous tissue.

chromaffin t. One composed mainly of chromaffin cells and a large supply of blood vessels and nerves; found in the adrenal medulla and the paraganglia.

connective t. (CT) A general term denoting any of the tissues that support and connect the various parts of the body except the nervous system. Also called interstitial tissue.

elastic t. Connective tissue composed chiefly of yellow elastic fibers; found in some ligaments and the walls of arteries and air passages.

epithelial t. See epithelium.

erectile t. Tissue containing an abundance of vascular spaces which, when distended with blood, render the part firm.

fibrous t. Connective tissue containing bundles of white fibers and a fluid ground substance; found in tendons, ligaments, aponeuroses, and such membranes as the dura mater.

granulation t. Tissue that appears in the early stages of wound healing; composed of different cell types and young blood vessels.

hemopoietic t. Tissue that is actively involved with the development of formed elements of the blood, as in the medulla of long bones.

interstitial t. See connective tissue.

lymphatic t. A network of fibers enclosing masses of lymphocytes.

lymphoreticular t. Tissue that carries out the functions of immunity through a variety of cell types, each performing a specific function, either by direct cell action or through the elaboration of antibody.

mesenchymal t. See mesenchyme.

metanephrogenic t. Portion of the intermediate mesoderm that eventually forms the excretory tu-

bules of the kidney.

muscular t. Tissue composed of threadlike fibers, either striated (skeletal) or nonstriated (smooth), which contract upon stimulation.

myeloid t. The red bone marrow that forms both red and white blood cells, consisting of the developmental and adult stages of erythrocytes, granulocytes, and megakaryocytes in a stroma of reticular cells and fibers.

nervous t. Tissue composed basically of nerve cells (neurons) supported by connective tissue (neuroglia).

osseous t. Connective tissue with a tough, rigid, fibrous matrix containing deposits of mineral salts. Also called bone tissue.

osteogenic t. A connective tissue forming the inner layer of periosteum, concerned with the formation of osseous tissue.

osteoid t. Bone matrix prior to calcification; uncalcified osseous tissue.

reticular t. The most delicate type of connective tissue, composed of a network of fine fibrils; it surrounds individual cells, the acini of glands, and muscle fibers.

subcutaneous t. The loose, generally fatty tissue immediately beneath the skin, attached to the dermis by coarse fibers (retinacula cutis).

target t. In immunology, the tissue against which antibodies are formed.

titanium A low-density, amorphous metallic element of the carbon group, symbol Ti, atomic number 22, atomic weight 47.90.

t. dioxide An exceptionally opaque white powder, TiO_2, used in creams and powders as a protectant against external irritations and solar rays. Also called titanic acid.

titer 1. In chemistry, the standard strength of a volumetric test solution determined by titration; assay value of an unknown measure by volumetric means. 2. The highest dilution of a material (serum or other body fluids) that produces a reaction in an immunologic test system.

titrate To analyze the concentration of a solution by titration.

titration The process of estimating the quantity of a substance in solution by adding to it a measured amount of standard test solution until a reaction of known proportion is reached (shown by a color change in a suitable indicator, the development of turbidity, or the change in electrical state); from this the unknown concentration of the substance is calculated. Also called titrimetry.

colorimetric t. Titration in which the end point is indicated by sudden change in color.

formol t. A process of titrating the amino group

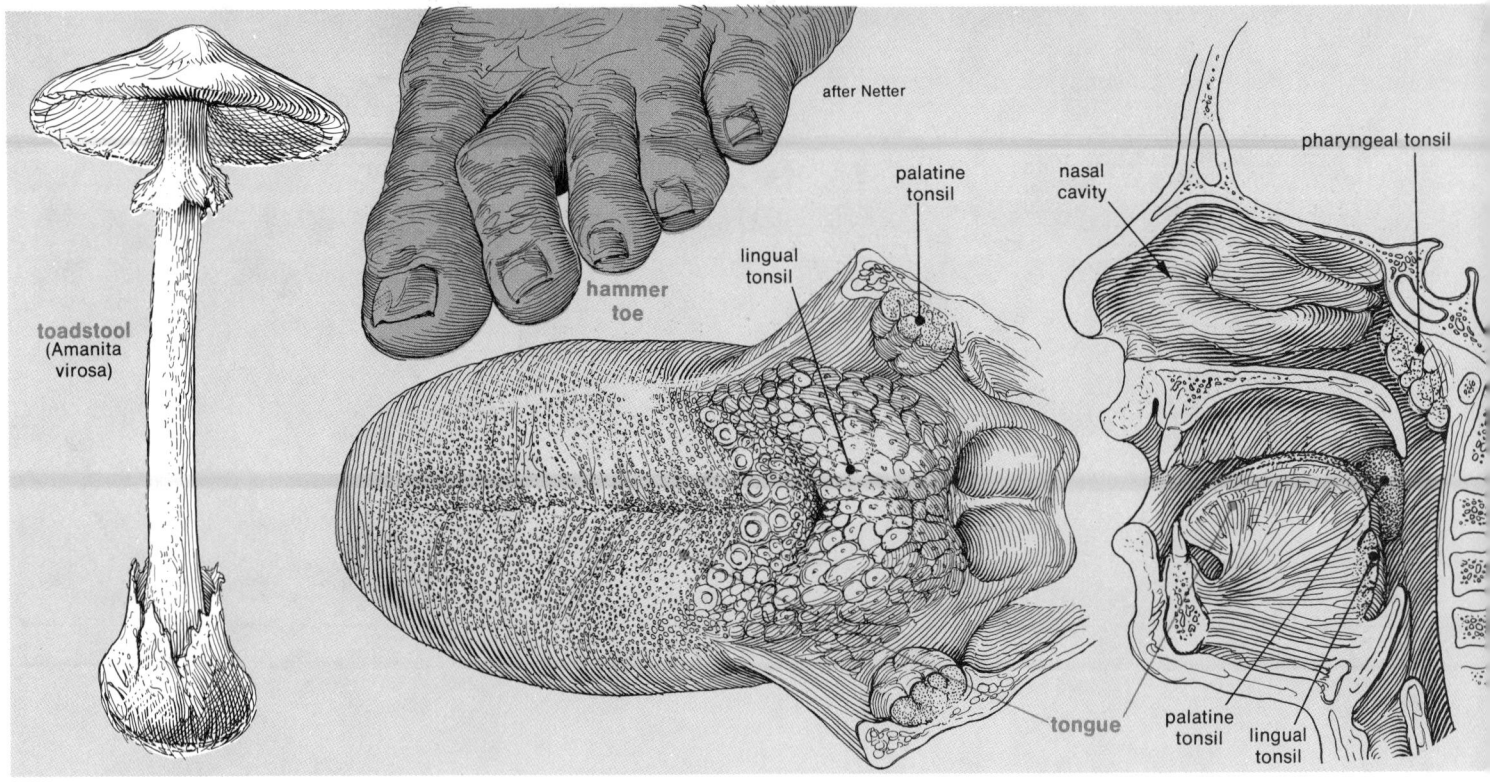

toadstool (Amanita virosa)

hammer toe

after Netter

lingual tonsil

palatine tonsil

nasal cavity

pharyngeal tonsil

tongue

palatine tonsil

lingual tonsil

of amino acids by adding formaldehyde to the standard test solution (reagent).

potentiometer t. Titration in which the pH is constantly monitored, with a specific pH value serving as end point.

TM-mode See M-mode.

toadstool Popular name for an inedible, umbrella-shaped mushroom; a poisonous mushroom.

tobramycin Antibiotic substance produced by *Streptomyces tenebrarius;* active against several types of bacteria, especially *Pseudomonas aeruginosa.*

tocodynamometer An instrument for measuring the force of uterine contractions. Also called tocometer; tokodynamometer.

tocopherol See vitamin E.

α-tocopherol (α-T) A derivative of vitamin E; a light yellow, completely fat-soluble substance that occurs in the fatty portions of food; it is stored in the adipose tissue of humans and functions in all tissues in the stabilization of the lipids of the cell's membranes; believed to play an important role in cellular metabolism.

toe One of the digits of the feet.

clawing t.'s An exaggerated dorsal contraction of the toes resulting from imbalance of the short intrinsic musculature and causing the toes to appear clawlike.

great t. Hallux.

hammer t. Deformity of a toe marked by dorsiflexion of the proximal phalanx with plantar flexion of the second phalanx; the second toe is most often affected.

mallet t. Deformity of a toe marked by plantar flexion of the distal phalanx.

pigeon t. See pigeon-toe.

webbed t.'s Adjacent toes abnormally connected by a fold of tissue at their base; a form of syndactyly.

toenail A horny plate on the dorsal surface of the tip of each toe. See also nail.

ingrown t., ingrowing t. A toenail, one edge of which is overgrown by the nail fold, producing a pyogenic granuloma; tight shoes, shrunken socks, and improper paring of the nail corners are common etiologic factors; trauma may also be a predisposing cause.

Togaviridae A large family of viruses (40 to 70 nm in diameter) that contain single-stranded RNA and replicate in cytoplasm; include viruses causing yellow fever, encephalitis and German measles.

toilet Local care and cleansing e.g., cleansing of a tracheostomy tube, of a wound and surrounding skin, of a patient after childbirth.

tolbutamide An oral hypoglycemic drug (sulfon-

amide derivative), used in the management of certain cases of diabetes; it stimulates the release of endogenous insulin; Orinase®.

tolerance, toleration The capacity to assimilate a drug continuously or in large doses, or to withstand increased physiologic activities without experiencing unfavorable effects.

acoustic t. The maximum sound pressure level (SPL) that can be endured without harmful effects.

cross t. Resistance to the effects of one drug resulting from an acquired tolerance to another, related drug.

g-t. Tolerance to certain forces resulting from either acceleration or deceleration.

glucose t. See test, glucose tolerance.

immunologic t. Inability to react to the stimulation of a specific antigen.

individual t. Unresponsiveness to a drug that the person has not received before.

species t. Unresponsiveness to a drug existing as a characteristic of a particular species.

vibration t. The maximum vibratory movements that a person can endure without pain.

tolerogen An antigen that causes the immune mechanisms of an organism to be unresponsive to itself, resulting in a state known as tolerance; the opposite of immunogen.

tolnaftate A topical antifungal agent effective against those species of *Epidermophyton, Microsporum,* and *Trichophyton* that cause dermatophytic infections (ringworms) in man; Tinactin®.

toluene A colorless volatile liquid, $C_6H_5 \cdot CH_3$, used in organic synthesis and the manufacture of explosives and dyes. Also called toluol; methyl benzene.

toluidine A derivative of toluene.

toluidine blue Methylene blue.

toluol See toluene.

tomogram A roentgenogram made by tomography.

tomograph An x-ray machine designed to take sectional roentgenograms (tomograms) of the body.

computed t. A tomograph that utilizes a computer to reconstruct a section of the patient's body from scanned x-ray profiles. Also called computerized axial tomograph.

tomography The radiographing of a selected level of the body while blurring structures in front of and behind this level; the x-ray tube and film move in opposite directions during exposure so that the roentgenographic shadow of a selected bodily plane remains stationary while the shadows of all other planes are in motion during exposure and therefore blurred. Also called body section roentgenography.

computed t. (CT) Tomography utilizing a computer-assisted tomograph. Also called computerized tomography; computerized axial tomography (CAT).

positron emission t. (PET) Direct visualization of physiologic and metabolic activities of living organs after administration of a biochemical substance (e.g., deoxyglucose) to which positron-emitting isotopes have been added; a computer interprets and produces data in the form of a color image; different shades of color indicate different concentrations of the substance.

tomomania 1. The tendency of certain surgeons to perform operations for minor ailments. **2.** A morbid desire to be operated upon.

tone 1. The tension of a muscle or state of an organ. **2.** The quality of sound or voice.

tongue The extremely mobile mass of striated muscle covered by mucous membrane that arises from the floor of the mouth; it serves as the principal organ of taste and aids in mastication, deglutition, and the articulation of sound. Also called lingua; glossus.

bifid t. A tongue that is split in its anterior portion by a longitudinal fissure. Also called cleft tongue.

black t., hairy t. Tongue with yellowish, brownish, or black furry patches on its dorsal aspect, made up of matted, overdeveloped papillae; the dark pigmentation is believed to be caused by microorganisms or by certain drugs. Also called furry tongue.

cleft t. See bifid tongue.

coated t. One having a whitish appearance due to deposits of food particles, inflammatory exudates, sloughed epithelial cells, or fungus growths; occurring when secretion of saliva is insufficient, or when special diets eliminate chewing or certain vitamins.

fissured t. See furrowed tongue.

furrowed t. A tongue with several longitudinal grooves. Also called fissured tongue.

geographic t. Tongue with patches of papillary atrophy which fuse at their borders suggesting the appearance of a map.

hairy t. See black tongue.

magenta t. A tongue with a magenta coloration; occurring in riboflavin deficiency.

strawberry t. A tongue with a whitish coat and enlarged red papillae, occurring in scarlet fever.

tongue-tie Condition in which tongue movements are restricted due to an abnormally short frenum.

tonic 1. A state of sustained muscular contraction. **2.** A remedy that is supposed to restore vigor.

tonicity 1. The normal condition of tension, as the slight continuous contraction of skeletal muscles. Also called tonus. **2.** The effective osmotic pressure,

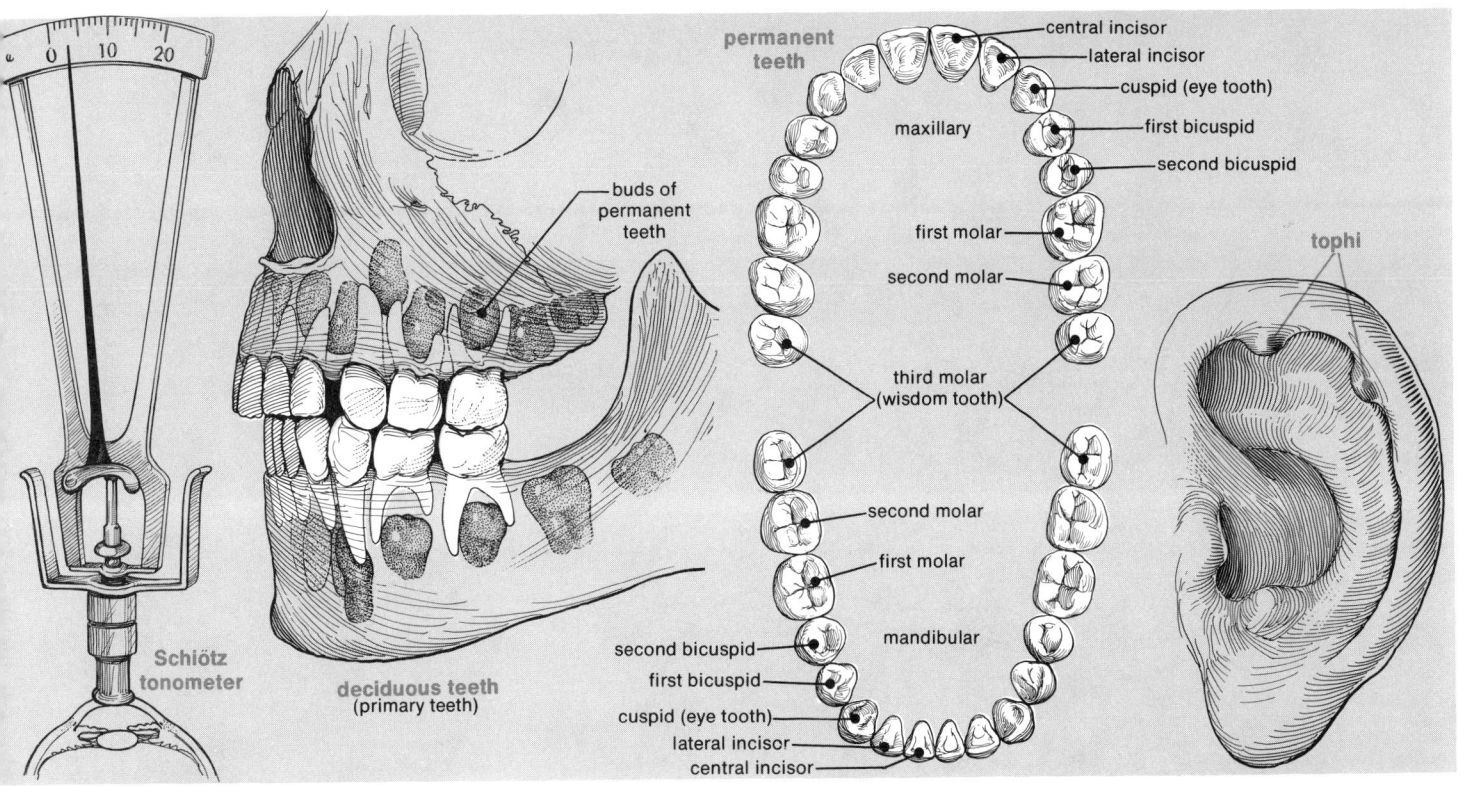

Schiötz tonometer

buds of permanent teeth

deciduous teeth (primary teeth)

permanent teeth

maxillary

central incisor
lateral incisor
cuspid (eye tooth)
first bicuspid
second bicuspid

first molar
second molar

third molar (wisdom tooth)

second molar
first molar

mandibular

second bicuspid
first bicuspid
cuspid (eye tooth)
lateral incisor
central incisor

tophi

usually compared to the osmotic pressure of plasma.

tonoclonic, tonicoclonic Denoting muscular spasms that are both tonic and clonic.

tonofibril One of the fine fibrils found in the cytoplasm of epithelial cells which gives a supporting framework to the cell.

tonofilament A structural cytoplasmic protein, bundles of which form a tonofibril.

tonography The continuous measuring and recording of changes in intraocular pressure with a tonometer.

tonometer An instrument for measuring tension or pressure.

Schiötz t. Tonometer that measures the intraocular pressure by determining the indentability of the cornea by a weighted plunger.

tonometry The determination of tension of a part, as of pressure within the eyeball by means of an instrument (tonometer).

tonsil 1. A small mass of lymphoid tissue, especially the palatine tonsil. 2. Any structure resembling a palatine tonsil.

cerebellar t. A lobule on the undersurface of each cerebellar hemisphere.

lingual t. An aggregation of lymphoid tissue on the posterior part of the tongue.

Luschka's t. See pharyngeal tonsil.

palatine t. One of two oval masses of lymphoid tissue, one on each side of the oral pharynx, between the pillars of the fauces.

pharyngeal t. A collection of lymphoid tissue on the posterior wall of the nasopharynx; when enlarged it is known as adenoids. Also called Luschka's tonsil.

tubal t. A collection of lymphoid tissue near the pharyngeal orifice of the auditory (eustachian) tube. Also called Gerlach's tonsil.

tonsillar, tonsillary Relating to a tonsil, especially the palatine tonsil.

tonsillectomy Surgical removal of the tonsils.

tonsillitis Inflammation of a tonsil or tonsils.

tonsilloadenoidectomy (T & A) The surgical removal of both the palatine tonsils and the adenoids.

tonsillolith A concretion or calculus in a tonsil.

tonsillotome An instrument, sometimes designed after a guillotine, for surgically removing a portion of a hypertrophied tonsil.

tonsillotomy The surgical removal of a portion of a hypertrophied tonsil.

tonus See tonicity (1).

tooth, *pl.* **teeth** One of the bonelike structures embedded in sockets in the jaws, used for chewing.

abutment t. See abutment.

buck teeth Prominent projecting maxillary anterior teeth; horizontal overlap in labioversion.

canine t. See cuspid.

dead t. Nonvital tooth.

deciduous teeth The 20 teeth that generally erupt between the 6th and 24th months of life, and are later replaced by the permanent teeth; they calcify partly before and partly after birth. Also called primary, temporary, or milk teeth.

eye t. See cuspid.

Hutchinson's teeth Permanent incisors in which the edge is notched and narrow; considered a sign of congenital syphilis. Also called notched teeth.

impacted t. A tooth that, due to its position in the jaw, is unable to erupt or to attain its normal position after it has erupted.

natal t. Tooth that has erupted prior to birth.

nonvital t. A tooth from which the pulp has been removed or one in which the pulp has died.

notched teeth See Hutchinson's teeth.

permanent teeth The 32 teeth that generally erupt from the ages of 6 to 21 years, belonging to the second or permanent dentition; they include 4 incisors, 2 cuspids, 4 bicuspids, and 6 molars in each jaw. Sometimes called succedaneous teeth.

primary teeth Deciduous teeth.

snaggle t. A tooth out of proper line in relation to the others in the arch.

spaced teeth Teeth that have shifted and lost proximal contact with adjacent teeth.

succedaneous teeth See permanent teeth.

temporary teeth Deciduous teeth.

unerupted t. A tooth prior to eruption through the gingiva.

wisdom t. Third permanent molar; erupts between the ages of 17 and 21 years.

toothache An aching pain in or about a tooth, usually due to caries, infection, or trauma. Also called odontalgia.

toothpick A wood sliver used to remove food particles from between the teeth.

balsa wood t. A triangular wedge of balsa wood used to stimulate the interdental gingival tissues and to cleanse the interproximal surfaces of the teeth.

topagnosis Inability to identify the exact place where the body is touched.

topalgia Pain localized at one spot without any lesion or trauma to account for it; a symptom sometimes occurring in neuroses.

topectomy Removal of a specific portion of the cerebral cortex in treating mental illness; a type of psychosurgery.

topesthesia Ability to determine which part of the skin is touched.

tophaceous 1. Gritty. 2. Having the features of a tophus.

tophus, *pl* **tophi** An accumulation of urate crys-

tals usually deposited in the articular and periarticular tissues in gout; it has a firm gritty consistency; the areas most vulnerable are those of the elbows, feet, hands, and the helix of the ear. Also called chalk stone.

topical Relating to a definite area.

topoanesthesia Inability to determine the location of a cutaneous sensation.

topognosis The ability to recognize the location of a sensation.

topogometer A movable fixation target attached to the front of a keratometer for measuring the curvature of the cornea in its periphery.

topography In anatomy, description of a limited area of the surface of the body.

toponarcosis Loss of sensation on a localized area of the skin.

torpor Sluggishness and slow response to stimuli.

torque A rotary force capable of producing torsion and rotation about an axis, as one applied to a denture base; a twisting force.

torsion The act of turning or twisting, or the condition of being turned or twisted, as the twisting of the spermatic cord.

torso The trunk.

torticollis Spasmodic contraction of the muscles of one side of the neck, causing the head to be drawn and usually rotated to that side. Commonly known as stiff neck; wryneck.

torulopsosis Yeast infection caused by *Torulopsis glabrata;* usually seen as an opportunistic disease in severely debilitated or AIDS patients.

torulus A small projection; a papilla.

torus 1. A protuberance or projection. 2. A benign, localized exostosis.

t. mandibularis A torus located on the lingual surface of the mandible in the cuspid-bicuspid region.

t. palatinus An overgrowth of bone usually located in the midline of the hard palate.

t. tubarius A ridge posterior to the pharyngeal opening of the auditory (eustachian) tube. Also called eustachian cushion.

totipotency The ability to regenerate a whole organism from a part.

touch 1. Special sense through which anything that comes in contact with the skin or mucous membrane is perceived. Also called the tactile sense. 2. To palpate or feel with the hands.

Tourette's disorder A rare form of generalized tic usually beginning in childhood, between 2 and 15 years of age; characterized by uncontrolled continuous gestures, facial twitching, foul language, and repetition of sentences spoken by other persons. Also called Gilles de la Tourette's disease or syndrome;

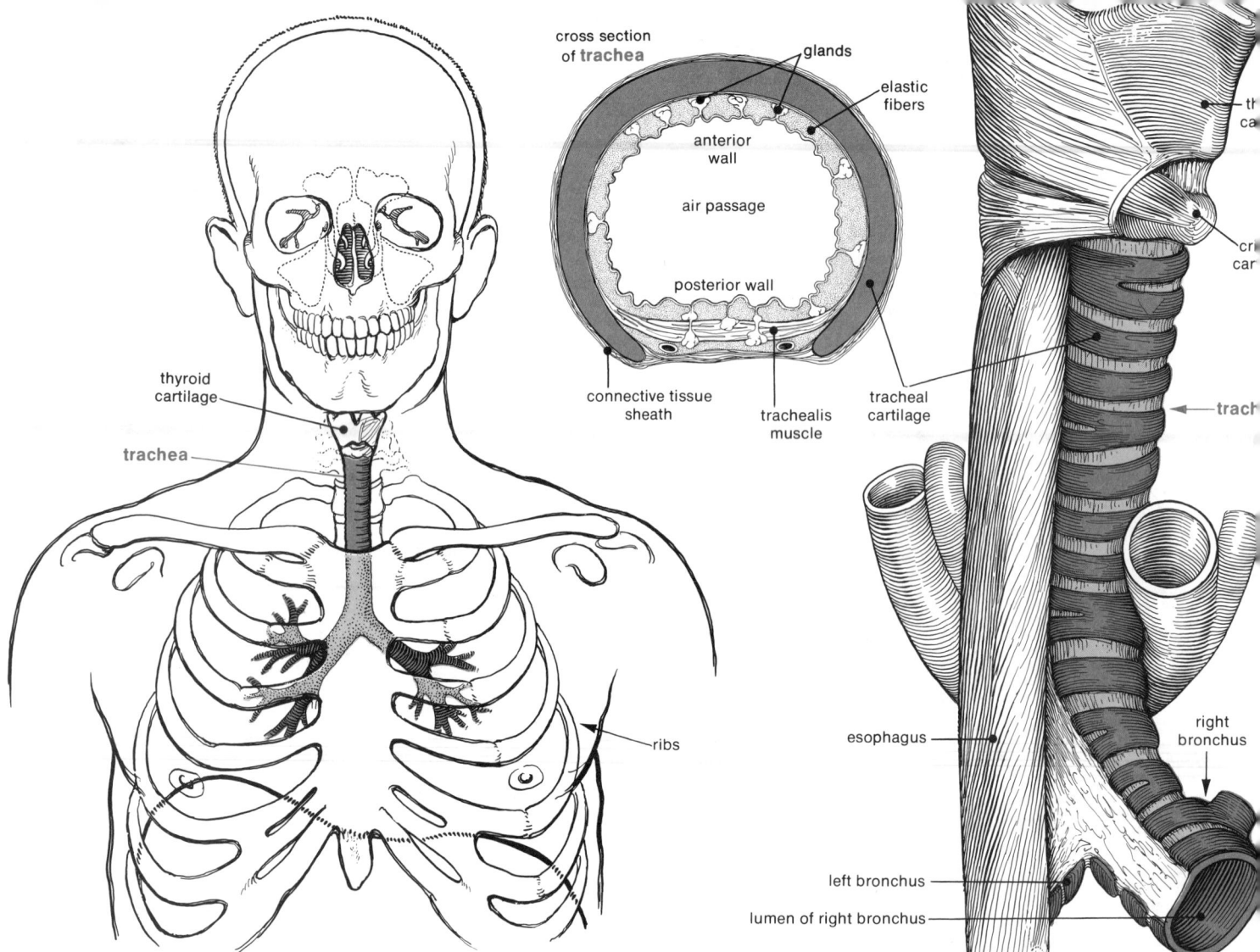

cross section of trachea

glands

elastic fibers

anterior wall

air passage

posterior wall

connective tissue sheath

trachealis muscle

tracheal cartilage

thyroid cartilage

trachea

ribs

esophagus

right bronchus

left bronchus

lumen of right bronchus

Tourette's syndrome; chronic multiple tic syndrome.

tourniquet Any device or constrictive wide band applied to an arm or leg for temporary compression of the blood vessels; used to stop arterial bleeding, prevent entry of a toxin into the body, or to distend the veins prior to venopuncture.

toxemia A condition caused by the presence in the blood of poisonous products of bacteria formed at a local site of infection.

　t. of pregnancy See preeclampsia.

toxic 1. Poisonous; harmful. **2.** Pertaining to a toxin. **3.** Caused by a poison.

　t. blood level See under level.

toxicant A poisonous or toxic agent; e.g., alcohol.

toxicity The quality of being poisonous.

Toxicodendron *Rhus.*

toxicoderma Any skin disease produced by a poison.

toxicodermatitis Skin inflammation produced by a poison.

toxicogenic 1. Producing a poison. **2.** Produced by a poison.

toxicoid Producing effects like those of a poison.

toxicologist An expert on poisons and their antidotes.

toxicology The study of the toxic or harmful effects of chemicals on the body; deals with the symptoms and treatment of poisoning as well as the identification of the poison.

　forensic t. Diagnosis and treatment of intentional and accidental poisoning and the attendant legal implications.

toxicopathy Any disease caused by a poison.

toxic shock syndrome Sudden onset of fever, muscle ache, vomiting, and diarrhea, accompanied by a peeling rash (especially of the palms and soles) and followed by low body temperature and shock; multiple organ involvement is common and may include kidneys, liver, mucous membranes, and cen-

tral nervous system; caused by staphylococcal endotoxin, especially from infection of the vagina associated with tampon use.

toxin A poisonous substance produced by certain microorganisms.

　extracellular t. Toxin produced and released by bacterial cells as a normal physiologic process. Also called exotoxin.

　intracellular t. Toxin produced and retained by bacterial cells and released only by destruction or death of the cells. Also called endotoxin.

toxipathy Any disease caused by a poison.

Toxocara A genus of parasitic roundworms of the family Ascaridae.

toxocariasis Infection with roundworms of the genus *Toxocara*.

toxoid A toxin that has been rendered nonpoisonous by chemicals or other agents but is still capable of producing immunity.

　tetanus t. The toxin from the tetanus bacillus, rendered nontoxic and used for immunization against the toxin produced by tetanus infection.

toxophore The group of atoms in the toxin molecule that is responsible for its poisonous action.

Toxoplasma gondii Intracellular protozoan parasite of the genus *Toxoplasma* causing toxoplasmosis in man.

toxoplasmosis Disease caused by infection with *Toxoplasma gondii*; it may resemble a mild cold or infectious mononucleosis in adults; a disseminated form may lead to hepatitis, pneumonitis, myocarditis, or meningoencephalitis; involvement of the eyes occurs in another form; an infected pregnant woman can spread the disease to her unborn child, causing eye or brain damage or even death; eating raw meat from infected animals is the most common way in which the disease is acquired.

trabecula, *pl.* **trabeculae** A supporting, anchoring fiber of connective tissue; a dividing band.

　septomarginal t. The moderator band that con-

nects the septal band with the anterior papillary muscle and the parietal wall of the right ventricle.

　trabeculae carneae Thick muscular bands on the inner walls of the ventricles of the heart.

trabecular Relating to, or marked by, the presence of trabeculae.

trabeculation The formation or the presence of trabeculae in a part.

trabeculectomy Microsurgery of the eye in which a small portion of the trabeculum and adjacent Schlemm's canal (scleral venous sinus) is removed to enhance drainage of aqueous humor, thus relieving intraocular pressure caused by open-angle glaucoma.

tracer 1. A substance that can be readily identified, such as a radioactive isotope, used to gain information. **2.** A device for recording the movements of the lower jaw.

trachea A cartilaginous and membranous tube extending from, and continuous with, the lower part of the larynx to the bronchi. Commonly known as windpipe.

tracheal Relating to the trachea.

trachealgia Pain in the trachea.

tracheitis Inflammation of the trachea.

trachelism, trachelismus Spasmodic backward bending of the neck.

trachelorrhaphy Repair of the uterine cervix, as from lacerations.

tracheobronchial Relating to the trachea and a bronchus or the bronchi.

tracheobronchitis Inflammation of the mucous membrane of the trachea and bronchi.

tracheobronchoscopy Visual inspection of the interior of the trachea and bronchi.

tracheocele Hernial protrusion of the mucous membrane through a defect in the wall of the trachea.

tracheosophageal Relating to the trachea and the esophagus.

tracheolaryngeal Relating to both the trachea

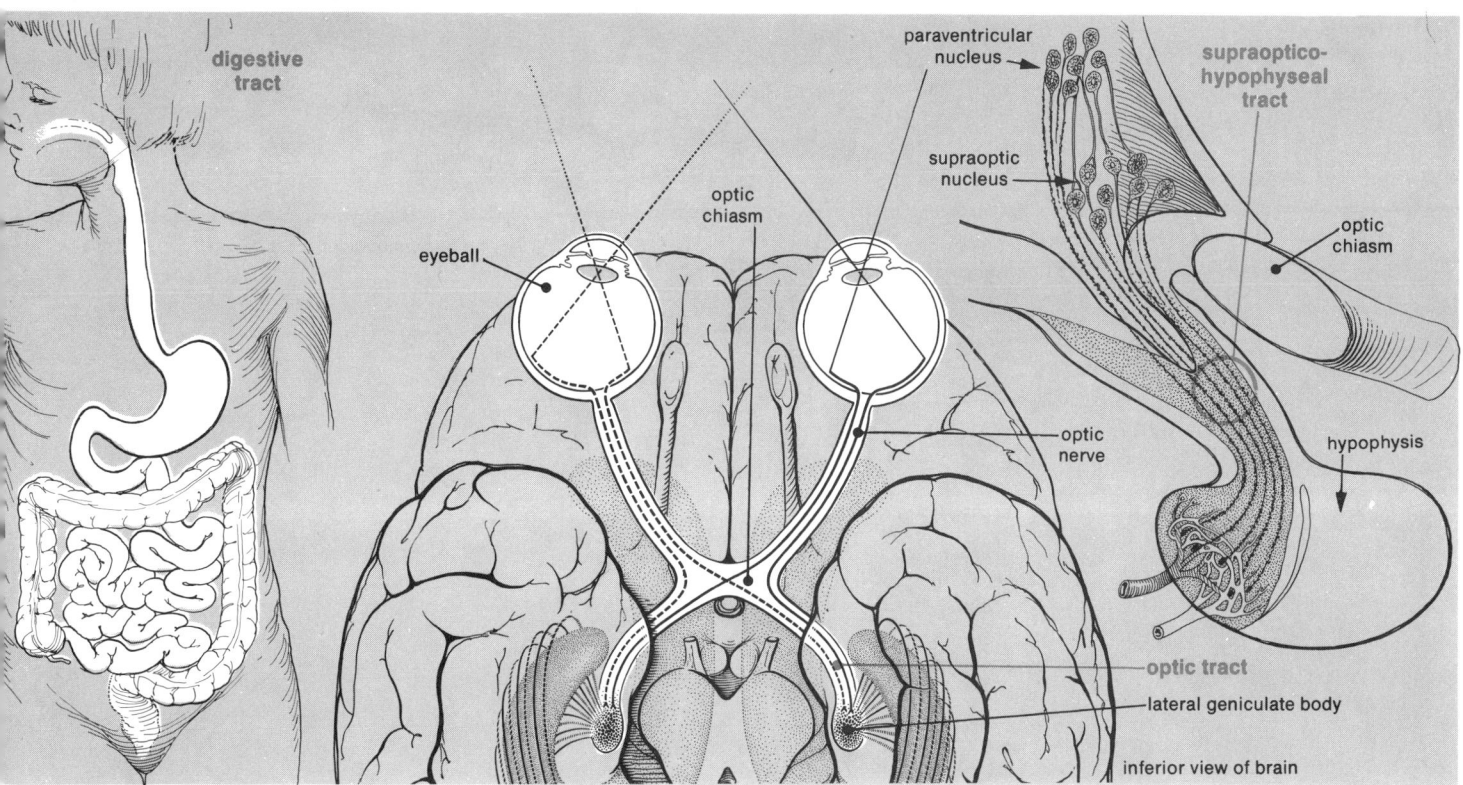

digestive tract

eyeball

optic chiasm

paraventricular nucleus

supraoptic nucleus

supraoptico-hypophyseal tract

optic chiasm

optic nerve

hypophysis

optic tract

lateral geniculate body

inferior view of brain

and the larynx.

tracheomalacia Softening and degeneration of the connective tissue of the trachea.

tracheopathy Any disease of the trachea.

tracheophony The hollow sound heard on auscultation over the trachea.

tracheoplasty Plastic surgery of the trachea.

tracheorrhagia Bleeding from the trachea.

tracheoscopy Visual examination of the interior of the trachea by means of a tracheoscope.

tracheostenosis Constriction of the trachea.

tracheostoma An opening into the trachea through the neck.

tracheostomy 1. A direct opening into the trachea through the neck to facilitate breathing or removal of secretions. 2. The artificial opening or stoma so produced.

tracheotome Tracheostomy knife.

tracheotomy Tracheostomy.

trachoma A contagious infection of the conjunctiva and cornea caused by *Chlamydia trachomatis*; at its onset the disease is characterized by inflammation followed by numerous follicles in the conjunctiva of the upper eyelid; after about six weeks these turn to large, red, hard papillae which last from several months to one or more years, ending with scar tissue formation which shortens and turns the eyelid inward and causes the conjunctiva and cornea to become dry; the disease is one of the chief causes of blindness in some parts of the world, especially the Middle East.

tracing A line or a pattern of lines made by a pointed instrument on thin paper or plate representing movement (e.g., cardiovascular activity, mandibular movements) or pertinent landmarks of a cephalometric x-ray picture.

tracks A slang expression for a series of tattoo-like needle scars from frequent narcotics injections.

tract 1. A system of structures, arranged in series, that perform one common function; e.g., the respiratory tract. 2. A collection of nerve fibers possessing the same origin, termination, and function.

  alimentary t. Digestive tract.

  ascending t. Any band of nerve fibers conveying impulses toward the brain.

  corticospinal t.'s Tracts composed of nerve fibers that originate from the cerebral cortex, pass through the medullary pyramid, and descend in the spinal cord.

  corticospinal t., anterior The portion of the corticospinal tracts that descends through the cervical segments adjacent to the anterior median fissure of the spinal cord (the fibers decussate at their level of innervation). Also called ventral corticospinal tract.

  corticospinal t., lateral The portion of the cor-

ticospinal tracts that upon decussation (at the junction of the medulla and spinal cord) descends the length of the lateral part of the spinal cord. Also called crossed pyramidal tract.

  descending t. Any band of nerve fibers conveying impulses from the brain downward.

  descending V t. See spinal trigeminal tract.

  digestive t. The mucous membrane-lined passage from the mouth to the anus.

  gastrointestinal t. The stomach and intestines.

  geniculocalcarine t. Nerve fibers that pass through the posterior limb of the internal capsule and terminate on the visual cortex of the occipital lobe. Also called optic radiation.

  genitourinary t. The urinary passageway from the pelvis of the kidney to the urinary orifice through the ureters, bladder, and urethra. Also called urogenital tract.

  iliotibial t. A strong, wide, thickened portion of the fascia lata of the thigh extending from the tubercle of the iliac crest to the lateral condyle of the tibia; it receives the greater part of the insertion of the gluteus maximus muscle.

  intestinal t. The part of the digestive tract between the pyloric end of the stomach and the anus.

  lemniscus t., lateral Lateral lemniscus.

  lemniscus t., medial Medial lemniscus.

  mamillotegmental t. Nerve fibers that arise from the mamillary nucleus and descend into the reticular formation of the brain stem, terminating in the dorsal and ventral tegmental nuclei.

  mamillothalamic t. Nerve fibers in the brain connecting the mamillary body to the anterior thalamic nuclear complex.

  olfactory t. A narrow band on the undersurface of the frontal lobe of the brain that connects the olfactory bulb to the cerebral hemisphere.

  optic t. A band of nerve fibers that extends from the optic chiasm to the lateral geniculate body, with some reflex fibers going to the spinal cord.

  pyramidal t. A term generally used to designate the corticospinal projections arising from the cerebral cortex and descending in the internal capsule, cerebral peduncle, and pons to the medulla oblongata; the term is restricted to mean nerve fibers that pass through the pyramid.

  respiratory t. The conducting airway consisting of the nose, mouth, pharynx, larynx, trachea, bronchi, bronchioles, and alveoli.

  rubrospinal t. A band of nerve fibers arising from the red nucleus (oval cell mass in the central part of the midbrain tegmentum); the fibers cross (decussate) and descend the length of the spinal cord.

  solitary t. A tract that begins in the upper medulla and extends to the cervical junction; it termi-

nates along the course of the solitary nucleus; formed primarily by visceral afferent and taste fibers from the vagus, glossopharyngeal, and facial (intermediate) nerves. Also called tractus solitarius.

  spinal trigeminal t., spinal V t. Afferent trigeminal root fibers that extend from the middle of the pons to the uppermost cervical spinal segments, where they terminate in the adjacent spinal trigeminal nucleus which forms a long cell column medial to the tract. Also called descending V tract.

  spinocerebellar t., anterior A band of nerve fibers that ascends along the lateral funiculus of the spinal cord to the cerebellum, via the superior cerebellar peduncle. Also called ventral spinocerebellar tract.

  spinocerebellar t., posterior A tract that lies in the lateral funiculus of the spinal cord and conveys nerve fibers from the thoracic nucleus to the cerebellum, via the inferior cerebellar peduncle. Also called dorsal spinocerebellar tract.

  spinothalamic t., anterior A band of nerve fibers in the anterolateral funiculus of the spinal cord that crosses over in the anterior white commissure before ascending to the ventral posterolateral (VPL) nucleus of the thalamus. Also called ventral spinothalamic tract.

  spinothalamic t., lateral A band of nerve fibers in the anterolateral funiculus of the spinal cord that ascends to the ventral posterolateral (VPL) nucleus of the thalamus, with some branches going to the reticular formation.

  supraopticohypophyseal t. A bundle of nerve fibers arising from the supraoptic and paraventricular nuclei of the hypothalamus and descending to the posterior lobe of the hypophysis (neurohypophysis), where these fibers branch profusely and form most of the bulk of the lobe.

  t. of Lissauer Poorly myelinated nerve fibers at the tip of the dorsal horn between the posteromarginal nucleus and the surface of the spinal cord, medial to the incoming dorsal roots; they are a continuation of the dorsal fibers that ascend and descend over two segments before terminating in the substantia gelatinosa. Also called dorsolateral fasciculus.

  tuberohypophyseal t. A bundle of nerve fibers arising from small cells (arcuate nucleus) around the floor of the third ventricle and projecting to the infundibular stem of the hypophysis. Also called tuberoinfundibular tract.

  urinary t. The urinary passageway from the pelvis of the kidney to the urinary orifice through the ureters, bladder, and urethra.

  urogenital t. See genitourinary tract.

  uveal t. See uvea.

messenger RNA (mRNA)

ribosome

translation of codon triplet (programs the proper aminno acid to be inserted into the growing protein chain)

transfer RNA (tRNA) with anitcodon triplet

amino acid complex

glutamic acid

transfer RNA (tRNA) with anitcodon triplet

lysine

glutamic acid

the appropriate acid is brought into proper alignment by the tRNA

the ribosome recognizes and pairs the mRNA and tRNA so that a peptide bond is formed

glutamic acid

proline

threonine

amino acids

leucine

peptide bond joining the amino acids to form the protein (polypeptide) chain

histidine

valine

tRNA separating from amino acid

the initial amino acid constituting the beta chain of hemoglobin

---

traction A method of treatment used in orthopedics to correct bone displacement by use of weights. Also called pulling or drawing.

skeletal t. Heavy traction delivered to a broken bone by pulling directly on a metal pin or wire inserted into or through a bone; capable of delivering a traction force of approximately 40 lb.

skin t. Light traction delivered to a bone by pulling on adhesive strips attached to the skin of an extremity; capable of delivering a traction force of approximately 10 lb; used frequently for the reduction of fractures in young children.

tractotomy Surgical severing of a nerve tract in the brain stem or spinal cord.

spinal t. Cordotomy.

trigeminal t. Severing of the descending root of the trigeminal nerve.

tractus Latin for tract.

tragacanth The dried gummy exudation from the thorny shrubs of the genus *Astragalus,* especially *Astragalus gummifer;* used in pharmacy as a suspending agent. Also called gum tragacanth.

tragus The small projection of cartilage in front of the opening of the external ear.

trait 1. In genetics, any inherited gene-determined characteristic; applied to any normal variation or to a disease, whether occurring in a recessive or a dominant condition. 2. A particular pattern of behavior.

autosomal t. Trait determined by a gene which is present on any chromosome other than a sex chromosome.

dominant t. Trait occurring when the responsible gene is present in a heterozygous state or single dose (i.e., having dissimilar alleles in corresponding loci of a pair of chromosomes).

recessive t. Trait occurring when the responsible gene is present in a homozygous state or double dose (i.e., having identical alleles at corresponding loci of a pair of chromosomes).

sickle-cell t. Term used in clinical medicine to denote a condition in which there is a tendency for the red blood cells to assume a sickle-like shape due to the presence of hemoglobin AS (the heterozygous state for hemoglobin S); individuals with the trait are usually asymptomatic but may manifest some of the complications of sickle cell disease.

trajector A device for following the path of a bullet in a wound.

trance A state of detachment from one's physical surroundings, characterized by diminished activity and consciousness, resembling sleep; e.g., the state seen in hypnosis.

tranquilizer A drug that allays anxiety and calms the patient.

transacetylation Metabolic reaction involving the transfer of an acetyl group.

transaction The reciprocal interaction between two or more individuals involving simultaneous stimulation and response.

transaminase Any enzyme that catalyzes the transfer of amino groups (a reversible reaction); present in body tissues and blood serum; released into the serum in increased quantities upon tissue injury. Also called aminopherase; aminotransferase.

glutamic oxaloacetic t. (GOT) Enzyme that catalyzes the transfer of the amino group of aspartic acid to α-ketoglutaric acid, forming glutamic and oxaloacetic acids; present in all body tissues, especially in heart, liver, and skeletal muscle; serum levels may be elevated in acute myocardial infarction, active liver disease, or some disorders of muscle. Also called aspartate aminotransferase; glutamate-aspartate transaminase.

glutamic pyruvic t. (GPT) Enzyme that catalyzes the transfer of the amino group of alanine to α-ketoglutaric acid, forming glutamic and pyruvic acids; present primarily in the liver and to a lesser extent in kidney and skeletal muscle; serum levels are elevated in certain liver disorders. Also called alanine aminotransferase; glutamate-alanine transaminase.

serum glutamic oxaloacetic t. (SGOT) Glutamic oxaloacetic transaminase present in blood serum; see glutamic oxaloacetic transaminase.

serum glutamic pyruvic t. (SGPT) Glutamic pyruvic transaminase present in blood serum; see glutamic pyruvic transaminase.

transamination The reversible process of amino group transfer, catalyzed by enzymes that have been called transaminases, aminopherases, and aminotransferases.

transcription 1. The process of transcribing, as in the transfer of the genetic code information from DNA to messenger RNA. 2. See signature.

transdiaphragmatic Across or through the diaphragm.

transducer A device that converts energy from one form to another.

Doppler ultrasonic t. A device that detects shift in sound (Doppler effect) from change in ultrasonic signal reflected from a bodily structure such as a blood vessel.

pressure t. A device that converts pressure differences into electric current, which can then be readily amplified and recorded.

transduction 1. The change in the genetic makeup of a cell by transfer of DNA from a virus to the cell. 2. The conversion of energy from one form to another.

transection 1. Cutting across. 2. A cross section.

transfection In genetic engineering, the artificial infection of a cell with an RNA tumor virus by adding DNA from a cell transformed by the virus; the virus (which has become integrated into the DNA of the transformed cell) is able to replicate in the transfected cell.

transferase An enzyme that catalyzes the transfer of a chemical grouping from one substance to another. Also called transferring enzyme.

transference 1. The shifting of symptoms from one part of the body to another. 2. In psychiatry, the unconscious shifting of an individual's feelings from people important in his early life to those important to him at a later time, as seen in the patient-analyst relationship during psychoanalysis.

transferrin Iron-binding beta globulin; it facilitates the transportation of iron to the bone marrow and tissue storage areas. Also called siderophilin.

transfer RNA A type of RNA (ribonucleic acid) that binds and transports amino acids to the ribosome; see under ribonucleic acid.

transfix 1. To pierce through with a pointed instrument. 2. To immobilize as with terror.

transformation 1. In chemistry, a change of form or structural arrangement of atoms. 2. In genetics, the genetic changes incurred by the incorporation into a cell of DNA purified from cells or viruses.

transfusion The introduction of a fluid, such as blood or plasma, into the bloodstream.

direct t. The transfer of blood directly from one person (donor) to another (recipient) without exposing it to air. Also called immediate transfusion.

exchange t. Removal of blood containing a toxic substance (e.g., removal of blood containing high levels of bilirubin from a newborn with erythroblastosis fetalis) coupled with blood replacement using donor blood. Also called substitution transfusion.

indirect t. Transfer of blood from a donor to a suitable container and thence to the recipient. Also called mediate transfusion.

reciprocal t. The transfer of blood from a person who has recovered from a contagious disease to a patient suffering with the same infection; an equal amount of blood is returned from the patient to the donor; used to confer passive immunity.

transient Short-lived.

transiliac Extending from one ilium to the other, as the transiliac diameter.

transillumination The examination of a body cavity by the passage of light through its walls.

translation The process whereby the genetic data present in a messenger RNA (mRNA) molecule direct the order of the specific amino acids during protein synthesis.

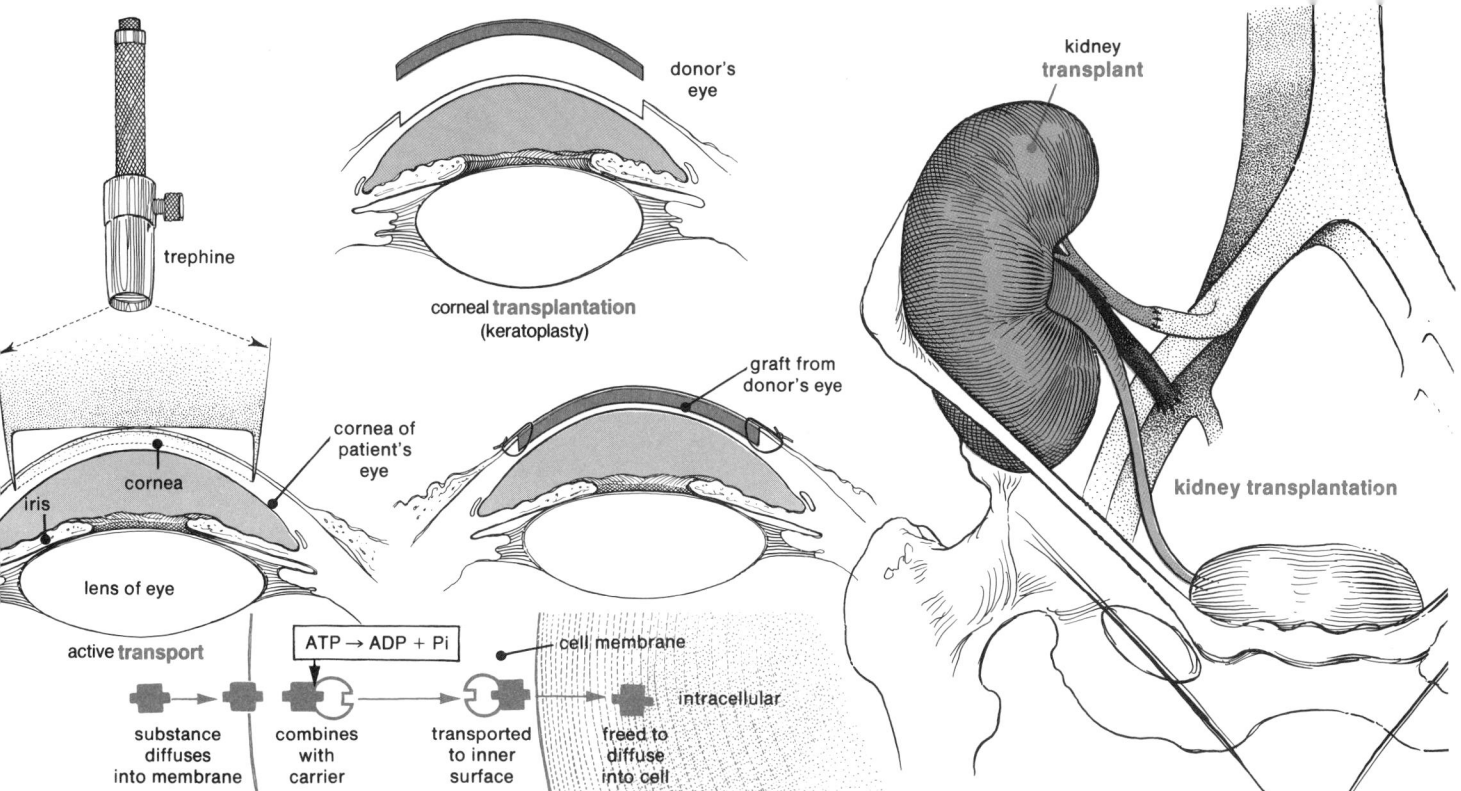

trephine

donor's eye

corneal **transplantation** (keratoplasty)

graft from donor's eye

cornea of patient's eye

cornea

iris

lens of eye

active **transport**

kidney **transplant**

kidney transplantation

ATP → ADP + Pi

cell membrane

intracellular

substance diffuses into membrane | combines with carrier | transported to inner surface | freed to diffuse into cell

translocation The transfer (often reciprocal) of segments of one chromosome to another, nonhomologous, chromosome.

translucent Partially transparent; permitting light to pass through with sufficient diffusion to obliterate distinct images.

transmethylase See methyltransferase.

transmethylation The process in which methyl groups are transferred to the precursors of methylated compounds, e.g., creatine, choline, and adrenaline.

transmigration The normal passage of blood cells through the capillary walls.

transmissible Capable of being passed from one person to another, as a disease.

transmission 1. Transfer, as of disease, from one person to another. 2. Conveyance.

  duplex t. Conveyance of impulses in both directions through one nerve.

  vertical t. Prenatal transmission from mother to child.

transmural Through or across a wall, as the wall of a hollow organ or cyst.

transmutation A change of a chemical element into another, resulting from radioactive decay or nuclear bombardment.

transpeptidase Enzyme that promotes the transfer of an amino acid residue or a peptide residue from one amino compound to another.

transphenoidal Through the sphenoid bone.

transphosphorylation Chemical reaction in which a phosphate group is transferred from one organic phosphate to another.

transpiration The passage of watery vapor or sweat through the skin or other tissue.

  pulmonary t. The passage of watery vapor from the circulating blood into the air of the lungs.

transpire To give off moisture through the skin or mucous membrane.

transplacental Denoting the movement of a substance through or across the placenta.

transplant 1. To transfer from one part to another, as in grafting. 2. The piece of tissue removed from the body for transplantation.

  Gallie t. Narrow strip of fascia lata from the thigh, used as suture material.

transplantar Extending across the sole of the foot; denoting muscular or ligamentous structures.

transplantation The transfer of tissue (graft) from one site to another.

  allogeneic t. Transplantation of tissue between genetically dissimilar members of the same species.

  autoplastic t. One in which the graft is taken from another part of the same individual.

  corneal t. Replacement of the cornea or a portion of it (whole or partial thickness) with a graft usually taken from an eye of an individual who has recently died. Also called keratoplasty.

  heart t. Replacement of a severely damaged heart with an entire organ from another person who has recently died.

  heterotopic t. Transfer of tissue from one area of the body of the donor to another site in the recipient.

  homotopic t. Orthotopic transplantation.

  kidney t. The transplantation of a kidney from one individual to another; the kidney transplant is usually obtained from a living relative with the same blood type or from a cadaver. Also called renal transplantation.

  orthotopic t. Transfer of tissue from an area of the body of the donor to an identical recipient site.

  renal t. See kidney transplantation.

  syngeneic t. Transplantation of tissues between genetically identical or near-identical animals, such as identical twins or highly inbred animals.

  syngenesioplastic t. The grafting of tissue to a recipient who is closely related to the donor, as from mother to her child.

  tendon t. The insertion of a slip from the tendon of a sound muscle into the tendon of a nonfunctioning (paralyzed) muscle.

  tooth t. The insertion of a tooth or tooth germ into a dental alveolus.

  xenogeneic t. Transplantation of tissue between two different species, such as the transplantation of a chimpanzee kidney into a human.

transport The conveyance of biochemical substances across cell membranes.

transposition 1. The moving of tissues or structures from one place to another. 2. The presence of an organ on the wrong side of the body.

transposon Any DNA sequence that may be transferred from one cell to another, resulting in rearrangement of the recipient cell's DNA.

transseptal Across a septum, as the transseptal fibers of the periodontal membrane, which go from the cementum of one tooth across the bony septum to the cementum of the adjacent tooth.

transsexual 1. An individual with an overpowering desire to be of the other sex. 2. An individual whose external sexual characteristics have been altered through surgery or hormonal intervention to resemble those of the other sex.

transsynaptic Denoting the transmission of a nerve impulse across a synapse.

transthoracic Across the chest or performed through the chest wall.

transtracheal Performed through the tracheal wall.

transudate A fluid that passes through a membrane, such as a capillary wall, as a result of differences in hydrostatic pressure.

transudation The passage of a fluid through a membrane, as when parts of the plasma pass through the capillary walls into the tissue spaces; it differs from osmosis in that the fluid passes with most of the substances held in solution or suspension.

transurethral Via or through the urethra.

transvaginal Through the vagina.

transverse Cross-wise.

transversion The eruption of a tooth in the wrong place or order.

transvestism, transvestitism 1. The practice of dressing in clothing of the opposite sex. 2. The overwhelming desire to be so dressed.

transvestite An individual who practices transvestism.

trapezium Name given to certain anatomic structures generally having a four-sided shape with no parallel sides.

trauma Injury or damage.

  occlusal t. Abnormal stresses and resulting pathologic changes on a tooth and surrounding tissues, caused by improper alignment of the teeth.

  psychic t. A painful emotional experience.

traumatic Caused by, or related to, injury.

traumatize To injure or wound either physically or psychologically.

traumatogenic Capable of causing injury or a wound.

traumatologist A physician with special knowledge in traumatology.

traumatology A surgical subspecialty concerned with the care and treatment of victims of violence or accidents.

tray A flat, shallow receptacle with raised edges used for carrying or holding various items.

  acrylic resin t. In dentistry, a custom-made impression tray of autopolymerizing acrylic resin for the individual patient.

  impression t. In dentistry, a metallic or acrylic receptacle consisting of a flanged body and a handle for use in carrying impression material to the mouth and holding it in position against the teeth or oral tissues while the material sets.

  surgical t. A tray for holding instruments in the operating room during a surgical operation.

treadmill A moving belt mechanism which permits individuals to walk or run in a stationary location under controlled conditions; used in studies of physiologic functions, particularly cardiac stress testing.

treat To give medical aid to an individual by medicinal, surgical, dietary, or other measures.

treatment The course of action adopted to care

trematode

trephine

Treponema

triamterene

H_2N —N—N—NH_2
—N—N—
NH_2

scrotum

superficial
transverse
perineal
muscle

urogenital
triangle

ischial
tuberosity

anal triangle

external
anal
sphincter

anus

coccyx

---

for a patient or to prevent disease.

conservative t. Treatment in which any radical therapeutic or surgical measures are avoided.

drug t. Treatment with medicines.

empirical t. Treatment based on experience rather than scientific data.

expectant t. Treatment aimed at the relief of symptoms until the nature of the illness is known. Also called symptomatic treatment.

heroic t. The use of aggressive measures to preserve the life of the patient.

medical t. 1. Treatment that employs medicines rather than surgical procedures. 2. Treatment rendered by medical personnel.

megavitamin t. The use of huge doses (megadoses) of vitamins in treating disorders, such as the use of vitamin B_3 (nicotinic acid) for the treatment of schizophrenia. Also called orthomolecular treatment.

palliative t. Treatment aimed at mitigating symptoms rather than curing the disease.

preventive t., prophylactic t. Treatment instituted to prevent a person from acquiring a disease to which he had been, or is expected to be, exposed.

root canal t. Removal of the pulp of a tooth followed by obliteration of the root canal.

shock t. A type of psychiatric treatment in which a convulsive or comatose state is produced by the administration of an electric current, carbon dioxide, or insulin.

supportive t., supporting t. Treatment aimed at maintaining the patient's strength.

surgical t. Treatment by any cutting operation.

symptomatic t. See expectant treatment.

Trematoda A class of flatworms (including flukes) of the phylum Platyhelminthes; parasitic in man and animals.

trematode, trematoid 1. A member of the class Trematoda; a fluke. 2. Relating to a fluke.

tremens See delirium tremens.

tremor Rhythmic, involuntary, alternating contraction of opposing muscle groups, fairly uniform in frequency and amplitude. Also called trembling.

essential t. High-frequency tremor, especially of the extremities, occurring during voluntary movement or when limbs are outstretched; tremor disappears when limbs are relaxed.

heredofamilial t. Essential tremor occurring as the only neurologic abnormality in several members of the same family; inherited as an autosomal dominant trait.

intention t. Tremor that is induced or intensified by a voluntary movement.

static t. A coarse rhythmic tremor occurring usually when the limb is at rest.

tremulous, tremulant, tremulent Quivering, trembling.

trench mouth Necrotizing ulcerative gingivitis; see under gingivitis.

Trendelenburg's sign See test, Trendelenburg's.

trephination Removal of a circular piece of skull with a trephine. Also called trepanation.

trephine A cylindrical saw for cutting a circular piece of bone or other tissue, e.g., the cornea.

trephining The cutting of a circular portion of tissue with a trephine.

Treponema A genus (family Treponemataceae) of spiral bacteria, several species of which are pathogenic.

T. pallidum The cause of syphilis in man.

T. pertenue The cause of yaws.

treponeme An organism of the genus Treponema.

treponemiasis Infection with bacteria of the genus Treponema.

triad A group of three closely related structures, signs, or symptoms.

adrenomedullary t. The symptoms produced by activation of the adrenal medulla; tachycardia, vasoconstriction, and perspiration.

Charcot's t. Nystagmus, tremor, and scanning speech, seen in multiple sclerosis.

hepatic t. See portal triad.

Hutchinson's t. Parenchymatous keratitis, labyrinthine disease, and Hutchinson's teeth, seen in congenital syphilis.

portal t. A triad at the angle of the liver lobule, consisting of a branch of the portal vein, a branch of the hepatic artery, and an interlobular bile ductule. Also called hepatic triad.

Saint's t. Hiatal hernia, diverticulosis, and gallstones occurring concomitantly.

t. of Luciani Manifestations of cerebellar disease: weakness (astenia), lack of normal tone (atony), and inability to stand (astasia).

triage The sorting of patients (as in a battlefield) to determine their priority for treatment.

triamcinolone A white crystalline powder, $C_{21}H_{27}FO_6$, used as an anti-inflammatory agent.

triamterene A drug that acts directly on renal tubules, producing sodium loss with potassium retention; when used in combination with thiazides, it enhances their hypotensive and diuretic effects; used to reduce edema associated with congestive heart failure, hepatic cirrhosis, and the nephrotic syndrome; Dyrenium®.

triangle A figure or area formed by connecting three points with straight lines; a three-cornered area.

Alsberg's t. A triangular space formed by a line through the long axis of the femoral neck, a second through the center of the diaphysis, and a third transversely at the level of the base of the femoral head.

anal t. A triangular space with the angles placed at both ischial tuberosities and at the tip of the coccyx.

anterior t. A triangular area in the neck, bounded by the mandible, the sternocleidomastoid muscle, and the midline of the neck.

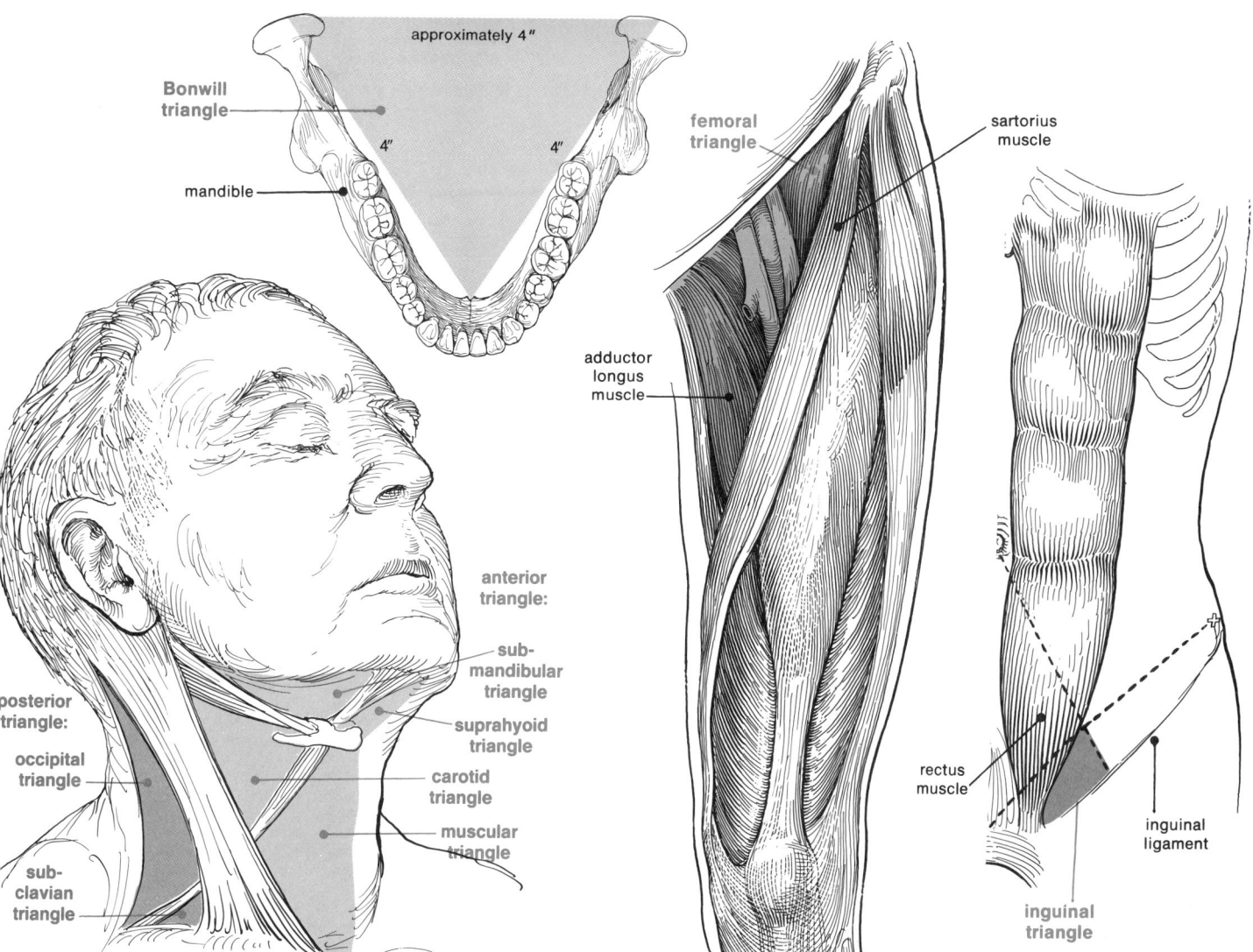

axillary t. The triangular area formed by the inner aspects of the arm, the axilla, and the pectoral region.

Bonwill t. An equilateral triangle with the angles placed at the center of each mandibular condyle and at the mesial contact areas of the mandibular central incisors.

Bryant's t. A triangle whose base is from the anterior-superior iliac spine to the top of the greater trochanter; its sides are formed, respectively, by a horizontal line from the anterior-superior iliac spine and a vertical line from the top of the greater trochanter.

carotid t. The triangle of the neck, bounded above by the stylohyoid muscle and posterior belly of the digastric muscle, behind by the sternocleidomastoid muscle, and below by the omohyoid muscle.

crural t. The triangular area formed by the inner aspect of the thigh and the lower abdominal, inguinal, and genital regions, with the base traversing the umbilicus.

cystohepatic t. The triangular area formed by the liver, the cystic duct, and the hepatic duct. Also called Calot's triangle.

Einthoven t. An imaginary equilateral triangle surrounding the heart, formed by lines representing the three standard limb leads of the electrocardiogram.

femoral t. A triangular space at the upper and inner part of the thigh, bounded by the sartorius and adductor longus muscles and the inguinal ligament; it is divided into two nearly equal parts by the femoral vessels. Also called Scarpa's triangle.

Hesselbach's t. Inguinal triangle.

inguinal t. A triangular area formed by the medial half of the inguinal ligament, the lateral edge of the abdominal rectus, and a line midway between the anterior-superior iliac spine and the pubic symphysis to the umbilicus; important area relating to inguinal hernia.

lumbar t. An area bounded by the edges of the latissimus dorsi and external oblique muscles and the crest of the ilium. Also called lumbar triangle of Petit.

muscular t. Triangle limited anteriorly by the median line of the neck from the hyoid bone to the sternum and posteriorly (above) by the superior belly of the omohyoid muscle and (below) by the anterior margin of the sternocleidomastoid muscle.

occipital t. The triangular area of the neck formed by the sternocleidomastoid, trapezius, and omohyoid muscles; the larger division of the posterior triangle.

olfactory t. A small triangular area just above the optic nerve near the chiasma, forming the posterior extremity of the olfactory tract where it diverges into the three roots. Also called trigonum olfactorium.

omoclavicular t. Subclavian triangle.

posterior t. A triangular area of the neck formed by the sternocleidomastoid muscle, the anterior margin of the trapezius muscle, and the middle third of the clavicle.

Scarpa's t. See femoral triangle.

subclavian t. The triangular area of the lower neck formed by the inferior belly of the omohyoid muscle, the clavicle, and by the posterior border of the sternocleidomastoid muscle; the smaller division of the posterior triangle.

submandibular t. The triangular area formed by the mandible, the stylohyoid muscle and posterior belly of the digastric muscle, and the anterior belly of the digastric muscle; it contains the submandibular gland.

submental t. Suprahyoid triangle.

suprahyoid t. Region bounded laterally by the anterior belly of the digastric muscle, medially by the middle of the neck from the hyoid bone to the mental symphysis, and inferiorly by the body of the hyoid bone. Also called submental triangle.

t. of auscultation Space bounded by the lower border of the trapezius muscle, the latissimus dorsi muscle, and the vertebral border of the scapula.

urogenital t. A triangular space with the angles placed at both ischial tuberosities and at the pubic symphysis.

vesical t. A triangular area in the bladder formed by the internal orifice of the urethra and the two orifices of the ureters. Also called trigonum vesicae.

triatomic 1. Denoting a molecule made up of three atoms. 2. Possessing three replaceable atoms or radicals.

tribasic Denoting a molecule with three replaceable hydrogen atoms; denoting an acid with a basicity of three.

tribe A taxonomic classification ranking just below a family or subfamily.

triceps Having three heads; denoting the muscle that extends the forearm.

trichatrophy, trichatrophia Atrophy of the hair bulbs, characterized by brittleness, splitting, and shedding of the hair; a deterioration of the hair apparatus.

trichiasis Inversion of hairs about an orifice, as eyelashes that turn in and cause irritation of the cornea.

trichina A larval worm of the genus *Trichinella*.

Trichinella A genus of nematode parasites in the aphasmid group, i.e., those lacking postanal phasmids (chemoreceptors); the cause of trichinosis in man.

T. spiralis An off-white, cylindroid worn about 1.5 mm in length; found coiled in a cyst in the striated muscle of various infected animals; a common cause of trichinosis in man. Also called trichina or pork worm.

trichiniasis, trichinelliasis See trichinosis.

trichinosis A disease caused by the parasite *Trichinella spiralis*, usually ingested with raw meat, especially infested pork; the parasites become lodged in muscle, producing muscular stiffness and painful

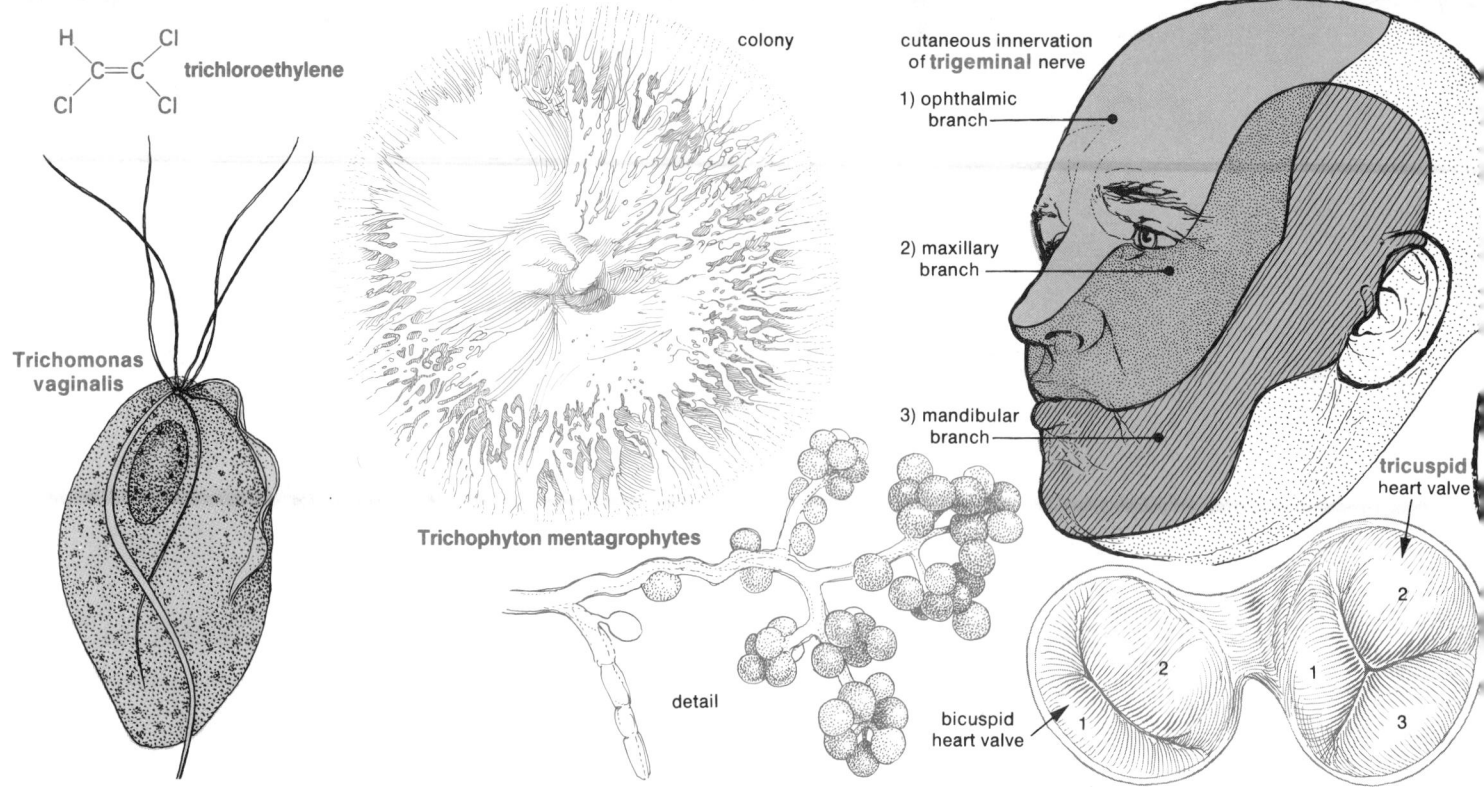

trichloroethylene

H   Cl
 \ /
  C=C   trichloroethylene
 / \
Cl   Cl

colony

Trichomonas vaginalis

Trichophyton mentagrophytes

detail

cutaneous innervation of **trigeminal** nerve

1) ophthalmic branch

2) maxillary branch

3) mandibular branch

tricuspid heart valve

bicuspid heart valve

---

swelling, accompanied by nausea, diarrhea, fever, and sometimes prostration. Also called trichiniasis; trichinelliasis.

trichloroethylene A sweet-smelling, nonflammable, volatile liquid with potent analgesic properties; used primarily as an analgesic in minor diagnostic surgical procedures and in obstetrics and dentistry; Trilene®.

trichloromethane Chloroform.

trichobezoar A compact mass of hair in the intestinal tract, frequently occurring in cats.

trichoclasia, trichoclasis Brittleness and eventual breakage of hair, as in monilethrix and trichorrhexis nodosa.

trichocryptosis 1. Ingrown hairs. 2. Any disease of the hair follicles.

trichocyst One of the minute elongated cysts, arranged radially around the periphery of certain protozoans, capable of ejecting a bristle-like extension.

trichoepithelioma A benign skin tumor originating in hair follicles; usually occurs on the face.

trichoesthesia The sensation felt when one of the hairs of the skin is touched.

trichogen Anything that stimulates hair growth.

trichoglossia Black tongue; see under tongue.

trichoid Resembling hair.

trichologia Compulsive plucking of the hair.

trichology The scientific study of hair: its anatomy, growth, and diseases.

Trichomonas A genus of parasitic protozoan flagellates (class Mastigophora), species of which are characterized by three to five anterior flagella, a posterior flagellum, and an undulating membrane.

   T. vaginalis A species found in the vagina and in the urinary tract of men, sometime causing inflammation.

trichomoniasis Inflammation of the vagina and urethra caused by infection with *Trichomonas vaginalis*.

trichomycosis Any infection of the hair with a fungus.

   t. axillaris Infection of the axillary (and occasionally pubic) hair with *Corynebacterium tenuis;* it affects the cortex of the hair, but not the roots or surrounding skin, and occurs in persons past puberty. Also called leptothrix.

trichonodosis A hair condition characterized by knots or bulges; results when new hairs are not permitted to grow naturally from their follicles. Also called beaded hair.

trichopathy Any abnormality of hair.

trichophobia 1. A morbid revulsion at the sight of loose hair on the clothing or elsewhere. 2. An unwarranted fear of hair in excess of that considered

normal for the area, especially on the face of women.

trichophytobezoar A hard ball composed of hair and vegetable fibers sometimes found in the stomach of man and animals.

Trichophyton A genus of pathogenic ringworm fungi (order Moniliales) possessing hyaline single-celled spores and being parasitic in the skin, nails, and hair follicles of man.

   T. ceratophagus *Trichophyton schonleini.*

   T. interdigitalis A variant of *Trichophyton mentagrophytes* that causes athlete's foot.

   T. mentagrophytes A superficial dermatophyte that causes ectothrix infections of scalp and beard hair (hyphae grow within and on the surface of hair shafts), and also of skin and nails; microconidia are numerous and occur in clusters at the ends of hyphae or singly alongside hyphae.

   T. rubrum A fungus with violet pigmentation of aerial mycelium; the cause of superficial infections in skin and nails.

   T. schonleini A fungus that causes favus, a severe form of chronic ringworm of the scalp, with destruction of hair follicles and permanent loss of hair in the infected area; in culture, the hyphae resemble reindeer horns and are sometimes referred to as favic chandeliers. Also called *Trichophyton ceratophagus.*

   T. tonsurans A yellowish ringworm fungus that causes endothrix infections of hair (the hyphae grow only within the hair shafts).

   T. violaceum A fungus with purple mycelia; the cause of simple tinea capitis, black-dot ringworm, or favic lesions.

trichophytosis A fungal infection caused by species of *Trichophyton.* See also tinea.

trichorrhea Abnormal shedding of hair.

trichorrhexis Condition in which the hair breaks easily.

   t. nodosa Nodular appearance of the hairs of the scalp, beard, and pubic area caused by transverse breakage of the shaft's cortex with subsequent longitudinal splitting into fine strands.

trichosis Any disease of the hair.

Trichosporon A genus of fungi which may infect the hair; it characteristically sporulates on hair or hairlike structures.

   T. beigelii Pathogenic species which is the cause of white piedra or trichosporosis.

trichosporosis Any mycotic infection of the hair caused by a pathogenic *Trichosporon.*

trichostasis spinulosa A common condition in which the hair follicle opening contains a dark plug of from 10 to 50 short fine hairs in a horny mass; usually seen in persons with acne and seborrheic dermatitis.

Trichostrongylus A genus of worms (class Ne-

matoda) which are intestinal parasites of herbivorous animals; they infest man only rarely and accidentally.

trichotillomania A compulsion to pull out or pluck one's own hair.

trichuriasis Infestation of the intestine with the whipworm *Trichuris trichiura.*

Trichuris A genus of worms of the class Nematoda.

   T. trichiura An intestinal parasite of man; the anterior three-fifths of the worm is whiplike, the posterior two-fifths is thicker; eggs are brownish and lemon-shaped with pluglike translucent polar prominences; infection is acquired by direct finger-to-mouth contact or by ingestion of food, water, or soil containing larvae. Also called whipworm.

tricuspid Having three cusps or points, as a valve in the heart or a tooth.

tricyclic Possessing three rings in the molecular structure; refers to one or more of a class of antidepressant drugs, such as, imipramine, amitriptyline, and doxepin hydrochloride.

triethylene glycol A compound $C_6H_{14}O_4$, used as an air disinfectant.

triethylenemelamine (TEM) A crystalline compound, $C_3N_3(NC_2H_4)_3$, used in the treatment of leukemia.

trifocal Having three focal lengths.

trifoliate Having three leaflike parts.

trifurcation Division into three branches or portions, as seen in the area of maxillary molars where the roots divide into three distinct portions.

trigastric Denoting a muscle with three bellies.

trigeminal 1. Triple. 2. Denoting the fifth cranial nerve.

trigeminal pulse See under pulse.

trigeminy A disturbance of the cardiac rhythm in which two premature beats follow each normal beat, or two normal beats are followed by a premature beat. Also called trigeminal rhythm.

triglyceride (TG) The most important of three groups of neutral fats; the basic unit consists of a molecule of glycerol in ester bond with three molecules of fatty acid; it serves as the major storage form of fatty acids and is practically the exclusive constitutent of adipose tissue.

trigonal 1. Relating to a trigone. 2. Triangular.

trigone Triangle; a triangular space, eminence, or fossa.

   collateral t. A somewhat triangular dilatation of the lateral ventricle of the brain between the posterior and descending horns.

   fibrous t.'s The two somewhat triangular masses of fibrous tissue that lie between the aortic arterial ring and the right and left atrioventricular rings.

   habenular t. A depressed triangular area of the

3,5,3 triiodothyronine (T₃)

trioses

glyceraldehyde   dihydroxyacetone

triplet

plano-concave lens   double-convex lens   negative meniscus lens

trilaminar wall

medullary cord of lymph node

trisomy D syndrome

chromosomes arranged according to size (karyotype)

brain between the habenula and the thalamus, rostral to the superior colliculus on each side.

interpeduncular t. The fossa at the base of the brain between the two cerebral peduncles.

olfactory t. The small grayish triangular eminence at the posterior extremity of the olfactory tract where it diverges into the three roots; it lies above the optic nerve near the chiasm.

t. of the bladder Vesical trigone.

vesical t. A triangular, smooth area at the base of the bladder, whose apices are the openings of the ureters and the internal urethral orifice; in this area the mucosa is closely adherent to the muscular layer of the bladder wall.

trigonitis Inflammation of the urinary bladder, localized in the mucous membrane of the trigone; it usually follows an uncomplicated course and in most instances responds well to antibacterial agents.

trihydrate Compound with three molecules of water.

trihydric Having three replaceable hydrogen atoms.

3,5,3′-triiodothyronine (T₃) A potent thyroid hormone containing three iodine atoms, normally present in the blood and thyroid gland; it usually represents about 5% of the total thyroid hormone in blood; it is three times as active on a weight basis as thyroxine and because of differences in binding and metabolism it contributes to tissue metabolism equally with thyroxine.

trilaminar Composed of three layers.

trill In speech, a sound produced by the vibration of a fluttering speech organ, most often the tongue; it causes a succession of closures and openings of the oral passage.

trilogy A group of three related symptoms.

t. of Fallot The combination of atrial septal defect, pulmonary stenosis, and ventricular hypertrophy.

trimester A period of three months; one-third of

the length of a pregnancy.

first t. The period of pregnancy from the first day of the last menstrual period before conception to the 98th day; the first 14 weeks of gestation.

second t. The term of pregnancy from the 15th through the 28th week of gestation.

third t. The term of pregnancy from the 29th through the 42nd week of gestation.

trimethoprim An antibacterial compound used, usually in conjunction with a sulfonamide, in the treatment of infections of the urinary tract, shigellosis, otitis media, and respiratory tract infections including pneumocystis carinii.

trimethylene See cyclopropane.

trimorphous Occurring in three forms.

trinitroglycerin See nitroglycerin.

trinitrophenol See picric acid.

trinitrotoluene (TNT) Explosive obtained by nitrating toluene.

triolein A colorless oily substance occurring in many natural fats and oils. Also called olein.

triose A three-carbon sugar; a monosaccharide, or sugar, possessing three carbon atoms in a molecule; e.g., glyceraldehyde and dihydroxyacetone; they represent the smallest carbohydrate molecules.

trip Term used by drug abusers meaning (a) to take a narcotic or a hallucinogenic drug; (b) the effects produced by such drugs.

acid t. A hallucinatory experience following ingestion of LSD (acid).

ego t. Anything done in order to boost one's self-esteem.

tripe The muscular wall of the stomach of cattle, used as food.

triphosphopyridine nucleotide (TPN) Old term for nicotinamide-adenine dinucleotide phosphate (NADP).

triplet **1.** One of three individuals born at one birth. **2.** Three lenses cemented or mounted together as a single lens system to correct aberration. **3.** Three

consecutive premature contractions of the heart. **4.** In molecular biology, a unit of three successive bases in DNA or RNA coding for a specific amino acid.

triploblastic Containing tissue derived from all three embryonic layers.

triploid A cell having three haploid sets of chromosomes in its nucleus.

triplopia Visual defect in which one object is perceived as three instead of one.

tripoli A mild abrasive derived from certain porous rocks, suspended in a greaselike medium; used in dentistry for finishing dental restorations.

triradius In dermatoglyphics, a point from which the dermal ridges course in three directions.

trisaccharide A carbohydrate with three monosaccharides in its molecule that upon hydrolysis yields three simple sugars; e.g., raffinose.

tris(hydroxymethyl)aminomethane (Tris) A buffer used in biologic preparations for in vitro studies, as with enzymes.

trismus Difficulty in opening the mouth due to tonic spasm of the muscles of mastication; usually the first symptom of tetanus; also called lockjaw.

trisomic Denoting a cell or an individual having an extra chromosome.

trisomy The presence of an additional chromosome, homologous with one of the existing pairs, so that one particular chromosome is present in triplicate; has been found for chromosome 21, 18, 13, 22, 8, and 9.

t. 13 See trisomy 13 syndrome.

t. 18 See trisomy 18 syndrome.

t. 21 Down's syndrome.

trisomy 13 syndrome Cleft lip and palate, extra fingers or toes, abnormalities of the heart, abdominal organs, and genitalia and defects of the central nervous system associated with mental retardation; the extra chromosome (the 13th) is a member of the D group. Also called Trisomy D; Patau syndrome.

trisomy 18 syndrome The presence of chromo-

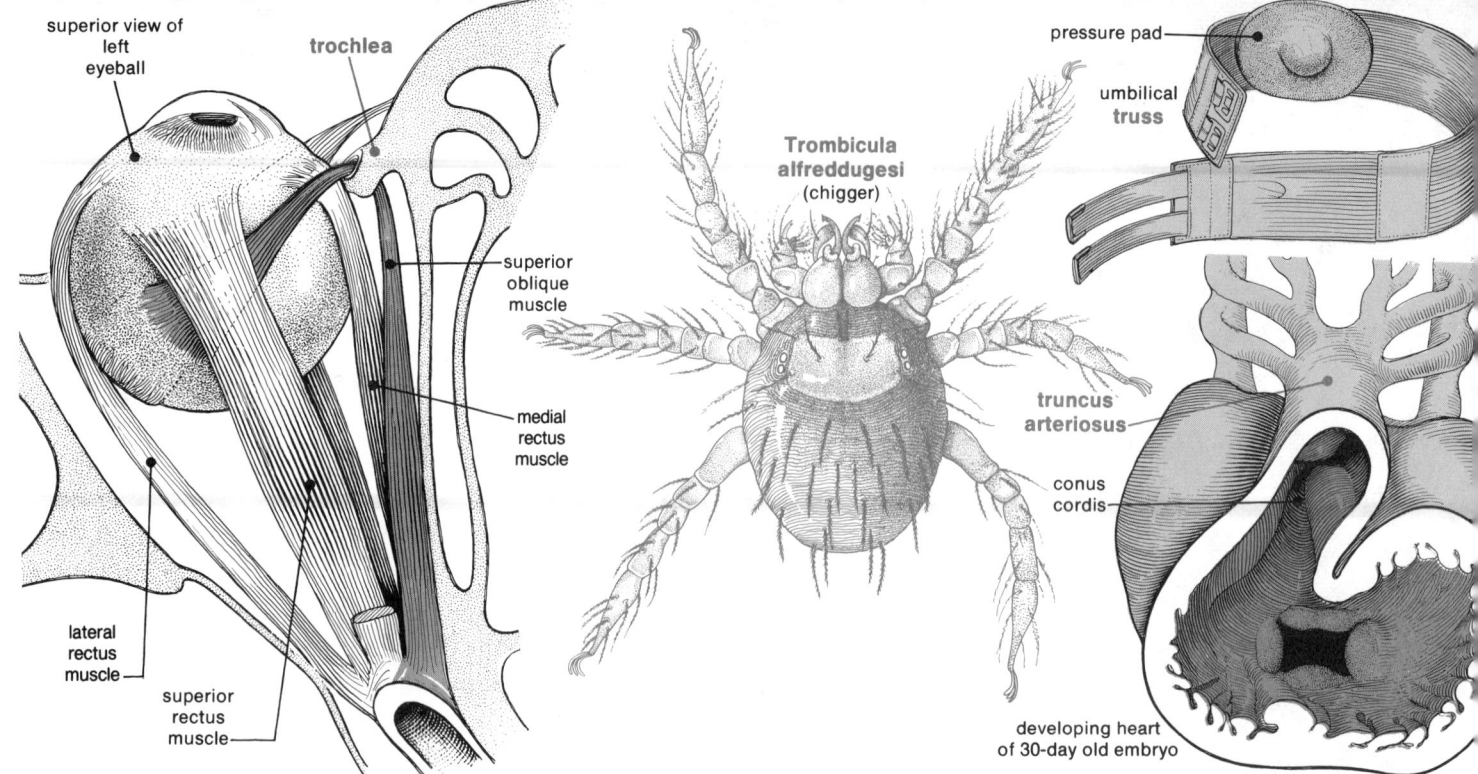

superior view of left eyeball

trochlea

superior oblique muscle

medial rectus muscle

lateral rectus muscle

superior rectus muscle

Trombicula alfreddugesi (chigger)

pressure pad

umbilical truss

truncus arteriosus

conus cordis

developing heart of 30-day old embryo

some 18 (group E) in triplicate rather than duplicate; characterized by mental retardation, skull deformities, abnormally small chin, low set ears, webbed neck, deafness, heart defects, and Meckel's diverticulum. Also called trisomy 18; Edwards' syndrome.

tritanopia Inability to perceive the color blue and reduced ability to perceive its combined forms (blue-greens and greens), except the violets; congenital tritanopia is rare; it occurs usually as a result of disease or detachment of the retina. Also called blue blindness; blue-yellow blindness; tritanopic vision.

tritium See hydrogen-3.

triturable Having the capability of being triturated.

trituratio (trit) Latin for triturate; used in prescription writing.

trituration 1. The process of reducing a solid to a fine powder by continuous rubbing, as the reduction of a drug to a fine powder (usually mixed thoroughly with milk sugar). **2.** In dentistry, the mixing of amalgam alloy either by itself or with mercury.

triturium A device used to separate immiscible liquids by virtue of their different densities.

trivalent Denoting an atom or radical with a valence of three. Also called tervalent.

trocar A sharp-pointed metal rod, used in a metal tube (cannula) for piercing the wall of a body cavity, after which it is withdrawn, leaving the cannula in place to permit evacuation of the fluid from the cavity. Also written trochar.

trochanter One of two prominences (major and minor) on the upper part of the femur.

trochar See trocar.

troche A small medicated tablet. Also called lozenge.

trochlea Any pulley-like structure, especially the fibrous loop in the orbital cavity through which passes the tendon of the superior oblique muscle of the eyeball.

trochlear 1. Relating to a trochlea or pulley. **2.** The fourth cranial nerve; the trochlear nerve.

Trombicula A genus of mites (family Trombiculidae) whose larvae have the ability to infest man.

   T. akamushi The kedani mite, a parasite of rodents; vector of rickettsial diseases.

   T. alfreddugesi A chigger; the larvae attack man, causing intensely irritating itching due to the injection of saliva into the skin.

trombiculiasis Infestation with mites of the genus Trombicula. Also called trombiculosis.

Trombiculidae A family of mites whose six-legged larvae (chiggers, red bugs, scrub mites, etc.) are parasitic on vertebrates, causing an irritating rash.

trophic Relating to nutrition.

trophoblast The outer layer of cells forming the wall of the blastocyst; it differentiates into two layers

(cytotrophoblast and syncytiotrophoblast) at the time of attachment to the uterus and eventually enters into formation of the placenta, but not the embryo.

trophoneurosis Alteration of any tissue due to interruption of nerve supply to the part.

   facial t. See hemiatrophy, facial.

trophopathia, trophopathy Any disorder of nutrition.

trophotropism Movement of living cells toward or away from nutritive material.

trophozoite The young, ameboid, undivided stage of a sporozoan organism, such as the malarial parasite, after it has been transmitted to man; the younger forms are ring-shaped; they eventually mature to form schizonts (the adult forms).

tropia Abnormal deviation of the eyes. See also strabismus.

tropine A poisonous alkaloid, 3α-tropanol; the major constituent of atropine and scopolamine, from which it is derived on hydrolysis; it possesses a tobacco odor and has medicinal value.

tropism Tendency for parts of a living organism (e.g., leaves) to turn toward or away from a stimulus.

tropocollagen The fundamental unit of collagen fibrils consisting of symmetric molecules with three helically arranged polypeptide chains.

tropometer 1. A device for measuring the degree of rotation of the eyeball. **2.** A device for measuring the torsion of the shaft of a long bone.

tropomyosin B A fibrous protein concentrated in the Z line of muscle that can be extracted from dry powdered muscle; it has a different molecular weight from myosin.

troponin A protein in muscle that heightens the dependence of the ATP-induced contraction of actomyosin.

trough A narrow shallow depression.

Trousseau's sign Muscular spasm of the hand elicited by compression of the upper arm (as with a blood pressure cuff); a sign of latent tetany.

truncal Relating to the trunk of the body or to any main branch.

truncate Cut at right angles to the main axis.

truncus Latin for trunk or stem.

   t. arteriosus The main arterial trunk of the fetal heart that gives rise to the aortic and pulmonary arteries.

trunk 1. The human body excluding the head and the extremities. Also called torso. **2.** The main part, usually short, of a nerve or vessel before its division. **3.** The main axis. **4.** A large collection of lymphatic vessels.

   brachial plexus t.'s The three trunks of the brachial plexus. See table of nerves.

   brachiocephalic t. The large artery coming off

the aortic arch that divides into the right subclavian and right common carotid arteries.

   celiac t. The large artery arising from the abdominal aorta just below the diaphragm; it divides into the left gastric, hepatic, and splenic arteries.

   intestinal lymphatic t. A short lymphatic vessel that drains lymph from the gastrointestinal tract and empties into the cisterna chyli.

   lumbar lymphatic t.'s Two large collecting lymphatic vessels, right and left, that drain lymph upward from the lumbar lymph nodes to the cisterna chyli.

   lumbosacral t. A large nerve formed by the union of the smaller part of the fourth and the entire fifth lumbar nerves; it enters into the formation of the sacral plexus.

   pulmonary t. Pulmonary artery. See table of arteries.

   root t. The part of the multirooted posterior tooth situated between the cervical line and the points of bifurcation or trifurcation of roots.

   sympathetic t.'s Two long chains of sympathetic ganglia on either side of the vertebral column extending from the base of the skull to the coccyx.

truss A device consisting of a belt and a pressure pad, used to retain a hernia in place after reduction or to prevent the increase in size of an irreducible hernia.

Trypanosoma A genus of parasitic protozoan flagellates (family Trypanosomidae), some of which are pathogenic.

   T. cruzi The species that causes Chagas' disease; endemic in Central and South America, especially in Brazil, Chile, Argentina, and Venezuela; found also in vectors in California, Arizona, and Texas.

   T. gambiense The species that causes West African or Mid-African sleeping sickness; transmitted by the tsetse fly. Also called *Trypanosoma hominis; Trypanosoma ugandense; Castellanella gambiense.*

   T. rhodesiense The species that causes Rhodesian trypanosomiasis (East African sleeping sickness); endemic in Rhodesia and Tanzania.

trypanosomiasis Any disease caused by infection with a protozoan parasite of the genus *Trypanosoma;* transmitted by the bite of the tsetse fly or by contamination of the bite wound of the kissing bug.

   African t. Disease of the central nervous system transmitted by several species of tsetse flies (genus *Glossinia*); the parasite (*Trypanosoma gambiense*) enters the circulation and becomes localized in the brain and lymph nodes; early manifestations include severe headache, fever, a feeling of oppression, and enlarged lymph nodes; wasting, mental deterioration, and drowsiness occur in the late stages and, if untreated, death occurs. Also called African sleeping

tryptophan

external auditory meatus

auditory tube

uterine tube

ovarian ligament

fundus of uterus

uterine tube

round ligament

ovarian ligament

fimbriated extremity of **uterine tube**

ovary

broad ligament

ureter

uterus

Coolidge tube

vagina

---

sickness.

American t. See Chagas' disease.

trypsin One of the protein-splitting (proteolytic) enzymes in the pancreatic juice derived from trypsinogen.

trypsinogen, trypsogen A substance secreted by the pancreas and converted, in the intestine, into trypsin by the enzyme enterokinase.

tryptic Relating to the proteolytic enzyme trypsin.

tryptophan (Trp) An essential amino acid present in varying quantities in common proteins; deficiency may result in the development of pellagra.

tsetse See *Glossina*.

tsutsugamushi disease Infectious disease occurring in Southeast Asia; caused by *Rickettsia tsutsugamushi* and transmitted by mites; characterized by painful swelling of the lymphatic glands, fever, headache, eruption of dark red papules, and blackish scab on the genitals. Also called mite-borne, scrub, or tropical typhus; island, tsutsugamushi, or Japanese river fever.

tubal Of, or relating to a tube, especially a uterine tube.

tube 1. A hollow cylinder. 2. A channel or canal.

auditory t. A channel connecting the cavity of the middle ear with the upper part of the throat (nasopharynx); it equalizes the pressure in the middle ear with the atmospheric pressure. Also called eustachian tube.

Cantor t. A 3.3 m rubber tube with a mercury filled bag at the extreme end, used for intestinal intubation; it is usually introduced via the nose and directed into the stomach; with proper positioning of the patient, the weight of the mercury bag helps to lead the tube through the duodenum and into the small intestine beyond.

cathode ray t. (CRT) One containing a filament which, when a low-voltage electric current is passed through it, becomes incandescent and produces a beam of electrons.

Coolidge t. A hot-cathode x-ray tube that develops its electrons from a heated filament.

Dominici t. A tube that allows the passage of only beta and gamma rays; used for the therapeutic application of radium.

drainage t. Tube placed in a wound or cavity to allow the escape of fluids.

endotracheal t. A rubber tube inserted in the trachea as an airway in endotracheal intubation.

eustachian t. See auditory tube.

fallopian t. See uterine tube.

Geiger-Müller t., Geiger t. A gas-filled tube containing a cylindrical cathode and axial wire electrode, used to detect radioactivity; radioactive particles penetrate the tube's envelope and produce momentary current pulsations in the gas.

Levin t. A flexible tube introduced into the duodenum or stomach, usually through the nose, after an operation.

Miller-Abbott t. A double lumen 3.3 m intestinal tube, used for diagnosing and treating obstructions of the small intestine.

neural t. The epithelial tube of the early embryo formed by the closure of the neural groove; it develops into the brain and spinal cord.

photomultiplier t. Apparatus used to amplify images of low intensity.

Sengstaken-Blakemore t. Device consisting of three tubes, two with an inflatable balloon and the third one attached to a suction apparatus; used to stop bleeding from the esophagus.

stomach t. A flexible 40 cm tube used for feeding or for washing out the stomach.

test t. Tube made of thin glass and closed at one end; used in a variety of laboratory procedures.

tracheotomy t. A metal or glass tube inserted into the trachea through a tracheotomy opening to facilitate breathing.

uterine t. One of two slender tubes, about 10 cm long, on either side leading from the uterus to the area of the ovary; it conveys the ovum from the ovary to the uterus and is usually where conception occurs. Also called fallopian tube; oviduct.

vacuum t. Glass tube from which air has been almost completely removed.

x-ray t. A vacuum tube used for the production of x-rays; the enclosed electrodes accelerate electrons and direct them to an anode, where their impacts produce high energy photons.

tubectomy See salpingectomy.

tube housing A lead-shielded container that provides radiation protection; it holds the x-ray tube, transformers, and insulating oils.

diagnostic protective t.h. One that reduces leakage radiation to 0.1 roentgens per hr at a distance of 1 m from the tube target when the tube is operating at its maximum rated voltage and current.

therapeutic protective t.h. One that reduces leakage radiation to 1 roentgen per hr at a distance of 1 m from the tube target when the tube is operating at its maximum rated voltage and current.

tuber, *pl.* **tubera** A prominence.

t. cinereum The small portion of the hypothalamus that protrudes into the floor of the third ventricle of the brain.

tubercle 1. The specific lesion of tuberculosis. 2. A rounded elevation on a bone. 3. A nodule on the skin.

tubercular Relating to or having tubercles; erroneously used instead of tuberculous to describe a person afflicted with tuberculosis. Also called nodular.

---

tuberculate, tuberculated Having nodules or tubercles.

tuberculation The formation or presence of nodules.

tuberculid A skin lesion caused by the toxins of tuberculosis.

tuberculin A substance made from the toxins of the tubercle bacillus, used in the diagnosis and, to some extent, in the treatment of tuberculosis.

old t. (O.T.) A concentrated filtrate made from a six-week-old culture of tubercle bacilli in glycerol broth; it contains only the soluble substance produced by the bacilli during growth, not the microorganisms.

purified protein derivative of t. (P.P.D.) An extract from tubercle bacilli prepared in the protein-free liquid medium.

tuberculoid 1. Resembling tuberculosis. 2. Resembling a tubercle.

tuberculoma A tumor-like mass of tuberculous origin.

tuberculosis (TB, tb, TBC) A communicable disease caused by any of several species of *Mycobacterium* referred to as the tubercle bacillus; it manifests itself by the formation of tubercles or lesions in the tissues affected, most commonly the lungs; tuberculosis in man is caused by the human variety of *Mycobacteria* (*Mycobacterium tuberculosis*) and the bovine variety (*Mycobacterium bovis*) as well as some atypical bacteria.

acute miliary t. A form of tuberculosis in which the tubercle bacilli are carried in the bloodstream throughout the body, thus affecting several organs simultaneously. Also called disseminated tuberculosis.

cutaneous t. A rare group of skin diseases caused either by the presence of microorganisms in the skin or by allergic reactions to a previous bacterial infection.

disseminated t. Acute miliary tuberculosis.

postprimary t. Tuberculosis of the lung occurring as a reinfection or a reactivation of a dormant infection.

primary t. The phase of a tuberculous infection immediately following invasion of tissues by the tubercle bacilli.

pulmonary t. Tuberculosis of the lungs, marked by ulceration and formation of cavities in the lungs, attended by fever and cough. Formerly called phthisis; consumption.

tuberculostatic 1. Denoting an agent that inhibits the growth of the tubercle bacillus. 2. Arresting the growth of the tubercle bacillus.

tuberculous Afflicted with tuberculosis.

tuberculum, *pl.* **tubercula** 1. An elevation on a bone. 2. A nodule on the skin.

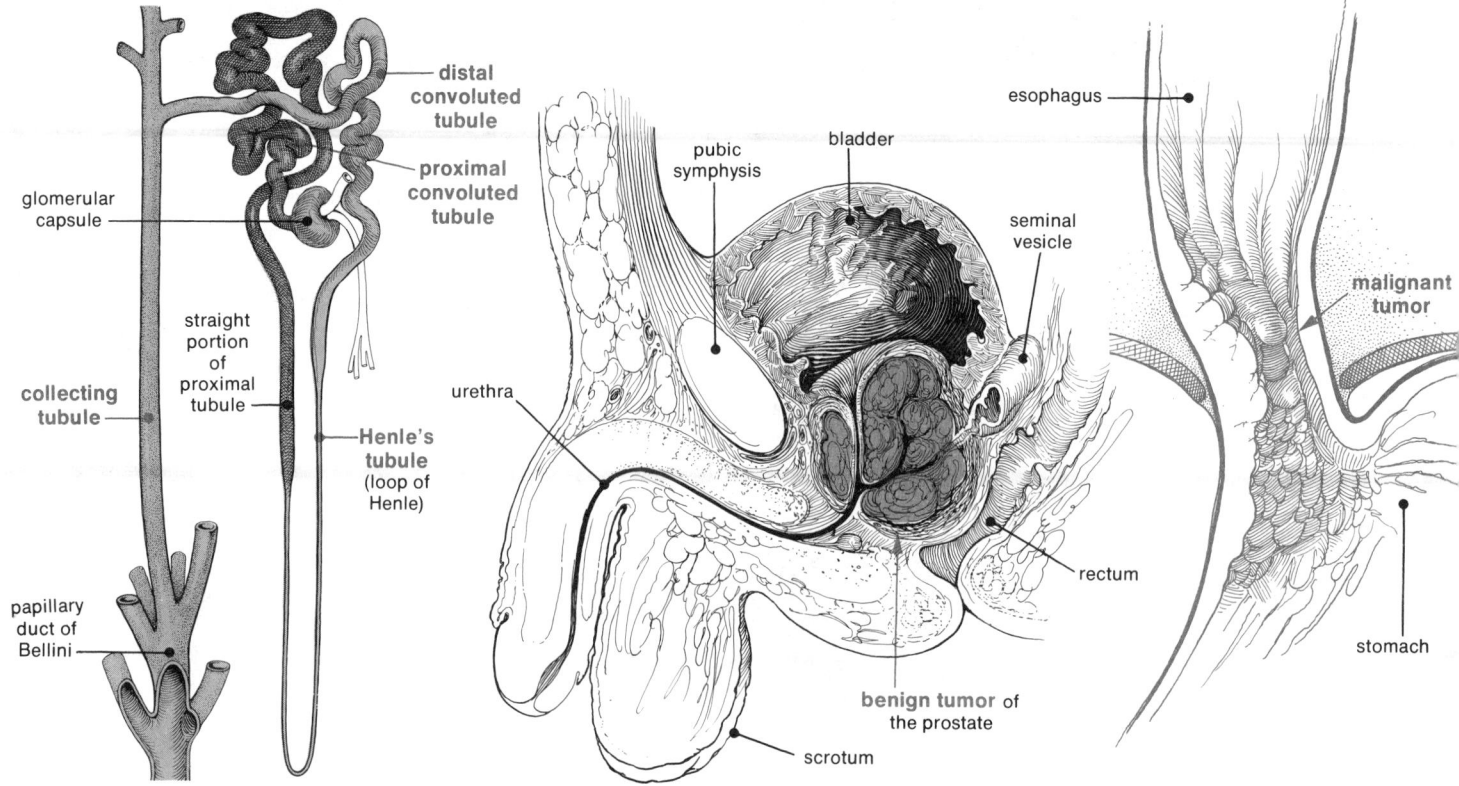

distal convoluted tubule

proximal convoluted tubule

glomerular capsule

straight portion of proximal tubule

collecting tubule

Henle's tubule (loop of Henle)

papillary duct of Bellini

pubic symphysis

bladder

esophagus

seminal vesicle

malignant tumor

urethra

rectum

stomach

benign tumor of the prostate

scrotum

tuberosity   A rounded protuberance from the surface of a bone or cartilage.

tuberous   Having many small rounded projections; lumpy. Also called nodular.

tubocurarine chloride   An active alkaloid derived from *Chondodendron tomentosum* that produces skeletal muscle paralysis by occupying the receptors at the neuromuscular junction, thereby blocking the action of the neurotransmitter acetylcholine; used to produce muscular relaxation during surgical operations and to reduce the severity of muscle spasms in severe tetanus.

tuboovarian   Relating to a uterine (fallopian) tube and ovary.

tubular   Relating to, shaped like, or consisting of a tube or tubes.

tubule   A small tube or canal. Also called tubulus.

  collecting t.   One of the straight tubules of the kidney (as opposed to the convoluted ones); it commences in the radiate part of the cortex, where it receives the distal convoluted tubule, and progresses to the renal pyramid in the medulla, where it empties into the papillary duct of Bellini. Also called straight tubule; excretory duct.

  convoluted t., distal   The tortuous portion of the renal tubule leading from the terminal part of the ascending limb of the nephronic (Henle's) loop to the collecting tubule.

  convoluted t., proximal   The tortuous portion of the renal tubule leading from the glomerular (Bowman's) capsule to the straight portion of the proximal tubule (pars recta) in the medullary ray. Also called pars convoluta.

  dental t.'s   Minute tubes or canals in the dentin of the tooth containing the dentinal fibers and extending radially from the pulp to the dentoenamel junction.

  Henle's t.'s   The straight descending and ascending limbs of a renal tubule which form the nephronic (Henle's) loop.

  malpighian t.'s   Slender tubular structures that emerge from the alimentary canal of some insects, usually between the midgut and hindgut.

  mesonephric t.'s   The tubules comprising the excretory organ (mesonephros) of the embryo; retained in the male beyond embryonic life as the epididymis and the deferent duct.

  proximal t.   The portion of the tubule leading from the glomerular capsule to the thin descending limb of the nephronic (Henle's) loop; it consists of a highly convoluted portion (pars convoluta) and a short straight segment (pars recta).

  renal t.   The part of the nephron responsible for conveying the glomerular filtrate to the renal pelvis and transforming it into the final urine product; it consists of the glomerular (Bowman's) capsule, proximal tubule, nephronic (Henle's) loop, distal tubule, and the collecting tubule.

  seminiferous t.'s   Long, threadlike, twisted tubules loosely packed in each lobule of the testis; the channels in which the spermatozoa develop and through which they are conveyed to the rete testis.

  transverse t.'s   Invaginations of the sarcolemma.

tubulization   Protection of an injured or sutured nerve with an absorbable cylinder to promote healing.

tubulorrhexis   Localized disintegration of epithelium and basement membrane of renal tubules; a characteristic lesion of acute tubular necrosis.

tuft   A cluster.

  malpighian t.   See glomerulus (1).

tularemia   An infectious disease caused by the bacterium *Pasteurella tularensis*, transmitted to man by the bite of infected animals and marked by a prolonged or remitted fever and swelling of the lymph nodes. Also called rabbit or deer-fly fever.

tumefacient   Causing a swelling.

tumefaction, tumescence   1. A swollen condition. 2. The process of swelling.

tumid   Swollen.

tumor   A neoplasm, an overgrowth of tissue.

  adenomatoid t.   Benign, slow growing, gray-white nodules of uncertain origin, occurring in both male and female genital tracts.

  adipose t.   See lipoma.

  benign t.   Tumor that does not metastasize or infiltrate and is unlikely to recur after its removal.

  blood t.   Tumor containing blood.

  carcinoid t.   One that arises from embryonic tissues (e.g., Wilm's tumor), occurs early in life and is usually malignant.

  carotid body t.   Chemodectoma.

  cellular t.   Tumor composed chiefly of cells of homogeneous stroma.

  desmoid t.   See desmoid.

  Ewing's t.   A malignant tumor occurring in the bones, especially the bones of the extremities, arising from medullary tissue; symptoms include fever, pain, and leukocytosis. Also called Ewing's sarcoma; diffuse endothelioma of bone.

  fibrocellular t.   See fibroma.

  fibroid t.   See fibroma.

  giant cell t. of bone   A soft, reddish-brown, usually benign tumor of long bones, composed chiefly of multinucleated giant cells and ovoid or spindle-shaped cells. Also called giant cell myeloma; osteoclastoma.

  glomus t.   An extremely painful, small, bluish-red benign tumor in the skin, arising from cells of a glomus body. Also called glomangioma.

  granular cell t.   A benign, usually small tumor of uncertain origin, often involving peripheral nerves in skin, mucosa, or connective tissue. Also called myoblastoma; granular cell myoblastoma.

  granulosa cell t.   A rare, benign (potentially malignant) tumor of the ovary, occurring most frequently during the active reproductive age; it elaborates estrogen and is sometimes the cause of precocious puberty.

  heterologous t.   A tumor composed of tissue different from the one in which it grows.

  homologous t.   Tumor made up of the same kind of tissue as the one from which it grows.

  Krukenberg t.   A malignant, usually bilateral, tumor of the ovary, secondary to a mucous carcinoma of the stomach.

  malignant t.   Tumor that forms metastases, may recur after removal, and eventually causes death if not treated early and appropriately. Also called cancer.

  mixed t.   Tumor composed of more than one tissue or cell type.

  mixed t. of salivary gland   Tumor believed to be derived from cells of salivary ducts or from embryonic cells of salivary glands; most frequently seen in the parotid gland. Also called pleomorphic adenoma.

  mucoid t.   See myxoma.

  osseous t.   See osteoma.

  papillary t.   See papilloma.

  phantom t.   An abdominal swelling, simulating an ovarian tumor or pregnancy; a form of neurosis.

  pontine angle t.   Tumor located in the proximal portion of the acoustic nerve.

  Pott's puffy t.   A circumscribed swelling of the scalp resulting from osteitis of the skull or from an extradural abscess.

  Schmincke t.   Tumor originating in the lingual and pharyngeal tonsils.

  Schwann's t.   See neurofibroma.

  theca cell t.   See thecoma.

  theca lutein cell t.   see thecoma.

  transition t.   A tumor originally appearing benign, recurring after removal, and then turning malignant.

  Warthin's t.   Papillary cystadenoma lymphatosum; see under cystadenoma.

  Wilm's t.   A malignant tumor of the kidney, occurring mostly in young children; composed of embryonic elements.

  Zollinger-Ellison t.   Tumor of the pancreas causing the Zollinger-Ellison syndrome.

tumorigenesis   The formation of a new growth.

tuning fork

tines

amniotic fluid

twin embryos

ossicles

internal ear

external auditory meatus

tympanum

$$HO- -CH_2-\underset{\underset{H}{|}}{\overset{\overset{NH_2}{|}}{C}}-COOH$$

tyrosine

tumorigenic Causing tumors.
tumorous Resembling a tumor.
tungsten A chemical element with a very high melting point used as the target material of an x-ray tube as well as in electric light filaments; symbol W, atomic number 74, atomic weight 183.86.
tunica A coat or enveloping layer of tissue.
  t. adventitia The fibrous outer layer of a blood vessel. Also called tunica externa.
  t. albuginea testis The thick, fibrous, bluish-white membrane covering the testis.
  t. dartos The highly vascular layer of smooth muscle in the scrotum; its deeper fibers form a septum which divides the scrotum in two halves.
  t. intima The inner, serous layer of an artery.
  t. media The middle muscular layer of an artery.
  t. vaginalis propria testis A closed serous pouch investing the testis; it consists of a parietal and a visceral layer.
tuning fork A forklike metal instrument with two prongs which, when struck, produce a sound of fixed pitch; used for testing hearing and vibratory sensation.
turbidimetric Relating to the measurement of turbidity.
turbidimetry Measurement of turbidity or cloudiness of a fluid.
turbidity Cloudiness caused by the stirring up of sediment or suspended foreign particles, resulting in a loss of transparency.
turbinate 1. Shaped like an inverted cone or a scroll. 2. A turbinate bone. See table of bones.
turbine A rotary instrument activated by a stream of water.
turbinectomy Surgical removal of a turbinate bone.
Turcot syndrome The presence of polyps in the colon combined with brain tumors; transmitted as an autosomal recessive trait.
turgescence The process of swelling; the state of being swollen.
turgid Congested; bloated.
turgor Fullness.
turista Colloquial term for traveler's diarrhea.
turn To move a fetus in the uterus from a malposition to one that will facilitate normal delivery.
Turner's syndrome Condition due to a chromosomal anomaly (only one X chromosome); absence of ovaries or possession of only rudimentary structures, infantile female genitalia, short stature, and webbed neck are some of the symptoms.
TURP Acronym for transurethral resection of prostate.
tussis A cough.
tussive Relating to or caused by a cough.
twin 1. One of two children born at one birth. 2.

Double; growing in pairs.
  cojoined t.'s Twins having varying degrees of connection or fusion with each other. Also called Siamese twins.
  dizygotic t.'s See fraternal twins.
  fraternal t.'s Twins developed from two separate ova; they may or may not be of the same sex. Also called dizygotic or heterozygous twins.
  heterozygous t.'s See fraternal twins.
  identical t.'s Twins resulting from a single fertilized egg that splits at an early stage of development; they are always of the same sex, have the same genetic constitution, and have pronounced resemblance to one another. Also called monozygotic or uniovular twins.
  monozygotic t.'s. See identical twins.
  Siamese t.'s Cojoined twins; originally applied to the publicized conjoined twins from Siam.
  uniovular t.'s See identical twins.
twinge A sudden, short, sharp physical or mental pain.
twitch 1. A brief involuntary or spasmodic contraction of a muscle fiber; usually phasic. 2. To move sharply and suddenly; to jerk.
two-carbon fragment The acetyl group CH_3CO-.
tyloma Heavy callus formation.
  t. conjunctivae A localized cornification of the conjunctiva.
tylosis 1. The formation of a callus. 2. A callosity.
tympanectomy Removal of the tympanic membrane.
tympanic Relating to the chamber of the middle ear.
tumpanites Distention of the abdomen due to accumulation of gas in the intestines. Also called meteorism.
tympanitic 1. Relating to tympanites, as the sound produced by percussing over the distended abdomen. 2. Tympanic or resonant.
tympanocentesis Aspiration of fluid from the middle ear with a needle inserted through the tympanic membrane; procedure used to identify organisms causing persistent middle ear infections.
tympanomastoiditis Inflammation of the middle ear and the mastoid cells.
tympanometry The measurement of the flow of sound energy in the external auditory meatus; a means of detecting middle ear disease.
tympanoplasty A general term denoting any of several operative procedures designed to restore hearing in patients with middle ear or conductive hearing loss.
  type I t. See myringoplasty.
tympanosclerosis Scarring of the tympanic membrane (eardrum), causing hearing impairment.

tympanosquamosal Pertaining to the tympanic and squamous portions of the temporal bone.
tympanotomy See myringotomy.
tympanum The chamber of the middle ear, a cavity in the temporal bone housing the chain of ossicles.
tympany A drumlike percussion sound.
type A pattern of characteristics common to a number of individuals, chemical substances, diseases, etc.
  blood t. See blood group.
  wild t. In genetics, the standard or the parent strain of an experimental microorganism; the most frequently observed form of an organism, or the one arbitrarily designated as normal.
typhoid Resembling typhus.
typhous Relating to typhus.
typhus An acute infectious and contagious disease caused by a *Rickettsia* and marked by sustained high fever, severe headache, and a characteristic rash. Also called typhus fever.
  endemic t. See murine typhus.
  epidemic t. Typhus caused by *Rickettsia prowazekii* and transmitted by body lice.
  murine t. Typhus caused by *Rickettsia mooseri* and transmitted by the rat flea. Also called endemic or flea-borne typhus.
  recrudescent t. Still Brill-Zinsser disease.
  scrub t. See tsutsugamushi disease.
typing Determination of the type category to which any entity belongs.
  DNA t. Test on a nucleated cell (e.g., of semen, blood, hair roots) to detect characteristics in genetic structure that are as unique to an individual as fingerprints. Also called DNA fingerprinting or profiling.
tyramine A colorless amine found in decayed animal tissue, certain cheeses, and ergot; produced by the decarboxylation of tyrosine; it has a weak sympathomimetic action but releases stored norepinephrine and has been used as a provocative agent in the diagnosis of pheochromocytoma.
tyrosinase A copper-containing oxidizing enzyme in bodily tissues which converts tyrosine into a red indole compound and thence to melanin; it catalyzes the oxidation of phenolic compounds. Also called monophenol oxidase.
tyrosine (Tyr) A crystallizable amino acid, $C_9H_{11}NO_3$, that is sparingly soluble in water; present in most proteins; an essential constituent of any diet; a precursor of melanin and thyroxin.
tyrosinosis A hereditary disease of tyrosine metabolism; believed to be caused by lack of p-hydroxyphenylpyruvic and oxidase, with resulting excessive excretion of p-hydroxyphenylpyruvic acid.

diabetic ulcer

ubiquinone

umbilical area of abdomen

umbilicus

ubiquinone 2,3-Dimethoxybenzoquinones, a hydrophobic compound that plays a role in electron transport in tissues. Also called coenzyme Q (for quinone).

udder The baglike mammary gland of animals such as cows, sheep, and goats.

ulcer A depressed lesion on the skin or mucous membrane.

aphthous u.'s Small whitish ulcers surrounded by a red border, occurring on the mucosa of the mouth in aphthous stomatitis.

Curling's u. Ulcer occurring in the duodenum as a result of severe bodily burns.

decubitus u. Ulcer of the skin, and sometimes muscles, occurring in pressure areas of bedridden patients allowed to lie in the same position for long periods of time. Also called bedsore; pressure sore.

dendriform u. Superficial ulcer of the cornea that spreads in a branching fashion in various directions; caused by the herpes simplex virus.

dental u. Lesion on the oral mucosa resulting from biting or friction from a rough edge on a tooth.

diabetic u. Ulcer associated with diabetes, occurring most frequently in the lower extremities, especially the toes.

duodenal u. Ulceration of the mucous lining of the duodenum.

esophageal u. Ulcer generally located at the lower end of the esophagus, frequently due to chronic regurgitation of gastric juice.

gastric u. Ulcer of the stomach usually on or near the lesser curvature.

gummatous u. Ulcer occurring during the late stage of syphilis.

indolent u. Ulcer that does not respond to treatment.

penetrating u. Ulcer that extends into the deep tissues of an organ, as a duodenal ulcer that penetrates into the pancreas.

peptic u. Ulcer of the mucous membrane of the stomach or duodenum caused by the digestive action of acid-pepsin gastric juice.

perforated u. Ulcer that has eroded through the wall of an organ, such as that of the stomach.

rodent u. Basal cell carcinoma of the skin.

roentgen u. Ulcer caused by overexposure to x rays.

stercoral u. Ulcer of the colon caused by impacted feces.

stomal u. Ulcer in jejunal mucosa following (and occurring near) the surgical union of the jejunum and stomach.

stress u. Peptic ulcer associated with other conditions.

transparent u. Ulcer occurring on the cornea and

healing without opacity.

trophic u. Ulcer due to impaired circulation to the part.

tropical u. Sloughing ulcer occurring usually on the legs as a bacterial infection superimposed on a scratch or insect bite; seen in tropical climates.

varicose u. Ulcer due to and overlying a varicose vein.

venereal u. Chancroid.

ulcerate To form an ulcer.

ulceration 1. The formation of an ulcer. 2. An ulcer.

ulcerative 1. Causing the formation of ulcers. 2. Marked by ulceration.

ulcerogenic Causing the formation of ulcers.

ulcerous Characterized by the presence of ulcers.

ulerythema An inflammatory process that ultimately results in atrophy or scarring.

u. ophryogenes Folliculitis of the eyebrows resulting in scarring and redness.

ulna The larger of the two bones of the forearm, extending from the elbow to the wrist on the side opposite to the thumb.

ulnar Relating to the ulna.

ulnoradial Relating to the ulna and radius (bones of the forearm).

ulotomy The cutting or sectioning of contracting scar tissue to relieve tension or deformity.

ultracentrifuge A convection-free high speed centrifuge (up to ±100,000 rpm); used in the separation of large molecules and for determinations of molecular weight.

ultrafilter A semipermeable membrane (collodion, fish bladder, or filter paper impregnated with gels) used for performing ultrafiltration.

ultrafiltration 1. Filtration through a filter capable of removing all but the smallest particles, such as viruses. 2. Filtration through a semipermeable membrane for the separation of colloids from their dispersion medium and dissolved crystalloids.

ultraligation Ligation or tying of a blood vessel beyond the point where a branch is given off.

ultramicrometer A micrometer with an extremely accurate gauge, capable of measuring to one millionth of a centimeter.

ultramicroscope A dark field microscope with high-intensity refracted illumination for viewing very minute objects or particles of colloidal size; the horizontal beam of light striking the particles is refracted and appears as bright spots against a black background.

ultramicroscopic Too small to be visible under the ordinary microscope.

ultramicrotome An instrument for cutting tissue into very thin sections (0.1μ thick, or less) for

electron microscopy.

ultrasonic Not perceptible to the human ear; relating to sound waves above 30,000 cycles per second.

ultrasonogram A record made by ultrasonography.

ultrasonograph An apparatus that sends sound impulses (at frequencies above the range audible to the human ear) toward an organ, which in turn bounces back or echoes the sounds; the patterns produced are graphically displayed on a fluorescent screen for interpretation. Also called ultrasonoscope.

ultrasonography The delineation of deep bodily structures by measuring the reflection of ultrasonic waves directed into the tissue. Also called sonography; echography.

Doppler u. Diagnostic technique to measure and visually record changes in the frequency of a continuous ultrasonic wave, indicative of the change in velocity of the blood-flow in underlying vessels.

gray-scale u. Amplification and processing of echoes (by a television video-scan converter) into a visual image ranging from white to different shades of gray, white representing the strongest echoes.

ultrasonoscope See ultrasonograph.

ultrasonosurgery The use of ultrasound (high frequency sound waves) to disrupt tissues or tracts, especially in the central nervous system.

ultrasonotomy A psychosurgical procedure in which discrete brain lesions are produced, generally in the prefrontal lobes, by high frequency sound waves; used in the treatment of certain severe psychiatric disorders.

ultrasound Sound waves of frequency higher than the range audible to the human ear, or above 20,000 cycles per second (hertz); the waves are propagated at a speed determined by the physical properties of the medium through which they travel.

ultrastructure The ultimate structure or organization of protoplasm, as seen with the aid of the electron microscope. Also called fine or submicroscopic structure.

ultraviolet (UV) Denoting a range of invisible radiation extending from the visible violet portion of the spectrum out to the low-frequency x-ray region of the electromagnetic spectrum.

ululation 1. The loud, inarticulate crying of emotionally disturbed persons, especially hysterical ones. 2. Loud lamentation.

umbilical Relating to or resembling the navel.

umbilicated, umbilicate Dimpled; having a pit or depression that resembles the navel.

umbilication A depression or pit resembling the navel.

umbilicus The depressed area of the abdominal

unguis

unilateral deformity

Units of Concentration			Units of Energy and Work		
molar (mol/liter)		M	joule		J
parts per million		ppm	calorie		cal
Units of Length			**Units of Temperature**		
meter		m	degree centigrade		°
micrometer (micron)		μm (μ)	thermodynamic temperature		K
Angstrom (0.1 nm)		Å	(Kelvin)		
Units of Volume			**Units of Radioactivity**		
milliliter		ml	counts per minute		cpm
microliter		μl	curie(s)		Ci
Units of Mass			**Miscellaneous Units**		
gram		g	revolutions per minute		rpm
microgram		μg	cycles per second (hertz)		Hz
			pascal (newton/meter$_2$)		Pa
Units of Time			lux		lx
hour		hr	candela		cd
minute		min	lumen		lm
second		s, sec			

Units of electricity		
ampere		amp
milliampere		mA
volt		V
ohm		Ω

Prefixes to Names of Units

exa	10^{18}	E	milli	10^{-3}	m
peta	10^{15}	P	micro	10^{-6}	μ
tera	10^{12}	T	nano	10^{-9}	n
giga	10^{9}	G	pico	10^{-12}	p
mega	10^{6}	M	femto	10^{-15}	f
kilo	10^{3}	k	atto	10^{-18}	a
centi	10^{-2}	c			

wall where the umbilical cord was attached to the fetus. Also called navel.

umbo, *pl.* **umbones 1.** A projection at the center of a rounded surface. **2.** The most depressed point on the outer surface of the tympanic membrane, formed by traction of the malleus on the inner surface of the membrane to which it is attached.

unciform Hook-shaped.

Uncinaria A genus of the class Nematoda, characterized by a hooklike structure.

   U. americana See *Necator americanus.*

   U. duodenalis See *Ancylostoma duodenale.*

uncinariasis Condition due to the presence of hookworms (species of Ancylostoma or Necator) in the intestine. Also called ancylostomiasis.

uncinate Hooked or shaped like a hook.

unconscious 1. Inability to respond to sensory stimuli. **2.** In Freudian theory, the part of the mind containing feelings, urges, and experiences of which the individual is only briefly or never aware.

uncoupler Any substance (such as dinitrophenol) that uncouples the usual linkage between oxidation and phosphorylation.

uncus The hooked anterior portion of the hippocampal gyrus.

undecylenic acid An antifungal proprietary agent, $CH_2CH(CH_2)_8COOH$, used in treating dermatophytic infections.

underachiever An individual, especially a student, who manifestly performs below his capacity as determined by tests of intelligence, aptitude, or ability.

undercut 1. The portion of a prepared tooth cavity that mechanically locks the restorative filling, such as amalgam, into place. **2.** The portion of a tooth that lies between the gingiva and the crest of contour. **3.** The contour of a dental arch which prevents the proper insertion of a denture.

undernutrition Any deviation below good nutrition; a condition resulting from a negative nutritive balance that occurs when metabolic utilization plus excretion of one or more essential nutrients exceeds the supply.

undescended Not descended to a normal position, as a testis that is retained in the abdomen.

undifferentiated Not differentiated; usually applied to cells.

undo Psychoanalytically, to act out in reverse an unacceptable prior action (a defense mechanism).

undulate 1. To fluctuate in wavelike patterns, as some fevers. **2.** Having an irregular, wavy border or appearance, as seen in the shape of a bacterial colony.

unerupted In dentistry, denoting a normal developing tooth or an impacted tooth that has not

emerged or perforated the oral mucosa.

ungual Relating to the nails. Also called unguinal.

unguent Ointment.

unguentum (ung., ungt.) Latin for ointment; used in prescription writing.

unguiculate Having nails or claws.

unguis, *pl.* **ungues** Latin for nail (either a fingernail or a toenail).

uniaxal 1. Possessing but one axis; e.g., a hinge joint. **2.** Developing chiefly in only one direction.

unicameral Consisting of a single cavity; characterized by one compartment only.

unicellular Consisting of one cell, as a protozoan.

unicuspid Denoting a tooth with one cusp.

uniform Consistent in appearance; without variation in form.

unigravida Primigravida.

unilaminar Possessing only one layer.

unilateral Occurring only on one side.

unilocular Having only one compartment.

uninuclear, uninucleate Having only one nucleus.

uniocular Relating to or having one eye.

union The process of joining together of tissues. Also called healing.

   delayed u. Healing of a fractured bone which appears to be unduly slow.

   faulty u. A condition where tissues have united but not in their proper positions.

   fibrous u. Formation of a fibrous callus on a bone at the site of a fracture without development of bone tissue.

   primary u. Healing that occurs without delay and without complicating infection. Also called healing by first intention.

   syngamic nuclear u. The uniting of the nuclei of spermatozoon and ovum during fertilization.

   vicious u. A faulty union that produces a deformity.

unipara Primipara.

unipennate Resembling one half of a feather; said of certain muscles with a tendon on one side. Also called unipenniform; demipenniform.

unipolar Having, produced by, or located at one pole.

uniport Transport of one substance across a cell membrane by a protein carrier.

unit (u) An entity regarded as an elementary constituent of a larger whole.

   Ångström u. (Å, AU, A) A unit of wavelength equal to .10 of a nanometer (millimicron).

   antigen u. The smallest amount of antigen that, in the presence of specific antiserum, will fix one unit of complement so as to prevent hemolysis.

   antitoxin u. The unit for expressing the amount

of antitoxin that will neutralize 100 minimal lethal doses of toxin.

   base u. Any one of the fundamental units of a system of measurement, such as those of the International System of Units (SI); i.e., the meter (m), kilogram (kg), second (s), ampere (A), kelvin (K), mole (mol), and candela (cd).

   British thermal u. (BTU) The amount of heat required to increase the temperature of one pound of water from 39° to 40°F.

   centimeter-gram-second u. (CGS unit) A metric unit denoting a rate of work.

   CGS u. Abbreviation for centimeter-gram-second unit.

   coronary care u. (CCU) A facility designed to provide maximal surveillance and optimal therapy for patients suspected of having acute myocardial infarctions and other acute cardiac disorders requiring intensive and continuous monitoring.

   dental u. An operative unit in which are assembled items used in dental procedures, such as saliva ejector, compressed air, dental engine, operatory light, water supply, cuspidor, etc.

   G-u. A coupling protein in the plasma membrane, between the hormone receptor and adenyl cyclase, which facilitates transmission of a hormonal signal.

   gravitational u. A unit equal to one pound of force divided by one pound of mass.

   Hounsfield u. Unit of x-ray attenuation used for CT scans, based on a scale in which air is -1000, water is 0, and bone is $+1000$.

   insulin u. See international insulin unit.

   intensive care u. (ICU) A specially equipped facility in a hospital operated by trained personnel for the care of critically ill individuals requiring immediate and continuous attention; also called medical intensive care unit (MICU); one designed to handle surgical problems is known as surgical intensive care unit (SICU).

   international insulin u. A unit of 0.045 milligram of pure international standard zinc-insulin crystals.

   international system of u.'s See under system.

   international u. (IU) A unit of biologic substance (e.g., vitamins) established by the World Health Organization (WHO).

   international u. of vitamin A The biologic activity of 0.3 micrograms of vitamin A (alcohol form).

   international u. of vitamin D The antirachitic activity of 0.025 micrograms of a standard preparation of crystalline vitamin D.

   King u. The amount of phosphatase which, acting upon disodium phenylphosphate at pH 9 for 30 minutes, liberates one milligram of phenol; a test of alkaline phosphatase activity; normal values in adult

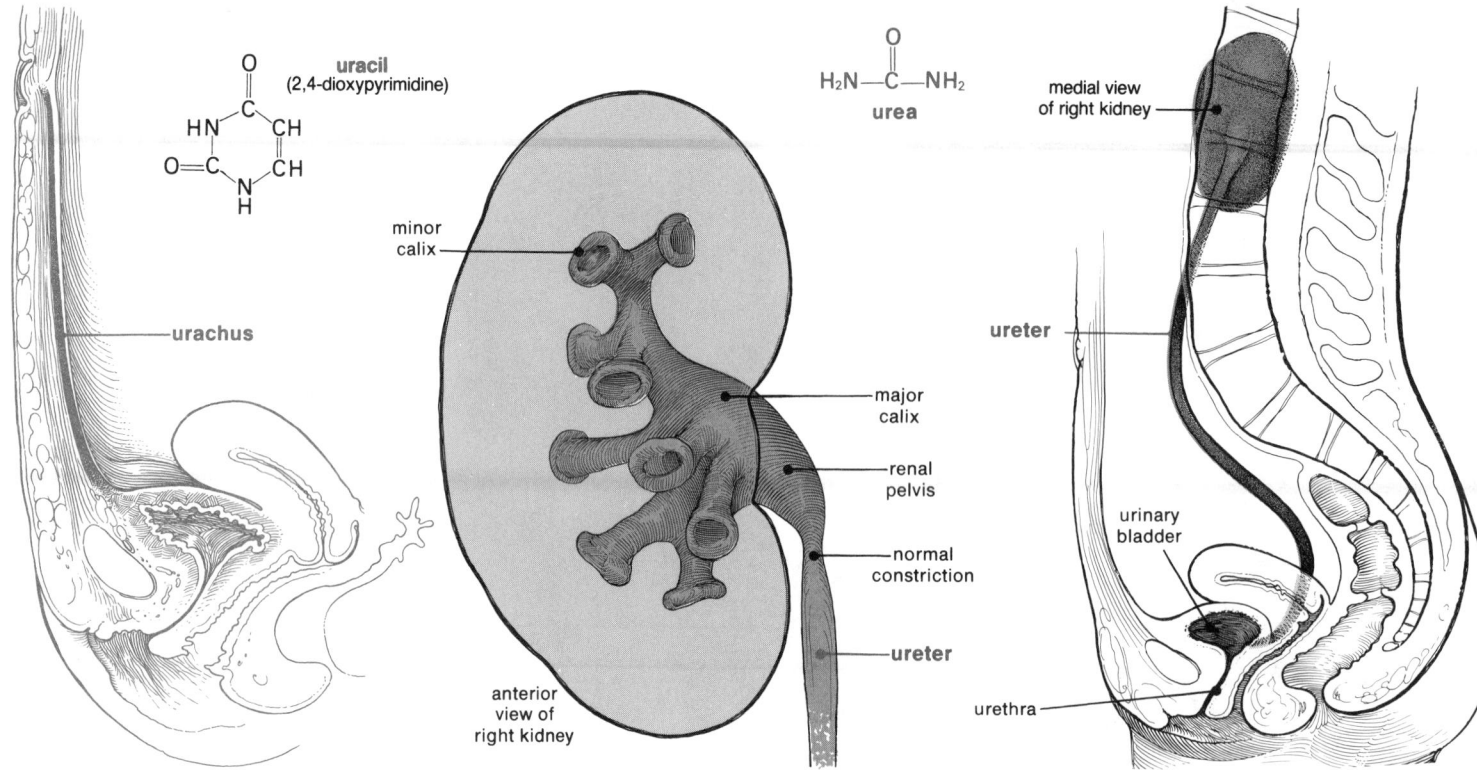

uracil
(2,4-dioxypyrimidine)

urea

medial view
of right kidney

urachus

minor
calix

major
calix

renal
pelvis

normal
constriction

ureter

anterior
view of
right kidney

ureter

urinary
bladder

urethra

serum are five to 13 units.

map u. The relative distance between two loci (specific gene sites) on a chromosome as determined by the frequency of crossing over (recombination). Also called map distance.

motor u. A motor nerve cell and the muscle fibers it innervates.

photofluorographic u. (PF unit) An apparatus consisting of an x-ray tube and a generator coupled to a photographic camera to record miniature radiographs.

rat u. (R.U.) The amount of a substance that under standardized conditions is just enough to produce a specified result in experimental rats.

SI u. Système International d'Unités; international system of units. See under system.

Svedberg u. A unit of time and velocity measuring the sedimentation constant of a colloid solution, equal to 10^{-13} seconds.

u. of force In the centimeter-gram-second (CGS) system, the dyne; the amount of force which accelerates a mass of one gram one centimeter per second.

u. of heat In the centimeter-gram-second (CGS) system, the calorie; the amount of heat required to raise one milliliter of water from 14.5 to 15.5°C.

u. of oxytocin The oxytocic activity of 0.5 milligram of the USP Posterior-pituitary Reference Standard; one milligram of synthetic oxytocin corresponds to 500 international units.

u. of penicillin The penicillin activity of 0.6 microgram of the Food and Drug Administration master standard.

u. of vasopressin The pressor activity of 0.5 milligram of the USP Posterior-pituitary Reference Standard.

USP u. A United States Pharmacopeia measure of the potency of any pharmacologic preparation.

United States Adopted Name Council (USAN) An enterprise that gives nonproprietary names to new drugs; it replaced the older AMA-USP Nomenclature Committee.

univalent Having a valence of one; having the combining power of one hydrogen atom. Also called monovalent.

unmyelinated Having no myelin sheath; a characteristic of some nerve fibers.

Unna's boot A flexible and porous occlusive dressing, similar to a plaster cast but consisting of gauze bandage impregnated with a gelatinous substance and a paste; applied primarily to the foot and leg, especially in treating dermatitides and ulcerated conditions.

unsaturated 1. Not saturated; denoting a solution capable of dissolving more solute at a given temperature. 2. Denoting an organic compound possessing

double or triple bonds, as ethylene. 3. Denoting a chemical compound in which all the affinities are not satisfied, thereby allowing other atoms or radicals to be added to it.

unsex To deprive of gonads or sexual attributes; to castrate.

unstable 1. Denoting emotional instability; psychologically maladjusted; not mentally fit to assume responsibility; unreliable. 2. Tending strongly to undergo spontaneous change, said of a solution. 3. Readily decomposing, as in radioactivity. 4. Not steady or consistent in action or performance.

unstriated Lacking striations; denoting the structure of the smooth muscle.

untoward Resistant to treatment.

upper Slang expression meaning an amphetamine pill or other substance which acts as a mood elevator.

uptake The amount of a substance, especially a radionuclide, absorbed by any tissue; e.g., radioiodine (^{131}I) by the thyroid gland.

urachal Of or relating to the urachus.

urachus A canal present in the fetus between the umbilicus and the apex of the bladder; after birth it normally persists as a solid fibrous cord.

patent u. A urachus which remains open after birth. Also called urachal fistula.

uracil 2,4-Dioxypyrimidine, a prevalent pyrimidine (base) found in nucleic acid.

uranium A heavy silvery-white, radioactive metallic element, occurring in several minerals, especially pitchblende; it has a half-life of 4.5×10^9 years; symbol U, atomic number 92, atomic weight 238.07.

^{235}U A uranium isotope with a half-life of 713 million years; the first substance shown capable of supporting a self-sustaining chain reaction.

^{238}U The most common uranium isotope, with a half-life of 4.51 billion years.

uranostaphyloplasty A surgical procedure for repairing a defect (usually a cleft) of both the soft and the hard palate. Also called uranostaphylorrhaphy.

uranostaphyloschisis Fissure or cleft of both the soft and hard palate.

uranyl The UO_2^{++} ion, as in such salts as uranyl nitrate, $UO_2(NO_3)_2$, and uranyl sulfate, UO_2SO_4.

urate A salt of uric acid; occurs commonly in urinary deposits and calculi.

urea 1. $CO(NH_2)_2$; chief end product of mammalian protein metabolism, formed in the liver from amino acids and compounds of ammonia; the chief nitrogenous component of urine; an average person, in steady state and consuming average amounts of dietary protein, excretes about 30 g of urea per day. 2. A preparation of hypertonic urea (30%) used intravenously to temporarily reduce intracranial or

cerebrospinal pressure in the control of cerebral edema; Ureaphil®.

urease An enzyme that promotes the breakdown of urea into ammonia and carbon dioxide; present in certain seeds and produced by certain microorganisms, especially *Proteus* bacteria.

urecchysis Escape of urine into the tissues; e.g., in rupture of the bladder.

uredema A swollen or edematous condition resulting from infiltration of extravasated urine into the tissues.

uredo 1. Urticaria. 2. A burning or itching sensation in the skin.

urelcosis Ulceration of any part of the urinary passage.

uremia A toxic condition caused by retention in the blood of waste substances normally excreted in the urine; the principal wastes that accumulate are products of protein metabolism; symptoms may include lethargy, loss of appetite, vomiting, anemia, blood clotting disorders, an abnormal mental state, pericarditis, and colitis.

uremic Relating to uremia.

ureolysis The breaking down of urea into carbon dioxide and ammonia.

uresis Urination.

ureter The long, slender, muscular tube that conveys urine from the pelvis of the kidney to the base of the bladder.

ureteral Relating to the ureter.

ureterectasia Distention of a ureter.

ureterectomy Surgical removal of a ureter or a segment of it.

ureteric Of or relating to a ureter or ureters.

ureterocele A cystlike dilatation at the lower end of a ureter, usually protruding into the bladder.

ureterocystostomy See ureteroneocystostomy.

ureteroenterostomy The surgical procedure of forming an anastomosis between a ureter and the intestine.

ureterogram A roentgenogram of a ureter after injection of a radiopaque substance.

ureterography The practice of x-raying the ureter after injection of a radiopaque substance.

ureterolith A stone in the ureter.

ureterolithiasis The presence of a calculus in a ureter.

ureterolithotomy Surgical removal of a stone from a ureter.

ureterolysis Rupture of a ureter.

ureteroneocystostomy Transplantation of the distal part of the ureter to a site in the bladder other than the normal one. Also called ureterocystostomy.

ureteronephrectomy Surgical removal of a kidney and its ureter.

uterus
urinary bladder
female urethra

CH2OH uridine diphosphate glucose

urinary bladder

uric acid

urinary bladder

male urethra

uterus
urinary bladder
urethrocele
cystocele

ureteropelvic Pertaining to a ureter and the adjoining renal pelvis.
ureteropyelitis Inflammation of a ureter extending up to and including the pelvis of the kidney.
ureteropyelogram Pyelogram.
ureteropyeloneostomy A surgical procedure for excising a portion of the ureter and inserting the remaining part through a new opening into the pelvis of the kidney.
ureteropyeloplasty Reparative surgery of the ureter and pelvis of the kidney.
ureteropyosis Accumulation of pus in a ureter.
ureterosigmoid Pertaining to the ureter and the sigmoid colon.
ureterosigmoidostomy Surgical implantation of the ureters into the sigmoid colon.
ureterostenosis Abnormal stricture of a ureter.
ureterostomy, cutaneous Attachment of the divided distal end of a ureter to the skin of the lower abdomen to create an external opening through which urine may be discharged when the bladder has been removed.
ureterotomy Any surgical division of a ureter.
ureteroureterostomy Surgical connection of the two ureters or of two sections of a ureter.
ureterovaginal Relating to or communicating with a ureter and the vagina.
ureterovesical Relating to a ureter and the bladder, as the junction of the two structures.
ureterovesicostomy Surgical division of a ureter and its implantation to another site in the bladder.
urethra The canal leading from the bladder and conveying urine to the exterior of the body.
  anterior u. The portion of the male urethra from the bulb to the tip of the glans penis; consisting of three parts: the bulbous, the pendulous, and the glandular parts.
  female u. A channel, about 38 mm long, extending from the bladder to the urinary opening behind the clitoris.
  male u. A channel, about 203 or 228 mm long, extending from the bladder to the opening at the tip of the glans penis; it conveys spermatic fluid as well as urine.
  posterior u. The portion of the male urethra extending from the neck of the bladder to the bulb; it consists of two parts: the prostatic and the membranous parts.
urethral Relating to the urethra.
urethralgia Pain in the urethra.
urethratresia Occlusion or atresia of the urethra.
urethrectomy Surgical removal of the urethra, or a segment of it.
urethremorrhagia Bleeding from the urethra.

Also called urethrorrhagia.
urethrism, urethrismus Irritability or chronic spasm of the urethra, usually associated with inflammation which may involve also the lower portion of the bladder.
urethritis Inflammation of the urethra.
  non-gonococcal u. (NGU) A sexually transmitted disease caused by various organisms, most commonly chlamydia; in males it usually produces a mild burning sensation on urination and a slight, grayish discharge, most commonly apparent before the first urination of the day; in females, it produces no symptoms although the organisms may be present in the cervix; a pregnant woman may transmit the infection to her newborn with serious complications. Also called non-specific urethritis.
  non-specific u. (NSU) See non-gonococcal urethritis.
urethrocele 1. Prolapse of the female urethra. 2. A sac or diverticulum of the wall of the female urethra.
urethrocystitis Inflammation of the urethra and bladder.
urethrocystopexy Operation for the relief of stress incontinence in which the urethrovesical junction is sutured to the back of the pubic bone.
urethrography The roentgenologic study of the urethra.
urethrometer An instrument for measuring the caliber of the urethra.
urethropenile Relating to the urethra and the penis.
urethrophyma Any circumscribed swelling or tumor of the urethra.
urethroplasty Surgical repair of a wound or a defect of the urethra.
urethroprostatic Relating to the urethra and the prostate gland.
urethrorectal Relating to or communicating with the urethra and the rectum.
urethrorrhagia Bleeding from the urethra.
urethrorrhea Abnormal discharge from the urethra.
urethroscope An instrument for inspecting the interior of the urethra.
urethroscopy Visual examination of the urethra with a urethroscope.
urethrospasm Spasmodic contraction of the urethra.
urethrostenosis Narrowing or stricture of the urethra.
urethrostomy Surgical formation of an opening into the urethra for temporary or permanent diversion of urine.
urethrotome An instrument for dividing a ure-

thral stricture.
urethrotomy Division of the urethra for treatment of a stricture or removal of a foreign body.
urethrovaginal Relating to the urethra and vagina.
urethrovesical Relating to the urethra and the bladder.
uric Relating to urine.
uric acid A white crystalline compound, $C_5H_4O_3$; a normal constituent of urine. Also called lithic acid.
uricolysis The splitting up of uric acid molecules.
uricosuria The passage of uric acid in the urine.
uricosuric An agent that tends to increase the excretion of uric acid in the urine.
uridine (Urd) $C_9H_{12}N_2O_6$, a ribonucleoside containing uracil; important in carbohydrate metabolism; 1-β-D-ribofuranosyluracil.
  u. diphosphate (UDP) A nucleotide important in glycogen and galactose metabolism and in nucleic acid synthesis.
  u. diphosphate galactose (UDP-galactose) A nucleotide derivative of galactose, resulting from the reaction of uridine diphosphate glucose (UDP-glucose) and galactose-1-phosphate. Also called diphosphogalactose.
  u. diphosphate glucose (UDP-glucose) A nucleotide derivative of glucose intermediary in glycogen synthesis; formed from the reaction of glucose-1-phosphate and uridine triphosphate (UTP). Also called uridine diphosphoglucose (UDPG).
  u. triphosphate (UTP) A high-energy nucleotide that participates in glycogen metabolism.
uridrosis The presence of urea or uric acid in the perspiration, sometimes deposited on the skin as minute crystals. Also written urhidrosis.
uridyltransferase See hexose-1-phosphate uridylyltransferase.
urinalysis Analysis of urine.
  routine u. Testing of the urine for the presence of abnormal amounts of protein or sugar, acidity, and specific gravity, and microscopic examination of the sediment from a centrifuged sample of urine.
urinary Relating to urine.
urinate To pass urine, to micturate.
urination The passing of urine. Also called micturition.
urine The fluid excreted by the kidneys, stored in the bladder, and discharged through the urethra; composed of approximately 96% water and 4% solid matter, chiefly urea and sodium chloride.
  residual u. The urine left over in the bladder after urination.
uriniferous Conveying urine, as the tubules in the kidney.
urinogenous Producing urine.

499

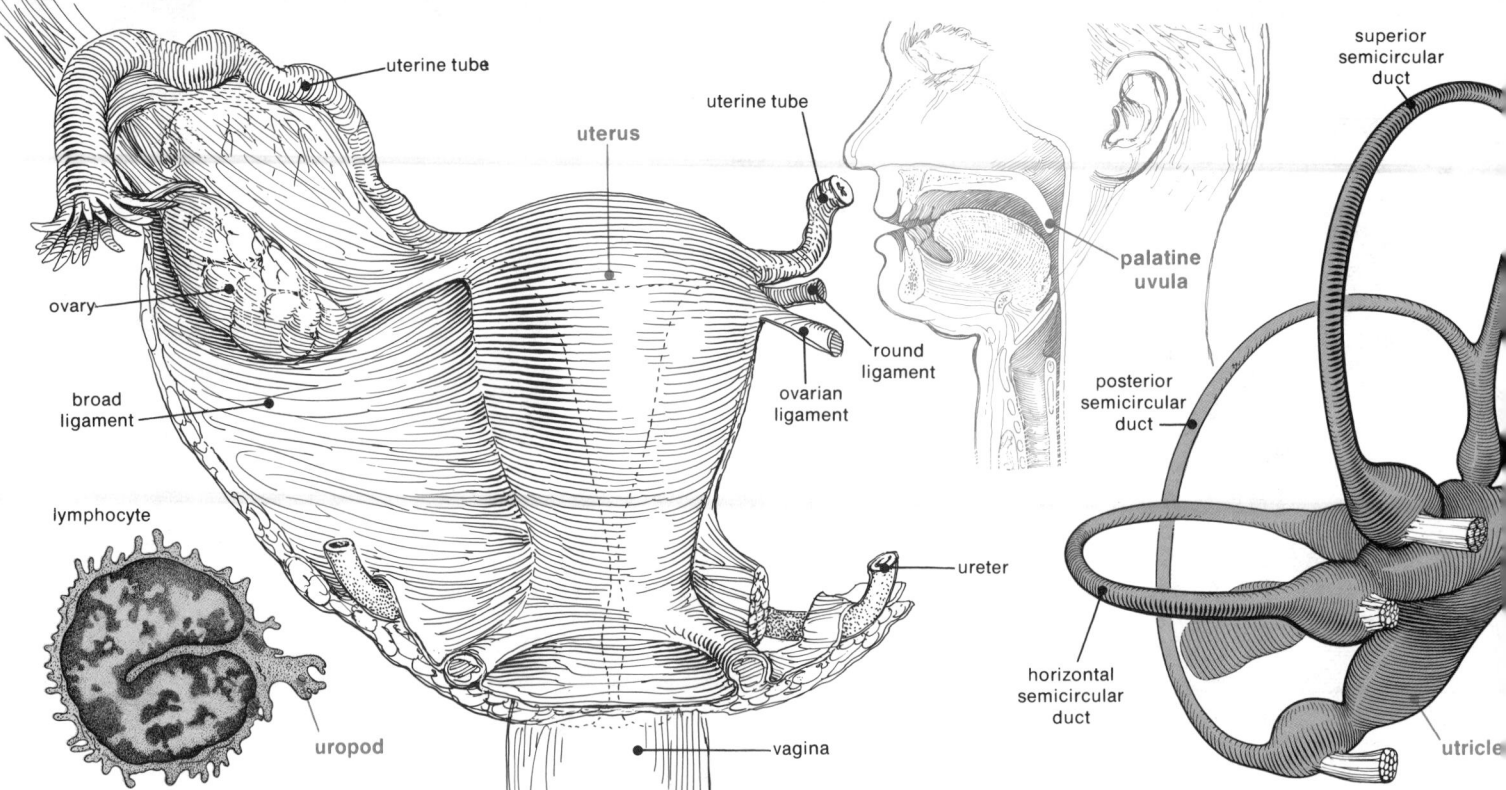

uterine tube

uterus

uterine tube

ovary

broad ligament

lymphocyte

round ligament

ovarian ligament

palatine uvula

superior semicircular duct

posterior semicircular duct

ureter

horizontal semicircular duct

uropod

vagina

utricle

urinometer A device used for determining the specific gravity of urine. Also called urometer; urogravimeter.

uroacidimeter An apparatus for estimating the degree of acidity of a sample of urine.

urobilin A pigment normally found in small amounts in urine; formed by the oxidation of urobilinogen.

urobilinemia The presence of urobilin in the blood.

urobilinogen A colorless compound present in large amounts in feces and in small amounts in urine; formed in the intestines by the reduction of bilirubin; upon oxidation it forms urobilin.

urocele Distention of the scrotal sac with extravasated urine.

urochrome A yellow or brownish substance believed to give urine its characteristic color.

urocystic Of or relating to the urinary bladder.

urodilatin A 32-amino acid polypeptide found in urine, believed to facilitate sodium excretion.

urodynia Urination accompanied by pain or discomfort.

uroerythrin A pigment sometimes present in urine; believed to be derived from melanin metabolism.

uroflometer An instrument for measuring and graphically recording the rate of urine flow by weighing it during voiding; rate of urination indicator.

urogastrone A polypeptide extractable from normal urine in man and dog which, when injected into the body, inhibits gastric secretions.

urogenital See genitourinary.

urogram X-ray image of the urinary tract obtained with the use of a radiopaque medium.

urography Roentgenography of any part of the urinary tract.

   excretory u. X-ray examination of the renal parenchyma, calices, pelves, ureters, and urinary bladder, following intravenous injection of a contrast medium which is rapidly excreted in the urine. Also called intravenous pyelography.

   retrograde u. Urography after injection of a contrast medium into the bladder or ureters.

urokinase A proteolytic enzyme in blood and urine that activates the fibrinolytic system by converting plasminogen to plasmin.

urolith, urolite A calculus in the urinary tract.

urolithiasis The formation of urinary calculi and the resulting disease condition.

urologic Relating to urology.

urologist A specialist in urology.

urology The branch of medicine concerned with the study, diagnosis, and treatment of diseases (especially by surgical techniques) of the urinary tract

of both male and female, and of the genital organs of the male.

uropathy Any disease of the urinary tract.

uroplania The escaping or extravasation of urine into the tissues.

uropod An enlarged cytoplasmic extension from the surface of a cell; it is usually capable of developing microspikes and pinocytotic vesicles.

uropoiesis The formation of urine.

uroporphyrin A porphyrin, usually found in small amounts in the urine; excretion of an excessive amount may be seen in heavy metal poisoning or in cutaneous porphyria or congenital erythropoietic porphyria.

uroschesis Urinary retention or suppression.

urosepsis Sepsis resulting from the absorption and decomposition of extravasated urine in the tissues.

ursodeoxycholic acid Drug prepared from the bile acid chenodiol; used to suppress symptoms of gallstones and other biliary tract diseases.

Urtica A genus of plants that have stinging hairs and secrete a poisonous fluid.

urticant 1. Any agent that causes itching or stinging. 2. Producing an itching or stinging sensation.

urticaria Eruption of transitory itchy wheals, often due to hypersensitivity to foods or drugs or to emotional factors. Also called hives.

   cholinergic u. Clusters of tiny itchy papules usually brought on by exercise or stress.

   cold u. Wheal formed upon exposure to cold.

   giant u. See edema, angioneurotic.

   papular u. A common and troublesome skin disease of childhood, characterized by the appearance of a wheal followed by a papule; although food allergy is widely accepted as a cause of the eruption, recent evidence favors a parasitic origin, such as bites from cat fleas and bedbugs.

   u. medicamentosa Urticaria occurring as a reaction to a drug.

   u. pigmentosa Disorder characterized chiefly by yellow-brown macules and papules on the skin; may involve only the skin (juvenile type) or occur with other systemic symptoms (adult type). Also called mastocytosis.

Usher's syndrome Profound childhood hearing impairment with retinitis pigmentosa; inherited as an autosomal recessive trait.

ut dictum Latin for as directed; used in prescription writing.

uterine Of or relating to the uterus.

uterocystostomy Surgical establishment of a communication between the cervix of the uterus and the bladder.

utero-ovarian Relating to the uterus and an

ovary.

uteroplasty Reparative surgery of the uterus.

uterosacral Relating to the uterus and the sacrum.

uterotonic 1. Overcoming relaxation of the uterine muscle. 2. An agent having such an effect.

uterotubal Relating to the uterus and its tubes.

uterovaginal Relating to the uterus and the vagina.

uterovesical Relating to the uterus and the bladder.

uterus A hollow, muscular organ of the female mammal situated in the pelvis between the bladder and rectum; its function is the nourishment of the developing young prior to birth; the mature human uterus is pear-shaped, thick-walled, and about 76 mm long, reaching adult size by the 15th year and diminishing after the menopause; the upper portion of the uterus opens on either side into the uterine tubes and the lower portion opens into the vagina. Also called womb.

   anomalous u. A malformed uterus.

   gravid u. A pregnant uterus.

   pubescent u. An underdeveloped uterus.

utricle The larger of the two sacs of the membranous labyrinth in the vestibule of the internal ear.

utricular Relating to or resembling a utricle.

utriculosaccular Relating to the utricle and the saccule of the internal ear.

utriculus Utricle.

uvea The middle, pigmented, vascular layer of the eye consisting of the choroid, the ciliary body, and the iris. Also called uveal tract.

uveal Relating to the uvea.

uveitis Inflammation of the uvea (choroid, ciliary body, and iris).

uveoparotitis Vascular inflammation of the uvea (middle coat of eye) and the parotid gland; a manifestation of sarcoidosis. Also called uveoparotid fever.

uviform Resembling grapes.

uvula From Latin, a small grape; any anatomic structure resembling a small grape; when used alone, the term designates the palatine uvula.

   palatine u. The conical, fleshy mass of tissue suspended from the free edge of the soft palate above the back of the tongue.

   vesical u. A mucosal ridge of the bladder just behind the internal urethral orifice, formed by the underlying median lobe of the prostate gland in the male.

uvulectomy Surgical removal of the uvula.

uvulitis Inflammation of the uvula.

uvulotomy Incision of the uvula or removal of a portion of it.

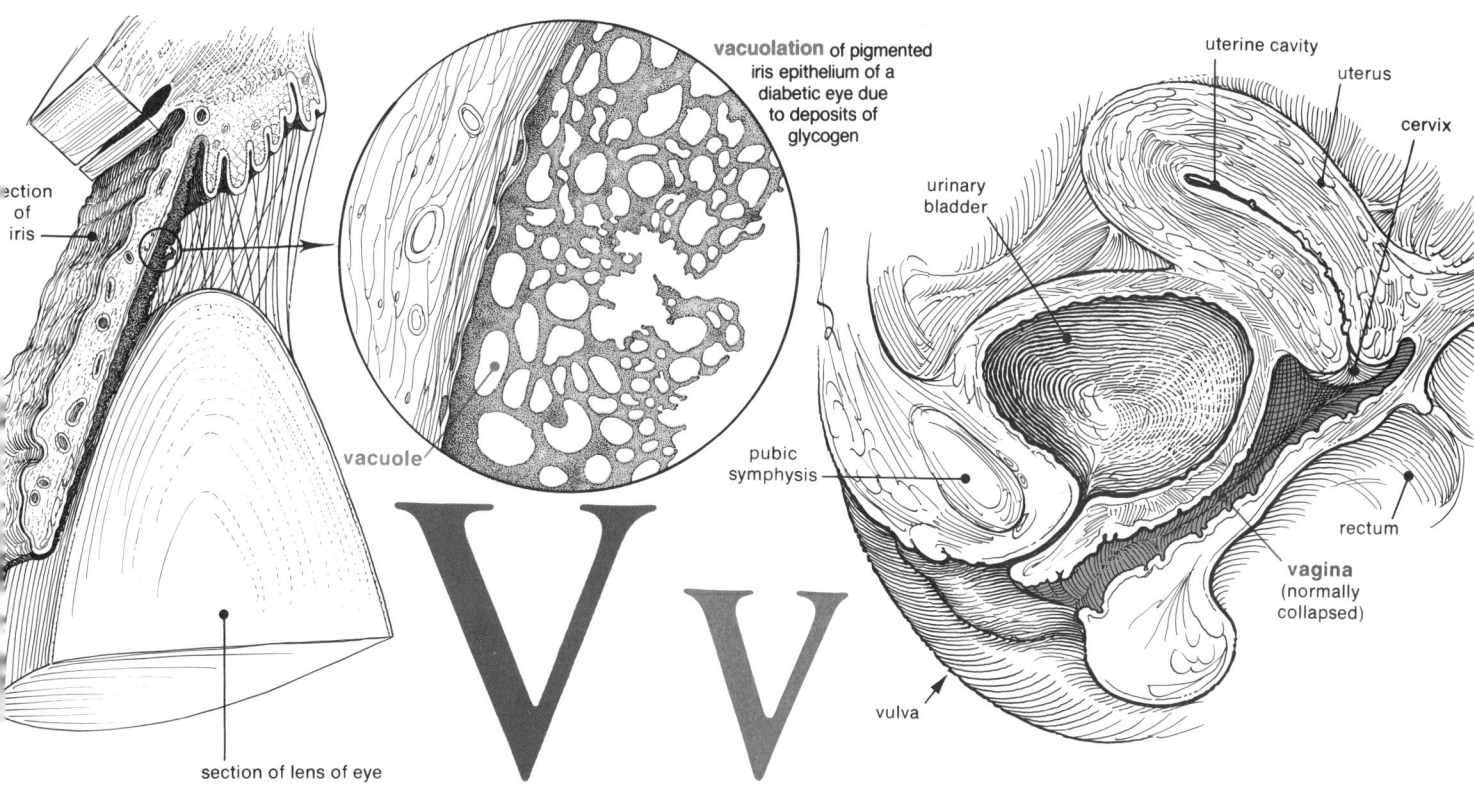

section of iris

vacuolation of pigmented iris epithelium of a diabetic eye due to deposits of glycogen

vacuole

pubic symphysis

section of lens of eye

uterine cavity

uterus

cervix

urinary bladder

rectum

vagina (normally collapsed)

vulva

V₁, V₂, V₃, V₄, V₅, V₆ Precordial leads; see under lead.

vaccinate To inoculate with a vaccine for the purpose of producing active immunity against a given infectious disease.

vaccination 1. Inoculation with the virus of cowpox, or vaccinia, as a means of producing immunity against smallpox. **2.** Injection or ingestion of an immunogenic antigen (vaccine) in order to produce active immunity against a given disease.

vaccinator 1. One who vaccinates. **2.** Instrument used in vaccination.

vaccine A preparation of dead, or live attenuated, viruses or bacteria for use in the prevention of infectious diseases by inducing active immunity.

autogenous v. Vaccine made from organisms obtained from the individual to be inoculated.

bacillus Calmette-Guèrin v. (BCG vaccine) An attenuated, viable bovine tubercle bacillus vaccine, which has proved to be highly effective in increasing the body's resistance against tuberculosis; possibly effective also in the treatment of certain neoplasms by a nonspecific stimulation of the body's immune system.

Calmette-Guèrin v. Bacillus Calmette-Guèrin vaccine.

cholera v. A sterile suspension of killed *Vibrio cholerae* organisms containing 8 billion organisms per ml; given intramuscularly or subcutaneously in two doses one week to one month apart.

diphtheria, pertussis, and tetanus v. (DPT) A triple vaccine for infants usually administered in three intramuscular injections 1 to 3 months apart, beginning at age 6 to 8 weeks.

influenza virus v. A sterile, aqueous suspension of inactivated influenza virus grown in egg allantoic fluid and killed with formalin.

live v. One prepared from live organisms whose virulence has been reduced.

measles v. Live, attenuated measles virus vaccine, given subcutaneously to children 1 year of age or older.

mixed v. One containing killed cultures of more than one species.

mumps v. A suspension of live attenuated mumps virus, given subcutaneously.

poliomyelitis v. Vaccine against paralytic poliomyelitis; available in two forms; live, attenuated oral poliovirus vaccine (Sabin), and the formaldehyde-inactivated poliomyelitis vaccine (Salk) given by injection.

rabies v. A sterile suspension of killed, fixed rabies virus; usually given after exposure to the virus in a series of 14 to 21 daily doses injected in separate sites.

Sabin v. (OPV) Live, oral poliovirus vaccine containing Types I, II, and III poliovirus strains; it produces a more rapid and longer lasting immunity than the Salk vaccine.

Salk v. A sterile suspension of formaldehyde-inactivated Types I, II, and III strains of poliovirus.

typhoid v. A killed suspension of typhoid bacilli (*Salmonella typhosa*).

typhus v. A sterile suspension of the killed rickettsial organisms (*Rickettsia prowazekii*), which are cultivated in the yolk sac of eggs and treated with formalin. Also called Cox vaccine.

yellow fever v. A live, attenuated strain of yellow fever virus grown in cell cultures and eggs.

vaccinia 1. A contagious disease of cattle caused by the vaccine virus. Also called cowpox. **2.** A local reaction induced in man by the introduction of the virus for the purpose of immunization against smallpox; the reaction is usually limited to a single lesion at the site of inoculation.

generalized v. Condition of secondary lesions of the skin following vaccination.

progressive v. Widespread vaccinal lesions following vaccination; a severe, often fatal condition occurring in individuals who fail to produce antibodies. Also called vaccinia gangrenosa.

v. gangrenosa See progressive vaccinia.

vaccinid Allergic reaction to vaccination marked by localized eruption of vesicles or papules.

vacciniform, vaccinoid Resembling cowpox.

vaccinogen A source of vaccine.

VACTERL Acronym for vertebral, anal, cardiac, tracheal, esophageal, renal, and limb; a pattern of congenital anomalies.

vacuant An agent that promotes emptying of the bowels.

vacuolate, vacuolated Containing vacuoles.

vacuolation The formation of vacuoles.

vacuole 1. A small space or cavity in the protoplasm of a cell. **2.** A small space in tissue.

vacuum A space devoid of gas or air; an empty space.

vagal Relating to the vagus nerve.

vagectomy Removal of a portion of the vagus nerve.

vagina 1. The musculomembranous tubular structure extending from the vulva to the uterine cervix. **2.** Any sheathlike structure.

vaginal 1. Of, or relating to, the vagina. **2.** Relating to, or resembling, a sheath.

vaginalectomy Surgical removal of a portion of the tunica vaginalis testis.

vaginalitis Inflammation of the tunica vaginalis testis.

vaginate 1. To form a sheath. **2.** Enclosed in a

sheath.

vaginectomy Partial or total excision of the vagina.

vaginismus Painful spasmodic contraction of the vaginal walls on slightest touch.

vaginitis Inflammation of the vagina.

emphysematous v. A form characterized by the presence of numerous small gas-filled cysts in the upper vagina.

mycotic v. A form caused by a fungus; particularly common during pregnancy and in diabetes.

senile v. Vaginitis occurring in elderly women, often causing adhesions which obliterate the canal.

vaginocele Hernia protruding into the vagina. Also called colpocele.

vaginodynia Vaginal pain. Also called colpodynia.

vaginofixation Suture of a prolapsed vagina to the abdominal wall. Also called colpopexy.

vaginolabial Relating to the vagina and the labia. Also called vulvovaginal.

vaginomycosis Vaginal infection due to a fungus.

vaginopathy Any vaginal disorder.

vaginoperineal Relating to the vagina and perineum.

vaginoperineorraphy Repair of the vagina and perineum, as in cases of perineal tears. Also called colpoperineorraphy.

vaginoperineotomy Enlarging the vaginal orifice by incising the vagina and perineum to facilitate childbirth.

vaginopexy Colpopexy.

vaginoplasty Surgical repair of the vagina. Also called colpoplasty.

vaginoscope See colposcope.

vaginoscopy Visual examination of the cervix and vagina, usually with the aid of a colposcope (vaginoscope).

vaginovesical Relating to the vagina and the bladder.

vaginovulvar Relating to the vagina and vulva. Also called vulvovaginal.

vagitis Inflammation of the vagus nerve (10th cranial nerve).

vagolysis The surgical destruction of a portion of the vagus nerve, usually the esophageal branch for the relief of cardiospasm.

vagolytic 1. Any agent that interferes with the transmission of impulses by the vagus nerve. **2.** Relating to, or causing, destruction of the vagus nerve.

vagomimetic Imitating the action of the vagus nerve.

vagotomy Interruption of the function of the va-after Netter

hallux **valgus**

palatine tonsil

dorsal surface of tongue

vallecula epiglottica

pulmonic valve

aortic valve

left atrioventricular valve

right atrioventricular valve

superior view of section of heart

NORMAL **VALUES** OF BLOOD PLASMA			THRESHOLD LIMIT VALUES OF SOME ENVIRONMENTAL CONTAMINANTS	
Base			Substance	
sodium (Na⁺)	142 mEq/1		ammonia	50 ppm
potassium (K⁺)	4 mEq/1		carbon monoxide	50 ppm
calcium (Ca⁺⁺)	5 mEq/1		carbon dioxide	5000 ppm
magnesium (Mg⁺⁺)	2 mEq/1		hydrogen sulfide	10 ppm
Acid			ozone	0.1 ppm
			mercury	0.1 mg/m³
HCO₃⁻	27 mEq/1		cement dust	30 mppcf
Cl⁻	103 mEq/1			
HPO₄⁻⁻	2 mEq/1			
SO₄⁻⁻	1 mEq/1			
organic acids	4 mEq/1			
protein	16 mEq/1			

gus nerve.

medical v. Interruption of the activity of the vagus nerve by drugs.

surgical v. Surgical division of the vagus nerve.

vagotonia Overaction or hyperexcitability of the vagus nerve.

vagus The 10th cranial nerve. See table of nerves.

valence, valency The combining power of one atom or group of atoms, using the hydrogen atom as the unit of comparison.

valgus Bent outward, or away from, the midline.

valine (Val) A naturally occurring amino acid, $C_5H_{11}NO_2$, constituent of many proteins; one of the amino acids essential for optimal growth.

vallate Surrounded by a depression and bounded by a circular elevation. Also called cupped.

vallecula In anatomy, a shallow groove, depression, or fossa.

v. cerebelli A deep hollow separating the inferior surface of the cerebellar hemispheres in which rests the medulla oblongata.

v. epiglottica The depression between the epiglottis and the root of the tongue, on either side of the median glossoepiglottic fold.

vallum, *pl.* **valla** Any raised surface surrounding a circular depression.

value A particular quantitative determination; a calculated numerical quantity; a number expressing a property.

caloric v. The measured heat evolved by a food when metabolized.

globular v. Color index; see under index.

threshold limit v. (TLV) The amount of a potentially noxious material to which individuals may be exposed without adverse effects; some values have been determined for a variety of atmospheric contaminants.

valvate Containing valves or valvelike parts.

valve A fold of the lining membrane of a tube or other hollow organ, so placed as to permit passage of fluid in one direction only.

aortic v. The valve between the left ventricle and the ascending aorta normally consisting of three semilunar cups.

Bianchi's v. The valve at the lower end of the nasolacrimal duct.

eustachian v. See valve of the inferior vena cava.

ileocecal v. The valve at the junction of the small and large intestines which regulates the flow of intestinal contents and prevents their backward flow.

left atrioventricular v. The bicuspid valve between the left atrium and the left ventricle of the heart. Also called mitral valve.

mitral v. See left atrioventricular valve.

pulmonic v. The valve located at the opening of the pulmonary trunk.

rectal v.'s Transverse folds of the rectum; see under fold.

right atrioventricular v. The valve between the right atrium and the right ventricle of the heart. Also called tricuspid valve.

semilunar v. One of the crescent-shaped segments or cusps that form the aortic valve and the pulmonic valve.

tricuspid v. See right atrioventricular valve.

v. of inferior vena cava The valve at the opening of the inferior vena cava in the right atrium of the heart. Also called eustachian valve.

v. of Kerckring See plica circularis.

venous v. One of a number of small cup-shaped valves found in many of the veins.

valviform Shaped like a valve.

valvoplasty Surgical reconstruction of a heart valve. Also called valvuloplasty.

valvotomy Surgical incision of a valve, such as one of the heart. Also called valvulotomy.

valvula, *pl.* **valvulae** A small valve.

valvular Relating to valves.

valvular disease of the heart (VDH) Any disease caused by abnormalities of the heart valves.

valvule A small valve.

valvulitis Inflammation of a valve, especially a valve of the heart.

valvuloplasty See valvoplasty.

valvulotome Instrument for cutting a valve.

valvulotomy See valvotomy.

valyl The radical of valine.

vanadium Metallic element; symbol V, atomic number 23, atomic weight 50.95.

vanilla 1. Any of several tropical orchids. 2. The fruit of such plants, especially *Vanilla planifolia,* which yields the aromatic substance vanillin.

vanillin Flavoring agent, $C_8H_8O_3$, derived from vanilla or prepared synthetically.

vanillylmandelic acid (VMA) 3-Methoxy-4-hydroxymandelic acid, the major urinary metabolite of adrenal and sympathetic catecholamines; the normal range for excretion is 2 to 10 mg per day; elevated levels of excretion suggest a pheochromocytoma.

vapor The gaseous state of any substance that is liquid or solid at ordinary temperatures.

vaporize To change into a vapor by heating.

vaporizer An apparatus for reducing fluids to vapor for inhalation.

vapotherapy The treatment of any disorder with vapor, steam, or spray.

variance 1. A difference. 2. The act of varying.

ball v. The changes occurring in the ball of a ballvalve prosthesis.

variant Tending to deviate from a standard.

L-phase v. A strain of bacteria with defective cell walls that has nutritive requirements similar to the strain from which it originated and is capable of reverting to its parental form. Also called L-form.

variceal Relating to a varix.

varicella See chickenpox.

Labels in figure:
deferent duct
internal spermatic vein
cirrhotic liver
varicose esophageal veins
glomerulus
nephron
arcuate vein and artery
pudendal plexus
variocele
vasa rectae
arteriola recta
venula recta
testis
glomerular (Bowman's) capsule
vas afferens glomeruli renis
juxtaglomerular cells
macula densa
distal convoluted tubule
after etter
proximal convoluted tubule
urinary space
glomerulus
nephronic (Henle's) loop
vas efferens glomeruli renis

varicelliform Resembling chickenpox.

varices Plural of varix.

varicocele Dilatation of the veins of the spermatic cord in the scrotum.

varicocelectomy Operation for removal of dilated veins of the spermatic cord (varicocele).

varicography Roentgenologic visualization of varicose veins achieved by introducing a radiopaque substance.

varicophlebitis Inflammation of varicose veins.

varicose Denoting abnormally dilated and tortuous vessels.

varicosity 1. The state of being abnormally swollen. **2.** A varicose vein.

varicotomy An operation for the removal of a varicose vein or varix.

varicula A varicose condition of small veins, especially of the conjunctiva.

varicule A small varicose vein.

variola See smallpox.

variolar Relating to smallpox.

varioliform In the shape or form of smallpox.

varioloid A mild case of smallpox occurring in partially immune persons.

varix, *pl.* **varices** A dilated and tortuous vessel, usually a vein.

  aneurysmal v. Varix resulting from the direct communication between a vein and an adjacent artery.

  esophageal varices Varicosities of the mucosal veins of the esophagus, usually the lower portion.

varnish A solution of a resin in a suitable solvent and an evaporating binder which when applied in a thin layer forms a hard, glossy, thin film.

  dental v. A solution of natural resins and gums in an organic solvent; it is applied over the walls and floor of the prepared tooth cavity; when the solvent evaporates, a thin film is left that protects the underlying tooth structure against the constituents of the restorative material and thermal shock.

varus Bent inward or toward the midline.

vas, *pl.* **vasa** A duct or canal through which a liquid, such as blood, lymph, chyle, or semen, is conveyed; a vessel.

  v. aberrans hepatis Any of the numerous, irregularly coursing, blind-ending bile ducts or associated blood vessels that are located in the coronary ligament, capsule, or fibrous appendix of the liver.

  v. afferens glomeruli renis The afferent arteriole that conveys blood toward the glomerulus of the kidney.

  v. afferens A vessel entering a structure such as the lymph node.

  v. brevia The small branches of the splenic artery supplying the greater curvature of the stomach.

  v. deferens Deferent duct; see under duct.

  v. efferens glomeruli renis The efferent arteriole that conveys blood away from the glomerulus of the kidney.

  v. efferens A vessel leaving a structure such as a lymph node.

  v. lymphaticum One that conveys lymph; there are two types; the afferent and efferent. Also called lymphatic vessel.

  v. previa An anomaly of the umbilical cord insertion in which the umbilical vessels traverse the lower uterine segment across the internal cervical os, and appear ahead of the fetal head at the opening of the uterus.

  vasa rectae The arterioles and venules that descend and ascend parallel to the nephronic (Henle's) loop in the pyramid of the kidney; the wider ascending limbs are often referred to as venulae rectae and the descending limbs are generally called arteriolae rectae.

  v. spirale ductus cochlearis The largest blood vessel in the basilar membrane just beneath the tunnel of Corti in the ear.

  v. vasorum One of many small blood vessels in the walls of larger arteries and their corresponding veins.

vascular Pertaining to, or containing, vessels.

vascularity The state of containing blood vessels.

vascularization The formation of blood vessels.

vasculature The system of blood vessels of an organ.

vasculitis Inflammation of a blood vessel or vessels.

vasculogenesis Formation of the system of blood vessels.

vasectomy Removal of the ductus (vas) deferens, or a segment of it; a means of male sterilization. Also called deferenectomy.

vasiform Tubular.

vasoactive Having an effect on blood vessels.

vasocongestion The state of being filled with blood.

vasoconstriction Narrowing of the lumen of blood vessels, especially of arterioles.

vasoconstrictor A drug or nerve that causes narrowing of the lumen of blood vessels.

vasodilation Widening of the lumen of the blood vessels, especially of the lumen of arterioles, leading to increased blood flow to a part.

  reflex v. Dilatation of a blood vessel due to a reflex response to a stimulus.

vasodilator A drug or nerve that causes widening of the lumen of blood vessels.

vasodistention Opposite of vasoconstriction. Also called vasodilation.

vasoganglion A glomus; a dense mass of blood vessels.

vasography Roentgenography of blood vessels.

vasohypertonic Causing increased tonicity in the smooth muscles of blood vessels; denoting increased arteriolar tension.

vasohypotonic Causing reduced tonicity in the

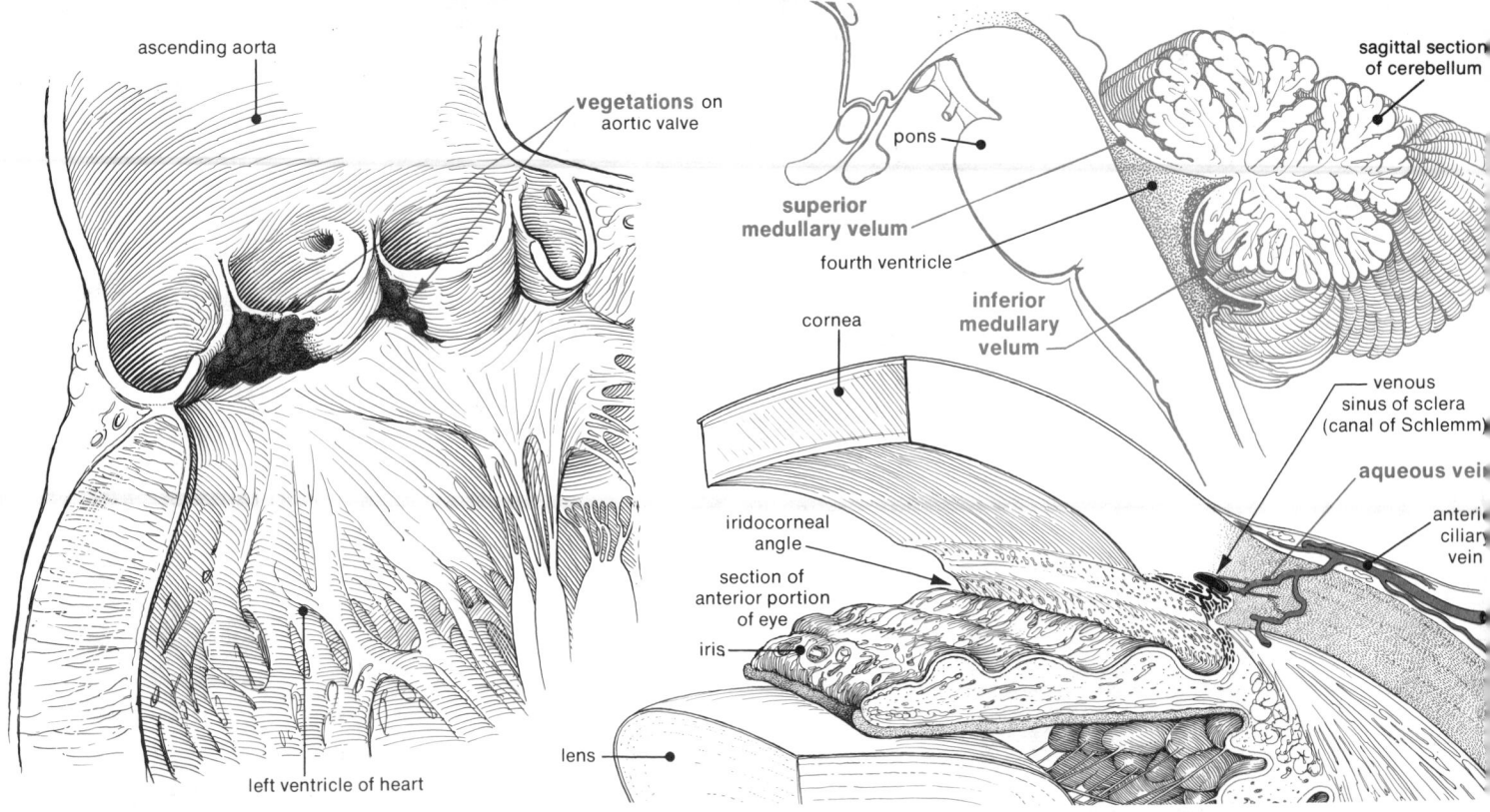

smooth muscles of blood vessels; denoting reduced arteriolar tension.

vasoinhibitor A drug that depresses the action of vasomotor nerves.

vasoinhibitory Restraining or reducing the action of the vasomotor nerves.

vasoligation Surgical ligation of the deferent duct (vas deferens).

vasomotion Dilatation and constriction of blood vessels. Also called angiokinesis.

vasomotor Causing constriction or dilatation of blood vessels; denoting the nerves that have this action.

vasoneuropathy Any disease affecting the blood vessels and nerves.

vasoparalysis Hypotonia of blood vessels. Also called vasomotor paralysis.

vasopressin Antidiuretic hormone; a hormone from the posterior lobe of the hypophysis having a potent antidiuretic action and some vasoconstrictive action on the splanchnic circulation.

vasopressor An agent that causes constriction of blood vessels and a rise in blood pressure.

vasosensory Denoting sensory nerves going to the blood vessels.

vasospasm Spasm or contraction of the muscular coats of blood vessels. Also called angiospasm.

vasostimulant 1. Exciting nerves that cause dilatation or constriction of blood vessels. 2. Any agent having such property.

vasotomy Cutting into the vas deferens (deferent duct).

vasotonic Relating to the tone of a blood vessel; an agent that increases tension of blood vessels.

vasotrophic See angiotrophic.

vasotropic Tending to act on blood vessels.

vasovagal Relating to the action of the vagus nerve upon blood vessels.

vasovasostomy Surgical union of the ends of a severed deferent duct.

vasovesiculectomy Surgical removal of a deferent duct and seminal vesicles.

VATER Acronym for vertebral, anal, tracheal, esophageal, and renal; a pattern of associated congenital anomalies.

vault Any arched anatomic structure resembling a dome.

vection Transmission of causative agents of disease.

vector 1. An organism that transmits pathologic microorganisms from one host to another. 2. Anything (electromotive force, velocity, etc.) that has a magnitude and a direction.

biological v. Vector (such as the Anopheles mosquito) in whose body an infective organism must

develop before becoming infective to its primary host.

mechanical v. Vector (such as the housefly) that simply transports an infective organism on its feet or mouth parts from one host to another and is not essential to the life cycle of the parasite.

vectorcardiogram (VCG) A graphic record of the magnitude and direction of the heart's action currents, displayed as a three-dimensional or spatial voltage loop.

vectorcardiography The determination of the direction and magnitude of the heart's electric forces at any point in time; represented by vector loops.

spatial v. Three-dimensional voltage loop produced by the heart's action current and projected on the frontal, horizontal, and sagittal reference planes.

vegan One who does not eat food derived from animals (meat, milk, eggs, etc.).

vegetarian One who does not eat meat or animal products; a strict vegetarian does not eat tubers. See also lactovegetarian.

vegetation An abnormal plantlike outgrowth of tissue; specifically, growth composed of fibrin and fused blood platelets adherent to a diseased heart valve; circulating bacteria tend to plant at these sites.

vegetative Having a role in the processes of growth and nutrition.

vehicle 1. In pharmacology, an inactive substance in which an active drug is dissolved or suspended; an excipient. 2. Any inanimate carrier of an infectious agent from one host to another.

veil Colloquial term for caul.

Veillonella A genus of anaerobic, gram-negative bacteria normally found in the mouth and intestinal, respiratory, and urogenital tracts of apparently healthy individuals.

vein (v) A vessel that carries blood toward the heart or one in the heart wall that returns blood to the right atrium. For specific veins, see table of veins.

aqueous v.'s Minute vessels that transport aqueous humor from the venous sinus of the sclera (canal of Schlemm) out of the eyeball to the episcleral, conjunctival, and subconjunctival veins.

cardinal v.'s The major embryonic vessels that drain the cephalic part (anterior cardinal vein) and caudal part (posterior cardinal vein) and empty into the heart (via the common cardinal vein).

emissary v.'s Veins that drain the intracranial venous sinuses and transport the blood to a vessel outside the skull; they serve as drainage channels in case of increased intracranial pressure.

large v. A vein, such as the inferior vena cava, characterized by having a tunica adventitia which is thicker than the tunica media and has many bundles of muscular fibers arranged longitudinally; the tun-

ica media is thin or may be absent.

medium v. A vein that characteristically has a thick tunica media composed of connective tissue with elastic fibers intermingled with circularly arranged muscle fibers; the tunica adventitia contains longitudinal elastic fibers.

pulmonary v.'s The four veins that return oxygenated blood from the lungs to the left atrium of the heart. See table of veins.

small v. A vein whose walls are thin, with poorly defined tunica which contain a network of longitudinal elastic fibers; some contain a few fibers of smooth muscle arranged circularly.

systemic v.'s All the veins that return venous blood to the right atrium of the heart; may be categorized into three groups: (a) veins of the heart; (b) veins of the head, neck, thorax, and upper extremities, all of which carry blood to the superior vena cava; (c) veins of the abdomen, pelvis, and lower extremities, all of which carry blood to the inferior vena cava.

varicose v.'s Abnormally dilated, tortuous veins produced by prolonged, increased intraluminal pressure; most commonly seen in the superficial veins of the leg; varicose veins along with phlebothrombosis account for approximately 90 percent of clinical venous disease.

vitelline v.'s Veins that return blood from the yolk sac of an early embryo; they form an anastomotic network around the duodenum and in the liver and empty directly into the sinus venosus of the primitive heart.

velopharyngeal Relating to the soft palate and the pharynx.

velum Any structure resembling a curtain.

inferior medullary v., posterior medullary v. A thin sheet forming part of the roof of the cerebral fourth ventricle; composed of the cellular lining of the ventricle on the inside and pia mater on the outside.

superior medullary v., anterior medullary v. A thin layer of white matter between the cerebellar peduncles, forming the anterior portion of the roof of the cerebral fourth ventricle.

v. palatinum Soft palate.

vena, *pl.* **venae** Latin for vein.

v. cava See table of veins.

venae comitantes, *sing.* **v. comitans** Veins (usually two) accompanying the corresponding artery.

venation The distribution of veins.

venectomy Phlebectomy.

veneer In dentistry, a porcelain or resin facing applied to a gold crown or pontic for esthetic purposes.

venenation Poisoning.

Figure labels (clockwise from top):
- internal jugular vein
- external jugular vein
- brachiocephalic vein
- subclavian vein
- axillary vein
- heart
- brachial vein
- inferior vena cava
- cephalic vein
- axillary vein
- superior vena cava

VEINS	LOCATION	DRAINS	EMPTIES INTO
alveolar v., inferior inferior dental v. *v. alveolaris inferior*	from mandibular canal it passes up the ramus of lower jaw	teeth of lower jaw	pyterygoid plexus
anastomotic v., inferior v. of Labbé *v. anastomotica inferior*	courses over temporal lobe of brain	superficial middle cerebral v.	transverse sinus
anastomotic v., superior v. of Trolard *v. anastomotica superior*	from lateral sulcus of brain across parietal lobe	superficial middle cerebral v.	superior sagittal sinus
angular v. *v. angularis*	anterior angle of orbit and root of nose	formed by union of frontal and supraorbital v.'s; receives infraorbital, superior and inferior palpebral and external nasal v.'s	facial v. (behind facial artery)
antebrachial v., median	see median vein of forearm		
appendicular v. *v. appendicularis*	along mesentery of vermiform appendix	appendix	ileocolic v.
v. of aqueduct of vestibule *v. aquaeductus vestibuli*	through aqueduct of vestibule (accompanied by endolymphatic duct)	internal ear	superior petrosal sinus
arcuate v.'s of kidney *vv. arcuatae renis*	in corticomedullary zone of kidney	interlobular v.'s, venulae rectae	interlobar v.
auditory v.'s, internal	see labyrinthine veins		
auricular v.'s, anterior *vv. auriculares anterior*	front part of ear	external ear	superficial temporal v.
auricular v., posterior *v. auricularis posterior*	side of head in back of ear	plexus on side of head, tributaries from back of ear, stylomastoid v.	external jugular v.
axillary v. *v. axillaris*	upper limb from lower border of teres major muscle to outer border of first rib	junction of basilic and brachial v.'s; cephalic v., deep brachial comitans	subclavian v. (at outer border of first rib)
azygos v. *v. azygos*	from front of first lumbar vertebra it passes to right side of fourth thoracic vertebra where it arches over right lung	ascending lumbar, right subcostal, intercostal, hemiazygos, esophageal, mediastinal, pericardial, and right bronchial v.'s	superior vena cava
azygos v., left	see hemiazygos vein		
basal v. *v. basalis*	from anterior perforated substance it passes posteriorly around cerebral peduncle	anterior perforated substance; anterior cerebral v., deep middle cerebral v., inferior striate v.'s	internal cerebral v.

VEINS	LOCATION	DRAINS	EMPTIES INTO
basilic v. *v. basilica*	from ulnar part of hand it passes up forearm and continues along medial border of the biceps	dorsal venous network of hand; tributaries from ulnar side of forearm	joins brachial v. to form axillary v.
basivertebral v.'s *vv. basivertebrales*	tortuous channels in substance of vertebrae	vertebrae	anterior external, and internal vertebral plexuses
brachial v.'s *vv. brachiales*	placed on either side of brachial artery	radial and ulnar v.'s, superior and inferior ulnar collateral v.'s, deep brachial v.	axillary v.
brachiocephalic v.'s innominate v.'s *vv. brachiocephalicae*	root of neck	*right side:* internal jugular, subclavian, internal thoracic, and inferior thyroid v.'s; *left side:* internal jugular, subclavian, and left highest intercostal v.'s	superior vena cava
bronchial v.'s *vv. bronchiales*	near bronchi	larger bronchi and roots of lungs	*right side:* azygos v.; *left side:* left highest intercostal or accessory hemiazygos v.'s
v. of bulb of penis *v. bulbi penis*	penis	expanded posterior part of the corpus spongiosum penis (bulb of penis)	internal pudendal v.
v. of bulb of vestibule *v. bulbi vestibuli*	vestibule	mass of erectile tissue on either side of vagina	internal pudendal v.
cardiac v.'s, anterior (three to four in number) *vv. cordis anterior*	ventral side of heart	ventral side of right ventricle	right atrium
cardiac v., great left coronary v. *v. cordis magna*	from apex of heart it ascends to front of heart	tributaries from left atrium and both ventricles; left marginal v.	left extremity of coronary sinus
cardiac v., middle *v. cordis media*	ascends up back of heart from apex	tributaries from both ventricles	right extremity of coronary sinus
cardiac v., small right coronary v. *v. cordis parva*	ascends up heart from back of right atrium and ventricle	back of right atrium and ventricle; right marginal v.	right extremity of coronary sinus or right atrium
cardiac v.'s, smallest (many minute veins) v.'s of Thebesius *vv. cordis minimae*	in muscular wall of heart	muscular wall of heart	mostly in atria, some in ventricles
cavernous v.'s of penis *vv. cavernosae penis*	penis	cavernous venous spaces in the erectile tissue of the penis (corpora cavernosae)	deep dorsal v. of penis, prostatic plexus
central v.'s of liver *vv. centrales hepatis*	middle of hepatic lobules	sinusoids in liver substance	sublobular v.
central v. of retina *v. centralis retinae*	from eyeball it passes out in optic nerve	retinal v.'s	superior ophthalmic v., cavernous sinus
cephalic v. *v. cephalica*	from radial part of hand it passes up forearm to groove along lateral border of biceps muscle of arm and more proximally between deltoid and pectoralis major muscles	radial side of dorsal venous plexus of hand; palmar and dorsal tributaries in forearm; thoracoacromial v.	axillary v. just caudal to clavicle
cephalic v., accessory *v. cephalica accessoria*	radial side of forearm	dorsal venous network of hand	cephalic v. at elbow
cerebellar v.'s, inferior *vv. cerebelli inferior*	bottom of cerebellum	inferior surface of cerebellum	transverse, superior petrosal, and occipital sinuses
cerebellar v.'s, superior *vv. cerebelli superior*	top of cerebellum (superior vermis)	upper surface of cerebellum	straight sinus and internal cerebral v.'s
cerebral v., anterior *v. cerebri anterior*	from upper surface of corpus callosum down through longitudinal fissure, above optic nerve to lateral cerebral sulcus	anterior perforated substance, lamina terminalis, rostrum of corpus callosum, septum pellucidum, striate v.	basal v.
cerebral v., deep middle deep Sylvian v. *v. cerebri media profunda*	lower part of lateral cerebral sulcus	tributaries from insula, neighboring gyri	basal v.

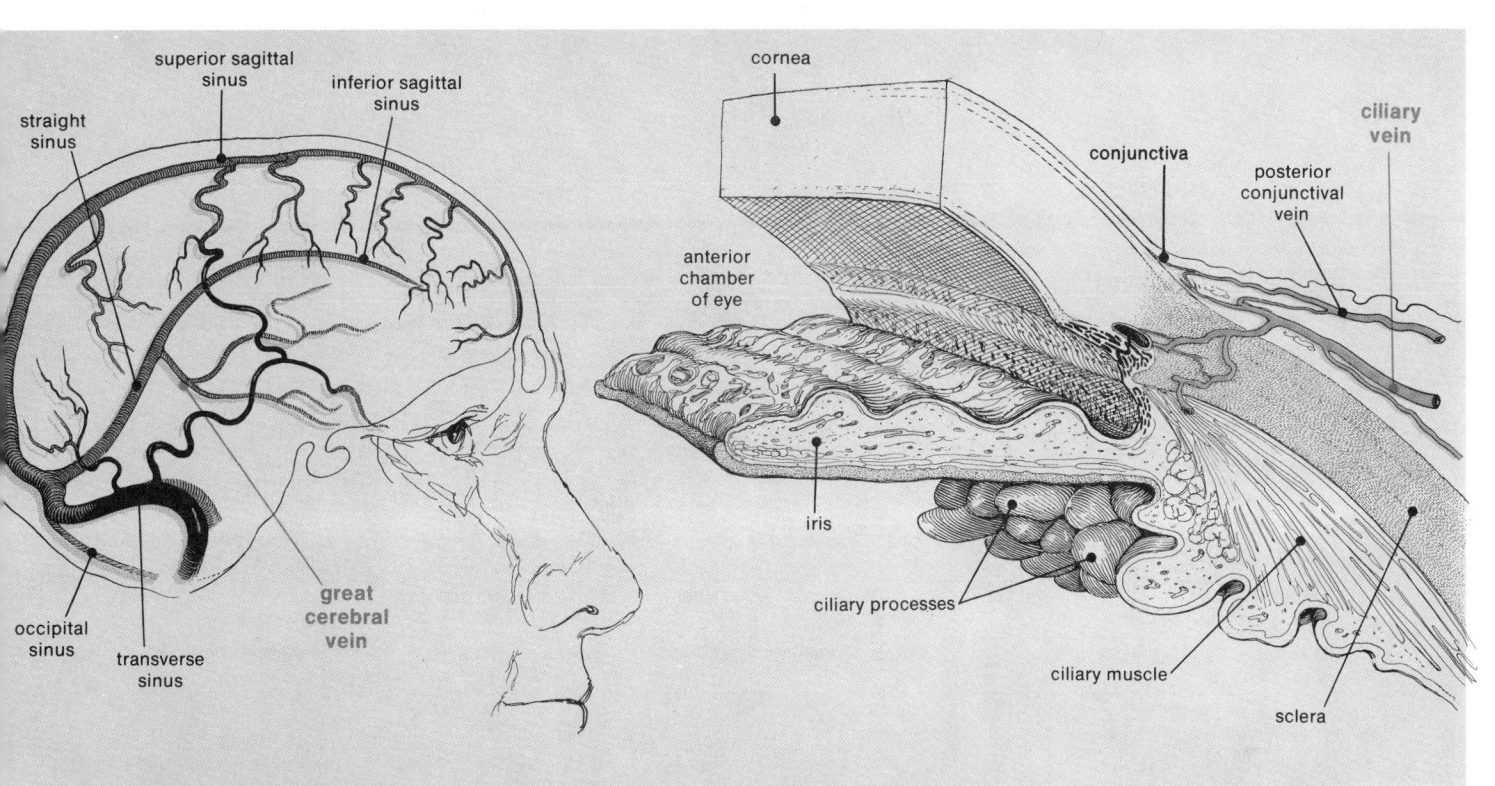

VEINS	LOCATION	DRAINS	EMPTIES INTO
cerebral v., great great v. of Galen *v. cerebri magna*	around back part of corpus callosum of brain	internal cerebral v.'s	anterior extremity of straight sinus
cerebral v.'s, inferior *vv. cerebri inferior*	bottom of brain	inferior surface of cerebral hemispheres	*frontal lobe portion:* superior sagittal sinus; *temporal lobe portion:* cavernous, superior petrosal, and transverse sinuses; *occipital lobe portion:* straight sinus
cerebral v.'s, internal (two in number) v.'s of Galen deep cerebral v.'s *vv. cerebri internae*	from interventricular foramen they pass backward between the layers of the tela choroidea of the third ventricle	the deep parts of the cerebral hemispheres; thalamostriate, choroid, and basal v.'s	great cerebral v.
cerebral v., superficial middle superficial Sylvian v. *v. cerebri media superficialis*	lateral surface of brain	lateral surface of cerebral hemispheres	cavernous and sphenoparietal sinuses
cerebral v.'s, superior (8–12 in number) *vv. cerebri superior*	brain	superior, lateral, and medial surfaces of cerebral hemispheres	superior sagittal sinus
cervical v., deep posterior deep cervical v. posterior vertebral v. *v. cervicalis profunda*	from suboccipital region it follows deep cervical artery down neck	plexus in suboccipital triangle, occipital v., deep muscles of back of neck, plexuses around spinal processes of cervical vertebrae	inferior part of vertebral v.
cervical v.'s, transverse *vv. transversae colli*	parallel to transverse cervical artery	trapezius muscle and neighboring structures	subclavian v. or external jugular v.
choroid v. *v. choroidea*	lateral ventricle of brain	lateral ventricle, choroid plexus, corpus callosum	internal cerebral v.
ciliary v.'s (anterior and posterior) *vv. ciliares*	from outer surface of choroidal layer of eyeball they pass through sclera	ciliary body, scleral venous sinus, conjunctiva	ophthalmic v.
cochlear v.'s *v. cochleares*	from lamina spiralis and basilar membrane to base of modiolus	cochlea	labyrinthine v.
colic v., left *v. colica sinistra*	alongside descending colon	descending colon and left colic (splenic) flexure	inferior mesenteric v.
colic v., middle *v. colica media*	transverse colon	transverse colon	superior mesenteric v.
colic v., right *v. colica dextra*	ascending colon	ascending colon	superior mesenteric v.
conjunctival v.'s *vv. conjunctivales*	eye	bulba conjunctiva	superior ophthalmic v.

VEINS	LOCATION	DRAINS	EMPTIES INTO
coronary v. gastric v. *v. gastrica dextra et sinistra*		see gastric vein	
coronary v., left		see cardiac vein, great	
coronary v., right		see cardiac vein, small	
coronary sinus (wide venous channel about 2.25 cm in length) *sinus coronarius*	posterior part of coronary sulcus (covered by muscular fibers from left atrium)	great, small, and middle cardiac v.'s, posterior v. of left ventricle, oblique v. of left atrium	right atrium between opening of inferior vena cava and atrioventricular aperture
cubital v., median *v. mediana cubiti*	passes obliquely across bend of elbow	cephalic v. below elbow	basilic v.
cystic v. *v. cystica*	in liver accompanying cystic duct	gallbladder	right branch of portal v.
digital v.'s, plantar *vv. digitales plantares*	plantar surface of toes	plexuses on the plantar surface of toes	unite to form four plantar metatarsal v.'s
diploic v., anterior temporal *v. diploica temporalis anterior*	middle layer (diploë) of frontal bone and parts of parietal bones of cranium	frontal bone and anterior part of parital bones	sphenoparietal sinus and deep temporal v.
diploic v., frontal *v. diploica frontalis*	middle layer (diploë) of frontal bone of cranium	frontal bone	supraorbital v. and superior sagittal sinus
diploic v., occipital (largest of the four diploic veins) *v. diploica occipitalis*	middle layer (diploë) of occipital bone of cranium	parietal bone	occipital v. or transverse sinus
diploic v., posterior temporal *v. diploica temporalis posterior*	middle layer (diploë) of parietal bone of cranium	parietal bone	transverse sinus
dorsal v. of clitoris, deep (unpaired) dorsal v. of clitoris *v. dorsalis clitoridis profunda*	dorsal midline of clitoris	body and glans of clitoris	primarily into the vesical plexus
dorsal v.'s of clitoris, superficial *vv. dorsales clitoridis superficiales*	clitoris	subcutaneous layers of clitoris	external pudendal v.
dorsal v. of penis, deep (unpaired) dorsal v. of penis *v. dorsalis penis profunda*	dorsal midline of penis	penis	prostatic plexus
dorsal v.'s of penis, superficial *vv. dorsales penis superficiales*	dorsal midline of penis	skin and subcutaneous layers of penis	external pudendal v.
dorsal v.'s of tongue		see lingual veins, dorsal	
emissary v., condylar *v. emissaria condylaris*	through condylar canal of cranium	area of foramen magnum	deep veins of neck
emissary v.'s, foramen lacerum (two or three in number) *vv. emissariae foraminis lacerum*	through foramen lacerum of cranium	cavernous sinus	pterygoid plexus
emissary v., foramen of Vesalius *v. emissaria foraminis Vesalii*	through foramen of Vesalius (when present)	cavernous sinus	pterygoid plexus
emissary v., mastoid *v. emissaria mastoidea*	through mastoid foramen of cranium	transverse sinus	posterior auricular v. or occipital v.
emissary v., parietal *v. emissaria parietalis*	through parietal foramen of cranium	scalp	superior sagittal sinus
epigastric v., inferior deep epigastric v. *v. epigastrica inferior*	from area of umbilicus it descends to deep inguinal ring area	abdominal wall; *in male:* ductus deferens; *in female:* round ligament	external iliac v. about 1.25 cm proximal to inguinal ligament
epigastric v., superficial *v. epigastrica superficialis*	from umbilicus it runs downward and laterally toward inguinal ligament	cutaneous part of lower and medial part of abdominal wall	great saphenous v.
epigastric v.'s, superior *vv. epigastricae superior*	from abdomen they ascend toward diaphragm	rectus muscle of abdomen; xiphoid process, diaphragm	internal thoracic v.
episcleral v.'s *vv. episclerales*	in sclera close to corneal margin	angle of eye, sclera, conjunctiva	anterior ciliary veins
esophageal v.'s (several in number) *vv. esophageae*	along the esophagus	esophagus	azygos, hemiazygos, gastric, and inferior thyroid v.'s

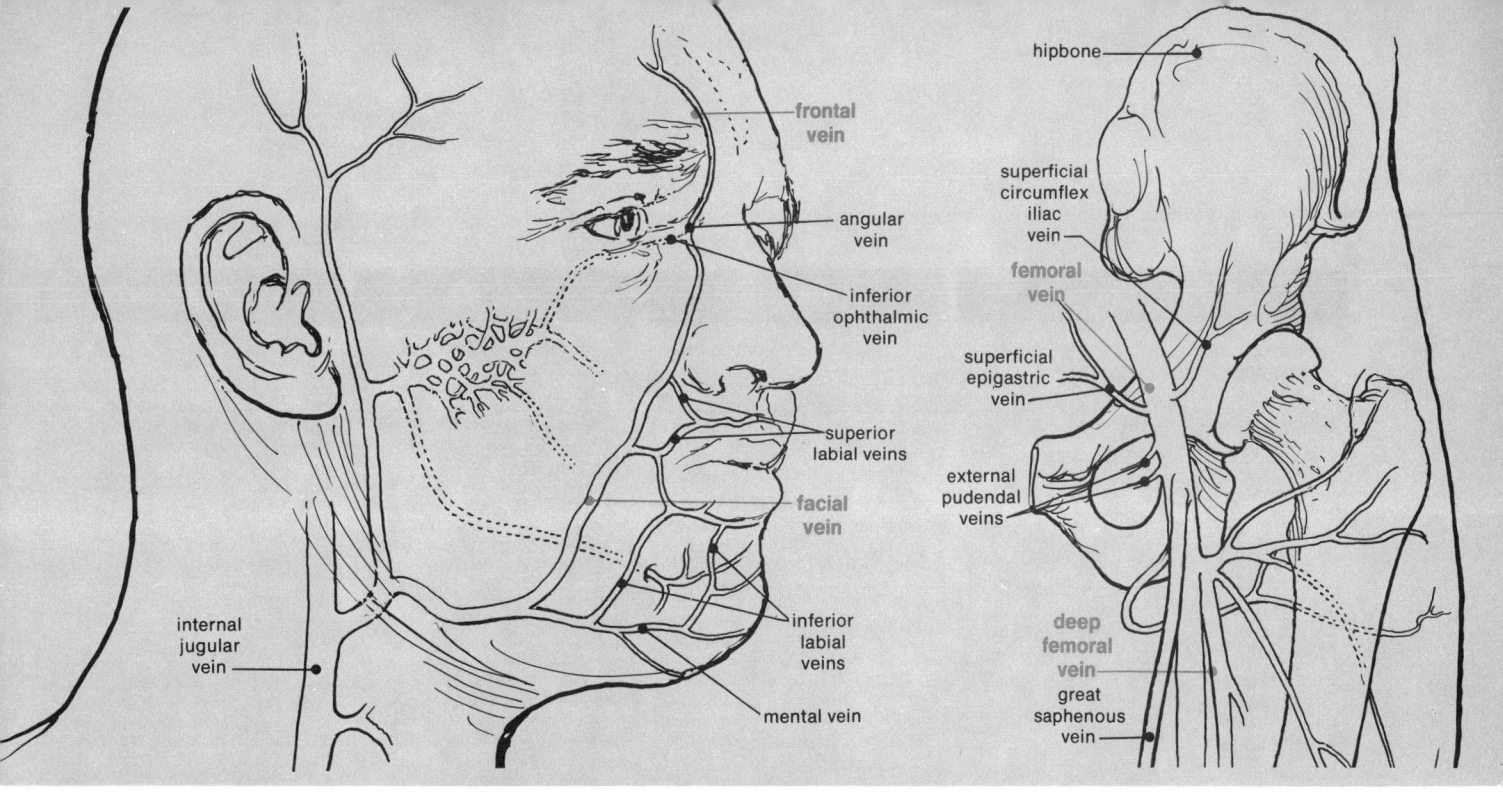

VEINS	LOCATION	DRAINS	EMPTIES INTO
ethmoidal v.'s *vv. ethmoidales*	ethmoidal sinuses	ethmoidal sinuses, frontal sinus, dura mater, walls and septum of nasal cavity	superior ophthalmic v.
facial v. anterior facial v. *v. facialis*	from medial angle of eye across face to neck	superficial structures of face; *tributaries include:* frontal, supraorbital, deep facial, superficial temporal, posterior auricular, occipital, and retromandibular v.'s	internal jugular v. or common facial v.
facial v., common	former term for the lower trunk of the facial vein (sometimes joined by retromandibular vein) which empties into the internal jugular vein		
facial v., deep *v. facialis profunda*	face	pterygoid plexus; small tributaries from buccinator, zygomatic, and masseter muscles	facial v.
facial v., transverse *v. facialis transversa*	from cheek it passes backward (just below zygomatic arch) to front of ear	muscles and related structures near the zygoma	superficial temporal v.
femoral v. *v. femoralis*	proximal two-thirds of thigh up to inguinal ligament	popliteal v., great saphenous v., profunda femoris v., muscular tributaries	external iliac v. at level of inguinal ligament
femoral v., deep profunda femoris v. *v. profunda femoris*	accompanies deep femoral artery	medial and lateral femoral circumflex v.'s; through muscular tributaries it anastomoses with popliteal v. distally and inferior gluteal v. proximally	femoral v.
femoral circumflex v.'s, lateral *vv. circumflexae femoris laterales*	winds around lateral side of upper femur	muscles of thigh, especially posterior muscles; lateral half of hip	femoral v.
femoral circumflex v.'s, medial *vv. circumflexae femoris mediales*	winds around medial side of upper femur	muscles of upper thigh, especially posterior muscles; hip joint	femoral v.
fibular v.'s	see peroneal veins		
frontal v. *v. frontalis*	from forehead to root of nose	plexus of forehead and scalp	facial v.
gastric v. coronary v. *v. gastrica*	from right to left along lesser curvature of stomach down peritoneum of lesser sac (omental bursa)	tributaries from both surfaces of stomach	portal vein
gastric v.'s, short (four or five in number) *vv. gastricae breves*	greater curvature of stomach	fundus and left part of greater curvature of stomach	splenic v.

vein | vein

VEINS	LOCATION	DRAINS	EMPTIES INTO
gastroepiploic v., left *v. gastroepiploica sinistra*	from right to left along greater curvature of stomach	tributaries from ventral and dorsal surfaces of stomach and greater omentum	splenic v.
gastroepiploic v., right *v. gastroepiploica dextra*	from left to right along greater curvature of stomach	tributaries from greater omentum and parts of stomach	superior mesenteric v.
gluteal v.'s, inferior sciatic v.'s *vv. gluteae inferior*	from the proximal part of posterior thigh they enter the pelvis through the greater sciatic foramen	skin and muscles of buttock and back of thigh; medial femoral circumflex and first perforating v.'s	internal iliac v.
gluteal v.'s, superior gluteal v.'s *vv. gluteae superior*	from buttock through greater sciatic foramen to pelvis	tributaries from buttock	internal iliac v.
hemiazygos v. left azygos v. inferior minor azygos v. *v. hemiazygos*	in thorax, it ascends on left side of vertebral column to ninth thoracic vertebra before horizontally crossing over vertebral column to join the azygos v.	left ascending lumbar v.'s, caudal four or five intercostal v.'s, left subcostal v., esophageal and mediastinal v.'s	azygos v.
hemiazygos v., accessory superior minor azygos v. *v. hemiazygos accesoria*	descends on left side of vertebral column in thorax and usually crosses over vertebral column at eighth thoracic vertebra	fourth to seventh posterior intercostal v.s	azygos v.
hemorrhoidal v.'s	see rectal veins		
hepatic v.'s *vv. hepaticae*	liver	substance of liver; central, intralobular, and sublobular v.'s	*upper group:* three large v.'s drain into the inferior vena cava below the diaphragm; *lower group:* several small v.'s drain into the inferior vena cava lower down
hypogastric v.	see iliac vein, internal		
ileocolic v. *v. ileocolica*	ileocolic area	terminal ileum, appendix, cecum, lower part of ascending colon	superior mesenteric v.
iliac v., common *v. iliaca communis*	from sacroiliac articulation, ascends to fifth lumbar vertebra	internal and external iliac v.'s; iliolumbar and lateral sacral v.'s (in addition, left common iliac v. receives middle sacral v.)	unites with its member of opposite side to form inferior vena cava
iliac v., external *v. iliaca externa*	from under inguinal ligament, along brim and lesser pelvis, to sacroiliac articulation	lower limb and lower abdominal wall; inferior epigastric, deep circumflex and pubic v.'s	common iliac v.
iliac v., internal hypogastric v. *v. iliaca interna*	from greater sciatic foramen it passes upward to brim of pelvis	continuation of femoral v.; superior gluteal, inferior gluteal, internal pudendal, obturator, lateral sacral, middle sacral, dorsal veins of penis, vesical, uterine, vaginal	common iliac v.
iliac circumflex v., deep *v. circumflexa ilium profunda*	inner aspect of ilium	venae comitantes of deep iliac circumflex artery	external iliac v. about 2 cm above inguinal ligament
innominate v.'s	see brachiocephalic veins		
intercostal v.'s, anterior (12 pairs) *vv. intercostales anterior*	lower border of each rib	ribs and intercostal muscles	internal thoracic and musculophrenic v.'s
intercostal v., left highest left superior intercostal v. *v. intercostalis suprema sinistra*	posterior wall of thorax across arch of aorta	first two or three left intercostal spaces, left bronchial v., and occasionally the left superior phrenic v. (it has a prominent anastomosis with the accessory hemiazygos v.)	left brachiocephalic v.
intercostal v., left superior *v. intercostalis superior sinistra*	across arch of aorta	left second, third, and fourth intercostal v.'s	left brachiocephalic v. or accessory hemiazygos v.

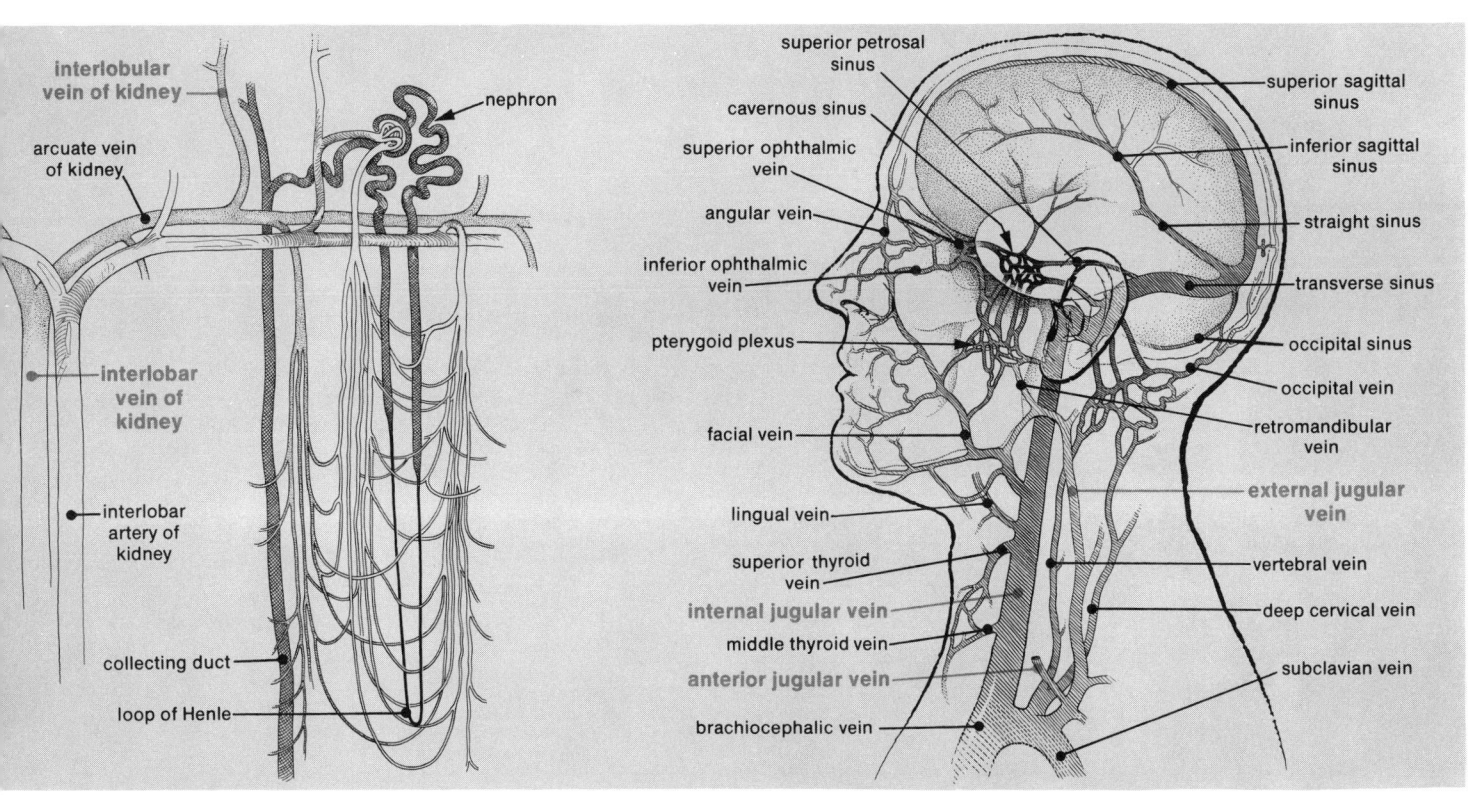

VEINS	LOCATION	DRAINS	EMPTIES INTO
intercostal v., right highest right superior intercostal v. *v. intercostalis suprema dextra*	posterior wall of upper thorax	upper two or three intercostal spaces	azygos v.
intercostal v.'s, posterior *vv. intercostales posterior*	one in each intercostal space	skin and muscles of back and spinal tributary from vertebral plexuses	*right side:* azygos v., right highest intercostal v.; *left side:* left brachiocephalic v., hemiazygos or accessory hemiazygos v.
intercostal v., right superior *v. intercostalis superior dextra*	posterior mediastinum	right second, third, and fourth intercostal spaces	azygos v.
interlobar v.'s of kidney *vv. interlobares renis*	between pyramids of kidney	arcuate v.'s	renal v.
interlobular v.'s of kidney *vv. interlobulares renis*	cortex of kidney	cortex of kidney; stellate, capsular, and perforating v.'s	arcuate v.'s of kidney
interlobular v.'s of liver *vv. interlobulares hepatis*	in substance of liver between lobules	central or intralobular and sublobular v.'s	hepatic v.'s
intervertebral v.'s *vv. intervertebrales*	vertebral column	internal and external vertebral plexuses; v.'s from spinal cord	vertebral, intercostal, lumbar, and lateral sacral v.'s
intestinal v.'s (usually 10–15 in number) jejunal and ileal v.'s *vv. intestinales*	run parallel with superior mesenteric artery between layers of mesentery	walls of jejunum and ileum	superior mesenteric v.
jejunal and ileal v.'s	see intestinal veins		
jugular v., anterior (usually two in number) *v. jugularis anterior*	from near hyoid bone it passes down anterior part of neck	laryngeal and thyroid v.'s, neck muscles	external jugular or subclavian v.
jugular v., external *v. jugularis externa*	from substance of parotid gland it runs perpendicularly down neck	deep parts of face, exterior of cranium, retromandibular and posterior auricular v.'s	subclavian v., internal jugular v., or brachiocephalic v.
jugular v., internal *v. jugularis interna*	from jugular fossa it descends side of neck lateral to internal carotid artery, and then lateral to common carotid artery	brain, face, and neck; transverse sinus, inferior petrosal sinus, facial, lingual, pharyngeal, superior and middle thyroid and at times the occipital v.'s	brachiocephalic v.
jugular v., posterior external *v. jugularis externa posterior*	from occipital region down to middle third of external jugular	skin and superficial muscles of back of head and neck	external jugular v.
labial v.'s, anterior *vv. labiales anterior*	vulva	anterior portion of labia majora; mons pubis	external pudendal v.

VEINS	LOCATION	DRAINS	EMPTIES INTO
labial v.'s, inferior *vv. labiales inferior*	edge of lower lip to angle of mouth	labial glands, mucous membrane and muscles of lower lip	facial v.
labial v.'s, posterior *vv. labiales posterior*	vulva	posterior portion of labia majora; vestibule, labia minora	internal pudendal v.
labial v.'s, superior *vv. labiales superior*	edge of upper lip between mucous membrane and muscle	upper lip, tributaries from nose, nasal septum	facial v.
labyrinthine v.'s internal auditory v.'s *vv. labyrinthi*	from internal ear through internal acoustic meatus	internal ear	inferior petrosal sinus or tranverse sinus
lacrimal v. *v. lacrimalis*	orbit	lacrimal glands, eyelids, conjunctiva	superior ophthalmic v.
laryngeal v., inferior *v. laryngea inferior*	dorsal part of larynx	muscles and mucous membrane of larynx	inferior thyroid v.
laryngeal v., superior *v. laryngea superior*	larynx	glands, mucous membrane, and muscles of larynx	superior thyroid v.
lingual v. *v. lingualis*	tongue	tongue by way of two or three tributaries	internal jugular or lower part of facial v.
lingual v., deep ranine v. *v. profunda linguae*	tongue	tip and deep part of tongue	vena comitans of deep lingual artery
lingual v.'s, dorsal *vv. dorsales linguae*	tongue	posterior part of tongue	lingual v.
lumbar v.'s (usually four in number on each side) *vv. lumbales*	lumbar walls	dorsal tributaries from skin and muscles of loin and by abdominal tributaries from abdominal wall; vertebral plexus	first and second drain into ascending lumbar v.; third and fourth drain into inferior vena cava
lumbar v., ascending *v. lumbalis ascendens*	ventral to transverse process of lumbar vertebrae	sacral and lumbar v.'s	*right side:* azygos v.; *left skin:* hemiazygos v.
maxillary v. *v. maxillaris*	short trunk between condyle of mandible and sphenomandibular ligament	pterygoid plexus	retromandibular v.
median v. of forearm median antebrachial v. *v. mediana antebrachii*	from base of thumb to middle of palmar forearm	venous plexus on palmar surface of hand	basilic v. and/or cephalic v., or median cubital v.
mediastinal v.'s anterior mediastinal v.'s *vv. mediastinales*	mediastinum	areolar tissue and lymph nodes of anterior mediastinum; pericardium	azygos v., brachiocephalic v., or superior vena cava
meningeal v.'s, anterior *vv. meningeae anterior*	over small wing of sphenoid bone	dura mater of anterior cranial fossa; cranium	ethmoidal and diploic v.'s, venous sinuses
meningeal v.'s, middle *vv. meningeae mediae*	from dura mater it leaves cranium via foramen spinosum of sphenoid bone	dura mater, internal surface of cranium, trigeminal ganglion	pterygoid plexus or parietosphenoidal sinus
mesenteric v., inferior *v. mesenterica inferior*	from rectum it ascends under cover of peritoneum to level of pancreas	rectum; sigmoid and descending parts of colon	splenic v.
mesenteric v., superior *v. mesenterica superior*	from right iliac fossa it ascends between two layers of mesentery to the level of pancreas	small intestine, cecum, appendix, and ascending and transverse parts of colon	portal v.
metacarpal v.'s, dorsal *vv. metacarpeae dorsales*	hand	dorsal metacrapal region	dorsal venous rete of hand
metacarpal v.'s, palmar *vv. metacarpeae palmares*	hand	palmar metacarpal region	deep palmar venous arch
metatarsal v.'s, dorsal dorsal interosseous v.'s of foot *vv. metatarseae dorsales*	run proximally in metatarsal spaces	dorsal digital v.'s at clefts of toes; metatarsal bones and neighboring muscles	dorsal venous arch of foot
metatarsal v.'s, plantar *vv. metatarseae plantares*	between metatarsal bones	plantar digital v.'s at clefts of toes; metatarsal bones and neighboring muscles	plantar venous arch of foot

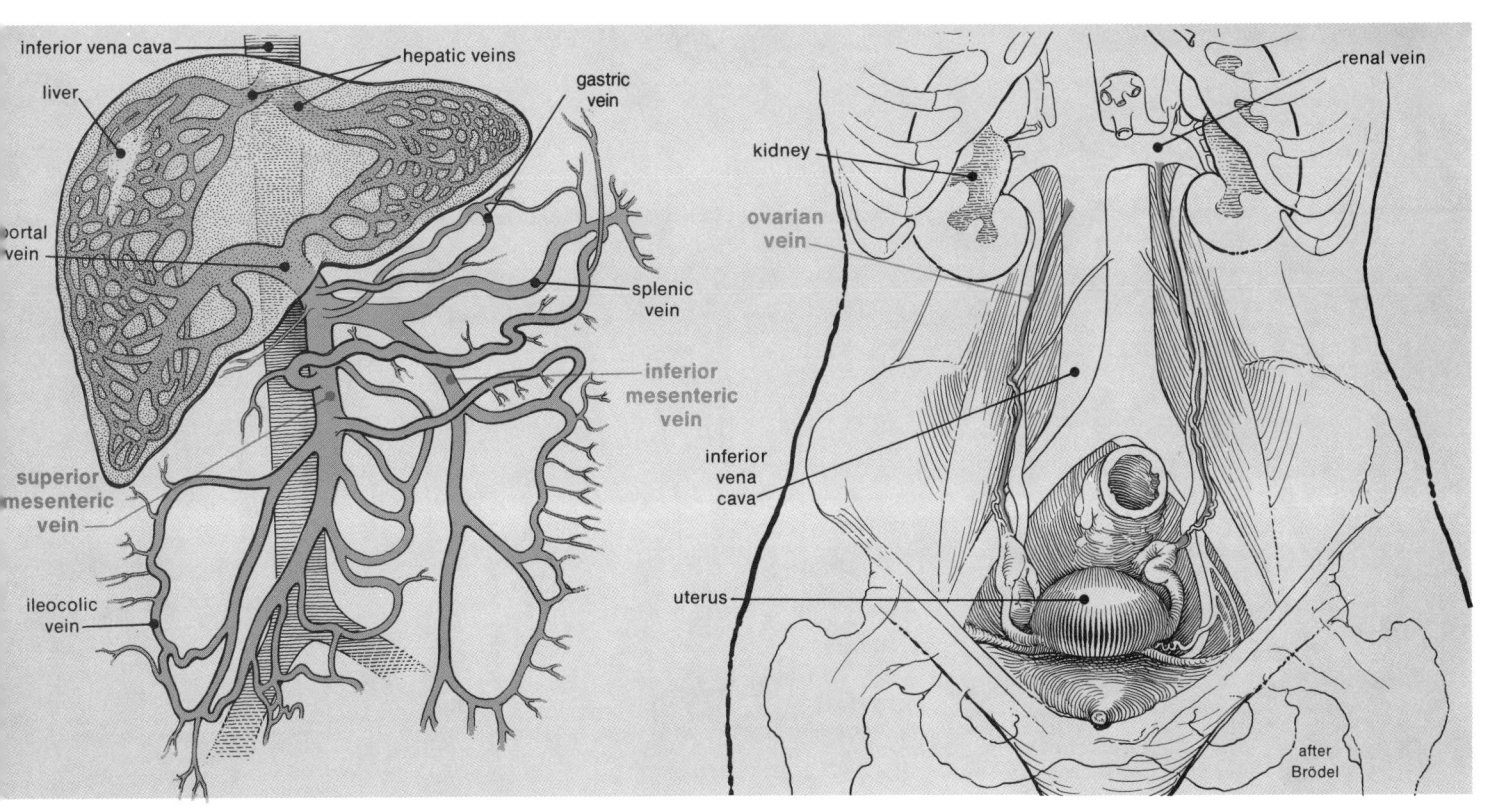

after Brödel

VEINS	LOCATION	DRAINS	EMPTIES INTO
musculophrenic v.'s *vv. musculophrenicae*	from diaphragm, along inner surface of costal cage at attachment of diaphragm, to sixth costal cartilage	diaphragm and lower intercostal spaces	internal thoracic v.
nasal v.'s, external (several in number) *vv. nasales externae*	from nose extending upward	external aspect of nose	angular and facial v.'s
nasofrontal v. *v. nasofrontalis*	anterior medial part of orbit	supraorbital and angular v.'s	superior ophthalmic v.
oblique v. of left atrium *v. obliqua atrii sinistri*	posterior wall of left atrium of heart	heart wall	coronary sinus
obturator v. *v. obturatoria*	from proximal portion of adductor region of thigh to pelvis through obturator foramen	hip joint and regional muscles	internal iliac v.
occipital v. *v. occipitalis*	from back part of scalp it passes into neck	plexus on posterior part of head; tributaries from posterior auricular and superficial temporal v.'s; parietal emissary, mastoid emissary, and occipital diploic v.'s	internal jugular or external jugular v.'s
ophthalmic v., inferior *v. ophthalmica inferior*	from floor of orbit it passes posteriorly to inferior back part of orbit	muscular and ciliary tributaries	cavernous sinus
ophthalmic v., superior *v. ophthalmica superior*	from inner angle of orbit, through orbit into cavernous sinus	eyeball, eye muscles, and eyelid	cavernous sinus
ovarian v.'s *vv. ovaricae*	in broad ligament near ovary and uterine tube	pampiniform plexus of broad ligament	*right side:* inferior vena cava; *left side:* left renal v.
palatine v., external *v. palatina externa*	palate region	tonsils and soft palate	pterygoid and tonsillar plexuses; facial v.
palpebral v.'s *vv. palpebrales*	eyelids	tributaries from palate	superior ophthalmic v.
palpebral v.'s, inferior *vv. palpebrales inferior*	lower eyelid	lower eyelid	facial v.
palpebral v.'s, superior *vv. palpebrales superior*	upper eyelid	upper eyelid	angular v. and superior ophthalmic v.
pancreatic v.'s *vv. pancreaticae*	at pancreas	tributaries from body and tail of pancreas	splenic v.
pancreaticoduodenal v.'s *vv. pancreaticoduodenales*	head of pancreas and proximal part of duodenum	pancreas and duodenum	upper part of superior mesenteric v.

vein | vein

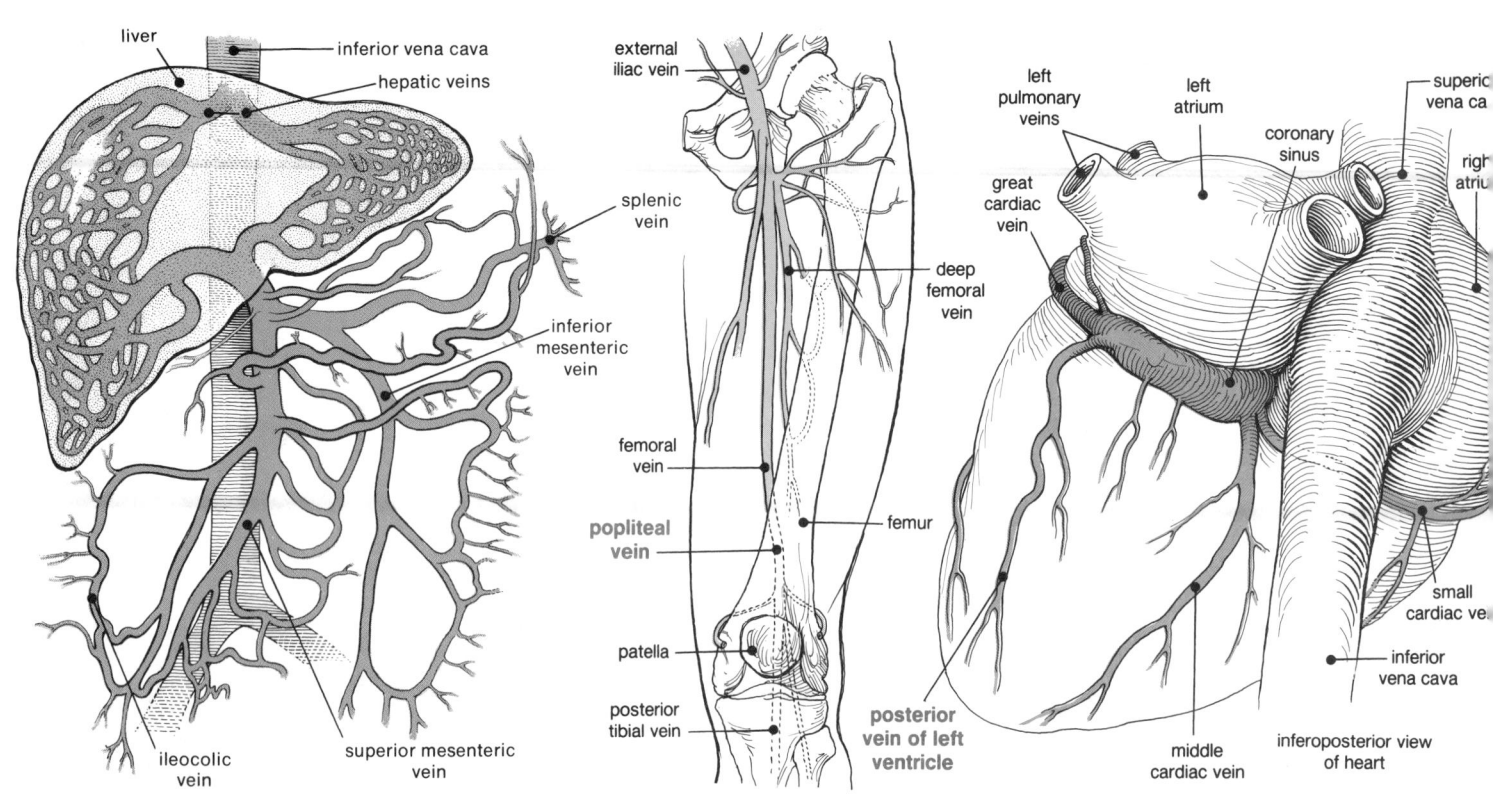

VEINS	LOCATION	DRAINS	EMPTIES INTO
paraumbilical v.'s parumbilical v.'s Sappey's v.'s *vv. paraumbilicales*	from umbilical area they pass along ligamentum teres to liver	cutaneous v.'s about the umbilicus	accessory portal v.'s in liver
parotid v.'s *vv. parotideae*	parotid gland	part of parotid gland	retromandibular v. or superficial temporal v.
peforating v.'s *vv. perforantes*	perforate great adductor muscle to reach back of thigh	thigh muscles, especially hamstrings	deep femoral v.
pericardiac v.'s (several in number) *vv. pericardiaceae*	membranous capsule of heart	pericardium	brachiocephalic v. or superior vena cava
pericardiacophrenic v.'s superior phrenic v.'s *vv. pericardiocophrenicae*	parallel to phrenic nerve between pleura and pericardium	diaphragm; tributaries from pericardium	brachiocephalic v.
peroneal v.'s *fibular v.'s* *vv. peroneae*	from lateral side of heel up back of leg just below knee	calcaneus, leg muscles, tibiofibular syndesmosis	posterior tibal v.
petrosal sinus, inferior *sinus petrosus inferior*	inferior petrosal sulcus	cavernous sinus, internal auditory v.'s, v.'s from medulla oblongata, pons, and inferior surface of cerebellum	bulb of internal jugular v.
petrosal sinus, superior *sinus petrosus superior*	superior petrosal sulcus in head	cavernous sinus	transverse sinus or sigmoid sinus
pharyngeal v.'s (several in number) *vv. pharyngeae*	outer surface of pharynx	posterior meningeal v.'s and v. of the pterygoid canal; pharyngeal plexus	internal jugular v.
phrenic v.'s, inferior *vv. phrenicae inferior*	undersurface of diaphragm	substance of diaphragm	*right side:* inferior vena cava; *left side:* left suprarenal v. (often a second vein on left side enters inferior vena cava)
popliteal v. *v. poplitea*	from lower border of popliteal muscle, through popliteal fossa to adductor hiatus	anterior and posterior tibial v.'s	femoral v. at adductor hiatus
portal v. (about 8 cm in length) *v. portae*	in abdomen behind neck of pancreas	superior mesenteric, splenic, gastric, pyloric, cystic, and paraumbilical v.'s	divides into right and left before emptying into substance of liver
posterior v. of left ventricle *v. posterior ventriculi sinistri*	from apex of heart it travels parallel to posterior interventricular sulcus	diaphragmatic surface of left ventricle	coronary sinus
prepyloric v. v. of Mayo *v. prepylorica*	pyloric end of stomach	pylorus	right gastric v.

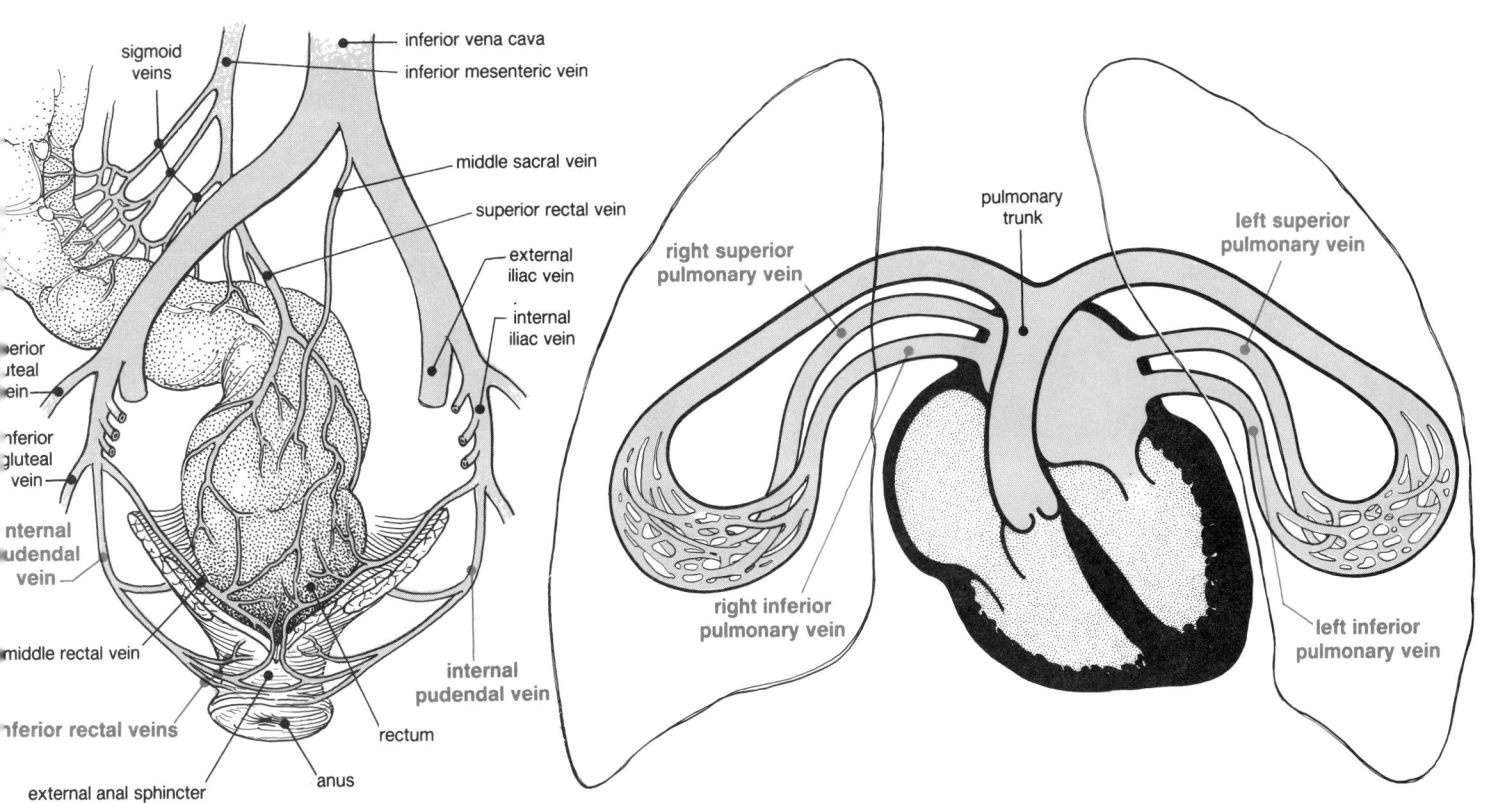

Labels (left diagram):
- sigmoid veins
- inferior vena cava
- inferior mesenteric vein
- middle sacral vein
- superior rectal vein
- external iliac vein
- internal iliac vein
- superior gluteal vein
- inferior gluteal vein
- internal pudendal vein
- middle rectal vein
- inferior rectal veins
- internal pudendal vein
- external anal sphincter
- rectum
- anus

Labels (right diagram):
- right superior pulmonary vein
- pulmonary trunk
- left superior pulmonary vein
- right inferior pulmonary vein
- left inferior pulmonary vein

VEINS	LOCATION	DRAINS	EMPTIES INTO
profunda femoris v.	see femoral vein, deep		
profunda linguae v.	see lingual vein, deep		
v. of pterygoid canal Vidian v. *v. canalis pterygoidei*	from ear and throat through pterygoid canal	sphenoid sinus	pterygoid plexus or cavernous sinus
pterygoid plexus *plexus pterygoideus*	infratemporal fossa	*tributaries from:* inferior alveolar, middle, meningeal, deep temporal, masseter, buccal, posterior superior alveolar, pharyngeal, descending palatine, infraorbital, pterygoid canal, and sphenopalatine v.s's	maxillary v.
pubic v. *v. pubis*	from dorsum of penis through obturator foramen to pelvis	pubic area	external iliac v.
pudendal v.'s, external external pudic v.'s *vv. pudendae externae*	from lower abdomen and genitalia to upper thigh	skin of lower part of abdomen; *in male:* anterior scrotal and superficial dorsal v.'s of penis; *in female:* anterior labial and superficial dorsal v.'s of clitoris	great saphenous v. or femoral v.
pudendal v.'s, internal internal pudic v.'s *vv. pudendae internae*	from perineum and genitalia to pelvis	perineum and genitalia	internal iliac v.
pulmonary v., left inferior *v. pulmonis inferior sinistra*	from left lung to heart	left lower lobe	left atrium of heart
pulmonary v., left superior *v. pulmonis superior sinistra*	from left lung to heart	left upper lobe	left atrium of heart
pulmonary v., right inferior *v. pulmonis inferior dextra*	from right lung to heart	right lower lobe	left atrium of heart
pulmonary v., right superior *v. pulmonis superior dextra*	from right lung to heart	right upper and middle lobe	left atrium of heart
pyloric v. *v. pylorus*	along pyloric portion of lesser curvature of stomach	pylorus and lesser omentum	portal v.
radial v.'s *vv. radiales*	from hand, winds around lateral side of carpus up forearm to elbow	dorsal metacarpal v.'s	joined by ulnar v.'s to form brachial v.'s
ranine v.	see lingual vein, deep		
rectal v.'s inferior inferior hemorrhoidal v.'s *vv. rectales inferior*	near anal canal and rectum	lower part of external rectal plexus	internal pudendal v.

VEINS	LOCATION	DRAINS	EMPTIES INTO
rectal v., middle middle hemorrhoidal v. *v. rectalis media*	rectal area	rectal plexus; tributaries from bladder, prostate gland, and seminal vesicle	internal iliac v.
rectal v.'s, superior superior hemorrhoidal v.'s *vv. rectales superior*	from rectum to brim of pelvis	upper part of rectal plexus	inferior mesenteric v.
renal v.'s *vv. renales*	at right angle to hilum of kidneys	kidneys; testicular, inferior phrenic, and suprarenal v.'s	inferior vena cava (right renal v. opens into inferior vena cava at a slightly lower level than left)
retromandibular v. posterior facial v. *v. retromandibularis*	from substance of parotid gland it passes alongside ramus of lower jaw	superficial temporal, maxillary, and tributaries from parotid gland and masseter muscle	external or internal jugular v.
sacral v.'s, lateral *vv. sacrales laterales*	anterior surface of sacrum	skin and muscles of dorsum of sacrum	internal iliac v.
sacral v., middle *v. sacralis media*	hollow of sacrum	region of posterior surface of rectum	left common iliac v.
saphenous v., accessory *v. saphena accessoria*	medial and posterior parts of thigh	inner and posterior parts of superficial thigh	great saphenous v.
saphenous v., great (longest vein in body) long saphenous v. *v. saphena magna*	from medial aspect of foot to 3 cm below inguinal ligament	tributaries from sole of foot; small saphenous v., anterior and posterior tibial v.'s, accessory saphenous v., superficial epigastric v., superficial iliac circumflex v., superficial external pudendal v.	femoral v.
saphenous v., small short saphenous v. *c. saphena parva*	from lateral ankle to middle of back of leg	lateral marginal v., deep v.'s of dorsum of foot, large tributaries from back of leg	popliteal v.
scrotal v.'s, anterior *vv. scrotales anterior*	scrotum	front part of scrotum	external pudendal v.
scrotal v.'s, posterior *vv. scrotales posterior*	scrotum	back part of scrotum	vesical venous plexus or internal pudendal veins
sigmoid v.'s (several in number) *vv. sigmoideae*	lower left side of colon	sigmoid colon and descending colon	inferior mesenteric v.
spinal v.'s *vv. spinales*	in pia mater of spinal cord where it forms a tortuous venous plexus	spinal cord and pia matter	internal vertebral venous plexus
spiral v. of modiolus *v. spiralis modioli*	modiolus of cochlea	cochlea	labyrinthine v.'s
splenic v. lienal v. *v. lienalis*	from hilum of spleen to vicinity of neck of pancreas	short gastric, left gastroepiploic, pancreatic, and inferior mesenteric v.'s	portal v.
stellate v.'s of kidney *vv. stellatae renis*	cortex of kidney near capsule	superficial part of cortex of kidney	interlobular v.'s of kidney
sternocleidomastoid v. sternomastoid v. *v. sternocleidomastoidea*	neck	sternocleidomastoid, omohyoid, sternohyoid, sternothyroid, and platysma muscles, skin of neck	internal jugular v.
striate v.'s, inferior *vv. thalamostriatae inferior*	corpus striatum	anterior perforated substance of cerebrum	basal v.
stylomastoid v. *v. stylomastoidea*	descends vertically from stylomastoid foramen	mastoid cells, middle ear chamber, semicircular canals	retromandibular v. or posterior auricular v.
subclavian v. *v. subclavia*	from outer border of first rib to sternal end of clavicle	continues from axillary v.; external jugular v., anterior jugular v. (occasionally)	joined by internal jugular to form brachiocephalic v.
subcostal v. *v. subcostalis*	in abdominal wall along caudal border of 12th rib	lower abdominal wall	*right side:* azygos v.; *left side:* hemiazygos v.
subcutaneous v.'s of abdomen *vv. subcutaneae abdominis*	abdominal wall	superficial layers of abdominal wall	thoracoepigastric, superficial epigastric, or deep v.'s of abdominal wall
sublingual v. *v. sublingualis*	below tongue	sublingual gland, mylohyoid and neighboring muscles, mucous membranes of mouth and gums, alveolar process of mandible	lingual v.

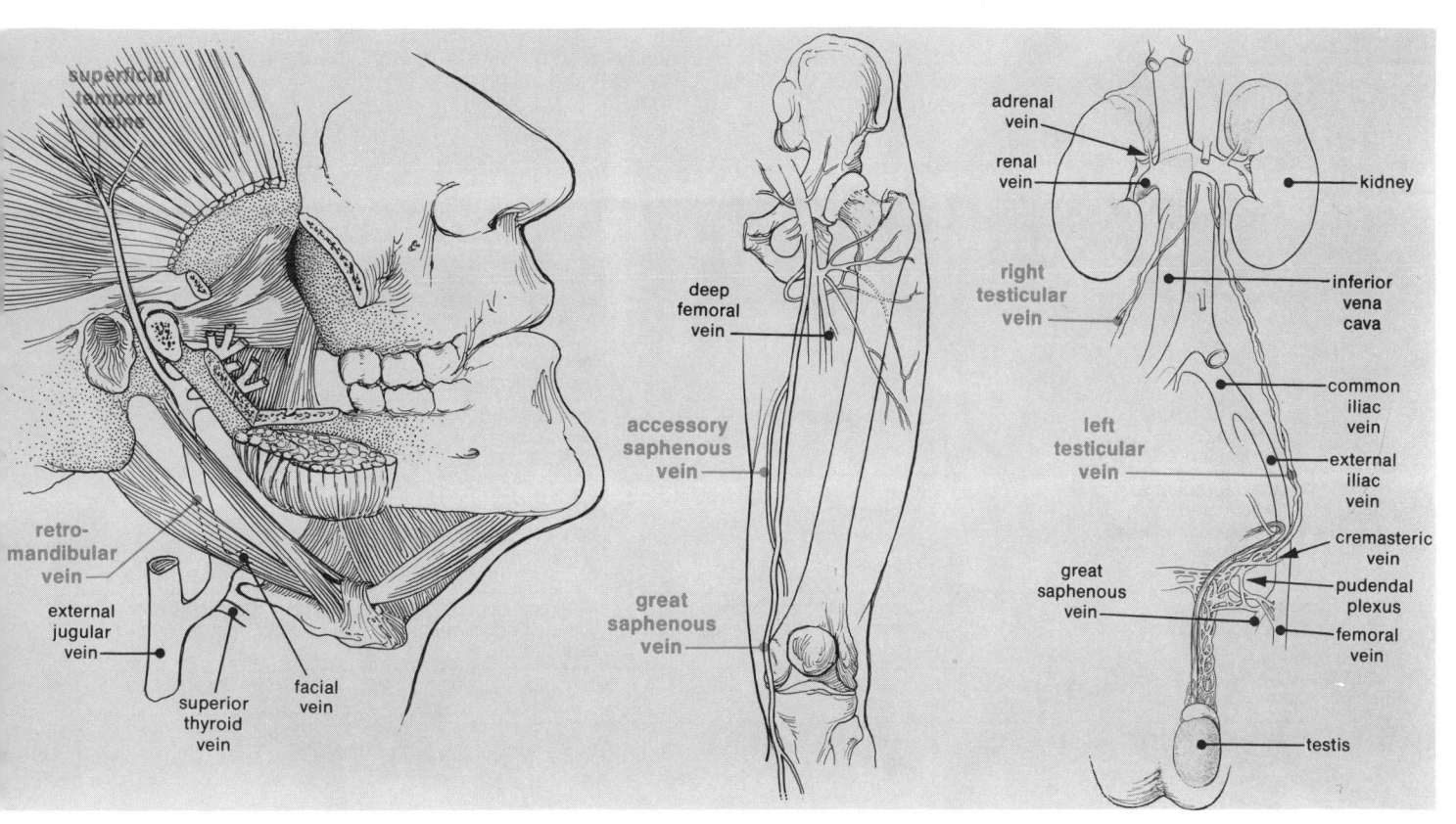

VEINS	LOCATION	DRAINS	EMPTIES INTO
submental v. *v. submentalis*	below margin of mandible	submandibular gland; mylohyoid, digastric, and platysma muscles	facial v.
supraorbital v. *v. supraorbitalis*	forehead	frontal muscle, frontal diploic v.	facial v. or superior ophthalmic v.
suprarenal v., left *v. suprarenalis sinistra*	hilium of left adrenal gland	left adrenal gland	left renal v. or left inferior phrenic v.
suprarenal v., right *v. suprarenalis dextra*	hilium of right adrenal gland	right adrenal gland	inferior vena cava
suprascapular v. transverse scapular v. *v. suprascapularis*	from posterior surface of scapula it passes through scapular notch, runs parallel with clavicle and then crosses over brachial plexus and subclavian artery	shoulder joint, scapula, clavicle, and neighboring muscles and skin	external jugular v. or subclavian v.
supratrochlear v.'s (usually two in number) *vv. supratrochleares*	front and top of head	venous plexus of forehead	angular v.
temporal v.'s, deep *vv. temporales profundae*	side of head	deep areas of temporal muscle	pterygoid plexus
temporal v., middle *v. temporalis media*	from lateral angle of orbit, it passes to side of ear	temporal muscle; zygomaticoorbital v.	retromandibular v. or superficial and deep temporal v.'s
temporal v.'s, superficial *vv. temporales superficiales*	from scalp on side of head down to parotid gland	plexus on side of head; transverse facial, anterior auricular, and middle temporal v.'s	retromandibular v.
temporomandibular v.'s *vv. temporomandibulares*	temporomandibular joint (TMJ)	area surrounding temporomandibular joint; tympanic v.'s	retromandibular v. or maxillary v.
testicular v., left left spermatic v. *v. testicularis sinistra*	from testis it ascends along spermatic cord through deep inguinal canal into abdomen	testis, epididymis	left renal v.
testicular v., right right spermatic v. *v. testicularis dextra*	from testis it ascends along spermatic cord through deep inguinal canal into abdomen	testis, epididymis	inferior vena cava
thalamostriate v. *v. thalamostriata superior*	deep part of brain	corpus striatum, thalamus, and corpus callosum	internal cerebral v.

VEINS	LOCATION	DRAINS	EMPTIES INTO
thoracic v., internal internal mammary v. *v. thoracica interna*	thorax	superior phrenic, superior epigastric, musculophrenic, perforating, anterior intercostal, sternal, thymic, mediastinal, and pericardiacophrenic v.'s	brachiocephalic v.
thoracic v., lateral long thoracic v. *v. thoracica lateral*	lateral thoracic wall	lateral thoracic wall; costoaxillary v.'s	axillary v.
thoracoacromial v.'s acromiothoracic v.'s *vv. thoracoacromiales*	parallel with thoracoacromial artery	acromion, coracoid process, sternoclavicular joint, tributaries from deltoid, subclavius, pectoralis major and minor muscles	subclavian v.
thoracoepigastirc v. *v. thoracoepigastrica*	anterior and lateral aspect of trunk (in subcutaneous tissue)	skin and subcutaneous tissue of anterolateral aspect of trunk	superiorly: lateral thoracic v.; inferiorly: superficial epigastric v.
thymic v.'s *vv. thymicae*	thymus gland	substance of thymus gland	left brachiocephalic and thyroid v.'s
thyroid v.'s, inferior (two to four in number) *vv. thyroideae inferior*	lower neck	venous plexus of thyroid gland; esophageal, tracheal, and inferior laryngeal v.'s	brachiocephalic v.'s
thyroid v.'s, middle *vv. thyroidea mediae*	from thyroid gland they pass laterally over common carotid artery	lower part of thyroid gland; tributaries from trachea and larynx	lower part of internal jugular v.
thyroid v.'s, superior *v. thyroidea superior*	from thyroid gland it passes up toward head	superior part of thyroid gland; superior laryngeal and cricothyroid v.'s	upper part of internal jugular v.
tibial v.'s, anterior *vv. tibiales anterior*	from foot and ankle joint up front of leg between tibia and fibula	venae comitantes of dorsal artery of foot; muscles and bones of anterior leg	popliteal v.
tibial v.'s, posterior (usually two in number) *vv. tibiales posterior*	from sole of foot to tibial side of leg where it ascends obliquely to back of leg just below bend of knee	muscles and bones of posterior leg	popliteal v.
tracheal v.'s (several in number) *vv. tracheales*	trachea	substance of trachea	thyroid venous plexus, brachiocephalic v., or superior vena cava
v. of tympanic cavity *v. cavum tympani*	middle ear	middle ear chamber (cavity), tympanic membrane, mastoid cells, auditory tube	pterygoid plexus and superior petrosal sinus
v.'s of tympanic membrane *vv. tympanicae membranae*	tympanic membrane (ear drum)	tympanic membrane	v.'s of tympanic cavity and external meatus
ulnar v.'s *vv. ulnares*	from hand it runs along border of wrist, up forearm to bend of elbow	deep palmar venous arches; superficial v.'s at wrist; palmar and dorsal interosseous v.'s	brachial v.'s
umbilical v. *v. umbilicalis*	accompanying umbilical cord	placenta	fetus
uterine v.'s *vv. uterinae*	sides and superior angles of uterus between two layers of broad ligament	uterine plexus	internal iliac v.
vaginal v.'s *vv. vaginales*	sides of vagina	vaginal plexus	internal iliac v.
vena cava, inferior (largest vein in body) vena cava inferior	from level of fifth lumbar vertebra it ascends along vertebral column to right side of heart	both common iliac v.'s; lumbar, renal, testicular (male), ovarian (female), suprarenal, inferior phrenic, and hepatic v.'s	right atrium of heart
vena cava, superior (second largest vein in body) vena cava superior	from close behind sternum to upper portion of right side of heart	cranial half to body via brachiocephalic v.'s	cranial part of right atrium
vertebral v. *v. vertebralis*	from suboccipital triangle through transverse foramina of first six cervical vertebrae	suboccipital venous plexus, occipital v., internal and external vertebral venous plexuses, anterior cerebral v., deep cervical v.'s, first intercostal v. (occasionally)	brachiocephalic v.

VEINS	LOCATION	DRAINS	EMPTIES INTO
vertebral v., accessory *v. vertebralis accessoria*	when present it accompanies vertebral vein and emerges through transverse foramen of seventh cervical vertebra	venous plexus of vertebral artery	brachiocephalic v.
vertebral v., anterior ascending cervical v. *v. vertebralis anterior*	from transverse processes of cervical vertebrae it descends between anterior scalene and longus capitis muscles (it accompanies ascending cervical artery)	plexus around transverse processes of cervical vertebrae	terminal part of vertebral v.
vesical v.'s *vv. vesicales*	back part of bladder and base of prostate gland	vesical plexus; anastomose with pudendal and prostatic plexuses	internal iliac v.
vestibular v.'s *vv. vestibulares*	internal ear	vestibule of internal ear	labyrinthine or internal jugular v.
vorticose v.'s (usually four or five in number) vortex v.'s *vv. vorticosae*	eyeball, midway between cribosa and sclerocorneal junction	choroid layer of eyeball	superior or inferior ophthalmic v.'s

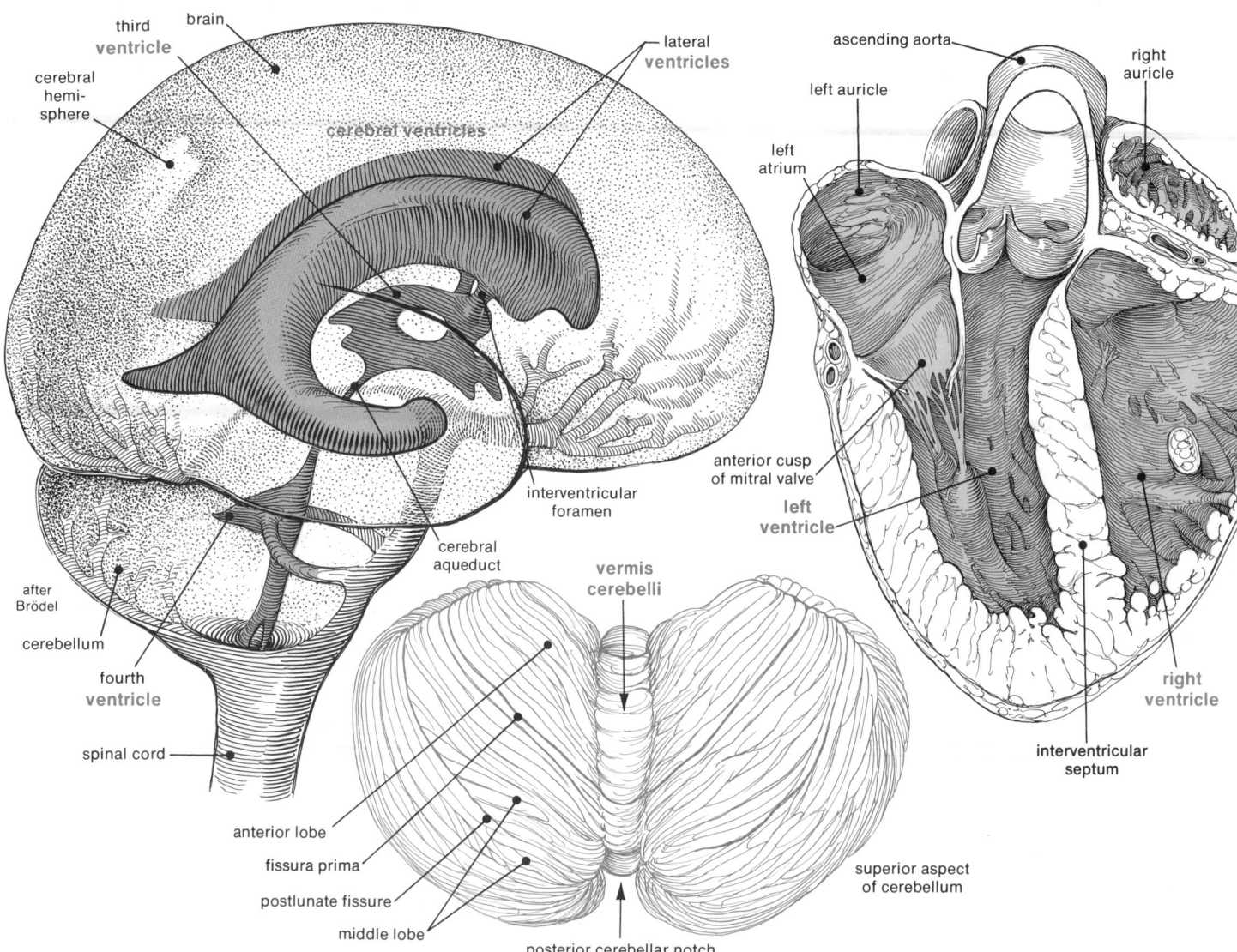

third ventricle · brain · cerebral hemisphere · cerebral ventricles · lateral ventricles · ascending aorta · left auricle · right auricle · left atrium · after Brödel · cerebellum · fourth ventricle · spinal cord · anterior lobe · fissura prima · postlunate fissure · middle lobe · interventricular foramen · cerebral aqueduct · vermis cerebelli · posterior cerebellar notch · superior aspect of cerebellum · anterior cusp of mitral valve · left ventricle · right ventricle · interventricular septum

veneniferous Bearing poison.

venenous Poisonous; toxic; venomous.

venereal Relating to, or resulting from, sexual intercourse; the term is derived from the Latin *venereus,* love.

venereology The study of venereal disease.

venesection Withdrawing of blood through an incision of a vein. Also called phlebotomy.

venipuncture The insertion of a needle into a vein.

venoclysis The continuous injection into a vein of a medicinal or nutritive fluid; intravenous infusion of fluids by slow gravity flow or intravenous drip.

venogram A roentgenogram of a vein or veins after intravenous injection of a radiopaque substance.

venography The making of a venogram. Also called phlebography.

venom A poisonous substance secreted by snakes or other animals.

venomotor Causing changes in the internal diameter of veins.

venopressor An agent which increases venous blood pressure by venoconstriction.

venostasis See phlebostasis.

venotomy See phlebotomy.

venous Relating to a vein.

venovenostomy Surgical connection of two veins.

ventilation Physiologic process in which air in the lungs is exchanged with atmospheric air; a cyclic process of inspiration and expiration in which alternately fresh air enters the respiratory tract and an equal amount of pulmonary gas is exhaled.

alveolar v. The amount of inspired gas which enters the alveoli each minute.

ventrad Toward the ventral side.

ventral Relating to (a) the belly; (b) the anterior part of a structure.

ventricle A cavity, especially in the heart or the brain.

cardiac v. One of the two lower and larger chambers of the heart.

cerebral v.'s The cavities within the brain (two lateral, the third, and the fourth ventricles).

left v. (LV) The left lower chamber of the heart.

right v. (RV) The right lower chamber of the heart.

ventricornu The anterior column of gray matter of the spinal cord.

ventricular Relating to any ventricle.

ventriculitis Inflammation of the lining of the ventricles of the brain.

ventriculocisternostomy Surgical establishment of communication between the ventricles of the brain and the subarachnoid space or cisterna magna.

ventriculocordotomy Removal of a portion of each vocal cord of a dog to reduce the sound of its bark.

ventriculogram A roentgenogram of the brain following the direct introduction of air or an opaque medium into the cerebral ventricles.

ventriculography The making of x-ray films of the brain after replacing the cerebrospinal fluid of the ventricles with a gas.

ventriculopuncture Introduction of a needle into a ventricle.

ventriculotomy Incision into a ventricle.

ventriculus, *pl.* **ventriculi** 1. Latin for ventricle. 2. The stomach.

ventrofixation of uterus An operation for the correction of a retroplaced uterus by suturing the uterine fundus to the anterior abdominal wall; this procedure is no longer used but is of historical interest in the evolution of uterine suspension. Also called hysteropexy; hysterorrhaphy.

ventroscopy Laparoscopy.

ventrotomy Laparotomy.

venula, *pl.* **venulae** Venule.

venulae rectae The numerous ascending venules that drain the medullary pyramids of the kidney and empty into arcuate veins.

venulae stellatae The stellate venules in the renal cortex near the capsule.

venule A minute vein; usually one less than 100 μm in diameter.

postcapillary v. Unique venule marked by elongated endothelial cells, situated in the lymph node cortex where it allows lymphocytes to pass from the blood to the lymph.

verapamil A calcium channel blocking agent used in the treatment of angina pectoris, especially variant angina.

verbigeration Repetition of meaningless words or phrases. Also called oral stereotypy.

verge Margin.

anal v. Area between the perianal skin and the anal canal.

vergence Movement of the eyes in opposite directions.

vermicide An agent that kills intestinal worms.

vermicular Wormlike.

vermiculation A wormlike motion.

vermicule 1. A small worm. 2. Wormlike.

vermiculose, vermiculous 1. Wormy. 2. Wormlike.

vermiform Having the shape of a worm.

vermifuge An agent that expels intestinal worms.

vermilionectomy Excision of the vermilion border of the lip; the exposed area is generally resurfaced by advancing the undermined labial mucosa.

vermin Parasitic insects.

verminous Infested with or caused by worms or any parasite.

vermis Latin for worm.

v. cerebelli The narrow median part of the cerebellum that connects the two cerebellar hemispheres.

cervical **vertebrae**

thoracic **vertebrae**

lumbar **vertebrae**

sacrum: 5 fused sacral **vertebrae**

coccyx: 4 fused coccygeal **vertebrae**

vertex

sinciput

occiput

ampulla of deferent duct

urinary bladder

seminal vesicle

ejaculatory duct

prostate

deferent duct

urethra

testes

vermix The vermiform appendix.

vernix Latin for varnish.

v. caseosa A fatty or cheesy substance on the skin of a newborn, consisting of stratum corneum, sebaceous secretions, and remnants of epithelium.

verruca Wart.

verruciform In the shape of warts or wartlike projections.

verrucose, verrucous Resembling or covered with warts or wartlike roughness; denoting wartlike projections or elevations.

verrucosis A condition characterized by the presence of multiple warts or wartlike elevations.

verruga Verruca.

verruga peruana The chronic form of bartonellosis; it usually, but not always, follows the anemic stage (Oroya fever); marked by a profuse skin eruption, chiefly on the face and limbs, which may persist from one month to two years. See also bartonellosis.

versicolor Marked by a variety of color; denoting turning or changing color.

version 1. Turning of a fetus in the uterus to alter its position to one more favorable for delivery. **2.** The state of an organ of being turned from its normal position. **3.** In ophthalmology, similar movement of the two eyes in the same direction.

bimanual v., bipolar v. Turning of the fetus with two hands; may be external or combined.

Braxton Hicks v. Seldom used procedure in which the forefinger and/or middle finger are introduced into the uterus to displace the presenting part of the fetus (often the shoulder) while the head is guided toward the birth canal by the operator's external hand.

cephalic v. Version performed in modern obstetrics only by external manipulations; each hand grabs one of the fetal ends and the head is gently pushed in the direction of the birth canal.

combined v. Version in which one hand is introduced into the uterus and the other is placed on the abdominal wall.

external v. Manipulation by placing the hands on the abdomen and applying force gently and intermittently.

Hicks v. Braxton Hicks version.

internal v. Direct turning of the fetus by introducing a hand into the uterus.

podalic v. Turning the fetus by seizing one or both feet and drawing them through the cervix.

spontaneous v. Version effected by contraction of the uterus alone.

vertebra, *pl.* **vertebrae** One of the 33 bones that form the spinal column; they are divided into 7 cervical, 12 thoracic, 5 lumbar, 5 sacral, and 4 coccygeal vertebrae.

vertebral Relating to a vertebra.

vertebrate 1. Having a backbone or vertebral column. **2.** Any member of the subphylum Vertebrata, characterized by having a segmented vertebral column.

vertebrectomy Surgical removal of a portion of a vertebra.

vertex 1. The uppermost part of the head. **2.** In obstetrics, the crown of the fetal head.

vertical Straight up and down; perpendicular, or at right angles, to the horizon.

verticil A whorl or circular arrangement; a collection of similar parts radiating about a point on an axis.

verticillate Characterized by, or forming, a whorl or whorls; circularly arranged.

vertigo Illusion of revolving motion, either of oneself or of one's surroundings.

auditory v. See Ménière's syndrome.

aural v. Vertigo caused by disease of the internal ear.

ocular v. Vertigo caused by errors in the refractive system of the eye or imbalance in the eye muscles.

organic v. Vertigo caused by brain damage.

verumontanitis Inflammation of the verumontanum (seminal colliculus).

verumontanum An elevation in the prostatic portion of the urethra, on either side of which open the prostatic and ejaculatory ducts. Also called seminal colliculus.

vesica Latin for bladder and blister.

vesical Of, or relating to, the bladder.

vesicant Any agent that produces blisters.

vesicate To blister.

vesication 1. The formation of a blister. **2.** A blister or blistered surface.

vesicle 1. A sac or hollow structure containing fluid or gas. **2.** A blister or circumscribed elevation on the skin containing serous fluid and ranging in size up to one centimeter, e.g., as in early chickenpox. Cf. bulla.

seminal v. One of the two sac-like glandular structures situated behind the bladder; its secretion is one of the components of semen.

synaptic v.'s A profusion of small spherical membrane-bound organelles in presynaptic nerve terminals that contain packages of protein-bound humoral transmitter substance; when released through the presynaptic membrane into the intercellular space, they cause changes in permeability and electric potential.

vesicobullous Describing blister-like lesions containing serum.

vesicocele See cystocele.

vesicoclysis Washing out of the bladder.

vesicoprostatic Relating to the bladder and prostate gland.

vesicorectal Relating to the urinary bladder and the rectum.

vesicotomy Surgical incision of the urinary bladder. Also called cystotomy.

vesicoureteral Relating to the bladder and the ureters.

vesicourethral Relating to the bladder and the

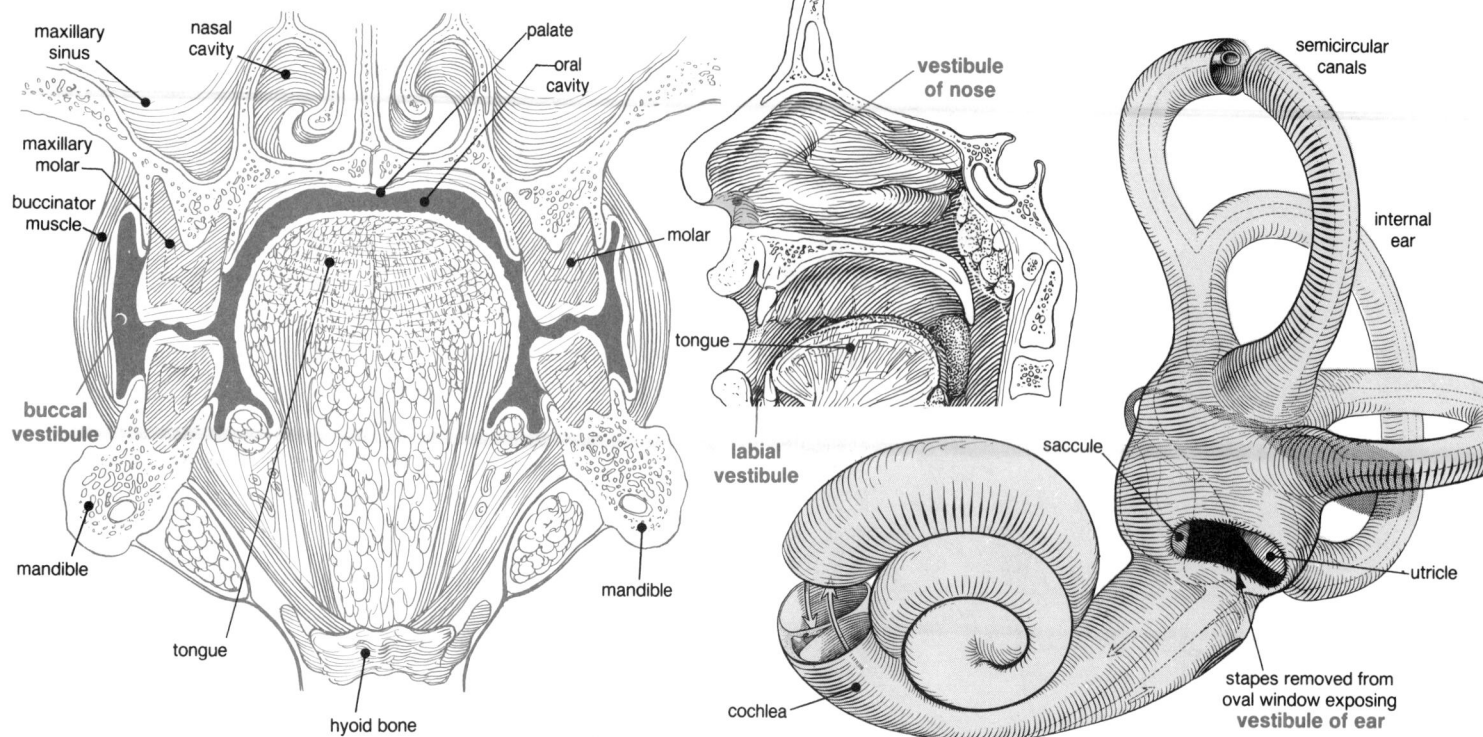

Labels on diagrams:
maxillary sinus, nasal cavity, palate, oral cavity, vestibule of nose, semicircular canals, maxillary molar, buccinator muscle, molar, internal ear, buccal vestibule, tongue, labial vestibule, saccule, mandible, tongue, hyoid bone, mandible, cochlea, utricle, stapes removed from oval window exposing vestibule of ear

urethra.

vesicouterine Relating to the urinary bladder and the uterus.

vesicouterovaginal Relating to the bladder, uterus, and vagina.

vesicovaginal Relating to the bladder and vagina.

vesicovaginorectal Relating to the bladder, vagina, and rectum.

vesicula, *pl.* **vesiculae** A small bladder-like structure.

vesicular 1. Of, or relating to, vesicles. 2. Containing vesicles.

vesiculation The formation of vesicles or the condition of having numerous vesicles.

vesiculectomy Removal of a seminal vesicle.

vesiculiform Having the shape of a vesicle.

vesiculitis Inflammation of a seminal vesicle.

vesiculopapular Relating to vesicles and papules.

vesiculoprostatitis Inflammation of the urinary bladder and the underlying prostate gland.

vesiculopustular Relating to vesicles and pustules.

vesiculotomy Incision into a seminal vesicle.

vessel Tubular structure that conveys fluids.

vestibular Of, or relating to, a vestibule, especially the vestibule of the internal ear where balance functions are governed.

vestibule A small chamber or space at the entrance to a canal.

  buccal v. The space between the teeth and gums and the cheek.

  labial v. The space between the teeth and gums and the lips.

  v. of aorta A small space within the left ventricle just below the aortic opening. Also called Sibson's aortic vestibule.

  v. of ear The oval cavity in the middle of the bony labyrinth.

  v. of nose The area just inside the nares.

vestibuloplasty Operative procedure to deepen the labial sulcus (especially of the maxilla) and increase ridge height.

vestibulotomy Surgical opening into the vestibule of the ear (labyrinth).

vestibulourethral Relating to the vestibule of the vagina and the urethra.

vestibulum, *pl.* **vestibula** A vestibule.

vestige 1. A rudimentary structure; usually a remnant of an organ or part. 2. An imperfectly developed organ that has ceased to function.

vestigial 1. Pertaining to a vestige. 2. A persisting rudimentary structure.

vestigium, *pl.* **vestigia** Remnant of a structure that was functional in the embryo.

veterinarian A person trained and licensed to diagnose and treat the diseases of animals, both domestic and wild.

veterinary Relating to the diagnosis and treatment of diseases of animals.

via, *pl.* **viae** Passage.

viability The condition of being viable.

viable Capable of living, as a fetus that has developed enough to be able to live outside of the uterus.

vial A small glass container for holding liquid medicines.

vibration The act of moving back and forth rapidly; the rapid movement in alternately opposite directions of an elastic solid or a particle about an equilibrium position. Also called oscillation.

  sonic v. Sound waves of ultrasonic frequencies used for disrupting cell structures in an aqueous medium.

vibrator A device that vibrates or causes vibrations.

Vibrio A genus of motile, gram-negative bacteria, occurring in salt and fresh water and in soil.

  V. cholerae A comma-shaped rod causing Asiatic cholera in man. Also called cholera bacillus; *Vibrio comma.*

  V. comma See *Vibrio cholera.*

vibrio Any bacterium of the genus *Vibrio.*

  El Tor v. Bacterium isolated from six pilgrims who died of dysentery and gangrene of the colon at the El Tor Quarantine Station on the Sinai peninsula.

vibrissa, *pl.* **vibrissae** One of the hairs within the nostrils.

vibrotherapeutics Therapeutic use of vibrating devices.

vicarious Acting as a substitute; occurring in a part of the body not normally associated with that specific function.

vicinal (v.) Relating to, or denoting, the adjoining or neighboring position of radicals in an organic compound, as the 1, 2, 3 positions in the benzene ring.

Victoria green Malachite green.

view See projection (4).

vigilambulism Condition, resembling sleepwalking but occurring in the wakeful state, in which the individual is unaware of his surroundings.

vigilance Morbid wakefulness; insomnia; the state of being at vigil.

villi Plural of villus.

villikinin One of a group of gastrointestinal hormones believed to be responsible for the contraction of villi during digestion.

villoma See papilloma.

villositis Inflammation of the villous aspect of the placenta.

villosity An aggregation of villi.

villous Covered with minute hairlike projections (villi).

villus, *pl.* **villi** A minute, vascular, hairlike projection from the surface of a membrane, such as the mucous membrane of the intestines.

  arachnoid villi Arachnoid granulations; see under granulation.

  chorionic villi Slender vascular projections of the chorion forming part of the placenta and through which all substances are exchanged between maternal and fetal circulations.

  intestinal villi Small projections on the surface of the mucosa of the small intestine; they are leaf-shaped in the duodenum and become finger-shaped, shorter, and sparser in the ileum; the sites of absorption of fluids and nutrients.

vinblastine sulfate A salt of an antineoplastic alkaloid extracted from the periwinkle plant, *Vinca rosea;* Velban®.

Vinca rosea See periwinkle.

Vincent's angina Fusospirochetal pharyngitis; see under pharyngitis.

Vincent's disease, Vincent's infection, Vincent's stomatitis Necrotizing ulcerative gingivitis; see under gingivitis.

vincristine sulfate A salt of an antineoplastic alkaloid extracted from the periwinkle plant, *Vinca rosea;* used primarily in the treatment of acute leukemias, lymphomas, and solid tumors in children; Oncovin®.

vinculum, *pl.* **vincula** A frenum or restricting bandlike structure.

vinegar An impure, dilute (approximately six per cent) solution of acetic acid formed by the fermentation of alcoholic liquids (wine, cider, malt, etc.), or by the distillation of wood.

vinegaroon The nonvenomous whip-scorpion, *Mastigoproctus giganteus,* of southern United States and Mexico that emits a vinegary odor when disturbed.

vinic Pertaining to, or derived from, wine.

violaceous Denoting a violet or purple discoloration, usually of the skin.

viper A venomous snake of the family Viperidae and sometimes of the closely related Crotalidae.

  European v. A common European viperine snake (*Vipera berus*), about 61 cm long with black markings patterned over a brownish-red to gray body. Also called adder.

  pit v. Any of various venomous snakes of the family Crotalidae, characterized by a hollow, heat-sensitive pit between the eye and nostril; includes rattlesnakes, copperheads, and water moccasins.

Viperidae A family of snakes that includes many

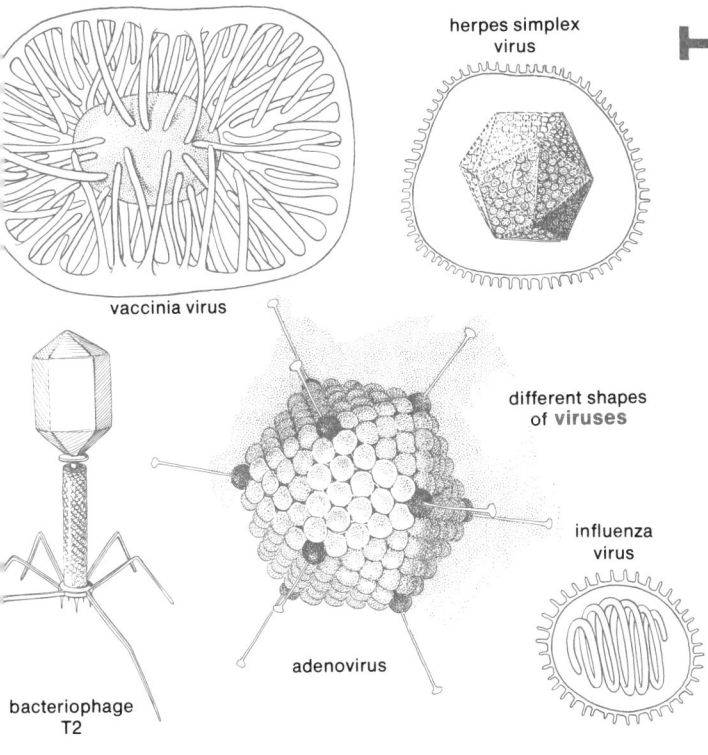

vaccinia virus

herpes simplex virus

relative sizes of various animal **viruses**
1000 nanometers (size of *Escherichia coli* for comparison)

vaccinia virus
(poxvirus)
200 by 250 nm

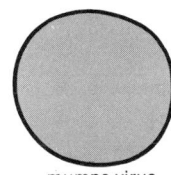

mumps virus
(paramyxovirus)
approx. 180 nm

bacteriophage
T2

adenovirus

different shapes
of **viruses**

influenza
virus

herpes simplex virus
(herpesvirus)
approx. 125 nm

influenza virus
(myxovirus)
approx. 100 nm

adenovirus
approx. 75 nm

reovirus
approx. 60 nm

poliovirus
approx. 25 nm

venomous species, characterized by movable, hollow, front fangs; included are the vipers and adders.

viral Relating to, or caused by, a virus.

viremia The presence of virus in the blood.

virgin A woman or man who has never had sexual intercourse.

virginity The state of not having experienced sexual intercourse.

virile 1. Relating to male sexual functions. **2.** Characteristic of masculine traits.

virilism The presence of male secondary sex characteristics in the female, caused usually by excessive amounts of androgenic hormones.

virility Masculine potency; manhood.

virilization The appearance of secondary male characteristics, especially in the female.

virion An elementary, morphologically complete virus particle.

viroid A folded, virus-like, single strand of low molecular replicating infectious RNA; the pathogen is smaller in size and simpler metabolically than a virus; it is thought to be linked to Creutzfeldt-Jakob disease.

virologist A specialist in virology.

virology The study of viruses and diseases caused by them.

viromicrosome An incompletely formed virus released during the premature disruption of the host cell.

viropexis A process of phagocytosis in which cells engulf virus particles.

virucide Any agent destructive to viruses.

virulence Denoting the degree of pathogenicity of parasites within a species or the disease-producing capability of a microorganism; the state of being poisonous.

viruliferous Conveying viruses.

viruria The presence of viruses in the urine.

virus An intracellular, infectious parasite, capable of living and reproducing only in living cells; virus particles usually range in size from 10 to 300 nm, are visible under the electron microscope, and are spherical, polyhedral, or rod-shaped in form; each particle is composed of a protein shell which usually encloses a single nucleic acid, either ribonucleic acid (RNA) or deoxyribonucleic acid (DNA).

attenuated v. A virus so modified as to be incapable of producing a disease.

common cold v. Any virus, especially of the genus *Rhinovirus*, associated with the common cold.

coxsackie v. See coxsackievirus.

dengue v. The causative agent of dengue, belonging to a group B arbovirus.

DNA v.'s A class of viruses having an inner core of DNA and multiplying chiefly in the nuclei of cells; included are those causing herpes simplex, herpes zoster, chickenpox, smallpox, warts, and certain malignant tumors.

EB v. (EBV) A virus (subfamily Gammaherpesvirinae, family Herpesviridae) that has specificity for B lymphocytes and causes infectious mononucleosis. Also called Epstein-Barr virus; herpesvirus 4.

ECHO v. Acronym for enteric cytopathogenic human orphan virus; see echovirus.

enteric v. A virus of the genus *Enterovirus*.

epidemic gastroenteritis v. The causative agent of epidemics of nonbacterial diarrhea.

epidemic keratoconjunctivitis v. A type 8 adenovirus causing epidemic inflammation of the conjunctiva at the border of the cornea (shipyard eye); also associated with swimming pool conjunctivitis.

Epstein-Barr v. EB virus.

equine encephalomyelitis v. A virus (genus *Alphavirus*, family Togaviridae) causing encephalomyelitis in horses and man; named by the region where it occurs, as eastern (EEE) virus, Venezuelan (VEE) virus and western (WEE) virus.

fitrable v. One small enough to pass through a porcelain filter or a filter of diatomaceous earths.

hepatitis A v. (HAV) A 27-nm RNA virus (genus Enterovirus, family Picornaviridae) causing hepatitis A, often as self-limited outbreaks in day-care centers and residential institutions; spread by contaminated food and water. Also called infectious hepatitis virus.

hepatitis B v. (HBV) A 42-nm DNA virus (family Hepadnoviridae) causing hepatitis B; found in body fluids, including saliva; spreads via transfusion, needle-stick accidents, shared needles, sexual route, or in childbirth. Also called serum hepatitis virus.

hepatitis C v. (HCV) A 10-kb RNA virus (family Flaviviridae), the cause of hepatitis C; spreads chiefly through transfusion and shared needles. Formerly classified as a non-A, non-B virus.

hepatitis D v. (HDV) A 37-nm RNA virus that requires the presence of the HBV to survive; spreads by infected blood or sexual contact. Also called delta agent.

hepatitis E. v. (HEV) A 7.5-kb RNA virus (family Caliciviridae); causes hepatitis E, mainly by contaminated water, via the gastrointestinal tract. Formerly classified as a non-A, non-B virus.

herpes v. See herpesvirus.

human immunodeficiency v. (HIV) A virus (subfamily Lentivirinae, family Retroviridae) causing acquired immune deficiency syndrome (AIDS); two types are known (HIV-1, HIV-2). Also called human T-cell lymphoma/leukemia virus type III; human T-cell lymphotropic virus type III.

human T-cell lymphotropic v. (HTLV) A virus (subfamily Oncovirinae, family Retroviridae) causing T-cell leukemia or lymphoma; two types are known (HTLV-I, HTLV-II). Also called human T-cell lymphoma/leukemia virus.

influenza v. A virus (genus *Influenzavirus,* family Orthomyxoviridae) causing influenza (flu).

lymphocytic choriomeningitis v. (LC virus) A virus (genus *Arenavirus*, family Arenaviridae) causing congenital lymphocytic choriomeningitis in mice; believed to be associated with other inapparent and influenza-like infections.

measles v. A virus (genus *Morbillivirus*, family Paramyxoviridae) that causes measles. Also called rubeola virus.

neurotropic v. One that thrives in nervous tissue.

oncogenic v. See tumor virus.

orphan v. One that has been isolated but not yet identified with any disease.

poliomyelitis v. See poliovirus.

rabies v. A virus (genus *Lyssavirus*, family Rhabdoviridae) that causes rabies.

respiratory syncytial v. (RSV, RS virus) A virus (genus *Pneumovirus*, family Paramyxoviridae) that causes pneumonia and bronchiolitis in infants; derives its name from its capacity to fuse cells into a multinucleated mass (syncytium).

RNA v.'s A large class of viruses having an inner core of RNA and multiplying chiefly in the cytoplasm of cells; included are those causing poliomyelitis, meningitis, yellow fever, encephalitis, mumps, measles, rabies, German measles, and the common cold. Also called riboviruses.

rubella v. A virus (genus *Rubivirus*, family Togaviridae) causing German measles (rubella).

slow v. Any virus causing a disease (e.g., kuru and subacute inclusion body encephalitis) characterized by a long, unremitting course and, once the symptoms appear, a gradual progression.

tumor v. One capable of producing tumors, either benign or malignant, under natural or laboratory conditions. Also called oncogenic virus.

varicella-zoster v. A virus (family Herpesviridae) morphologically identical to herpes simplex virus; causes chickenpox (varicella) and shingles (herpes zoster). Also called herpesvirus 3.

viscance A measure of the dissipation of energy in the flow of bodily fluids within cells and tissues or in tubes.

viscera Plural of viscus.

visceral Pertaining to the internal organs.

visceroinhibitory Restricting the function of the viscera.

visceromegaly Abnormal enlargement of the viscera.

VITAMIN	Sources	Functions	Deficiency
A	green and yellow vegetables, liver, eggs, dairy products	helps maintain normal body growth and health of specialized tissues especially retina	nightblindness, skin lesions, xerophthalmia (keratinization and dryness of tissues of the eye)
B$_1$ (thiamine)	yeast, meat, bran coat of cereals	involved in carbohydrate metabolism	beriberi
B$_2$ (riboflavin)	milk, egg yolk, fresh meat	hydrogen transfer from metabolites to blood stream	proliferation of blood vessels around cornea, abnormal reddening of lips, ulceration of corners of mouth, inflammation of tongue
B$_6$ (pyridoxine)	meat, vegetables	involved in protein metabolism	convulsions, muscular weakness, dermatitis of face
B$_{12}$	foods of animal source	involved in nucleic acid metabolism	pernicious anemia
C (ascorbic acid)	citrus fruits, green leafy vegetables, new potatoes	development of normal bones, cartilage and collagen	scurvy
D	fish liver oil	essential in formation of bone	rickets in children, osteomalacia in adults
E	green leafy vegetables, wheat germ, rice	antioxidant	impairment of fat absorption
K	fish, cereal	involved in clotting of blood	tendency to hemorrhage

visceromotor Causing functional activity of the viscera.

visceroparietal Relating to the abdominal organs and the abdominal wall.

visceroptosia, visceroptosis Downward displacement of the abdominal organs.

viscerosensory Relating to sensations in the viscera.

viscerotropic Affecting the organs.

viscid Sticky.

viscidity Stickiness.

viscosimeter Apparatus used to measure the viscosity of a fluid.

viscosity The resistance to flow by a substance caused by molecular cohesion.

viscosurgery Surgery of structures in front of the anterior chamber of the eye, performed after injecting a viscous fluid into the chamber; the fluid facilitates the operation by maintaining the shape of the chamber.

viscous Possessing a relatively high resistance to flow. Also called sticky; glutinous.

viscus, *pl.* **viscera** Any large internal organ, especially in the abdomen.

vision (V) Sight.

  binocular v. Vision in which both eyes contribute to the formation of one fused image.

  near v. Ability to see objects clearly at normal reading distances (from 33 to 40 cm).

  night v. Ability to see clearly in reduced illumination.

  peripheral v. Ability to perceive objects outside of the direct line of vision.

  scotopic v. Lack of ability to distinguish colors and small details, without diminution of the ability to detect motion and low luminous intensities.

  stereoscopic v. Depth perception; see under perception.

  tunnel v. Vision in which the visual field is severely contracted. Also called tubular vision.

visual Relating to vision.

visualize 1. To make a mental image. 2. To view.

visual purple See rhodopsin.

visual violet See iodopsin.

visual yellow All-*trans*-retinal; see retinal.

visuoauditory Relating to both vision and hearing.

visuopsychic Relating to the visual association areas of the occipital cortex of the brain, concerned with the interpretation or judgment of visual impressions.

visuosensory Relating to perception of visual impressions.

visuscope Instrument designed to identify the fixation characteristics of a partially blind (amblyopic) eye.

vita Latin for life.

vital Relating to life.

vitality 1. Vigor, vital force, or energy. 2. The capacity to live, grow, or develop.

vitallium A platinum-white, extremely hard cobalt-chromiumalloy; used for orthopedic appliances and for cast dentures.

vitalometer An electrical device used to determine the vital condition of a dental pulp; it could be either of high or low frequency. Also called pulp tester.

vitals 1. Viscera. 2. Bodily parts and organs necessary for life.

vitamer Substance performing a vitamin function.

vitamin (V) General term for any of several organic substances essential for normal metabolic processes and which, when absent in the diet, produce deficiency states.

  v. A A fat-soluble vitamin necessary for normal bone development and the health of certain specialized epithelial tissues, especially the retina for production of visual purple; present in green and yellow vegetables as a provitamin or precursor, which the body transforms into its active form; occurs in its preformed state in animal products (liver, eggs, and dairy products).

  v. A$_1$ See retinol.

  v. B A member of the vitamin B complex.

  v. B$_1$ See thiamine.

  v. B$_2$ See riboflavin.

  v. B$_6$ See pyridoxine.

  v. B$_{12}$ A protein complex occurring in foods of animal source; lack of vitamin B$_{12}$ causes pernicious anemia. Also called cyanocobalamin; antipernicious anemia factor; extrinsic factor.

  v. C See ascorbic acid.

  v. D A group of fat-soluble sterols that promote retention of calcium and phosphorus, thus aiding in bone formation; lack of vitamin D causes rickets in children and osteomalacia in adults; present primarily in fish liver oils; can be formed in the body upon exposure of the skin to sunlight. Also called the sunray vitamin; antirachitic factor.

  v. D$_2$ An irradiation product of ergosterol used as an antirachitic vitamin. Also called ergocalciferol; calciferol.

  v. D$_3$ A sterol of the vitamin D group formed by ultraviolet irradiation of the provitamin 7-dehydrocholesterol. Also called cholecalciferol.

  v. E A group of naturally occurring fat-soluble substances which have antioxidant properties; in experimental animals, a lack of vitamin E may lead to sterility and muscular degeneration. Also called tocopherol.

  v. K A group of fat-soluble compounds essential for clotting of blood; produced in the body by normal intestinal bacteria. Also called antihemorrhagic factor.

  v. P Capillary permeability factor; citrin.

vitamin B complex See complex, vitamin B.

vitellin The main protein present in the yolk of eggs.

vitelline Relating to, or resembling, the yolk of an egg.

vitellogenesis Formation of yolk.

vitellus The yolk of an egg.

vitiliginous Characterized by vitiligo.

vitiligo Sharply demarcated, milky-white patches on the skin, usually on the face, neck, hands, lower abdomen, and thighs, caused by absence of melanin. Also called acquired leukoderma.

vitrectomy The surgical removal of the formed vitreous body from the eye.

  closed v. Vitrectomy performed via minute incisions; a miniaturized surgical instrument is introduced to gain access to the diseased vitreous body. Also called pars plana vitrectomy.

  radical anterior v. The surgical removal of the vitreous body within the eye's anterior half, usually performed during a full-thickness corneal graft procedure.

vitreoretinopathy Disease of the eye involving the vitreous body and the retina.

vitreous 1. Glassy. 2. See body, vitreous.

vitrification Conversion of dental porcelain into a glassy substance.

vitriol 1. Any of various sulfates of heavy metals. 2. Sulfuric acid.

  blue v. Cupric sulfate.

  green v. Ferrous sulfate.

  oil of v. Sulfuric acid.

  salt of v. Zinc sulfate.

  white v. Zinc sulfate.

vivarium Quarters in which animals are kept for observation or medical research. Also called animal house.

vividialysis Dialysis through a living membrane, as in lavage of the peritoneal cavity.

vividiffusion The passage of blood through a membrane and its return to the living body without exposure to air; the principle used in the artificial kidney.

vivification Assimilation and utilization of protein by the living cell.

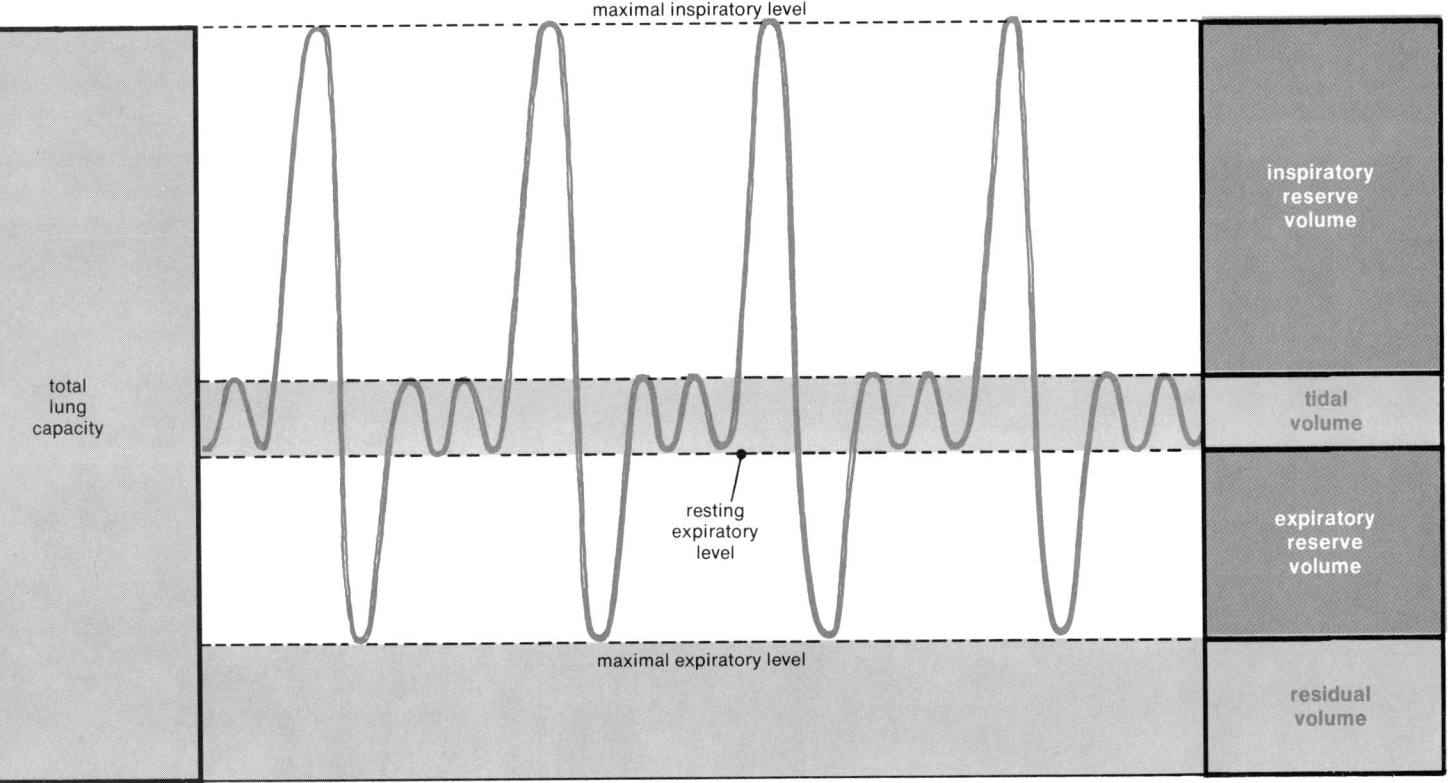

maximal inspiratory level

total lung capacity

inspiratory reserve volume

tidal volume

resting expiratory level

expiratory reserve volume

maximal expiratory level

residual volume

---

vivipara Denoting all forms of life whose eggs are developed within the body, thereby giving birth to living young.

viviparous Giving birth to living young developed within the mother's body. Also called zoogonous.

viviperception Study of vital processes in a living organism.

vivisection The performance of surgery on living animals for the purpose of experimentation.

vocal Relating to the voice.

voice The sound produced by air passing through the larynx, upper respiratory tract, and oral structures of vertebrates, especially humans.

void 1. To discharge a bodily waste, especially urine; to evacuate. 2. Empty. 3. Having no legal or binding effect or force; null.

vola Latin for the palm of the hand or the sole of the foot.

volar Denoting the palmar surface of the hand or the plantar surface of the foot.

volatile Having a tendency to evaporate rapidly at normal temperatures and pressures.

volatilization Evaporation.

volatilize To cause evaporation or to pass off in vapor.

volley A group of synchronous impulses.

volt (v) A unit of measure of electricity; a unit of electric potential necessary to cause one ampere of current to flow against one ohm of resistance on a conducting wire; named after the Italian physicist Allessandro Volta.

voltage Electromotive force expressed in volts.

voltammeter An apparatus for measuring the strength and quantity of current.

voltampere A unit of electric power, equal to one volt times one ampere; one watt.

voltmeter An electronic apparatus for measuring the potential differences in volts between two points.

volume (v, V) The space occupied by matter in any state or form.

  blood v. The quantity of blood present in the vascular compartment of the body.

  closing v. Lung volume at which airways at the bases of the lungs begin to close during expiration and airflow from the lungs is mainly from the upper portions (apices).

  expiratory reserve v. (ERV) The quantity of air that can be expelled from the lungs after a normal expiration. Formerly called supplemental air.

  forced expiratory v. (FEV) Maximal volume of air exhaled from the lungs during a particular time interval, starting from maximal inspiration.

  inspiratory reserve v. (IRV) The quantity of air

that can be inspired after a normal inspiration. Formerly called complemental air.

  minute v. 1. The volume of air expelled from the lungs per minute. 2. The volume of blood pumped by the left ventricle in one minute, normally 4 to 5 liters at rest.

  packed cell v. (PCV) Hematocrit (1); the volume of blood cells in a centrifuged blood sample, expressed as a percentage.

  residual v. (RV) The quantity of air remaining in the lungs after a maximal expiration. Also called residual air and residual capacity.

  standard v. The volume of a perfect gas at standard temperature and pressure, measured at 22.414 liters.

  stroke v. The quantity of blood expelled from each cardiac ventricle with each heartbeat.

  tidal v. The volume of air inspired and expired in a normal breath.

  v. of distribution The volume of fluid in which a test substance is distributed evenly. By measuring the concentration of the test substance after equilibrium, an estimate can be made of the volume of a fluid compartment, e.g., extracellular fluid.

volumenometer Instrument for measuring the volume of a body.

volumetric Relating to measurement of, or by, volume.

voluntary Initiated by one's own free will; not obligatory. Also called intentional.

volute Rolled up.

volvulosis See onchocerciasis.

volvulus Twisting of a segment of intestine, causing obstruction.

vomer See table of bones.

vomica A pus-containing cavity, as in the lung.

vomit 1. To expel the contents of the stomach forcibly through the mouth. 2. The matter expelled from the stomach. Also called vomitus.

vomiting The forceful expulsion of the stomach contents through the mouth.

  cyclic v. Periodic or recurrent vomiting.

  pernicious v. Persistent, uncontrollable vomiting.

  projectile v. Expulsion of the stomach contents with great force, often not preceded by nausea.

  v. of pregnancy Vomiting occurring during pregnancy, especially in the early morning.

vomitus Vomited material.

von Gierke's disease Type 1 glycogenosis; see under glycogenosis.

von Graefe's sign See Graefe's sign.

von Hippel-Lindau disease An inherited dis-

order of children marked by hemangiomas of the retina and hemangioblastoma of the cerebellum, medulla oblongata, and spinal cord; sometimes associated with cysts of several organs, especially the kidneys and pancreas. Also called Hippel-Lindau or Lindau's disease; retinocerebral angiomatosis.

von Recklinghausen's disease See neurofibromatosis.

von Willebrand's disease Inherited hemorrhagic disorder in which deficiency of factor VIII/von Willebrand's factor decreases platelet adhesion to vessel walls, resulting in prolonged bleeding time in the presence of normal platelet count and clot retraction; a common cause of minor bleeding, especially from the gums, gastrointestinal tract and uterus. Also called angiohemophilia; constitutional thrombopathy.

vortex, *pl.* **vortices** Latin for whirlpool; a general anatomic term designating a pattern involving rotation about an axis; a whorled design.

  v. coccygeus The whorl of hairs sometimes present in the coccygeal region.

  v. cordis The whorl of muscular fiber bundles at the apex of the heart.

  v. lentis The whorl or star-shaped pattern of light lines visible on the surface of the lens of the eye.

  vortices pilorum Hairs arranged about an axis, as at the crown of the head. Also called hair whorls.

vorticose Having a whorled appearance, as the vorticose veins of the choroid layer of the eye.

vox Latin for voice.

voyeur One who practices voyeurism; French for one who sees.

voyeurism The practice of deriving sexual gratification from witnessing sexual acts of others or by observing the naked body.

vulcanize To combine rubber with sulfur or other additives under high temperature and pressure in order to improve its strength and resiliency.

vulgaris Of the usual type; belonging to the multitude. Also called ordinary; common.

vulva The external female genitalia.

vulvar, vulval Of, or relating to, the vulva.

vulvectomy Partial or complete removal of the vulva.

vulvitis Inflammation of the vulva.

vulvocrural Relating to the vulva and the crura of the clitoris.

vulvouterine Relating to the vulva and the uterus.

vulvovaginal Relating to the vulva and the vagina. Also called vaginovulvar.

vulvovaginitis Inflammation of the vulva and vagina.

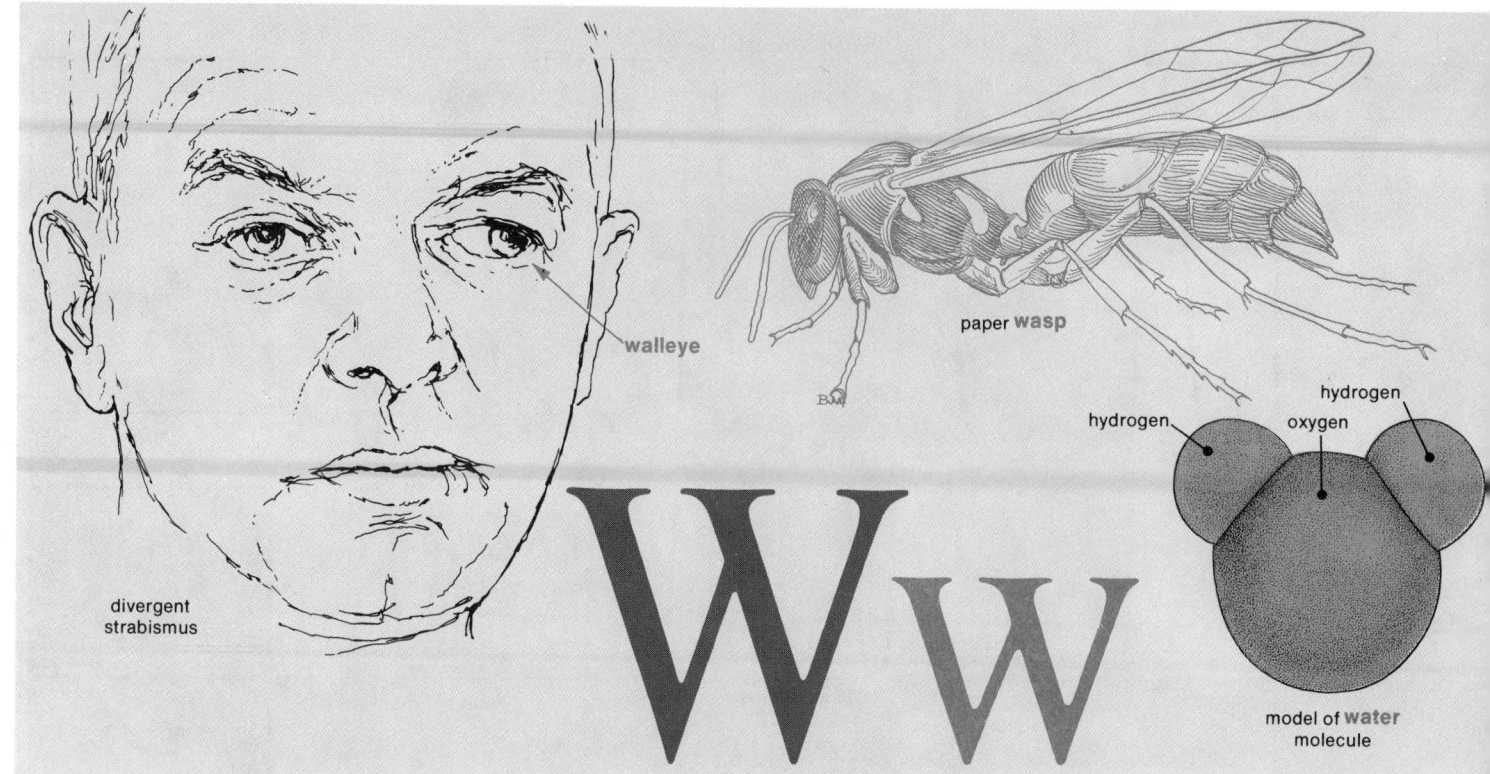

walleye

paper wasp

hydrogen

hydrogen

oxygen

divergent strabismus

Ww

model of water molecule

Waardenburg's syndrome A genetic defect characterized by anomalies of certain facioskeletal structures, congenital deafness, and pigmentary disorders; an estimated five percent of individuals with congenital deafness have this genetic disorder.

wadding A soft layer of fibrous cotton or wool, used for surgical dressings.

waddle To walk with short steps that cause the body to sway from side to side, as a duck; occurring in pseudohypertrophic muscular dystrophy and certain other nervous conditions.

waist The part of the trunk between the bottom of the rib cage and the hips.

waisting Shape of a bone in which the middle is narrower than the ends in transverse diameter.

Waldenström's syndrome Macroglobulinemia.

wale A linear skin wheal. Also called welt.

walk 1. To move on foot. 2. The manner in which one moves when going on foot. See also gait.

wall An investing structure that serves to enclose, divide, or protect an anatomic part; a part enclosing a cavity or space.

  cavity w. One of the enclosing surfaces bounding a prepared cavity in a tooth.

  enamel w. The part of the wall of a prepared cavity consisting of enamel.

walleye 1. A dense, whitish opacity (leukoma) of the cornea. 2. The eye that diverges in divergent strabismus.

walleyed Having divergent strabismus.

ward 1. A large room in a hospital usually with several beds for patients. 2. A section of the hospital for special care and treatment of a particular group of patients.

  accident w. Emergency room; see under room.

  isolation w. A ward in a hospital or institution where persons having or suspected of having a contagious disease are placed in quarantine.

  locked w. A ward in which mental patients are confined by locked doors.

  open w. A ward which is not locked.

  psychopathic w. A ward in a general hospital for the reception and treatment of mental patients.

warfarin A colorless crystalline compound, 3-(α-acetonylbenzyl)-4-hydroxycoumarin, widely used as an anticlotting drug and rat poison; an acronym for Wisconsin Alumni Research Foundation + (Coum)arin.

warm-blooded Having a relatively high and constant body temperature independent of surrounding temperature. Also called homothermal.

warp To distort out of shape.

wart A small horny outgrowth on the skin, usually of viral origin. Also called verruca.

  common w. A rough horny lesion varying in size from 1 mm to 2 cm in diameter; usually occurring on the hands. Also called verruca vulgaris.

  filiform w. A long, horny, fingerlike projection, usually occurring in multiples; seen most commonly in adult males, in the bearded area of the face; also occurring on the eyelids and the neck.

  flat w. A small, smooth, skin-colored wart occurring in clusters; commonly seen on the face, neck, and dorsum of the hands.

  moist w. A soft, moist, pink to red mass, occurring as a single lesion or in clusters that resemble a cauliflower; usually seen around the genitalia and anus, less often between the toes and at the corners of the mouth; not usually of venereal origin. Also called condyloma acuminatum; acuminate, venereal, or fig wart.

  plantar w. A wart occurring on the sole of the foot. Also called verruca plantaris.

  venereal w. See moist wart.

wash A lotion, often containing solid matter in suspension.

  eye w. See eyewash.

  mouth w. See mouthwash.

  red w. A lotion of zinc sulfate in compound tincture of lavender.

  yellow w. A suspension of mercuric oxide derived by precipitating a solution of mercuric chloride with calcium hydroxide.

wasp An insect of the superfamilies Vespoidea and Sphecoidea, having a slender spindle-shaped body with elongated waist; it is second only to the bumblebee in frequency of reported fatalities from its sting.

waste 1. To emaciate; to grow thin. 2. The undigested residue of food voided from the bowels. Also called feces.

wasting Emaciation.

water A clear, colorless liquid, H_2O, present in all organic tissues and essential for life.

  alkaline w. Water that contains appreciable amounts of the bicarbonates of calcium, lithium, potassium, or sodium.

  bound w. Water in bodily tissues tenaciously held to colloids.

  distilled w. Water purified by the heat-dependent process of distillation.

  free w. 1. Water in the body that is not attached to colloids; it can be removed by ultrafiltration. 2. That amount of dilute urine formed per minute which can be considered free of solute, assuming that the remainder of the urine is isotonic; C_{H_2O} (free water clearance) = V (urine flow in ml/min − C_{osm} (osmolar clearance).

  hard w. Water containing ions, such as Mg^{++} and

Ca^{++}, that form insoluble salts with fatty acids, especially water with more than 90 parts per million of calcium carbonate; it generally resists the action of soap to form a lather.

  heavy w. A compound analogous to water in which most of the hydrogen atoms are deuterium (heavy hydrogen); it differs from ordinary water in having higher boiling and freezing points. Also called deuterium oxide (D_2O).

  lime w. A solution of calcium hydroxide.

  metabolic w. See water of metabolism.

  mineral w. Water that has appreciable amounts of mineral salts in solution.

  potable w. Drinkable water free from contamination.

  saline w. Water that contains neutral salts (chlorides, bromides, iodides, sulfates) in appreciable amounts.

  soft w. Water that contains few or no ions that form insoluble salts with fatty acids, especially water with less than 80 parts per million of calcium carbonate; ordinary soap can lather in it easily.

  total body w. (TBW) The total water content of the adult human body; equal to 50–70% of the body weight.

  w. of combustion See water of metabolism.

  w. of crystallization Water in chemical combination with a crystal, necessary for the maintenance of crystalline properties but capable of being separated by adequate heat.

  w. of hydration Water chemically united with a substance to form a hydrate, which can be removed, as by heating, without substantially changing the chemical composition of the substance.

  w. of injection Water purified by distillation for parenteral use.

  w. of metabolism The water in the body derived from the oxidation of the hydrogen of a food element such as starch, glucose, or fat; the largest amount is produced in the metabolism of fat, approximately 117 g per 100 g of fat. Also called metabolic water; water of combustion.

water-borne Conveyed by drinking water; describing certain diseases transmitted by contaminated water, such as cholera and typhoid fever.

water brash The filling of the mouth with refluxed fluid from the esophagus, usually associated with heartburn.

Waterhouse-Friderichsen syndrome A disorder of rapid onset marked by an extensive purpuric rash, bilateral adrenal hemorrhage, shock, and circulatory collapse. Also called acute fulminating meningococcemia.

water on the brain Colloquialism for hydrocephalus.

brain waves
(normal adult electroencephalogram)

frontal-central

central-occipital

frontal-temporal

temporal-occipital

cannon wave

jugular venous tracing

R wave

P wave

T wave

U wave

Q wave

S wave

normal electro-cardiogram

|← wavelength →|

wavetrain

waters Colloquial term for amniotic fluid, the fluid that surrounds the fetus.

watershed The region of diminished blood circulation around a vascular bed.

watt (W) The amount of electrical power produced by one volt with one ampere of current.

wattage Amperage multiplied by voltage.

wave A periodic increase and subsidence, as an oscillation propagated from point to point in a medium, characterized by alternate elevations and depressions.

alpha (α) w.'s Waves in the electroencephalogram with a frequency band from 8 to 13 cycles per second. Also called alpha rhythm.

arterial w. A wave in the jugular phlebogram due to the vibration produced by the carotid pulse.

beta (β) w.'s Waves in the electroencephalogram that have a frequency band from 18 to 30 cycles per second. Also called beta rhythm.

brain w.'s Electrical potential waves of the brain.

cannon w. A large positive venous pulse wave produced by atrial contraction; it occurs when the right atrium contracts at the same time the tricuspid valve is closed by right ventricular systole, as in complete heart block and ventricular premature beats.

delta (δ) w.'s **1.** Waves in the electroencephalogram that have a frequency band from ½ to 3 cycles per second. Also called delta rhythm. **2.** The slow-rising, slurred, initial portion of the upstroke of the electrocardiographic R wave seen in the Wolff-Parkinson-White (W-P-W) syndrome, caused by preexcitation of a part of the ventricular myocardium.

dicrotic w. The second notch in the tracing of the normal arterial pulse.

f w.'s Small irregular waves or oscillations of the atria, characteristically seen in atrial fibrillation.

F w.'s Regular rapid undulating atrial waves seen in atrial flutter; thought to represent the manifestation of atrial depolarization and repolarization occurring in rapid succession from an ectopic focus.

fluid w. A sign of free fluid in the abdominal cavity; percussion on one side of the abdomen transmits a wave that is felt on the opposite side.

microelectric w. See microwave.

P w. The initial deflection of the electrocardiogram, representing depolarization of the atria; if retrograde or ectopic, it is labeled P'.

pulse w. A wave originated by the impact of ejection of blood from the left ventricle into the full aorta and propagated to the periphery through the column of blood and the arterial walls.

Q w. The initial deflection of the QRS complex when such deflection is downward (negative).

R w. The first upward deflection of the QRS complex in the electrocardiogram (ECG).

radio w.'s Electromagnetic waves with wavelengths between 1 mm and 30 km. Also called hertzian rays.

random w.'s Brain waves in the encephalogram produced by irregular changes of electric potential.

retrograde w. A distorted P wave pattern in the electrocardiogram, inverted in several leads where it should be upright, caused by an ectopic impulse from the ventricle spreading backward into the atria.

S w. A downward (negative) deflection of the QRS complex following an R wave.

sound w. System of longitudinal pressure waves passing through any medium; may or may not be audible.

T w. The deflection of the normal electrocardiogram which follows the QRS complex; it represents ventricular repolarization.

theta (θ) w. Brain wave in the encephalogram having a frequency between 4 and 7 cycles per second. Also called theta rhythm.

tidal w. The second and lesser of the two waves forming the main systolic arterial pulse wave.

U w. A minor deflection of the normal electrocardiogram which occasionally occurs in early ventricular diastole following the T wave; especially prominent in persons with electrolyte imbalance.

ultrasonic w. A high frequency sound wave, greater than 20,000 Hz; it cannot be heard by humans; used in diagnostic imaging and therapeutically.

waveform The mathematical graphic representation of a wave.

wavelength (λ) One of three measurements of the vibration of a sound wave (others are amplitude and frequency); the longitudinal distance between the crests of two successive sound waves.

wavetrain A series of waves sent along the same axis by a vibrating body.

wax A plastic, heat-sensitive substance secreted by insects, or obtained from plants or petroleum; consists essentially of high molecular weight hydrocarbons or esters of fatty acids; characteristically insoluble in water but soluble in most organic solvents.

baseplate w. A hard wax for making baseplates and occlusion rims.

bone w. Wax used for filling sterile bone cavities.

boxing w. A soft wax for boxing impressions for dental prostheses.

carnauba w. A hard wax with a high melting point used for the control of the melting range of various waxes; it is derived from the fine powder on the leaves of certain tropical palms.

casting w. A compound of various waxes with controlled properties of thermal expansion and contraction; used in making patterns which represent the exact reproduction of the missing tooth structure; it allows a mold to be made, into which the alloy is cast.

ear w. Cerumen.

inlay w. Wax used in making patterns for dental restoration from which an inlay is cast.

paraffin w. A white or colorless wax derived from the high-boiling fractions of petroleum; composed chiefly of a complex mixture of hydrocarbons of the methane series. Also called paraffin.

sticky w. An adhesive wax used in dentistry for attaching a sprue pin to a wax restoration pattern.

whipworm
(Trichuris trichuria)

anus

anterior
end

♀

♂

infective egg
containing
larva

whorls of fingerprint

simple whorl

central pocket whorl

double loop whorl

accidental whorl

semicircular
duct

semicircular
canals

left internal
ear

cochlea

endolymphatic
duct

utricle

saccule

oval window

round window

---

wean To discontinue the breast feeding of an infant, with substitution of other nourishment.

web A membrane or membranous fold.

esophageal w. A condition marked by the presence of one or more membranous folds in the esophagus.

Weber-Christian disease A disease of unknown cause marked by recurring fever and formation of subcutaneous nodules and plaques with atrophy of subcutaneous fat; the thighs and trunk are most frequently affected. Also called relapsing febrile nodular nonsuppurative panniculitis.

weight (wt.) The measured heaviness of a specific object; the force with which a body is pulled toward the earth by gravity.

atomic w. (at. wt.) The weight of an atom of any element compared with the weight of an atom of carbon-12 (^{12}C), which is taken as 12.00000; tables of atomic weights list a value of the element's isotopic weights.

avoirdupois w. A system of weights and measures in which a pound equals 16 ounces, 7,000 grains, or 453.59 grams.

combining w. Gram equivalent; see under equivalent.

equivalent w. See equivalent, gram.

gram-molecular w. The numerical molecular weight of a substance expressed in grams; an amount of substance containing a weight in grams numerically equal to its molecular weight.

molecular w. (mol. wt., MW) The sum of the atomic weights of all the atoms that make up a molecule.

weightlessness The state of experiencing no gravitational pull.

Weil's disease Severe leptospirosis with jaundice, caused by *Leptospira icterohemorrhagiae* transmitted to man by rats; characterized primarily by continued fever and hepatic disturbances, associated with jaundice, renal manifestations, and congestion of the conjunctiva. Also called infectious spirochetal jaundice; icterohemorrhagic fever; leptospirosis icterohemorrhagica.

Weiss' sign See Chvostek's sign.

welt A linear wheal, usually raised on the skin by a lash, blow, or flog. Also called wale.

wen Sebaceous cyst, especially of the scalp.

Wernicke-Korsakoff syndrome Disorder of the central nervous system caused by abusive intake of alcohol and nutritional depletion, especially of thiamine; characterized primarily by sudden weakness and paralysis of eye muscles, double vision, and inability to stand or walk unaided; followed by derangement of mental functions, e.g., confusion, apathy, loss of retentive memory, and confabulation; it may terminate in death.

wet nurse A woman who breast-feeds another woman's child.

wheal A round or ridgelike transitory swelling on the skin; e.g. hives.

wheeze 1. To breathe with difficulty, producing a whistling sound, usually due to bronchiolar constriction as in asthma. 2. The sound thus produced.

whey The watery part of milk that separates from the casein or coagulated part. Also called serum lactis.

whiplash See injury, whiplash.

Whipple's disease A rare systemic disorder characterized by anemia, increased skin pigmentation, arthritis, steatorrhea, and other signs of malabsorption; the intestinal wall and lymphatics are infiltrated by macrophages filled with glycoproteins; occurs predominantly among middle-aged men. Also called lipophagic intestinal granulomatosis; intestinal lipodystrophy.

whipworm A small whiplike roundworm, parasitic in the large intestine of man; the cause of trichuriasis. Also called *Trichuris trichuria.*

whitehead 1. A vernacular alternate for milium. 2. Term colloquially used for a superficial skin lesion with a white purulent content.

whites Colloquial term for leukorrhea, a thick whitish vaginal discharge.

whiting A pure grade of chalk, $CaCO_3$; used in polishing metal and plastic structures, especially dental prosthetics.

whitlow Painful, suppurative inflammation of a finger tip, especially under or around the nail.

herpetic w. A recurrent cluster of blisters caused by a herpesvirus transmitted through abrasions on the finger.

melanotic w. A malignant tumor of the nail bed.

thecal w. Infection of the distal phalanx of a finger, involving the synovial sheath of the flexor tendon.

whoop The shrill, noisy, paroxysmal gasp characteristic of whooping cough.

systolic w. See honk, systolic.

whooping cough See under cough.

whorl A spiral twist, such as any of the circular ridges of a fingerprint, the arrangement of muscular fibers at the apex of the heart, or the area of hair growing in a radial manner.

widow's peak A V-shaped point formed by the hairline at the middle of the forehead; term derived from the superstition that it is a sign of early widowhood.

Wilson's disease 1. (Samuel A. Kinnier Wilson) Hepatolenticular degeneration: see under degeneration. 2. (Sir William J. E. Wilson) Exfoliative dermatitis; see under dermatitis.

windburn Skin irritation due to excessive exposure to wind.

window An opening in a wall. Also called fenestra.

aortic w. A radiolucent area below the aortic arch formed by the bifurcation of the trachea and traversed by the left pulmonary artery, visible in the left anterior oblique roentgenogram.

oval w. An oval opening in the medial wall of the middle ear chamber, which leads into the vesti-

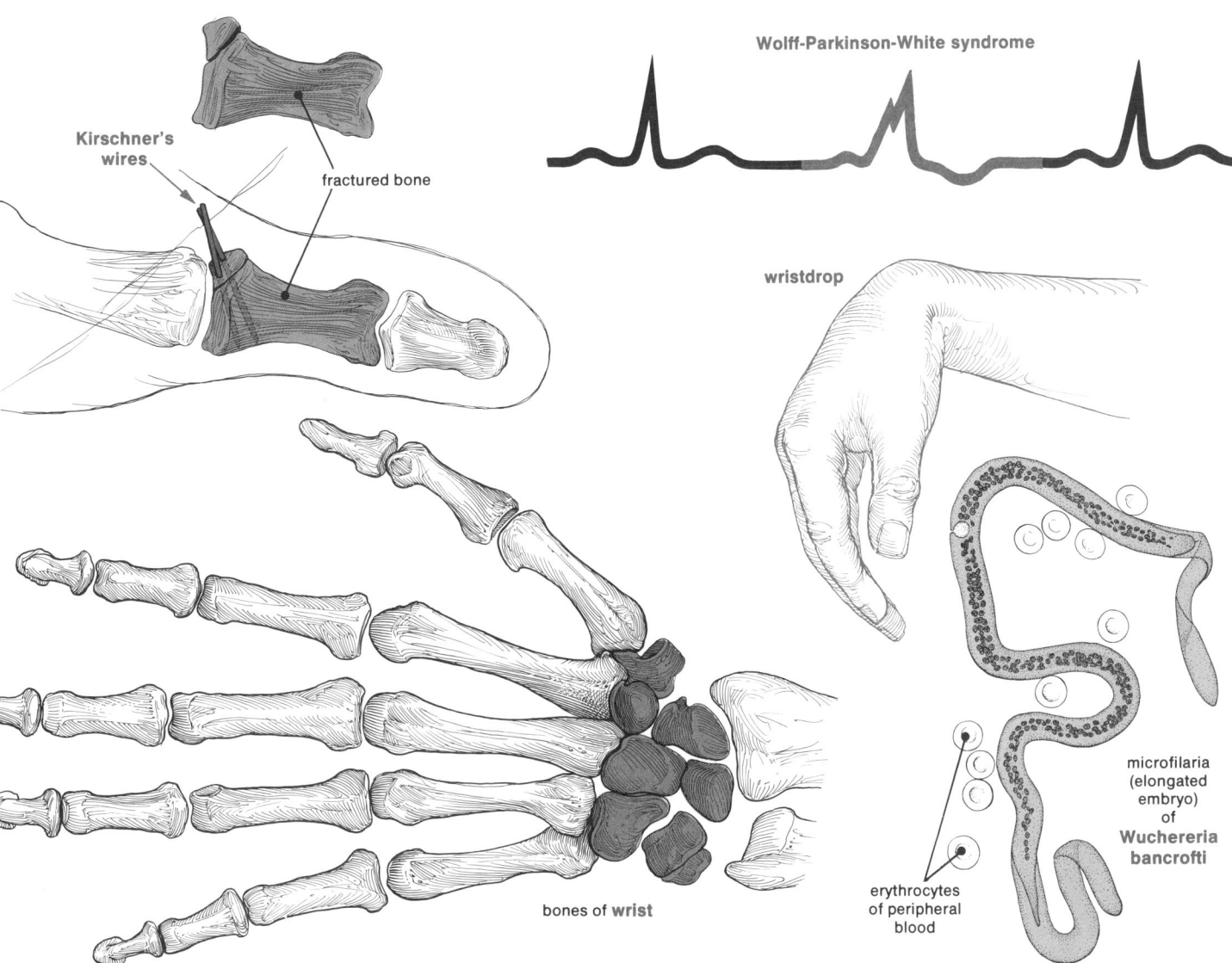

Wolff-Parkinson-White syndrome

Kirschner's wires

fractured bone

wristdrop

bones of **wrist**

microfilaria (elongated embryo) of **Wuchereria bancrofti**

erythrocytes of peripheral blood

bule of the internal ear; it houses the baseplate of the stapes. Also called fenestra vestibuli.

round w. A round opening in the lateral wall of the internal ear, which leads from the scala tympani of the cochlea to the middle ear chamber; it is closed by the secondary tympanic membrane. Also called fenestra cochleae.

windpipe Common term for trachea.

wing Any anatomic structure resembling the wing of a bird.

winking The rapid closing and opening of the eyelids.

Winterbottom's sign Swelling of the posterior cervical lymph nodes; indicative of early stages of African sleeping sickness.

wintergreen A low-growing evergreen plant of eastern North America, *Gaultheria procumbens.*

oil of w. See under oil.

wire 1. A slender, pliable, metallic strand, used in surgery and dentistry. 2. To bind structures with a wire or wires.

arch w. An orthodontic wire attached to molar bands positioned around the dental arch; used to provide tooth stabilization and/or maintain controlled pressure for tooth movement.

Kirschner's w. A heavy gauge steel wire used for applying traction in long bone fractures and for transfixation of fractured bones.

ligature w. A soft slender wire used to tie an arch wire to the band attachment around a tooth.

wiring Fixation of the ends of broken bones by means of wire.

Wiskott-Aldrich syndrome An X-linked recessive inherited syndrome of males, characterized by eczema, low platelet count, and increased susceptibility to infections due to a defect in cellular immunity; present primarily in infants and early childhood; bloody diarrhea is a common feature. Also called Aldrich syndrome.

witch hazel A liquid extract obtained from the

dried bark and leaves of the plant *Hamamelis virginiana*; used as an astringent.

withdrawal A pathologic detachment or retreat from emotional involvement with people or the environment; seen in its extreme in schizophrenics.

withdrawal syndrome Intense physiologic disturbances when abruptly discontinuing the administration of a drug that, by its prolonged use, induced physical dependence. Also called abstinence syndrome.

Wolff-Parkinson-White syndrome (WPW) Anomalous atrioventricular excitation; congenital heart condition marked by irregular heart beat and distorted patterns of the electrocardiogram (shortened P-R interval and prolonged QRS complex). Also called preexcitation syndrome.

womb See uterus.

wood alcohol See alcohol, methyl.

wool fat The fatlike substance obtained from sheep's wool, used in the preparation of ointments. Also called anhydrous lanolin.

workaholic A person who suffers from an abnormal, uncontrollable, habitual desire to work excessively.

working through In psychoanalysis, all the processes in which a problem is actively explored by patient and therapist until a satisfactory solution has been found or until a symptom has been traced to its unconscious sources; it generally involves the recapture of infantile, repressed, unconscious material and its conversion into conscious thoughts and strivings.

World Health Organization (WHO) An agency of the United Nations concerned with health on an international level.

worm Common name for any of various elongated invertebrates, as those of the phyla Annelida, Nematoda, or Platyhelminthes.

eye w. See *Loa loa.*

flat w. See flatworm.

guinea w. See *Dracunculus medinensis.*

heart w. See *Dirofilaria immitis.*

lung w. See lungworm.

Medina w. See *Dracunculus medinensis.*

pin w. See pinworm.

pork w. See *Trichinella spiralis.*

seat w. See pinworm.

serpent w. See *Dracunculus medinensis.*

trichina w. See *Trichinella spiralis.*

wound Injury or trauma in any tissue.

contused w. Injury to the tissues without a break in the skin.

incised w. A cut made with a knife or any sharp instrument.

lacerated w. A tear.

open w. One with an exposed opening.

penetrating w. One that enters a body cavity.

puncture w. A narrow wound made by a spiked instrument or weapon.

wrinkle 1. A crease in the skin, especially one caused by habitual frowning or by atrophy of the corium, as in old age. 2. A furrow or crevice on a normally smooth surface.

wrist The carpal bones and adjoining structures between the hand and the forearm.

wristdrop Paralysis of the extensor muscles of the hand and digits.

wrist sign The distal phalanges of the first and fifth fingers of one hand overlap when wrapped around the opposite wrist, as seen in individuals with the Marfan syndrome.

wryneck See torticollis.

Wuchereria A genus of parasitic nematode worms of the superfamily Filarioidea.

W. bancrofti The bancroftian filaria, a parasite of the lymphatic vessels and the cause of elephantiasis. Formerly called *Filaria bancrofti; Filaria nocturna.*

wuchereriasis Infestation with worms of the genus *Wuchereria.*

Xenopsylla cheopis

xanthopterin

xanthurenic acid

xanthine

xanthelasma of the eyelids

xanthoma tuberosum

xylulose

---

xanthelasma A form of xanthoma; yellow, wrinkled, slightly raised patches on the skin, occurring on the eyelid, usually bilaterally near the inner angle of the eye. Also called xanthelasma palpebrarum.

xanthemia See carotenemia.

xanthene A crystalline compound that is the basic structure of many dyestuffs.

xanthic 1. Yellow. 2. Of or relating to xanthine.

xanthine A white purine base present in most of the body tissues; sometimes found in urinary stones; converted by xanthine oxidase to uric acid.

xanthinuria Passage of excessive amounts of xanthine in the urine.

xanthochromia A yellow discoloration of spinal fluid, usually an indication of a previous bleeding episode within the central nervous system.

xanthochromic, xanthochromatic Yellow colored.

xanthocyanopsia Abnormal color vision marked by inability to perceive red and green hues; vison is limited to yellow and blue.

xanthodont One who has yellowish teeth.

xanthogranuloma Infiltration of tissue by lipid-laden macrophages.

xanthoma Slightly raised, yellow skin plaque, due to a disorder of fat metabolism.

  eruptive x. Clusters of small xanthomas that appear suddenly on the elbows, knees, back, and buttocks; associated with high serum lipid levels and, occasionally, with cases of severe diabetes.

  x. diabeticorum, diabetic x. See eruptive xanthoma.

  x. tuberosum, x. tuberosum multiplex The eruption of xanthomas in the form of yellow nodules of varying size chiefly of the knees, elbows, palms, and soles.

xanthomatosis The presence of multiple xanthomas. Also called lipoid or lipid granulomatosis; xanthoma multiplex.

  cerebrotendinous x. Genetic disorder transmitted as an autosomal recessive inheritance; characterized by the formation of cholesterol deposits in tendons, lungs and the brain, causing pulmonary insufficiency and neurologic dysfunction; it usually develops after puberty. Also called cerebrotendinous cholesterinosis.

  essential x. Lipid metabolism disturbance with deposit of lipids in various tissues and characterized by gingivitis, bone defects, diabetes insipidus, and retardation of growth.

xanthomatous Relating to a xanthoma.

xanthophyll A yellow carotenoid pigment in plants and egg yolk; also seen in human plasma as

a result of ingesting food containing the pigment.

xanthopsia Condition in which everything appears yellow. Also called yellow vision.

xanthopterin A yellow pigment present in many sources including butterfly wings and the integument of wasps and hornets; an inhibitor of xanthine oxidase.

xanthosine A nucleoside, xanthine-9-ribofuranoside, $C_{10}H_{12}O_6N_4$; formed by the deamination of guanosine.

xanthosis A yellow discoloration of the skin, sometimes seen in patients afflicted with cancer.

xanthurenic acid 4,8-Dihydroquinaldic acid, large amounts of which are excreted during pregnancy and by pyridoxine-deficient individuals.

xanthyl The monovalent radical $C_{13}H_9O$ which occurs in xanthene.

xenobiotic Any chemical substance not produced by, therefore foreign to, living organisms (e.g., carcinogens, drugs, insecticides).

xenogeneic Relating to individuals of different species.

xenogenic Originating outside the body or in a foreign substance within the body.

xenograft A graft derived from a species different from that receiving it. Also called xenogeneic graft; heterograft; heterotransplant.

xenology The study of the relationship between a parasite and its host.

xenon An odorless inert gaseous element found in minute proportions in the atmosphere; symbol Xe, atomic number 54, atomic weight 131.30.

xenon-133 (^{133}Xe) A gamma-emitting radioactive inert gas with a physical half-life of 5.27 days; used to measure blood flow and regional pulmonary ventilation.

xenophobia An undue fear of strangers.

xenophthalmia Inflammation of the conjunctiva due to injury or to the presence of a foreign body.

Xenopsylla A genus of fleas.

  X. cheopis The rat flea; vector of *Pasteurella pestis*, the causative bacillus of plague.

xeransis Loss of moisture in the tissues.

xerantic Causing dryness.

xerocheilia Dryness of the lips.

xeroderma A skin disease marked by roughness, dryness, and discoloration of the skin.

  x. pigmentosum A congenital condition of the skin marked by extreme sensitivity to light which causes skin inflammation, freckles, superficial ulcerations, glossy white spots due to thinning of the skin, and keratoses that become malignant. Also called

atrophoderma pigmentosum.

xerography A dry photographic process in which an image formed by a resinous powder on an electrically charged photoconductive surface is transferred and developed on paper with carbon powder that adheres only to the electrically charged areas.

xeromammography A dry, totally photoelectric process of producing x-ray images of the female breast.

xeromenia Occurrence of the usual general symptoms of menstruation without a blood flow.

xerophthalmia Xerosis of the conjunctiva; a degenerative condition, marked by extreme dryness and thickness of the conjunctiva with diminished secretions. Also called ophthalmoxerosis.

xeroradiography The making of nontransparent black and white prints of densities produced by x rays on a specially coated plate.

xerosis Abnormal dryness of the skin, conjunctiva, or mucous membranes.

xerostomia Abnormal dryness of the mouth, caused by diminished or arrested secretion of saliva.

xerotic Affected with abnormal dryness of the skin or conjunctiva.

xiphisternum The xiphoid process or cartilage.

xiphocostal Relating to the xiphoid cartilage and the ribs.

xiphodynia Pain in the area of the xyphoid cartilage.

xiphoid Sword-shaped. See table of bones.

X linkage See under linkage.

X-linked Determined by a gene located on the X chromosome. Also called sex-linked.

x ray See under ray.

XXY syndrome See Klinefelter's syndrome.

xylene A flammable hydrocarbon obtained from wood and coal tar, used as a solvent. Also called xylol.

xylometazoline Compound used to reduce congestion of the nasal mucosa.

xylose A pentose sugar (the molecule of which has five carbon atoms), $C_5H_{10}O_5$, found in beechwood, straw, etc.; the absorption of xylose from the intestine is used as a test in suspected cases of malabsorption syndrome. Also called wood sugar.

xylulose A pentose sugar found in two forms.

  D-x. An intermediate in pentose metabolism.

  L-x. An abnormal constituent of urine seen in essential pentosuria.

xylyl The hydrocarbon radical, $C_6H_4(CH_3)CH_2$, consisting of xylene minus a hydrocarbon atom.

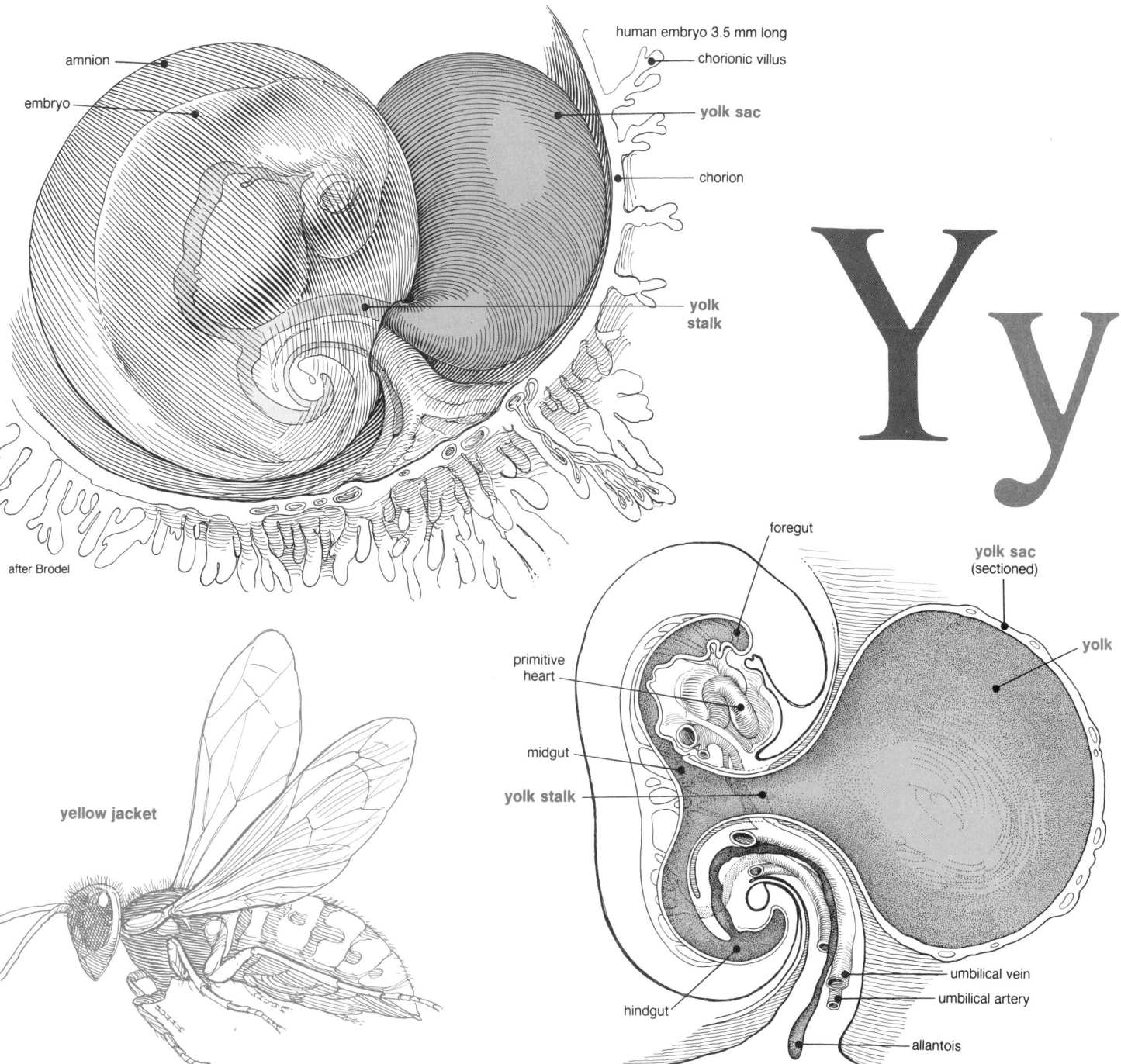

amnion

embryo

human embryo 3.5 mm long

chorionic villus

yolk sac

chorion

yolk stalk

after Brödel

foregut

yolk sac (sectioned)

yolk

primitive heart

midgut

yolk stalk

yellow jacket

hindgut

umbilical vein

umbilical artery

allantois

yabapox Smallpox of nonhuman primates. Also called tanapox; monkeypox.

yaw One of the lesions of the eruption of yaws.

yawn A usually involuntary gaping of the mouth accompanied by a deep inspiration.

yaws An infectious skin disease of tropical regions, marked by papular eruptions on the face, hands, and feet, and around the external genitals; caused by a spirochete, *Treponema pertenue*. Also called frambesia; tropica; piăn; bouba.

yeast 1. Any of several fungi of the genus *Saccharomyces* capable of fermenting carbohydrates. 2. A commercial preparation, in either dry or moist form, used as a leavening agent or as a dietary supplement.
  brewer's y. A by-product of the brewing of beer; used as a source of protein and vitamin B-complex.

yellow 1. The hue of the spectrum between green and orange; evoked in the normal observer by radiant energy stimulation of wavelength approximately 580 nm. 2. A dye or stain of this hue.

yellow fever See under fever.

yellow jacket Any of various small wasps of the family Vespidae, having yellow and black markings and usually constructing round, paper-like nests in the ground under logs or rocks; next to the honeybee,

it is the most common stinging insect. Also called yellow hornet.

Yersinia Genus of coccoid, oval or rod-shaped, gram-negative bacteria (family Enterobacteriaceae).
  Y. enterocolitica Species found in feces and lymph nodes of animals and humans; the cause of yersiniosis.
  Y. pestis Causative organism of plague in man and rodents; transmitted by the rat flea. Formerly called *Pasteurella pestis*.
  Y. pseudotuberculosis A gram-negative, aerobic, non-spore forming bacillus that is coccobacillary when virulent and bacillary when avirulent; a ubiquitous animal pathogen, now recognized as a potentially significant human pathogen, causing mesenteric lymphadenitis. Formerly called *Pasteurella pseudotuberculosis*.

yersiniosis Infection with *Yersinia enterocolitica*, characterized by diarrhea, inflammation of lymph nodes, especially in the abdomen, and arthritis of several joints.

yoga A system of exercises aimed at promoting the control of the body and mind.

yogurt, yoghurt Curdled milk produced by the action of a ferment containing a lactic acid bacillus.

yohimbine An alkaloid; the active principle of the bark of the African tree *Corynanthe yohimbi*, similar in structure to reserpine; a relatively selective inhibitor of alpha$_2$-adrenergic receptors.

yolk 1. The nutrient portion of an ovum, especially the yellow mass of the egg of a bird or a reptile. 2. The fatty substance present in the unprocessed wool of sheep which, when purified, becomes lanolin.

yolk sac The highly vascular umbilical vesicle enveloping the nutritive yolk of an embryo. Also called vitelline sac.

yolk stalk The narrowed passage between the intraembryonic gut and the yolk sac. Also called omphalomesenteric duct.

ytterbium A bright silvery rare-earth element that has the ability to vary its valence in different environments; symbol Yb, atomic number 70, atomic weight 173.04.

yttrium A silvery metallic element; symbol Y, atomic number 39, atomic weight 88.90; always occurs with the rare earth minerals.

yttrium-90 (^{90}Y) A radioactive isotope of yttrium (radioyttrium); has been used in the treatment of breast and prostatic cancer.

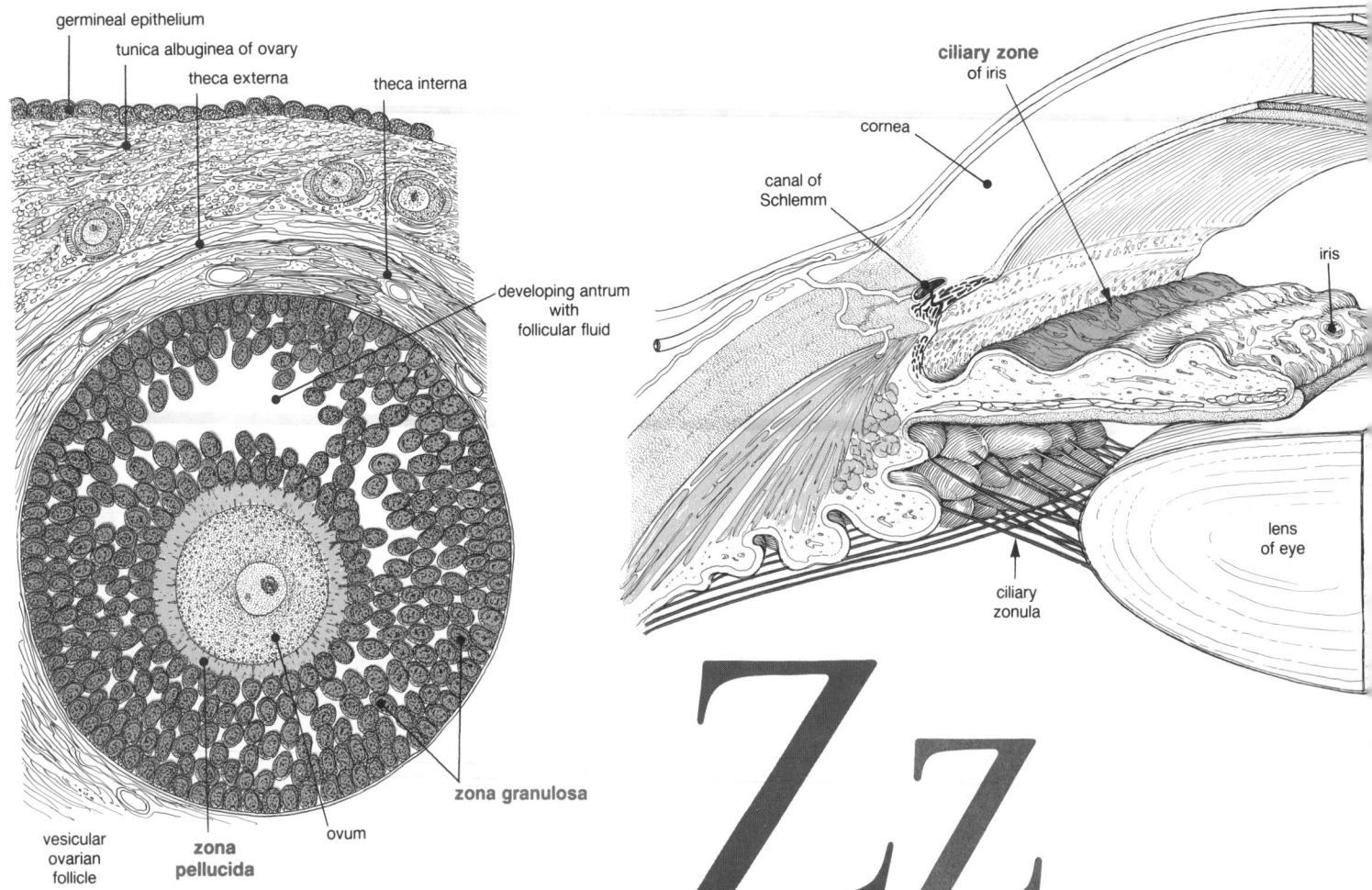

germineal epithelium
tunica albuginea of ovary
theca externa
theca interna
developing antrum with follicular fluid
zona granulosa
vesicular ovarian follicle
zona pellucida
ovum

ciliary zone of iris
cornea
canal of Schlemm
iris
lens of eye
ciliary zonula

Zz

zeaxanthin A carotinoid found in yellow corn, egg yolk, and cetain seaweed (*Fucus vesiculosus*) of the North Atlantic Ocean; used as a coloring agent.

zero (z) The point on a thermometer scale from which the graduations are numbered in either direction; in the centigrade scale, the freezing point for distilled water.

  absolute z. The hypothetical point in a temperature scale in which there is complete absence of heat; in kinetic theory, absence of relative linear molecular motion, postulated as $-273.2°C$.

zidovudine A drug used in the management of acquired immune deficiency syndrome (AIDS); adverse effects include anemia and gastrointestinal intolerance. Formerly called azidothymidine.

zinc A malleable and ductile metallic element; symbol Zn, atomic number 30, atomic weight 65.38.

  z. carbonate A white amorphous powder with mild astringent properties; chief constituent of calamine lotion.

  z. chloride A water-soluble caustic powder, $ZnCl_2$; used locally to destroy tissues.

  z. gelatin See under gelatin.

  z. ointment A compound made of 20% zinc oxide with beeswax and petrolatum; used as a salve.

  z. oxide A white powder, ZnO, insoluble in water; a mild astringent and antiseptic incorporated in ointments, lotions, and dusting powders; used to prevent sunburn and to treat skin disorders (eczema, ringworm, psoriasis, varicose ulcers, and ivy poisoning); the main ingredient of calamine lotion.

  z. oxide and eugenol (ZOE) Compound used widely as a base material beneath tooth restorations, a temporary filling, an impression paste, and root canal filling; also used as a hardening agent for demineralized dentin.

  z. permanganate Dark brown, water-soluble crystals, used in solution as a germicide.

  z. peroxide (ZPO) A yellowish powder, ZnO_2, insoluble in water; used as a wash for oral infections (suspended in four parts of water) and to disinfect, deodorize, and promote healing of wound infections.

  z. peroxide, medicinal A mixture of zinc peroxide, zinc carbonate, and zinc hydroxide; used, as a local disinfectant, astringent, and deodorant.

  z. stearate White greasy granules, insoluble in water; an antiseptic in dusting powder form, used to protect epithelial surfaces and wounds.

  z. sulfate White water-soluble powder, used in solution as an eyewash to treat mild eye irritations and as a lotion (white lotion) to treat skin diseases and infections (acne, impetigo, and ivy poisoning). Also called salt of vitriol; white vitriol.

  z. white Zinc oxide.

zirconium A metallic element, symbol Zr, atomic number 40, atomic weight 91.22.

Z line See under line.

zoacanthosis Any dermatitis following the skin penetration of foreign bodies such as bristles, hairs, and stingers derived from insects and animals.

zoetic Relating to life.

Zollinger-Ellison syndrome (Z-E syndrome) Syndrome caused by a gastrin-secreting tumor of the pancreas, producing a high concentration of hydrochloric acid in the stomach; ulcers are formed in the esophagus and upper intestinal tract; symptoms include malabsorption, diarrhea, pain, and nausea; often associated with other endocrine abnormalities, especially hyperparathyroidism.

zona A zone, especially an encircling region distinguished from adjacent parts by some distinctive feature.

  z. adherens See zonula adherens.

  z. dermatica An area of thick, elevated skin surrounding the protrusion of a meningocele.

  z. fasciculata The intermediate layer of radially arranged cell cords in the cortex of the adrenal gland, between the zona glomerulosa and zona reticularis; together with the zona reticularis, it is the site of formation of adrenal steroids other than aldosterone.

  z. glomerulosa The thin outermost layer of the cortex of the adrenal gland just below the capsule; the site of aldosterone production.

  z. granulosa A mass of stratified cuboidal epithelium surrounding the ovum within a vesicular ovarian (graafian) follicle.

  z. hemorrhoidalis The part of the anal canal that contains the rectal (hemorrhoidal) venous plexus.

  z. incerta The narrow zone of gray matter between the lateral nucleus of the thalamus and the subthalamic nucleus.

  z. occludens See zonula occludens.

  z. orbicularis of the hip joint The deeper, circularly-arranged fibers of the articular capsule of the hip joint which encircle the neck of the femur.

  z. pellucida A refractile, gel-like neutral glycoprotein formed around the developing ovum; it is about 4 μm thick and is formed by the mutual interaction of the ovum and follicular granulosa cells; it degenerates and disappears just prior to implantation to the endometrium.

  z. reticularis The inner layer of the cortex of the adrenal gland where the cell cords form an irregular network; together with the zona fasciculata, the site of production of adrenal steroids other than aldosterone.

  z. spongiosa 1. Horizontal strata; see under stratum. 2. Older term for the most posterior layer of the dorsal horn of the spinal cord, now known as Rexed's lamina I.

  z. vasculosa of Waldeyer The highly vascular stroma in the center of the ovary. Also called medullary substance.

zone (z) Any area or space with specific characteristics.

  ciliary z. The peripheral region of the anterior surface of the iris. Cf. pupillary zone.

  comfort z. A range of environmental temperature in which the body heat is maintained in equilibrium, without sweating or shivering; 28 to 30°C (82 to 86°F) for the naked body and 13 to 21°C (55 to 70°F) for the clothed body.

  erogenous z. An area of the body which on appropriate stimulation produces sexual sensations. Also called erotogenic zone.

  extravisual z. The anterior portion of the retina outside the visual zone; it is too far forward for images to fall upon it.

  Golgi z. The portion of the cytoplasm, near the cell nucleus, which contains the Golgi apparatus; in

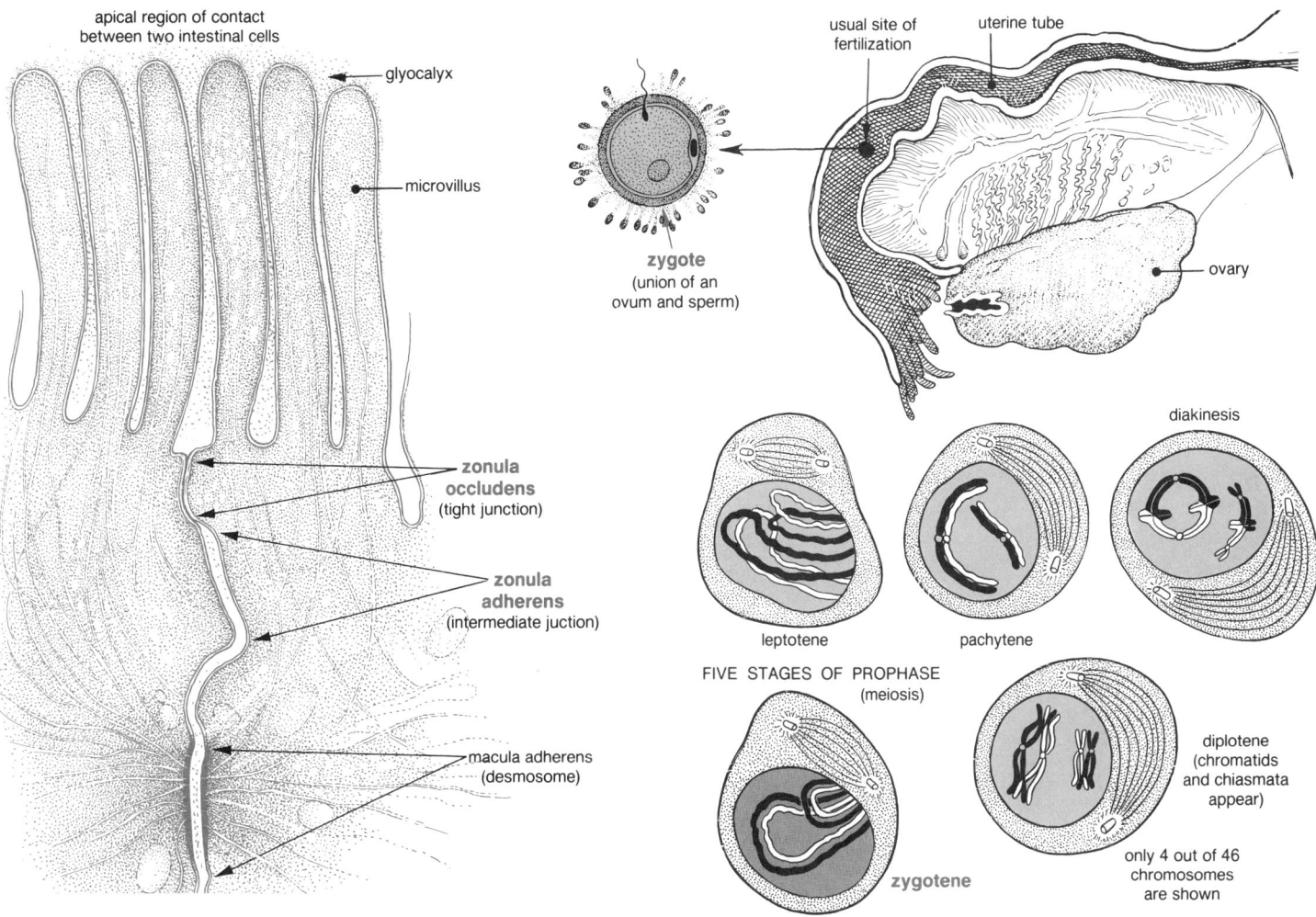

apical region of contact between two intestinal cells

glyocalyx

microvillus

zonula occludens (tight junction)

zonula adherens (intermediate juction)

macula adherens (desmosome)

usual site of fertilization

uterine tube

ovary

zygote (union of an ovum and sperm)

diakinesis

leptotene

pachytene

FIVE STAGES OF PROPHASE (meiosis)

zygotene

diplotene (chromatids and chiasmata appear)

only 4 out of 46 chromosomes are shown

a secretory cell it is the area between the nucleus and the luminal side of the cell through which expulsion of the secretion takes place.

visual z. The area of the retina that receives light rays passing through the center of the pupil without any significant spherical aberration.

optical z. of cornea The central third of the cornea of the eye.

pupillary z. The central region of the anterior surface of the iris, around the pupil. Cf. ciliary zone.

transitional z. 1. The region of the lens of the eye where the anterior epithelial capsule cells develop into the fibers which constitute the lens substance. **2.** The border of a scleral contact lens which joins the scleral and corneal sections.

z.'s of discontinuity Concentric zones of varying optical density seen in the lens of the eye with the aid of the slit lamp.

zonesthesia A constricting sensation, as by a girdle.

zonula A small zone, usually a circular one.

ciliary z. The suspensory apparatus of the lens of the eye, consisting of numerous delicate fibers that originate in the ciliary body and attach to the anterior and posterior surface of the capsule of the lens; as the ciliary muscle contracts, the tension of the fibers accomodates, thus determining the degree of convexity of the lens. Also called zonula of Zinn.

z. adherens That part of the junctional complex of epithelial cells where the adjacent cells have a narrow (~200 Å) space between apposing membranes. Also called zona adherens.

z. occludens That part of the junctional complex of epithelial cells where adjacent cell membranes are fused, with obliteration of the intercellular space. Also called zona occludens.

z. of Zinn See ciliary zonula.

zonular Relating to a zonula.

zonulolysis Dissolving of the ciliary zonule by an enzyme, such as chymotrypsin, to facilitate removal of the lens in some cases of cataract extraction.

zooanthroponosis A disease of vertebrates that can be naturally acquired from humans when they are the maintenance host; e.g., human tuberculosis.

Cf. anthropozoonosis; amphixenosis.

zoochemistry The chemistry of animal tissues.

zoogenic, zoogenetic Caused by animals.

zoogonous Giving birth to living animals which derive nutrition directly from the maternal organism. Also called viviparous.

zooid 1. An animal cell capable of independent movement within a living organism; e.g., spermatozoon and ovum. **2.** Resembling an animal.

zoological 1. Relating to animals. **2.** Relating to the science of zoology.

zoologist One who specializes in zoology.

zoology The branch of biology concerned with the study of animals.

comparative z. the comparative study of the structure and function of different animals.

zoonosis Any disease acquired from animals or shared by man and other vertebrates.

zoonosology The study of diseases of animals.

zoonotic 1. Pertaining to zoonosis. **2.** Describing a disease transmitted to man from an animal.

zooparasite An animal parasite.

zoopathology Veterinary pathology; the study of diseases which affect animals.

zoophilic Denoting a preference for animals.

zoophobia Abnormal fear of animals.

zoophyte An invertebrate animal that superficially resembles a plant, such as a sponge.

zoospore A motile, flagellated, asexual spore, as of certain fungi. Also called swarm spore.

zootoxin A substance found in snake venom and the secretions of certain insects.

zoster An encircling belt or pattern; a girdle.

herpes z. See under herpes.

zosteroid Resembling herpes zoster.

Z-plasty A technique for repairing contracted scar tissue.

zwieback Bread made of rich, sweetened dough that is baked as a loaf, sliced and toasted. Also called "twice-baked (bread)."

zwitterion An ion that possesses both negative and positive charges. Also called dipolar ion.

zygodactyly Fusion of the skin and connective tissue between fingers or toes without fusion of

bones.

zygoma 1. The zygomatic process of the temporal bone. **2.** The zygomatic arch. **3.** Term sometimes applied to the zygomatic bone (cheekbone).

zygomatic Relating to the zygoma.

Zygomycetes A class of fungi that reproduce by the union of gametes of equal size.

zygosis Fusion of two unicellular organisms, including exchange of nuclear material.

zygosity The condition of being developed from one or more eggs; said of multiple births.

zygote The single fertilized cell formed by the union of two gametes.

zygotene In meiosis, the second stage of prophase in which the homologous chromosomes approach each other and begin to pair.

zymase Obsolete term for enzyme.

zymogen See proenzyme.

zymogenesis The formation of an active enzyme from a proenzyme (inactive precursor).

zymogenic, zymogenous 1. Pertaining to a proenzyme or to zymogenesis. **2.** Producing a fermentation.

zymogram A graphic representation of electrophoretically separated enzymes.

zymoid Resembling an enzyme.

zymology Enzymology.

zymolysis Chemical process or fermentation brought about by means of an enzyme.

zymolytic Fermentative.

zymophore The active portion of an enzyme molecule.

zymoplastic Participating in the formation of enzymes.

zymosan An insoluble anticomplementary factor derived from the walls of yeast cells and used in the assay of the protein properdin; composed of lipids, polysaccharides, proteins, and ash of variable concentrations.

zymose Invertase.

zymosis 1. Fermentation. **2.** The development of infectious diseases.

zymotic 1. Relating to or caused by fermentation. **2.** Denoting any infectious disease.

ABOUT THE AUTHORS

IDA G. DOX, PH.D. is an internationally known medical communicator, co-author of the award-winning book, *Melloni's Illustrated Review of Human Anatomy* (J.B. Lippincott). Her many private consulting services have included working for the U.S. House of Representatives, on the medical panel of the Select Committee on Assassinations investigating the assassinations of President John F. Kennedy and Dr. Martin Luther King, Jr. She is listed in Marquis *Who's Who of American Women* and *Who's Who in the World*. She resides near the National Institutes of Health in Bethesda, Maryland.

B. JOHN MELLONI, PH.D. is the co-author of several books, including: *Anatomy & Physiology* (McGraw-Hill), *Databases: A Primer For Retrieving Information By Computer* (Prentice-Hall), and *Melloni's Illustrated Review of Human Anatomy* (J.B. Lippincott). Over the years, he has served as a Professorial Lecturer in Human Anatomy, Chairman of a Department of Medical Communication, Editor-in-Chief of a medical magazine, Reviewer of grant proposals for the Public Health Service, and private consultant to a host of non-profit and profit organiza-

tions, including HarperCollins Publishers. Now retired from the National Institutes of Health, where he served as Special Expert in Biomedical Communication, he continues to be co-director of the Archives of Medical Visual Resources at the Francis A. Countway Library of Medicine at Harvard Medical School.

GILBERT M. EISNER, M.D. is a graduate of Harvard College, cum laude, and Yale Medical School. He served as an intern at the Grace New Haven Hospital in New Haven, Connecticut, spent two years in the U.S. Army as a captain in the Medical Corps, then was a resident and a fellow in renal disease at Mt. Sinai Hospital in New York City. He completed his medical residency at Georgetown University Hospital in Washington DC. Since 1962 he has been on the part-time faculty of Georgetown University Medical Center and in the private practice of internal medicine and nephrology. He served for 25 years as assistant editor of *American Family Physicians* and his bibliography includes 60 scientific papers. He has held offices in numerous local and national professional organizations.